Advanced EMT

A Clinical-Reasoning Approach

Melissa Alexander, Ed.D., NREMT-P

- Lake Superior State University
  Sault Sainte Marie, MI

Richard Belle, BS, NREMT-P

- Acadian Ambulance/National EMS Academy
  Lafayette, LA

Steven Weiss, MD, MS, FACEP, FACP, *Medical Editor*

D1569261

PEARSON

Boston Columbus Indianapolis New York San Francisco Upper Saddle River Amsterdam
Cape Town Dubai London Madrid Milan Munich Paris Montreal Toronto Delhi
Mexico City São Paulo Sydney Hong Kong Seoul Singapore Taipei Tokyo

Library of Congress Cataloging-in-Publication Data

Alexander, Melissa.
Advanced EMT : a clinical-reasoning approach / Melissa Alexander, Richard Belle ;
medical editor, Steven Weiss.
   p. ; cm.
   Includes bibliographical references and index.
   ISBN-13: 978-0-13-503043-1
   ISBN-10: 0-13-503043-9
I. Belle, Richard. II. Title.
[DNLM: 1. Emergency Medical Services—methods—Handbooks. 2. Critical Care—methods—Handbooks.
3. Emergencies—Handbooks. 4. Emergency Medical Technicians—Handbooks. 5. Emergency Treatment—
methods—Handbooks. WX 39]
LC classification not assigned
616.02'5—dc23

2011029783

Publisher: Julie Levin Alexander
Publisher's Assistant: Regina Bruno
Editor-in-Chief: Marlene McHugh Pratt
Acquisitions Editor: Sladjana Repic
Senior Managing Editor for Development: Lois Berlowitz
Project Manager: Jo Cepeda
Assistant Editor: Jonathan Cheung
Director of Marketing: David Gessell
Marketing Manager: Brian Hoehl
Marketing Specialist: Michael Sirinides
Managing Editor for Production: Patrick Walsh
Production Liaison: Faye Gemmellaro
Production Editor: Heather Willison, S4Carlisle Publishing Services
Manufacturing Manager: Ilene Sanford
Editorial Media Manager: Amy Peltier

Media Project Manager: Lorena Cerisano
Art Director: Christopher Weigand
Interior and Cover Design: Wanda Espana/Wee Design
Section-Opener Images: 1: Shutterstock, #543665;
   2: Shutterstock, #70093495; 3: Thinkstock, #200274650;
   4: Superstock, 1647R-100295; 5: Thinkstock, 200248739;
   6: Thinkstock, #86479750
Cover Images: Thinkstock, Superstock, Shutterstock
Managing Photography Editor: Michal Heron
Photographers: Nathan Eldridge , Ray Kemp/Triple
   Zilch Productions, Kevin Link
Composition: S4Carlisle Publishing Services
Printer/Binder: RR Donnelley
Cover Printer: Lehigh-Phoenix Color/Hagerstown

Credits and acknowledgments borrowed from other sources and reproduced, with permission, in this textbook appear on the appropriate pages within the text.

Notice on Trademarks Many of the designations by manufacturers and sellers to distinguish their products are claimed as trademarks. Where those designations appear in this book, and the publisher was aware of a trademark claim, the designations have been printed in initial caps or all caps.

Notice on Care Procedures It is the intent of the authors and publisher that this textbook be used as part of a formal Advanced EMT education program taught by qualified instructors and supervised by a licensed physician. The procedures described in this textbook are based upon consultation with Advanced EMT and medical authorities. The authors and publisher have taken care to make certain that these procedures reflect currently accepted clinical practice; however, they cannot be considered absolute recommendations.

The material in this textbook contains the most current information available at the time of publication. However, federal, state, and local guidelines concerning clinical practices, including, without limitation, those governing infection control and universal precautions, change rapidly. The reader should note, therefore, that the new regulations may require changes in some procedures. It is the responsibility of the reader to become thoroughly familiar with the policies and procedures set by federal, state, and local agencies as well as the institution or agency where the reader is employed. The authors and the publisher of this textbook and the supplements written to accompany it disclaim any liability, loss, or risk resulting directly or indirectly from the suggested procedures and theory, from any undetected errors, or from the reader's misunderstanding of the text. It is the reader's responsibility to stay informed of any new changes or recommendations made by any federal, state, or local agency as well as by the reader's employing institution or agency.

Notice on Gender Usage The English language has historically given preference to the male gender. Among many words, the pronouns "he" and "his" are commonly used to describe both genders. Society evolves faster than language, and the male pronouns still predominate in our speech. The authors have made great effort to treat the two genders equally, recognizing that a significant percentage of Advanced EMTs are female. However, in some instances, male pronouns may be used to describe both males and females solely for the purpose of brevity. This is not intended to offend any readers of the female gender.

Notice on "Case Studies" The names used and situations depicted in the case studies throughout this text are fictitious.

Notice on Medications The authors and the publisher of this book have taken care to make certain that the equipment, doses of drugs, and schedules of treatment are correct and compatible with the standards generally accepted at the time of publication. Nevertheless, as new information becomes available, changes in treatment and in the use of equipment and drugs become necessary. The reader is advised to carefully consult the instruction and information material included in the page insert of each drug or therapeutic agent, piece of equipment, or device before administration. This advice is especially important when using new or infrequently used drugs. Prehospital care providers are warned that use of any drugs or techniques must be authorized by their medical director, in accord with local laws and regulations. The publisher disclaims any liability, loss, injury, or damage incurred as a consequence, directly or indirectly, of the use and application of any of the contents of this book.

Brady
is an imprint of

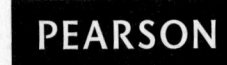

www.bradybooks.com

10 9 8 7
ISBN 13:   978-0-13-503043-1
ISBN 10:   0-13-503043-9

Dedicated with love to my family for their support and encouragement for this and other projects. To Lindsay, Chris, and Asher Giroux; Brittany, Brandon, Ethan, and Grant Moore; and Eleanor Shook. And to the EMS students and patients who continue to inspire me to be at my best in my work always.

—M. A.

This book is dedicated to my fellow EMS professionals whom I have had the opportunity to work with and my family, past and present, who has provided me with unwavering support and inspiration. To my wife Rhonda, for your extraordinary patience, support, and willingness to sacrifice so that I could complete this textbook. I couldn't have done it without you. Mom, Dad, Aunt Gwen, and Uncle Warren, thank you for teaching me the value of hard work and self confidence. To my children James, Victoria, and Allison: dream big, work hard, and never compromise who you are. I am very proud of you and I love you.

—R. B.

I want to dedicate my work to my wife, Amy, my daughter, Natalie, and to the rest of my family whom I have rarely seen over the years because I moved so far away to pursue a career. I want to send my best wishes to our family's next generation: Natalie, Scott, Sara, Max, Oliver, Lucy, and Zack in the often difficult pursuit of careers of their own. And I want to thank all of the EMS providers and students who helped and inspired me along the way on this interesting path.

—S. W.

Brief Contents

Detailed Contents

Photo Scans

Welcome, students!

You are beginning an exciting learning experience with which this textbook will assist you. We have designed it to help you learn facts, principles, and concepts in EMS. But we have gone beyond simply presenting facts, principles, and concepts. This textbook contains features that help you learn critical thinking and problem solving, which are highly desired skills in the health care professions. The process of using critical thinking to solve patient care problems is called *clinical-reasoning*. The clinical-reasoning process is a cornerstone of safe, excellent patient care and we have made it a foundation of this textbook.

We, as authors, educators, and clinicians, are excited about the unique focus of our textbook on clinical reasoning. Each chapter begins with a Case Study and Problem-Solving Questions to frame the material in the chapter in a way that establishes its importance. Beginning each chapter with a specific problem in mind helps you read the chapter for deeper understanding of how the material can be applied in your real-life Advanced EMT practice. After the chapter material is presented, the Case Study Wrap-Up with Clinical-Reasoning Process helps you understand how the Advanced EMTs in the Case Study determined and solved the problems, providing you with a model for transferring what you have learned from the classroom to the work environment.

Congratulations on your decision to further your professional development in EMS by becoming an Advanced EMT. We are glad to have you among our peers in the profession. We welcome your questions and correspondence. Please don't hesitate to contact us at the e-mail addresses provided. If you have the opportunity to attend professional conferences, we hope we will have the chance to meet you in person!

Melissa Alexander, EdD, NREMT-P

melalexander1@gmail.com

Richard Belle, BS, NREMT-P

rbelle2024@yahoo.com

Steven Weiss, MD, MS, FACEP, FACP

sweiss@salud.unm.edu

Preface

Advanced EMT: A Clinical-Reasoning Approach was developed with your success in mind. Its purpose is to assist you in successfully completing your Advanced EMT course and ultimately obtaining your licensure. Advanced EMT is a new level of EMS provider, thus warranting a first-edition textbook with the National EMS Education Standards as its foundation. Special care was taken to ensure that the latest applicable research was reviewed during the development of this textbook, resulting in our ability to deliver the latest information on evidence-based patient care to you.

You will increase your likelihood of being successful in class if you utilize proper study habits, learning tools, note taking, preclass preparation, and test preparation. This Preface provides you with tips to study and prepare efficiently and effectively.

An Introduction to Your Course of Study

No doubt you are beginning your Advanced EMT course with both excitement and anxiety, as every student does. Students are excited at the prospect of learning new information and skills, meeting new people, having new experiences, being mentally challenged, and being prepared for a new step in their careers. One of the main sources of anxiety comes from wondering if you will be successful in the course. Being successful means completing the class, having met all of the standards of your program and being prepared to pass the high-stakes examinations required for licensure. Most of all, successful completion of your Advanced EMT course means having the knowledge, skills, empathy, and confidence it takes to provide emergency care to a wide variety of patients. Most students are willing to put in the tremendous amount of work this takes, but they may not use their study time as efficiently and effectively as possible. There are no short cuts: Learning takes time and work. However, there are a number of ways to make sure you are using your time and effort in the best ways possible.

Academic success relies on a number of factors aside from desire and aptitude. In addition to committing to attending every scheduled class and putting in your clinical experience time, you must be ready to commit substantial time outside of class to prepare. You must have good time management and organizational skills. You also must develop learning habits that give the best results for the time and effort you put into them. As a general rule, students must spend 3 hours outside class for every hour in lecture to learn the content required. Often, students wait until just before the first exam, or worse, after not doing so well on the exam, to ask their instructor, "What is the best way to study for the test?"

The best way to study for any test is to *not* study for the test but, instead, to study for understanding. Understanding can only develop incrementally over time, not in the last days and hours before a test. You must spend time every day immersing yourself in the course content in order to build understanding. This is where your excitement comes in: It gives you the motivation and energy required to keep going even when you might feel somewhat discouraged or anxious. Beyond motivation, though, there are a number of concrete actions and tools that will help you organize the content for understanding.

Because time is at a premium for everyone, you should use your study time to your best advantage. The following offers you some basic information about how learning occurs, to what degree learning styles play a role in how you should approach studying, and some specific skills, tips, and tools you can use to help yourself acquire the knowledge and problem-solving skills needed to successfully complete your course.

The Nature of Advanced EMT Learning

Whether or not you are taking your course for college credit, the complexity of concepts in Advanced EMT courses are college level. However, the information in most college classes is memorized for a short period of time, regurgitated on a test, and then largely forgotten. As an Advanced EMT, you must maintain the required knowledge in a useful form throughout your career. This requires a different approach than you might have used in other learning situations.

Readiness for Learning

The nature, situation, and experience of each student are different. Those differences have an impact on learning. Whether you are a working professional, a parent, or a college student with other courses to take, everyone has responsibilities outside of Advanced EMT class. For some, the load is heavier than for others. It is important that you assess the meaning this class has for you, how it fits with your other priorities, whether the current time is the right time for you, and how you can allow sufficient time to not only attend class, but to commit the time needed outside of class in order to succeed. Time and effort are things you must bring to the learning situation that your instructor cannot provide for you.

Learning Styles

There are a variety of instruments that measure different aspects of learning styles. The most important thing to know about learning styles is that they are preferences for the way people take in and process information. People may or may not be better at learning when using their preferred style. One of the most popular tools for measuring learning style tells people whether they prefer a visual, auditory, or kinesthetic (hands-on) learning process. Those designations are not meant to label learners or give them an excuse for not taking full advantage of learning situations that do not match their preferences. Everyone can and does learn by all of those means.

In truth, the most effective way to learn something has more to do with what is being learned than how people prefer to learn it. Most complex concepts have components that are better learned in one way than another. For example, the concepts behind measuring

xix

Sunday	Monday	Tuesday	Wednesday	Thursday	Friday	Saturday
• Review previous class notes • Prepare for class (Ch. 4)	• Class, 6:00 pm • Review & summarize class notes	• Review Ch. 4 notes • Prepare for class (Ch. 5)	• Class, 6:00 pm • Review & summarize class notes	• Do homework for Ch. 4 & Ch. 5	• Study group, 7:00 pm	

FIGURE 1

Plan your study time.

blood pressure are best learned through reading and lecture, often with accompanying figures and diagrams. However, the skill of taking a blood pressure is best learned by demonstration and hands-on practice.

Study Habits

There are many prescriptions for effective study habits. Some of the key ideas behind effective study habits include being organized, planning study time, and having an environment that is conducive to focusing and learning. An example of being organized is making sure that everything you need, such as a pen or pencil, paper, computer, textbook, and perhaps a drink or snack are readily at hand. This prevents an interruption in your thinking process to retrieve needed items. Commit to study time. Block out specific time in your schedule to study (Figure 1). For the period of time you are taking your Advanced EMT course, consider your study time a necessary appointment with yourself. Depending on your work schedule and lifestyle, the time that works best for you to study may vary. Intervals between classes, or between work and class, or even 20 minutes in the car spent waiting to pick up your child from school serve as planned study time. Learning occurs best when you study for short periods of time with a small break between segments. For example, you might study for 20 to 50 minutes and take a 5-minute break before resuming study. Take some time to reflect on what study environment works for you. Some people prefer to study with a partner or in a group, while others prefer to study alone. Create a comfortable place as free from distractions as possible. Many of the specifics of these factors are individual preferences.

The Nature of Learning

Not only must you learn for the short-term goals of testing, but you also must be able to transfer knowledge and skills to the job. This requires learning in three domains: cognitive (facts, concepts,

thinking, and problem solving), psychomotor (hands-on skills), and affective (values and professionalism). The main focus of this Preface is the cognitive domain.

Knowledge is arranged in hypothetical mental structures called *schemas*. A schema is a collection of related information that helps in making sense of what we see, hear, read, and experience in other ways. When you can relate new information to an existing schema, learning is easier and more effective. A schema provides a context and framework for interpreting and storing information. Much of the rest of the information in this Preface takes advantage of how schemas work and the ideas that learning occurs in small increments over time, and with repetition.

Graphic Organizers

Graphic organizers are learning tools that help arrange information in ways that make it more easily processed and learned. You are most likely familiar with graphic organizers, even if you have not heard them called by this name. Tables, flow charts, and Venn diagrams are common types of graphic organizers (Figures 2 and 3). Graphic organizers are powerful learning tools because they allow you to see how information is organized in a way that goes beyond words. By using graphic organizers, you can better understand overall relationships between concepts and ideas.

This text contains many graphic organizers to help structure your learning process. However, creating your own graphic organizers as part of your study process adds even more to your learning power. The Resource Central website that accompanies this text contains a number of graphic organizer ideas and templates for your use.

KWL (know, want, learn) charts are effective because they help identify what you do not yet know (Figure 4). This is critical because learning cannot take place until you recognize the boundaries of your current knowledge. (A variation of a KWL chart is shown in Figure 5.)

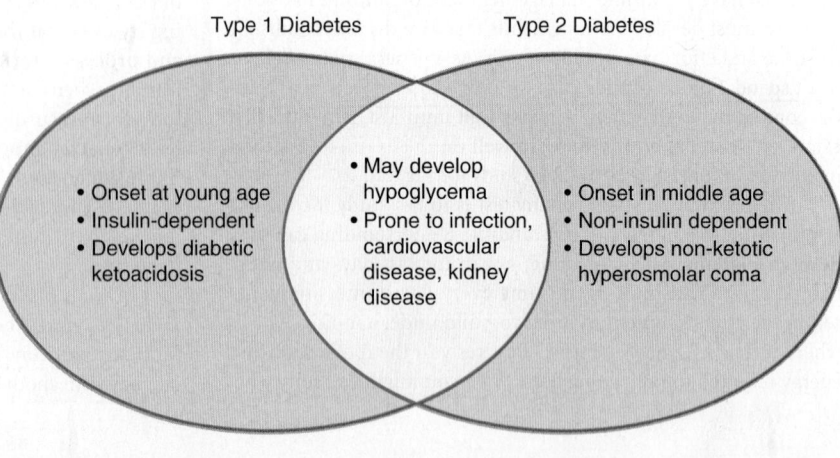

FIGURE 2

Venn diagrams are used to compare and contrast the features of two or three related items. The organization of overlapping circles allows information to be organized according to what features are unique each item and which features are shared. The example below shows a Venn diagram for type I and type II diabetes.

Feature	Cushing's Syndrome	Addison's Disease
Cause	Excess adrenal cortical hormones due to glucocorticoid therapy (steroid medications) or pituitary tumor resulting in increased ACTH.	Insufficient secretion of adrenal cortical hormones due to destruction of adrenal cortex. Adrenal insufficiency may occur due to sudden withdrawal of corticosteroid therapy.
Associated conditions	COPD, asthma, cancer, or inflammatory conditions requiring steroid therapy. Diabetes, infection. Increased risk of cardiovascular disease and stroke.	Inability to respond to stressors such as infection, surgery, trauma, or illness.
Signs and symptoms	Weight gain in the trunk, often with thin extremities. "Moon face" appearance, accumulation of fat in the upper back ("buffalo hump"). Thin, easily bruised skin. Delayed wound healing. Development of facial hair in women.	Hyperpigmentation of the skin and gums, fatigue, weakness, and weight loss.
Emergencies	Increased risk of MI, stroke, and infection.	Adrenal crisis (Addisonian crisis). May be present with hypoglycemia, hypotension, and cardiac rhythm disturbances due to electrolyte abnormalities.

FIGURE 3

Tables can be used to organize and summarize information for side-by-side comparison. This example compares the features of two adrenal-gland disorders.

KWL Chart: Advanced EMT Chapter 2 EMS Systems		
What I Know About EMS Systems	What I Want to Know About EMS Systems	What I Learned About EMS Systems

FIGURE 4

KWL Chart. KWL stands for know, want, learn. Information is organized by what you already know, what you want to know, and what you then learned.

A variety of configurations can be used to create mind maps or webs, cause–effect diagrams, processes, timelines, and other ways of summarizing and representing information (Figures 6, 7, and 8). If you prefer to use computer-based tools rather than drawing those structures in your notes, Microsoft Word has a number of graphic organizer templates in its online resources.

Note Taking

Taking notes on both your assigned reading and your instructor's lectures is a way of creating study materials for later use. An effective method is that of Cornell notes, which is explained in the following section (Figure 9). When taking notes in class, do not write word-for-word what your instructor is saying, or what he might have on a slide. Writing things word for word is rote, requiring

little thinking, and interferes with listening for meaning. Mentally summarizing what is said and writing in your own words helps you develop understanding. Approaching note taking in this way helps you listen for meaning as you translate your instructor's words into your own.

An effective way of preparing is discussed in the following section. As you listen to your instructor, write only those things that you do not already have in your reading notes, or those that bear special emphasis. If you have not prepared for class and are being exposed to the material for the first time, you will not be able to determine what to write, and will attempt to write down everything. Attempting to write everything down causes you to fall behind the pace of the lecture and miss a great deal of information. Don't do it.

Instead, use the Cornell notes method. Cornell notes are a simple, effective and widely used note-taking structure that you

FIGURE 5

The KWHL chart is a variation of the KWL chart that includes a "how" section for listing references for information.

KWHL Chart: Advanced EMT Chapter 2 EMS Systems	
1. What I Know About EMS Systems	**2. What I Want to Know About EMS Systems**
• History of modern EMS began in 1966 with the White Paper • Much of what is known about prehospital care is based on military experience • The EMS Agenda for the Future outlines goals for EMS system development	• What are the specific goals of the EMS Agenda for the Future?
3. How I Learned About EMS Systems	**4. What I Learned About EMS Agenda Goals**
• National Highway Transportation Safety Administration, The EMS Agenda for the Future at www.ems.gov	• Integration of health services • EMS research • Legislation and regulation • System finance • Human resources • Medical direction • Education systems • Public education • Prevention • Public access • Communications systems • Clinical care • Information systems • Evaluation

FIGURE 6

Vocabulary sheet.

Vocabulary Sheet Chapter 1		
Vocabulary Term	**Defnition**	**Relevance to Chapter**
Advanced Emergency Medical Technician (Advanced EMT)	A prehospital emergency care provider who uses basic and limited advanced life support skills to care for acutely ill and injured patients.	1 of the 4 nationally recognized levels of EMS providers.
Advanced life support (ALS)	Complex patient care assessments and interventions that require in-depth training.	Advanced EMTs provide basic and limited advanced life support.

can use to take notes while reading and during class. You can use the Cornell notes template provided in Resource Central, or create your own. The steps are to divide, document, write, review and clarify, summarize, and study. First, divide your paper as shown in Figure 9. Document the course name and the date at the top of the page. Write your notes in the main section of the paper. Learn to use abbreviations and symbols to help you write your notes more quickly and concisely. (Once you read Chapter 7, Medical Terminology, you will have an ample supply of symbols and abbreviations at your disposal.) Review and clarify the notes by

Scene Size-Up
Initial Impression
Primary Assessment
Patient Priority
Secondary Assessment
Treatment
Reassessment
• Scene safety
• Situation
• Airway
• Breathing
• Circulation
• History
• Vital signs
• Physical exam
• Primary assessment
• Aspects of secondary assessment
• Effects of treatment

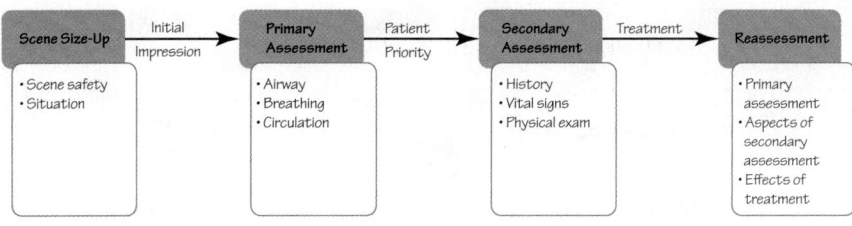

FIGURE 7

A variety of charts and graphs can illustrate the steps in a process, such as a skill, or the steps of a physiological or pathophysiological process. The example here shows the main steps in patient assessment.

Pathophysiology of Asthma			
Inflammation and constriction narrow the bronchioles. It requires more work to move air past the obstruction, especially on exhalation. Oxygen and carbon dioxide exchange are impaired.			
Inspection (See)	**Palpation (Feel)**	**Auscultation (Hear)**	**Smell**
• Increased work of breathing: use of accessory muscles. • Impaired gas exchange: signs of hypoxia, such as cyanosis and increased respiratory rate • Decreased oxygen saturation.	• Air movement at mouth and nose may be decreased • Pulse may be increased.	• Patient complaints: difficulty breathing, chest tightness, history of asthma • Wheezing breath sounds • Chest may be silent in severe attack	• None expected

FIGURE 8

A pathophysiology and presentation graphic such as this can be used to show the relationship between disease pathophysiology and the signs and symptoms it causes in the patient.

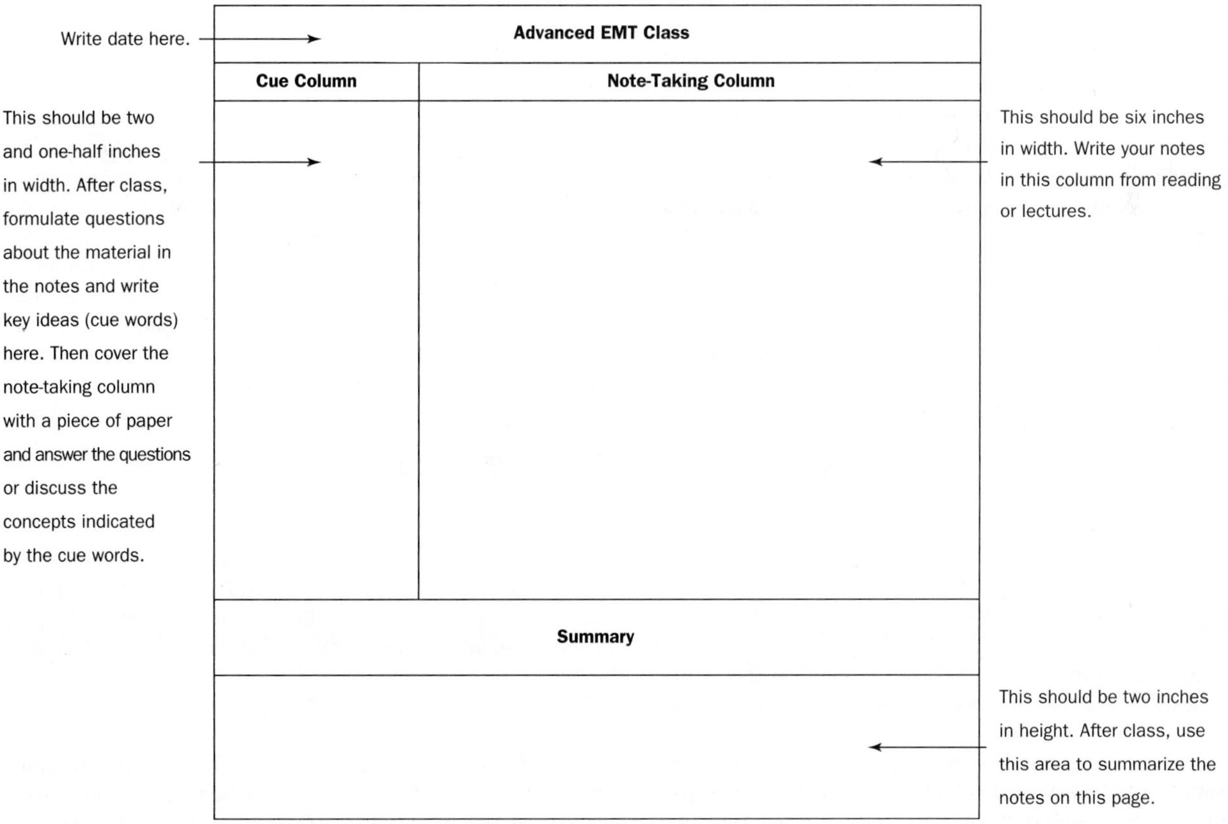

Write date here.
Advanced EMT Class
Cue Column
Note-Taking Column
This should be two and one-half inches in width. After class, formulate questions about the material in the notes and write key ideas (cue words) here. Then cover the note-taking column with a piece of paper and answer the questions or discuss the concepts indicated by the cue words.
This should be six inches in width. Write your notes in this column from reading or lectures.
Summary
This should be two inches in height. After class, use this area to summarize the notes on this page.

FIGURE 9

Cornell notes is a note-taking system that allows for effective organization of information and recognition of key points.

FIGURE 10
Study process.

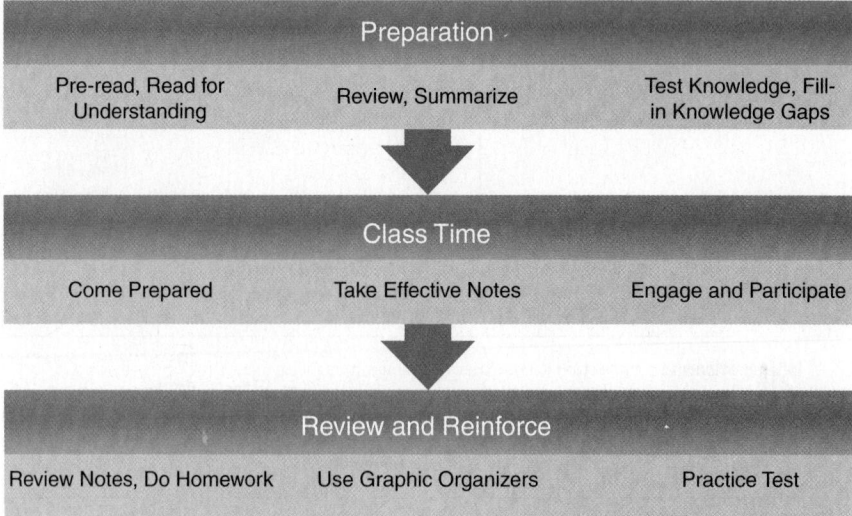

pulling out main concepts and key ideas and writing them in the cue column on the left side of the paper. Also write any questions you have in that column. Summarize your notes at the bottom of the page, and then study from the page.

Three Time Frames for Learning Activities

Learning for each concept in the course can be divided into three time frames: preparation for class, time in class, and review and reinforcement after class (Figure 10). None of these three time periods can be sacrificed. The use of these three time periods underscores the importance of repetition in learning. It is rarely possible, even with simpler concepts, to fully grasp a concept on first exposure. Each time you are exposed to the same concept, you will pick up additional understanding of it. Repetition allows you to correct misconceptions, fill in gaps in knowledge, and develop deeper and more sophisticated understanding of concepts.

The variety of different ways in which you are exposed to a concept through repetition also enriches your understanding of it. Just reading about vital signs will not give you a complete understanding. You will learn more by also hearing your instructor talk about vital signs, working on case studies in which patients' vital signs have different meanings, seeing your lab instructor demonstrate the skills, practicing hands-on skills in lab, seeing other health care providers perform the skill, and incorporating the skills into practice scenarios and clinical experience. Being exposed to the same concept in various settings helps in being able to transfer learning from one context to another (such as from in the classroom to on the job).

Preparing for Class

Preparation is important for a couple of reasons. First, it provides a framework for making sense of the information that will be provided when you are in class (recall the concept of *schema* introduced earlier). Preparation allows you to be an active, and therefore more effective, participant in the learning process. This allows you to fully participate, both mentally and in interaction with your instructor and classmates. Coming to class prepared with questions helps focus your attention during lecture so that you can begin to fill in gaps in understanding. Preparation consists, at a minimum,

of fully reading what has been assigned and reviewing your previous notes. Effective reading of assigned material requires pre-reading, reading for understanding, review, summarization, testing to identify gaps in knowledge, and filling gaps in knowledge. The design of this textbook helps you in these activities.

Pre-Read the Assigned Text Chapter

Begin pre-reading the chapter by reading the chapter introduction and summary. Next, review the objectives, key terms, and subject headings. Each of those items serves as a preview of the content to come, helping you prepare mentally to receive the information. The features are turned into even more powerful learning tools when you phrase each of them as a question to be answered. For example, when you see a chapter learning objective that says "*After reading this chapter, you should be able to identify signs and symptoms of stroke,*" turn it into a question to be answered in your reading, "*What are the signs and symptoms of stroke?*" If one of the key terms in the chapter is *aphasia*, ask yourself, "*What is aphasia*"? If a subject heading is "*Pathophysiology of Type I Diabetes,*" turn it into a question, "*What is the pathophysiology of type 1 diabetes?*" Read each of the chapter review questions to get an idea of the answers you will look for in your reading. Reading for answers is an effective way of reading for meaning.

Reading for Understanding

Begin a chapter by reading the case study presented at the beginning. The case studies and questions that accompany them are specifically designed to prime your thinking to read for understanding and problem solving. Read for meaning by looking for material that answers each of the questions posed by objectives, key terms, and subject headings. Take notes on your reading.

Using a highlighter, either on paper or electronically, is rarely effective. The nature of textbooks is that all of the information presented is important. As a result, students often end up highlighting almost everything in the text. Features in the textbook, summarized in the *Guide to Features* section of this textbook's front matter, help draw your attention to key ideas. by using a bold typeface for key terms and using "Pediatric Care" notes, "Geriatric Care" notes, case studies, tables to summarize concepts, and at the end of each chapter, review material including "Critical-Thinking Questions." The highlighted features are as follows:

- *Key Terms.* Terms that are important for you to know are listed at the beginning of each chapter and placed in bold face type to draw your attention. The terms are boldfaced the first time they are used or defined in the textbook. All subsequent uses of the term in a chapter are not boldfaced.
- *"Pediatric Care" notes.* In some cases, the assessment and management of pediatric patients differs from that of adults. "Pediatric Care" notes are used throughout the textbook to draw attention to key pediatric information within the context of the chapter.
- *"Geriatric Care" notes.* As with pediatric patients, there are differences in the assessment and management of geriatric patients. "Geriatric Care" notes are used throughout the textbook to draw attention to key geriatric information within the context of the chapter.
- *Case Study with Problem-Solving Questions.* A case study at the beginning of each chapter introduces you to the kinds of problems you will encounter in Advanced EMT practice and frames the importance of the chapter content that follows. This feature is used to assist you in developing critical-thinking skills following a systematic assessment approach while utilizing resources available to you. Case studies guide you through an emergency situation emphasizing the process of making good decisions after analyzing all information gathered. The solution to each case study is presented at the end of the chapter in the Case Study Wrap-Up, which explains the Advanced EMT's clinical-reasoning process. In lengthier chapters, the case study unfolds with further information given throughout the chapter.
- *Tables, Figures, and Scans.* When it is important for you to learn multiple concepts that are related to one another, it is sometimes best to see the information in an organized table. Tables are placed throughout the textbook to assist you in learning and understanding specific information. Figures and Scans provide visual material to enhance the explanations of concepts and procedures presented in the text.
- *Chapter Summary.* The chapter summaries include a synopsis of the main ideas of the chapter and multiple-choice and critical-thinking questions. Multiple-choice questions test your recall of chapter information and simple application of concepts. Your goal is to not just learn the information presented in the textbook and in class, but also to understand it. Critical-thinking questions are intended to test your knowledge by requiring you to think your way through the question using the information provided and your previous knowledge to identify the most correct answer.

Reviewing and Summarizing

Review your reading by again reading the introduction, the subject headings, and summary. Summarize the chapter in your own words. It helps to do this in writing, but you can also do it mentally or by talking with a classmate or mentor.

Testing Your Knowledge and Identifying Learning Gaps

Test your knowledge by answering the question form of each of the objectives and subject headings. Use the review questions at the end of the chapter to further test your knowledge. Identify gaps in knowledge by making a note of anything you were not able to answer. Go back and read for the answer. Before class, write any questions you have from your reading in the *Cues* column of a fresh page of notes to be used in class. Listen for the answers to those questions, and ask for clarification if you do not hear the answers you are looking for.

In Class

Your time in class allows repetition and explanation of key information, an opportunity for your instructor to elaborate on concepts and give examples, and it provides you with opportunities for critical thinking and asking questions. Creating and taking advantage of those opportunities is a joint responsibility of you and your instructor. To do your part, begin by attending class prepared and well rested. Be ready to fully focus and engage with the instructor, content, and your classmates. An important step in doing this is avoiding distractions. If your instructor does not have a policy regarding phone calls, texting, and Internet use during class, avoid those temptations voluntarily. The ability to multitask effectively is a myth. When two tasks are undertaken simultaneously, they will both suffer.

Take the perspective of cooperation, rather than competition, in learning with your classmates. Form working relationships with them, because it is important for your learning and theirs. Also form a good working relationship with your instructor. Mutual trust and respect are key components in a successful learning experience. Keep an open mind about the information you receive. Ideas that seem to be in conflict often can be reconciled. At earlier levels of learning, complex concepts can be presented very simply. When presented at a more complex level, there can at first seem to be a contradiction when, in reality, there is not. It is helpful to ask your instructor how your previous understanding of the concept relates to the current explanation.

Reviewing and Reinforcing

After class, while the lecture is still fresh, review or rewrite your notes to fill in any gaps. Use graphic organizers to summarize and clarify information. As you study your notes on a daily basis, focus more and more on the main ideas in the *Cues* column, moving back to the detailed notes or the text when you are unable to fully explain the main ideas to yourself or a study partner. Prior to quizzes and tests, repeat your pre-reading of the chapter, answering each of the questions developed from objectives, key terms, and headings. For anything you are not able to answer, go back and re-read that section of the chapter.

Testing and Practice Testing

An effective supplement to your study regimen is frequent practice testing. A number of resources, including the end-of-chapter reviews in this text and quizzes in Resource Central, as well as other commercial test preparation products (electronic, Web-based, and print) allow you to test yourself. Practice testing provides you with feedback on your learning process and guides you to specific areas in which you need more work. The process also helps you prepare for your in-class and licensing exams.

There are a few strategies to keep in mind when taking graded exams. Everyone experiences some level of anxiety regarding exams. To a point, that anxiety provides motivation that improves performance. However, performance declines when anxiety levels are high. At such levels, you may have difficulty reading and understanding test instructions and test items. You may experience the phenomenon of drawing a blank on a test item, only to remember it as soon as you turn in your test. Some of things that lead to test anxiety are under your immediate control. Understanding the material well enough to recall it when you are under stress is a key way to decrease test anxiety. This kind of understanding develops over time. Putting off reading and studying until the night before the exam is a sure way to increase your anxiety level.

To decrease anxiety during the test, focus on one item at a time. Do not worry about how many questions you have answered or how many questions you still need to answer. Do not entertain thoughts about poor performance on the exam and do not worry about how long it takes other people to finish the exam. There is little correlation between test performance and how long it takes to complete the test. In general, do not change your answers on multiple-choice items. If you are not sure of the answer, stay with your first choice. Only change your response if you mismarked the answer or you misread the question or one or more of the responses to it.

If possible, first answer the questions you find easiest, then come back to the harder ones. This makes the most efficient use of the limited time you have to take a test. However, a drawback is the possibility of skipping a question or mismarking the answer. Whether you answer questions in order or not, take a few minutes at the end of the exam to check your answers. Make sure you have answered all of the questions and that you have marked your answer sheet correctly.

Finally, test anxiety is reduced and mental performance is enhanced by taking good care of yourself. Get a full night's sleep prior to the exam. Eat nutritious foods and avoid excessive sugar and caffeine.

In Summary

By taking this class, you have set a high but achievable goal for yourself. Achieving any important goal requires planning, time, and work. Being successful in your Advanced EMT class is no different. Study skills provide you with tools you can use to make the most efficient use of the time you are dedicating to this class. By using them, you will be able to organize the considerable amount of information you are about to receive in ways that make it easier to learn.

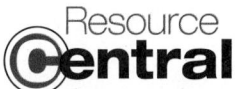
Resource Central

This robust Web site has all your instructor resources in one location! It provides chapter support materials and all your teaching resources: PowerPoint program with embedded media links, visuals, instructor's notes with teaching tips, skills slides and objectives; Instructor's Resource Manual that includes a book-specific curriculum, lesson plans, and reinforcement and assessment handouts; and an updated testing program, with critical-thinking questions. To access Resource Central, go to www.bradybooks.com and select Resource Central. The following teaching resources can be accessed on Resource Central:

Instructor's Resource Manual

Available electronically, this new package is available for download from Resource Central. It includes a book-specific curriculum, lesson plans, media assets, and reinforcement and assessment handouts.

PowerPoint Presentation with Instructor Notes

This resource includes more than 2,000 customizable lecture slides and 100 skills slides that are truly visual supplements for your lectures that will hold student interest. Lecture slides present key concepts of a chapter with important photographs and illustrations from the text. Instructor's Notes reinforce content on the slides, provide expanded lesson presentation tools, as well as provide teaching tips, discussion questions, and additional resources. Skills slides summarize and present key information and step-by-step procedures.

MyTest Program

This program contains over 1,800 multiple-choice questions that support and reinforce textbook content. MyTest software can be used to customize your tests chapter-by-chapter and provide questions electronically or on paper. You can also add your own questions to the database. Answer keys are provided.

CourseCompass

CourseCompass is a dynamic, interactive, online learning environment. You can easily create a course and customize it with your own materials. All instructor resources for this edition are already loaded to enable you to run your online course with ease.

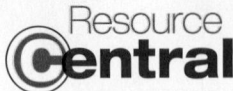
Resource
Central

This online study aid provides chapter support materials and interactive resources in one location. Students can prepare for class and exams with skills and objective checklists, multiple-choice questions, case-study activities, interactive exercises, games, audio glossary, web links, animations and videos, study aids, and more! At the beginning of each chapter, students are prompted to visit Resource Central to access resources that reinforce or enhance text material.

To access Resource Central, students follow directions on the Student Access Code Card provided with the text. If there is no card, go to www.bradybooks.com and follow the Resource Central link to Buy Access from there.

Workbook for Advanced EMT: A Clinical-Reasoning Approach (0-13-503106-0)

This self-paced workbook contains matching exercises, multiple-choice questions, short-answer questions, labeling exercises, and case studies with questions. This workbook is available for purchase at www.bradybooks.com.

Acknowledgments

The hard work and expertise of many people go into transforming an idea into a textbook. The professionalism, guidance, expertise, and support of those individuals make the work of the authors better, more meaningful, and more personally rewarding. We thank the following people for their long hours and dedication to making this the best text possible.

We are grateful to the Brady editorial staff for their trust in us and their leadership and guidance. Thank you to Marlene Pratt, Editor-in-Chief; Lois Berlowitz, Senior Managing Editor for Development; Sladjana Repic, Acquisitions Editor; Jonathan Cheung, Assistant Editor; Faye Gemmellaro, Production Liaison; and Pat Walsh, Managing Editor for Production.

Thank you to Josephine Cepeda, our developmental editor, with whom we have had almost daily contact during the development process. It has been a pleasure to work with Jo. Her tireless work, attention to detail, and expertise have been invaluable.

We also acknowledge the extraordinary attention to every nuance of scientific and medical accuracy provided by our medical editor, Steven Weiss, MD. Dr. Weiss held our work to the highest levels of scrutiny, providing his incomparable medical expertise to the preparation of this textbook. His time, effort, and dedication to EMS education are greatly appreciated.

Thank you to Heather Willison, Senior Project Editor, at S4Carlisle Publishing Services for expert production management.

Content Contributors

Becoming an Advanced EMT requires study in a number of content areas ranging from airway to medical and trauma emergencies to pediatrics and rescue. To ensure that each area is covered accurately and in the most up-to-date manner, we enlisted the help of several expert contributors. We are grateful for the time and energy each put into his or her contribution.

Dan Batsie, BA, NREMT-P
Education Coordinator
North East Maine EMS
Bangor, ME

John Grassham, BS (in EMS)
EMS Educator
University of New Mexico School of Medicine
Albuquerque, NM

Patrick Hardy, MSc, LLM, NREMT
President
Hytropy, LLC
Baton Rouge, LA

Dustin Hillerson, BS
Paramedic, Medical Student
University of New Mexico School of Medicine
Albuquerque, NM

Sean M. Kivlehan, MD, MPH, NREMT-P
Emergency Medicine Resident
University of California - San Francisco
San Francisco, CA

Lt. J. Harold "Jim" Logan, BS, EMT-P I/C
EMS Consequence Management
The Fire Department of Memphis
Memphis, TN

Christopher L. Mixon, AAS, NREMT-P
Education Coordinator
Acadian Ambulance / National EMS Academy
Lafayette, LA

Greg Mullen, MS, NREMT-P
EMS Program Manager
National EMS Academy
Lafayette, LA

Charles "Harry" Murphy, Jr., NREMT-P, CCEMT-P
Education Coordinator
National EMS Academy
Lafayette, LA

Phillip T. Sanderson, NREMT-P, BS, MHA
Manager, EMS Operations
Methodist Le Bonheur Healthcare Systems Methodist
    University Hospital
Memphis, TN

David J. Turner, NREMT-P, IC
EMS Educator
University of New Mexico School of Medicine, EMS Academy
Albuquerque, NM

Steven Weiss, MS, MD
Professor of Emergency Medicine
University of New Mexico
Albuquerque, NMSteven Weiss, MS, MD

Scott Oglesbee, BA, EMT-P
Research Coordinator, Department of Emergency Medicine
University of New Mexico School of Medicine
Albuquerque, NM

We wish to thank the following reviewers for providing invaluable feedback and suggestions in preparation of the first edition of *Advanced EMT: A Clinical-Reasoning Approach.*

Jeffrey L. Barnes, EMT-P
Instructor, Operation's Manager, Firefighter, Haz Mat Tech
Weatherly, PA

Lauri Beechler, RN, MSN, CEN, NREMT-B
Loyola University Medical Center
Maywood, IL

George Blankinship, EMT-FP
Flight Paramedic
Moraine Park Technical College
Fond du Lac, WI

David Bryant, BS, EMT-P
Associate Professor, Health Related Professions
Northeast State Community College
Blountville, TN

David Burdett, NREMT-P
Training Officer/ Clinical Coordinator
Hamilton County EMS and Chattanooga State
    Community College
Chattanooga, TN

Rebecca Burke, BS, RN, NREMT-P
Wallace Community College
Dothan, AL

Helen T. Compton, NREMT-P
Paramedic
Mecklenburg County Rescue Squad
Clarksville, VA

Steve Creech, BA, MMin (NC), EMT-P
National Director
Nazarene Disaster Response
Lenexa, KS

Lyndal M. Curry, MA, NREMT-P
University of South Alabama
Mobile, AL

Glenn Faught, AAS, BS, MS
Program Chair and Associate Professor
Emergency Medical Technology SW Tennessee CC
Memphis, TN

James W. Fogal, MA, NREMT-P
EMS Instructor
Opelika, AL

David C. Harrington, AS, NREMT-P
City of Oak Ridge Fire Department
Oak Ridge, TN

James F. Jones, NREMT-P
Program Director
Southeastern Technical College
Vidalia, GA

Kevin F. Jura, NREMT-P
Lead ALS Instructor
DC Fire & EMS
Washington, DC

Deb Kaye, NREMT, BS Health Education, Physical Education
Director/Instructor Dakota County Technical College
EMT – Sunburg Ambulance, Lakes Area Rural Responders
Rosemount, MN

Robin Kinsella, NECEM I/C
Mad River Valley Ambulance Service
Waitsfield, VT

Peggy Lahren, NREMT-P
Regional EMS Coordinator
Arizona Bureau of EMS and Trauma System
Phoenix, AZ

Jim Massie, BS, NREMT-P
Instructor, EMS Program
College of Southern Idaho
Twin Falls, ID

M. Allen McCullough, PhD
Fire Chief / Director of Public Safety
Department of Fire & Emergency Services
Fayetteville, GA

Deborah Poskus Medley, RN-BC, MSN, CCRN
Excela Health Westmoreland
Greensburg, PA

Elizabeth E. Morgan, NREMT
Mt. Hood Community College
Gresham, OR

Tom Nevetral, BS, NREMT-P
ALS Training Coordinator
Virginia Department of Health Office of Emergency
    Medical Services
Glen Allen, VA

Steve Nguyen, MS, NREMT-P
Tulsa Technology Center
Tulsa, OK

Mark Podgwaite, NREMT-I, NECEMS I/C
Training Coordinator
VT EMS District 6
Berlin, VA

Warren J. Porter, MS, BA, LP, NREMT-P
Director, Clinical and Education American Medical Response-
    South Region
Arlington, TX

Barry Reed, MPA, RN, EMTP, CCRN, CEN, CCEMTP
EMS, Fire, AHA Programs Director
Northwest Florida State College
Niceville, FL

Douglas P. Skinner, BS, NREMTP, NCEE
Training Officer
Loudoun County Fire Rescue
Leesburg, VA

Dale Trusty, EMT-P
Paramedic/ Instructor
North Georgia Technical College
Clarkesville, GA

Rebecca Valentine, BS, CCEMT-P, I/C
EMS Instructor
Natick, MA

Kelly Weller, MA, GN, LP, EMS-C
EMS Program Coordinator
Lone Star College-Montgomery
Conroe, TX

Randy Williams, NREMT-P
Instructor of Paramedic Technology/EMS Programs Coordinator
Bainbridge College
Bainbridge, GA

Photo Advisor and Sources

Special thanks to Eric Wellman, Southern Maine Community College EMS Program and Tim Nagle, Portland Maine Fire Department.

About the Authors

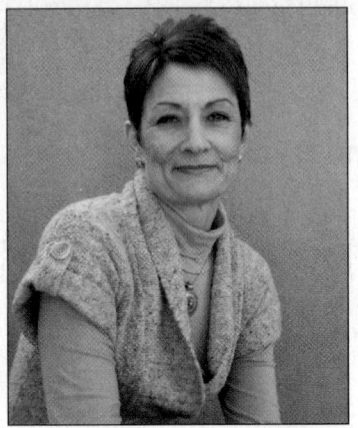

Melissa Alexander, EdD, NREMT-P

Melissa Alexander began her career in EMS in 1982 and has worked in various prehospital, hospital, and educational settings throughout the United States over the years. She has a BA in Community Health Education from Purdue University, an MS in Health Sciences Education from Indiana University, and an EdD in Human Resources Development from the George Washington University. Dr. Alexander is an assistant professor in the School of Criminal Justice, Fire Science, and EMS at Lake Superior State University in Sault Sainte Marie, Michigan. She has authored and contributed to several EMS texts. Dr. Alexander's research and advocacy interests are in various aspects of EMS education, including improving clinical-reasoning skills, and EMS workforce issues. She has three daughters, Lindsay, Brittany, and Eleanor; and three grandsons, Asher, Ethan, and Grant. She enjoys spending time with family, organic gardening, and hanging out with her dogs Sabrina, Benito, and Winston.

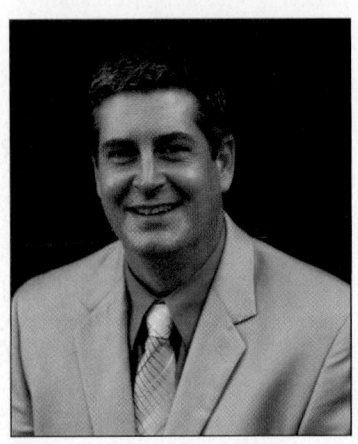

Richard Belle, BS, NREMT-P

Richard Belle, a native of New Orleans, LA, began his EMS career in 1996 after completing EMT-Basic and Paramedic training at Nicholls State University in Thibodaux, Louisiana. Richard has worked throughout south Louisiana as a field paramedic, new employee preceptor, student preceptor, and as a flight paramedic. He has been actively involved in EMS education since 1999. Richard served as Education Coordinator for Acadian Ambulance's southeastern district while he returned to Nicholls State University and earned a Bachelor of Science Degree. After four years of teaching EMT Basic and Paramedic courses, he transferred to Lafayette, Louisiana, to serve as Acadian Ambulance's Continuing Education Coordinator where he was responsible for providing refresher training and continuing education opportunities to medics across Louisiana, Texas, and Mississippi. Currently, Richard works in Lafayette, Louisiana as Continuing Education Manager for Acadian Ambulance and the National EMS Academy. Richard lives in south Louisiana with his wife Rhonda and their three children: James, Victoria, and Allison.

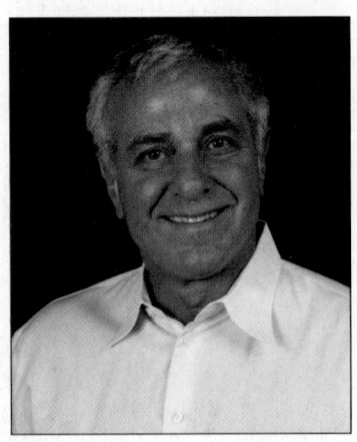

Steven Weiss, MD, MS, FACEP, FACP, *Medical Editor*

Dr. Weiss was first drawn to EMS as a working EMT in the mountains of Colorado. After completing medical school, he trained and received board certifications in both Emergency and Internal Medicine at Charity Hospital in New Orleans. He is a fellow of the *American College of Emergency Physicians* and the *American College of Physicians*. His career has spanned a great diversity of emergency medicine and EMS systems from Louisiana, Tennessee, California, and now New Mexico. Over the 20 years working in EMS, he has worked as a medical director of numerous EMS services and EMS training programs. During his time in Tennessee, he was the State EMS medical director.

Dr. Weiss has always been involved in training residents, physicians, and EMTs in EMS concepts and practice. He has published over 30 articles relating to EMS and presented over 20 abstracts at national meetings. Most recently, he spent four years as the medical director for the *EMS Academy* in Albuquerque, which trains all levels of EMS providers throughout the state. Presently, Dr. Weiss is a tenured professor of Emergency Medicine at the University of New Mexico where he works as a research director with the EMS fellows and with the ambulance services. He is on the editorial board of *Prehospital and Emergency Care*. He is married to Amy Ernst, a fellow emergency physician with an interest in injury prevention and intimate partner violence. His only daughter will be working as an intermediate EMT next year and plans to use this textbook to upgrade herself to an Advanced EMT.

SECTION 1

Preparing for Advanced Emergency Medical Technician Practice

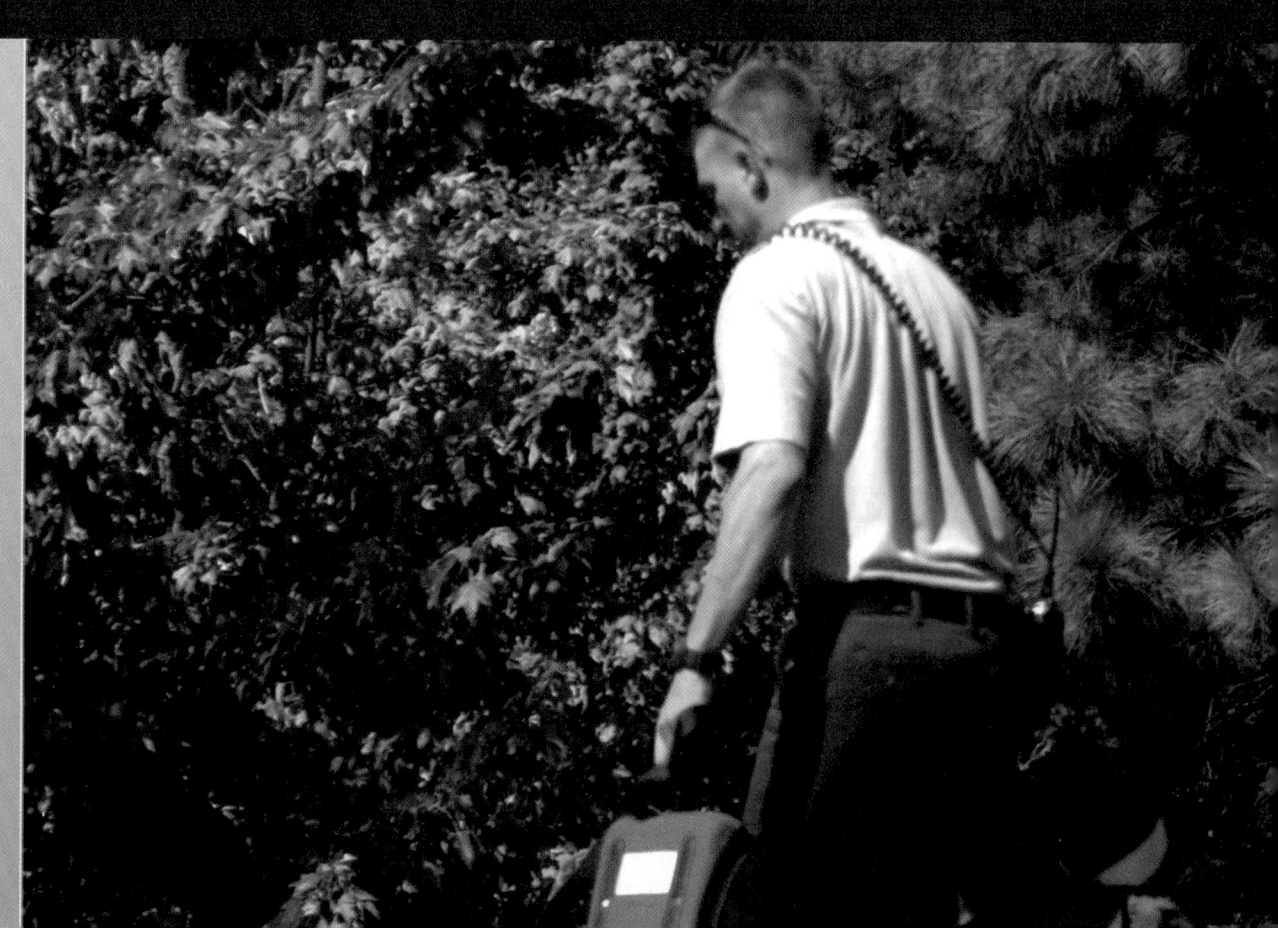

1 Introduction to Advanced Emergency Medical Technician Practice

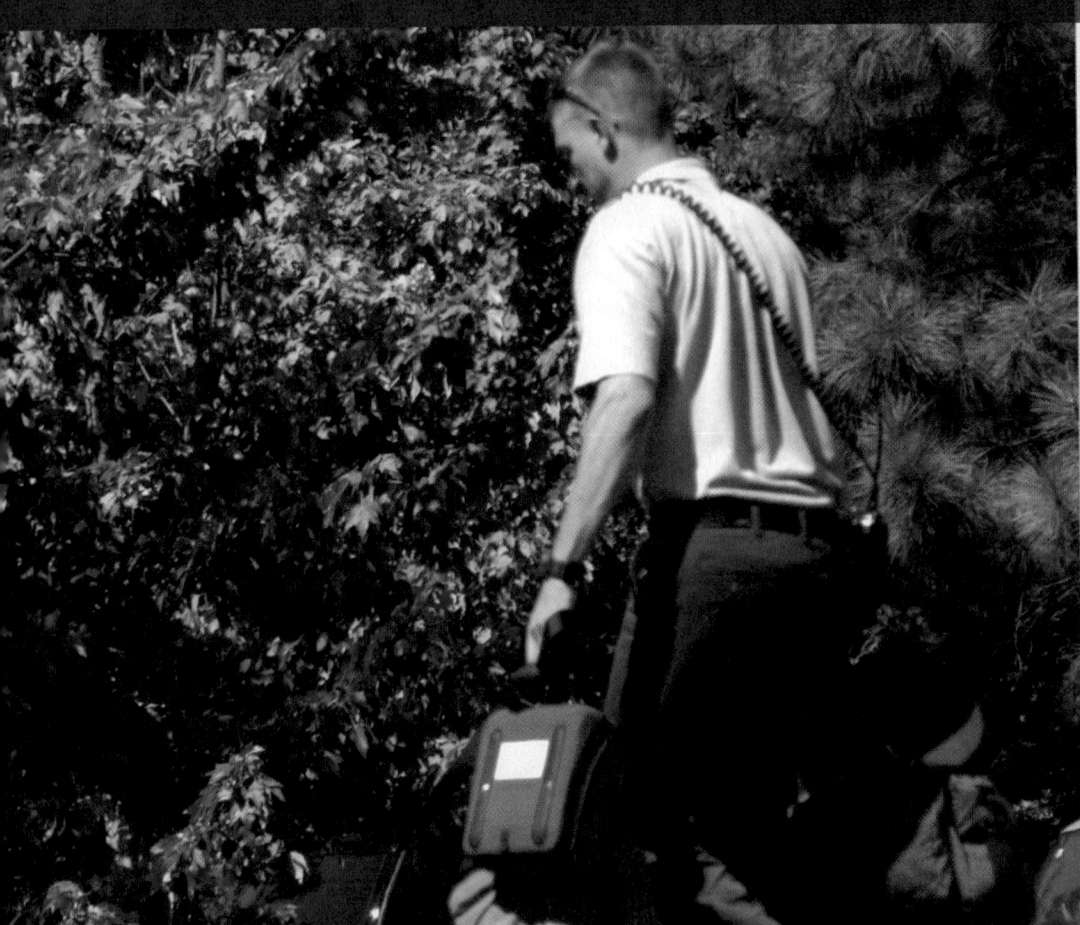

Content Area: Preparatory

Advanced EMT Education Standard: Applies fundamental knowledge of the EMS system, safety/well-being of the Advanced EMT, and medical/legal and ethical issues to the provision of emergency care.

Objectives

After reading this chapter, you should be able to:

1.1 Define key terms introduced in this chapter.

1.2 Describe the competencies, roles, responsibilities, and professional characteristics of the Advanced Emergency Medical Technician (Advanced EMT).

1.3 Describe the scope of practice of the Advanced EMT.

1.4 Place the roles and responsibilities of the Advanced EMT in the larger contexts of emergency medical services (EMS), health care, and public health.

1.5 Discuss key issues in the contemporary practice of the Advanced EMT, including professionalism, the focus on patient safety, research, and evidence-based practice.

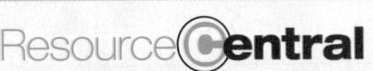

Resource**Central**

To access Resource Central, follow the directions on the Student Access Card provided with this text. If there is no card, go to www.bradybooks.com and follow the Resource Central link to Buy Access. Under Media Resources, you will find:

• *EMS Labor Force.* Compare EMS to other occupations.

• *The Future of Emergency Care.* See how EMS impacts the health care crisis.

• *The Winding Road of EMS.* Watch a video about the history and future of the EMS profession.

Advanced EMTs Jane McFadden and Kevin Breen are enjoying a few minutes of downtime at a city park, watching a soccer game, when their radios sound with a dispatch. "Ambulance 14, respond to 1025 West Bluff Street for difficulty breathing. That's one-zero-two-five West Bluff Street for difficulty breathing. Coordinates 400 north, 1025 west." Kevin moves from his position at the front of the ambulance toward the driver's seat, and pushes the "responding" status button on the front of the radio panel. Jane climbs into the passenger seat, fastens her seat belt, and readies a pair of vinyl gloves.

Three minutes later, as they park along the curb in front of the residence, Kevin pushes the "at scene" status button on the radio panel. This is a quiet, well-kept neighborhood, and the arrival of the ambulance has attracted the attention of some neighbors. Jane and Kevin deliberately scan the house, yard, and surrounding area. They notice nothing out of the ordinary that could pose a danger to them, so they walk up the steps and onto the porch. Before they can ring the bell, an anxious-looking woman in her late 30s opens the door. "I'm glad you're here," she says. "It's my son, Justin. He's wheezing and his inhaler isn't helping. He's getting worse. This is the second asthma attack he's had this week. He's back here, in the kitchen."

Problem-Solving Questions

1. How should Jane and Kevin proceed?
2. What are their overall goals in managing this situation?
3. What knowledge and skills do you think Jane and Kevin will be calling on?

Introduction

Students, welcome to the ranks of the Advanced Emergency Medical Technician (Advanced EMT)! Reading this chapter marks the beginning of an exciting journey in advancing your status as a health care provider. Taking this step gives you a greater array of career opportunities and settings in which to care for sick and injured patients. Advanced EMTs comprise a critical part of the **emergency medical services (EMS)**. As an Advanced EMT, you will provide comfort, emergency medical care, and transportation for a variety of ill and injured patients. While carrying out your **roles** and **responsibilities** as an **EMS provider**, you will provide a link between patients and the health care and public health systems.

EMS and EMS Providers

Advanced EMTs comprise one of the four nationally recognized levels of health care providers who work in EMS systems. EMS systems were developed to provide essential lifesaving care and emergency transportation to critically ill and injured patients. Initially, training focused on treating patients who were injured in motor vehicle crashes (MVCs) and those in cardiac arrest. But, over time, the larger health care system and the public have come to rely on EMS in a variety of situations. EMS providers respond to patients with an assortment of injuries and illnesses in emergency

situations. EMS providers also routinely provide **interfacility transportation** for patients with both chronic and acute illness. In addition to these roles, EMS providers engage in community health education and promotion efforts, respond to disasters, and work in a variety of settings. Those settings include emergency departments, fire departments, industrial settings, and even movie sets (Figure 1-1).

The scope of knowledge and skills required of EMS providers has changed over time to reflect the diversity of situations in which EMS providers may find themselves. This chapter summarizes the contemporary practice of EMS, the roles of EMS providers, and the practice of Advanced EMTs.

The Contemporary EMS Profession

A **profession** is an occupation or vocation with particular characteristics, and it is defined by a specialized set of knowledge. In EMS, that knowledge is defined in documents published by the National Highway Transportation Safety Administration (NHTSA) of the U.S. Department of Transportation (DOT), such as the *National EMS Core Content, National EMS Scope of Practice,* and *National EMS Education Standards.* Professions are considered self-regulating. This means that a profession is directed and guided by people who are in the profession, rather than by an external group. Professions have codes of conduct or ethics. The EMT Oath (Figure 1-2) and EMT Code of Ethics (Figure 1-3) describe

FIGURE 1-1

Advanced EMTs work in a variety of settings. (© Craig Jackson/In the Dark Photography)

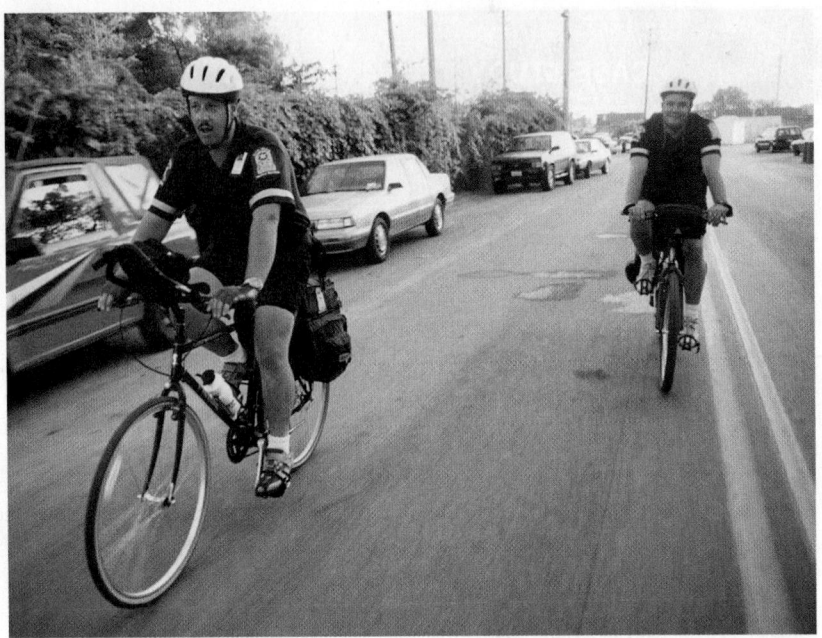

The EMT Oath

Be it pledged as an Emergency Medical Technician, I will honor the physical and judicial laws of God and man. I will follow that regimen which, according to my ability and judgment, I consider for the benefit of patients and abstain from whatever is deleterious and mischievous, nor shall I suggest any such counsel. Into whatever homes I enter, I will go into them for the benefit of only the sick and injured, never revealing what I see or hear in the lives of men unless required by law.

I shall also share my medical knowledge with those who may benefit from what I have learned. I will serve unselfishly and continuously in order to help make a better world for all mankind.

While I continue to keep this oath unviolated, may it be granted to me to enjoy life, and the practice of the art, respected by all men, in all times. Should I trespass or violate this oath, may the reverse be my lot.

So help me God.

Written by Charles B. Gillespie, MD
Adopted by the National Association of Emergency Medical Technicians, 1978.

FIGURE 1-2

The EMT Oath. (Reprinted with permission of National Association of Emergency Medical Technicians)

the professional conduct expected of EMS personnel. Finally, professionals are more motivated by the desire to provide service than the desire to achieve a high income.

The self-regulating characteristic of EMS also means that EMS providers have a professional obligation to be aware of the current issues in the profession. EMS providers must be aware of the activities and agendas of the major state and national professional agencies and organizations in EMS (Table 1-1). Those desiring leadership positions in EMS must take an active role in those organizations.

EMS providers constitute a link for patients between the **prehospital** setting and the hospital and are an important part of the health care team. The roles of EMS providers in public health are still emerging, with the potential for EMS providers to have a significant impact on public health. The *EMS Agenda for the Future* (NHTSA, 1996) envisions EMS providers as playing important roles in health assessment, health education, and health services (Figure 1-4).

EMS Provider Levels

The four nationally recognized levels of EMS providers are **Emergency Medical Responder (EMR)**, **Emergency Medical Technician (EMT)**, **Advanced Emergency Medical Technician (Advanced EMT)**, and **Paramedic**. In some areas, the titles may vary slightly. Many states are in transition between an older model of EMS provider designations and the newer one. For example, EMRs may be called First Responders, EMTs may be called EMT-Basics,

The EMT Code of Ethics

Professional status as an Emergency Medical Technician and Emergency Medical Technician-Paramedic is maintained and enriched by the willingness of the individual practitioner to accept and fulfill obligations to society, other medical professionals, and the profession of Emergency Medical Technician. As an Emergency Medical Technician-Paramedic, I solemnly pledge myself to the following code of professional ethics:

A fundamental responsibility of the Emergency Medical Technician is to conserve life, to alleviate suffering, to promote health, to do no harm, and to encourage the quality and equal availability of emergency medical care.

The Emergency Medical Technician provides services based on human need, with respect for human dignity, unrestricted by consideration of nationality, race, creed, color, or status.

The Emergency Medical Technician does not use professional knowledge and skills in any enterprise detrimental to the public well being.

The Emergency Medical Technician respects and holds in confidence all information of a confidential nature obtained in the course of professional work unless required by law to divulge such information.

The Emergency Medical Technician, as a citizen, understands and upholds the law and performs the duties of citizenship; as a professional, the Emergency Medical Technician has the never-ending responsibility to work with concerned citizens and other health care professionals in promoting a high standard of emergency medical care to all people.

The Emergency Medical Technician shall maintain professional competence and demonstrate concern for the competence of other members of the Emergency Medical Services health care team.

An Emergency Medical Technician assumes responsibility in defining and upholding standards of professional practice and education.

The Emergency Medical Technician assumes responsibility for individual professional actions and judgment, both in dependent and independent emergency functions, and knows and upholds the laws which affect the practice of the Emergency Medical Technician.

An Emergency Medical Technician has the responsibility to be aware of and participate in matters of legislation affecting the Emergency Medical Service System.

The Emergency Medical Technician, or groups of Emergency Medical Technicians, who advertise professional service, do so in conformity with the dignity of the profession.

The Emergency Medical Technician has an obligation to protect the public by not delegating to a person less qualified, any service which requires the professional competence of an Emergency Medical Technician.

The Emergency Medical Technician will work harmoniously with and sustain confidence in Emergency Medical Technician associates, the nurses, the physicians, and other members of the Emergency Medical Services health care team.

The Emergency Medical Technician refuses to participate in unethical procedures, and assumes the responsibility to expose incompetence or unethical conduct of others to the appropriate authority in a proper and professional manner.

Written by: Charles B. Gillespie, MD
Adopted by the National Association of Emergency Medical Technicians, 1978.

FIGURE 1-3

The EMT Code of Ethics. (Reprinted with permission of National Association of Emergency Medical Technicians)

Advanced EMTs may be called EMT-Intermediates, and paramedics may be called Emergency Medical Technician-Paramedics or EMT-Ps. With time, it is anticipated that there will be greater uniformity in EMS titles across the country.

Emergency Medical Responder

Emergency Medical Responders (EMRs) are trained in very basic skills. They use minimal equipment to provide immediately lifesaving care to critically ill and injured patients while awaiting the arrival of more highly trained EMS personnel. EMRs also provide basic first-aid measures to less critically ill and injured patients. The basic nature of EMR training makes it possible for rural communities to train EMRs who can arrive quickly at the scene of an injury or illness to provide care while awaiting an ambulance.

EMR training can be completed in 48 to 60 hours. The training is ideal for those who do not want to make a career of EMS, but who want to provide a critical service to their communities. Industrial workers may obtain

TABLE 1-1   National EMS Agencies and Professional Organizations

Organization	Purpose	Website
National Association of Emergency Medical Technicians	Represents and serves all EMS practitioners through quality education, membership, and national advocacy	www.naemt.org
National Registry of Emergency Medical Technicians	Provides assurance through testing and recertification processes that EMS personnel are competent	www.nremt.org
National Association of State EMS Officials	Provides support in developing EMS policy and oversight and provides vision, leadership, and resources in the development and improvement of state, regional, and local EMS and emergency care systems	www.nasemsd.org
National Association of EMS Physicians	An organization of physicians and other professionals who provide leadership and foster excellence in prehospital emergency medical services	www.naemsp.org
National Highway Transportation Safety Administration, Emergency Medical Services	Website provides background and updates on federal EMS initiatives and programs	www.ems.gov

The Vision

Emergency medical services (EMS) of the future will be community-based health management that is fully integrated with the overall health care system. It will have the ability to identify and modify illness and injury risks, provide acute illness and injury care and follow-up, and contribute to treatment of chronic conditions and community health monitoring. This new entity will be developed from redistribution of existing health care resources and will be integrated with other health care providers and public health and public safety agencies. It will improve community health and result in more appropriate use of acute health care resources. EMS will remain the public's emergency medical safety net.

FIGURE 1-4

EMS is developing and growing to include additional components of health care and public health. (From *National Highway Transportation Safety Administration (1996). EMS Agenda for the Future*)

EMR training so they can assist injured coworkers while awaiting help. Law enforcement officers, who are often the first to arrive on the scene of injured patients, also may be EMRs.

EMRs can perform simple assessments to identify and manage life threats. They use basic airway management and ventilation skills, cardiopulmonary resuscitation (CPR), automatic external defibrillators (AED), and simple methods to control bleeding. EMRs are trained to recognize injuries that require immobilization, and other conditions that can be treated in the EMR scope of practice. For example, EMRs can provide initial care for patients who have a foreign substance in the eye, and treat themselves or peers for nerve agent poisoning, using an antidote auto-injection kit. As an Advanced EMT who may be interacting with EMRs, it is important that you know the scope of practice of EMRs. (See Table 1-2 for EMS providers' scopes of practice.)

Emergency Medical Technicians

Emergency Medical Technicians (EMTs) provide emergency medical care and transportation to the ill and injured, using the basic equipment supplied on an ambulance. EMTs play a variety of roles in EMS systems. Some EMTs act in a first-response capacity, arriving at the scene prior to more highly trained EMS personnel to provide immediately lifesaving care. Many EMTs provide the primary transporting EMS service in a community. Other EMTs work for ambulance services that primarily perform interfacility transports. The EMT may work with a partner at the same level, or may work with an Advanced EMT or paramedic partner.

Like EMRs, EMTs may work in industry or public safety agencies. Some EMTs work in emergency departments and urgent care centers where they use their skills to assist nursing and medical staff.

TABLE 1-2	EMS Provider Descriptions and Scopes of Practice	
Provider Level	**Description**	**Minimum Psychomotor Skills**
Emergency Medical Responder (EMR)	Provides simple, noninvasive treatments to reduce morbidity and mortality from illness and injury while awaiting arrival of more highly trained personnel	Use of simple airway devices designed for placement in the oropharynx Positive pressure ventilation (bag-valve mask) Upper airway suctioning Oxygen administration Self- or peer-administration of nerve agent antidote kit Automatic external defibrillation Manual stabilization of suspected spinal and musculoskeletal injuries Bleeding control Emergency moves
Emergency Medical Technician (EMT)	Provides basic, noninvasive interventions at the scene and during transportation of patients to the hospital	All EMR skills Nasopharyngeal airways Manually triggered and automatic transport ventilators Assisting patients in taking their own medications Oral glucose for hypoglycemia Aspirin for chest pain Pneumatic antishock garment for fracture stabilization
Advanced Emergency Medical Technician (Advanced EMT)	Provides basic and limited advanced skills focused on the acute management and transportation of critical and emergent patients Functions at an emergency scene, en route from an emergency scene to a health care facility, between health care facilities, or in other health care settings	All EMT skills Airways not intended to be placed in the trachea Tracheobronchial suctioning of an already intubated patient Peripheral IVs and administration of nonmedicated IV fluids Intraosseous access in pediatric patients Sublingual nitroglycerin for chest pain Subcutaneous of intramuscular epinephrine for anaphylaxis Glucagon and 50 percent dextrose for hypoglycemia Inhaled bronchodilators for wheezing Narcotic antagonist for suspected narcotic overdose Nitrous oxide for pain relief
Paramedic	Provides basic and advanced skills for acute management and transportation of a broad range of patients Functions at an emergency scene, en route from an emergency scene to a health care facility, between health care facilities, or in other health care settings	All Advanced EMT skills Endotracheal intubation Percutaneous cricothyrotomy Decompression of the pleural space Intraosseous infusion in adults Administration of various approved medications by a variety of routes Maintenance of blood or blood product infusions Synchronized cardioversion, transcutaneous pacing, and manual defibrillation

EMTs are trained to assess patients, performing a basic history and physical examination to identify patient's problems and complaints, and monitor them for changes. In addition to all of the knowledge and skills of the EMR, EMTs are expected to be able to identify a wider range of patient conditions, and can administer or assist a patient in self-administering some basic emergency medicines. These wider scopes of knowledge and practice are reflected in a longer course length of 150 to 190 hours. In addition to classroom and skills laboratory components, EMT courses are expected to include hospital/emergency department and ambulance experience as part of the educational program.

Advanced EMTs

As an Advanced EMT, your training will include all of the knowledge and skills of EMRs and EMTs. You will gain a greater breadth and depth of understanding of many of the topics introduced at lower levels of training, and will be able to provide a limited number of **advanced life support (ALS)** interventions. These interventions are primarily geared toward meeting the needs of critically ill patients who have problems with their airway, breathing, and circulation. Like all EMS providers, you must practice within the **scope of practice** approved by your state and your EMS service **physician medical director**. Understanding Advanced EMT authorization to practice is crucial. It will be discussed in detail in Chapters 2 and 4.

Advanced EMTs may be the highest level providers available in some communities or work in conjunction with paramedics. They may work for ambulance services, fire departments, volunteer public safety agencies, hospital emergency departments or urgent care clinics, and industrial or other settings.

Prior EMS training is not a prerequisite for EMRs and EMTs. However, Advanced EMT students must either have completed EMT training or it must be incorporated into their program. Advanced EMT training requires approximately 150 to 250 hours beyond the time required to complete EMT training. Training includes classroom and laboratory education plus **clinical training** and **field training**. By the time you complete Advanced EMT training, you will have completed between 300 and 440 hours of education as a health care provider.

Paramedics

Paramedics are **allied health care professionals** who provide complex assessments and interventions for critical and emergent patients. Paramedic education prepares them to integrate EMS operational knowledge with complex understanding of anatomy, physiology, pathophysiology, and treatment modalities. This knowledge prepares them to assess and manage patients with a variety of illnesses and injuries.

Because of the depth and breadth of knowledge and skill expected of paramedics, their education programs are often based in institutions of higher education. The Commission on Accreditation of EMS Programs (CoAEMSP) accredits paramedic education programs to ensure that they meet minimum standards. Students should apply only to paramedic programs that are accredited.

The core portion of paramedic programs ranges from about 1,000 to 1,500 hours beyond the EMT level. Many institutions offer associate's degrees for paramedics. Several offer bachelor's degree programs in EMS that include paramedic training. The commitment of time and money required to complete paramedic training means that paramedics are not available in all communities.

Advanced EMT Roles and Responsibilities

An Advanced EMT's authorization to practice is based on state legislation, employer policies and procedures, and the guidance provided by a physician medical director. Each state has legislation that defines the scope of practice of licensed EMS personnel. Your specific scope of practice is available through your state EMS office. **Protocols** and **standing orders** for your EMS service are available through your employer. You must practice only within the boundaries specified by your state scope of practice and your EMS service medical director, policies, and procedures. However, there are roles and responsibilities that define Advanced EMT practice, regardless of the specific patient care skills or employer procedures used to carry out these roles and responsibilities.

Emergency Vehicle Readiness and Operations

Before patient care can begin, you and other EMS providers must safely reach the scene of the emergency. This means your emergency vehicle must be in good mechanical repair, its warning devices must be working properly, and it must be driven safely for the sake of the EMS crew and the public. If your vehicle is not properly maintained and does not start or breaks down on the way to the scene, you cannot provide emergency care for the patient. Similarly, if you are involved in a vehicle collision, you will not reach the scene. If you and your crew are injured in a collision, additional emergency medical resources will be needed to care for both the original patient and you. Your training as an Advanced EMT includes basic instruction in ambulance operations. Your state and employer will likely have additional specific requirements for emergency vehicle operations training (Figure 1-5).

In addition to performing a daily maintenance check on your vehicle, you also will be responsible for having an adequate amount of required equipment and supplies. Once you arrive at the scene, the equipment and supplies you need

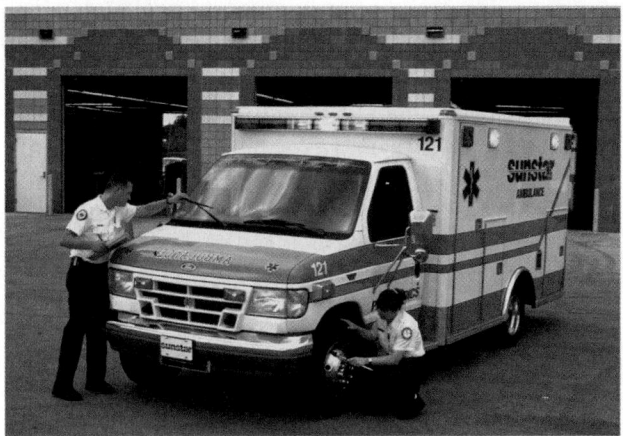

FIGURE 1-5

Advanced EMT responsibilities include making sure equipment and the emergency vehicle are prepared to respond to emergency calls.

TABLE 1-3	Select EMS Tasks with High Risk for Errors and Patient Injury

- Transferring care from one provider to another at the scene or at the hospital
- Communicating, either in writing or verbally
- Identifying and using medications
- Assessing and managing the airway
- Lifting and moving patients
- Responding and transporting by ambulance
- Assessing the need for, and performing, spinal immobilization

TABLE 1-4	Ways to Minimize the Risk of Mistakes and Patient Injury

- Maintain current knowledge and competence in skills.
- Make the environment as conducive as possible to quality care (maximize space and light, minimize distractions).
- Have a clear understanding of protocols.
- Organize drugs to minimize mistakes.
- Reflect on actions and question assumptions.
- Obtain feedback on performance.
- Ask for help when needed (contact medical direction, consult with your partner).

to assess, treat, lift, and move your patient must be available in the proper quantities and sizes, be in good repair, and be organized so you can locate them easily.

Safety

EMS providers have substantial responsibility for their own safety, and the safety of coworkers, patients, and others. Your safety and that of your coworkers includes many things. You must drive safely and avoid dangers at the scene. Such dangers include highway traffic, leaking chemicals, downed power lines, and violent patients and bystanders. You also must avoid exposure to communicable diseases by using Standard Precautions (Chapter 3), including appropriate personal protective equipment.

Patient safety involves many considerations. The same scene hazards that pose a threat to you also pose a threat to your patient. Errors by medical personnel account for between 44,000 and 98,000 patient deaths annually (Institute of Medicine [IOM], 1999). Tens of thousands of additional patients are harmed by medical errors each year. The costs associated with medical errors are between $17 billion and $29 billion dollars annually.

Many medical errors occur in the administration of medications. This points to the importance of the Advanced EMT's adherence to safe medication administration practices. Patients can be harmed in ambulance collisions as well. They can be dropped or improperly handled during lifting and moving. They may be improperly assessed or managed (O'Connor, Slovis, Hunt, Pirallo, & Sayre, 2002) (Table 1-3.) Harm also can come to patients when there is a miscommunication about a patient's condition and treatment. This text places great emphasis on the knowledge, skills, and attitudes required for safe Advanced EMT practice (Table 1-4).

You must be aware of the safety of the public while operating an emergency vehicle and the safety of others at the scene of an emergency. Family members and bystanders who are distraught or distracted by the emergency may not be aware of any nearby danger. You must provide direction in order to keep them out of harm's way.

Scene Leadership, Management, and Teamwork

The patient and others at the emergency scene will look to you to bring order to a stressful, perhaps even chaotic, situation. You must be confident and in control. You also must be empathetic to the medical and emotional needs of patients and family members. In conjunction with your coworkers, you will need to determine the nature of the problem, decide what must be done about it, and then carry out your plan to address the problem.

A consistent goal on all EMS calls is to transport your patient to the most appropriate hospital. Patient assessment, patient care, and patient transportation must be integrated into a smooth process. Your success in gaining the patient's cooperation, and that of the family, bystanders, and other personnel depends upon the development of professional characteristics and learning key skills in communication, leadership, and teamwork (Figure 1-6).

of high-quality emergency medical care requires command of a body of specialized knowledge and skills. As the body of **research** in emergency medical care increases, our knowledge of the best ways to assess and manage illnesses and injuries changes. You must always be aware of the most current trends and practices in EMS in order to provide the best care possible for your patients.

Research gives us new tools and methods for assessing and treating patients, but it also challenges previously unquestioned practices. Health care providers must always be as willing to discard outdated knowledge and practices as they are to add new ones. The reliance on research findings to guide medical practice is called **evidence-based practice**, or evidence-based medicine. For example, full immobilization of the spine has been unquestioned for years. It was widely assumed to be necessary to prevent a spine injury from turning into permanent paralysis. However, emerging research suggests that, not only may there be no substantial benefit to spinal immobilization, but there also may be serious consequences associated with the procedure. Currently, spinal immobilization is a standard of care for most trauma patients, but this is one area of practice, among others, that may change.

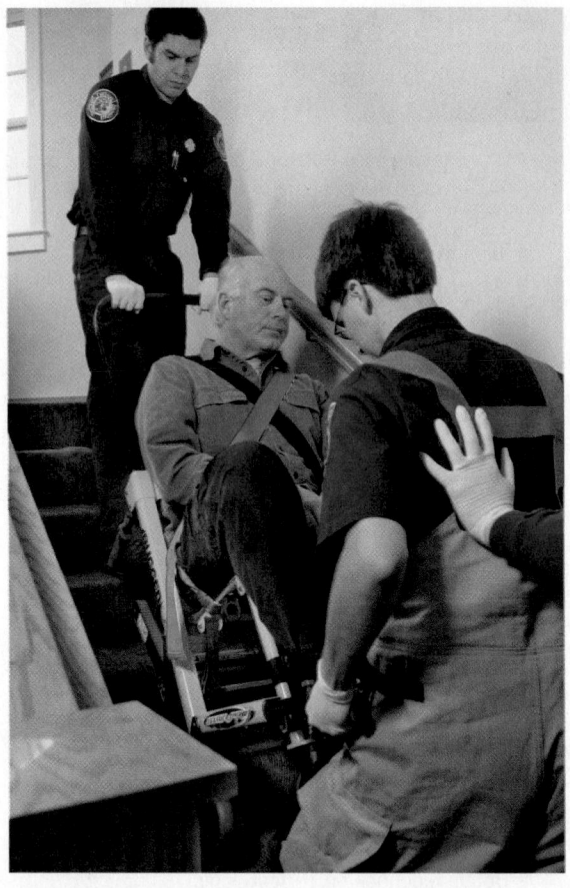

FIGURE 1-6

Teamwork is required to integrate the tasks of patient care and patient transportation.

Patient Assessment and Management

The foundation of Advanced EMT practice is the ability to assess and manage patients who have a variety of illnesses and injuries, ranging from minor to critical. The delivery

Maintaining Certification or Licensure

Maintaining current knowledge is an ethical responsibility for those entrusted with patient care. It also is generally a legal requirement for continued certification or licensure. In order to continue practicing as an EMS professional, one of your responsibilities is to meet your state's requirements. Requirements typically include documentation of mandatory continuing education activities, medical director verification of skills, submission of a CPR card, and payment of a fee. Maintaining licensure is an individual professional obligation of each health care provider, not a responsibility of employers or educational institutions.

PERSONAL PERSPECTIVE

Advanced EMT Mike Twain: I've been in EMS since I graduated from high school. That's 25 years ago this month, believe it or not! When I took my EMT class, things were taught in a very black-and-white manner. The thought of changes in the way we were doing things never entered my mind. One of the things that was drilled into us was how important it was to quickly get the antishock trousers on critical trauma patients. We thought they worked like magic. We saw unconscious patients with low blood pressures wake up and start talking to us. There was no doubt in our minds that we saved lives using the shock pants. It turns out some folks were researching shock pants and found out that they weren't effective. How could that be,

you know? A lot of us were angry. We knew they worked. Research and evidence-based medicine weren't part of what we were taught at the time. Our medical director, Doc Brown, did a good job of calming us down and explaining the research. Even though we saw a temporary increase in blood pressure, it turns out that there was no difference in survival, whether patients had shock pants put on or not. In fact, the time we were taking at the scene to put the things on was probably time better spent getting the patient to surgical care more quickly. Well, a lot of other things have changed since then, too. I understand why change is needed now, but I sure wish we'd been taught with the idea that things would change.

IN THE FIELD

Certification can be granted by any entity to recognize achievement, but it does not give legal permission to practice. Licensure is permission from a governmental agency to engage in a profession.

Working with Other Public Safety and Health Care Personnel

Emergency medical services are cross-disciplinary. They are both public safety and health care personnel. They interact with other public safety personnel and health care providers to provide patient care. It is in the best interests of the patient for Advanced EMTs to always strive to maintain cooperative relationships with other professionals. On any single shift, you may find yourself interacting with emergency medical dispatchers, firefighters (or if you are a firefighter, with transporting ambulance personnel), EMS personnel from other agencies, law enforcement officers, home health care providers, and a variety of health care technicians, nurses, and physicians. Good communication, an orientation toward teamwork, and keeping the patient's best interests at the forefront are essential in ensuring continuity of patient care (Figure 1-7).

Advanced EMT Professional Characteristics

Have you always been treated as you think you should be treated when seeking health care? Have encounters with the health care system left you feeling satisfied? Health care professionals have an opportunity to impact the lives of others in many ways. One way in which you can positively impact the experience of your patients is to follow the golden rule: Do unto others as you would have them do unto you. This is one of the core tenets of professional ethics. Professionalism is conveyed through adherence to a set of values and behaviors that are accepted as defining features of a given occupation.

Professional characteristics are defined by the expectations of the public, the professional group itself, and other related professional groups. The most visible way in which patients and their families can judge your professionalism is through your interactions with them. Patients may not know if you have the most up-to-date information or if you are providing the correct treatment, but they are very aware of your appearance and demeanor. Your peers, other health care providers, and public safety providers will judge your professionalism as well.

The level of professionalism you convey to others is not just a reflection on you, but on EMS providers as a group. If one of your family members required emergency medical assistance at this moment, what would you expect of the EMS personnel arriving to help? What are some of the behaviors that would convey to you that a caring, competent professional has arrived to manage the situation?

Integrity

Integrity encompasses such behaviors as honesty, honor, reliability, and being upstanding. It is often described as doing the right thing when no one is looking. An example of integrity in EMS is being thorough, accurate, and honest on your daily vehicle and equipment checklists. You must be able to be trusted with a patient's well-being, information, and belongings.

Empathy

Empathy means showing compassion and understanding for others. In other words, it means putting yourself in someone else's shoes, so to speak. Patients may be reluctant or uncooperative because they are frightened. It is important to understand the emotions behind the behavior in order to decide the best way to interact with them. At times you may feel that a patient has called 911 for something that is not an emergency. One reason for this is that you and patients do not have the same understanding of what an emergency is. Rather than being impatient or judgmental, look at things from the patient's point of view.

Self-Motivation

Self-motivation means doing things that need to be done based on your initiative, rather than waiting to be told to do them. If your vehicle is dirty, make sure it is washed before your supervisor has to remind you. If your oxygen cylinder is

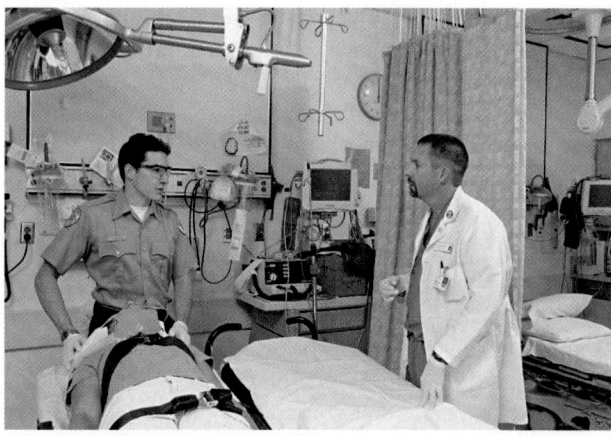

FIGURE 1-7

Advanced EMTs work closely with other health care and public safety providers.

low, replace it. Obtain your continuing education before your supervisor sends you a memo to remind you that it is due. In short, stay on top of the things that are your responsibility.

Appearance and Personal Hygiene

EMS personnel wear uniforms so that they can be recognized by the public as individuals who are there to help. The uniform represents you as a professional and represents the service you work for. Lack of care in personal appearance and hygiene indicates to others a lack of regard for professionalism. Can the Advanced EMT who does not take the time to clean his uniform be trusted to properly clean the patient's skin before starting an intravenous (IV) line? Although it may be argued that no one should be judged by appearance, the truth is that everyone is judged on appearance to some degree. Present yourself so as to be recognized immediately by others as a professional (Figure 1-8).

Self-Confidence

Being self-confident means that you have reasonable and realistic faith in your abilities. Self-confidence is displayed through poise, by being calm and in control. Your demeanor should reassure patients. Being uncertain of yourself will cause patients to doubt your abilities. Of course, keep in mind that overconfidence is a leading factor in making mistakes and is a cause of interpersonal friction between coworkers. The best way to become self-confident is to learn well the knowledge, skills, roles, and responsibilities of Advanced EMTs. Perfection is not always possible, but competence is essential. Naturally, you will be nervous at first as you venture into the field as an Advanced EMT. It is the employers' obligation to orient

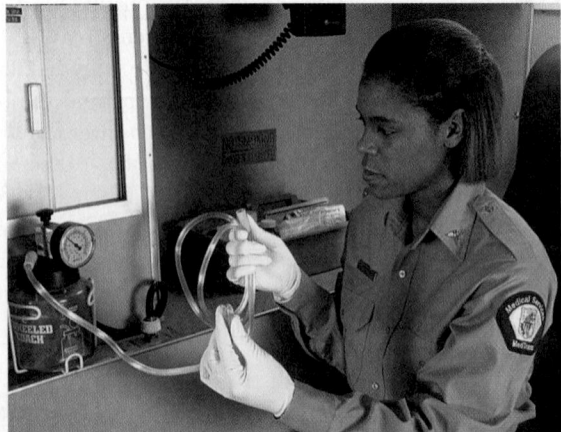

FIGURE 1-8

Appearance and demeanor are critical elements of professionalism.

new providers to the job, and to provide them with a field training officer, senior partner, or mentor.

Communications

A very large proportion of the Advanced EMT's working time is spent in some kind of communication. You communicate with supervisors, coworkers, dispatchers, patients, family members, and other public safety and health care personnel. Communication is required for effective teamwork and patient care. The messages you convey and how you convey them tell much about your professionalism. For example, people judge your intelligence, and therefore your trustworthiness, as a health care provider by your grammar, diction, and vocabulary. You will communicate over the radio and in person with personnel at receiving hospitals, and will leave them with a written report of your patient assessment and management. Your competence as a health care provider will be judged on your ability to convey your patient's story accurately, completely, concisely, and coherently.

Time Management

Time management as an EMS provider has many facets. It includes getting to work on time, taking care of responsibilities in a timely manner, and being able to prioritize tasks.

Teamwork, Diplomacy, and Respect

Completing a call with the feeling that great teamwork allowed things to go smoothly is a satisfying feeling. Teamwork requires a common understanding of the goals of a situation and of the methods and techniques used to achieve the goals. Each person on a team, including the team leader, must understand and fulfill his role. To be effective, a team must always keep the patient's best interests at the forefront.

Simply put, diplomacy means tact. Diplomacy is required for effective communication and teamwork.

Respect means having regard for the innate value of others. You must respect the dignity of all human beings in order to provide the highest quality care possible. Lack of respect is easily communicated and is detrimental to communication and teamwork.

Patient Advocacy

Advocacy means to support or promote something. In this case, it means to support or promote the needs and rights of patients. Imagine that you are walking through a busy emergency department after delivering your patient to his assigned bed. You hear a feeble voice call out from behind a closed curtain, "Help me, please. Can somebody help me?" The nurses and technicians are all busy with other patients. Are you obligated to see what you can do for this patient? Ethically and professionally, you are. Perhaps it is something simple you can take care of yourself, like getting an extra blanket from the linen cart. Maybe the patient has an urgent need that needs to be communicated to a hospital staff member, or maybe he just needs reassurance that there is someone there, outside the curtain. Remember empathy. How would you feel if you were isolated behind a curtain in a strange setting and needed something, but no one responded?

Careful Delivery of Service

The careful delivery of service as a professional characteristic includes making sure your vehicle and equipment are in working order. It also includes driving safely, lifting and moving patients with care, listening carefully to make sure you get the patient's history right, and adhering to proper procedures and safety precautions when caring for patients. Remember, patient safety is one of the most critical current issues in health care.

CASE STUDY WRAP-UP

Clinical-Reasoning Process

Advanced EMTs Jane McFadden and Kevin Breen are on the scene of a 13-year-old patient, Justin Wallace, who has a history of asthma. They have a number of overall goals to accomplish. They've responded safely to the scene, communicated with dispatch, and checked for hazards as they approached the house. They must now interact with Justin and his mother, determine what Justin's problems are, provide the right treatment, and safely transport Justin to the hospital.

Kevin responds to Justin's anxious mother, "Let's take a look and see how he's doing." Jane notes that Justin is sitting up, leaning forward with his hands on his knees. She immediately recognizes the signs of respiratory distress. Kevin is already pulling an oxygen mask from the equipment bag.

"Hi, Justin," says Jane. "Let's see if we can get you feeling a little better before we get you on your way to the hospital." As Kevin administers oxygen, Jane turns to Justin's mother. "Ma'am, I'd like to give Justin some medication. I just need to ask you a few questions while I'm getting it ready." Meanwhile, Kevin listens to Justin's lungs with a stethoscope and checks his oxygen level with a finger probe. Continuing to reassure Justin, Kevin takes an initial set of vital signs.

As Jane prepares a breathing treatment for Justin, she asks Justin's mom when the asthma attack started, what medications he takes, and how much medication he has taken today. She asks if he has any allergies or other medical problems, and what hospital she wants Justin to go to. While Jane begins the breathing treatment, Kevin brings the stretcher inside and positions it next to Justin. "Mrs. Wallace, will you be okay to drive to the hospital, or would you like to ride with us and call someone to meet you there?"

"I want to stay with Justin," she responds.

"No problem," replies Kevin. "We'll get Justin ready to go while you make sure you've got everything you need to take with you."

En route to the hospital, Jane's reassessment reveals some improvement in Justin's breathing and oxygen level. "You're wheezing less, Justin," she says. "How are you feeling?"

"A little bit better," he replies.

"Great," says Jane. "I'm going to call the hospital on the radio now and let them know you're coming."

CHAPTER REVIEW

Chapter Summary

Advanced EMTs are an essential part of EMS and of the health care and public health systems. Advanced EMTs are health care professionals of whom the public has high expectations. Your responsibilities are great, but so are the rewards and pride that come with providing safe, high-quality professional services to patients in the prehospital setting.

Review Questions

Multiple-Choice Questions

1. Who are the EMS providers trained to administer basic lifesaving care while awaiting arrival of more highly trained EMS providers who will transport the patient?
   a. Emergency Medical Responders
   b. First-aid assistants
   c. Emergency Medical Technicians
   d. Basic Emergency Medical Technicians

2. En route to the hospital, your patient says she really needs to use the restroom. As the triage nurse assigns your patient a bed, you ask if it is okay if you help the patient to the restroom before helping her into bed. Which one of the following professional characteristics is best represented by your actions?
   a. Careful delivery of service
   b. Integrity
   c. Patient advocacy
   d. Time management

3. Which one of the following is within the scope of practice of Advanced EMTs?
   a. Giving medications to stop preterm labor
   b. Starting IVs
   c. Manual defibrillation
   d. Endotracheal intubation

Critical-Thinking Questions

4. List two specific characteristics that allow EMS to be defined as a profession.

5. Give an example of behavior that is consistent with the professional characteristic of self-motivation.

6. List two EMS tasks with high potential for mistakes or patient injury.

7. Explain the relationship between EMS providers and other health care providers.

References

Institute of Medicine (IOM). (1999). *To err is human: Building a safer health system*. Washington, DC: National Academies Press. Retrieved May 22, 2010, from http://www.nap.edu/catalog.php?record_id=9728

National Highway Transportation Safety Administration (NHTSA). (1996). *EMS agenda for the future*. Washington, DC: Author.

O'Connor, R. E., Slovis, C. M., Hunt, R. C., Pirallo, R. G., & Sayre, M. R. (2002). Eliminating errors in emergency medical services: Realities and recommendations. *Prehospital Emergency Medicine*, 6, 107–113.

2 Emergency Medical Services, Health Care, and Public Health Systems

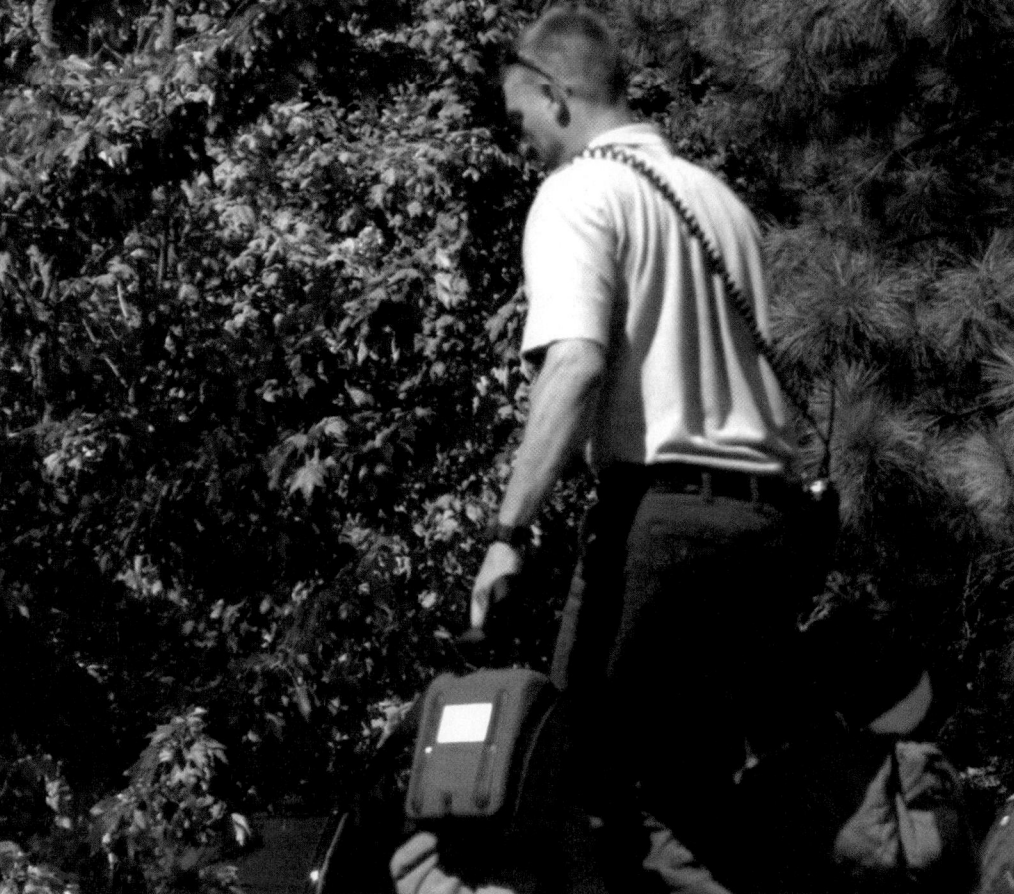

Content Areas: Preparatory; Public Health

Advanced EMT Education Standards:
- Applies fundamental knowledge of the EMS system, safety/well-being of the Advanced EMT, and medical/legal and ethical issues to the provision of emergency care.
- Uses simple knowledge of the principles of the role of EMS during public health emergencies.

Resource Central

To access Resource Central, follow the directions on the Student Access Card provided with this text. If there is no card, go to www.bradybooks.com and follow the Resource Central link to Buy Access. Under Media Resources, you will find:
- *Scope of Practice.* See how your Scope of Practice compares to other levels of EMS.
- *Educate to the Standard.* Find out more about the education of an Advanced EMT.
- *The Heart of EMS.* Learn ways to ensure your heart health.

Objectives

After reading this chapter, you should be able to:

2.1 Define key terms introduced in this chapter.

2.2 Describe key historical events that have shaped the development of EMS systems.

2.3 Briefly explain each of the components of the Technical Assistance Program Assessment Standards.

2.4 Describe the components of an EMS system that must be in place for a patient to receive emergency medical care.

(continued)

CASE STUDY

Arthur Schultz, a 57-year-old factory worker, doesn't feel well. "My head is killing me, Martha," he tells his wife of nearly 40 years. "It just came on like a bomb went off in my head. I think I need a doctor," he says, as he heads to the sofa to lie down.

Martha, who doesn't drive, is immediately worried. Arthur had a couple of what the doctor called "light strokes" about six months earlier. He looks sicker now than he did then. Martha calls their daughter, Sandy, who lives about 20 minutes away. "Sandy, I'm worried about your dad. I think he needs to go to the hospital."

After hearing the story, Sandy tells her mom to call the ambulance. Martha opens a drawer in the kitchen to find the phone book. She wonders briefly if she should call Auffenberg's or Heiny's for the ambulance. "Art, who do you want?" she asks. Receiving no answer, she realizes that Mr. Schultz is unconscious. Fingers shaking, she dials a number.

"Auffenberg's Funeral Home. How can I help you?"

"This is Martha Schultz. My husband Arthur is having an attack of some kind. He needs an ambulance."

"You live out by the lake, don't you, Mrs. Schultz?"

"Yes, that's right. Go past the county airport and the stone barn, then down the hill. It's the second road on the left. We're all the way down on the right." Mrs. Schultz waits by her husband's side, not knowing what else to do but pat his hand. His breathing isn't right, she can tell, and tears start to roll down her cheeks. Fifteen minutes later, a sleek, gray, Cadillac hearse with a red bubble light on top pulls into the driveway, followed by Sandy's pickup truck. Two men in dark suits with ties follow Sandy into the living room. One of the men, John Auffenberg, the son of the funeral home owner, says, "This doesn't look good, ma'am. We are going to get our litter so we can get on our way. Call your doctor and have him meet us at the emergency room."

Both men leave, and return a minute later with a portable canvas stretcher. Grabbing Mr. Schultz under the arms and knees, they place him on the stretcher and carry him to the hearse. After sliding the stretcher in the back, both men get in front and head to the hospital, 15 minutes away. On the way, the second attendant, Stephan Polanski, pulls a hard-backed ledger out and records the date: April 3, 1972.

Problem-Solving Questions

1. How does this differ from what you would expect when you call an ambulance today?
2. How did ambulance transportation move away from family-owned funeral homes to the municipal and large private ambulance services of today?
3. Who were some of the people and agencies that helped bring these changes about?

(continued from previous page)

2.5	Discuss the features and benefits of 911 and enhanced 911 emergency access systems.
2.6	Explain the importance of Advanced EMTs understanding the health care and public-health resources available in the community.
2.7	Discuss the role of EMS as part of the health care system.
2.8	Describe the scope of concerns of a public-health system.
2.9	Describe the relationship between EMS and public health.
2.10	Discuss the purposes of medical direction and medical oversight in the EMS system.
2.11	Give examples of offline, online, prospective, concurrent, and retrospective medical direction.
2.12	Describe the purpose of continuous quality improvement (CQI) programs in EMS, and the Advanced EMT's role in CQI.
2.13	Identify current issues and trends in EMS.
2.14	Identify resources for learning about issues and trends in EMS.
2.15	Given an issue or problem in EMS, suggest changes that could be implemented.

Introduction

Many students do not remember a time when there was not an organized system of EMS. The history of the creation of the system that exists today is crucial to understanding the modern EMS system and the goals for its future. Many key events and documents can help you understand the history, components, context, relationships, current issues, and goals of EMS. Understanding these things is an important step in developing your professional identity. As a profession, we must know where we came from, how we got where we are, and what directions we should follow to create our future.

In its infancy, EMS was guided by physicians and nurses, based on principles of in-hospital care. Today's leaders in EMS (including those who are nurses and physicians) have backgrounds as EMS providers, making EMS a self-regulating occupation. There is now an emphasis on research to determine what practices are best in EMS, rather than assuming that what works in the hospital is what helps patients in the prehospital setting.

Research results help direct changes in practice and change has become a constant in the profession. Professionals are not passive recipients of changes in their profession. They are active in assessing the need for changes and making the changes happen. To understand what changes will benefit the public, the health care system, and practitioners of the profession, you must understand EMS as a system that currently exists at the intersection of public safety and health care, with a yet unrealized potential for contribution to public health (Figure 2-1). You must be aware of the goals for the future of EMS and how you can contribute to your profession.

Evolution of the EMS System

The publication of a **white paper** entitled *Accidental Death and Disability: The Neglected Disease of Modern Society*, by the National Academy of Sciences (NAS) National Research Council (NRC) in 1966, marks the beginning of the modern history of EMS. This report called attention to the high number of preventable highway traffic injuries and deaths.

Deficiencies in prehospital care were cited as one reason, among several, for the unacceptably high number of deaths and disabilities resulting from highway traffic injuries. These deficiencies included training requirements for ambulance personnel and the lack of a systems approach to prehospital emergency care.

Publication of the white paper, lessons from military history, and research and advocacy by early EMS leaders launched a series of events that moved EMS along its path to the present.

Transportation of the Sick and Injured

Until relatively modern times, all medical care took place outside the hospital. Although the history of medicine dates back to the ancient Greeks, Romans, and Sumerians, hospitals were created much later. The first U.S. hospital was Bellevue Hospital in New York. It was founded in 1736 (National Highway Traffic Safety Administration [NHTSA], 1996). However, hospitals were not commonplace, and people did not use hospitals as they do today. Therefore, civilian ambulance transportation was not perceived as a need in the United States until there was a rapid increase in the number of hospitals in the 19th century.

Although there are earlier reports of methods of transporting patients, the need to move injured patients to a place where they could be cared for was highlighted in the Napoleonic wars. In 1797 Napoleon's surgeon-in-chief, Dominique-Jean Larrey, implemented a system of specially designed carriages to quickly retrieve the injured from the battlefields and bring them to surgeons for care (NHTSA, 1996).

Military ambulances were used in the United States during the Civil War, and the first civilian ambulance services in the country were established in large cities about the same time. Hospitals, such as Commercial Hospital in Cincinnati (in 1865) and Bellevue Hospital in New York (in 1869), began using horse-drawn ambulances to bring patients to the hospital (Figure 2-2) (NHTSA, 1996). With the advent of the automobile, horse-drawn ambulances were phased out.

In the last century, prior to the beginning of organized EMS, hearses provided a convenient vehicle in which sick and injured patients could be transported while lying down. Because the public did not rely on ambulance transportation to the degree we do now, the services tended to be part of local, family-owned funeral homes. Often, the patient was transported unattended in the back of the hearse. The focus was on transportation, not on caring for the patient prior to arriving at the hospital.

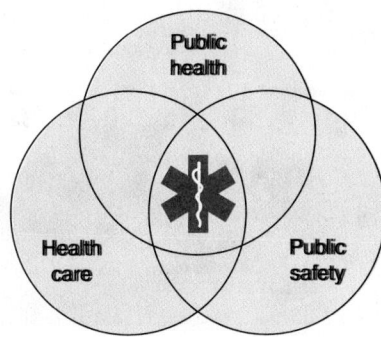

FIGURE 2-1

EMS is at the intersection of health care, public health, and public safety.

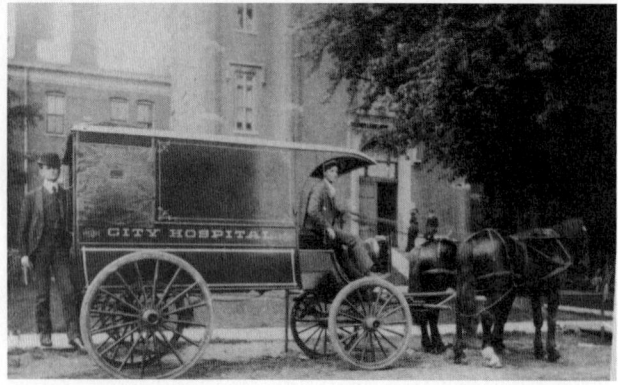

FIGURE 2-2

An ambulance parked at the entrance of City Hospital, which would later become Wishard Memorial Hospital, circa 1901–1903. The first City Hospital ambulance began carrying sick and injured Indianapolis-area patients in 1887. (Photo used with permission of Wishard Health Services)

Emergency Prehospital Care

The first volunteer rescue squads began on the East Coast in the 1920s. Beginning in the 1950s there were scattered attempts at improving and standardizing emergency prehospital care. However, EMS would not see rapid development until after the publication of the white paper and institution of the **National Highway Traffic Safety Administration (NHTSA)** in 1966. The first **National Standard Curriculum (NSC)** for training EMTs (called EMT-Ambulance) was published in 1971 (NHTSA, 1998).

As prehospital providers began to acquire patient care skills, including CPR, airway management, spinal immobilization, splinting, and bandaging skills, hearses could no longer accommodate the equipment or space needed for patient care. Modern ambulances were developed to carry equipment and allow space for patient care (Figure 2-3). Even so,

it took time to implement the changes, and hearse transportation continued in some places into the 1970s.

Military Influence

Much of what we know about prehospital care, especially about trauma, comes from military experiences. The death and disability of so many men and women is a tragedy that cannot be forgotten. To fail to learn from it would be an even greater tragedy.

From the beginnings of helicopter transport in the Korean War in the 1950s, to field and surgical experiences in the Vietnam War in the 1960s and 1970s, to present-day experience in trauma management in Iraq and Afghanistan, military experience has contributed to the development of civilian EMS systems (Figure 2-4).

One of the most recent military lessons incorporated into civilian EMS is the increased emphasis on the use of tourniquets to control hemorrhage. In the past, tourniquets were discouraged. However, recognition that many soldiers were dying from hemorrhage from otherwise survivable wounds has given tourniquets a new place in EMS (Figure 2-5).

Key Events in EMS

Through the years, many key events have influenced the development of EMS (NHTSA, 1996).

1960s–1990

The Highway Safety Act of 1970 established NHTSA within the U.S. Department of Transportation (DOT) to lead the development of EMS systems from the federal level. The Highway Safety Act also required each state to establish a highway safety program, including emergency medical services, according to federal standards.

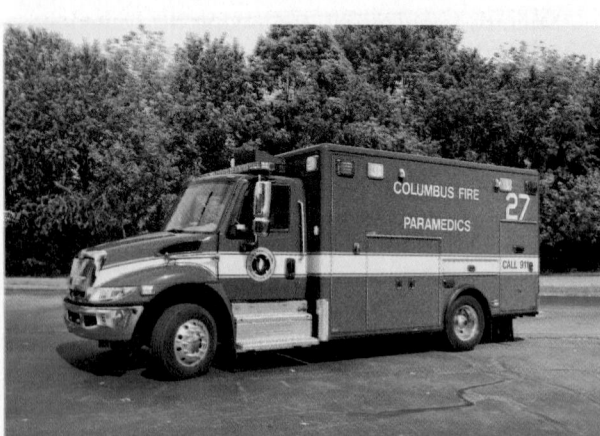

FIGURE 2-3

Modern ambulances allow EMS providers to carry emergency equipment and provide patient care en route to the hospital.

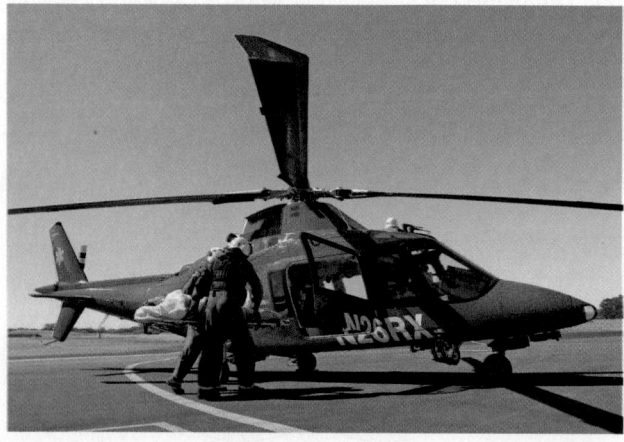

FIGURE 2-4

Civilian air medical transport systems developed after the military used helicopters to transport injured soldiers in the Korean and Vietnam wars.

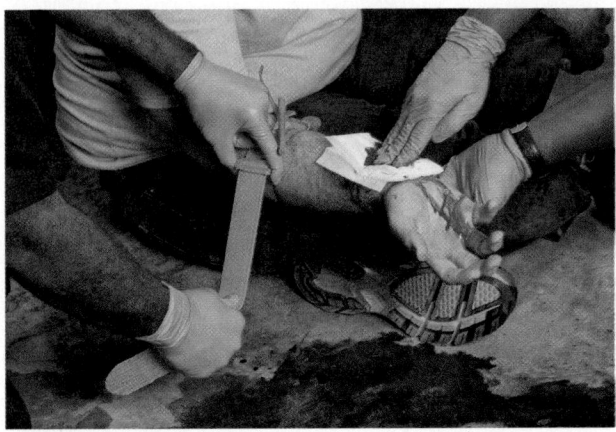

FIGURE 2-5

Lessons learned from military experience include renewed recognition of the role of tourniquets in life-threatening hemorrhage.

Substantial progress in the development of EMS systems began with the Emergency Medical Services Act of 1973, which provided federal funding for EMS system development and implementation. The $300 million allocated by the EMS Act of 1973, along with grants from other sources, allowed tremendous progress in the growth and development of EMS systems. However, the Omnibus Budget Reconciliation Act (OBRA) of 1981 called for consolidation of health care funding into block grants that allowed each state to allocate the funds as it saw fit. In many cases, this meant that little funding was available to continue the development of EMS systems.

At the national level, a number of events occurred, both as a part of the National Highway Transportation Safety and Emergency Medical Services Acts, and independently of them. These events include:

- *1960s.* The **American Heart Association (AHA)** begins teaching public CPR classes.
- *1970.* **National Registry of Emergency Medical Technicians (NREMT)** is formed to develop uniform standards for credentialing ambulance attendants.
- *1972.* The U.S. Department of Health, Education, and Welfare provides $16 million for EMS system demonstration projects in five states.
- *1973.* $15 million in funding is offered by the Robert Wood Johnson Foundation for regional EMS system development.
- *1970s.* NBC's *Emergency!* is the first television show about EMS, based on two fictional Los Angeles County firefighter/paramedics. The show increased public awareness (and expectations) of EMS.
- *1973.* Emergency Medical Services Act establishes 15 components of EMS systems.
- *1970s.* First national standard curricula for EMS training are published by NHTSA (EMT-Ambulance, 1971; EMT-Paramedic, 1977; First Responder, 1979).

- *1975.* American Medical Association (AMA) recognizes EMT-Paramedic as an allied health occupation.
- *1978.* AMA establishes essentials for the **accreditation** of EMT-Paramedic programs; adopted by the Joint Review Committee on Education for the EMT-Paramedic (now called the Committee on Accreditation of EMS Programs [CoAEMSP]).
- *1981.* OBRA eliminates specific federal funding for EMS.
- *1984.* EMS for Children (EMSC) Act focuses attention on specific prehospital care needs of pediatric patients.
- *1988.* NHTSA publishes the Statewide EMS Technical Assessment program; replaces 15 components of an EMS system with a list of 10 components.
- *1990.* Trauma Care Systems and Development Act focuses on development and implementation of trauma systems.
- *1980s–1990s.* Revisions of national standard curricula.

1990s–Present

As EMS has evolved, EMS providers have taken greater ownership of their own profession. This is reflected in the move toward greater planning for the future of EMS.

- *1993.* National EMS Practice and Education Blueprint is developed.
- *1996.* NHTSA publishes the EMS Agenda for the Future.
- *2000.* NHTSA publishes the EMS Education Agenda for the Future.
- *2006.* Institute of Medicine (IOM) publishes EMS at the Crossroads.
- *2007.* NHTSA publishes the National Scope of Practice Model.
- *2009.* NHTSA publishes EMS Education Standards to replace national standard curricula.

Key Documents in EMS

In addition to *Accidental Death and Disability: The Neglected Disease of Modern Society* (NAS, 1966), a number of other documents have steered the course of EMS. A few of them are listed here:

- *National Standard Curricula (NSC) (NHTSA, 1995, 1998, 1999).* The NSC documents provided very detailed information on the required hours and content for each level of EMS training. The level of detail made them very rigid, prone to rapid obsolescence, and difficult and expensive to update.
- *Emergency Medical Services at the Crossroads (Institute of Medicine [IOM], 2006).* A panel convened by the IOM to examine and make

recommendations about all aspects of emergency medical care published a report that expressed concerns over the future of EMS, including:

- The evolving role of EMS as an integral component of the overall health care system
- EMS system planning, preparedness, and coordination at the federal, state, and local levels
- EMS funding and infrastructure investments
- EMS workforce trends and professional education
- EMS research priorities and funding

- *EMS Agenda for the Future (NHTSA, 1996).* The "Agenda," as it is referred to, was published to set goals for systematic development of EMS systems, and envisioned a greater role for EMS in the health care system.

- *EMS Education Agenda for the Future: A Systems Approach (NHTSA, 1998).* The "Education Agenda" was published to flesh out the educational goals established by the *EMS Agenda for the Future.* It called for the development of National EMS Core Content (NHTSA, 2007, the National EMS Scope of Practice Model (NHTSA, 2006), and EMS Education Standards (NHTSA, 2009).

- *National EMS Core Content.* This promotes a universal (consistent from state to state) set of knowledge and skills for EMS providers.

- *National EMS Scope of Practice Model.* This established four levels of nationally recognized EMS providers: Emergency Medical Responder (EMR), Emergency Medical Technician (EMT), Advanced EMT, and Paramedic.

- *National EMS Education Standards.* This replaced the NSC with a more general description of the types of knowledge and skills expected of EMS providers at each level.

Key People in EMS   *Sam Stone*

The development of today's EMS system could not have taken place without the hard work of thousands of individuals. However, some especially remarkable people have contributed immeasurably to EMS. Many of the things done

IN THE FIELD

Although the federal government issues standards and models, it cannot compel states to adopt them. Most states eventually do adopt the federal standards, with or without modification. The adoption process is slow, because many states must change legislation to make the adoption. There also will be a transition period for providers trained under older levels of practice. Therefore, provider levels, scopes of practice, and the process of reciprocity may still vary from state to state.

today in EMS are done because of the pioneering efforts of those individuals (Barishansky, 2008).

Just as nurses know who Florence Nightingale and Clara Barton are, and physicians know who Hippocrates is, you should know about some pioneers in EMS. They and many other individuals have contributed, and continue to contribute, to the development of EMS. Their contributions are far more in-depth than can be described here. For more on EMS history, visit the National EMS Museum website at *http://www.emsmuseum.org.*

- *Nancy Caroline, MD.* Dr. Caroline was committed to the idea that people who were not physicians could be taught to deliver lifesaving emergency care outside the hospital. She was involved with one of the first paramedic programs in the country, and authored the first paramedic textbook in the 1970s.

- *Jeff Clawson, MD.* Dr. Clawson developed the first set of standardized dispatch protocols in 1978, which have evolved into the widely used Medical Priority Dispatch System.

- *R. Adams Cowley, MD.* Dr. Cowley, after whom the renowned shock trauma center in Baltimore is named, recognized the need for rapid treatment of patients in shock. He developed the concept of the "Golden Hour" and was instrumental in the development of one of the first air EMS services in the country through the Maryland State Police.

- *Joseph D. "Deke" Farrington.* In the 1950s, Dr. Farrington promoted vehicle extrication and established a first aid training curriculum that served as a prototype for the first EMT-Ambulance curriculum.

- *Norman McSwain, MD.* Dr. McSwain, the director of trauma surgery at Charity Hospital in New Orleans, was instrumental in the development of the Pre-Hospital Trauma Life Support (PHTLS) course through the National Association of EMTs (NAEMT). Dr. McSwain remains the PHTLS medical director today.

- *Rocco Morando.* Mr. Morando was the founding executive director of the NREMT and instrumental in developing the NAEMT.

- *James O. Page, JD.* Mr. Page was an EMS pioneer in the Los Angeles County Fire Department, founder of the *Journal of Emergency Medical Services (JEMS),* and technical consultant to the television show *Emergency!.*

- *Peter Safar, MD.* Dr. Safar introduced the concept of airway, breathing, and circulation (ABCs) in CPR in the 1950s. He founded the Freedom House Ambulance Service and Training Program in Pittsburgh, and continued research in hypothermic therapy in resuscitation until his death in 2003.

Components of an EMS System

Beyond the ability to call for and receive help in an emergency, there are many requirements for a functional EMS system. In 1988, the NHTSA published Statewide Technical Assistance Program Assessment Standards that specify the components of state EMS systems (NHTSA, 1996). The ten components are:

- *Regulation and Policy.* Each state must have a lead EMS agency. Each state must also have legislation, regulations, policies, and procedures to govern the operation of EMS. Cities and counties also have policies governing EMS.

- *Resource Management.* Each state must ensure that every locality within the state has access to an acceptable level of emergency care. This requires coordination among different hospitals in the state.

- *Human Resources and Training.* All personnel who staff ambulances must be trained to at least the EMT level.

- *Transportation.* An EMS system must provide safe and reliable transportation. Depending on population density and geographical location, transport may include ground ambulances, air medical helicopters, and fixed-wing air ambulance transportation.

- *Facilities.* Patients must be transported to an appropriate facility in a timely manner. Rural areas may have critical access hospitals that can stabilize critical patients for later transportation to a hospital with greater capabilities.

- *Communications.* A communications system must be in place to allow public access to EMS and to allow communication among dispatchers, EMS providers, and hospital personnel.

- *Public Information and Education.* EMS should participate in activities to educate the public and prevent injuries in their communities.

- *Medical Direction.* A licensed physician medical director is required in every EMS system to oversee patient care.

- *Trauma Systems.* Trauma systems must exist in each state to provide care for trauma patients.

- *Evaluation.* There must be an EMS quality improvement system in each state to assess and improve prehospital care.

This list of components serves as a checklist to evaluate statewide EMS systems. Local EMS services must be aware of the structure of the statewide system, and must have structures and processes in place to contribute to the function of the statewide system. You must understand why these system components are necessary and how they work (Figure 2-6).

Legislation and Regulation

State legislation and regulations address standards in EMS education, licensure, communication, medical direction, provision of services, and other aspects of EMS. You must know and be in compliance with the state regulations that affect you. You should be able to access your state's laws and regulations either through your state EMS office or by searching for online access to your state's administrative code. The NHTSA's website for EMS, *http://www.ems.gov*, has a link to state EMS offices under the *EMS System* tab.

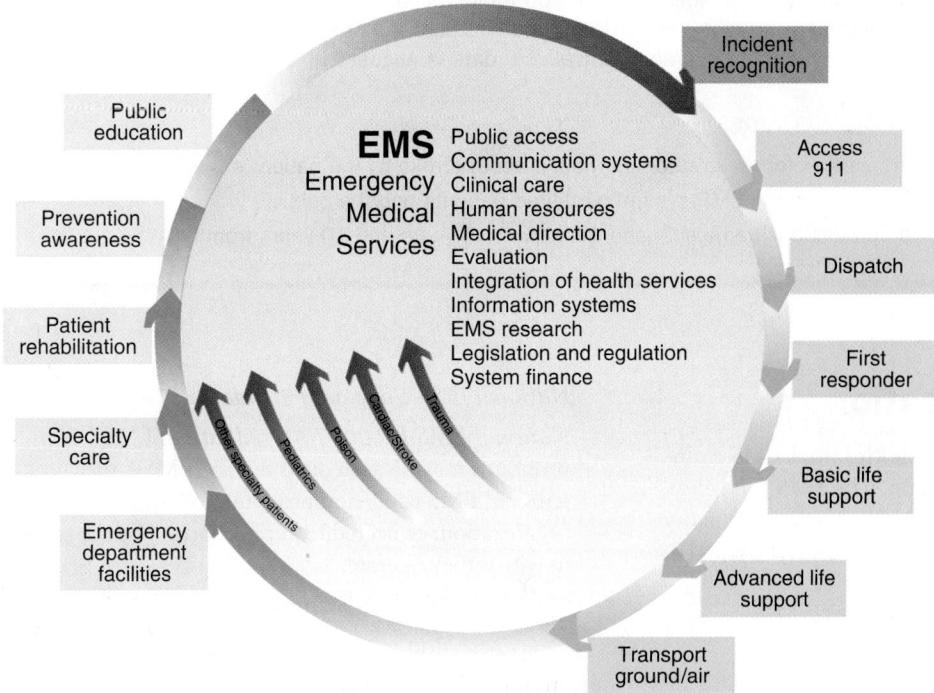

FIGURE 2-6

Components of an EMS system. (From the National Highway Transportation Safety Association at www.ems.gov)

CASE STUDY (continued)

Arthur Schultz, a 57-year-old factory worker, doesn't feel well. "My head is killing me, Martha," he tells his wife of nearly 40 years. "It just came on like a bomb went off in my head. I think I need a doctor," he says, as he heads to the sofa to lie down. With the memory of Arthur's two recent minor strokes fresh in her mind, Martha recognizes some additional warning signs. Arthur's speech seems slurred and the right side of his face is drooping. Martha dials 911.

"911. What is your emergency?"

"I think my husband is having a stroke."

"Is he conscious?"

"Yes, but he has a severe headache. His speech is slurred and his face is drooping. He's had two strokes in the past."

"Ma'am, I show the address you are calling from as three-seven-oh-one Freeman Drive. Is that correct?"

"Yes. Oh, hurry! I think he's unconscious now."

"I'm sending the ambulance now, ma'am. Please stay on the line. Is your husband breathing?"

"Yes. He's snoring like he's asleep but I can't wake him up."

"I am going to stay on the phone with you and give you some instructions, okay?" Martha remains on the phone with the dispatcher for a few more minutes as the dispatcher guides her through opening Mr. Schultz's airway. She waits by his side, following the dispatcher's instructions to monitor him. Within three minutes a rescue squad pulls into the driveway. Two EMTs in uniforms knock on the door and Mrs. Schultz calls for them to come in.

"I'm EMT Sam Snell and this is my partner, Rick. What happened, ma'am?" As Mrs. Schultz explains, the EMTs carry equipment to Mr. Schultz's side. Sam begins an assessment, while Rick keeps Mr. Schultz's airway open and prepares to administer oxygen.

A moment later, an ambulance pulls up to the residence and Advanced EMTs Nick Callais and Terri Secatero enter the home with more equipment and the ambulance stretcher.

While Nick goes to Mr. Schultz's side, Terri places her hand on Mrs. Schultz's arm and says, "Ma'am, let's step over here so I can ask you some questions."

After gathering information about Mr. Schultz's medical history, Terri says, "Mrs. Schultz, you can ride with us to the hospital. Who can we call to meet you there?"

Meanwhile, Nick, Sam, and Rick have completed their on-scene assessment and care, and are wheeling Mr. Schultz to the ambulance on their stretcher. Rick agrees to accompany Nick in the back of the ambulance to help care for Mr. Schultz.

After making sure Mrs. Schultz is buckled up, Terri gets behind the wheel and pushes a button on the radio console to let dispatch know they are on their way to the hospital. En route, Nick switches control of the radio to the patient compartment and contacts the hospital to give a report on the patient's condition and an estimated time of arrival. The date is August 27, 2010.

Problem-Solving Questions

1. What would account for the greater knowledge about stroke by the patient's wife?
2. How have changes in the EMS system benefited patients and the public?
3. How do you predict this same scenario will play out 5 years and 10 years from now?

EMS Provider Education

EMS provider education includes both initial EMS training courses and continuing education. The *EMS Education Agenda for the Future* (NHTSA, 1998) spelled out many goals for EMS education to be accomplished by 2010. These include:

- *National EMS Core Content.*
- *National EMS Scope of Practice Model.*

- *National EMS Education Standards.*
- *National EMS Program Accreditation.* EMS programs may be accredited by CoAEMSP, the national EMS education program-accrediting organization, or accredited or authorized by the state in which they operate.
- *National EMS Certification.*

In most health professions, the state **licensure** procedure requires that applicants have completed a national credentialing exam (**certification** process) to be eligible for state licensure. This ensures consistency in the level of provider competence between states. Most people expect to receive the same level and quality of medical, dental, or nursing care no matter where in the country they live. In EMS, the national credentialing exam offered by the NREMT is not required in all states. Where it is required, it is mostly at the paramedic level and does not include lower EMS licensure levels.

Ongoing national registration requires both **continuing education (CE)** and **refresher education**. The intent of CE is to build on entry-level professional knowledge and to keep informed about trends and research in EMS. Refresher education is intended to ensure that providers remain competent in entry-level knowledge and skills.

States that do not require ongoing national registration have their own CE and refresher requirements. Requiring CE and refresher programs for continued licensure intuitively makes sense. However, there is a lack of evidence for their effectiveness in maintaining competence (Studnek, Fernandez, & Margolis, 2009). There are several possible reasons for this, but it does not mean EMS should abandon the idea of CE.

Research is needed to determine the most effective ways of ensuring continued competence and professional development. Recently, for example, the NREMT began offering an option to reregister through testing instead of through CE and refresher education. Providers must demonstrate minimum competency, just as they did to become registered initially.

EMS System Configuration and Workforce

Not all EMS systems operate in the same way. Different types of agencies, different levels of EMS service, different combinations of staffing, and other factors make each EMS system unique in many ways (Table 2-1).

To make any EMS system work, employers must be able to attract and retain a qualified workforce. You must understand how the specific system in which you work is configured.

Types of EMS Systems

The components of an EMS system can exist in a fire-based system, hospital-based system, private services

contracted by local governments, municipal third services, or some combination of these (Williams & Ragone, 2010). In some communities, EMS is a part of the fire service. Personnel may serve a dual role of both firefighting and providing EMS, or separate EMS and fire divisions may exist within the same department. Some fire service organizations provide all EMS services within a community, and others act to provide first response or additional personnel when needed.

An EMS system that has a larger number of basic life support EMS vehicles located throughout the community to reach a patient quickly while awaiting ALS arrival is called a **tiered response**. A tiered response can be used whether the fire department provides all services, or works cooperatively with a private, hospital-based, or **third service** in a community.

Hospital-based EMS services may be separate hospital departments, or may operate as part of the emergency department. The hospital may be a taxpayer-supported public hospital, or a private hospital that has contracted with the city to provide care, in a privatization model. In a privatization model, rather than providing a service itself, a local government requests bids for an outside company to provide the service. Private ambulance services place competitive bids to be awarded the contract.

A municipal third service is a public safety model of EMS. In this model, the local government operates EMS as a city or county service that is independent of the other two public safety branches—fire and law enforcement. These systems can coexist. For example, a fire-based system may provide first response using nontransporting vehicles, while a private, hospital-based, or third service responds to provide transportation.

EMS System Staffing

EMS system staffing configurations can vary. Some states require that EMS services provide the same level of care 24 hours a day, seven days a week. Other states allow provisional Advanced EMT or paramedic services. This means that the service typically provides a lower level of care, but if an Advanced EMT or paramedic is available, he or she can respond to provide a higher level of care than is otherwise provided by the service.

Ambulances most often are staffed with two providers. Some services have different levels of provider staffing on different vehicles, whereas others have the same level of providers on all vehicles. For example, EMS Service A may have 13 BLS ambulances, each staffed by two EMTs, and eight additional ambulances, each staffed by a paramedic and an Advanced EMT. Meanwhile, EMS Service B has 21 ambulances, all staffed with two Advanced EMTs. Depending on regulations and policies, a service may staff with two crew members of the same level (for example, two Advanced EMTs), or may use crews with one partner who is licensed at a higher level, and one at a lower level (for example, an Advanced EMT and an EMT).

TABLE 2-1   Examples of EMS System Configurations

	Geography/Population	System Description
System A	This system is in a midwestern county with a population of 25,000 and an area of 500 square miles. The county seat, a city of 6,000, is in the far southeastern corner. There are eight smaller cities and towns of between 500 and 1,800 people.	The county seat's fire department provides the only ALS service and the only paid EMS service in the county. The fire department has two ambulances in service at all times: one staffed with two paramedics and one staffed with two EMTs. It can take the service up to 25 minutes to reach the furthest areas of the county. One of the smaller towns has a BLS transporting ambulance. The others have nontransporting first responders at the EMR and EMT levels. The only hospital in the county is a critical access hospital in the county seat. The nearest level II trauma center is 30–45 minutes away; the nearest level I trauma center is 90 minutes away by ground ambulance. Once requested, a medical helicopter can be at the critical access hospital in 50 minutes.
System B	This system is in a rural southwestern county with a population of 13,000 and an area of 4,200 square miles. More than half the population lives in the county seat.	The fire department in the county seat provides one paid and one volunteer Advanced EMT on a transporting ambulance 24 hours a day. There are volunteer EMRs and EMTs in the county, but their availability to respond varies. Ambulance response times can be up to 50 minutes. Because of mountainous terrain, residents in the southwestern portion of the county must often rely on a private EMS service from a neighboring county. The nearest critical access hospital is 75 miles away, and the nearest trauma center is 150 miles away. A medical helicopter can be at the critical access hospital in an hour.
System C	This system is in a midwestern county with a population of 150,000 and an area of 500 square miles. The central metropolitan area, consisting of two cities, has a combined population of 90,000. Five cities and towns of 500 to 1,500 people are located throughout the county.	Two hospital-based ambulance services work under an agreement with the county to provide transporting ALS service in the county. Four ALS, two Advanced EMT, and two BLS ambulances are available 24 hours a day. The Advanced EMT and BLS ambulances are also used for interfacility transports. When tiered emergency response is required, it is provided by sending two ambulances in the metropolitan area. First response using EMRs and EMTs is provided by a variety of volunteer fire departments in the smaller towns and rural areas of the county. There are three hospitals in the county, with two level II trauma centers. A level I trauma center can be reached in 60 minutes by ground, and a helicopter can land on the scene or at one of the hospitals within 35 minutes.
System D	This system is in a large east coast metropolitan area with an overall population of 5.5 million.	Large, urban fire departments, some with dual-role personnel and some with separate EMS divisions, provide tiered response and transport within the different cities of the metropolitan area. BLS rescue engines or squads respond within 2 to 3 minutes, and transporting ALS is on the scene in 5 to 6 minutes. Full-service hospitals are available within a few miles of nearly any location, but helicopter transport is used for critical patients when traffic prevents efficient ground ambulance transport. A number of private ambulances are available for interfacility transfers.

Advanced EMT Mallory Henley: I looked at a lot of different career options before I started working in EMS. The health sciences advisor at my college was really helpful. She had a lot of information about different careers, and a shadowing program to allow students to spend time with different health care professionals.

Every career has its pros and cons. I looked at the education needed, the pay and benefits, the number of jobs available, the work environment, who I would be working with, types of schedules, what a typical day was like—lots of things. One of the things that really helped me decide was when my advisor said you have to love what you do to be happy with your career. I loved my ride-along experience in EMS! I've been doing this for 10 years now, and I don't have any regrets. I've seen so many positive changes in the profession, and I'm excited for the future!

The EMS Workforce

EMS work requires excellent clinical knowledge and skills, interpersonal skills, physical health, and specific intrapersonal characteristics. EMS services must recruit, hire, and retain an adequate number of qualified employees in order to provide services to the community. The Bureau of Labor Statistics (BLS) *Occupational Outlook Handbook* (2009) projects a growing need for EMS personnel into the future.

There are a few recognized issues facing the EMS workforce. However, the profession is working to address those issues. EMS provider pay is lower compared to other public safety and health care providers (NHTSA, 2008). Improvements in **reciprocity** will provide greater geographic mobility within the profession. Research is needed to identify ways to attract more women and minorities, who are currently underrepresented, to the profession. EMS providers should be well informed about these issues so they can bring about positive change.

Communication and System Access

The public must be aware of the telephone number used to access EMS in their communities. The number 911 is widely used to request all emergency services in an area. A call to 911 is answered at a **public safety answering point (PSAP)**. The 911 operator may handle all calls, or may route requests for law enforcement, EMS, and the fire department to different dispatchers. **Enhanced 911,** or E-911 systems, identify the caller's location and provide the information to the dispatcher's console, as long as the call is coming from a fixed telephone line. The ability to quickly and precisely identify the location of a cellular phone is not widely developed. Gaps in cellular phone coverage still exist in rural areas, which may cause delays in reporting incidents and requesting help.

EMS vehicles are selected to respond depending on whether the system uses **system status management**—with or without vehicle global positioning system (GPS) information—or assigned districts or response areas. System status management allows vehicles to be continually moved to be positioned in close proximity to where EMS calls are expected to occur at certain times of day, based on historical statistics for the system.

System status management also allows a system to have fewer or more EMS units available at different times of day, based on **peak load** data. Other systems assign vehicles to designated geographic regions and provide the same amount of staffing 24 hours a day.

System status management was developed to make most efficient use of resources while providing the needed level of service within a specified amount of time. A common system standard for ALS service is to respond to 80 percent of calls in eight minutes or less. However, whether this benchmark affects patient outcomes, and how system status management affects EMS crews, is currently being questioned.

Medical Direction

A physician medical director is an essential and required part of an EMS system. Physicians provide expert input into the clinical operations of an EMS system. States have an EMS medical director or medical direction committee to oversee EMS issues at a statewide level. Local governments also may have a medical director or medical direction committee to ensure consistency in practices among several services in an area.

Each individual EMS service also has a physician medical director who provides specific protocols and standing orders, participates in provider education, and oversees the continuous quality assurance process. The exact scope of the medical director's involvement varies according to state law and job description, but he or she should be actively involved with the leadership of the EMS system or service. The medical director is typically responsible for approving EMS providers to practice within the system.

A common misconception is that EMS providers operate under the license of the physician medical director. This is not true. The medical director supervises, directly or indirectly, the care given by EMS providers. EMS providers function under their own licenses.

The supervision provided by the physician medical director can be classified as **prospective medical direction**, **concurrent medical direction**, and **retrospective medical direction**. Prospective medical direction is also called **offline** or **indirect medical direction**, and concurrent medical direction is called **online** or **direct medical direction**.

Prospective medical direction takes place in the form of protocols and standing orders that are already in place before an EMS provider responds to a particular patient. In concurrent medical direction, the physician has real-time contact with the EMS provider by radio, cellular phone, or less commonly, by on-scene supervision.

Retrospective medical direction is part of the **continuous quality improvement (CQI)** process. The medical director reviews medical care provided by EMS personnel and provides feedback to improve the overall delivery of care in the system.

The medical director should be actively involved in the EMS system and should be accessible to EMS providers to give feedback and answer questions. An EMS medical director should be an advocate and supporter of EMS providers, representing their interests to the broader emergency medicine community. Ideally, he or she will have a background in emergency medicine or emergency medical services, and will have taken a medical direction course to better understand his or her roles and responsibilities within an EMS system (NHTSA, 2001).

Evaluation

Evaluation is the process of measuring the performance of a system against predetermined benchmarks. Some benchmarks in EMS systems include response times, scene times, transport times, and out-of-service times; compliance with protocols; completion of required paperwork; and patient satisfaction.

Evaluation results must be used to continually improve the system in order to offer high-quality, safe, efficient patient care. In continuous quality improvement (CQI), there is a specific plan that includes what benchmarks to measure, how to measure them, what the acceptable levels of performance are, how to address deficiencies, and when to reassess interventions to improve deficiencies. CQI is not a system designed to discipline personnel who do not meet benchmarks. The goal of CQI is to improve the performance of the system. Each EMS provider has an obligation to strive to meet system benchmarks, and to work to implement the feedback provided by evaluation.

Beyond the improvement of a single EMS system, data reported to the National EMS Information System (NEMSIS) can be used for research to improve EMS practices nationwide.

Health Care and Public Health

EMS, health care systems, and systems of public health all exist to protect and improve the health of communities, and must interact with one another to do so effectively. These services are more integrated in some states, and less so in others. The EMS office for many states exists within the state's department of public health, but may or may not be involved with activities of the other branches of the department. Some hospitals recognize their hospital-based EMS services as an integral part of their health care system; others allow their services to exist somewhat independently.

The *EMS Agenda for the Future* (NHTSA, 1996) and the IOM report (2006) both call for greater roles for EMS providers in health care and public health, and better integration of EMS into these systems. There have been some demonstration projects using community paramedics in a broader role, but the current overall level of EMS integration into the health care and public health systems is marginal. This remains an opportunity for development in EMS.

The Health Care System

Hospitals, clinics, treatment and diagnostic centers, physicians' offices, rehabilitation centers, and extended-care facilities are all part the health care system. As part of this system, EMS providers interact with many of the facilities in the course of both emergency calls and interfacility transfers.

Smaller cities and rural areas usually offer a limited range of health care services. In an emergency, **critical access hospitals** and smaller community hospitals can stabilize a patient and prepare him for transport to a more specialized facility for definitive care. Larger cities provide full-service hospitals that offer a range of specialty services, such as:

- Intensive and critical care units
- Trauma centers
- Burn centers
- Cancer centers
- Cardiac care centers
- Centers for high-risk obstetric and neonatal patients
- Emergency mental health services
- Pediatric hospitals
- Poison centers
- Stroke centers

The idea that EMS providers can reduce the burden of overcrowding in emergency departments has received attention in the past several years. However, more research must be done to establish how EMS providers can safely make decisions about health care alternatives with the limited resources and information available in the prehospital setting. Other possibilities, yet to be implemented on a widespread basis, include following up on patients after hospital discharge and providing health screening visits in the community.

In addition to better integrating EMS into the overall health care system, states must cooperate to allow out-of-state EMS providers to practice in disasters, such as hurricanes, floods, and earthquakes. These events overwhelm local health care systems, but state laws may prevent out-of-state EMS providers from providing care in these situations.

The Public Health System

Public health systems exist to prevent, identify, and find solutions for health problems in communities (Table 2-2 and Table 2-3). Public health can be protected through laws (such as communicable disease reporting and seatbelt laws), preventive programs (such as vaccines and child safety seat fitting programs), educational programs (such as drug, tobacco, alcohol, and sexually transmitted disease awareness), monitoring programs (such as food safety and water testing), and responses to public health problems (such as disease outbreaks). Visit your state's public health department website to find out what services are offered. Search "public health department" and your state's name.

EMS personnel can contribute to the health of their communities in many ways. EMS personnel access many neighborhoods and areas of communities and can identify and report potential health hazards, such as substandard housing, children riding bicycles without helmets, and other issues.

EMS personnel can provide information to patients about public health resources and educate them about

TABLE 2-2	Examples of Public Health Functions and Programs

- Agricultural and environmental health
- Behavioral health programs
- Disease prevention and immunization
- Emergency management/emergency response
- Emergency medical services
- Epidemiology/disease surveillance
- Food and water safety monitoring
- Health facility licensure
- Health promotion and injury prevention
- Issuing birth and death certificates
- Lead and radon detection programs
- Medical error reporting program
- Oral health programs
- Professional licensure
- Radiologic safety
- Trauma programs
- Women, children, and minority health programs

TABLE 2-3	Ten Great Public Health Achievements from 1900 to 1999

- Vaccination
- Motor vehicle safety
- Safer workplaces
- Control of infectious disease
- Decline in deaths from coronary heart disease and stroke
- Safer and healthier foods
- Healthier mothers and babies
- Family planning
- Fluoridation of drinking water
- Recognition of tobacco use as a health hazard

Source: From Centers for Disease Control and Prevention [CDC], 1999

health issues and injury prevention measures. You may be able to participate in vaccination and health screening programs in your community. For example, many EMS providers worked in vaccination clinics to provide immunization for the H1N1 influenza outbreak in 2009 and 2010.

Getting to the Future

You have just learned about some of the current issues and goals in EMS. They are often attributed to the growing pains of a relatively young profession. However, other young health care professions moved beyond some of those issues much earlier in their histories. One reason for this is that those health care professionals are a unified body of individuals who have agreed that national standards are in the best interest of their profession.

EMS has competing interests within it, making for unique political situations within EMS. The mix of paid and volunteer, urban and rural, fire-based, hospital-based, private, and third-service EMS systems are often at odds with one another. One of EMS's greatest challenges as it moves into the future will be the development of new leaders who can continue to move the profession forward.

You do not have to be a supervisor or manager to be a leader. Anyone who is passionate and knowledgeable about a cause can make a difference. Realize that there is a "big picture" in EMS and that much has happened over the past 40 years. Become knowledgeable about issues that interest you. Do you want to make a difference in setting education program standards, EMS and public health, initial and continuing licensure, or pay and benefits?

Find out what sources of information are available about the issue and what is already known about it. Become active in EMS professional organizations, attend conferences, and visit the websites of state and national EMS agencies and organizations. Subscribe to industry publications and professional journals. Know who the decision makers and leaders are in your area of interest. Know what the politics of the issue are at local, state, and national levels. Find out how your peers feel about the issue so you can anticipate reactions to your ideas.

Do not be discouraged if not everyone sees the issue as you do. Advancing the profession requires change, and change is not always well received. Find out more about the issue and find out reasons for resistance to change. This is *your* profession now. Be an advocate for its success, growth, and development.

CASE STUDY WRAP-UP

Clinical-Reasoning Process

It is January 15, 2015. Advanced EMTs Nick Callais and Terri Secatero pull into the driveway at the home of Arthur Schultz. It is not an emergency, though. Mr. Schultz, a 57-year-old factory worker, was released from the hospital yesterday after suffering a mini-stroke—what the doctor called a *transient ischemic attack,* or TIA.

Mr. Schultz's regular physician cannot see him for three months. Nick and Terri are going to teach Mr. Schultz how to check his blood pressure and make sure that the Schultzes recognize the signs and symptoms of stroke.

Nick and Terri have been certified to teach patients and their families some ways to decrease their risk of stroke. They enjoy this part of the job (and the freshly baked oatmeal cookies Mrs. Schultz greets them with). For the next several years, Nick and Terri see Mr. and Mrs. Schultz in town occasionally and always stop to talk. Mr. Schultz reaches retirement age, and in 2020 he and Mrs. Schultz move out of state to be near their grandchildren.

As access to and cost of health care continue to present issues, the framework of the traditional system of health care that emerged in the 20th century will be challenged. Key documents, legislation, events, and people continue to accelerate the pace of change in EMS, allowing EMS to be poised to take a larger role in public health and health care.

CHAPTER REVIEW

Chapter Summary

EMS evolved from the need to reduce preventable highway traffic deaths and manage out-of-hospital cardiac arrest. Today, EMS is a complex system of private and public agencies that provide coordinated delivery of emergency medical care. The system is integrated with public safety, health care, and public health.

EMS is guided nationally by NHTSA, but each state has laws and regulations that structure its EMS system. Effective EMS requires an educated public that can recognize emergencies, and a communication system through which they can report them. The communication must allow EMS providers to be dispatched and communicate with hospital personnel.

Highly trained EMS professionals work under the guidance of a physician medical director to provide care for patients with a variety of problems at the scene of the emergency and en route to the hospital. EMS providers transport patients to health care facilities for emergency and ongoing specialty care. Evaluation programs are used to continuously improve the quality of EMS.

The contributions of thousands of individuals have allowed EMS to make great strides since 1966. However, EMS has the potential to contribute even more to the health and safety of communities. The *EMS Agenda for the Future* has set the current direction of the profession. Related documents detail the goals of the Agenda and provide guidance on the steps required to meet them. Meeting those goals and determining future goals require continuous development of passionate, well-informed advocates and leaders from within the ranks of EMS professionals like you.

Review Questions

Multiple-Choice Questions

1. Which one of the following events marks the history of present-day EMS system development?
   a. The Emergency Medical Services Systems Act
   b. Publication of *EMS at the Crossroads*
   c. Publication of *Accidental Death and Disability: The Neglected Disease of Modern Society*
   d. The Omnibus Budget Reconciliation Act

2. The origins of the modern EMS system arose from public concern over:
   a. infectious disease.
   b. deaths from terrorism incidents.
   c. maternal and infant mortality.
   d. highway traffic deaths.

3. Goals for the development of the EMS system were published in 1996 in the:
   a. *EMS Agenda for the Future.*
   b. National Standard Curriculum.
   c. Statewide Technical Assistance Program Standards.
   d. *EMS Scope of Practice.*

4. Dr. Jeff Clawson is recognized for his contribution to the development of:
   a. automobile extrication techniques.
   b. EMS dispatch standards.
   c. shock recognition and management.
   d. the National Registry of EMTs.

5. An EMS education program that has been evaluated by an official third-party organization and meets certain standards is:
   a. registered.
   b. certified.
   c. licensed.
   d. accredited.

6. An Advanced EMT who attends a program to learn about a new medication that will be introduced for use in his EMS service is participating in _____ education.
   a. continuing
   b. remedial
   c. initial
   d. refresher

7. In the city of Avon, a BLS rescue squad that can reach a patient in 2 to 3 minutes is dispatched at the same time as a transporting Advanced EMT ambulance that can reach the patient in 5 to 7 minutes. This is best described as:
   a. a third service.
   b. tiered response.
   c. dual role.
   d. system status management.

8. A centralized location at which all requests for emergency services in a certain area are received is called a(n):
   a. medical priority dispatch center.
   b. system status management hub.
   c. public safety answering point.
   d. enhanced 911 nucleus.

9. Which one of the following is an example of concurrent medical direction?
   a. Protocols
   b. Scope of practice
   c. Continuous quality improvement
   d. Medical treatment orders over the radio

10. A small, rural hospital that meets certain criteria and can stabilize critical patients for transfer to a facility with a higher level of care is a _____ hospital.
    a. critical access
    b. specialty
    c. trauma
    d. resource

Critical-Thinking Questions

11. What is the importance of the medical direction component required of EMS systems?

12. What is the relationship between battlefield medicine and civilian EMS systems?

13. How did EMS come to be under the direction of the National Highway Traffic Safety Administration? If EMS was to be placed under the direction of a different agency, what should it be, and why?

14. How does the Institute of Medicine influence the direction of EMS?

15. What roles can EMS play in public health?

16. What are some ways you can find out about issues in EMS and make a difference in its future?

References

Barishansky, R. (2008). Founding fathers of EMS. *EMS Magazine.* Retrieved August 25, 2010, from http://www.emsresponder.com/print/EMS-Magazine/Founding-Fathers-of-EMS/1-6014

Bureau of Labor Statistics. (2009). *Occupational outlook handbook.* Retrieved August 31, 2010, from http://www.bls.gov/oco/ocos101.htm#outlook

Centers for Disease Control and Prevention. (1999). Ten great public health achievements: United States, 1900–1999. *Morbidity and Mortality Weekly Report, 48*(12), 241–243. Retrieved September 2, 2010, from http://www.cdc.gov/mmwr/preview/mmwrhtml/00056796.htm

Institute of Medicine (IOM). (2006). *Emergency medical services: At the crossroads.* Washington, DC: National Academy Press.

National Academy of Sciences (NAS), National Research Council (NRC). (1966). *Accidental death and disability: The neglected disease of modern society.* Washington DC: National Academy Press.

National Highway Traffic Safety Administration (NHTSA). (2001). *Guide for preparing medical directors.* Washington, DC: Author.

National Highway Traffic Safety Administration (NHTSA). (2006). *National EMS scope of practice model.* Washington, DC: Author.

National Highway Traffic Safety Administration (NHTSA). (2007). *National EMS core content.* Washington, DC: Author.

National Highway Traffic Safety Administration (NHTSA). (2008). *EMS workforce for the 21st century: A national assessment.* Washington, DC: Author.

National Highway Traffic Safety Administration (NHTSA). (2009). *National EMS education standards.* Washington, DC: Author.

National Highway Transportation Safety Administration (NHTSA). (1995). *Emergency medical technician-basic national standard curriculum.* Washington, DC: Author.

National Highway Transportation Safety Administration (NHTSA). (1996). *EMS agenda for the future.* Washington, DC: Author.

National Highway Transportation Safety Administration (NHTSA). (1998). *Paramedic national standard curriculum.* Washington, DC: Author.

National Highway Transportation Safety Administration (NHTSA). (1999). *Emergency medical technician-intermediate national standard curriculum.* Washington, DC: Author.

Studnek, J. R., Fernandez, A. R., & Margolis, G. S. (2009). Assessing continued cognitive competence among rural emergency medical technicians. *Prehospital Emergency Care, 13*(3), 357–363. doi:10.1080/10903120902935355

Williams, D. M., & Ragone, M. (2010). JEMS 200 city survey: Zeroing in on what matters. *JEMS.* Retrieved August 31, 2010, from http://www.jems.com/article/2009-jems-200-city-survey

3 Workforce Wellness and Personal Safety

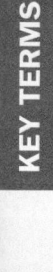

Content Area: Preparatory

Advanced EMT Education Standard: Applies fundamental knowledge of the EMS system, safety/well-being of the Advanced EMT, and medical/legal and ethical issues to the provision of emergency care.

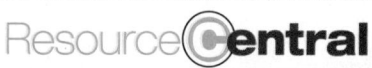

Objectives

After reading this chapter, you should be able to:

3.1 Define key terms introduced in this chapter.

3.2 Identify aspects of work in EMS that can pose a risk to the health and well-being of EMS providers.

3.3 Identify specific measures Advanced EMTs can take to protect their health and safety, both on and off the job.

3.4 Discuss the leading health indicators in the United States.

3.5 Describe the components of wellness, including considerations for nutrition and physical fitness.

3.6 List specific communicable diseases of concern to health care providers.

(continued)

To access Resource Central, follow the directions on the Student Access Card provided with this text. If there is no card, go to www.bradybooks.com and follow the Resource Central link to Buy Access. Under Media Resources, you will find:

- *Your Risk at Work.* Read how you can reduce your risk of injury or illness.

- *Get unstressed!* Discover stress prevention for EMS workers.

- *The Hands Tell All.* Learn more about the Centers for Disease Control and Prevention (CDC) guidelines for hand washing.

CASE STUDY

Although he was hoping for a day shift, Advanced EMT Ryan Mitchell is thrilled that he has just been hired by Seeley County EMS. His schedule is 7:00 PM to 7:00 AM in a pattern of six days on and seven days off. During his first rotation of shifts, Ryan has difficulty staying awake through the night, so he has been drinking more coffee than usual.

When he gets home in the morning he can't get to sleep, but he is too tired to go to the gym. After he gets to sleep it is hard to wake up. By the time he showers he doesn't have time to eat at home, so he has been going through a drive-through fast-food restaurant on the way to work. By the fifth night, he's starting to feel like a zombie. He hopes there will be some donuts at the hospital emergency department—all the caffeine is making his stomach churn. Still, he is excited about the job, although he is looking forward to sleeping at night like a normal person during his days off.

Problem-Solving Questions

1. How does shift work impact individuals and the EMS system?
2. What steps can Ryan take to adapt to his new schedule?
3. What are the short-term and long-term consequences of frequent fast-food meals and excess caffeine?
4. How would you advise Ryan concerning making healthier choices?

(continued from previous page)

3.7	Discuss factors that influence the transmission of communicable diseases.
3.8	Take appropriate Standard Precautions to protect against communicable diseases in specific situations.
3.9	Recognize situations that may be stressful for EMS providers.
3.10	Describe the effects of stress on performance.
3.11	Explain the effects of stress hormones and the sympathetic nervous system in response to stressors.
3.12	Explain the general adaptation syndrome model of stress.
3.13	Recognize signs of stress in yourself and others.
3.14	Identify healthy mechanisms for coping with stress.
3.15	Explain the benefits and characteristics of moderate intensity exercise and vigorous exercise.
3.16	List steps that can reduce the impact of long and irregular shifts on wellness.

Introduction

To be your best at your job—as well as in other important aspects of your life—you must enjoy a high level of personal wellness. Wellness is an optimal state of living that includes well-being in all components of life (University of Illinois at Champaign-Urbana, 2010). Different models of wellness include slightly different components, but some generally agreed-upon areas of well-being are emotional, social, spiritual, occupational, intellectual, physical, and environmental.

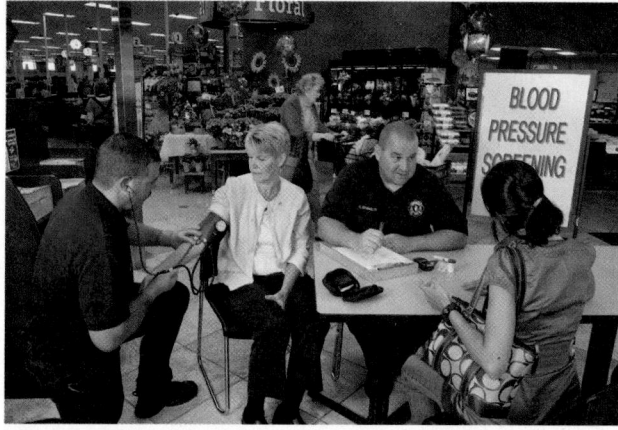

FIGURE 3-1

Advanced EMTs play an important role in health promotion in their communities.

Health and wellness are closely related concepts. The World Health Organization (WHO) defines **health** as "a state of complete physical, mental, and social well-being and not merely the absence of disease or infirmity" (1948).

There are two reasons you must be well informed about health and wellness. First, as a nation, the United States faces a number of challenges to the health of its population, such as high rates of obesity, trauma, diabetes, heart disease, smoking, and cancer, and lack of universal access to high-quality, affordable health care (Table 3-1). Health care providers are role models for health and healthy behavior, and have an obligation to educate patients about health issues. Two guiding documents in EMS, the *EMS Agenda for the Future* (National Highway Traffic Safety Administration [NHTSA], 1996) and *EMS at the Crossroads* (Institute of Medicine [IOM], 2006), call for EMS providers to have an active role in health promotion and public health (Figure 3-1).

Second, the nature of work in EMS creates additional challenges to some aspects of wellness. The way you experience your job affects all other aspects of your life, and other aspects of your life affect your job. Striving to achieve wellness and balance in all life aspects is critical to your health and happiness, and the success and longevity of your career.

Health of the Nation

Unfortunately, health and physical education classes have been cut from many public schools in recent years, and the general public is not always well informed about health issues. Currently, there are a number of health concerns for Americans. The U.S. Department of Health and Human Services (DHHS) issues a report on the health of the Nation and goals for the future every 10 years. *Healthy People 2010* (U.S. Department of Health and Human Services

[DHHS], 2000) is the most current report, although goals for *Healthy People 2020* have already been drafted. The two overall goals of *Healthy People 2010* are increasing the quality and years of healthy life, and eliminating health disparities. There are 28 focus areas that address those goals (Table 3-2). The current leading health indicators include:

- Physical activity
- Overweight and obesity
- Tobacco use
- Substance abuse
- Responsible sexual behavior
- Mental health
- Injury and violence
- Environmental quality
- Immunizations
- Access to health care

Advocating healthy behaviors requires more than just being a role model. As an EMS provider, you can take an active role in the health of your community through organized health education and screening and injury prevention activities. You also must be aware that changing health-related behaviors is not as simple as it might seem.

Health and health behaviors are determined by a variety of complex and interrelated factors such as genetics, environment, cultural beliefs, level of education, socioeconomic status, and more. Educating, coaching, encouraging, and other positive actions are much more effective in changing behaviors than simply telling someone that he needs to change.

Wellness and Emergency Medical Services

A career in EMS can affect the components of **wellness**, both positively and negatively. Understanding the interaction between your job and other aspects of your well-being is important to minimize risks and maximize satisfaction in all areas of life.

Wellness and Maslow's Hierarchy of Needs

Many components of health are closely related to Maslow's hierarchy of needs (Figure 3-2). Maslow's hierarchy is used to explain motivation, but deprivation or threat in any of the areas of the hierarchy creates **stress** and affects wellness.

Abraham Maslow proposed that for human beings to reach their full potential, a series of lower-level needs must first be satisfied, at least to some degree. The most basic of human needs are physiologic. When people do not have adequate food, sleep, or shelter, it is difficult to focus on

| TABLE 3-1 | | Diseases and Risk Factors | | |

Risk Factor	Diseases/Conditions	Actions	Additional Information
Obesity	Heart attack Stroke High blood pressure Cancers Type 2 diabetes Liver and gallbladder disease Arthritis High cholesterol and triglycerides Obstetrical/gynecologic problems Sleep apnea	Achieve and maintain a normal body mass index (BMI) and waist circumference through healthy nutrition and exercise	Centers for Disease Control and Prevention Obesity Fact Sheet http://www.cdc.gov/obesity/causes/health.html
Diabetes	Heart attack Stroke High blood pressure High cholesterol and LDL levels Blindness Kidney disease Peripheral vascular disease Neuropathy Amputation	Prevent and manage type 2 diabetes through healthy body weight, diet, and exercise; manage type 1 and type 2 diabetes through careful monitoring and control of blood glucose levels	American Diabetes Association http://www.diabetes.org/diabetes-basics/diabetes-statistics/
High blood pressure	Heart attack Heart failure Stroke Kidney failure Peripheral artery disease Aortic aneurysm	Achieve and maintain a resting blood pressure of 120/80 or less through diet, exercise, and if needed, medication	eMedicine Health http://www.emedicinehealth.com/high_blood_pressure/article_em.htm
High cholesterol/ high LDL/ low HDL	Heart attack Stroke	Target lipid levels: cholesterol <200 mg/dL, LDL <100 mg/dL, HDL >60 mg/dL, triglycerides <150 mg/dL Achieve and maintain healthy body weight through diet (low in saturated fat) and exercise, do not smoke, take medications if prescribed	National Heart, Lung, and Blood Institute http://www.nhlbi.nih.gov/health/public/heart/chol/wyntk.htm
Lack of exercise	Obesity Heart attack Stroke High blood pressure Type 2 diabetes Cancers High cholesterol Depression/anxiety Osteoporosis	Engage in 30 minutes of moderate physical activity most days of the week	*Healthy People 2010*
Smoking and tobacco use	Heart attack Stroke Aortic aneurysm Peripheral artery disease Lung cancer Chronic obstructive pulmonary diseases (emphysema and chronic bronchitis) Cancers of the kidney, pancreas, bladder, larynx, oral cavity, pharynx, cervix, stomach, esophagus, and uterus; leukemia Pregnancy complications and SIDS	Do not smoke or use smokeless tobacco; avoid secondhand smoke	Centers for Disease Control and Prevention Smoking and Tobacco Use Fact Sheet http://www.cdc.gov/tobacco/data_statistics/fact_sheets/health_effects/effects_cig_smoking/

TABLE 3-2	*Healthy People 2010* Focus Areas		
Access to quality health services	Educational and community based programs	Injury and violence prevention	Oral health
Arthritis, osteoporosis, and chronic back conditions	Environmental health	Maternal, infant, and child health	Physical activity and fitness
	Family planning		Public health infrastructure
Cancer	Food safety	Medical product safety	Respiratory diseases
Chronic kidney disease	Health communication	Mental health and mental disorders	Sexually transmitted infections
Diabetes	Heart disease and stroke		
	HIV	Nutrition and overweight	Substance abuse
Disability and secondary conditions	Immunizations and infectious disease	Occupational safety and health	Tobacco use
			Vision and hearing

Source: *Centers for Disease Control and Prevention Healthy People 2010 Focus Areas at a Glance*, http://www.cdc.gov/nchs/healthy_people/hp2010/hp2010_focus_areas.htm

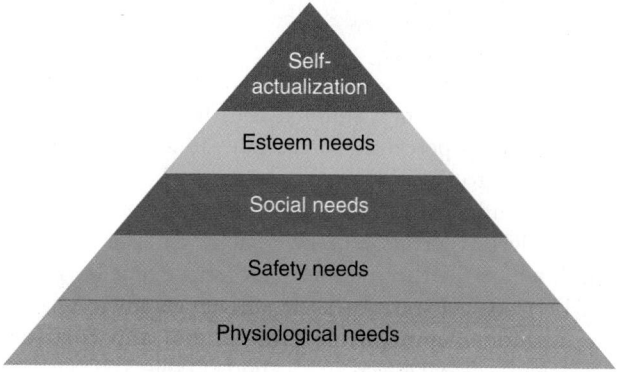

FIGURE 3-2

Maslow's hierarchy of needs.

relationships, learning, and achievement. People must next have a safe, secure environment, free from threats to physical and emotional well-being, before they can focus on the next level of needs. Safety needs include job security, a safe neighborhood, adequate finances, and access to health care.

People become more aware of their social needs once physiologic and safety needs are adequately addressed. People must have relationships to others—family, friends, and coworkers—and feel a sense of belonging to groups.

Esteem needs refer to our innate need to feel worthwhile and to be recognized as worthwhile by those around us. To accomplish this, our contributions and achievements must be recognized and appreciated.

Once these lower-level needs are satisfied, people strive for self-actualization by seeking truth, justice, wisdom, and meaning. Maslow believed that very few individuals ever reach self-actualization.

It is the need to try for self-actualization that provides motivation for learning, challenging work, and progress toward other goals. Without the challenge and motivation to action caused by gaps between our current state and optimal state, we suffer from boredom, which is in itself a stressor that affects wellness.

Stress

From a biologic standpoint, stress is simply the body's response to any demand. The demand, or **stressor**, is the stimulus that produces a stress response. In popular usage, we have come to view stress as distress—a negative impact arising from a stimulus. However, a little stress can be a good thing.

Up to a certain point, an increase in stress improves performance (Figure 3-3). When stress improves performance

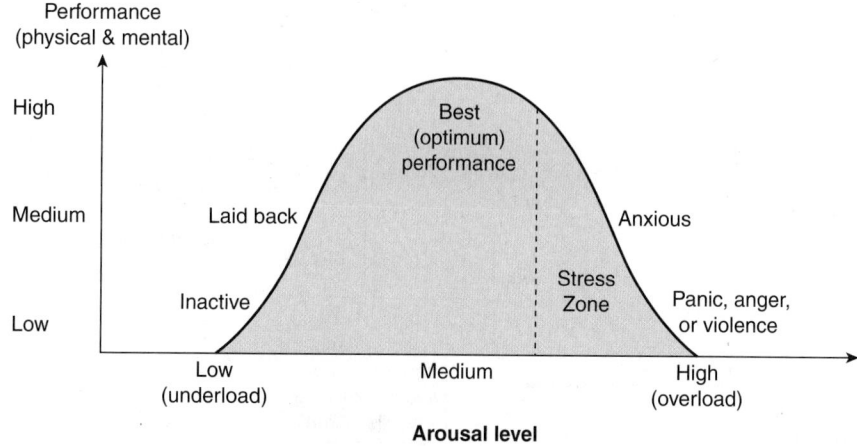

FIGURE 3-3

The relationship between stress and performance.

and has an overall positive effect, such as the effect of moderate physical exercise or a challenging problem to solve, it is called *eustress*. When a stressor results in a negative impact on functioning, it is called *distress*. Even though the emotions experienced may be different, the body's reaction to stressors—whether negative or positive—is similar. However, the severity and duration of the reaction are different.

The Stress Response

A widely accepted model of stress is **general adaptation syndrome (GAS)**, described by the endocrinologist Hans Selye in 1926. GAS divides the stress response into three phases (Figure 3-4). The initial response is the alarm

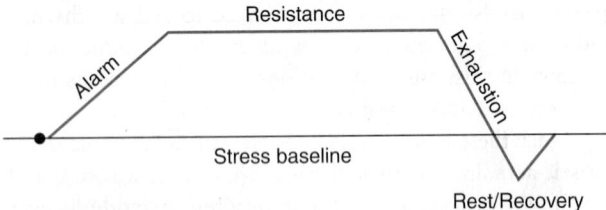

FIGURE 3-4

Phases of stress in the general adaptation syndrome model. (Mitchell, Jeff; Bray, Grady, Emergency Services Stress: Guidelines on Preserving the Health and Careers of Emergency Services Personnel, 1st edition, © 1990. Reprinted by permission of Pearson Education, Inc., Upper Saddle River, NJ)

phase, which prepares the body to respond to the stressor. If an anticipated stressor does not materialize, the normal response is for the body to return to a resting state.

If the stressor materializes, the next phase, resistance, involves actively coping with the stressor and repairing damage done by the stressor. During resistance, the initial physiologic responses brought about in the alarm state may return to normal. As long as the stressor continues, you may alternate between the alarm and resistance phases.

Once the stressor is removed, the body returns to normal. However, if the stressor cannot be managed and the stress response continues, the body enters the third phase of response to stress, exhaustion. When exhaustion occurs, a period of rest and recovery are needed for the body to return to a state of wellness. (It should be noted that this model was developed to describe the biologic, rather than psychological, response to stress.)

In the alarm phase of the stress response, the sympathetic nervous system is stimulated by hormonal secretion (Figure 3-5). A perceived threat causes the limbic system in the brain to signal the hypothalamus. The hypothalamus responds by secreting corticotropin-releasing hormone (CRH). CRH acts on the adjacent anterior pituitary gland, which then secretes **adrenocorticotropic hormone (ACTH)**. ACTH stimulates the adrenal glands to release the hormones **epinephrine** (adrenaline) and **cortisol**, which have several effects on the body (Table 3-3). The response to epinephrine, called the **fight-or-flight response,**

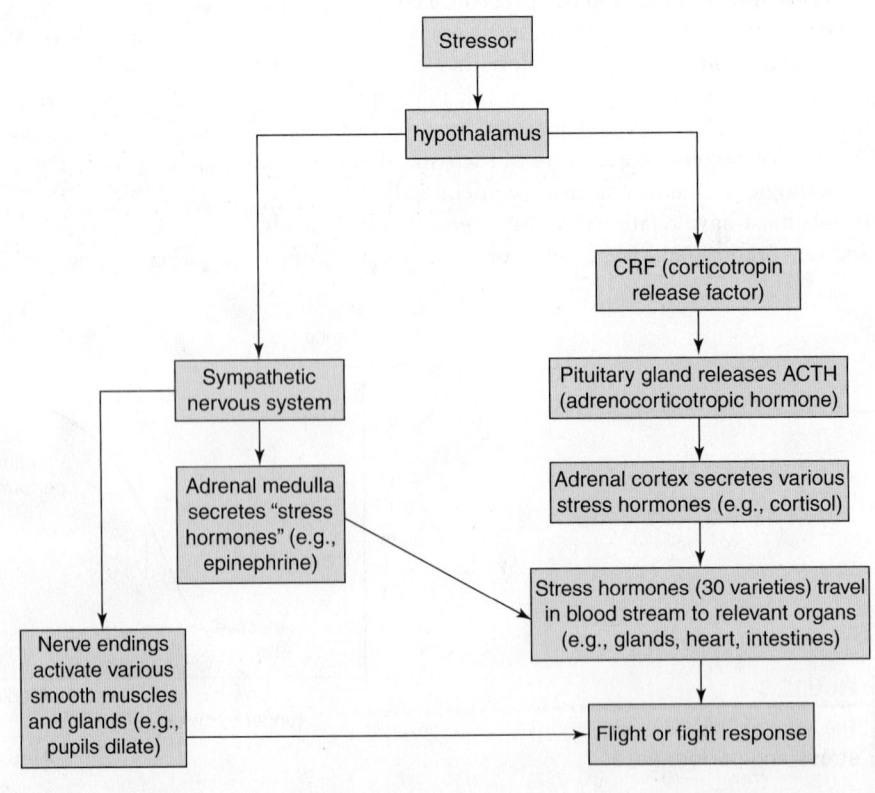

FIGURE 3-5

Hormonal regulation of stress.

TABLE 3-3	Signs and Symptoms of Acute Stress		
Physical	**Cognitive**	**Emotional**	**Behavioral**
Nausea/vomiting	Confusion, difficulty with calculations and logic	Anxiety (in anticipation of event, during, or immediately afterward)	Increase or decrease in activity
Tremors/shaking	Poor concentration	Denial	Withdrawal/silence
Feeling uncoordinated	Poor memory of events	Fear, panic	Inappropriate humor
Profuse sweating	Difficulty making decisions	Feeling overwhelmed or lost	Crying
Chest pain or tightness, palpitations	Disorientation	Anger	Suspiciousness
Difficulty breathing/rapid breathing		Numbness	Change in appetite
Diarrhea			Increased smoking
Dry mouth			
Headache			
Sleep disturbances			
Vision disturbance			

prepares the body to fight against or flee from the stressor (alarm phase).

The release of epinephrine is critical when faced with a physical threat. This allowed our ancestors to survive the dangerous conditions in which they existed and serves us well today when we realize, for example, that a tornado is about to hit. However, much of the stress experienced in modern life does not require physical fight or flight. As a result, the effects of epinephrine physiologically stress the body without protecting us from harm.

You immediately notice the effects of epinephrine when you develop palpitations and sweating palms, but cortisol is the primary hormone that regulates the stress response over time (resistance phase). The body uses cortisol (and epinephrine) to maintain **homeostasis** under normal circumstances. Usually, when the level of cortisol rises to a certain level, it signals the hypothalamus to stop producing CRH. Under significant stress, this regulatory mechanism appears to be overridden and cortisol production continues.

Prolonged and excessive exposure to cortisol has negative effects on the body (exhaustion phase). The immune system is suppressed, wound healing and tissue maintenance are impaired, blood glucose levels are high, and excess fat is deposited. In the presence of excess cortisol, you may experience fatigue, irritability, anxiety, problems with concentration and memory, and depression.

Chronically increased cortisol levels may be linked to several diseases, including cancer, diabetes, cardiovascular disease, and memory impairment.

Duration and Timing of Stress Reactions

The response to stress can be acute, chronic, or cumulative. An **acute stress reaction** occurs during or immediately after exposure to a stressful incident. You may experience, or note in your partner or others involved with the call, changes in cognition (thinking and processing information), behavior, emotions, and physical signs and symptoms (Table 3-4).

In an acute stress reaction, individuals have difficulty focusing attention and receiving and processing information. Your patient, for example, may have difficulty following your directions. Emotions may seem inappropriate for the situation, and behavior may not make sense. Physiologic response to acute stress includes increased heart rate and breathing, a sense of anxiety or nervousness, increased

TABLE 3-4	Signs and Symptoms of Cumulative Stress and Burnout		
Physical	**Cognitive**	**Emotional**	**Behavioral**
Fatigue	Poor memory and concentration	Anxiety	Irritability
Headaches	Disturbing dreams	Boredom	Increased smoking or alcohol intake
Gastrointestinal problems	Difficulty thinking and making decisions	Apathy	Increased or decreased food intake
Changes in appetite		Emotional exhaustion, loss of emotional control	Withdrawal, avoidance
Joint and muscle aches		Feelings of guilt	Substance abuse
		Depression	
		Paranoia	
		Suicidal thoughts	

TABLE 3-5   Signs and Symptoms of Delayed Stress Reaction and Post-Traumatic Stress Disorder

Physical	Cognitive	Emotional	Behavioral
Fatigue	Poor memory and concentration	Anxiety	Irritability
Headaches	Nightmares	Boredom	Increased smoking or alcohol intake
Gastrointestinal problems	Flashbacks	Apathy, feelings of detachment	Increased or decreased food intake
Changes in appetite	Difficulty thinking and making decisions	Difficulty in interpersonal relationships	Withdrawal, avoidance
Joint and muscle aches		Emotional exhaustion, loss of emotional control	Substance abuse
		Feelings of guilt	
		Depression	
		Paranoia	
		Suicidal thoughts	

blood pressure, pale skin, sweating, and dilated pupils. An acute stress reaction can last up to four weeks.

Often, we do not have the luxury of being able to remove one stressor before another affects us. Repeated exposure to stressors over time results in **cumulative stress** (Table 3-5). When stressors continue unabated, the individual enters the third phase of the stress response, exhaustion, or **burnout**. You are no longer able to respond to additional stressors, and you become susceptible to psychological problems (such as depression) and physical problems (infection, weight gain, and others). At this point, you must have a period of rest and recovery to restore well-being.

Individuals subjected to traumatic events can suffer a delayed response, or **post-traumatic stress disorder (PTSD)**. PTSD can significantly interfere with normal functioning, including social relationships, memory, sleep, and emotional response. The public often thinks of PTSD as a problem that affects military personnel who have served in combat. In fact, combat was the situation in which PTSD was recognized, but is just one of a number of events that can lead to PTSD. Any event that is life-threatening, severely compromises emotional well-being, causes intense fear, or constitutes a devastating life change can lead to PTSD. Examples of such events also include being involved in a natural disaster or severe collision, terrorist attacks, rape, assault, and abuse.

Although the signs and symptoms of PTSD are similar to those of an acute stress reaction, they persist for more than one month (Table 3-6). Complex PTSD (C-PTSD) results from prolonged exposure to a severe stressor and is long lasting, with a severe impact on functioning.

Stressors

Whether a particular individual experiences an event negatively or positively depends on several factors. Someone else may perceive something you perceive to be a welcome challenge as a threat. Those differences can be explained by individual personality factors and an individual's cognitive appraisal of the situation (Li, 2009).

TABLE 3-6   Effects of Epinephrine and Cortisol

Epinephrine	Long-Term Effects of Excess Cortisol
Increased heart rate and strength of contraction	Weight gain/increased body fat
Increased blood flow to skeletal muscles	Decreased tissue repair and regeneration (skin, connective tissue, bone, muscle)
Pupil dilation	Decreased immune system function
Increased blood glucose level and breakdown of fat	Increased blood glucose levels, higher insulin resistance
Constriction of blood vessels in the skin and digestive tract	Increased blood pressure
Increased blood pressure	Reduced size of hippocampus in brain, impairs memory
Increased respiratory rate	Impaired production of other hormones
Increased diameter of airways	
Feelings of anxiety	
Tremors	
Nausea/vomiting	

Cognitive appraisal is a process of determining whether or not we perceive a situation as a threat. How you perceive a situation is affected by past experiences, values and expectations, and belief that you can manage the threat. In fact, consciously reframing your cognitive appraisal of a situation is an effective way of managing stress. However, there are some types of events that are likely to produce stress in most people. Many of those stressors are "everyday" stressors, whereas some arise from infrequent, but dramatic, events.

EMS personnel have the same stressors that most people have in their jobs and lives, but some aspects of health care and public safety create unique stressors. In EMS, some of those stressors are:

- Issues with work hours, workload, and pay
- Conflict with coworkers or supervisors
- Failure of other drivers to respond to emergency vehicle lights and sirens
- Confrontational or difficult patients
- Fear of making the wrong decision or making mistakes
- Calls involving dead or dying patients
- Calls involving abuse and neglect
- Calls involving children
- Multiple-casualty incidents
- Injury or death of a coworker
- Seeing severe or disfiguring traumatic injuries

Coping and Stress Management

EMS providers can be put in overwhelmingly stressful situations in which they still must perform their jobs. You may experience any of the physical, cognitive, emotional, or behavioral reactions previously described.

To maintain control in such situations, focus on accomplishing the tasks at hand. You must temporarily put aside intrusive thoughts and feelings, with the understanding that you will need to examine and manage them later. One of the most important things you can do to manage stressful calls is to be competent in your knowledge and skills. The better you know things and the more practiced you are, the more easily they will come to you under stress. Conversely, being poorly prepared and lacking confidence will add to your stress.

In the past, EMS training emphasized a technique called critical incident stress debriefing (CISD) as part of an overall approach to critical incident stress management (CISM). Research has shown, however, that the CISM approach (including CISD) is not effective in reducing the impact of stress on EMS personnel involved in stressful incidents, and, in fact, may interfere with the normal healing process. As a result, CISM is no longer recommended.

Mental health personnel do have a critical role to play in the response to disasters and in counseling EMS personnel suffering from significant stress-related symptoms. Instead of CISM, disaster mental health services and principles of psychological first aid are used. Disaster plans should include planning for having mental health professionals available to assess and assist all those affected by a disaster, including EMS, fire, and law enforcement personnel, as well as disaster victims.

Given the stressors of life, additional stressors of EMS, and negative health effects of stress, it is important to learn and use effective strategies for coping with stress. Individuals use various **coping mechanisms** to address the stressful situation (Table 3-7). More unconscious methods of responding to stress work in the short term, but may cause additional problems. Other ways of responding, called *mature defenses,* are learned and are more helpful in solving problems. Learning and using mature defenses contribute to emotional resilience and can help individuals grow from adversity.

Mental health professionals can be very helpful in developing effective coping strategies. Emotional wellness, physical wellness (including good nutrition and regular exercise), and a strong social support network (family, friends, coworkers) are important in stress management. Some additional stress management techniques include massage therapy, developing time management and organizational skills, meditation, tai chi, yoga, guided imagery, and counseling.

Abusing recreational drugs, alcohol, or prescription medications is not an effective way of relieving stress. In addition to the health risks of substance abuse, the underlying problems are not solved and additional problems may be created.

An arrest for substance abuse–related infractions or a report by a supervisor, colleague, patient, or other person to your state's EMS licensing board will result in investigation and possible revocation of licensure. Many states have impaired provider programs that allow providers with substance abuse issues to provisionally retain their licenses under certain circumstances, which typically include documentation of receiving substance abuse treatment.

Physical Wellness

Aspects of physical wellness include disease and injury prevention, adequate sleep, maintaining a healthy body weight, good nutrition, and physical fitness. Some of the risks and

TABLE 3-7	Stress Coping Mechanisms
SHORT-TERM, LESS-HELPFUL MECHANISMS	
Denial	Inability or refusal to accept what is happening or what has happened
Acting out	Impulses are acted on without restraint (yelling, hitting, running away)
Trivializing	Making light of a situation to avoid distress (such as inappropriate humor)
INTERMEDIATE MECHANISMS	
Displacement	Placing blame for something that is happening or that has happened on a "safe" target, rather than acknowledging the cause, such as blaming only the intoxicated driver and not the pedestrian who was walking along a dark road, dressed in black
Intellectualization	Taking feelings and thoughts out of context and isolating their meaning, such as excessively reading about shock to avoid thinking about your reaction to a patient's death
Reaction formation	Suppressing what you believe are unacceptable feelings and recognizing only what you believe are acceptable feelings, such as recognizing only sympathy for an injured intoxicated driver rather than acknowledging anger
Workaholism/escapism	Involving yourself excessively in work or activities to avoid dealing with the problem, such as working overtime, exercising, studying, hobbies
MATURE MECHANISMS	
Suppression	Consciously choosing to put distressing thoughts and feelings aside temporarily until there is a more favorable time for dealing with them, such as you are angry with something your partner did on a call but you wait until the call is over to address it
Distraction	Temporarily involving oneself in activity to redirect distressing thoughts or feelings, such as focusing on patient care to distract yourself from distressing thoughts until the call is over
Active problem solving	Actively seeking a positive way to improve the situation

challenges to physical fitness experienced by EMS providers include:

- Motor vehicle collisions
- Back injuries
- Violence
- Exposure to communicable diseases
- Sleep disruptions and unusual schedules
- Lack of healthy food choices while on duty
- Long periods of sedentary activity

Motor Vehicle Safety

The most common cause of severe injury and death among on-duty EMS personnel is motor vehicle collisions (MVCs) (Figure 3-6). Fortunately, a number of actions can reduce your risks of MVC-related injury and death. Ambulances handle differently and operate in different circumstances than your personal vehicle. EMS personnel should take special emergency vehicle operation training to learn the skills necessary for driving safety.

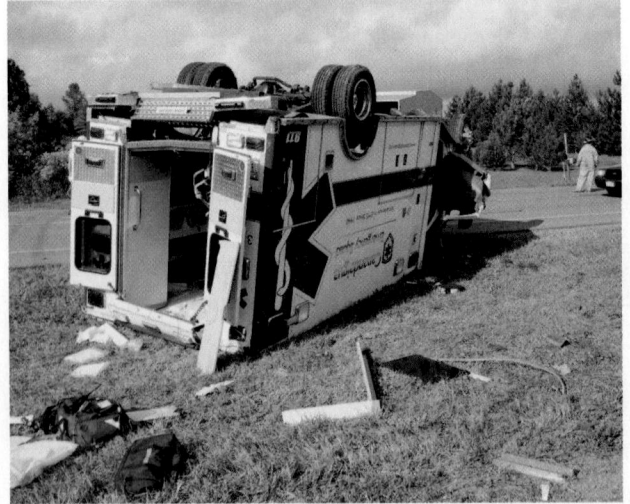

FIGURE 3-6

Motor vehicle collisions pose the greatest safety risk to EMS providers. (Courtesy of Canandaigua Fire and Rescue)

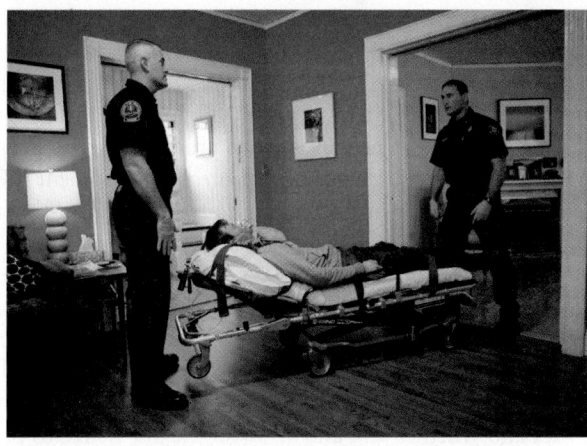

1. Get into position. Keep your feet about shoulder-width apart, turned slightly outward, and flat on the ground.

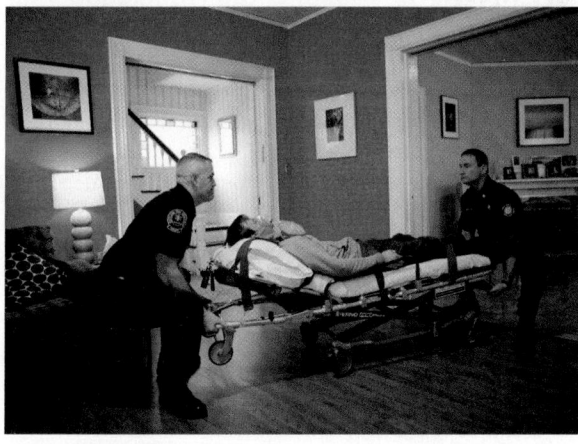

2. As lifting begins, keep your back locked and keep your feet flat. Tighten the muscles of your back and abdomen to splint your lower back.

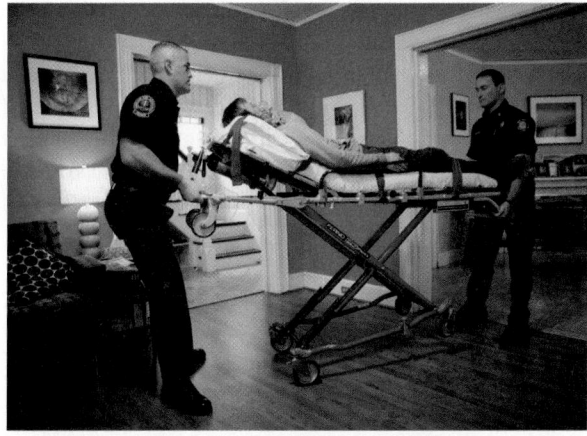

3. As you return to a standing position, make sure your back is locked in and your upper body comes up before your hips.

Outside of work, remember that MVCs are the most common cause of traumatic deaths in people under 44 years old. Many of those deaths can be prevented by wearing seatbelts, avoiding driving under the influence of substances that affect judgment and physical skill, obeying speed limits and other traffic laws, and adjusting driving habits for night time and inclement weather. A substantial part of Chapter 5 is dedicated to giving you more details about reducing those risks.

Back Safety

Advanced EMTs routinely lift and move patients and equipment, making back injuries a common cause of lost work time. Lifting safely requires adhering to proper **body mechanics** and following some simple guidelines (Scan 3-1). Muscular strength is key in lifting safely. The muscles that support your spine and your abdominal muscles must be in good condition.

Proper lifting (Table 3-8) relies on the strength of the large muscles of thighs, and your arms must be able to hold the weight. Correct posture (Figure 3-7), good nutrition, and normal body weight are essential to back health as well. Ideally, employee orientation programs will include back safety education.

Scene Safety

EMS providers respond to situations in which there can be an increased likelihood of violence and injury. Because you

TABLE 3-8   Proper Lifting Technique

- Keep your palms up when possible.
- Don't rush; take time to position yourself properly.
- Use a wide base of support, with one foot slightly in front of the other.
- Bend at the knees, lower your buttocks, and keep your chin up to maintain proper spine position.
- Work as a team when lifting with others; only one person gives the commands.
- Inhale and tighten your abdominal muscles.
- Exhale while using the large leg muscles (quadriceps) to do the work.
- Do not twist or turn; take short steps if you must carry the weight, walking forward whenever possible.

IN THE FIELD

Your personal safety is the highest priority on every call.

are a professional committed to helping others, your initial impulse may be to go directly to the patient. However, the safety of you and your coworkers comes first. If you or your coworkers are injured, you cannot provide care for the patient. Additional EMS responders will be needed to care for you, as well as for the patient. The process of **scene size-up** and selecting adequate **personal protective equipment (PPE)** are essential parts of protecting yourself from on-the-job injuries.

Any time you respond to a scene where someone else has been injured, you must consider whether the risk to your safety still exists, or whether other risks have been created. When responding to MVCs, you must check whether traffic in the area has been controlled to prevent further injuries and whether you and your vehicle are visible to passing traffic. You also must consider whether the vehicles involved are stable, whether there are damaged or downed power lines, chemical spills, broken glass, jagged metal, and other hazards.

Industrial settings, farm settings, construction sites, domestic violence situations, and other situations all have specific hazards that should be anticipated. Some dangers are more insidious. A routine call can result in injury, for instance, if you slip on ice or trip over a loose rug or electrical cord. A call for a sick person might turn out to involve

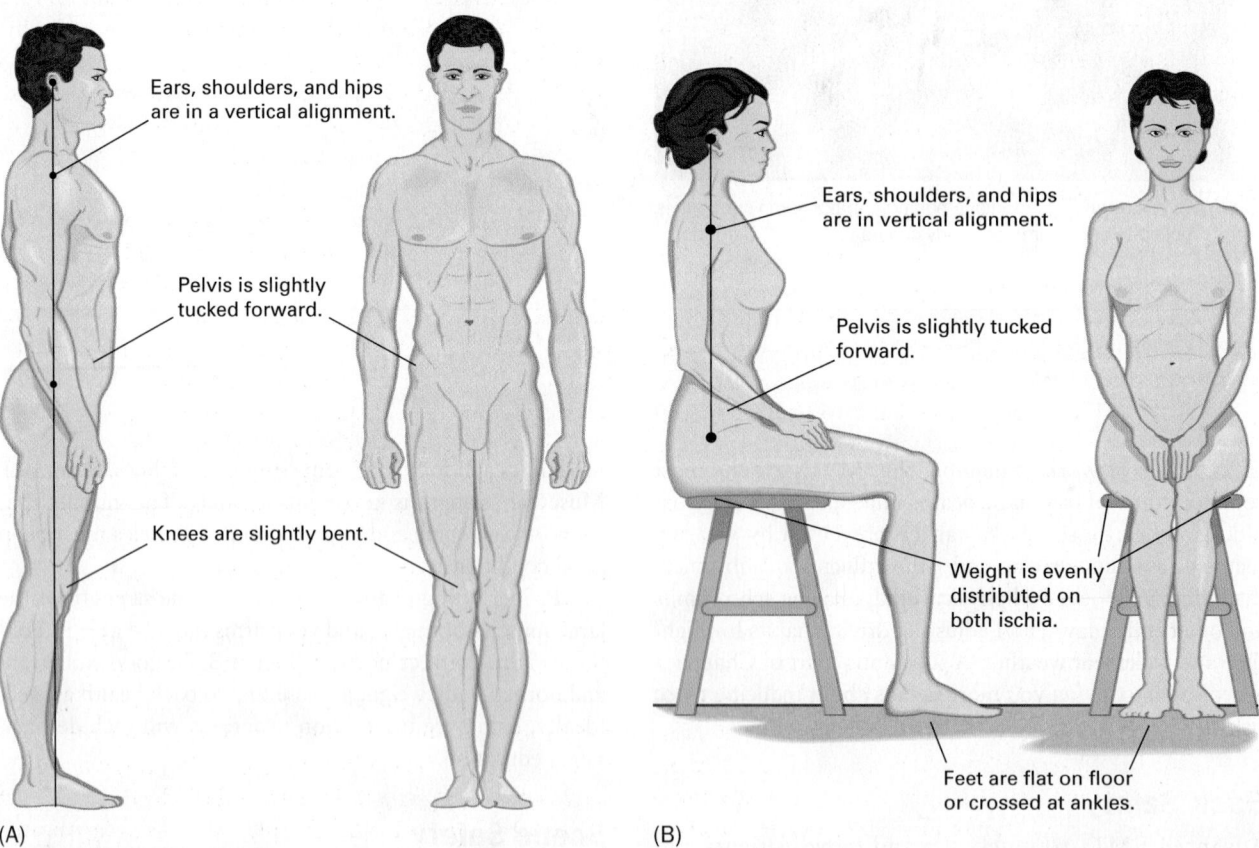

(A)   (B)

FIGURE 3-7

Correct standing (A) and sitting (B) posture.

carbon monoxide exposure. You must always be vigilant for hazards.

If you can make the situation safe without unreasonable risk, do so before caring for the patient. If you cannot make the situation safe, do not approach the scene. Request the resources you need, such as law enforcement, the power company, or animal control.

In situations in which violence has already occurred, you must anticipate the possibility of additional violence toward you, the patient, or others at the scene. Patients experiencing a behavioral emergency, because of either situational factors or psychiatric illness, also pose a danger to EMS personnel. You must wait for law enforcement to establish the safety of the scene before approaching. Sometimes a scene that initially seemed to pose no risk of violence can change.

Experiencing an emergency can provoke a number of emotional and behavioral responses. Patients, family, and bystanders can become confrontational under stress. Using principles of therapeutic communication, you can often defuse the other person's anger. However, you must recognize when you are in jeopardy and be prepared to leave the scene until it is safe. You will learn more about how to recognize signs of impending violence and respond to it throughout this text.

Infectious Disease Prevention

Advanced EMTs work to care for the sick and injured in a variety of environments. As a result, you will be exposed to **infectious illnesses** (infectious diseases) and patients with **communicable illnesses** (communicable diseases). Infectious illnesses are caused by **micro-organisms**, or what are commonly referred to as *germs*. Communicable illnesses are a subset of infectious illnesses that are contracted from other human beings. For example, tetanus is an infectious illness that can be contracted when a wound is contaminated with *Clostridium tetani* bacteria by the instrument that caused the wound. Influenza is a communicable illness. It is caused by various viruses that are spread from person to person.

We share our environment with a multitude of micro-organisms, most of which are not harmful to human beings. In fact, many micro-organisms are beneficial to human beings. For example, a strain of bacteria found in the intestinal tract is important in producing vitamin K, which is essential to blood clotting. Micro-organisms that cause disease are called **pathogens**. Pathogens include bacteria, viruses, parasites, fungi, and prions.

Some communicable diseases pose greater health risks than others, and particular actions are taken by health care providers to prevent them. (Additional infectious diseases are discussed in Chapter 28.) Minimizing your chances of contracting infectious diseases is largely a matter of knowing your enemy. Knowledge of how diseases are transmitted and factors that influence whether an exposure leads to illness allows you to understand how you can reduce your chances of illness (Table 3-9).

Routes of Transmission

Communicable diseases can be spread via direct or indirect routes. In **direct transmission**, the infected person and a noninfected person must be in close proximity or direct contact with each other. HIV-AIDS, for example, is spread primarily by direct contact with the blood or **body fluids** of an infected person. Despite the fact that HIV-AIDS is a very serious, noncurable disease, the human immunodeficiency virus (HIV) that leads to acquired immune deficiency syndrome (AIDS) is fragile outside the body, and dies quickly.

In contrast, the hepatitis B virus (HBV) can be spread by direct transmission, but also survives on surfaces for a long period of time, which can lead to **indirect transmission**. With indirect transmission, there is a nonhuman intermediary between the infected and noninfected individuals. An animal intermediary is called a vector. Mosquitoes are vectors for a number of diseases, such as malaria, West Nile virus, and other viruses that cause encephalitis. An inanimate intermediary, such as a contaminated piece of medical equipment, is called a fomite.

Communicable diseases also are classified by the routes by which they leave and enter the body. Tuberculosis is spread through the respiratory route. *Mycobacterium tuberculosis* is contained in the sputum of individuals with active infection in the lungs. Coughing allows droplets containing the bacteria to become airborne. The airborne particles can then be inhaled into the respiratory tracts of nearby individuals.

Bloodborne pathogens are transmitted from one person to another through exposure of **mucous membranes** and nonintact skin to infected blood or body fluids. HBV and HIV are both transmitted this way.

Pathogens can leave and enter the body through the gastrointestinal tract. Hepatitis A can be spread by daycare workers who change diapers and do not adequately wash their hands. Some diseases, such as chlamydia and gonorrhea, are spread primarily through sexual contact (sexually transmitted diseases [STDs] or sexually transmitted infections [STIs]), but can be spread in select other ways, such as from mother to newborn during childbirth.

Not all contacts with pathogens result in disease. A number of factors determine whether or not contact will lead to infection. The agent, host, and environment all have characteristics that influence whether or not illness occurs.

Characteristics of the agent, or pathogen, that influences disease include virulence and dose. Virulence is the strength of the organism. Dose is the number of micro-organisms that come in contact with the potential host. Host factors include the immune status, behaviors (such as hand washing), and general health of the individual.

An environment that is inhospitable to micro-organisms decreases the chances of disease transmission. For example, the spread of tuberculosis bacteria is reduced greatly by good ventilation and exposure to sunlight.

TABLE 3-9 Infectious Diseases of Particular Concern to the Advanced EMT

Disease	Agent	Description	Transmission	Prevention
HIV-AIDS	Virus (human immunodeficiency virus)	Suppresses T-cells in the immune system; patient is susceptible to infections	Contact with blood or body fluids, including through intravenous drug use and sexual contact. Rarely transmitted via needle stick	Standard Precautions for anticipated contact with blood or body fluids
Hepatitis B Hepatitis C	Viruses (HBV and HCV)	Cause inflammation of the liver, decreasing liver function	Blood, body fluids, contaminated objects	Standard Precautions for anticipated contact with blood or body fluids; disinfection of contaminated equipment surfaces; hepatitis B vaccination
Tuberculosis (TB)	Bacteria	Can infect many body tissues, but usually affects the lungs. TB is spread when active disease is present. Antibiotic-resistant forms exist	Primarily by respiratory droplets. Can be present on contaminated surfaces. Transmission often requires prolonged close proximity to infected patient (prevalent in prisons, homeless populations, extended care facilities)	Standard Precautions; use of N-95 respirator for known or suspected active TB (high-risk patient with cough, fever, weight loss). Disinfection of surfaces and equipment. Routine TB skin testing to check for exposure
Bacterial meningitis (meningococcal)	Bacteria	Inflammation of the lining surrounding the brain and spinal cord. Can be fatal or result in permanent disability	Oral and nasal secretions	Standard Precautions, including face mask, for suspected disease (fever, malaise, stiff neck, light sensitivity, decreased level of responsiveness, rash). Vaccine recommended for high-risk populations
Pneumonia	Viruses, bacteria, fungi	Infection results in areas of infiltrate (pus) in lungs, causing coughing and shortness of breath	Respiratory; oral and nasal secretions	Standard Precautions for suspected cases, including face mask. Vaccine (pneumococcal bacteria only) available for high-risk populations
Staphylococcal skin infection, including impetigo, methicillin-resistant Staphylococcus aureus (MRSA)	Bacteria	Infection of wounds, skin lesions. Patients or health care providers may culture positive without signs of active disease. Staphylococcal bacteria can also cause wound infection, sepsis, and food poisoning	Skin contact with open wounds or contaminated objects	Standard Precautions. Disinfection and frequent hand washing to prevent nosocomial infection
Influenza	Viruses (H1N1, influenza B, and others)	Group of respiratory viral illnesses that range from mild to fatal (usually from complications, such as pneumonia in susceptible populations). Results in fever, cough, muscle and joint pain	Primarily seasonal; respiratory droplets or direct contact	Standard Precautions with suspected infection, hand washing, disinfection. Vaccines given annually to ensure immunity to predicted prevalent strains

TABLE 3-9	**Infectious Diseases of Particular Concern to the Advanced EMT—continued**			
Disease	**Agent**	**Description**	**Transmission**	**Prevention**
German measles (rubella)	Virus	Usually mild in children (rash, headache, fever, runny nose), may be more severe in adults; Of particular concern in the first 20 weeks of pregnancy	Respiratory droplets	Standard Precautions; Vaccination, usually combined with measles and mumps (MMR)
Pertussis (whooping cough)	Bacteria	Causes characteristic severe, persistent coughing; Currently increased incidence in some U.S. areas	Respiratory, airborne	Standard Precautions, including face mask; Vaccination available, usually combined tetanus, diphtheria, and pertussis (Tdap)
Severe acute respiratory distress syndrome (SARS)	Virus	An outbreak in 2003 caused concern about global spread; There has not been a SARS outbreak since 2004, but the severity of the disease warrants ongoing preparedness and surveillance	Respiratory, airborne, direct contact	Standard Precautions, including face mask

Preventing Exposure

The general controls against infectious disease exposure include:

- Training and administration, such as classes and policies
- Engineering controls, such as equipment and environmental design
- Work practice controls, such as good habits
- Personal protective equipment (PPE)

Some specific measures include being in good general health, having appropriate immunizations, hand washing, properly handling sharps and contaminated items, **cleaning** and **disinfecting** the ambulance, and wearing personal protective equipment (PPE). Keep in mind that sick and injured patients are more susceptible to infection and many infections are acquired in health care settings. Infection control practices protect not only you, but your patients as well.

The Occupational Safety and Health Administration (OSHA) enforces regulations that require employers to provide specific types of PPE to workers in certain jobs. The Centers for Disease Control and Prevention (CDC) issues guidelines for health care workers for immunization (Table 3-10) and in the use of PPE and **Standard Precautions** against contracting infectious diseases.

Standard Precautions are based on the assumption that any patient's blood or body fluids could be infectious. This

TABLE 3-10	**CDC Recommended Health Care Provider Immunizations**

- Hepatitis B (three-vaccine series; subsequent boosters not currently recommended).
- Influenza (annually).
- Measles (if born in 1957 or later and have not had prior vaccination or disease).
- Mumps (recommended for susceptible individuals born in 1957 or later who have not had prior vaccination or disease).
- Rubella (if born in 1957 or later and have not had prior vaccination or disease).
- Varicella zoster (chickenpox) (for those without reliable history of disease or laboratory evidence of immunity).
- Tetanus and diphtheria (every 10 years after initial vaccination series; for wound management).
- Additional vaccines may be recommended for health care providers or laboratory personnel in certain settings, and for postexposure management.

assumption is particularly important in prehospital and emergency care, because a patient's infectious disease status is not likely to be known. Contact with sweat and tears are exceptions to the need for PPE.

There currently are no immunizations—or, in some cases, no widely available or advisable immunizations—for some communicable diseases. Those diseases include HIV-AIDS and tuberculosis (TB), among others. PPE, hand washing, carefully handling contaminated sharps, and disinfection are key in preventing transmission of these diseases.

In all cases of exposure to communicable disease, you must follow your employer's postexposure plan. The specific actions will depend on the pathogen and type of exposure received. Check your employer's policies for immunization and infection control. The 2009 reauthorization of the 1990 Ryan White Comprehensive AIDS Resources Emergency Act requires that emergency response personnel, including EMS providers, must be notified when they have been exposed to a patient who has an infectious, potentially fatal disease, such as HIV-AIDS.

Gloves

Gloves are the most frequently used PPE in Standard Precautions. You must wear gloves any time you are performing a procedure with high likelihood of coming into hand contact with blood, other body fluids, mucous membranes, or nonintact skin. This includes handling contaminated patient care equipment, as well as direct patient contact. For example, you must wear gloves when starting an IV, controlling bleeding, or decontaminating bloody equipment. However, it is not necessary to wear gloves to take vital signs if you will not come in contact with mucous membranes, blood, or open wounds.

OSHA does *not* require gloves for giving intramuscular or subcutaneous injections, because the risk of coming into contact with blood is negligible. However, your state or employer may require the use of PPE for these procedures.

Nonsterile exam gloves are used for routine prehospital patient contact. You will use sterile gloves for some patient care procedures, such as endotracheal suctioning.

Some health care providers and patients have allergies to the latex used in some gloves. Gloves made of other materials, such as vinyl and nitrile, are widely available. Select gloves that are the best fit for you so that you can perform your work without getting your gloves caught or tearing them.

Put on the gloves before engaging in activities with risk for exposure to blood, body fluids, or nonintact skin. Change gloves between patients, if caring for more than one patient, and before performing other tasks, such as touching equipment and driving, to avoid contaminating other surfaces.

Remove gloves as shown in Scan 3-2. Always wash your hands after patient contact, even when gloves were worn.

Hand Washing

Hand washing is the single most important method of reducing the spread of communicable disease (Figure 3-8). The high rate of **nosocomial infections** is one of the most significant concerns in health care settings today. Those infections are greatly reduced when health care providers use proper

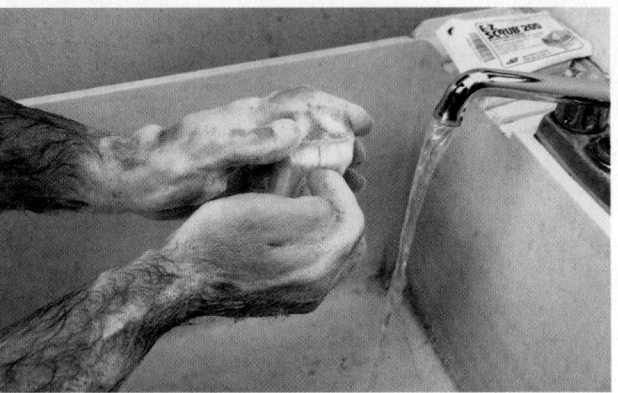

FIGURE 3-8

Hand washing is the most important step in preventing the spread of communicable disease.

hand washing as soon as possible after each patient contact or contact with contaminated equipment (Table 3-11). When soap and water are not available, a waterless alcohol-based gel hand sanitizer can be used until soap and water are available. Any time the hands are visibly soiled, soap and water are required. Plain soap works as well as antibacterial soap for hand washing.

Good hand hygiene includes keeping nails trimmed and clean, avoiding artificial nails, and wearing jewelry that can trap micro-organisms. Frequent hand washing can cause the skin and cuticles to crack, which can be uncomfortable, as well as allowing microbial growth and providing a route of entry for infection. Using hand lotion will help keep your skin healthy and intact.

Masks, Eye Protection, and Gowns

Respiratory and eye protection and fluid-impervious gowns are used when there is the possibility of airborne droplet contact (from coughing, sneezing, or airway management procedures) or being splashed or sprayed with blood and body fluids (Figure 3-9). Prescription eyeglasses and sunglasses do not provide adequate protection against splashed or sprayed fluids. Goggles used for PPE must fit snugly around the eyes or over eyeglasses.

TABLE 3-11 **Hand-Washing Steps**

1. Wet your hands with warm water.
2. Apply liquid soap.
3. Rub hands together with soap for 20 seconds.
4. Include wrists, palms, backs of hands, between fingers, and under fingernails.
5. Rinse soap from hands.
6. Dry hands with a paper towel.
7. Use paper towel to turn off faucet.
8. Dispose of paper towel.

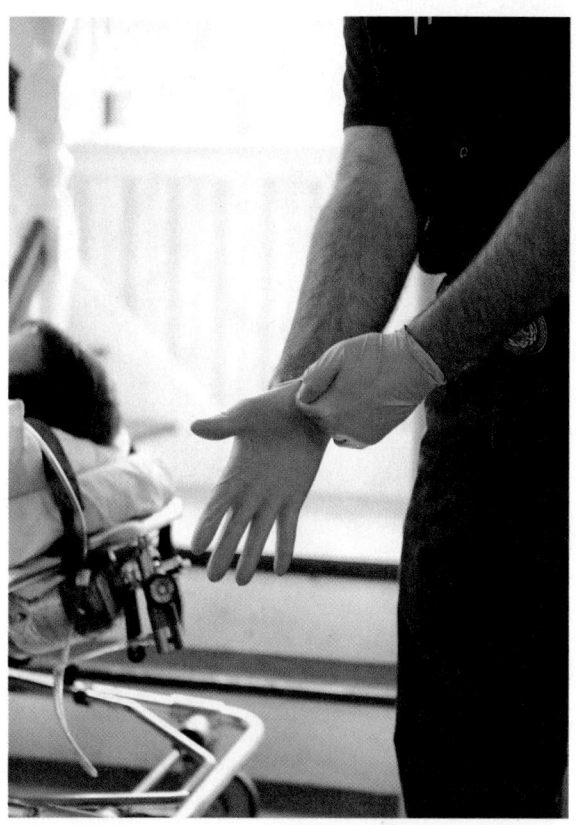

1. Use a gloved finger to pull a cuff out and down on the other glove. Do not touch the inside of the glove.

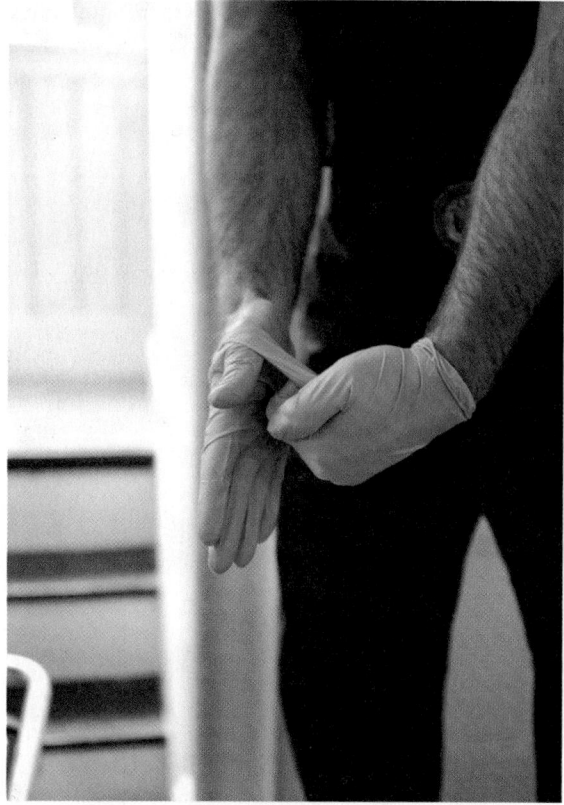

2. Without touching the inside of the glove, continue pulling it downward.

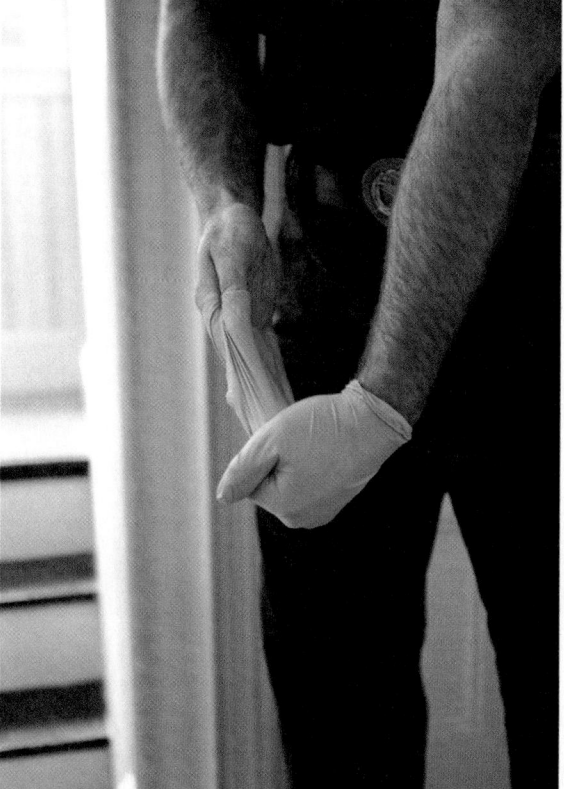

3. Pull until the glove is inside-out and off all but the tips of the fingers and thumb.

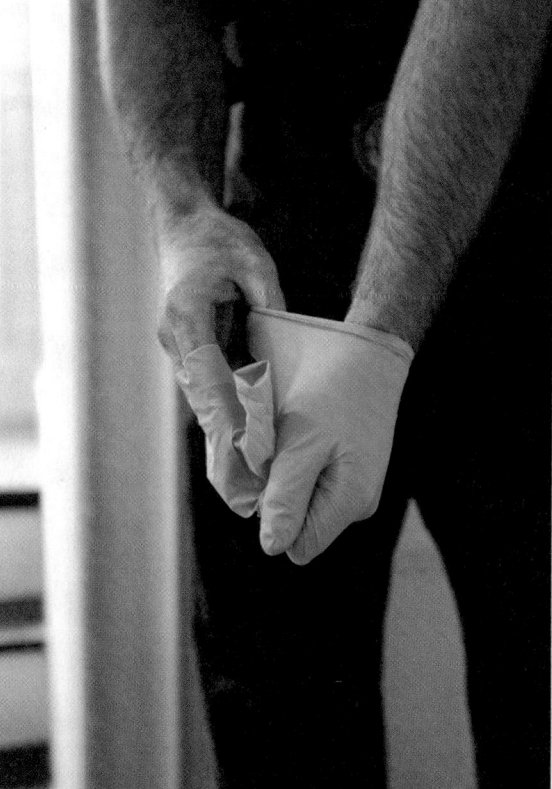

4. Hook the clean inside surface of the partially removed glove into the clean inside of the other glove.

(continued)

Proper Technique for Removing Gloves (continued)

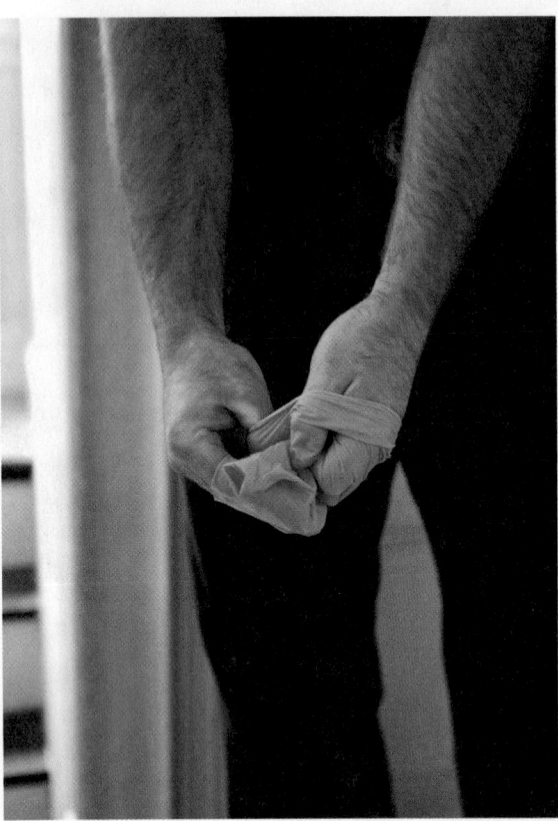

5. Use the clean inside surfaces of the partially removed glove to pinch and pull down on the other glove.

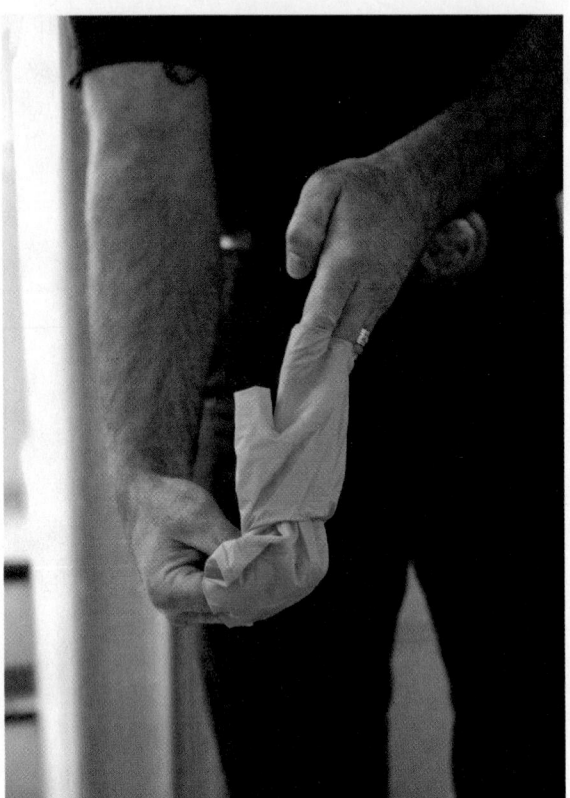

6. Finish pulling the second glove downward. Use the clean inside surfaces to finally pull off both gloves.

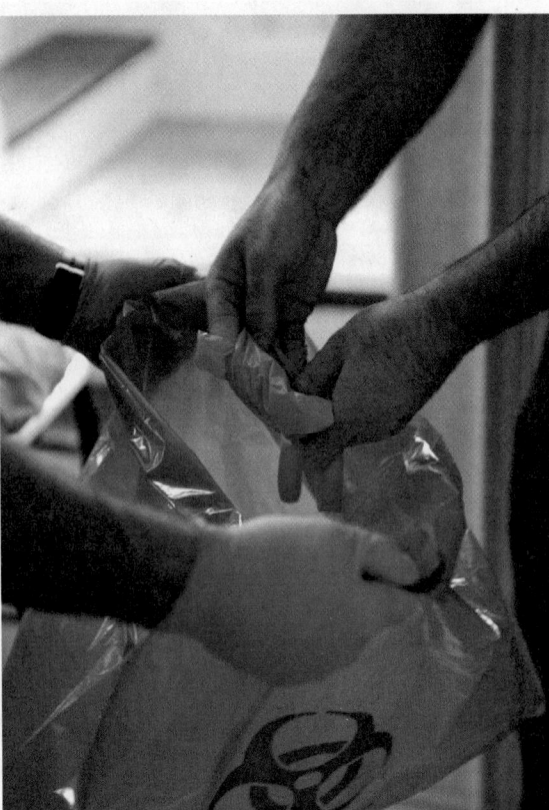

7. Drop the contaminated gloves into a biohazard container.

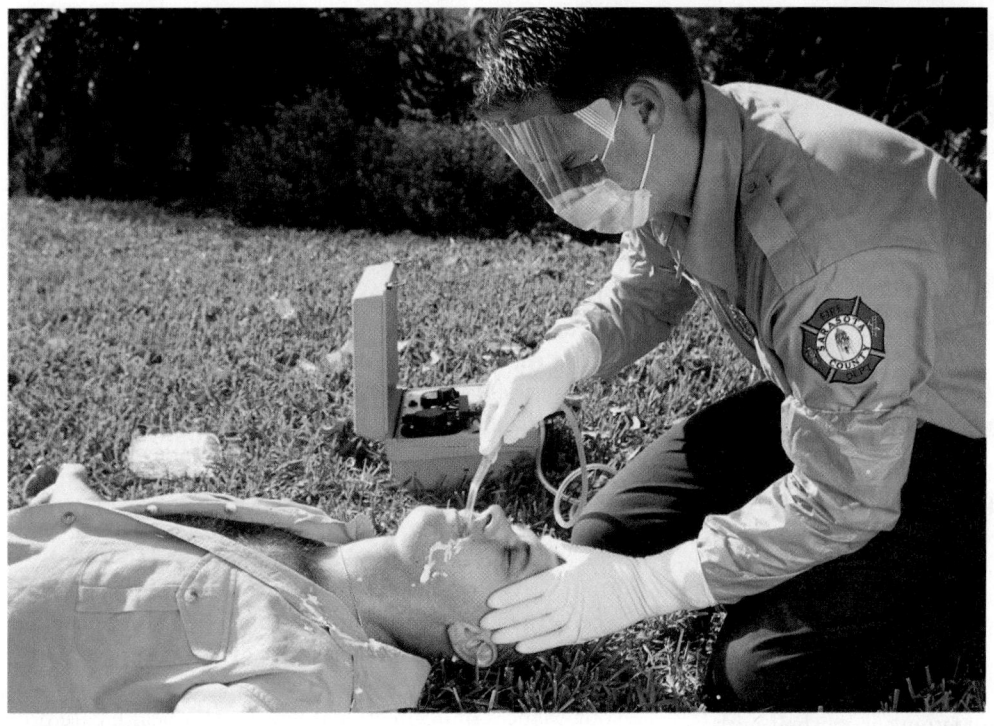

FIGURE 3-9

Protect the eyes, face, and clothing when spraying or splashing of blood or other body fluids is anticipated.

TABLE 3-12	**Signs and Symptoms of Active Pulmonary Tuberculosis**

- Productive cough
- Fever
- Loss of appetite
- Weight loss
- Night sweats
- Chest pain
- Shortness of breath

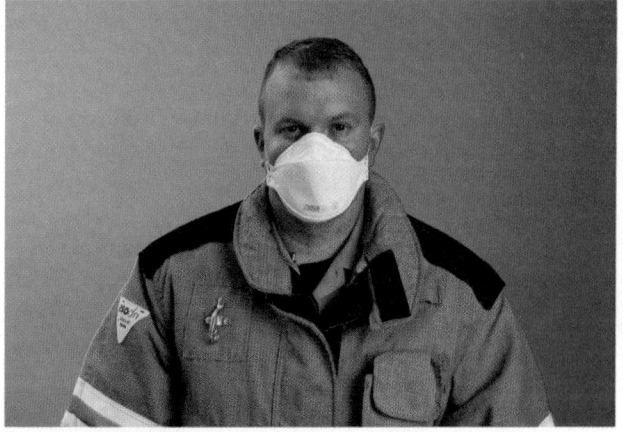

FIGURE 3-10

N-95 respirators are worn when in contact with a patient with known or suspected active pulmonary tuberculosis.

Face masks are designed to protect the nose and mouth. A flexible nose piece allows the masks to be fitted snugly. For patients with suspected active tuberculosis (Table 3-12), a specially fitted N-95 respirator is used (Figure 3-10). This type of mask filters smaller particulates than typical face masks. A face shield can be used in place of goggles and mask.

Gowns are used in situations such as childbirth and major trauma with significant bleeding to protect your clothing from being soaked with blood or body fluids. Make sure the gown you select is large enough to close in back. Secure the gown with ties at the neck and waist.

When you have completed patient care, carefully remove PPE, avoiding skin contact with its contaminated surfaces. Place used PPE in proper disposal receptacles. In many cases, PPE can be disposed of with regular trash in the ambulance or emergency department. PPE that is heavily contaminated or capable of leaking liquid blood or body fluids is disposed of in specially labeled **biohazard** waste bags.

Managing Contamination and Exposure

Any time your skin is contaminated with potentially infectious material, you must wash with soap and water. If your clothing is contaminated, you must remove and bag it, shower, and put on a clean uniform. The contaminated uniform must be laundered according to your service's guidelines. Contaminated uniforms must not be laundered at home. Your service may provide a washer and dryer at your station, or may use a laundry service to wash contaminated clothing.

An **exposure** occurs if potentially infectious material comes in contact with mucous membranes or nonintact skin. Nonintact skin includes contamination of existing wounds, as well as needle sticks and other injuries (for example, cutting your hand on a bloody piece of glass during vehicle extrication). Immediately wash the area with soap and water. If your eyes are splashed, irrigate them with water or saline. Report the exposure according to your employer's guidelines and seek a medical evaluation.

Equipment Decontamination

Contaminated equipment and surfaces are handled by disposal, cleaning, disinfecting, or **sterilizing**. Many patient care items—for example, IV catheters, airway devices, needles, syringes, dressings and bandages, and suction catheters—are disposable and meant for a single use. Sharp objects ("sharps"), such as used needles and disposable surgical instruments, must be discarded in special puncture-resistant biohazard disposal containers (Figure 3-11).

Cleaning means that something is washed with detergent and water to remove gross debris. Disinfection is intended to kill many micro-organisms on the surface of nonporous items. Disinfection is appropriate for items that are not used for invasive procedures, such as backboards, the stretcher mattress, and splints, and for cleaning up spilled or splashed blood and body fluids. Disinfection requires the use of a commercial hospital-grade disinfectant or a solution of one part household bleach (6 percent sodium hypochlorite) to 10 parts water.

Sterilization uses pressurized steam or chemical sterilization solutions to kill all micro-organisms on an object. Items that are reusable and will come in contact with mucous membranes or nonintact skin or will be used for invasive procedures must be sterilized between uses.

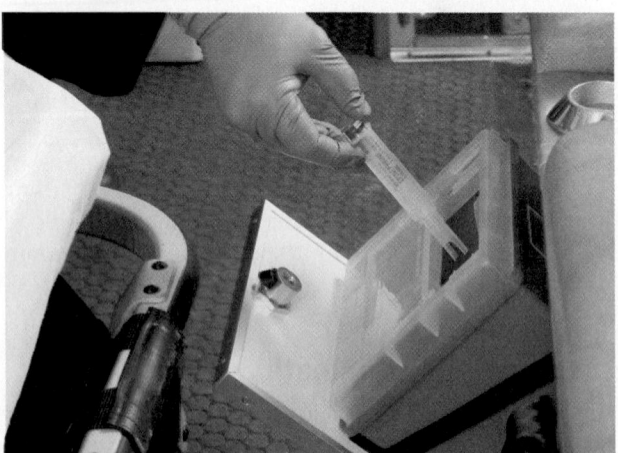

FIGURE 3-11

Sharps, such as used needles, are placed in a puncture-resistant container after use.

Laryngoscope blades, used by some prehospital personnel to see the vocal cords and pass a tube through them, are an example of equipment that must be sterilized. EMS personnel clean and disinfect, but your service likely has a contract with a hospital supply service for sterilization.

Other Preventive Measures

Avoid eating, chewing gum, applying lip balm or cosmetics, touching your face, eating and, of course, smoking in patient care areas. If you have any open wounds that could be contaminated, check with your supervisor about your employer's policies. If you are sick with signs and symptoms of an infectious illness, such as diarrhea, conjunctivitis (pink eye), or influenza, you should not be involved in patient care activities.

Sleep

People in the United States are chronically sleep deprived, receiving far less than the recommended seven to eight hours per night. Sleep deprivation is associated with several adverse health outcomes, including more than doubling your chances of occupational injury. As a health care provider, your lack of sleep will not just affect you, but also can jeopardize your patient, your partner, and the public.

There is a significant association between sleep deprivation and patient care mistakes. Falling asleep or inattention while driving has been implicated in many ambulance collisions as well.

There are a number of reasons that you may be short on quality sleep, including work hours, staying out late, insomnia, or sleep apnea. Inadequate sleep, even for one night, results in significantly decreased alertness and task performance. Sleep deprivation affects your ability to process and remember information and to sustain attention. Driving safety is decreased substantially in sleep-deprived individuals, contributing to tens of thousands of injuries annually. There is a relationship between chronic sleep deprivation and high blood pressure, heart attack, obesity, depression, and other chronic health problems.

Insomnia is a common complaint in the United States. In EMS, several additional factors can interfere with the quality and quantity of sleep. Many EMS providers work night shifts or are on duty for 24 to 48 hours at a time. Because sleep-wake cycles are part of your **circadian rhythm**, it is difficult to change them or adapt to interruptions. It is recommended that those who regularly work night shifts do not try to switch back to a daytime routine.

There are several suggestions for "sleep hygiene" (Table 3-13). If none of these suggestions works and you frequently suffer from poor sleep, see your physician.

Nutrition

Healthy nutrition is important for maintaining a normal **body mass index (BMI)** (Table 3-14), as well as for maintaining the health of body tissues and decreasing the risk of

TABLE 3-13	Tips for Healthy Sleep Behavior (Sleep Hygiene)

- Go to bed only when you are sleepy. If you are not asleep in 20 minutes, get up and do something quietly, such as reading, until you are sleepy. If you wake up during the night, do not look at the clock.
- Do not nap throughout the day. If you must nap, limit your nap to less than 1 hour.
- Maintain your sleep–wake schedule on days off.
- Do not exercise in the 4 hours before bedtime.
- Develop a ritual, such as having a bath, a cup of caffeine-free tea, or a few minutes of recreational reading (not studying).
- Do not use your bedroom for studying, working, or watching TV.
- Avoid caffeine and alcohol for 6 hours before bedtime.
- Do not eat a heavy meal before bed, although a light snack may be helpful.
- Make sure your bed and bedroom are comfortable and dark. A cooler room with more blankets is better than a warmer room. Use an eyeshade, ear plugs, or a white noise machine if needed.

TABLE 3-14	Calculating Body Mass Index

- Find your weight in kilograms (kg) by dividing your weight in pounds (lb) by 2.2 (example: 175 lb/2.2 = 79.5 kg).
- Find your height in meters (m) by multiplying your height in inches (in.) times 2.54 and dividing by 100 (example: (70 in. × 2.54)/100 = 1.8 m).
- Find the square of your height in meters (m^2) (example: 1.8 m × 1.8 m = 3.24 m^2).
- Divide your weight in kg by your height in m^2 (example: 79.5 kg/3.24 m^2 = 24.5).
  Underweight: BMI < 18.5
  Normal: BMI 18.5–24.9
  Overweight: BMI 25–29.9
  Obese: BMI > 30

Note: You can also use the website to calculate body mass index: http://www.cdc.gov/healthyweight/assessing/bmi/adult_bmi/english_bmi_calculator/bmi_calculator.html

many diseases. To achieve and maintain ideal body weight, you must have the right balance between caloric intake and caloric expenditure.

To get the nutrition you need from a relatively limited number of calories, you must choose lower-calorie, nutrient-rich foods. Unfortunately, the majority of those in the United States fall far short of recommendations for healthy nutrition (Figure 3-12). Most people do not get enough fruits, vegetables, and whole grains in their diets, and consume too much fat and sodium and too many calories.

Fruits, vegetables, and whole grains provide dietary fiber, vitamins, minerals, and a variety of **phytonutrients** (such as those found in green tea, whole grains, fruits, and vegetables). Many phytonutrients have **antioxidant** properties that protect against cellular damage caused by **inflammation**. Inflammation and cellular damage have been

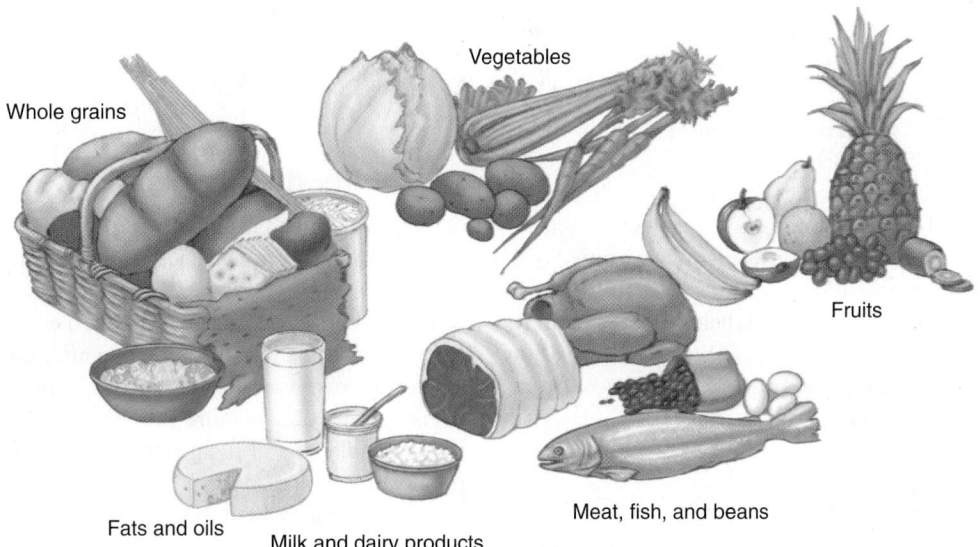

FIGURE 3-12

Whole grains, vegetables, fruits, dairy products, meats, and fats are all part of a healthy diet.

implicated in a number of disease processes, including heart disease, dementia, and cancer.

Research is ongoing into the health benefits of a number of nutrients. Current areas of research include the effects of antioxidants from phytonutrients, **omega fatty acids**, dietary fiber, calcium, and vitamin D.

The amount of information can be overwhelming. Good nutrition is best obtained by eating a variety of plant-based, minimally processed foods on a regular basis, rather than focusing on a single nutrient. The *Dietary Guidelines for Americans* (U.S. Department of Health and Human Services, 2005) makes recommendations in several areas of nutrition.

The U.S. Department of Agriculture (USDA) uses the *My Plate* system, based on the *Dietary Guidelines*, to recommend intake from selected food groups. The USDA website, http://www.choosemyplate.gov, has a number of interactive tools to help you find your recommended intake from each food group, based on your age, gender, weight, and activity level. The site provides a wide variety of suggestions for meeting these recommendations.

Labels and Serving Sizes

The food portions served in restaurants are not typically a single serving. They are usually several times larger than one serving. The use of larger serving plates makes the amount of food even more deceiving. Portion control is critical in any effort to lose or maintain weight. Check food labels carefully to see what a serving size is. Food labels also contain information about calories and nutrient content, helping you make healthier food choices.

Read the lists of ingredients on food products. The ingredients are listed in descending order of quantities in the food. For example, "multigrain bread" and "wheat bread" do not mean "whole grain" bread unless the first ingredient listed is a whole grain, such as "whole wheat." Be aware of ingredients and food additives, such as high fructose corn syrup, sodium, monosodium glutamate (MSG), trans fats (partially hydrogenated oils), sulfites, food colors and dyes, nitrites, and nitrates that are associated or thought to be associated with health problems.

Unfortunately, other food contaminants, such as hormones, pesticides, and antibiotics present in commercially farmed products, do not appear on the label. Know your food terminology. Some terms, such as "organic," have no agreed-upon definitions. Foods labeled as organic may vary in how "organic" they truly are. Other terms may not sound like what they really are. For example, sucrose, fructose, maltose, and dextrose are all sugars.

Eating Well at Work

Fast foods, convenience foods, and restaurants are all temptations in a hectic lifestyle. Although it is possible to make some healthy food choices when faced with these temptations, you must be able to make informed choices. Recent

IN THE FIELD

Do not try to overhaul your entire lifestyle all at once. Sudden, dramatic changes are difficult to sustain. Implement a few small but important changes at a time. Set reasonable, specific goals so you can measure your progress. For example, an initial goal of bringing your meal every day may not be feasible, so start with a goal of packing a healthy meal to take to work four days out of seven. If you set an unrealistic goal, failure to meet it can be discouraging. On the other hand, success in meeting a reasonable goal provides motivation to set additional ones.

legislation requires that fast-food restaurants display nutrition information about their products (the exact regulations guiding the implementation of the legislation have not yet been implemented). Would you still eat a bacon double cheeseburger, a large order of fries, and a large soda if you knew that the meal would approach, or even exceed, your daily recommended caloric intake while offering nothing nutritionally?

Whether you bring your food with you or pick up something during the course of your shift, eating healthier foods at work requires a little planning and commitment. If you do not have time to prepare food to take with you, you can still make healthier choices. Instead of stopping for fast food, stop at the grocery store to pick up fresh foods that do not require preparation, such as fruits, unsalted nuts, whole grain crackers, prepackaged fresh vegetables, and yogurt.

Deli-style sandwiches can be a healthier choice than typical fast-food burgers and chicken sandwiches. Choose whole grain breads and low-fat meats such as turkey, pile on the vegetables, and top it with mustard or a drizzle of vinegar and oil dressing instead of mayonnaise or heavier dressings.

Instead of soda, choose bottled water or unsweetened brewed iced tea. (Bottled teas and teas from soda fountains contain high amounts of sugar and may not have the same nutritional benefits as freshly brewed tea.)

Alcohol and Caffeine

Despite widespread negative information about alcohol and caffeine, there is also evidence that moderate intake of these substances can have some health benefits. Drinking a cup or two of coffee each day because you enjoy it is much different, however, than drinking cup after cup to try to stay awake because you are not getting enough sleep. Energy drinks often contain more caffeine than coffee, as well as other stimulants and sugar or sweeteners. Those drinks are not healthy choices.

Enjoying a cocktail, beer, or glass of wine is fine, but relying on alcohol as a stress reliever is not healthy. Research continues on both sides of the issue for these substances, so make sure you stay up to date on the latest information and recommendations.

Food Safety

The safety of our nation's food supply in terms of contaminants, additives, and genetically modified organisms is a current concern. Several recent foodborne outbreaks of *E. coli* and *Salmonella* have received national attention. One step you can take to avoid those health risks is selecting, preparing, and storing food properly.

People often associate foodborne illnesses, or food poisoning, with raw, undercooked, or improperly stored animal products, such as meat and eggs. These are, in fact, important sources of foodborne illness. But raw fruits and vegetables and processed foods can be contaminated with bacteria, too. Much of the contamination occurs in the fields and during processing and transportation.

The skins of fruits and vegetables can help prevent bacteria from entering the food if they are intact. Wash fruits and vegetables, especially those that will be eaten raw, prior to use. Peeling fruits and vegetables can remove some bacteria, but fruit and vegetable peels are often high in nutrients.

Cooking destroys bacteria in food, and refrigeration prevents the growth of existing bacteria. However, overcooking vegetables destroys many nutrients. Meat, seafood, and eggs, though, must always be cooked for safety (Table 3-15).

TABLE 3-15	Safe Temperatures for Meat
Poultry (whole)	180°F
Poultry (ground)	165°F
Pork, eggs, ground meats	160°F
Beef steaks and roasts, veal, lamb	145°F
Holding temperature for hot foods	140°F

Always check the "use by" dates on food you are purchasing. Keep your refrigerator temperature at no more than 40 degrees Fahrenheit. Store frozen foods at 0 degrees Fahrenheit or less. Use refrigerated leftovers within three to four days.

Prepare leftovers for refrigeration by placing smaller portions in individual containers and letting them come to room temperature before refrigerating. Discard food left at room temperature for more than two hours. When it comes to food, live by the adage, "When in doubt, throw it out."

Use clean surfaces and utensils to prepare and store food. For example, never use the same knife with which you cut raw meat, poultry, or fish to cut vegetables for your salad. Although cooking will destroy the bacteria in the meat, the bacteria that were transferred to the salad vegetables will not be destroyed.

Wash your hands before preparing and eating food. Ensure that cooked foods reach the appropriate temperature. Maintain foods that will be served hot at a temperature of at least 140 degrees Fahrenheit.

Physical Fitness

Physical fitness includes healthy body weight, muscular strength, flexibility, and cardiovascular endurance. Physical fitness offers several health advantages. It is important in decreasing the risk of cardiovascular diseases and several cancers, and in improving blood glucose levels in diabetes, among other benefits. Physical exercise is also important to psychological health. It is associated with improvement in mood in depressed patients and reduction in stress.

Depending on the nature of your job, you may feel like you are busy all day, while you are actually getting very little physical activity. At a minimum, to reduce the risk of chronic disease and promote physical and psychological health, engage in at least 30 minutes of moderate intensity physical activity most days of the week.

PERSONAL PERSPECTIVE

Advanced EMT Ike Murphy: My partner, Todd, and I had just turned over a very sick elderly patient to the emergency department. One of the techs commented that he would rather die young than get old. "I don't want to take a dozen meds, limp around on arthritic hips, and schedule my life around doctors' appointments."

It is not age that most people fear. It is the loss of control that comes with illness and disability. Personally, I don't want to die young. I want to live a long, healthy life. You can't guarantee your future health. No one can. But you have a lot more control over it than you think. There is so much information now on the risk factors for chronic diseases, and how you can reduce the risk. The way we live and the choices we make have a huge impact on our health, both short term and long term.

I had a health scare a couple of years ago. My doc sent me for some tests for cancer. There is a lot of cancer in my family and I was scared. It wasn't cancer, but the experience gave me a wake-up call about my risk factors. I did a lot of reading and research while I was waiting for the test results. Some of the same risk factors increase your chances of a lot of diseases. I started making some changes. Little changes led to bigger changes.

I guess I didn't realize that I felt bad until I started feeling good. Once I felt good, I wanted to feel better. Some of my friends tease me about having some kind of health nut gene, but honestly, I'm far from perfect as far as that goes. But I feel better than I ever have, and it is because of the choices I make.

Check with your physician before beginning an exercise program if you are obese, take medication to treat an illness, have arthritis or a joint injury, have any chronic illness, smoke or recently stopped smoking, are pregnant, have had chest pain or shortness or breath, or are a male over 45 years or female over 55 years of age.

Moderate intensity exercise means increasing your heart rate to 60 to 73 percent of your peak heart rate. (If you do not regularly exercise, begin at 50 percent of your peak heart rate and gradually increase the intensity of exercise.) Estimate your peak heart rate by subtracting your age in years from 220. Moderate exercise for a 20-year-old would be increasing the heart rate to between $(220 - 20) \times 0.60$ and $(220 - 20) \times 0.73$, or between 120 and 146 beats per minute. Include activities you enjoy. Some options are walking, hiking, swimming, running, cycling, yard work, or circuit training.

To lose weight or prevent age-related weight gain, 60 minutes of moderate to vigorous exercise most days of the week is recommended. Vigorous activity means increasing your heart rate to 74 to 88 percent of your peak heart rate. If you can, build physical activity into your routine by walking or riding your bike to work.

Aerobic activity, such as swimming, bicycling, and jogging, contributes to cardiovascular endurance. Resistance exercises using weights builds muscular strength. Stretching is required to achieve and maintain flexibility. All three types of exercise are required for physical fitness. Stretch before both aerobic activity and resistance exercises to prevent muscle injury.

When engaging in aerobic activity, warm up with a lesser-intensity activity before increasing activity to reach your target heart rate. After achieving your goal for your aerobic workout, cool down with another period of lesser-intensity physical activity.

Other Physical Health Considerations

There are a number of recommendations for reducing the risk of illness and injury and early detection of health problems. Some additional health and safety tips include:

- Do not use tobacco in any form or expose yourself to secondhand smoke.

- If you use alcohol and caffeine, do so in moderation. Never drive or perform potentially dangerous tasks under the influence of any substance that can alter judgment or reaction time.

- Install and regularly test smoke detectors in your home.

- Wear sunscreen with at least SPF 30 when outdoors, even when outdoors for only short periods of time (including when going on calls).

- Use protective equipment during recreational activities (life vests when boating, bicycle and motorcycle helmets, and other appropriate sports equipment).

- Seek medical advice promptly for any health concerns.

- Have an annual physical exam and follow your physician's advice for health screenings based on your personal and family health history, age, and gender (such as a skin exam, Pap test, prostate cancer screening, cholesterol and triglyceride levels).

- See your dentist twice a year for examination and cleaning. (Poor dental health has recently been associated with increased risk of heart disease.)

Other Aspects of Wellness

Social wellness exists when we have positive relationships with friends, family, and coworkers. Family and friends sometimes do not understand EMS work, and EMS providers can sometimes let their work lives get out of balance with their social lives. However, maintaining this social support network is important in reducing work-related stress.

Most people with families experience conflict between work and family, and this can be exacerbated in EMS. EMS must be available 24 hours a day, seven days a week, every day of the year. As an EMS provider, you will likely be scheduled to work on at least some holidays and may miss other family functions. This can affect both social and occupational wellness. Take time for family and friends, and maintain relationships outside of EMS.

Emotional wellness means understanding yourself and acknowledging and effectively coping with emotions. Feelings experienced in each aspect of life can affect the others. Work in EMS can bring about feelings you have not experienced before. You must learn to cope with them to maintain emotional wellness. Events that can provoke those feelings include the death of a patient, being injured on the job, and changes in relationships with coworkers. If you experience ongoing symptoms of stress that interfere with any aspect of your life, seek assistance in managing your response to stressors.

EMS work brings many opportunities for intellectual wellness. Lifelong learning and pursuit of new knowledge and skills contribute to your professional development, as well as personal intellectual wellness. Sharing knowledge with others also contributes to our intellectual wellness. Continued learning can be formal or informal. In addition to required continuing education activities, seek information in other areas of interest through reading, Internet searches, lectures, or classes.

Environmental wellness exists when you pay attention to, and make a positive impact on, the environment around you. The environment can be as small as the ambulance you work on, or as large as the planet. Your home, workspace, and community are all part of your environment. Keeping areas clean, organized, and healthy are all part of environmental wellness. The environment extends beyond the physical to include the emotional environment as well. An emotionally safe environment at home and work, and in other aspects of life, is critical to your well-being.

Spiritual wellness can exist either through or independently of religious beliefs. Optimal spiritual wellness exists when you are aware of your values and are able to make decisions that are consistent with them, and when you find meaning and purpose in life. Spiritual wellness allows you to feel at peace with yourself and the world. Spiritual wellness can be affected any time someone must act in ways that are not congruent with his values and beliefs.

If you work full-time (40 hours per week) until mandatory retirement age, you will work more than 100,000 hours in your lifetime. This is around one-fifth of the total hours of your life, making occupational wellness an essential component of overall wellness. Human beings need meaningful work to be happy, and their identities are profoundly shaped by their work and their beliefs about how successful they are in it.

Occupational wellness exists when you are well matched to your occupation and your employer. Occupational wellness is achieved by being able to use your knowledge and skills to make a positive impact on society and your organization while maintaining balance in other areas of life. However, 69 percent of all employees say that work is a significant source of stress, affecting other areas of their lives (American Psychological Association [APA], 2009).

Do your homework before accepting a job offer. One of the primary sources of work stress is an employee's immediate supervisor (Bock, 2010). Immediate supervisors have an impact on productivity, satisfaction, morale, and individual well-being. Until recently, such issues have received little attention outside academia. However, there is currently growing support for healthy workplace legislation to hold employers accountable for civility in the workplace (Yamada, 2010).

Employers who have a psychologically healthy workplace have higher employee satisfaction, and thus lower turnover rates (9 percent versus 41 percent) (APA, 2009). Characteristics of such workplaces include exciting and challenging work, opportunities for career growth, competent coworkers, fair pay, and supportive management.

CASE STUDY WRAP-UP

Clinical-Reasoning Process

Advanced EMT Ryan Mitchell has just started working the night shift at his new job. When he clocks in on the last night of his first rotation, his partner Belinda Hogan says, "You are looking a little tired, partner."

"Wow. That's an understatement!" replies Ryan. "How do you get used to this routine?"

"Well, as long as you are on this shift, give up the thought of changing your routine back and forth between rotations. I used to do that, but it was killing me. Even on my days off I sleep from 9:00 AM to 2:00 PM.

"The other thing is, I had to adjust my thinking about food. With all of the junk I was eating for convenience and failing to get out and ride my bike, I gained 15 pounds the first year I worked nights! Now, I cook a few healthy dishes on the last day I'm off each rotation and put them in freezer containers. I stop by the store a few times a week for fresh fruits and vegetables to bring to work with me and, if you've noticed, I don't drink coffee after 2:00 AM. From that point on, it's water or caffeine-free tea. It makes a big difference. Trust me, partner!"

CHAPTER REVIEW

Chapter Summary

Maintaining overall wellness, achieving balance between various aspects of life, and taking action to minimize work-related injuries and illness are critical to professional and personal satisfaction in all occupations. You must be aware of emotional, environmental, intellectual, occupational, physical, social, and spiritual areas of wellness. You also are a role model to the public for wellness. As a health care professional, you have an obligation to act in ways that protect and improve the health of those in your community.

Although you face the same health issues the general population faces, a career in EMS also poses some particular health risks and challenges. However, you have a great deal of control over both general and work-related health risks. Some of the particular risks facing EMS providers include MVCs, scene hazards, long periods of sedentary activity, long or irregular shifts, frequent heavy lifting, unique stressors (such as MCIs), and exposure to communicable diseases.

There are many things you can do to minimize those risks. This includes using effective strategies for coping with stress, maintaining physical fitness and good nutrition, receiving recommended immunizations, and using appropriate PPE. Make time for friends and activities outside EMS and engage in personal and professional learning activities. Stay well informed on issues of health and safety, and make good choices with regard to your own personal health and safety. By doing those things, you can enjoy a long and satisfying career in EMS.

Review Questions

Multiple-Choice Questions

1. The document published every 10 years that describes health goals for the nation is:
   a. *EMS Agenda for the Future.*
   b. *Accidental Death and Disability: The Neglected Disease of Modern Society.*
   c. *Healthy People.*
   d. *EMS at the Crossroads.*

2. According to Maslow's hierarchy of needs, the most basic needs of human beings are _____ needs.
   a. physiologic
   b. safety
   c. esteem
   d. social

3. When exposure to a stressor results in improved performance, this is best described as a state of:
   a. delayed stress.
   b. distress.
   c. eustress.
   d. cumulative stress.

4. The hormone directly responsible for the signs and symptoms of the fight-or-flight response is:
   a. cortisol.
   b. adrenocorticotropic hormone.
   c. insulin.
   d. epinephrine.

5. The stress hormones cortisol and epinephrine are released from the:
   a. hypothalamus.
   b. adrenal glands.
   c. limbic system.
   d. pituitary gland.

6. An Advanced EMT experiences nightmares, flashbacks, anxiety, and depression six weeks after caring for a badly burned child who later died. What he is experiencing is best described as:
   a. an acute stress reaction.
   b. burnout.
   c. general adaptation syndrome.
   d. post-traumatic stress disorder.

7. A dam breaks during heavy rains, causing sudden severe flooding. In a town with a population of 6,000, dozens of families are trapped and need rescuing, 19 people are killed, and at least 60 are injured. Part of the response to this situation should include:
   a. critical incident stress debriefing.
   b. psychological incident management.
   c. post-traumatic stress debriefing.
   d. disaster mental health services.

8. The most common cause of severe injury and death to EMS providers is:
   a. motor vehicle collisions.
   b. violent patients.
   c. work partner violence.
   d. communicable disease.

9. The muscle group used to do the work of heavy lifting is in the:
   a. arms.
   b. thighs.
   c. abdomen.
   d. back.

10. Micro-organisms that cause disease are called:
    a. pathogens.
    b. hosts.
    c. vectors.
    d. fomites.

11. Routinely recommended immunizations for health care providers include immunization against:
    a. tuberculosis.
    b. SARS.
    c. hepatitis B.
    d. MRSA.

12. Which one of the following is a healthy body mass index?
    a. 12
    b. 21
    c. 28
    d. 32

Critical-Thinking Questions

13. What are at least three effects of chronically increased levels of cortisol?

14. How can the process of reframing help manage a stressor?

15. A patient has a cut on his arm that has a slow but steady amount of bleeding. What is the appropriate PPE for BSI in this situation?

16. You used a long backboard to transport a patient who had a bleeding cut. Before returning the backboard to service, what level of decontamination is required?

17. What resources can you use to create wellness goals for yourself?

18. How can you apply the components of wellness to your life?

References

American Psychological Association (APA). (2009). *Stress in America 2009*. Retrieved September 8, 2010, from http://www.apa.org/news/press/releases/stress-exec-summary.pdf

Bock, W. (2010). You can't have a healthy workplace with a toxic boss. *Good Company* e-newsletter, *4*(8). Retrieved September 10, 2010, from http://www.phwa.org/resources/goodcompany/newsletter/article/213

Institute of Medicine (IOM). (2006). *Emergency medical services: At the crossroads.* Washington, DC: National Academy Press.

Li, M. (2009). *Cognitive appraisal and/or personality traits: Enhancing active coping in two types of stressful situations.* Paper based on a program presented at the American Counseling Association Annual Conference and Exposition, Charlotte, NC.

National Highway Traffic Safety Administration (NHTSA). (1996). *EMS agenda for the future.* Retrieved November 22, 2010, from http://www.ems.gov

U.S. Department of Health and Human Services (DHHS). (2005). *Dietary guidelines for Americans 2005.* Retrieved September 8, 2010, from http://www.healthierus.gov/dietaryguidelines

U.S. Department of Health and Human Services (DHHS). (2000). *Healthy people 2010*, 2nd ed. Retrieved September 9, 2010, from http://www.healthypeople.gov/

University of Illinois at Champaign-Urbana. (2010). *What is wellness?* Retrieved September 8, 2010, from http://www.mckinley.illinois.edu/units/health_ed/wellness.htm

World Health Organization (WHO). (1948). *Preamble to the Constitution of the World Health Organization as adopted by the International Health Conference, New York, 19–22 June 1946.*

Yamada, D. (2010). *Healthy workplace bill.* Retrieved September 9, 2010, from http://www.healthyworkplacebill.org/

Additional Reading

Centers for Disease Control and Prevention (CDC). (1998). *Guideline for infection control in health care personnel, 1998.* Retrieved September 8, 2010, from http://www.cdc.gov/hicpac/pdf/InfectControl98.pdf

Centers for Disease Control and Prevention. (2009). Healthy people 2010 focus areas at a glance. Retrieved September 10, 2010, from http://www.cdc.gov/nchs/healthy_people/hp2010/hp2010_focus_areas.htm

Occupational Safety and Health Administration (OSHA). (2010). *Blood borne pathogens and needle stick prevention.* Retrieved September 8, 2010, from http://www.osha.gov/SLTC/bloodbornepathogens/index.html

4 Ethical and Medical/Legal Considerations in Advanced EMT Practice

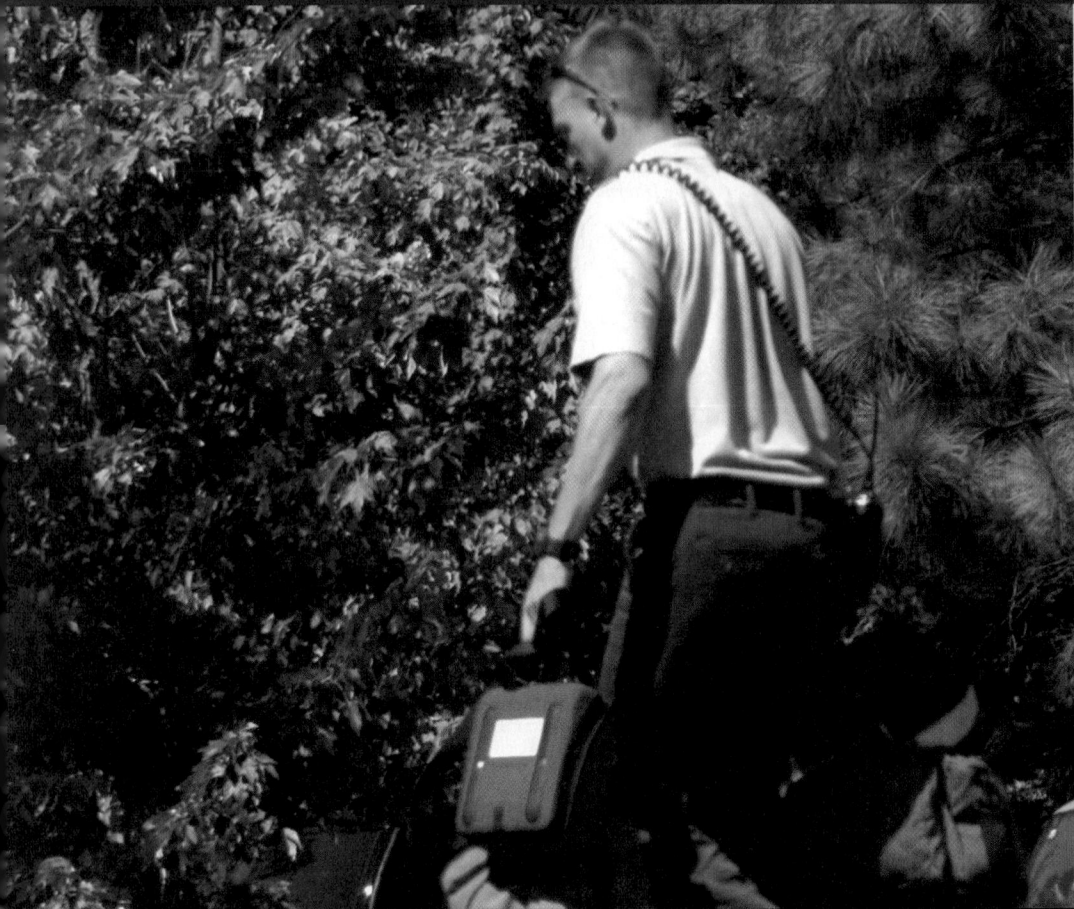

Content Area: Preparatory

Advanced EMT Education Standard: The Advanced EMT applies fundamental knowledge of the EMS system, safety/well-being of the Advanced EMT, and medical/legal and ethical issues to the provision of emergency care.

Objectives

After reading this chapter, you should be able to:

4.1 Define key terms introduced in this chapter.

4.2 Describe your responsibilities as an Advanced EMT with respect to scope of practice, standard of care, and medical direction.

4.3 Given a variety of ethical dilemmas, discuss the issues that must be considered in each situation.

4.4 Discuss the application of the EMT Oath and professional ethics to the practice of EMS.

4.5 Give examples of federal and state laws affecting the practice of EMS.

4.6 Give examples of legal situations involving tort and criminal issues.

Resource Central

To access Resource Central, follow the directions on the Student Access Card provided with this text. If there is no card, go to www.bradybooks.com and follow the Resource Central link to Buy Access. Under Media Resources, you will find:

- *The Ethics of Resuscitation.* Read ethical recommendations from the American Heart Association (AHA).

- *Your Professional Ethics.* Discover the EMT Code of Ethics and how it applies to you.

- *The Call for Privacy.* Learn more about the Health Insurance Portability and Accountability Act (HIPAA).

CASE STUDY

"Ambulance 412, Squad 441. Respond to 30 Gold Finch Court for a person with difficulty breathing."

Advanced EMTs Lieutenant Lydia Blume and Firefighter Adam Grolier notify dispatch that they are responding. They are three minutes away from the address, while Ambulance 412 is eight minutes away. As Lt. Blume and Firefighter Grolier pull in front of the residence, dispatch notifies them that the patient is now reported to be in cardiac arrest. Grabbing their gear from the side compartment of the squad, the crew approaches the front door. A distraught woman in her 60s opens the door as they step onto the porch. "He's gone. I know he's gone. I don't know what to do. What should I do?"

"Where is the patient, ma'am?" asks Lt. Blume.

"It's my husband, Luther. He's in the TV room," replies the woman, turning to lead the crew to the patient.

"What happened?" asks Lt. Blume.

"He's been getting steadily worse for months. It is his heart. He has heart failure. He just started struggling to breathe and turned gray. Then he just passed out and I think his heart stopped."

Reaching the TV room, Lt. Blume and Firefighter Grolier find an apparently unresponsive male in his late 80s in a recliner. He is cyanotic and not breathing. Firefighter Grolier quickly pulls the recliner out from the wall and reaches under the patient's arms from behind while Lt. Blume places her hands beneath his knees. "One, two, three, lift." Firefighter Grolier and Lt. Blume lift the patient and place him on the floor. Grolier positions his hands to start chest compressions as Lt. Blume reaches for the defibrillator.

"Oh, no!" the woman cries out. "Don't do that. He doesn't want any CPR or machines or breathing tubes."

Problem-Solving Questions

1. How should the crew respond to the wife's declaration?
2. What are the crew's legal obligations?
3. What are the crew's ethical obligations?
4. What additional information could clarify how they should handle the situation?

4.7	Describe the purpose of and typical protections afforded by Good Samaritan Laws.
4.8	Given a scenario, identify circumstances that may allow a claim of negligence to be established.
4.9	Discuss several ways to defend yourself against claims of negligence.
4.10	Given a scenario, determine the type of patient consent that applies.
4.11	Evaluate factors that should be considered when determining a patient's decision-making capacity and in situations where the use of force or patient restraint are being contemplated.
4.12	Apply the concept of the right to self-determination to issues of consent and advance directives.
4.13	Describe how to avoid claims of assault, battery, abandonment, false imprisonment/kidnapping, and defamation.
4.14	Identify situations in which Advanced EMTs may be mandatory reporters of suspected crimes or other legally reportable situations.
4.15	Differentiate between instances in which you can and cannot legally share a patient's protected health information.

(continued)

(continued from previous page)

4.16   Discuss the application of EMTALA and HIPAA legislation to the practice of EMS.

4.17   Identify presumptive signs of death.

4.18   Discuss considerations in transport and resuscitation for patients who may be organ donors.

4.19   Identify situations in which law enforcement or the medical examiner's office should be notified.

4.20   Discuss legal considerations in the response to crime scenes and the care of both crime victims and suspects.

4.21   Identify items that may be considered evidence at a crime scene.

Introduction

There are legal and ethical aspects to every EMS call. You must have a patient's consent for assessment, treatment, and transport. You must provide care that is within your scope of practice. You must keep the patient's protected health information private and do no harm in the course of caring for him. Those principles and guidelines seem clear and, in most cases, their application is straightforward. At times, though, the application of what seem to be unambiguous laws and ethical principles becomes muddled. You are required to use your judgment in those cases. To do so, you must have a working understanding of the types of laws that apply to emergency medical care and the principles of medical ethics.

The delivery of health care is highly regulated. The same legal concepts apply from state to state, but the way the concepts are enacted varies. To gain a full understanding of what is required of you, you must be aware of your state's laws and the rules that govern their implementation. Laws are constantly added, changed, and repealed. It is your responsibility to maintain current knowledge of your obligations under federal, state, and local laws.

Ethics describe the code of conduct expected of members of a profession. Laws and ethics in EMS are both intended to protect the public. It is possible, however, for an act to be legal yet unethical, or illegal yet ethical. Such situations, while not the norm, create dilemmas in which each option carries risks and confers benefits that are difficult to weigh against one another. In addition, you do not have the benefits of time and consultation with an ethics committee, as doctors and nurses would for a hospitalized patient. You must make the best decisions possible quickly and without the benefit of all of the information that could influence the decision.

Ethics

Ethics is a branch of philosophy that tries to answer questions about notions of what is good and bad and what is right and wrong. More specifically, ethics are the guidelines for the expected conduct of members of a profession. Ethics are similar to morals, but morals apply more broadly to all of human conduct. You were introduced to the EMT Oath and EMT Code of Ethics in Chapter 1. Those documents provide the standards of conduct for the EMS profession. Knowing the standards is straightforward. Applying them in context can be complicated.

Because application of ethics can be difficult, it is helpful to keep several guiding principles in mind. They include the principles of:

- Beneficence (doing good)
- Nonmalfeasance (the medical principle of *primum non nocere*, or first do no harm)
- Justice
- Concern for the well-being of others
- Respect for others
- Advocacy for others
- Patients' rights to self-determination
- Objectivity (remaining nonjudgmental)
- Avoiding conflicts of interest
- Full disclosure (including informed consent)
- Due diligence or duty of care
- Confidentiality
- Adhering to professional responsibilities

Again, those principles may seem clear cut. Of course, Advanced EMTs should strive to do good and not harm and respect others, following the Golden Rule: Do unto others, as you would have them do unto you. But what about caring for the registered sex offender who was injured while being taken into custody, or the intoxicated driver who survived a vehicle collision that left a family of five dead? What about the obviously ill or injured patient who refuses transport, or refuses a component of treatment you consider essential? What about the partner whom you know has a substance abuse issue?

Regardless of the strong feelings you will have about such situations, you must adhere to the ethics of the EMS profession. You have an obligation to the public to provide and promote safe, effective emergency medical care and promote health. You must respect the patient's dignity and autonomy. You also have an obligation to report incompetence or unethical conduct of others in an appropriate and professional manner.

As we continue cognitive moral development through adulthood, experiences and reflections change the way we see situations and the way we act in them. (See Chapter 9 for more on cognitive moral development.) Still, most of us have what is called an *espoused theory* (what we say we would do in certain circumstances) and a *theory in use* (what we actually do in those circumstances) (Argyris & Schön, 1974). There almost always is a gap between the two theories. What we must do is be conscious of whether our behavior in each situation is truly reflective of our belief system, and always strive to decrease the gap.

With time, the gap between the espoused theory and the theory in use becomes smaller. In fact, there is some evidence that ethical behavior can be learned, and that we are much more a product of the environment created by those around us than we would like to think. The predominant attitudes and behaviors of those around us can profoundly influence us, for better or for worse. What is often called "burnout" in EMS may not be burnout at all, but a product of socialization by other EMS providers. Burnout is an *individual's* psychological and physical state of exhaustion from overexposure to stress, which may be reflected in behavior. Burnout can lead to many maladaptive behaviors, including irritability. Sometimes, though, burnout is used as an excuse for a poor organizational culture that accepts poor work attitudes and interactions with patients. Before accepting a job, consider the attitudes of those with whom you will be working. Is it acceptable to be apathetic or discourteous toward patients? Or, are providers in the service expected to be conscientious and empathetic?

Branches of Government and General Areas of Law

Laws that affect Advanced EMT practice may be federal, state, or local. Laws are created and upheld through the three branches of government: legislative, executive, and judicial. All three branches exist federally, and in each state. The legislative branch is Congress at the federal level and is usually called the legislature at the state level. In both cases, the legislative branch is comprised of a House of Representatives and a Senate, elected by voters. The legislative branch writes and votes on bills, which, when enacted, are called statutes or laws. This is called *legislative law,* and it provides direction to the various oversight agencies of the federal and state government.

Some examples of federal statutes are the **Emergency Medical Treatment and Active Labor Act (EMTALA),** the **Health Insurance Portability and Accountability Act (HIPAA),** the Ryan White CARE Act, and the Social Security Act, which created Medicare. State statutes include areas of EMS regulation, mandatory reporting situations, family law, motor vehicle law, and some areas of employment law.

The executive branch executes the laws enacted by Congress, and serves as part of the system of checks and balances in government. It consists, at the federal level, of the president and the secretaries of the many government agencies, such as the Department of Transportation, the Department of Health and Human Services, and the Department of Labor. At the state level, the executive branch consists of the governor and state-level agencies, such the department of health, department of education, and other offices that often mirror federal level of offices.

The executive branch writes regulations or rules (called *administrative law* or *regulatory law*) that provide specific language to guide the implementation of statutes, which are written more broadly. A committee within the state legislature may write a bill that requires a criminal background check for all health care providers. Both the state house of representatives and the state senate must approve the bill, and the governor must approve it for it to become law. The state secretary of health is tasked with writing the specific requirements to implement the background check. The task is usually assigned to a committee and input of communities of interest is solicited before the secretary approves the regulations or rules that implement the statute.

The judicial branch of government, at both the federal and state levels, is made up of various levels of courts that make rulings and decisions related to laws. Criminal and civil cases are argued before judges and juries and decisions are made as to whether the **defendant** was in compliance with the law. Decisions are initially rendered in trial courts. If one party disagrees with the ruling and believes he or she has a cause to appeal the decision, the case goes to an appellate court. In fewer cases, if a party disagrees with the appellate court ruling, the case may go to a state or federal supreme court. In some cases, judicial decisions become case law or common law, setting a precedent that guides subsequent legal decisions.

Three types of law can affect Advanced EMT practice. Administrative law applies to issues such as requirements for initial and continuing licensure. **Civil law** pertains to family court matters and legal issues in which one person is liable for damage to another. This second area of civil law is called **tort law.** Slander, libel, and negligence are examples of matters of civil law. **Criminal law** addresses actions that constitute crimes against society, such as homicide, reckless driving, assault, and battery. In some cases, all three types of law may apply. For example, consider the following: An Advanced EMT driving to an emergency call is exceeding the speed limit and runs a red light, colliding with a vehicle crossing the intersection. The driver of the car is killed. Under criminal law, the Advanced EMT is charged with manslaughter. The victim's family sues him for damages in civil court, and under administrative law, he loses his Advanced EMT license.

Authorization to Practice

State laws govern the requirements to become and remain a licensed health care provider and what each type of licensed health care provider is permitted to do, and under what circumstances. For example, although EMS providers are licensed, they may only provide care under the supervision (direct or indirect) of a physician medical director. **Licensure** is the granting of official permission by a governmental agency to practice in a regulated occupation or profession. Boards or panels within a government agency typically oversee licensure. Eligibility for licensure may be based on **certification** or **registration**.

Any entity can provide a certificate, such as a certificate of course completion. In some cases, regulations determine who can grant specific certificates and under what conditions. For example, the state EMS agency may determine the requirements for an institution to grant an EMS course certificate. Registration means that your name and relevant information is maintained in a database. In the case of the National Registry of EMTs (NREMT), you must meet certain education and testing requirements to be listed in the database.

EMS personnel must be licensed and authorized by their EMS system medical director to practice. Each EMS provider practices only the skills that he is trained to do, that are within the legal scope of practice, and that are authorized by the medical director.

Scope of Practice

The scope of practice legally defines what a health care provider is permitted do in the course of his duties. In some states, the scope of practice is spelled out specifically in legislation (laws). This makes any change in scope of practice difficult to achieve, because the legislation must be amended. In other states, the scope of practice regulation refers to a document that is not part of the legislation to define the scope of practice. The document can be amended as needed without requiring a change in the law.

The National EMS Scope of Practice Model (National Highway Traffic Safety Administration [NHTSA], 2006) is just what the name denotes: a model after which states can pattern their scope of practice. It is desirable to have as much consistency in scope of practice from state to state as possible to permit reciprocity and decrease confusion in disasters, when EMS providers may cross state lines. However, each state defines its own scope of practice and may modify the National Model to meet its needs.

Medical Direction

There are several layers of EMS medical direction in each state. Each state has a state medical director, who is instrumental in determining the state scope of practice. Each state also may have a medical direction committee that consists of representatives of various regions or communities of interest. Each locality, such as a metropolitan area, county, or region, may have a medical director, and a medical direction committee may exist at that level, as well. Finally, each EMS service has a medical director. EMS medical directors are licensed physicians who should have a background in emergency medicine and emergency medical services. The service medical director provides indirect medical direction, which means that he or she is not acting at the moment during which patient care is occurring. Instead, he or she is responsible for quality assurance/quality improvement, continuing education, writing protocols, and management of inappropriate medical conduct by service EMTs.

As an EMS provider, you must be authorized by your EMS service medical director to provide patient care. You must follow the protocols and standing orders approved by your medical director. The term *medical direction* also is used to refer to consulting with the physician who is at the receiving emergency department and who helps at the moment care is being provided. That physician is not your medical director, but provides medical direction for the care of an individual patient. Still, you must apply that direction within your scope of practice and the protocols approved by your EMS service medical director.

Consent and Refusal of Emergency Medical Care

All of the skills you perform as an Advanced EMT have one thing in common: They may only be done with the patient's consent. In theory, asking the patient's permission to treat him is easy. It would be easy in practice, too, if you worked in a clinic setting where patients made appointments, registered upon arrival, and signed a consent form before seeing you for treatment. In EMS, you often respond to care for patients for whom care was requested by another party. The patient may not want medical treatment, or may have an altered mental status and be unable to provide consent. The patient may be a minor whose parents cannot be immediately reached for consent. With a critically ill patient, it is not likely to be feasible to have him sign a consent form.

You must obtain informed consent from all **competent** adult patients before providing care. All competent adult patients also have the right to refuse all emergency care, or any aspect of it. Competence, in this context, means that the patient is capable of understanding what he is consenting to, as well as the consequences of not consenting. In some cases, it can be difficult to make a determination about the patient's competence. Can an elderly patient who does not know the date make an informed decision? What about a patient who smells of alcohol and has slurred speech? What about a patient who is pale and diaphoretic with severe chest pain who refuses treatment and transportation?

Transporting a competent patient against his will could result in a claim of kidnapping or false imprisonment. Failing to transport a patient who is not competent can result in a claim of negligence. Your best protection against both claims lies in adherence to several principles. Within the limitations of the situation, determine the patient's competence. If you are unclear about the patient's level of competence, it is always better to err on the side of the treatment, rather than nontreatment, in an emergency situation.

Always follow your protocols and procedures. Failure to do so puts you at risk of liability. Contact law enforcement, if necessary, when a patient with a behavioral emergency refuses care. Involve medical direction and supervision when faced with an unclear situation. Always act in the patient's best interest. Finally, document all relevant information about the situation, including how you determined whether or not the patient was competent, what you said to attempt to get the patient's cooperation and consent, what the patient said to you, and who you contacted for assistance (medical direction, supervisor, law enforcement, family member) and what action was taken.

Determining Competence

The general rule is that a competent adult may refuse care even if the refusal seems unreasonable to the health care provider. If an adult has been found legally incompetent in a court hearing, the judge will appoint another adult to be his legal guardian. In many cases, though, the patient's incapacitation is of a sudden nature and may be temporary. There will be no legal guardianship in those cases. This puts the onus on you, as an Advanced EMT, to make a decision. Only courts can determine legal competence, but medical personnel can make a determination about a person's decision-making capacity in an emergency.

Several things can impair a person's decision-making capacity, including mental illness, a behavioral emergency, intoxication by drugs or alcohol, a medical emergency, such as a stroke or diabetic emergency, or trauma that alters the patient's mental status. Alcohol is a common intoxicant, but there are levels of intoxication and not all patients who have had something to drink have lost their decision-making capacity. The same is true with both legal and illegal drugs. Also consider the patient's intellectual capacity. The patient must have the ability to understand what he is consenting to or refusing, and the consequences of the decision.

When you determine that a patient is not competent to consent to or refuse care, document the patient's mental status and be specific about why you believe he can or cannot make decisions for himself. Give examples of things he says or how he reacts to his surroundings. If the patient incorrectly believes that you are his niece, or that you are a government spy, or that there are spiders crawling all over his

IN THE FIELD

People who seldom go outside the home or who are not engaged in work, such as elderly individuals, may not be aware of the exact day, or even month, because they may not follow a calendar or regular schedule. They should, however, be able to tell you what season and year it is.

body, your argument that the patient is not competent to consent will be credible. If the patient has an odor of alcohol on his breath, it should be documented, but it is not sufficient to successfully argue that he cannot make decisions. But, if you also document that his speech is slurred and he is unsteady on his feet, it supports the argument that the patient is unable to consent to or refuse care.

Similarly, if a patient refuses treatment and you are not going to transport him, you must paint a picture that leaves no doubt of his decision-making capacity to refuse treatment. Consider the following situation: You are called to a family function where a 25-year-old female injured her knee playing volleyball after drinking three beers. Important factors to consider include whether she can speak clearly and coherently, and knows where she is, what happened, the date, and the people around her. Further, consider whether she conveys an appropriate level of concern for the injury and whether she has an alternate plan for seeking treatment, such as having a (nonintoxicated) family member drive her to an urgent care center. Also determine and document whether there is a responsible adult present that can monitor the patient and, if needed, call again for help.

An important concept of decision-making capacity is that it can depend on the importance of the decision. For instance, the decision not to be transported may require a different degree of capacity if the injury is a sprained ankle than if it is severe chest pain and shortness of breath. Additionally, a diagnosis alone does not determine the ability to make a decision, as many schizophrenic patients have good decision-making capacity.

Informed Consent

When a patient acknowledges verbally, nonverbally, or in writing that he will accept treatment, this is known as **expressed consent**. When you ask a patient, "May I take your blood pressure?" and the patient nods his head, says, "Yes," or extends his arm to you, he has given expressed consent. Informed consent means that you must provide the patient with information about the nature of the treatment, why it is needed, what it is expected to do, any potential for side effects or complications, and the consequences of not receiving the treatment. This information must be delivered in a format the patient can understand and the patient must have the opportunity to ask questions. In an emergency, when time is of the essence, this may be as simple as saying, "Your blood pressure is low. I would like to start an IV and give you some fluids. It will sting a bit when I put the needle in, but the fluids will bring your blood pressure up. Is it alright if I go ahead and put in an IV?"

The more urgent the situation, the less information you will be able to provide, but most situations allow you plenty of time to explain to the patient what you are planning to do and why you are planning to do it, and give the patient an opportunity to ask questions. Whenever possible, have the patient sign to indicate consent. A place is available on the patient care report (PCR) for that purpose.

Refusal of Consent

When a patient refuses to consent to treatment or transportation, first attempt to understand the patient's reasons for refusal. He may be concerned about the cost involved, or he may be the caretaker of someone else in the home who cannot be left alone. There can be many reasons for a patient's reluctance to be transported to the hospital. Understanding the reluctance will help you address those concerns in the best way you can. When you can give the patient reassurances about his concerns, or explain why, regardless of his concerns, he should receive treatment, you may be able to obtain consent. Most services require consultation with medical direction in at least some circumstances involving a refusal of treatment.

Just as consent to treatment must be informed, so must refusal of treatment. Your documentation of the circumstances, your attempts to obtain consent, and the patient's response to the attempts must be meticulous. Remember, patients have the right to refuse some or all of your care. For example, a patient can accept transport to the hospital but refuse an IV. Some agencies provide checkboxes to remind you of key points to explain to the patient, as well as a checklist to help you determine the patient's competence to refuse treatment (Figure 4-1). You must obtain the patient's signature and most protocols require that you try to have a witness, other than your partner or other EMS personnel, to the patient's refusal. You also must inform that patient that he may request EMS at any time he changes his mind (Figure 4-2).

Implied Consent

In some cases, circumstances do not allow the patient to consent. A patient who is unresponsive needs immediate intervention, but is not able to give consent. An elderly patient who is confused because of Alzheimer's disease and has pneumonia needs treatment and transport, but may not be competent to either consent to treatment or to refuse it. In such situations, EMS providers rely on the doctrine of implied consent. In essence, implied consent means that you assume that, if the patient were able, he would give his consent for emergency treatment. That is, it is implied that he would give consent. Implied consent applies to patients in cardiac arrest, who are unresponsive, or otherwise incapacitated.

Minor's Consent

Although there are a few exceptions, patients under the age of 18 are not legally permitted to consent to or refuse medical treatment. The patient's parent or guardian must give permission for medical treatment. This situation may arise when a teenager is involved in a motor vehicle collision (MVC) or when a minor is at home alone, at school or daycare, or with a babysitter. In all cases, make every attempt to contact the parents. If you must transport before they can arrive at the scene, verify as best you can that you are speaking to the patient's parent or legal guardian and obtain verbal consent. If the parent or guardian cannot be contacted, get the consent of the closest relative, such as a

IN THE FIELD

Minors who may be emancipated include those who are legally married or in the military. It may also include minors who are parents. In some cases, a judge may have legally granted emancipation, but the patient generally is not required to carry documentation of his status. Be aware of the laws in your state.

REFUSAL OF TREATMENT AND TRANSPORTATION

I, THE UNDERSIGNED HAVE BEEN ADVISED THAT MEDICAL ASSISTANCE ON MY BEHALF IS NECESSARY AND THAT REFUSAL OF SAID ASSISTANCE AND TRANSPORTATION MAY RESULT IN DEATH, OR IMPERIL MY HEALTH. NEVERTHELESS, I REFUSE TO ACCEPT TREATMENT OR TRANSPORT AND ASSUME ALL RISKS AND CONSEQUENCES OF MY DECISION AND RELEASE GOLD CROSS AMBULANCE COMPANY AND ITS EMPLOYEES FROM ANY LIABILITY ARISING FROM MY REFUSAL.

_____
SIGNATURE OF PATIENT

_____
WITNESSED BY

_____
DATE SIGNED

FIGURE 4-1

A sample checklist used by EMS personnel when a patient refuses treatment and transport.

EMS PATIENT REFUSAL CHECKLIST

PATIENT'S NAME: _____ AGE: _____

LOCATION OF CALL: _____ DATE: _____

AGENCY INCIDENT #: _____ AGENCY CODE: _____

NAME OF PERSON FILLING OUT FORM: _____

I. ASSESSMENT OF PATIENT (Check appropriate response for each item)

1. Oriented to: Person? ☐ Yes ☐ No
              Place?   ☐ Yes ☐ No
              Time?   ☐ Yes ☐ No
              Situation? ☐ Yes ☐ No

2. Altered level of consciousness? ☐ Yes ☐ No

3. Head injury? ☐ Yes ☐ No

4. Alcohol or drug ingestion by exam or history? ☐ Yes ☐ No

II. PATIENT INFORMED (Check appropriate response for each item)

☐ Yes ☐ No Medical treatment/evaluation needed

☐ Yes ☐ No Ambulance transport needed

☐ Yes ☐ No Further harm could result without medical treatment/evaluation

☐ Yes ☐ No Transport by means other than ambulance could be hazardous in light of patient's illness/injury

☐ Yes ☐ No Patient provided with Refusal Information Sheet

☐ Yes ☐ No Patient accepted Refusal Information Sheet

III. DISPOSITION

☐ Refused all EMS assistance

☐ Refused field treatment, but accepted transport

☐ Refused transport, but accepted field treatment

☐ Refused transport to recommended facility

☐ Patient transported by private vehicle to_____

☐ Released in care or custody of self

☐ Released in care or custody of relative or friend

  Name: _____ Relationship:_____

☐ Released in custody of law enforcement agency

  Agency: _____ Officer: _____

☐ Released in custody of other agency

  Agency: _____ Officer: _____

IV. COMMENTS: _____

_____

_____

_____

FIGURE 4-2

A sample form signed by patients who refuse care to release the EMS provider and system from liability.

grandparent or older sibling (18 years or older). If you are not able to obtain consent in a time that is reasonable, given the circumstances, treat under the assumption of implied consent, assuming that if the parents or guardian could be contacted, they would want the child to be treated.

Legal Issues Related to Consent

The legal consequences of failing to obtain proper consent for treatment include claims of abandonment, assault, battery, and false imprisonment. **Abandonment** is termination of the patient–provider relationship by the provider without turning over care to an appropriately credentialed health care provider, when the patient is still in need of care and desires that care be continued. A claim of abandonment could occur in the following situations:

- You initiate advanced life support care, such as an IV or administering medications, and then turn patient care over to a provider who is licensed at a lower level.

- You leave a patient at the hospital without providing an appropriate transfer of care to nursing or medical staff.

- You stop to provide care at the scene of an emergency while off-duty and then leave before other EMS providers arrive.

Attempting to treat a patient without proper consent can lead to a claim of assault or battery. **Assault** is an act that places a person in fear of impending physical harm. **Battery** is unlawful physical contact with another person without his consent. Assault and battery also may occur even when a patient has given consent. Picture the following scenario: A 16-year-old female claims to have taken an overdose of over-the-counter medication after a fight with her parents. The Advanced EMT on scene does not believe that the patient is truly unresponsive, but that she is feigning unresponsiveness to scare her parents. Her airway is open and her breathing and pulse are normal. There is no indication of an immediate threat to life. However, the patient does not respond to a loud voice or sternal rub. The Advanced EMT states, "If you don't open your eyes, I'm going to stick a big needle in your arm." This could be considered assault. After the patient still fails to respond, the Advanced EMT applies an unnecessarily forceful sternal rub. This is battery.

Actions that amount to assault and battery need not be so blatant as the previous example. Starting an IV or performing other treatments without the patient's consent can constitute battery, as well.

False imprisonment occurs when there is deliberate detainment of an individual without his consent in the absence of a valid reason. Always consider the possibility of a false imprisonment claim when a patient refuses treatment. It is sometimes a difficult decision when you have a patient who seems to be under the influence of alcohol or drugs, but whether or not he is incapable of making decisions is unclear. If the patient refuses treatment, you may be liable if harm comes to him after your departure. If you transport the patient against his will, he may claim false imprisonment. If you remain in doubt about the patient's competence after a careful evaluation, you should err on the side of treatment and transport, rather than leave the patient at the scene.

Also consider the case when there is a discrepancy between the facility to which a patient requests to be transported and the facility that you believe to be in the patient's best interest, or a better destination for operational reasons. When possible, honor the patient's request. In many cases, his medical records are available at his chosen destination and his insurance may reimburse at a higher rate. On the other hand, in true emergencies, insurance companies often pay for the patient's care at the closest appropriate facility.

Always try to resolve the issue with the patient. Explain why another facility is a better choice in a particular situation. For instance, the patient's choice of hospitals may be ideal for caring for medical emergencies and minor trauma, but may not be a trauma center. If the patient requires a trauma center, explain the benefits to the patient. If there are operational policies that prevent you from transporting to facilities further away than a specified boundary, let the patient know that this is so that the ambulance can be available in a reasonable amount of time for other emergencies.

Excellent documentation of the facts and observations supporting your decision will help you in the event that the patient makes a claim of false imprisonment. In many EMS systems, EMS providers are encouraged or compelled by policy to consult with medical direction or supervision when confronted with situations that pose a high risk of legal consequences.

Resuscitation Decisions and Recognizing Death

In most cases, resuscitation must be performed for patients who present in cardiac arrest. There are times, though, that resuscitation attempts are not appropriate. This includes instances where death is obvious, according to accepted criteria, and when patients have an advance directive or present directive that you are legally allowed to recognize, according to your protocols.

Advance Directives

An advance medical directive is a written statement of a patient's wishes regarding end-of-life issues. A **living will** is a document written by an individual that states either generally or specifically the types of medical care he does and does not want at the end of life. For example, the document may state that if the patient suffers a condition, such as a devastating stroke, that leaves him dependent on artificial life support without chance of recovery, that he would want those life-sustaining interventions discontinued. Other issues addressed include a patient's request to die at home,

Dr. Caitlin Ferguson: I was caring for a patient in her 50s who had COPD and developed pneumonia. She was decompensating and going into respiratory failure, but she insisted that she did not want to be "kept alive by machines." The patient was only in her 50s and still had several years ahead of her, as well as having a family who loved her very much. I didn't think she understood that intubating her and placing her on a ventilator would help her get better, and was not a futile attempt at prolonging life. I talked to her several times over the next hour, as she continued to deteriorate. She insisted that she did not want to be kept alive by machines. She went into respiratory failure and I had to think quickly. I truly believed that the patient did not understand the consequences of what she was asking. I intubated her, and she was admitted to the intensive care unit. A few days later, she had been extubated and antibiotics were taking care of the pneumonia. I sat down next to her bed and said, "You must be really angry with me. You said you did not want to be kept alive by machines, but I put a tube in your throat and put you on a ventilator."

"Oh, that's okay," she replied.

I was dumbfounded. She had asked me to withhold treatment without which she would have died and truly had no understanding of the consequences. It was a difficult situation and it still makes me wonder how much patients really understand when they are consenting to treatment or refusing treatment. I acted in what I thought was the patient's best interest, and I'm glad I did. That is my standard for evaluating my patient care decisions: What is in the best interest of the patient?

and not in the hospital. Follow your protocols and applicable state or local laws with respect to living wills, and consult with medical direction.

A **health care proxy** and a **durable power of attorney** are documents in which the patient has given, or in which the court has awarded, authority to another individual to make health care decisions on the patient's behalf if the patient is incapacitated. As an EMS provider, you usually may rely on those documents for obtaining consent, but it is generally not advisable to rely on them to make determinations about refusing care or terminating resuscitation in the prehospital setting.

Present Directives

Do not resuscitate (DNR) orders (also called *do not attempt resuscitation [DNAR] orders*) are generally legally recognized in the prehospital setting. A DNR is a signed, dated physician's order to withhold resuscitative efforts (Figure 4-3). The order may request that all resuscitative effort be withheld, or that only specific measures, such as advanced airway management, be withheld. Most protocols require consultation with medical direction concerning the DNR.

In addition, DNRs must meet certain criteria to be honored. You cannot rely just on the word of the patient's family or extended care facility staff that a DNR exists. You must actually see the signed, dated order. The state may have a specific form on which DNRs must be recorded and, in general, DNRs are not valid for an indefinite period of time. DNRs are usually issued for patients with terminal illnesses. If the patient has not died within a specific period of time, the DNR issue should be revisited by the patient and his physician. Because of the legal implications associated with honoring or not honoring a DNR, most protocols require that you consult with medical direction when presented with one.

A DNR does not mean that you cannot provide any care. Patients with terminal illnesses are often in need of comfort care, such as providing oxygen for shortness of breath or analgesia for painful conditions. If a living will or DNR is not clear about what treatments are acceptable to the patient, communicate with the patient and family to make decisions about care.

Presumptive Signs of Death

Most EMS systems provide a list of situations in which resuscitation should not be implemented. If the patient has a DNR, presumptive signs of death include absence of pulse and breathing, unresponsiveness to all stimuli, no eye movement or pupil response, and absence of reflexes. If death occurred more than just a very short time before, the patient's skin may be cold and he may have **dependent lividity (livor mortis)** or **rigor mortis** (Figure 4-4).

Generally, in the absence of a DNR, resuscitation should begin if the patient is warm. It also should begin if the patient is cold but the suspected cause is hypothermia. Resuscitation is not begun if there are signs that are incompatible with life. They include:

- Decapitation
- Transsection of the body
- Decomposition
- Charring
- Rigor mortis
- Livor mortis

PREHOSPITAL DO NOT RESUSCITATE ORDERS

<u>ATTENDING PHYSICIAN</u>

In completing this prehospital DNR form, please check Part A if no intervention by prehospital personnel is indicated. Please check Part A and options from Part B if specific interventions by prehospital personnel are indicated. To give a valid prehospital DNR order, this form must be completed by the patient's attending physician and must be provided to prehospital personnel.

A) _____ **Do Not Resuscitate (DNR):**
No Cardiopulmonary Resuscitation or Advanced Cardiac Life Support to be performed by prehospital personnel

B) _____ **Modified Support:**
Prehospital personnel administer the following checked options:
_____ Oxygen administration
_____ Full airway support: intubation, airways, bag/valve/mask
_____ Venipuncture: IV crystalloids and/or blood draw
_____ External cardiac pacing
_____ Cardiopulmonary resuscitation
_____ Cardiac defibrillator
_____ Pneumatic anti-shock garment
_____ Ventilator
_____ ACLS meds
_____ Other interventions/medications (physician specify)
_____

Prehospital personnel are informed that (print patient name)_____
should receive no resuscitation (DNR) or should receive Modified Support as indicated. This directive is medically appropriate and is further documented by a physician's order and a progress note on the patient's permanent medical record. Informed consent from the capacitated patient or the incapacitated patient's legitimate surrogate is documented on the patient's permanent medical record. The DNR order is in full force and effect as of the date indicated below.

_____   _____
Attending Physician's Signature

_____   _____
Print Attending Physician's Name   Print Patient's Name and Location
                                          (Home Address or Health Care Facility)

_____
Attending Physician's Telephone

_____   _____
Date   Expiration Date (6 Mos from Signature)

FIGURE 4-3

A sample do not resuscitate (DNR) order.

Withholding or Terminating Resuscitation

In some systems, resuscitation is not begun in cases of traumatic cardiac arrest, particularly those with blunt trauma. Always follow your system's protocols regarding when resuscitation should be started and when it should be withheld. Many EMS systems, particularly those with paramedics, have protocols for terminating resuscitation in the field. Such protocols issue guidelines for deciding when

further resuscitation efforts would be futile. Decisions to terminate resuscitative efforts are made in consultation with medical direction.

Your service will have a policy for who should be contacted in the event that you respond to a patient who has died, and what your obligations are at death scenes. You may be required to notify the coroner or medical examiner's office in cases where death appears to be natural, but was not expected, as well as in other cases. In cases where there is any suspicion that death was not due to natural causes,

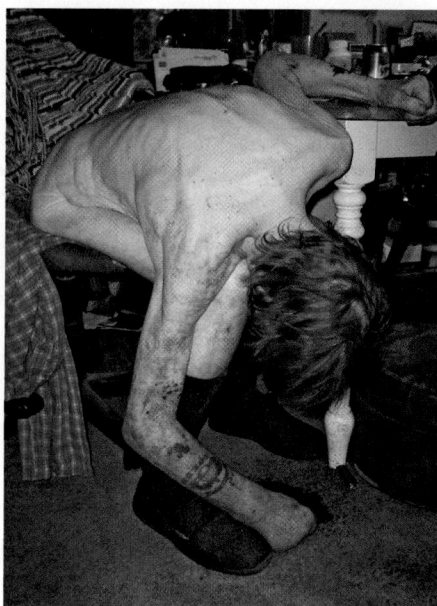

FIGURE 4-4

Livor mortis, or dependent lividity, occurs after death as blood pools in the tissues due to gravity. (© Skye Carpenter)

you should request law enforcement at the scene. Examples include suspected homicide, suicide, or other violent death, including deaths that may be due to child or elder abuse. Violent deaths that are reported to be accidents, such as accidental shootings or falls, and the presence of unusual circumstances at the scene should be investigated by law enforcement, as should vehicular deaths. Law enforcement is also generally required for suspected sudden infant death syndrome (SIDS).

Matters of Civil Law

When a patient or another person experiences damages as a result of an EMS provider's actions, the injured party may have sufficient cause to sue the provider, seeking a monetary award in compensation for damages. A patient, or someone on behalf of the patient, such as his family, may sue a health care provider if he believes there was a negligent action on the part of the provider, or another action that caused damages, such as defamation of character. The patient or family making the claim will seek the advice of an attorney, who will investigate the incident and decide whether the claim has merit. If the attorney believes the case has merit, he will file a claim with the court on behalf of the patient or his family, now called the **plaintiff**. A copy of the complaint will be provided to the EMS provider and other parties thought to be at fault (such as the provider's employer), now called the *defendant*. The defendant must seek representation by an attorney, who will answer the complaint.

Prior to a trial, all relevant information about the incident is sought and documented in a process called *discovery*. During the trial, both sides present their arguments and evidence in front of a jury. The jury then receives instructions about deliberations and comes to a decision about the defendant's **liability** and the amount of damages (if the defendant is liable) that the plaintiff is entitled to. Either party may appeal the decision in a higher-level court in the event of procedural errors in the legal proceedings. The parties may agree on a settlement at any point in the proceedings. Usually, the plaintiff settles for a lesser amount on the condition that he drops further proceedings.

Establishing the Elements of Negligence

Although a patient may believe that he is entitled to monetary compensation from a poor outcome of medical treatment, there are four elements that must be established to prove negligence:

- There was a duty to act.
- There was a breach of duty.
- Actual damages occurred.
- There is proximate cause.

First, the health care provider must have a **duty to act** as defined by law. For example, as an Advanced EMT, you have the duty to respond to calls and provide care within your scope of practice and to the standard of care. You must obey all applicable laws, such as motor vehicle laws, and operate with due regard for the safety of others. You must provide transportation and act in compliance with your employer's policies and your medical director's protocols and standing orders.

Second, there must be a **breach of duty**, such as deviating from the accepted standard of care, either through an act or omission of an act. A provider may give an unnecessary medication, constituting an act that violates the standard of care, or may fail to properly splint a badly injured extremity, constituting an omission that violates the standard of care. The breach of duty may be categorized as **malfeasance, misfeasance, or nonfeasance** (Table 4-1).

In a civil case, the defendant need not be proven guilty beyond a reasonable doubt. Instead, it must only be proven that it is more likely than not that negligence occurred. In most cases, the burden of proof is on the plaintiff. However, if the plaintiff invokes the doctrine of *res ipsa loquitur*, the burden of proof shifts to the defendant. *Res ipsa loquitur* means, "the thing speaks for itself." To rely on *res ipsa loquitor,* it must be argued that the damages would not have occurred but for the defendant's actions, that the instrument that caused the damages was under the defendant's control at all times, and that the plaintiff in no way could have contributed to the damages.

The third element required to establish negligence is that actual damages occurred. That is, harm must have

TABLE 4-1   Negligent Acts

Type of Act	Definition	Example
Malfeasance	Performance of an improper act	An Advanced EMT performs a skill that is not within his scope of practice, or performs a skill that is within his scope of practice but not indicated for the patient; for example, inserting an advanced airway into a patient with a gag reflex, causing vomiting and aspiration of stomach contents
Misfeasance	Improper performance of a legitimate act	An Advanced EMT is caring for a patient who needs an IV and intravenous dextrose, but fails to recognize that the IV is infiltrated; he administers the dextrose, which enters the tissue and causes tissue damage
Nonfeasance	Failure to perform an act that should be performed	An Advanced EMT should apply an automatic defibrillator to patients in cardiac arrest, but fails to do so

occurred that can be remunerated monetarily. It must be proven that physical, psychological, or financial damages occurred as a result of the provider's actions. Even if a provider has a duty to act and commits a breach of duty, unless damages occur, he is not held liable for negligence. If a provider's actions were a result of **gross negligence** (acting with disregard for the welfare of the patient) or willful and wanton misconduct, the plaintiff may also seek punitive damages.

The last element necessary to support a claim of negligence is **proximate cause**. The plaintiff's attorney must establish a causal link between the act or omission committed by the provider and the damages suffered by the plaintiff. Not every poor medical outcome is the result of medical error. In some cases, the patient's underlying condition or even the patient's own actions are causes of a poor outcome. In some cases, a combination of the patient's actions and the provider's actions may have resulted in harm. For example, failure to administer nitroglycerin to a patient with chest pain may worsen damage to the heart, but if the patient delayed calling for help, this also may have contributed to more damage than otherwise would have occurred.

Your scope of practice defines what you legally are allowed to do as an Advanced EMT. The **standard of care** defines what level and quality of care are expected, within the scope of practice, in a particular situation. It is a measure of whether or not an Advanced EMT applied the knowledge and skills within his scope of practice in the manner expected of similarly trained providers. This is known as the *reasonable person standard*. The underlying question is, did you act as a reasonable person with the same training would have acted in the same situation? This concept considers *whether* you provided the appropriate assessment and care and the *quality* with which you provided the assessment and care. The standard of care is established by referencing several sources, including recognized and accepted Advanced EMT textbooks, local and state protocols, EMS system policies and procedures, and the care that would be expected by other Advanced EMTs, as established by expert testimony.

Other Civil Claims

Negligence is not the only civil claim for which a patient (or others) may sue an EMS provider. If a patient experiences damages from a breach of confidentiality or defamation, he also may sue. Consider the case in which an Advanced EMT transports a well-known public figure and learns in the course of taking his history that he has hepatitis C, which is often (but not always) transmitted through needles shared between intravenous drug abusers. The Advanced EMT is overheard discussing the information, clearly insinuating that IV drug abuse is the cause of the disease, with an individual not involved in the patient's care. A third party hears the information and posts it on a popular political blog. The once-promising figure is now considered undesirable as a candidate within his political party. The Advanced EMT may be sued for invasion of privacy and defamation of character.

Keep in mind that the patient does not have to be a public figure to suffer defamation of character. **Defamation** is the intentional false communication of information that damages a person's reputation. The communication of false and injurious information may occur through spoken language, called **slander**, or through written communication, called **libel**.

IN THE FIELD

Use only professional communication in spoken and written statements, including communication with coworkers and other health care providers, patients, family and bystanders, and in your patient-care documentation. Not only is it unethical to do otherwise, but you may find yourself facing a claim of defamation.

High-Risk Situations

Some situations bear a higher risk of patient harm than others, and some situations have a higher risk of creating circumstances in which a patient will sue. Many lawsuits arise, not from the fact that damages were or were not incurred, but from the patient's perception of being treated badly by the health care provider. Patients often do not have the background to assess the quality of medical care you are providing, but everyone knows when they are being treated disrespectfully or in a dismissive manner. One way to minimize your risk of being involved in a lawsuit is to be empathetic, compassionate, and respectful to all patients, in addition to adhering to the standard of care.

Medication errors are a common cause of patient injury. You must always use the utmost care when administering medications, following all safety precautions. Whether or not injury occurs, the patient is entitled to know that a mistake was made. In fact, admitting an error to the patient does not necessarily make him more likely to sue. You also must follow your employer's procedures for reporting errors and documenting the error.

Other high-risk areas of EMS care include patient injury from dropping or improper handling and injury from emergency vehicle collisions. Exercise due regard in handling patients and in transportation.

Patients may, on occasion, need to be physically restrained to prevent them from hurting themselves or others (see Chapter 31). Never use restraint punitively, and always use only the amount of force needed to control the patient to prevent the patient from harming himself or others. The use of excessive force can lead to claims of assault and battery. Only use accepted methods of restraint, follow your protocols, and clearly document why restraint was required. Describe what the patient was doing or saying that indicated self-harm or harm to another was imminent. Also document how the patient was restrained and your reassessment of the potential for injury resulting from restraint.

Criminal Law Issues

Some infractions are punishable by fines or imprisonment, in addition to causing damages to patients. HIPAA specifies the instances in which protected health information (PHI) may be legally provided to others. Unauthorized disclosure of such information may result not only in a lawsuit filed by the patient, but in fines imposed by the court, as well. HIPAA includes the following provisions regarding PHI:

- Information may be shared if the patient consents in writing. The patient or his parent or legal guardian can request the release of medical records for any reason, and can direct that the information be provided to a third party, such as an attorney. As an Advanced EMT, it is *not* your duty to provide this information. Your agency will have a policy and procedure

IN THE FIELD

HIPAA is often misunderstood by health care providers. For example, it is not uncommon for hospital or nursing home personnel to refuse to release patient information to EMS providers who are transporting the patient from one facility to another. However, PHI disclosure is permitted and required to provide continuity of care. If you find yourself in a situation in which patient information that is important to your assessment and care is being withheld, the issue should be addressed between your management and management of the facility.

designating who handles requests for release of information.

- Information may be shared, without the patient's written consent, to other medical care providers who have a need to know. It is permissible to share the information during your radio report to the receiving hospital or upon transferring care of the patient to another provider.

- Information may be released when there is a court order compelling its release. Again, this request will be handled according to your agency's policies.

- Information may be released for billing purposes. Information can be released to insurance companies, Medicare, and Medicaid programs. It is preferable that patients sign an authorization to release this information. An authorization form is sometimes included on the patient care record.

- Patients are permitted by law the right to inspect their medical records and request amendments, and to request an accounting of disclosures of PHI, other than PHI released for legal authorized purposed.

EMTALA gives all patients, regardless of the ability to pay, the right to an appropriate screening examination and emergency medical care, and treatment (or appropriate emergency transfer) for patients in active labor. EMTALA arose from the Consolidated Omnibus Budget Reconciliation Act (COBRA) and is also referred to as the anti-dumping statute.

Legal Protections

The best way to avoid legal liability is to fully understand and adhere to the standard of care and to exercise due diligence in all activities. Those actions do not make you immune to civil claims, but if you act in good faith and adhere to the standard of care, the chances that you will be found liable are greatly reduced. Professionalism in appearance and actions are also important. A sloppy appearance conveys inattention to details. If the provider does not attend to the details of his appearance, what other details does he omit? If a provider is not professional in his interactions with a patient, it is not a stretch to believe that he was unprofessional in his assessment and treatment.

Protection can be provided in some circumstances by **Good Samaritan laws, governmental immunity,** and **statutes of limitations.** Good Samaritan laws generally do not apply to anyone being paid to provide medical care. But they may apply to EMS providers who provide care while off-duty, such as stopping to help at the scene of a collision or caring for a patient who collapses while waiting in line in front of you in the supermarket. Good Samaritan laws do not provide protection against gross negligence. Governmental immunity may apply in limited cases, but are not designed to offer protection to individual providers. A statute of limitations is a law that specifies the time in which a legal claim can be made or in which charges can be filed. After the specified time has passed, legal action cannot be pursued. Statutes of limitations vary from state to state and according to the legal issue. Contributory negligence on the part of the patient or another party can reduce the amount of liability of an EMS provider.

Your patient care documentation and documentation of any supplemental reports can provide tremendous protection, or lack thereof, depending on its quality. Your documentation can be subpoenaed in either a criminal or civil case. Documentation provides the best protection when you:

- Complete the documentation immediately after the call to ensure accurate recall.

- Write the report to support your decision making, as well as including all relevant details. The report should provide a picture of how the patient presented so that it leaves no question as to what the correct course of action was. If you do not record findings or procedures, you cannot prove that you found all relevant information and provided necessary treatments.

- Present information objectively. Do not make value judgments or assumptions. For example, do not document, "The patient was drunk." Instead, document, "The patient stated he drank seven margaritas between 7:00 PM and 9:00 PM. His speech was slurred, his gait was unsteady, and there was an odor of alcohol on his breath."

- Write neatly and accurately, using proper grammar, sentence structure, terminology, and abbreviations. Your documentation is a direct reflection on you as a professional.

- Make any corrections promptly and in an acceptable manner. Never scribble out, obliterate, or delete after the fact any documentation. If your documentation is in error, cross it out with a single line (for paper documentation), and date and initial the correction. If necessary, attach supplemental documentation and identify it clearly as an amendment or addendum.

Crime Scenes

When an injury or illness occurs during the commission of a crime, EMS providers have obligations in addition to protecting their own safety and caring for the patient. EMS providers are sometimes heard saying that evidence preservation and collection are not their concern. However, if the crime victim is the patient, you have an ethical obligation to act in the patient's best interest, which includes not destroying evidence that may lead to conviction of the perpetrator (Figure 4-5). In cases where the patient is a crime suspect, you still are obligated to do your utmost to preserve evidence.

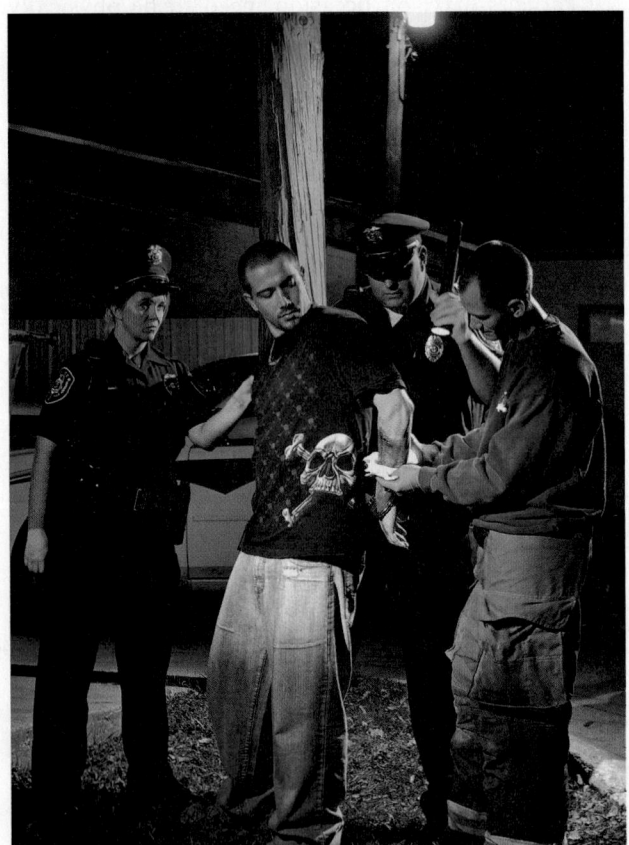

FIGURE 4-5

Work with law enforcement to preserve evidence when caring for a patient who has been involved in a crime.

Some key considerations in preserving evidence at crime scenes include:

- Disturb as little as possible. If you must move something, make a note of it and communicate what was moved to law enforcement.

- Follow the same path out of the crime scene as you took into it and have all providers take the same path.

- Use the minimum number of providers needed to care for the patient.

- Avoid, if possible, cutting through holes in clothing that may be from gunshots or weapons used in stabbing.

- If the patient is clearly dead, do not enter the crime scene.

- If you must remove anything from the scene (such as a weapon impaled in the patient), notify law enforcement.

- Document your observations and actions.

Other Legal Situations

In some states, relatives must be asked about the possibility of organ donation. It may or may not be the EMS provider's obligation to do so, so you must be aware of the laws in your area. Follow your protocols in the treatment of patients who are potential organ donors.

Although patient confidentiality is of utmost importance, there are some situations in which you are legally required to make a report of the patient's situation. Mandatory reporting laws vary, but generally include such things as gunshot wounds, child abuse and elder abuse, and animal bites. Some communicable diseases may be reportable, as well. In cases where individuals are designated as mandatory reporters, there is often protection from being sued by the person accused, as long as the report was made in good faith. In suspected abuse situations, you have not only a legal obligation, but an ethical obligation to protect and advocate for your patient.

In the course of caring for a patient, if you violate his civil rights, you may be legally liable. All patients, regardless of gender, ethnicity, marital status, age, sexual identity, or disability ethically and legally are entitled to the same standard of care.

The borrowed servant doctrine may be an issue in some cases of negligence. If you provide direction and supervision to someone with a lower level of licensure and they fail to uphold the standard of care, you may be held responsible. Ensure that the tasks you delegate are within that provider's scope of practice and provide adequate supervision of his actions.

CASE STUDY WRAP-UP

Clinical-Reasoning Process

Advanced EMTs Lieutenant Lydia Blume and Firefighter Adam Grolier are first on the scene for a person reported to be in cardiac arrest. They find the patient in his recliner, cyanotic and not breathing. As they place the patient on the floor to begin CPR and prepare to apply the defibrillator pads, his wife cries out, "Don't do that. He doesn't want any CPR or machines or breathing tubes."

Lt. Blume asks the patient's wife, "Do you have anything in writing? A living will or do not resuscitate order from his doctor?"

"Oh, yes. We have papers. They are in the office," she replies.

"We need to see them, ma'am, and consult with our doctor at the emergency department by radio. Can you bring me the papers?"

The patient's wife moves quickly to another a room and returns a few seconds later with a form signed by the patient's physician. The information on the DNR looks complete. Lt. Blume speaks into her radio, "Dispatch, Squad 441, requesting contact with University Hospital for medical direction."

Lt. Blume speaks with the on-line physician, concisely explaining the situation and relaying the information on the DNR. The physician agrees that the DNR is valid and confirms that resuscitation should not be attempted. Firefighter Grolier places his hand on the wife's shoulder and tells her he is sorry that her husband has died. He walks her to a chair and asks if she needs to call any family members or friends.

Later, after returning to service, Adam tells Lydia, "I'm glad the wife was able to find the DNR orders. I wouldn't have felt right starting resuscitation against their wishes, but without the DNR, it would have been a dilemma."

"You're right about that," replies Lydia. "It places us at legal risk if we don't resuscitate when there is no DNR, but ethically, it is difficult to go against the patient's and family's wishes."

CHAPTER REVIEW

Chapter Summary

Advanced EMTs operate within a legal and ethical structure that requires having authorization to practice, awareness of issues of patient consent, adhering to the standard of care, maintaining patient confidentiality, and exercising due diligence in all actions and decisions. Often, the issues are relatively uncomplicated. In other cases, the patient's ability to consent to or refuse care may be in question, the patient may pose a danger to himself or others, or you may suspect that a crime has been committed. You must be aware of your legal and ethical obligations and apply good judgment to avoid claims of assault, battery, false imprisonment, or abandonment. To protect yourself from liability, if such a claim is made, you must document the objective facts of the situation in a manner that justifies your actions.

Claims of negligence may arise when a patient experiences a poor outcome. But, to establish negligence, it must be proven that you had a duty to act, that you breached that duty, that the patient suffered harm, and that your actions or omissions were the proximate cause of the patient's harm. To protect yourself against successful litigation, ensure that you are competent in all of the knowledge and skills required of Advanced EMTs and treat patients compassionately and respectfully.

Review Questions

Multiple-Choice Questions

1. As you are returning from a call, a homeless man flags down the ambulance and tells you he is cold and hungry. While your partner arranges transportation for him to a homeless shelter, you place him in the back of the ambulance where it is warm and offer him an apple and a sandwich from your lunch. This best demonstrates the ethical principle of:

   a. nonmalfeasance.
   b. a patient's right to self-determination.
   c. beneficence.
   d. avoiding conflicts of interest.

2. Which one of the following actions would be in violation of federal law?

   a. Refusing to transport an uninsured patient with chest pain
   b. Failing to stop at the scene of an emergency while off-duty
   c. Not reporting a suspected case of child abuse
   d. Failing to maintain licensure and not reporting it to your employer

3. Negligence is a concept of what type of law?

   a. Criminal
   b. Civil
   c. Administrative
   d. Case

4. A 25-year-old male experienced a seizure while attending a hockey game. When you arrive, he responds to pain but is incoherent. He is with a friend, but there are no family members present. To obtain consent to treat him, you should:

   a. call a family member.
   b. request law enforcement.
   c. contact medical direction.
   d. rely on implied consent.

5. You tell a patient you would like to check her blood glucose level and she holds out her hand so that you can perform a finger stick. This is an example of _____ consent.

   a. expressed
   b. implied
   c. informed
   d. involuntary

6. You believe your patient is intoxicated and does not show appropriate concern for his injuries, but he states he does not want to go to the hospital. If you do not transport him, he could later claim:

   a. false imprisonment.
   b. battery.
   c. abandonment.
   d. assault.

7. You are on the scene of a patient reported to be not breathing at a nursing home. The nursing staff presents you with a document, signed by the patient's physician, that states you may apply oxygen and use a bag-valve-mask device, but you may not use CPR, defibrillation, start an IV, or give medications. This document best fits the description of a:

   a. durable power of attorney.
   b. health care proxy.
   c. living will.
   d. do not resuscitate (DNR) order.

8. You have arrived on the scene of a patient who is not breathing and does not have a pulse. Which one of the additional findings, on its own, would be the most defensible reason for not starting resuscitation?
   a. The patient has an apparently self-inflicted gunshot wound that has destroyed his head above the lower jaw, with massive amounts of brain matter missing.
   b. The patient's adult children plead with you to withhold resuscitation so that their father does not suffer any more.
   c. The patient's skin is cold to the touch.
   d. The patient has a past medical history of cancer.

9. Which one of the following death circumstances would be least likely to require you to notify the office of the medical examiner?
   a. Three-year-old found submerged in a swimming pool
   b. Motor vehicle collision with two fatalities, but no suspicion of involvement of alcohol
   c. Patient with terminal cancer who has a DNR
   d. 26-year-old found hanging from a support beam in the basement and appears to have left a suicide note

10. An Advanced EMT responds to an unresponsive patient with an unknown history. He does not check the patient's blood glucose level. At the hospital, the patient is determined to have a low blood glucose level. He is given dextrose intravenously and released later that afternoon. Which one of the following would be the most difficult to establish in this case?
    a. Advanced EMT's duty to respond
    b. Damages suffered by the patient
    c. Breach of duty by the Advanced EMT
    d. Standard of care

11. Upon which one of the following should you rely most heavily for protection from liability?
    a. Governmental immunity
    b. Good Samaritan laws
    c. Documentation
    d. Your employer's malpractice insurance coverage

12. In which one of the following cases would you most likely be legally obligated to make a report to law enforcement or other authorities?
    a. Patient suffers a panic attack after smoking marijuana
    b. Patient with a gunshot wound to his foot says it was an accident and refuses transport
    c. Minor patient has an odor of alcohol on his breath
    d. 17-year-old mother refuses treatment for her 10-month-old child, who hit his lip on a tile floor, causing a small laceration

Critical-Thinking Questions

13. A patient with chest pain refuses treatment and transport. How should you respond? How should you assess his competence to make that decision?

14. Upon arriving at the scene for a person down, you recognize the patient as a homeless alcoholic who is frequently found passed out in public places. Your partner uses the toe of his boot to kick the patient in the buttocks several times, yelling at him to "get your worthless butt up off the ground." What are the legal and ethical issues here? What actions should you take?

15. You are dispatched for an injured person at a high school wrestling meet. As you enter the gymnasium, a wrestling coach approaches you and says you are not needed. You can see a student athlete holding a bloody cloth to his nose sitting on a bench in the gym. What are the issues to be considered in this situation? How should you respond?

16. When you arrive at the scene of the emergency, a law enforcement officer tells you there is a badly injured patient in the apartment and that she was beaten in a domestic dispute. You see that tables are knocked over, the phone is off the hook, and the handset is covered with blood. Generally, things are in disarray and several objects are between you and the patient. What actions can you take to disturb the crime scene as little as possible? What communication should you have with law enforcement at the scene?

References

Argyris, C., & Schön, D. (1974). *Theory in practice: increasing professional effectiveness.* San Francisco: Jossey-Bass Publishers.

National Highway Transportation Safety Administration (NHTSA). (2006). *National EMS scope of practice model.* Retrieved December 14, 2010, from http://www.ems.gov

Additional Reading

Bledsoe, B. E., Porter, R. S., & Cherry, R. A. (2009). *Paramedic care: Principles and practice* (3rd ed., Vol 1). Upper Saddle River, NJ: Pearson.

Mistovich, J. J., & Karren, K. J. (2010). *Prehospital emergency care* (9th ed.). Upper Saddle River, NJ: Pearson.

5 Ambulance Operations and Responding to EMS Calls

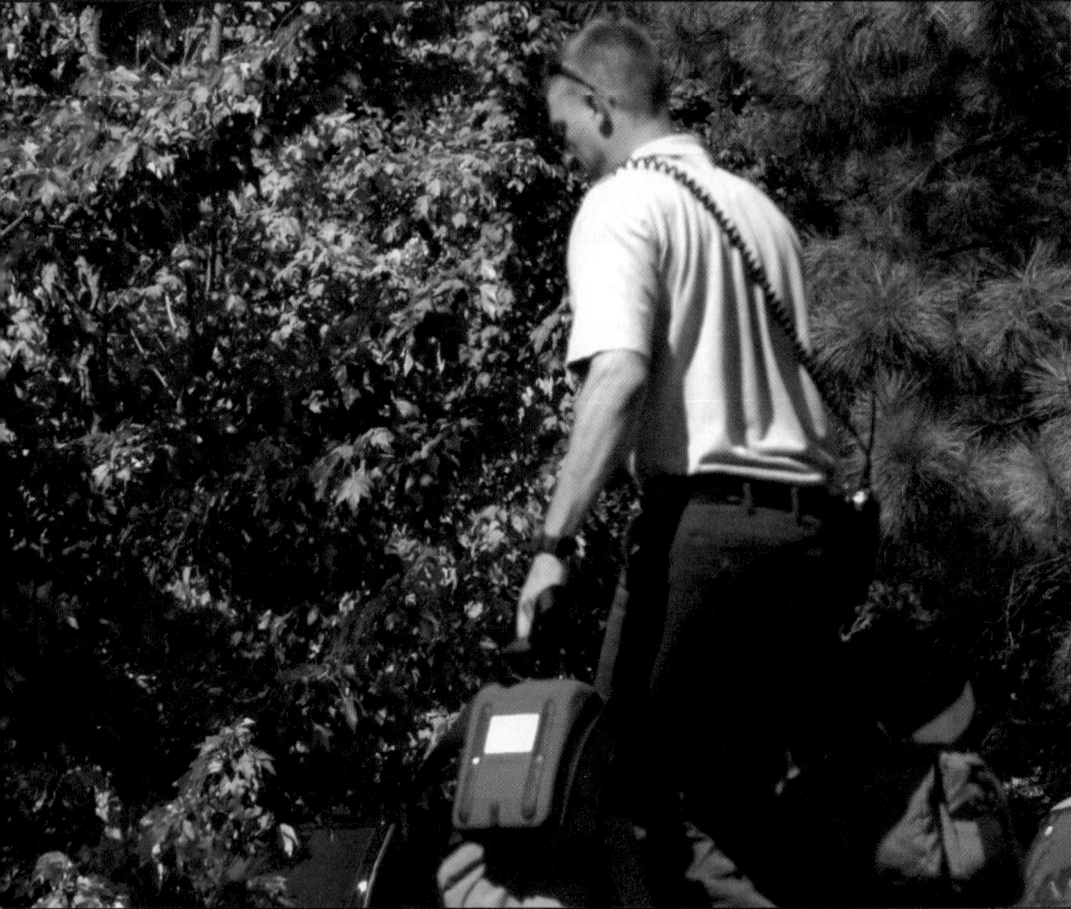

Content Area: EMS Operations

Advanced EMT Education Standard: The Advanced EMT applies knowledge of operational roles and responsibilities to ensure patient, public, and personal safety.

Objectives

After reading this chapter, you should be able to:

5.1 Define key terms introduced in this chapter.

5.2 Give examples of the Advanced EMT's responsibilities during each of the major phases of an ambulance call.

5.3 Describe the recommendations of the National Association of EMTs with respect to EMS provider security and safety.

5.4 Describe the legal responsibilities and privileges afforded to Advanced EMTs operating ambulances, and the precautions that must be observed while using those privileges.

5.5 Give examples of habits and behaviors that improve driving safety.

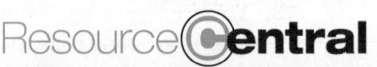

Resource **C**entral

To access Resource Central, follow the directions on the Student Access Card provided with this text. If there is no card, go to www.bradybooks.com and follow the Resource Central link to Buy Access. Under Media Resources, you will find:

• *Be the Safe Driver.* Read how to avoid collisions by applying defensive driving techniques.

• *Your Body in Motion.* Learn safe body mechanics and patient lifting strategies.

• *The Air Ambulance.* Learn about the unique challenges faced by air medical service providers.

CASE STUDY

Advanced EMT Gary Noonan is checking and stocking the supplies and equipment in the back of the ambulance, while his partner, Mercede Farmer, does a mechanical inspection of the vehicle. Just as Mercede writes in the fuel level on the vehicle log, they are dispatched for a trench collapse at a construction site: "Ambulance 53, respond to 3600 East on North County Line Road for a person entrapped in a trench collapse. Enter the construction site from the west entrance. Security will meet you there."

Problem-Solving Questions

1. How will Mercede and Gary decide on the best route of travel to the dispatch location?
2. What actions must they take to minimize their chances of being in a collision during their emergency response?
3. Once at the scene, what should they look for?
4. When the patient is freed, what is the best way to get him to the ambulance for transportation?
5. How should the patient's condition affect decisions about driving while en route to the emergency department?

5.6	Discuss factors that can affect your ability to maintain control of an ambulance.
5.7	Explain precautions that should be taken when operating an ambulance at night or in inclement weather.
5.8	Describe the appropriate use of emergency warning devices, such as lights and sirens.
5.9	Describe the safety precautions to be taken when working at scenes on and near roadways.
5.10	Explain precautions to avoid exposing yourself and others to increased levels of carbon monoxide from vehicle exhaust.
5.11	Compare the relative risk of ground ambulance operation to other potential risks faced by EMS providers.
5.12	Relate features of ambulance design to both hazards and safety in ambulance crashes.
5.13	Given a high-risk ambulance operation situation, such as negotiating intersections or highway driving, describe actions to reduce the risk as much as possible.
5.14	Explain the impact of speed on both emergency response time and safety.
5.15	Describe the ways of minimizing distractions while driving.
5.16	Explain the impact of fatigue and shift work on the safety of ambulance operations.
5.17	Discuss situations in which air medical transportation should be considered, disadvantages of air medical transport, and guidelines for setting up a landing zone and interacting with the air medical crew.
5.18	Apply principles of proper body mechanics to lifting and moving patients and equipment.
5.19	Describe the importance of teamwork and communications in lifting and moving patients.
5.20	Differentiate among situations that call for emergency, urgent, and nonurgent moves.
5.21	Demonstrate the steps required to properly package a patient for transport by ground or by air.

(continued)

(continued from previous page)

5.22   Describe the proper use, advantages, disadvantages, and techniques for using each
of the following:
- Armpit forearm drag
- Backboard
- Blanket drag
- Devices for bariatric patients
- Direct carry
- Direct ground lift
- Draw sheet method
- Extremity lift
- Log roll
- Neonatal isolette
- Portable stretcher
- Power grip
- Power lift
- Pushing and pulling
- Rapid extrication
- Scoop or basket stretcher
- Shirt drag
- Squat lift
- Stair chair
- Wheeled stretcher

5.23   Given a scenario involving any of the following types of patients, demonstrate
proper patient positioning:
- Chest pain or difficulty breathing
- Geriatric, pediatric, pregnant, or physical disability
- Known or suspected spine injury
- Nausea or vomiting
- Shock
- Unresponsive

Introduction

The prehospital environment is a unique setting for health care. Before you apply knowledge of anatomy, physiology, patient assessment, and emergency care, you must understand how to anticipate and respond to the challenges of working outside the walls of a traditional health care setting. Your professional roles and responsibilities, aside from direct patient care, are the operational aspects of the job. One of the most visible operational tasks of Advanced EMTs is emergency vehicle operations. Most EMS calls require thorough patient assessment and basic patient care. A few will require advanced lifesaving care, and a few will result in no patient care at all. Yet every call will require operation of a vehicle.

An ambulance is by far the most complex and potentially lethal piece of equipment used by EMS providers. The first rule of medicine is to do no harm. Yet, emergency vehicle operations pose a very real risk of injury or death to providers, their patients, and the public. Just as excellence in patient care knowledge and skills protects patients from harm, knowledge of and respect for principles of emergency vehicle operations substantially reduces the risk.

In addition to emergency vehicle operations, there are many other operational aspects of EMS. You must know what equipment you need and how it works. You must quickly recognize when a scene presents special challenges or risks, such as an entrapped patient or person with a weapon, and know what actions to take and what resources to request. In addition to vehicle-related injuries, lifting injuries are a common cause of lost work and disability in EMS.

Many challenges of the job are related not to medical care, but to issues such as how and when to move patients, how to get through traffic during rush hour, and where to set up a landing zone for a medical helicopter. Anticipating and responding to the operational challenges of working in the prehospital setting have as significant an impact on patients as the medical care you provide. This chapter addresses operational aspects of EMS with emphasis on safety of EMS providers, patients, and the public.

Phases of EMS Calls

EMS providers have duties and responsibilities from before a call is received to putting the ambulance back in service after a call. Some details may vary slightly at your particular service, or at the different levels of care. However, most calls progress through six phases: preparation, receiving and responding, on-scene care and preparation for transport, transporting the patient, transferring patient care, and terminating the call.

Preparation

The modern ambulance is nearly a mobile emergency room, and contains many pieces of specialized equipment (Figure 5-1). The vehicle must be in good mechanical repair with an adequate amount of fuel for response. All emergency warning devices, communication devices, and patient care equipment must be checked and verified to be in working order before it is needed on a call. The many disposable supplies used in EMS must be stocked, and the patient compartment must be clean and safe for the patient and EMS provider. Advanced EMTs must be prepared for their work by being highly knowledgeable and skilled, well rested, and emotionally and physically prepared for the job.

Receiving and Responding

Advanced EMTs must be ready to receive and respond to calls at all times while on duty. Most EMS services have policies that spell out the amount of time that is acceptable between being notified of a call, acknowledging the call, and beginning the response to the call. You must operate the responding vehicle with regard for your, your partner's, and the public's safety while arriving at the scene in a timely manner. You must be able to determine the best route of travel to the scene, and know how to use maps and navigation devices. The receiving and responding phase also includes selecting the best location to park the ambulance for safety and efficiency.

Before making contact with the patient, a scene size-up is performed to determine the nature of the call, the presence of hazards, the number of patients, and the need for additional resources. The communication that is required during this process, and the rest of the EMS call, is described in Chapter 6.

On-Scene Care and Preparation for Transport

The scene size-up begins as you arrive at the scene and continues as you make initial contact with the patient. You then conduct a primary and secondary patient assessment, perform needed care, and prepare the patient for transportation to the hospital. Skilled therapeutic communication

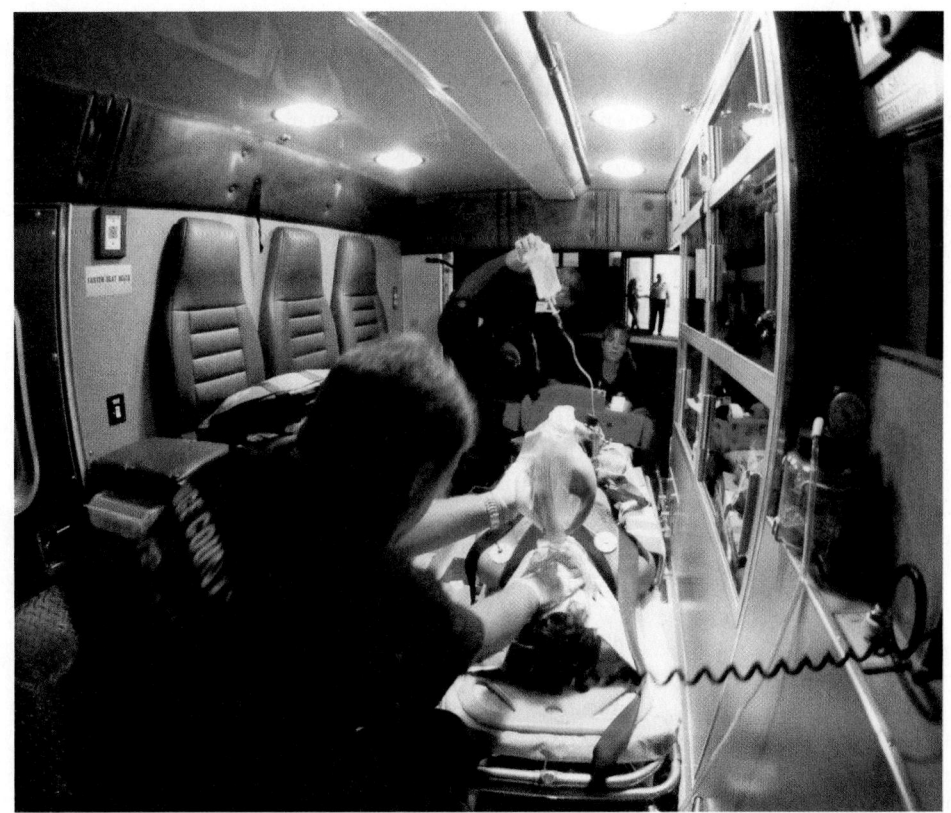

FIGURE 5-1

A modern ambulance has many of the capabilities of a hospital emergency department.
(© Craig Jackson/In the Dark Photography)

and teamwork are required to establish rapport with the patient and others, obtain needed information, and interact effectively with all EMS providers, law enforcement, and others at the scene. You must have excellent patient assessment, clinical reasoning, and patient care skills to identify the problem and respond to it. A unique aspect of EMS is the need to integrate patient assessment and care with **packaging** the patient in preparation for transport.

Transporting the Patient

Acutely ill or injured patients are transported to the emergency department for definitive care. In small communities, there may be only one hospital within a reasonable transport distance. In larger communities there are other considerations in determining the transport destination. Critically ill and injured patients are transported to the closest hospital that can provide the level of care they need. Noncritical patients are generally transported to the hospital of their choosing, as long as it is within a reasonable distance.

In some cases, your role will be to transfer care of the patient to an advanced life support (ALS) unit or air medical crew for transportation. On a typical call, one crew member drives the ambulance and the other rides in the patient compartment to continue assessing and treating the patient. Both crew members have critical responsibilities during patient transportation. The driver must select the best route to the hospital, maneuver the large vehicle through traffic, and provide a ride that is comfortable for the patient and allows safe ongoing care. The driver must communicate with dispatch and make decisions about the use of warning lights and sirens. Safe and efficient emergency vehicle operation requires proper training and many hours of practice. Meanwhile, the other crew member (sometimes called the *tech* or *attendant*) reassesses the patient, continues care, communicates with the receiving facility and medical direction when needed, and documents information for the **patient care report (PCR)**.

Transferring Patient Care

Once you have arrived at the patient's destination, you must transfer his care to the staff of the receiving facility. Failure to appropriately transfer care can result in a claim of patient abandonment. In most cases, you may transfer patient care only to someone of an equal or higher level of medical training. Usually, you will transfer care to a registered nurse (RN), although you also may transfer care to a physician, physician's assistant, or paramedic, depending on the facility.

Often, your first stop in the emergency department will be the **triage desk**, where you will give a brief report that allows the triage nurse or technician to make a decision about where to place the patient. Often with critical patients, you will be given a room destination over the radio so that you can transfer the patient without delay. You will take the patient to his assigned room or bed and give a hand-off report to the staff who will be caring for the patient. Ideally, you will leave a copy of the PCR with patient care staff before you leave the hospital.

Terminating the Call

Terminating the call, which is also called "returning to service," includes all steps necessary to prepare for the next call. You and your partner clean and disinfect equipment, replace supplies used, complete necessary paperwork, and inform the dispatch center that you are back in service.

Prehospital Environment and Types of Calls

EMS providers are called upon at all times of the day and night, to many types of locations, and for many different reasons. There may be busier times, or more common call types, but there is no way to predict when a call will come, or what type of care may be needed. Different types of calls and locations require different approaches and offer different challenges. Advanced EMTs must be well prepared and able to respond in a variety of circumstances.

Nonemergency Calls

Nonemergency calls typically involve **interfacility transfers**, often referred to simply as "transfers." Often, transfers are scheduled ahead of time, but can be requested urgently to transfer a patient admitted at one hospital to another hospital that offers a higher level of care. Typically, transfers involve nonambulatory patients who cannot be transported by another means. They are transported by ambulance from their home or residential care facility for procedures, such as computerized tomography (CT) scans or magnetic resonance imaging (MRIs), outpatient procedures, dialysis, or for doctor appointments, and then returned to their home or care facility. Such nonemergency calls are scheduled through the EMS service, not through the 911 system.

Depending on your EMS system and geographical location, some nonemergency transfers involve long distances.

Nonemergency patients receive a brief assessment, including vital signs prior to transport. Patients may require monitoring of oxygen administration or intravenous drips during transfer. Depending on the length of the transfer, you will reassess the patient as needed.

The role of Advanced EMTs on nonemergency calls includes high-quality, compassionate care and ensuring the patient's safety. The patient must be delivered on time and to the correct location. A PCR is completed for nonemergency calls, just as it is for emergency calls. For nonemergency calls, reimbursement from insurance or Medicare may depend on your documentation of the patient's need for ambulance transport. Follow your employer's guidelines for documenting nonemergency calls.

Emergency Calls

Emergency calls can be stressful for EMS providers. They can require emergency driving techniques, rapid patient assessment, quick decision making, advanced treatment, and safe, prompt transport. While many calls come in as emergencies, you will often determine, through your assessment of the patient, that the situation is not immediately life threatening. Your approach to noncritical and critical emergency patients will differ.

Most emergency calls will be received through the 911 system, and require immediate dispatch of the appropriate resources. The response time should be kept at a minimum, but safe emergency vehicle operation is required for the unit to arrive at the scene at all. Responding without delay does not mean responding recklessly or driving too fast. Emergency scenes can be uncontrolled and hazardous. Response by many public safety units to the same call can increase the risk of collisions and complicate decisions about how and where to park the ambulance at the scene. For example, if you arrive first on the scene of a house fire, it might seem like a good idea to park close to the house so you can get patients into the ambulance quickly. However, later arriving fire apparatus or news vehicles could block your departure from the scene.

Although you could encounter hazards on any call, the uncontrolled and sometimes emotional nature of emergencies increases the risk of injury to EMS providers. In addition to hazards associated with driving, you must assess the scene for other dangers. Check for uncontrolled traffic at the scene of motor vehicle collisions. Look for indications of violence when responding to crime scenes, domestic violence calls, or behavioral emergencies. In various situations you could be faced with the presence of hazardous chemicals, downed electrical lines, unstable structures or vehicles, and other dangers. A stressed pet dog trying to protect its owner from an intruder (you) may present a danger. Some dangers are more mundane, such as a loose handrail on the stairs or an icy sidewalk. The operational aspects of scene size-up, including determining the safety of the scene, are discussed later in this chapter.

Medical Calls

Many requests for EMS involve patients who have **acute** or **chronic** illnesses. Because the incidence of many diseases increases with age, many of the patients encountered on medical calls are elderly. However, illness affects people of all ages, including infants. In order to plan and implement the correct treatment for a patient, you must determine the nature of a patient's illness and form a field impression of the problem. You must take a thorough medical history and conduct a proper assessment to determine what treatment (such as oxygen or medication administration) is required. The tasks of medical care are integrated with decisions about how to move the patient to the ambulance and provide safe transport to an appropriate facility. Advanced EMTs reassess patients and continue care during transport. When required by the patient's condition, the receiving hospital is notified and physician's orders are requested.

Trauma Calls

Many EMS calls are for patients who have been injured. Trauma occurs in patients of all ages, but younger patients are more likely to need EMS because of trauma than because of a medical problem. Many injuries are accidental, but some are a result of intentional violence. In cases of intentional violence or preventable injuries, you must concentrate on patient care and not become distracted from your priorities by frustrations about the person or actions responsible for the incident.

Most injuries are not immediately life or limb threatening, but a critical trauma patient requires a number of the Advanced EMT skills. In addition to determining the mechanism of injury and performing a thorough assessment, you may need to perform critical airway and ventilation skills, control serious bleeding, immobilize the spine, splint fractured extremities, and start an intravenous line. Patients with critical traumatic injuries can be stabilized and packaged for transport by EMS, but repairing their injuries often requires surgery. The role of the EMS provider in caring for critical trauma patients is to provide immediate interventions to ensure the patient has an open airway, is being ventilated, and to control bleeding while packaging the patient for transport. The goal for critically injured trauma patients is to be on the scene for 10 minutes or less. However, having multiple patients or patients who are entrapped or difficult to access sometimes complicates this goal. The time to transport the patient to a trauma center must be considered and, where available, the feasibility, risks, and benefits of air medical transport should be weighed.

Responding to a Residence

Many calls for service will be to a patient's residence, which poses unique opportunities, responsibilities, and challenges. EMS providers see the patient's environment and take it

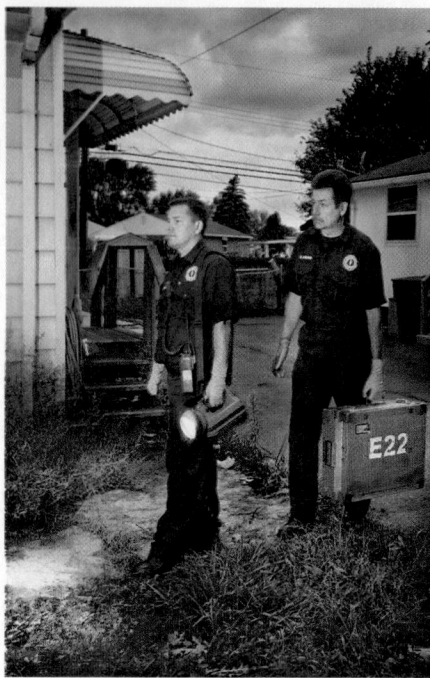

FIGURE 5-2

When responding to residences, observe the patient's environment.

into consideration in making decisions about the patient's needs (Figure 5-2). Other health care providers do not usually have access to this information. Always keep in mind that you are entering the home of another person. Treat his property with care and respect. Remember, this is his home, and you are a complete stranger. Treat patients, as well as their homes and belongings, with the respect you would expect to receive, while keeping what you see and hear confidential.

In certain circumstances, you may be required to gain access to a patient's home by breaking through a locked door or window. This should be done in the presence of police and with as little damage as possible. You also should take care to leave a patient's home safe and secure by turning off lights, appliances, closing and locking windows and doors, and bringing necessary keys. Although a home may seem a relatively safe place to enter, dangers can be well hidden in and around homes. Some common concerns are sounds of violence (screaming, yelling, banging walls or furniture), barking dogs, unusual odors, unsafe steps or stairs, and inadequate lighting.

Responding to Roadway Scenes

Calls on roadways have the highest potential for provider and patient injuries and fatalities. *Extreme caution must be observed at all times.* Be careful to position the ambulance so providers do not exit or enter the vehicle from a lane of traffic. Vehicles should be positioned so providers do not have to cross traffic to get to patients. Personnel and

patients should be moved away from lanes of travel as soon as possible. If care must be rendered in or near a travel lane, traffic must be blocked. Reflective clothing must be worn whenever standing or walking on or near a roadway. Providers should have part of their attention on nearby moving traffic at all times, and have a plan of escape already formulated. Other hazards at roadway scenes include rolling or unstable vehicles, sudden deployment of airbags that were not activated in the original collision, leaking vehicle fluids, downed electrical lines, and involvement of a vehicle carrying hazardous cargo.

Rescue Situations

Rescue calls require the planned removal of patients from enclosed areas or locations that are difficult to access. Part of the scene size-up as you first arrive is determining if any additional resources, such as specialized rescue teams, are required. Rescue may include removing patients from crashed vehicles, collapsed buildings, bodies of water, steeply angled locations such as cliffs or ravines, and industrial and farm machinery. Rescues require specialized training and equipment and should only be performed by those who have been specially trained for the specific situation at hand.

Operation at rescue scenes may allow only one provider to access the patient. For example, assessment and treatment may need to be done in difficult situations such as inside an overturned vehicle (Figure 5-3) or on a cliff side. The safety of providers and the patient must always be considered before attempting any access to or movement of the patient. Your cooperation with rescue personnel is essential to the outcome of the call. If you are caring for a patient in a rescue situation, wear appropriate protective equipment and follow the instructions of rescue personnel. Additional information on rescue operations is discussed in Chapter 47.

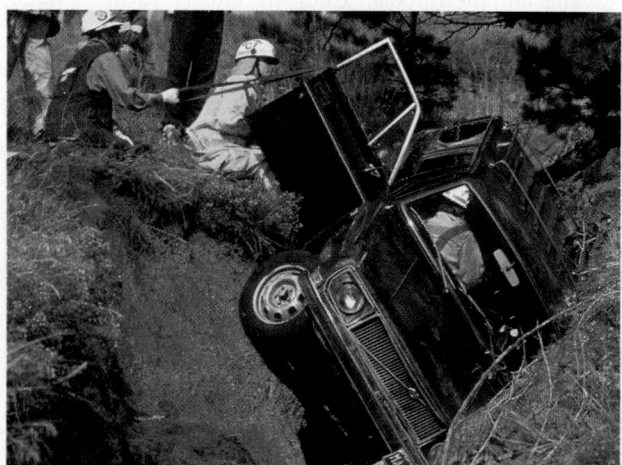

FIGURE 5-3

Special training is required for rescue situations.
(© Howard M. Paul/Emergency! Stock)

Hazardous Materials Situations

Commonly referred to as "hazmat incidents," hazardous materials situations involve possible exposure to toxic chemicals or substances. Your primary role is to recognize the potential involvement of hazardous materials and request specialized resources to respond and determine the nature of the situation. Advanced EMTs provide care to patients who have been exposed to hazardous materials only after trained personnel have properly decontaminated them. Only highly trained and specially equipped personnel are permitted to enter areas that are potentially contaminated by hazardous materials. EMS providers should never hesitate to contact hazmat teams (usually fire department based) whenever they suspect a contaminated scene. Hazmat response is discussed in more detail in Chapter 48.

Multiple-Casualty Incidents

The **multiple-casualty incident (MCI)**, as the name implies, involves multiple patients (Figure 5-4). The number of patients considered to be an MCI depends on the availability of local resources and the assistance that can be expected from surrounding agencies. MCIs are, by definition, overwhelming to available services. A large service might consider 10 or 12 patients to be an MCI, whereas a small service might consider three patients to be an MCI.

An MCI has the potential to be chaotic, with multiple services interacting in a small area, and transporting multiple patients to emergency departments, which may be underequipped for the number of patients or nature of injuries. It is extremely important for areas to have an **incident command system (ICS)** and conduct MCI drills and training sessions. Those drills will familiarize providers with MCI operations, how to best communicate with other responding agencies, and how to work within an ICS.

In MCIs, triage is used to categorize patients according to the severity of their conditions. Triage prioritizes them for orderly transport to area hospitals. MCIs, ICS, and triage are addressed in more detail in Chapter 33.

Ambulance Design

Ambulances are not built by the automotive industry, and do not handle like automobiles. They begin as an automotive industry–produced heavy-duty truck chassis. An ambulance manufacturer then extensively modifies the chassis. While these modifications allow for patient care during transportation, they also provide driving and safety challenges. Ambulance manufacturers produce four standard types of ambulances:

- *Type I ambulance.* This ambulance is built on a pick-up truck chassis. The cab is left intact, and a large box modification is added to the frame (Figure 5-5).

- *Type II ambulance.* This ambulance is built on a van chassis. Most of the original vehicle is left intact, but the roof is removed and a fiberglass extension is added to increase the height. This modification allows providers to stand in the back while providing care (Figure 5-6).

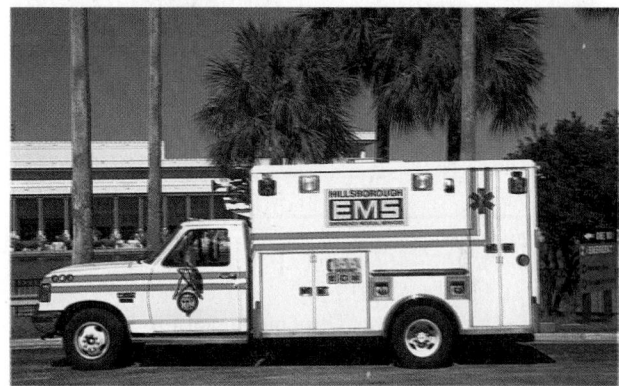

FIGURE 5-5

A type I ambulance.

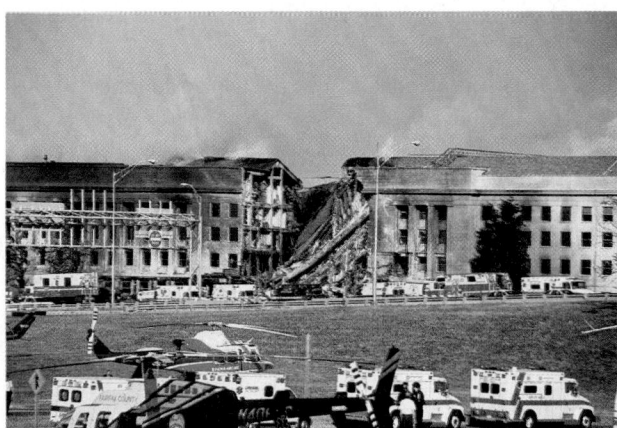

FIGURE 5-4

A multiple-casualty incident exists when the number of patients exceeds the resources available to care for them.
(© Rob Crandall/Image Works)

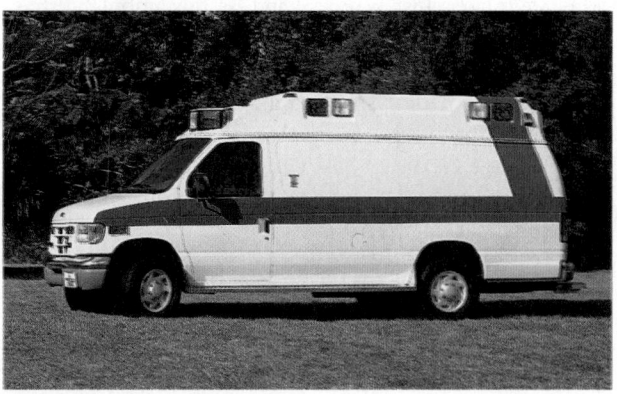

FIGURE 5-6

A type II ambulance.

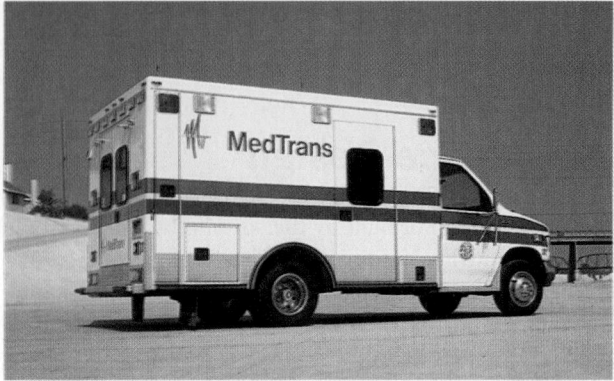

FIGURE 5-7

A type III ambulance.

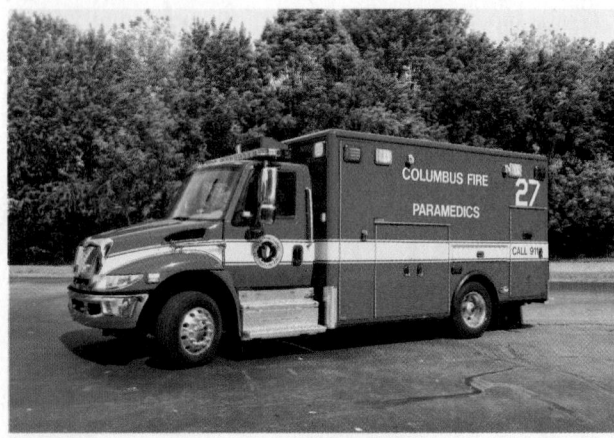

FIGURE 5-8

A medium-duty ambulance.

- *Type III ambulance.* This ambulance also is built on a van chassis, but has had extensive modification. As in type I, the type II cab is left intact and a large box modification is added (Figure 5-7).

- *Medium-duty ambulance.* This ambulance is built on a large truck chassis, such as International or Freightliner. Just as types I and III, this ambulance has an intact cab with a large box modification. Due to the taller loading height, many medium-duty ambulances have pneumatic suspension that allows them to "kneel" or lower to permit loading of stretchers. The large, heavy ambulances are primarily used by fire departments looking to carry large amounts of equipment (Figure 5-8).

Ambulance design is dictated by federal specifications. The specifications document, KKK-1822-E (known as the triple K specifications), is written by the General Services Administration (GSA) of Federal Supply Services (a division of the U.S. Department of Transportation). It should be noted that the triple K specifications are purchase specifications, required for vehicles displaying a **Star of Life** symbol.

They are not construction or safety standards. The lack of safety standards is a factor in ambulance collision injuries. However, EMS personnel can take many actions to reduce their risk of injury in ambulance collisions (discussed later in this chapter).

Vehicle Readiness

Before responding to calls, ambulances must be in safe working order and completely stocked with supplies and equipment. Your ambulance, and the equipment in it, is your responsibility. If the previous crew forgot to refill the oxygen tank, and you arrive on scene without oxygen, it is not their fault. It is yours. There are many items that must be checked, including mechanical items and medical supplies. Most EMS services have a vehicle inspection checklist and a policy requiring its completion prior to the start of each shift.

Exterior Vehicle and Mechanical Readiness

Large EMS services may have mechanics on duty who perform repairs and preventive maintenance, but you are still ultimately responsible for ensuring that your vehicle will make it safely to your destination. The following are some mechanical items that should be checked:

- *Engine.* Check the oil, coolant, and washer fluid levels, and top off if necessary.

- *Brakes.* Report any difficulty braking, such as a soft pedal, vibration, or noise.

- *Lights.* Headlights, high beams, turn signals, brake lights, hazards, and running lights, must all be activated and checked.

- *Tires.* Check the tread depth, wear, and air pressure of all tires. (Do not forget the inner tires of dual rear wheels.)

- *Windshield wipers.* Check the wipers and the condition of the blades.

- *Emergency warning devices.* Check all emergency lights: lightbar, strobes, flashers, loading lights, scene lights, grill lights, headlight flashers (wig-wags), and so on. Check the siren (all tones) and the horn.

- *Radios.* Check the mobile radio and the function and battery power of portable radios and pagers.

Patient Care Equipment and Supplies

The medical equipment and the quantities carried may vary between services, but are based on recommended medical equipment standards from several agencies. The American

College of Surgeons (ACS) Committee on Trauma (COT) publishes a list of "Essential Equipment." The National Institute for Occupational Safety and Health (NIOSH) and the Occupational Safety and Health Administration (OSHA) both have safety equipment recommendations. The National Fire Protection Association (NFPA) recommends equipment for fire service vehicles. Services accredited by the **Commission on Accreditation of Ambulance Services (CAAS)** follow their guidelines.

Emergency Vehicle Operations

Before learning the basics of operating an ambulance, you need to know the risks. Ambulance accidents are not rare and they are not just an inherent risk of EMS. In fact, most are not "accidents" at all. They are predictable and preventable crashes.

Unfortunately, a centralized database of ambulance crash data does not exist. Conservative estimates put the number of annual ambulance crashes in the United States at about 6,500 (Zagaroli & Taylor, 2003). That is nearly 20 each day. It also is estimated that those crashes injure up to four people per day, and kill up to four people per month (Becker, Zaloshnja, Levick, & Miller, 2003). This means that one in 300 ambulance services will experience a fatal crash each year. The estimated number of injuries and fatalities occurring in and around ambulances, compared to other types of vehicles, make ambulances one of the most dangerous vehicles on the road.

NIOSH did a study of EMS provider fatalities and discovered that the fatality rate of EMS workers is 12.7 per 100,000 workers, which is double the national average of all other occupations. The primary cause of the line-of-duty

deaths is vehicle crashes (Maguire, Hunting, Smith, & Levick, 2002). They looked specifically at 300 fatal ambulance crashes, and found that more fatalities (60 percent) occurred in the front of the ambulance, likely due to the frequency of front-end collisions and impact with the steering wheel.

NHTSA's research on EMS provider injuries found that the ambulance crash injury rate is 10 to 20 times that of civilian vehicles (Levick & Mener, 2009; U.S. Department of Transportation, 2008). Their research showed two primary facts. First, most injuries occurred in the patient compartment and were caused by improperly restrained occupants and equipment. Second, the cause of most crashes was human error by the ambulance operator, commonly due to speed, distractions, and fatigue. This alone should indicate the importance of a comprehensive emergency vehicle operations training program.

Defensive Driving

A key factor in any driver education program, **defensive driving** refers to a constant state of awareness and the ability to avoid an adverse situation with evasive maneuvers. The driver of an emergency vehicle needs to be able to avoid other drivers' mistakes and actively prevent collisions. A good defensive driver must always be aware of his surroundings, able to predict potential problems, and prepared to take action to maintain control of the vehicle and prevent crashes. A crash caused by another driver is still a crash, will still cause injuries or fatalities, and must be avoided. Defensive driving tactics are important in crash prevention and include constant scanning and cushion of safety.

The emergency vehicle driver must constantly scan the surroundings. The scan should include everything outside

PERSONAL PERSPECTIVE

Advanced EMT Hector Torres: I've been reading lately about hospitals creating a culture of safety. It turns out that a lot of the ideas come from the airline industry. People are concerned about airline safety because when something goes wrong, it's well publicized, but overall, the airline industry has achieved a remarkable safety record. That's not the case with EMS yet. In the industry, we hear a lot about crashes, but the public isn't aware of the problem. There are so many reports of air medical crashes and ground ambulance collisions. It's tragic. It seems like almost all of my colleagues know of someone who has been injured or killed in an on-duty crash.

There are some really good ideas for airline safety that we could adopt in EMS. First, it is against regulations for pilots to fly without a certain amount of "down time." In EMS, too often, we have people pulling so much overtime that they haven't slept more than a few hours in two or three days. I know I want my driver to be well rested, to be capable of making good

judgments, and to have quick reactions. Second, a flight never takes off without completing a preflight checklist. In EMS we check the ambulance at the beginning of the shift, and we restock, but we don't do a safety checklist for each call.

Hospitals are using safety checklists in a lot of ways, too. I'm not talking about pages of check boxes. Maybe five or seven critical things should be checked before we put the ambulance in drive.

The third thing is the right of anybody on the team to speak up without fear of retaliation or ridicule if they think something is unsafe. They are doing this in medicine, too. Traditionally, nurses have been afraid to speak up to surgeons in the OR if they have concerns. Progressive hospitals have put policies in place so that everyone is expected to speak up about their concerns. I guess my next step is to talk to other people, to get some momentum behind this. It sure doesn't do any good for me to just think about these things. I'd really like to see some changes, and I think I can help make them happen.

the front windshield, windows, all mirrors, and blind spots. Drivers must be aware of everything happening outside the ambulance.

The cushion of safety is an area of clear space on each of the four sides of the ambulance that can provide room for error or evasive action. Drivers should ensure that there are no other vehicles within this space, and attempt to clear this space whenever possible.

The front cushion is the easiest to maintain because you are in control of your own vehicle. Simply do not follow other vehicles too closely. If the vehicle in front of you slows or stops suddenly and you hit it, it is your fault. The stopping distance of cars at 30 mph is 106 feet, at 60 mph it is 292 feet. The stopping distance of an ambulance, depending on type and weight, can be up to three times that distance. Keep a two- to four-second following distance, increasing that in inclement weather. When stopping in traffic, be sure to leave enough room in front for you to leave the lane of traffic if necessary.

Detecting vehicles at your side cushions requires constant scanning of your side mirrors. Simple maneuvers, such as speeding up for a few seconds (without exceeding the posted speed limit), slowing down, or changing lanes, can easily clear the cushion of safety on the sides of your vehicle.

Be especially alert for tailgaters. They may be difficult to see because of the blind spot created by the size of your vehicle. The vehicle following too closely may not see traffic ahead and can easily rear-end your ambulance. The most common tailgater is the patient's family. You should instruct the family not to follow the ambulance. This is particularly important if you will be transporting the patient with lights and sirens activated, if you go through a red light, they will, too. Ask the family to leave the scene before the ambulance. Give them directions to the hospital if necessary. When being followed too closely, slow down or move over to allow the vehicle to pass. Never tap your brakes or flash your loading lights at them.

Speed

Speed kills, and ambulance speed is no exception. Speed exponentially increases kinetic energy, greatly increasing crash forces. Speed increases reaction distance and reduces the time available to make evasive maneuvers. Driving too fast for conditions is the primary factor in loss of control of vehicles. Ambulances traveling with lights and sirens are allowed to disregard certain traffic laws, including speed limits. But to reduce the possibility of crashes, operators should cap their speed at 10 mph over the limit, and never exceed 75 mph.

Due Regard

Most states require emergency vehicle operators to drive with **due regard** for the safety of others. This means drivers must have appropriate concern for others on the road.

For example, imagine you are driving to an emergency on a residential street at 40 mph. At this speed, known stopping distance would not allow you to avoid a collision with a vehicle that pulled out of a driveway 100 feet in front of you. Even if the other driver was cited for failure to yield, you did not operate with due regard and are not likely to be protected under state motor vehicle laws.

Emergency Driving

For the most part, everything learned in driver's education classes applies to emergency vehicles. However, there are additional concerns due to the size, weight, and blind spots of an ambulance. For example, to maintain safety:

- *Scan 12–15 seconds ahead.* To find all hazards early, look as far ahead as possible. In urban areas, this is at least one to two blocks. You should be watching for signs such as pedestrians, other vehicle's angled front wheels, turn signals, brake lights, and so on.

- *Avoid other vehicles' blind spots.* Ambulances are larger than many other vehicles on the road, but still can be invisible to inattentive drivers or if you are in another driver's blind spot. Be aware of where you are in relation to other vehicle's blind spots, and try to avoid them.

- *Avoid sudden stops and lane changes.* Pay close attention and prepare early for stops and turns. Last-minute maneuvers are rough on patients and providers in the back, and are unexpected by other drivers. Signal early and be courteous. Allow other vehicles to pass or turn in front of you, and wait for them to allow you to do the same. Remember, your vehicle is a billboard for EMS and for your service. Changing lanes in an ambulance can be difficult. Think ahead and move into turn lanes well in advance of the turn.

- *Smooth ride for patient and crew.* Although modified, ambulances are still trucks and do not provide a smooth ride. Rear occupants are bumped and jolted even with cautious driving. A patient on a backboard or with a fracture will certainly be put in additional pain. Providing a ride that is as smooth as possible requires thought, but is not difficult.

Turns are notorious for causing increasing forces in the patient compartment. Take turns slowly and cautiously. Swinging out to round the corners of turns provides the smoothest ride, but may not be possible at some intersections. If a sharp turn is necessary, proceed very slowly. Due to the length of an ambulance, pull forward far enough to ensure the rear wheels clear the curb. A curb strike can cause significant injury to rear occupants. Any sudden movements of the ambulance are multiplied and felt in the patient compartment.

Avoid sudden movements of the gas and brake pedals, and of the steering wheel. Remove your foot from the pedals slowly, and apply your foot to the pedals slowly. Also, turn the steering wheel slowly and smoothly. When stopping, avoid the jolt of the stop by letting up on the brake pedal slightly just before coming to a complete stop. Lastly, with the ambulance in park, and before removing your foot from the brake pedal, apply the parking brake to avoid the slight roll and jerk of the transmission engaging into the locked position.

Safe Backing

Backing accidents are the most common type of ambulance crash, and often the most costly for ambulance services. Backing should be avoided when possible. Avoid backing into patient's driveways or into parking spaces. The stretcher has wheels and can be used to carry equipment and patients to and from the ambulance. If you must back the ambulance, certain rules must be followed.

■ *Observe your surroundings.* Make sure you know what obstacles, if any, are around your ambulance. This is extremely important if you were not the person who drove the ambulance to its current location. In this case, before getting to the driver's seat, look around the vehicle for obstacles.

■ *Open windows.* This allows you to hear any potential verbal instructions from those outside the vehicle, and may permit you to look further into your blind spot without striking your head on the driver's window.

■ *Use a spotter.* A **spotter** is your partner or other personnel, who directs your backing progress from outside the ambulance. You must never back without a spotter, regardless of the weather or the distance of the travel in reverse. The spotter should position himself at the left rear of the vehicle, visible to the driver in the left side mirror. The spotter must be active and provide specific directions, not just warnings.

■ *Hand signals.* In order to ensure perfect communication with your spotter, you must use hand signals. Many services train employees in universal hand signals or in their own approved signals. You must communicate, and agree on hand signals with your spotter before backing.

■ *Scan mirrors constantly.* You must be able to see the path of your vehicle to avoid a crash, so you constantly scan all mirrors. If you need to look away from your spotter to look at the right side mirror, or evaluate clearance at the front of the vehicle, stop backing up. Continue backing up only when directly visualizing your spotter.

Night Driving

Driving at night reduces your visual acuity. You must adjust your speed and following distance accordingly. Due to the height of your ambulance, oncoming drivers may be temporarily blinded by your headlights. For this reason, you should never activate your high beams when other vehicles are approaching. This includes high beam flashers and emergency lights during emergency responses at night.

Highway Driving

Highway or freeway driving involves high speed and high risk. Crashes may be less common on freeways but they frequently result in fatalities. It is extremely important to monitor your speed, and drive with due regard. Increase your following distance, especially in high traffic areas or adverse weather conditions. You should be scanning far ahead; 12 to 15 seconds now becomes a half mile. Using the center lane of freeways may be smoother, and may allow you to avoid extremely slow and extremely fast drivers. The force of sudden movements will be multiplied at high speeds, so remember to change lanes slowly and smoothly. A six-second lane change is recommended. If it is necessary to pass another vehicle, do not do it with a sudden acceleration or exceed the speed limit in the process.

Emergency Response and Use of Warning Devices

Although emergency driving is exciting and a draw for many adrenaline seekers, it is the most deadly part of an EMS provider's job. Most crashes happen during **emergency responses**. In fact, you are five times more likely to be involved in a collision as compared to **nonemergency responses**. There are two primary reasons for this increased risk: civilian driver confusion and ambulance operator adrenaline. There is some evidence that the use of sirens actually causes the driver to increase speed.

Adrenaline and Emotions

With emergency driving, the dispatch information can be the source of inattentive emotional driving. When responding to a call for a child ejected in a motor vehicle collision, you will drive differently than you would to an elderly patient with a headache. This is human nature. Awareness is the key. Be aware of your emotions and your actions while driving. Be aware of your speed. Check the speedometer. Chances are you are driving faster than you realize. Always drive safely, cautiously, and with due regard, regardless of the call type.

Lights and Sirens

Most state laws allow emergency vehicles with *both* visual and audible warning devices activated to exceed the posted speed limit, disregard a traffic control device, and drive against the flow of traffic. However, you must still drive with due regard for the safety of others on or near the road. This includes coming to a complete stop before proceeding through a stop sign or red light.

If you are found to be at fault for an ambulance crash, you will likely be held personally liable. The fact that you are a professional care provider en route to an emergency will not protect you. Your employer will likely not protect you. Providers are increasingly being held legally responsible for crashes. Many providers have been convicted of charges such as traffic violations, reckless driving, and even involuntary manslaughter and vehicular homicide, as a result of ambulance crashes.

Emergency responses are considered either emergent or nonemergent. Warning lights and sirens are not used on nonemergent calls. Responding to emergency calls or transporting critical patients carry the expectation that your response time or transport time will be expedited. Therefore, you must use warning lights and sirens to alert other drivers that you are requesting the right of way. Many state laws prohibit a "lights only" response, requiring that both lights and sirens be used on emergency responses. Remember: The purpose of lights and sirens are to make the ambulance conspicuous, and to ask other drivers to pull over and let you pass. Warning devices do not give permission to drive fast, and they do not guarantee you a clear path through traffic. Many drivers are distracted, not paying attention, or unable to hear the siren. Do not assume other vehicles will yield or pull over, just be thankful for the ones that do. An important aspect of emergency response is not necessarily to be fast, but to be smooth. In a smooth emergency response, your ambulance will be able to avoid much of the stop and go of normal traffic flow and proceed relatively unimpeded to your destination.

Improvements to EMS systems, such as **system status management (SSM)** and **medical priority dispatch systems (MPDS)**, serve to limit the number and distance of emergency responses. When transporting a patient to the hospital, the decision to use lights and siren is made by the Advanced EMT in charge of patient care. Reserve emergency transports for patients with truly life-threatening or unstable conditions. The driver also has responsibility in this decision. After all, the driver is ultimately responsible for the safe operation of the vehicle, and has the greatest sense of road and traffic conditions. If for any reason, during an emergent response or transport, the driver senses a safety risk, he or she has the right to downgrade to nonemergent driving. Once the risk has subsided, the response can be upgraded again to emergency driving. The following are examples of when to downgrade emergency driving:

- *When traffic has nowhere to go.* If the vehicles you are approaching are unable to pull to the right and stop, you should not be asking them to try. This may cause panic and frustration in drivers and cause them to make dangerous maneuvers. You may encounter this situation in construction zones or on narrow rural roads.

- *When approaching a blocked intersection at a red light.* A blocked intersection is one where all lanes in your direction of travel are occupied by a stopped vehicle. In order for the vehicles to pull to the right to let you through, they would need to pull forward, into the intersection. This is essentially "pushing" vehicles into the intersection, and must not be done to avoid putting them in the path of cross traffic. If the lanes of your travel are separated from oncoming traffic by a double yellow line, your service may allow you to cross over, into the oncoming traffic lanes and oppose traffic or travel against the flow of traffic. This procedure can be extremely dangerous, and may not be permitted by some EMS services. The safest method, or the only method when there is a solid median separating traffic, is the following: Upon realizing the upcoming intersection is blocked, the driver should immediately downgrade to nonemergent driving, and wait with the other traffic until the light turns green. After the light turns green, it will be safe for the then-moving vehicles to safely pull to the right. Return to emergency mode, and proceed safely through the intersection.

- *When entering or exiting a freeway.* If an ambulance responding emergently is entering a freeway by way of an on-ramp, vehicles correctly pulling to the right will be entering the path of the ambulance. The ambulance should employ nonemergency driving upon entering the on-ramp, proceed onto the freeway, signal as usual to advance into the far left lane, then return to emergency response mode. The same applies to exiting the freeway by way of a right-side exit ramp. Exiting using emergency driving will be asking vehicles to pull to the right, into your path. Downgrade to nonemergency driving, signal your intentions, proceed to the right, and enter the ramp. Once safely on the exit ramp, return to emergency mode.

- *When approaching school zones and school buses.* Children are fascinated with emergency vehicles and are eager to see them pass by. They may run toward the lights and siren, disregarding their surroundings and putting themselves at risk. Therefore, when responding through a school zone, you should downgrade to nonemergency driving. Once you are through the school zone and clear of children, return to emergency status. The situation is similar when passing a school bus that is stopped with its lights flashing. Downgrade to nonemergency driving and stop as all vehicles should. Once all children are clear and the bus has turned off its lights, you may return to emergency driving and pass the bus. Some services may allow emergency vehicles to stop behind the school bus with only their emergency lights on, to alert the school bus driver of the emergency response. In this case, wait for the bus driver to signal you to pass before you proceed. Once clear of the bus, return to emergency driving.

Always Pass on the Left

When traveling in emergency mode, you are asking other vehicles to pull to the right and stop. Therefore, you should always be passing them on the left. Civilian drivers often receive mixed messages from emergency vehicles. They may have seen other emergency responders go around vehicles to the right, or travel down the center of traffic, or pass on the right shoulder. This leads to civilian driver confusion, and an increased risk of a crash. A civilian driver may suddenly remember his driver education course, and pull abruptly to the right into the path of an ambulance passing on the right.

You must be consistent, and communicate your intentions clearly. Your ambulance should always be positioned in the far left lane or at the far left side of the road. If a vehicle in your lane slows down or pulls left to let you pass, remain behind it, do not pass on the right (Figure 5-9). Make sure your intention to pass on the left is clear. Pull as far to the left as possible, increase your audible warnings by changing the siren tone or activating the horn. The vehicle should get the idea and pull to the right. If the civilian driver still refuses to do the right thing, pass them slowly and cautiously on the right, being alert for him to move suddenly to the right at any time. After any move from the left lane, such as passing a vehicle or turning right, always immediately return to the left lane.

Emergency Patient Transportation

Driving emergently with a patient onboard is a particularly stressful and dangerous situation. The patient will be seriously ill or injured and unstable. In these cases, there may be one or more EMTs caring for the patient, in various positions, attempting to perform treatment. Smooth emergency driving is imperative to reduce the chance of provider and patient injury. It is also important for emergency vehicle operators to have their attention on the road, and not on the patient care occurring behind them.

Intersections

Intersections are the most dangerous place for emergency vehicles. Most crashes occur there. It is extremely important to always use safe intersection practices. Varying the tone of the siren can increase other driver's awareness of your presence at intersections. When traveling emergently through an intersection with a green light, you should be at or below the posted speed limit, with your foot covering the brake pedal. When proceeding through a red traffic light, *you must first come to a complete stop.* When the intersection is clear, proceed slowly and cautiously through. A clear intersection is one in which all lanes are either blocked by a stopped vehicle or not occupied at all. If the intersection has multiple lanes, treat each lane as a separate intersection. Come to a complete stop at the intersection and evaluate all lanes. Proceed only across clear lanes, stopping before any unclear lane until you are sure it is clear. Do this for each unclear lane. When the last lane is clear, proceed as usual. If all lanes are clear, proceed slowly and cautiously across all lanes (Figure 5-10).

The provider in the passenger seat should assist the driver by evaluating the lanes on the right side of the intersection. The assistant should give a verbal signal such as "all clear" or "clear right" when all lanes are clear. Be careful to avoid communicating with words that could be misinterpreted, the word "no" can be heard as "go." Even with assistance from a partner, the driver should never proceed forward without first looking.

Following Other Emergency Vehicles

Multiple emergency vehicles traveling together to a scene should be avoided. Civilian drivers may hear sirens and mistakenly believe that one emergency vehicle is approaching. They may pull over, and then after the first vehicle has passed, pull back into the lane, into the path of the second

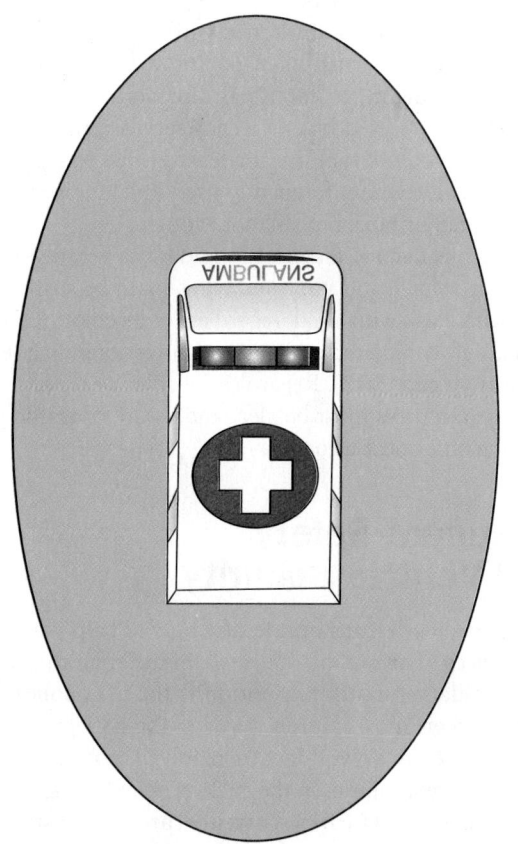

FIGURE 5-9

Cushion of safety. This shows distance that should be maintained between ambulance and other vehicles.

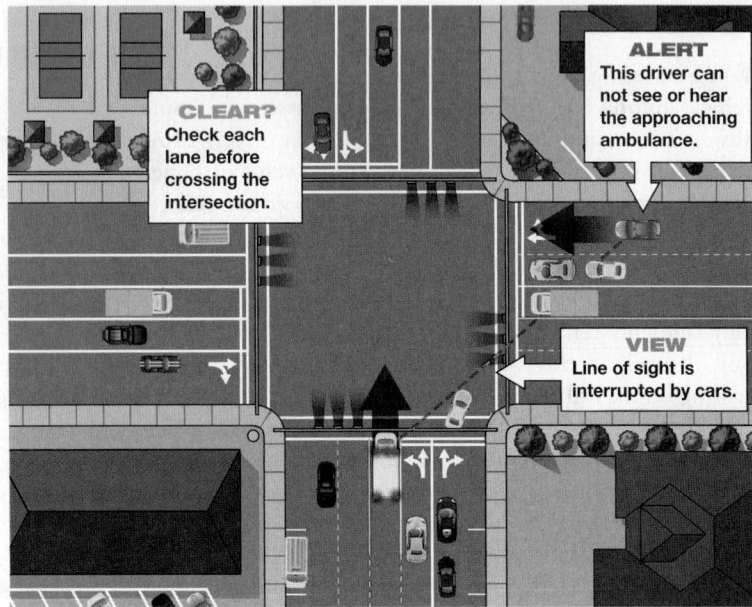

FIGURE 5-10

Clear each lane of traffic as you proceed through an intersection.

emergency vehicle. When traveling with other units, be sure to leave enough space between vehicles so that it is obvious there is more than one. If possible, avoid the situation entirely by taking a slightly different route.

Parking on the Scene

Parking on scene is an extremely important part of the safety of an EMS response. Emergency vehicles must be positioned to permit the best access to patients, while providing a safe location for all in and around them. A vehicle crashing into a parked ambulance with a patient and providers inside or nearby can cause a multitude of injuries or fatalities. As discussed earlier, backing up to park should be avoided. Remember, the stretcher and equipment can be rolled or carried to the patient, and the patient can be rolled or carried to the ambulance. As you approach the scene, evaluate the surroundings for the best location to park the vehicle. At a residence, it should be as close as possible to the front door, driveway, or sidewalk.

On a highway it gets a little more complicated. The safest place is on the same side of the road, ahead of the scene, off the road, with an obstacle between the ambulance and traffic (Figure 5-11). The larger the obstacle, the better. Examples include a fire truck, a police car, or the crash vehicles themselves. In this position, the back doors of the ambulance are easily accessible for providers and patients. It also allows for easy egress, or exit, when leaving the scene. In the event you are the first to arrive, and the crash scene is exposed to traffic, you may wish to park behind it to protect patients and providers on scene. Position your ambulance well before the scene to provide a buffer zone, and turn the wheels to prevent it from being pushed into the scene in the event it is struck from behind. Vehicles arriving later should

be positioned as an obstacle to protect the ambulance, or the ambulance should be moved as soon as possible.

Even when parked appropriately on scene, ambulances and providers can be struck by passing vehicles. This is a common cause of provider injuries and fatalities. EMS providers must always be concerned with the visibility of their vehicles and uniforms when positioned near roadways, especially at night. Research has discovered that the most common colors used by emergency services, red and blue, are the two colors that are the least visible to the human eye. The color white, frequently used in EMS, is more visible than red or blue, but still not enough.

Retro-reflective material provides the greatest visibility. Your vehicle and your uniform should be striped with this highly visible material, regardless of its color. Reflective vests are now required for any person working on a federal highway (Figure 5-12). Regardless of color or reflective material, you always must be alert and aware of traffic when working on or near a roadway.

Occupant Safety and Vehicle Security

The preceding lessons in safe driving will help you reduce the chances of an ambulance crash. In the event that a crash is unavoidable, injury prevention is the next concern. As stated earlier, most injuries occur in the patient compartment. There are several factors involved in understanding how to prevent injuries in the back of ambulances.

Unfortunately, there currently are no construction, safety, or crash test standards for U.S. ambulances. The standards that apply to all other motor vehicles, Federal Motor Vehicle Safety Standards (FMVSS), do not apply to the back of ambulances. In ambulances, everything from

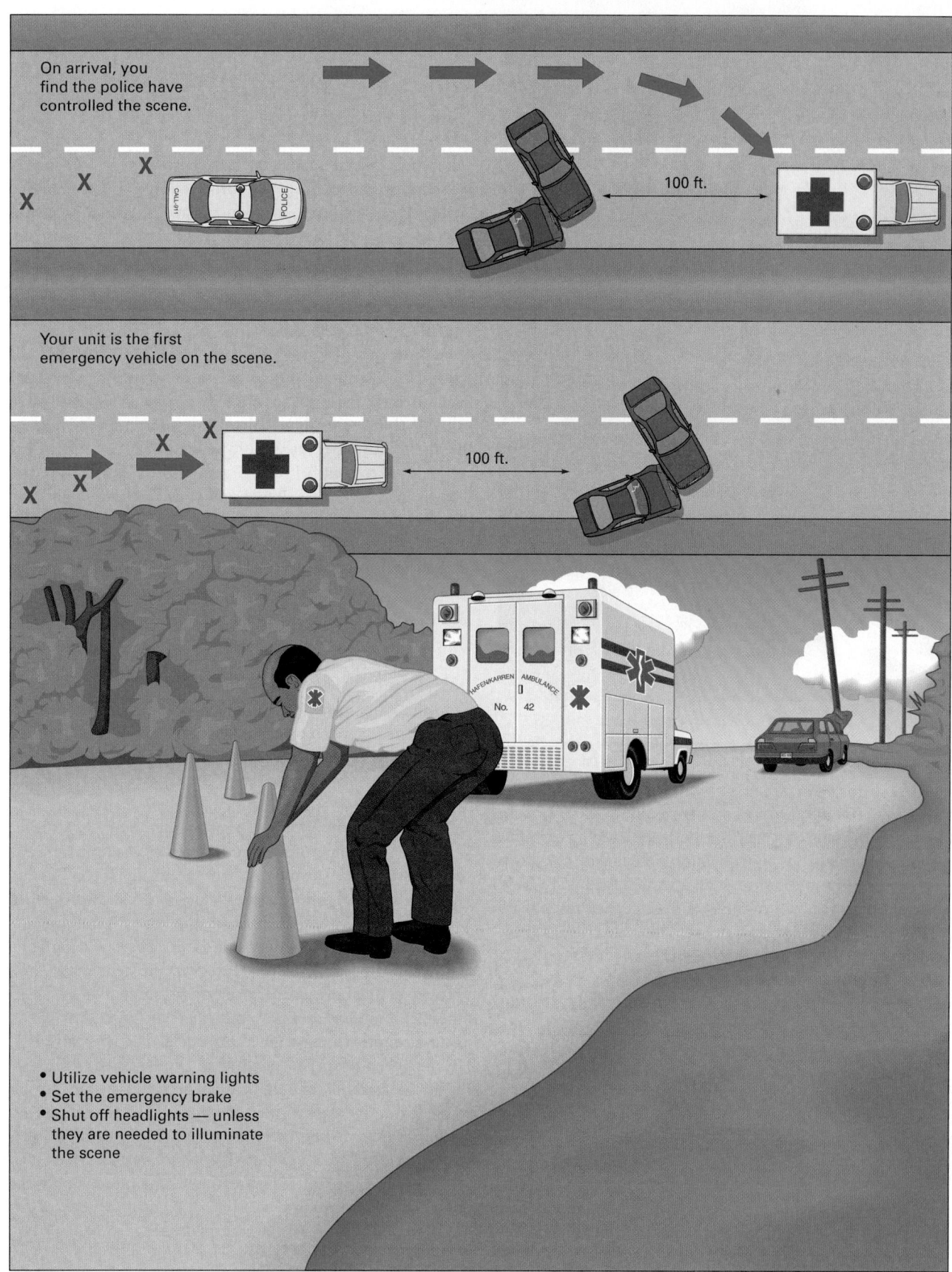

On arrival, you find the police have controlled the scene.

100 ft.

Your unit is the first emergency vehicle on the scene.

100 ft.

- Utilize vehicle warning lights
- Set the emergency brake
- Shut off headlights — unless they are needed to illuminate the scene

FIGURE 5-11

Proper parking position at roadway scenes.

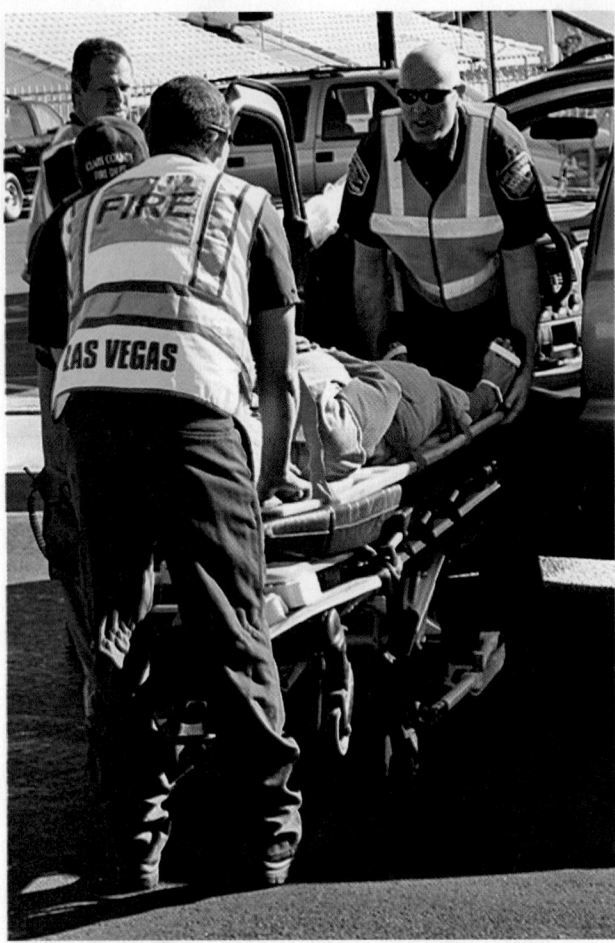

FIGURE 5-12

A safety vest with retro-reflective material. (© Daniel Limmer)

stable wall or cabinet. This includes all small loose supplies, oxygen tanks, cardiac monitors, and suction units.

All occupants must be appropriately restrained at all times while the vehicle is in motion. Patients must be secured to the stretcher with at least three safety belts, including a shoulder harness. Belts alone will not prevent patients from being ejected from the stretcher. If the shoulder harness interferes with a procedure such as an ECG, remove it for the procedure, and then replace it. Stretcher manufacturers include harnesses with their stretchers because the harnesses have been proven to eliminate patient ejection from stretchers. Also, ensure that the stretcher is locked into place, and that the stretcher mounts are securely affixed to the floor of the ambulance.

Providers also must be appropriately restrained at all times. Unrestrained providers are injuring themselves, as well as their patients, in ambulance crashes. Studies have shown that fewer than half of providers report wearing seatbelts during transport. In reality, very few providers regularly wear seatbelts. This trend must change. As future Advanced EMTs, you must begin your career the right way and set an example for others. If you regularly wear your seat belt in your car, why would you not wear it in your ambulance? It is a motor vehicle, traveling on the same roads, but with an increased risk of crashes and injuries. Being properly restrained is the best way to protect yourself and your patient from injury.

In most situations you should plan your patient care so that it is primarily done on scene. Once you begin transport, you should be properly restrained for the duration. If treatment is necessary en route, unbelt and provide care. As soon as treatment is complete, fasten your safety belt again.

10 inches behind the driver's seat is exempt from those standards. Manufacturers construct the ambulance box modification primarily from plywood and sheet metal. They then test the integrity of the box with a static test, by lowering a weight onto the roof of the box. This type of test has no bearing on how the box will perform in a real crash. In fact, dynamic tests, like crash tests, have proven that these boxes cannot withstand real-world crash forces.

Manufacturers claim their ambulances are safe, but very few have actually been dynamically crash tested. Until the federal government or other body develops ambulance standards, providers need to be extra vigilant about reducing injuries in the event of a crash.

Restraints

The single most important factor in reducing injuries in ambulance crashes is proper restraint of occupants and equipment. The large open area of the patient compartment allows loose objects to become deadly projectiles. This includes loose occupants. Everything in the back of an ambulance must be properly secured.

All equipment must be either stored in a cabinet that can be latched closed, or securely fastened to a structurally

Seating Positions

The safest seating position in the back of the ambulance is on the stretcher. The most dangerous position is on the side facing the bench seat. A side-facing seat is not present in any other motor vehicle, because it is not safe and not permitted under federal safety standards. Therefore, patients should not be transported seated on the bench seat, and providers must always be properly restrained when seated there. Manufacturers now offer nets at the end of bench seats to capture unrestrained providers. The nets can be effective when properly constructed and installed. Arm rests or partial walls should not be used, because they are responsible for an increase in hip, abdomen, and kidney injuries. A few manufacturers offer the ultimate in provider safety: a forward-facing attendant seat. Crash tests have proven that forward- or rear-facing seating configurations offer the best crash protection.

A child must never be transported in a caregiver's lap. Children must always be properly restrained. Children need increased crash protection in cars and the back of the ambulance is no different. If a child is at an age where he would be in a car seat, he needs to be in a car seat in an ambulance. When possible, use the child's own car seat; he will be more comfortable and it is already properly sized and adjusted. When using the patient's car seat, it must be securely attached to the stretcher or captain's chair. It should *never* be attached to the side-facing bench seat. It may help to secure the seat to the stretcher when it is empty. You can kneel into it while securing it, to ensure it is held tightly.

If the child's car seat is not available, you must provide one. A car seat should be standard equipment in your ambulance. Several manufacturers offer a child seat integrated into the rear-facing attendant seat or "captain's chair." These seats have not been tested by the automotive industry and may not be as safe, but they are very convenient and far safer than a small child secured to a large stretcher or in a parent's lap.

Carbon Monoxide in Ambulances

One final safety concern for EMS providers is carbon monoxide (CO). EMTs are at an increased risk of exposure to this potentially deadly gas because they frequently work in and around motor vehicles. CO is a colorless, odorless, and tasteless product of combustion. In the EMS environment, it could come from the ambulance exhaust; the exhaust of other vehicles nearby, such as fire engines; and from any gasoline, diesel, kerosene, or propane-powered vehicles or equipment, such as power saws or generators. You should be familiar with the symptoms of carbon monoxide exposure, such as headache, dizziness, nausea, and vomiting. If anyone in or near your ambulance experiences the symptoms of CO poisoning, immediately remove them from the ambulance to an area free from exhaust, and administer high-flow oxygen. (CO poisoning is discussed in detail in Chapter 32.)

The following are recommendations to prevent or reduce CO exposure:

- Ensure your ambulance has appropriate preventive maintenance, including tune-ups.
- Ensure vehicle exhaust exits beyond the side of the vehicle, not under it.
- Keep ambulance windows shut.
- Ensure that all doors and windows close tightly.
- Cover any opening to the outside, such as vents.
- Keep the heater or air conditioner on at all times. This creates continuous interior positive pressure.
- Do not use fuel-powered supplemental equipment inside the ambulance.

Carbon monoxide testers and monitors are available, and should be used to protect patients and providers from this deadly gas.

Operational Security

Recent incidents of domestic terrorism have prompted additional security measures for EMS personnel. There is a potential risk for ambulances to be stolen and used to gain access to protected or sensitive areas. To reduce this risk, the National Association of Emergency Medical Technicians (NAEMT) has established recommended guidelines for improved safety and security of EMS vehicles.

- Security briefings should be conducted prior to the start of shifts. They may be meetings, information sheets, or postings.
- EMS crews need to be well informed of, and should participate in, the development of operational security measures.
- EMS vehicles should be tracked at all times, including out-of-service vehicles. Random audits should be performed to account for all vehicles.
- EMS vehicles should not be left running or unattended with the key in the vehicle.
- Out-of-service vehicles should be properly secured to eliminate access to unauthorized persons. Audits should be conducted to account for these vehicles.
- A key log must be kept to account for all keys to restricted buildings and vehicles. Keys that are not accounted for should be considered a security breach.
- Ensure that vehicles off premises for repairs or other reasons are properly secured.
- Vehicles that are to be permanently out of service should have all EMS markings and warning devices removed.
- EMS patches, badges, and ID cards must be safeguarded against theft and unauthorized distribution.
- EMS badges and ID cards should be counterfeit resistant and include a photo of the bearer.
- EMS uniforms must be sold only to authorized EMS personnel.

Scene Size-Up

Scene size-up is your initial evaluation of the unique situation you are about to encounter. This initial evaluation gives you both operational and patient assessment information. The operational purposes of scene size-up are:

- To determine the general nature of the situation
- To determine the safety of the situation for you, your team, the patient, and the public
- To determine the number of patients
- To determine if additional resources are required to deal with the situation

One of the biggest mistakes an EMS provider can make is to fail to perform an adequate scene size-up. Failing to size up the scene can result in injury or death to you, your partner, or the patient from a variety of hazards. You may fail to find additional patients, causing a delay in their care or causing them to be overlooked completely. Failure to take a moment to assess the need for additional resources can result in delays of critical assistance in securing the safety of the scene, extrication, lifting, or transportation of patients.

EMS situations are dynamic. A situation that seemed to be safe can deteriorate for many reasons. The scene size-up begins before patient contact and continues throughout the call. Consider the following in the scene size-up: nature of the situation, scene safety, number of patients, additional resources, and, to a certain degree, patient assessment.

Nature of the Situation

Dispatch information provides a general idea of the nature of the call. However, keep in mind that the dispatcher can only give you information received from the caller. The situation may involve elements other than those shared by the caller, so avoid getting tunnel vision about the nature of the call. Use the dispatch information and initial information gathered as you approach the scene to determine the general **nature of the illness** or **mechanism of injury (MOI)**. The nature of the illness or MOI helps you start anticipating how you will approach the scene, what additional resources you may need, what hazards may be present, and how you will assess and manage your patient. Many other clues can be observed while determining the nature of the situation. You may discover that a patient is living in a house without electricity, or that he appears to be unable to care for himself. These observations can be useful in helping you determine the patient's story and how you can best help him.

Scene Safety

An injured EMS provider cannot care for patients and takes additional resources away from the original situation. Regardless of the nature of the call or what you see or hear as you approach the scene, you must never rush in without

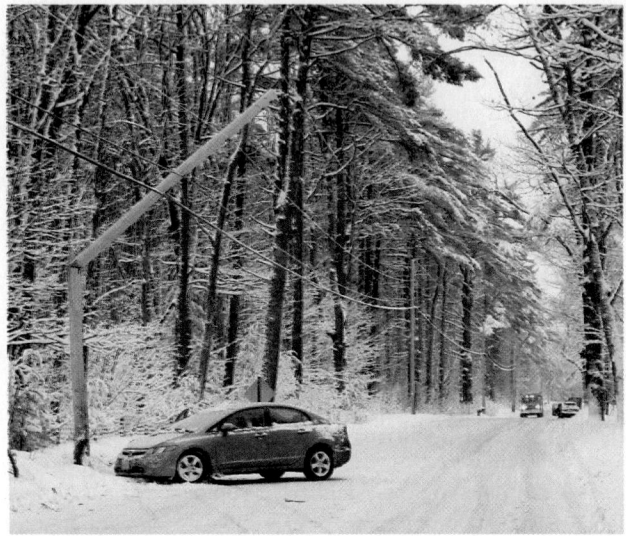

FIGURE 5-13

Assess the safety of the scene. (© Daniel Limmer)

making an assessment of potential dangers at the scene (Figure 5-13). Start thinking about the location and nature of the call before you arrive. Think about the potential hazards of roadway incidents and issues anticipated in certain neighborhoods and on certain types of calls. Think about the level of personal protective equipment (PPE) you should anticipate. Then as you arrive on the scene, check your suspicions, and be alert to other potential hazards. What do you see, hear, or smell? Look at the big picture, and scan around 360 degrees. Is there anything that could potentially be unsafe for anyone involved? If the scene is not safe and cannot be made safe without risking harm to yourself, your partner, or the patient, do not approach the scene. Request the resources needed to make the scene safe. If a patient or bystander poses a threat to you, stay in the ambulance or return to it and request law enforcement assistance. If you smell an odor of natural gas in a business or residence, do not enter and request the fire department and gas company to investigate. If you see downed electrical lines, avoid them and call the power company to assist.

Number of Patients

You may end up with more than one patient in a number of circumstances. It is not unusual for a family member of the critically ill patient you are caring for to faint or have chest pain. Violent situations often result in more than one person being injured. Motor vehicle collisions (MVCs) very often involve more than one patient. A call for a sick person in an office building may turn into an MCI if the cause of the initial patient's symptoms is a chemical leak or similar problem. Determine if you have only one patient, or if there are multiple patients. Look around, ask your patient, or ask witnesses or bystanders. Pay particular attention to vehicle crashes, account for each empty seat (including empty child seats), because patients may have walked away or been

IN THE FIELD

Crime scenes, including domestic violence scenes, and calls involving behavioral emergencies pose an increased risk for violence against EMS providers. Signs of agitation include an increasing volume of speech, pacing, shouting, anger, frustration, hitting or kicking things, making threats, and profanity. Always stay between the potentially violent person and a way out. If you cannot de-escalate the situation and law enforcement has not yet arrived, leave the scene until it can be made safe.

ejected. If the number of patients and the nature of their illnesses or injuries exceed your abilities to adequately care for and transport them, request additional transporting units.

Additional Resources

The presence of hazards, multiple patients, patients in need of specialized rescue, and other situations evaluated in the scene size-up tell you what additional resources you need. Additional resources may include more ambulances, advanced life support, police, fire department, heavy rescue, air medical transportation, electrical power or gas company, or animal control. Request these resources as soon as you know you need assistance.

Patient Assessment Aspects of Scene Size-Up

Information from the operational phases of scene size-up is combined with your initial impression when you first see the patient and the patient's **chief complaint**. When you first make contact with the patient, you are trying to get a general idea of how sick he is in order to make decisions about your next steps. The patient assessment aspects of the scene size-up are discussed in detail in Chapter 15.

Lifting and Moving Patients

An operational aspect of nearly every EMS call is the need to lift and move patients and carry equipment. These activities pose a risk of injury to both you and the patient if performed improperly. (Body mechanics were discussed in Chapter 3.) Proper lifting techniques are one of the keys to protecting the longevity of your career. Lifting-related injuries often include the back, resulting in both short-term and long-term disability. Beyond prematurely ending your career in EMS, chronic back pain can significantly impact your quality of life in other ways. Patients may need to be moved immediately to avoid further harm (**emergency moves**) or as a routine part of preparing the patient for transport (**nonemergency moves**). A variety of techniques and equipment are used to lift and move patients emergently and nonemergently. Proper lifting techniques and skilled use of the proper equipment for each situation are important aspects of patient safety. Dropping a patient can result in serious injury or death, and is a source of liability for EMS providers.

Back Safety

As an EMT you are committed to care for and protect your patients, and ensure they are transported safely to their destination. Before you can do that, you need to guarantee your own safety. You need to come home each day, safe and uninjured, to enjoy a long and satisfying career. Injury prevention must be a priority in your daily responsibilities.

So, before lifting, know your personal limit, and do not be afraid to request additional help. Never let your ego cause you to injure yourself or your patient.

When lifting with an assistant, be sure to communicate throughout the lift. Plan the lift, including who will lead or initiate the lift, and how it will be directed (1–2–3-lift, or 1–2-lift on 3). Proper lifting techniques include: planting your feet shoulder distance apart, positioning hands with palms foreword, lifting with your legs not your back, and never leaning or twisting as you lift. Practice those techniques to ensure they become habits. Specialized techniques and equipment are used to prevent injury to providers and patients and provide comfort to patients in different lifting situations.

Equipment and Techniques Used to Lift and Move Patients

The most common piece of equipment used to move patients is the wheeled ambulance stretcher. Ambulance stretcher design has evolved over the years to require less lifting and support greater patient weight. You must be familiar with the type of stretcher used in your service. Know how to release the stretcher from its locking mechanism in the patient compartment, how to ensure the stretcher is in locked position to prevent it from collapsing under the weight of the patient, know how to lower and raise the stretcher, and how to place it in the back of the ambulance and lock it into place. You also must know how to change the position of the stretcher to elevate the patient's head or feet, and know how to brake the wheels. Use a power grip and power lift (Figure 5-14) or squat lift (Figure 5-15) to lift the stretcher.

A variety of techniques can be used to place a patient on the stretcher, depending on the circumstances. These include the draw sheet method, direct ground lift, extremity lift, and direct carry methods. Position the patient according to his condition and comfort. Most noncritical medical patients are placed in **Fowler's position** (head of the stretcher greater than 45 degrees) (Figure 5-16) or **semi-Fowler's position** (head of the stretcher between 30 and 45 degrees). Patients with respiratory distress usually prefer Fowler's position. Unresponsive patients without spinal trauma who are breathing adequately can be placed in the **recovery (left**

IN THE FIELD

There is a risk of injury for both EMS providers and patients while lifting and moving patients. To minimize chances of injury, be thoroughly familiar with the operation of all lifting and moving devices used in your service. Properly secure patients using the safety straps (or other features) intended for use with each device. Follow the principles of safe lifting and moving, including using an adequate amount of help. Communicate with your patient and lifting partners. Never leave a patient unattended on a device used for lifting and moving.

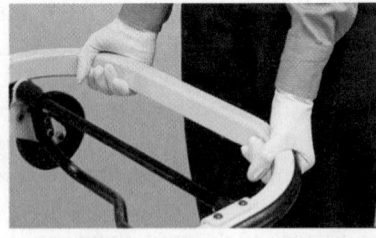

(A)

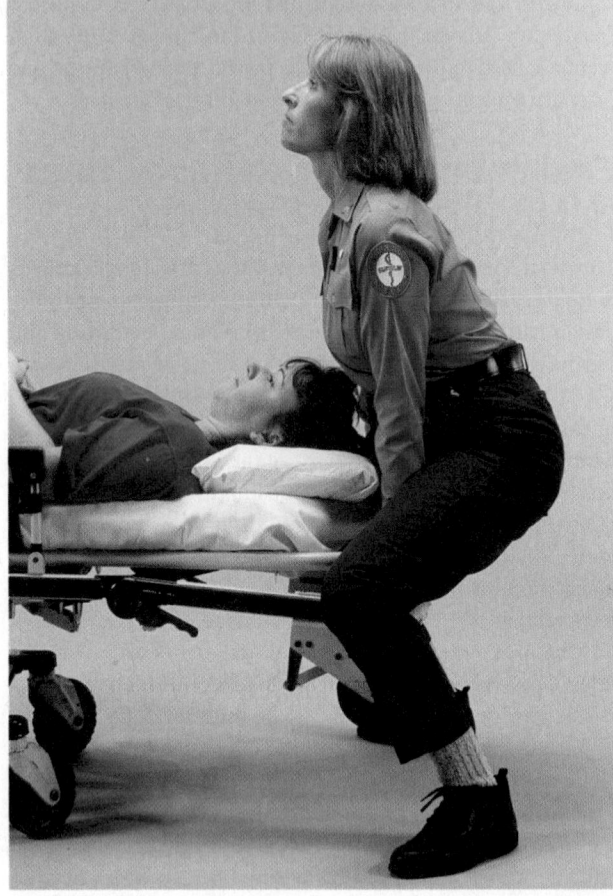

(B)

FIGURE 5-14

(A) Using a power grip and (B) a power lift.

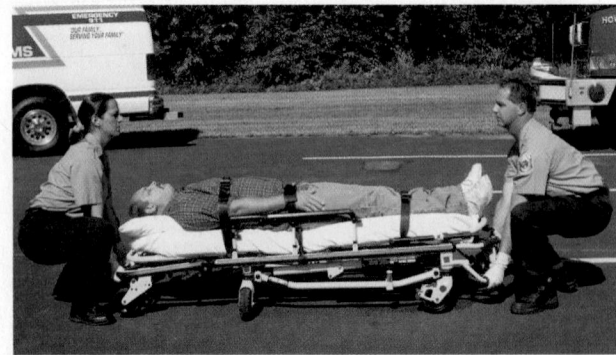

FIGURE 5-15

Squat-lift technique.

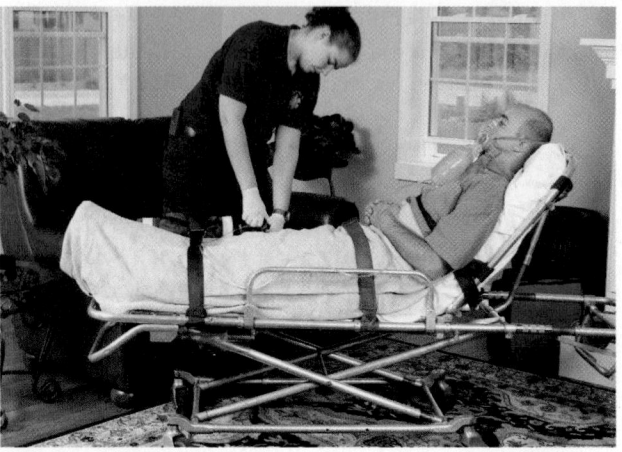

FIGURE 5-16

Fowler's position.

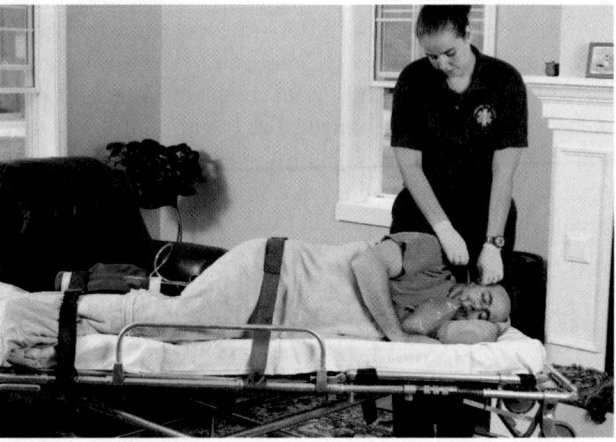

FIGURE 5-17

Recovery position.

lateral recumbent) position (Figure 5-17) to assist in maintaining an open airway. Patients with abdominal discomfort may prefer to lie in a lateral recumbent position with the legs drawn up to relieve tension on the abdominal muscles and reduce pain. By necessity, patients who are immobilized to a long backboard will be supine. However, if necessary, a folded towel or blanket can be used to elevate the head of the backboard (for example, in a patient with difficulty breathing). This may be particularly useful in elderly patients, who may have a difficult time lying flat due to the effects of chronic illnesses. Patients in the third trimester of pregnancy must not be placed in a supine position. If they must be placed on a backboard, use a folded blanket or towels under the right side of the board to slightly tip it to the left.

It is important to communicate with all patients when positioning them for transport. Communication is particularly important when positioning patients with a physical disability. Consider the patient's comfort, his chronic conditions, and acute condition when selecting a position for transport.

Patients with inadequate perfusion are placed in a **supine** position to maximize circulation to the vital organs.

Shock (Trendelenburg) position is no longer recommended. In the past, it was thought that lowering the patient's head and elevating the lower extremities would increase blood flow to the vital organs. However, since the peripheral vasculature is already maximally constricted in shock, it is unlikely that blood from the lower extremities is returned to the central circulation. In addition, and more concerning, placing a patient in this position causes the abdominal organs to move upward, which restricts the motion of the diaphragm. This, in turn, compromises ventilation in a patient who needs all of the ventilatory capacity he has. In some cases, such as when shock is caused by vasodilation, it may be beneficial to place a rolled towel or blanket under the patient's feet to elevate them no more than 12 inches.

Cover the patient with a sheet and, as conditions dictate, a blanket. Always secure the patient using the safety straps on the stretcher (placed over the sheet and blanket, so you can access them), and put the side rails up after you have positioned the patient on the stretcher. Take care that you do not pinch the patient's arms or hands when raising and lowering the side rails. Never leave a patient unattended on a stretcher. When possible, move the stretcher so that the patient is looking in the direction you are moving him, instead of facing backward. When going up or down steps, the patient should be facing the top of the steps, not the bottom, so that he does not slide toward the foot of the stretcher (Figure 5-18). Walk forward (not backward) when pushing the stretcher, whenever possible. When going up or down steps, it is usually necessary for the provider at one end of the stretcher to walk backward. You must always move slowly and use a spotter when walking backward. Communicate with the patient about the moves and lifts you will be doing. Sudden, unexpected movements can cause the patient to shift his position and the stretcher can become unbalanced and tip. The wheels on ambulance stretchers are not intended for rough terrain or surfaces. Look where you are going when pushing the stretcher to avoid bumps and holes that cause the stretcher to tip.

After each call, clean the stretcher mattress with an approved disinfectant solution and allow it to dry. If the mattress cover is torn, cut, or punctured, the mattress must be replaced, because the damaged cover will allow blood and body fluids to seep into the mattress cushion, which cannot be cleaned. Clean any soiled parts of the stretcher frame as needed, and use an approved disinfectant for any part of the frame that is contaminated with blood or body fluids. Remove, clean, and disinfect contaminated straps. Place clean linens on the stretcher for your next patient.

Portable stretchers (Figure 5-19) are seldom used in routine situations, but may be useful in MCIs or when the terrain over which the patient must be carried makes the use of a wheeled stretcher difficult or dangerous. Scoop baskets or stretchers (Figure 5-20) also are useful in these situations. An advantage to a scoop stretcher is that the two sides can be separated, placed under the patient, and locked back into place so that the patient does not have to be log rolled or lifted onto the device. Another advantage is that the contours of the device minimize patient movement during lifting and carrying.

Long backboards are used for spinal immobilization (Chapter 40), but also are useful devices for lifting and moving patients in other circumstances (Scan 5-1). If the patient is to remain on the backboard during transport, you must

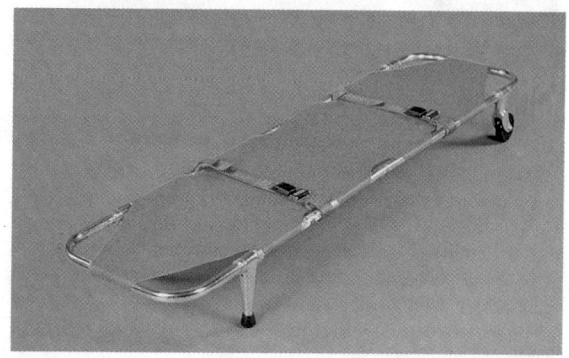

FIGURE 5-19

A portable stretcher.

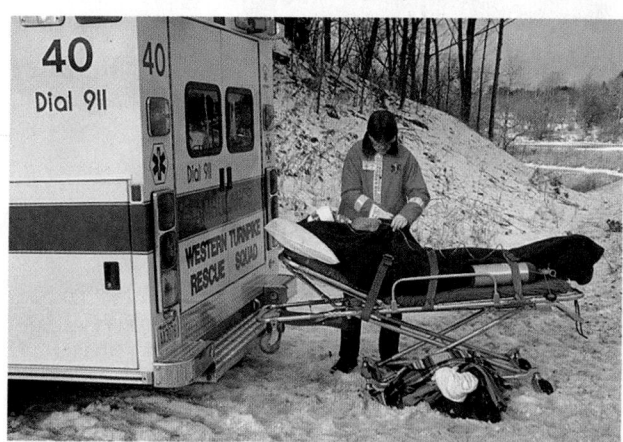

FIGURE 5-18

Position the patient on the stretcher with straps secured and side rails raised. Never leave the patient unattended.

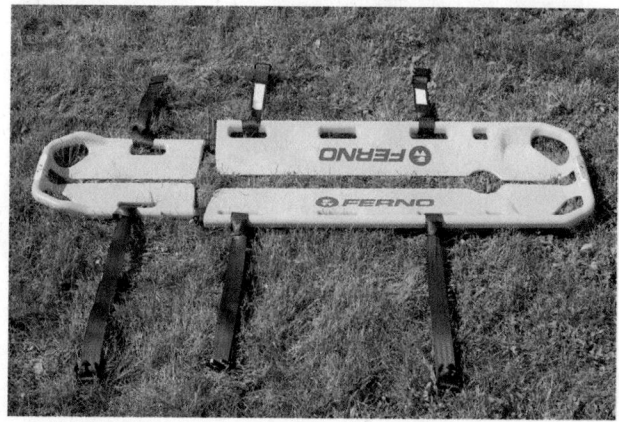

FIGURE 5-20

A scoop stretcher.

Log Roll onto a Long Backboard

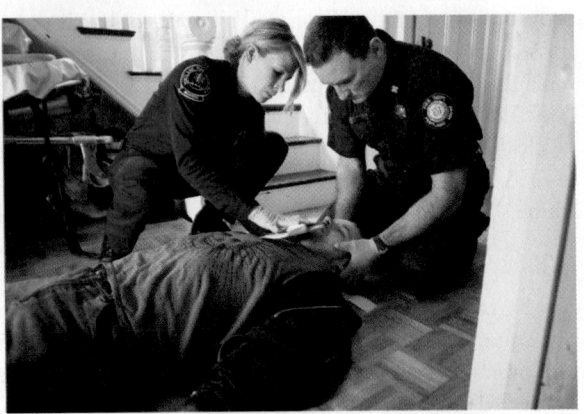

1. If spine injury is suspected, ensure that a cervical collar is in place prior to the log roll. Ensure that one EMS provider manually stabilizes the patient's head and neck.

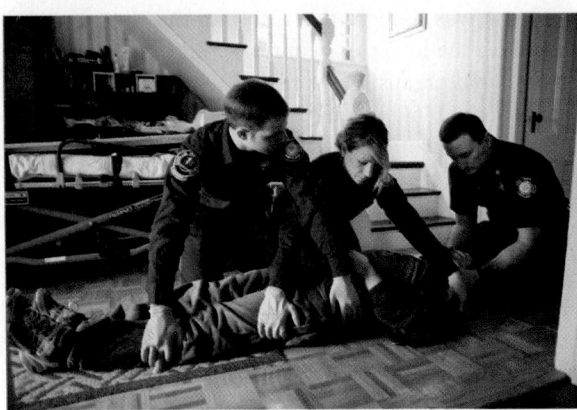

2. Providers must be positioned to support the patient at the head, torso, and legs during the log roll.

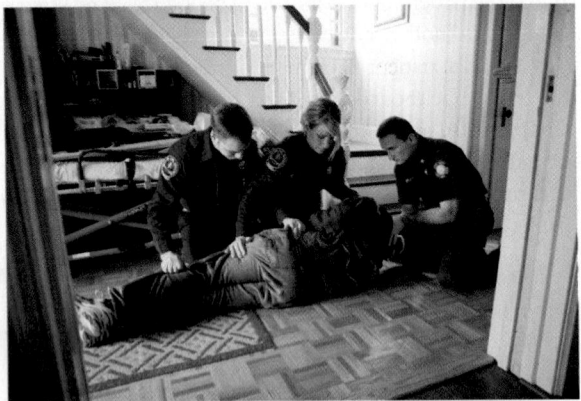

3. The EMS provider at the patient's head instructs the assistants to roll the patient on his command (for example, "Roll on the count of three. One. Two. Three). The patient is rolled toward the providers' knees. Roll the patient slightly forward of center so that he is resting against the providers' knees.

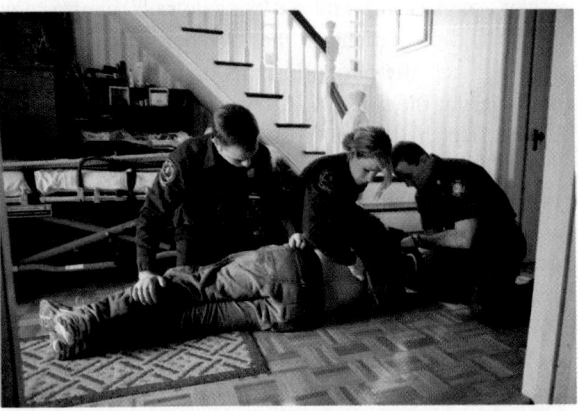

4. Assess the patient's back, if indicated, for signs of injury or illness.

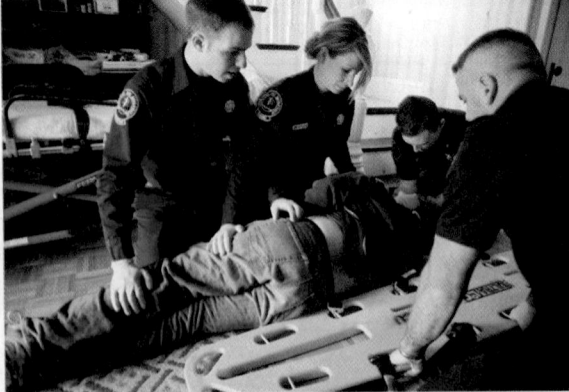

5. Another EMS provider positions the backboard flat on the ground, as close to the patient as possible, with the foot end of the board even with the backs of the patient's knees.

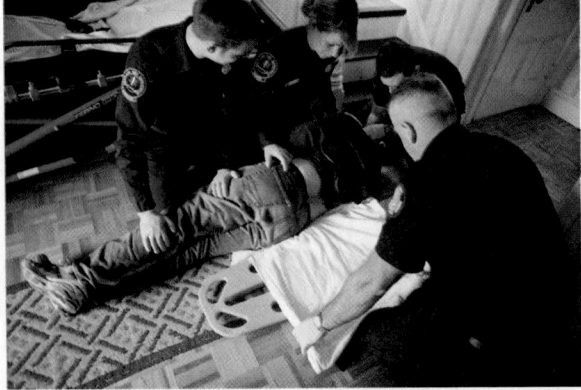

6. Ensure that the backboard straps will not be trapped under the patient or the board during the log roll. Place padding, such as a folded blanket, on the backboard. Have additional padding ready to place under the patient's head and, if necessary, lower back.

(continued)

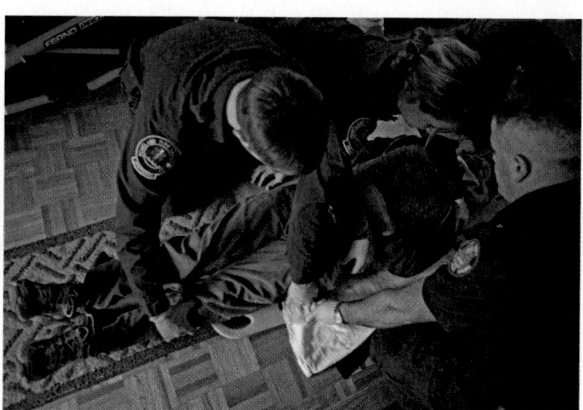

7. The EMS provider behind the patient holds the backboard in place. The patient is lowered onto the board on the command of the Advanced EMT at the patient's head.

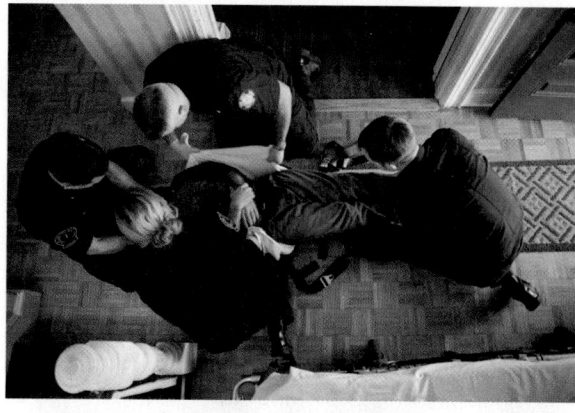

8. The blanket beneath the patient is used to smoothly pull him into position on the board. EMS providers on each side of the patient grasp the blanket at the shoulder level. For large patients, an additional provider can straddle the patient and grasp the blanket at the hips to assist in pulling the patient into place.

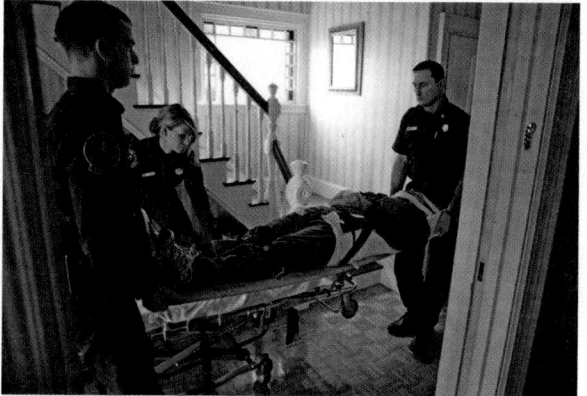

9. Pad under the head and secure the patient to the backboard before lifting him onto the stretcher.

pad it to prevent pain and potential tissue injury from the pressure of the hard material of the backboard. Always secure the patient to the backboard with straps before lifting it (Figure 5-21).

A stair chair is useful for moving patients up and down stairs and for maneuvering in tight spaces that will not accommodate a stretcher or backboard (Figure 5-22). A disadvantage to the stair chair is that patients must be able to sit up.

Various other devices for lifting, moving, and immobilizing patients, such as vacuum immobilization devices, may be available in your service. Always know the indications, contraindications, and proper use of each device. Clean, and when necessary, disinfect these lifting devices after use.

Special devices are used for **bariatric** patients and for interfacility transportation of **neonates**. Very obese patients can exceed the weight capacity of standard wheeled stretchers, and may be too large for the width of standard equipment. Many EMS services have bariatric equipment available, but

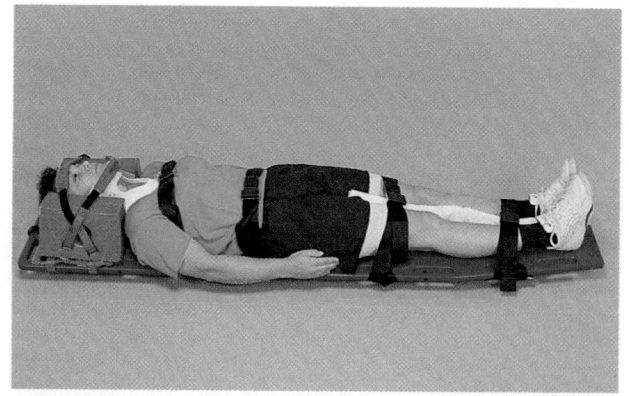

FIGURE 5-21

Use padding and straps to properly secure a patient to a long backboard.

not on every ambulance (Figure 5-23). The use of such devices can be planned for interfacility transfers. On emergency calls, you may need to contact dispatch or your supervisor to have specialized equipment brought to the scene. Always ensure that you have an adequate amount of lifting help when managing bariatric patients. In extreme cases, special rescue equipment and personnel may be required.

Sick newborns often require the services of a neonatal intensive care unit. Most small, or even midsized, hospitals do not have the resources to care for sick newborns, which means they must be transported to a higher-level facility by ground or by air. When neonates are transported, you will be primarily responsible for facilitating care by a team of specialized personnel who will accompany the patient. This team includes, at a minimum, a neonatal nurse, but often also includes a respiratory therapist and neonatologist (pediatrician specializing in newborn care). Special neonatal isolettes are modified to be secured into the ambulance using the bracket that locks the wheeled stretcher into place (Figure 5-24).

Occasionally, a sick or injured patient must be moved quickly out of harm's way before you can safely assess and manage him. Examples of situations requiring emergency moves (sometimes called *urgent moves*) include imminent threat of fire, flood, violence, or traffic hazards. You should not approach the patient unless it is safe to do so. However, once you make contact with the patient, you may realize that the situation has become unsafe. It would then be appropriate to use an emergency move.

Emergency moves are used only when the risks of moving the patient without first assessing or treating him are outweighed by the risks of *not* moving him. In such cases, you may use the armpit-forearm drag (Figure 5-25), shirt drag (Figure 5-26), or blanket drag (Figure 5-27). If assistance is available, you also may use the extremity lift (Figure 5-28). In most circumstances, patient moves are considered nonemergent (sometimes called *nonurgent moves*). This gives you a moment to coordinate lifting and moving with other team members for the patient's comfort and safety. Techniques used for nonemergency moves include the log roll, direct ground lift (Figure 5-29), direct carry (Figure 5-30), extremity lift, and draw-sheet method (Scan 5-2).

Significant MVCs provide a mechanism of injury for spinal trauma. With noncritical trauma patients, take time to very carefully limit motion of the spinal column while extricating (removing) the patient from the vehicle. However,

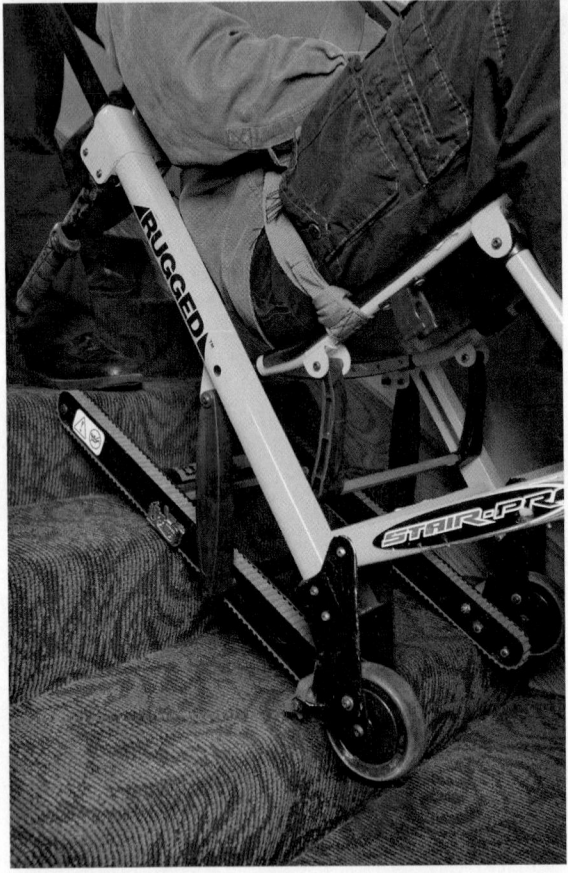

FIGURE 5-22
A stair chair.

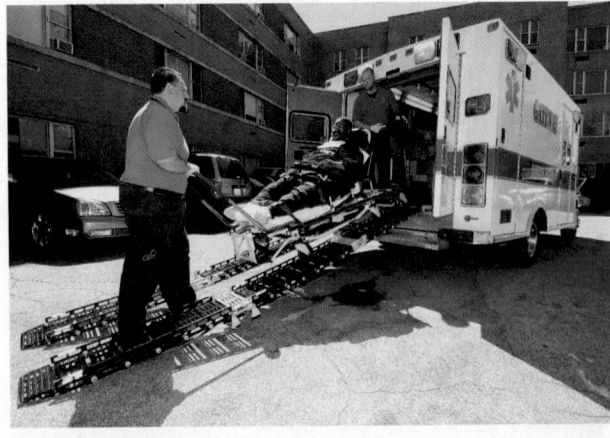

FIGURE 5-23
Special equipment may be needed for very large patients.
(© Ray Kemp/Triple Zilch Productions)

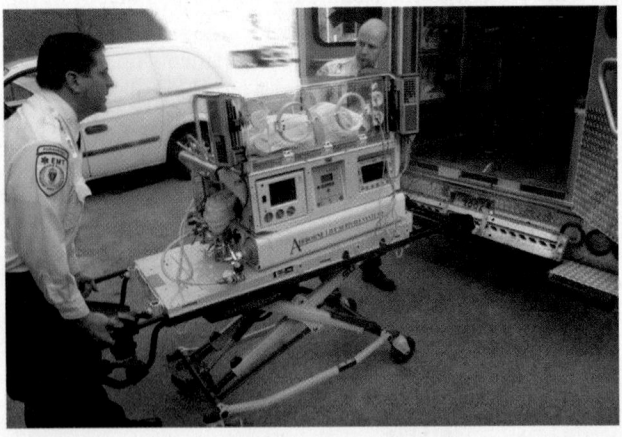

FIGURE 5-24
A neonatal isolette. (© Mark C. Ide)

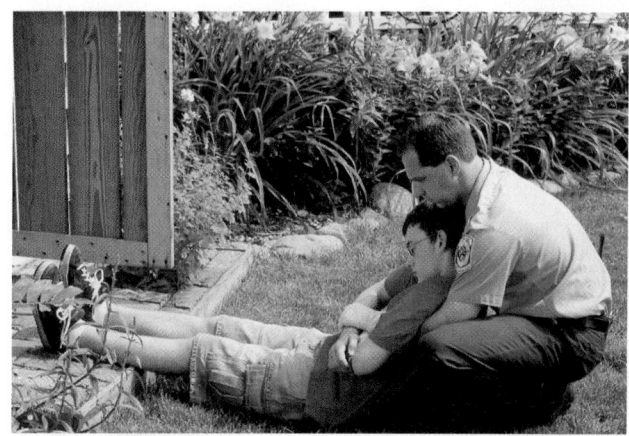

FIGURE 5-25

Armpit-forearm drag.

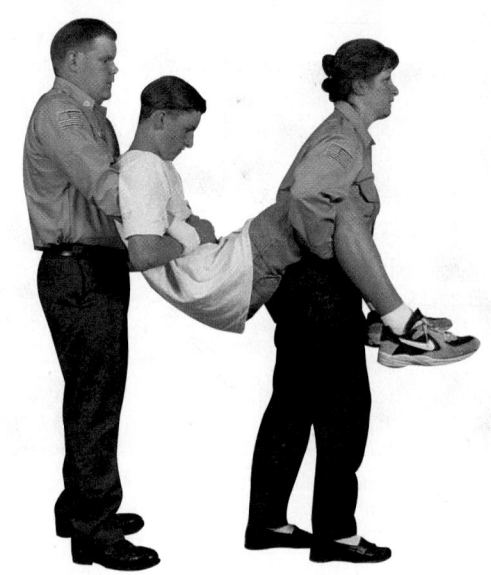

FIGURE 5-28

Extremity lift.

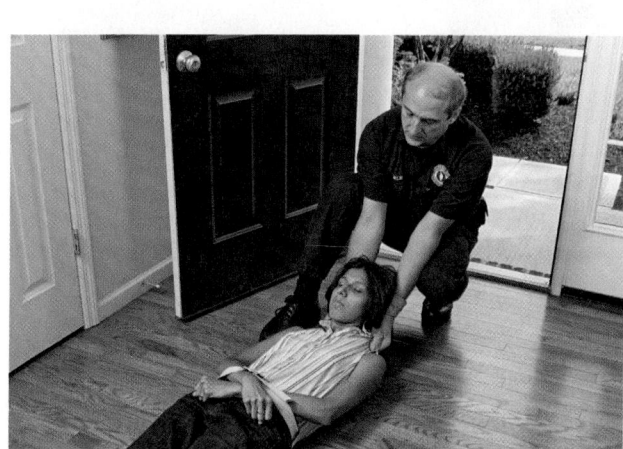

FIGURE 5-26

Shirt drag.

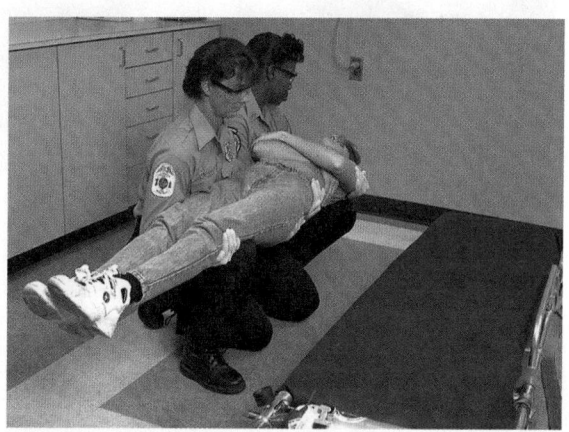

FIGURE 5-29

Direct ground lift.

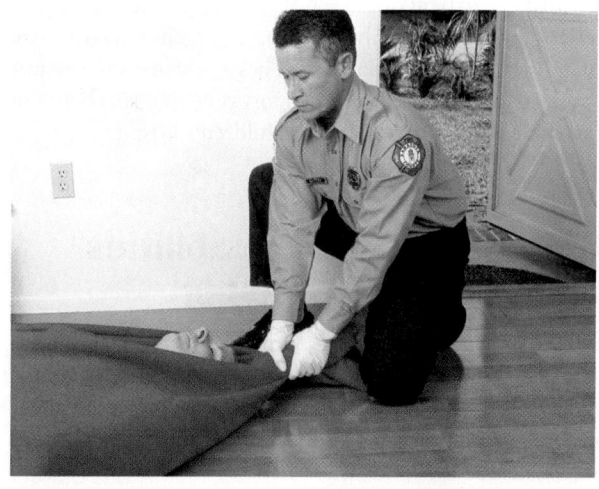

FIGURE 5-27

Blanket drag.

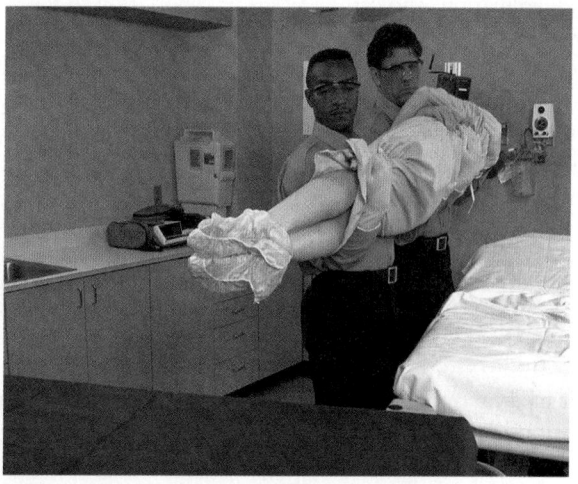

FIGURE 5-30

Direct carry.

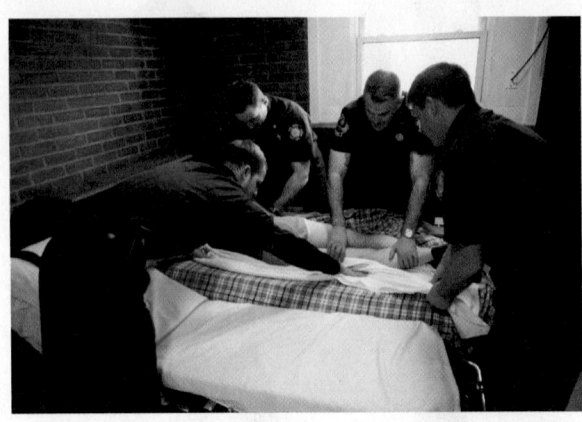

1. Log-roll the patient. Lay a sheet or blanket along the back of the patient's body. Bunch up the edge of the sheet closest to the patient and tuck it underneath the length of his body.

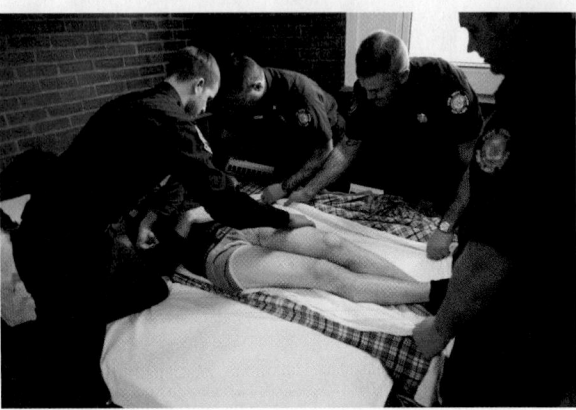

2. Lower the patient and then log roll him to the opposite side. Straighten the edge of the blanket that was tucked beneath the patient.

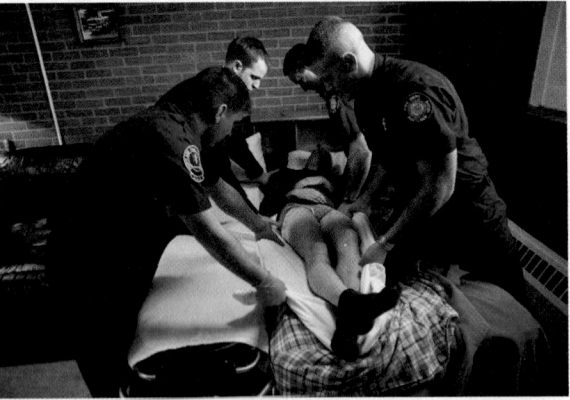

3. Lower the patient onto his back and position the stretcher next to the bed. Roll the edges of the sheets up next to the patient. Grasp the edges of the sheet to support the patient's head, torso, and legs.

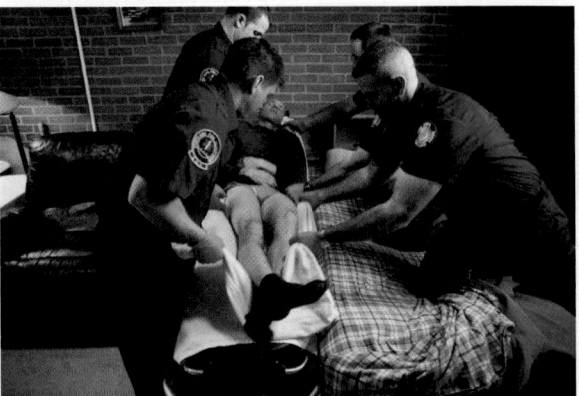

4. One EMS provider gives the command to move. The patient is lifted from the bed to the stretcher.

taking those extra moments for a critical trauma patient can delay adequate management of his airway, breathing, and circulation, and can delay his transportation to the appropriate facility. Techniques of **rapid extrication** are used for critical MVC trauma patients, and to move less severely injured patients who are blocking access to a critical trauma patient. The principle of rapid extrication is to stabilize the cervical spine as well as possible while quickly removing the patient from the vehicle. Approaches to rapid extrication are covered in Chapter 40.

Air Medical Transport

Air medical transport is considered an extension of the hospital intensive care unit (ICU). They are usually staffed by a nurse (RN), and a paramedic, and have extended capabilities and equipment for a higher level of care. Air medical transport consists of **fixed-wing aircraft** (airplanes) and **rotor-wing aircraft** (helicopters). Fixed-wing aircraft are

typically used for long-distance critical care transports between hospitals. Those transports require an ambulance to transport patients between the hospital and the airport. Helicopters are typically used for emergency transport of critically ill or injured patients. These patients often require advanced care with a long transport time to a specialty hospital such as a trauma center or children's hospital.

Advantages and Capabilities of Air Medical Transport

Air medical transport units are capable of an advanced level of care above that of ground EMS services. Providers in air medical transport have additional education in critical care and often neonatology. The additional equipment and capabilities include the following:

- Administration of blood products
- Insertion of central lines and umbilical lines

- Invasive monitoring such as central arterial pressure and pulmonary arterial pressure
- Cardiac balloon pumps
- Rapid sequence intubation/pharmacologically assisted airway management
- Blood chemistry and blood gas metering
- Ventilators
- IV pumps
- Chest tubes
- 12-lead ECGs
- Capnography
- Additional medications (typically cardiac, sedatives, and paralytics)

Limitations of Air Medical Transport

Air medical transport can be very useful in saving patients' lives, but there are a few disadvantages and limitations:

- *Weather.* Inclement weather such as wind, rain, snow, or fog may prevent air medical units from flying or landing at your destination. Once requested, the flight service will check current weather conditions at their origin, the scene, and the destination. If conditions are poor at any of these locations, they will not respond.
- *Altitude.* Smaller aircraft may have difficulty flying at extremely high altitudes, such as mountain peaks, due to the thin air. Also, patients with certain conditions such as lung injuries or diving injuries may suffer adverse effects from transport at high altitude.
- *Aircraft cabin size.* Most medical aircraft cabins are very small. Patients who are obese, have extensive deformities, or impaled objects may not be candidates for transport.
- *Weight limit.* Small aircraft may have a weight limit. They will often only transport one patient, and may calculate crew and patient weight before agreeing to transport. Some services may decide to leave a crew member on scene to conserve weight. Space and weight limitations usually mean that the patient's family will need to find ground transportation to the hospital.
- *Terrain.* Irregular ground terrain may not allow for a safe landing zone. In many cases, ground ambulances can rendezvous with the aircraft at another, more appropriate location.

Requesting Air Medical Transport

In addition to the high cost of operating air medical transport, air medical crashes are not uncommon and can be catastrophic. Therefore, their use must be weighed against the risks. They should only be used when deemed absolutely necessary by patient condition, transport time, and destination. When considering transport time, keep in mind the *total* time it will take for the air medical unit to respond, load the patient, and transport to their destination.

Consider the following:

- Unlike with a ground ambulance, the air medical crew is probably not standing by in a running aircraft. It may take several minutes to prepare for liftoff. The pilot needs to start and prepare the aircraft, obtain clearance for liftoff, and gather flight and weather information. Also, the crew may be working in a hospital unit, and may take a few minutes to get to the aircraft. This preparation would not be necessary if the aircraft is already in the air returning from another mission.
- Unlike with a ground ambulance, an aircraft cannot just stop and put it in park. They will need to assess the landing zone, and set the aircraft down slowly.
- Once on scene, patients must be transferred to the aircraft stretcher, and other monitoring equipment, and securely packaged before being loaded into the aircraft.
- Once the aircraft reaches the destination hospital, the patient must be transported to the emergency department, often traveling from the roof and down an elevator.

In addition to your protocol, ask the following questions when considering air medical transport: Is transport time critical, and will air transport clearly save time? Does the patient require transport to a specialty hospital, such as a trauma center, that is not local? Is the patient located in a remote area, not accessible by ground units? Does the patient need specialized medical procedures or monitoring that is not available with ground ambulances?

Each EMS system has its own individual procedures for contacting air medical services. Some will allow direct radio contact, while others require a telephone call. Most EMS services have providers request air medical transport through their dispatch center. When requesting a helicopter, you should be prepared to provide the following information:

- Your service name and unit number
- Nature of the incident
- Brief patient condition report, including patient weight
- Exact scene location or landing zone location, including surrounding hazards
- Radio frequency and call signs of the ground contact person

Setting Up a Landing Zone

The landing zone must be a large, flat area, free of obstacles and hazards, at least 150 feet from the scene (Figure 5-31). It should be clearly visible from the air. Provide the pilot with large landmarks, cross streets, or GPS coordinates. Use the following guidelines for specific landing zone setup:

- The size may be aircraft dependent, but is usually at least 100 feet by 100 feet.
- The ground should be flat, or less than a five-degree incline.
- The surface must be free of loose debris. If landing on a dirt or grassy surface, the fire department should wet it down to reduce dust.
- The landing zone should be marked at each corner by highly visible devices, such as large traffic cones, or vehicles. At night, markers should be lighted, and it is ideal to have vehicles with their headlights or other lights aimed into the landing zone. Never direct any lights upward, toward the aircraft, because this may blind the pilot.

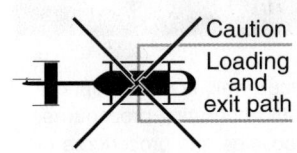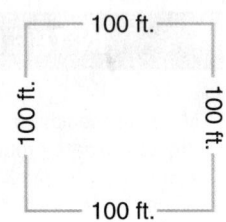

FIGURE 5-31

Helicopter landing zone.

Air and Ground Crew Safety

Due to the rapidly spinning rotors of a helicopter and the extreme wind of the down draft, the landing zone can be extremely dangerous. When operating at or near the landing zone, the following safety precautions must be taken:

- Advise the pilot by radio of wind direction and any power lines or other obstacles near the landing zone.

CASE STUDY WRAP-UP

Clinical-Reasoning Process

Advanced EMTs Mercede and Gary have just been dispatched for a trench collapse at a construction site with one patient entrapped.

To decide on the best route of travel to the scene, Gary checks the GPS navigation system for directions and advises Mercede of the route. Gary and Mercede know there are a variety of ways to decrease their chances of vehicle-related injury. With seat belts fastened, Mercede starts the ambulance and pulls out of the bay. At the end of the approach, she activates the lights and sirens and waits for traffic from both directions to stop before pulling onto the street. Traffic is heavy, and Mercede must navigate carefully around it. Gary assists in observing for traffic at intersections. Arriving at the security booth on the scene, Mercede follows the security vehicle to the patient's location.

A scene size-up is critical to further decision making. Gary and Mercede make several observations:

- Heavy rescue is on the scene, determining how to best extricate the patient.
- Because the trench is not secured, Gary and Mercede stay back and get a report on the patient's condition from the rescue team. The patient is a 49-year-old male who is buried up to the lower chest in heavy clay soil. He is awake, but is having difficulty breathing.
- The trench site is in jeopardy of further collapse, and rescue crews cannot begin treatment until they've secured it from further collapse.

The rescue and ambulance crews work together to ensure the patient will be smoothly and efficiently transferred to the ambulance when he is extricated, without aggravating any of his injuries. The rescue team has BLS equipment and a long backboard ready for the patient, and Mercede and Gary are standing by with the wheeled ambulance stretcher. The rescue team advises that extrication time will be about 45 minutes. Mercede and Gary prepare the back of the ambulance for the patient's arrival, awaiting further communication with the rescue crew.

When the patient is freed and secured to the backboard, he is loaded into the ambulance on the stretcher. Gary requests a firefighter/EMT to ride along to the hospital to help care for the patient. Gary communicates with his partner so she can make decisions about the drive to the emergency department.

Leaning through to the driver's compartment, he tells Mercede, "He's critical. We need to transport emergently to St. John's Trauma."

"Okay," she replies. "The security road out to the highway is bumpy. I'll take it nice and slow." She puts the vehicle in gear, knowing that patient care and the safety of the crew and patient depend on the quality of her driving.

- If the landing zone is on a divided freeway, stop traffic in both directions to minimize distractions for drivers and the pilot.

- Ensure that the patient and crew are 100 to 200 feet away from the landing zone during landing to avoid high winds and flying debris.

- Do not enter the landing zone, or approach the helicopter, until instructed to do so by the pilot.

- Always approach the helicopter from the front, while making eye contact with the pilot (Figure 5-32).

- Post a tail guard, in a fixed position near the rear of the helicopter to prevent anyone from approaching the tail. The tail rotor spins very quickly and may not be visible.

- Always approach the helicopter in a crouched position to avoid the main rotor. The pilot may or may not shut down the rotors before allowing you to approach.

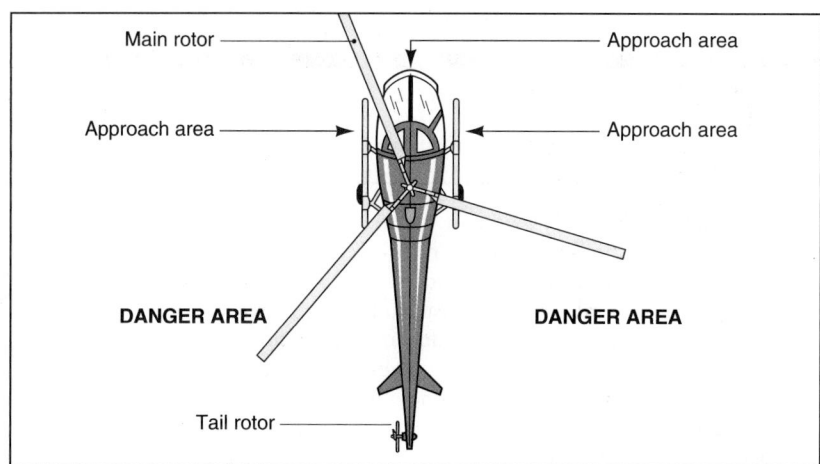

(A)

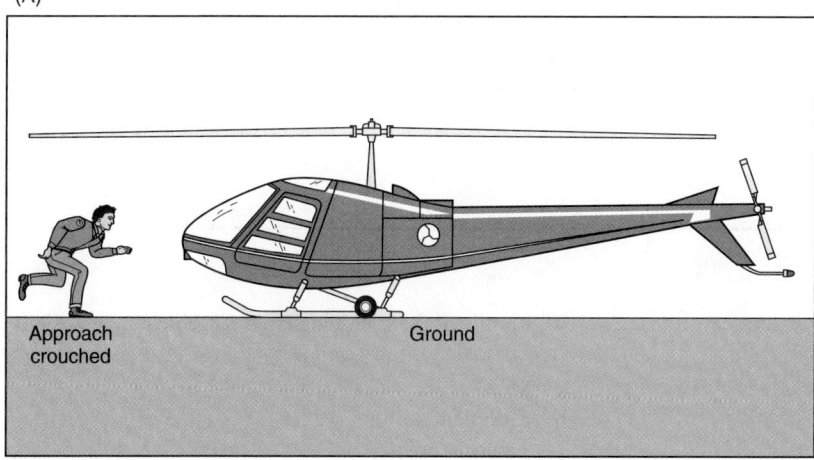

(B)

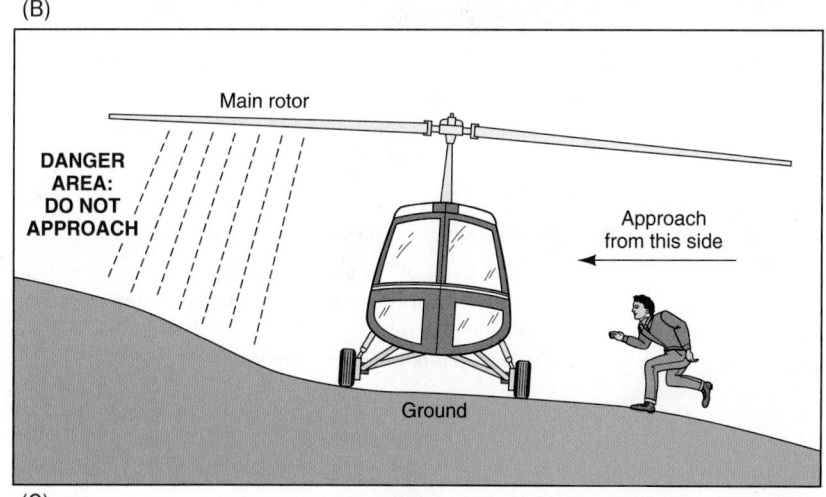

(C)

FIGURE 5-32

Correct approach to the aircraft.
(A) The area around the tail rotor is extremely dangerous. A spinning rotor cannot be seen.
(B) A sudden gust of wind can cause the main rotor of a helicopter to dip to a point as close as four feet from the ground. Always approach a helicopter in a crouch when the rotor is moving.
(C) Approach the aircraft from the downhill side when a helicopter is parked on a hillside.

As the rotor slows, the blades will droop downward, but may still be moving too quickly to see.

- If landing on a slight incline, always approach from the downhill side.
- Secure all loose personal clothing and equipment such as hats, coats, and stethoscopes before approaching the helicopter.

- Ensure that the patient is packaged securely before approaching the helicopter, then cover the patient and secure all equipment, blankets, IVs, clothing, and so on.
- Clear all personnel from the landing zone during liftoff.

CHAPTER REVIEW

Chapter Summary

EMS providers work in a unique patient care environment that requires attention to multiple tasks and sources of information. This unique environment has risks and considerations that are different from those of any other type of health care provider. The special risks of the prehospital care environment can be substantially reduced by careful attention to the operational aspects of the job. The operational aspects include vehicle operations, driving safety, scene size-up, lifting and moving patients, and interacting with air medical services.

Before providing care, EMS providers are responsible for ensuring that their vehicle is fully stocked, clean, safe, and mechanically capable of responding to the scene. EMS providers must be aware of the special risks posed by driving a large, modified vehicle under emergency conditions and must drive defensively to maintain safety. As an Advanced EMT, you must be able to size up each unique scene to determine the nature of the problem, the safety of the situation, the number of patients, the need for additional resources, and the patient's general condition. You must know how and when to move patients, and how to safely operate each and every piece of equipment on the ambulance. You must know how to transport patients under emergency and nonemergency situations, and when to consider air medical transport. When air medical transport is indicated and feasible, you must know how to safely interact with the air medical crew.

Review Questions

Multiple-Choice Questions

1. The time from dispatch to when a unit arrives on the scene of an emergency is called:
   a. on-scene time.
   b. elapsed time.
   c. response time.
   d. platinum time.

2. The incident command system (ICS) should be activated by:
   a. an EMS supervisor.
   b. a fire department officer.
   c. a police officer.
   d. the first arriving EMS unit.

3. A typical emergency response to a motor vehicle collision in a city includes police, a BLS fire department engine, and an ALS private ambulance. This is an example of a:
   a. mutual aid response.
   b. multijurisdictional response.
   c. two-tiered system.
   d. three-tiered system.

4. Which one of the following types of vehicle carries the greatest risk of injury on the road?
   a. Motorcycle
   b. Ambulance
   c. Tractor-trailer
   d. Passenger vehicle

5. Ambulance crash fatalities occur more frequently:
   a. in the front of the ambulance (cab).
   b. in the rear of the ambulance (patient compartment).
   c. to occupants of other vehicles.
   d. to pedestrians.

6. Ambulance crash injuries occur more frequently:
   a. in the front of the ambulance (cab).
   b. in the rear of the ambulance (patient compartment).
   c. to pedestrians.
   d. to occupants of other vehicles.

7. Ambulance crashes occur most commonly:
   a. while backing.
   b. on freeways.
   c. in intersections.
   d. at stop signs.

8. Which one of the following is NOT a principle of safe backing?
   a. Use a spotter.
   b. Open windows.
   c. Turn on emergency lights.
   d. Activate the siren.

9. Scanning 12 to 15 seconds ahead on a highway, is about:
   a. ¼ mile.
   b. ½ mile.
   c. 1 mile.
   d. 2 miles.

10. When driving an ambulance on a freeway, a smooth lane change should take about _____ seconds.
    a. 2
    b. 4
    c. 6
    d. 12

11. Ambulance crashes resulting in injuries and fatalities, most commonly occur:
    a. on wet roads.
    b. at stop signs.
    c. in intersections.
    d. while backing.

12. An intersection in which all lanes are either occupied by a stopped vehicle, or not occupied at all, is called:
    a. a clear intersection.
    b. clear right.
    c. an open intersection.
    d. a blocked intersection.

13. When parking at the scene of a motor vehicle crash, the ambulance should be positioned:
    a. ahead of the scene.
    b. in the opposite lanes of traffic.
    c. behind the scene.
    d. next to the crashed vehicles.

14. An ambulance built on a van chassis without an added box is called a type _____ ambulance.
    a. I
    b. II
    c. III
    d. IV

15. Ambulance design and construction standards:
    a. are written by the auto industry.
    b. address the safety of the crew.
    c. specify what is necessary to display the Star of Life.
    d. address the safety of patients.

16. Real-world crash forces and their outcomes are best predicted by what kind of testing?
    a. Dynamic
    b. Static
    c. Conditional
    d. Highway

17. The safest position for transporting an infant is:
    a. in a car seat secured to the bench seat.
    b. in the arms of a restrained caregiver.
    c. seat belted and lying on the stretcher.
    d. in a car seat secured to the stretcher.

18. You and your partner are in your running vehicle standing by upwind from the scene of an industrial fire. You both become very sleepy, and your partner complains of a headache. You should suspect:
    a. fatigue due to shift work.
    b. carbon monoxide poisoning from ambulance exhaust.
    c. hazardous materials in the industrial fire.
    d. that your last patient exposed you to an infectious disease.

Critical-Thinking Questions

19. You have just arrived at a high-rise senior citizens' housing complex. What safety concerns can you anticipate in this situation?

20. How would you determine if a situation meets criteria for a multiple-casualty incident?

21. What are some actions you can take to prevent vehicle-related injuries and back injuries on the job?

22. You have been dispatched for a report of an injured football player at a high school. Explain how you will approach the scene size-up.

23. You are driving on a divided street with four lanes of traffic in each direction to return to your station after a call. It is rush hour and traffic is heavy. Explain how you will apply the "Cushion of Safety."

24. Your route to an emergency call will involve driving through congested streets, entering an interstate highway and then exiting it in approximately 3 miles. Do you anticipate the possibility of having to downgrade the response? Why or why or not?

25. What are some conditions you should anticipate in order to make emergency patient transports safer for patients and providers?

References

Becker, L. R., Zaloshnja, E., Levick, N., & Miller, T. R. (2003). Relative risk of injury and death in ambulances and other emergency vehicles. *Accident Analysis and Prevention, 35*, pp. 941–948.

Levick, N., & Mener, D. (2009). *"Searching for ambulance safety: Where is the literature?"* Paper presented at the annual meeting of the National Association of EMS Physicians, Registry Resort, Naples, FL. Retrieved May 25, 2009, from http://www.allacademic.com/meta/p64904_index.html

Maguire, B., Hunting, K., Smith, G., & Levick, N. (2002). Occupational fatalities in emergency medical services: a hidden crisis. *Annals of Emergency Medicine, 40*, pp 625–632.

U.S. Department of Transportation, Federal Motor Carrier Safety Administration. (2008). *All motor vehicle injury crash statistics.* Retrieved August 23, 2010, from http://www.fmcsa.dot.gov/facts-research/LTBCF2008/tbl8.htm

Zagaroli, L., & Taylor, A. (2003, January 27). *Ambulance driver fatigue a danger: Distractions pose risks to patients, EMTs, traffic.* Detroit News Washington Bureau.

6 Communication and Teamwork

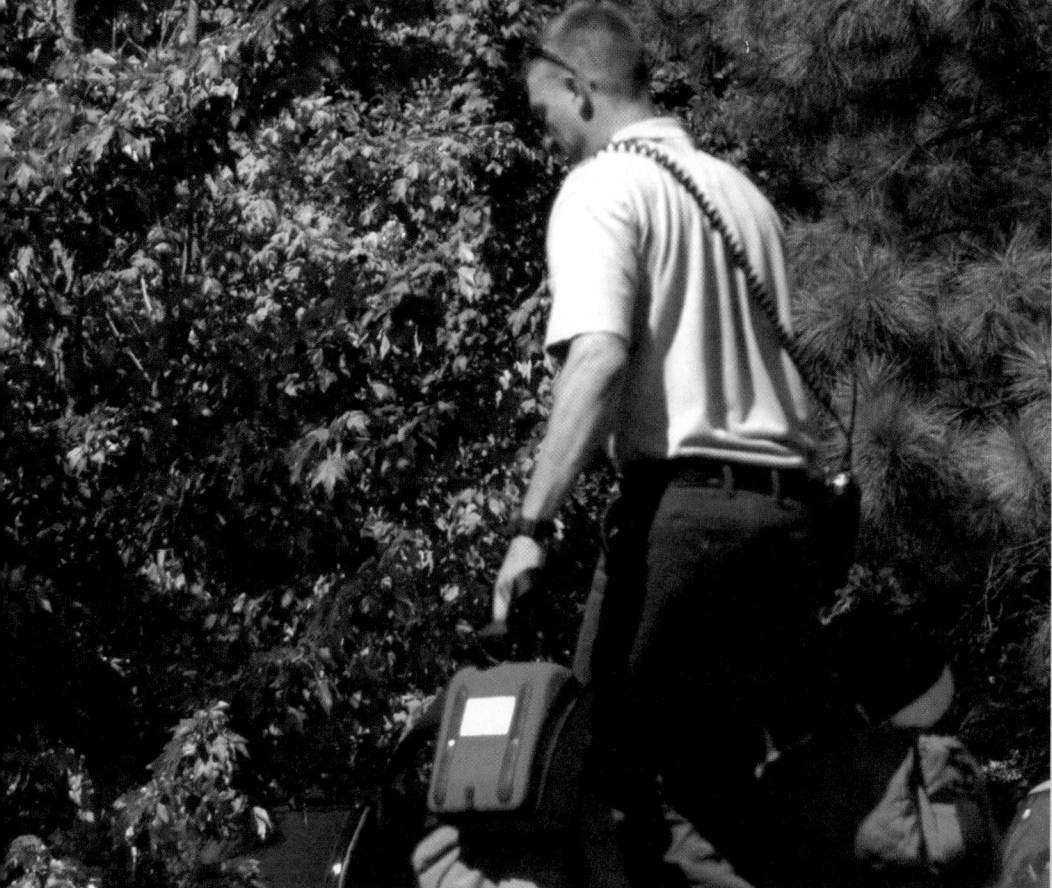

Content Area: Preparatory

Advanced EMT Education Standard: The Advanced EMT applies fundamental knowledge of the EMS system, safety/well-being of the Advanced EMT, and medical/legal and ethical issues to the provision of emergency care.

Objectives

After reading this chapter, you should be able to:

6.1   Define key terms introduced in this chapter.

6.2   Describe the components of the communication process, including factors that can interfere with effective communication.

6.3   Identify the potential impact of the perceptions of nonverbal behaviors on communication.

6.4   Demonstrate effective communications that promote continuity and safety in patient care when communicating with EMS crew members, other public safety personnel, and receiving hospital personnel.

6.5   Given a scenario, demonstrate effective communication that improves team dynamics.

(continued)

Resource Central

To access Resource Central, follow the directions on the Student Access Card provided with this text. If there is no card, go to www.bradybooks.com and follow the Resource Central link to Buy Access. Under Media Resources, you will find:

- *Be Therapeutic in Your Communication.*

- *Your Cultural Compass.* View effective cross-cultural communication methods.

- *Communication with Children.* Learn more about unique age-related communication obstacles and techniques.

CASE STUDY

As he stands in line at the convenience store to pay for his bottle of water, Advanced EMT Stan Tetzloff's portable radio sounds a tone, followed by dispatch information. "Rescue 15 and Engine 29 respond to one-seven-two-five East Washington Street for a report of a person down in front of the residence. Law enforcement is on the scene." Placing his money on the counter, Stan heads toward the rescue unit, where his partner, EMT Lucas Brown, is obtaining the same information from the mobile data terminal in the vehicle. Lucas pushes the "Responding" status button on the radio console, switches on the emergency lights and sirens, and waits for traffic to stop before proceeding into the street. Three minutes later, Lucas pulls to a stop in front of the address, just behind Engine 29. One police officer is talking to a man lying in the grass, and another is talking to a man and woman on the porch of the residence.

Problem-Solving Questions

1. What additional communication will Rescue 15 need to have with dispatch?
2. How should Stan and Lucas interact with the engine crew, law enforcement officers, and bystanders?
3. What actions should the crew take to establish rapport with the patient and gain his trust?
4. What written documentation must be completed on this call?

(continued from previous page)

6.6 Describe the responsibilities of the Federal Communications Commission with respect to EMS communication.

6.7 Discuss the purpose and characteristics of each of the following EMS system communication components:
- Base station
- Cellular phones
- Digitized radio equipment
- Interoperability
- Mobile data terminals
- Mobile radios
- Portable radios
- Repeater

6.8 List the key points in an EMS call at which you should communicate, and with whom you should communicate.

6.9 Demonstrate standard rules of radio communications.

6.10 Deliver a concise, organized radio report that clearly communicates essential information to medical direction or the receiving facility.

6.11 Demonstrate the ability to receive and confirm an order for medical treatment over the radio.

6.12 Discuss the advantages and disadvantages of using radio codes.

6.13 Convert back and forth between standard clock and 24-hour (military) time.

6.14 Explain the importance of establishing rapport with patients and their families in the therapeutic communication process.

6.15 Given a scenario, engage in effective, empathetic, culturally sensitive communication.

6.16 Give examples of the appropriate use of the following communication behaviors:
- Clarification
- Closed-ended questions
- Confrontation

(continued)

(continued from previous page)

- – Empathy
- – Explanation
- – Open-ended questions
- – Reflection
- – Silence
- – Summary

6.17 Analyze your communication to avoid the pitfalls of:
- – Leading or biased questions
- – Interrupting the patient
- – Talking too much
- – Providing false reassurance or inappropriate advice
- – Implying blame

6.18 Given a scenario, demonstrate modifications in communication for the following situations:
- – Communicating with a patient's family
- – Getting a noncommunicative patient to talk
- – Interviewing a hostile patient/using verbal defusing strategies
- – Cross-cultural communication and language barriers
- – Communicating with children, elderly patients with sensory deficits, and patients with cognitive impairment

6.19 Explain the purposes and importance of documenting patient care.

6.20 Describe the elements of the U.S. Department of Transportation (DOT)/National EMS Information System (NEMSIS) minimum data set for patient care reports (PCR).

6.21 Accurately complete the contents of each section of a PCR to include:
- – Administrative data
- – Patient demographic data and other patient data
- – Vital signs
- – Narrative
- – Treatment

6.22 Give examples of each of the following types of PCR narrative data:
- – Chief complaint
- – Pertinent history
- – Subjective information
- – Objective information

6.23 Explain the importance of using proper abbreviations and terminology in the PCR.

6.24 Describe the SOAP, CHART, and CHEATED methods of PCR narrative documentation.

6.25 Explain each of the following legal concerns with respect to the PCR:
- – Confidentiality
- – Documentation of consent and refusal to consent
- – Correction of errors
- – Falsification of PCR information

6.26 Discuss how to handle each of the following situations with respect to documentation:
- – Transfer of patient care when returning to service before the PCR is complete
- – Multiple-casualty incidents
- – Supplemental reports for special situations, such as exposure to infectious disease and injury to a patient in the course of treatment and transport

Introduction

It is not possible to perform any of the roles of an EMS provider without engaging in communication and teamwork. Communication is required to initiate the EMS call and for every phase of the call that follows. You must communicate with your coworkers and supervisor in other work-related activities, too. Being a successful Advanced EMT requires teamwork to coordinate efforts and achieve the common goal of high-quality patient care. Effective teamwork and communication do not always come naturally. You must be aware of principles of the communication process in general, understand how to effectively communicate as a health care professional, and understand how to use specialized EMS system communication equipment. Understanding principles of teamwork is vital to an enjoyable work experience and excellent patient care. This chapter introduces fundamental concepts in communication and teamwork that you will continue to build upon, particularly as you learn patient assessment and history taking.

Communication

Communication takes place when a message is exchanged between a **sender** and a **receiver** (Figure 6-1). The process is far more complex than it sounds. There are many characteristics of the environment, sender, receiver, message, and channel or medium through which the message is sent. These characteristics can impact the effectiveness of communication. Being aware of the **feedback** you receive when communicating with others and frequently reflecting on how to improve communication will help you develop your professional communication skills.

Sender Characteristics

Your characteristics and the way you are perceived affect the amount of influence you have when communicating and, therefore, impact the effectiveness of your communication efforts. One of the most important professional characteristics impacting communication is the **credibility** others perceive you have. **Verbal** and **nonverbal cues** provide others with information about your credibility. Others' perceptions of your expertise and trustworthiness are important in establishing credibility.

One way to immediately establish your credibility is to communicate your credentials. Your uniform, patches, and name badge should clearly identify you as an Advanced EMT. You must also speak and act confidently to convey that you are a credible professional. Introduce yourself to your patient, using your credentials and stating that you are there to help. For example, "Good morning, sir. My name is Jack. I'm an Advanced EMT with the fire department. How can I help you today?"

Initially, others may determine your trustworthiness based on your appearance, but you will need to continue to earn trust by being honest and following through on what you say. Do not tell a patient that the IV you are going to start will not hurt, and do not make false promises that things will be fine, when they clearly may not be. Do not promise your partner that you will take care of a task, but not keep your promise.

The perceived authority of medical and public safety personnel can intimidate patients. The patient must see you as someone who is easy to talk to (Figure 6-2). Look at the patient, and focus your attention on him. Physically place yourself at the patient's level, rather than standing over him. Ensure that your facial expression, body language, and tone of voice convey **empathy** and respect.

Also keep in mind how you perceive others as senders. Keep an open mind about their credibility and knowledge.

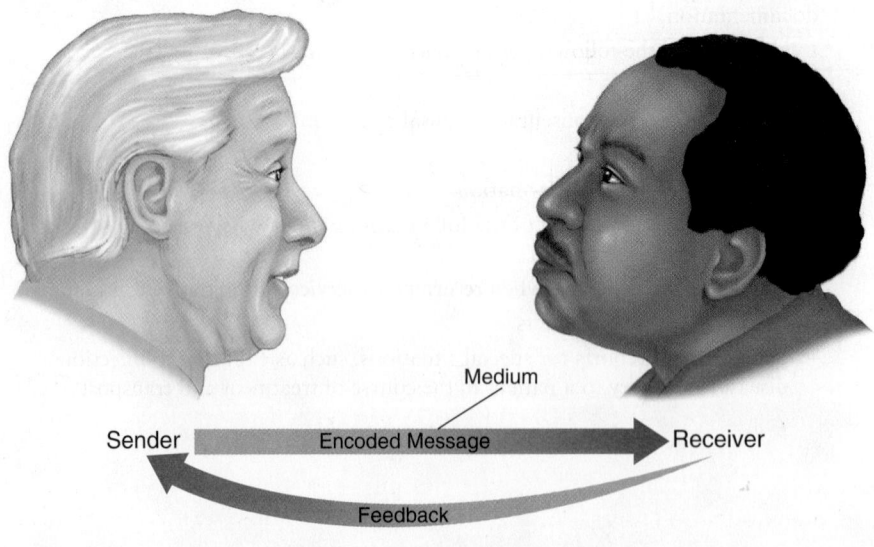

FIGURE 6-1
An overview of the communication process.

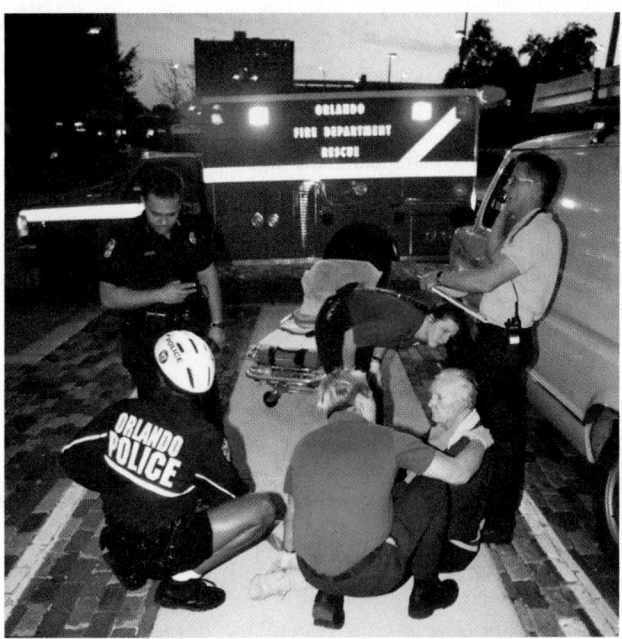

FIGURE 6-2

Being at the patient's eye level helps establish rapport.
(© Craig Jackson/In the Dark Photography)

Take care that you do not make judgments that interfere with your ability to listen and understand the message being sent. Patients' stressful circumstances can interfere with their ability to communicate. Sometimes patients, or even other health care providers, communicate in ways that may make you feel disrespected or angry. The professional response is to maintain your composure.

Receiver Characteristics

Personality characteristics, intelligence, self-esteem, and language skills affect how receivers understand and react to messages. As noted, stressful circumstances, such as those surrounding an emergency situation, interfere significantly with the ability to process information. This applies to you, your coworkers, and the patient. It is critical to communicate clearly and seek feedback on understanding in such situations.

Active listening improves your chances of understanding messages. It is an important way of establishing trust and rapport. Active listening means listening to completely appreciate the sender's meaning, rather than just hearing the words and taking them at face value. A number of responses, discussed later in the chapter, demonstrate to others that you are actively listening.

Message Characteristics

The goal of communication is to exchange information in a way that is understood by both parties. The language used to convey the message can obscure the intended meaning. Medical terminology and technical jargon can improve communication between people with similar backgrounds,

but can be unclear to patients. On the other hand, many patients are well-educated and well-informed about their health and medical conditions. Do not assume that patients understand medical terms, but listen for indications of the patient's level of education and understanding. Adjust your communication to the patient's level.

Communication Channels, Interference, and Feedback

Advanced EMTs use many **communication channels**, or mediums, and must be familiar with their advantages and disadvantages. **Interference** can occur with any channel, and also can be caused by characteristics of the sender and receiver, and the interaction between the two. Communication channels may either be verbal or nonverbal. Advanced EMTs communicate by radio, cellular phones and text devices, computers, written reports, and of course, by speaking directly with others.

Interference is anything that gets in the way of communication. Some of these factors are under your control, while others are not. Sources of interference include poor radio or cellular phone reception, a patient's malfunctioning hearing aid, sloppy handwriting, poor vision, poor diction, intruding thoughts and feelings, environmental noise, cultural differences, language barriers, and many other sources.

A variety of intended, and sometimes unintended, messages are sent through communication channels. While your words convey one thing, your facial expression, tone of voice, eye contact, body language, and other nonverbal behaviors may convey something different. Patients may communicate mixed messages, too. Consider the patient who says he is fine and does not need your care, but who keeps rubbing his hand over his chest.

Feedback is a general term that means information about a system's output is returned to its source to modify further output. Many homeostatic mechanisms in the body, such as blood glucose regulation, use feedback loops. In the case of communication, the receiver sends information back to the sender about his understanding of the message. Feedback is not foolproof, though. A person who is hard of hearing, not fluent in English, or simply is not sure what you mean may indicate understanding by nodding his head in order to avoid embarrassment or inconveniencing the sender. Solicit feedback as specifically as possible to minimize misunderstanding. It can be helpful in some situations to have the patient summarize back to you what you have communicated to ensure understanding.

Team Dynamics and Communication

A **team** is a group of individuals with specific common goals. EMS providers form teams with other public safety and health care providers. All health care teams have the

Lucas pushes the "on-scene" button as Stan sizes up the scene. Because Rescue 15 is the transporting unit and they have arrived at the same time as the engine, the rescue crew is in charge of patient care. As the ranking EMS provider on the rescue unit, Stan is responsible for assessing the patient to determine what level of care the patient requires. In what seems like a well-choreographed routine, Captain Miller from Engine 29 begins taking down information about the call, while Lucas ensures needed equipment is taken to the patient's side. One of the EMTs from the engine prepares to take vital signs.

Problem-Solving Questions

1. How do the team members each know what their roles are?
2. How would the scenario be affected by a poor team leader or poor team members?

common goal of providing safe, efficient, high-quality patient care. EMS teams have the additional goal of transporting the patient from the scene of the emergency to the hospital.

A number of different tasks are required to meet goals. Everyone on the team must have a common understanding of these goals and the ways in which they are achieved. Each team member must understand the roles and responsibilities of the others. Individuals on a team may change from call to call, but the roles of various types of providers are consistent. Effective communication before, during, and after EMS calls is essential to smooth teamwork.

At times, you will be a team leader. Other times, you will take direction from a team leader. Clear policies and protocols must be in place to ensure individuals know what roles and responsibilities they are expected to fulfill in various situations. Whether you are a leader or a team member, two-way communication and cooperation are required for patient safety.

Teamwork and team communication extend beyond the immediate group physically present at the scene. Dispatchers, medical direction physicians, and others with whom you communicate through technology are also part of the team. Communication through technology is usually devoid of the nonverbal cues that contribute to understanding face-to-face verbal communication. Always confirm that you have correctly heard information received through technology by repeating back key points. In particular, whenever you receive medical orders over the phone or radio, repeat them back to the physician to make sure you understood correctly.

EMS System Communication

Communication technology is rapidly evolving. The exact configuration of individual EMS communication systems varies. Your particular system may or may not have all of the features discussed here, but you must have

a basic understanding of EMS communication system components and be proficient in the use of the communication technology in your system and guidelines for radio communication.

Oversight, Maintenance, and Coordination

The **Federal Communications Commission (FCC)** is responsible for oversight of many different types of communication systems, including EMS radio communication. Some of the responsibilities of the FCC include approving radio equipment, assigning broadcast frequencies, licensing **base stations**, and assigning radio call signs. The FCC also issues regulations concerning interference with emergency medical broadcasts, and bars the use of profane language.

EMS communication system maintenance and availability of back-up systems and equipment are essential to preventing breakdowns in communication. At the least, such breakdowns are inconvenient, but, more importantly, patients may not get proper care. At a minimum, EMS providers are responsible for charging and changing **portable radio** or cellular phone batteries and conducting a radio check each shift to ensure that they can send and receive transmissions. EMS systems should have regular maintenance schedules for radio equipment to be tested and maintained by qualified experts.

EMS communication system components are ideally part of an overall system of public safety communication, allowing integrated delivery of emergency services. The importance of communication system **interoperability** between multiple agencies and jurisdictions has been highlighted through communication difficulties in recent disaster situations. Project 25 is a large, collaborative interoperability effort involving the communication industry and public sector and private agencies. The purpose of Project 25 is to establish uniform standards and processes for interoperability. The goal is to ensure that communication between systems is possible.

Radio Frequencies and Traffic

Radio systems in EMS operate on assigned **radio frequencies,** or channels. Dispatch frequencies are often available to the public, but frequencies over which patient information is transmitted should be secure. **Digital radio equipment** can assist with security, but the security of a radio system should never be taken for granted. Information that could be used to identify a patient is not given over the radio. EMS radio systems use a push-to-talk (PTT) system, in which a button on the radio is depressed to open the channel for transmission. Your radio cannot receive a transmission from someone else while the PTT button is depressed. The length of any single transmission should not exceed 30 seconds. Many radio systems have a "time-out" feature that limits the length of time you can transmit at one time. Radio frequencies are shared with other EMS units in your area. Keep your calls short and to the point to keep the frequencies clear for other communication.

The messages sent back and forth in radio communications are called *traffic*. Some systems use radio codes or "signals" to streamline radio traffic. Codes and signals can communicate some types of information concisely or securely. However, this practice also creates an opportunity for miscommunication if the codes or signals have not been memorized. For example, "Signal 10," may be used to communicate that you are responding with lights and siren. In a "ten-code" system, sequential numbers are preceded by the number 10. The code "10-2" may indicate that a transmission was clear or well-received, while "10-9" can be a request to repeat your last communication. In general, it is best to use plain language in radio communications. Some other terms are frequently used in radio communication, such as "copy," to indicate receipt and understanding of a message (Table 6-1).

Communicating and Documenting Times

Times are used in EMS system communication for a number of reasons. You must track response times, on-scene times, times that communication took place, and times that patient care interventions were performed. The recorded times serve as a legal record that can provide you with protection from claims that it took too long to respond or that you were on the scene too long. Time synchronization between communication devices, clocks, or watches used to note the time of patient care interventions, and patient care devices, such as automatic external defibrillators (AEDs) helps avoid discrepancies that could inaccurately reflect the time from arrival to treatment. These times also provide your EMS service with important data for continuous quality improvement. Often, the dispatcher will end any radio transmission by stating the time.

Rather than using the standard 12-hour clock times followed by "AM" or "PM," most dispatch centers and hospitals use a 24-hour clock, or military system. The relationship between standard and military time is simple. The 24-hour clock starts at midnight (12:00 AM), which is designated as 0000 hours, or "zero-hundred hours." Each of the first 12 hours of the 24-hour clock corresponds with the "AM" time. For example, 1:00 AM is 0100 hours ("oh-one-hundred hours") until noon, which is 1200 hours ("twelve-hundred hours"). Instead of starting over again at 1:00 PM, add 12 to each hour after noon. So 1:00 PM is 1300 hours, and 11:00 PM is 2300 hours. To designate minutes after the hour, 3:21 AM is 0321 hours, and 4:06 PM is 1606 hours.

Communication Equipment

EMS communication system components include base stations, **mobile radios**, portable radios, **repeaters**, digital equipment, and cellular phones (Figure 6-3). In some cases, such as for scheduled interfacility transports, you may receive faxed or electronic patient information. A base station

TABLE 6-1	Radio Terminology

RADIO COMMUNICATION TERMS

Term	Meaning
Affirmative	Yes
Clear	End of transmission
Copy	Message received and understood
ETA	Estimated time of arrival
Go ahead	Continue with your transmission
Landline	Telephone
Negative	No
Over	End of transmission, waiting for response
Repeat	Message not understood
Stand by	Wait
10–4	Message received and understood

LANGUAGE TO AVOID

Slang or jargon
"Please" and "Thank you" (Courtesy is implied.)

CLARIFICATION AND DIFFICULT-TO-UNDERSTAND TERMS

- Numbers with more than one digit can be misunderstood. Say the number, then the individual digits (for example, "231 Dexter Place, two-three-one Dexter Place").
- Words that are difficult to understand or that must be spelled out are clarified using standard words that start with the letter (for example, "725 Gilpin Street, Apartment B, as in boy").
- Echo orders and directions to ensure understanding.

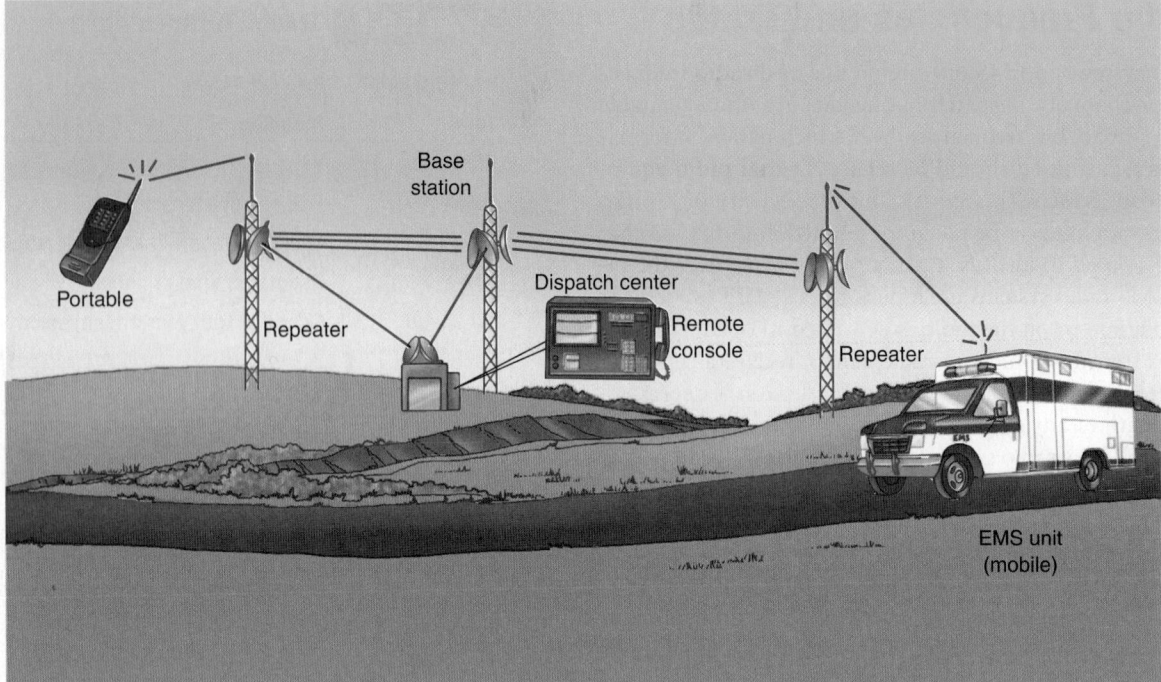

FIGURE 6-3

An overview of an EMS communication system.

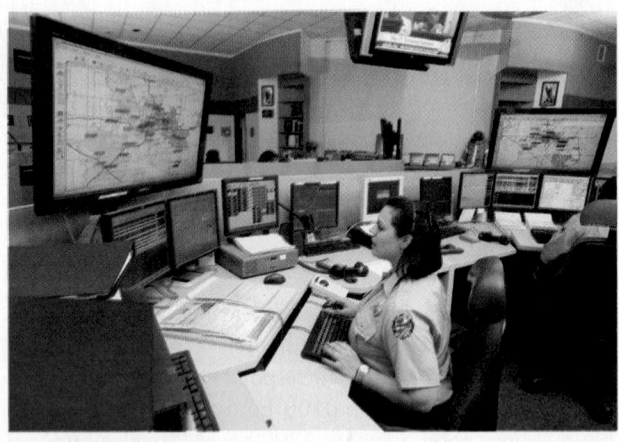

FIGURE 6-4

An example of a base station radio.

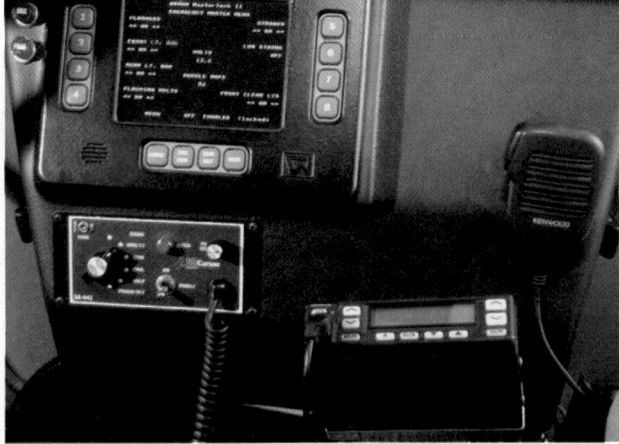

FIGURE 6-5

An example of a mobile radio with status buttons and data screen.

is a high-power (up to 150 **watts**), two-way radio at a fixed site, such as a dispatch center or hospital (Figure 6-4). Base stations have a fixed antenna to facilitate transmission and reception. A mobile radio is radio mounted inside a vehicle (Figure 6-5). It has lower power (20 to 50 watts) than a base station. The range from which the radio can receive and transmit is affected by the power of the radio, the type of radio frequency used, and the geography of the area. The

typical range of mobile radios is 10 to 15 miles. Portable radios are low-power (1 to 5 watts), two-way radios with a limited range and are carried by EMS personnel to enable communication from outside the vehicle (Figure 6-6).

Repeaters enhance transmissions from mobile and portable radios by picking up the lower-power transmissions of portable and mobile radios and retransmitting them at a

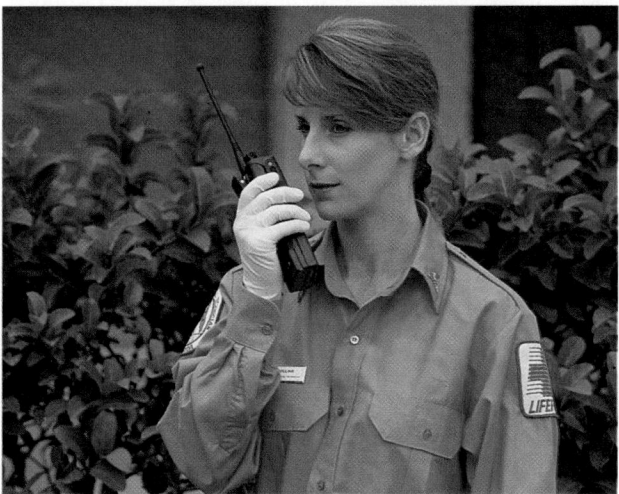

FIGURE 6-6

Portable radios allow communication away from the vehicle.

TABLE 6-2	Guidelines for Radio Communication

- Make sure the radio is powered on and you have selected the correct frequency.
- Listen before transmitting to avoid interrupting other transmissions.
- Press the "PTT" button and wait one second to avoid cutting off the first part of your transmission.
- Hold the microphone two to three inches away from your mouth. Speak clearly and in a normal volume. Control voice inflection, and aim for a neutral, professional tone.
- First state the name of the entity or unit you are calling, followed by your unit identification. If you are Medic One and you are contacting Methodist Hospital, say, "Methodist Hospital, Medic One."
- Wait for the unit being called to respond. "Go ahead," means proceed with your transmission. "Stand by," means wait for the unit to let you know they are ready for your transmission.
- Transmit for no more than 30 seconds without a pause.
- Deliver information in a concise, organized format.

higher power on a different frequency. Repeaters may either be fixed or mobile.

A disadvantage to all radio systems is the limited range of transmission. This disadvantage can sometimes be overcome by using cellular telephones. However, in some rural and mountainous areas, subways, and other locations, neither radios nor cellular equipment can send or receive. In such cases, you must change locations to communicate.

Digital radio equipment encodes and decodes sound waves into digital format. Digital radio equipment allows more data to be sent over the limited number of available radio frequencies. **Mobile data terminals**, digital pagers, and cellular phones are also capable of receiving digitized information. Digital radio systems also allow the use of radio status buttons to streamline communications. Instead of speaking to dispatch over the radio, the push of a button on the radio console indicates the unit status, such as responding, on scene, leaving scene, at the hospital, and in service. Digital systems can encrypt information for added security.

Guidelines for Radio Communication

Although practices vary slightly from system to system, there are some basic ground rules that apply to EMS communication (Table 6-2). There is a typical progression of radio communication transmissions throughout an emergency call (Figure 6-7). Also be aware that most EMS system communication is recorded for legal and quality assurance reasons. There is a typical format for providing information to the receiving hospital and requesting orders from medical direction (Table 6-3). When you arrive at the hospital, you will summarize the information given in your radio report, add any relevant information, and advise receiving staff of any additional treatment given, or changes in the patient's condition.

Therapeutic Communication and Interviewing Patients

Patient assessment and obtaining a medical history are among the Advanced EMT's primary skills. You must establish rapport with the patient and efficiently obtain specific pieces of information. Conducting an interview to successfully complete those tasks requires special techniques of **therapeutic communication** in addition to knowledge of the general principles of communication. Cultural differences can present possibilities of misunderstanding and must be considered, too.

Intercultural and Language Considerations

We live in increasingly culturally diverse communities (Figure 6-8). Many areas have growing Hispanic, Asian, and Middle Eastern communities. The differences in perception

IN THE FIELD

You will develop your skills in interviewing and giving verbal and written reports as you increase your understanding of patient assessment, pathophysiology, and patient management.

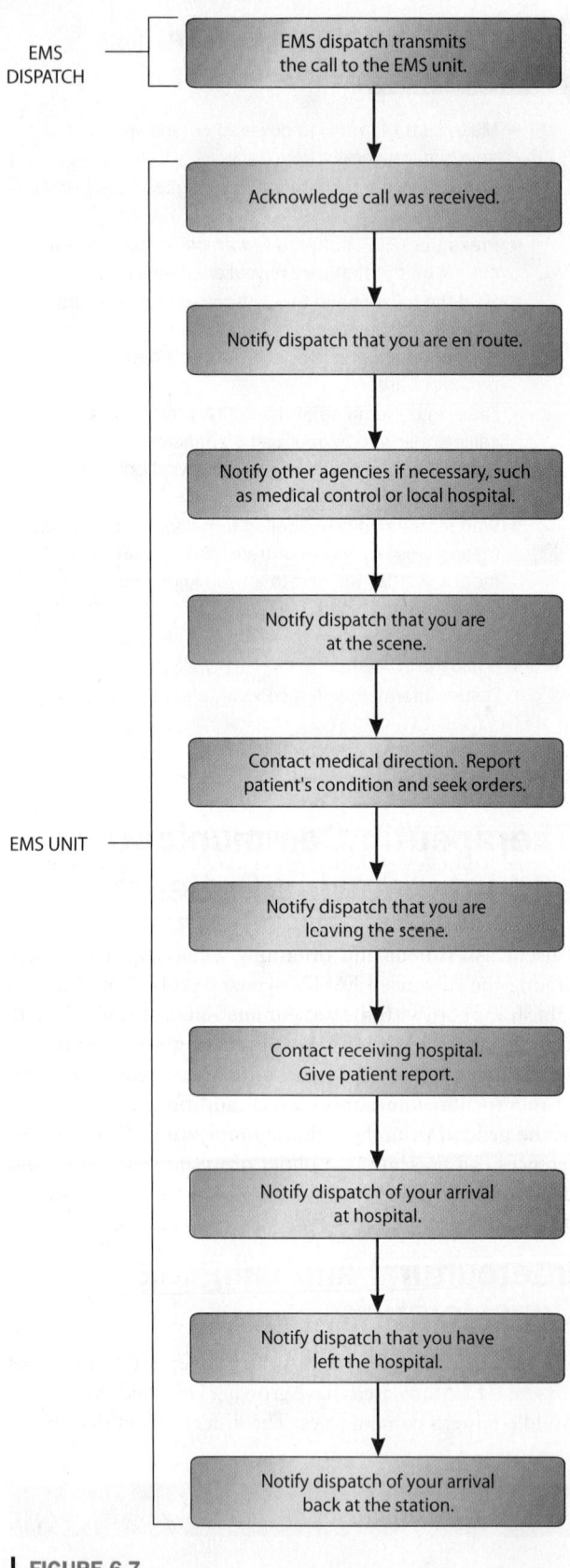

EMS DISPATCH

EMS dispatch transmits the call to the EMS unit.

EMS UNIT

Acknowledge call was received.

Notify dispatch that you are en route.

Notify other agencies if necessary, such as medical control or local hospital.

Notify dispatch that you are at the scene.

Contact medical direction. Report patient's condition and seek orders.

Notify dispatch that you are leaving the scene.

Contact receiving hospital. Give patient report.

Notify dispatch of your arrival at hospital.

Notify dispatch that you have left the hospital.

Notify dispatch of your arrival back at the station.

FIGURE 6-7

Typical progression of communications for an EMS call.

TABLE 6-3   Radio Report Format

SAMPLE RADIO REPORT WITH REQUEST FOR ORDERS

You: "Marshal County Hospital, Ambulance 2."

Hospital: "This is Marshal County, we copy you loud and clear Ambulance 2. Go ahead."

You: "We're requesting a physician for orders. Over."

Hospital: "Stand by."

Dr. Rashad: "Ambulance 2, this is Dr. Rashad. Go ahead."

You: "We are en route with a 27-year-old male diabetic. He was found unresponsive at his desk at work. On our arrival he was unresponsive to painful stimuli. Initial vital signs: pulse 100, blood pressure 122/78, respirations 16, pulse ox 98 percent on room air. We obtained a blood glucose level of 40 mg/dL, but have been unable to obtain IV access to administer 50 percent dextrose. The patient has no other known medical problems, no known allergies, and no medications. There are no signs of trauma. We are requesting an order for IM glucagon. Our ETA is 15 minutes. Over."

Dr. Rashad: "Copy, Ambulance 2. Give 1 mg of glucagon, IM, and advise us of further problems."

You: "Copy, Marshall County. That is 1 mg of glucagon, IM, and advise of further problems. Ambulance 2 clear."

Dr. Rashad: "See you in about 15 minutes. Marshall County clear."

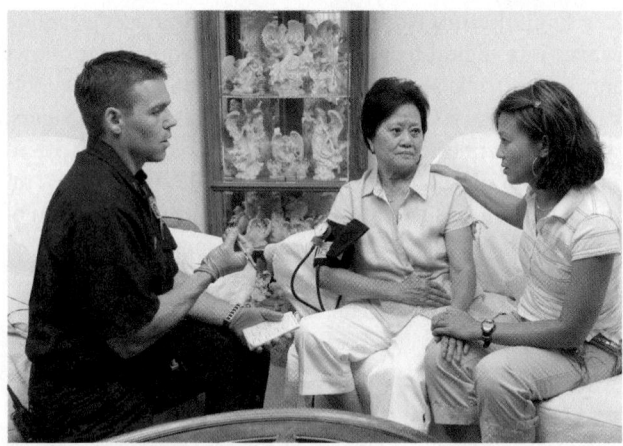

FIGURE 6-8

Cultural differences and language barriers can present communication challenges.

of communication behaviors by people of different cultures can be surprising. It is easy to take for granted that communication behaviors have the same meaning in all cultures. When responding to patients whose culture is different from yours, examine any biases or stereotypes you may hold that can impact communication. Evaluate how your actions may be perceived, and how you can best understand the patient's behavior before proceeding.

CASE STUDY (continued)

As Stan approaches the patient, he recognizes him as a homeless man who frequently is found sleeping in public places during the day. He notes dried vomit in the patient's beard and that the patient's words are slurred as he talks with the police officer. Lowering himself on one knee, Stan says, "Hi Mr. Gregory, I'm an Advanced EMT with the rescue squad. My name is Stan, do you remember me?"

"I sure don't need to go to the hospital with you!" Mr. Gregory says grumpily. "Why don't you just go on and get out of here?"

Problem-Solving Questions

1. What can Stan do to improve rapport with Mr. Gregory?
2. What should Stan avoid doing as he attempts to establish rapport?

Language barriers are frustrating to EMS providers and patients. Hospitals generally have interpreter services that can provide impartial, accurate translation in both directions. These services are typically not an option in the prehospital setting. Although family or EMS crew members who speak more than one language can be helpful, there is still opportunity for misunderstanding. If a language other than English is common in your community, consider learning the language well enough to interact with patients.

Trust and Rapport

A patient's first impression of you sets the tone for the rest of the call. Consider the following example:

Advanced EMT: "Hello, ma'am. My name is David Smith. I'm an Advanced EMT with Reynolds Ambulance Service. This is my partner, Sam. What's your name?"

Patient: "I'm Sharon Lieb. Everyone calls me Shar."

Advanced EMT: "How can we help you today, Mrs. Lieb?"

Patient: "Oh, call me Shar, everyone does. I got so dizzy when I got up from my chair I thought I was going to fall."

Advanced EMT: "We're here to help. I'd like to ask you some questions while Sam takes your pulse and blood pressure. Is that okay?"

While it is important to convey respect to your patient by addressing him formally and using his name, too-frequent use of the patient's name or title such as "ma'am" or "sir" can seem condescending. Never address a patient with terms of endearment or nicknames, such as "dear," "cupcake," "dude," "partner," "hon," "sweetheart," or similar terms. It diminishes the patient's dignity at a time when he already fears loss of dignity and autonomy.

Not all patients will be as cooperative and willing to accept your help as well as the patient in the previous example. Embarrassment, fright, denial, concern over the cost of services, and other factors can create resistance. Attempt to overcome resistance by respectfully persisting. For example, "You've got a cut on your forehead. Can I take a look at it for you?" Or, "You don't need to decide at this moment about going to the hospital. Is it alright if I just ask you a few questions?"

PERSONAL PERSPECTIVE

Advanced EMT Kevin Schute: A couple of months ago I had outpatient surgery to clean up some cartilage in my knee. They use techs in the day surgery center, and I couldn't tell what kind of training they had, but my experience that day wasn't a good one. When they called me back to the prep area, this really young tech said, "Ok, hon, I need you to take off all your clothes and put them in this bag and then put on this hospital gown." I think the hair on the back of my neck actually stood up. Being called "hon" like that really irked me. "Mr. Schute" would have been appropriate. I could even have dealt with "Kevin." To make it worse, when she came back to start my IV, her cell phone rang. When she answered it, I thought it must be a work call. But when she said, "Hi baby. No, I'm at work. I'll call you on my break. Love you, too!" I just about flipped out. How rude and unprofessional! A couple of weeks later I got a survey in the mail that asked me about my surgery experience. I filled it out. I hope it did some good. Anyway, I never used to give it much thought when I heard coworkers calling patients, "sweetie," or "bud," or whatever. Now I say, "Hey, I've got a story to tell you."

Tone, volume, inflection, and rate of speech are important. Your tone should convey courtesy, compassion, and respect. The stress of the situation may make it difficult for the patient to focus on what you are saying. So, speak clearly, calmly, and deliberately. Take care not to speak too rapidly. Speak with a normal volume unless attempts to do so reveal that the patient is having difficulty hearing. Even then, raise your voice only to a "loud-normal" volume to avoid the distortion of words that occurs with yelling or shouting.

Control the Environment

Provide privacy for the patient as much as allowed by the situation. Keep bystanders at a distance from the patient during the interview. Even the presence of family members and friends may cause the patient to be self-conscious and prevent him from answering honestly. The presence of too many EMS and public safety personnel can be overwhelming to the patient, too. So, keep the number of providers in the patient's immediate vicinity to the number needed to provide effective care.

If possible, control noise from the environment. If a television is on in the background, ask if you can turn it off. It is sometimes best to move patients out of the noisy environment created by street noise and the engines of emergency response vehicles before conducting an interview. Keep the volume on your portable and mobile radios at an acceptable volume.

Nonverbal Communication

In addition to your general appearance and facial expressions, other nonverbal behaviors communicate messages. Many times people are unaware of the nonverbal messages they are sending. Sometimes, nonverbal messages can undercut the rapport you are trying to establish.

Posture, Gestures, and Facial Expressions

It is commonly held that standing with your arms crossed or hands on your hips can convey negative emotion. However, research on this perception is not convincing. Nonetheless, the overemphasis on this aspect of nonverbal communication in many classes and texts may cause some people to interpret this posture negatively, rather than neutrally.

Pay attention to your patient's facial expression as you approach. This is an important piece of information in forming a general impression of the patient's condition. Although facial expressions are not completely foolproof, they are usually easy to recognize and consistent among cultures. A smile is a smile in all cultures. Your patient's facial expressions can tell you whether he is afraid, apprehensive, in pain, angry, or sad (Figure 6-9).

Your patient also will recognize the meaning behind your facial expressions, and attribute meaning to your

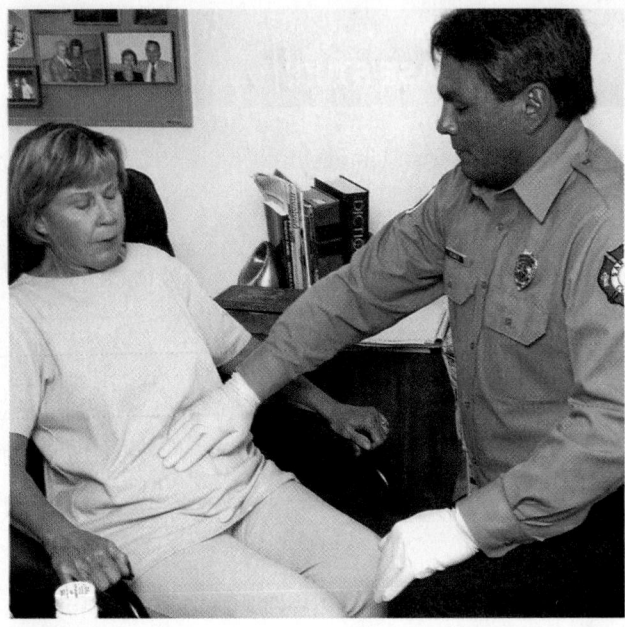

FIGURE 6-9

Pay attention to the nonverbal communication of the patient's facial expressions.

gestures. A wink can indicate a familiarity that may make the patient uncomfortable. Depending on circumstances, it could be interpreted as flirting. Rolling your eyes can indicate disbelief or disrespect. The meaning of gestures has more variability among cultures, and they must be used cautiously.

Making eye contact provides an important piece of information about a patient. Eye contact is considered a respectful gesture in Western society. It indicates to your patient that you are confident and that you are paying attention to him. Discomfort with eye contact among Westerners may indicate poor self-esteem, embarrassment, general emotional discomfort, or even that you are too close to the patient. Eye contact can signify disrespect or aggressiveness in other cultures, particularly in some Asian, Indonesian, Native American, and Arab cultures. If your eye contact makes a patient of a different culture uncomfortable, adjust your approach.

Space and Touch

The amount of personal space considered acceptable varies among cultures and individuals. A space of less than 18 inches can be threatening or disconcerting to many people. Although the nature of EMS work requires physical contact with patients, it is best to remain a distance of two to four feet from patients while interviewing them. When you need to move closer or touch the patient, explain what you are going to do. Read your patient's nonverbal communication to determine if you are too close. If the patient seems uncomfortable, give him more space.

Touch is a similarly sensitive issue. Placing your hand on the shoulder, hand, or forearm can be an effective way to display empathy and compassion to some patients. Other patients are not comfortable being touched in this manner by strangers, even strangers with a professional role to play. Again, read your patient's body language. If he is not comfortable with you being close to him, he will probably be uncomfortable with your touch.

A handshake is a socially acceptable, and often overlooked, gesture in EMS. Naturally we are concerned with protecting ourselves from communicable diseases, so we wear gloves in many situations. Think about your last visit to your primary care provider. Most likely, the nurse or medical assistant who took your vital signs was not wearing gloves. Your health care provider most likely was not wearing gloves when he shook your hand or performed most aspects of your examination. OSHA requires gloves only when there is a likelihood of contact with blood or body fluids. Gloves are not required for much of the contact you have with patients, unless blood or body fluids are present or you are performing an invasive procedure. However, good hand washing is essential after patient contact, whether or not you are wearing gloves.

Verbal Communication

Several techniques of verbal communication can be used to conduct an effective patient interview. Active listening is listening beyond the words to understand the meanings conveyed in messages. Sometimes those meanings are subtle and are learned with experience. For example, the elderly patient who asks, "Do I really need to go to the hospital?" may not be asking about the seriousness of his condition as much as he is expressing fear or anxiety about leaving his home unattended, or about his ability to afford health care. Active listening is required for empathy. The techniques below demonstrate active listening and other ways to improve communication.

Being Available

Make yourself available to your patient for communication. If possible, sit next to the patient in the ambulance, not behind him where he cannot see you. If you must sit behind him, explain the reason. You might say, "I need to sit behind you for a few minutes to use the radio to let the hospital know how you're doing." Another way of being available is to let the patient know you want to hear from him: "If your pain comes back or you have any concerns, let me know."

Asking Questions

The interview process involves asking questions. **Open-ended questions** do not have a limited range of options. They are designed to ensure that patients have an opportunity to tell you their concerns in their own way. Generally, the interview begins with an open-ended question such as, "How can we help you today?" Begin the medical history with an open-ended question, such as, "What medical problems have you had?" This opens up the conversation for the patient to tell you about the problems that concern him. Do not interrupt the patient while he is answering, and do not become distracted by other tasks, family members, or team members unless absolutely necessary. Focus on listening to the patient's answers.

Closed-ended questions have a narrow range of expected responses, but limit the patient's ability to give you additional information. Closed-ended questions are important when you need a specific answer, or to follow up on information from open-ended questions. For example, "How long have you had this cough?" or "Do you have a history of high blood pressure?" Closed-ended questions also can be used to direct a patient who is overly talkative or providing excess detail.

Ask only one question at a time and wait for the answer. If you ask, "Do you have a history of diabetes or heart problems?" the response, "Yes," may mean that the patient has a history of either or both of the conditions. Listen to the patient's answer. The answer will affect your selection of the next question. Having an overly rigid approach to the patient interview can result in not following up on the patient's answers. Providers who rely too much on a "checklist" approach to history taking are often more focused on the next question than on listening to the patient's answer. In fact, a common cause of poor listening in any communication is focusing on what you want to say, rather than listening to what the other person is saying. You must be prepared to explore the answer to a question before moving on to the question you originally had planned to ask next.

Leading questions are questions that suggest an answer to patients, instead of allowing them to answer as they otherwise might have. Leading questions indicate assumptions on your part, rather than active listening. Avoid leading questions such as, "You probably want some medication for pain, don't you?"

Checking Understanding

Checking your understanding of what the patient has told you, sometimes called *interpretation*, demonstrates active listening. This technique also allows you to check the accuracy of your understanding. Example: "Let me see if

I understand. You have a history of high blood pressure and you are concerned that your headache might be a symptom of a stroke?"

Clarifying

Ambiguous information must be clarified. **Clarification** can be used when a patient has given a lot of information and you are not sure exactly what his complaint is, or when you are otherwise unclear about an aspect of the patient's story. You could ask, "I'm not sure I understand. Are you having chest pain now, or is the chest pain something you experienced in the past?"

Confronting

In the common use of the word **confrontation**, people are often referring to a disagreement or argument. In the therapeutic sense, confrontation means pointing out inconsistencies in the patient's communication. For example, "You said that you don't have a headache, but you keep rubbing your forehead."

Facilitating

Facilitation helps the patient move past a difficult point in the conversation. The patient may become hesitant in some aspect of his story. Perhaps the patient is uncertain if the information he is relating is important, or he is embarrassed, or has become distracted by another thought. Acknowledge what you've heard the patient say, and encourage him to go on. ("You were saying you were on your way to work when this happened. Go on.")

Reflecting

Reflection is a technique used to check for understanding by repeating the patient's words back to him. If a patient says, "This pain is the worst I've ever had. I took five aspirin this morning," you would say, "You took five aspirin this morning?" Of course, it would be important to follow up if the patient confirms that he took five aspirin.

Silence

Silence can seem awkward in social situations, but is a useful therapeutic communication technique. Silence allows the patient time to organize his thoughts. Ensure that you leave enough time for patients to think before answering questions.

Summarizing

Use **summarization** to make sure that you heard everything the patient is concerned about. An example of summarization is, "Let me make sure I have all the information. You were running on the treadmill when the chest pain started. It was just to the left of your breastbone and felt like someone was pressing in on your chest. You rated the pain an 8 on a scale of 1 to 10, but the pain went away a minute or so after you stopped running." This gives the patient an opportunity to correct any misunderstanding and add any information he did not initially think of.

Pitfalls in Communication

Just as you must make a conscious effort to use specific techniques of therapeutic communication, you must make an attempt to avoid actions that interfere with communication. One cause of poor listening is that the speed of thought is many times faster than the speed at which people can speak. In social situations, this can lead to wandering thoughts while trying to listen to someone speaking.

In EMS the need to multitask and divide your attention challenges the ability to listen and make sense of information. You must split your attention between the environment around you, what the patient is saying, interpreting vital signs, and thinking ahead to the next steps of assessment, treatment, and transport. New EMS providers must think much more consciously about each step of the job, while certain aspects of the job have become more automatic for experienced providers. You can improve listening by learning patient care tasks well. This way, conscious thought about things like how to use a blood glucose meter do not take up space in working memory that should be devoted to collecting and analyzing patient information. One pitfall for more experienced providers is that they have heard similar stories many times. Instead of obtaining specific information about the current patient, there is a tendency toward unconscious substitution of information that is typical of similar calls.

Specific types of verbal statements can inhibit therapeutic communication. Requesting an explanation from a patient ("Why didn't you call 911 sooner?" or, "Why did you call 911 for this?") implies blame or disapproval. These judgments are destructive to rapport with your patient. Overloading the patient with too much information or too many questions at once can cause confusion. Avoid unwarranted opinions and advice. A patient who is depressed may tell you that he is unhappy with his job. It would be inappropriate to say, "It sounds like your boss is a jerk. You should quit." An appropriate, empathetic response would be, "That sounds like a really frustrating situation." Changing the subject while the patient is giving you information conveys that you are not interested in, or are uncomfortable with, what he is saying. Providing false reassurance diminishes your trustworthiness to the patient. Interrupting your patient conveys that what he has to say is not important.

Special Patient Communication Situations

The communication principles discussed in this chapter generally apply to all patients. In some cases, there are special considerations or challenges. Age-related psychosocial characteristics that affect communication are introduced in Chapter 9. The application of these principles to patient interaction is further discussed in Chapters 44 and 45. Communication with patients with special challenges, such as sensory deficits or cognitive impairment, is discussed in Chapter 46. When interacting with any of these groups, direct your attention to the patient, rather than assuming he cannot communicate. Begin by communicating with the patient directly. You can verify or obtain additional information from family or caregivers later, if needed. Assist the patient in obtaining hearing aids, dentures, or eyeglasses if needed for effective communication. Patients with difficulty speaking due to a stroke may be able to write down their responses for you to read. Similarly, you may need to write out questions for patients with hearing deficits.

Involve family members in communication as much as the patient desires. Some patients may be comforted by the presence of family, while others may not share information with you in front of family members. Sometimes, a family member may try to dominate the conversation, speaking for the patient instead of allowing the patient to speak for himself. This is often a display of anxiety and concern about the patient. In some cases of abuse, this behavior can be an indication that the family member is attempting to control the information given by the patient. In most circumstances, it is not desirable to shut the family member out of the process, particularly with pediatric patients. A typical way of addressing the family member who is speaking for the patient is to say, "I know you have information for me, but I need to hear the answers to these questions from him." In some cultures, a large group of family and perhaps friends or neighbors may surround the patient. A possible response is, "I can see that you are all concerned, but we need some room to work. Could all but one or two of you please wait outside?"

The first consideration in communicating with a patient who shows signs of hostility is your own safety. If a patient is agitated or angry but his behavior has not escalated to the point where your safety is at risk, verbal defusing strategies may be effective. These strategies are discussed in detail in Chapter 31. Let the patient know you are there to help, and acknowledge his feelings. Stay calm and professional, but take care not to seem condescending, which can provoke an angry patient.

There are many reasons a patient may be uncommunicative with you. He may be depressed, afraid, or uncertain that he can trust you. If the patient seems overwhelmed by open-ended questions, try closed-ended questions and let the patient know that his response is important. For example, if your patient responds affirmatively that he has a history of high blood pressure, you could say, "You have a history of high blood pressure. That's important for me to know. I'm glad you told me that."

Documentation

There are several types of **documentation** that are important in EMS. You must document your vehicle and equipment check, fill out patient care report for each call, and document any special circumstances, such as being injured on the job, or injuries to patients. The focus of this section is patient care documentation.

Patient care is documented on a **patient care report** (**PCR**), which may be paper or electronic (Figures 6-10 and 6-11). The PCR serves several functions. It is an essential part of continuity of patient care. The assessments, history, treatments, and other information in the PCR communicate critical information to hospital personnel. This information can prevent duplicate doses of medications and giving a patient a medication to which he is allergic. It also provides a baseline against which to measure changes in the patient's condition.

Administrative uses of PCRs include providing information for billing, insurance claims, and statistical information about the operation of the EMS service. The PCR is a legal document, as well, that may be subpoenaed in criminal or civil cases involving you or the patient. PCRs provide data for research and education, and are a key component of the continuous quality improvement process.

Standardized Data Collection

Standardization of the data collected by EMS systems provides the possibility of greater understanding of the nature of EMS through research. Data can be used to understand the types of patients who seek EMS, the types of care provided, and the outcomes of patients, as well as allow many other types of EMS research. This information, in turn, provides support for changes in EMS systems and EMS provider scopes of practice and education. The National EMS Information System (NEMSIS) provides assistance to establish local and state EMS databases and link them to a national database. For the database to work, systems must collect the same kind of information and record it in the same ways. NEMSIS has a minimum standard data set that serves this purpose. The two categories of information in the minimum data set are patient information and administration information (Table 6-4).

IN THE FIELD

Signs of impending violent behavior include yelling, profanity, rapid speech, rapid physical movement, possession of a weapon, hitting, kicking, or throwing objects, and threats of violence. Maintaining your own safety is your first priority in these situations.

IN THE FIELD

PCRs provide information for five functions: continuity of patient care, administrative functions, education and research, and continuous quality improvement.

MAINE ⚡EMS   PRESS DOWN, YOU ARE MAKING THREE COPIES.

RUN REPORT # 746118	Mo.	Day	Year	M T W Th / F S Sun	SERVICE NAME		SERVICE NO.	VEHICLE NO.	ALS ☐ Performed ☐ Back-up called	SERVICE RUN NO.

NAME	BILLING INFORMATION

STREET OR R.F.D.

CITY/TOWN	STATE	ZIP

AGE/DATE OF BIRTH	☐ Male ☐ Female	PHONE

INCIDENT LOCATION:	ADDRESS	CITY/TOWN

TRANSPORTED TO:	TREATING/FAMILY PHYSICIAN	CREW LICENSE NUMBERS

TRANSPORTATION/COMMUNICATIONS PROBLEMS

☐ Medical
  ☐ Cardiac
☐ Poisoning/OD
  ☐ Respiratory
☐ Behavioral
  ☐ Diabetic
☐ Seizure
  ☐ CVA
☐ OB/Gyn
  ☐ Other _____

☐ Trauma
  ☐ Multi-Systems Trauma
☐ Head
  ☐ Spinal
☐ Burn
  ☐ Soft Tissue Injury
☐ Fractures
  ☐ Other _____

☐ Code 99

R L LUNG SOUNDS
☐ ☐ CLEAR
☐ ☐ ABSENT
☐ ☐ DECREASED
☐ ☐ RALES
☐ ☐ WHEEZE
☐ ☐ STRIDOR

TYPE OF RUN
☐ Emergency Transport
☐ Routine Transfer
☐ Emergency Transfer
☐ No Transport
☐ Refused Transport

☐ MEDICATIONS   ☐ ALLERGIES

CHIEF COMPLAINT:

	TIME	CODE		ODOMETER
Call Received				
Enroute				
At Scene				
From Scene				
At Destination				
In Service				

TIME	PULSE	RESP	BP	PUPILLARY RESPONSE	SKIN	VERBAL RESPONSE	MOTOR RESPONSE	EYE-OPENING RESPONSE	CAPILLARY REFILL
						5 4 3 2 1	6 5 4 3 2 1	4 3 2 1	☐ Normal ☐ None ☐ Delayed
						5 4 3 2 1	6 5 4 3 2 1	4 3 2 1	☐ Normal ☐ None ☐ Delayed
						5 4 3 2 1	6 5 4 3 2 1	4 3 2 1	☐ Normal ☐ None ☐ Delayed

☐ MVA ☐ Concern AOB/ETOH   SEAT BELTS: ☐ Used ☐ Not Used ☐ N/A ☐ Helmet Used

MUTUAL AID: Assisted/Assisted by Service # _____ Time Called: _____

PATIENT'S SUSPECTED PROBLEM: 746118	☐ Medication Administered	☐ Defib Lic.# _____	MEDICAL CONTROL	☐ Written Order/Protocol ☐ Verbal Order/Protocol
	☐ Monitor	☐ Chest Decomp	IV ☐ SUC LIC.# _____	Total Attempts
	☐ Pacing	☐ Caricothyrotomy	☐ UNSUC LIC.# _____	

		EOA	Total Attempts	ET	Total Attempts
Cleared Airway	Extrication				
Artificial Respiration/BVM	Cervical Immobilization				
Oropharyngeal Airway	KED/Short Board	☐ SUC LIC.# _____		☐ SUC LIC.# _____	
Nasopharyngeal Airway	Long Board	☐ UNSUC LIC.# _____		☐ UNSUC LIC.# _____	

CPR–Time:	Restraints	LIC #	EKG RHYTHM	TIME	MEDS/DEFIB/C-VERT	DOSE W/S	ROUTE
Bystander CPR	Traction Splinting						
AED	General Splinting						
Suction	Cold Application						
Oxygen–L/min ___ ☐ Nasal ☐ Mask	MAST Inflated						
Pulse Oximetry							
Autovent							

NAME OF E.D. TREATING PHYSICIAN   SIGNATURE OF CREW MEMBER IN CHARGE   COPY 1 HOSPITAL

FIGURE 6-10

A paper patient care report (PCR) form.

TABLE 6-4 Minimum EMS Data Set
MINIMUM DATA SET FOR PATIENT INFORMATION ■ Chief complaint ■ Level of responsiveness/mental status ■ Blood pressure (patients > three years old) ■ Skin perfusion ■ Skin color, temperature, and condition ■ Pulse rate ■ Respiratory rate and effort ■ Patient demographics (age, gender, ethnicity, weight)
MINIMUM DATA SET: ADMINISTRATIVE INFORMATION (TIMES) ■ Incident reported ■ Unit notified ■ Arrived at patient ■ Unit left scene ■ Unit at hospital (or other destination) ■ Patient care transferred
Source: National EMS Information Systems Technical Assistance Center, Office of Emergency Medical Services, National Highway Traffic Administration, Department of Transportation

TABLE 6-5 Sections of the Patient Care Report
ADMINISTRATIVE INFORMATION (RUN DATA) ■ EMS unit ■ Crew names ■ Key times ■ Dispatched address
PATIENT DATA AND DEMOGRAPHICS ■ Name, age, gender, ethnicity, date of birth ■ Home address ■ Location where patient was found ■ Insurance and billing information ■ Care provided before EMS arrival
VITAL SIGNS (MINIMUM OF TWO SETS) ■ Pulse ■ Respirations ■ Blood pressure ■ Other information may be included in this section, such as pulse oximetry, blood glucose level, pupil assessment, and so on.
PATIENT CARE NARRATIVE ■ Written account of the call ■ Follows one of several standard formats

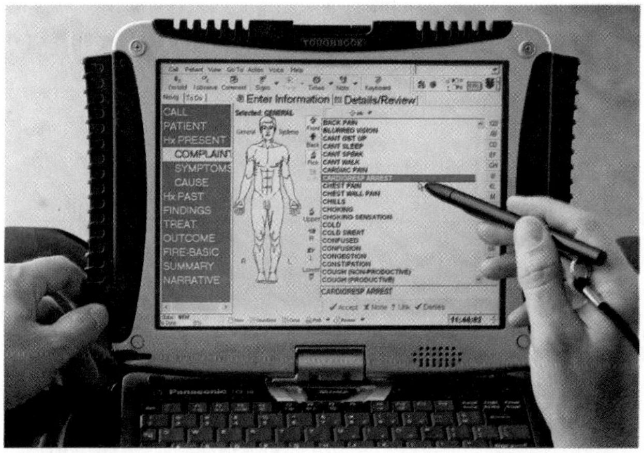

FIGURE 6-11

Electronic PCR systems eliminate some of the disadvantages of paper forms, such as poor handwriting and difficulty in database reporting.

Sections of the Patient Care Report

The elements of the minimum data set and other information needed by the EMS system are recorded in PCR sections for administrative information, patient demographic data, vital signs, a **narrative report** of the call, and treatment provided (Table 6-5). All information recorded in these sections must be recorded using standard terminology and abbreviations, and entered with the utmost attention to accuracy and completeness.

The narrative section can be structured in several ways to ensure that all relevant information is included (Table 6-6). Narratives are a form of technical writing that use a factual, straight-forward style. They are objective, contain all relevant information, include **pertinent negatives,** and omit irrelevant information. Advanced EMTs do not state opinion, draw conclusions, or make assumptions in the narrative. For instance, you should never state that a patient was "drunk" or "intoxicated." Instead, it would be acceptable to document, "The patient stated he drank six beers in a two-hour period" or "The patient's speech was slurred and there was an empty 750 mL bottle of vodka on the table next to him."

Legal Considerations in Documentation

PCRs are legal medical records protected by HIPAA. Therefore, PCR information is only provided to other medical personnel involved in the patient's care, such as receiving hospital staff, and for approved administrative purposes, such as filing insurance claims and billing. Shield all

TABLE 6-6 Patient Care Report Narrative Formats

SOAP

- *Subjective:* Information about the problem as it is given by the patient, including the chief complaint, history of the present illness, and symptoms.

  Example: Pt. c/o difficulty breathing that started 90 min. ago. Hx: asthma. States he has used his albuterol inhaler × 2 s̄ relief of symptoms.

- *Objective:* Information observed in some way by the Advanced EMT, such as vital signs, pupil reaction, response to pain, and other physical findings. Also includes description of the circumstances in which the patient was found.

  Example: Pt. found prone on living room floor c̄ pool of emesis next to his face. Did not respond to painful stimuli, but was breathing spontaneously at a rate of 12 breaths per minute.

- *Assessment:* Your field impression of the patient's problem, based on subjective and objective information.

  Example: Suspected hypoglycemia.

- *Plan:* Treatment provided and transport information.

  Example: Airway opened with a head-tilt/chin-lift. Pt. unable to tolerate OPA. O₂, 15 L/min by NRB. IV NS TKO, lt. forearm. 25 g dextrose, IVP. LOC ↑ within 2 minutes. Pt. remained A&O × 3 throughout transport to Cass County Hospital.

CHART

- Usually starts with an introductory statement.

  Example: 48 yowf found LLR on sofa with empty emesis basin on floor.

- *Chief complaint (CC):* Describes the patient's chief complaint; also includes associated complaints and pertinent negatives.

  Example: Pt. c/o RUQ abd pain radiating to rt. Shoulder × 2 hours, with no provoking or alleviating factors. Pain described as "sharp and crampy," and constant. Pt. rates pain 7/10. Pt. c/o nausea, but denies vomiting.

- *History:* Includes history of the present illness (HPI) and pertinent past medical history (PMH).

  Example: Pt. states the pain has been increasing in severity and becoming more constant over the past 2 hrs. PMH: NKDA, no medications, no major illnesses or surgeries, last oral intake: catfish, fries, cole slaw, and soda at 1230 hrs. Pt. felt well until onset of pain at 1600 hrs.

- *Assessment:* Information from primary and secondary assessments and reassessment.

  Example: Pt. A&O ×3, initial VS above. Skin warm, moist, normal color. RUQ tender to palpation. No guarding, masses, or discoloration noted.

- *Rx (treatment):* Lists treatments provided and the patient's response to them.

  Example: Pt. placed in position of comfort (LLR) on stretcher.

- *Transport:* How and where patient was transported, changes in transport, transfer of care.

  Example: Transported nonemergent to Douglas Medical Center s̄ Δ in condition. Released with report to RN in room #6.

CHEATED (VARIATION ON CHART)

- *Chief complaint*
- *History*
- *Exam:* Information from primary and secondary assessments.
- *Assessment:* Field impression, based on chief complaint, history, and exam.
- *Treatment*
- *Evaluation:* Information from on-going assessment.
- *Disposition:* Transport and transfer of care information.

(Refer to Chapter 7 for symbols and abbreviations.)

protected health information (PHI), whether in electronic or paper format, from the view of anyone not directly involved in patient care. PCRs may be subpoenaed through your employer for civil and criminal legal actions. Because PCR documentation is used for legal purposes, it must be complete, accurate, neat, and unaltered. The PCR also must be completed as soon as possible after the call to ensure accurate recall. The correct way for correcting an error on a written PCR is to draw a single line through the error, initial it, and write the correct information (Figure 6-12). Falsification of information on a PCR is a serious violation that can lead to patient harm and disciplinary action against you, including revocation of your license. It is not acceptable to document assessments or treatments that you did not do, knowingly provide inaccurate information, or omit information from the PCR.

COMMENTS PATIENT COMPLAINS OF PAIN IN HIS ~~RIGHT~~ ᴰᴸ LEFT SHOULDER THAT RADIATES TO THE LEFT ARM.

FIGURE 6-12

Correct errors with a single line drawn through them. Initial the correction.

GUIDELINES

REFUSAL INFORMATION SHEET

PLEASE READ AND KEEP THIS FORM!

This form has been given to you because you have refused treatment and/or transport by Emergency Medical Services (EMS). Your health and safety are our primary concern, so even though you have decided not to accept our advice, please remember the following:

1) The evaluation and/or treatment provided to you by the EMS providers is not a substitute for medical evaluation and treatment by a doctor. We advise you to get medical evaluation and treatment.

2) Your condition may not seem as bad to you as it actually is. Without treatment, your condition or problem could become worse. If you are planning to get medical treatment, a decision to refuse treatment or transport by EMS may result in a delay which could make your condition or problem worse.

3) Medical evaluation and/or treatment may be obtained by calling your doctor, if you have one, or by going to any hospital Emergency Department in this area, all of which are staffed 24 hours a day by Emergency Physicians. You may be seen at these Emergency Departments without an appointment.

4) If you change your mind or your condition becomes worse and you decide to accept treatment and transport by Emergency Medical Services, please do not hesitate to call us back. We will do our best to help you.

5) DON'T WAIT! When medical treatment is needed, it is usually better to get it right away.

I have received a copy of this information sheet.

PATIENT SIGNATURE: _____ DATE: _____

WITNESS SIGNATURE: _____ DATE: _____

AGENCY INCIDENT #: _____ AGENCY CODE: _____

NAME OF PERSON FILLING OUT FORM: _____

G 11A

FIGURE 6-13

Patient refusals require careful documentation.

Special Documentation Circumstances

You may be required to return to service before completing your PCR. In some systems, an abbreviated form or a copy of partial PCR information is left with hospital staff to provide as much information as possible. Your protocols and documentation system determine how the completed report is added to the patient care record. In any case, ensure that you have given a complete verbal report of patient care information to hospital staff. When a patient refuses care, there is typically a special additional section of the PCR to be completed (Figure 6-13).

Another situation that complicates documentation of patient care is a multiple-casualty incident. The number of patients may not allow completion of a traditional PCR. Typically, a limited amount of information gained in triage, major injuries, and treatments is provided in abbreviated form (Figure 6-14). System protocols dictate how to complete abbreviated documentation in such cases.

Occasionally, events take place for which complete documentation is outside the scope of the PCR. For example, if you are injured on a call, this is not usually documented in the PCR, unless the patient's behavior caused the

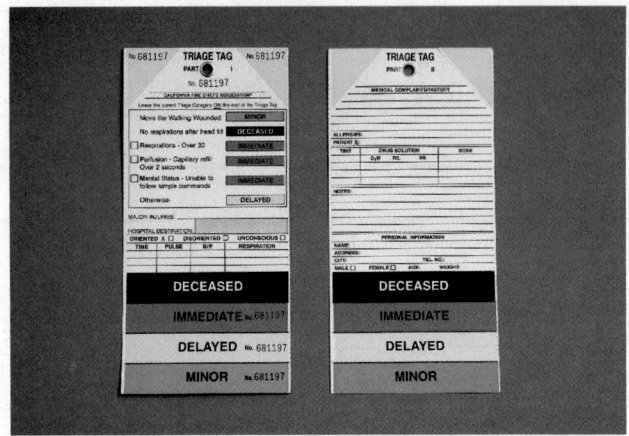

FIGURE 6-14

Abbreviated documentation is used in multiple-casualty incidents.

injury. You would use a separate incident form provided by your employer (Figure 6-15). Patient injuries and patient care mistakes are mentioned in the PCR, but complete documentation of the circumstances usually requires additional explanation.

CASE STUDY WRAP-UP

Clinical-Reasoning Process

Each member of the team knows that he has an important role to play, whether it is leading or following. Operating procedures and advance planning and communication make the roles of each provider clear. They all respect the fact that deviating from expected roles can lead to confusion, inefficiency, and mistakes. All of the team members know their roles, yet they do not make unwarranted assumptions and they recognize that clear communication is a key part of good teamwork.

Stan realizes that responding in kind to Mr. Gregory's demeanor is unprofessional, unproductive, and would likely lead to an escalation of his disagreeable conduct. He knows that patience, empathy, and focusing on the patient's needs are much more likely to gain his cooperation.

"The folks who live here called us because they were concerned about you. You were asleep in their yard and they couldn't wake you up," Stan explains. "How are you feeling right now?"

"I could feel better, I'll tell you that," replies Mr. Gregory.

"I see. In what way are you not feeling well?"

"My gut is killing me. Feels like somebody stuck a knife in there."

"How about letting my partner check your blood pressure while I ask you some questions about your stomach?"

Mr. Gregory agrees, although impolitely. After transporting Mr. Gregory to the hospital and giving a report to the triage nurse, Stan completes the PCR.

Special Incident Report

Town of Colonie
Department of Emergency Medical Services ────────────

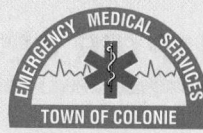

Date of Incident: _____ Time: _____ REMO #: _____

Town Run #: _____ Reported by: _____ Zone: _____

Type of Incident: ☐ MCI ☐ Rescue ☐ Personnel Matter ☐ Injury ☐ Collision with an EMS vehicle
☐ Infectious Disease Exposure ☐ Scene Conflict ☐ Other _____

Total # of Patients: ☐ #P-1: ____ ☐ #P-2: ____ ☐ #P-3: ____ ☐ #P-0: ____
Elapsed Scene Time: *(First unit arrival to last unit to hospital)* _____
Total Time of Incident: _____

Describe the Incident Below:
Attach any additional documentation such as news clipppings and the prehospital care report.
Attach additional sheets if necessary.

_____

_____

_____

_____

_____

_____

_____

_____

_____

_____

_____

_____

_____

_____

_____

_____

_____

_____

Signature: _____ Date: _____

- -

Office Use Only
This incident relates to: ☐ Day Operation: TOT ☐ Night Operations: TOT: ☐ Administration: TOT:

_____ _____ _____

Disposition: _____

_____

_____ Date: _____

Notifications/Copies: ☐ Director ☐ Deputy Director ☐ Supervisors
☐ Deputy Supervisors ☐ Senior Medics ☐ Zone Coordinator(s)
☐ Other _____ Zone: ☐ 2 ☐ 3 ☐ 4

FIGURE 6-15

Employers have forms for documentation of incidents, such as employee or patient injury on a call.

CHAPTER REVIEW

Chapter Summary

Effective communication is essential to every aspect of the EMS provider's job. You communicate with dispatch, team members, patients, patients' families, and other health care providers. Be aware of your verbal and nonverbal communication and the affect it has on others. Strive to improve communication and teamwork. Establish rapport with patients and use therapeutic communication techniques to obtain the information you need to make good treatment decisions. Keep in mind that cultural differences, language barriers, and other patient factors require you to adjust your communication strategies.

Make sure that you are proficient in the use of EMS communication equipment and adhere to guidelines for effective radio communication and patient care documentation. Communication skills are every bit as important as other Advanced EMT skills. Breakdowns in communication can jeopardize your safety and the patient's, as well as make your job more difficult and less satisfying.

Review Questions

Multiple-Choice Questions

1. A high-power, two-way radio in a fixed location, such as a hospital or dispatch center, is a(n):

   a. base station.
   b. repeater.
   c. antenna.
   d. transmitter.

2. The ability for multiple agencies and jurisdictions to communicate with each other using access to shared radio frequencies is called:

   a. facilitation.
   b. reflection.
   c. interoperability.
   d. mutual aid.

3. Your partner tells you he is a New York Yankees fan. You give him a puzzled look. Your behavior is an example of:

   a. a verbal cue.
   b. confrontation.
   c. interference.
   d. feedback.

4. As you are interviewing a patient who became ill in the train station, a man walks by with loud music playing. This is an example of:

   a. interference.
   b. modulation.
   c. feedback.
   d. reflection.

5. Which one of the following is a characteristic of a team?

   a. Common goals
   b. Identical training and qualifications
   c. Always consists of the same individuals
   d. Work for the same agency

6. The government agency with oversight responsibility for EMS radio use is the:

   a. Department of Transportation.
   b. Federal Communications Commission.
   c. Department of Homeland Security.
   d. National Registry of EMTs.

7. You are leaving the ambulance to go inside the grocery store. Which one of the following should you carry with you?

   a. Mobile radio
   b. Repeater
   c. Mobile data terminal
   d. Portable radio

8. Radio system equipment that offers the ability to transmit more traffic over limited frequencies and makes transmissions more secure through encryption is _____ radio equipment.

   a. cellular
   b. ultra–high-frequency
   c. amplitude modulated
   d. digital

9. On a 24-hour clock, 6:00 PM is _____ hours.

   a. 0600
   b. 1200
   c. 1800
   d. 2400

10. Which one of the following is an example of patient demographic data on the patient care report?

    a. Gender
    b. Chief complaint
    c. Treatment given
    d. Vital signs

Critical-Thinking Questions

11. Decide which part of the CHART narrative format each option represents by identifying the CHART letter to which it corresponds.

    a. The patient states he has the worst headache he's ever had.

    b. Gave the patient 0.4 mg nitroglycerin sublingually.

    c. Transferred to bed #9 with a verbal report to Dr. Simmons.

    d. The patient is allergic to sulfa and shellfish.

    e. Wheezing was heard in all lung fields.

12. You are on the scene of a charter bus crash, working the triage sector. You have assessed 15 patients. How would you document your findings?

13. Which therapeutic communication technique is demonstrated in the following exchange?

    Patient: "I haven't taken very good care of this house or myself since my wife died last year."

    You: "I'm sorry your wife died. It must be hard for you to take care of everything yourself."

14. Describe the initial approach to communicating with an elderly, pediatric, or challenged patient.

15. Every time you ask Mr. Legatutta a question, his daughter answers for him. How should you handle this situation?

16. Mr. Amos says his wife took an overdose of pills. You follow him to the bedroom where Mrs. Amos is standing on the bed. She is holding a liquor bottle in one hand and yelling profanities at you and her husband. How should you proceed?

Human Development, Health, and Disease

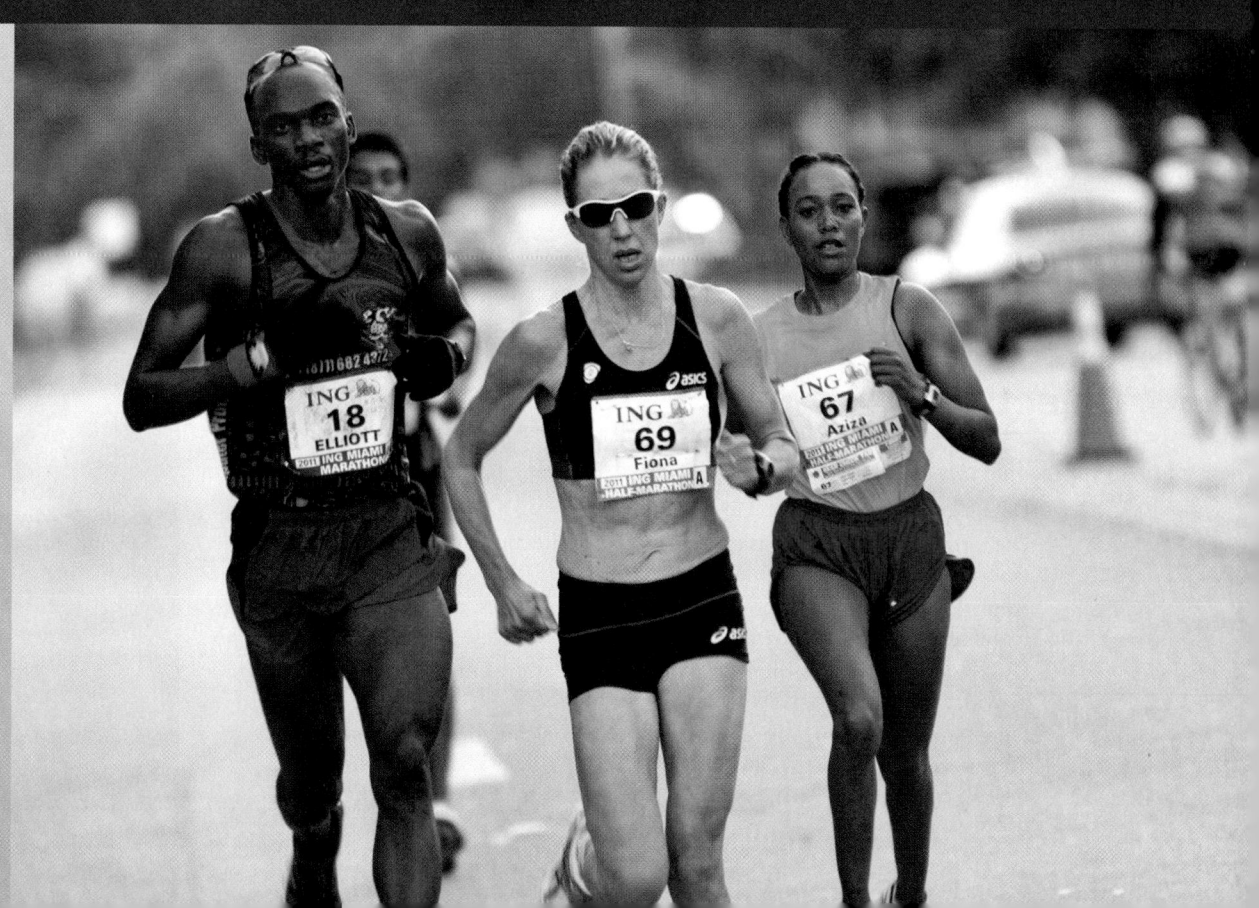

7

Medical Terminology

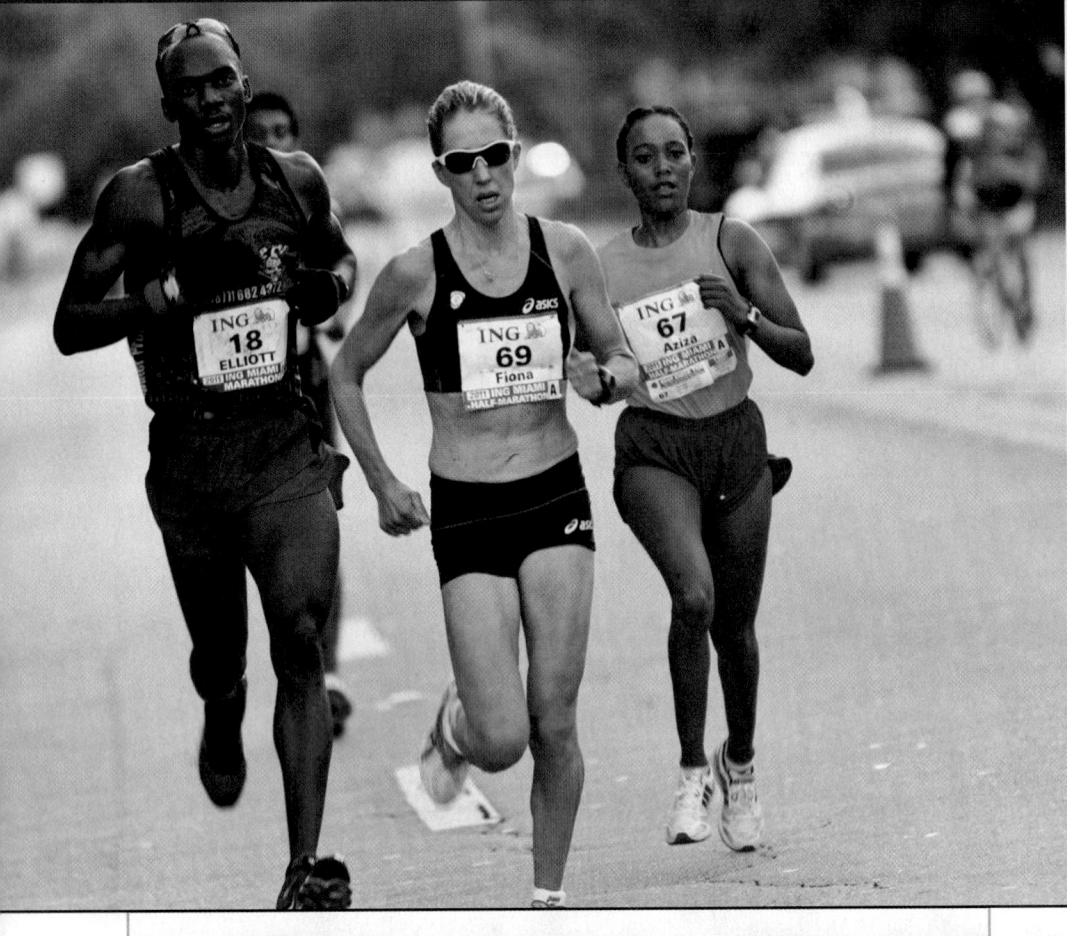

Content Area: Medical Terminology

Advanced EMT Education Standard: The Advanced EMT uses foundational anatomical and medical terms and abbreviations in written and oral communications with colleagues and other health care professionals.

Objectives

After reading this chapter, you should be able to:

7.1   Define key terms introduced in this chapter.

7.2   Use terms of anatomical position, planes, and direction and movement to describe the anatomy of the body.

7.3   Apply knowledge of common medical prefixes, suffixes, and roots (combining forms) to determine the meaning of medical terms.

7.4   Use common medical terminology in communication with other health care providers, including inpatient care documentation.

7.5   Differentiate between accepted standard and nonstandard medical symbols and abbreviations.

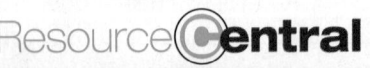

Resource **Central**

To access Resource Central, follow the directions on the Student Access Card provided with this text. If there is no card, go to www.bradybooks.com and follow the Resource Central link to Buy Access. Under Media Resources, you will find:

• *Are We Speaking the Same Language?* Watch to see why EMS professionals should use medical language.

• *Medical Abbreviations.* Read about the role of medical abbreviations and why some should be avoided.

• *It's Quiz Time!* Engage in an interactive medical language quiz to evaluate your knowledge.

Advanced EMT Cameron Baldwin is writing the narrative of a patient care report. The physical examination portion is as follows:

The patient is awake and he knows where he is, what day it is, and who the people are around him. His skin is warm, moist, and normal in color. His vital signs are blood pressure 118/72, pulse 84 regular, breathing rate 16. He has minor cuts and scrapes on the palms of both hands. There is a deformity on the front of his right lower leg about 3 inches above his ankle. His lower leg is swollen and bruised. He has feeling and movement in his toes and there is a pulse present in the top of the foot.

Problem-Solving Questions

1. How could this section of Cameron's report be rewritten using medical terms?
2. What are the advantages of using medical terms in patient care documentation?
3. What are some possible disadvantages of using medical terms?
4. What should you do if you cannot remember or are unsure of a medical term when communicating orally or in writing?

Introduction

Every profession has a unique language that allows precise and efficient transmission of meaning among individuals who are fluent in the language. Medical terminology, the language of health care professionals, has its roots in Latin and ancient Greek. The language has evolved over the years as science has contributed to the scope of knowledge and technology in health care. Although the number of terms used can seem overwhelming, there are common prefixes, root words, and suffixes that are combined to create terms. Knowing the meanings of the most common prefixes, root words, and suffixes allows you to understand the meaning of words you may not have seen or heard before. The language of medicine also includes common symbols, abbreviations, and conventions for writing numbers. (Writing numbers properly is covered in Chapter 6 and in the pharmacology chapters of the text.)

In addition to a basic understanding of medical terminology, an up-to-date medical dictionary is an essential tool for all health care providers. Most medical dictionaries are now available in paper and electronic formats. Programs that can be downloaded to smart phones are a great way to have a medical terminology reference at your fingertips.

Medical Terminology Basics

A large number of medical terms follow a pattern. The pattern usually starts with a **prefix**, which is attached to a **root word** or its **combining form**, and ends in a **suffix**. A root word is the foundation of a medical term. A prefix is placed at the beginning of a root word to modify its meaning. A suffix is placed at the end of the root word also to modify its meaning.

A combining vowel is used to connect the root word (turning the root word into its combining form) to the suffix, or to combine two root words. For example, the root *gastr* means "stomach," and the suffix *-itis* means "inflammation." The term *gastritis* means "inflammation of the stomach." Now that you know the suffix *-itis*, you will recognize it when it is used to modify other roots. Another example is the root *pharyng*, which refers to the throat. So, the term *pharyngitis* means "inflammation of the throat," or a sore throat.

Similarly, whenever you see the root *gastr* again, you will know it means "stomach." The prefix *epi-* means "above or over," and the suffix *-ic* means "characteristic of or related to." Therefore, the term *epigastric* refers to something that is in the region over the stomach. When you hear or read that a patient has epigastric pain, you now know that the pain is in the region above the stomach. Tables 7-1 through 7-4 list commonly used root words and combining forms, prefixes, and suffixes.

Spelling and pronunciation are always important—even more so in medical terminology. A misspelled or mispronounced medical term can look or sound like a term that means something completely different. For example, *ileum* is part of the small intestine, whereas *ilium* is a bone of the pelvis. The consequences of misunderstanding can result in patient care errors. Whenever you are in doubt about a term, look it up. If you are not able to look it up, use plain language to avoid confusion. In verbal communication, ask for clarification if you have any doubt about meaning.

The rules for pluralizing medical terms are based on the letter(s) in which the term ends (Table 7-5). Keep in mind, though, that there are exceptions to every rule.

TABLE 7-1   Commonly Used Root Words with Combining Forms

Root/Combining Form	Meaning	Example
aden (adeno)	gland	adenoma (glandular tumor)
carcin (carcino)	cancer	carcinogenic (causes cancer)
cardi (cardio)	heart	cardiomegaly (enlargement of the heart)
cyt (cyto)	cell	cytology (study of cells)
derma (dermato)	skin	dermatitis (inflammation of the skin)
enter (entero)	small intestine	gastroenteritis (inflammation of the stomach and intestine)
gastr (gastro)	stomach	gastric (pertaining to the stomach)
gyne (gyneco)	female	gynecology (study of females; particularly of problems of the female reproductive system)
hema (hemato)	blood	hematoma (blood tumor [literally], referring to a collection of blood within a tissue)
hydr (hydro)	water	hydrostatic (pressure exerted by nonmoving water)
necr (necro)	death	necrosis (condition of death, such as death of tissues)
somat (somato)	body	somatic (pertaining to the body)
path (patho)	disease	pathogenic (disease causing)

TABLE 7-2   Numeric/Quantitative Prefixes

Prefix	Meaning	Example
nulli-	none	nullipara (a woman who has not given birth)
hemi-	half	hemithorax (half of the thoracic [chest] cavity)
semi-	half or partial	semilunar (half-moon shaped)
uni-	one	unilateral (one side)
mono-	one	monocular (pertaining to one eye)
bi-	two	biphasic (occurring in two phases)
poly-	many	polycythemia (too many blood cells)
multi-	many	multipara (woman who has given birth more than once)
tri-	three	triceps (muscle with three heads)
tetra-	four	tetralogy (combination of four symptoms)
quad-	four	quadrisect (cut into four pieces)

TABLE 7-3 Common Prefixes

Prefix	Meaning	Example
a-	without	afebrile (without fever)
an-	without	anuria (without urine)
ante-	before, in front (of)	antemortem (before death)
anti-	against	anticoagulant (against clotting)
brady-	slow	bradycardia (slow heart rate)
con-	together or with	congenital (present at birth; literally, "born together")
dys-	painful or difficult	dyspnea (difficulty breathing)
epi-	above or upon	epidural (above the dura, the outermost lining of the brain)
eu-	normal	eupnea (normal breathing)
hyper-	above, over	hypertension (blood pressure above normal)
hypo-	under, below	hypotension (blood pressure below normal)
inter-	between	intercostal (between the ribs)
intra-	within	intraocular (within the eye)
macro-	large	macroscopic (large, visible to the eye)
micro-	small	microvasculature (small blood vessels, not visible to the eye)
neo-	new	neoplasm (new growth of cells)
par- para-	equal; pair beyond, alongside	paranasal (alongside the nose) sinuses; paraplegic (paralysis of both lower extremities)
per-	through	percutaneous (through the skin)
peri-	around	periumbilical (around the navel)
post-	after	postoperative (after surgery)
pre-	before	prenatal (before birth)
pseudo-	false	pseudomembrane (false membrane)
retro-	backward, behind	retrosternal (behind the sternum)
sub-	below, under	subcutaneous (below the skin)
supra-/super-	above, over	supraventricular (above the ventricles of the heart)
tachy-	rapid, fast	tachypnea (rapid breathing)

TABLE 7-4 Common Suffixes

Suffix	Meaning	Examples
-ac, -al, -an, -ar, -ary, -eal, -iac, -ic, -ical, -ile, -ior, -ory, -ose, -ous, -tic	pertaining to	cardiac (pertaining to the heart) renal (pertaining to the kidney) hepatic (pertaining to the liver) cervical (pertaining to the neck) optic (pertaining to vision)
-algia	pain	arthralgia (joint paint)
-cise	cut	excise (cut out, cut away)
-cyte	cell	hepatocyte (liver cell)
-ectasis	dilation	atelectasis (imperfect dilation [collapse] of the alveoli of the lungs)
-ectomy	surgical removal of	pulmonectomy (surgical removal of a lung)
-genic	produces, produced by	cardiogenic (produced by the heart, such as cardiogenic shock)
-gram	picture or recording	electrocardiogram (recording of the activity of the heart)
-graph	instrument for recording	electrocardiograph
-graphy	process of recording	capnography (measuring the level of carbon dioxide)
-ia	state, condition	tachycardia (state of having a fast heart rate)
-iasis	abnormal condition	lithiasis (condition of having stones, such as cholelithiasis, or gallstones)
-ism	state of	bruxism (state of grinding the teeth)
-itis	inflammation of	stomatitis (inflammation of the mouth)
-ology	study of	hematology (study of the blood)
-ostomy	surgically created opening	tracheostomy (surgically created opening into the trachea)
-lysis	destruction, break down	lipolysis (break down of fat cells)
-megaly	enlargement	splenomegaly (enlargement of the spleen)
-meter	instrument for measuring	thermometer (instrument for measuring heat)
-metry	process of measuring	oximetry (measuring oxygen levels)
-oma	tumor, mass	angioma (tumor consisting of blood vessels)
-osis	abnormal condition	cyanosis (abnormal condition of being blue [an indication of lack of oxygen])
-otomy	cutting into	hysterotomy (cutting into the uterus)
-pathy	disease	cardiopathy (disease of the heart)
-plasia/plasm	growth or formation	hyperplasia (growth above normal, such as tissue hyperplasia)
-plasty	surgical repair of	rhinoplasty (surgical repair of the nose)
-rrhage	excessive or abnormal flow	hemorrhage (abnormal bleeding)
-rrhea	discharge or flow	rhinorrhea (discharge from the nose)
-sclerosis	hardening	arteriosclerosis (hardening of the arteries)
-scope	instrument for viewing	laryngoscope (instrument for viewing the larynx)
-scopy	process of viewing	otoscopy (process of using an instrument to view the structures of the ear)
-stenosis	narrowing	mitral stenosis (narrowing of the opening of the mitral valve of the heart)
-trophy	development	dystrophy (absence of development, such as muscular dystrophy)

TABLE 7-5	Rules for Pluralizing Medical Terms	
Singular Word Ending in	**Examples**	**Plural Form**
-a	aorta	aortae, aortas
	vertebra	vertebrae
-ax	thorax (chest)	thoraces
-en	foramen (opening, such as the foramen magnum at the base of the skull)	foramina
-ex or -ix	cortex (rind, meaning the outer portion of a structure, such as the adrenal cortex of the adrenal gland)	cortices
	appendix	appendices
-is	pelvis	pelves
	diagnosis	diagnoses
-ma	hematoma	hematomata
-nx	phalanx	phalanges
	salpinx ([Fallopian] tube)	salpinges
-on	phenomenon	phemonena
-us	viscus (organ)	viscera
	locus	loci
-um	ilium (bone of the pelvis)	ilia
	ovum	ova
-y	autopsy (postmortem exam; literally, "to see for oneself")	autopsies

IN THE FIELD

The continuous quality improvement process in medicine has allowed discovery of symbols and abbreviations that have frequently led to medical errors. As a result, changes are sometimes made in what is considered acceptable for documentation. Always use your employer's most up-to-date list of accepted symbols and abbreviations.

IN THE FIELD

Work with your clinical and field experience preceptors to learn and practice documentation.

Medicine also uses its own set of abbreviations and symbols for writing medical orders and completing patient care documentation (see the last two tables in this chapter). If used incorrectly, they can lead to confusion. Hospitals and other health care organizations often have a list of approved abbreviations and symbols.

In addition to official medical terms, health care and public safety personnel tend to use jargon that can sound a bit odd compared with conversational English. Jargon is a way of sharing meaning within a particular group. It uses acronyms and idiomatic expressions that are not understood outside the group, which can lead to misunderstanding. For example, in patient histories, a health care provider might say or write that a patient *denies smoking*. In everyday English, *denies* is a loaded word that insinuates that someone is doing something but refuses to admit it. In medical jargon, *denies* simply means that the patient answered negatively to the question, "Do you smoke?"

There is overlap between medical terminology and jargon, but jargon includes slang, too, which you should avoid when talking with patients. For example, your patient will likely not appreciate that taking him to the "bus" or loading him into the "truck" means that you will be putting him into the ambulance.

Medical documentation also uses a rather stilted form of English that you will get used to. For example, rather than writing, "The patient is a 68-year-old male with a past medical history of emphysema, who was found sitting at the kitchen table," you would more likely see, "68 yom, PMH: emphysema. Found sitting at table."

Anatomical Terms

Terms of position and direction (Table 7-6 and Figure 7-1) are useful in describing the location of body structures and abnormal findings, such as injuries or **lesions**. Those terms use the **anatomical position** (Figure 7-2) and **body planes** (Figure 7-3) as points of reference. Terms that relate to the tissues, organs, primary body cavities (Figure 7-4), and body regions (Figure 7-5) are used frequently, as well.

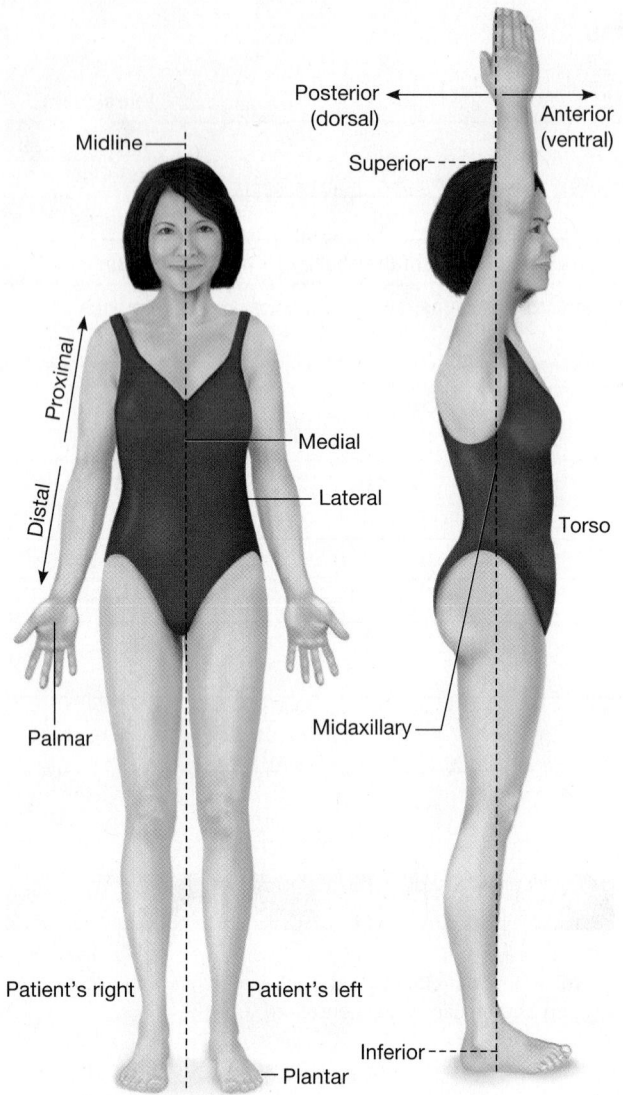

FIGURE 7-1

Terms of position and direction.

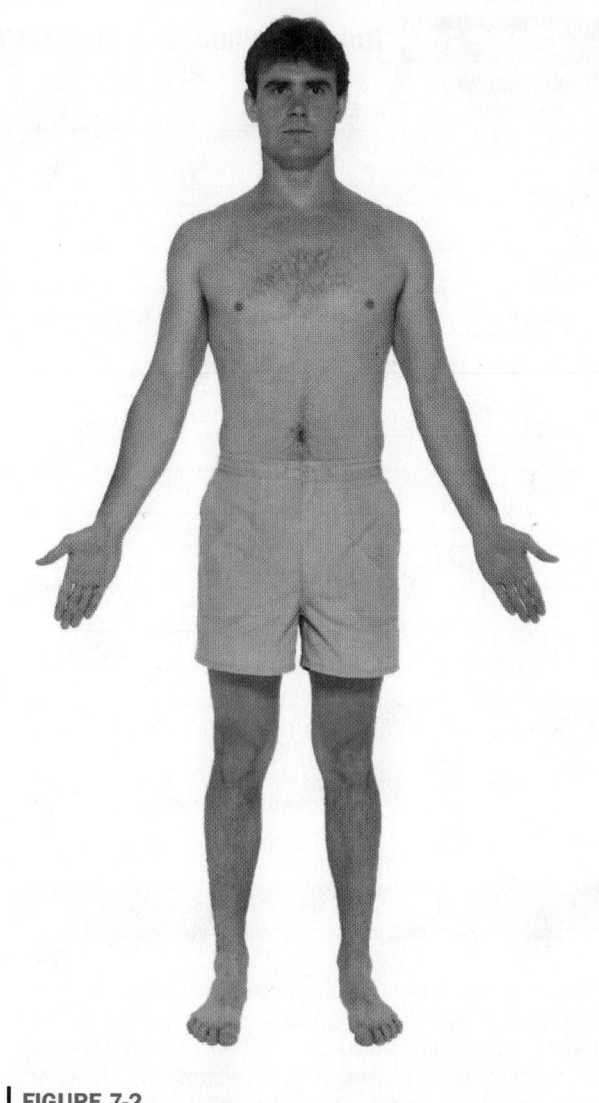

FIGURE 7-2

As a point of reference, the body is assumed to be in the anatomical position, standing up, facing forward, with the palms turned forward.

TABLE 7-6 Terms of Position and Direction

Term	Meaning	Example
abduction	movement away from the midline	Lifting the arm out to the side.
adduction	movement toward the midline	Lowering the arm back to the side of the body.
anterior	toward the front	The umbilicus (navel) is on the anterior aspect of the body.
apex	the tip of a structure	The apex of the heart points downward.
base	the lower part of a structure	The bases of the lungs rest against the diaphragm.
caudal	toward the tail (in humans, the feet)	Moving from head to toe is the same as moving in a caudal direction.
cephalad	toward the head	Moving from toe to head is the same as moving in a cephalad direction.
deep	toward the inside of the body	The muscles are deep with reference to the skin.
distal	away from the midline or other point of reference	The foot is distal to the knee.
dorsal	toward the back (posterior)	A shark's dorsal fin is on its back.
extension	straightening a joint to move the two parts further apart	When you straighten the knee, you are extending it.
flexion	bending a joint to bring the two parts closer together	Bending the elbow is the same thing as flexing the elbow.
inferior	below	The inferior vena cava brings blood from the areas below the heart back to the right atrium of the heart.
lateral	toward the side (away from the midline)	The thumb is on the lateral aspect of the hand.
medial	toward the midline or middle	The inside of the leg is the medial aspect.
midline	vertical line dividing the body into equal left and right sides	The nose is in the midline.
posterior	toward the back (dorsal)	The shoulder blades (scapulae) are on the posterior aspect of the body.
prone	lying face down	Sleeping on your "stomach" is sleeping in a prone position.
proximal	near the midline or point of reference	The elbow is proximal to the hand.
superficial	toward the outer surface of the body	The skin is superficial with respect to the muscles.
superior	above	The superior surface of the tongue rests against the roof of the mouth.
supine	lying on the posterior aspect of the body	When you sleep on your back, you are in a supine position.
ventral	toward the front (anterior)	The sternum is on the ventral aspect of the body.

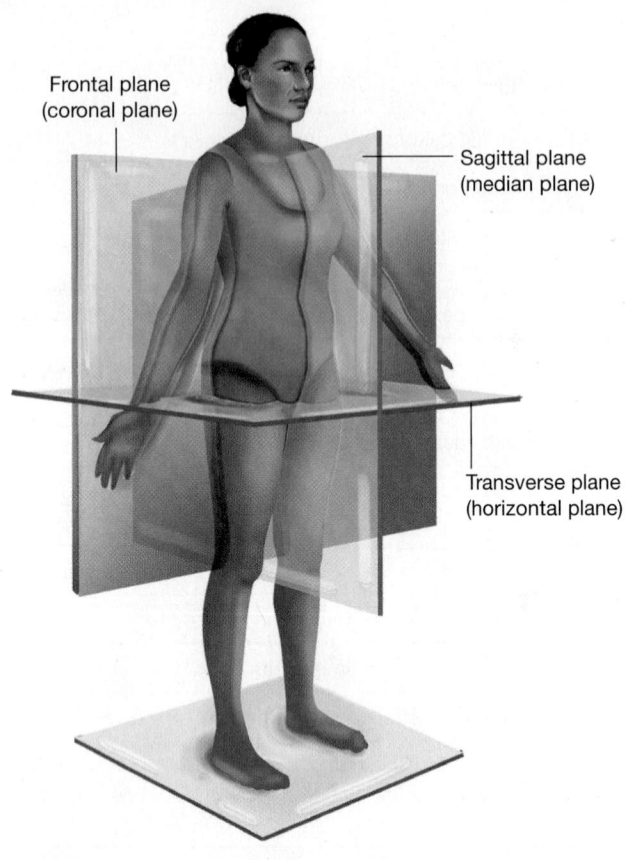

Frontal plane
(coronal plane)

Sagittal plane
(median plane)

Transverse plane
(horizontal plane)

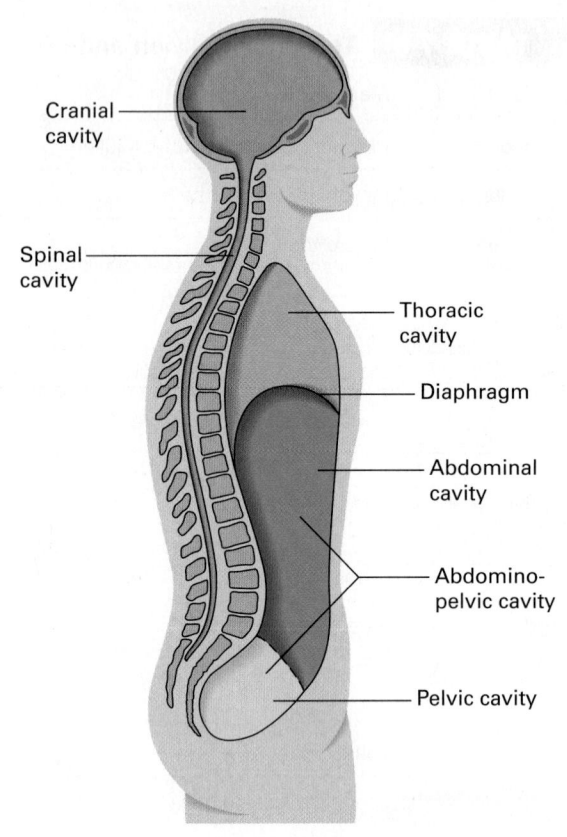

Cranial
cavity

Spinal
cavity

Thoracic
cavity

Diaphragm

Abdominal
cavity

Abdomino-
pelvic cavity

Pelvic cavity

FIGURE 7-3

For reference, the body, or any of its parts, can be divided
by imaginary planes.

FIGURE 7-4

Many medical terms refer to the main body cavities.

TABLE 7-7	Selected Terms Associated with the Musculoskeletal System
Term	**Meaning**
arthritis	inflammation of a joint
arthroscopy	procedure to view the inside of a joint with a special instrument
cervical	pertaining to the neck
myeloid	pertaining to bone marrow
osteoporosis	porous bones
orthopedics	branch of medicine specializing in treating disorders of the musculoskeletal system

TABLE 7-8	Selected Terms Associated with the Cardiovascular System
Term	**Meaning**
angiogram	X-ray recording (image) of the blood vessels
cardiologist	physician specializing in treatment of disorders of the heart
pericardium	sac around the heart
phlebitis	inflammation of a vein
thrombosis	condition of blood clotting
vasodilation	dilation of the blood vessels

Terms by Body System

Each body system has particular terms associated with it.
A variety of sample terms associated with each body system are offered in Tables 7-7 through 7-12. Understanding
those terms will help you in your upcoming reading in this

text, as well as in your clinical experience. However, the
language of medicine is extensive. Therefore, this chapter
can give only an introduction to common terms. Continue
to learn additional vocabulary throughout the text and,
most importantly, throughout your career.

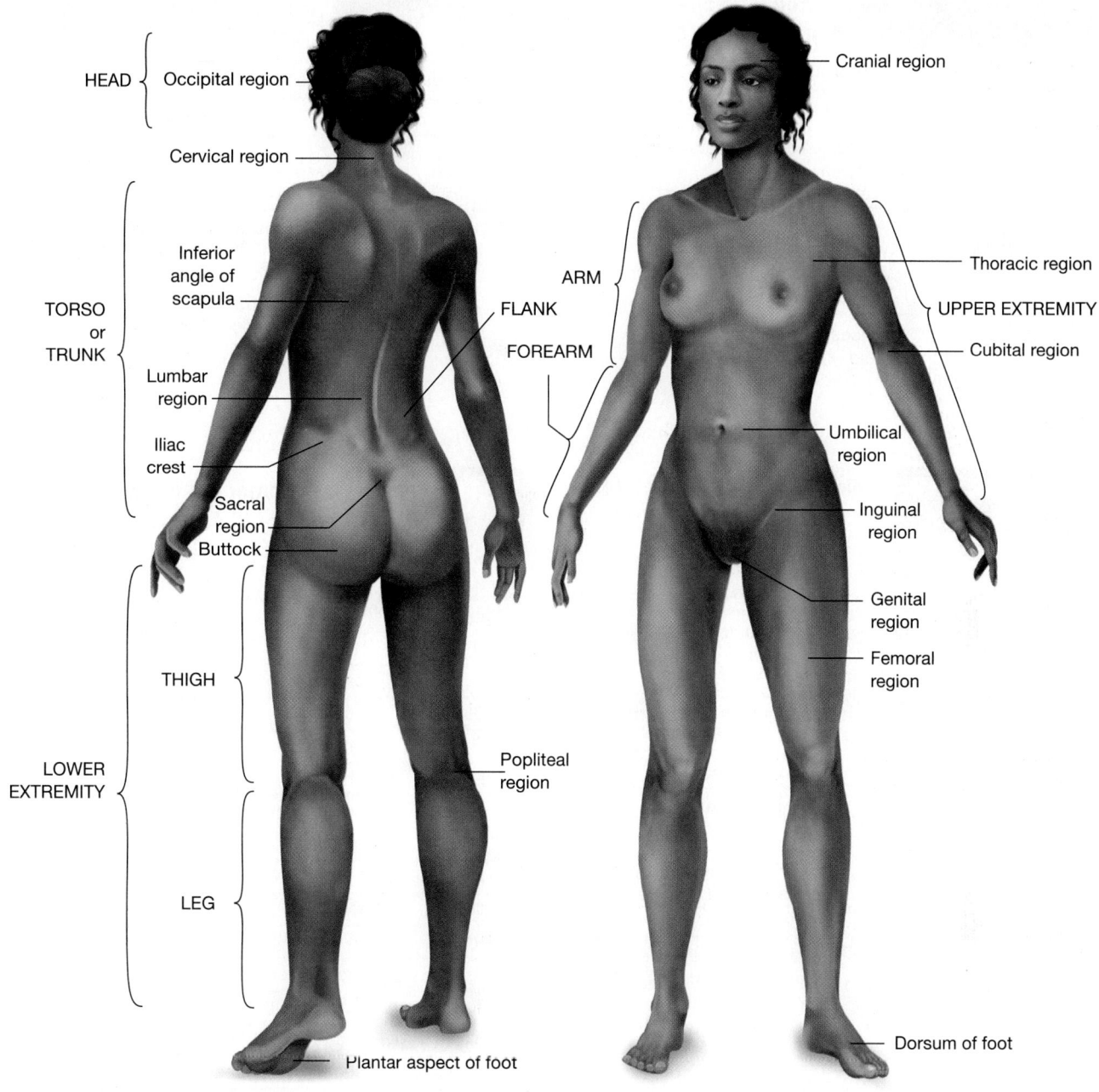

HEAD { Occipital region

Cervical region

Inferior angle of scapula

TORSO or TRUNK

Lumbar region

Iliac crest

Sacral region

Buttock

THIGH

LOWER EXTREMITY

LEG

Plantar aspect of foot

FLANK

FOREARM

ARM

Cranial region

Thoracic region

UPPER EXTREMITY

Cubital region

Umbilical region

Inguinal region

Genital region

Femoral region

Popliteal region

Dorsum of foot

FIGURE 7-5

Many medical terms refer to the main regions of the body.

TABLE 7-9 Selected Terms Associated with the Blood and Immune System

Term	Meaning
erythrocyte	red (blood) cell
exsanguination	condition of blood outside the body (bleeding)
fibrinolytic	substance that breaks down fibrin; a substance in blood clots
leukocytosis	condition of too many white blood cells
lymphadenopathy	disease (in this case, swelling) of the lymph glands

TABLE 7-10 Selected Terms Associated with the Respiratory System

Term	Meaning
apnea	absence of breathing
bronchoconstriction	narrowing of the bronchioles, as in asthma
dyspnea	difficulty breathing
hypercapnia	high level of carbon dioxide
hypoxia	low level of oxygen
oropharyngeal	pertaining to the oral cavity and throat
pneumothorax	air within the chest cavity but outside the lung (collapsed lung)
pulmonologist	physician who specializes in disorders of the lungs

TABLE 7-11 Selected Terms Associated with the Gastrointestinal System

Term	Meaning
anorexia	absence of appetite
bariatric	pertaining to a patient's weight (obesity)
cholecystectomy	surgical removal of the gallbladder
laparotomy	surgical incision into the abdomen
hematemesis	vomiting blood
polyphagia	excessive eating/swallowing

TABLE 7-12 Selected Terms Associated with the Nervous System

Term	Meaning
analgesia	absence of pain
anesthesia	absence of sensation
ataxia	absence of coordination
encephalitits	inflammation of the brain
hemiparesis	weakness on one side of the body
meningitis	inflammation of the membranes surrounding the brain and spinal cord
neuropathy	nerve disease/disorder
quadriplegia	paralysis of all four extremities

TABLE 7-13 Commonly Accepted Medical Abbreviations and Symbols

$\bar{a}$	before
$\bar{c}$	with
NTG	nitroglycerin
O_2	oxygen
OB	obstetrics
$\bar{P}$	after
PE	physical exam, pulmonary embolism
PO	orally, by mouth
Pt	patient
q	every
QID	four times a day
R/O	rule out
Rx	prescription
$\bar{s}$	without
s/s	signs/symptoms
SIDS	sudden infant death syndrome
SL	sublingual
SOB	shortness of breath
stat	immediately
Sx	symptoms
TIA	transient ischemic attack
TID	three times a day
TKO	to keep open
Tx	treatment
X	times
y/o	years old
↑	increased
↓	decreased

TABLE 7-14 Standard Medical Charting Abbreviations

PATIENT INFORMATION/CATEGORIES

African American	AA
Asian	A
Black	B
Chief complaint	CC
Complains of	c/o
Current health status	CHS
Date of birth	DOB
Differential diagnosis	DD or DDx
Estimated date of confinement	EDC
Family history	FH
Female	♀
History	Hx
History and physical	H&P
History of present illness	HPI or HOPI
Impression	IMP
Male	♂
Medications	Med
Newborn	NB
Past history	PH or PMH
Patient	Pt
Physical exam	PE
Private medical doctor	PMD
Signs and symptoms	S/S
Vital signs	VS
Weight	Wt
Year-old	y/o

BODY SYSTEMS

Abdomen	Abd
Cardiovascular	CV
Central nervous system	CNS
Ear, nose, and throat	ENT
Gastrointestinal	GI
Genitourinary	GU
Gynecological	GYN
Head, eyes, ears, nose, and throat	HEENT
Musculoskeletal	M/S
Obstetrical	OB
Peripheral nervous system	PNS
Respiratory	Resp

COMMON COMPLAINTS

Abdominal pain	abd pn
Chest pain	CP
Dyspnea on exertion	DOE
Fever of unknown origin	FUO
Gunshot wound	GSW
Headache	H/A
Lower back pain	LBP
Nausea/vomiting	n/v
No apparent distress	NAD
Pain	pn
Shortness of breath	SOB
Substernal chest pain	sscp

DIAGNOSES

Abdominal aortic aneurysm	AAA
Abortion	Ab
Acute myocardial infarction	AMI
Adult respiratory distress syndrome	ARDS
Alcohol	ETOH
Atherosclerotic heart disease	ASHD
Chronic obstructive pulmonary disease	COPD
Chronic renal failure	CRF
Congestive heart failure	CHF
Coronary artery bypass graft	CABG
Coronary artery disease	CAD
Cystic fibrosis	CF
Dead on arrival	DOA
Delirium tremens	DTs
Deep vein thrombosis	DVT
Diabetes mellitus	DM
Dilation and curettage	D&C
Duodenal ulcer	DU
End-stage renal disease	ESRD
End-stage renal failure	ESRF
Epstein–Barr virus	EBV
Foreign body obstruction	FBO
Hepatitis B virus	HBV
Hiatal hernia	HH
Hypertension	HTN
Infectious disease	ID

(continued)

TABLE 7-14 **Standard Medical Charting Abbreviations—continued**

Inferior wall myocardial infarction	IWMI	Diphtheria–pertussis–tetanus	DPT
Insulin-dependent diabetes mellitus	IDDM	Hydrochlorothiazide	HCTZ
Intracranial pressure	ICP	Lactated Ringer's, Ringer's lactate	LR, RL
Mass casualty incident	MCI	Nitroglycerin	NTG
Mitral valve prolapse	MVP	Nonsteroidal anti-inflammatory agent	NSAID
Motor vehicle crash	MVC	Normal saline	NS
Multiple sclerosis	MS	Oral birth control pill	OBCP
Non–insulin-dependent diabetes mellitus	NIDDM	Penicillin	PCN
		Phenobarbital	PB
Organic brain syndrome	OBS	Potassium	K^+
Otitis media	OM	Sodium bicarbonate	$NaHCO_3$
Overdose	OD	Sodium chloride	NaCl
Paroxysmal nocturnal dyspnea	PND	Tylenol (acetaminophen)	APAP
Pelvic inflammatory disease	PID	**ANATOMY/LANDMARKS**	
Peptic ulcer disease	PUD	Abdomen	Abd
Pregnancies/births (gravida/para)	G/P	Antecubital	AC
Pregnancy-induced hypertension	PIH	Anterior axillary line	AAL
Pulmonary embolism	PE	Anterior cruciate ligament	ACL
Rheumatic heart disease	RHD	Anterior–posterior	A/P
Sexually transmitted infection	STI	Dorsalis pedis (pulse)	DP
ST elevation myocardial infarction	STEMI	Gallbladder	GB
Transient ischemic attack	TIA	Intercostal space	ICS
Tuberculosis	TB	Lateral collateral ligament	LCL
Upper respiratory infection	URI	Left lower lobe	LLL
Urinary tract infection	UTI	Left lower quadrant	LLQ
Wolff–Parkinson–White syndrome (disease)	WPW	Left upper lobe	LUL
		Left upper quadrant	LUQ
MEDICATIONS		Left ventricle	LV
Angiotensin-converting enzyme	ACE	Liver, spleen, and kidneys	LSK
Aspirin	ASA	Lymph node	LN
Bicarbonate	HCO_3^-	Midaxillary line	MAL
Birth control pills	BCP	Posterior axillary line	PAL
Calcium	Ca^{++}	Right lower lobe	RLL
Calcium channel blocker	CCB	Right lower quadrant	RLQ
Calcium chloride	$CaCl_2$	Right middle lobe	RML
Chloride	Cl^-	Right upper lobe	RUL
Digoxin	Dig	Right upper quadrant	RUQ
Dilantin (phenytoin sodium)	DPH	Temporomandibular joint	TMJ
Diphenhydramine	DPHM	Tympanic membrane	TM

TABLE 7-14 **Standard Medical Charting Abbreviations—continued**

PHYSICAL EXAM/FINDINGS

Arterial blood gas	ABG
Bilateral breath sounds	BBS
Blood glucose level	BGL
Breath sounds	BS
Cerebrospinal fluid	CSF
Chest X-ray	CXR
Complete blood count	CBC
Computed tomography	CT
Conscious, alert, and oriented	CAO
Costovertebral angle	CVA
Deep tendon reflexes	DTR
Dorsalis pedis (pulse)	DP
Electrocardiogram	EKG, ECG
Electroencephalogram	EEG
Expiratory	Exp
Extraocular movements (intact)	EOMI
Fetal heart tones	FHT
Full range of motion	FROM
Full-term normal delivery	FTND
Heart rate	HR
Heart sounds	HS
Hemoglobin	Hgb
Inspiratory	Insp
Jugular venous distention	JVD
Laceration	lac
Level of consciousness	LOC
Level of responsiveness	LOR
Moves all extremities (well)	MAEW
Nontender	NT
Normal range of motion	NROM
Palpation	Palp
Passive range of motion	PROM
Point of maximal impulse	PMI
Posterior tibial (pulse)	PT
Pulse	P
Pupils equal and reactive to light	PEARL
Pupils equal, round, reactive to light and accommodation	PERRLA

Range of motion	ROM
Respirations	R
Temperature	T
Unconscious	unc
Urinary incontinence	UI

MISCELLANEOUS DESCRIPTORS

After (post-)	$\bar{p}$
After eating	pc
Alert and oriented	A/O
Anterior	ant.
Approximate	≈
As needed	prn
Before (ante-)	$\bar{a}$
Before eating (*ante cibum,* before meal)	a.c.
Body surface area (%)	BSA
Celsius	°C
Change	Δ
Decreased	↓
Equal	=
Fahrenheit	°F
Immediately	stat
Increased	↑
Inferior	inf.
Left	Ⓛ
Less than	<
Moderate	mod.
More than	>
Negative	−
No, not, none	Ø
Not applicable	n/a
Number	No or #
Occasional	occ
Pack years	pk/yrs, p/y
Per	/
Positive	+
Posterior	post.
Postoperative	PO
Prior to arrival	PTA
Radiates to	→
Right	®

(continued)

TABLE 7-14 Standard Medical Charting Abbreviations—continued

Rule out	R/O	Treatment	Tx
Secondary to	2°	Turned over to	TOT
Superior	sup.	Verbal order	VO
Times (for 3 hours)	× (× 3h)	**MEDICATION ADMINISTRATION/METRICS**	
Unequal	≠	Centimeter	cm
Warm and dry	W/D	Cubic centimeter	cc
While awake	WA	Deciliter	dL
With (*cum*)	c̄	Drop(s)	gtt(s)
Within normal limits	WNL	Drops per minute	gtts/min
Without (*sine*)	s̄	Every	q
Zero	0	Grain	gr
TREATMENTS/DISPOSITIONS		Gram	g, gm
Advanced cardiac life support	ACLS	Hour	h or hr
Advanced life support	ALS	Hydrogen-ion concentration	pH
Against medical advice	AMA	Intracardiac	IC
Automated external defibrillator	AED	Intramuscular	IM
Bag-valve mask	BVM	Intraosseous	IO
Basic life support	BLS	Intravenous	IV
Cardiopulmonary resuscitation	CPR	Intravenous push	IVP
Continuous positive airway pressure	CPAP	Joules	j
Do not resuscitate	DNR	Keep vein open	KVO
Endotracheal tube	ETT	Kilogram	kg
Estimated time of arrival	ETA	Liter	L
External cardiac pacing	ECP	Liters per minute	lpm, L/min
Intermittent positive-pressure ventilation	IPPV	Microgram	mcg
Long spine board	LSB	Milliequivalent	mEq
Nasal cannula	NC	Milligram	mg
Nasogastric	NG	Milliliter	mL
Nasopharyngeal airway	NPA	Millimeter	mm
No transport—refusal	NTR	Millimeters of mercury	mmHg
Nonrebreather mask	NRM	Minute	min
Nothing by mouth	NPO	Orally	PO
Oropharyngeal airway	OPA	Subcutaneous	SC, SQ
Oxygen	O_2	Sublingual	SL
Per square inch	psi	To keep open	TKO
Physical therapy	PT	**CARDIOLOGY**	
Positive end-expiratory pressure	PEEP	Atrial fibrillation	AF
Short spine board	SSB	Ventricular fibrillation	VF
Therapy	Rx	Ventricular tachycardia	VT

CASE STUDY WRAP-UP

Clinical-Reasoning Process

Advanced EMT Cameron Baldwin is writing the narrative of a patient care report. The physical examination portion is as follows:

Pt. A&O x3. Skin warm, moist, normal in color. VS: BP 118/72, P 84R, RR 16. PE: Superficial lacerations and abrasions to palmar surfaces of hands, bilaterally. Deformity to anterior lt. leg 3 in. proximal to ankle, with edema and discoloration. Distal pulse, motor, and sensory function intact.

PERSONAL PERSPECTIVE

Mrs. Jenny Foster: I went to my doctor's office last week because I thought I had a really bad chest cold. After the doctor took my temperature, checked my oxygen level, and listened to my lungs, she said she thought I had a bad pneumonia. She called 911 and the ambulance arrived a few minutes later. I was really worried about being a lot sicker than I thought I was. As Dr. Shaw talked to the EMTs, I couldn't understand most of what she said to them. She told them I was hypoxic and that my sats were low. One of the young men on the ambulance, Perry, who said he was an Advanced EMT, explained.

"Mrs. Foster", he said, "the pneumonia is preventing oxygen from getting from your lungs into your bloodstream. That means the oxygen level in your blood is a little on the low side. That's what Dr. Shaw meant when she said you were hypoxic. I'm going to give you some oxygen through your nose, though, to increase your oxygen level."

I'm glad Perry took the time to explain. I still felt lousy, but I relaxed a little bit when I understood what was happening and how the EMTs were going to help me.

CHAPTER REVIEW

Chapter Summary

Part of what identifies particular professions is the unique language used by its members. Proper use of medical terminology, symbols, and abbreviations is required of all health care providers as a way of efficiently and precisely sharing meaning. A large number of medical terms can be identified with ease by learning common root words, prefixes, and suffixes. The meaning of unfamiliar terms can be determined using knowledge of those word parts. Always take care to use the proper term, proper spelling, and accepted symbols and abbreviations in communications using medical terminology. When in doubt, use a medical dictionary to confirm meanings. If you cannot find clarification, use plain language to express your ideas.

Review Questions

Multiple-Choice Questions

1. Myocardium refers to:
   a. skeletal muscle.
   b. chambers of the heart.
   c. bone marrow.
   d. heart muscle.

2. A midsagittal plane divides the body into:
   a. four quadrants.
   b. right and left halves.
   c. trunk and extremities.
   d. top and bottom.

3. Which one of the following is characteristic of the anatomical position?
   a. Lying face down
   b. Palms turned forward
   c. Legs crossed
   d. Arms folded across the chest

4. The spinal cord is contained within the _____ cavity of the body.
   a. cranial
   b. ventral
   c. dorsal
   d. thoracic

5. Which one of the following statements is accurate with respect to terms of position and direction?
   a. The foot is distal to the hip.
   b. The elbow is proximal to the shoulder.
   c. The outside of the leg is the medial aspect.
   d. Cephalad means moving in a head-to-toe direction.

6. Which one of the following terms means that the spleen has been surgically removed?
   a. Splenomegaly
   b. Splenotomy
   c. Splenectomy
   d. Splenoplasty

7. A physician who specializes in the treatment of blood disorders is a:
   a. hematologist.
   b. pathologist.
   c. dermatologist.
   d. gastroenterologist.

8. Tissue that is dead has undergone:
   a. cytology.
   b. necrosis.
   c. hemolysis.
   d. myopathy.

9. Hemiplegia means:
   a. weakness in the lower body.
   b. paralysis of all extremities.
   c. weakness of one side of the body.
   d. paralysis of one side of the body.

10. To describe rapid breathing, you should use the term:
    a. bradycardia.
    b. bradypnea.
    c. tachypnea.
    d. tachycardia.

Critical-Thinking Questions

11. Each person on your ambulance service is required to review patient care reports every few months as part of the continuous quality improvement process. You notice that several of your peers are having trouble with the plural forms of medical terms, so you are going to put together a handout that includes the plural forms of common terms. Write the plural form of each of the terms listed below:
    a. Cervix
    b. Renal calculus (kidney stone)
    c. Corpus (body)
    d. Index

12. The conditions below came up in your exam and history of a patient. Write the term that fits each definition correctly.
    a. Surgical incision into the stomach
    b. Enlarged liver
    c. Inflammation of cartilage
    d. Low oxygen in the blood

13. While reading a continuing education article, the following terms come up. Write what each one means.
    a. Hypocapnia
    b. Thrombocyte
    c. Pericarditis
    d. Epidermis

8

Human Body Systems

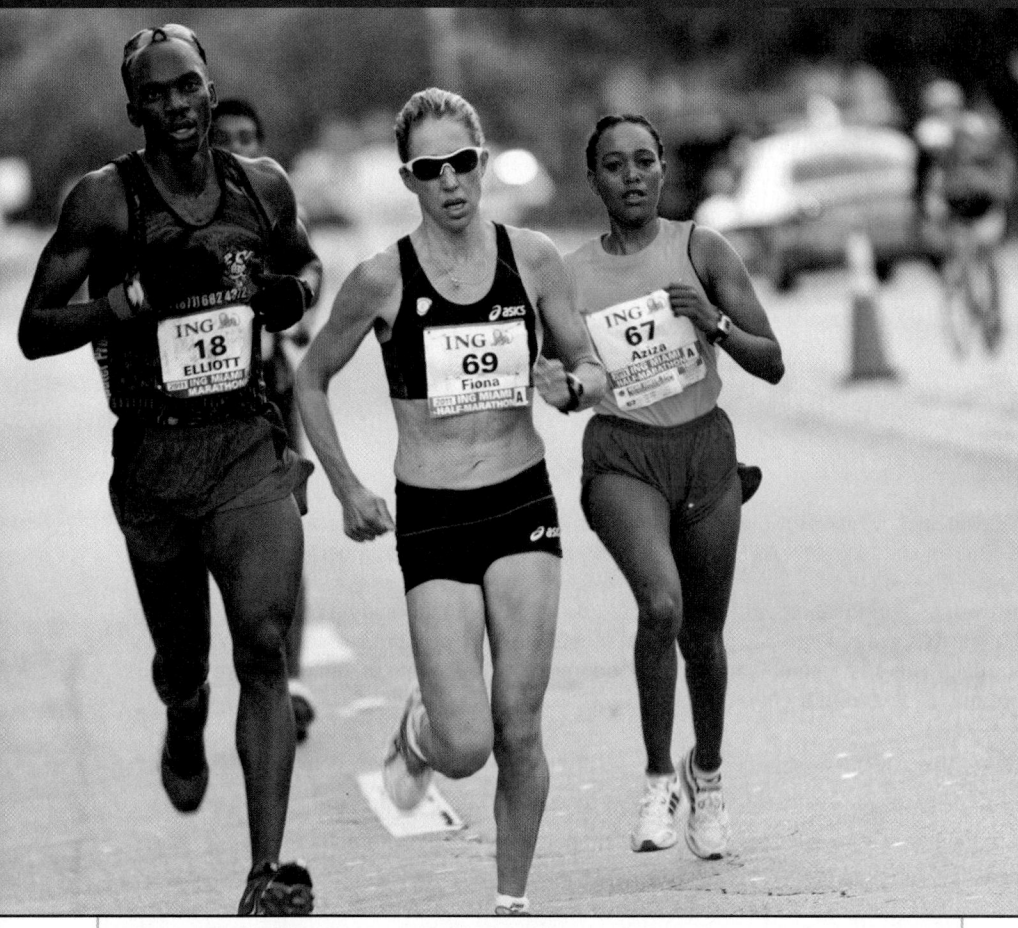

Content Area: Anatomy and Physiology

Advanced EMT Education Standard: Integrates complex knowledge of the anatomy and physiology of the airway, respiratory, and circulatory systems to the practice of EMS.

Objectives

After reading this chapter, you should be able to:

8.1   Define key terms introduced in this chapter.

8.2   Explain the concepts of metabolism and homeostasis.

8.3   Describe each of the levels of organization of the human body.

8.4   Describe the anatomy and physiology of a typical body cell.

8.5   Explain the physiology and distribution of fluids and electrolytes in the body.

8.6   Describe the regulation of acid–base balance and blood gases.

(continued)

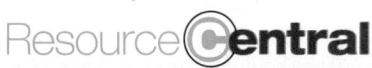

To access Resource Central, follow the directions on the Student Access Card provided with this text. If there is no card, go to www.bradybooks.com and follow the Resource Central link to Buy Access. Under Media Resources, you will find:

- *Glands and More Glands.* View an animation to learn about the structure and function of the many endocrine organs.

- *Osmosis and Diffusion.* Read and learn about the roles of osmosis and diffusion.

- *It's a Small World!* View the exciting and complex world inside the living cell.

KEY TERMS (continued)

gradient *(p. 156)*

hemoglobin *(p. 174)*

hemostasis *(p. 181)*

histamine *(p. 181)*

homeostasis *(p. 155)*

hormones *(p. 199)*

hydrostatic pressure *(p. 155)*

insulin *(p. 201)*

ion *(p. 153)*

Krebs cycle *(p. 157)*

lumen *(p. 187)*

mean arterial pressure (MAP) *(p. 191)*

metabolism *(p. 157)*

millimeters of mercury (mmHg) *(p. 174)*

neurotransmitters *(p. 191)*

osmolarity *(p. 156)*

osmosis *(p. 155)*

osmotic pressure *(p. 156)*

oxidative phosphorylation *(p. 157)*

partial pressure (Pa) *(p. 174)*

perfusion *(p. 188)*

pH *(p. 158)*

pulse pressure *(p. 191)*

repolarization *(p. 160)*

respiration *(p. 173)*

respiratory membrane *(p. 176)*

serous fluid *(p. 176)*

surfactant *(p. 176)*

sutures *(p. 166)*

tidal volume (TV) *(p. 178)*

ventilation *(p. 173)*

villi *(p. 202)*

zygote *(p. 206)*

CASE STUDY

Advanced EMTs Elaine Jacoby and Atul Singh have just arrived on the scene of a patient with multiple gunshot wounds. The patient, 17-year-old Edward Lampey, has wounds to his upper right chest, upper right abdomen, and left groin.

In their primary assessment, Elaine and Atul find that Edward is confused and has pale, cool, sweaty skin. He is having difficulty breathing. They cannot feel a pulse in his wrist, but the carotid pulse in his neck is weak and rapid. There is a small amount of blood from the abdominal and chest wounds, but a significant amount of bleeding from the groin wound.

Problem-Solving Questions

1. What organs do you suspect may have been injured by each of the gunshot wounds?
2. How can the patient's injuries explain the weak, rapid pulse and difficulty breathing?
3. What mechanisms is the patient's body using to try to compensate for the effects of the injuries?
4. How could the patient's injuries lead to death?

(continued from previous page)

8.7   Identify the anatomy and explain the basic physiology of the following body systems:
   - Gastrointestinal
   - Genitourinary
   - Integumentary
   - Male and female reproductive
   - Musculoskeletal

8.8   Identify the anatomy and explain the functions, including mechanisms for maintaining homeostasis, of the following systems:
   - Cardiovascular, with particular attention to cardiac electrophysiology, cardiac output, hemodynamics, and perfusion
   - Endocrine, with particular emphasis on the regulation of glucose
   - Nervous, with particular focus on the autonomic nervous system and its sympathetic and parasympathetic receptors and neurotransmitters
   - Respiratory, with particular attention to the mechanics of ventilation, and external and internal respiration

Introduction

As an Advanced EMT, you will assess patients for abnormal conditions that may require intervention. In order to recognize what is *abnormal*, though, you must first have a thorough understanding of what is *normal*. As a health care provider, you are expected to have a high level of health literacy, including basic knowledge about the body in both health and disease.

This chapter focuses on two interdependent subjects: anatomy and physiology. *Anatomy* is the study of the structures of the human body. The study of anatomy includes gross anatomy, the study of structures as they appear to the naked eye, and microscopic anatomy. In both cases, structures are precisely designed to efficiently carry out specific functions in the body. *Physiology* is the study of the functions of the body.

The interrelated nature of anatomy and physiology makes it difficult to consider one without the other. There are special considerations in the anatomy and physiology of pediatric and geriatric patients, which you must understand to properly assess and anticipate their needs. Those special considerations are discussed in detail in Chapter 9. *Pathophysiology*, the study of the effects of illness and injury on the human body, can be understood only after normal functioning is understood. (See Chapter 10.)

All structures within the human body are comprised of the same basic building blocks of chemical elements and compounds. At the foundation of body structure is the cell, often referred to as the basic building block of life. Each microscopic cell has its own miniature environment contained within a cell membrane.

The cell membrane is more than just a simple boundary between the cell and the environment surrounding it. It is a complex structure that performs many critical functions. Each cell is filled with specialized fluid called *cytoplasm* (also called *cytosol*) surrounding a nucleus. The viscous cytoplasm gives the cell its shape and provides a medium within which various molecules can interact. A variety of specialized structures called *organelles* are suspended in the cytoplasm. Some functions of the organelles are common to all cells, and some are unique to certain types of cells.

Groups of cells form tissues, which in turn form organs and body systems. These function together to support metabolism and maintain homeostasis, which is the overall inner balance maintained within the body despite environmental changes.

Anatomy and physiology are extensive topics, yet a solid foundation is required for successfully studying the subsequent information in the text. For that reason, this chapter takes a unique approach to allow you the best opportunity to organize and assimilate the critical information in it. It is divided into six sections:

- General Concepts in Anatomy and Physiology
- Support, Movement, and Protection
- Respiration and Circulation
- Control, Communication, and Integration
- Nutrition and Excretion
- Reproduction

General Concepts in Anatomy and Physiology

Chemical Basis of Life

The basic building block of life is the cell, but before you learn about cells, you must understand them and their environment on an even more basic level. Cells are surrounded by a chemical environment and, in fact, are composed of chemicals.

Chemistry involves the study of the composition of substances and the interactions between various elements and compounds. It is chemistry that allows cells to engage in metabolism and maintain homeostasis. The chemistry of life is complex, but understanding just a few principles goes a long way toward understanding anatomy, physiology, and pathophysiology. The body relies on those principles in the function of every body system.

Basic Principles of Chemistry

A chemical *element* is a substance that cannot be broken down further into simpler components. Oxygen, hydrogen, iron, and calcium are examples of elements. All known chemical elements are listed in the periodic table of the elements.

The simplest unit of an element is an atom. Atoms consist of three types of subatomic particles: neutrons, protons, and electrons (Figure 8-1). Electrons have a negative electrical charge, protons have a positive electrical charge, and neutrons are electrically neutral.

An electrical charge is a physical property of the subatomic particles such that particles with a like charge will repel each other and particles with opposite charges will attract each other. The electrical charge is either positive or negative. An electrical current flows from an area of positive electrical charge to an area of negative electrical charge.

The attraction of oppositely charged particles and various other properties of atoms explains the ability of certain substances to combine. Knowing those properties allows you to predict what happens under certain conditions in the body. One application of this knowledge is in understanding how the body uses oxygen and why it is important to life.

Electrons, which are in the outermost portion of atoms, are usually balanced with protons, so the overall electrical charge of the atom is neutral. However, some atoms are capable of either gaining or losing electrons, so they are either positively or negatively charged. An atom (or group of atoms) that can carry a positive or negative electrical charge is called an **ion**. A positively charged ion is called a *cation* and a negatively charged ion is called an *anion*.

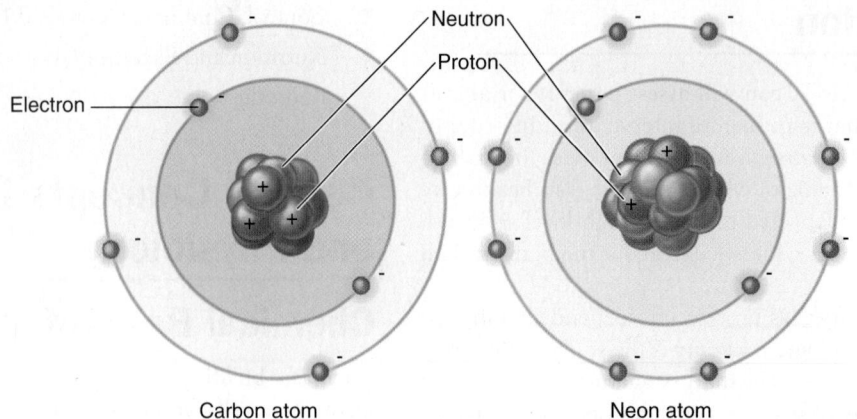

FIGURE 8-1

Typical structure of atoms.

An **electrolyte** is a substance that dissociates into negatively and positively charged ions (anions and cations) when placed in water (Figure 8-2). For example, sodium chloride, or table salt (represented chemically by NaCl, which is electrically neutral), dissociates into sodium cations (Na^+) and chloride anions (Cl^-) when placed in water.

The body uses a small set of electrolytes in many of its functions (Table 8-1). One such function is the conduction of electrical impulses along nerve cells.

IN THE FIELD

The same sodium and chloride found in table salt are abundant in the body and comprise the most commonly used intravenous (IV) fluid used in the prehospital setting. Normal saline is an IV solution containing 0.9 percent NaCl in water.

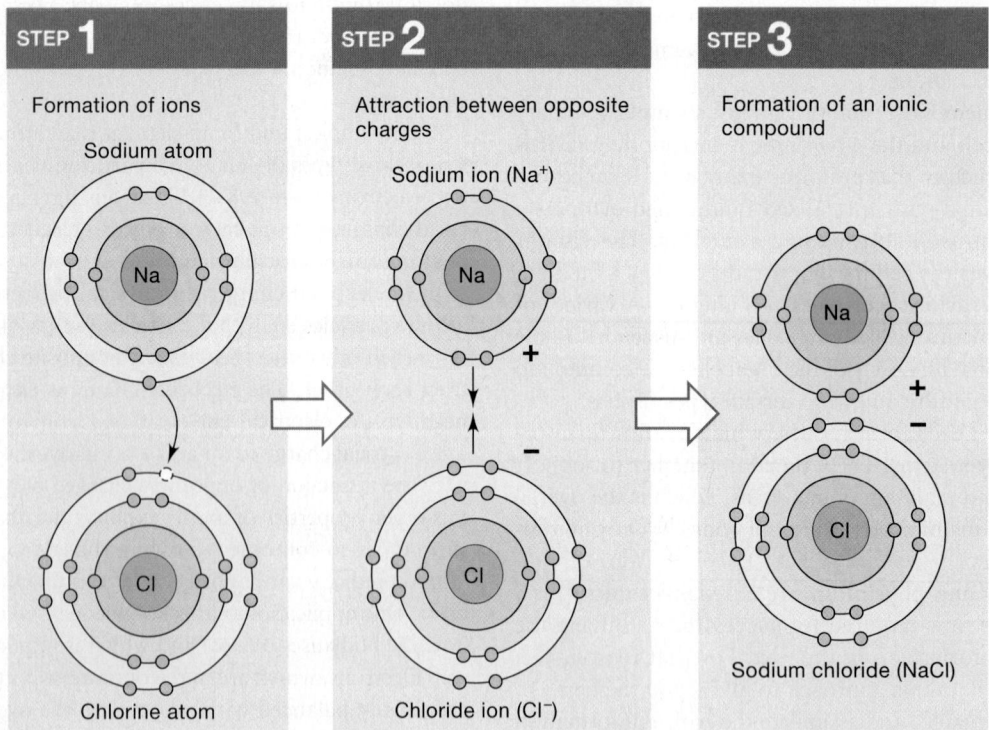

FIGURE 8-2

Electrolytes are compounds made of a positively charged ion (cation) and a negatively charged ion (anion). When an electrolyte is placed in a solution, it will dissociate into charged ions. (Bledsoe, Bryan E.; Martini, Frederic H.; Bartholomew, Edwin F.; Ober, William C.; Garrison, Claire W.; Anatomy & Physiology for Emergency Care, 2nd Edition, © 2008. Reprinted with permission of Pearson Education, Inc., Upper Saddle River, NJ)

TABLE 8-1 Most Common Ions in Body Fluids

Cations	Anions
Na^+ (sodium)	Cl^- (chloride)
K^+ (potassium)	HCO_3^- (bicarbonate)
Ca^{++} (calcium)	HPO_4^{2-} (biphosphate)
Mg^{++} (magnesium)	SO_4^{2-} (sulfate)

IN THE FIELD

As an Advanced EMT, you will make decisions about starting IVs and administering IV fluids. You must understand how adding fluids and solutes to the body affects the fluid balance within the fluid compartment. This requires a basic understanding of how the concentrations of certain substances inside and outside cells affect water movement.

TABLE 8-2 Principal Chemical Elements in the Body

Element (Percent of Body Weight)	Significance
Oxygen, O (65)	A component of water and other compounds; oxygen gas is essential for respiration
Carbon, C (18.6)	Found in all organic molecules
Hydrogen, H (9.7)	A component of water and most other compounds in the body
Nitrogen, N (3.2)	Found in proteins, nucleic acids, and other organic compounds
Calcium, Ca (1.8)	Found in bones and teeth; important for membrane function, nerve impulses, muscle contraction, and blood clotting
Phosphorus, P (1.0)	Found in bones and teeth, nucleic acids, and high-energy compounds
Potassium, K (0.4)	Important for proper membrane function, nerve impulses, and muscle contraction
Sodium, Na (0.2)	Important for membrane function, nerve impulses, and muscle contraction
Chlorine, Cl (0.2)	Important for membrane function and water absorption
Magnesium, Mg (0.06)	Required for activation of several enzymes
Sulfur, S (0.04)	Found in many proteins
Iron, Fe (0.007)	Essential for oxygen transport and energy capture
Iodine, I (0.0002)	A component of hormones of the thyroid gland

Four chemical elements comprise more than 99 percent of the body's atoms. These four elements are hydrogen (H), oxygen (O), carbon (C), and nitrogen (N). A limited number of trace elements account for the rest of the atoms in the body (Table 8-2). Different arrangements of these elements form the wide array of different proteins, enzymes, minerals, carbohydrates, and lipids that provide the structure of the body and allow it to perform the functions needed for metabolism and homeostasis.

Water

The body is composed largely of water, which is a molecule consisting of two hydrogen atoms and one oxygen atom, represented as H_2O. The adult body is about 60 percent water by weight. Water is contained within two major compartments in the body.

Intracellular fluid (ICF) is the total amount of water within cells, accounting for the greatest proportion of water

(about 75 percent) in the body. **Extracellular fluid (ECF)** is the fluid outside of cells. ECF is further compartmentalized as either intravascular or interstitial fluid. Intravascular fluid is the fluid within the blood vessels. Interstitial fluid is the fluid that surrounds cells within the tissues.

The interstitial compartment is sometimes called the "third space," with the intracellular and intravascular compartments as the first two spaces. Water can move among these three spaces to maintain **homeostasis**.

Abnormal conditions in the body can cause problems with the balance of fluid in each of the three spaces. For example, edema (swelling) is an abnormal increase in interstitial fluid. Fluids can move between compartments by **osmosis** and under the force of **hydrostatic pressure**.

Solutes

Water serves as a solvent that contains varying amounts of different solutes in the body. Solutes are formed particles, such as electrolytes, carbohydrates, proteins, lipids, drugs, and other substances. The concentration of solutes in the three fluid compartments influences the movement of water in and out of them.

The concentration of solutes is measured as the mass (amount of matter in an object, roughly translated as the weight) of particles per a given volume of fluid. When two solutions of different concentrations are separated by a membrane that allows water to move through it but not the solutes (a semipermeable membrane), water will move from the less concentrated solution to the more concentrated solution until the two solutions are equal in solute

concentration. The movement of water across a semipermeable membrane along a **gradient** from lower to higher solute concentration is called osmosis. The difference in concentration of solutes creates **osmotic pressure**, which can be thought of as the ability to "pull" water across the cell membrane from the less concentrated solution to the more concentrated solution to equalize the two solutions.

Oncotic pressure is a portion of the total osmotic pressure that is created by the concentration of large protein molecules that cannot pass through the capillary walls. Because the capillaries are very permeable to small ions, the oncotic pressure is equivalent to the total osmotic pressure in those vessels. Oncotic pressure returns fluid to the bloodstream when it is forced out through the capillary walls under the hydrostatic pressure created by the force of blood. The higher concentration of proteins (albumin) in the bloodstream "pulls" the water back into the capillaries, preventing edema.

Osmotic pressure of IV fluids also is called *tonicity*. When a fluid is equal to body fluids in its amount of solutes, it is said to be *isotonic*. The concentration of IV fluids is measured in milliosmols (mOsm) per liter of fluid.

The **osmolarity** of body fluids is between 280 and 310 mOsm/L. In terms of the electrolytes Na^+ and Cl^-, a 0.9 percent solution of NaCl (called *normal saline solution*) has a concentration of 310 mOsm/L and is considered isotonic (Figure 8-3). When it is given, it has no immediate net effect on the movement of water between the extravascular and intravascular compartments (Figure 8-4).

A more concentrated solution, higher in solutes, is *hypertonic* (has higher osmotic pressure; >350 mOsm/L). Hypertonic IV fluid, such as 2 percent NaCl, causes water to move from within red blood cells to the intravascular compartment (crenation of red blood cells). A less concentrated solution, such as 0.45 percent NaCl, is *hypotonic* (has lower osmotic pressure; <250 mOsm/L). A hypotonic solution added to the blood would cause water to leave the bloodstream and enter the interstitial fluid and cells. As a general rule, a way to remember how the concentration of solutes affects water movement is *wherever sodium goes, water follows*. However, keep in mind that this general rule

FIGURE 8-3

Fluids with the same osmolarity as body fluids are isotonic. In comparison, fluids with higher osmolarity are hypertonic and fluids with lower osmolarity are hypotonic. The net movement of water across a semipermeable membrane, such as a cell membrane, is called *osmosis*. Water moves from an area of lower solute concentration (lower osmolarity) to an area of higher solute concentration (higher osmolarity) until the concentration of solutes has equilibrated.

FIGURE 8-4

In the presence of a hypotonic environment, water moves into cells. In the presence of a hypertonic environment, water moves out of cells.

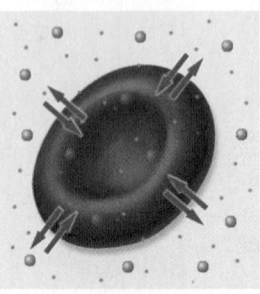

Isotonic

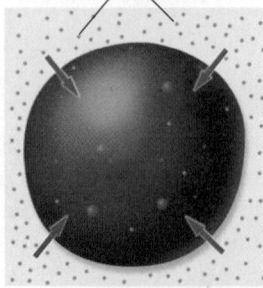

Hypotonic

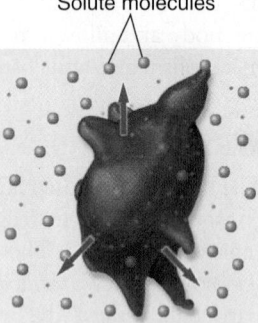

Hypertonic

applies to osmosis. The movement of sodium and water is affected at the cellular level by active transport mechanisms.

The sodium/potassium pump is a protein on cell membranes that provides a mechanism to keep the ions at their proper levels inside and outside the cell (Figure 8-5). The principal intracellular cation is potassium (K^+), and the principal extracellular cation is Na^+, although both ions are present to some degree on both sides of the cell membrane. Na^+ is able to enter the cell from the extracellular fluid. However, it does not leave the cell because its concentration is greater on the outside of the cell.

If Na^+ is not removed from the cell, water will enter the cell in sufficient quantities that the cell will burst and die (lysis). The sodium/potassium pump moves three Na^+ out of the cell for every two K^+ it moves into the cell. The difference in the concentration of ions creates a negative electrical charge within the cell, relative to the charge provided by the greater concentration of Na^+ outside cell. This difference in charges creates a membrane potential (discussed later in this section).

The sodium/potassium pump requires energy to move Na^+ against its gradient to maintain normal Na^+ balance. Without oxygen, the cell is unable to produce enough energy to fuel the sodium/potassium pump, and the result is cell death. When a sufficient number of cells die, the individual dies.

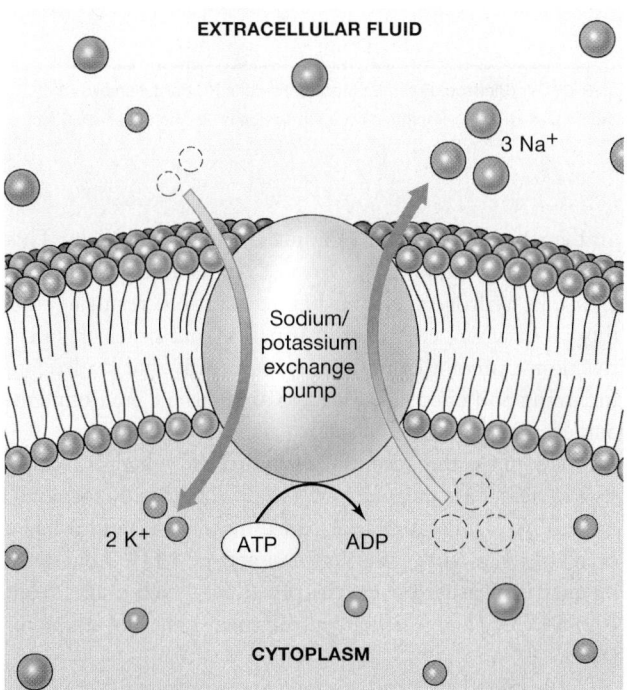

FIGURE 8-5

The sodium/potassium pump on the cell membrane uses energy to move sodium and potassium ions across the membrane. (Bledsoe, Bryan E.; Martini, Frederic H.; Bartholomew, Edwin F.; Ober, William C.; Garrison, Claire W.; Anatomy & Physiology for Emergency Care, 2nd Edition, © 2008. Reprinted with permission of Pearson Education, Inc., Upper Saddle River, NJ)

Energy

The work of the body, like all work, requires energy. Energy production in cells is a chemical process of breaking down glucose (which consists of carbon, hydrogen, and oxygen) into molecules that can be used as energy in cellular process.

Cells require energy to carry out the functions needed to maintain their own chemical integrity, such as the work of the sodium/potassium pump. Cells also require energy to produce substances needed by the body, such as the proteins needed to develop and maintain tissues. In order to produce the greatest amount of energy with the least amount of toxic byproducts, the cell needs glucose and oxygen.

The cells require a constant supply of both glucose and oxygen for survival. Some cells, such as those of the brain and heart, are more sensitive to deprivation of those substances than other cells.

The body receives glucose, as well as other nutrients, through the digestive tract. Glucose that is not used immediately is stored in complex form for use between meals. Sufficient oxygen must enter the blood through the work of the respiratory system. The cardiovascular system must be able to pump blood throughout the body to deliver oxygen and nutrients to the cells and to deliver wastes to the kidneys, liver, and lungs for removal.

The collection of chemical processes that allow the body to grow, reproduce, maintain and repair itself, and respond to its environment is called **metabolism** (Figure 8-6). Metabolism takes two forms: anabolism and catabolism. Anabolism occurs when the body manufactures (synthesizes) more complex substances from simpler ones. For example, amino acids are used to form a variety of proteins in the body. Anabolic processes require energy.

Catabolism occurs when the body breaks down complex substances into simpler ones, releasing energy in the process. The desired end product of cellular catabolism is the creation of energy in the form of a molecule called *adenosine triphosphate (ATP).*

Cells create ATP in a process called **oxidative phosphorylation.** Energy production takes place inside the cell in two phases. In the first phase, which occurs in the cytoplasm of the cell, glucose is broken down into pyruvic acid in a process called **glycolysis.** This step does not require oxygen, and is called **anaerobic metabolism.** It produces only a small amount of ATP (two moles).

When oxygen is present, a second phase of cellular energy production, **aerobic metabolism,** by way of the **Krebs cycle** (also called the *TCA cycle*), takes place in organelles called *mitochondria.* Aerobic metabolism is a complex process that results in a larger amount of ATP (36 moles). The process releases heat, which contributes to maintaining the body's temperature, and allows the breakdown of pyruvic acid (through a series of reactions) into carbon dioxide and water. Carbon dioxide and water are both easily eliminated from the body.

Without oxygen, an insufficient amount of energy is produced to sustain cell function and pyruvic acid is

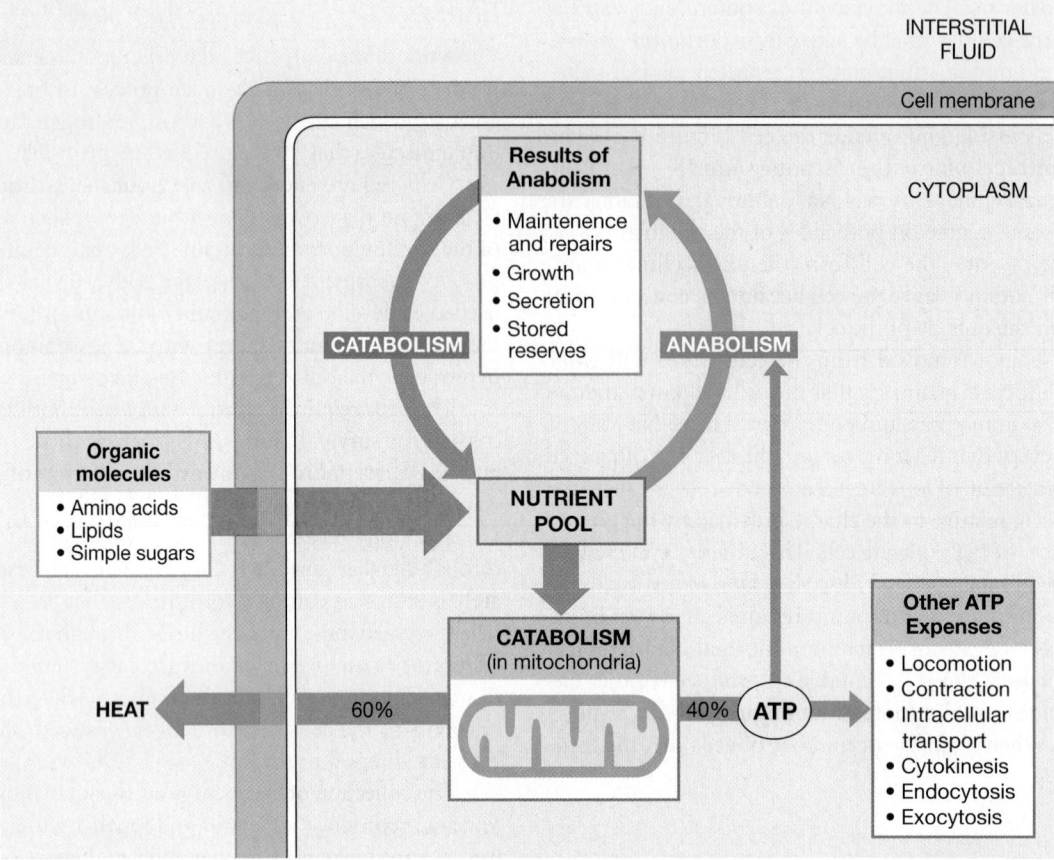

FIGURE 8-6

Metabolism is the sum of all chemical and physical changes in the body. (Bledsoe, Bryan E.; Martini, Frederic H.; Bartholomew, Edwin F.; Ober, William C.; Garrison, Claire W.; Anatomy & Physiology for Emergency Care, 2nd Edition, © 2008. Reprinted with permission of Pearson Education, Inc., Upper Saddle River, NJ)

IN THE FIELD

One of the most critical actions you can take as an Advanced EMT is providing oxygen to a patient whose cells are not receiving enough of it. The presence of an adequate amount of oxygen allows the patient's cells to keep functioning aerobically, and prevents accumulation of lactic acid in the body.

converted to lactic acid, a toxic byproduct that accumulates in the body. If oxygen levels are not quickly restored, cell death and death of the individual will occur.

Acid–Base Balance

The breakdown of glucose results in pyruvic acid. A series of steps called *oxidation* changes pyruvic acid into series of different **acids** that are eventually reduced into water and carbon dioxide.

In an anaerobic environment, ATP production is greatly reduced and acids cannot be converted into water

and carbon dioxide for elimination from the body. This lack of energy and accumulation of metabolic acids (an increase in hydrogen ion [H^+] concentration) result in conditions in which cells cannot function and other chemical reactions cannot take place. It is in this way that inadequate breathing and circulation lead to an anerobic environment, and eventually, death.

The **pH** is the potential of hydrogen, which is a measure of acid–base balance in the body. Chemically speaking, an acid is a substance that can donate a H^+ and a base, or **alkali**, is a substance that can accept a H^+. Acid–base balance is measured using the pH scale, which ranges from 0 to 14. A pH of 7 is neutral (neither acidic nor alkaline) (Figure 8-7).

The pH scale can be somewhat confusing because it is an inverse measurement in which each unit is calculated logarithmically. This means that as the H^+ concentration increases, the number on the pH scale decreases. A pH of 5 is more acidic than a pH of 6, and pH of 4 is more acidic than a pH of 5. The most acidic pH is 0 and the most alkaline pH is 14.

The logarithmic calculation means that a pH of 5 represents an H^+ concentration 10 times that of a pH of 6,

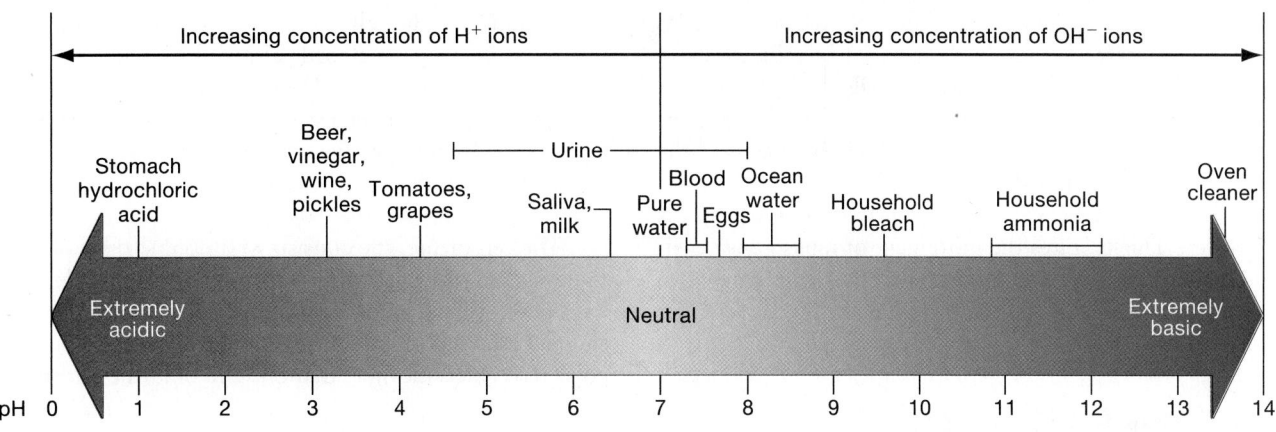

FIGURE 8-7

An increase in hydrogen ion concentration results in a lower, more acidic pH. A decrease in hydrogen ion concentration results in a higher, more alkaline pH. (Bledsoe, Bryan E.; Martini, Frederic H.; Bartholomew, Edwin F.; Ober, William C.; Garrison, Claire W.; *Anatomy & Physiology for Emergency Care*, 2nd Edition, © 2008. Reprinted with permission of Pearson Education, Inc., Upper Saddle River, NJ)

and a pH of 4 represents an H^+ concentration 100 times that of a pH of 6. Therefore, very small changes in pH actually represent very large changes in H^+. The normal pH of body fluids is within a very narrow range, between 7.35 and 7.45.

When oxygen is present in sufficient quantities, the H^+ produced in metabolism combines with it, so each oxygen atom combines with two hydrogen atoms, resulting in H_2O, or water. The other product created in this process is carbon dioxide, CO_2, which is carried in the blood back to the lungs, where it is exhaled.

When increased energy metabolism results in increased H^+, and therefore increased carbon dioxide, the rate and depth of breathing increase to bring more oxygen to the cellular level, and to deliver the increased amount of carbon dioxide to the lungs for elimination. In addition, the heart rate increases to circulate more oxygen to the cells and deliver more carbon dioxide to the lungs.

The mechanism by which excess hydrogen ion is converted into substances that prevent acid accumulation, thereby maintaining acid–base balance, is called a **buffer system**. A simple buffer system used in the body is the bicarbonate–carbonic acid buffer system, which is used to convert excess H^+ into carbon dioxide and water. (This is discussed in more depth in Chapter 10.)

The kidneys also play a role in acid–base balance, but the adjustments made by the renal system are not as immediate as those made by the respiratory system.

Membrane Potential

Membrane potential is a chemical phenomenon that is reflected by a difference in the concentration of electrically charged particles (ions) on the inside and outside of the cell.

All chemical elements contain various numbers of electrically charged particles. The electrical charge of ions is determined by their ability to gain or lose electrons. Electrical current is essentially the movement of ions that have too few or too many electrons. Ions move from an area in which electrons are more abundant to an area in which they are less abundant.

This concept of movement along a gradient is the same as the concept of the gradient for movement of water and solutes. Without the sodium/potassium pump, the concentration of ions (along with their electrons) would tend to equilibrate across the cell membrane. The sodium/potassium pump maintains a relatively negative charge within the cell. When there is a difference in electrical charge across the cell membrane, the cell is said to be *polarized*.

When the imbalance reaches a certain point, electrolytes begin to move across the cell membrane to equalize the charge (equilibrate). This is called **depolarization**, which stimulates adjacent cells, which then repeat the process. As

IN THE FIELD

When patients have increased breathing or heart rates, suspect an increased cellular need for oxygen and increased carbon dioxide production. Provide supplemental oxygen.

IN THE FIELD

The flow of ions across the membranes of cells in the electrical conduction system of the heart is recorded as the various waves on an electrocardiogram (ECG) or cardiac monitor. The waveforms of the ECG or cardiac monitor provide information about the electrical activity in the heart. An imbalance in electrolytes can affect cardiac conduction and is often reflected by characteristic changes in the waveforms of the ECG or cardiac monitor.

the electrolyte balance changes from cell to cell (that is, as electrons as part of atoms move from cell to cell), electrical current flows through a pathway of cells. The positive and negative electrical charges of ions allow the flow of electricity from one cell to another—most notably in cells of the nervous system and cardiac conduction system.

Repolarization occurs as the difference in charges is restored. This requires the movement of ions against their gradient, in the opposite direction that they would move on their own. Cells must use energy to fuel the mechanism that allows this.

Cellular Basis of Life

The life-sustaining chemical processes that take place within cells mean that cells must have certain structures that allow these processes to occur. The cell membrane, cytoplasm, and organelles work together to maintain the cellular environment needed to perform cellular work (Figure 8-8; Table 8-3).

The Cell Membrane

Cell membranes must allow some substances to move in and out of the cell, while preventing others from doing so. That is, the cell membrane must be semipermeable, allowing water and small molecules, but not larger molecules, to move through it. The physical and chemical structures of the cell membrane make this possible (Figure 8-9).

Channels in the cell membrane, which are sometimes open and sometimes closed, allow substances to move through it at certain times. The channels are constructed of proteins; some require energy to operate (active transport) and others do not (passive transport). The movement of other substances through the cell membrane is regulated by the electrical charge of the molecules that comprise it.

The cell membrane consists of a double layer of molecules called *phospholipids*. This is called a *lipid bilayer*. Each phospholipid molecule has a phosphate portion on one end and a lipid portion on the other end. Phospholipids are polar molecules, meaning that one end of it (the phosphate

IN THE FIELD

Some proteins on the cell membrane and within the cell have a shape that is a specific match to certain substances, such as hormones or drugs. These substances can affect a cell's function only when a specific receptor for them is present on the cell. This mechanism works like a lock and key. The concept of cellular receptors helps explain the effects of the medications you give your patients. *For instance, the proteins on cell membranes that allow glucose into the cell require insulin to unlock them. Therefore, a person's blood sugar level can be very high, but without insulin, the cells will not have any glucose to use and will starve even while being bathed in glucose.*

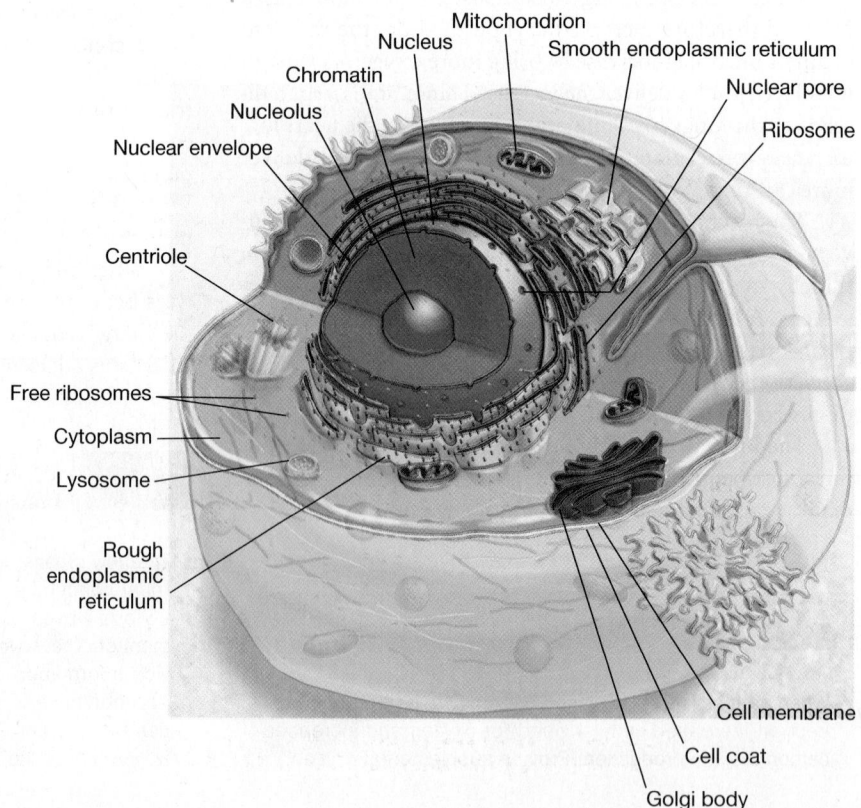

FIGURE 8-8

The cell is the basic unit of the body, consisting of organelles suspended in cytoplasm, and is separated from its environment by a cell membrane.

TABLE 8-3	Cellular Components
Component	**Function**
Cell membrane	Serves as the boundary of the cell. Selectively allows substances to move in and out of the cell
Cytoplasm (cytosol)	The fluid substance in which the organelles are suspended; allows substances to move within the cell by diffusion
Cytoskeleton (composed of microtubules and microfilaments)	Provides support
Centrioles	Allow movement of chromosomes during cell division
Ribosomes (free ribosomes within cytoplasm and ribosomes bound to the rough endoplasmic reticulum)	Synthesize protein
Endoplasmic reticulum	Smooth endoplasmic reticulum synthesizes lipids and carbohydrates Rough endoplasmic reticulum is lined with ribosomes; packages proteins
Golgi apparatus	Stores and packages substances that will be secreted from the cell
Lysosomes	Contain powerful enzymes to rid the cell of damaged organelles and pathogens
Mitochondria	Produce ATP
Nucleus	Contains RNA and DNA

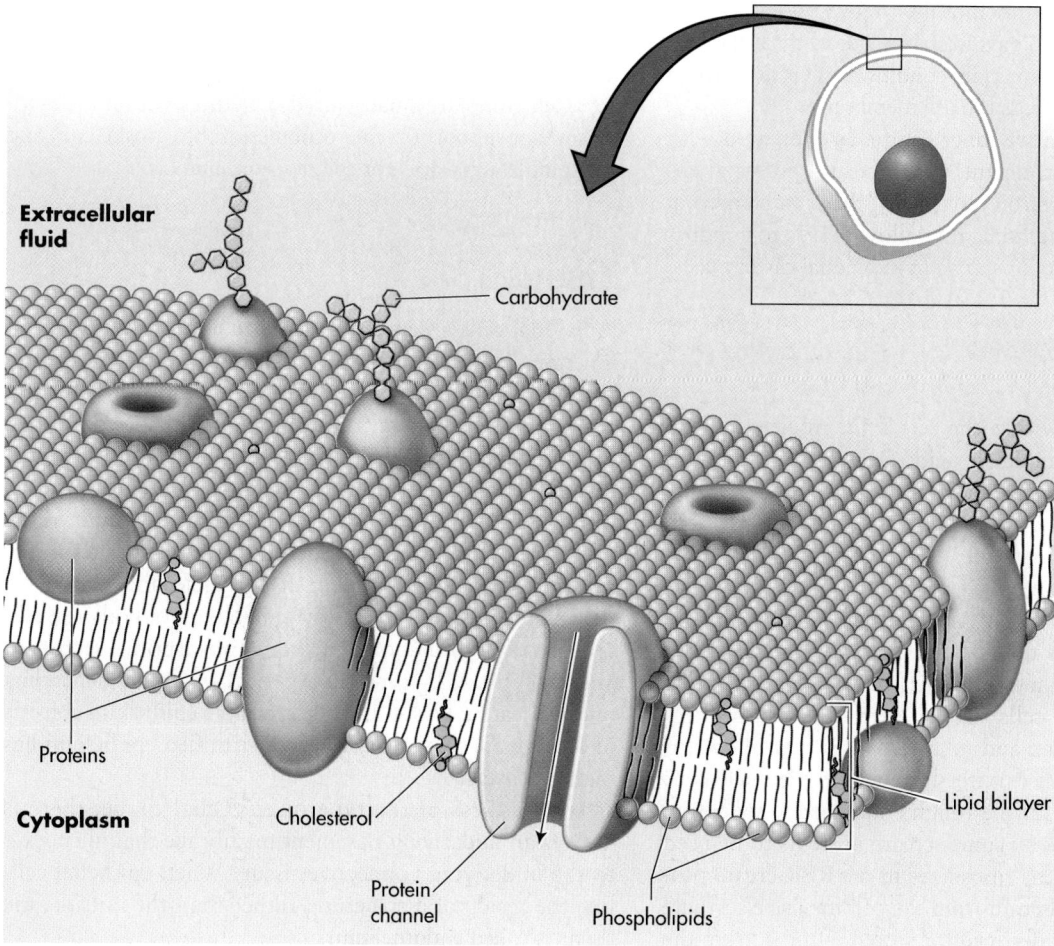

Extracellular fluid

Carbohydrate

Proteins

Cytoplasm

Cholesterol

Protein channel

Phospholipids

Lipid bilayer

FIGURE 8-9

The cell membrane.

portion) has an electrical charge and the other (the lipid portion) does not have an electrical charge.

The two rows of phospholipids that comprise the cell membrane are arranged so that the uncharged lipid portions face each other. This occurs because the uncharged end is not attracted to water (hydrophobic, or water hating) and the charged phosphate end is attracted to the watery environment inside and outside the cell (hydrophilic, or water loving). The charged phosphate ends are oriented toward the cytoplasm on one side of the membrane and the interstitial fluid on the other side.

The structure of the lipid bilayer allows free transit of certain small charged and uncharged molecules, but not larger or more strongly charged ones. Water can move freely, but electrolytes such as sodium and potassium are too strongly charged to pass through the hydrophobic inner layer of the membrane. This feature allows osmosis and the electrical differences that exist across the cell membrane, called the membrane potential.

Because osmosis is an attempt by a fluid to equalize concentrations across a membrane permeable only to water, abnormal concentrations of solutes inside or outside the cell affect the movement of water, which can cause the cell to shrink (crenate) or swell to the point of bursting (lyse).

The membrane potential results from the inability of electrolytes, which are positively or negatively electrically charged ions, to freely traverse the membrane. There are channels in the cell membrane that allow controlled amounts of these ions to pass from one side of the cell membrane to the other under certain conditions. This leads to an imbalance of charge across the cell membrane.

Cells have a negative inner charge as compared with the extracellular environment, which creates potential energy (potential for electron movement) that can be used in the form of **action potentials** that allow nerves to conduct messages and electricity to spread to individual cardiac cells, causing them to contract.

The Organelles

The core organelle within the cell is the nucleus, which houses the deoxyribonucleic acid (DNA) that comprises chromosomes, creating the body's genetic code. It is inside the nucleus that DNA is transcribed to ribonucleic acid (RNA), which then exits into the cytoplasm to be transcribed by ribosomes into proteins.

Proteins are comprised of amino acids and go on to serve many functions throughout the body, ranging from membrane transport mechanisms, to serving as chemical messengers to other cells (in the form of hormones), to formation of the bone and muscle tissues that allow for movement. Ribosomes can free-float within the nucleus or attach to the surface of the rough endoplasmic reticulum (RER). Free-floating ribosomes create proteins to be used within the cell, whereas ribosomes in the RER create proteins destined for secretion from the cell for use elsewhere in the body. Proteins destined for secretion move from the RER to the Golgi apparatus, which modifies the protein prior to secretion.

Smooth endoplasmic reticulum (SER) in the cytoplasm plays roles in drug detoxification and steroid metabolism. A variation of SER called the *sarcoplasmic reticulum* is found within the cytoplasm of muscle cells, where it is involved in storing calcium ions used in muscle contraction.

Mitochondria are scattered throughout the cell and produce energy in the form of ATP through oxidative phosphorylation. This process uses oxygen molecules to release energy from carbohydrate molecules (glucose) through a series of chemical reactions. This process begins when glucose enters the cytoplasm of the cell and undergoes glycolysis to be converted into pyruvic acid (anaerobic metabolism). Pyruvic acid then enters the mitochondria and participates in the Krebs cycle, which generates the ATP used to fuel the cell's activities.

Lysosomes and vacuoles are small cavities within cells that are surrounded by their own membranes. Lysosomes function to destroy waste and toxins within the cell, and possess powerful enzymes. When lysosomes within the cell rupture, their enzymes break down the structures of the cell itself, resulting in cellular death.

Vacuoles function to store and transport proteins within the cell. Cells have a scaffolding network that consists of long chains of proteins called *microtubules, intermediate filaments,* and *microfilaments*. This network creates a cytoskeleton ("cell skeleton") that maintains cell structure, allows for transport of materials within the cell, and can be rearranged to allow for cell movement.

Centrioles are small paired structures within the cytoplasm that support the microtubules of the cytoskeleton and the spindle apparatus for cell division, mitosis.

Tissues

Individual cells are grouped together both structurally and functionally to create tissues. Tissues are a group of specialized cells surrounded by a matrix. The nature of the matrix ranges from the mineral-dense matrix that makes bone hard to the fluid substance of plasma, in which various types of blood cells are found. Tissues function as a unit to achieve a certain purpose. Various types of tissue can be found within each organ. There are four general types of tissues in the human body: epithelial, connective, muscle, and nervous.

Epithelial tissue creates the thin linings of body surfaces and has many functions, including absorption, secretion, and protection. It comes in a variety of forms, depending on the location within the body. Simple epithelium consists of a single layer of cells, whereas stratified epithelium has multiple layers.

Regardless of the type of epithelial tissue, there is always an underlying basement membrane that anchors it to the underlying connective tissue. When epithelial cells line the inside of a structure, rather than the outside, the tissue is called **endothelium**.

Connective tissue consists of fibers such as collagen and elastin and provides structure and strength to the body. Bones, cartilage, and adipose tissue (fat) are three of the most common types of connective tissue. Adipose tissue is found beneath the skin and around organs. It provides protection, gives the body shape, and serves as a form of stored energy.

Muscle tissue consists of cells with proteins that can change in length (contract and relax). There are three sub-types of muscle tissue: skeletal, smooth, and cardiac.

Nervous tissue consists of specialized nerve cells that generate, receive, and transmit electrical impulses throughout the body. Those cells comprise the brain, spinal cord, and peripheral nerves.

Anatomical Terminology and Topographic Anatomy

A common language is spoken in the fields of medicine and science to avoid confusion when describing the anatomy and physiology of the human body. You must be fluent in this terminology to effectively communicate a patient's complaints and your physical exam findings to other health care providers, both orally and in your documentation. (See Chapter 7 for a general review of medical terminology.) A subset of this terminology is used to describe the surface features of the body, which serve as landmarks for procedures and points of reference for other structures. Those landmarks are the topographical anatomy of the body.

Anatomical terms of position and direction use the body's anatomic position as a point of reference. In the anatomic position the body is standing upright, looking forward, with feet together and arms at the sides with palms facing forward.

Three imaginary planes are drawn through the body in this position to allow for better description of locations (Figure 8-10). The frontal, or coronal, plane runs vertically from head to toe, dividing the body into anterior and posterior sections. The sagittal plane also runs from head to toe, but at a 90-degree angle to the frontal plane. This divides the body into left and right sides.

The transverse or axial plane passes horizontally through the body, dividing it into superior, or cephalad (toward the head) and inferior, or caudal (toward the tail or feet) sections. The transverse plane is particularly important in computed tomography (CT) scanning, because this is the orientation of the primary images produced.

Standardized lines of reference are used to describe locations within the trunk of the body, locations that are not well described by the terms *proximal* and *distal*. In the chest, the midaxillary line refers to a line drawn vertically from the center of the armpit, or axilla, to the waist. The midclavicular line refers to a line drawn vertically from the middle of the collarbone, or clavicle, to the waist. The anterior and posterior axillary lines can be used to further define the area, referring to vertical lines parallel to the midaxillary

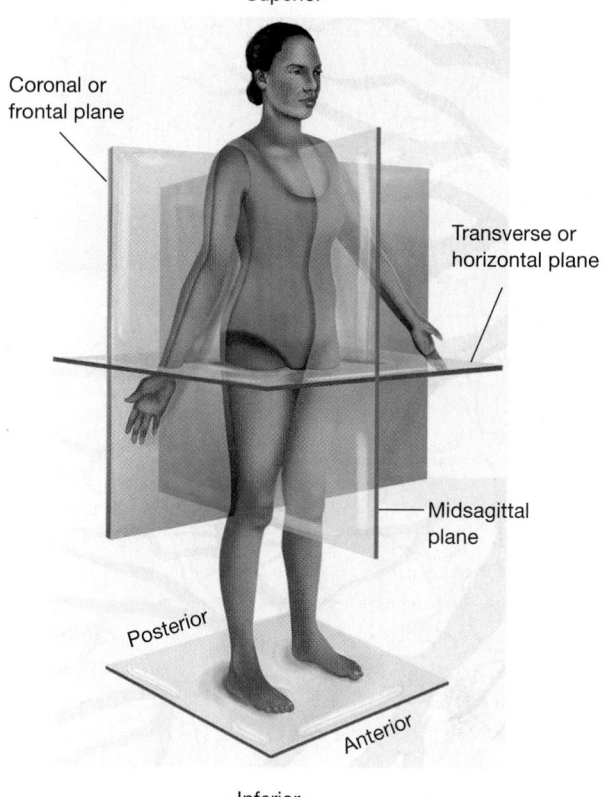

FIGURE 8-10

The anatomical position.

line. Those two lines are at the anterior and posterior axillary skin folds, one to two inches anterior and posterior to the midaxillary line, respectively.

The abdomen has its own frame of reference that involves drawing vertical and transverse lines through the anterior torso. For anatomical purposes, the abdomen is divided into nine regions (Figure 8-11). For the purposes of physical examination and documentation, two intersecting lines are drawn directly through the belly button, or umbilicus (Figure 8-12). This divides the abdomen into four quadrants: the left upper quadrant (LUQ), right upper quadrant (RUQ), left lower quadrant (LLQ), and right lower quadrant (RLQ). Knowledge of which organs are associated with each quadrant aids in developing differential diagnoses for patients complaining of abdominal pain.

Body Cavities

The body is divided into cavities within which internal organs are contained (Figure 8-13).

The cranial cavity contains the brain and connects inferiorly with the spinal cavity, which contains the spinal cord. Together, those two cavities are called the *dorsal body cavity*. Its contents are bathed in cerebrospinal fluid. The ventral body cavity consists of the thoracic and

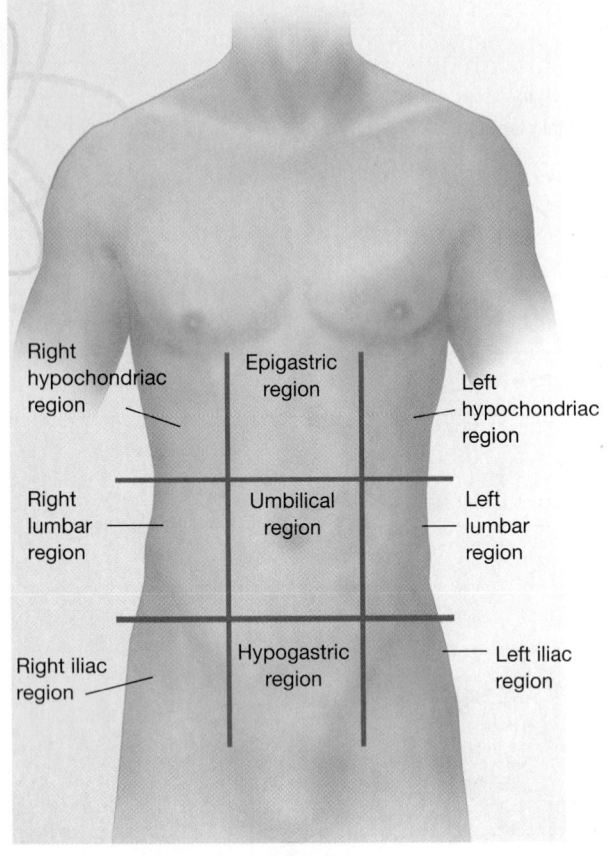

FIGURE 8-11

Anatomically, the abdomen is divided into nine regions.

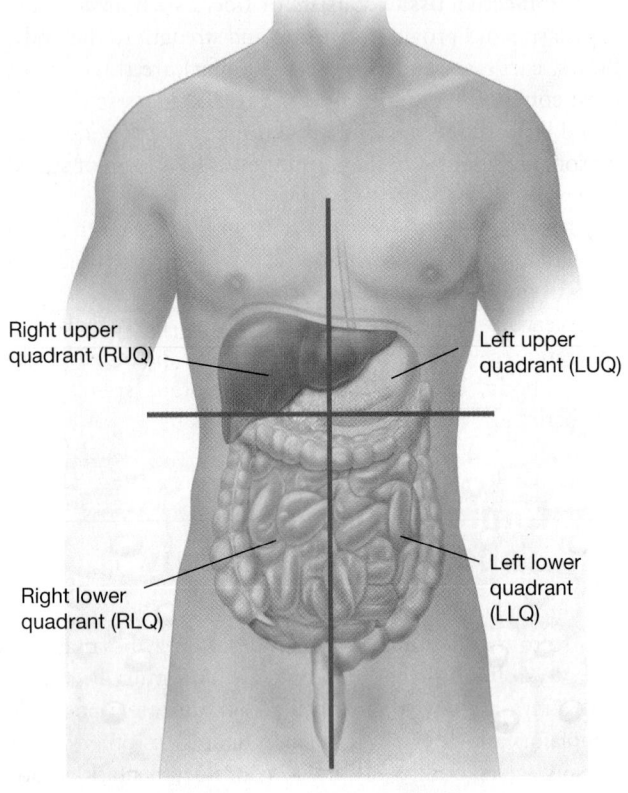

FIGURE 8-12

Medically, the abdomen is divided into four quadrants.

abdominopelvic cavities, the latter being further divided into the abdominal and pelvic cavities.

The thoracic cavity contains the heart, lungs, great vessels, and esophagus, and is bordered laterally by the rib cage, posteriorly by the spine, anteriorly by the sternum, superiorly by the base of the neck, and inferiorly by the diaphragm. The mediastinum is a specific section of the thorax between the lungs, containing the heart, roots of the great vessels, esophagus, trachea, nerves, and lymphatic structures.

The abdominal cavity is inferior to the diaphragm and contains the abdominal viscera (organs), including the stomach, liver, spleen, pancreas, and intestines. The abdominal cavity is continuous inferiorly with the pelvic cavity, which contains the reproductive and urinary organs as well as the distal parts of the large intestine. The pelvic cavity is surrounded by the bones that comprise the pelvic girdle.

Organs and Body Systems

Tissues come together to form organs, which work together in systems to serve specific functions. Most organs consist of a variety of tissues: For example, the heart consists of muscular tissue that contracts, nervous tissue that stimulates the muscle to contract, connective tissue that organizes its overall structure, epithelial tissue that lines the cavities, and fatty tissue that pads the external surface of the heart.

Systems are collections of organs and tissues that interact to carry out a complex set of functions. For example, the skeletal system provides structure to the entire body, and the cardiovascular system works with the respiratory system to perfuse the body tissues.

Support, Movement, and Protection

Skeletal System

The skeletal system consists of the bones, cartilage, tendons, and ligaments that provide the body with structure, support, and protection. Bones are also an important reservoir of calcium and house bone marrow, wherein new blood cells are created.

The skeletal system works in conjunction with the skeletal muscles to allow movement. The skeleton consists of 206 bones that are classified as long, short, or flat.

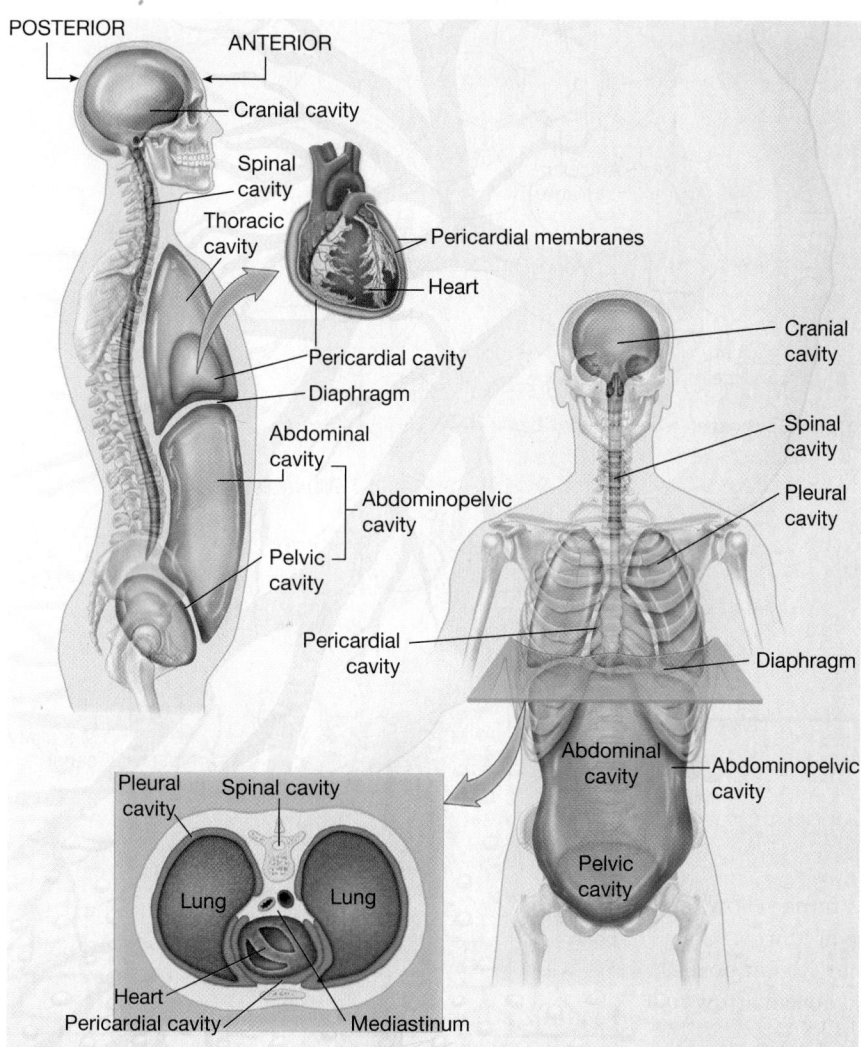

FIGURE 8-13

The body cavities.

Cartilage, Ligaments, and Tendons

Cartilage is a connective tissue that supports the skeleton in many areas. It is found at the surfaces of bones that come together to form joints, and it connects ribs to the sternum in the thoracic (chest) cavity, and provides structure to part of the nose and to the ears. Cartilage is stiff but has more flexibility than bone. It pads many of the joints in the body (Figure 8-14). One such example is the intervertebral disks that provide a cushion between the bones of the spine.

Cartilage that covers the ends of bones at joints is smooth and lubricated by synovial fluid produced within the joint. This type of cartilage is called *articular cartilage* and provides for smooth joint movement.

Tendons are bands of connective tissue that connect bones to muscles. It is this connection of a muscle to an adjacent bone that allows movement of that bone when the muscle contracts.

Ligaments are bands of connective tissue that connect bones to bones, providing stability and support to joints. Many joints contain synovial fluid, a connective tissue that lubricates and protects the bone ends from injury.

IN THE FIELD

Injuries and chronic inflammation and destruction (from disease or overuse) of joints are common and range from mild to debilitating. An injury to a tendon is called a *strain*, whereas one to a ligament is called a *sprain*. Inflammation of the joint is called *arthritis*.

Bones

Short bones comprise the wrist and ankle and are roughly cube shaped. Flat bones include the sternum, ribs, scapula, pelvis, and ribs. Long bones, such as the femur in the thigh, are found in the extremities.

Most of the flat and long bones have a central cavity, the medullary cavity, which contains bone marrow (Figure 8-15). At birth, all bone marrow is red and capable of producing new blood cells. As a person ages,

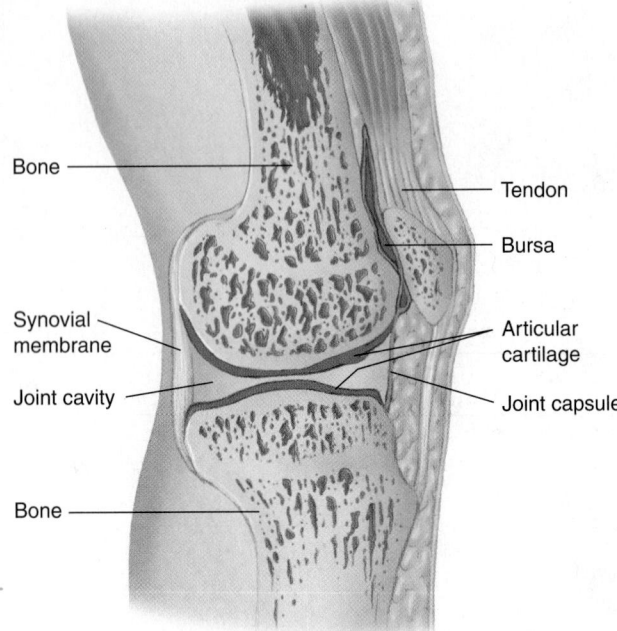

FIGURE 8-14

Structure of a joint.

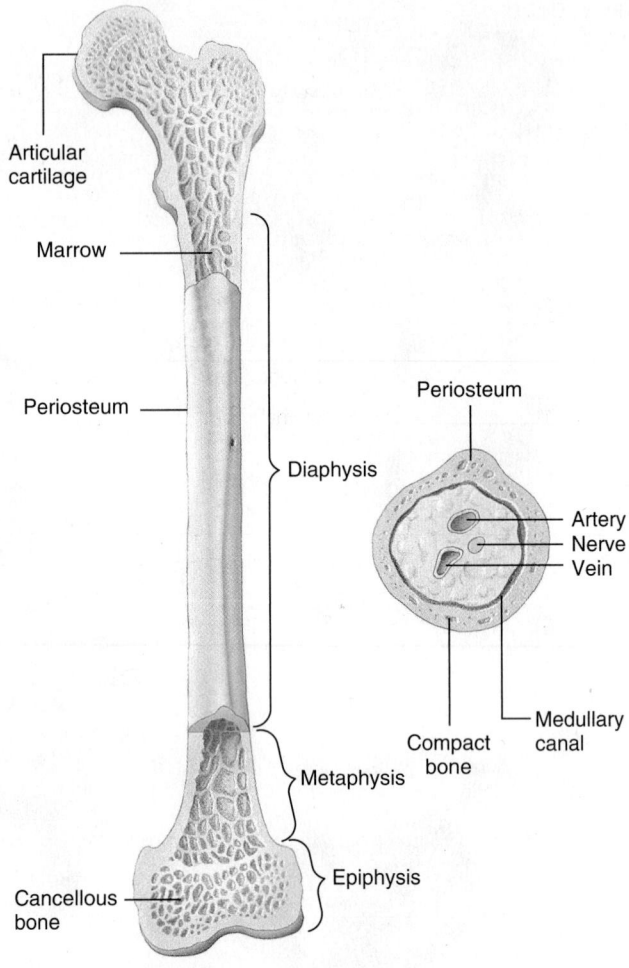

FIGURE 8-15

Structure of a typical long bone.

the marrow in the middle of long bones turns yellow, an inactive and fatty version. However, the need to produce blood cells remains throughout life, and certain bones, such as the sternum and pelvis, retain red bone marrow to serve this purpose.

A typical long bone has a number of identifiable features (Table 8-4). The diaphysis is the shaft of the bone. The epiphyses are at the ends, and the metaphysis is the area that connects the diaphysis and epiphyses. In children, the epiphyseal plate, commonly called the *growth plate*, is where longitudinal bone growth occurs. When anatomical features of bones can be detected on the surface of the body, this allows them to serve as anatomical landmarks.

Bone consists of collagen and a mineral compound of calcium and phosphate. Sheets of bone tissue are called *lamellae*. They are arranged to surround the blood vessels in the bone.

Bone cells called *osteoblasts* are scattered throughout bone tissue. They secrete the bone matrix that eventually surrounds them. Once surrounded with their own matrix, they become osteocytes, which manage nutrition and waste disposal within bone. Another type of cell, the osteoclast, destroys excess bone.

The Skeleton

The bones of the skeleton are categorized into two divisions. The axial skeleton is in a straight line at the core of the body. It consists of the skull, spine, ribs, and sternum. The appendicular skeleton consists of the bones of the upper and lower extremities (the appendages), including the bones of the shoulder and pelvis that connect them with the axial skeleton (Figure 8-16).

Axial Skeleton

The skull is divided into two portions: the cranium, which surrounds and protects the brain, and the face.

The cranial bones are flat bones connected by immovable joints called **sutures**, which hold them tightly together. The bones of the cranium include the frontal, temporal, parietal, occipital, sphenoid, and ethmoid bones (Figure 8-17).

The bones of the middle ear, known as the *auditory ossicles* (malleus, incus, and stapes), are found within the temporal bone. The orbits, formed by several of the cranial and facial bones, are the depressions in the anterior skull that hold the eyes.

TABLE 8-4   Surface Features of Bones

General Description	Anatomical Term	Definition
Elevations and projections (general)	Process	Any projection or bump
	Ramus	Extension of a bone that makes an angle with the rest of the structure
Processes formed where tendons or ligaments attach	Trochanter	Large, rough projection
	Tuberosity	Smaller, rough projection
	Tubercle	Small, rounded projection
	Crest	Prominent ridge
	Line	Low ridge
	Spine	Pointed process
Processes formed for articulation with adjacent bones	Head	Expanded articular end of an epiphysis, separated from the shaft by a neck
	Neck	Narrow connection between the epiphysis and the diaphysis
	Condyle	Smooth, rounded articular process
	Trochlea	Smooth, grooved articular process shaped like a pulley
	Facet	Small, flat articular surface
Depressions	Fossa	Shallow depression
	Sulcus	Narrow groove
Openings	Foramen	Rounded passageway for blood vessels or nerves
	Canal	Passageway through the substance of a bone
	Fissure	Elongate cleft
	Sinus	Chamber within a bone, normally filled with air

The bones that comprise the inferior portion of the cranium, forming the floor of the cranial cavity, are called the **basilar skull** (Figure 8-18). The opening at the base of the skull, through which the spinal cord descends from the brainstem into the spinal canal, is called the **foramen magnum.**

The cranial cavity (or vault) is almost completely filled by the brain. The remainder of the cavity is filled with the **cerebrospinal fluid (CSF)** that bathes and cushions the brain from impact with the skull bones.

The 14 facial bones include the paired maxilla, temporal, nasal, palatine, lacrimal, and inferior nasal concha bones, along with the mandible and vomer.

IN THE FIELD

Because the cranium cannot expand in size, any bleeding within it or swelling of the brain increases pressure within the cranial cavity, exerting pressure on the brain. The increased pressure interferes with the function of the brain and, if not relieved, interferes with brain function and can push the brainstem through the foramen magnum.

The mandible, or jawbone, is the only movable bone of the face. It articulates (forms a joint) with the maxilla to form the *temporomandibular joint.* Thirty-two permanent teeth (16 upper and 16 lower) are embedded in the maxilla and mandible. Below the face, situated anteriorly in the neck and serving as an attachment for the muscular tongue, is the hyoid bone. The hyoid bone is unique in that is the only bone in the body that is not connected to other bones.

The spinal column consists of 33 bones, called *vertebrae*, divided into five anatomical sections (Figure 8-19). From superior to inferior, these are the cervical, thoracic, lumbar, sacral, and coccygeal regions of the spine.

Most of the vertebrae are ring-shaped bones that form a central column through which the spinal cord passes (Figure 8-20). The spinal canal is continuous with the cranium and the spinal cord within it is bathed in the same CSF that bathes the brain. The vertebrae form joints (called *facet joints*) with each other to allow movement. Strong ligaments and muscles surround the spinal column, keeping it in alignment.

The posterior portion of each vertebra, the spinous process, can be felt under the skin of the neck and back. Openings (foramina) within the vertebral arches allow nerves to enter and exit the spinal column to communicate between the spinal cord and the rest of the body. The bodies

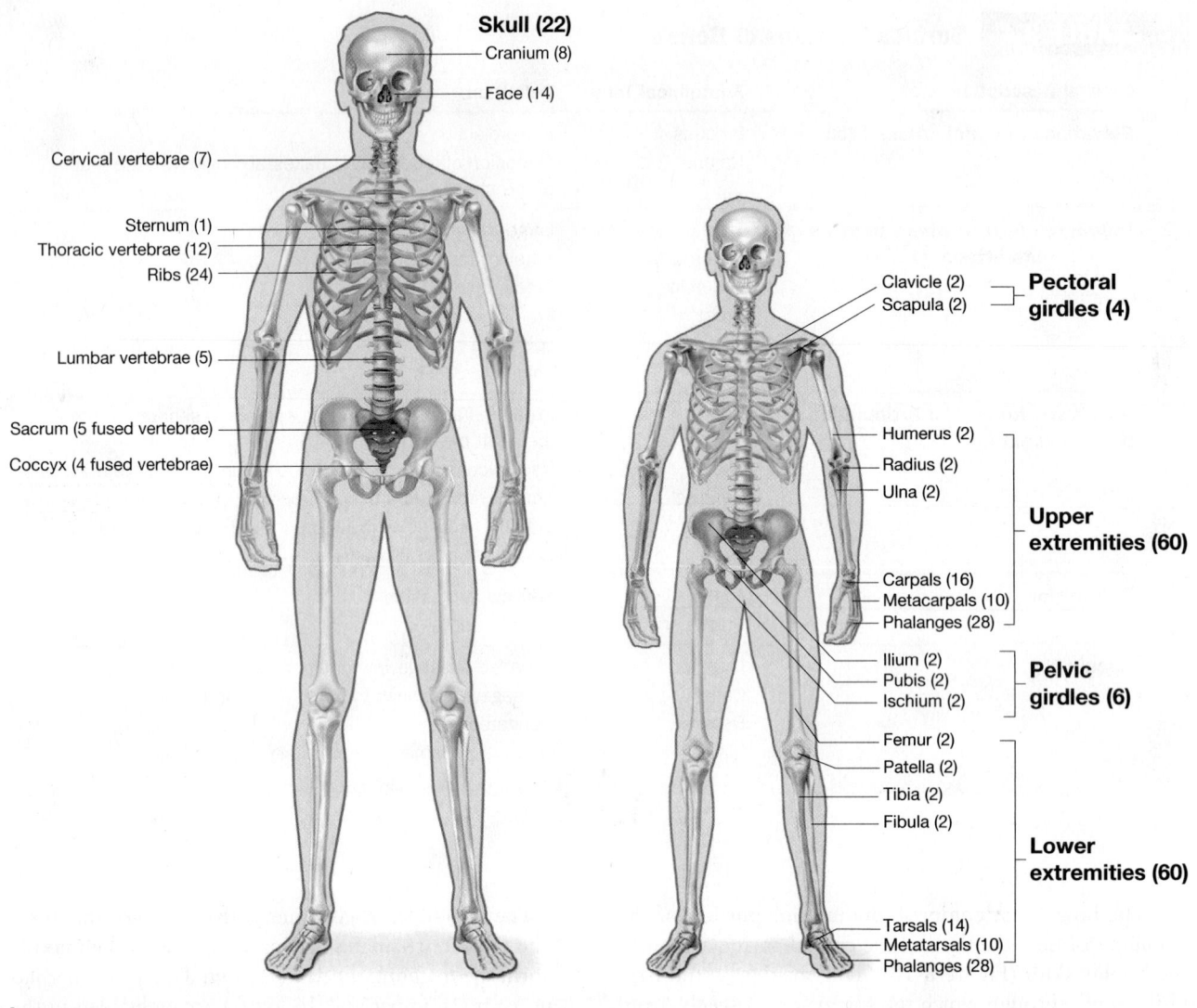

Skull (22)
— Cranium (8)
— Face (14)

Cervical vertebrae (7)

Sternum (1)
Thoracic vertebrae (12)
Ribs (24)

Lumbar vertebrae (5)

Sacrum (5 fused vertebrae)
Coccyx (4 fused vertebrae)

Clavicle (2)
Scapula (2)
} **Pectoral girdles (4)**

Humerus (2)
Radius (2)
Ulna (2)

Upper extremities (60)

Carpals (16)
Metacarpals (10)
Phalanges (28)

Ilium (2)
Pubis (2)
Ischium (2)
} **Pelvic girdles (6)**

Femur (2)
Patella (2)
Tibia (2)
Fibula (2)

Lower extremities (60)

Tarsals (14)
Metatarsals (10)
Phalanges (28)

FIGURE 8-16

The skeleton consists of 206 bones divided between its axial and appendicular divisions. The axial skeleton consists of the skull, spine, and thorax. The appendicular skeleton consists of the bones of the extremities, including the bones that allow them to attach to the axial skeleton.

of the vertebrae are separated by thick intervertebral disks that act as shock absorbers. Viewed laterally, the spine has prominent curves that are designed to support the weight of the body.

The seven cervical vertebrae of the neck are small and delicate compared with the larger, thicker thoracic and lumbar vertebrae. The first cervical vertebra, C1, also called the *atlas*, articulates with the occipital bone of the skull (Figure 8-21). The second cervical vertebra, C2, which is also called the *axis*, articulates with C1 by way of a projection called the *odontoid process*. This feature allows the head to turn from side to side. The seventh cervical vertebra, C7, which is the most inferior of the cervical vertebrae, has a prominent spinous process

that can be felt at the back of the neck, just above the shoulders.

Each of the 12 thoracic vertebrae, T1 through T12, articulates with a pair of ribs, one on each side.

Five lumbar vertebrae (L1 through L5) form the curve of the lower back. The spinal cord ends at approximately L2. The nerves that exit the spinal cord at this level continue down the spinal canal. They are arranged so that they resemble a horse's tail, and are called the *cauda equina*.

The five sacral and four coccygeal vertebrae are fused, forming the posterior aspect of the pelvis (sacrum) and the "tailbone," (coccyx) respectively.

The thoracic (rib) cage, consisting of the sternum and 12 pairs of ribs, comprises the remainder of the axial

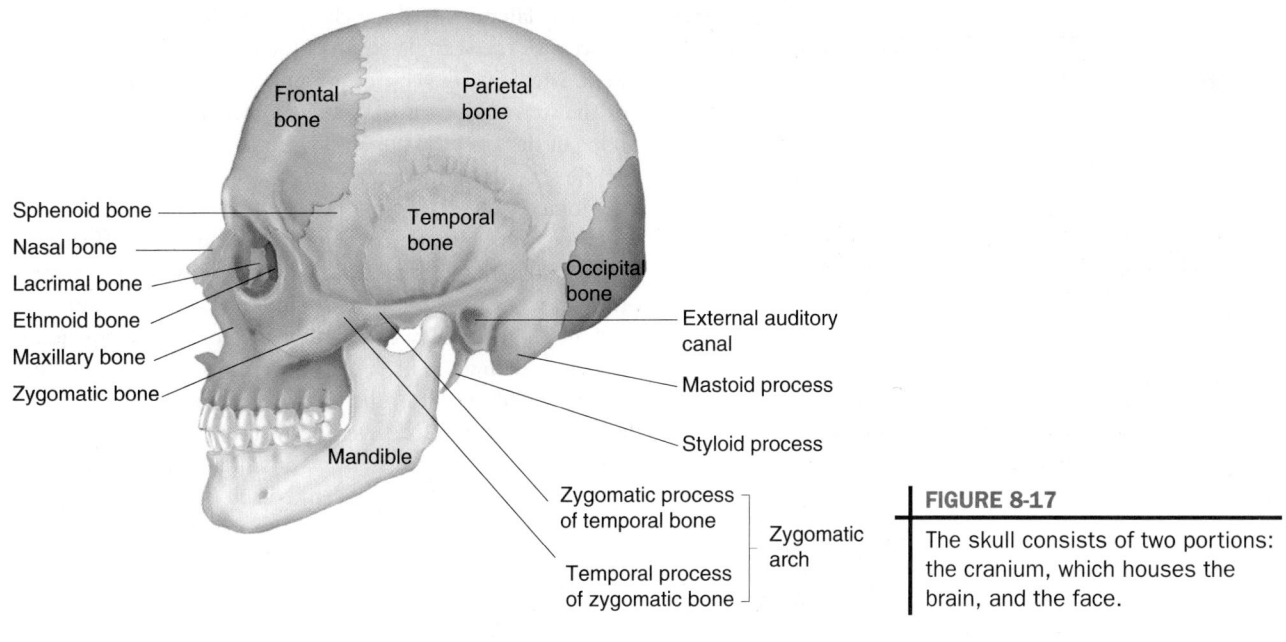

Frontal bone
Parietal bone
Sphenoid bone
Nasal bone
Lacrimal bone
Ethmoid bone
Maxillary bone
Zygomatic bone
Temporal bone
Occipital bone
External auditory canal
Mastoid process
Styloid process
Mandible
Zygomatic process of temporal bone
Temporal process of zygomatic bone
Zygomatic arch

FIGURE 8-17

The skull consists of two portions: the cranium, which houses the brain, and the face.

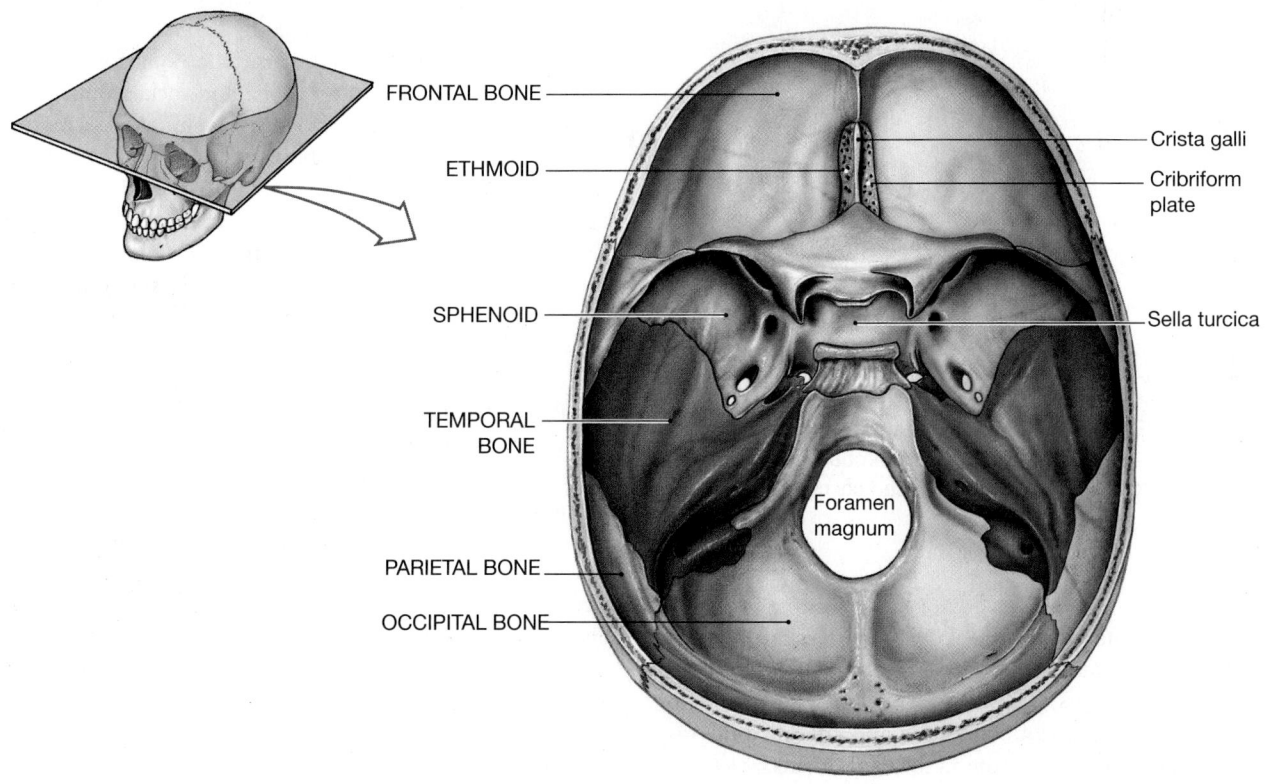

FRONTAL BONE
ETHMOID
SPHENOID
TEMPORAL BONE
PARIETAL BONE
OCCIPITAL BONE
Crista galli
Cribriform plate
Sella turcica
Foramen magnum

FIGURE 8-18

The basilar skull comprises the floor of the cranial cavity. (Bledsoe, Bryan E.; Martini, Frederic H.; Bartholomew, Edwin F.; Ober, William C.; Garrison, Claire W.; Anatomy & Physiology for Emergency Care, 2nd Edition, © 2008. Reprinted with permission of Pearson Education, Inc., Upper Saddle River, NJ)

skeleton (Figure 8-22). The sternum has three sections. The most superior portion is the manubrium, with which the clavicles (collarbones) articulate to form part of the shoulder girdle. The depression at the top edge of the manubrium, called the *sternal notch*, serves as a useful anatomic landmark for medical procedures. The body of the sternum is the longest portion, and the distal tip is called the *xiphoid process*.

Each rib is connected posteriorly to its corresponding thoracic vertebrae. The first rib lies under the clavicle

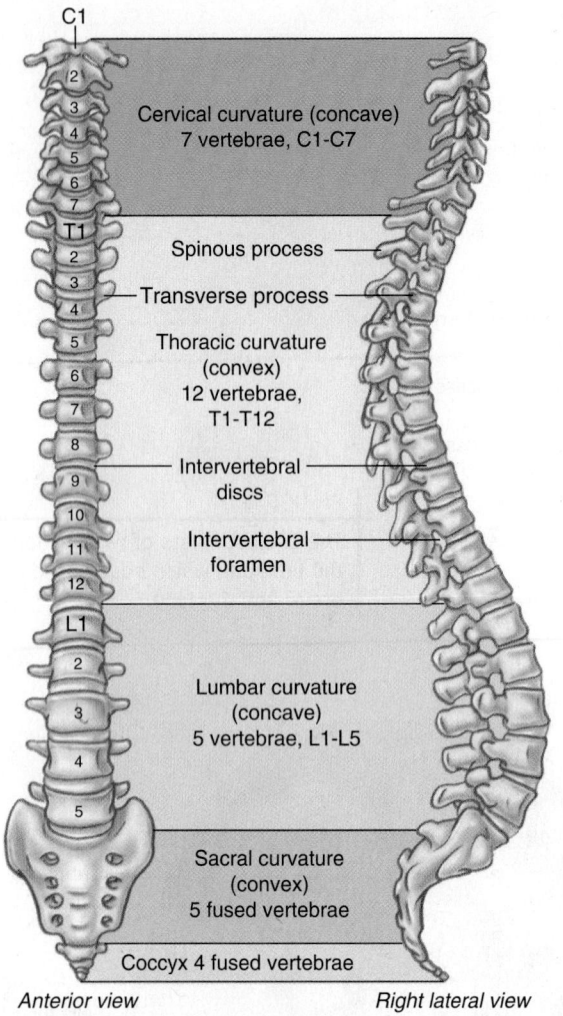

C1

Cervical curvature (concave)
7 vertebrae, C1-C7

Spinous process
Transverse process

Thoracic curvature
(convex)
12 vertebrae,
T1-T12

Intervertebral
discs

Intervertebral
foramen

Lumbar curvature
(concave)
5 vertebrae, L1-L5

Sacral curvature
(convex)
5 fused vertebrae

Coccyx 4 fused vertebrae

Anterior view   *Right lateral view*

FIGURE 8-19

The 33 vertebrae of the spine are arranged in five
sections. From superior to inferior, there are 7 cervical
vertebrae, 12 thoracic vertebrae, 5 lumbar vertebrae,
5 fused sacral vertebrae, and 4 fused coccygeal vertebrae.

(collarbone) and cannot be felt through the skin. The first
10 pairs of ribs are connected to the border of the sternum
by varying amounts of cartilage. The last two pairs of ribs
do not have an anterior connection and are called *floating
ribs*. The thoracic cage protects the vital organs of the cardiovascular and respiratory systems and plays a vital role in
ventilation—the process of moving air into and out of the
lungs.

Appendicular Skeleton

The appendicular skeleton includes the shoulder girdle and
the pelvic girdle, from which the upper and lower extremities extend. The shoulder girdle consists of the scapula, or
shoulder blade, and clavicle, or collarbone. This arrangement results in three shoulder joints.

The lateral end of the clavicle attaches to the acromion
process of the scapula to form the acromioclavicular (AC)
joint. Medially, the clavicle articulates with the manubrium
of the sternum (sternoclavicular joint). The proximal long
bone of the arm, the humerus, inserts into the glenoid fossa
of the scapula to form the glenohumeral, or "true," shoulder joint.

As a ball-and-socket joint, the shoulder is afforded a
tremendous range of motion. The four muscles of the rota-
tor cuff work to stabilize the shoulder. Distally, the humerus
articulates with the radius and ulna to form the elbow joint,
which is a hinge joint. The olecranon process of the ulna
forms the bony part of the elbow. Together, the radius and
ulna comprise the forearm and distally articulate with the
wrist. The wrist consists of eight small carpal bones. Five
metacarpal bones form the hand, each of which in turn articulate with a phalange to comprise the fingers. Each of the
fingers has three phalanges, and the thumb has two.

The pelvic girdle consists of two halves, each formed
of three fused bones: the ilium, ischium, and pubis. The sacrum articulates with the ilium at the sacroiliac joint and
the two pubic bones articulate anteriorly at the pubic symphysis. The acetabulum is formed by parts of all three fused
pelvic bones, and provides the insertion point for the head
of the femur. The hip joint is a ball-and-socket joint analogous to the shoulder and provides a wide range of motion
as well, but less so than the shoulder.

The femur, which is the longest bone in the body, articulates distally with the tibia to form the knee joint. The
patella, or kneecap, is anterior to the knee joint and is connected superiorly to the quadriceps muscles and inferiorly
by the patellar tendon to the tibia. The knee joint is a hinge
joint that is held together by a variety of supporting ligaments: the anterior and posterior cruciate ligaments (ACL
and PCL), and the medial and lateral menisci, among others.

Distal to the knee, the fibula runs posterior and lateral
to the larger tibia. Along with the tibia, it articulates with
the talus to form the ankle joint. As a central bone in the ankle, the talus also articulates posteriorly and inferiorly to the
calcaneus, which forms the heel. The talus, calcaneus, na-
vicular, cuboid, and cuneiform bones comprise the tarsals.
Five metatarsals comprise the bones of each foot, which in
turn articulate with phalanges to form the toes in a fashion
analogous to the hand.

Muscular System

Muscle tissue is built from cells that have unique proteins (actin and myosin) arranged in filaments that can
contract (shorten) and relax, thereby allowing movement.
Contraction occurs in response to nervous stimulation
and requires a complex chemical interaction within the
muscle cell.

There are three types of muscle tissue in the body. Each
type has a specific function and appears different under the
microscope. Skeletal muscle (also called *striated* muscle, for

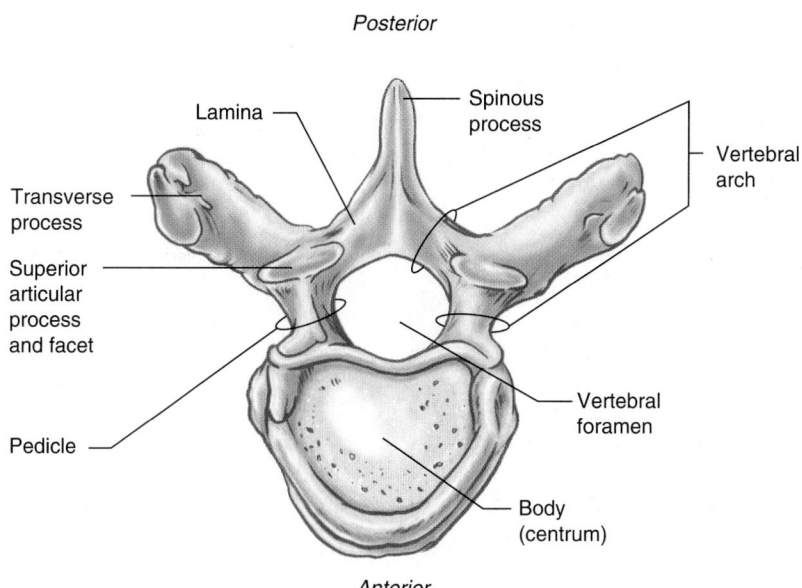

Posterior

Lamina — Spinous process

Vertebral arch

Transverse process

Superior articular process and facet

Pedicle

Vertebral foramen

Body (centrum)

Anterior

FIGURE 8-20

Typical vertebral structure.

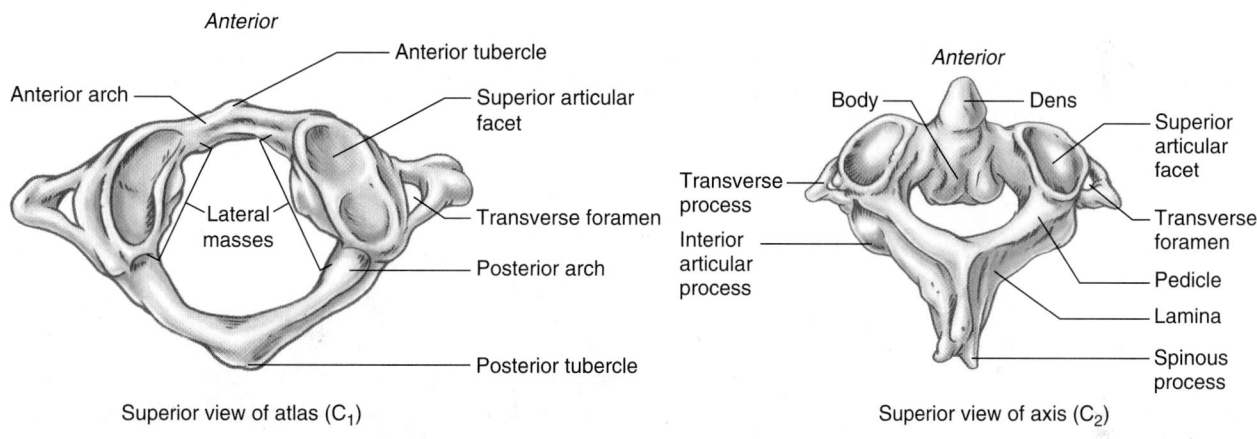

Anterior

Anterior arch —

— Anterior tubercle

— Superior articular facet

Lateral masses

— Transverse foramen

— Posterior arch

— Posterior tubercle

Superior view of atlas (C₁)

Anterior

Body — — Dens

— Superior articular facet

Transverse process

Interior articular process

— Transverse foramen

— Pedicle

— Lamina

— Spinous process

Superior view of axis (C₂)

FIGURE 8-21

The atlas (C1) and axis (C2) allow for rotation of the head.

its striped appearance under the microscope) attaches to bones and allows movement by way of tendons. Skeletal muscle can be controlled voluntarily, but also moves by way of reflex.

Each skeletal muscle has an origin and an insertion. For example, the biceps brachii of the arm has its origins on the scapula and inserts on the radius. When the biceps contract and shorten, the elbow flexes, decreasing the angle between the forearm and the arm.

Smooth muscle is under involuntary control and is found in the organs. Smooth muscle in the walls of blood vessels can constrict, decreasing the diameter of the vessel, and relax, increasing the diameter to control the amount of blood that flows through the vessels. Smooth muscle in the digestive tract contracts rhythmically to propel digestive contents along its length. Smooth muscle in the tiny

bronchioles of the lungs can constrict and dilate, changing the amount of air that can flow in and out of the alveoli (air sacs) of the lungs.

Cardiac muscle looks somewhat similar to skeletal muscle, but is under involuntary control and is adapted to its unique function of allowing the heart to pump blood throughout the body. The unique properties and function of cardiac muscle are considered again later in the chapter.

Integumentary System

The skin, or integument, is the largest organ in the human body. It has the crucial tasks of maintaining body warmth and protecting from external pathogens. Through its oil and sweat glands, it also plays an important role in maintaining

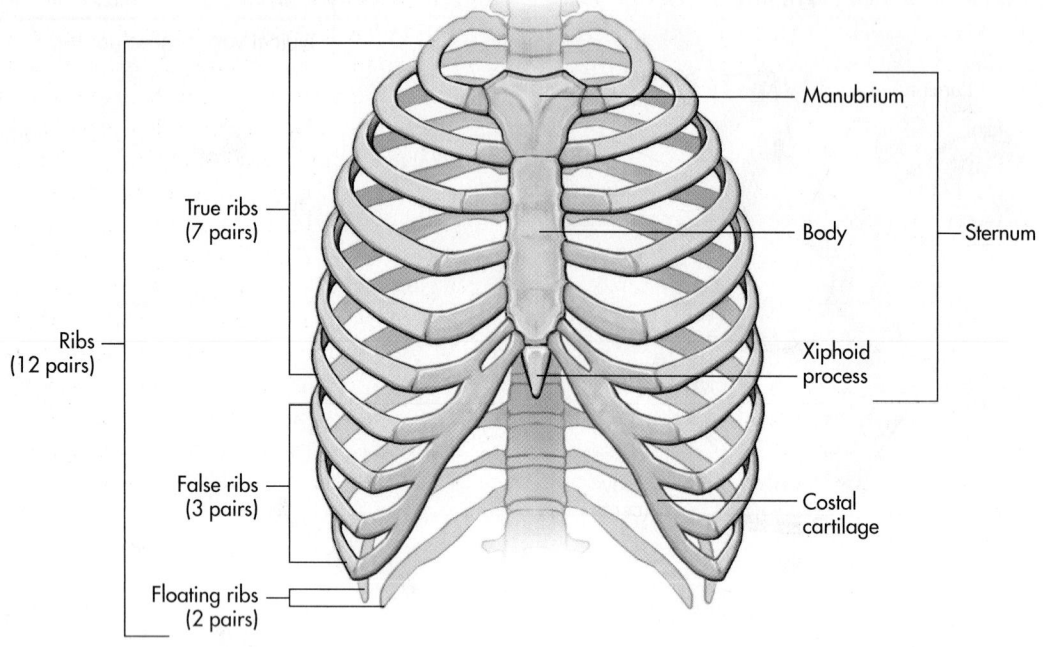

FIGURE 8-22

The thorax consists of 12 pairs of ribs that articulate posteriorly with the thoracic vertebrae and anteriorly with the sternum, which is divided into three sections: the manubrium, body, and xiphoid process.

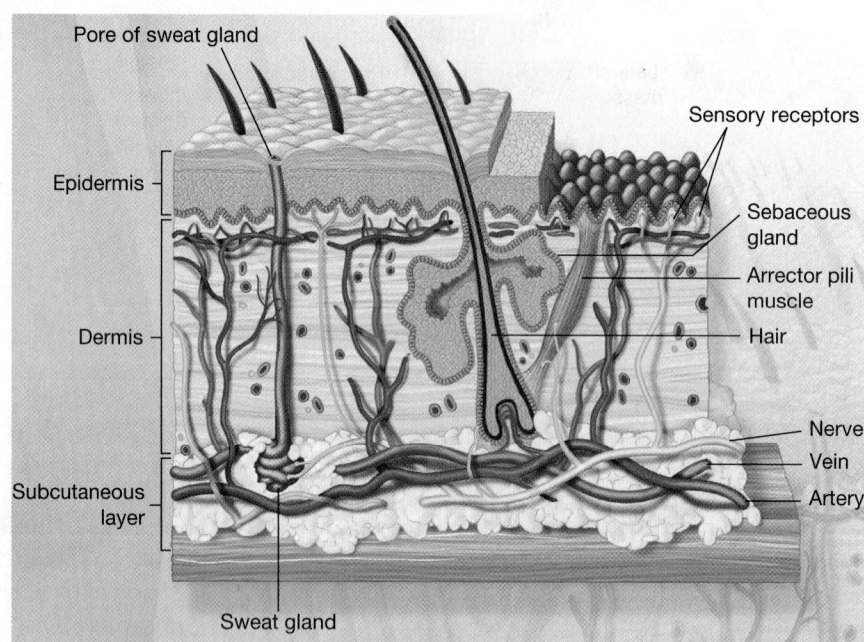

FIGURE 8-23

The skin consists of an outer protective layer called the *epidermis*, and an inner layer that contains the glands, nerves, and blood vessels, called the *dermis*.

the overall fluid balance in the body. The hair and nails are also part of the integumentary system.

The skin is composed of three layers, the outermost of which is called the *epidermis* (Figure 8-23). The epidermal layer consists of several thin layers of dead epithelial cells. Many of those cells contain a pigment called *melanin*, which protects the skin from the ultraviolet rays of the sun and produces coloration. Epidermal cells also contain keratin, a protein that provides the strength required to withstand the external environment.

The dermis lies just beneath the epidermis. It is a thicker layer of connective tissue that contains most of the structures of the skin. The dermis contains blood vessels, nerves, sweat glands, oil glands, and hair follicles. This layer plays a major role in the maintenance of body temperature through the use of blood vessels and sweat glands. When the body needs to lose heat, the **cutaneous** blood vessels dilate and increased perspiration is produced by the sweat glands. When the body needs to preserve heat, blood vessels constrict and perspiration decreases.

The subcutaneous layer, or hypodermis, lies beneath the dermis and consists mainly of fat. That layer also contains blood vessels and nerves and plays a role in body heat preservation. The majority of excess fat in the body is stored as subcutaneous fat.

Respiration and Circulation

Respiratory System

The function of the respiratory system is to obtain oxygen needed for cell metabolism and eliminate carbon dioxide produced by cell metabolism. The interface of microscopic blood vessels (capillaries) with the microscopic air sacs of the lungs (alveoli) allows the exchange of gases between the atmosphere and each individual cell in the body.

The conduit for air to enter and leave the lungs is called the *airway*. The airway is a series of passages that begin with the mouth and nose and end at the alveoli. The process of moving air in and out of the lungs is a mechanical process called **ventilation**. The exchange of the gases oxygen and carbon dioxide is called **respiration** (Figure 8-24). In other words, ventilation is required for respiration.

Respiration is divided into external respiration, which occurs in the alveoli, and internal respiration, which occurs at the cellular level. Ventilation relies on basic principles of physics to create the conditions for air to flow in and out of the lungs. The process further relies on the way the lungs are structured and situated in the thoracic cavity.

Respiration relies on the microscopic anatomy of the alveoli and capillaries, as well as the principle of gradients—differences in the concentrations of gases from one area to another.

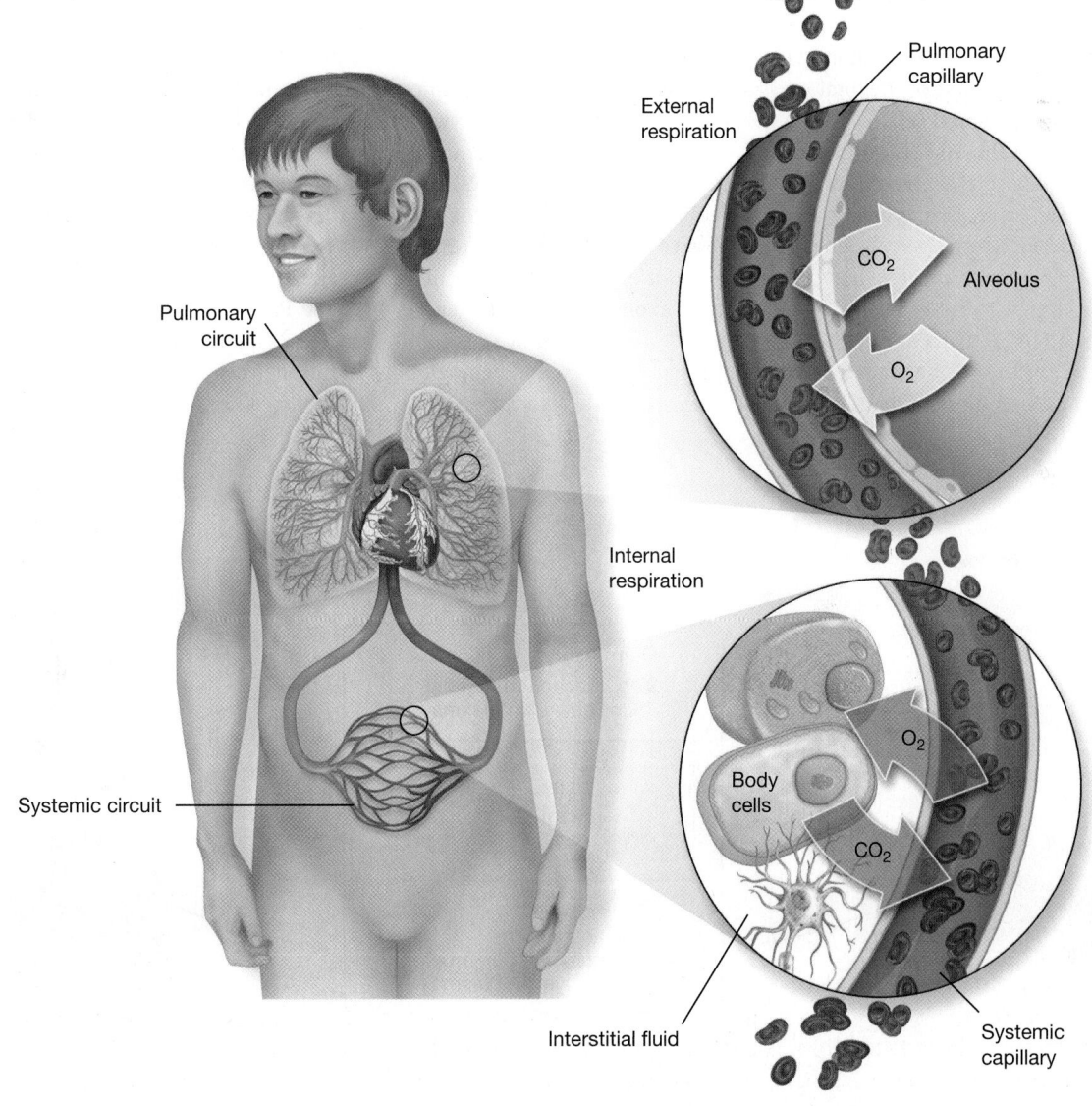

FIGURE 8-24

Respiration is the exchange of gases between the body and the environment.

Gases

The atmosphere that surrounds the earth is a mixture of gases. Each gas in a mixture exerts a certain amount of pressure, contributing to the total pressure of the mixture of gases.

The most familiar example of the measurement of the pressure of gases is barometric pressure, which is the total pressure exerted on the earth by the atmosphere. When this measurement is given in the weather forecast, the units used are inches of mercury. A barometric pressure of 29.92 inches of mercury, which is the normal pressure at sea level, is equivalent to 760 **millimeters of mercury** (**mmHg**), also called *torr* (for physiologic measurements). Barometric pressure varies slightly according to atmospheric conditions and elevation.

The amount of pressure that an individual gas contributes to the total pressure is known as the **partial pressure (Pa)** of the gas. For example, the pressure exerted by oxygen in a mixture of gases is the PaO_2. The air we breathe is approximately 79 percent nitrogen and 21 percent oxygen, along with a variety of trace gases present in very small quantities. Because the atmosphere is about 21 percent oxygen, it contributes to 21 percent of the total pressure of the atmosphere, or about 160 mmHg.

As air enters the alveoli on inspiration it mixes with the gases already in the alveoli, mostly water vapor and carbon dioxide. Therefore, the PaO_2 in the alveoli is about 100 mmHg. Not all the oxygen inhaled is able to cross the respiratory membrane. The body uses only about one-quarter of the oxygen from inspired air. Therefore, expired air contains about 16 percent oxygen.

It is the difference between the partial pressures of oxygen and carbon dioxide that determine the direction in which they will **diffuse**. Gases diffuse along a gradient from an area of higher pressure to lower pressure. It is hard to imagine the concept of gases in the blood. However, they exist in dissolved form in the bloodstream so they can be transported. Of the oxygen molecules that enter the blood, 98.5 percent bind to **hemoglobin** in red blood cells, and the rest is dissolved in plasma.

Carbon dioxide is carried in three different ways (Figure 8-25). Most of it is in the form of **bicarbonate**, some is bound to hemoglobin, and a smaller amount is dissolved in plasma.

Because oxygen is used at the cellular level, the amount of oxygen in the blood that returns to the heart is low. This deoxygenated blood is pumped from the heart to the lungs. When the blood enters the capillaries surrounding the alveoli, the PaO_2 is about 40 mmHg. As oxygen diffuses from the alveoli to the capillaries, the PaO_2 of the blood increases to 100 mmHg. The $PaCO_2$ of blood returning from the body to the heart is 45 mmHg. The level decreases to 40 mmHg as carbon dioxide diffuses into the alveoli to be exhaled.

The amount of oxygen that can bind to hemoglobin and how well it can be released at the cellular level depend on several factors. One of the most important factors is the PaO_2. When the PaO_2 is higher, more oxygen can be carried by hemoglobin. That is, each hemoglobin molecule can be more saturated with oxygen. The more saturated hemoglobin is, the more oxygen that it can deliver to the cells. At the cellular level, where the PaO_2 is lower, oxygen is released more readily to the cells. This relationship between PaO_2 and hemoglobin saturation is called the *oxyhemoglobin dissociation curve*.

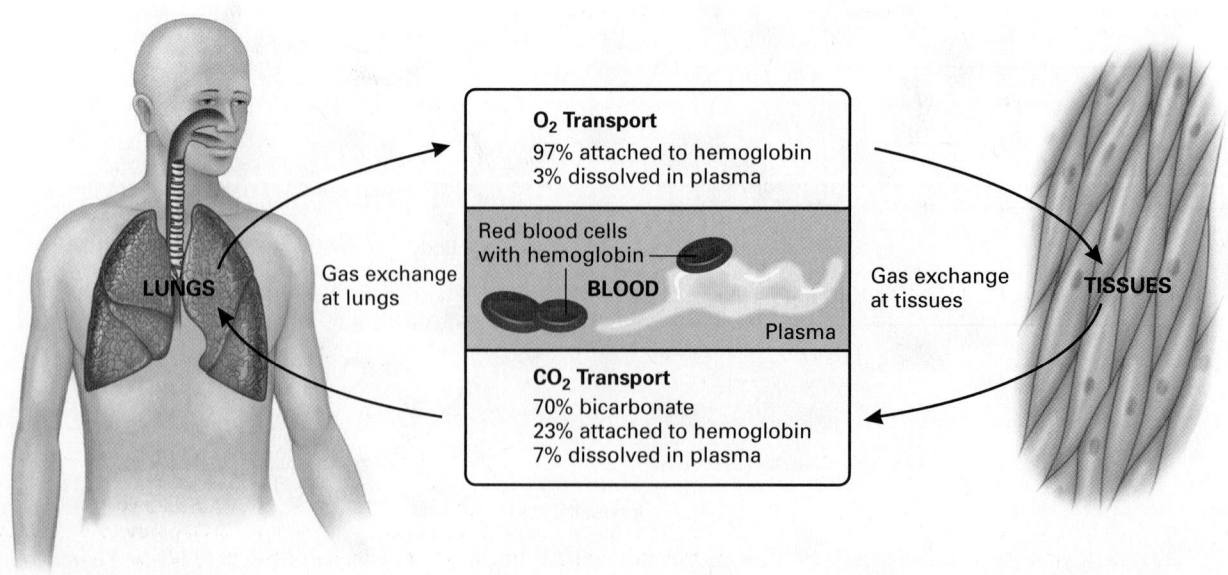

FIGURE 8-25

Carbon dioxide produced by aerobic metabolism is transported to the lungs for elimination, primarily within red blood cells.

Gases follow laws of physics that explain how the body creates the conditions that move air into and out of the lungs. **Boyle's law** states that the pressure of a fixed quantity of gas varies inversely with its volume. This means that the same amount of gas will be under less pressure if its container becomes larger, and will be under greater pressure if its container becomes smaller. Air flows due to differences in pressure. Specifically, air moves from areas of higher pressure to areas of lower pressure.

Movement of the ribs and diaphragm increases and decreases the size of the thoracic cavity, and the lungs within it, producing pressure gradients that cause air to flow into and out of the lungs (Figure 8-26).

Respiratory Anatomy

Before reaching the gas exchange surface of the alveoli, inhaled air must first traverse a variety of passageways. Those passageways are divided, both functionally and anatomically, into the upper and lower airways (Figure 8-27). The upper airway warms and humidifies air while filtering out particulate debris. The lower airway, which begins at the vocal cords, allows air to reach the alveolar beds so gas exchange can occur.

Upper Airway

The mouth and nose serve as the body's entry portals for inspired air, which moves quickly into the oropharynx and nasopharynx, respectively. The nasopharynx is particularly important in warming, humidifying, and filtering air, with the use of its three pairs of nasal turbinates, or *conchae*. The turbinates slow down the air and circulate it around the mucous membrane lining the nasopharynx.

The mucous membranes are warm and moist, allowing the air to be warmed and humidified. The mucus secreted from this lining traps debris. The action of hairlike projections, called *cilia*, of the epithelial cells prevents the debris from entering lower portions of the airway. The cilia work to filter any debris inhaled in the air.

Olfactory receptors within the nasal cavity provide the sense of smell. Those receptors communicate with the brain by way of the first pair of cranial nerves, the olfactory nerves.

Openings to the paranasal sinuses are found within the walls of the nasal cavity, and lead to the four pairs of sinuses: maxillary, frontal, ethmoid, and sphenoid. The sinuses are hollow cavities within the bones of the skull that make the skull lighter and provide resonance to the voice. They are lined with mucous membranes that can become inflamed and swollen from infection or allergies, creating the familiar "nasal" sounding voice associated with colds.

The oral cavity, which contains the teeth and tongue, is continuous with the posterior oropharynx lying behind it. The base of the tongue meets the base of the epiglottis at an angle called the *vallecula*. The roof of the mouth is formed anteriorly by the hard palate, which is formed by processes of the maxillae and the palatine bones of the skull.

The hard palate transitions posteriorly to the boneless soft palate, from which the uvula hangs. The tonsils are

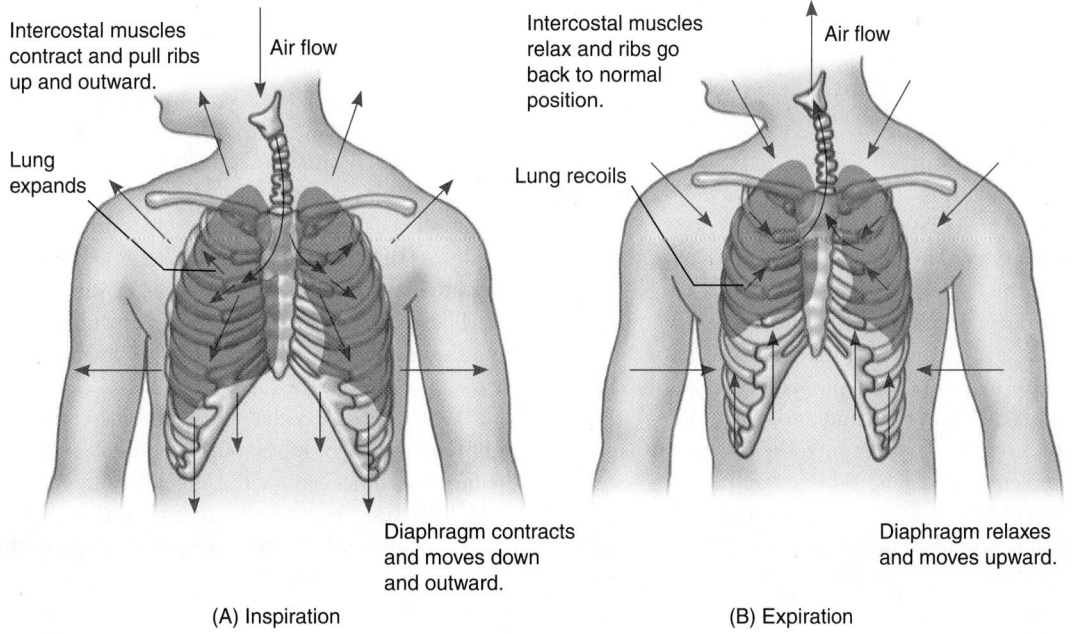

FIGURE 8-26

Ventilation is the mechanical process that allows air to enter and exit the lungs. It consists of two phases. (A) Inspiration is an active muscular process of enlarging the thoracic cavity to decrease the intrathoracic pressure. (B) Expiration is a passive process by which the muscles of ventilation relax, allowing the thoracic cavity to return to the smaller size of its resting state.

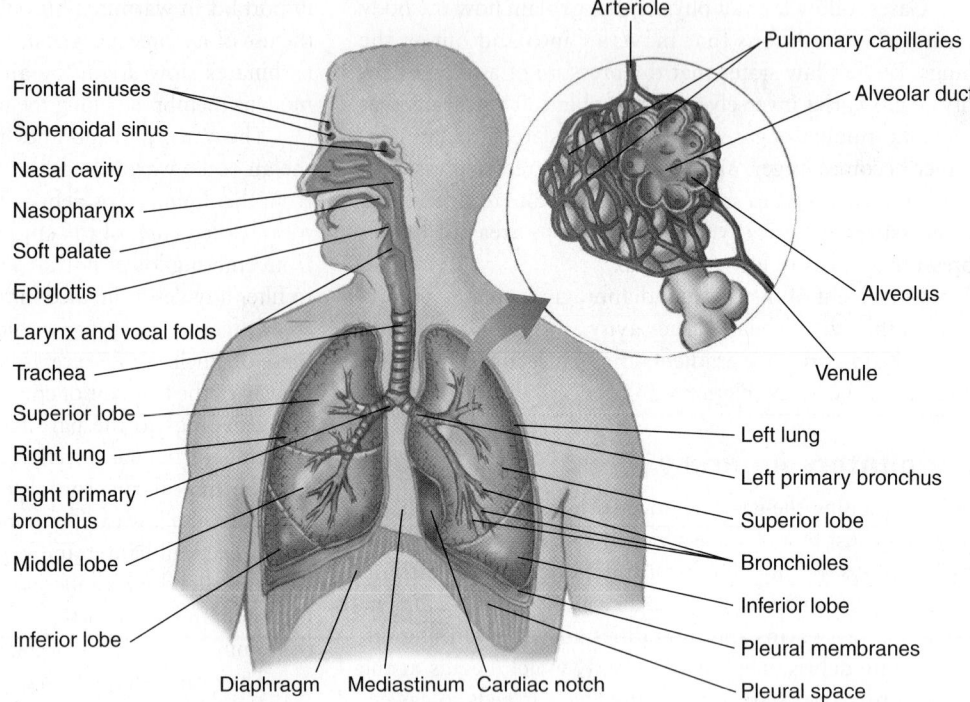

Arteriole
Pulmonary capillaries
Alveolar duct
Alveolus
Venule

Frontal sinuses
Sphenoidal sinus
Nasal cavity
Nasopharynx
Soft palate
Epiglottis
Larynx and vocal folds
Trachea
Superior lobe
Right lung
Right primary bronchus
Middle lobe
Inferior lobe

Left lung
Left primary bronchus
Superior lobe
Bronchioles
Inferior lobe
Pleural membranes
Pleural space

Diaphragm   Mediastinum   Cardiac notch

FIGURE 8-27

The upper and lower airways serve as a conduit for gases to reach the alveolar level for gas exchange.

along the lateral aspects of the posterior oropharynx, where they serve to pick up pathogens that enter the area.

The nasal and oral pharynges communicate posteriorly and traverse inferiorly into the neck to become the laryngopharynx. The laryngopharynx is the final common pathway for food and air, ending at the openings of the esophagus and larynx. The epiglottis is a cartilagenous flap of tissue that covers the opening of the larynx during swallowing to prevent aspiration of food into the lungs.

Lower Airway

The larynx, commonly called the *voice box*, is the entrance to the lower airway. It is anterior to the esophagus, and the thyroid cartilage covers its anterior aspect. The vocal cords lie within the larynx. The opening between the vocal cords is called the *glottis*.

The larynx is continuous with the trachea (windpipe). The trachea is a pipe that is roughly 13 cm (five inches) long, held open by up to 20 C-shaped cartilage rings. The length of the trachea and the number of rings varies directly with a person's height. The first ring, the cricoid cartilage, is the only complete ring. Each of the remaining rings is completed posteriorly by a strip of smooth muscle. The inside of the trachea is lined by epithelial tissue, which is specialized to remove inhaled debris that becomes trapped by the mucus it secretes. The cilia beat uniformly to slowly push debris upward so it can be expelled.

The trachea divides, or bifurcates, into the left and right mainstem bronchi at the carina. The right mainstem, or primary, bronchus is wider in diameter and follows a straighter path off of the trachea than its counterpart, making it more susceptible to foreign body aspiration. The

bronchi continue to divide, more than 20 times in all, becoming smaller in diameter, as they progress through the lung tissue. The smaller divisions of bronchi are called *bronchioles*, which then give rise to the respiratory bronchioles that lead to the alveolar ducts and, ultimately, alveoli.

Lungs

Alveoli are small sacs that are only one cell thick. The alveoli are kept open by a secretion called **surfactant**. Without surfactant, the walls of the alveoli collapse. Networks of pulmonary capillaries, the walls of which are also a single cell thick, closely surround the alveoli.

The area of contact between the alveolar wall and capillary wall is called the **respiratory membrane** (Figure 8-28). It is across this thin membrane that gas exchange occurs between the respiratory system and the cardiovascular system.

There are about 170 alveoli per cubic millimeter of lung tissue. Together, the roughly 300 million alveoli in each lung comprise the lung parenchyma (functional tissue).

Each lung is divided into sections called *lobes*. The right lung has three lobes, but the left has only two because the heart occupies part of the left side of the thoracic cavity.

The lungs are covered with a thin membrane called the *visceral pleura*, which folds over itself to form the parietal pleura that lines the inner thoracic cavity. A small amount of **serous fluid** is secreted into the potential space between the two pleural layers. The pleural fluid provides lubrication to allow smooth movement of the lungs with inspiration and expiration.

The pleura allow for a single opening, called the *hilum*, on the medial aspect of each lung. The hilum admits the bronchus, bronchial artery and vein, pulmonary artery and

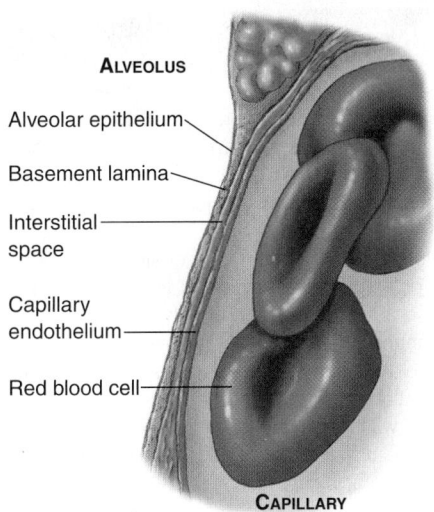

ALVEOLUS

Alveolar epithelium

Basement lamina

Interstitial space

Capillary endothelium

Red blood cell

CAPILLARY

FIGURE 8-28

The respiratory membrane consists of the single-celled walls of the alveoli and pulmonary capillaries, which are in close proximity to allow the exchange of gases.

vein, and lymphatic vessels that serve each lung. The pulmonary and bronchial vessels differ in their functions: The pulmonary vessels carry blood between the heart and alveoli for the purpose of gas exchange, whereas the bronchial vessels carry oxygenated blood from the aorta to the lung parenchyma and return to the vena cava.

Ventilation

Ventilation consists of two phases: inspiration and expiration. Inspiration is an active (energy-requiring) process that begins with a signal from the brain to breathe. This signal originates from stimulation of **chemoreceptors** in the respiratory control centers of the medulla oblongata in the brainstem.

The carbon dioxide produced by cellular metabolism combines with water (H_2O) to create carbonic acid (H_2CO_3), which then dissociates into H^+ and bicarbonate (HCO_3^-) for transport to lungs. The increase in H^+ decreases the pH. Chemoreceptors in the medulla sense an increase in carbon dioxide (by way of a decrease in the pH of blood and CSF), which stimulates inspiration. Inspiration brings in more oxygen and is followed by expiration. The reaction that created bicarbonate is reversible, allowing it to be converted back to carbon dioxide and water so that carbon dioxide is eliminated with expiration.

The inspiratory signal from the medulla is transmitted by nerve tracts in the spinal cord to the phrenic nerve, which originates in the spinal cord at the C3 to C5 level. The phrenic nerve stimulates the diaphragm, the dome-shaped muscle at the inferior aspect of the thoracic cavity, to contract. The intercostal muscles between the ribs are simultaneously stimulated to contract. When the intercostal muscles contract, the ribs are lifted upward, which enlarges

IN THE FIELD

An injury of the spinal cord above the level of C5 affects communication between the CNS and the phrenic nerve, paralyzing the diaphragm. A significant injury below C5 paralyzes the intercostal muscles that raise the ribs but leaves the diaphragm intact, so the patient may exhibit "diaphragmatic" breathing, where only the movement of the abdomen is apparent in the breathing process.

the volume of the thoracic cavity. When the diaphragm contracts, it flattens and moves downward, also enlarging the space within the thoracic cavity.

Just prior to inspiration, the pressure within the lungs (intrapulmonary pressure) is the same as the typical atmospheric pressure, 760 mmHg. When the thoracic cavity increases in size, the potential space between the parietal and visceral pleura also becomes larger, creating negative intrapleural pressure. The negative pressure causes the volume of the lungs to increase. The increased volume of the lungs results in intrapulmonary pressure that is slightly lower than atmospheric pressure. Air moves from the higher pressure of the atmosphere into the area of lower pressure within the lungs.

Air stops moving once intrapulmonary pressure is equal to atmospheric pressure, completing inspiration. At this point, a portion of the inhaled air has reached the alveoli and gas exchange is occurring. When the diaphragm and intercostal muscles relax, the intrapleural and intrapulmonary volumes decrease, which causes pressure within the lungs to increase. Once again, air moves from the higher area of pressure to the lower area, this time causing air to flow out of the lungs in the process of expiration. When the pressures are again equalized, expiration is complete.

IN THE FIELD

Inspiration uses the external intercostal muscles to some degree, but relies mainly on the diaphragm. Expiration is passive, relying on relaxation of the diaphragm and intercostal muscles. When there is an increased demand for oxygen, the body can recruit accessory muscles of respiration to further increase the intrathoracic volume.

In diseases that cause resistance to airflow out of the lungs, such as chronic obstructive pulmonary disease (COPD) and asthma, expiration becomes an active process to further increase intrathoracic pressure to enhance the flow of air against the resistance of narrowed airways.

Various accessory muscles can be used to aid ventilation in times of respiratory distress, and can often be used as indicators of the level of distress. The internal intercostal muscles, rectus muscles of the abdomen, and the sternocleidomastoid and scalene muscles in the neck all have a role in enhancing thorax movement when required.

Tidal volume is the total amount of air moved through the upper and lower airway with each breath. Of this air, 150 mL is above the level of the respiratory bronchioles and alveoli and therefore cannot participate in gas exchange. This 150 mL is contained in what is called the *anatomical dead space*. Only 350 mL of the tidal volume is available for alveolar ventilation. The amount of dead space does not change. If respirations are shallow, decreasing the tidal volume, it is alveolar ventilation that is reduced, not dead space. Always consider the depth of a patient's ventilation, as well as the rate.

Two aspects of respiratory physiology have led to recent changes in the way CPR is performed. In the past, airway and breathing were the first priorities. Current thinking is that the residual volume in the lungs contains enough oxygen to provide the cells with adequate oxygenation for a short period of time if chest compressions are begun to circulate blood through the lungs and to the brain. Therefore, for laypersons and in cases in which a health care provider is alone, chest compressions are now the first priority.

Another aspect that contributes to a decreased focus on early ventilation in CPR is that the compression and release of the chest wall produce changes in intrathoracic pressure, similar to the changes produced by movement of the diaphragm and thoracic cage during inspiration and expiration.

Under normal conditions, a respiratory cycle occurs once every 3 to 5 seconds, giving a respiratory rate of 12 to 20 breaths per minute. The respiratory rate increases when there is increased carbon dioxide production or another cause of low pH. Anything that increases cellular metabolism (and thus carbon dioxide), such as an illness that produces fever or exercise, increases respiratory rate.

A secondary stimulus to breathe is decreased oxygen levels in the blood. When diffusion of oxygen from the alveoli to the blood is impaired, as in pneumonia, the low level of oxygen results in an increased respiratory rate as well. Under conditions of slowed metabolism, such as hypothermia (decreased body temperature), the respiratory rate decreases.

Lung Volumes

Pulmonary air volumes can be measured with spirometry, a pulmonary function test that measures the amount of air inhaled and exhaled. Normal values predicated for adults are helpful in assessing the extent of disease processes as well as for planning interventions, such as using a mechanical ventilator.

Tidal volume (TV) is the volume of air inhaled in a typical breath, generally around 500 mL (5 to 7 mL per kg of body weight). The minute respiratory volume (MRV), sometimes simply called *minute volume*, is the volume of air exchanged over a minute. It is calculated by multiplying the TV by the respiratory rate. A typical respiratory rate of 12 produces the predicted MRV of 6 liters.

The vital capacity is the volume of air exchanged in a single maximal inspiration and expiration, typically around 4 liters. Residual volume is the amount of air that remains in the lungs after maximal exhalation and is about 1.2 liters.

Cardiovascular System

The cardiovascular system consists of the heart, blood, and blood vessels that provide blood with access to the tissues and organs of the body for the exchange of gases, nutrients,

and other substances (Figure 8-29). It is a closed system, within which oxygenated blood is pumped out of the left side of the heart, into arteries, and then into capillary beds in the tissues. Capillaries lead into veins, which return blood to the right side of the heart. The right side of the heart pumps blood to the lungs for gas exchange. The oxygenated blood returns to the left side of the heart and the cycle repeats.

Blood

Blood is a tissue that consists of a liquid medium, plasma, in which a variety of formed elements are suspended. Generally, there is 70 mL per kg of blood in the adult male and 65 mL per kg in an adult female. In an average-size adult, this amounts to about 5 liters of blood.

Plasma is a straw-colored liquid that comprises slightly more than half the volume of blood. Plasma serves as a transport medium for proteins (such as albumin), nutrients, elements, gases, chemical messengers, and wastes.

Erythrocytes, or red blood cells (RBCs), give blood its characteristic color. There are several types of leukocytes, or white blood cells (WBCs), including macrophages, neutrophils, basophils, eosinophils, and lymphocytes. Those cells serve a variety of roles in protecting the body from disease and in responding to injury.

Platelets are cell fragments that are attracted to injured tissues to initiate the blood clotting process.

All blood cells begin in the red bone marrow as undifferentiated stem cells, which can be stimulated to develop into the different types of blood cells. This general process is called *hematopoiesis*.

Red Blood Cells

The process by which RBCs are developed is a form of hematopoiesis called *erythropoiesis*. The color of RBCs is provided by hemoglobin, a protein molecule that contains iron. When oxygen molecules bind to hemoglobin to be

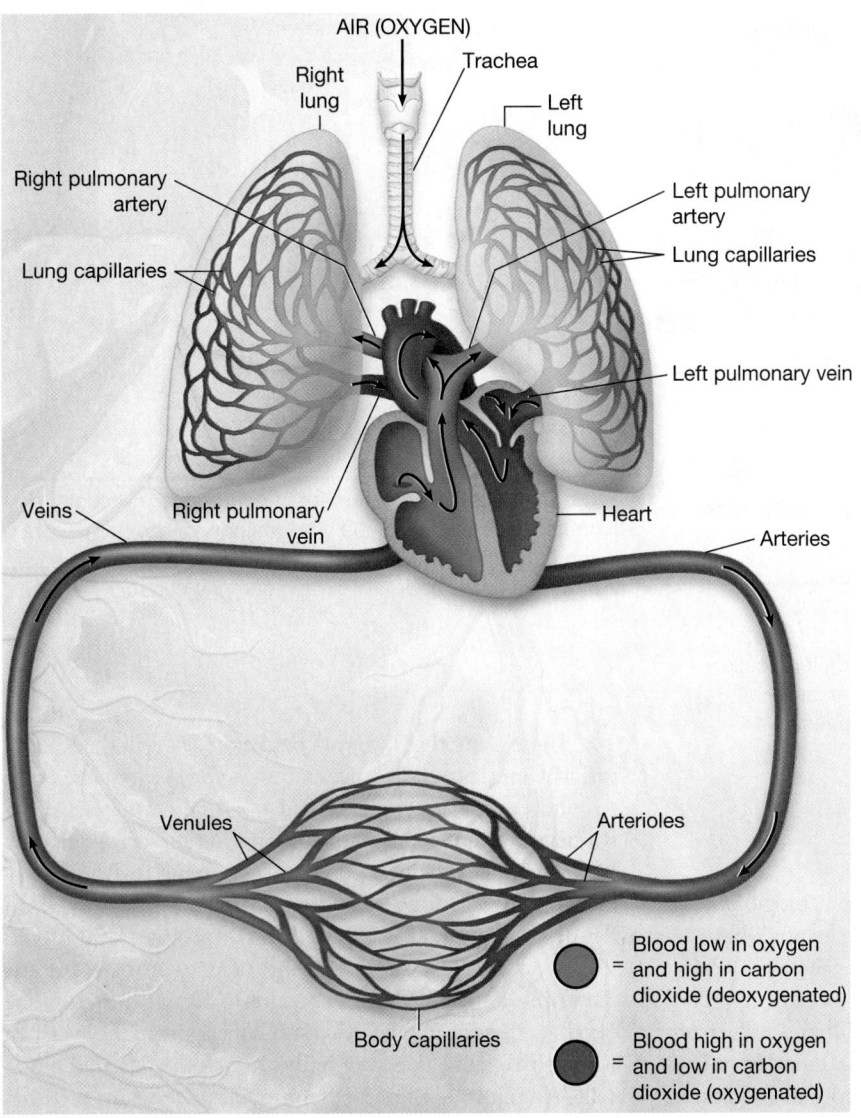

AIR (OXYGEN)

Trachea

Right lung

Left lung

Right pulmonary artery

Left pulmonary artery

Lung capillaries

Lung capillaries

Left pulmonary vein

Veins

Right pulmonary vein

Heart

Arteries

Venules

Arterioles

Blood low in oxygen and high in carbon dioxide (deoxygenated)

Body capillaries

Blood high in oxygen and low in carbon dioxide (oxygenated)

FIGURE 8-29

The cardiovascular system consists of the heart, blood vessels, and blood. The heart is a two-sided pump that pumps blood to the lungs for oxygenation, and then pumps the returning oxygenated blood to the body. Blood travels through three types of vessels: arteries, capillaries, and veins. Blood is a liquid medium that transports blood cells, proteins, nutrients, drugs, wastes, and other substances throughout the body.

carried throughout the body, hemoglobin has a bright red color. When the molecules are deoxygenated, they are a darker, blue red-color.

Mature RBCs have no nucleus, which allows them to be filled with hemoglobin (Figure 8-30). They are disk-shaped, with a central depression on both sides. This shape, along with their small size, allows RBCs to flow single-file through capillaries so gas exchange can occur.

The typical life span of RBCs is 120 days. Most of the cell components are recycled for reuse. A pigment in hemo-globin breaks down into a waste product called *bilirubin*, which is normally transported in the blood to the liver, where it is broken down further for excretion. However, if the liver is not functioning, such as in hepatitis or cirrho-sis, bilirubin accumulates, causing yellowing of the eyes and skin known as *jaundice*.

The hematocrit (Hct) is the percentage by volume of formed elements in the blood, the majority of which con-sists of RBCs (Figure 8-31). To obtain the Hct, a vial of

blood is centrifuged so the formed elements settle at the bot-tom, allowing a measurement of percentage by volume. The normal value is slightly lower in females (36 to 48 percent) than in males (42 to 52 percent).

Another way of quantifying the number of RBCs is by their number per cubic millimeter of blood, which is roughly 5 million. A high Hct indicates an increased num-ber of RBCs (as in chronic hypoxia) or a decreased plasma volume relative to the normal total number of RBCs (as in dehydration). A low Hct can indicate anemia or blood loss.

Whenever the body is hypoxic, the kidneys increase se-cretion of a hormone (erythropoietin) that acts on the bone marrow to increase the production of RBCs. In patients who have chronic lung disease or who live at high altitudes, this mechanism results in a higher Hct, increasing the over-all oxygen-carrying capacity of the blood.

Hemoglobin is the essential component of red blood cells that allows them to transport oxygen. The bond between oxygen and hemoglobin is reversible, with some

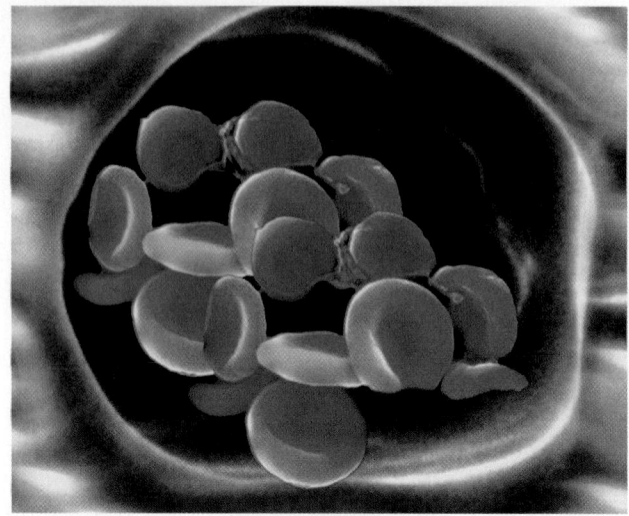

FIGURE 8-30

Mature red blood cells do not have a nucleus, allowing them to be filled with hemoglobin for oxygen transportation. The size and shape of red blood cells is specially designed to allow maximum areas of contact between them and the capillary beds.
(© SPL/Photo Researchers, Inc.)

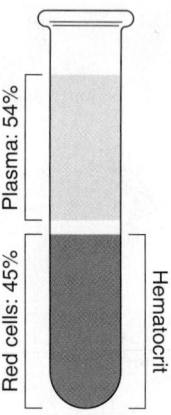

FIGURE 8-31

The hematocrit is the percentage of formed elements (cells) by volume of blood. The majority of the hematocrit consists of red blood cells. The hematocrit provides a way of assessing a patient's oxygen-carrying capability.

factors favoring onloading of oxygen onto hemoglobin and others favoring the release of oxygen from hemoglobin.

One of the primary factors involved is the blood PaO_2. When the PaO_2 is high, more oxygen is onloaded. Whenever the PaO_2 is above 60 mmHg, hemoglobin is 80 percent saturated with oxygen. At PaO_2 levels of 50 mmHg or less, such as occurs in the body tissues under normal conditions, oxygen is very readily offloaded. Oxygen is more easily bound when the pH is high and body temperature is lower, and more easily released when the pH is low and the body temperature is higher. This is best remembered by recalling that the tissue needs more oxygen during anaerobic metabolism and fever.

ABO and Rh Blood Groups

Small proteins called **antigens**, which establish an A, B, AB, or O blood type, are present on the surface of red blood cells. Type A cells have the A antigen, B have the B antigen, AB have both, and O have neither.

Antibodies are created within the body to attack any blood type other than a person's own, which is why blood typing prior to transfusion is important. For example, people with type B blood will have antibodies to type A blood and cannot receive either type A or type AB blood. They could receive type B (for which they have no antibodies) and type O (which has no antigens). Following this logic, type O is the universal donor because the donated blood has no antigens and type AB is the universal recipient because the recipient has no antibodies.

There is another layer of complexity as well, the Rh factor. The presence or absence of this factor is what is referred to when a blood type is called *positive* or *negative*. An Rh-negative individual does not have antibodies against the Rh factor unless he is exposed at some point to Rh-positive blood. This becomes most important in pregnancy, if an Rh-negative mother is exposed to Rh-positive fetal blood. In the first pregnancy, the mother does not have anti-Rh antibodies, but upon exposure to fetal Rh factor, she develops these antibodies. In a subsequent pregnancy with an Rh-positive fetus, these antibodies attack the fetal red blood cells. An injection of anti-Rh antibodies (Rhogam) prevents this immune response from occurring. Rhogam is given following pregnancy or if there is a suspected contact between Rh positive fetal blood and Rh negative maternal blood.

White Blood Cells

WBCs provide protection from invading antigens and support the development of inflammation resulting from injury or infection. An antigen is any foreign substance (usually a protein) that produces an immune response. Pathogens, or disease-producing organisms, are one source of antigens, as are allergens and transplanted tissues and organs.

The immune system can be grossly divided into two functional components: innate and adaptive. The innate immune system recognizes materials as either part of the self or foreign (nonself), and responds automatically and quickly to protect the body from substances that are not a part of it (Figure 8-32). This process occurs on an ongoing basis throughout the body. The innate immune system also plays a role in inflammation, which is necessary for tissue healing. Neutrophils and macrophages ingest invading bacteria while the inflammatory process increases blood flow to the area to enhance the immune response.

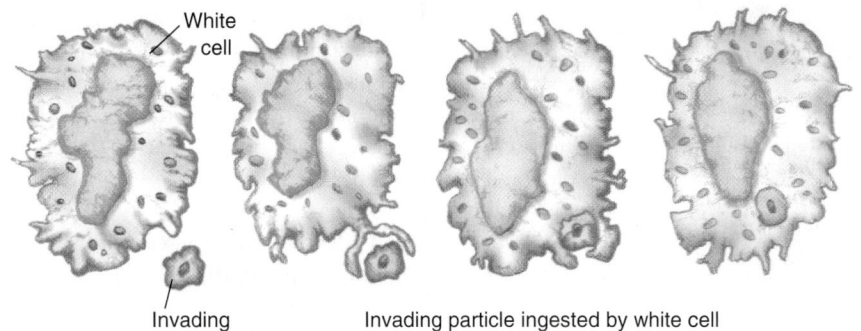

White cell

Invading particle

Invading particle ingested by white cell

FIGURE 8-32

Several types of white blood cells provide a variety of functions in defending the body against illness.

The adaptive system uses B lymphocytes and T lymphocytes, as well as antibodies, to tailor the immune response to specific antigens, allowing a more direct attack on them. After the immune system develops specific antibodies for an antigen, it essentially has a memory for the antigen (immunologic memory). However, this process takes time to develop. This is why, with many illnesses, a person becomes sick with the first exposure, but is immune when exposed to the same illness again. During the first exposure, the person does not have specific antibodies, but is triggered to produce them. With a second exposure, the antigen is quickly recognized and suppressed by the immune system.

That same mechanism is used to prevent future illness. Often, the antigen can exist, even when the pathogen is killed. For example, some influenza viruses can be killed and injected into the body. Even though the virus cannot cause illness, the body develops antibodies to the antigen carried by the virus. When a live virus later enters the body, its antigen is recognized and the body attacks it, killing the virus. Some vaccines require a live pathogen, but weakened so it does not cause illness (live vaccine).

Allergies occur when an individual develops antibodies to an antigen, such as a protein in shellfish or bee venom, to which most people do not develop antibodies. Those antibodies are carried on the surface of white blood cells called *basophils* and result in a response that produces the signs and symptoms of allergies. Basophils circulate in the blood but also can enter tissues, where they become known as *mast cells*.

When a specific antigen interacts with a specific antibody on the surface of a cell, basophils and mast cells release **histamine** and other substances. Histamine has a variety of effects that lead to the signs and symptoms of allergies. In some cases, this allergic response is greatly exaggerated (called *anaphylaxis*) and can result in death.

Platelets and Coagulation

Platelets are small cell fragments that arise from the break up of larger cells and are responsible for part of the process called **hemostasis** (not to be confused with homeostasis). Platelets circulate in an inactivated form until they are activated by chemical events that occur in response to injury to blood vessels (Figure 8-33).

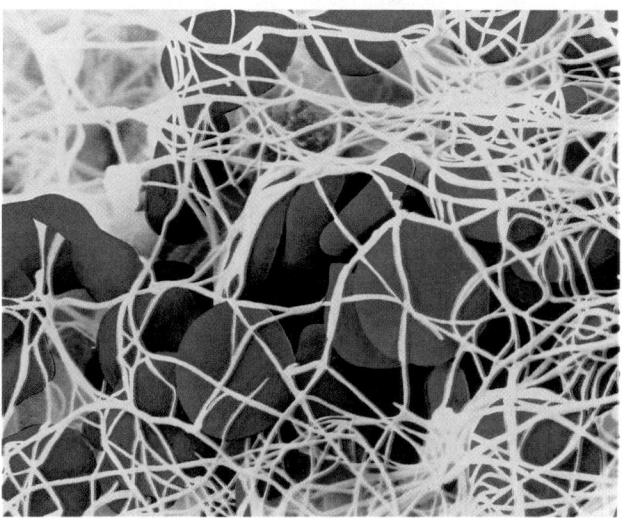

FIGURE 8-33

Hemostasis consists of three phases. First, vasoconstriction decreases the diameter of the blood vessel to decrease blood flow through it. Second, platelets are activated by factors from the exposed collagen of the damaged vessels. Platelets clump together at the site to form a platelet plug. Third, the clotting cascade results in formation of a stable blood clot. (© SPL /Photo Researchers, Inc.)

When activated, platelets are attracted to the site of injury and become sticky, adhering to the injured site and to each other to form a platelet plug to stop bleeding. This platelet plug serves as a precursor to the formation of a stable blood clot. Activated platelets release a variety of chemicals that cause the complex clotting cascade to progress. The end result of this process is the creation of a fibrin clot, which is a solid meshwork of proteins, platelets, and other cells around the injury site. Many of the other factors involved are produced by the liver and require vitamin K for their proper function.

Although effective clot formation, or coagulation, is important for survival, an overactive response can lead to a number of life-threatening conditions, such as myocardial infarction (MI) (heart attack), pulmonary embolus

(PE) (blood clot in the lung), and **disseminated intravascular coagulation (DIC)**. To keep the system in balance, the body has a number of anticlot molecules, such as tissue plasminogen activator (t-PA), which breaks down formed clots, and antithrombin III, which slows the clotting cascade progression.

Anatomy of the Heart

The heart is the muscular central pump that circulates blood throughout the vessels of the cardiovascular system. The specialized cardiac muscle is supported by fibrous connective tissue that forms a cardiac skeleton.

The heart is roughly the size of a human fist and is located within the mediastinum in the center of the chest between the lungs (Figure 8-34). It lies slightly to the left behind the sternum and is surrounded by the pericardium, which is a doubled-over epithelial membrane analogous to the pleura. The visceral pericardium (also called the *epicardium*) lies directly on the heart muscle. The parietal pericardium is folded over and adherent on its outer surface to the fibrous pericardium (pericardial sac) that encases the entire heart. A small amount of serous pericardial fluid between the visceral and parietal pericardium lubricates the heart as it contracts.

The heart has four chambers that function as two side-by-side pumps. The right side of the heart serves as a pump for the pulmonary circulation and the left side serves as a pump for the systemic circulation (Figure 8-35). The right atrium receives deoxygenated blood from the body via the large inferior and superior venae cavae. The right ventricle receives blood from the right atrium and pumps it through the pulmonary artery into the lungs, where it circulates around the alveoli. Oxygenated blood from the lungs travels through the pulmonary vein into the left atrium.

The left ventricle receives blood from the left atrium and pumps it into the aorta, the largest artery in the body. From the aorta, oxygenated blood is distributed through a network of arteries, arterioles, and capillaries. After circulating through the tissues in the capillaries, blood enters the venous system, beginning with venules, which empty into veins, eventually reaching the vena cava and returning to the right side of the heart.

Cardiac tissue consists of three layers: a thin internal endocardial lining that coats the chambers to allow for

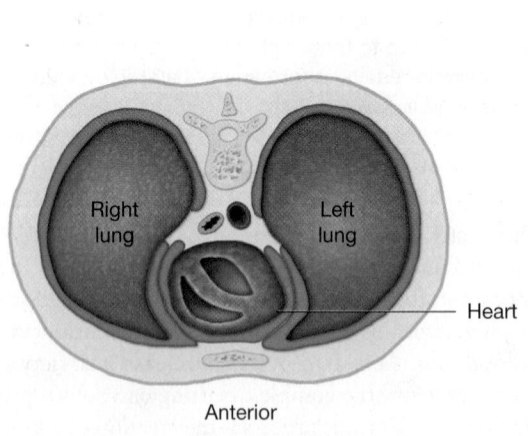
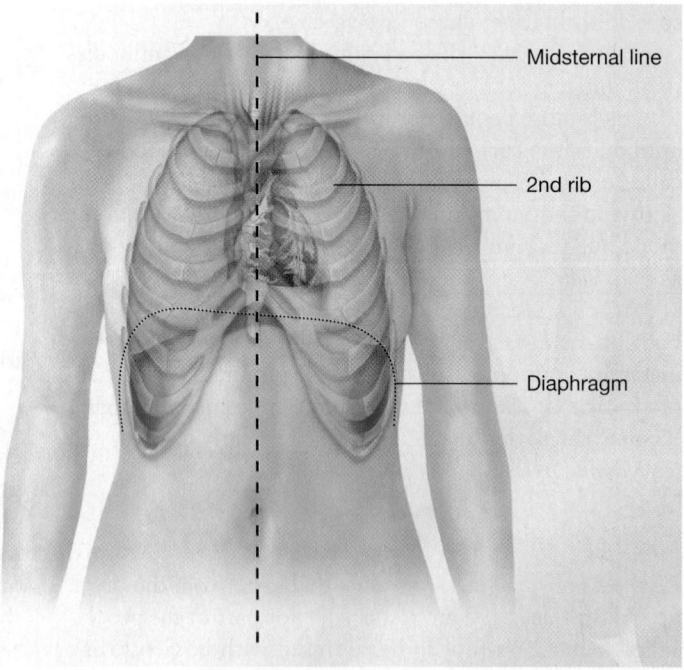

FIGURE 8-34

The heart is located in the mediastinum in the center of the chest. It is oriented so that it points toward the left side.

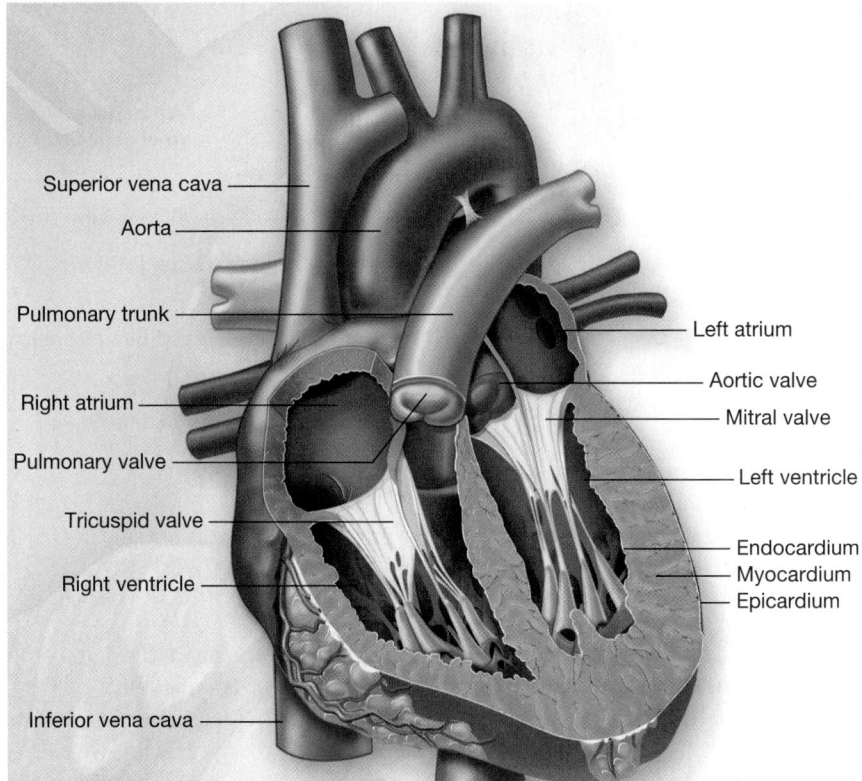

- Superior vena cava
- Aorta
- Pulmonary trunk
- Right atrium
- Pulmonary valve
- Tricuspid valve
- Right ventricle
- Inferior vena cava
- Left atrium
- Aortic valve
- Mitral valve
- Left ventricle
- Endocardium
- Myocardium
- Epicardium

FIGURE 8-35

Internal anatomy of the heart.

smooth blood flow, a thick myocardial muscle layer, and an external epicardial layer that forms the visceral pericardium. The portion of myocardium that comprises the atria is thinner. The atria require little muscular strength to pump blood to the ventricles sitting just below them. A thin wall called the *interatrial septum* separates the atria.

The muscle of the right ventricle is somewhat thicker than that of the atria, but not as thick as that of the left ventricle, which must contract with enough force to circulate blood through the entire systemic circulation. A more substantial interventricular septum separates the ventricles.

Valves in the heart direct the flow of blood as the chambers contract. When the ventricles contract, valves between each atrium and ventricle keep the blood from being forced backward into the atrium. This allows blood to be ejected into the pulmonary artery and aorta. The mitral (bicuspid) valve sits between the left atrium and left ventricle. The tricuspid valve sits between the right atrium and right ventricle. Both valves are attached to the papillary muscles inside the ventricles by chordae tendoneae, which are small fibrous bands that hold the valves in place. Pressure in the aorta and pulmonary artery would allow blood to flow backward into the ventricles during ventricular relaxation if there were not valves to prevent this.

After blood is pumped from the left ventricle into the aorta, the aortic semilunar valve closes to prevent blood from flowing from the aorta into the left ventricle. After blood is pumped from the right ventricle into the pulmonary artery, the pulmonic or pulmonary semilunar valve

closes to prevent blood from flowing back into the right ventricle from the pulmonary artery.

The heart is stimulated to contract by autonomic nervous system tissue embedded within it, called the *cardiac conduction system* (Figure 8-36). The cardiac conduction system begins with the sinoatrial (SA) node in the right atrium, which generates impulses and sends them along conductive pathways to the muscle of both atria and to a group of cells at the junction of the atria and ventricles called the *atrioventricular (AV) node*.

From the AV node the impulse spreads down a bundle of tissue, called the *bundle of His*, along the interventricular septum. The bundle splits into left and right bundle branches, which divide into the Purkinje fibers that stimulate the cells of both ventricles.

The special properties of the myocardium allow it to contract in a uniform, rhythmic fashion to pump blood throughout the circulatory system. The two atria contract simultaneously during atrial systole, followed by simultaneous contraction of the ventricles during ventricular systole. The relaxation phase of each cardiac cycle is called *diastole*.

In addition to pumping blood to the rest of the body, the heart also requires its own blood supply for every individual cardiac cell. Oxygenated blood is delivered to the myocardium by the coronary arteries, which originate at the base of the aorta. When the left ventricle contracts, the aortic semilunar valve is open, blocking the entrance of the coronary arteries. When the valve closes during diastole, blood from the aorta flows into the coronary arteries.

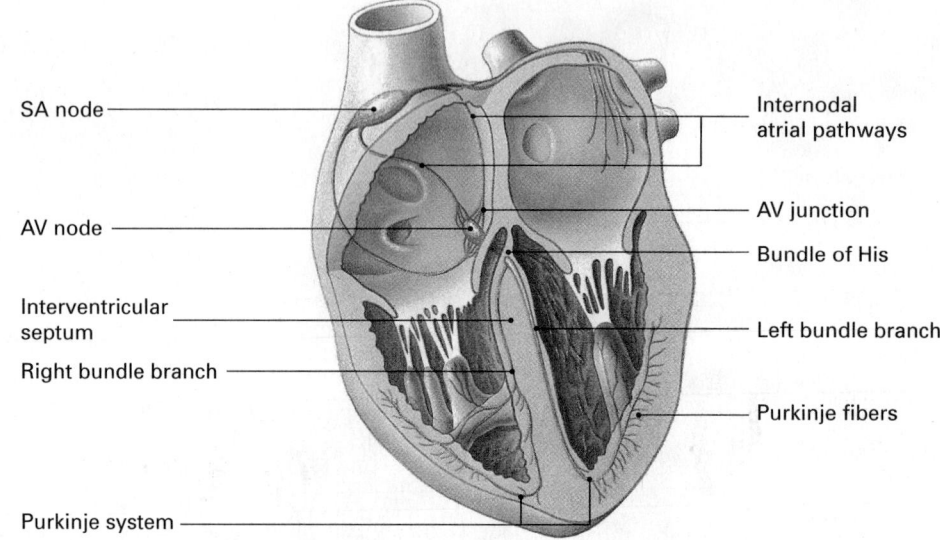

SA node

Internodal atrial pathways

AV node

AV junction

Bundle of His

Interventricular septum

Left bundle branch

Right bundle branch

Purkinje fibers

Purkinje system

FIGURE 8-36

The cardiac conduction system.

The left and right main coronary arteries emerge from the aorta. The left coronary artery and its branches supply the left atrium and left ventricle and the interventricular septum. The right coronary artery and its branches supply the right atrium and portions of both ventricles. The left main coronary artery quickly bifurcates into the left anterior descending artery that supplies blood to the left ventricle and the interventricular septum, and the circumflex artery, which also supplies the left ventricle. The right coronary artery supplies the right ventricle, and later gives off the posterior descending artery that provides blood supply to the inferior wall of the heart. The SA and AV nodes are supplied by the right coronary artery in most people. Venous return from the heart is provided by the coronary sinus, which is an opening into the right atrium that returns deoxygenated blood draining from the coronary veins.

Cardiac Physiology

The heart follows a regular cycle of events with each beat, called the *cardiac cycle*. During this cycle, a series of electrical events produces the mechanical contraction of the heart muscle. The electrical activity involves the exchange of Na^+, K^+, and other ions across cell membranes in the electrical

conduction system, and the movement of Ca^{++} into the myocardial (muscle) cells to produce contraction.

Mechanically, this cycle is divided into two phases: diastole and systole. Electrically, the cycle is known as the *cardiac action potential*, which consists of the movement of ions and the associated differences in electrical charge across the cell membranes.

The electrical current produced can be detected by placing electrodes on the surface of the body. The ability to view this electrical activity allows cardiac monitoring to detect abnormalities. The mechanical function of the heart is reflected by the patient's pulse and blood pressure.

The cycle begins at the conclusion of diastole (from the previous cardiac cycle), when the atria have completed filling with blood (Figure 8-37). During diastole, the mitral and tricuspid valves are open, so the ventricles are receiving some of the blood that is filling the atria. The ventricles receive a substantial amount of blood this way, but a contraction of the atria finishes the filling process. This is atrial systole, which marks the beginning of cardiac systole.

Atrial systole is stimulated by an action potential produced by the SA node, which travels across both atria to stimulate the myocardium to contract. Once the ventricles have filled with blood, the mitral and tricuspid valves close and the aortic and pulmonary valves open. The action potential, which was slightly delayed at the AV node, now travels down a portion of the electrical pathway called the *bundle of His* and into the Purkinje system. The action potential results in mechanical contraction of the ventricles, or ventricular systole. Blood is squeezed out of the heart and into the aorta and pulmonary artery.

The human heart really functions as two hearts in one. The left heart receives oxygenated blood from the lungs and pumps it out to the entire body for use. The right heart receives blood from the body, now deoxygenated after being used by the tissues, and pumps it into the lungs to become oxygenated again. The blood from the lungs, now

IN THE FIELD

Obstruction of any portion of the coronary arterial system prevents the myocardial cells beyond that point from receiving blood. The lack of blood to the tissues is called *ischemia*. If not quickly reversed, the cells become injured, and then die. The death of myocardial tissue is called *myocardial infarction*. The necrotic (dead) tissue cannot be regenerated. Subsequent heart function depends on the location and extent of damage.

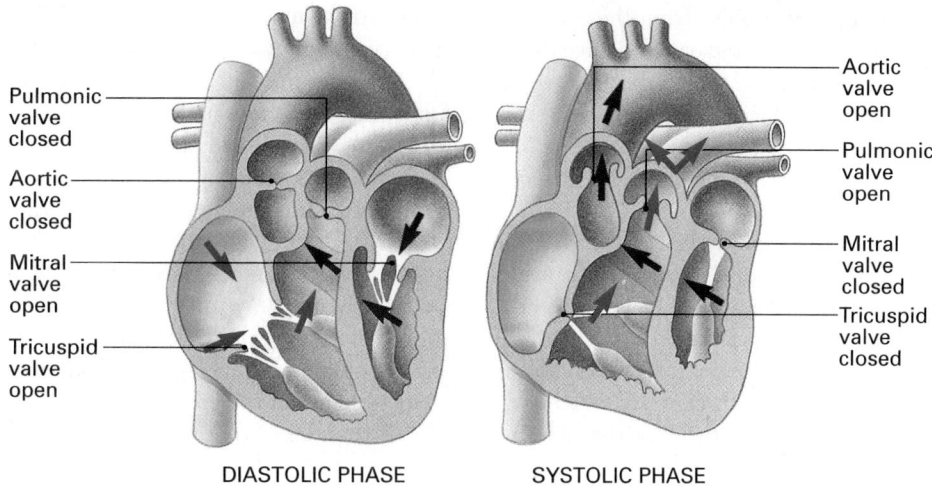

FIGURE 8-37

The cardiac cycle consists of two mechanical phases. In diastole, the chambers of the heart are relaxed, allowing them to fill with blood. In systole, the chambers contract to eject blood. Atrial systole occurs first, to finish filling the ventricles. Ventricular systole occurs immediately afterward, to eject blood into the pulmonary artery and aorta.

oxygenated, returns to the left heart and the cycle continues. Despite this functional separation, the heart beats as one, with the left and right atria contracting together followed by simultaneous contraction of the left and right ventricles.

The simultaneous contraction of the atria followed by simultaneous contraction of the ventricles means that the heart valves close in pairs. It is this closing of each pair of heart valves that are heard as "lub-dub" when listening for heart sounds with a stethoscope. The first sound (S1), which sounds like "lub," marks the beginning of ventricular systole. S1 is the result of the closure of the mitral and tricuspid valves as the ventricles begin to contract.

The second sound (S2), which sounds like "dub," occurs shortly after, as the aortic and pulmonic valves close at the completion of ventricular systole. A variety of abnormal conditions can result in changes to the character of the heart sounds or produce additional sounds.

Cardiac Electrophysiology

In addition to the property of contractility possessed by all muscle cells, myocardial cells have three unique properties that allow them to function the way they do.

Automaticity is the ability of the heart to self-depolarize in order to initiate its own electrical activity. Typically, it is the SA node that sets the pace of the heart at 60 to 100 beats per minute. The two divisions of the autonomic nervous system can influence the intrinsic rate of the SA node. Sympathetic nervous system stimulation increases the heart rate (positive chronotropy), rate of conduction (positive dromotropy), and strength of contraction (positive inotropy). Parasympathetic nervous system stimulation via the vagus nerve slows the SA node and has the opposite effects.

The influences of the sympathetic and parasympathetic divisions of the autonomic nervous system allow fine-tuning of the heart rate to meet the needs of the body. When there is a need for increased cardiac output, the sympathetic nervous system dominates and when the body is at rest, the parasympathetic system dominates.

Excitability allows the myocardial cells to respond to an electrical impulse and contract. **Conductivity** is the ability of those cells to allow an electrical impulse to move quickly from one to another. A special feature at the ends of cardiac muscle cells called an *intercalated disk* allows this action.

Electrical impulses originating in the SA node must travel a relatively long distance in a short period of time during each cycle. Although the action potential can move from cell to cell, specialized conduction pathways exist that serve to rapidly move the action potential between areas.

IN THE FIELD

The vagus nerve supplies many organs and can be stimulated in many ways, such as by a full stomach or vomiting. In certain individuals, the vagus is especially sensitive and, when stimulated, can slow the heart rate (bradycardia). Medical treatment of certain types of rapid cardiac dysrhythmias takes advantage of the sensitivity of the vagus nerve to slow the heart rate, using a technique called the *Valsalva maneuver*. In the Valsalva maneuver, the patient is instructed to bear down against a closed glottis in the same way as if they were having a bowel movement. This stimulates the vagus nerve and can sometimes terminate certain rapid dysrhythmias.

At the same time that an impulse from the SA node spreads throughout the atria, a bundle of conductive tissue allows the action potential to travel simultaneously to the AV node. The AV node delays the impulse for a brief moment, allowing the atria to complete depolarization. The impulse is then transmitted through the bundle of His and left and right bundle branches.

The fibrous tissue of the cardiac skeleton serves as a barrier to prevent any movement of electrical activity from the atria and ventricles except by way of the bundle of His. The numerous Purkinje fibers penetrate the muscle of the ventricle, allowing stimulation of myocardial cells. When cardiac muscle is stimulated, the cells contract together as a single unit, allowing the atria and then the ventricles to contract smoothly.

The aging process, effects of drugs, genetic problems with ion channels, or ischemia can disrupt the cardiac conduction system. Resulting abnormalities can block or delay conduction of impulses or result in rapid, repetitive depolarizations. This abnormal electrical activity affects the mechanical activity of the heart, which can cause a decrease in the amount of blood the heart can provide to the body.

The myocardial cells maintain an electrical potential across their cell membrane that leaves the interior of the cell relatively negatively charged. That is, the membrane is polarized. As described earlier, this gradient is maintained by the sodium/potassium pump, which places three sodium ions out of the cell for every two potassium ions it takes in. As a result, there are many sodium ions and few potassium ions outside of the cell. In contrast, there are few sodium ions and many potassium ions within the cell.

When the imbalance of ions across the membrane reaches a certain point, channels in the cell membrane open, allowing sodium to rapidly enter the cell. This influx of positive ions turns the interior of the cell membrane that was previously negative into a positively charged environment in a process called *depolarization*.

These fast sodium channels remain open for only a few milliseconds, and as they close potassium and calcium channels open. The calcium channels allow an influx of calcium ions into the cell. Once inside the cell, calcium interacts with the special proteins inside muscle cells that allow them to contract.

Potassium channels permit a slow leak of potassium ions out of the cell, bringing the overall membrane charge back to negative. The return of the cell to its resting state is called *repolarization*.

The ECG is a representation of those electrical changes within the heart during the cardiac cycle. The characteristic pattern of ECG waves is discussed in Chapter 21.

Cardiac Output

Cardiac output (CO) is the amount of blood ejected from the heart, determined as the volume of blood leaving the left ventricle each minute. CO is determined by two factors: the stroke volume (SV) and the heart rate (HR).

SV is the amount of blood, in milliliters, that is ejected from the ventricle with each contraction, and is about 70 mL for a normal adult male. SV is multiplied by HR to determine the volume of blood ejected from the heart in one minute, measured in liters per minute. At an average HR of 70 with a SV of 70 mL, the typical CO is 4.9 L/min.

The nature of the relationship between heart rate and stroke volume allow one variable to compensate for the other when needed. For example, if a person has a low stroke volume due to a high afterload (resistance in the vascular system that the left ventricle must overcome to eject blood), an increased heart rate can compensate and maintain a normal cardiac output. A situation such as this is often observed in hypertensive patients.

In patients who have lost blood volume, the preload (amount of blood returning to the heart) is decreased, which thereby decreases stroke volume. In response, the heart rate increases, producing tachycardia, a classic sign of shock.

Stroke volume is not the total volume of blood in the ventricle, but is only about 55 to 70 percent of the volume in the ventricle at the end of diastole (end-diastolic volume). This percentage is called the *ejection fraction*. The ejection fraction can be significantly reduced in heart failure, making it difficult for the heart to meet the needs of the body.

The stroke volume is adjusted by several factors to maintain homeostasis. Those factors include preload, contractility of the heart, and afterload. Preload is the amount of blood that is returned to the heart in diastole, and this is the volume of blood present in the ventricle just prior to contraction.

Contractility is affected by preload. The Frank–Starling's law states that the more the myocardium is stretched from the preload, the more force with which the myocardium will contract, and the larger the stroke volume will be. This effect can be compared to the increased force with which a rubber band will contract when it is stretched. However, just as this effect is limited in a rubber band, it is also limited in the heart. Contractility also is affected through the inotropic property of the myocardium, which is the ability of the myocardium to physically contract more strongly in response to certain stimuli, such as the release of epinephrine.

Afterload is the resistance against which the heart must contract with each beat, and is determined primarily by systemic vascular resistance (SVR), most of which is provided by the diameter of the peripheral arterioles. If the peripheral vasculature is constricted, afterload will increase and stroke will decrease. Alternatively, a decreased SVR will decrease afterload and therefore allow for an increase in stroke volume.

All the compensatory mechanisms just described can maintain homeostasis to a point. However, in illness and injury, if a severe underlying problem, such as blood loss, is not corrected, the body's compensatory mechanisms become overwhelmed.

Vasculature

The "vascular" part of the cardiovascular system refers to the blood vessels. There are three types of blood vessels, the characteristics of which reflect their functions (Figure 8-38).

Arteries are thick-walled elastic vessels that carry blood away from the heart. Because the blood leaving the heart is under higher pressure, the arteries are built to withstand this force. The walls of arteries are constructed of three layers, called *tunics*. The tunica intima (or tunica interna) is the smooth inner lining of endothelial cells (epithelium that lines the internal aspect of structures) that allows blood to flow with minimal friction through the **lumen** of the vessel.

The tunica media is the thicker middle layer, which consists of varying degrees of elastic tissue and smooth muscle, depending on the size of the vessel. For example, the aorta is composed mostly of elastic tissue and does not have the ability to constrict. Arterioles, the smallest arteries, have a substantial layer of smooth muscle, allowing them to selectively constrict and dilate to control blood flow into the capillary beds.

The smooth muscles of both arteries and veins have **alpha$_1$ receptors,** cellular receptors for epinephrine and norepinephrine (secreted by the sympathetic nervous system), which cause the smooth muscle to constrict. Smooth muscle constriction controls the diameter of the blood vessels, and thus the blood flow through them.

The tunica externa (or tunica adventitia) is the outer layer of collagen connective tissue that provides strength and stability.

In most cases, arteries carry oxygenated blood. One exception to this is the pulmonary artery, which pumps deoxygenated blood from the right ventricle to the lungs.

Arteries divide into smaller and smaller branches as they travel away from the heart. The smallest of the branches are the arterioles, which lead into the capillary beds.

Capillaries are microscopic vessels traversing the tissues to provide cells a means for exchanging oxygen and carbon dioxide and receiving nutrients and other substances. The walls of capillaries are a single cell thick (consisting only of tunica intima), allowing for efficient exchange of substances between the blood within them and the interstitial fluid surrounding them. The internal diameter of capillaries is just sufficient to admit red blood cells in single file so each one has maximum opportunity to release its oxygen to the tissues.

Because fluid exerts pressure, called *hydrostatic pressure,* which is slightly greater within the capillaries than in the surrounding interstitial fluid, the tendency is for fluid to leave the capillaries at their arterial ends. However, the concentration of protein molecules in the blood, which constitutes its oncotic pressure, serves to "pull" fluids back into the capillaries at their venous end. Fluid not returned to the capillaries is captured by the lymphatic vessels and returned to the circulation.

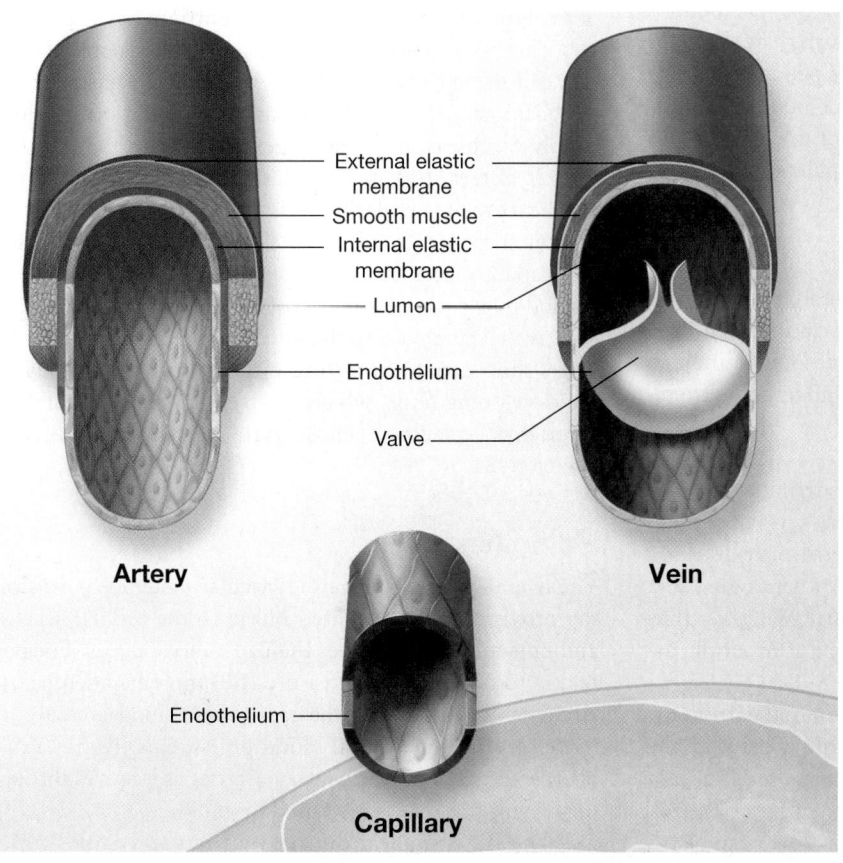

Artery

Vein

External elastic membrane
Smooth muscle
Internal elastic membrane
Lumon
Endothelium
Valve
Endothelium

Capillary

FIGURE 8-38

Both arteries and veins consist of three tissue layers. Capillaries consist of only one layer of endothelial cells.

Veins carry blood that is lower in pressure and thus are thinner-walled than arteries. Nonetheless, they consist of the same three layers as arteries. Venules receive blood from capillary beds, emptying into successively larger veins as blood returns toward the heart. Veins carry unoxygenated blood, except for pulmonary veins, which bring the oxygenated blood from the lungs to the left atrium.

Because venous pressure is so low and blood is traveling against gravity, two features assist in the return of blood to the heart. First, veins contain one-way valves that prevent the backflow of blood. Second, blood in the lower extremities is assisted in its movement by the contraction of skeletal muscle in the legs.

The importance of the skeletal muscle pump is illustrated by a phenomenon called "parade square faint," after the tendency of some military personnel to faint after standing at attention for a prolonged period of time, particularly in warm weather. The absence of skeletal muscle movement in the lower extremities results in less blood being returned to the heart. Decreased preload translates to decreased cardiac output. Under lower pressure, a sufficient amount of blood cannot overcome gravity to circulate to the brain. The absence of oxygen and glucose causes the brain cells responsible for maintaining consciousness to stop functioning. When the person collapses and blood no longer has to overcome the force of gravity to reach the brain, circulation of oxygenated blood is restored to it and the person regains consciousness.

The blood vessels are arranged into two main circuits: the pulmonary circuit and the systemic circuit. The pulmonary circuit begins with the pulmonary artery at the right ventricle, which divides into right and left pulmonary arteries that subdivide to carry deoxygenated blood to capillaries surrounding the alveoli in each lobe of the lungs. Once blood is oxygenated in the pulmonary capillaries, it empties into pulmonary veins that converge to empty oxygenated blood into the left atrium.

The systemic circulation begins at the aorta, which receives blood from the left ventricle (Figure 8-39). The aorta first ascends (ascending aorta), then arches (aortic arch) into the descending aorta. Large arteries that later branch to provide blood to the head, neck, chest, and upper extremities arise from the aortic arch.

The subclavian arteries run beneath the clavicles, branching into the arteries of the upper extremities. The internal carotid arteries and vertebral arteries provide blood to the brain, and the external carotid arteries provide blood to the scalp and face. Although the larger arteries are deep, some of the smaller branches are superficial. Wherever they pass over firmer underlying tissue, the pulsation of the artery can be felt.

For example, the pulsation of the external carotid arteries is felt in the anterior neck in the groove between the thyroid cartilage and the sternocleidomastoid muscle. The brachial arteries can be felt along the anterior surface of the elbow in the antecubital fossa, and the radial artery can be felt on the anterior aspect of the wrist at the base of the thumb.

IN THE FIELD

Being able to locate distal pulses is important in the assessment of an injured extremity. If injury or associated swelling obstruct blood flow to the distal extremity, the tissues beyond the obstruction will become ischemic.

The descending aorta is divided into the thoracic aorta and abdominal aorta. Numerous branches arise from the descending aorta to provide blood flow to the trunk. The aorta bifurcates at about the level of L4 to form the right and left common iliac arteries. In turn, the common iliac arteries further divide to provide blood flow to the lower extremities.

The pulsation of the femoral arteries can be felt at the groin. The popliteal artery runs behind the knee, the dorsalis pedis can be felt on the dorsum of the foot, and the posterior tibial artery can be felt just posterior to the tibial tuberosity on the medial aspect of the ankle.

The location of the smaller veins is somewhat variable, as you will note when you learn to start IVs. However, their locations are more consistent as the branches become larger. The veins of the upper extremities, head, and neck empty into the subclavian veins, which lead to the superior vena cava (Figure 8-40). The veins of the trunk and lower extremities empty into the inferior vena cava. Both portions of the vena cava empty into the right atrium of the heart.

There is an important sidetrack to the systemic circulation called the *hepatic portal circulation*. The gastrointestinal (GI) system receives a substantial portion of the blood supply to absorb nutrients ingested through the GI tract. Instead of returning directly to the systemic venous system and heart for recirculation, this blood first travels through the hepatic portal vein to the liver, where it enters a second capillary bed. The liver cells (hepatocytes) remove toxins and nutrients before the blood is returned to the hepatic vein, which empties into the inferior vena cava.

Other variations of the circulatory system exist in the developing fetus, which receives oxygen and nutrients through the placenta. Those variations are considered in Chapter 43.

Hemodynamics

The overall goal of the cardiovascular system is **perfusion**, the provision of oxygenated blood to the cellular level in amounts adequate to meet their metabolic needs. For perfusion to occur, blood pressure (BP) must be adequate to circulate blood through the capillaries. Blood pressure, or more specifically, arterial blood pressure, is the force that blood exerts against the walls of arteries as it moves through them. This pressure is measured in mmHg.

The BP is highest during ventricular systole, which causes a wave of increased pressure to move throughout

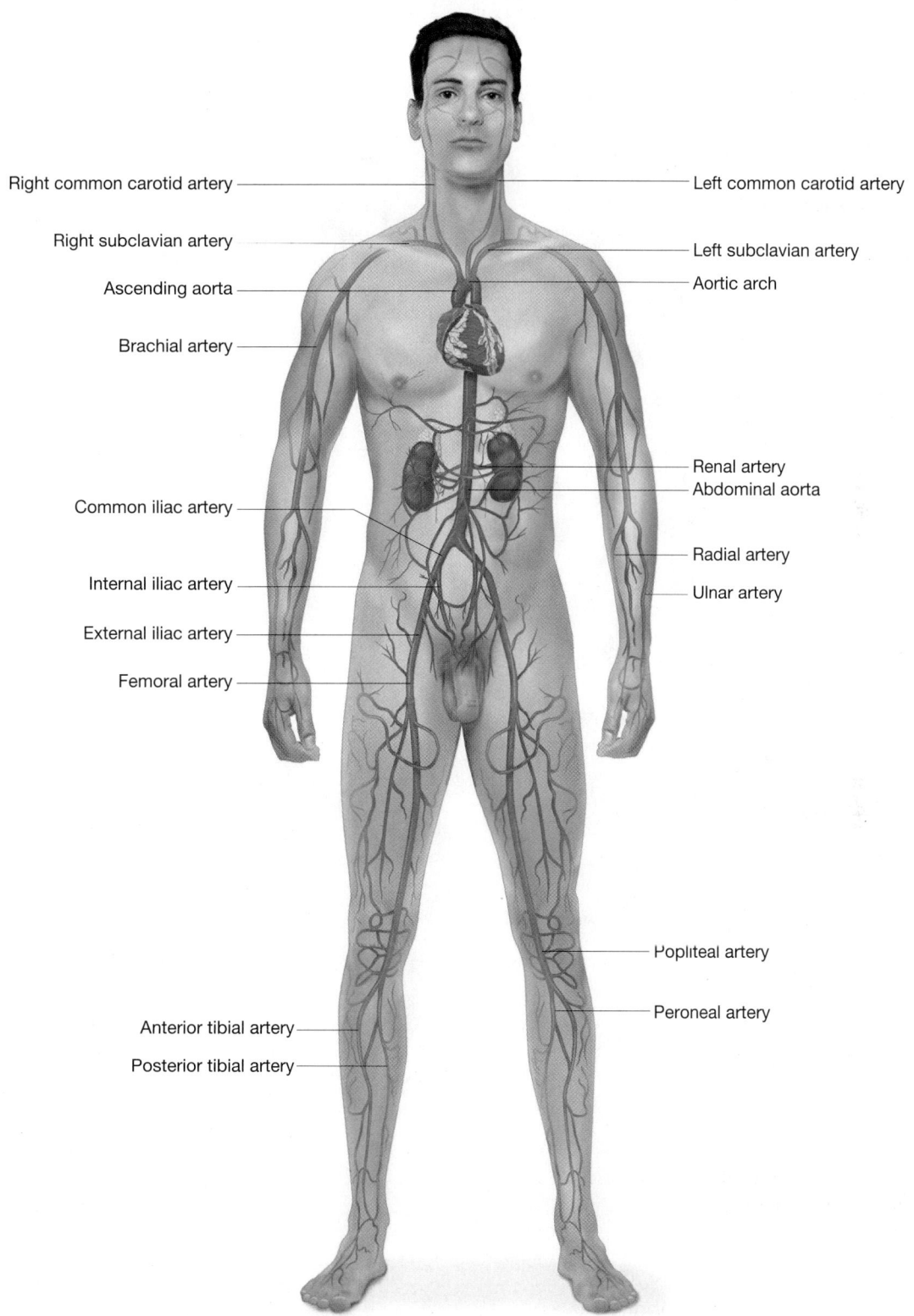

Right common carotid artery

Right subclavian artery

Ascending aorta

Brachial artery

Left common carotid artery

Left subclavian artery

Aortic arch

Renal artery

Abdominal aorta

Common iliac artery

Internal iliac artery

External iliac artery

Femoral artery

Radial artery

Ulnar artery

Popliteal artery

Peroneal artery

Anterior tibial artery

Posterior tibial artery

FIGURE 8-39

Arteries carry blood away from the heart. Arteries carry oxygenated blood, with the exception of the pulmonary artery, which carries deoxygenated blood from the right ventricle to the lungs.

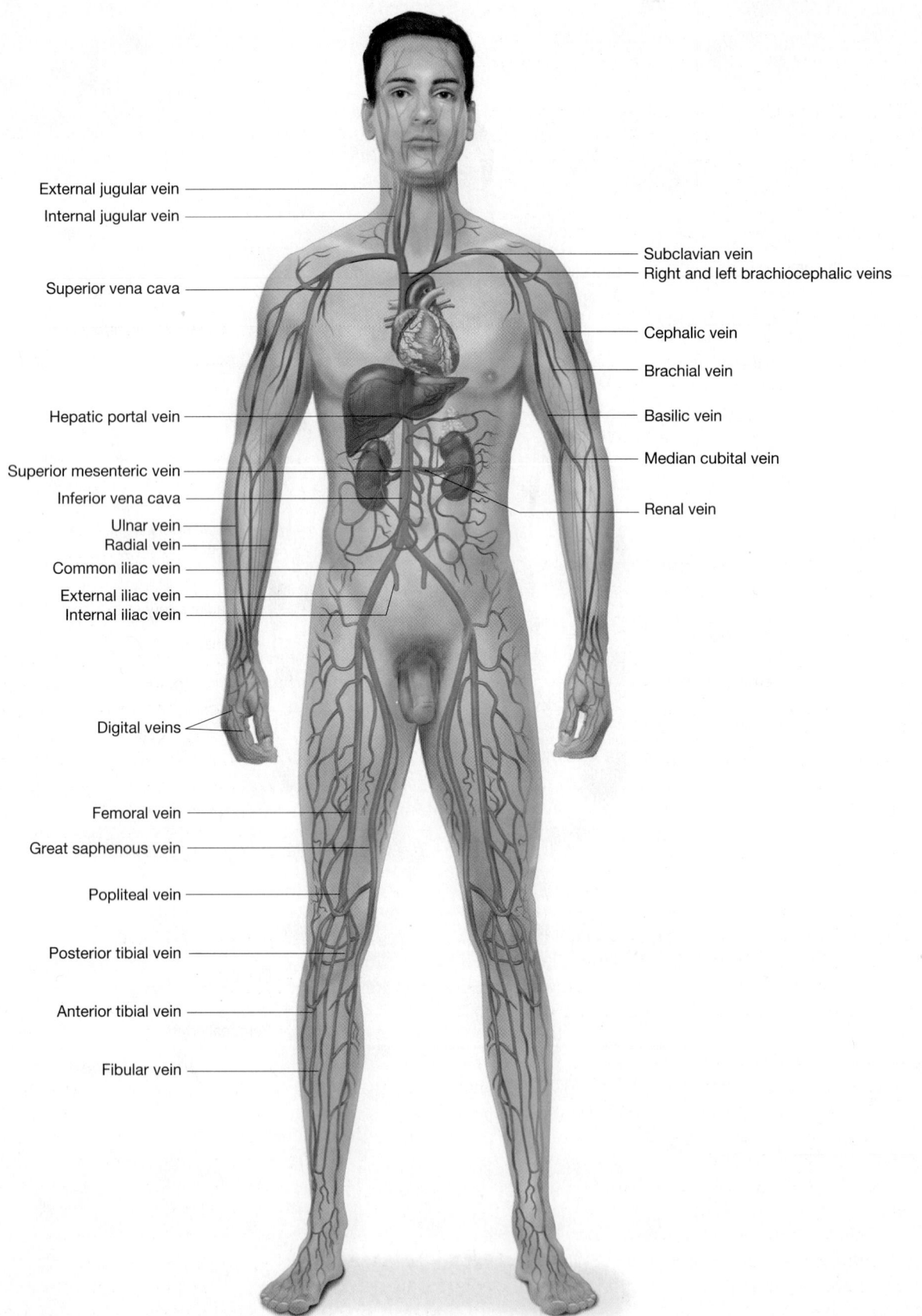

External jugular vein

Internal jugular vein

Superior vena cava

Hepatic portal vein

Superior mesenteric vein

Inferior vena cava

Ulnar vein

Radial vein

Common iliac vein

External iliac vein

Internal iliac vein

Digital veins

Femoral vein

Great saphenous vein

Popliteal vein

Posterior tibial vein

Anterior tibial vein

Fibular vein

Subclavian vein

Right and left brachiocephalic veins

Cephalic vein

Brachial vein

Basilic vein

Median cubital vein

Renal vein

FIGURE 8-40

Veins return blood to the heart. Veins carry deoxygenated blood, with the exception of the pulmonary vein, which carries freshly oxygenated blood from the lungs to the left atrium.

the arterial system. This is called the *systolic blood pressure (SBP)*. The lower pressure exerted against the walls of the arteries during diastole is the *diastolic blood pressure (DBP)*.

When BP is measured, both SBP and DBP are obtained and recorded as the SBP over the DBP. For example, a BP of 116/74 mmHg means that the SBP is 116 mmHg and the DBP is 74 mmHg. The American Heart Association considers normal adult BP to be <120 mmHg systolic and <80 mmHg diastolic. (The measurement of BP is described in Chapter 18.)

Because the BP varies with each heartbeat, the **mean arterial pressure (MAP)** is used to determine the overall adequacy of perfusion. Calculating MAP requires another value, the **pulse pressure**, which is the difference between the SBP and DBP. Using the BP in the previous paragraph, 116/74 mmHg, the pulse pressure is 42 mmHg (116 − 74 = 42). MAP is the DBP plus one third of the pulse pressure. Continuing with the same example:

$$MAP = 88 \text{ mmHg } (74 + (1/3 \times 42) = 88)$$

The relationship between blood pressure, cardiac output, and systemic vascular resistance is represented by the following formula:

$$MAP = CO \times SVR$$

Several factors influence blood pressure, including the function of the heart, the volume of blood, and the capacity of the vascular system. A problem with any of those factors can reduce blood pressure and, therefore, the ability of blood to circulate to the cellular level and return to the heart. When one factor is affected, the others can compensate to maintain an adequate blood pressure, but only to a degree.

Together, the volume of the blood and the function of the heart determine cardiac output. The greater the cardiac output, the greater the blood pressure. The capacity of the blood vessels is determined by their degree of constriction or relaxation. The more constricted the vessels, the greater the resistance they provide to blood flow, thus the term *systemic vascular resistance (SVR)*. The greater the SVR, the greater the blood pressure.

The way those factors work together is reflected in the changes that occur to maintain homeostasis when one of them changes. For example, a loss of blood volume results in decreased blood volume returning to the heart (preload), which results in decreased cardiac output, and decreased blood pressure. However, an increase in heart rate will increase cardiac output, and an increase in systemic vascular resistance will further increase blood pressure. Therefore, two signs of shock associated with blood loss are tachycardia and the pale, cool skin that results from vasoconstriction.

The body also responds to an overall increase in the volume of fluid in the body, because fluid overload in the vascular space increases the blood pressure. When blood pressure increases, preload increases, which increases the

stretch on the atria. When the atria stretch, cells secrete a substance called *atrial natriuretic peptide (ANP)*, which has two effects. The immediate effect is to stimulate vasodilation to lower blood pressure. The second effect suppresses a mechanism that causes fluid retention, called the *renin–angiotensin–aldosterone system*.

The renin–angiotensin–aldosterone system regulates blood pressure by affecting how much fluid the kidneys retain. This is a complex system that involves the detection of fluid levels by special cells in the kidney, the juxtaglomerular apparatus. States of low kidney perfusion stimulate a cascade of effects that lead to the release of a potent vasoconstrictor, angiotensin II, which increases blood pressure. Angiotensin II also stimulates the adrenal cortex to secrete aldosterone. Aldosterone acts on the kidneys, causing them to retain more Na$^+$. By retaining more Na$^+$, the kidneys retain more water to increase the intravascular volume.

Control, Communication, and Integration

The Nervous System

The body receives a constant supply of sensory input from both its internal and external environments, to which it must respond. The nervous system allows integration of sensory input and coordination of responses to it. Together with the endocrine system, the nervous system allows for control and communication in the body.

The nervous system encompasses all the nerve cells, or neurons, in the body. Neurons are the basic unit of structure and function of the nervous system. Neurons come in a variety of forms suited to their specific functions, but they have basic features in common (Figure 8-41). These characteristics allow neurons to communicate by way of chemicals called **neurotransmitters** and to conduct action potentials.

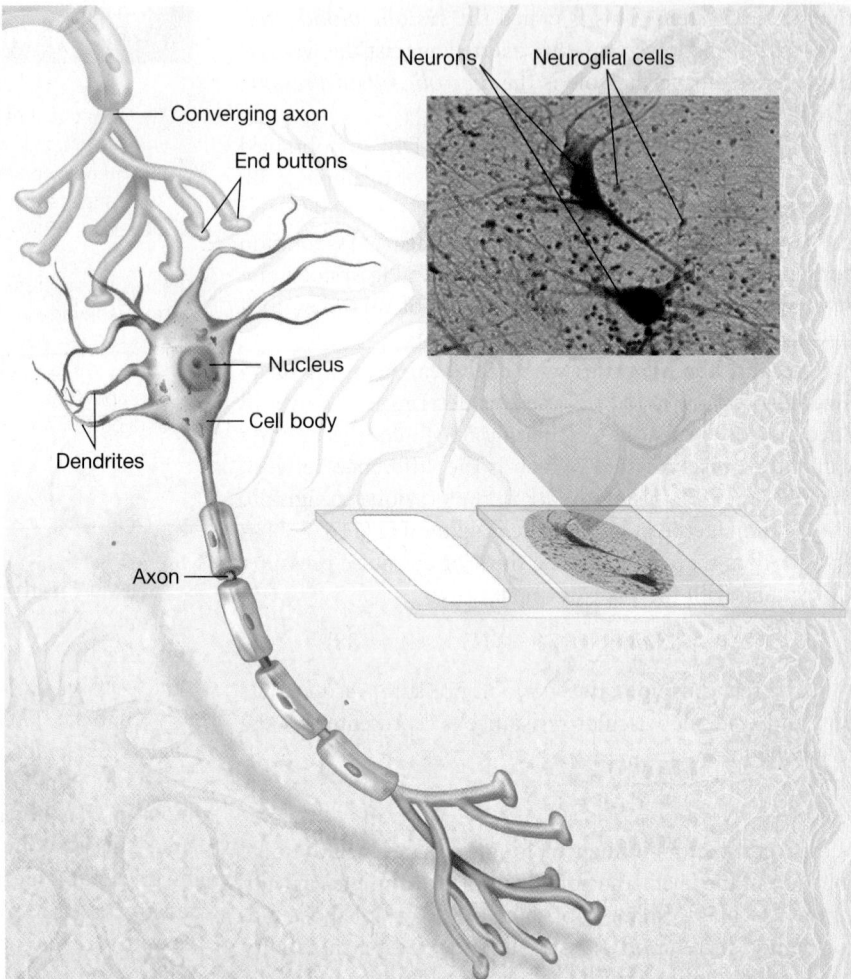

FIGURE 8-41

Neurons may take on different shapes, but have the same basic features in common: dendrites that receive input, a cell body, and an axon that carries information to adjacent cells.

The neurons within the brain and spinal cord comprise the central nervous system (CNS), and all neurons outside the brain and spinal cord comprise the peripheral nervous system (Figure 8-42).

The CNS and peripheral nervous system work together to allow both voluntary (somatic) functions and involuntary (autonomic) functions. Autonomic functions are further classified into actions of the sympathetic nervous system and parasympathetic nervous system.

The actions of these two divisions of the autonomic nervous system oppose each other to provide both balance and the ability to respond to stimuli to maintain homeostasis. The general function of the sympathetic nervous system is to mediate the "fight-or-flight" response to stressors. The general function of the parasympathetic nervous system is to manage the everyday functions of life, such as digestion and sexual functions.

Neuron Structure and Function

A typical neuron consists of a cell body (soma) with two specialized ends. Dendrites at one end of the cell allow the cell to receive messages. When a message is received, an action potential is generated and travels along the cell's axon to its synaptic terminals. A synapse is the microscopic gap that serves as the junction between two neurons, or between a neuron and a target tissue, such as a muscle or gland.

When the action potential reaches the synaptic terminals, it causes the release of neurotransmitters. The neurotransmitters cross the synapse, where they bind with receptors on the dendrites of an adjacent neuron or tissue cell receptors.

Special structures in neuron bodies, called *Nissl bodies*, are responsible for the appearance of gray matter. A special insulating layer around the axons of neurons, called *myelin*, is responsible for the appearance of white matter. The myelin sheath allows for rapid conduction of nerve impulses.

There are three main functional classifications of neurons: sensory neurons, motor neurons, and interneurons. Different types of sensory neurons receive a variety of different types of input, such as visual, auditory, tactile (touch), olfactory (smell), and gustatory (taste) stimuli, as well as input that aids in maintaining balance, blood pressure, and chemical composition of the body.

When the dendrites of sensory neurons are activated, the neuron generates an action potential that travels toward

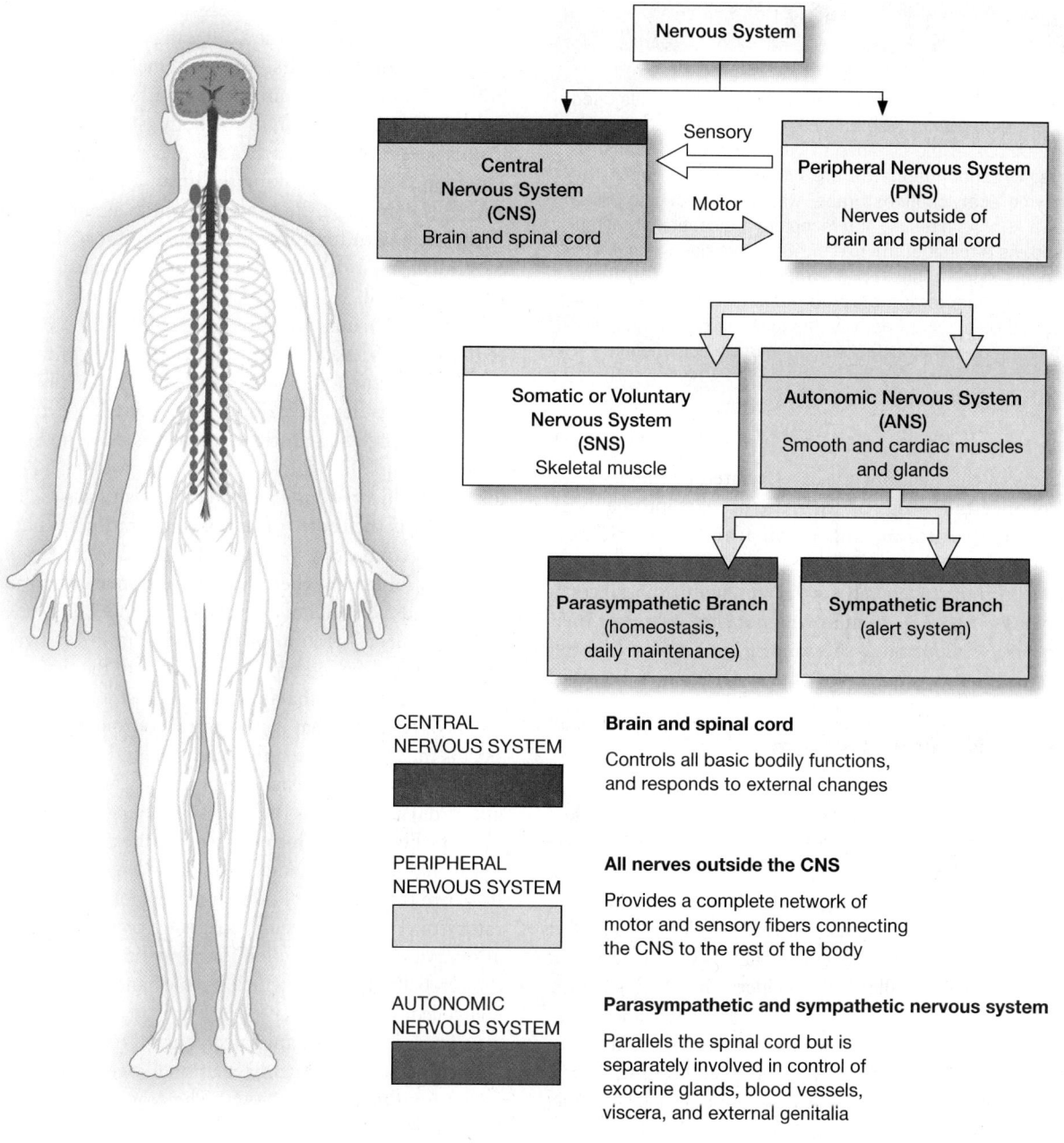

FIGURE 8-42

Functional divisions of the nervous system.

the CNS. Motor neurons arise in the CNS, where they await voluntary or involuntary stimuli. When stimulated, their action potential travels out of the CNS, toward a target tissue (effector).

Interneurons are connecting neurons in the CNS that allow communication between neurons to integrate sensory information and coordinate a motor response. Neurons are supported by specialized cells called *neuroglia*. Different types of neuroglia, or glial cells, perform functions as diverse as secreting CSF, engulfing pathogens, and providing a selective barrier between the brain and the blood (the blood–brain barrier).

Neurotransmitters

A variety of substances in the body serve as chemical messengers between the synaptic terminals of neurons and adjacent receptors. The neurotransmitters act only on cells that have specific receptors for them. The response by the cell depends on the particular function for which the cell is designed.

Acetylcholine (ACh) plays roles in the somatic nervous system and in both the sympathetic and parasympathetic divisions of the autonomic nervous system. In addition to ACh, there are more than 50 other neurotransmitters. Some of them that are especially relevant to EMS providers, either in terms of their actions, diseases related to them, or the effects of certain drugs on them are norepinephrine (NE), dopamine, serotonin, and gamma aminobutyric acid (GABA).

Neurotransmitters rely on the presence of substances at the synapse to break them down after they stimulate their receptors. Without these substances, the neurotransmitter causes continuous stimulation of the adjacent nerve or cells.

Central Nervous System

The brain is the central integrating organ of the nervous system, and is itself comprised of many nerve bodies packed together. The brain is contained within the cranium, where it is cushioned by CSF and surrounded by three layers of membranes called the *meninges* (Figure 8-43).

The innermost meningeal layer, which is adherent to the brain, is called the *pia mater*. The middle layer is the *arachnoid layer*, so called for its spiderweb-like appearance. The subarachnoid space between the pia mater and arachnoid layer contains the CSF that surrounds the brain.

The tougher outermost layer is called the *dura mater*, which is continuous with the periosteum that lines the inner surface of the skull. Blood vessels called *bridging vessels* traverse the space between the skull and brain.

The brain tissue itself is extremely fragile, and the brain has only limited movement within the skull. However, sudden deceleration of the body (such as would occur from a severe blow to the head or when the body comes to a sudden stop upon striking the ground during a fall from a height) can cause the brain to collide against the inside of the skull with force, producing brain injury. During this movement, the bridging veins can be torn, causing bleeding within the skull.

The cerebrum, which is part of the forebrain, is the center of consciousness and higher thought, and is where decision making takes place (Figure 8-44). It is divided into several regions that have distinct functions. The frontal lobe is where thoughts are formed, emotions arise, and decision making occurs. It is the location of the primary motor cortex from which voluntary physical activity arises. The parietal lobe is the center of sensory integration and home to pathways connecting various other parts of the brain. The temporal lobes are where hearing and memory formation occurs, and the occipital lobe houses the mechanics of vision.

The deeper portion of the forebrain lies between the brainstem and the cerebrum and consists of the thalamus and hypothalamus. The thalamus is an egg-size structure in the center of the brain that is the central coordination center for signals traveling between the cerebrum and spinal cord. The hypothalamus projects into the pituitary gland and has a role in coordinating various hormones of the endocrine system.

The brainstem, which sits beneath the cerebrum, consists of the midbrain, pons, and medulla oblongata (Figure 8-45). It is here that the core bodily functions of heart rate, respiratory rate, and body temperature are controlled. The pons also serves as the connection for the brain and spinal cord to the cerebellum, within which balance and coordination are controlled.

Twelve pairs of cranial nerves arise from the inferior aspect of the brain, exiting through small openings in the bone called *foramina* (Figure 8-46). The cranial nerves function

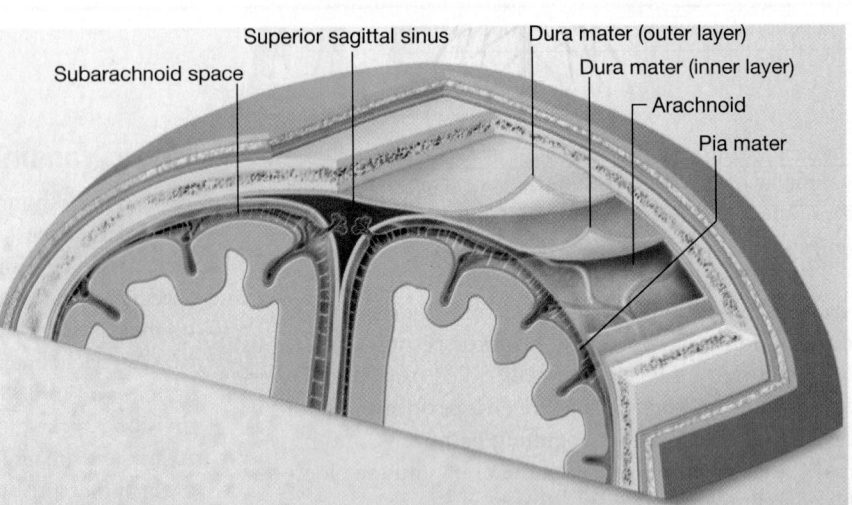

FIGURE 8-43

The brain is protected by the skull, cerebral spinal fluid, and three layers of tissue collectively called the *meninges*. From external to internal, these layers are the dura mater, arachnoid, and pia mater.

Subarachnoid space
Superior sagittal sinus
Dura mater (outer layer)
Dura mater (inner layer)
Arachnoid
Pia mater

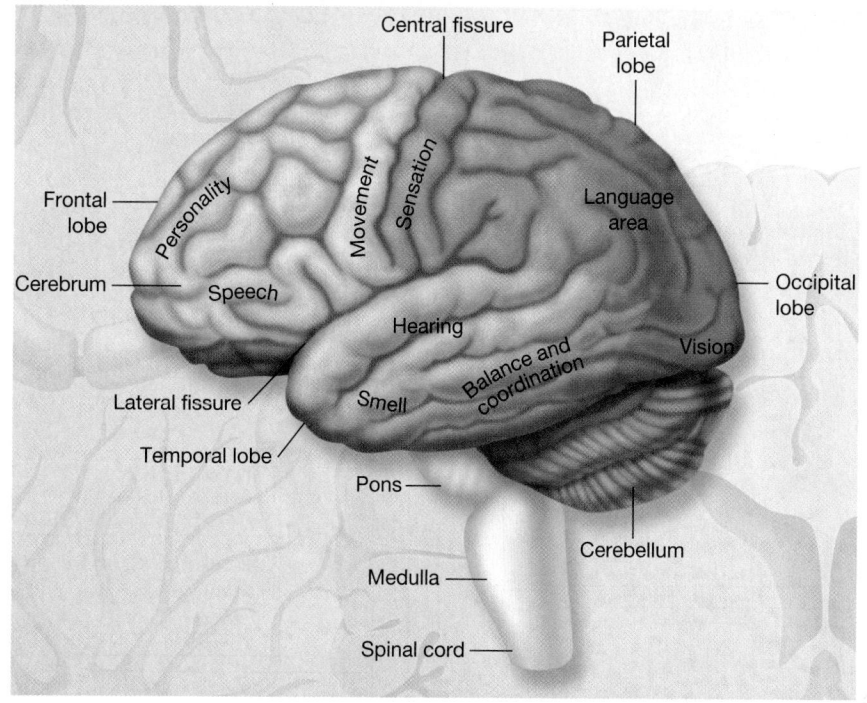

FIGURE 8-44

The cerebrum is the seat of higher brain functions.

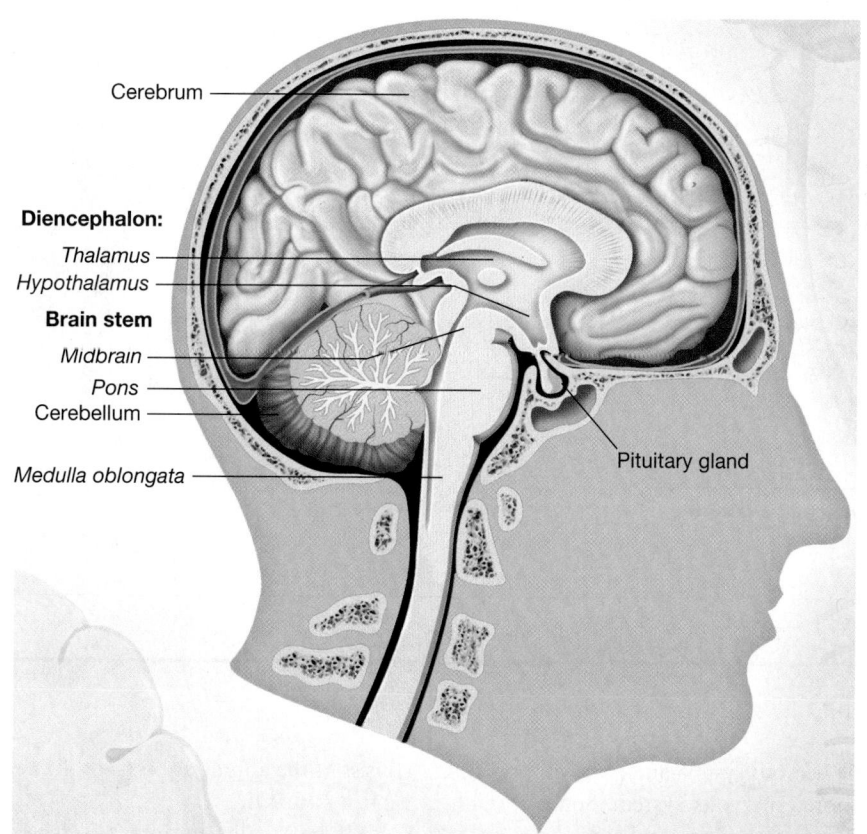

FIGURE 8-45

The brainstem, consisting of the medulla oblongata and pons, is responsible for control of vital functions.

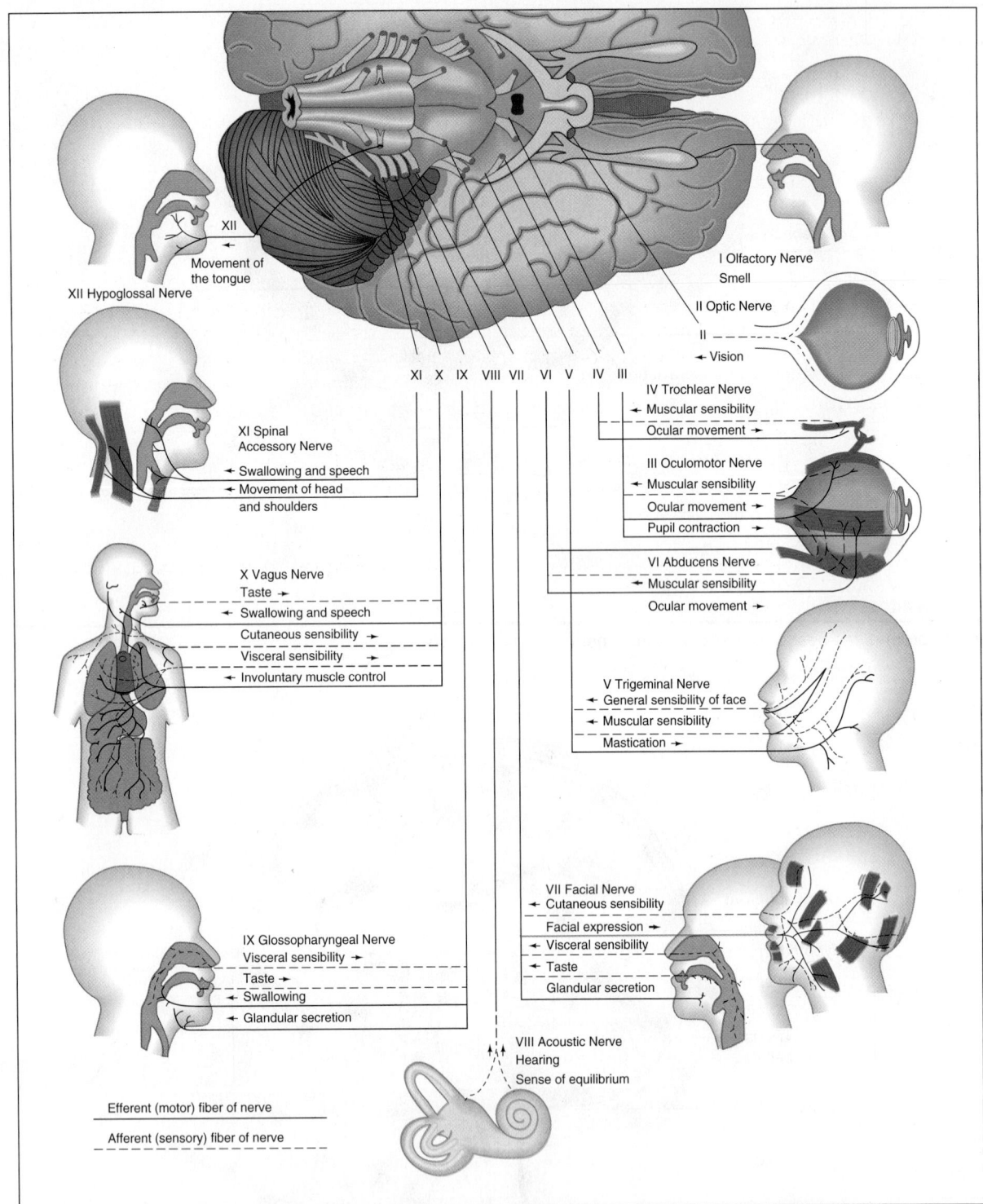

FIGURE 8-46

The cranial nerves.

as parts of the somatic nervous system and parasympathetic division of the autonomic nervous system. Some cranial nerves are sensory, others are motor, and some have both sensory and motor functions.

Each pair of cranial nerves has both a name and a number, as well as serving specific functions. The numbers

consist of the abbreviation *CN* followed by Roman numerals from I to XII.

Of particular importance to Advanced EMTs are CN III, the oculomotor nerve, and CN X, the vagus nerve. CN III functions to produce constriction of the pupils. When pressure increases inside the cranium because of swelling of the brain or bleeding, the function of CN III can be impaired, producing dilation of the affected pupil.

CN X serves a variety of functions, among them reducing the function of the SA node of the heart. When CN X is abnormally stimulated, the heart rate can slow to a level that decreases cardiac output enough to cause hypotension and altered mental status.

The reticular activating system (RAS) is an interconnected network of neurons in the brainstem, thalamus, and cerebrum that is responsible for consciousness, sleep–wake cycles, and attention. Although it is still incompletely understood, it is known to use both cholinergic and adrenergic receptors, and is implicated in the evolution of many psychiatric conditions, such as schizophrenia, attention deficit hyperactivity disorder (ADHD), Alzheimer's and Parkinson's diseases, and narcolepsy.

The spinal cord is a long bundle of nerve bodies and myelin sheaths that continues from the brainstem to the level of the L2 vertebra. The meninges are continuous, covering the spinal cord as well as the brain. The spinal cord is bathed in cerebral spinal fluid within the vertebral canal. During its

course, the spinal cord gives rise to 31 pairs of spinal nerves, which are part of the peripheral nervous system.

At the termination of the spinal cord, the remaining spinal nerves still travel inferiorly before exiting and create a horsetail-like design, called the *cauda equina*. The layered arrangement of pairs of spinal nerves accounts for the sensory dermatomes that are observed in the body (Figure 8-47). These are specific areas of spinal nerve innervation found on the skin that can be used to detect the level of a cord injury (Figure 8-48).

The neural tissue of the spinal cord is arranged into bundles called *tracts*. Each of the tracts carries different

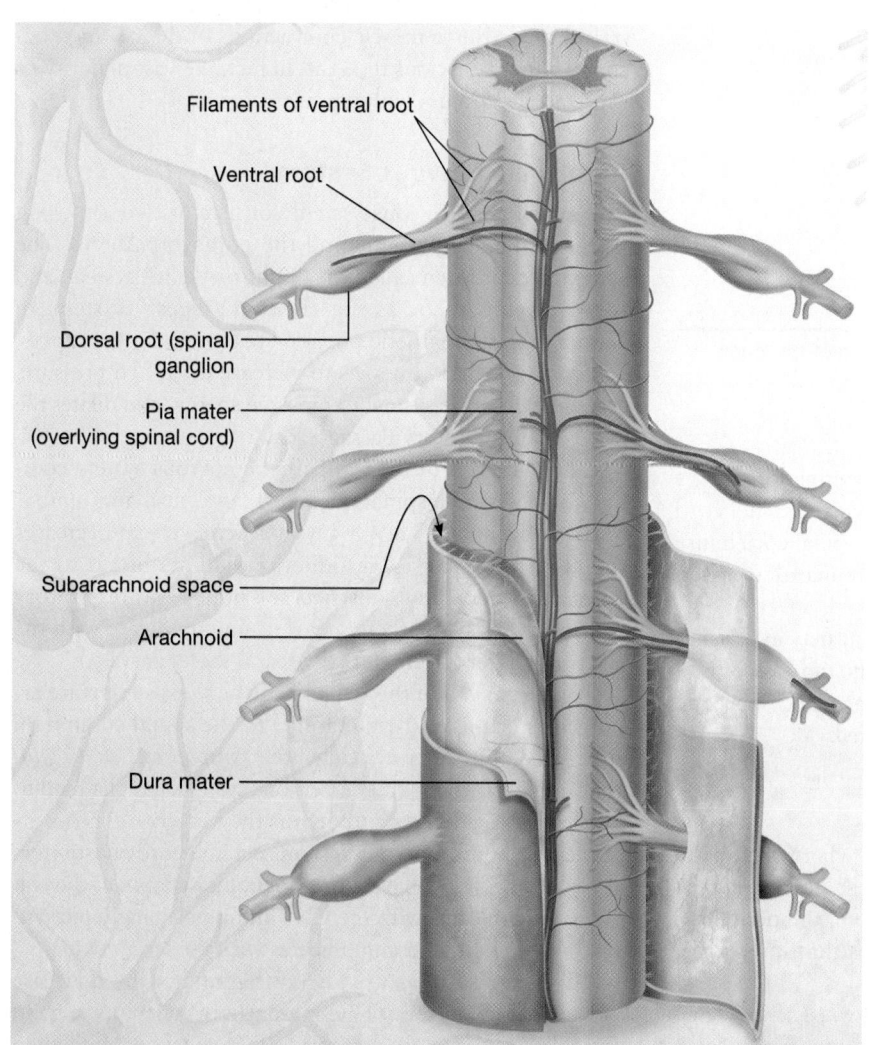

Filaments of ventral root

Ventral root

Dorsal root (spinal) ganglion

Pia mater (overlying spinal cord)

Subarachnoid space

Arachnoid

Dura mater

FIGURE 8-47

The spinal cord consists of tracts of tissue that ascend toward the brain and tracts of tissue that descend toward the spinal nerves.

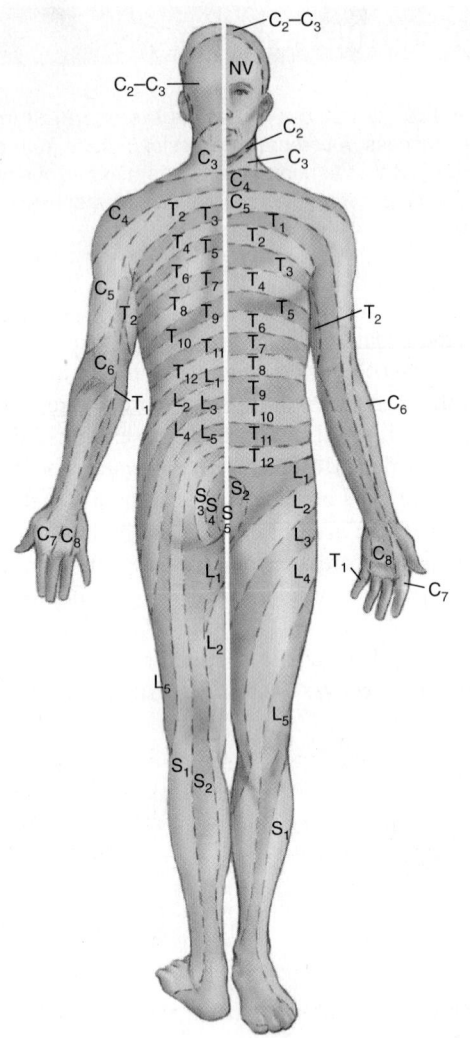

FIGURE 8-48

Each spinal nerve supplies a specific area of the body with sensation and motor function.

types of information. In some cases, the information crosses over so information is carried up or down the spinal cord on the opposite side of the body. When a spinal cord injury completely severs the spinal cord, all communication ceases. In some cases, a spinal cord injury is partial, affecting only one of the tracts. In such cases, the patient may experience loss of sensation on one side of the body and loss of motor function on the opposite side. The particular signs and symptoms depend on which tract is affected.

Peripheral Nervous System

The peripheral nervous system begins where the spinal nerves and cranial nerves enter and exit the meningeal coverings of the spinal cord and brain. Often, the peripheral nerves emerge from the cord in bundles that intertwine, called a *plexus*.

There are two types of peripheral nerves: sensory and motor. Sensory nerves are also called *afferent nerves* because

they travel toward the spinal cord, and motor nerves are also called *efferent nerves* because they travel away from the spinal cord. The motor nerves emerge anteriorly from the spinal nerve root, and the sensory nerves return posteriorly, through the dorsal root ganglia.

A ganglion is a collection of nerve cell bodies. Some ganglia of the sympathetic nervous system are arranged in chains that run parallel to the spinal column on either side of it. These are called the *sympathetic chain ganglia*. In the parasympathetic nervous system, ganglia tend to be closer to the tissues and organs that they innervate.

Neurons of the autonomic nervous system secrete neurotransmitters at two points. They have a preganglionic synapse at the end that communicates with the CNS and a postganglionic synapse at the end that communicates with the target tissue.

Voluntary Nervous System

Functionally, the nervous system can be divided into the voluntary (somatic) and involuntary, or autonomic, nervous systems. The voluntary system encompasses any nerve that is involved in an action that the brain must consciously think about to initiate. For example, picking up an object from a table is controlled by voluntary motor neurons. Peristalsis, or rhythmic muscle contractions of the GI tract, occurs without conscious thought. In fact, the vast majority of nerve activity occurs without awareness.

Autonomic Nervous System

The autonomic nervous system consists of two opposing systems: the sympathetic and the parasympathetic. The sympathetic is often called the "fight-or-flight" system, and the parasympathetic as the "rest-and-digest" system. In general, the sympathetic portion speeds up the heart rate, vasoconstricts blood vessels to increase the blood pressure, slows the digestive system to preserve energy, and dilates the pupils and respiratory passages.

The neurons of the sympathetic nervous system communicate with the spinal cord in the thoracic and lumbar areas of the spine. The parasympathetic system decreases the heart rate, causes vasodilation, shunts blood to the digestive system, and constricts the pupils and respiratory passages. Parasympathetic neurons communicate with the CNS by way of the cranial nerves and sacral nerves.

Some ganglia of the sympathetic nervous system are arranged in chains that run parallel to the spinal column on either side of it. They are called the *sympathetic chain ganglia*. In the parasympathetic nervous system, ganglia tend to be closer to the tissues and organs they innervate. Neurons of the autonomic nervous system secrete neurotransmitters at two points. They have a preganglionic synapse at the end that communicates with the CNS and a postganglionic synapse at the end that communicates with the target tissue.

The two systems are also differentiated by their use of neurotransmitters. The sympathetic nervous system secretes ACh into the preganglionic synapses, and then

TABLE 8-5	Effects of the Sympathetic Nervous System

Cellular Receptor Type	Effects
Alpha$_1$	Vasoconstriction, pupil dilation
Alpha$_2$	Regulates alpha$_1$ effects
Beta$_1$	Increases heart rate, conductivity, contractility, and automaticity
Beta$_2$	Smooth muscle relaxation allowing bronchodilation and arteriolar dilation

IN THE FIELD

The substances released by the body's cells during a severe allergic reaction cause constriction of the bronchioles, creating restricted air flow and wheezing, and dilation of the blood vessels, which results in low blood pressure. Epinephrine is used to treat these effects. Its alpha$_1$ adrenergic effects cause constriction of smooth muscle in the blood vessels to raise the blood pressure. Epinephrine's beta$_1$ adrenergic effects increase the force (and rate) of cardiac contraction to increase cardiac output, further increasing blood pressure, and its beta$_2$ adrenergic effects cause relaxation of the smooth muscles of the bronchioles.

norepinephrine into the postganglionic, or target tissue, synapses. The parasympathetic system also uses ACh for preganglionic synapses, but then continues to use ACh in the target tissues as well.

Neurons and cellular receptors are often referred to by the neurotransmitter that they secrete or react to: *cholinergic* for those that secrete or react to acetylcholine, and *adrenergic* for those that secrete or react to norepinephrine.

The term *adrenergic* comes from the relationship between the sympathetic nervous system and the adrenal glands. Adrenergic receptors are further categorized as alpha$_1$, alpha$_2$, beta$_1$, and beta$_2$ receptors. Different types of tissues have one or more types of these receptors. When activated, each of these receptors is responsible for different cellular effects that facilitate the fight-or-flight response (Table 8-5).

Some substances are capable of binding with different types of receptors, whereas others bind with only one type of receptor. For example, epinephrine has alpha$_1$, beta$_1$, and beta$_2$ effects, whereas norepinephrine produces predominantly alpha$_1$ effects.

Endocrine System

Whereas the nervous system is an immediate means of communication within the human body, the endocrine system provides an equally important, but slower, means of communication.

The endocrine system is a collection of ductless glands that secrete various chemicals, called **hormones**, into the bloodstream. Various cells throughout the body have different types of receptors to which specific hormones can bind (Figure 8-49).

Hypothalamus and Pituitary Gland

The pituitary gland is a master gland that secretes tropic hormones that control the secretion of other hormones throughout the body. Anatomically, the pituitary is divided into anterior and posterior sections, both of which hang from the hypothalamus in the center of the skull. In fact, the posterior hypothalamus, or neurohypophysis, is a direct extension of the hypothalamus.

PERSONAL PERSPECTIVE

Advanced EMT Tommy Isom: I enjoyed learning about anatomy and physiology as an Advanced EMT student. Well, I mostly enjoyed it. It was difficult at times, but it is amazing stuff, really. Even so, I would wonder sometimes how the information was going to help me as an Advanced EMT.

Sooner or later, as we got to the parts of class where we talked about different kinds of emergencies, it made sense that we had to have the A&P background to understand what was wrong with patients and what to do about it. Still, there were some things that seemed a little obscure. Until I met Mrs. Creswell.

Mrs. Creswell was unresponsive with depressed breathing, slight bradycardia, and cool, dry skin. Her oxygen and glucose levels checked out fine. There were no signs of trauma.

When we got her list of medications, I noticed that thyroid hormone was among them. I started thinking: the thyroid gland regulates metabolism. If she is taking thyroid hormone, her body must not be making enough of it. If she took too much thyroid hormone, her energy production would be increased and everything would speed up. But if her supplement wasn't enough, energy production would be decreased and everything would slow down.

It seemed like a reasonable hypothesis. We provided supportive treatment for Mrs. Creswell and transported her to the hospital. It turns out that her thyroid hormone level was low. I was pretty amazed at having been on the right track. It is great how a little knowledge of how the body works can give you clues about what is wrong with patients!

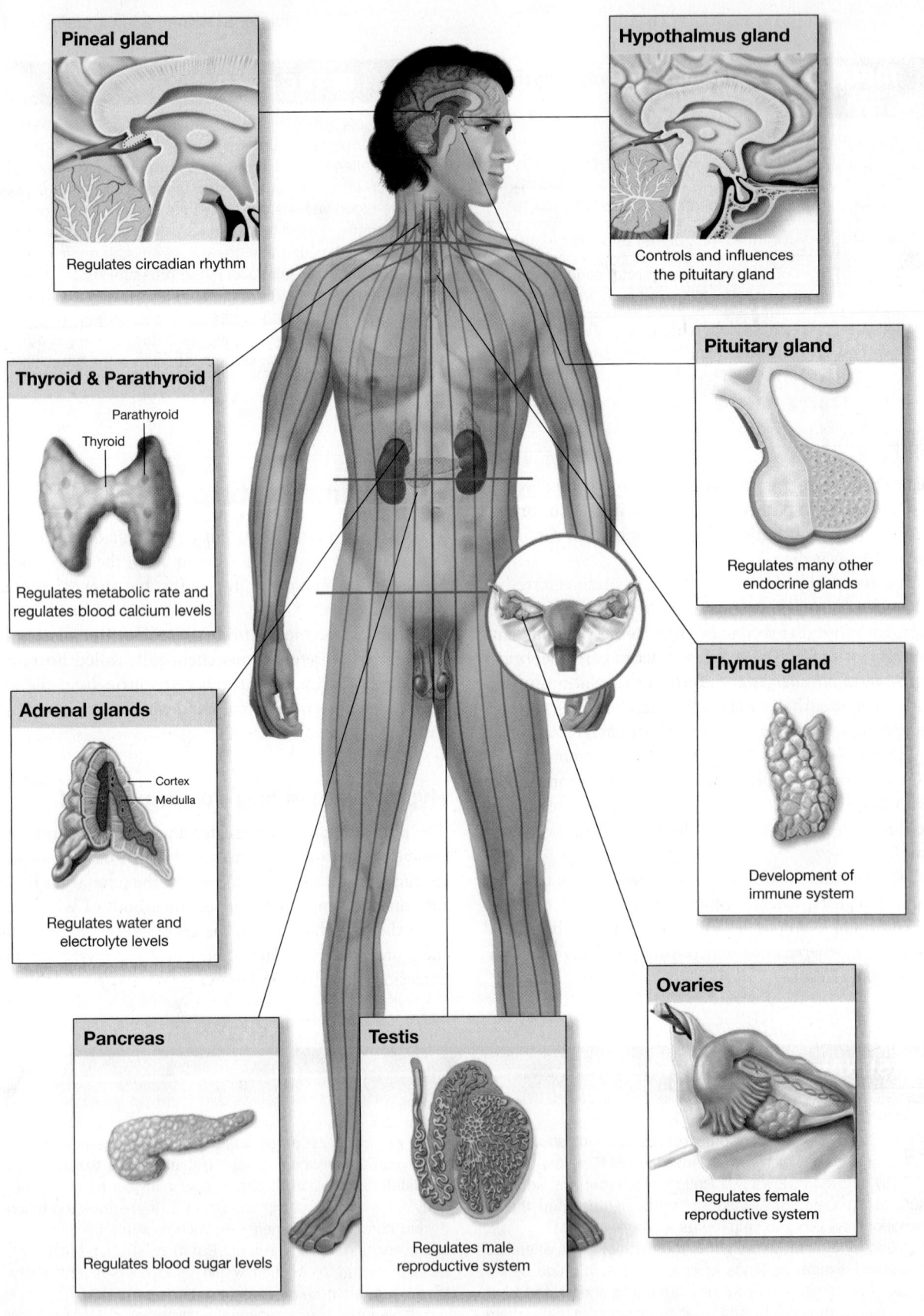

Pineal gland

Regulates circadian rhythm

Hypothalmus gland

Controls and influences the pituitary gland

Thyroid & Parathyroid

Parathyroid

Thyroid

Regulates metabolic rate and regulates blood calcium levels

Pituitary gland

Regulates many other endocrine glands

Adrenal glands

Cortex

Medulla

Regulates water and electrolyte levels

Thymus gland

Development of immune system

Pancreas

Regulates blood sugar levels

Testis

Regulates male reproductive system

Ovaries

Regulates female reproductive system

FIGURE 8-49

The endocrine system is a collection of ductless glands that secrete hormones, which are carried in the bloodstream to target cells that have specific receptors for the hormone. The hormone acts as a chemical messenger that regulates the function of the cell.

Two hormones are secreted from the posterior pituitary: antidiuretic hormone (ADH), also called *vasopressin*, and oxytocin. ADH, as may be assumed by the name, prevents diuresis (loss of fluid through the urinary system). It is released in volume-depleted states and works on the collecting tubules of the kidneys to allow increased resorption of water. Oxytocin is secreted during and after labor: first to stimulate the contraction of uterine muscles during childbirth, and later to stimulate milk ejection from the lactating breast.

The anterior pituitary, also called the *adenohypophysis*, secretes a number of hormones that affect a variety of body functions. Adrenocorticotropic hormone (ACTH) works on the adrenal glands to increase secretion of glucocorticoids, including steroids.

Thyroid-stimulating hormone (TSH) stimulates the thyroid gland to release thyroid hormone, which in turn can increase the metabolic rate of the body, increase the heart rate, and increase the body temperature.

Follicle-stimulating hormone (FSH) and luteinizing hormone (LH) are secreted in response to stimulation from gonadotropin-releasing hormone (GnRH) released from the hypothalamus. FSH and LH stimulate the reproductive system to grow and develop, as well as cause the ovaries or testes to produce and secrete estrogen, progesterone, and testosterone.

Growth hormone (GH) stimulates the growth of bones, muscles, and other tissues within the body. Its secretion is regulated by growth hormone–releasing hormone (GHRH) secreted from the hypothalamus. Prolactin (PRL) stimulates the production of milk in the lactating woman's breasts.

Pancreas

The pancreas is a dual-function organ, located in the upper abdomen, with both endocrine and exocrine roles. Endocrine systems work by secreting molecules into the bloodstream without the use of ducts. Exocrine systems always use ducts to reach their target organ directly. The exocrine functions of the pancreas act on the digestive system, and are discussed along with the gastrointestinal system.

Three types of endocrine cells are found within the islets of Langerhans of the pancreas. Alpha cells (not to be confused with the alpha receptors of the sympathetic nervous system) secrete the hormone **glucagon** in response to low blood sugar levels. Glucagon stimulates breakdown of glycogen, a complex carbohydrate in the liver, to glucose.

Beta cells (not to be confused with the beta receptors of the sympathetic nervous system) secrete **insulin**. Insulin opposes the actions of glucagon. It is secreted in response to high glucose levels. Once in the bloodstream, it promotes the uptake of glucose by cells to use in metabolism. Insulin also promotes conversion of excess glucose into glycogen for storage in the liver.

Delta cells secrete somatostatin, which inhibits the release of digestive hormones and insulin and glucagon.

Adrenal Glands

The adrenal glands are small pyramid-shaped structures on top of each kidney. Each adrenal gland has two parts: the outer cortex and inner medulla.

The cortex has three layers, each secreting a different class of molecules. The outermost layer secretes aldosterone. The middle layer secretes glucocorticoids such as cortisol, and the inner layer secretes androgens.

The adrenal medulla contains cells that are actually specialized postganglionic neurons controlled directly by the autonomic nervous system. These cells release epinephrine and norepinephrine in response to sympathetic stimulation. These two hormones have a variety of effects throughout the body consistent with sympathetic nervous system stimulation, such as an increased heart rate and bronchodilation.

Nutrition and Excretion

Gastrointestinal System

The gastrointestinal (GI) system receives and digests food, absorbing nutrients into the body, and excretes waste (Figure 8-50). The GI system consists of a long tract, essentially a tube, that runs from the mouth to the anus. When food enters the mouth, both mechanical and chemical digestion begin.

Mechanical digestion takes place through chewing, which crushes the food, and chemical digestion begins as enzymes secreted by the salivary glands begin to break down food. After chewing, food is swallowed, passing into the esophagus by way of the pharynx.

The esophagus is a muscular tube that runs from the oropharynx through the mediastinum and diaphragm to connect with the stomach. Food is moved down the esophagus by peristalsis, which is a series of rhythmic smooth muscle contractions that push food through the GI tract.

Stomach

The stomach is a muscular container found in the left upper quadrant of the abdomen. Small when empty, the stomach expands to accommodate food and liquid intake and then uses its strong muscles to continue mechanical digestion.

Cells in the lining of the stomach secrete large amounts of hydrochloric acid to continue chemical digestion. The lining of the stomach secretes other hormones important in digestion, as well: gastrin, which increases stomach secretions and movement; and intrinsic factor, which is important in vitamin B_{12} absorption.

Pepsinogen is an enzyme secreted by the stomach in inactive form. When pepsinogen encounters the acidic stomach environment, it is converted to pepsin, a powerful

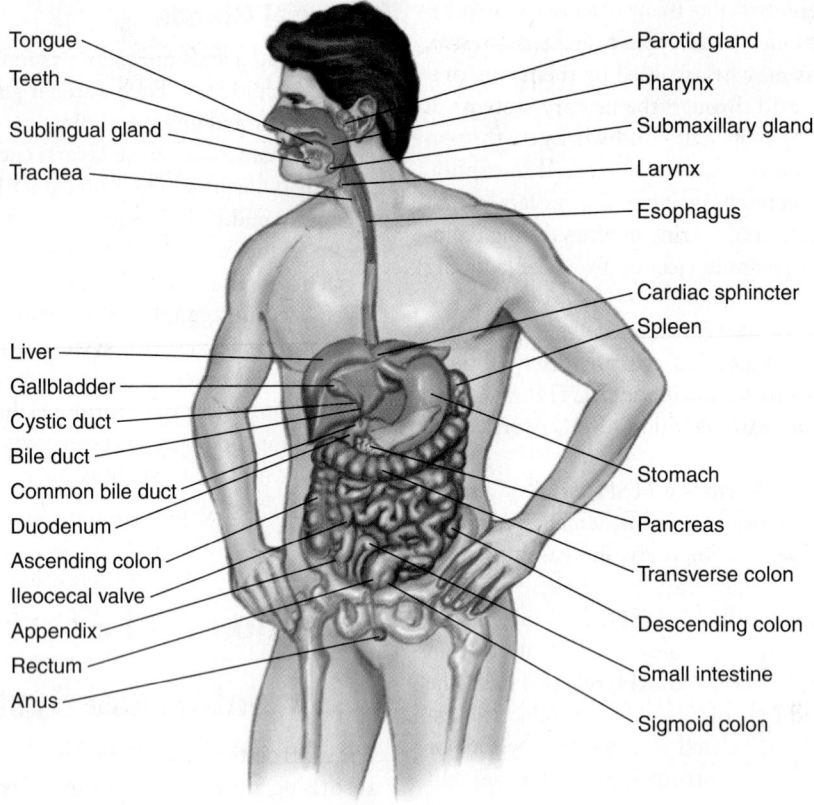

Tongue
Teeth
Sublingual gland
Trachea
Liver
Gallbladder
Cystic duct
Bile duct
Common bile duct
Duodenum
Ascending colon
Ileocecal valve
Appendix
Rectum
Anus

Parotid gland
Pharynx
Submaxillary gland
Larynx
Esophagus
Cardiac sphincter
Spleen
Stomach
Pancreas
Transverse colon
Descending colon
Small intestine
Sigmoid colon

FIGURE 8-50

The gastrointestinal system consists of the alimentary canal and accessory organs of digestion. The alimentary canal consists of the mouth, pharynx, esophagus, stomach, small intestine, large intestine (colon), rectum, and anus. The accessory organs include the salivary glands, liver, gallbladder, and pancreas.

enzyme that breaks down proteins. Ultimately, the stomach drains its semidigested contents, called *chyme*, into the first part of the small intestine, the duodenum.

Small Intestine

The small intestine begins at the outlet of the stomach, winding a 6-meter course through the abdomen. The small intestine is divided into three parts: the duodenum, jejunum, and ileum. Overall, the function of all three sections is to further chemically digest food and absorb nutrients across its border into the bloodstream. However, there are some specializations.

Each section of the small intestine accomplishes its function in a slightly different manner. The duodenum secretes cholecystokinin, a hormone that stimulates the release of enzymes and bile from the pancreas. Both substances enter the intestine through the common bile duct. Cholecystokinin also inhibits the stomach from producing more acid and digestive enzymes and induces a feeling of fullness, or satiety, in the person.

The jejunum and ileum make up the bulk of the small intestine and have major roles in absorbing nutrients. A large surface area that comes into contact with capillaries is needed to efficiently absorb nutrients. The endothelial lining

of these structures folds over itself and contains projections called **villi**. Both the folds and the villi increase the surface area for absorption. To even further increase surface area, the villi contain microvilli, another layer of folding.

Peristaltic contractions continue through the small intestine to continue to advance food to the next portion of the GI tract, the large intestine.

Large Intestine

The ileum of the small intestine connects to the large intestine by way of the ileocecal valve. The large intestine has six regions. It functions less to digest food than to absorb water and form and store stool. The appendix projects as a blind pouch from the first section, the cecum. The ascending colon follows, traveling up the right abdomen.

The colon makes a 90-degree turn, called the *hepatic flexure*, and continues across the abdomen from right to left as the transverse colon. At the splenic flexure, it again turns 90 degrees and travels down the left side of the abdomen as the descending colon. Finally, it travels posteriorly along a winding path as the sigmoid colon, which then transitions into the rectum.

Colonic tissue is different from that of the small intestine, reflecting its functional needs. Instead of being relatively narrow chambered with villi and microvilli to maximize surface area, the large intestine bulges in a series of sacs called *haustra*. Haustra store feces as it forms and slowly moves toward the rectum. Three strings of muscular tissue, the teniae coli, travel the lengths of the large intestine and pull the material into the haustra.

Accessory Organs of Digestion

The alimentary canal, or digestive tract, serves as both the conduit by which food passes through the body and a compartment for digestion to occur in. However, many of the enzymes used in digestion are produced by and stored in a variety of other abdominal organs, which are discussed here.

The accessory organs, along with the stomach and intestines, are held in place within the abdomen by mesenteries, which are folds of tissue that carry arteries and veins to and from the organs as well.

The peritoneum, a thin epithelial lining, surrounds most of the abdominal organs. Similar to the pleura and pericardium, the peritoneum consists of a visceral layer that is fixed to the organ surfaces and folds over itself to create a parietal layer. There is a small amount of peritoneal fluid between the two layers that lubricates the movements of the organs.

Some organs, such as the kidneys, part of the duodenum and pancreas, and the ascending and descending colon, are retroperitoneal and not within the peritoneal cavity.

Liver and Gallbladder

The liver is a large, solid organ in the right upper quadrant with a number of important functions. As discussed earlier, it receives all the blood returning from the digestive tract via the hepatic circulation to sort the absorbed nutrients, identify any pathogens, and eliminate toxins. Further, the cells of the liver store glucose in the form of glycogen and produce the **bile** that is used to emulsify (break up) fats.

Hepatocytes are the functional cells of the liver, performing the many tasks of the liver. They are arranged in a way that maximizes cell exposure to vessels for both blood and bile. A hepatic venule at the center of each lobule drains filtered blood into the hepatic vein for transport to the inferior vena cava. The hepatic artery delivers oxygenated blood to the liver cells. The hepatic portal vein brings nutrient-filled blood for filtration. The small bile duct serves as the avenue for bile produced and secreted by the hepatocytes to drain into the main bile duct.

The main bile duct travels inferiorly to the duodenum, but soon after exiting the liver, it puts off a branch called the *cystic duct* that travels to the gallbladder. The gallbladder is a small pouch tucked under the liver that stores bile for later use. Cholecystokinin secreted from the duodenum in response to fatty food intake stimulates the gallbladder to contract and release bile.

Pancreas

The exocrine tasks of the pancreas are performed by clusters of acini ducts that secrete digestive enzymes for transportation into the duodenum. The enzymes travel through the pancreatic duct, which empties into the common bile duct, allowing the secretions to share a passageway with bile.

The pancreas also secretes substantial amounts of bicarbonate into the duodenum to neutralize the acidity of the chyme.

Urinary System

The urinary system is considered in two parts: the kidneys, which comprise the renal system, and the urinary tract (Figure 8-51).

The kidneys function to maintain fluid and electrolyte balance, maintain blood pressure, and filter waste products from the blood. They accomplish this by filtering out large amounts of water and solutes, and then selectively allowing a portion of the water and some of the solutes to be reabsorbed into the body. The concentrated fluid that remains is eliminated from the kidney through the urinary tract as urine.

In males, some structures of the urinary tract and reproductive system are shared, while in females, they are separate.

Kidneys

The kidneys lie retroperitoneally in the flanks and are roughly 12 cm (4.5 to 5 inches) long. They are encapsulated organs, similar to the liver and spleen. Each has a hilum, or opening, on the medial aspect that allows the entry and exit of the vasculature and ureters.

The renal arteries, arising from the aorta, supply the kidneys with blood. Blood returns from the kidneys through the renal veins, which empty into the inferior vena cava. The kidney parenchyma is arranged into an outer cortex and inner medulla, along with functional divisions called *pyramids* that are packed with nephrons (Figure 8-52).

The peak of each pyramid points inward into one of several renal calyces, which in turn deposit urine into the renal pelvis. From the renal pelvis, urine drains into the ureters, which carry the urine to the bladder for storage. The bladder is emptied via the urethra, which is a short tube-like structure in females and a longer, winding structure in males.

Nephrons

Each kidney contains more than a million microscopic units called *nephrons*, whose responsibility is to filter blood, manage electrolytes, and excrete waste as urine. The majority of each nephron is found within the renal cortex, although parts of it dip deep into the medulla to concentrate the **filtrate** that becomes urine.

Each nephron is supplied by an arteriole (afferent arteriole) that arises from the branches of the renal artery

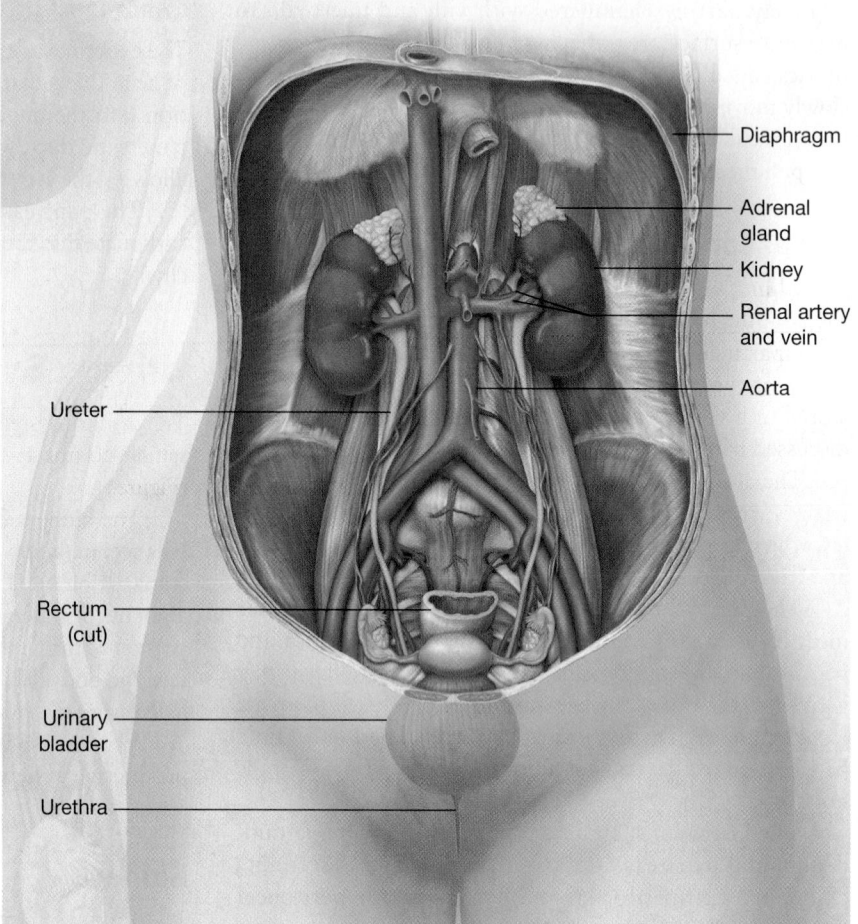

Diaphragm

Adrenal gland

Kidney

Renal artery and vein

Aorta

Ureter

Rectum (cut)

Urinary bladder

Urethra

FIGURE 8-51

The urinary system consists of the kidneys (renal system) and urinary tract (ureters, bladder, and urethra).

(Figure 8-53). This arteriole branches into a meshwork of capillaries called the *glomerulus* within a structure called the *Bowman capsule*, and then emerges as the efferent arteriole. This vascular arrangement is unique in that the capillary bed converges to form an arteriole, rather than a venule.

Fluid and solutes are filtered from the capillaries that form the glomerulus and then enter the system of tubules that handle the filtrate, allowing selective reabsorption of substances in the process of forming urine.

Together, the mesh of capillaries and the Bowman capsule is called the *renal corpuscle*. It is here that waste is filtered from the blood. The Bowman capsule receives the filtrate, and drains it into the proximal tubule, where significant reabsorption of molecules and electrolytes not meant to be excreted occurs. The tubule then shoots into the medulla as the descending limb of the loop of Henle, which eventually turns 180 degrees and returns to the cortex as the ascending loop. Once back in the cortex, the tubule becomes the distal convoluted tubule, which empties into the collecting duct.

Several nephrons drain filtrate into one collecting duct, which again travels deep into the medulla, where it connects with increasing numbers of other collecting ducts to eventually empty into a renal **calyx**.

The efferent arteriole that emerged from the glomerulus continues to travel alongside the proximal tubule and loop of Henle to allow for reabsorption of material from the filtrate. As it penetrates into the medulla around the loop, the blood vessels are called the *vasa recta*.

Just before the afferent arteriole enters the renal corpuscle, it forms the juxtaglomerular apparatus, along with the distal convoluted tubule that runs alongside it. Specialized cells in this region monitor blood pressure and fluid status of the body and secrete renin to manage blood pressure as described previously in the cardiovascular system.

Bladder and Urethra

The ureters insert into the bladder, a hollow and muscular organ found in the lower pelvis. Upon urination, the bladder contracts and urine passes through the urethra, a single tube that allows urine to exit the body.

In males, the urethra passes through the prostate, a gland that secretes a liquid medium in which sperm travels during ejaculation. Due to its anatomical location, enlargement of the prostate can impede urine flow in men. After passing through the prostate, the urethra travels the length

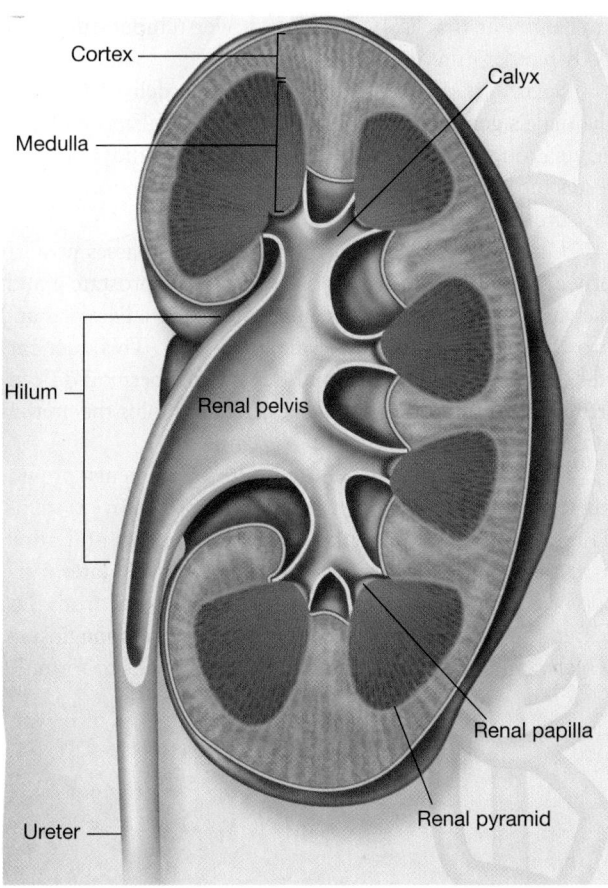

FIGURE 8-52

Internal anatomy of the kidney.

of the penis to open on its distal end. In females, the urethra is much shorter and opens to the environment just anterior to the vagina.

Acid–Base Buffer System

Similar to the way that respiratory rate changes affect the pH of the bloodstream by altering the amount of carbon dioxide retained, the kidneys affect pH through the secretion of bicarbonate.

Recall the chemical reactions of the carbonic acid buffer system that describe the transport of carbon dioxide in the blood:

$$CO_2 + H_2O \leftrightarrow H_2CO_3 \leftrightarrow H^+ + HCO_3^-$$

If the blood pH is decreased (meaning that there are too many free hydrogen ions, resulting in acidosis), the kidney will decrease excretion of bicarbonate from the blood. The bicarbonate binds to the excess hydrogen ions, thereby reducing free hydrogen ions and increasing pH.

In alkalotic states, the kidney allows excretion of excess bicarbonate, thereby allowing an increase in free hydrogen ions. The acid–base balancing systems of the respiratory system and kidneys balance each other, allowing for compensation and maintenance of homeostasis.

Respiratory rates can change quickly, and the blood levels of carbon dioxide can increase or decrease to modify the pH within minutes. However, the kidneys respond more slowly, changing the pH by increasing or decreasing bicarbonate excretion, which can take hours or even days.

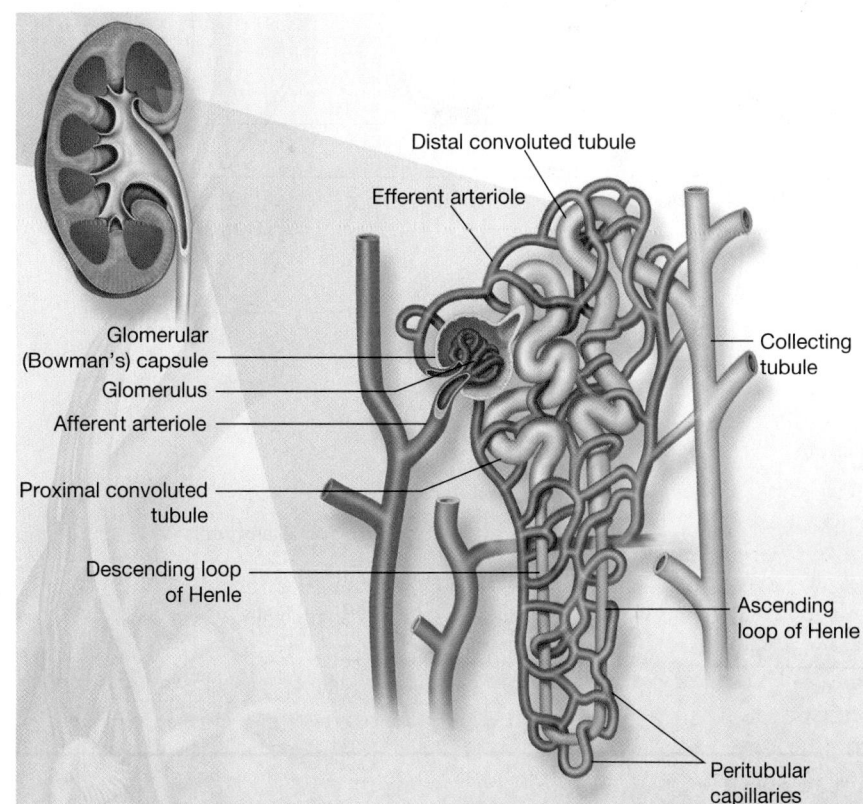

FIGURE 8-53

The basic functional unit of the kidney is the nephron.

Reproduction

Reproductive System

The reproductive system consists of the organs that allow for the storage of human DNA in the male and female sex cells, the sperm and egg. These highly specialized cells each carry one set of 23 chromosomes that will combine upon fertilization to become a full set of 46, which direct the development of a **zygote** to an **embryo**, to a **fetus** and beyond. Because of some sharing of structures with the urinary system in men, this reproductive system is often called the *genitourinary system*.

Male Reproductive System

The male reproductive system consists of the testicles, which produce the specialized sperm of the male, and various ducts that provide the fluid within which they travel (Figure 8-54). The testes are paired olive-size organs that reside within the scrotum. The scrotum is a sac of skin that hangs from the pelvis to provide the testes with an ideal sperm-producing

environment that is at a slightly lower temperature than body temperature.

Sperm are unique flagellated cells that deliver a copy of the male's genome to the female egg for fertilization. Upon ejaculation, the sperm are ejected from the epididymis of the testes into the vas deferens, which passes superiorly out of the scrotum and into the abdomen.

Once in the abdomen, the vas deferens passes posteriorly around the bladder. Upon reaching the prostate gland, the vas deferens receives ducts from the seminal vesicles and prostate, and becomes the ejaculatory duct. This duct carries the now complete seminal fluid, with sperm and fluids from the prostate and seminal vesicles, and joins the urethra at the base of the penis.

The urethra runs the entire length of the penis, providing functions for both the urinary and reproductive systems. Three distinct components comprise the penis and allow it to function. The corpora cavernosa are two lateral tissue beds that engorge with blood during sexual arousal to stiffen the penis. Between them lies the corpus spongiosum, which contains the urethra and distally expands to form the

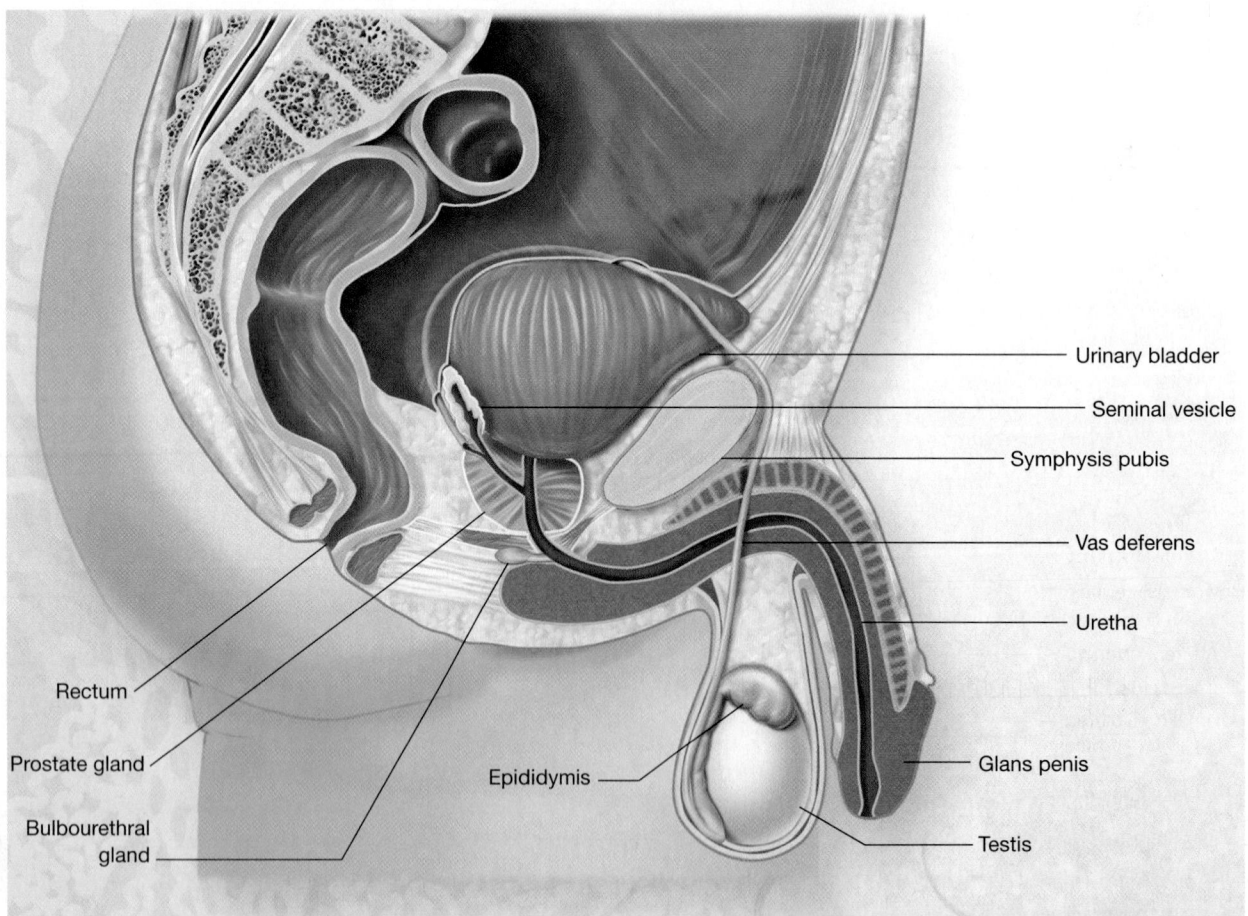

FIGURE 8-54

The male reproductive organs.

glans penis. The glans penis is the most distal end and is the site of the urethral opening.

Testosterone is a steroid (cholesterol-based) hormone secreted from the testes that stimulates the growth of male sexual organs and secondary sex characteristics, such as facial and body hair. Testosterone also supports the growth of muscle and bone both in puberty and throughout adult life.

Female Reproductive System

The female reproductive system not only must produce the female gamete, but also must carry and support the development of a fetus for roughly 40 weeks after fertilization (Figure 8-55). The ovaries are two small oval organs situated bilaterally in the lower abdomen. Each ovary contains oocytes (egg cells) that carry a copy of the female genome. Each month, an oocyte will mature into an egg under the influence of hormones from the pituitary gland.

During each month of childbearing years a mature egg, or ovum, will be ejected from an ovary into one of the two fallopian tubes (Figure 8-56). The tubes are paired structures that collect the egg after release with its fimbriae, long fingerlike projections. The fimbriae pass the egg into the tube, within which the rhythmic beating of cilia push the egg into the uterus.

The uterus is a muscular organ situated in the center of the pelvis. The fallopian tubes enter the uterus at each side, superiorly. The inferior portion of the uterus, the cervix, projects into the upper portion of the vagina.

The inner layer of the uterus is called the *endometrium*, which undergoes a monthly cycle of growth in preparation of possible fertilization. If fertilization does not occur, the tissue sloughs off, resulting in menstrual flow, which lasts three to five days.

The myometrium is a smooth muscle layer, which is surrounded by the perimetrium and then visceral peritoneum. The myometrium undergoes additional development during pregnancy to allow the strong, regular contractions that expel the fetus from the birth canal. The uterus and fallopian tubes are supported by a number of ligaments within the lower abdomen and pelvis.

The vagina is a canal that extends from the inferior pole of the uterus to its external orifice between the anus and urethral opening. The vagina receives the penis during intercourse, allows discharge of shed endometrium and blood during menstruation, and serves as the birth canal during childbirth. The area surrounding the

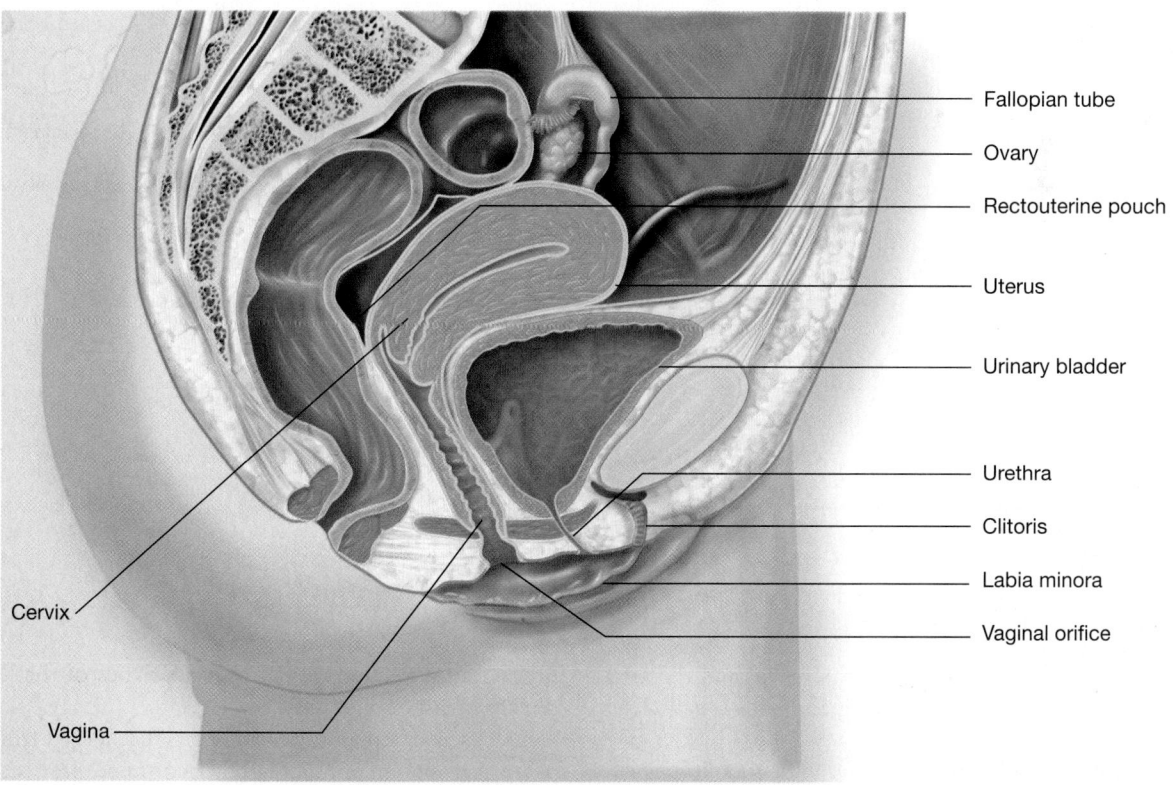

FIGURE 8-55

The female reproductive organs.

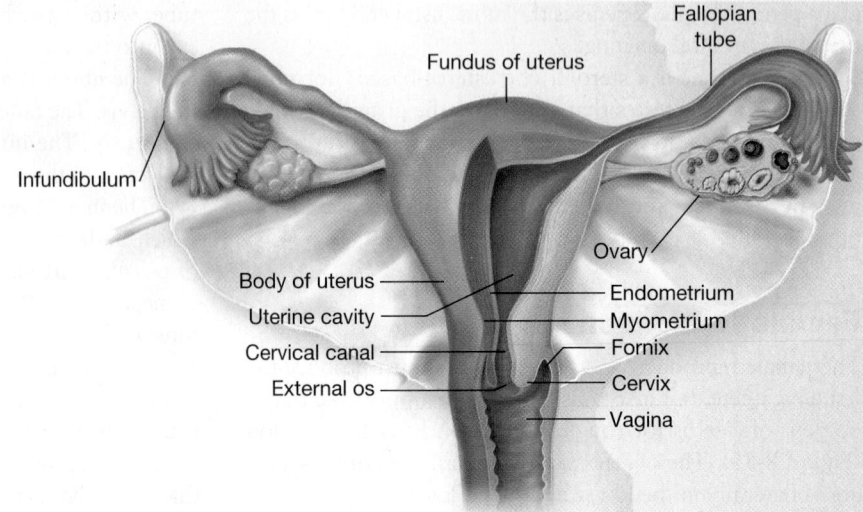

FIGURE 8-56

The uterus and ovaries.

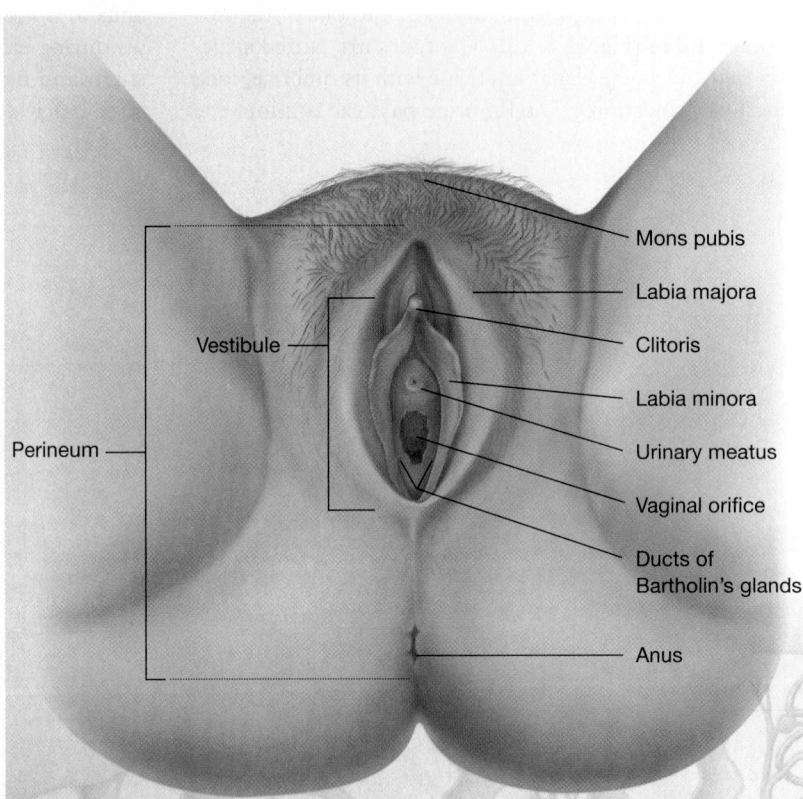

FIGURE 8-57

Female external genitalia.

external opening of the vagina is the vulva, and the area of skin between the vaginal opening and anus is called the *perineum* (Figure 8-57).

The ovaries and testes both have endocrine functions, as well as the ability to produce gametes (ova and spermatazoa, respectively). The ovaries produce estrogen, a steroid hormone, in response to stimulation from anterior pituitary hormones. Analogous to testosterone in males, estrogen produces the secondary sex characteristics of the female such as breast development.

Cells that remain after an egg is discharged from the ovary at ovulation produce another hormone, progesterone. Progesterone stimulates the uterine walls to thicken in preparation for possible fertilization and zygote implantation. If fertilization does not occur, progesterone levels drop each month to allow for menstruation.

CASE STUDY WRAP-UP

Clinical-Reasoning Process

Advanced EMTs Elaine and Atul are caring for 17-year-old Edward Lampey, who has multiple gunshot wounds. Edward is confused and has pale, cool, sweaty skin. He is having difficulty breathing and has a weak, rapid carotid pulse. The most significant external blood loss is coming from the wound in his left groin, but he also has wounds to his upper right chest, and upper right abdomen.

Elaine and Atul use their knowledge of anatomy to suspect that Edward's upper right chest wound could have injured the right lung, which is one explanation for his difficulty breathing. They also know that major blood vessels and nerves lie in the thoracic cavity. The upper right abdomen contains the liver, which has a significant blood supply, as well as blood vessels and portions of other organs. Therefore, Edward's total blood loss could be much greater than the amount noted from the groin wound. The groin wound itself is concerning because the femoral artery, vein, and nerve run through this area.

Edward has lost a lot of blood, and therefore the ability to carry enough oxygen to his cells. The body initially attempts to compensate for decreased blood volume by increasing the heart rate and constricting blood vessels in nonvital areas of the body. The respiratory rate is increased in response to decreased oxygen levels in the blood. However, the ongoing blood loss eventually outpaces the body's ability to compensate. The low blood volume results in a weak pulse.

Elaine and Atul recognize that Edward has immediate threats to life. The lack of oxygen means that less cellular energy is produced and acidic waste products are accumulating. Without sufficient energy to maintain cells, they will start to die. When enough cells die, tissues, organs, and systems begin to fail. Without intervention, death will follow. Edward needs more oxygen at the cellular level. He needs supplemental oxygen and, perhaps, assistance with ventilation. The wound in Edward's chest must be covered to prevent air from being sucked into the chest on inspiration. The external bleeding must be controlled and Elaine and Atul must treat Edward for shock. Most of all, Edward needs rapid transport to a trauma center, where he can receive blood and undergo surgery to repair his injuries.

CHAPTER REVIEW

Chapter Summary

The human body is remarkable in its complex structure and function. Its systems work together, allowing it to maintain homeostasis despite the effects of illness and injury and changes in the environment. Your ability to distinguish abnormal structure and function from normal is the first step in recognizing that a patient is sick or injured.

Interruptions in some of the body's structures and functions can result in immediately life-threatening conditions. You must be able to picture how such impairments lead to cell damage and death and, ultimately, the patient's death. This understanding makes learning what you will need to do as an Advanced EMT to attempt to restore homeostasis much easier than if you were to simply try to memorize lists of treatments. Understanding the roles of the respiratory, nervous, cardiovascular, and endocrine systems is particularly critical, because you must recognize specific emergencies involving these systems and formulate appropriate treatment plans for them.

Review Questions

Multiple-Choice Questions

1. The simplest unit of a chemical element is a(n):

a. molecule.

b. compound.

c. atom.

d. proton.

2. A substance that separates into its component ions when placed in a solution is a(n):

a. cation.

b. electrolyte.

c. phospholipid.

d. atom.

3. The largest proportion of water in the body is located:
   a. within cells.
   b. between cells.
   c. in the lymphatic system.
   d. in the blood vessel.

4. Which one of the following saline solutions is hypertonic with respect to body fluids?
   a. 0.25 percent
   c. 0.9 percent
   b. 0.45 percent
   d. 2 percent

5. When a red blood cell is placed in a solution, water moves into the cell. Therefore, the surrounding solution must be:
   a. hypertonic.
   c. bradytonic.
   b. hypotonic.
   d. isotonic.

6. The primary substance used by cells to create energy in the form of ATP is:
   a. fats.
   c. alcohol.
   b. proteins.
   d. glucose.

7. A decrease in pH (acidosis) occurs when there is excess:
   a. hydrogen.
   c. sodium.
   b. potassium.
   d. bicarbonate.

8. The state in which there is a difference in electrical charge on either side of the cell membrane, creating a membrane potential, is called:
   a. depolarization.
   c. isopolarization.
   b. repolarization.
   d. polarization.

9. The fluid that fills the inside of cells is called:
   a. endoplasmic reticulum.
   b. cytoplasm.
   c. phospholipid.
   d. centriole.

10. The spinal cord is contained in the _____ cavity.
    a. dorsal
    c. thoracic
    b. cranial
    d. ventral

11. The tissue that covers bone ends at joints to cushion them and provide for smooth movement is called:
    a. tendon.
    c. cartilage.
    b. ligament.
    d. endothelium.

12. The end of a long bone is called the:
    a. medullary cavity.
    c. metaphysis.
    b. epiphysis.
    d. diaphysis.

13. The uppermost portion of the spine is the _____ spine.
    a. sacral
    c. cervical
    b. coccygeal
    d. lumbar

14. The joint in the midline of the anterior pelvis is the:
    a. symphysis pubis.
    c. acetabulum.
    b. sacroiliac.
    d. glenoid fossa.

15. In which one of the following structures would you find smooth muscle?
    a. Heart
    c. Spinal cord
    b. Thigh
    d. Intestine

16. In which one of the following ways is most of the carbon dioxide in the body transported?
    a. As $PaCO_2$
    b. Dissolved in plasma
    c. Bound to hemoglobin
    d. In the form of bicarbonate

17. The mechanical process by which air moves in and out of the lungs is:
    a. external respiration.
    c. inspiration.
    b. internal respiration.
    d. ventilation.

18. For the average person, what is the amount of air available for gas exchange in normal ventilation?
    a. 150 mL
    c. 500 mL
    b. 350 mL
    d. 650 mL

19. Which one of the following occurs to allow long-term adaptation to living at a higher altitude?
    a. Increased red blood cells
    b. Increased respiratory rate
    c. Increased tidal volume
    d. Increased residual volume

20. The heart valve between the left atrium and ventricle is the _____ valve.
    a. bicuspid (mitral)
    c. left semilunar
    b. tricuspid
    d. pulmonic

21. Cardiac impulses normally originate in the:
    a. medulla oblongata.
    b. sinoatrial node.
    c. atrioventricular node.
    d. Purkinje fibers.

22. The amount of blood ejected from the heart every minute is the:
    a. stroke volume.
    c. preload.
    b. pulse pressure.
    d. cardiac output.

23. The phenomenon in which increased return of blood to the heart results in more forceful contraction of the heart is called _____ law.
    a. Boyle's
    c. Newton's first
    b. Frank–Starling's
    d. Cushing's

24. The neurotransmitter for the voluntary nervous system, preganglionic sympathetic nervous system, and pre- and postganglionic parasympathetic nervous system is:
    a. ADP.
    c. norepinephrine.
    b. serotonin.
    d. ACh.

25. The gap between axon terminals of a neuron and the cell adjacent to it is the:
    a. Nissl body.
    c. synapse.
    b. myelin sheath.
    d. interneuron.

26. The area of the brain in which decision-making functions occur is the:

   a. cerebellum.
   b. frontal lobe.
   c. reticular activating system.
   d. thalamus.

27. The gland that serves as the master gland of the endocrine system, secreting hormones that control other endocrine glands, is the _____ gland.

   a. thyroid   c. pituitary
   b. pineal   d. thymus

28. The pancreatic hormone secreted in response to low blood glucose levels is:

   a. glucagon.   c. somatostatin.
   b. aldosterone.   d. insulin.

29. The first portion of the small intestine is the:

   a. cecum.   c. ileum.
   b. duodenum.   d. sigmoid colon.

30. The basic unit of the kidney is the:

   a. nephron.   c. papilla.
   b. calyx.   d. medulla.

31. Sperm are produced by the:

   a. vas deferens.   c. scrotum.
   b. urethra.   d. testes.

32. During menstruation, the _____ is shed.

   a. perimetrium   c. myometrium
   b. endometrium   d. fertilized ovum

Critical-Thinking Questions

33. Explain how failure of the sodium/potassium pump, as would occur in the presence of inadequate oxygen, leads to cell death.

34. Why is oxygen required for metabolism?

35. Explain how the contraction of skeletal muscle results in movement.

36. Explain how the relationship between changes in thoracic volume and air pressure result in ventilation.

37. What is the respiratory membrane?

38. Why is it important to have a high PaO_2 in the alveoli?

39. What is the relationship between antigens and antibodies?

40. What are the factors that determine blood pressure?

41. What is the hepatic portal circulation? What is its purpose?

42. Contrast the actions of the sympathetic nervous system with those of the parasympathetic nervous system.

43. What is the role of the pancreas in digestion?

44. What is the kidney's role in blood pressure regulation?

Additional Reading

Martini, F. H., Bartholomew, E. F., & Bledsoe, B. E. (2008). *Anatomy and physiology for emergency care.* Upper Saddle River, NJ: Pearson Prentice Hall.

Moore, K. L., & Agur, A. M. (2007). *Essential clinical anatomy* (3rd ed.). Philadelphia, PA: Lippincott, Williams, & Wilkins.

Netter, F. H. (2006). *Atlas of human anatomy* (4th ed.). Philadelphia, PA: Saunders/Elsevier.

9 Life Span Development and Cultural Considerations

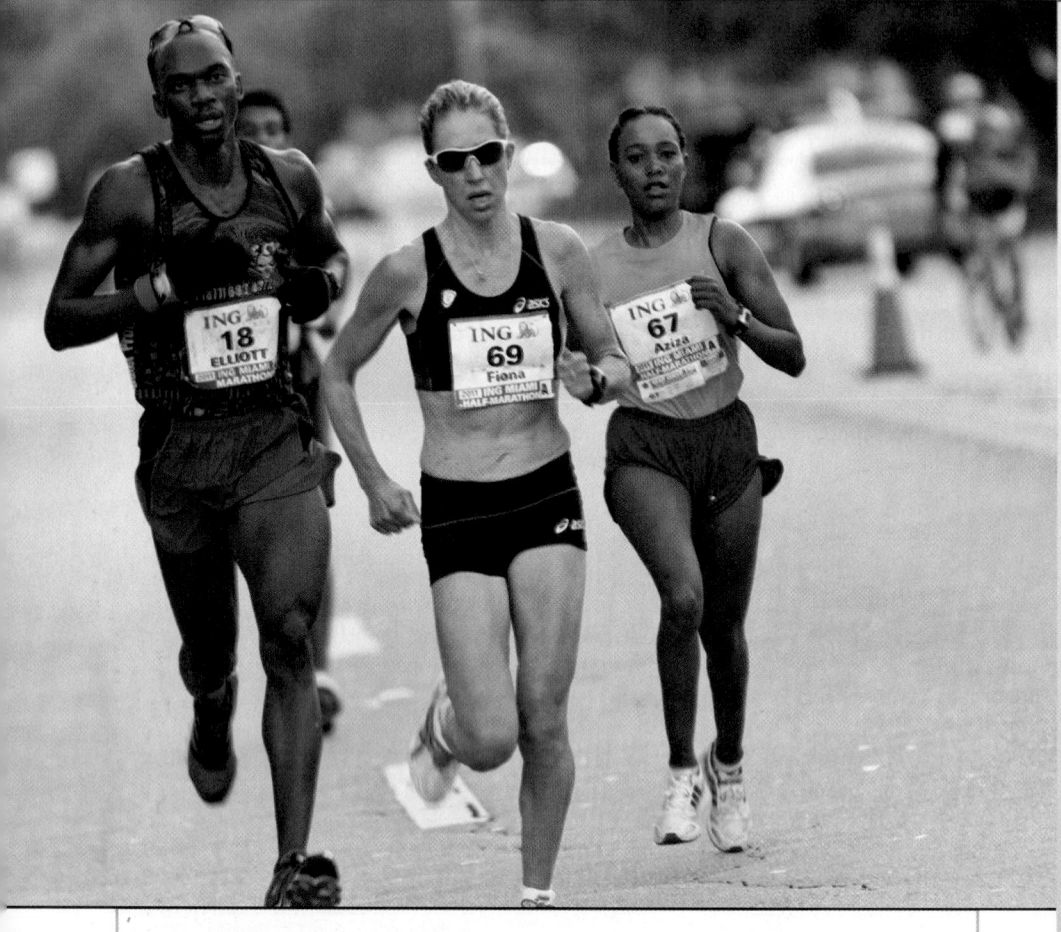

Content Areas: Preparatory; Life Span Development

Advanced EMT Education Standards:
- The Advanced EMT applies fundamental knowledge of the EMS system, safety/well-being of the Advanced EMT, and medical-legal and ethical issues to the provision of emergency care.
- The Advanced EMT applies fundamental knowledge of life span development to patient assessment and management.

Objectives

After reading this chapter, you should be able to:

9.1   Define key terms introduced in this chapter.

9.2   Identify the age ranges associated with each of the following age classifications: neonate, infant, toddler, preschooler, school age, adolescent, early adulthood, middle adulthood, and late adulthood.

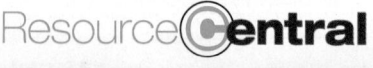

To access Resource Central, follow the directions on the Student Access Card provided with this text. If there is no card, go to www.bradybooks.com and follow the Resource Central link to Buy Access. Under Media Resources, you will find:
- *The Changing Brain.* Watch a video and discover how the remarkable brain changes throughout the lifespan.
- *School-Age Children.* Learn the importance of fostering healthy living from a young age.
- *They Grow Like Weeds!* View the rapidly changing first year of life as an infant achieves major milestones.

CASE STUDY

Advanced EMTs Jeremy House and Dee Ann Pointer are responding to Klondike Elementary School for an injured eight-year-old child on the playground. After confirming the call with dispatch, Jeremy says, "I feel so awkward on calls with kids. I never know what to say to them."

"You'll do fine," responds Dee Ann. "If you get stuck, I'll help you. This kiddo is a school ager. As long as you explain things so she can understand them, she is likely to be cooperative and I'm pretty sure she won't bite you!"

Arriving on the scene, Jeremy and Dee Ann look for potential hazards. The principal, Ms. Baldridge, meets them at the front of the school and leads them to the playground. "The student's name is Emma Rand. She fell with her arms out when she jumped off the swings. It looks like her left arm is broken. Her dad is on the way. He should be here in 5 or so minutes."

Jeremy approaches Emma, who is sitting on the ground, holding her left arm against her chest with her right hand. Emma is visibly upset, but her skin color is good and there are no other obvious signs of injury. Squatting down to Emma's level, Jeremy says, "Hi Emma. I'm Jeremy and this is my partner, Dee Ann. We work on the ambulance and we're here to take a look at your arm. Can you tell me what happened?"

Problem-Solving Questions

1. What communication strategies will be most helpful for Jeremy and Dee Ann in gaining Emma's trust and cooperation?
2. What do you anticipate Emma's greatest concerns might be?
3. How do you expect Emma's vital signs to compare with those of an adult?

9.3	Describe the physiologic adaptations that occur immediately after birth.
9.4	Discuss the key physical and psychosocial characteristics and concerns of individuals in each age classification.
9.5	Describe reactions to loss, death, and dying, including stages of grief.
9.6	Demonstrate awareness of health beliefs of different cultures.
9.7	Adapt communication strategies to patients of different cultural backgrounds.
9.8	Display cultural sensitivity in interactions with patients of different ethnicities.

Introduction

Author Anais Nin said, "We don't see things as they are, we see them as we are." Each person has a unique life history and circumstances that shape who he is and how he sees things. This makes it difficult for us to see things exactly the way another person sees them. Fortunately, for all our uniqueness, we also share similarities that allow us to make sense of the world and those around us. If we were not able to see things at all as others see them, we would not be able to relate to other people or share ideas with them. The way we see things is shaped not only by our individual personalities and biographies, but also by predictable changes in perspective that occur at various stages in life. The cultures with which each person identifies also shape his beliefs, values, and expectations for the behavior of others.

As a health care provider, you must establish rapport with patients and their families, as well as with coworkers and others with whom you interact. It is critical to understand how psychosocial development and culture affect how patients interpret your actions, and how your background affects your interpretation of their actions.

Most of the discussion in EMS textbooks focuses on the average patient: a 70-kg adult male. In many ways, that knowledge serves you well. But patients vary anatomically and physiologically, as well as psychosocially and culturally. What is true on the average is not necessarily true for a given individual. Certain differences are anticipated based on gender, size, and age. In particular, newborns, infants, and children are not just smaller versions of adults. Their anatomical proportions are different. In some ways, their bodies are physiologically very efficient; in others, they lack the maturity to adjust as well as adults do. Later in life, age-related decline of body structures and functions affect the body's ability to maintain homeostasis in the face of injury and illness, the way drugs are metabolized, types of injury patterns expected, and many other variables.

This chapter presents you with information about some of the variations among people that can affect your interactions with them and your assessment and differential diagnosis processes.

Psychosocial Development

Psychosocial development is the psychological maturation that takes place through a person's interactions in a social context. It describes the relationship between a person and his social environment at different points in the lifespan. Aspects include how information is perceived, the mental operations we perform to make sense of the information, how we communicate with others, and how we decide whether things are right or wrong. Two of the most well-known theories of psychosocial development are those of the Swiss psychologist Jean Piaget and the psychoanalyst Erik Erikson.

Piaget's theory explains stages of development from birth to adulthood, but does not account for continued psychosocial development throughout adulthood. Because Piaget's theory focuses on children, it gives emphasis to cognitive development as well as moral and other aspects of development. Erikson's theory explains the stages of development from infancy through adulthood, focusing on a psychosocial conflict that must be resolved at each stage. Lawrence Kohlberg's theory of moral development enhances understanding of psychosocial development. It extends Piaget's theory and explains continued moral development throughout the life span.

Piaget's Theory of Cognitive Development

As with all patients, it is important to see things from the child's perspective to establish rapport. Piaget's theory divides childhood development into four stages that are based on how the child understands the world (Table 9-1). At each stage, children have different explanations for how things occur, based on their level of cognitive development. Some of Piaget's key concepts include schemas (mental representations of categories of knowledge) and assimilation (fitting new information to what is already known).

Children understand things in terms of what they currently know, as illustrated by the following anecdote: A young child hears his mother say she plans to buy something for the garden, which she calls a crape myrtle (a tree). Having no familiarity with a tree by this name, the child interprets the word in terms of what he and other young children do know about (his schema), and tells his father that they are going to buy a "great turtle" to put in the garden. The child assimilated the words said by his mother and made them fit his schema. You have most likely had similar experiences with children in which their understanding of something you took for granted takes you by surprise. Although it is difficult to anticipate exactly how a child's schema might look, it is still important to have awareness that they may have a very different understanding than you do about what is going on.

Erikson's Theory of Psychosocial Development

In Erikson's eight-stage theory, each stage occurs sequentially, but is less strictly tied to specific ages, especially in adulthood (Table 9-2). Personality develops throughout life, and is shaped by the resolution of basic psychosocial

---

TABLE 9-1   Piaget's Stages of Cognitive Development

Stage	Age	Description
Sensorimotor	Birth to two years (infancy)	The infant has limited but developing knowledge and understanding of the world. The primary way of interacting with the world is through senses and motor skills. Toward the end of the sensorimotor period, the use of symbols to communicate (language skills) develop.
Preoperational	Two to seven years (toddler, preschooler, early school age)	Language skills continue to develop and memory and imagination develop. Thoughts occur in relationship to oneself (egocentric and illogical thought).
Concrete operational	Seven years to adolescence (school age to early adolescence)	The child uses symbols to think about concrete concepts, such as measurements.
Formal operational	Adolescence and adulthood	Many adults do not reach this stage and do not think abstractly in adulthood.

TABLE 9-2	Erikson's Stages of Psychosocial Development	
Psychosocial Stage/Outcome	**Approximate Age**	**Description**
Trust vs. mistrust	Infancy (birth to 1½ years)	Infants must have their physical and emotional needs met in order to develop trusting relationships. If needs are not met, the individual is less able to feel hope. Overprotectiveness can lead to misplaced trust.
Autonomy vs. shame	Toddler (1 to 3 years)	Toddlers must learn the right balance between self-reliance and limits, based on parental reactions. The sense of confidence and independent thought develops if the conflict is resolved successfully and the child develops self-control, resourcefulness, and courage. Without successful resolution, the individual may lack confidence and a sense of self.
Initiative vs. guilt	Preschooler (3 to 6 years)	The approval or disapproval of parents and others either give individuals the ability to take initiative to create and accomplish tasks, or make them feel guilty or incompetent about their ideas and efforts. There must be a balance between allowing the child to experiment and learn through trial and error and keeping the child safe and giving him a realistic view of the consequences of mistakes. Successful resolution at this stage of development leads to a sense of purpose.
Industry vs. inferiority	School age (5 to 12 years)	Children who are allowed to find and develop talents and learn skills (including skills needed for academic success) develop a sense of competence, unique strengths, and potential. Children who are denied opportunities feel inferior and develop low self-esteem. Parents remain important at this stage, but children also must be accepted by peers to develop confidence and self-esteem.
Identity vs. role confusion	Adolescence (onset of puberty to 18 years)	Adolescents strive to develop a sense of who they are and their place in the world. Acceptance by peers and others is important, yet adolescents must develop a sense of independence. Developing morality and a lack of life experience can lead to periods of idealism.
Intimacy vs. isolation	Young adult (18 to 40 years)	This is the stage in life in which individuals seek a significant other and start families. Failure to secure stable relationships results in feelings of loneliness and isolation.
Generativity vs. stagnation	Middle adult (40 to 65 years)	The focus is on successful parenting as children mature, and finding satisfying work and ways to express creativity. The challenge is to contribute back to family and society and to avoid becoming self-absorbed and self-indulgent. Without an outlet through which to give back, growth stagnates.
Integrity vs. despair	Older age (>65 years)	Successful resolution of the psychosocial conflict results in feelings of satisfaction and accomplishment in life. Without successful resolution, there is a sense of bitterness over lost opportunities.

conflicts at each of the eight stages. For example, in the first stage, during about the first year of life, the conflict to be resolved is that of trust versus mistrust. The infant whose needs for comfort, food, and so on are met will develop the ability to trust. The infant whose needs are not met will become mistrustful. A significant event in life, such as divorce or loss of a job can bring up a conflict that was resolved in the past.

Kohlberg's Theory of Moral Development

Theories of moral development help in understanding certain behaviors. Kohlberg's theory explains the reasoning behind moral decisions at various stages of development.

According to this theory, moral development occurs in three levels, each with two stages (Table 9-3). The theory is loosely tied to age, but not all adults progress through all stages of moral development. People only move from one stage to the next when they realize that their current way of thinking about moral dilemmas is inadequate.

Physical Development

After about 40 weeks of gestation, the **neonate**, or newborn, must make immediate physiologic adjustments at birth. He has been dependent on his mother for oxygen, elimination of carbon dioxide, and delivery of nutrients directly to the bloodstream. (See Chapter 43.) At birth, the lungs must

TABLE 9-3   Kohlberg's Stages of Moral Development

LEVEL I: PRECONVENTIONAL MORALITY

Stage 1: Obedience and punishment	At this stage, actions are either good or bad, based on their physical consequences. For example, throwing rocks at the neighbor's house is not considered wrong unless a window was broken in the process. Decisions are made to avoid punishment and show deference to power and authority. For example, a certain behavior is done, "Because Mom said so."
Stage 2: Individualism and exchange (instrumental relativist)	What an individual views as right is determined by what he perceives as good for him, and sometimes what is good for others. Decisions about actions toward others are guided by a *quid pro quo* (you scratch my back and I'll scratch yours) mentality, but the exchange must be very concrete and relatively immediate.

LEVEL II: CONVENTIONAL MORALITY

Stage 3: Interpersonal relationships (interpersonal concordance)	Whether behavior is judged right or wrong is based on what is perceived as approved by the social group ("Everyone else is doing it"). Approval is achieved by "being nice," and doing what is helpful or pleasing to others.
Stage 4: Maintaining social order (law and order orientation)	There is loyalty to the structures that maintain social order. Actions are judged according to whether they are within or against the law or rules in place. Rules are important for determining acceptable conduct.

LEVEL III: POSTCONVENTIONAL MORALITY

Stage 5: Social contract and individual rights	Right and wrong are determined by what has been agreed upon by society, but there is awareness that, through proper procedure, laws and rules can be changed.
Stage 6: Universal principles	Decisions are made according to abstract, self-chosen, ethical principles. The guiding principles at this level are respect for the dignity of human beings, justice, reciprocity, and equality.

begin to take in air, and blood that was once diverted from the pulmonary circulation must now flow through the lungs for oxygenation and carbon dioxide elimination. Blood that once largely bypassed the gastrointestinal tract must now circulate through it to pick up nutrients and deliver them to the liver for processing.

In the first months of life, the **infant** continues to develop at an astounding rate cognitively, emotionally, and physically (Table 9-4). Children continue in their social, emotional, cognitive, and physical development through **toddler, preschooler, school-age,** and **adolescent** years.

The body functions well through young adulthood. Some age-related changes become noticeable in middle adulthood, and they become more pronounced in late adulthood. With age-related decline of body systems, we become less able to maintain homeostasis. The same illnesses and injuries the body could easily overcome in young adulthood pose a greater risk of morbidity and mortality to older adults. The maximum **life span** of human beings is about 120 years. However, our **life expectancy** is much lower, currently 77.9 years on the average in the United States (Centers for Disease Control and Prevention, National Center for Health Statistics, 2010). Life expectancy is affected by gender, genetics, environment, and behavior. Life expectancy is different for different cohorts of individuals, depending on their year of birth, and is influenced by cultural differences, such as diet and other health behaviors.

Through the life span, anatomy and physiology differ in significant ways. Knowledge of the differences in normal vital signs and other findings between age groups helps you determine whether there is cause for concern in the findings of your assessment (Table 9-5). The heart rate of a newborn is expected to be between 100 and 160 beats per minute immediately after birth. Whereas a heart rate of 160 might lead to heart failure in an elderly patient, a heart rate of 80 cannot provide adequate cardiac output for a newborn.

Neonates and Infants

A neonate, or newborn, is a child from the time he is born until he is one month of age (Figure 9-1). From one month of age to one year of age, the child is referred to as an infant (Figure 9-2). During the first year, the rapidly growing infant is expected to achieve several developmental milestones (Table 9-6). The average birth weight is 3.0 to 3.5 kg (6.6 to 7.7 lb). In the first week, newborns lose 5 to 10 percent of their birth weight, in large part due to the loss of excess body fluids. Overall, neonates and infants have immature body systems. Developmental priority is given to the organ systems that need to be more fully developed at birth. The kidneys and liver do not function the same way they will as the child continues to grow and develop. The liver is large for the size of the abdomen, meaning that

TABLE 9-4 Average Heights and Weights by Age

Age	MALE Height in Inches	MALE Weight in Pounds	FEMALE Height in Inches	FEMALE Weight in Pounds
Birth	19.75	8	19.5	7.5
3 months	24	13	23.5	12
6 months	26.5	17.5	25.5	16
12 months	29.5	22.5	29	21
18 months	33	26	32	24.5
2 years	34.5	28	34	27
3 years	39.5	31.5	37.5	30.5
4 years	40	36	40	34
5 years	43	41	42	40
6 years	45.5	46	45	44
7 years	58	51	48	50
8 years	50.5	56	50	56
9 years	52.5	62	52	64
10 years	55	70	54	72
11 years	56.5	80	57	82
12 years	59	90	59	92
13 years	61	100	62	100
14 years	64.5	112	63	110
15 years	67	124	64	115
16 years	68.5	135	64	120
17 years	69	142	64	122
18 years	69.5	149	64	125
19 years	69.75	152	64	126
20 years	69.75	156	64	128

TABLE 9-5 Normal Vital Signs for Each Age Group

Age Group	Respiratory Rate (per minute)	Heart Rate (per minute)	Systolic Blood Pressure in mmHg	Temperature in °F
Newborn	30 to 60	100 to 180	70 to 90	98 to 100
Infant	25 to 40	100 to 160	70 to 90	98 to 100
Toddler	24 to 30	80 to 130	72 to 100	98.6 to 99.6
Preschooler	22 to 34	80 to 120	78 to 104	98.6 to 99.6
School age	18 to 30	70 to 110	80 to 115	98.6
Adolescent	12 to 20	60 to 105	88 to 120	98.6
Adult	16 to 20	60 to 100	≤120	98.6

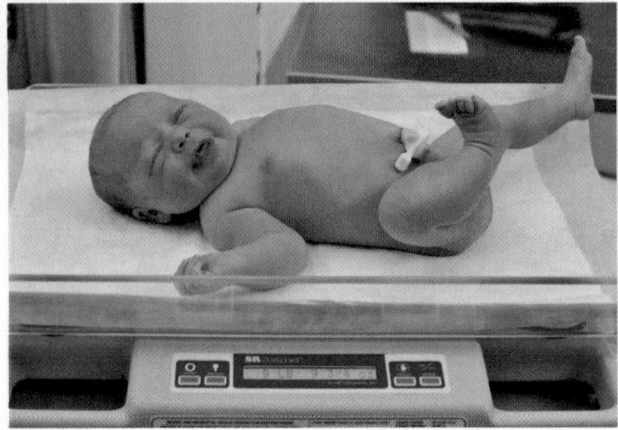

FIGURE 9-1

A neonate.

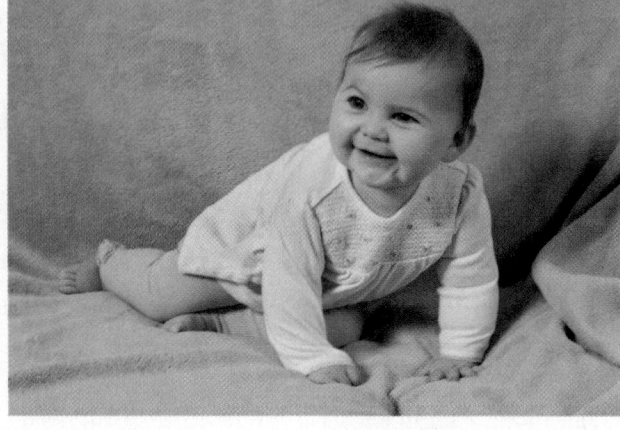

FIGURE 9-2

An infant.

TABLE 9-6 **Developmental Milestones**

Birth	3 Months	7 Months	12 Months	24 Months	36 Months
Reflexes: startle (moro), grasping, rooting, sucking	Has a social smile Raises head when lying on stomach Supports upper body with arms when lying on stomach Stretches out legs and kicks Watches faces and recognizes familiar objects from a distance Reaches for toys Turns head toward sounds	Enjoys social play Responds to others' emotions Interested in mirror images Struggles to get objects out of reach Responds to name and "no" Babbles chains of sounds Rolls over Sits without support	Shy or anxious around strangers Cries when separated from parents Crawls Walks (alone or with help) Says "mama" and "dada" Feeds self finger foods Begins to use objects (hair brush, telephone, etc., correctly) Uses a pincer grasp Bangs objects together	Excited about company of other children Imitates behavior Demonstrates more independence, some defiant behavior Sorts objects Begins make-believe play Uses simple sentences Pulls toys Kicks a ball Scribbles	Affectionate Plays make-believe Puts together simple puzzles Climbs Pedals a tricycle More developed language and fine motor skills

abdominal muscles and ribs do not protect it as well as in adults. The kidneys do not efficiently concentrate urine. The bones are softer and less well formed. The skeletal muscle mass is small, providing less strength, protection, and heat production.

At birth and throughout infancy, the head is disproportionately large. The neck is weak, and newborns are not able to hold up their heads on their own. The head comprises about 25 percent of the body weight at this age. Two **fontanels** can be felt beneath the scalp. They are membranes that allow the skull to be compressed during birth and permit rapid growth of the brain and head. The posterior fontanel closes at about three months of age and the larger, diamond-shaped anterior fontanel closes at between 12 and 18 months of age. The soft fontanels do not provide the protection to the brain that the harder bones of the skull will provide as the infant grows.

Neonates and infants have a greater surface area to volume ratio. That means neonates and infants have a large surface area for their body size, which allows for increased heat loss from the body. Heat loss is also increased with increased respiration. The heat transferred to air as it passes through the airway is lost at a greater rate when respiratory distress causes an increase in ventilatory rate. Combined with an immature thermoregulatory system, neonates and infants are prone to hypothermia and must be kept warm.

Covering the head prevents heat loss from the large surface area of the scalp.

The tongue takes up a relatively larger portion of the oral cavity. The airway is slightly funnel shaped, with the narrowest point at the cricoid ring. The airway is proportionately shorter and softer. The nose is small and soft, and neonates are primarily nose breathers. The tiny nares can easily be obstructed by mucus during a respiratory infection. The occipital region of the skull is prominent compared to the torso. When an infant is supine, the large occiput causes flexion of the neck. Older infants learn to grasp objects and put them in their mouths. Each of those differences means that airway obstruction can occur very easily in this age group (Figures 9-3 and 9-4).

There are fewer alveoli in the lungs and the lungs are fragile and easily damaged. The tidal volume is small, approximately 6 to 8 mL per kg. With an average birth weight of 3.0 to 3.5 kg (6.6 to 7.7 lb), this means that average tidal volume is 18 to 28 mL, compared to the 500 mL average tidal volume of an adult. By one year of age, the tidal volume increases to about 10 mL/kg. The chest wall is pliable and the ribs have a more horizontal orientation, increasing reliance on the diaphragm for breathing. The respiratory muscles are immature and glycogen stores are minimal. Respiratory failure and respiratory arrest can occur quickly in a neonate or infant with respiratory distress.

The water vapor lost with every breath leads to dehydration with increased respirations during respiratory

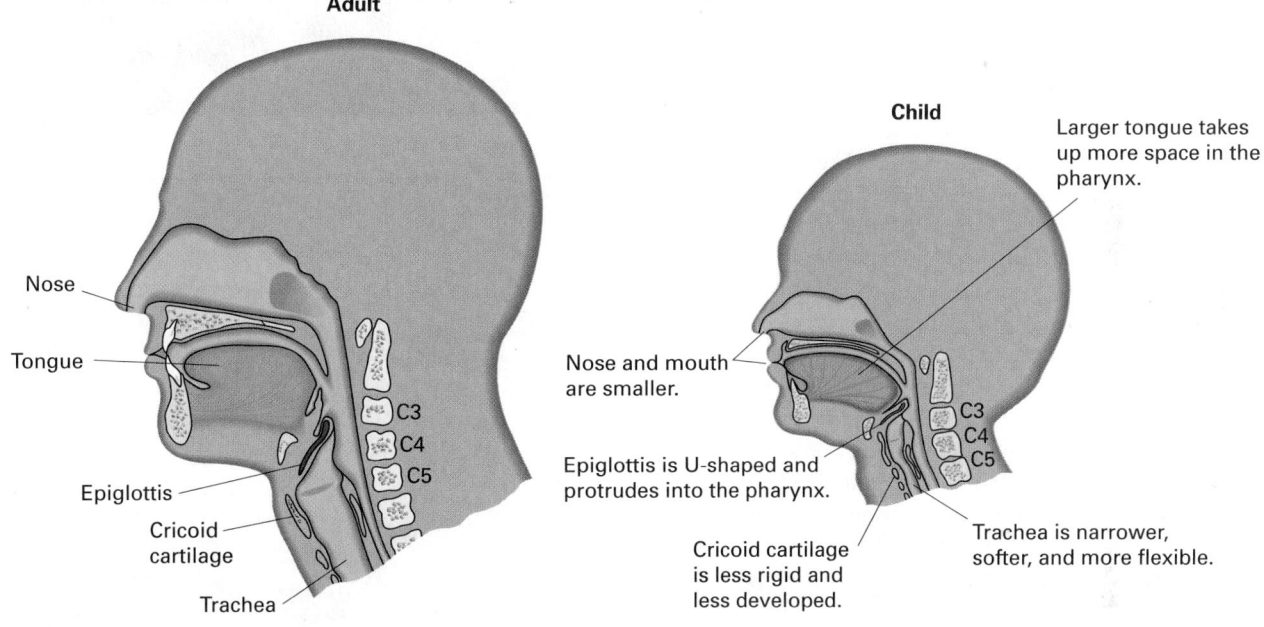

Adult

Nose
Tongue
Epiglottis
Cricoid cartilage
Trachea
C3
C4
C5

Child

Larger tongue takes up more space in the pharynx.
Nose and mouth are smaller.
Epiglottis is U-shaped and protrudes into the pharynx.
Cricoid cartilage is less rigid and less developed.
Trachea is narrower, softer, and more flexible.
C3
C4
C5

FIGURE 9-3

Several features of the pediatric airway make it more prone to obstruction than that of adults.

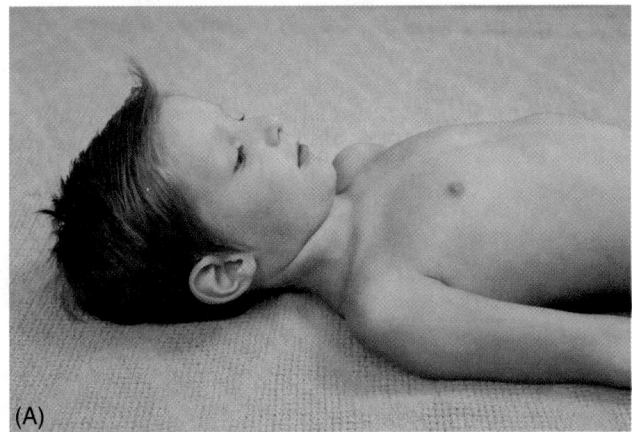

(A)

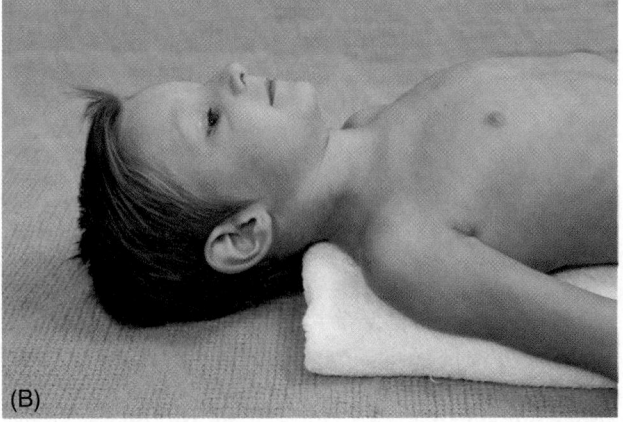

(B)

FIGURE 9-4

(A) The large occiput in pediatric patients can flex the neck, resulting in airway obstruction. (B) Proper positioning may require padding beneath the shoulders.

distress. The blood volume of neonates and infants is small. Just a few milliliters of fluid loss can lead to shock. Poor feeding, vomiting, diarrhea, and fever can result in significant dehydration.

Fetuses receive maternal antibodies through the placenta prior to birth, offering limited immunity in infancy. The infant's immune system is immature and less able to fight infection. Immaturity of the nervous system means that a young infant may not have a high fever, even with serious infection. Fevers in neonates and infants are always concerning. Breast-fed neonates and infants receive antibodies through breast milk, providing additional protection against infection. The passive immunity conferred by the mother's antibodies is limited, though, and children must develop active immunity (make their own antibodies) through vaccinations and exposure to pathogens. Childhood immunizations are required to provide immunity against a number of potentially life-threatening illnesses, such as tetanus, diptheria, hepatitis B, measles, mumps, rubella, pertussis, and others. The ability to develop active immunity develops slowly over the first three months. Therefore, with the exception of the hepatitis B vaccine, vaccines are not recommended until the infant is at least three months old.

Crying is the newborn's and young infant's only way of communicating. They may cry from pain, fear, being cold, overstimulation, or hunger, or because they need a diaper change. Teething, or the eruption of the baby teeth, which begins at about four months and can continue until two years of age, can lead to pain and fever. Parents and caregivers often recognize the difference in cries for different reasons. Parents may be concerned because of a change in the infant's cry or because the infant is inconsolable. Crying is normal response to being separated from a parent or other primary caregiver. The best way to prevent crying from separation is to allow the parent to hold the child while you examine him. If an infant does not cry when he is separated from his parents, consider the possibility of illness, injury, or developmental issues.

Toddlers and Preschoolers

A toddler is a child from one to three years of age (Figure 9-5). Preschoolers are three to six years of age (Figure 9-6). The head is still proportionally large, but not as disproportionate as an infant's. As physiologic development continues, children also become more social and curious about the world and experience dramatic psychosocial and cognitive development. Gross and fine motor skills develop as children learn to walk, play with toys, scribble and draw, and ride tricycles.

Levels of maternal antibodies decrease and toddlers and preschoolers are exposed to more people, making them vulnerable to communicable diseases. The vast majority of those diseases are minor and are an important part of developing immunity. Ear infections and upper and lower respiratory tract infections are common. Some diseases, such as croup, respiratory syncytial virus (RSV), and epiglottitis can lead to respiratory distress in this age group. (See Chapter 44.)

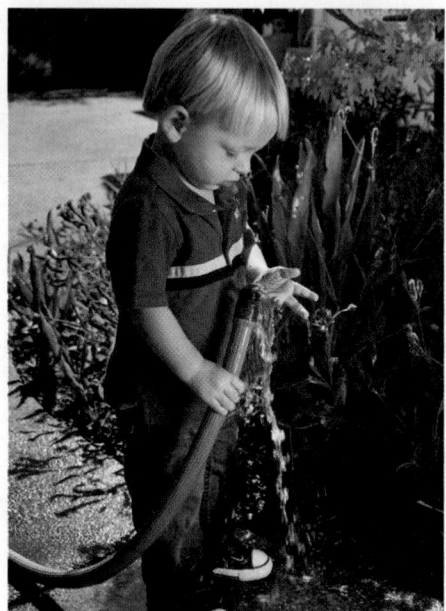

FIGURE 9-5

A toddler.

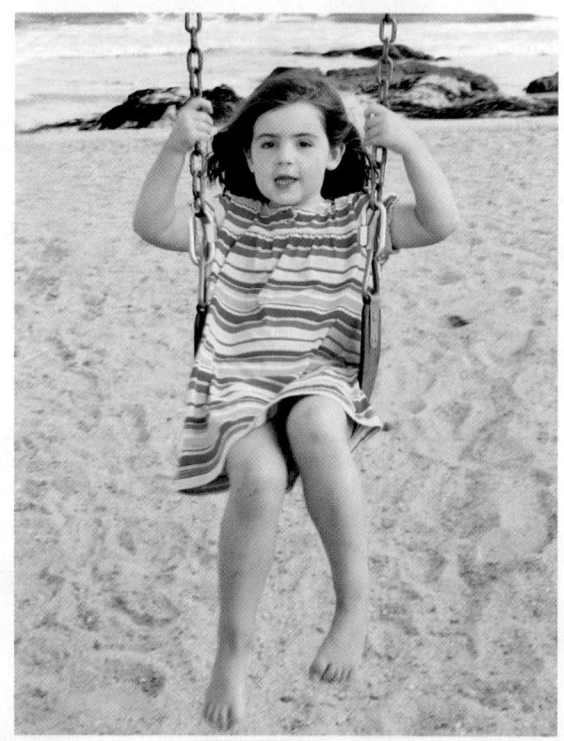

FIGURE 9-6

A preschooler. (© Daniel Limmer)

Toilet training is usually complete as the child transitions from toddler to preschooler (at an average age of 28 months), but he may continue to have nighttime enuresis (bed wetting) through the preschool years. Language skills and vocabulary develop rapidly. Children may continue to cry when separated from parents, or cling to parents when they are left in the care of someone else, but they also express increasing independence. Toddlers and preschoolers take great pride in being able to do things for themselves. Strangers, including health care providers, can provoke anxiety in children this age. Establish rapport and gain the child's trust and communicate with them in a way they can understand. Demonstrating the techniques of assessment you plan to use on a doll or stuffed animal can decrease anxiety, as can allowing the child to handle the equipment, if appropriate, before you use it.

At this age, children express much of what is on their minds through play. Toddlers engage in magical thinking to explain things they are not yet able to understand and enjoy playing make-believe. Understanding is concrete and interpretations are literal. When someone says they have butterflies in their stomach, toddlers and preschoolers believe that there literally are butterflies in the person's stomach. Competitive behavior begins to emerge.

School-Age Children

The school-age years are from 6 through 12 years of age (Figure 9-7). Physical proportions become more adult-like. School-age children begin losing the primary teeth that emerged in infancy and the toddler years, and permanent teeth erupt in their place. In these years, children continue to develop more relationships outside of the family, and are developing self-esteem. As a part of identity development, school-age children compare themselves to their peers. Approval and acceptance are important. Problem-solving ability is developing, but reasoning skills remain relatively concrete. Children in this age

group are beginning to develop an understanding of illness, loss, death, and dying, but still need adults' assistance in coping with the fears associated with those issues. Modesty and the need for privacy are developing and must be kept in mind when caring for school-age children.

Adolescents

Between 12 and 18 years of age, children's vital signs approach adult values, and toward the later years physical growth is nearly complete. It is during this period of development that children complete puberty (development of secondary sex characteristics) (Figure 9-8). Girls have their first menstrual periods (menarche) between the ages of 9 and 16 years, with an average of 12.5 to 13 years. Adolescents typically experience a two- to three-year period of rapid growth. The increased rate of growth begins with the extremities, often giving adolescents a gangly appearance.

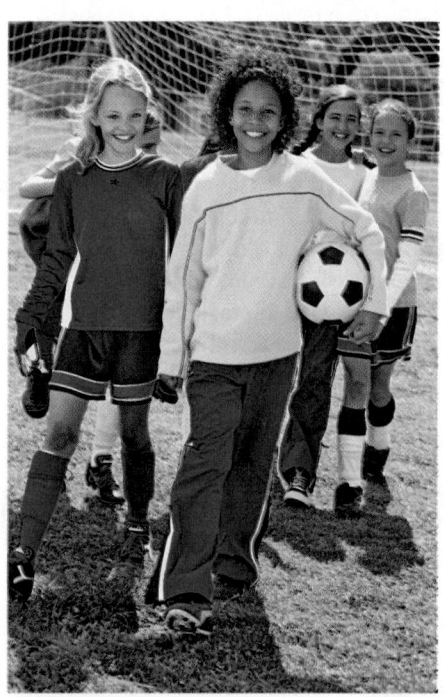

FIGURE 9-8

Adolescents. (© JJ Getty Images)

IN THE FIELD

Approximately 17 percent of U.S. children between the ages of 2 and 19 years are obese. Childhood obesity increases the risks of cardiovascular disease, diabetes, and adult obesity. Obese children are often the targets of bullying and discrimination. The result may be low self-esteem, which can affect academic performance and social development. Childhood obesity results from a combination of genetic, behavioral, and environmental factors.

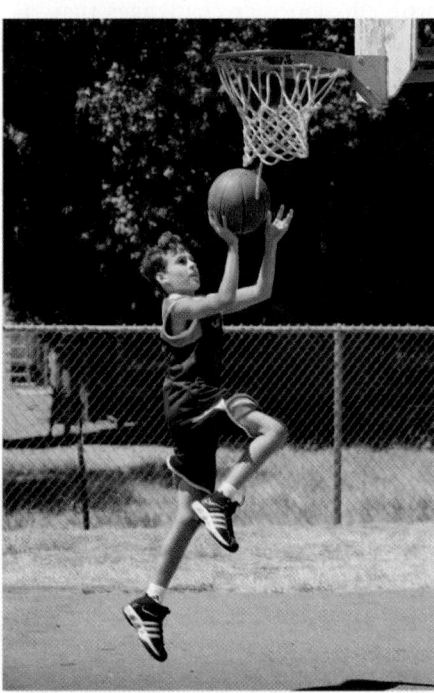

FIGURE 9-7

School-age children.

Adolescents have an increased interest in the opposite sex and begin to develop romantic relationships. They want to be regarded as adults, but are not legally capable of making medical decisions. The teenage brain has not yet developed adult judgment and handles emotions differently than the adult brain. Adolescents become more challenging to parental authority and family conflict often increases with an adolescent in the home. Teens can have a sense of invulnerability. This, along with immature judgment and the experimentation that emerges during identity development, can lead to risky behaviors, including unsafe driving; use of tobacco, alcohol, and drugs; and unsafe sexual behavior. Rates of depression and suicide increase in this age group.

Adolescents are self-conscious and concerned with appearance and body image. An injury may cause anxiety at the thought of scarring or disfigurement. Eating disorders often surface at this age, particularly in girls, but increasingly in boys, as well. Anorexia nervosa is a body image disorder in which the individual perceives herself as being obese, despite often being very thin. The individual takes extreme measures to lose and control weight, including minimal food intake and engaging in excessive exercise. Bulimia is an eating disorder in which the individual induces vomiting after eating to rid the stomach of food. Often, she binges, eating a large amount of food, and then induces vomiting. Laxatives are often abused in this disorder, as well, to speed the elimination of food through the digestive tract. Both disorders lead to malnutrition and other complications, which can be life threatening.

Young Adulthood

Young adulthood is the period from 19 to 40 years of age. Peak physical condition occurs between 19 and 26 years of age, and all body systems function well through young adulthood. The leading cause of death is trauma, with a significant proportion due to motor vehicle collisions. Mature romantic relationships develop and childbirth is most common at this age. Job stress can be high and conflicts between career and family are common.

Middle Adulthood

From 41 to 60 years of age, body systems continue to function at fairly high levels, but age-related changes start to become apparent. In some classification schemes, middle adulthood continues until age 65. There is not a specific age at which people invariably have an onset of age-related conditions. Aging is a process that takes place over time. Although the incidence of certain conditions statistically increases at a given age, it does not mean that every person of that age has the same level of health. For example, the onset of age-related hearing loss depends on many factors, including exposure to occupational and other sources of noise.

In middle adulthood, there commonly are changes in vision as the lens of the eye loses ability to focus (presbyopia), creating problems in seeing objects close-up. Some age-related hearing loss may occur, as well (presbycusis). The incidence of cardiovascular disease and risk factors increases, hypercholesterolemia and hypertension are more common, and cardiac output declines. Weight control becomes more difficult and obesity is associated with the onset of type II diabetes. There also is an increase in the incidence of cancer. Menopause occurs in women in their late 40s to early 50s, with an average age of 51 years.

During middle adulthood, individuals have learned to face problems more as challenges than as threats. Middle-aged adults may face financial pressures related to costs of having children at home, sending children to college, and caring for aging parents. Children leaving home presents both opportunity and challenge (empty-nest syndrome).

PERSONAL PERSPECTIVE

Advanced EMT Sadik Muhammad: As a college student, it is hard to remember the way I thought about things as a small child. Still, there are memories and I can relate to some degree to the way kids think. I remember being scared of getting in trouble when I got hurt, and that kind of thing. It is much harder to relate to someone whose age you have never been though. It is hard to see things from the perspective of an older person. My Advanced EMT class instructor, Walter Mason, opened up my eyes a little bit. He brought in a box of items to class one day that he had us use to simulate some of the changes that occur with aging. We wore glasses with yellow lenses, which made it hard to tell one color from another. I could see then how easy it would be to mix up pills based on their color. He had us wear garden gloves and glasses smeared with petroleum jelly and then asked us to thread a needle. It was so frustrating! It was such a simple task, but we all struggled with it. Half of us kept on the glasses and put cotton balls in our ears. Then Walter handed us copies of patient care reports and had our partners try to explain to us what we were signing and why. It was confusing and I had to have my partner repeat things a couple of times. We wrapped elastic bandages around our elbows and knees and tried to walk around and do various tasks around the classroom. I don't know exactly what it is like to live with those changes on a daily basis, but I gained a new understanding of how I can be a little more helpful and patient with elderly patients.

Late Adulthood

From age 61 years (65 years in some classification schemes) onward, body systems continue to decline, including worsening of the vision and hearing changes that began in middle age (Figure 9-9). Thickening of the blood vessels increases systemic vascular resistance and organ perfusion decreases. Those changes increase the workload of the heart (Table 9-7). At the same time, the heart functions less efficiently, is less able to respond to increased physical activity, and becomes less tolerant of tachycardia. Anemia and decreased response to infection can occur. Some forms of leukemia are more prevalent in this age group.

Decline in the respiratory system puts older adults at risk for health problems, including decreased ability to increase oxygenation to meet increased demands during illness and injury. Lung capacity decreases, as does gas diffusion through the respiratory membrane. Respiratory muscle function declines and the chest wall becomes less compliant. Ribs and costal cartilage become weakened and brittle. The cough and gag reflexes are diminished, providing less protection to the lower airway. The gastrointestinal system becomes less efficient at processing nutrients, and appetite can decrease. Decreased senses of taste and smell, along with isolation and decreased mobility and financial means can lead to decreased food intake. Diminished salivation and gastric secretions decrease digestive function and nutrients are not as well absorbed, leading to vitamin and mineral deficiencies. A lifetime of dental issues may creep up on the elderly, leading to poor dentition and tooth replacement with dentures.

Constipation is common and bowel impaction and obstruction may occur. Diminished activity of the endocrine system results in less insulin production and decreased glucose metabolism. Liver function decreases as well, and substances (including medications) may not be efficiently eliminated from the body.

Loss of nephrons (up to 50 percent) and glomerular abnormalities result in decreased urine production, and substances that normally are excreted through the kidneys may accumulate. Changes in the nervous system include decreased sensory function, reaction time, and **proprioception** (sensation of the orientation of the body or body parts without visual input). A common scenario involving elderly drivers related to the decrease in proprioception is the driver mistakenly pressing the accelerator instead of the brake, leading to a collision.

Pain perception decreases and even serious injury and illness may not produce the expected degree of pain. Neurons function less efficiently and problem-solving ability and new knowledge assimilation can slow. Overall, cognitive decline, including Alzheimer's disease and other forms of dementia, is not a normal consequence of aging, but of pathologic processes. The sleep–wake cycle may become impaired as levels of melatonin drop, and is common in patients with dementia.

The view of the aged varies by culture. They may be seen as a source of wisdom, or may be disregarded or seen as a burden. The elderly person may doubt his self-worth. Losses of function, independence, and companionship and financial burdens are common in this age group. Depression is common among the elderly and suicide may occur.

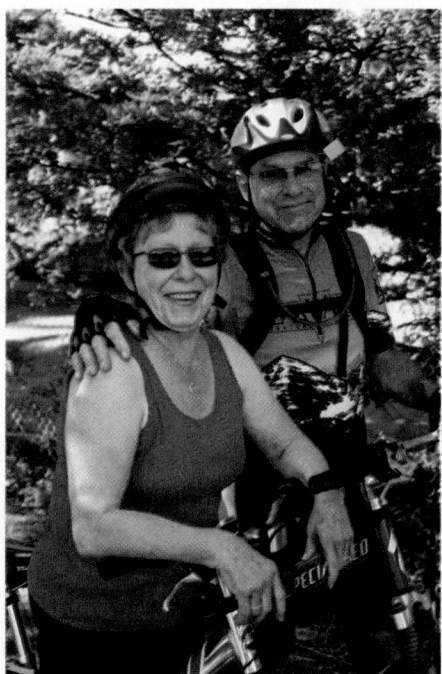

FIGURE 9-9

An older adult.

IN THE FIELD

Elderly patients often take several medications for several different conditions. Sometimes, they obtain prescriptions from different physicians and get them filled at different pharmacies, making it difficult for their health care providers to prevent medication interactions. People of any age may be using over-the-counter or herbal remedies that their doctors or pharmacists do not know about, without realizing that serious interactions can occur between those remedies and their prescription medications. In addition, forgetfulness, confusion, and the small print on prescription bottles can result in medication errors. As the function of the liver and kidneys decline with age, medications are not eliminated as quickly from the body. All of those factors put the elderly at risk for complications related to medication interactions and toxicity. Patients may present with confusion, dizziness, falling, cardiac problems, and a variety of other conditions. Always ask specifically about over-the-counter and herbal remedies used in addition to asking about prescription medications.

TABLE 9-7   Physiologic Changes Associated with Aging

System	Change
Cardiovascular system	Heart valves become calcified with narrow openings (stenosis). Hypertension is common. Maximum heart rate decreases. Decreased cardiac output and ability to compensate for loss of volume or vascular tone. Cardiac dysrhythmias. Arteriosclerosis. Decreased sensitivity of baroreceptors.
Respiratory system	Diminished cough and gag reflexes, weaker coughing effort. Decreased gas exchange. Increased incidence of respiratory infections.
Nervous system	Decreased brain mass. Degenerative changes (such as plaques) may occur. Slowed cognitive responses. Slowed reflexes. Decreased pain perception. Disturbances in sleep–wake cycles. Depression is common.
Senses	Diminished senses of vision, especially night vision and near vision; cataracts. Decreased hearing acuity, especially for higher pitched sounds. Decreased senses of taste and smell.
Gastrointestinal system	Decreased appetite. Decreased nutrient absorption. Constipation is common. Decreased liver function.
Renal system	Decreased efficiency due to loss of nephrons; may contribute to drug toxicity.
Musculoskeletal system	Loss of bone mass. Decreased skeletal muscle mass and strength.
Integumentary system	Thin, fragile skin. Slow healing. Loss or thinning of hair. Brittle nails.
Endocrine system	Decreased hormone amount and target organ sensitivity impairs water and electrolyte balance, glucose metabolism, sleep, and thyroid and other functions.
Immune system	Decreased defenses against infection. Fever may not be present, even with severe infection.

Nonetheless, the majority of elderly patients live independently, with minimal assistance, or with family members. A minority of the elderly live in nursing homes.

Cultural Differences

Our experiences and cultures are such fundamental elements of our identities that it is difficult to realize how the way we see the world has been shaped by them. It does not seem like these things have influenced us; instead, we tend to think that the way we see things is objectively the way things are. When there is conflict between groups or individuals, it is often because of differences in worldviews. A worldview is the set of assumptions that affect our beliefs and interpretations of reality, which in turn affect our behavior and expectations of others. A part of the worldview is shared among members of the same culture, while some aspects remain individual. The shared expectations and beliefs shape everything from beliefs about death, disease, justice, education, and the role of elders in society, to expectations for how to greet someone and what behaviors are and are not allowed in public. Keep in mind that things you take for granted may be seen as rude or disrespectful in other cultures.

Health Disparities

The Institute of Medicine (Smedley, Stith, and Nelson, 2002) reports that there are many health disparities among racial and ethnic minorities in the United States, even among those with higher incomes and health care insurance. Bias, stereotypes, and lack of understanding by health care providers contribute to the disparities.

Health Care Beliefs and Social Interactions

Some similarities are common within cultural groups, but there is variation within groups, as well as between groups. The following information is not intended to stereotype or overgeneralize, but to create understanding when differences in beliefs and behaviors are encountered. Health and medical beliefs of every culture are rich and complex, and difficult to summarize (Figure 9-10). In contrast to the dominant U. S. culture, minority groups tend to place more emphasis on the value of family, including extended family, the community (social group, tribe, village, neighborhood), and respect and deference to elders. Multigenerational families living under the same roof are more common than among White Americans (U.S. Department of Health and Human Services [HHS] Office of Minority Health [OMH], 2010).

There is a more holistic view of health and medicine, and many cultures prefer, or even mandate, same-sex health care providers. People of many cultures expect that health care providers will offer some kind of treatment in the form of medications or procedures, rather than just consultation. A number of cultures believe in the importance of prayer by and for the ill, and value the use of plant-based traditional medicines and other alternative and complementary approaches. Many recent immigrants have fled political

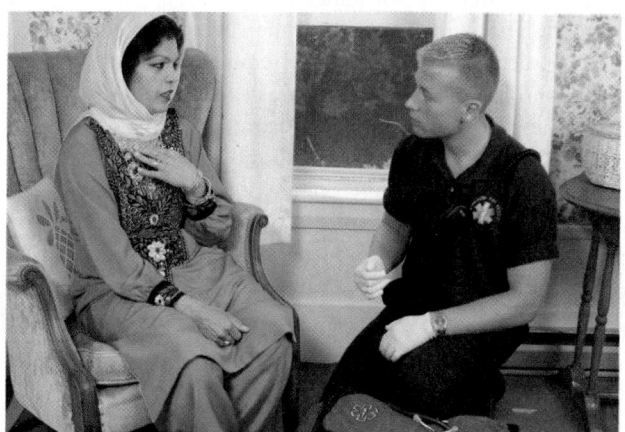

FIGURE 9-10

Patients from different cultures have differing beliefs about health and different expectations for interactions with health care providers.

There is a growing trend for people to use forms of complementary and alternative medicine approaches. They include reflexology, acupressure, acupuncture, traditional Chinese herbal medicine, the use of any number of herbal supplements and natural remedies, aromatherapy, massage, chiropractic, and many other approaches. There is increasing acknowledgement of those therapies by mainstream medical practitioners and research into their use continues.

unrest, corrupt governments, war, and other conditions that may make them distrustful of those in authority.

Hispanic/Latino Culture

Hispanics/Latinos have cultural origins in more than 40 countries in the Caribbean and Latin America in which Spanish is the most commonly spoken language. There are over 46.9 million Hispanic/Latino Americans, comprising 15 percent of the U.S. population (HHS OMH, 2010). Of this number of Hispanics/Latinos, 21.5 percent live in poverty. In Hispanic/Latino culture, maintaining eye contact is important and friendly physical contact, such as a hand on the shoulder, is widely accepted. It is often expected that health care providers will position themselves closer than they might otherwise. Treating others with respect is highly valued, as is the recognition paid to those with official titles. Spending time with family is a regular part of life. Hispanics/Latinos tend to have higher rates of obesity and diabetes, with cardiovascular disease and cancer comprising the leading causes of death.

African American Culture

African Americans comprised about 13.5 percent of the U.S. population in 2008, with 80 percent living in 16 states (HHS OMH, 2010). African Americans disproportionately live in high-poverty areas, with 24.5 percent of families living in poverty. Those living in urban areas are more subject to certain health problems, such as violence. Female heads of household are common. Economic and educational disparities accompany the health care disparities. Many African Americans are very involved in religious institutions.

African Americans tend to have a distrust of the health care system. The most significant cause of death among African Americans is hypertension, with high rates of cardiovascular disease, stroke, and cancer. The rate of death for cardiovascular disease is more than twice that of Whites. Health problems include high rates of smoking, lung cancer, HIV, obesity, and diabetes with kidney failure and lower extremity amputation. Many barriers to preventive health care exist. Although still rare, sickle cell disease is more common in this group, with 8 percent having sickle cell trait, and 0.2 percent having sickle cell disease.

American Indian/Native Alaskan Culture

There are 562 federally recognized American Indian and Native Alaskan tribes in the United States with over 200 families of languages, some of which have no written form. Many other tribes are recognized at the state level, or not recognized at all by state and federal governments. There are more than 4.9 million American Indians/Native Alaskans in the United States, comprising 1.6 percent of the population, with the greatest proportions living in the West and South (HHS OMH, 2010). About 25 percent of this group lives in poverty, and many of the health issues are those associated with poverty and lack of access to health care. There are disproportionate death rates from alcoholism, tuberculosis, type II diabetes, injuries, suicide, and murder. The infant mortality rate is 40 percent higher than that of White infants.

Particularly among those who live on reservations (about 30 percent), obligations to tribe and family are part of everyday life. Health is viewed holistically, with emphasis on physical, spiritual, social, and psychological health. There are many systems of healing within the American Indian/Native Alaskan population, with emphasis on the spiritual aspect of healing and the role of imbalance in some aspect of life as the cause of illness. The use of traditional healers and medicines is common.

Some general things to keep in mind in communication are that a softer handshake may be seen as more respectful or humble (Management Sciences for Health, 2010). A comfortable communication distance is several feet and unnecessary contact may not be welcome, especially among elders. Make eye contact, but extended eye contact can be seen as disrespectful. Many medical terms do not have a translation in American Indian/Native Alaskan languages. Silence and slower speech patterns are valued. Listen carefully and do not interrupt.

Asian Culture

Asians are a very diverse group, with diverse religious beliefs. Most Asians in the United States are from China, Vietnam, India, and the Philippines, although more than 20 countries are represented with 100 languages. There are about 15.5 million Asian Americans and Pacific Islanders in the United States (HHS OMH, 2010). The majority of Asians and Pacific Islanders in the United States live in urban areas, with 55 percent living in California, Washington, and Hawaii. Despite higher incidences of some diseases among specific subgroups, Asians and Pacific Islanders are generally healthier than the population as a whole, with lower rates of obesity, stroke, and heart disease. Asian American women have the longest life expectancy of any group at 85.8 years. Adoption of Western dietary habits is associated with negative impact on health status.

Self-control, respect for elders, and family loyalty are important. Negative emotions, such as anger, are sometimes not expressed openly and politeness is highly valued. Patients may prefer a same-sex health care provider. Smiling and nodding may be used out of politeness, despite lack of understanding. Generally, there is no contradiction between science and spirituality or holistic medicine. There are several systems of Asian medicine, including Ayurveda and traditional Chinese medicine.

Middle Eastern Culture

Islam is the most common religion for people from Western Asia and the Middle East, but there are other religious groups as well. Judaism and Christianity are important, as are Baha'i and Zoroastrianism. People from this region are proud of family and cultural heritage and value honor. While not usually a concern in the prehospital setting, dietary restrictions are common. Pork is not eaten, for example, and observant Jews follow a Kosher diet. Same-sex health care providers are preferred (sometimes mandated). In many countries, both men and women cover the head. Women may further be expected to cover the face and not expose the arms or legs. The use of alcohol may be discouraged or forbidden. Muslims may pray several times a day at given times.

Grief, Dying, and Death

People can die at any age and can suffer losses and the death of loved ones throughout the life span. A person's cognitive and emotional development affects how they understand loss and death. Amongst older children and adults, there is a common sequence of reactions to loss, while younger children are less able to comprehend death.

Bereavement is the state of having experienced a loss. **Grief** is the emotional reaction to bereavement, while **mourning** is the expression of grief. Beliefs about death and mourning rituals vary greatly between cultures.

Until relatively recently in the history of the United States, death usually occurred at home, and a wake was held in the home, not in funeral homes. People were much more familiar with death. With the advent of medical technology, death more and more frequently occurred in the hospital, rather than in the home. People became estranged from the process of death. This estrangement is reflected in the use of euphemisms to talk about it. More recently, the futility and lack of dignity often associated with end-of-life care have resulted in **hospice** programs, do not resuscitate orders, and living wills, allowing individuals and their loved ones more control over the ends of their lives.

Elisabeth Kübler-Ross Stages of Dying

There are several theories about how human beings react to death and dying, but one of the most familiar is Elisabeth Kübler-Ross's theory (Copp, 1998). Kübler-Ross's theory proposes that the reaction to death and dying proceeds through five stages. Those reactions may occur in response not only to death and dying, but also to any significant loss, such as divorce or job loss. The five stages are denial, anger, bargaining, depression, and acceptance.

Advanced EMTs often deal with the families of patients who have died and with terminally ill patients. Understanding the patient's and family's reactions can help you better respond to their needs. The stages are described as follows:

- *Denial.* The initial reaction to the news of death of a loved one, or of one's own impending death, is disbelief. A family member in denial may seem to have minimal response to the news that a loved one has died. Though it may seem uncomfortable, it is essential that you use the words *death, dead,* or *died.* Euphemisms leave room for misunderstanding about what has happened. It is better to say, "I'm so sorry, Mr. Thornton, but your mother has died," than it is to say, "I'm so sorry, but your mother is no longer with us," or "Your mother has gone to a better place." In particular, the latter statement makes assumptions about the family's beliefs about death.

- *Anger.* Once the reality of death or dying is clear, the person becomes angry. Family members may lash out at health care providers, punch walls or throw things, or become angry with the deceased. Terminally ill patients also become angry as part of the dying process. Anger is an expected response. Keep in mind that the family member is overwhelmed, shocked, and in tremendous pain. Although you must take measures to protect your own safety, compassion and empathy toward the family member will go a long way toward defusing the situation.

- *Bargaining.* The dying patient or his family make promises in an attempt to find out that the diagnosis was a mistake, or to buy more time. A family member may state that they would gladly change places with the dying loved one. A dying patient may vow to be a better parent to his children, to be nicer to others, or to make any number of changes.

- *Depression.* Sadness and cognitive and physical symptoms of depression appear as it becomes clear that death is approaching, or that the death of a loved one has occurred.

- *Acceptance.* If the dying person has enough time, or with time after the death of a loved one, the situation is finally accepted.

Although Kübler-Ross's model is presented linearly (one stage follows the other), those who deal often with terminally ill patients and their families suggest that the person moves back and forth between stages, sometimes more hopeful and sometimes less so (Copp, 1998). This model is not to be seen as a prescription for how people should act, but as a description of how people often act. Knowing how long it takes for a person to pass through each of the stages is difficult and may depend on the suddenness of the situation, and whether or not the death was expected.

Children and Grief

Before the age of six years, children seldom understand the permanence of death. They may believe that the person who has died will wake up or come back. The use of euphemisms, such as, "passed" may be confusing to the literal mind of a child this age. Infants as young as six months may become irritable and show changes in eating, sleeping, and crying patterns. School-age children begin to understand the permanence of death and may develop fears about the possibility of death, including their own. They may be curious about the physical process of death. In early adolescence, developing abstract thought allows children to think more about spiritual aspects of death. They may feel especially vulnerable and insecure at this age (Lyles, 2010). Often, the death of a pet is the child's introduction to the death process. Older adolescents may feel more comfortable talking to peers, rather than adults, about their feelings, and may engage in risk-taking behavior in response to the death of someone close.

Children may react to death by becoming anxious at separation from loved ones. Crying and sadness are common. Grieving children may overeat or lose their appetites, develop physical symptoms such as a stomachache or headache, fear doctors or hospitals, have difficulty sleeping, and have trouble concentrating at school and on homework. Children may fear that they are somehow responsible for death and feel guilt. They may have feelings of abandonment, insecurity, and fear. Some children's behavior may regress and they may act younger than they are (American Academy of Child and Adolescent Psychiatry, 2008).

Children may have nightmares in response to a loved one's death and, in the beginning, may think about the person almost constantly. It is common for children to report feeling the presence of the person who has died, as if they are being watched over.

Cross-Cultural Perspectives on Death and Dying

The United States is populated by members of diverse cultures, whose rituals surrounding death differ. Beliefs and funeral practices are heavily influenced by religious beliefs, particularly about the soul and the afterlife. Even amongst those who do not practice organized religion, the rituals and beliefs surrounding death are influenced by the religious traditions of the culture. The following descriptions of beliefs are general. Recognize that there are many variations within each of the major world religions.

Hinduism

Hinduism is widely practiced in India and by those of Indian descent. Hindus strive to achieve freedom from eternal reincarnations that result from karma, which is the accumulation of the person's actions in present and past lives (Kemp & Bhungalia, 2002). Hindus may believe that illness is a result of karma. Taking care of unfinished business in relationships and other matters is an important concern for Hindus at the end of life. Chanting, meditation, prayer, and incense are important parts of the dying and mourning processes. It is preferred that only family touch the body of the deceased, and health care providers should touch the body as little as possible. In the home, pictures are turned toward the wall and mirrors may be covered. Embalming and organ donation are prohibited and cremation is preferred.

Judaism

There are three primary branches of Judaism in the United States: Orthodox, Conservative, and Reform, with Reform Jews being the largest group and the most liberal in the interpretation of religious teachings. The eyes of the deceased should be closed, preferably by a relative. It is preferred that a family member remain with the body until burial. Cremation, embalming, the use of cosmetics or restorative procedures, public viewing, and lavish caskets are forbidden. Autopsy may be performed if required by law. Organ donation may be allowed in conference with a rabbi. Burial should take place within 24 hours, but should not be done on the Sabbath. The initial period of mourning is called *shivah,* and extends from death until seven days after the burial. Traditionally, family members sit only on low benches or the floor during shivah.

Buddhism

Buddhism is the major religion of East Asian countries, including Cambodia, China, Japan, Thailand, Vietnam, and Tibet, but practices vary from country to country. Beliefs regarding the requirements for attaining Nirvana, a state of freedom from rebirth (karma or kamma), vary. In Buddhism, it is believed that separation and suffering—such as birth, illness, and death—are inevitable, and that suffering results from desire, or attachments. Following the Eightfold Path (eight steps for belief and conduct) ends desire and suffering, and leads to Nirvana. Prescriptions for how to handle the body after death, and whether autopsy or organ donation is allowed, are not specific in Buddhism.

Islam

Islam is a widely practiced religion with two primary branches (Sunni and Shi'a) and various sects within each branch. Those who practice Islam are called *Muslims,* and the Qur'an, God's word to the Prophet Muhammad, provides their laws. The Qur'an does not provide strict guidance on matters of illness, death, and burial. Important facets of Islam are ritual cleanliness before prayers, prayer while facing Mecca (to the east), dietary guidance, fasting (especially during the holy period, Ramadan), and modesty. It is strongly preferred that health care providers are the same gender as the patient. At death, the patient should be facing Mecca and after death the body should not be touched by non-Muslims. Autopsy is allowed if required by law and organ donation may be permitted.

Christianity

Though there are various beliefs and interpretations of the Bible among Christians, the common belief is that Jesus Christ is the Son of God. Christians believe that baptism and forgiveness for sins are required for everlasting life after death. The two main branches of Christianity are Protestantism and Catholicism. Depending upon particular beliefs, there are many end-of-life Sacraments or rites that are desired to be performed by a priest or minister. They may include Baptism, Confession, Holy Communion, and Last Rites (Anointing of the Sick). Dying patients may wish to read or have read to them passages from the Bible and may wish to pray. Most Christian churches do not forbid autopsy or organ donation, but a few denominations forbid specific medical procedures.

Within Christianity, the reaction to death varies greatly between and within ethnicities and denominations. The practice of eulogizing the deceased is common in many denominations. In the United States, it is common practice to spend large sums of money on elaborate caskets and watertight burial vaults. The deceased may have ornate headstones or monuments to mark their graves or may be placed in mausoleums.

In contrast, the Amish funeral focuses not on eulogizing the deceased, but on praising God and reminding the community to prepare for the afterlife. In keeping with a simple lifestyle, the deceased is embalmed only if required by state law and placed in a handmade wooden casket. The casket is plain and unpadded. There are no photos of the deceased, flowers, music, or hymns at the funeral, and the hand-dug grave is marked by a simple headstone with the individual's date of birth and death.

In the United States, different ethnic groups have different norms surrounding the reaction to the news of death. Those of some Asian and European backgrounds are very reserved and stoic in response, while some Asian, Hispanic/Latino, and African American groups are more demonstrative (Lobar, Youngblut, & Brooten, 2006). In some groups, there are different expectations of the reactions of men and women, with men expected to be less demonstrative. To each group, the reaction of the others may seem odd. One group may seem cold and unfeeling in response to the news that a loved has died, while the expression of emotion may make others uncomfortable. Keep in mind that the differences are expected and normal, and must be accepted.

Death in the Field

Once a patient has died, the well-being of the family becomes one of the Advanced EMT's primary concerns. It is often difficult to know what to say to someone whose loved one has just died. It is not necessary to say something profound. Simply let the family know that you care and that you are sorry for their loss. A few words of comfort are important, and often the family needs assistance in taking the first steps.

It can be helpful to ask if the family needs to make particular phone calls, and if there is anything you can do at that moment. Unless the scene is a known or potential crime scene, family members may be permitted to sit with the deceased until arrangements are made to move him. If it is appropriate (the case is not a medical examiner's case or crime scene), you may cover the patient with a clean sheet up to the chin, wipe away any secretions, and close the eyes in preparation for the family to sit with their loved one. Always follow your EMS system's protocols and procedures, which differ in directing the roles of EMS providers at the scene.

In some systems, you must return to service as quickly as possible. In others, you may have additional time to spend with the family. (See Chapter 4 for information on the legalities surrounding death in the field.)

Hospice and Palliative Care

Hospice is a relatively recent addition to health care that exists to assist terminally ill patients and their families in preparation for the patient's death. Hospice patients often receive **palliative care**, which is aimed at making the patient as comfortable as possible. Palliative care may include pain medication and medications for nausea, as well as other comfort measures.

CASE STUDY WRAP-UP

Clinical-Reasoning Process

Advanced EMTs Jeremy House and Dee Ann Pointer are responding to Klondike Elementary School for an injured eight-year-old child on the playground.

Jeremy sees that Emma looks frightened and in pain. He knows he must gain her trust in order to treat her effectively. He squats down, bringing himself to her level to avoid towering over her and intimidating her. He introduces himself and his partner to Emma, and lets her know that they are there to help her.

After establishing rapport with Emma, Jeremy tells her that they need to take a look at her arm and check her pulse. Her pulse is 94 and regular, respirations are 24, and blood pressure is 102/68—all normal for nine-year-old Emma.

Jeremy is honest with Emma and tells her that they will be very careful, but it might hurt when they place her arm in a splint. He tells her the splint is important because, after it is on, it will keep her arm from moving and it will not hurt as much. He knows that if he makes a promise he cannot keep, such as telling Emma that it will not hurt, he will lose her trust and cooperation.

Emma's father arrives and asks if he can ride to the hospital with Emma in the ambulance. Dee Ann tells him he can, and she and Jeremy place Emma on the stretcher and place her in the ambulance. During the ride to the hospital, Jeremy asks her what her favorite subject is in school and what she likes to do when she is not school. Jeremy reassesses Emma en route and reassures her that she is doing just fine.

CHAPTER REVIEW

Chapter Summary

One of the most challenging aspects of work in EMS is communicating with and effectively caring for patients who come from diverse backgrounds and present in some of the most stressful circumstances of their lives. To be effective, you must understand the cognitive, psychosocial, and physical characteristics of patients from birth to old age. People of different ages have different fears and concerns. Physically, children are not just smaller, they are proportioned and their bodies work differently. The elderly are less able to compensate for illness and injury and may present differently from younger adults with the same problems. You must understand how the differences affect your assessment and management strategies.

Not only do health issues and expectations differ by patient age, they also differ by cultural and ethnic background. Cardiovascular disease, cancer, and stroke are leading causes of death in the United States among all ethnicities, but affect some cultures disproportionately. Higher rates of poverty among some ethnic groups create barriers to health care access. Health care providers' lack of understanding of the health beliefs of diverse groups can lead to distrust and inability to establish effective therapeutic relationships. For example, the firm handshake you usually offer may be seen as aggressive by some American Indian cultures and the eye contact you have learned is important may be viewed as disrespectful by some from Asian backgrounds. While it is not always possible to know the expectations of every patient, an attitude of seeking to understand the other person's expectations is universally important.

Review Questions

Multiple-Choice Questions

1. According to Piaget's stages of cognitive development, a child from birth to two years of age is in the _____ stage.
   - a. preoperational
   - b. concrete operational
   - c. formal operational
   - d. sensorimotor

2. A child from approximately 5 to 12 years of age, according to Erikson's theory of psychosocial development, is trying to resolve which one of the following conflicts?
   - a. Trust vs. mistrust
   - b. Autonomy vs. shame
   - c. Initiative vs. guilt
   - d. Industry vs. inferiority

3. The average life expectancy in the United States is about _____ years.
   - a. 60
   - b. 80
   - c. 100
   - d. 120

4. At birth, the average infant in the United States weighs approximately _____ kg.
   - a. 1
   - b. 3
   - c. 5
   - d. 7

5. Which one of the following is a characteristic of the pediatric airway that can lead to airway obstruction?
   - a. Uniform cylindrical shape of the airway
   - b. Small tongue
   - c. Prominent occipital skull
   - d. Rigid tracheal cartilage rings

6. The maximum normal heart rate for a neonate immediately after birth is _____ beats per minute.
   - a. 100
   - b. 120
   - c. 140
   - d. 160

7. Which age group listed below characteristically includes children who express their thoughts and frustrations through play?
   - a. Infant
   - b. Preschooler
   - c. School age
   - d. Adolescent

8. Which one of the following is a primary feature of the thought process of preschoolers and toddlers?
   - a. Literal
   - b. Logical
   - c. Abstract
   - d. Conceptual

9. Body image becomes a significant concern in which age group?
   - a. School age
   - b. Adolescent
   - c. Young adulthood
   - d. Middle adulthood

10. The leading cause of death for young adults is:
    - a. cardiovascular disease.
    - b. cancer.
    - c. stroke.
    - d. trauma.

11. The most significant cause of death among African Americans as a whole is:
    - a. cancer.
    - b. trauma.
    - c. hypertension.
    - d. HIV.

12. According to the stages of grief model by Elisabeth Kübler-Ross, which one of the following is the initial reaction to the news of death?
    - a. Bargaining
    - b. Anger
    - c. Denial
    - d. Depression

13. Engaging in risk-taking behavior during the mourning process is most likely in the _____ age group.
    - a. school-age
    - b. adolescent
    - c. young adult
    - d. older adult

14. Shivah is a mourning ritual in the _____ religion.
    - a. Jewish
    - b. Hindu
    - c. Buddhist
    - d. Muslim

15. Providing comfort measures at the end of life is known as _____ care.
    - a. hospice
    - b. terminal
    - c. palliative
    - d. definitive

Critical-Thinking Questions

16. How could Kohlberg's theory of moral development be applied to ethical decision making in EMS?

17. How might you anticipate the findings of shock to differ in an 80-year-old patient as compared to a 25-year-old patient?

18. What are some of the behaviors and feelings you should anticipate from a child who recently suffered the death of a close family member?

19. How can you interact more effectively with a patient who has age-related hearing and vision changes?

20. Your patient is a middle-aged woman from Saudi Arabia. What are some cultural considerations you should keep in mind in interacting with this patient?

21. What are some reasons ethnic minority groups might distrust the U.S. health care system?

References

American Academy of Child and Adolescent Psychiatry. (2008). *Children and grief* (fact sheet). Retrieved December 27, 2010, from http://aacap.org/page.ww?name=Children+and+Grief&section=Facts+for+Families

Centers for Disease Control and Prevention, National Center for Health Statistics. (2010). Retrieved December 27, 2010, from http://www.cdc.gov/nchs/fastats/lifexpec.htm

Copp, G. (1998). A review of current theories of death and dying. *Journal of Advanced Nursing, 28*(2), 382–390.

Kemp, C., & Bhungalia, S. (2002). Culture and the end of life: A review of major world religions. *Journal of Hospice and Palliative Nursing, 4*(4), 235–242.

Lobar, S. L., Youngblut, J. M, & Brooten, D. (2006). Cross-cultural beliefs, ceremonies, and rituals surrounding the death of a loved one. *Pediatric Nursing, 32*(1), 44–50.

Lyles, M. M. (2010). *Children's grief responses.* Children's Grief Education Association. Retrieved December 27, 2010, from http://www.childgrief.org/howtohelp.htm

Management Sciences for Health. (2010). *The provider's guide to quality and culture.* Retrieved June 7, 2011, from http://erc.msh.org/mainpage.cfm?file=1.0.htm&module=provider&language=English

Smedley, B. D., Stith, A. Y., & Nelson, A. R. (Eds). (2002). Unequal treatment: Confronting racial and ethnic disparities in health care. *Institute of Medicine Report.* Washington, DC: The National Academies Press.

U.S. Department of Health and Human Services (HHS) Office of Minority Health (OMH). (2010). (*Think cultural health: Bridging the healthcare gap through cultural competency continuing education programs.* Retrieved June 7, 2011, from https://www.thinkculturalhealth.hhs.gov/cccm/

10 Pathophysiology: Selected Impairments of Homeostasis

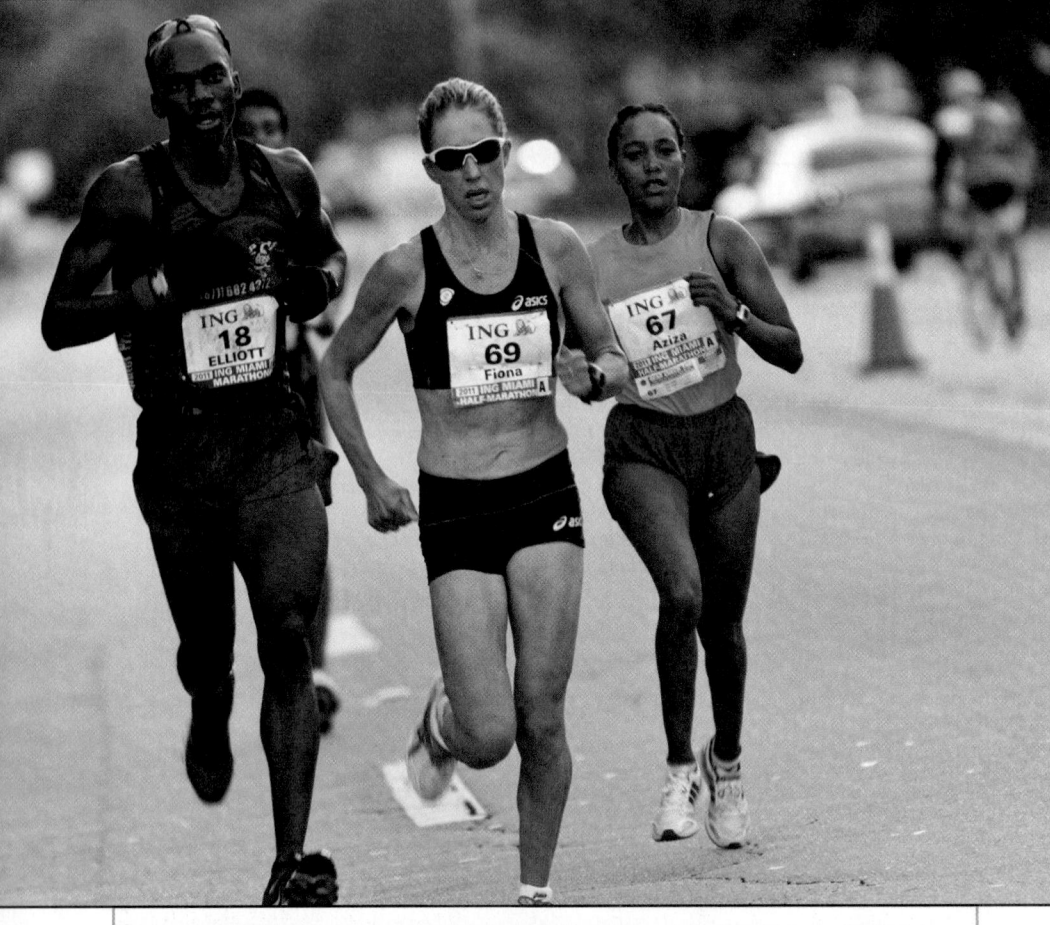

Content Area: Pathophysiology

Advanced EMT Education Standard: The Advanced EMT applies comprehensive knowledge of the pathophysiology of respiration and perfusion to patient assessment and management.

Objectives

After reading this chapter, you should be able to:

10.1 Define key terms introduced in this chapter.

10.2 Explain the importance of understanding basic pathophysiology.

10.3 Give examples of mechanisms that cause disease and injury in the human body.

10.4 Describe the composition of ambient air as it relates to ventilation and respiration.

10.5 Explain how changes in the compliance of the lungs and chest wall and in airway resistance can affect ventilation.

10.6 Explain how common disease processes can interfere with ventilation and with external and internal respiration.

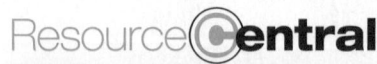

To access Resource Central, follow the directions on the Student Access Card provided with this text. If there is no card, go to www.bradybooks.com and follow the Resource Central link to Buy Access. Under Media Resources, you will find:

• *CO_2—The Other Gas.* Watch an animation and see how CO_2 moves in and out of cells.

• *Cardiac Output.* Read and learn about the factors that influence cardiac output and regulate blood pressure.

• *Acid-Base Imbalances.* Discover the causes of acid-base abnormalities and how those changes affect cellular function.

CASE STUDY

Colin Lear and Tyler Erb, Advanced EMTs with Bayside EMS, have just arrived on the scene of a report for a person down, unknown problem, at an outdoor café on the boardwalk. From 20 feet away, the patient, a woman in her 30s, appears to be unresponsive and pale. Passersby noticed her slumped over a table, but no one witnessed what happened. Employees of the café report that the patient purchased her food and sat down to eat about 15 minutes before a bystander reported a problem. As they near the patient, Colin and Tyler hear the stridorous sounds of a partial airway obstruction and notice cyanosis of the lips, ears, and nail beds. The patient's skin is cool and diaphoretic.

Problem-Solving Questions

1. What are the patient's immediate problems?
2. What body system or systems may be involved?
3. What mechanisms of illness or injury should Colin and Tyler explore as underlying causes of the problems?
4. Why is it important that Colin and Tyler look for explanations, rather than just treating obvious problems?

10.7   Describe the homeostatic mechanisms that attempt to correct for changes in ventilation and perfusion.

10.8   Explain the consequences of impaired tidal volume, respiratory rate, and minute volume, as well as increases in anatomical dead space.

10.9   Explain the concept of ventilation–perfusion mismatch.

10.10   Explain the pathophysiology of shock (hypoperfusion), including the consequences of cellular hypoxia and death.

10.11   Compare and contrast aerobic and anaerobic cellular metabolism, including consideration of the amount of ATP produced and the removal of byproducts of energy metabolism.

10.12   Describe the consequences of failure of the cellular sodium/potassium pump.

10.13   Describe how inadequate vascular volume, inadequate heart function, and decreased peripheral vascular resistance can each lead to shock.

10.14   Give examples of conditions that can lead to the following:
- Loss of vascular volume
- Inadequate heart function
- Decreased peripheral vascular resistance

10.15   Explain the mechanisms and pathophysiology of each of the following types of shock:
- Hypovolemic (hemorrhagic and nonhemorrhagic)
- Distributive (anaphylactic, septic, neurogenic)
- Cardiogenic
- Obstructive

(continued)

(continued from previous page)

10.16 Explain how mechanisms such as exposure to carbon monoxide and cyanide can lead to shock.

10.17 Explain the body's compensatory reactions to hypoperfusion and how they manifest in the early signs and symptoms of shock.

10.18 Describe the progression of shock through the compensated, decompensated, and irreversible stages.

10.19 Discuss the rationales behind the priorities and goals of prehospital management of patients with hypoperfusion.

10.20 Given a series of scenarios:
- Recognize patients who are at risk for shock.
- Explain the influence of age on the assessment and management of patients with hypoperfusion.

10.21 Describe the pathophysiology of cardiac arrest.

10.22 Differentiate between the electrical, circulatory, and metabolic phases of cardiac arrest.

10.23 Explain the dependence of cells upon glucose as a source of energy.

10.24 Explain the consequences of untreated hypoglycemia.

10.25 Explain how disruptions of electrolyte balance and pH impact body functions.

10.26 Explain the consequences of inadequate temperature regulation in the body.

Introduction

Homeostasis is the physiologic steady state achieved by the body's complex regulatory mechanisms. The body operates only within narrow ranges of temperature, pH, oxygen levels, glucose levels, electrolyte levels, and other parameters. When disease, environmental conditions, or trauma threaten to disrupt homeostasis, the body responds, correcting for the disruption. It is in this way that the body routinely, and usually without our awareness, protects itself against invading pathogens, prevents itself from bleeding to death from minor injuries, maintains internal temperature despite changes in environmental temperature, and keeps blood composition and characteristics within narrow parameters.

In some cases, the disruption of homeostasis is severe. The body's compensatory mechanisms respond, but are not sufficient to restore the conditions necessary to sustain life. Noticeable signs and symptoms appear, yet they are only superficial indications of what is happening at the cellular level. A patient's respiratory rate increases, but that is not the underlying problem. It is the lack of oxygen at the cellular level that triggers the increased respiratory rate. The skin appears cyanotic (bluish), but cyanosis is not the problem. It is a visible indicator that the hemoglobin within red blood cells is not adequately saturated with oxygen. The desaturated hemoglobin gives blood a dark, dusky color that shows beneath the skin as the hue of cyanosis. In treating a patient with cyanosis, you are not working to correct cyanosis. Instead, you are working to provide oxygen to be carried by hemoglobin to the cellular level. You must recognize signs and symptoms, but you must also understand what causes them.

Whereas physiology is the study of the function of the body, and **pathology** is the study of disease, the study of the effects and progression of disease and injury is called **pathophysiology**. All diseases and injury affect the body at a cellular level. A laceration disrupts cellular integrity of the skin and its associated blood vessels and other structures. The blood that flows from the laceration contains red blood cells. The loss of a critical mass of red blood cells translates into a decrease in the oxygen available for each and every cell in the body. The impaired cellular function can result in visible signs and symptoms, such as weakness, because the diminished amount of oxygen reduces the amount of energy cells can produce; pale, cool skin as the body attempts to compensate for blood loss by constricting peripheral blood vessels to divert blood to the vital organs; or hypotension as the loss of blood becomes so great that the body's compensatory mechanisms are no longer sufficient to maintain pressure within the vascular system.

The body responds in predictable ways to specific threats to homeostasis. The tangible, objectively observable results of these responses, and the direct effects of the disease or injury itself, are **signs** of the disease process. The patient's subjective sensations of the body's responses are **symptoms**. Signs and symptoms, along with information about the patient's medical history or the mechanism of injury, allow you to develop an informed **clinical impression** of the patient's problem. It is only with a clinical impression that you can appropriately plan the patient's treatment.

Anaphylaxis (severe allergic reaction), pneumothorax (a collapsed lung), and **pulmonary edema** (fluid in the lungs) from heart failure all cause difficulty breathing. **Hypoxia** and resulting impaired cellular energy production is the final common pathway for all of those problems. Yet, the mechanisms that cause each problem and the treatment needed to correct each mechanism are very different. All of the patients require supplemental oxygen and, perhaps, assisted ventilations. Basic attention to the airway, breathing, and circulation are necessary for patients, but are not sufficient to address the underlying causes of those problems. You must be able to think beyond hypoxia to its root causes to determine specific treatment needed. Epinephrine is potentially lifesaving for the patient with anaphylaxis, but potentially fatal for the patient with heart failure.

A number of emergencies affect cellular energy production. Any condition that disrupts tissue perfusion, interferes with the use of available oxygen, or leads to a decrease in glucose available to the cell decreases cellular energy production. In some circumstances, cells can briefly adapt to adverse conditions to maintain vital functions, but their adaptations are limited and come at a cost. Without immediate restoration of homeostasis, cells cannot carry out their functions and body systems begin to fail. In cases of hypoxia, **shock**, hypoglycemia, and other acute, life-threatening conditions, the window of opportunity to intervene and restore the cellular environment to normal is brief. You must understand the pathophysiology leading to disruption of the cellular environment in order to plan treatment to best correct the cellular environment.

Mechanisms of Disease and Injury

There are several mechanisms by which homeostasis can be disrupted. They include hypoxia, nutritional imbalance, genetic diseases, cancer, physical injury, toxins, infections, environmental extremes, and inflammation (Table 10-1). Many emergencies share a common consequence: impaired

TABLE 10-1   Selected Mechanisms of Disease

Disease Mechanism	Example	Pathophysiology
Hypoxia	A narcotic overdose depresses the respiratory centers in the central nervous system.	Decreased respiratory center function causes slow, shallow ventilations. An inadequate amount of air reaches the alveolar level for gas exchange, resulting in poor oxygenation of the blood returning to the lungs. Inadequately oxygenated red blood cells cannot deliver sufficient oxygen to the cellular level. Without oxygen, the cells engage in anaerobic metabolism, producing less ATP. Without ATP, cellular mechanisms fail and cell death occurs.
Nutritional imbalance	A diabetic patient takes his insulin, but does not eat.	The increased amount of insulin quickly facilitates the entry of the available glucose into cells. Without an additional source of glucose from the digestive tract, the blood glucose level quickly falls. The remaining glucose is inadequate to fuel the metabolic needs of the cell. ATP is not produced and cellular mechanisms begin to fail.
Physical trauma	A patient falls from a second-story roof. When he lands, a screwdriver in his tool belt impales him in the right side, lacerating his liver. The liver begins to bleed profusely.	With a decreased number of red blood cells, inadequate oxygen and glucose are delivered to the cells to fuel metabolism and cellular mechanisms begin to fail. Unless the bleeding is stopped quickly and red blood cells are restored, the patient will die.
Infection	A patient develops pneumonia.	Cellular debris and fluid fill the alveoli in the affected lobe, preventing oxygen from diffusing across the respiratory membrane and into the blood. Less oxygen reaches the cellular level, impairing cellular metabolism.
Toxin	A faulty gas furnace releases carbon monoxide into a residence.	Carbon monoxide binds to hemoglobin, preventing oxygen from binding to it. Oxygen is not delivered to the cellular level, impairing cellular metabolism.
Environment	A person locks his keys in his car and is unable to get back into his car or into his house. It is 2°F with a 20-mph wind. His closest neighbor is 3 miles away.	The body loses heat to the cold air, and this effect is increased substantially by the wind. Despite shivering and the exercise of walking to get help, the body is unable to generate enough heat to maintain the core temperature. The electrical system of the heart becomes irritable, the nervous system begins to malfunction, and less oxygen is released to the cells in the tissues.

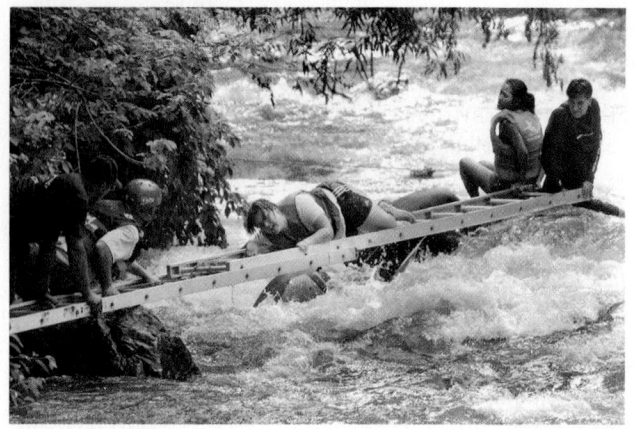

FIGURE 10-1

Homeostasis can be disrupted in a number of ways. This patient may have received trauma in the event that caused her to enter the water, aspirated water may impair breathing, immersion in water can quickly lead to hypothermia, and the patient may have pre-existing diseases. You must be able to anticipate the many ways in which homeostasis can be disrupted, and be able to intervene in pathophysiologic processes.

(© AP Photo/Standard Examiner, Brian Nicholson)

cellular energy production. Energy production may be impaired by low levels of glucose or insulin, or by a lack of oxygen or poor perfusion. The causes of those conditions are varied, ranging from an overdose of narcotics that depresses

the respiratory system to massive hemorrhage from a gunshot wound. Other causes of emergencies related to disruptions of the cellular environment include changes in pH, electrolyte balance, and temperature.

Though there are a variety of ways to categorize mechanisms of cellular dysfunction and injury, for the purposes of this chapter, they will be categorized as hypoxic cellular injury, shock, impaired glucose metabolism, electrolyte and pH disturbances, or environmental disorders. As you will see, there is considerable overlap among mechanisms, reflecting the interdependence of the body's systems on each other (Figure 10-1).

Compensation and Adaptation

The human body is capable of remarkable adaptation under stress, allowing it to withstand significant challenges to homeostasis. For example, the body can adapt by using alternative forms of fuel when glucose is not available and by creating energy anaerobically when oxygen availability is limited. The body adjusts heat production and loss to the temperature of the environment. The immune system reacts quickly to neutralize invading pathogens, and the cardiovascular system can compensate for fluid losses and changes in the size of the vascular system.

In the long term, cells can adapt to a variety of conditions (Table 10-2). For example, squamous cells that can

TABLE 10-2 Types of Cellular Adaptation

Adaptation	Description
Atrophy	Reduction in the size of cells of a tissue. For example, skeletal muscle atrophy occurs when an extremity has been immobilized in a cast for several weeks. Cells adapt to the lack of use by decreasing in size.
Metaplasia	A change in the type of cells that comprise a tissue into a different type of cell that is not normal for that tissue in order to adapt to changes in the environment. For example, cells that line the esophagus (squamous epithelium) can change into a different type (columnar epithelium) to adapt to chronic exposure to stomach acids (Barrett's esophagus).
Hyperplasia	Increase in the number of cells of a tissue. An example is benign prostatic hypertrophy in middle-aged men. The prostate increases in size and can obstruct the urethra, interfering with urine flow.
Hypertrophy	Increase in the size of cells of a tissue. The best example of this is the growth of a muscle following weight lifting. The number of skeletal muscle cells remains constant, but cell size increases.
Anaplasia	Loss of cellular differentiation. This is an indication of malignant tumors.
Dysplasia	Cell maturation and differentiation are delayed, resulting in the loss of uniformity of cells within a certain tissue. This is often a precursor to cancer. For example, a Pap smear may show dysplasia of cells of the cervix, indicating a need for further examination and treatment to prevent cancer.
Neoplasia	New or expanded growth in an area of the body where it is not expected. Neoplasia can be accompanied by anaplasia. This, and the degree to which the neoplasm invades normal tissues, determines whether or not the tumor is benign or malignant. An example of a benign neoplasm is uterine fibroid tumors. An example of a malignant neoplasm is osteosarcoma, a cancerous bone tumor.
Apoptosis	The genetic instructions provided by DNA can command cellular self-destruction, either as part of a normal process, or to destroy damaged cells that are a threat to the body.

better withstand smoke toxins replace the pseudociliated columnar epithelial cells lining the trachea of a cigarette smoker. This process is called *metaplasia*, and it is not without cost. Although the squamous cells resist smoke better, they lack the ability to secrete mucus that traps debris and the cilia that remove it. Ultimately, this is a major contributor to the development of both chronic bronchitis and the frequent pneumonias that smokers experience.

Hypoxic Cellular Injury

Despite its amazing abilities, the body can compensate only within limits. Eventually, if the insult is overwhelming or prolonged, damage occurs. Early cell damage sometimes can be reversed if the conditions causing it are corrected. If **ischemia** (lack of blood flow to tissue, resulting in hypoxia) is reversed by restoring perfusion, or if hypoxia is corrected by adequate ventilation and supplemental oxygen, permanent cellular injury may be averted. In hypoxic conditions, cells initially can adapt to the lack of oxygen by switching from aerobic to anaerobic metabolism (Figure 10-2). But, this backup method can only support the cell for a limited time. Depending on the tissue type, cells without adequate oxygen can become irreversibly injured in as little as 5 minutes.

Hypoxic cellular injury occurs any time that oxygen delivery to, or utilization by, cells is disrupted. The normal PaO_2 of human arterial blood is 85 to 100 mmHg. This level is required for hemoglobin to be adequately saturated with oxygen molecules, which are then delivered to cells. Oxygen molecules are released from hemoglobin under

the conditions that exist at the cellular level. Oxygen then diffuses across the cell membrane, and finds its position on the end of the electron transport chain within the inner membrane of the mitochondria.

Aerobic Metabolism

The *electron transport chain* is the series of enzymes within all aerobic cells that receive the end products of glycolysis (sugar breakdown) and extract energy from them in the form of hydrogen ions. In order to extract this energy in a controlled fashion, electrons must be transferred from one enzyme to another along the chain. Oxygen, a very electronegative element, is the driving force of this chain reaction by attracting the electrons to it.

When working properly, the force of oxygen pulling the electrons through the chain results in numerous hydrogen ions being extracted into the intermembrane space of the mitochondria (Figure 10-3). The ions build up within this space to create a concentration gradient that forces them into the inner mitochondria through a small exit. The ATP synthase enzyme sits within this exit, and it uses the energy of the hydrogen ion concentration gradient passing through it to create ATP molecules. Overall, this process is called *oxidative phosphorylation*, and the ATP molecules go on to fuel the many metabolic reactions of the cell. Without oxygen, the electron transport chain halts activity because the electrons no longer are subject to a force that pulls them along. As a result, the hydrogen ion gradient is not created and ATP is not generated. Without ATP, the cells cannot power their reactions and activities, including the function of the **sodium/potassium pump**, which maintains the electrolyte balance across the cell membrane.

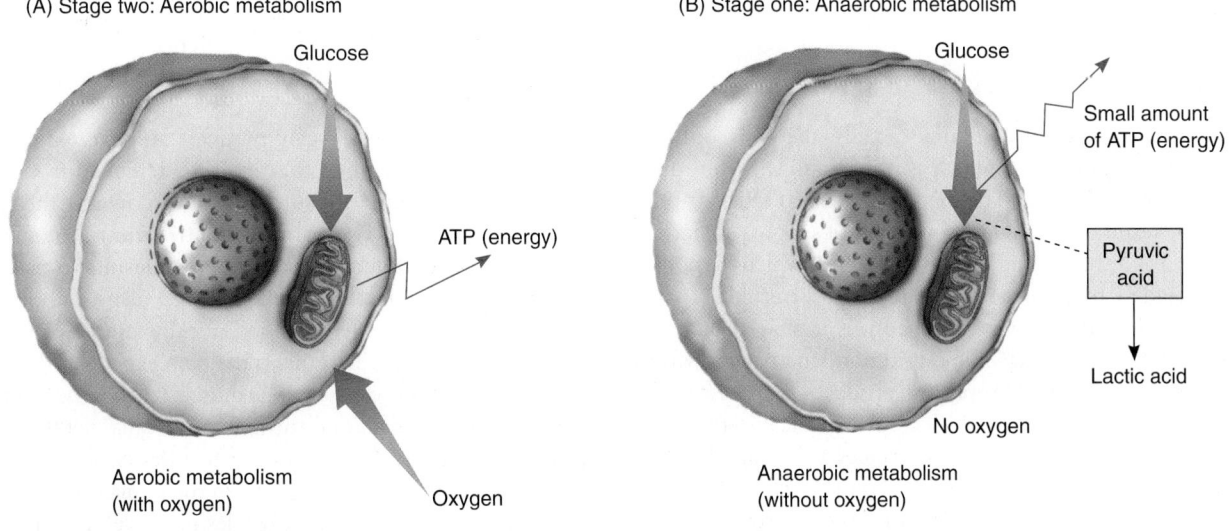

(A) Stage two: Aerobic metabolism

Glucose

ATP (energy)

Aerobic metabolism (with oxygen)

Oxygen

(B) Stage one: Anaerobic metabolism

Glucose

Small amount of ATP (energy)

Pyruvic acid

Lactic acid

No oxygen

Anaerobic metabolism (without oxygen)

FIGURE 10-2

(A) Aerobic metabolism. Glucose broken down in the presence of oxygen produces a large amount of energy (ATP).
(B) Anaerobic metabolism. Glucose broken down without the presence of oxygen produces pyruvic acid that converts to lactic acid and only a small amount of energy (ATP).

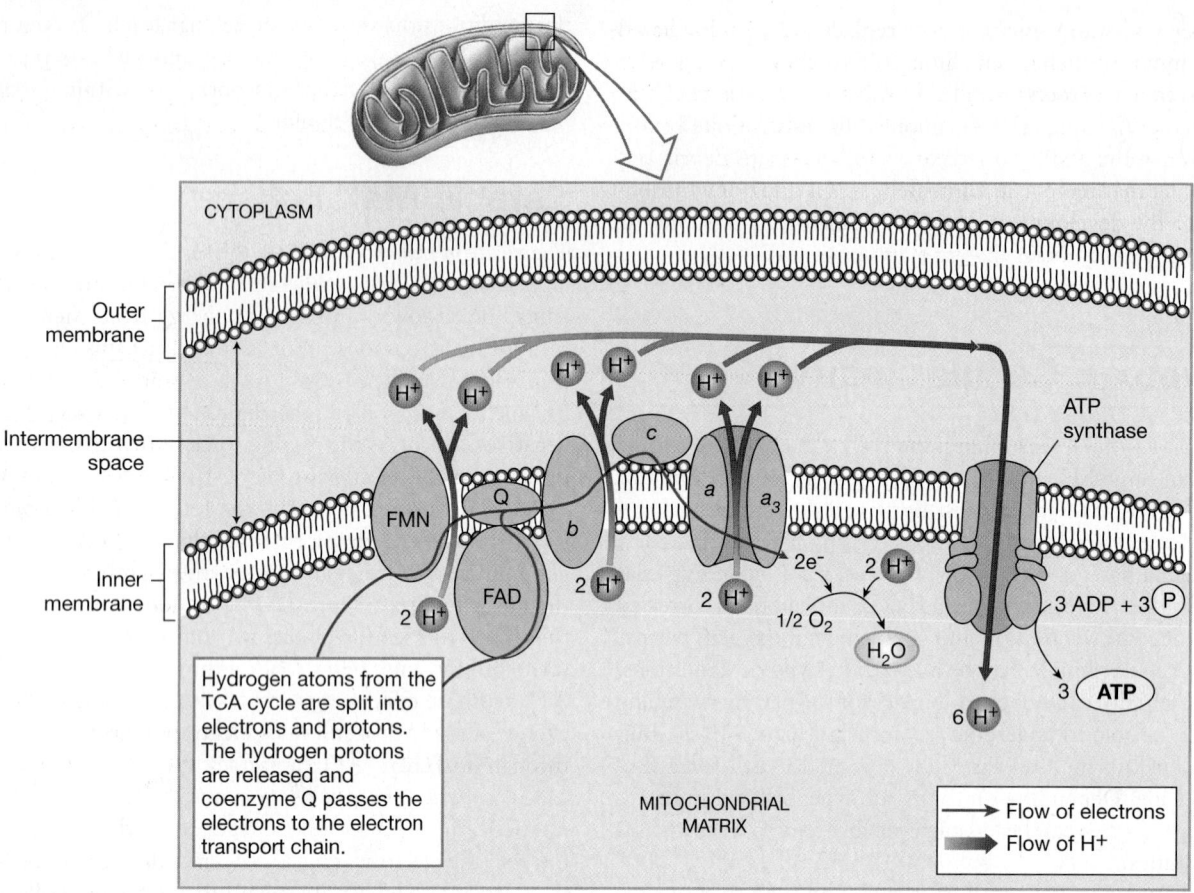

CYTOPLASM

Outer membrane

Intermembrane space

Inner membrane

ATP synthase

FMN

Q

c

b

a a_3

FAD

$2\,H^+$

$2\,H^+$

$2\,H^+$

$2e^-$

$2\,H^+$

$1/2\,O_2$

H_2O

$3\,ADP + 3\,(P)$

$6\,H^+$

3 **ATP**

Hydrogen atoms from the TCA cycle are split into electrons and protons. The hydrogen protons are released and coenzyme Q passes the electrons to the electron transport chain.

MITOCHONDRIAL MATRIX

→ Flow of electrons
⇒ Flow of H^+

FIGURE 10-3

The electron transport system (ETS) and ATP formation. The diagrammatic view shows the locations of the coenzymes and the electron transport system in the inner mitochondrial membrane. The electrons of hydrogen atoms from the TCA cycle are transferred by coenzyme Q to the ETS (a series of cytochrome molecules), and the hydrogen ions (H^+) remain in the matrix. The energy-carrying electrons are passed from one cytochrome to another. Energy released by the passed electrons is used to pump H^+ from the matrix into the intermembrane space. This creates a difference in the concentration of H^+ across the inner membrane. The hydrogen ions then diffuse through ATP synthase in the inner membrane, and their kinetic energy is used to generate ATP. (Bledsoe, Bryan E.; Martini, Frederic H.; Bartholomew, Edwin F.; Ober, William C.; Garrison, Claire W.; Anatomy & Physiology for Emergency Care, 2nd Edition, © 2008. Reprinted with permission of Pearson Education, Inc., Upper Saddle River, NJ)

Anaerobic Metabolism

When oxygen is not available to cells, they rely only on anaerobic respiration, which is a mechanism to produce ATP without oxygen. The method is far less efficient than aerobic respiration, however, and cannot support life indefinitely. It is a short-term adaptation, during which the conditions leading to cellular hypoxia must be corrected.

The initial pathway of glycolysis is shared between both aerobic and anaerobic respiration, and occurs within the cell's cytoplasm. This process produces four ATP molecules by breaking down one glucose molecule into two molecules of **pyruvate**. Two ATP molecules are required to fuel the reaction, so the net gain in ATP is only two.

In aerobic respiration, pyruvate is converted to acetyl coenzyme A, which enters the mitochondria and participates in the Krebs cycle. This ultimately produces 36 ATP molecules through oxidative phosphorylation. In anaerobic metabolism, the cell must function on less than one

tenth of the ATP that is normally available in the presence of oxygen.

In the absence of oxygen, pyruvate is converted to **lactic acid**, a waste product that must be removed from the cell. Lactic acid cannot be further broken down by the cells and accumulates in tissues. This contributes to the **metabolic acidosis** that accompanies hypoxic insults to tissues. Therefore, blood lactate levels are used as an important marker of tissue-level hypoxia in critically injured or ill patients. A good example of this is the pain experienced by all of us during muscle overuse. The muscle reaches the limit of oxidative metabolism and turns to anaerobic metabolism, producing lactic acid, which causes muscle aches.

The largest consumer of ATP in the human body is the sodium/potassium pump that resides in the cell membrane. This pump is responsible for maintaining the chemical and electrical gradient across the cell membrane, which allows for functions such as depolarization, transport, and signaling. During each cycle of the sodium/potassium pump, it moves three sodium ions out of the cell and takes in two potassium ions, at the cost of one ATP molecule. This unequal movement of molecules is critical in maintaining the osmotic gradient across cells. When ATP production is diminished, function of this pump decreases or stops. The buildup of sodium ions within the cells increases water intake into the cell by osmosis. In turn, cellular edema, and eventually, lysis, occurs. As the structural architecture of the cell is disrupted, the cell may undergo **apoptosis**, or cellular-directed death, and release lysosomal enzymes that will further the destruction of not only that cell, but surrounding cells.

Causes of Hypoxia

Oxygen delivery to the cells relies on the following components (Figure 10-4):

- Adequate onloading of oxygen onto the hemoglobin in red blood cells
- Circulation of red blood cells through the microvasculature (capillary beds) to perfuse the tissues of the body
- Adequate offloading of oxygen to the tissues once red blood cells reach the microvasculature

The components can be disrupted in four general ways: oxygen delivery to the bloodstream, oxygen transport within the bloodstream, oxygen transport from the bloodstream to the cells, and oxygen utilization by the cells.

Oxygen Delivery to the Blood

A prerequisite for oxygen to reach the lungs is an atmosphere that contains an adequate amount of oxygen. The air we breathe contains about 21 percent oxygen, 79 percent nitrogen, and trace amounts of other gasses. When a patient is in an atmosphere deficient in oxygen, hemoglobin within red blood cells cannot be fully saturated. Oxygen-deficient environments may occur when a patient is trapped in a toxic environment in an enclosed space, or at high altitudes.

Ventilations must produce an adequate tidal volume and minute volume to provide oxygen to the blood. With each breath, the average 70-kg person inspires about 500 mL of air (about 7 mL/kg). This volume of air constitutes the tidal volume. Of the 500 mL, 150 mL remains in the conducting portions of the airway and is not available to participate in gas exchange. This portion of the airway is called **anatomical dead space**. No matter how much or how

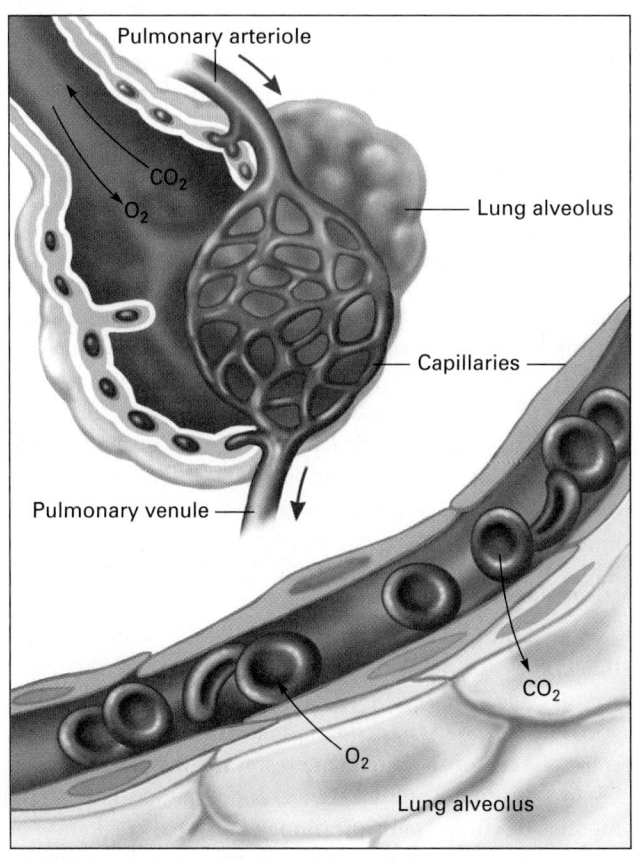

(A)

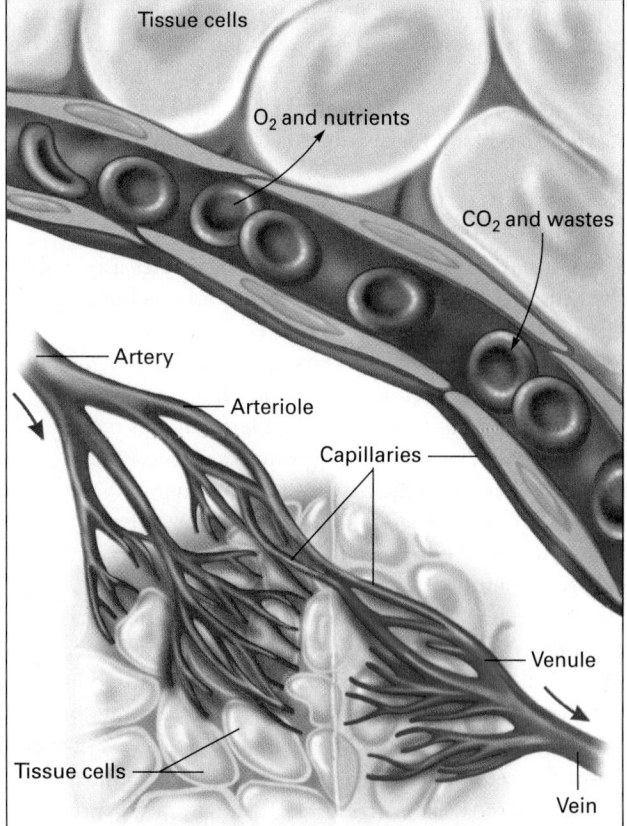

(B)

FIGURE 10-4

(A) Alveolar/capillary gas exchange. Oxygen moves from the lung alveolus into the capillary. Carbon dioxide moves from the capillary into the lung. (B) Capillary/cell gas exchange. Oxygen and nutrients move from the capillary into the cell. Carbon dioxide and other wastes move from the cell into the capillary.

little air is inspired, the volume of the dead space does not change. With normal tidal volume, 350 mL of air is available for gas exchange (alveolar air). If breathing becomes shallow and the tidal volume decreases to 300 mL, only 150 mL is available for gas exchange.

The body can compensate for decreased tidal volume by increasing the respiratory rate. Remember that the tidal volume multiplied by the respiratory rate is the minute volume. With an average tidal volume of 500 mL and a respiratory rate of 12 breaths per minute, the minute volume is 6 liters (6,000 mL). Of this air, 4.2 liters (4,200 mL) reaches the alveoli for gas exchange. If the tidal volume decreases to 400 mL, a respiratory rate of 15 breaths per minute still produces a minute volume of 6 liters. However, the amount of air reaching the alveoli decreases to 3.75 liters (3,750 mL). Theoretically, a tidal volume of 200 mL could produce a minute volume of 6 liters at a respiratory rate of 30 per minute. But keep in mind that only 50 mL of the 200 mL is reaching the alveoli. Even at a respiratory rate of 30, only 1,500 mL of air is reaching the alveoli, an amount insufficient to meet the body's needs. Likewise, although an increase in tidal volume can compensate for a decrease in respiratory rate, if the respiratory rate slows beyond a certain point, an increase in tidal volume can no longer maintain alveolar ventilation.

Unfortunately, conditions that cause shallow breathing often also cause slow breathing, resulting in inadequate ventilation. Any condition that affects tidal volume or respiratory rate can prevent an adequate amount of oxygen from reaching the blood for distribution throughout the body.

Effects of Altitude

The normal composition of ambient air creates a pressure gradient that allows oxygen to diffuse from its higher concentration in the ambient air that enters the alveoli to the lower concentration in the deoxygenated blood of the pulmonary capillaries. At the cellular level, the higher concentration of oxygen in the tissue capillaries allows oxygen to diffuse across the capillary membrane to the lower concentration of oxygen in the tissues. If the amount of oxygen in the atmosphere decreases and becomes closer to levels in the body, the ability of oxygen to diffuse into the blood and tissues is impaired.

The relative proportions of atmospheric gases remain fairly constant at any altitude humans can reach, up to 80,000 feet. Atmospheric pressure is measured as the amount of force exerted by the atmosphere per unit of area. Essentially, it is the weight of the air above the level at which it is measured. At sea level, the pressure of the atmosphere is 760 mmHg (which corresponds to a barometric pressure of 29.92 inches of mercury). The total amount of the pressure exerted is the combined pressures exerted by each gas in the mixture. The proportion of the total pressure exerted by each gas is the partial pressure (Pa) of the gas. Because there is 21 percent oxygen in the atmosphere, oxygen exerts 21 percent of the total pressure of the atmosphere.

This means that the partial pressure of oxygen (PaO_2) at sea level is 159.6 mmHg (760 mmHg × 0.21).

At higher altitudes, as the total amount of atmosphere pressing downward decreases, the atmospheric pressure decreases. Although the percentage of oxygen in the air remains constant at 21 percent, at an elevation of 5,000 feet (just under 1 mile) the atmospheric pressure is about 640 mmHg. The PaO_2 is 134.4 mmHg (640 mmHg × 0.21). At sea level, the normal PaO_2 of arterial blood is between 85 and 100 mmHg and the PaO_2 of blood returning to the lungs is about 40 mmHg.

The gradient created between the atmosphere and the blood is significant (159.6 mmHg versus 40 mmHg). At an altitude of 5,000 feet, the gradient is less (134.4 mmHg – 40 mmHg). However, the PaO_2 of alveolar air is somewhat lower than that of the atmosphere, about 90 to 100 mmHg because the air in the alveoli is fully saturated with water vapor, and because carbon dioxide is diffusing into the alveoli.

At elevations over 8,000 feet, the symptoms of altitude sickness can begin to develop due to a combination of the decreased oxygen availability and dehydration from the much drier air. Above 10,000 feet, oxygen pressure begins to decrease even more dramatically and will often cause shortness of breath. At still higher altitudes, life-threatening conditions such as high-altitude pulmonary edema (HAPE) and high-altitude cerebral edema (HACE) can occur. For this reason, flight crews must work within a pressurized cabin, or wear oxygen at altitudes above 14,000 feet, or if at altitudes of 12,500 feet for more than 30 minutes. (See Chapter 41.)

Airway Obstruction

The passageways through which air must travel to reach the alveoli must be unobstructed. If the airway is obstructed at any level, air cannot reach the respiratory bronchioles and alveoli, and hemoglobin is not saturated with oxygen. Causes of airway obstruction include swelling from infection, allergic reaction, or trauma. Causes of mechanical obstruction are from relaxation of the tongue and throat muscles, and foreign bodies lodged in the airway.

Neurologic Impairment

The respiratory centers in the medulla and pons must be functioning to stimulate inspiration and regulate the respiratory cycle (Figure 10-5). Stroke, traumatic brain injury, and narcotic overdoses are among causes of decreased respiratory center function. The respiratory centers must be able to communicate with the diaphragm and intercostal muscles to stimulate inspiration. The spinal cord and peripheral nerves leading to the diaphragm and intercostal muscles must be intact. Spinal cord injury above the level of C5 can sever communication between the spinal cord and diaphragm by way of the phrenic nerve. Thoracic spinal injuries can affect communication between the intercostal muscles and the spinal cord.

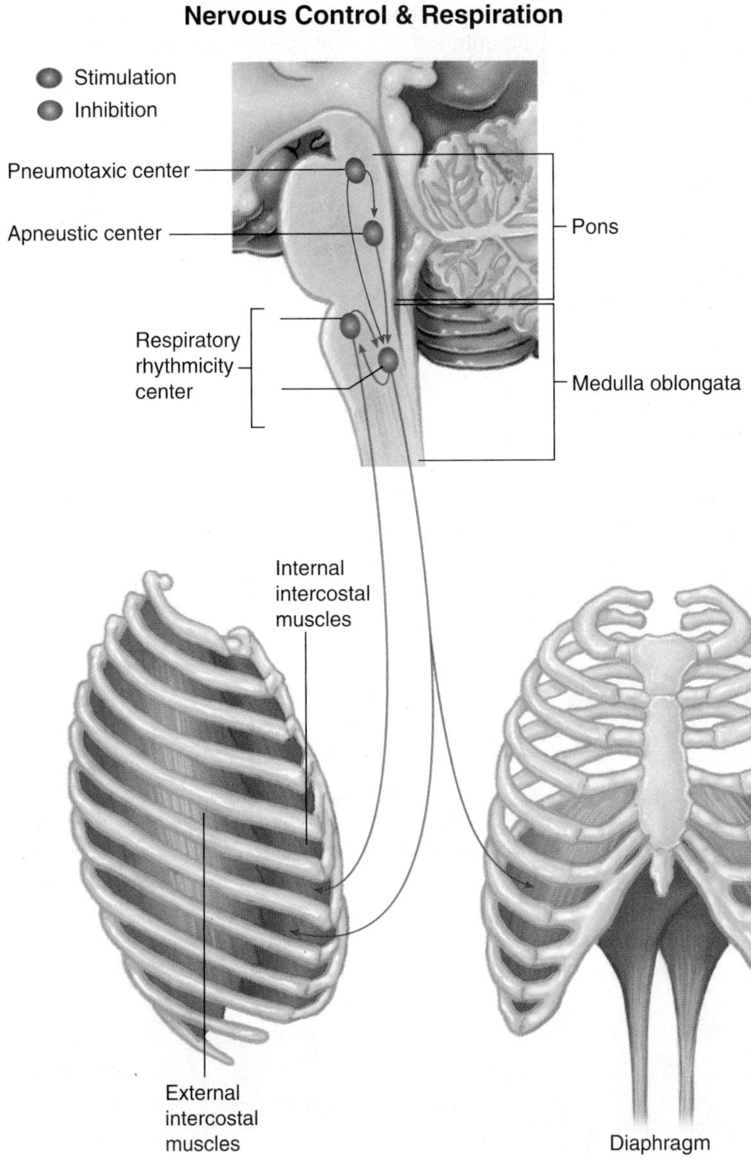

Nervous Control & Respiration

FIGURE 10-5

Nervous control of respiration.

- ● Stimulation
- ● Inhibition

Pneumotaxic center

Apneustic center

Pons

Respiratory rhythmicity center

Medulla oblongata

Internal intercostal muscles

External intercostal muscles

Diaphragm

Chest Wall Integrity

The chest wall and pleura must be intact to create negative intrapulmonary pressure. An accumulation of fluid or air in the pleural space interferes with the negative pressure that allows the lungs to expand when intrathoracic pressure decreases. Fractures of multiple ribs, or of the sternum, interfere with chest wall movement, also decreasing ventilation (Figure 10-6). Anything that restricts chest wall movement also decreases pulmonary ventilation, decreasing the amount of air that reaches the alveolar level. For example, severe burns result in a thick, leathery consistency of the skin, called *eschar*. Eschar is inelastic and if it encircles the chest, prevents the chest wall from expanding. A patient with severe burns around the thorax may require an escharotomy: an incision through the burned tissue that allows the chest wall to expand.

Bronchoconstriction, Atelectasis, and Diffusion Distance

Once air reaches the bronchioles and alveoli, they must be open for gas exchange to occur. The alveoli must be in close contact with the pulmonary capillaries surrounding them to allow oxygen to diffuse from the alveoli into the capillaries, where it can cross the red blood cell membranes and bind to hemoglobin. Asthma, chronic obstructive pulmonary disease (COPD), and anaphylaxis (severe allergic reaction) result in constriction of the bronchioles by various mechanisms (Figure 10-7). For example, in asthma, bronchoconstriction is caused by a combination of bronchiolar smooth muscle spasm and inflammation and swelling of the lining of the bronchioles. Bronchoconstriction initially impairs expiration more than inspiration, resulting in air trapping in the alveoli. As the oxygen in the trapped air is used and

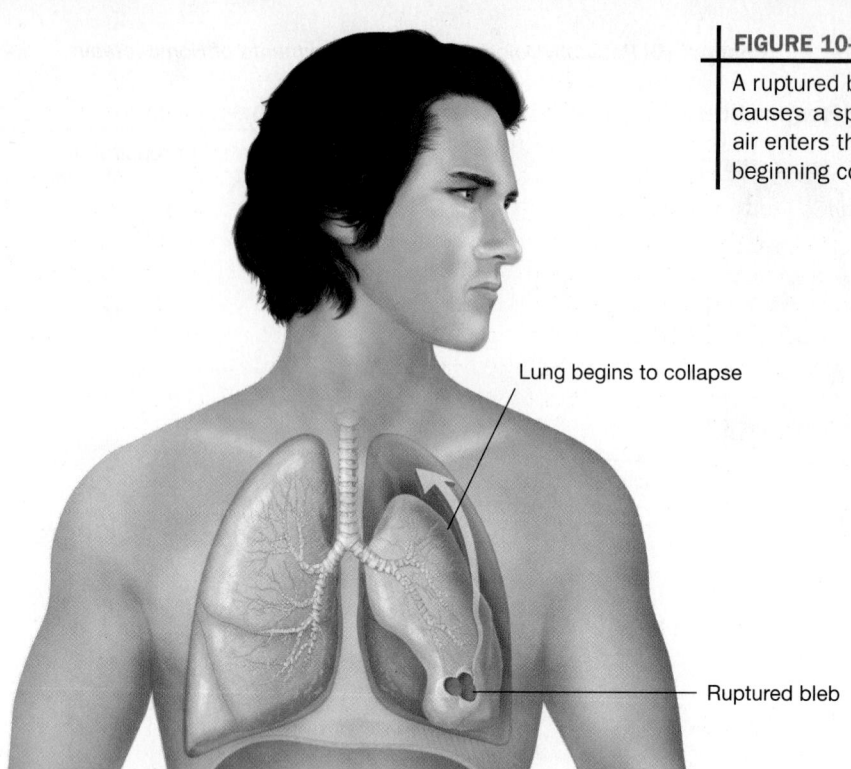

FIGURE 10-6

A ruptured bleb, or weakened area of lung tissue, causes a spontaneous pneumothorax in which air enters the pleural cavity and travels upward, beginning collapse of the lung from the top.

Lung begins to collapse

Ruptured bleb

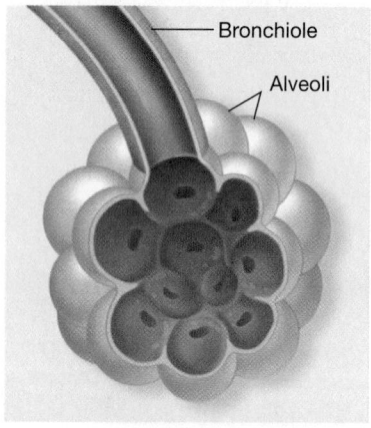

Bronchiole

Alveoli

(A) Normal

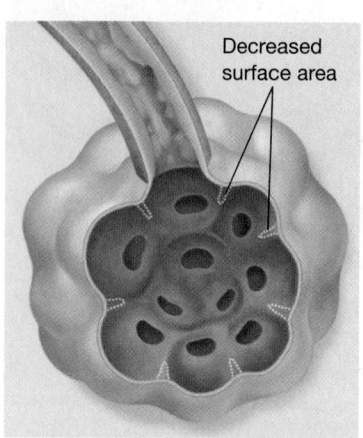

Decreased surface area

(B) Emphysema

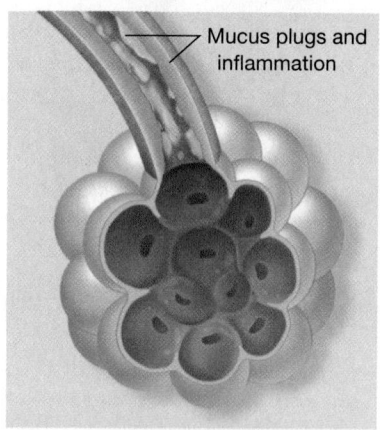

Mucus plugs and inflammation

(C) Chronic Bronchitis

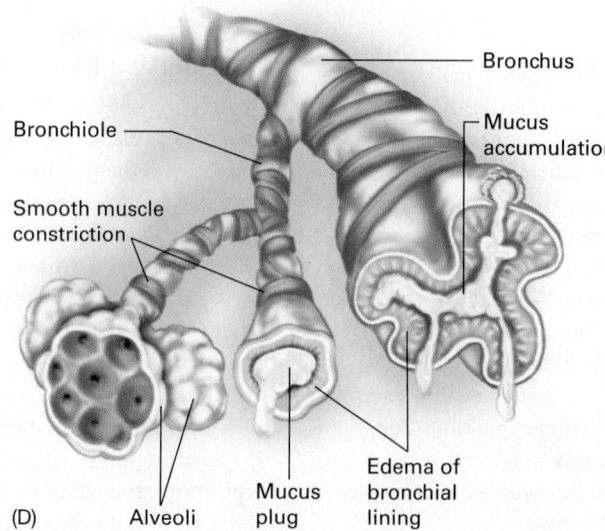

Bronchus

Bronchiole

Mucus accumulation

Smooth muscle constriction

FIGURE 10-7

(A) Normal alveolus.
(B) Alveous in emphysema.
(C) Alveolus in chronic bronchitis. (D) Alveoli in asthma.

(D)   Alveoli

Mucus plug

Edema of bronchial lining

carbon dioxide diffuses from the capillaries into the alveoli, the deoxygenated air serves as a barrier to oxygenated air.

The alveoli are kept from collapsing by surfactant (a wetting agent that allows fluid to spread across a surface). Surfactant is secreted by specialized cells in the alveoli and increases the surface tension of the alveoli, which allows them to stay open. A loss of surfactant causes alveoli to collapse and become airless, a condition called **atelectasis**. Surfactant production begins late in fetal development. Premature infants often lack surfactant, resulting in respiratory distress. Surfactant production also can be affected by acute respiratory distress syndrome (ARDS) and severe blunt trauma to the lung.

A number of conditions can increase the distance between the air in the alveoli and the red blood cells in the pulmonary capillaries. In pulmonary edema, fluid within the alveoli forces inspired air to traverse a greater distance to undergo gas exchange (Figure 10-8). In pneumonia, an infiltrate of mucus and debris in the affected lobe physically prevents air from accessing the alveoli for gas exchange.

Lung compliance, the amount of resistance to air movement, can be affected by decreased surfactant and a number of lung diseases. Compliance in the lungs must be maintained within a certain range: Too much or too little compliance will result in ventilatory compromise. Chronic exposure to chemical irritants such as coal, asbestos, or silicone, among others, can damage the alveolar walls and cause scarring, ultimately stiffening the lung. This stiffening causes a decrease in compliance that prevents effective inhalation.

Excessive compliance is detrimental to ventilation and is the result of the chronic obstructive lung diseases (COPD). Loss of lung elasticity decreases the ability of the lung to recoil following inhalation. This leads to air trapping. The anatomical dead space in the lungs increases, reducing the effectiveness of ventilation. The physical result of this constant lung expansion is a barrel chest, which can be readily seen on physical examination. The inability to properly exhale causes a chronically increased carbon dioxide level in the body. Over time, the chemoreceptors that respond to increased carbon dioxide levels become insensitive to them. To breathe, the patient must then rely on the secondary stimulus–decreased oxygen levels.

Ventilation–Perfusion Mismatch

In general, the observed results of most pulmonary disease states can be traced to a **ventilation–perfusion (VQ) mismatch**. The initiating problem may be a decrease in ventilation, lung perfusion, or both. Decreases in ventilation affect the ability of air to get to the alveoli for gas exchange. Examples of this include pulmonary edema, atelectasis, pneumonia, aspirated foreign bodies, and **pneumothorax**. A pneumothorax results in a collapse of a portion or even all of a lung. The volume available for gas exchange decreases, and mismatch occurs. Decreased lung perfusion is

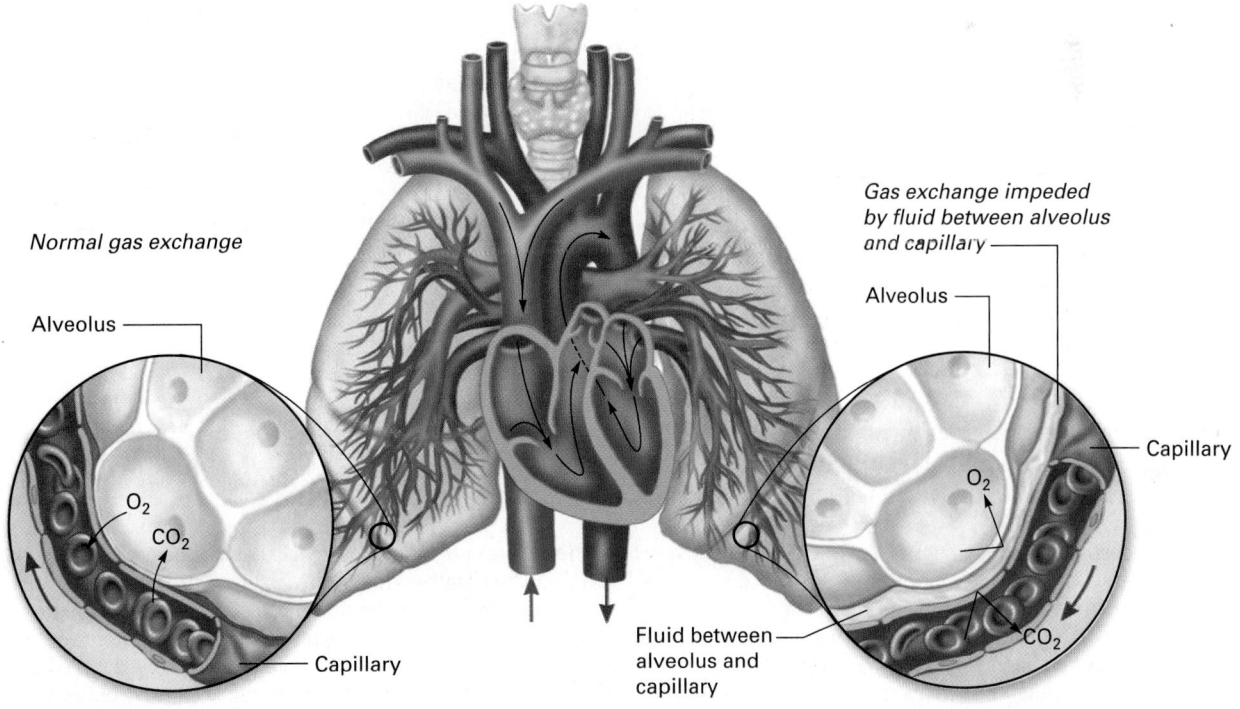

Normal gas exchange

Alveolus

O_2
CO_2

Capillary

Gas exchange impeded by fluid between alveolus and capillary

Alveolus

Capillary

O_2

CO_2

Fluid between alveolus and capillary

FIGURE 10-8

Fluid that collects between the alveoli and capillaries, preventing normal exchange of oxygen and carbon dioxide. The fluid also may invade the alveolar sacs.

illustrated by **pulmonary embolism**, an obstruction to blood flow through the pulmonary circulation. In this case, the lung is ventilated, but the portion of lung beyond the obstruction does not receive circulation. In effect, the surface area for gas exchange is reduced.

Respiratory Failure and Arrest

The body can compensate to some degree for problems that interfere with the ability of oxygen to reach the red blood cells. The respiratory rate increases, and tidal volume may increase. In long-standing hypoxia, the number of red blood cells is increased to provide more hemoglobin for oxygen transport. Depending on the severity of the underlying problem, varying degrees of hypoxia, acidosis, and hypercapnia (high carbon dioxide levels) develop. The body requires more oxygen to fuel the increased work of ventilation at a time when the availability of oxygen to the cells is decreased. If the underlying problem progresses or is not corrected, respiratory failure occurs. Untreated, **respiratory failure** progresses rapidly to **respiratory arrest**. Untreated respiratory arrest leads to cardiac arrest and death.

Patients with any level of ventilatory compromise require immediate intervention, both supportive and specific. Supportive treatment consists of ensuring that the patient's airway is open, providing supplemental oxygen, and, if needed, assisting ventilations or providing artificial ventilation. Advanced EMTs may administer some specific treatments in the prehospital setting. For example, inhaled bronchodilators for asthma and COPD, and epinephrine for anaphylaxis. In other cases, paramedics can initiate treatment in the prehospital setting, or you may need to transport the patient without delay for treatment in the hospital. You must make decisions about how to get the right care to the patient in the right amount of time.

Oxygen Transport in the Blood

Once oxygen is in the alveoli, it requires sufficient circulating blood volume and hemoglobin and favorable biochemical conditions to be transported to the tissue beds for use. Any of the variables can be negatively affected by pathologic conditions. In states of shock, oxygenated blood volume delivery to tissues is inadequate, and tissue hypoxia ensues. This occurs regardless of the type of shock; hypovolemic, obstructive, distributive, and neurologic shock all have the same end result despite differing mechanisms.

Anemia and Acidosis

Deficient hemoglobin despite an adequate blood volume affects oxygen delivery. In anemic states, regardless of the cause, the number of red blood cells is decreased with an accompanying decrease in hemoglobin. The result is reduced oxygen-carrying capacity, causing insufficient oxygen to reach the tissues. Patients with anemia can become short of breath, even with mild exertion, reflecting the inadequate amount of tissue oxygen.

Both acidosis and alkalosis alter the ability of oxygen to bind with, and release from, hemoglobin. Toxic chemicals also can diminish the oxygen-carrying ability of hemoglobin. A classic example is carbon monoxide (CO) poisoning: the carbon monoxide molecule binds hemoglobin with 200 times the affinity of oxygen, displacing oxygen from hemoglobin.

IN THE FIELD

When hemoglobin binds to carbon monoxide, it has a bright red color, just as it does when it binds to oxygen. Because hemoglobin is saturated, although with carbon monoxide instead of oxygen, the patient may not appear cyanotic, despite life-threatening hypoxia. Pulse oximetry estimates the oxygen level essentially by measuring its color. Pulse oximetry passes beams of infrared light through the tissue (such as a finger or earlobe) and measures the light absorbed. The bright red color of hemoglobin saturated with carbon monoxide gives a falsely high oxygen saturation reading. To avoid this error, some devices also emit additional wavelengths of light to differentiate between oxyhemoglobin (hemoglobin saturated with oxygen) and carboxyhemoglobin (hemoglobin saturated with carbon monoxide).

PERSONAL PERSPECTIVE

Advanced EMT Kim Tranh: Despite the descriptions of patients in shock and the lists of signs and symptoms in my textbooks, nothing prepared me for the reality of the appearance of a patient in shock. The first patient I had who was in shock had been stabbed in the thigh and had an arterial bleed. The patient was barely conscious when we arrived. He was shivering uncontrollably. His skin was more pale than I could have imagined, and it had a waxy, shiny appearance. He was completely without color. It was striking. I will never forget the coldness of his skin when I checked his pulse. Calling the increased breathing that occurs with shock "air hunger" is no exaggeration. No matter how much air he was getting into his lungs, there were not enough red blood cells to transport the oxygen to the cells. His cells were literally starved for oxygen. Luckily, we reached the patient within 3 minutes of the injury and were able to control bleeding. He received blood right away in the emergency department and was taken to surgery to repair the wound.

Cardiac Arrest

When the heart stops beating, oxygen delivery to the cells has ceased. In many cases, cardiac arrest occurs as a result of known disease and may be expected. It also may occur when the body has sustained unsurvivable trauma. In those cases, cardiopulmonary resuscitation (CPR) is typically not indicated and not likely to lead to a successful outcome. Cardiac arrest may follow **asphyxiation**, such as in drowning or respiratory failure; or as a result of drug overdose, **hypothermia**, or other acute conditions. **Sudden cardiac arrest (SCA)** occurs due to a sudden cardiac rhythm disturbance, most often a result of disease of the coronary arteries.

It is important to have a fundamental understanding of the pathophysiologic basis of cardiac arrest. The specifics of the assessment and management of cardiac arrest is discussed elsewhere. This section serves as an overview.

The most common initial rhythms in SCA are pulseless ventricular rhythms, either **ventricular fibrillation** or **ventricular tachycardia**. In both rhythms, there is electrical activity in the heart, but it is not the normal electrical activity produced by the sinoatrial node. In ventricular fibrillation, multiple cells in the ventricles are randomly generating electrical activity. The activity does not spread normally throughout the heart and produce rhythmic contraction. Instead, the myocardium quivers ineffectively, producing no cardiac output. In ventricular tachycardia, there is typically a single ectopic pacemaker in the ventricles, overriding the normal function of the sinoatrial node. In some cases ventricular tachycardia produces a pulse and in some cases it does not.

Both rhythms can be successfully terminated with **defibrillation** (passing an electrical current through the heart). Defibrillation works by simultaneously depolarizing a critical mass of myocardial cells, allowing them to repolarize in an organized fashion. If the sinoatrial node has not been damaged by the event that led to cardiac arrest or by the ensuing ischemia, it may be able to take over again as the pacemaker of the heart.

In cardiac arrest, there is no cardiac output and no cell perfusion. Cells become hypoxic and stop functioning. Cells with high ischemic sensitivity (such as brain, heart, and lung cells) begin to suffer irreversible damage in just 4 to 6 minutes. Unless circulation is restored, death is almost certain in 10 minutes. Yet, in patients with SCA, survival rates can be increased substantially when all components needed for successful resuscitation are immediately available and applied properly.

Pediatric Care

The most common cause of cardiac arrest in pediatric patients is respiratory failure.

Sudden cardiac arrest can be divided into three distinct phases that are helpful in guiding management approaches: the electrical phase, circulatory phase, and the metabolic phase (Ali & Antezano, 2006). The first 4 minutes of a cardiac arrest is the electrical phase. During this time, the myocardium is still relatively well-perfused and likely to respond to defibrillation. Once this time period has passed, the patient enters the circulatory phase of cardiac arrest, which lasts for approximately 6 minutes. At this point, the cells of the myocardium have become hypoxic through the mechanisms discussed earlier and are unlikely to respond to defibrillation. In those cases, CPR prior to defibrillation may help restore perfusion to the heart, allowing successful defibrillation.

Once a patient has been in cardiac arrest for 10 to 15 or more minutes, he transitions to the metabolic phase of cardiac arrest. At this point, cells have been hypoxic for a considerable time throughout the body and begin to breakdown. During this breakdown, inflammatory factors are released into the body that further myocardial and cerebral depression. Therapeutic hypothermia is one modality that attempts to mitigate this phase. In theory, cooling the patient to a lower core temperature will slow or halt the detrimental cell breakdowns and metabolic reactions, creating a better resuscitation environment. In some cases, prehospital protocols may allow the use of chilled intravenous fluids to initiate hypothermia after resuscitation.

The American Heart Association (AHA) Chain of Survival consists of five links, each of which must be present and effective to provide cardiac arrest patients with increased chances of survival. The five links are:

- Immediate recognition of cardiac arrest and EMS notification
- Immediate CPR with emphasis on chest compressions
- Rapid defibrillation
- Early advanced life support
- Integrated postresuscitation management

With each minute that passes without intervention, the patient's chances of survival diminish rapidly. Hypoxic cells can engage in anaerobic metabolism for a brief period of time, but as described previously, energy production is limited and acidosis occurs quickly. Cellular sodium/potassium pumps fail, allowing massive amounts of sodium and water to enter the cell, resulting in lysis. Release of cellular lysozymes increases damage.

In the first minutes following cessation of circulation, some oxygen remains in the blood and lungs, but is not being delivered to the cells. If chest compressions are begun immediately, the remaining oxygen can be delivered to the cells of the brain, heart, and lungs. In addition, the compression and release of the thoracic cage alternatively increases and decreases pressure within it, allowing for some passive air movement in and out of the respiratory system. When EMS arrives on the scene, ventilation and oxygenation are implemented, further increasing oxygenation.

CPR is intended to limit cellular damage while awaiting an intervention that can restore the heart's normal rhythm and cardiac output, but is unlikely to restore cardiac function by itself. Rapid defibrillation is required to terminate ventricular fibrillation or pulseless ventricular tachycardia. Other abnormal rhythms may respond to medications. Once a perfusing cardiac rhythm is restored, the focus is on stabilizing the rhythm to prevent its recurrence, ensuring adequate perfusion, and minimizing cellular damage in the aftermath of hypoxia.

Oxygen Delivery to the Cells

Even if oxygen-saturated red blood cells arrive at the tissue bed, there are disease processes that can prevent the effective offloading of oxygen. In very alkalotic states, the hemoglobin binds oxygen with greater affinity, preventing it from dissociating at the tissue level. The result of this situation is a diminished ability of hemoglobin to deliver the oxygen to the tissues that need it.

Cellular Oxygen Utilization

Certain chemicals can reduce the ability of the cell to utilize oxygen for ATP production, even when ATP reaches the cellular level. Cyanide is one of the substances that can prevent the cell from using oxygen. Cyanide is found in the pits of some stone fruits, such as peaches and apricots. It also is released from burning synthetic materials, silk, and wool, and is commonly present in the smoke from structure fires. Cyanide is used in some industrial applications (electroplating and fumigation). Cyanide exists in many forms and there is some concern that it could be used in a terrorist attack.

Cyanide binds to molecules (cytochrome oxidase) that are part of the electron transport chain in the mitochondria of cells, disabling oxidative phosphorylation. Despite the presence of oxygen, the cell is unable to use it. Aerobic metabolism cannot occur, and cells switch to anaerobic metabolism. In the absence of oxidative phosphorylation, pyruvic acid is converted to lactic acid, resulting in lactic acidosis (Leybell, Borron, & Roldan, 2010). If untreated, cyanide poisoning rapidly causes death from asphyxia.

One of the barriers to treating cyanide poisoning is being able to detect its presence. In the prehospital setting, the primary clue to cyanide poisoning is the patient's history, such as having been in an enclosed spaced with burning synthetic materials. Often, cyanide poisoning is complicated by simultaneous exposure to carbon monoxide and other chemicals. An older type of cyanide antidote kit uses sodium nitrite, sodium thiosulfate, and amyl nitrite. More recently, hydroxycobalamin has been introduced as a treatment for cyanide poisoning. Cyanide combines with hydroxycobalamin to create cyanocobalamin (vitamin B_{12}). Cyanocobalamin can then be excreted through the kidneys.

Cellular Glucose Use

Cells require glucose to produce ATP. It is through glycolysis, the breakdown of glucose, that ATP is produced through anaerobic and aerobic metabolism. The body is adept at storing glucose, and can survive for some time without new intake. Some cells can adapt for brief periods of time using alternative mechanisms of energy production. Alternative energy production methods are not as efficient in producing ATP and are all associated with byproduct waste buildup that eventually has toxic effects. The brain, however, is unable to quickly adapt to using alternate fuels. A sudden and significant drop in blood glucose level can quickly lead to brain cell damage and death.

In order for glucose in the blood to enter most cells in sufficient quantities, insulin must be present to facilitate its passage across the cell membrane. In states of poor insulin production or use, such as diabetes mellitus, cells are deprived of glucose despite high blood glucose levels. Notably, glucose does not require insulin to enter brain cells. Other cells must derive energy from fatty acids in the absence of insulin. When fatty acids are used for energy, ketones are produced as a byproduct. Ketones are an acidic substance, and the lack of insulin eventually results in **diabetic ketoacidosis (DKA)**. In DKA, the patient is in a state of metabolic acidosis and, in some patients, the ketone level rises to a point where an odor of ketones can be detected on the breath.

Normal glucose levels are generally considered to be between 80 and 120 mg/dL, and in healthy patients the body tightly regulates this level under the influence of insulin and glucagon. The action of insulin is to lower the blood glucose level by facilitating cellular uptake of glucose and promoting glucose storage in the form of glycogen (glycogenesis) in the liver. Glucagon opposes the action of insulin by promoting the breakdown of glycogen back into glucose (glycogenolysis) when blood glucose levels are low, and by promoting gluconeogenesis (formation of glucose from amino acids).

By far, the most common cause of hypoglycemia is an excess of insulin in relation to the amount of glucose available in diabetic patients. When glucose levels decrease below normal, predictable signs and symptoms manifest as cells are deprived of glucose. The brain is the largest consumer of glucose and requires a constant supply for its proper functioning.

IN THE FIELD

The preferred prehospital treatment of hypoglycemia is administration of sugars that are metabolized by the body for energy, such as sucrose (given orally) or dextrose (given intravenously). When you cannot start an IV in a patient with a decreased level of responsiveness, glucagon can be given intramuscularly. However, the patient must have adequate glycogen stores in the liver to be broken down into glucose for this treatment to be effective.

Decreased blood glucose levels are a threat to survival and, as such, stimulate the sympathetic nervous system. The initial signs and symptoms of hypoglycemia reflect dysfunction of the cerebral cortex and the effects of epinephrine on body functions. For this reason, many of the initial symptoms of hypoglycemia are neurologic in nature (Table 10-3).

As blood glucose levels begin to drop, confusion is one of the first symptoms. That will progress to lethargy and unconsciousness as levels decrease to less than 30 mg/dL, and ultimately progresses to coma if left untreated. In an effort to increase energy production by alternative methods, a catecholamine (epinephrine) release will occur and a number of sympathetic signs are observed. The skin becomes cool, pale, and diaphoretic as peripheral vasoconstriction shunts blood to the core. Heart rate increases. Hypoglycemic seizures are common as neuron function is disrupted, and in contrast to epileptic seizures are easily treated by increasing the blood glucose level.

TABLE 10-3 Signs and Symptoms of Hypoglycemia

- Anxiety
- Sweating
- Tremor
- Extreme hunger
- Rapid heartbeat
- Irritability
- Confusion, difficulty thinking
- Anger
- Weakness
- Blurred vision
- Slurred speech
- Staggering, poor coordination
- Seizures
- Unresponsiveness (coma)

Hypoglycemia is treated by increasing the blood glucose level through administering simple sugars orally or intravenously. For patients who are unable to take anything by mouth, an intravenous solution of dextrose (50 percent for adults, 25 percent for children, 10 percent for newborns) is given. If an IV or intraosseous access cannot be established, glucagon is given intramuscularly. But, to be effective, the patient must have adequate glycogen stores in the liver that can be converted to glucose.

Acid-Base and Electrolyte Disturbances

Hypoxia is one cause of acidosis. Diabetic ketoacidosis (DKA) is another cause, one that also leads to fluid and electrolyte disturbances. Acute aspirin (salicylic acid) overdose, chronic aspirin toxicity, and overdose of other salicylates, such as oil of wintergreen (methyl salicylate) can lead to acidosis, as well. Ethylene glycol, a primary component of automotive antifreeze solution, is sometimes ingested accidentally or intentionally, either for intoxicating effects or in suicide attempts, and also causes profound acidosis.

Metabolic acidosis is defined by an arterial pH of less than 7.35, generally with an accompanying bicarbonate level less than 24 mmHg. However, in the presence of more than one problem, such as diabetic ketoacidosis with severe vomiting, the bicarbonate level can be higher. In an effort to buffer the pH, these patients often present with increased ventilatory depth and rate to remove excess carbon dioxide from the body and raise the pH. Remember:

$$CO_2 + H_2O \leftrightarrow H_2CO_3 \leftrightarrow H^+ + HCO_3^-$$

As pH decreases, hemoglobin becomes less effective at binding oxygen (Figure 10-9). At the tissue level, this is desirable, and forms part of the basis of the oxyhemoglobin

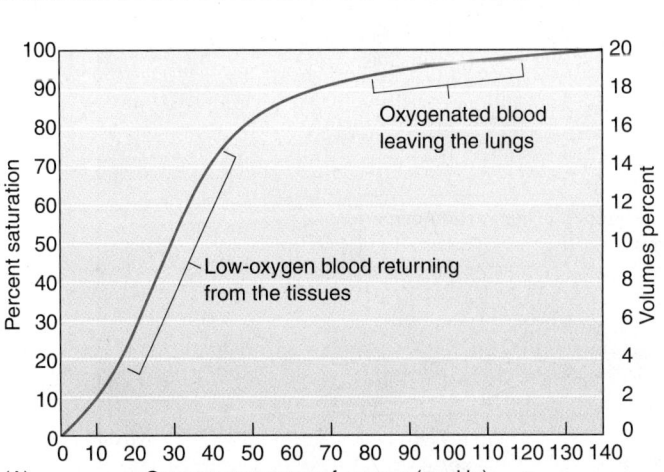
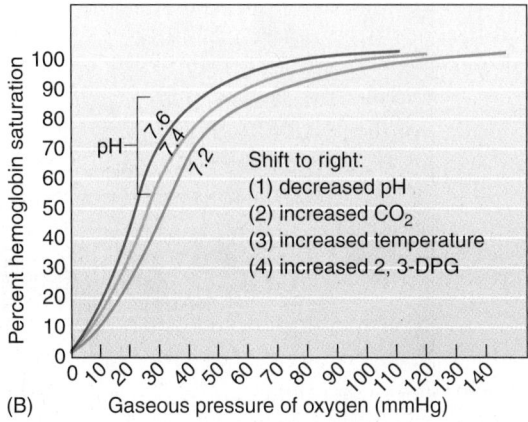

FIGURE 10-9

(A) The oxygen–hemoglobin dissociation curve. (B) Effects of pH, increased carbon dioxide, and temperature on the oxygen–hemoglobin dissociation curve.

dissociation curve. When the pH is decreased systemically, it becomes a problem. As hemoglobin saturation decreases, the overall oxygen availability to tissues will decrease, as well. This will force cells to utilize anaerobic metabolism to an extent and therefore produce less ATP. In the setting of hypoxia, this only further worsens the state of oxygen deprivation and acidosis. In alkalosis, the reverse situation occurs: Oxygen is not as easily released at the cellular level.

Dependent upon the cause of the acidosis, certain electrolyte abnormalities may be present. In acidosis resulting from hypoxia, electrolyte levels are typically normal. In other cases such as ingestion of acidic substances (aspirin, methyl alcohol, ethylene glycol) and diabetic ketoacidosis, potassium levels can be elevated. Cardiac abnormalities can result from both the increased potassium as well as the acidosis itself if severe enough.

Alkalosis can occur in patients who have taken excess amounts of sodium bicarbonate or magnesium hydroxide as antacids, in patients who have lost large amounts of H^+ through vomiting, and in patients taking certain diuretics. Signs and symptoms of metabolic alkalosis are nonspecific, but hypoventilation can occur in severe cases. The mortality rate of significant, uncorrected metabolic alkalosis is high.

The critical function of electrolytes in the cell and in fluid balance means that the levels of electrolytes must be maintained within narrow ranges for normal cellular function and fluid balance. Cardiac rhythm, electrical conduction, and contraction can be affected by disturbances in sodium, potassium, magnesium, and calcium. Hyperkalemia (increased potassium levels) and hypokalemia (decreased potassium levels) are considered when determining an underlying problem for patients in cardiac arrest. Patients at risk for electrolyte disturbances include those with kidney failure, vomiting, diarrhea, burns, and those taking certain medications, such as diuretics (medications to promote fluid loss through the kidneys).

Shock

All forms of shock share a final common pathway of inadequate cellular perfusion to meet metabolic needs (Figure 10-10). However, there are different mechanisms that lead to the final common pathway. Conditions affecting adequate onloading of oxygen to hemoglobin, adequate

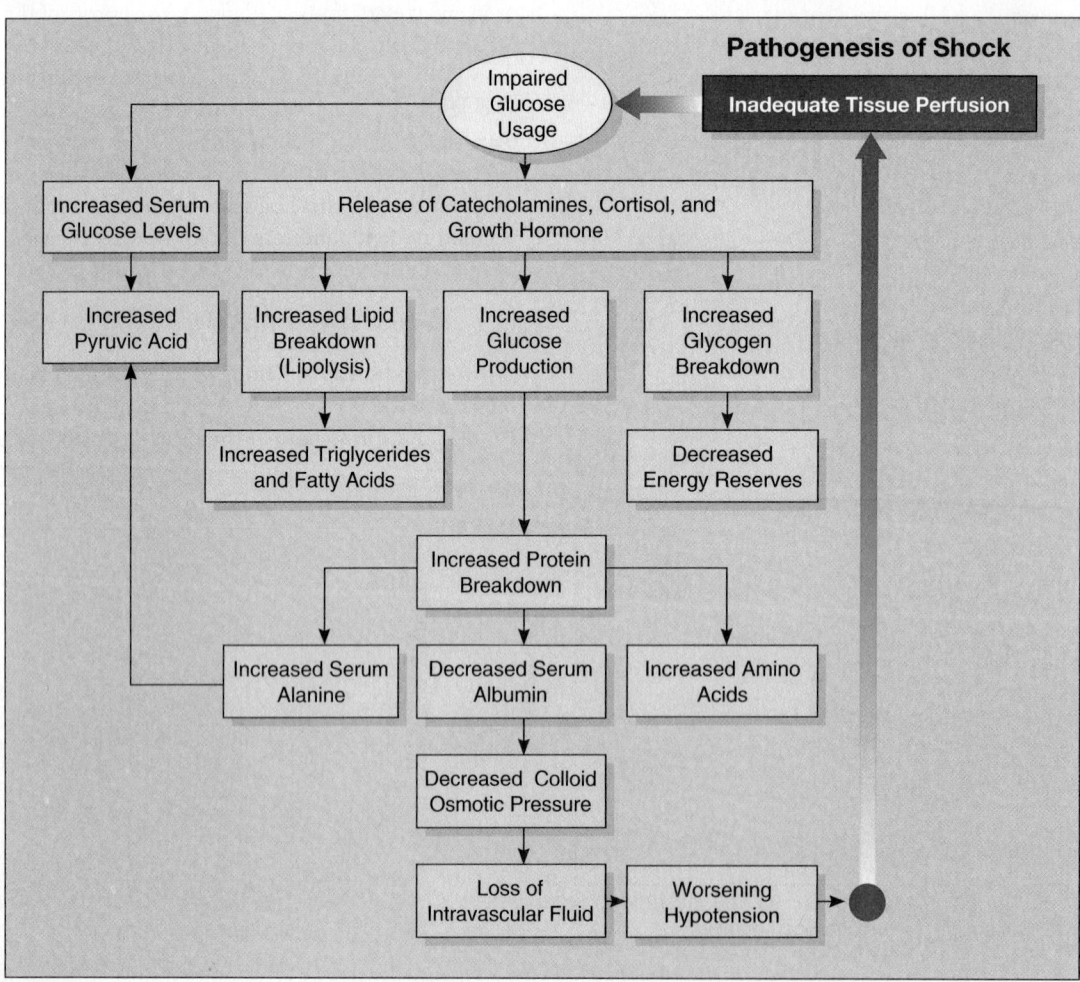

FIGURE 10-10

Progression of inadequate perfusion to cellular death.

circulation to the tissues, and adequate offloading of oxygen at the cellular level can result in cellular hypoxia. But the underlying problem may be a traumatic injury that causes an obstruction to the return of blood to the heart, blood loss, loss of nervous control over the diameter of the arterioles, or a number of other problems.

There are four general classifications of shock: cardiogenic, hypovolemic, distributive, and obstructive. Each describes failure of a different component of the cardiovascular system: the heart, the volume of blood, peripheral vascular resistance, and mechanical impediment of blood flow, respectively. Simply stated, shock is a case of inadequate oxygen

supply to meet the demand for oxygen at the cellular level. When any part of the supply chain becomes inadequate, the other components can compensate for the weak component, but only to a degree. When compensation fails, blood pressure begins to drop, the brain, heart, and lungs are no longer adequately perfused, and **irreversible shock** follows.

Hypovolemic Shock

Hypovolemic shock is the result of a loss of blood volume (Figure 10-11). This can occur suddenly, as in the case of a severe laceration to a large artery, or slowly, such as happens

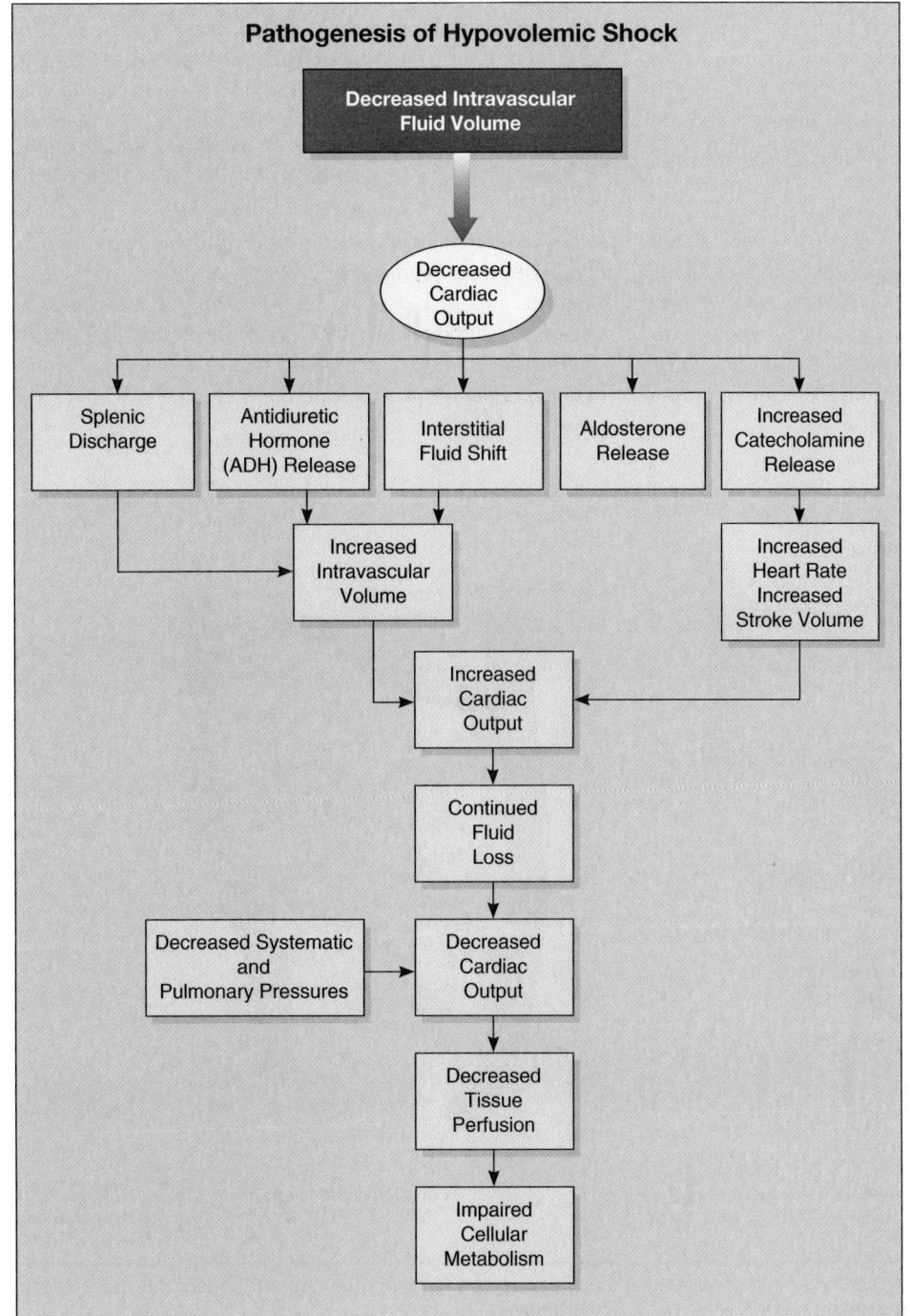

FIGURE 10-11

Progression of hypovolemic shock.

with moderate gastrointestinal bleeding. Hypovolemic shock may occur from severe dehydration or the loss of fluids through extensive burns. In that case, there is not a loss of red blood cells, but a loss of water from the vascular space. In some cases, fluid is not lost from the body, but is distributed in fluid compartments other than the vascular space.

Regardless of the cause, the outcome is that an insufficient blood volume within the vascular space prevents tissues and organs from being adequately perfused. The decrease in perfusion results in stimulation of the sympathetic nervous system, the actions of which are intended to restore perfusion through compensatory mechanisms. Under sympathetic nervous system influence, the heart rate increases, the heart is stimulated to contract more forcefully, and the peripheral vasculature constricts to increase peripheral vascular resistance. The mechanisms allow maintenance of blood pressure in the early stage of shock, called **compensated shock**. This means that the blood pressure does not drop until the compensatory mechanisms fail and the patient enters **decompensated shock**.

If shock is not reversed before extensive cell death and tissue damage occurs, the patient enters irreversible shock. At that point, regardless of treatment, the patient will die. Death may occur immediately or may be delayed. In some cases, bleeding is stopped and circulation is restored, but the organs have sustained significant damage. Though the organs may provide minimal function, they cannot sustain

life beyond a few days. The patient dies from failure of the lungs, blood clotting disorders, or multiple organ failure.

Early in shock, the precapillary sphincters of the arterioles leading into peripheral capillary beds and postcapillary sphincters of the venules leading out of the peripheral capillary beds both constrict (Figure 10-12). Blood is diverted away from tissues with higher tolerance for ischemia, such as skin and skeletal muscle. At the vascular level, this phase of shock is called the **ischemic phase**. If shock is not corrected, the resulting acidosis (from anaerobic metabolism) and hypoxia cause the precapillary sphincters to fail. Blood can enter the capillary beds, but cannot leave. Red blood cells clump together and microscopic blood clots form because the blood is stagnant in the capillaries. Shock has now progressed to the **stagnant phase**. As the cycle of shock continues, the postcapillary sphincters fail. The stagnant blood, with accompanying microscopic blood clots and lactic acid, washes out of the capillaries and re-enters the circulation. This is called the **washout phase**, and is irreversible.

Signs and symptoms of hypovolemic shock include what is often thought of as the classic presentation of shock. The symptoms predictably progress in severity as increasing amounts of blood are lost. Although hemorrhage as a cause of hypovolemic shock is due to blood loss (called **hemorrhagic shock**), the blood loss may not be obvious. There are many spaces within the body that can hold large

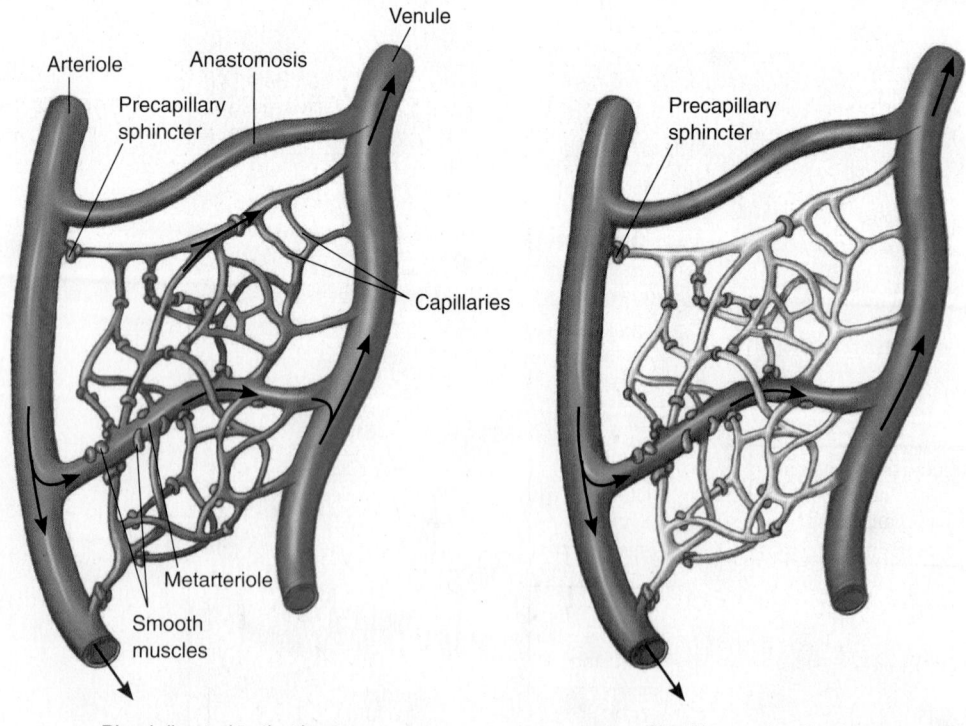

Blood directed to the tissue.   Blood bypassing the tissue.

FIGURE 10-12

The precapillary and postcapillary sphincters close in the ischemic phase of shock. In the stagnant phase, the precapillary sphincters open. The postcapillary sphincters open in the washout phase.

Pediatric Care

Children often can compensate very well in early stages of shock, and the signs and symptoms may be attributed to fear or anxiety. Despite effective early compensation, children in shock deteriorate very quickly once decompensation begins. It is critical to anticipate and look for shock in pediatric patients with a history or mechanism of injury that may lead to shock.

Geriatric Care

The effects of aging include decreased response of the sympathetic nervous system. Elderly patients may not exhibit some of the expected signs of shock, such as tachycardia, despite significant blood loss.

amounts of blood from internal bleeding. The chest cavity, abdomen, pelvis, and thigh can all hold more than enough blood to result in shock. Maintain a high index of suspicion whenever there is a significant mechanism of injury, or in patients with a medical history that is consistent with a risk for bleeding. Otherwise unexplained tachycardia can be an early clue to the presence of internal bleeding.

The severity of hemorrhagic shock is classified into four stages based on estimated blood loss (Table 10-4). The evolution of signs and symptoms is predictable because the body recruits an increasing number of compensatory mechanisms in response to continued blood loss and as the compensatory mechanisms start to fail. Decreased blood pressure is a very late sign of shock, requiring a loss of at least 25 to 35 percent of the blood volume.

Cardiogenic Shock

Cardiogenic shock occurs when the heart cannot pump a sufficient amount of blood to maintain an effective cardiac output (Figure 10-13). The most common cause of cardiogenic shock is a large myocardial infarction. When a portion of the myocardium dies, it can no longer contract or propagate an electrical impulse. The effects of this are twofold:

The affected areas of the heart wall cannot contribute to the physical pumping of blood and the overall electrical coordination of the heart becomes disrupted. If the size of the infarct affects a large enough area of the left ventricular wall, stroke volume can decrease to levels that cannot maintain an adequate blood pressure. Various electrical abnormalities such as blockage of electrical conduction through the branches of the bundle of His can occur if the infarct affects the electrical pathways. Other causes of cardiogenic shock include cardiac **dysrhythmia**, **cardiomyopathy**, and cardiac valve malfunction.

Keeping in mind that cardiac output is a product of the stroke volume and heart rate, it is easy to see how an abnormality of either one can produce cardiogenic shock. In the same way that tidal volume and respiratory rate compensate to maintain minute volume, stroke volume and heart rate can compensate for each other to maintain cardiac output. Again, compensation has its limits. With an average stroke volume of 70 mL and heart rate of 70 beats per minute, typical cardiac output is 4.9 liters (4,900 mL) per minute. If the heart rate drops below about 50 (except in well-conditioned athletes), the stroke volume can no longer compensate and hypotension occurs. When the heart rate increases over about 150 beats per minute, the diastolic period is shortened, causing two problems. First, there is insufficient time between contractions for the ventricles to

TABLE 10-4	Stages of Hemorrhagic Shock	
CLASSIFICATION OF HEMORRHAGE		
Class	**Blood Volume Loss in 70-kg Adult**	**Signs**
Class I hemorrhage	Up to 15 percent (750 mL)	Usually well-tolerated Can lead to mild tachycardia
Class II hemorrhage	15–30 percent (750–1,500 mL)	Moderate tachycardia Pale skin Delayed capillary refill
Class III hemorrhage	30–40 percent (1,500–2,000 mL)	Tachycardia Failure of compensation Hypotension
Class IV hemorrhage	40–50 percent (2,000–2,500 mL)	Profound hypotension End-organ failure (for example, bradycardia, anuria) Death

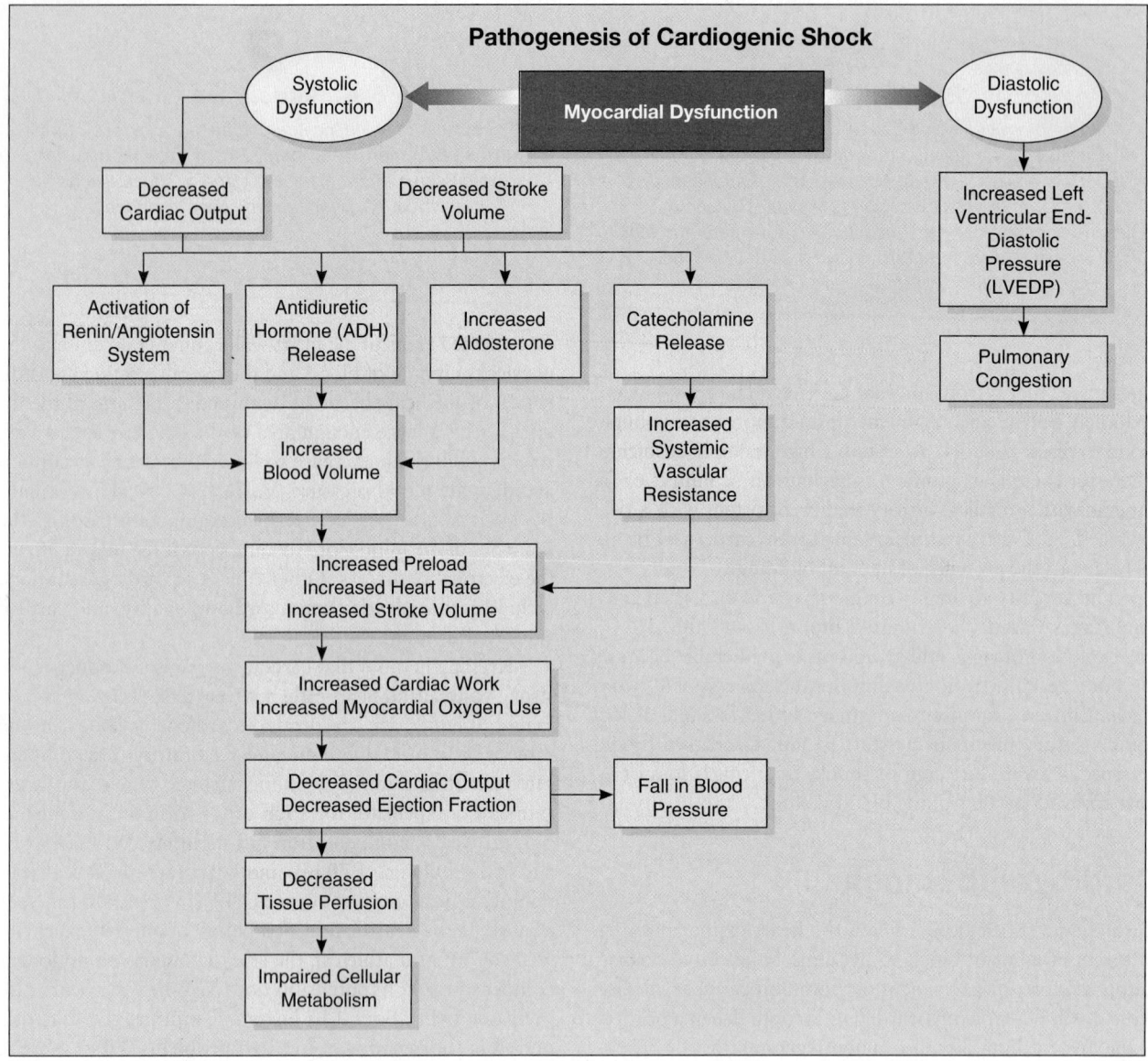

FIGURE 10-13

Progression of cardiogenic shock.

fill adequately, decreasing stroke volume. Second, since the coronary arteries are underperfused during the shortened ventricular diastole, the myocardium becomes ischemic.

The signs and symptoms of cardiogenic shock are similar to other forms of shock: anxiety, tachycardia (unless the underlying cause is a slow heart rate), pallor, and diaphoresis. The effects of the sympathetic nervous system stimulate the heart to beat harder and faster, increasing the demand on an already failing myocardium. Initially, the peripheral vascular resistance will increase to compensate and maintain a blood pressure, but it cannot be maintained indefinitely. Because the most common cause of cardiogenic shock is a myocardial infarction, patients often present with chest pain. The patient also may have pulmonary edema, which is often severe.

Pulmonary edema occurs because the left ventricle cannot accept all of the blood trying to return from the lungs.

Blood backs up into the pulmonary circulation. As hydrostatic pressure in the pulmonary circulation increases, fluid is forced through the walls of the capillaries and into the interstitial spaces around the alveoli. This creates conditions that decrease the ability of oxygen to diffuse from the alveoli to the capillaries, resulting in hypoxia. In severe cases, fluid enters the alveoli and the patient may have frothy, pink sputum. The external jugular veins in the neck can become distended as blood from the right ventricle backs up into the systemic circulation. This is called *jugular venous distention* (*JVD*).

Prehospital treatment of cardiogenic shock is aimed at supporting the airway, breathing, and circulation. Definitive treatment requires medications, electrical therapies, and other interventions to correct the underlying cause. Even with treatment, the mortality rate for cardiogenic shock is high.

Distributive Shock

The mechanism of distributive shock is uncontrolled vaso-dilation, creating a vascular container that is too large for the amount of blood in the body. Even when the blood volume is normal, it cannot exert the force needed to maintain blood pressure. There are three mechanisms of distributive shock: neurogenic, anaphylactic, and septic.

Neurogenic Shock

The sympathetic nervous system always exerts some amount of influence on body functions. Basal sympathetic tone maintains varying amounts of peripheral vasoconstriction, constantly making dynamic adjustments to maintain blood pressure and adjust blood flow to the needs of the tissues. The nerve pathways from the sympathetic ganglia travel through the spinal cord en route to their blood vessel targets, and can be interrupted by severe high–spinal cord injuries. The loss of sympathetic tone results in an uncontrolled vaso-dilatation below the injury site that can result in a sudden on-set of hypotension, called *neurogenic shock* (Figure 10-14).

In contrast to the pale, cool skin observed in hypovolemic and cardiogenic shock, massive vasodilation results in redistribution of blood to the peripheral tissues. The skin is warm and color may be normal. In addition, because the sympathetic nervous system pathways are disrupted, other components of the sympathetic nervous system response to shock are absent. The heart rate is normal, perhaps even slow, without input from the sympathetic nervous system. The heart, therefore, cannot compensate for the low blood pressure caused by vasodilation. Diaphoresis, the copious perspiration resulting from sympathetic nervous system stimulation, is absent. Sometimes a line of demarcation can separate the areas of the body above the level of spinal cord impairment from those below it at the dermatome level of the injury.

Impaired ventilations may complicate the condition of patients in neurogenic shock. The diaphragm is innervated by cervical spinal nerves three, four, and five, so a fairly high injury is required to disrupt this. The intercostal muscles that raise the thoracic cage during ventilation are innervated by spinal nerves exiting the cord at levels corresponding to their location. Muscles innervated by nerves exiting the spinal cord below the level of injury are paralyzed.

Prehospital treatment includes immobilization of the spine, airway management, supporting ventilations, providing supplemental oxygen, keeping the patient warm, and administering IV fluids according to your protocol.

Anaphylactic Shock

Anaphylaxis is the result of an exaggerated immune response to an antigen (foreign protein). The most common causes of anaphylaxis are antibiotics such as penicillin, iodine including IV contrast, hymenoptera (bee or wasp) stings, and peanuts. An antigen binds an antibody (IgE immunoglobulin)

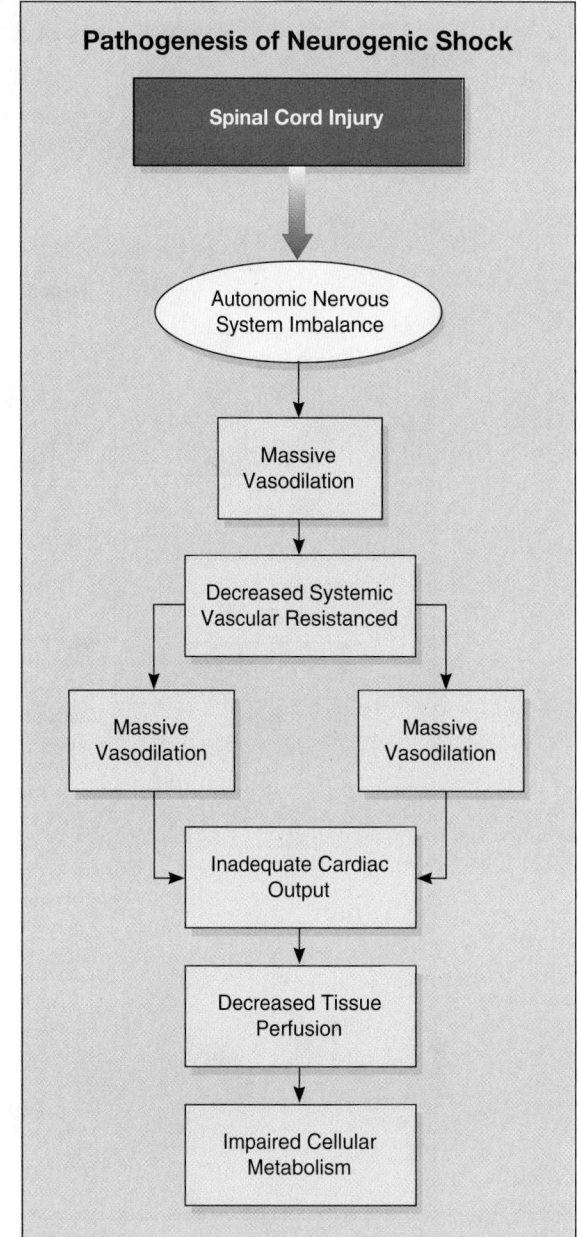

FIGURE 10-14

Progression of neurogenic shock.

on mast cells (basophils that have migrated to the tissues), which causes a release of histamine and other chemicals that mediate the immune response. The effects of histamine include vasodilation, increased gastrointestinal activity, and constriction of the bronchioles (Figure 10-15). While reactions such as this occur normally in controlled responses to foreign agents in the body, the response in anaphylaxis is uncontrolled and systemic. In anaphylaxis, as the inflammatory reaction progresses, the blood vessels not only dilate but also leak plasma into the interstitial spaces, adding a hypovolemic component to this type of shock. As the peripheral vascular resistance decreases, the blood pressure drops. Reactions can progress quickly, leading to death in minutes

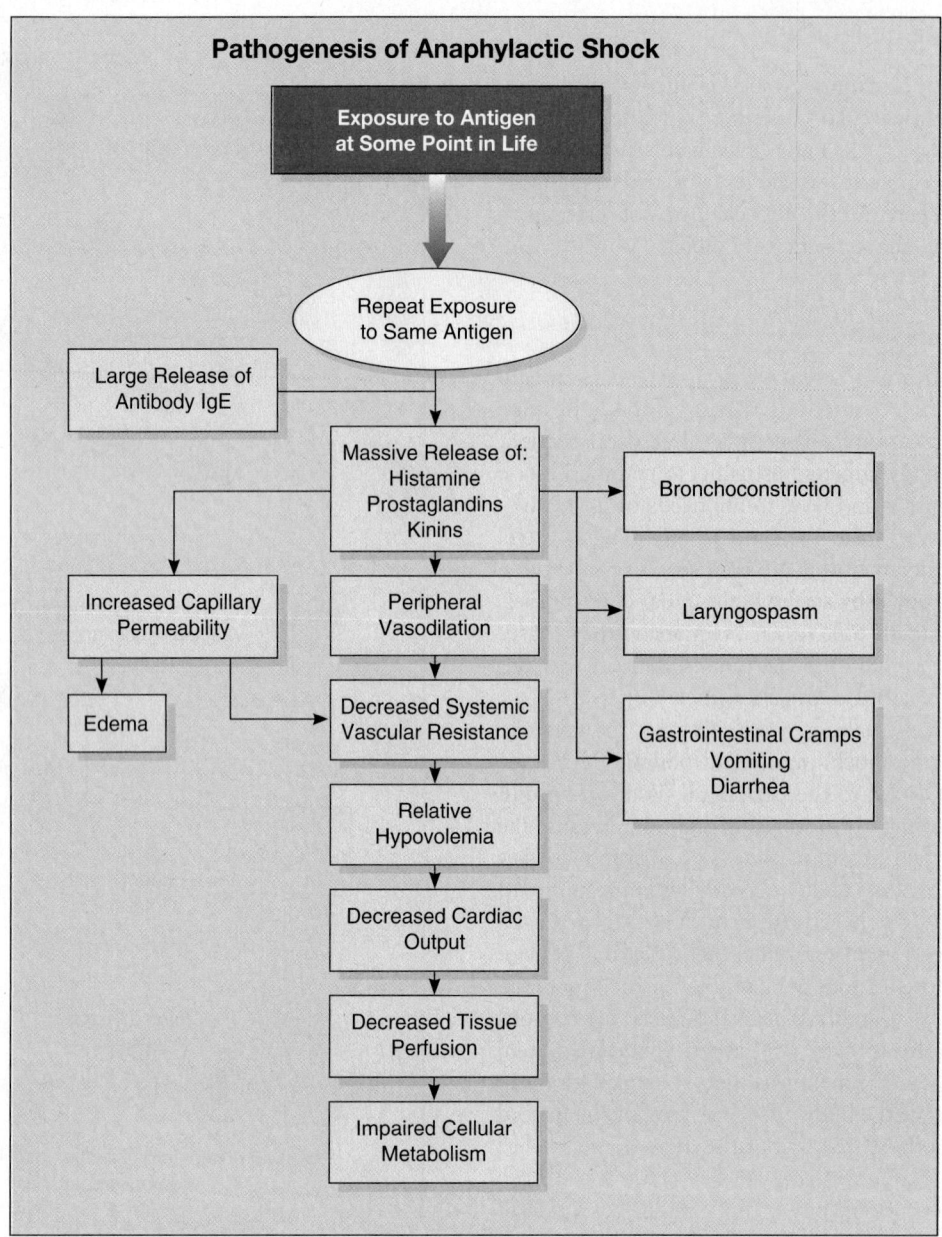

FIGURE 10-15

Progression of anaphylactic shock.

and worsen over a susceptible person's lifetime with each new exposure.

In addition to the typical signs and symptoms of shock, patients in anaphylaxis can present with hives, complaints of itching in the throat, stridor, wheezing, and abdominal cramping. Airway swelling can rapidly worsen leading to obstruction. Airway management and ventilation are critical, but will not be effective if the patient's airway is obstructed due to swelling, or if his bronchioles are severely constricted. The immediate treatment of anaphylaxis is administration of epinephrine to relieve the vasodilation that causes many of the life-threatening problems associated with anaphylaxis.

Patients with a known anaphylactic history will have been prescribed an epinephrine auto-injector (such as an EpiPen) that they should carry with them at all times. Epinephrine causes vasoconstriction, relaxes bronchial smooth muscle, and increases cardiac output. Even if the patient carries an epinephrine auto-injector, additional intramuscular administration of epinephrine may be required, because epinephrine has a short duration of action. Additional prehospital treatment includes administration of IV fluid, according to protocol and, if in your scope of practice, administration of the antihistamine diphenhydramine (Benadryl).

Septic Shock

Septic shock is the result of a systemic inflammatory response to a pathogen (Figure 10-16). Localized inflammation is a normal and protective response to pathogen invasion, but overstimulation of this mechanism is problematic. In a normal inflammatory response, local vasodilation occurs to increase blood flow to the area so more white blood cells and chemical messengers can enter the area. Think about the redness, heat, and swelling that surround the site of a cat scratch. Much of this is due to vasodilation.

When vasodilation occurs systemically, the blood pressure decreases as the size of the container holding the blood volume increases dramatically. Further, the permeability of capillaries to fluid increases, allowing intravascular fluid to enter the interstitial spaces, adding a hypovolemic component.

Septic shock can present dramatically, with a high fever, tachycardia, respiratory distress, decreased mental status, and hypotension. In some patients, especially the elderly, fever is absent. In fact, the patient may be

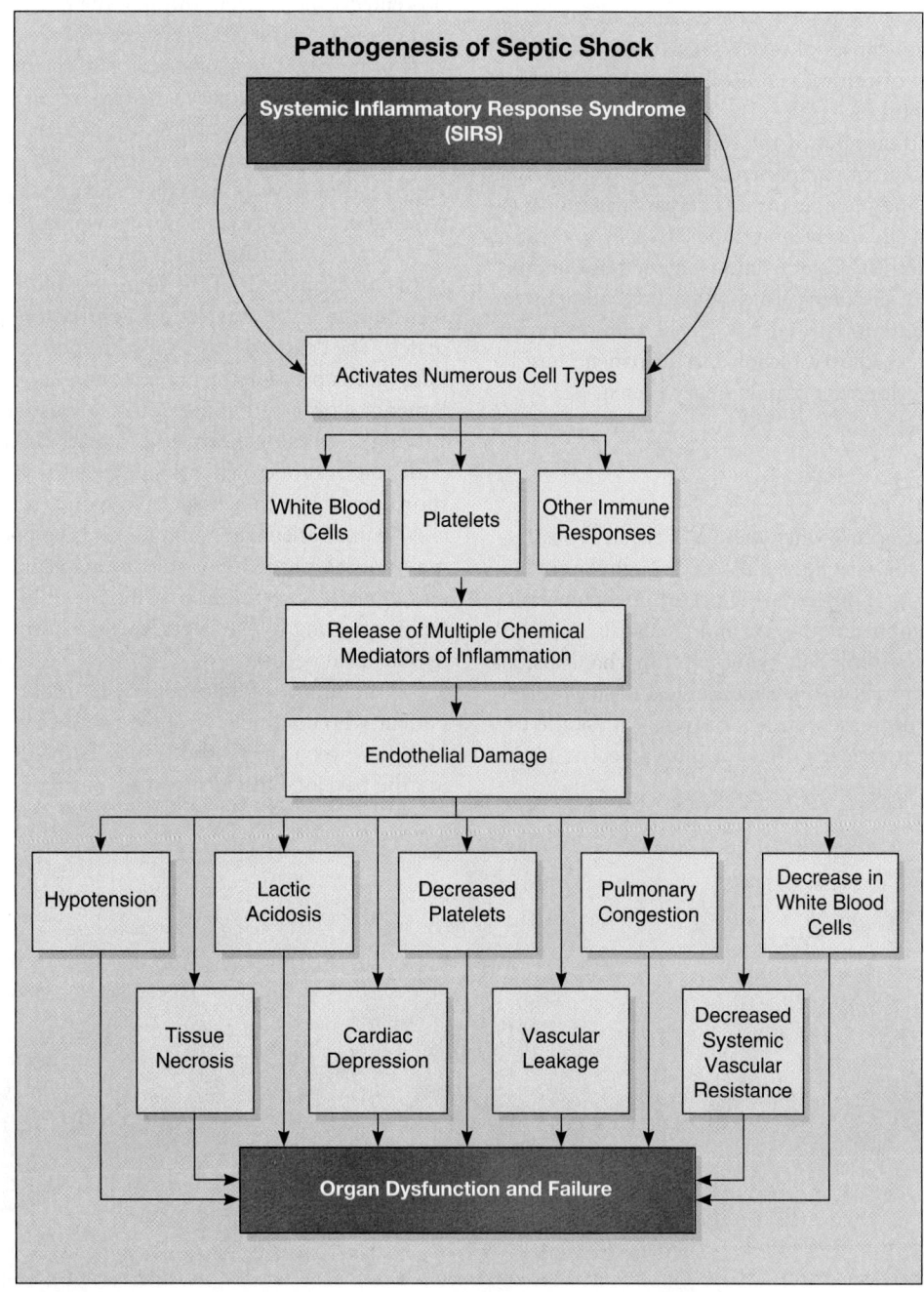

FIGURE 10-16

Progression of septic shock.

Geriatric Care

Aging can result in poor function of temperature regulation mechanisms. That means elderly patients sometimes do not have a fever, even with serious infection.

hypothermic. Vasodilation results in increased heat loss from the body and the core temperature may drop significantly. History is important in the assessment of a septic shock patient; it can help identify the source of infection. The most common causes of severe sepsis are infection introduced by way of central venous lines, Foley catheters, and endotracheal tubes.

Prehospital treatment of the septic shock patient includes management of the patient's airway, ventilation, circulation, and body temperature. The patient needs supplemental oxygen and intravenous fluids. However, because the patient's underlying health status may be poor and because of increased vascular permeability, fluid administration may cause pulmonary edema. Fluid administration must be guided by medical direction and the patient must be monitored for development of pulmonary edema.

Obstructive Shock

Obstructive shock occurs when there is a physical obstruction blocking the forward flow of blood through the circulatory system. Causes of obstructive shock include pulmonary embolism, tension pneumothorax, and pericardial tamponade (Figure 10-17). Although by different mechanisms, all three of the conditions create a mechanical obstruction to blood flow that decreases cardiac output. Unless the obstruction is quickly relieved, the mortality associated with the conditions is high.

Pulmonary Embolism

An embolus is a mass, usually a blood clot, that forms in one area of the body but travels through the circulatory system, eventually lodging in a vessel too small to allow it to pass. Emboli also can be created by bone marrow from a fractured bone, air bubbles, clumps of infectious material, or foreign bodies. Pulmonary embolism occurs when an embolus, or perhaps a shower of smaller emboli, lodges in the pulmonary vasculature. Blood ejected from the right ventricle cannot flow past the obstruction. If only a small pulmonary vessel is obstructed, circulation is not impaired. If a large vessel is obstructed, a significant amount of blood is prevented from flowing through the pulmonary circulation and returning to the heart. A large embolus can cause a complete or near-complete obstruction of the pulmonary artery.

The pulmonary vasculature is often affected because that is the first point where the vasculature narrows after returning from the venous system. Clots often arise in the large veins of the legs and pelvis and are able to travel unobstructed until they reach this narrow point in the circulation.

Because a portion of the blood is not able to circulate to the alveolar level of the lung, less blood is oxygenated, resulting in hypoxia from a ventilation–perfusion mismatch. The degree of hypoxia corresponds to the amount of lung that is prevented from receiving deoxygenated blood. Patients with a pulmonary embolus usually present with varying degrees of shortness of breath. In severe cases, the patient is cyanotic or the skin appears mottled. Sometimes, shortness of breath is associated with a complaint of sharp chest pain. Patients are anxious and the body's attempts at maintaining perfusion result in tachycardia, diaphoresis, and anxiety. If a significant amount of blood is prevented from returning to the heart, cardiac output decreases and hypotension occurs.

A hallmark of significant pulmonary embolism is a patient who continues to get worse despite treatment with high-flow oxygen. IV fluids may be beneficial in increasing the patient's blood pressure, but they do not treat the

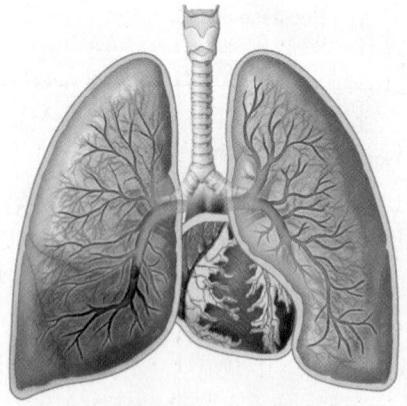 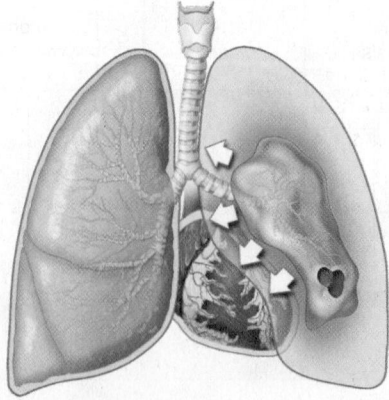 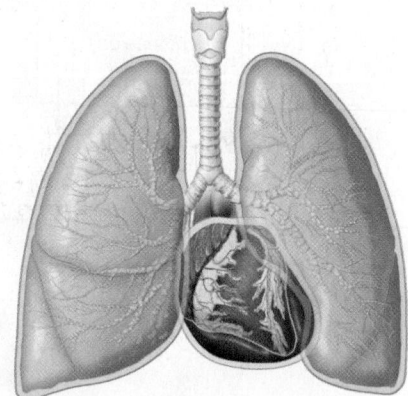

(A) Pulmonary embolism   (B) Tension pneumothorax   (C) Pericardial tamponade

FIGURE 10-17

Causes of obstructive shock. (A) Pulmonary embolism. (B) Tension pneumothorax. (C) Pericardial tamponade.

underlying problem. Treatment in the hospital is directed at removing the embolus, either with drugs that break down the clot (fibrinolytics) or a surgical procedure to remove the clot (embolectomy).

Tension Pneumothorax

A tension pneumothorax occurs when damage to the lung allows air to leak from the lung into the pleural space. Air accumulates within the pleural space, taking up space normally occupied by lung tissue. In most cases, the defect to the lung is small enough that, as the lung collapses, the defect is sealed off, and air stops leaking into the pleural space. Sometimes the defect to the lung is large, allowing air to continue to accumulate under pressure in the pleural space. With each breath, additional air enters the pleural space. The lung on the affected side collapses, and then increasing pressure pushes the heart, great vessels, and other structures in the mediastinum toward the opposite side. Eventually, the other lung is compressed.

When the structures of the mediastinum are shifted, the vena cava may become obstructed, preventing blood from returning to the right side of the heart. In addition, because the normal pressure in the vena cava is very low, blood return through it depends on the negative intrathoracic pressure created on inspiration. Blood flow through the vena cava cannot overcome the increased intrathoracic pressure caused by a tension pneumothorax, further reducing blood return to the heart. Preload is decreased, which decreases cardiac output. The condition worsens as the blood pressure gets lower, but intrathoracic pressure gets higher.

Patients with a tension pneumothorax present with severe shortness of breath and hypotension, often with a history of penetrating trauma to the neck, chest, back, or abdomen. Jugular venous distention (JVD) occurs due to the pooling of blood in the venous system behind the obstruction. Subcutaneous emphysema (air trapped beneath the skin) can sometimes be noted as the high levels of air pressure within the chest wall force air into the skin of the chest and neck. In severe cases, tracheal deviation away from the affected side will occur secondary to mediastinal shift. Lung sounds will be diminished or absent on the affected side.

In addition to the standard treatment for shock in trauma patients, an opening must be made in the patient's thorax to release the air accumulating under pressure. This can be done by paramedics, using a large-gauge IV catheter, or by a physician in the emergency department, using a chest tube inserted through a small incision in the chest. Whenever you suspect a patient has a tension pneumothorax, you must decide what the quickest way is to make thoracostomy (creating an opening in the chest wall) available to the patient.

Pericardial Tamponade

The heart is surrounded by a fibrous pericardium that folds upon itself to form visceral and parietal layers. Between the layers is a small amount of serous pericardial fluid that lubricates the heart as it contracts and expands during the cardiac cycle. If a disease process increases the secretion of serous fluid, the amount of fluid in the space can increase, compressing the heart so that it cannot adequately fill during diastole. When the accumulation of fluid occurs over a longer period of time, the pericardium can stretch slightly to accommodate the fluid. However, the capacity of the pericardium to stretch is limited. If a traumatic event lacerates or ruptures a coronary vessel, or the myocardium itself, blood rapidly fills the pericardial space, significantly decreasing cardiac output.

Traumatic pericardial tamponade occurs most often due to low-velocity, penetrating chest trauma, such as a stab wound. A mechanism such as this creates a small laceration of the pericardial sac and damages the heart. A coronary vessel may be damaged, or penetration of the myocardium may allow blood from the chambers of the heart to leak into the pericardial space. The laceration to the pericardial sac is small, and either may seal itself or allow far less blood to leak out of the pericardium than is entering it from the injured heart.

Blunt trauma that rapidly and forcefully compresses the heart, such as impact from a high-speed motor vehicle collision (MVC), may increase the pressure within the heart to such a degree that it lacerates or ruptures the myocardium, leaving the pericardial sac intact. The pericardial sac must be punctured and blood withdrawn from it, or cardiac arrest will quickly follow. This procedure, called *pericardiocentesis*, cannot be performed in the prehospital setting. The patient must be transported without delay to the closest facility at which the procedure can be performed. Ultimately, the damage to the heart must be repaired surgically to prevent additional blood from accumulating in the pericardial sac.

Pathophysiology of Shock

Regardless of the underlying cause, the initial signs and symptoms of shock are the external manifestations of the body's compensatory reactions to hypoperfusion. As shock progresses, signs and symptoms begin to reflect the failure of compensatory mechanisms. Release of epinephrine and norepinephrine from the sympathetic nervous system response accounts for many of the signs and symptoms of shock. The patient is anxious, and tachycardia occurs as the heart rate attempts to maintain adequate cardiac output. The body shunts blood away from the skin and gastrointestinal system through vasoconstriction to the core organs most required for life—the heart, brain and lungs. The skin becomes pale and cool, when the color and warmth provided by the circulation of blood has disappeared. Gastrointestinal tract upset—nausea, vomiting, and sometimes bowel incontinence—occurs because the stomach and intestines are deprived of blood. The increase in sympathetic activity causes diaphoresis, as well.

Thirst occurs when renal and hypothalamic mechanisms for volume replacement are triggered by low blood pressure. The anxiety produced by sympathetic nervous system stimulation progresses to agitation, lethargy, confusion, decreased responsiveness, and unresponsiveness as compensatory mechanisms become unable to maintain brain perfusion and the brain is deprived of oxygen and glucose to fuel its metabolic needs.

The respiratory rate increases for two reasons. First, increased energy needs for the tissues to respond to sympathetic nervous system stimulation increases oxygen demand. Second, anaerobic metabolism in ischemic tissues results in acidosis. The respiratory system attempts to correct acidosis by making more oxygen available and ridding the body of the increased amount of carbon dioxide produced. Cyanosis occurs as hypoxia progresses.

Without intervention to correct the underlying cause of hypoperfusion, compensatory mechanisms will fail and the patient enters a state of decompensated shock. In decompensated shock, the blood pressure can no longer be maintained despite maximal efforts and it begins to fall. Although even decompensated shock can be reversible with immediate intervention, it quickly progresses to irreversible shock. Organ damage from hypoperfusion becomes so severe that, even with proper resuscitation, recovery is not possible.

As an Advanced EMT, your role is to anticipate and recognize shock quickly, provide appropriate field interventions, and provide transportation to the closest facility capable of providing the care the patient needs.

Heat and Cold Emergencies

The homeostatic mechanisms of the body constantly adjust to changes in both the internal and external environment to maintain a normal core body temperature of about 98.6°F (37°C). Because heat is a byproduct of aerobic energy metabolism, increased physiologic activity generates heat. When the amount of heat becomes excessive, the body adjusts to dissipate it. The peripheral vascular system dilates to bring more blood to the skin, where excess heat can be transferred to the environment. When the core temperature drops below a certain point, the body adjusts to increase heat production and decrease heat loss. Shivering uses energy, which generates that heat. The peripheral vasculature constricts to prevent loss of the heat to the environment.

Those mechanisms are critical. The body's physiologic activities can only occur within a narrow range of core temperature. When the body cannot compensate for environmental extremes, or its temperature regulation mechanisms are impaired, death can occur. Hypothermia causes a shift in the oxygen–hemoglobin dissociation curve. Less oxygen is offloaded at the tissue level. Blood-clotting mechanisms become impaired, and the heart and central nervous system malfunction. **Hyperthermia**, whether environmental or exertional, and **hyperpyrexia** have significant consequences for the central nervous system.

CASE STUDY WRAP-UP

Clinical-Reasoning Process

Advanced EMTs Colin Lear and Tyler Erb have just arrived at an outdoor café where a woman in her 30s is unresponsive and pale. There were no witnesses to the collapse, and the patient was last seen 15 minutes before being discovered. Colin and Tyler also note stridor and cyanosis, along with cool, diaphoretic skin.

The patient has signs of airway obstruction, hypoxia, and shock. Colin and Tyler recognize that those are the patient's priority problems and that they must take immediate action to open the airway, assist with breathing, and provide oxygen. With the assistance of rescue squad personnel, they implement airway management, oxygen, and ventilation. There is no indication of external bleeding or trauma, so they must search for something else that explains the patient's presentation before deciding on specific treatment.

Signs of hypoxia (stridor, cyanosis, unresponsiveness) and poor circulation (pale, diaphoretic skin, unresponsiveness) indicate impairment of the respiratory system and circulatory system. The patient is in shock and cellular energy metabolism is severely impaired. Colin and Tyler begin comparing their mental framework for different pathophysiologic presentations of shock to the patient's presentation.

- Respiratory failure is possible. The patient just sat down to eat and may have choked on food or developed a sudden respiratory problem. The finding of stridor is consistent with partial airway obstruction. However, there are other causes of upper airway obstruction than foreign bodies. A quick check of breath sounds reveals that the patient also has wheezing in the lungs. It is less likely that a foreign body would cause wheezing. Asthma can cause wheezing, but is less likely to cause stridor. Colin and Tyler begin considering things that would cause both stridor and wheezing.

- Hypoglycemia is possible. The patient may have been seeking food because she knew her blood glucose level was dropping. There is no medical history immediately available, and no medical identification jewelry indicating diabetes. The presence of hypoglycemia is easily determined, and Tyler prepares to obtain a blood glucose level. In a few seconds, the blood glucose level is determined to be 97 mg/dL, which is within normal limits.
- External hemorrhage can be ruled out, but internal hemorrhage could be present. The patient could be hypovolemic from dehydration, but dehydration does not appear suddenly and the patient was at the boardwalk and ordering food. Neither type of shock would explain the stridor and wheezing.
- Cardiogenic shock is less likely in a patient in her 30s. In the primary assessment, the patient had a weak but regular carotid pulse of 132. The patient has neither bradycardia nor tachycardia enough to cause shock. There were no specific indications of fluid in the lungs when Colin listened to breath sounds. Wheezing can occur with fluid in the lungs, but the stridor is unexplained by this mechanism. Cardiogenic shock cannot be eliminated as a cause, but seems less likely than other causes.
- Distributive shock could be caused by a spinal cord injury, anaphylaxis, or sepsis. The scene size-up and known history are not consistent with spinal cord trauma. Sepsis develops more slowly, as a result of systemic infection and also is not likely. However, anaphylaxis comes on suddenly and there are two findings in the history and scene size-up that are consistent with anaphylaxis: The patient just began eating food, and she is outdoors. Could she have a food allergy or have been stung by a bee or wasp? Colin and Tyler determine that the patient has hives. Hives, airway swelling leading to stridor, and bronchoconstriction leading to wheezing are consistent with anaphylaxis. So is the poor perfusion, which could be explained as the vasodilation and increased capillary permeability caused by anaphylaxis.
- Obstructive shock can be caused by tension pneumothorax, pericardial tamponade, or pulmonary embolism. The most likely cause of tension pneumothorax in a patient of this age is trauma, which does not appear to be the case. In addition, though wheezing was present, there were breath sounds present in both lungs. In the physical exam, Colin noted that there was no jugular venous distention. Unless caused by trauma, a pericardial tamponade is unlikely to develop as suddenly as the patient's problem developed. Again, there is no jugular venous distention. Pulmonary embolism occurs suddenly and may occur in patients of this age group. However, it does not explain stridor, wheezing, or hives, making it less likely.

Colin and Tyler decide anaphylaxis is the most likely reason for the patient's presentation. While Tyler starts an IV, Colin quickly consults with medical direction. The on-line physician, Dr. McGraw, agrees with the assessment and consents to Colin's request to administer a 0.3 mg dose of epinephrine intramuscularly. With continued airway management and oxygenation, intravenous fluids for volume replacement, and epinephrine for airway obstruction, wheezing, and vasodilation, the patient begins to improve en route to Bayside Memorial Hospital.

CHAPTER REVIEW

Chapter Summary

The myriad diseases and injuries suffered by human beings often present as emergencies when the pathophysiology results in inadequate cellular energy production to maintain cell functions. Although the initial mechanisms of illness and injury can be diverse, prehospital treatment often comes down to ensuring the delivery of oxygen and glucose to the cells, and maintaining a normal body temperature. As an Advanced EMT, you are able to provide general, supportive treatments to maintain the patient's airway, breathing, and circulation; and some specific treatments aimed at reversing the pathophysiologic processes (or at least some components of them) causing the patient's problem. In order to appropriately select specific treatments and avoid causing harm to patients, you must understand the pathophysiology of the patient's problem. Now that you have a basic background in the pathophysiology of common emergency conditions, you will build upon your understanding in upcoming chapters.

Review Questions

Multiple-Choice Questions

1. Shock is best defined as:
   a. pale, cool, diaphoretic skin.
   b. metabolic alkalosis.
   c. hypotension with tachycardia.
   d. inadequate perfusion to meet cellular needs.

2. A change from the normal cell type of a tissue to a type of cell not expected in that tissue is called:
   a. apoptosis.
   b. metaplasia.
   c. necrosis.
   d. hyperplasia.

3. Which one of the following occurs during anaerobic metabolism?
   a. Increased ATP production
   b. Efficient glycolysis
   c. Conversion of pyruvate to acetyl coenzyme A
   d. Accumulation of lactic acid

4. Which one of the following changes occurs when altitude above sea level increases?
   a. The partial pressure of oxygen decreases.
   b. The partial pressure of nitrogen increases.
   c. The percentage of oxygen in the atmosphere decreases.
   d. The percentage of nitrogen in the atmosphere increases.

5. Which one of the following would you expect from a loss of pulmonary surfactant?
   a. Atelectasis
   b. Increased mucus production
   c. Swelling of bronchial epithelium
   d. Fluid in the alveoli

6. What is the mechanism by which carbon monoxide causes asphyxia?
   a. It displaces oxygen from hemoglobin.
   b. It causes pulmonary edema.
   c. The cytochrome oxidase system is impaired.
   d. Oxygen is converted to carbon dioxide.

7. Under which one of the following conditions is oxygen more readily released from hemoglobin at the cellular level?
   a. Decreased body temperature
   b. Acidosis
   c. Decreased H^+
   d. Decreased $PaCO_2$

8. Hypoxia of the myocardium sufficient to prevent defibrillation begins in the _____ phase of cardiac arrest.
   a. electrical
   b. alkalotic
   c. circulatory
   d. metabolic

9. Which one of the following would most likely occur due to a decrease in insulin availability?
   a. Increased blood glucose level
   b. Inability of brain cells to use glucose
   c. Metabolic alkalosis
   d. Increased glycogen storage

10. Which one of the following would you expect to see in patients in metabolic acidosis?
    a. Low potassium levels
    b. Increased bicarbonate levels
    c. Shivering
    d. Increased respiratory rate

11. Hypotension is first noted when a patient enters _____ shock.
    a. compensated
    b. decompensated
    c. irreversible
    d. stagnant

12. The mechanism common to all forms of distributive shock is:
    a. decreased heart rate.
    b. severe infection.
    c. vasodilation.
    d. loss of sympathetic nervous system function.

13. Which one of the following marks the onset of the stagnant phase of shock?
    a. Constriction of the precapillary sphincters
    b. Constriction of the postcapillary sphincters
    c. Relaxation of the precapillary sphincters
    d. Relaxation of the postcapillary sphincters

14. The most common cause of cardiogenic shock is:
    a. poisoning.
    b. pericardial tamponade.
    c. myocardial infarction.
    d. dysrhythmias.

15. The substance responsible for vasodilation and bronchoconstriction in anaphylaxis is:
    a. epinephrine.
    b. histamine.
    c. norepinephrine.
    d. bacterial toxins.

Critical-Thinking Questions

16. You have a diabetic patient with a blood glucose level of 20 mg/dL. Explain how this condition can lead to death if left untreated.

17. A patient has severe pneumonia and his arterial oxygen levels are low. Explain why he is presenting with confusion.

18. A patient with a normal tidal volume of 500 mL has taken a narcotic overdose and is presenting with a tidal volume of 350 mL. Is oxygenation likely to be affected? Why or why not?

19. Explain how each of the following leads to a ventilation–perfusion mismatch: pneumothorax and pulmonary embolism.

20. Why is it important for an Advanced EMT to differentiate among the types of shock?

References

Ali, S., & Antezano, E. S. (2006). Sudden cardiac death: Management of out-of-hospital cardiac arrest (OHCA). *Southern Medical Journal, 99*(5), 502–510. Retrieved December 17, 2010 from http://www.medscape.com/viewarticle/533755_10

Leybell, I., Borron, S. W., & Roldan, C. J. (2010). *Cyanide toxicity.* eMedicine.com. Retrieved December 14, 2010 from http://emedicine.medscape.com/article/814287-overview

Additional Reading

Bledsoe, B. E., Porter, R. S., & Cherry, R. A. (2009). *Paramedic care: Principles and practice* (3rd ed., vol. 1). Upper Saddle River, NJ: Pearson.

Keyes, D. C. (2010). *Ethylene glycol toxicity.* eMedicine.com. Retrieved December 14, 2010 from http://emedicine.medscape.com/article/814701-overview

11

Principles of Pharmacology

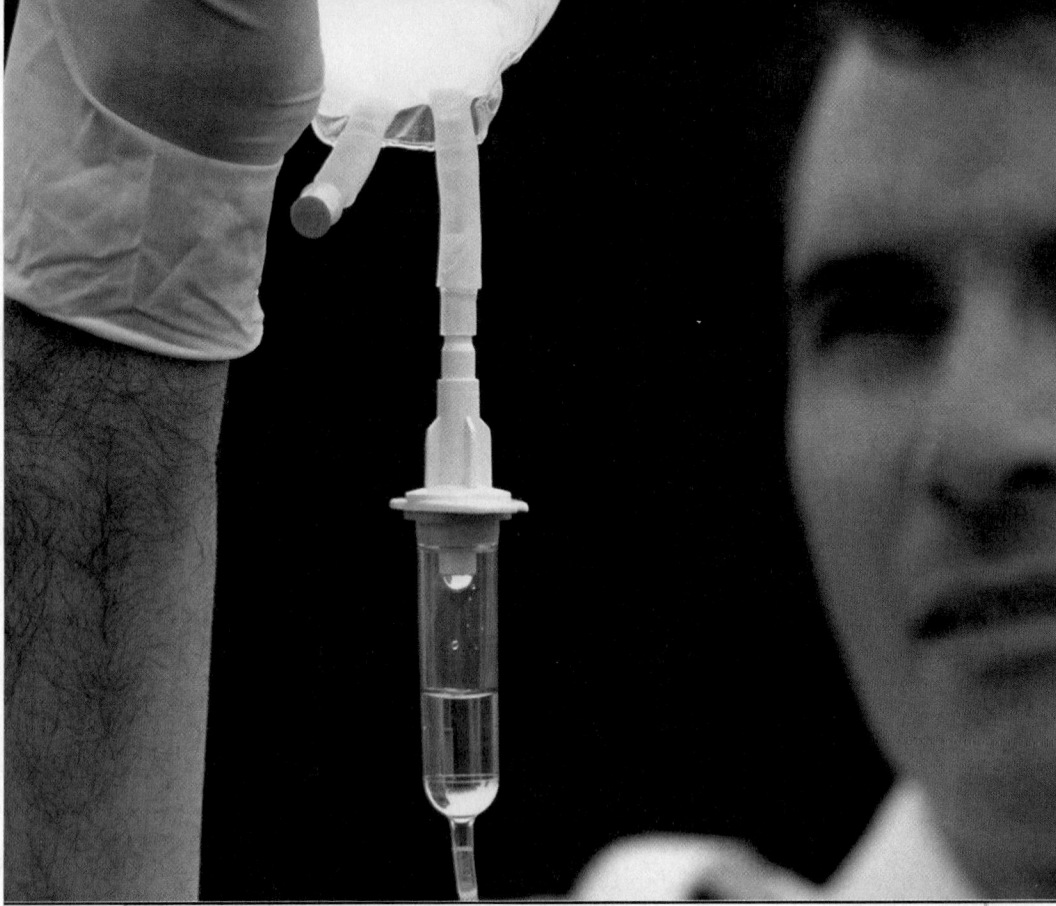

Content Area: Pharmacology

Advanced EMT Education Standard: The Advanced EMT applies fundamental knowledge of medications in the Advanced EMT scope of practice to patient assessment and management.

Objectives

After reading this chapter, you should be able to:

11.1 Define key terms introduced in this chapter.

11.2 Give examples of each of the four sources of drugs.

11.3 Explain the role of the U.S. Food and Drug Administration in the development and continued oversight of drugs.

11.4 Discuss relevant legislation regarding the administration of prescription medications, including controlled substances.

11.5 Identify the official, generic, and trade names of drugs in the Advanced EMT scope of practice.

11.6 Describe the various forms in which drugs are supplied.

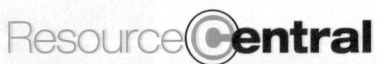

CASE STUDY

Advanced EMTs Matt Flynn and Mike Reilly have just begun their shift. While inventorying their equipment, they are dispatched to respond to an unknown emergency. En route, dispatch reports an unresponsive woman in a department store parking lot. When they arrive, they find a middle-aged woman in the driver's seat of a car that has apparently just stopped in the middle of a parking lot against a parking divider. There is no visible damage to the vehicle and the airbags have not deployed. She is wearing a seatbelt. A police officer approaches Mike and tells him that the car was not in a collision but simply rolled to a stop when it struck a curb. There is no one on the scene who knows the patient.

Mike approaches the car and determines that the driver has no apparent external injury. Her skin is pale, moist, and cool to the touch. She opens her eyes to questions but does not respond. A painful stimulus causes her to withdraw and she moves all extremities. Mike determines that her pupils are equal and reactive to light while Matt obtains baseline vital signs. Vital signs are pulse, 120 strong and regular; respirations, 22 normal; blood pressure, 130/90; pulse oximetry, 99 percent at room air; $EtCO_2$, 35 mmHg.

Mike finds a prescription bottle of phenytoin (Dilantin) between the front seats in the car. The medication is prescribed to the patient, who has been identified as Jaimie Callahan.

Problem-Solving Questions

1. What are some initial hypotheses about causes of the patient's condition?
2. What additional information would assist Mike and Matt in determining the cause of the patient's condition?
3. What initial steps in management should the crew take as they continue their assessment?

11.7 Describe the various types of medication packaging.
11.8 Explain each of the components of a drug profile.
11.9 Explain each of the following with respect to pharmacology:
– Drug absorption
– Drug distribution
– Mechanism of action
– Drug elimination
11.10 Explain the roles of the kidneys and liver in drug metabolism and excretion.
11.11 Explain factors that can affect the concentration of a drug in a patient's body.
11.12 Describe the concepts of drug receptor sites and protein binding of medications.
11.13 Identify special populations in whom the administration of drugs may need to be modified.

Introduction

As an Advanced EMT, you will have the responsibility to administer medications to ill and injured patients. This is a responsibility that must not be taken lightly because some medications, when administered under the wrong circumstances, produce life-threatening consequences. So, before administering any medication to a patient, you must have a general understanding of pharmacology. **Pharmacology** is the study of the origin, nature, properties, and actions of drugs and their effects on living organisms. In this chapter you will obtain a working knowledge of the principles of pharmacology, enabling you to appropriately administer pharmacologic treatment to your patients.

This chapter offers basic information about the sources of medications, how medications are regulated and supplied, and how the body absorbs, distributes, and excretes them.

Medication Sources

Medications have four basic sources: plant, animal, mineral, and synthetic. Plants are the oldest source of medications, many of which are still used today. Atropine, a medication that blocks the parasympathetic nervous system, is an extract of the belladonna plant. Morphine, a very potent painkiller, is a product of the opium poppy. Digitalis is produced from the purple foxglove plant. One very common EMS medication, 50 percent dextrose, is made from sugar cane.

Nearly all animal sources of medication have been replaced by synthetic sources. Historically, animals have provided many different hormones, such as oxytocin and insulin, that were a close enough match to human hormones to have the same effect on the body. Today, many different vaccines are produced using chicken eggs as an incubating source.

Salts and other inorganic materials are a common source of medications, especially those used to treat mineral deficits in the body. Sodium bicarbonate is an example of a medication that is produced from a mineral source. Others include calcium chloride, saline (sodium chloride) solutions, and potassium chloride.

With the advances in recombinant DNA technology over the last two decades, many of the medications that were once derived from animal or plant sources are now created in the laboratory with recombinant DNA technology. Recombinant DNA medications include Humulin (human insulin), and tissue plasminogen activator (tPA), a fibrinolytic (a substance that breaks down blood clots). Other medications are designed by pharmaceutical researchers to meet a specific need. Lidocaine (an antidysrhythmic and local anesthetic) and diazepam (a benzodiazepine sedative–hypnotic drug) are examples of synthetic drugs developed in a laboratory to achieve specific effects within the body.

Medication Reference Material

Before administering any drug, you must know the basic information about it. What is known about drugs and their effects changes, so you must keep current by reviewing new information regularly. There are many different printed and electronic sources of medication reference material. Be familiar with reliable and up-to-date sources that are available to you and use them when necessary.

The *Physician's Desk Reference (PDR)* and the *American Medical Association (AMA) Drug Evaluations* are publications that provide in-depth information about medications. Other reliable sources of medication information include drug inserts, which are included in the packaging of the medication, and the *Hospital Formulary,* which is a listing of medications currently available to hospitals and pharmacies. Many sources of medication information can be accessed online free of charge. However, check with your medical director about the reliability of specific sources.

Medication doses may be slightly different from source to source. Many sources list a range of dosages, but your protocols usually give a specific dosage within that range. For example, a reference guide may list the dose of epinephrine for anaphylaxis as 0.3 to 0.5 mg of a 1:1,000 solution, to be given subcutaneously or intramuscularly. Your protocol might specifically state that you should administer 0.3 mg subcutaneously. You must follow your protocol and administer the 0.3 mg of medication as directed.

Medication Profile

A medication profile describes the key information needed in order to administer a medication safely. A typical medication profile includes the following information:

- *Medication name.* The medication name includes the generic name, trade name, and chemical name of the medication.
- *Classification.* The classification of a medication is the type of medication it is. A number of different classification schemes are used. Drugs may be classified by their mechanism of action or by the body system on which they are intended to act. As an example, nitroglycerin USP is a vasodilator, but it also can be classified as a cardiovascular medication.

- *Mechanism of action.* The **mechanism of action** is the way in which a medication achieves its intended effects. For example, epinephrine stimulates $alpha_1$, $beta_1$, and $beta_2$ cellular receptors in the sympathetic nervous system. It causes an increase in cardiac contractile force, speed of cardiac electrical conduction, and rate of cardiac contraction. It causes dilation of the bronchiolar smooth muscle, but causes constriction of peripheral vascular smooth muscle.

- *Indications.* The **indications** are the conditions that the medication is intended to treat. For example, 50 percent dextrose is indicated for hypoglycemia. Your protocols may define a specific glucometer reading as an indication for the drug.

- *Pharmacokinetics.* **Pharmacokinetics** describe how a drug is absorbed, distributed to the tissues, and eliminated from the body.

- *Side effects.* Side effects are unintended effects of the medication. For example, one side effect of nitroglycerin administration is headache. An *untoward effect* is a side effect with a negative impact on the body, such as hypotension.

- *Route of administration.* The route of administration is the way in which a medication is introduced into the body. Many medications have more than one route of administration. For example, nitroglycerin may be given by sublingual and transdermal routes, depending upon the form prescribed.

- *Contraindications.* **Contraindications** are conditions that make administration of the drug harmful, even though it is otherwise indicated for the patient's medical problem.

- *Dose.* The dose is the amount of medication to be administered and the frequency with which it should be administered. For example, 0.4 mg nitroglycerin can be administered sublingually (SL) every 3 to 5 minutes up to a total of three doses.

- *How supplied.* This portion of the profile describes the forms of packaging and concentrations that are available. For example, epinephrine is packaged as 1 mg in 1 mL (1:1,000 concentration) and as 1 mg in 10 mL (1:10,000 concentration). Each concentration is supplied for different routes of administration and indications. The 1:1,000 concentration is administered intramuscularly and subcutaneously, and the 1:10,000 concentration is administered intravenously.

- *Special considerations.* This section of the medication profile describes any changes in dosage, administration, or other aspects of the medication for pediatric, geriatric, or pregnant patients, or patients with particular medical conditions, such as renal failure. It also describes any special precautions to be observed when administering the drug to special patient populations.

Medication Oversight and Regulation

Pharmaceutical manufacturers in the United States must adhere to many laws and regulations that are in place to protect the consumer from harm. Think of a medication commercial that you have seen on television. Do you recall the narrator listing the potential side effects of the medication? The manufacturer is required to provide the public with information in all marketing of the medication so that the consumer can make an informed decision about using it. Additionally, manufacturers are required to follow strict standards to ensure that medications produced by different manufacturers are the same strength and are safe for use. Further information on U.S. drug regulations can be accessed through the National Formulary and the United States Pharmacopeia (USP).

Legislation

Medication legislation is intended to protect the public from unsafe and mislabeled medications. The Pure Food and Drug Act of 1906 was enacted to ensure the proper medication labeling. The Harrison Narcotic Act of 1914 placed regulations on the importation, manufacture, sale, and use of medications, including the addictive drugs opium and cocaine. Violations of the Act result in penalties up to and including imprisonment. The Food, Drug, and Cosmetic Act of 1938 was enacted to provide additional protection to the public. The Act was revised twice, in 1952 and 1962. The Food, Drug, and Cosmetic Act of 1938 provides the following more comprehensive regulations:

- Authorized the formation of the U.S. Food and Drug Administration (FDA)

- Mandated that addictive and harmful medications are dispensed with a prescription by a medical doctor, dentist, or veterinarian

- Required manufacturers to label their medications when they include addictive drugs and to list potential side effects of the medication

In 1958, the Durham-Mumphrey Amendments were added to the act of 1938. Those amendments required pharmacists to dispense certain medications only with a written or verbal prescription by a physician. The amendments also defined the **over-the-counter (OTC) medication** category.

The Comprehensive Drug Abuse Prevention and Control Act of 1970, known as the Controlled Substances Act, replaced the Harrison Narcotic Act of 1914. To further protect the public, five schedules of controlled substances were created with each having its own regulations regarding level of control (Table 11-1). Drugs are assigned to a schedule based on their potential for abuse: Schedule I drugs have the greatest potential for abuse and Schedule V drugs have the least potential for abuse. Controlled substances used in

TABLE 11-1   Schedules of Controlled Substances

SCHEDULE I Schedule I medications have a high potential for abuse and do not have any recognized medical use in the United States.	Examples: heroin, LSD, mescaline, methaqualone
SCHEDULE II Schedule II medications have a high potential for abuse and a recognized medical use in the United States. These medications require a written prescription, are restricted from phone renewals, and require oversight by a physician. Abuse may result in severe physical or psychological dependence.	Examples: morphine, codeine, meperidine, hydrocodone, and a host of very addictive stimulants and depressants
SCHEDULE III Schedule III medications have less abuse potential than Schedule II medications and an accepted medical use. Abuse can result in moderate to low physical or psychological dependence.	Examples: anabolic steroids, nonprescription painkillers combined with small amounts of Schedule II substances such as acetaminophen with codeine or hydrocodone. Also medications that contain small amounts of opiates.
SCHEDULE IV Schedule IV medications have less abuse potential than Schedule III medications and an accepted medical use. Abuse can result in less physical or psychological dependence than drugs in Schedule III.	Examples: benzodiazepines, some barbiturates, steroids, stimulants
SCHEDULE V Schedule V medications have less abuse potential than Schedule IV medications and an accepted medical use. Abuse can result in less physical or psychological dependence than drugs in Schedule IV.	Examples: over-the-counter (OTC) medications for cough or antidiarrheal medications that contain small amounts of controlled substances

the prehospital environment include morphine and fentanyl for pain relief and benzodiazepines, such as midazolam and diazepam, for seizures.

Most of the other medications used in EMS, although they are not controlled substances, have been identified as dangerous enough to require a prescription. When you administer a medication to a patient according to protocol, you are doing so under direct order by your medical director, which means the medication is being prescribed to the patient by the medical director. Even though the physician is prescribing the medication, he is doing so based on your assessment of the patient. It is your responsibility to perform a thorough assessment to identify the need for proper medication administration.

OTC medications are medications that present a low risk to the user, as long as the medication is used as directed on the label. Because the risk is low, OTC medications can be purchased without a prescription at pharmacies and other retailers.

Regulations outlining the proper storage, tracking, and distribution of medications in the prehospital setting can vary from state to state. You must be familiar with the regulations of your state and employer.

IN THE FIELD

As an Advanced EMT, you will be responsible for the administration of some over-the-counter (OTC) medications. Even though they are OTC medications, they still may be used only as directed by protocol. In fact, in some cases, you may be required to obtain a direct physician's order to administer the medication.

Medication Safety and Regulation

Before 1938, medication testing was not always required. In fact, before the creation of the FDA, there was little or no oversight of what could be sold to the public as a medication. Today, developing a new medication is a very stringent and controlled process that takes years to accomplish. The FDA is responsible for the testing of each new medication offered for sale in the United States and for continuing to collect data about its safety after it is on the market. The

FDA is also responsible for food safety, the testing of new medical devices, and cosmetics safety in the United States.

In order to obtain FDA approval for a medication, manufacturers must participate in a rigorous and very expensive process. In the initial phases of this process, a new medication must be proven safe using animal and laboratory testing over several generations of test animals. During this time, researchers determine the safe dose and how the medication enters and leaves the body. If the medication is proven safe to administer after several cycles of lab testing, it can enter clinical trials for evaluation in humans. The clinical trial process is tightly controlled and can take years to complete.

In phase I testing, researchers attempt to determine the safe dose and how the medication is both absorbed and eliminated from the body. This is usually conducted on a limited number of healthy volunteers. Phase II consists of the drug being tested on a small number (usually 300 or less) of people with the illness or condition the drug is designed to treat. In this phase, researchers attempt to determine the needed level of drug to obtain the desired effect without causing undesirable side effects.

In phase III, the trial is expanded to include a large sample size, usually in the thousands of individuals, and establish the overall safety and effectiveness of the drug. Risk versus benefit for using the medication is determined during this phase. At the conclusion of phase III, the FDA may approve marketing the medication for sale.

Phase IV trials compare the medication to other medications on the market.

Because there are strict guidelines regarding testing drugs on pediatric and pregnant patients, the safety of drugs in those groups often has not been established.

Special Considerations

Medications can affect patients differently. Some special considerations to be kept in mind include those for patients who are pregnant, patients who are infants or children, and patients who are elderly.

Medications and Pregnancy

Prior to administering a medication to a woman of childbearing age, consider the possibility of her being pregnant. Ask her about it during your assessment. If she is pregnant, you will be treating two patients. This is particularly true when administering medications because some will affect the fetus by crossing the placental barrier. Even some OTC medications pose a risk to a developing fetus and should be avoided by the mother. You must consider the risk versus benefit of administering the medication. If the patient's condition is life threatening, you must treat her. When unclear about how you should proceed, you will contact medical direction for instructions.

When treating a pregnant patient, consider the following:

- *Changes in anatomy and physiology.* In order to support the fetus, the mother's heart rate, cardiac output, and blood volume increase. Additionally, metabolism in the liver is decreased. Those alterations can affect the onset, duration of action, and rate of elimination of medications.

- *Risk to the fetus.* **Teratogenic** medications are those that potentially can deform, injure, or kill the fetus. In order to provide direction to health care providers, the FDA created FDA Pregnancy Categories for medications (Table 11-2). Drugs also are rated for their safety during breast feeding.

Pediatric Patients

In addition to the obvious physical differences between the adult and pediatric patient, there are also differences in how medications affect children. Pediatric drug dosing is usually

---

TABLE 11-2   FDA Pregnancy Categories

Category	Description
A	Studies have not identified a risk to the fetus during pregnancy.
B	Animal studies have not identified a risk to the fetus but there are no adequate human studies. OR Adequate studies in humans have not demonstrated a risk to the fetus during pregnancy but animal studies have produced adverse effects.
C	Animal studies have demonstrated adverse effects but there are no adequate studies in pregnant women; however, benefits may be acceptable despite the potential risks. OR No adequate animal studies or adequate studies of pregnant women have been performed.
D	Studies have shown risk to the fetus. In some situations, benefits could outweigh the risks.
X	Studies have shown risk to the fetus. This risk outweighs any potential benefit to the mother. Avoid using these medications in pregnant or potentially pregnant patients.

Geriatric Care

Geriatric patients are prone to medication interactions for many reasons, including changes in physiology, taking multiple drugs, and memory impairment.

based on the patient's weight (amount per kilogram), so the dosage varies from patient to patient, even between patients of the same age. Because it takes infants longer to absorb, metabolize, and eliminate medications than it does adults, doses must be adjusted according to the patient's body weight to prevent toxicity. Older children can absorb and metabolize some medications faster than an adult; therefore, they also require adjustments in dose and frequency of administration.

Geriatric Patients

The effects of a medication in geriatric patients are often different from that of a younger adult. As people age, a steady decrease of muscle mass, renal and hepatic function, and oral absorption rates occur. Each of those affects important processes, including the **absorption**, distribution, metabolism, and elimination of a medication.

Geriatric patients may have multiple medical conditions that require the use of multiple medications. When some medications are used together, they can produce life-threatening conditions. For example, administering nitroglycerin to a patient who has taken an erectile dysfunction medication such as Cialis or Viagra may cause severe hypotension. During your assessment, identify which medications the patient is taking and avoid administering medications that will interact with the others, resulting in an adverse effect.

Medication Names

Most medications have four names: trade name, chemical name, generic name, and the official name. Each describes the medication in a different way and for a different purpose. Manufacturers create a proprietary, or trade name, for a medication under which they can trademark and market the drug. For example, the medication Proventil is the

trade name for albuterol (the generic name) of a popular medication used to treat asthma. Trade names are capitalized and, in drug packaging and marketing, followed by either the trademark symbol (™) or the registered symbol (®). Often, the trade name of a new medication is the one that most people recognize because those drugs are heavily marketed to the public. The same drug may be marketed under different trade names by different companies. Once a pharmaceutical company's patent on a drug expires, it is often sold primarily under its generic name.

The chemical name is a precise description of the chemical composition and molecular structure of the medication. Usually, it is a complex formula and most likely only recognizable and usable by a pharmacist. However, a common example is acetylsalicylic acid, the chemical name for aspirin.

The official and generic names for a medication are often identical and are often very familiar to the public. In many cases, the medication is referred to only by the generic name due to the long established use of the medication. For example, the generic and official medication names albuterol sulfate and albuterol sulfate USP are usually more familiar to people as their trade name Proventil. The official name of a medication is assigned by the USP and can be identified by the letters USP that appear after the name.

The following is an example of how each name is published:

- Trade name: Proventil
- Chemical name: α_1 [(tert-butylamino) methyl]-4-hydroxy-m-xylene-α, $\acute{\alpha}$-diol sulfate (2:1) (salt)
- Generic name: albuterol sulfate
- Official name: albuterol sulfate USP

Medication Forms

Medications are supplied in a variety of forms and, in many cases, dictate the route by which you will administer the medication. Be familiar with the following medication forms: solids, liquids, semisolids, and gases.

Solid Medications

The majority of medications that are administered by mouth to a patient are in solid form as either a tablet or a capsule. A *tablet* consists of the medication, along with other substances, all of which are compressed into shape under high pressure. Some tablets are designed to dissolve rapidly and increase rate of absorption. An example of this is sublingual nitroglycerin tablets. The tablets are rapidly dissolved and absorbed in the highly vascular sublingual region beneath the tongue. In some situations, medications are ground into a powder or chewed in order to increase absorption rates. Other tablets are designed to be swallowed whole and dissolved in the gastrointestinal (GI) tract.

A *capsule* is a liquid or powdered medication held within a gelatin casing. Capsules are designed to be ingested and absorbed in the GI tract.

Solid medications also may be fine powders that are administered for inhalation, such as medications in many metered-dose inhalers.

Liquid Medications

Liquid medications are usually solutions of a solid medication dissolved in a solvent. A *solution* is a liquid mixture of one or more substances that does not separate as a result of standing or filtering. Solutions may be administered by ingestion, intravenous injection, intramuscular injection, subcutaneous injection, intranasal, topically, sublingually, or inhaled. In addition to solutions, liquid medications are available in various forms, as follows:

- *Suspensions.* These consist of substances that do not dissolve well in liquids. The substances are ground into fine particles that can be well distributed in a liquid when shaken or stirred.
- *Tinctures.* Prepared by using an alcohol extraction process, these are usually made for topical application.
- *Spirits:* Meant to be taken orally, these are solutions of a medication and alcohol.
- *Elixirs.* These are produced by mixing medication with sweeteners and flavorings for oral administration.
- *Syrups.* These mixtures of a medication with a thick, sweet flavored liquid improve the taste of the medication.
- *Emulsions.* A combination of two liquids that are not soluble, these are typically emulsions that consist of an oil and water.

Semisolid Medications

Semisolid medications are lotions, creams, gels, ointments, and medicated adhesive patches that can be applied to the skin or mucous membranes. Some are designed for their topical effects on the skin, while others are designed to be absorbed through the skin (transcutaneous or transdermal medications) or mucous membranes. Because lotions, creams, and ointments contain different amounts of water and oil, they have different absorption rates.

The amount of water in the mixture is directly related to the rate of absorption. Simply stated, the more water the mixture contains, the faster it is absorbed. Lotions contain the most water and are absorbed fastest. Creams contain more water than ointments and therefore have a faster absorption rate than ointments. Nitroglycerin paste and morphine patches are examples of transcutaneous medications.

Gases

Some medications are designed to be breathed into the lungs where they are almost immediately absorbed. Gaseous medications used in the prehospital environment include oxygen and nitrous oxide.

Classifications of Medications

Medications are classified in many different ways, such as mechanism of action, target tissue, how they treat a condition, and the body system affected by the drug. For example, ibuprofen, a common nonprescription pain reliever, may be classified as any of the following:

- Analgesic, because it reduces the symptom of pain
- Nonsteroidal anti-inflammatory, for how it treats a problem
- Cyclo-oxygenase inhibitor (COX-1, COX-2), for its specific mechanism of action

All of these classifications describe the same medication in ways that help you understand its uses.

Medications That Affect the Nervous System

The autonomic nervous system (ANS) regulates and makes frequent, rapid changes in involuntary functions by constantly balancing its sympathetic and parasympathetic divisions. The sympathetic nervous system is responsible for the "fight-or-flight" responses of the body.

The sympathetic responses of the body are called **adrenergic** (pertaining to the adrenal glands) because nerve fibers trigger the release of the neurotransmitters epinephrine and norepinephrine from the adrenal glands. Epinephrine and norepinephrine stimulate adrenergic cellular receptors in various tissues, such as those in the lungs and cardiovascular system. Adrenergic receptors are divided into four categories (Table 11-3).

Stimulation of the parasympathetic nervous system results in effects that are opposite that of the sympathetic nervous system using the neurotransmitter acetylcholine. Parasympathetic stimulation results in a decrease in heart rate, decrease in blood pressure, constriction of pupils, and an increase in GI system activity.

Pediatric Care

Many drugs appropriate for topical administration in adults are not appropriate for pediatric administration. Pediatric patients have thinner skin and a larger body surface-to-volume ratio. In pediatric patients, topically administered drugs may be absorbed to a greater degree and result in a higher concentration than intended.

TABLE 11-3	Adrenergic Receptors and Their Responses to Stimulation
Alpha$_1$	Peripheral vasoconstriction
Alpha$_2$	Peripheral vasodilation Little or no bronchoconstriction
Beta$_1$	Increased heart rate Increased automaticity Increased myocardial contractility Increased conductivity
Beta$_2$	Bronchodilation Vasodilation

Sympathetic Nervous System Medications

Some of the medications administered by Advanced EMTs produce the same effects as those produced by the neurotransmitters of the sympathetic nervous system. Those medications are called **sympathomimetics** or *adrenergic agonists* because they mimic the effects of the sympathetic nervous system. An example is the administration of an adrenergic beta$_2$-selective medication (such as albuterol sulfate) to treat asthma. Because the medication is beta$_2$ specific, only beta$_2$ effects will be produced. Medications that inhibit the sympathetic nervous system are called **sympatholytics**. For example, some patients take beta blocker medications to control hypertension and some cardiac arrhythmias. Beta blockers work by binding to beta receptor sites, preventing them from being stimulated by epinephrine, norepinephrine, or symphthomimetic medications. Some beta blockers are selective for beta$_1$ receptors, some are selective for beta$_2$ receptors, and some are nonselective, and block both beta$_1$ and beta$_2$ receptor sites.

Parasympathetic Nervous System Medications

Parasympathetic nervous system **agonists** are also called **parasympathomimetics** or **cholinergics**, while parasympathetic antagonists (drugs that block parasympathetic effects) are called **parasympatholytics**, or **anticholinergics**.

Parasympathomimetic medications stimulate the cholinergic receptors that are normally stimulated by the neurotransmitter acetylcholine (ACh). Direct-acting cholinergic medications simulate the effects of ACh by binding with cholinergic receptors. Indirectly acting cholinergic medications affect acetylcholinesterase, the substance that breaks down acetylcholine in the synapse to prevent continuous stimulation of the receptors. By inhibiting the breakdown of ACh, indirect agents prolong cholinergic effects. Parasympatholytic medications block the action of ACh at the

receptor site. The prototypical medication in this class is atropine, which blocks acetylcholine effects and decreases the impact of the parasympathetic nervous system. Atropine is used as an antidote to nerve agents that work by blocking acetylcholinesterase.

Analgesics

Analgesics are medications that reduce pain. When you are called to care for an injured patient who is in pain, you may administer an analgesic to him if your protocols allow. A common type of analgesic used in prehospital advanced life support care is the opioid agonist. Opioid agonists are chemically similar to opium, which is extracted from the poppy plant. Morphine and fentanyl are both opioid agonists. Opioid **antagonists** are used to reverse the effects of opioid medications by binding to opioid receptors, thereby blocking the opioid molecules. Opioid agonist–antagonists have both agonist and antagonist properties. They often are preferred for use because they can effectively reduce pain without the side effects of opioid agonists such as CNS and respiratory depression. The analgesic in the National Scope of Practice Model for Advanced EMTs is nitrous oxide, an inhaled gas that is not in the opioid class.

There are many different analgesics available through physician prescription and for OTC purchase. Analgesics that are not derived from opium are called *nonopioid analgesics*. This class of medications includes several OTC medications. Some of the most common nonopioid analgesics include: **nonsteroidal anti-inflammatory drugs (NSAIDs)** such as ibuprofen, salicylates (the most common of which is aspirin), and para-aminophenol derivatives such as acetaminophen.

Antianxiety and Sedative– Hypnotic Medications

While the administration of anti-anxiety and sedative–hypnotic medications is not included in the National Scope of Practice Model for Advanced EMTs, you are likely to encounter patients who are using them. Those medications are designed to reduce anxiety. During medical procedures, they are used for sedation and to produce short-term amnesia. Specific medications you should know are barbiturates, benzodiazepines, and nonbarbiturate hypnotics.

Barbiturates are sedatives whose mechanism of action includes the increase in affinity between the gama-aminobutyric acid (GABA) receptor sites and GABA, the neurotransmitter that binds with the receptor sites.

Benzodiazepines are the most commonly prescribed sedatives. Their mechanism of action is similar in some ways to that of barbiturates because of their affinity for GABA receptors.

Nonbarbiturate hypnotics are used for sedation and have a mechanism of action very similar to the barbiturates and benzodiazepines but produce fewer side effects. One example is the commonly prescribed sleeping medication zolpidem (Ambien®). Other nonbarbiturate hypnotic medications are used in the hospital setting but are usually only encountered by EMS personnel during interfacility transfers.

Stimulants

Stimulants are medications that produce central nervous system excitation. This is accomplished in one of two ways: by increasing excitatory neurotransmitter activity, or decreasing the release of inhibitory neurotransmitters. Stimulants cause an increase in awareness while reducing the subjective sensation of fatigue. Other, potentially harmful, effects of stimulants include tachycardia, hypertension, and seizures. Some common stimulants that you should be familiar with include: caffeine, cocaine, and amphetamine, including methamphetamine. Because of the feeling they produce, stimulants are widely abused.

Depressants

Depressants are medications that slow CNS activity and are commonly used to treat anxiety, muscle tension, stress, pain, and insomnia. Examples of depressants include benzodiazepines (such as diazepam, alprazolam, and midazolam), barbiturates, and narcotics.

Anticonvulsants

Anticonvulsants, also called *antiseizure* or *antiepileptic* medications, are used to treat seizures. Their mechanism of action is thought to be the result of inhibiting the influx of sodium into the cells. In doing so, the cell's ability to depolarize is inhibited, resulting in a decrease in the likelihood of seizure activity.

Psychotherapeutic Medications

Psychotherapeutic medications are used to treat mental illness (such as depression), anxiety disorders, and psychotic disorders (such as schizophrenia). They achieve their effects by enhancing or blocking the effects of various neurotransmitters, including dopamine. In many cases, they are effective in treating the conditions for which they are prescribed, but they produce several side effects including orthostatic hypotension and sedation. Antipsychotics, in particular, can produce extrapyramidal symptoms, including acute dystonic reactions (a condition involving involuntary muscle spasms).

Unfortunately, some antipsychotic medications are misrepresented on the street as mood altering drugs. You may see a patient with extrapyramidal symptoms who just ingested a street drug that he thought was valium or LSD. Extrapyramidal symptoms (EPS) include involuntary muscle movements such as jerking, tremors, muscle rigidity, and changes in heart and respiratory rates.

Patients with schizophrenia can function quite well as long as they are compliant with their antipsychotic medications. Unfortunately, compliance with medications is sometimes difficult because of their unpleasant side effects. However, noncompliance with medications results in a return of the signs and symptoms of schizophrenia.

Antidepressants are very commonly prescribed, not only to treat depression, but to treat chronic pain, obsessive-compulsive disorders, and other problems. Antidepressants include selective serotonin reuptake inhibitors (SSRIs), selective serotonin and norepinephrine reuptake inhibitors (SNRIs), cyclic antidepressants and monoamine oxidase inhibitors (MAOIs). Cyclic antidepressants and MAOIs are less frequently prescribed because of their side effects and because of the availability of newer, safer medications.

PERSONAL PERSPECTIVE

Advanced EMT Gwen Hillman: My partner, Jimmy, and I were called for an unresponsive patient at a department store. When we got there, the store manager told us that an employee found a young man in a restroom, unconscious on the floor. The manager stated that he made an announcement over the store PA system to see if anyone in the store was with the young man, but no one responded.

The patient was in his mid-20s and the employee had rolled him from a prone position onto his back. He had snoring respirations with a lot of oral secretions, and responded to painful stimuli by moaning. We opened the airway and suctioned the patient. His respirations were adequate, so we put oxygen on him by nonrebreather mask. As part of our assessment, we found a medication bottle in his backpack. Jimmy showed it to me and said, "Are you thinking what I'm thinking?"

"Carbamazepine. I think that's an anticonvulsant," I said, and quickly checked my field drug guide to confirm. The name of the medication, along with the patient's presentation, made us think that the patient had suffered a seizure and was in a postictal state. We continued our assessment to make sure we weren't missing something else that could be causing the patient's condition. There was no trauma and his blood glucose level was normal. His pupils were normal in size, equal, and reacted to light. His perfusion was normal.

Within a few minutes, the patient's level of responsiveness began to increase. En route to the hospital, as the patient became more alert and oriented, he confirmed that he had a seizure disorder and had suffered a seizure in the restroom in the store. Identifying the medication and confirming it were important clues to figuring out what was going on with this patient.

Respiratory Medications

People take a wide variety of OTC medications that affect the respiratory system, including nasal decongestants, expectorants (medications that make coughs more productive), cough suppressants, and mucolytics (medications that decrease the viscosity of mucous secretions).

Prescription respiratory medications include beta$_2$ agonists used to treat the bronchospasms that occur in asthma and chronic obstructive pulmonary disease (COPD). Corticosteroids, such as methylprednisolone, and other types of anti-inflammatory drugs are used to decrease the inflammatory response associated with asthma and COPD.

Cardiovascular Medications

Since cardiovascular disease is common, cardiovascular medications are among some of the most frequently prescribed medications. Several classes of cardiovascular medications are prescribed to treat hypertension, heart failure, and dysrhythmias, and to reduce the chances of acute coronary syndrome (ACS). In emergency situations, a variety of medications are administered for the previously described effects and for other reasons, such as to raise the blood pressure and increase cardiac output.

Antidysrhythmic Medications

Antidysrhythmic medications are used to treat abnormal heart rhythms. The medications are classified by their mechanism of action on the heart, as follows:

- Sodium channel blockers slow the electrical conduction down (negative dromotropic effect).
- Beta blockers reduce adrenergic stimulation of the beta receptors.
- Potassium channel blockers cause a positive inotropic effect on the heart.
- Calcium channel blockers cause negative inotropic and dromotropic effects by slowing the influx of calcium back into the cells of the heart.

Antihypertensive Medications

According to the Centers for Disease Control and Prevention (CDC), hypertension affects over 30 percent of people in the United States (Sung Sug (Sarah) Yoon, 2010) (CDC). Those individuals rely on antihypertensives to keep their blood pressure under control. Drugs used as antihypertensives include diuretics, vasodilators, and sympatholytics.

Blood pressure and water volume are directly related in the body. When the body has too much intravascular water volume, blood pressure increases. **Diuretics** are medications that increase urine production to reduce excess water volume. Vasodilators, such as nitroglycerin, which relaxes vascular smooth muscle, increase the size of the vascular container to lower blood pressure.

Angiotensin-converting enzyme (ACE) inhibitors reduce blood pressure by preventing the conversion of angiotensin I to angiotensin II in the renin-angiotensin-aldosterone system.

Drugs with sympathetic alpha and beta blocking effects also are used to treat hypertension.

Antiplatelet and Anticoagulant Agents

Patients who suffer from coronary artery disease, particularly those who have required some sort of previous medical intervention, are often prescribed antiplatelet or anticoagulant agents. Those medications reduce the potential for blood clots to form in the coronary arteries.

Antiplatelet agents inhibit platelet aggregation. Aspirin and clopidogrel (Plavix®) are the principle medications used for this purpose. Antiplatelet agents do not break down existing blood clots. Instead, they inhibit the platelet aggregation phase of blood clotting to reduce the likelihood of abnormal blood clot formation.

Anticoagulant agents prevent coagulation of blood by interfering with one or more steps in the clotting cascade. Warfarin (Coumadin®) is a commonly prescribed anticoagulant. The blood levels of anticoagulant medications must be carefully monitored. The same mechanisms that prevent abnormal coagulation also prevent the normal coagulation of blood in response to injury when medication levels are too high.

Fibrinolytics

Fibrinolytic agents breakdown the fibrin network of existing blood clots. Fibrinolytics are administered in the hospital to some patients with stroke, acute coronary syndrome, or pulmonary embolism. Fibrinolytics include tissue plasminogen activator (tPA), which is a naturally occurring substance in the body, and agents derived from certain strains of bacteria, such as streptokinase.

Diabetic Medications

As of 2010, diabetes affects over 25 million people in the United States (Centers for Disease Control and Prevention, 2011). Diabetics either cannot secrete insulin, or have increased cellular resistance to insulin. Since insulin is the hormone that facilitates the entry of glucose into cells, diabetics must rely on medications to control their blood sugar. Type 1 diabetics take insulin injections to replace the insulin that is no longer manufactured by the pancreas. Type 2 diabetics take medications that either promote production of insulin by the pancreas or help overcome the cellular resistance to insulin.

Immunosuppressant Medications

People who have an autoimmune disease or undergo organ transplantation take immunosuppressants to inhibit the actions of the immune system. Immunosuppressants decrease the body's attack on its own tissues in autoimmune disease, and reduce the likelihood that the patient's body will reject a transplanted organ.

Medication Packaging

Medication manufacturers package medications in various ways. Since medications can be administered by different routes, they are packaged to accommodate their intended use. For example, since epinephrine is administered by injection, it is commonly supplied in a prefilled syringe. *Unit dose packaging* is used to help avoid medication errors. This means that the medication is supplied in the amount given in a typical dose. When epinephrine is used in cardiac arrest, 1 mg of 1:10,000 concentration is given intravenously every three to five minutes. A 10 mL solution of 1:10,000 equals 1 mg of epinephrine. The manufacturer supplies individual prefilled syringes with 1 mg of medication in 10 mL of solution. The usual dose for 50 percent dextrose for hypoglycemia is 25 to 50 grams. Each prefilled syringe contains 25 grams.

When a drug dose you have calculated requires multiple units (such as more than one prefilled syringe) or substantially less than is the amount provided in one unit, you should recheck your calculations before administering the drug.

Packaging also protects the medication during storage. Some medication vials are clear glass or plastic, while others are dark brown glass or plastic. The dark brown color protects medications that are particularly susceptible to breakdown when exposed to light. Medications intended for intravenous (IV), intraosseous (IO), intramuscular (IM), or subcutaneous (SQ) administration must be sterile; thus, their packaging must maintain the sterility of the medication.

Medications may be packaged as vials, ampules, prefilled syringes, or nebules:

- *Prefilled syringe.* Prefilled syringes consist of a barrel with a needle or adapter attached and a prefilled glass or plastic tube containing the medication. They are a common form of packaging used for EMS medications. Some prefilled syringes use a needleless system for intravenous injection to reduce the risk of needle-stick injuries (Figure 11-1).

- *Vials.* These consist of a glass or plastic container with a sealed rubber stopper that can be pierced by a needle to withdraw the medication (Figure 11-2).

- *Nonconstituted medications.* These medications are packaged in separate vials to extend the shelf life of certain medications that would have a shorter shelf life if stored as solution. For example, glucagon is a medication that is packaged in two separate vials—one has the medication in a powdered form and the other has a liquid solvent used to reconstitute or mix the medication prior to administration (Figure 11-3).

- *Ampules.* These are sealed glass containers with a thin, breakable neck (Figure 11-4). Once the top is removed by breaking it at the neck, the medication is drawn into a syringe using a needle or filter straw (needleless system).

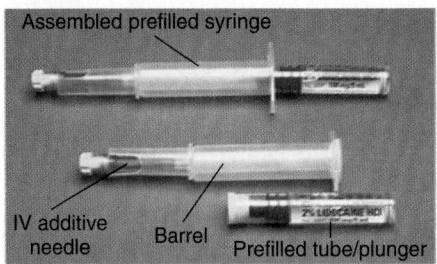

Assembled prefilled syringe

IV additive needle Barrel Prefilled tube/plunger

FIGURE 11-1

Example of a prefilled syringe.

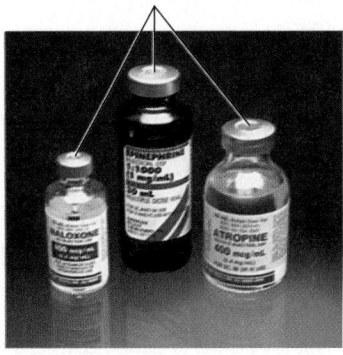

Self-sealing rubber top

FIGURE 11-2

Examples of medication vials.

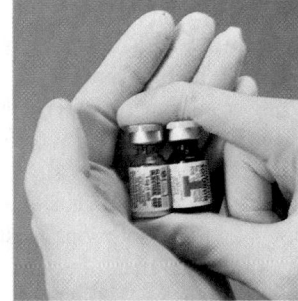

FIGURE 11-3

Examples of nonconstituted medication vials.

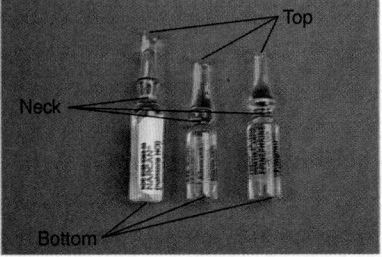

Top

Neck

Bottom

FIGURE 11-4

Examples of ampules.

■ *Nebule.* A nebule is similar to an ampule, but it is a plastic container designed so that the top can be torn off and the medication squeezed out. Nebules are commonly used for medications administered by small volume nebulizer, such as albuterol sulfate or ipratropium bromide.

Pharmacokinetics

Pharmacokinetics is the branch of pharmacology concerned with the way drugs are absorbed, distributed, metabolized, and eliminated from the body. Medications are designed to create specific effects by modifying existing natural functions of the body.

Absorption

When a medication is introduced to the body, it must first enter into the body's circulatory system through a process called *absorption*. Several factors can affect absorption. Medications are absorbed at a faster rate when introduced in highly vascular regions of the body. For example, injecting a medication into a muscle will provide a faster absorption rate than injecting it into the subcutaneous tissue of the skin. This is because the muscles are more vascular then the subcutaneous layer of the skin, allowing the medication in the tissue to more readily come into contact with blood vessels. With this in mind, consider how hypothermia and shock will affect the absorption of medication. When a patient is hypothermic or is in shock, he experiences a decrease in peripheral blood flow, thereby decreasing the rate of absorption in peripheral circulation. The opposite is true as well. When a patient is suffering from hyperthermia, peripheral blood flow increases, which will result in a faster absorption rate.

When a medication is taken orally, it is absorbed through the gastrointestinal mucosa. The lining of the stomach is not well-designed for absorption. Most drug absorption from the gastrointestinal tract does not occur until the drug reaches the duodenum. Some oral medications have an enteric coating that slowly dissolves and releases the medication over time. This is sometimes called a *time-released medication* or a *controlled-release medication.*

Absorption from the gastrointestinal tract is also affected by the interaction of the medication with acidic environment of the stomach or the more alkaline environment of the duodenum.

Geriatric Care

Individuals over the age of 60 begin to experience a decrease in GI motility, which may result in a slower absorption rate.

The rate of absorption is directly related to the amount of surface area available for absorption to take place. The more surface area available, the more potential for absorption to occur. Consider the following: The alveoli in the lungs provide a tremendous amount of highly vascular surface area, thus providing a very rapid rate of absorption when a medication is inhaled. However, the medication must consist of extremely fine particles or droplets in a relatively small amount, making most medications unsuitable for this route of administration. The same principle applies to drugs that are administered by nasal spray, since the nasal mucosa is highly vascular. Naloxone, a narcotic antagonist, is supplied in a liquid form with a mucosal atomizer device (MAD) to administer naloxone to patients with suspected narcotic overdose when an IV cannot be established.

Drugs given intravenously are administered directly into the bloodstream, and do not require absorption.

The concentration of a medication also affects absorption. Drug molecules diffuse from an area of higher concentration to an area of lower concentration. For example, in a patient who applies a nicotine patch, nicotine will diffuse from the higher concentration in the patch, through the skin and into the circulation until the patch no longer contains a higher level of nicotine than the body. Medications present in higher concentrations will be absorbed more rapidly than medications present in lower concentrations.

Distribution

Once a medication enters the circulation, it must be distributed to the target tissues on which it is intended to act. After absorption, some medications bind to plasma proteins in the blood and are referred to as *bound drug.* When a medication binds with a plasma protein (primarily albumin), it is not available for use at the target tissue. Medication that is not bound to proteins is called *free drug* and is available to bind with target tissue cellular receptor sites. There is a balance between bound drug and free drug.

If a patient is taking a drug that binds to plasma proteins, but begins taking a second drug that also binds to the same plasma proteins, the drugs will compete to bind to the available plasma proteins. As a result, the level of free drug of one or both medications may be higher than otherwise anticipated. Competing for protein binding sites is one mechanism by which drug interactions can occur.

Medications also may have a strong binding affinity with body tissues such as fat, bone, or muscle, reducing the amount available for immediate use by the target tissue.

There are also physical barriers to distribution, even when there is excellent blood flow at the site of administration. Medications that easily diffuse across the capillary wall are distributed faster than those that require active transport. The blood–brain barrier in the central nervous system prevents some types of medications from entering the brain and spinal cord. The placenta also can act as a barrier to prevent some medications from reaching the fetus or drastically reduce the total amount of drug that reaches the baby.

Biotransformation

Some medications are active immediately after administration and then become inactive as they are metabolized. Other drugs must be metabolized from the inactive form in which they are administered to an active form. This process of chemically changing a medication through metabolism is called **biotransformation.**

The primary organ in the human body for metabolizing and biotransforming medications is the liver. If the patient has decreased liver function, he may experience a delay in drug metabolism that prolongs both the time the drug takes to have an effect and to be broken down after administration. In such cases, a risk for the accumulation of a medication to toxic levels exists.

Bioavailability is the amount of a drug that is still active when it reaches its target tissues. An adequate amount of a medication must be administered to provide for the amount of drug that may be broken down before it reaches the target tissue. Bioavailability is affected by the route of administration of a drug. For example, beta blockers have different bioavailability when administered by mouth than they do when administered intravenously and are therefore dosed according to the route of administration.

Some drugs are affected by *first pass metabolism* when given enterally, or through the gastrointestinal tract. Drugs given enterally are absorbed into the hepatic portal circulation and are acted upon by the liver before entering the systemic circulation. Some drugs are no longer bioavailable after this process and cannot be given by the enteral route.

Elimination

Medications, whether unchanged or broken down into other substances called *metabolites,* are excreted from the body. Because most medications are excreted in the urine, they depend on adequate renal function for elimination. Renal failure or decreased renal perfusion, such as in states of shock, impair drug excretion. As people age, renal efficiency begins to decline. Geriatric patients, and any other patient with inadequate kidney function, may not be able to eliminate medications adequately, placing them at risk for accumulation of medications to toxic levels.

In addition to elimination through urination, medications are also eliminated through respiration, feces, perspiration, and the mammary glands during lactation.

Many drugs are metabolized in the liver in a process that uses various forms of the enzyme cytochrome P450. Some drugs enhance the effects of cytochrome P450 and others decrease its effects. When more than one drug that is metabolized by the cytochrome P450 system is administered, the rate at which the drugs are metabolized can be increased or decreased. The medicinal components of many herbal supplements use the cytochrome P450 system, explaining some of the interactions between herbs and other medications.

Pediatric Care

Nursing mothers should be familiar with medications to avoid in order to protect their infants from harm.

Pharmacodynamics

Pharmacodynamics, also called *mechanism of action*, is the way in which specific medications achieve their desired effect. Most drugs have their effects by binding with cellular receptors.

Receptor Sites

The easiest way to conceptualize a receptor site is by thinking of it as a lock. If the key fits in the lock, it will open the door when turned. If the key does not fit, it will not unlock the door.

Receptor site theory states that there are specific receptor sites on cells that when activated by substances that have an affinity for that particular type of receptor, inhibit or enhance the functions of the cell. The more receptor sites in a tissue or organ, the stronger the effect when the receptor sites are activated. A drug that can cause an effect at a specific receptor site is known as an *agonist* (Figure 11-5). Agonists can either enhance or inhibit a cell's normal function when a receptor site is occupied. When one agonist has a greater effect than another when it occupies a receptor, it is said to have greater *efficacy*. Antagonists bind to receptor sites and prevent another substance having an effect on the cell (Figure 11-6). It is possible for a medication to be both an agonist and antagonist. Some medications can cause an effect at the receptor site and, at the same time, block other agonists from occupying the same type of sites.

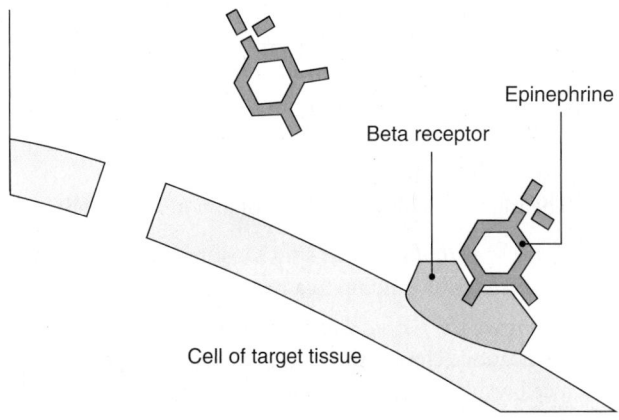

FIGURE 11-5

Receptor site binding.

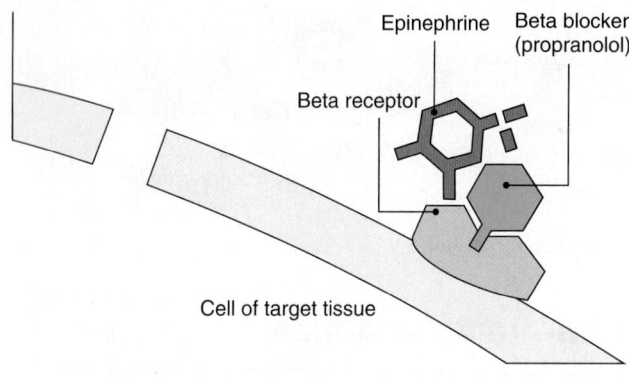

FIGURE 11-6

Receptor site blocked by medication with greater affinity to site.

IN THE FIELD

Naloxone has a shorter duration of effect than a narcotic. If repeated doses are not used, the narcotic will reoccupy the site when the naloxone is metabolized and the effects of the narcotic will reoccur.

Affinity

Drugs have an **affinity** or attraction to a receptor site. The stronger the attraction, the greater the affinity. For example, naloxone does not have any narcotic effects in the body, but it has a greater affinity for opiate receptor sites than most narcotic pain relievers. When an overdose of a narcotic is suspected, naloxone will displace the narcotic drug that is occupying the sites, because it has a greater affinity for the receptor sites.

Mechanism of Action

The effects of a medication may be local, systemic, or both. Local effects result from the direct application of a medication to an area. Systemic effects involve more than one organ. For example, epinephrine is a naturally occurring endocrine hormone that has its effect by binding to specific receptor sites in the body; in this case, alpha (α) and beta (β) receptors in the sympathetic nervous system.

The four types of mechanisms of action are as follows:

- *Binding with a receptor site.* Most medications cause their effects by binding to a receptor.
- *Changing the physical properties of a cell.* Some medications change the specific physical properties of a cell resulting in an effect such as changing osmotic balance.
- *Combining with another chemical substance.* Some medications combine with other chemical

substances and change its chemical structure. For example, the alkalotic medication sodium bicarbonate is administered intravenously to neutralize acids in the bloodstream in an attempt to correct acidosis.

- *Changing metabolic pathways.* Medications such as those used to treat forms of cancer can be introduced into the body with the intent to block or disrupt the formation of additional cancer cells.

Dose–Response Relationship

When administering a medication, you must provide enough to cause the desired effect without administering too much. Too much of a medication can result in undesired side effects or even death. For some drugs, a loading dose must be administered to raise the level of the medication in circulation to a point where the desired effect occurs. This is known as the **therapeutic threshold** (Figure 11-7). Until the levels of the drug in circulation reach this point, there is not enough in the bloodstream to cause the desired effect. Maintaining a therapeutic dose of a medication requires the administration of additional doses. The time between each dose is determined by how long it takes for the body to metabolize 50 percent of the peak concentration. This is known as the drug's **half-life**.

Therapeutic index is the ratio of dose of medication that is lethal in 50 percent of the population (LD_{50}) and the dose that is effective in 50 percent of the population (ED_{50}). Drugs that have a greater difference between the therapeutic and lethal doses have a wide therapeutic index and are considered safer to administer than those with a smaller difference between the effective and lethal doses. Medications in which the lethal and therapeutic doses are very close together have a *narrow therapeutic index* and the danger of a lethal dose in the attempt to achieve therapeutic results is much higher.

Factors Influencing Medication Effects

Many factors influence the effects of drugs on the body. Table 11-4 outlines some factors that influence the effects of medication. The therapeutic effects of a medication are the effects that the medication is intended to produce to treat a disease. Side effects are not intended to occur, but are expected to occur. For example, atropine commonly produces dilation of the patient's pupils, a predictable side effect. **Idiosyncratic reactions** are unusual reactions that are known to occur in a small number of individuals, but which are not predictable. For example, a drug may result in a decreased white blood cell count in a small number of individuals. Idiosyncratic reactions are thought to be caused by genetic variations in the way a person responds to a drug or its metabolites.

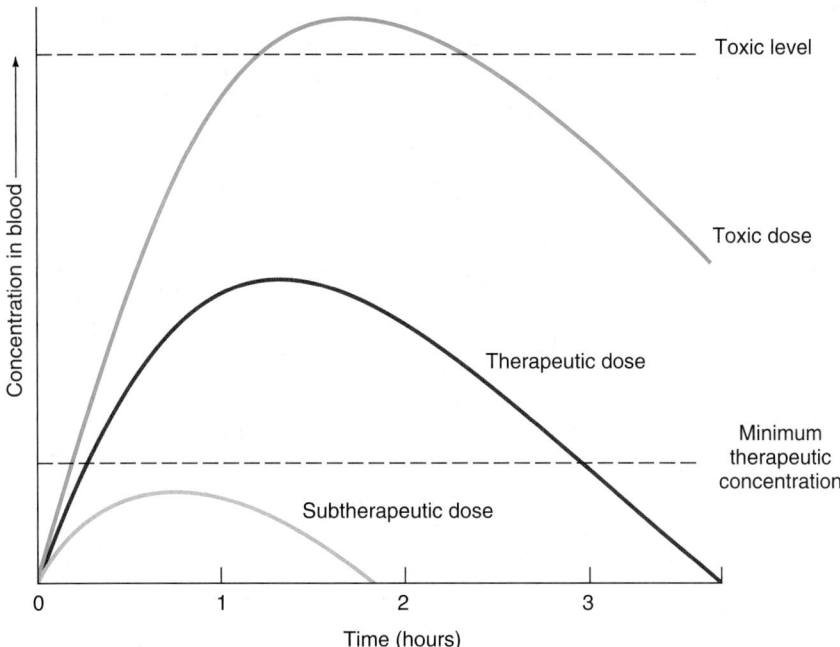

FIGURE 11-7

Minimum and maximum dose for a medication over time.

| **TABLE 11-4** | **Factors That Influence Medication Effects** |

Factor	Description of Altered Response
Age	Patients at the extremes of age have different responses to medications that might be expected. Infants do not have mature organ systems and often their liver is not mature enough to process and metabolize drugs efficiently. Their kidney function may not remove the medication from the body as quickly. Elderly patients often have other multiple medical conditions such as liver and kidney dysfunction that result in the same effect, they are unable to metabolize drugs efficiently due to liver damage and they cannot filter and eliminate medications as rapidly because the kidneys no longer function at peak efficiency.
Gender and body mass	Larger patients require more of a given medication to achieve the therapeutic dose. You will determine the amount of medication to be administered to the patient based on their body weight. Because men tend to have a greater weight and muscle mass, they tend to require a higher dose than women. If the weights are equal, you still may need to make a specified change in the dose due to the different fat-to-muscle ratio for women.
Pathologic state	Patients with significant liver disease or kidney failure will not experience the same drug response as an otherwise healthy individual. You may need to make adjustments when the patient has any significant renal or hepatic disease because he will not be able to metabolize or eliminate the drug efficiently.
Genetic factors	Patients who have a genetic disorder that affects either thyroid hormone function or growth hormone secretion may require a dose adjustment. Any disease that affects metabolic rate will significantly alter the expected response to the medication. Idiosyncratic reactions are thought to be due to genetic variations in the way patients respond to drugs or their metabolites.
Time of administration	This is primarily of concern when the medication is administered orally. The presence or lack of food in the digestive tract has a dramatic impact on the rate of absorption. Medications are absorbed more rapidly on an empty stomach and more slowly when food is present.
Psychological effects	Psychological stress may alter the rate at which the body is able to metabolize a medication. It has been known for a long time that a patient will get a greater effect if they believe that the medication will help them. Imagine the difference between telling the patient "this is not very strong, but it is all I can give you for pain" and telling them "I am going to give you a medication to reduce your pain. It works very quickly so I need you to tell me as soon as it starts to work so I can monitor the effect and not give you too much." One statement enhances the patient's expectation of how well the drug will work and the other diminishes it significantly.

Individuals who have experienced an allergic reaction to a substance have a **hypersensitivity** and are likely to experience subsequent reactions that are more severe than the first. Drugs commonly implicated in hypersensitivity reactions include antibiotics, the narcotic analgesic codeine, and aspirin.

An **iatrogenic** effect is any adverse condition resulting from treatment provided, and includes infections at an IV site and medication dosage and administration errors.

Some medications, when taken regularly for a long period of time, produce less of an effect as the person develops **tolerance** to the medication. The person often must take a larger dosage of the medication to obtain the original effect. In some cases, tolerance to one medication results in **cross-tolerance** to medications of the same classification. For example, individuals who take the benzodiazepine diazepam on a regular basis may have developed a tolerance to the medication and require a higher than normal dose of midazolam, another benzodiazepine, to achieve the desired effect.

The prolonged use of medications that have addictive properties can lead to a dependence on the medication. *Drug dependence* is a physical and/or psychological need to use a drug in order to function normally. Suddenly stopping the use of some medications can lead to "withdrawal" symptoms severe enough to be life threatening. **Habituation** is the term used to describe the increase in tolerance to a drug following repeated doses.

A drug interaction occurs when the effects of a medication are affected by the presence of another medication. When two or more medications with a similar mechanism of action are taken at the same time, the combination of the effects resulting from each medication is called a *summation effect.*

Some medications can therapeutically or non-therapeutically enhance the effects of another medication.

The enhancement of one medication as a result of being combined with another is called **potentiation**. For example, the consumption of alcohol will potentiate the effects of barbiturates. Other medications, when combined, enhance the effects of one another. That enhancement is called **synergism**.

Medication Storage

Most medications that you carry as an Advanced EMT require a physician's prescription. It is for this reason that you must properly secure all medications when not in use. Your employer will have specific policies and procedures in place regarding storing and accounting for medications.

Controlled substances must be tracked closely and accounted for following strict guidelines set forth by the U.S. Drug Enforcement Agency (DEA). When you administer a controlled substance, you are required to complete separate documentation that includes the way the unused portion of the controlled substance was disposed.

The stability of medications depends on their storage environment. Medications must be stored at a controlled temperature and protected from light and exposure to air and moisture. Prehospital conditions often make storing medications in ideal conditions difficult. EMS services must have policies concerning the amount of drug stored in the ambulance, the storage conditions, and the frequency with which drugs must be replaced. Some ambulances are equipped with an electrical cord that allows the heater and air conditioner to be used while the ambulance is parked at a station. When it is not possible to control the temperature of the patient compartment while the ambulance is parked, it may be necessary to bring the medications inside.

CASE STUDY WRAP-UP

Clinical-Reasoning Process

Advanced EMTs Mike and Matt are on the scene of a patient found in her car in a parking lot. By observing the scene, assessing the patient, and talking to bystanders, they have determined that there are no indications of trauma, and the patient's perfusion and oxygenation are adequate. Keeping in mind the most common causes of altered mental status, Mike checks the patient's blood glucose level. He finds it's 30 mg/dL, providing a likely cause for the patient's altered mental status. Recognizing that untreated hypoglycemia can lead to serious adverse outcomes, including death, Mike sets up equipment to start treatment as Matt, with the help of an engine crew, places the patient on the stretcher and in the ambulance.

Mike starts an IV and, just before departing the scene, administers 25 grams of 50 percent dextrose. A few moments later, as they are en route to the hospital, the patient becomes more alert. Mike is able to obtain a complete history, including the facts that she has a seizure disorder and is an insulin-dependent diabetic.

CHAPTER REVIEW

Chapter Summary

You must not only know what medications you can give to patients and in what dosages, but you also must know how medications act on the body, and how the body processes medications. You must know what laws and regulations apply to the approval and administration of medications.

Pharmacology is a dynamic field that changes constantly. New medications are constantly being developed while older ones are removed from use. It is your responsibility to remain current on medications you might encounter in the field and those that you will administer to patients.

Review Questions

Multiple-Choice Questions

1. The reason that a specific medication should be given to a patient is known as a(n):
   a. indication.
   b. effect.
   c. mechanism of action.
   d. protocol.

2. Fifty percent dextrose is an example of a medication derived from what source?
   a. Synthetic
   b. Natural
   c. Plant
   d. Mineral

3. The Federal Food, Drug, and Cosmetic Act established which one of the following?
   a. Food and Drug Administration
   b. Drug Enforcement Agency
   c. Public Health Service
   d. National Formulary

4. Morphine is an example of a drug listed in which one of the following schedules?
   a. I
   b. II
   c. III
   d. IV

5. Lasix® is an example of which one of the following drug names?
   a. Trade
   b. Official
   c. Generic
   d. Chemical

6. Aspirin USP is an example of which one of the following drug names?
   a. Trade
   b. Official
   c. Generic
   d. Chemical

7. When a medication is dissolved in alcohol, it is known as a(n):
   a. elixir.
   b. syrup.
   c. tincture.
   d. suspension.

8. Which one of the following glass drug packages has the advantage of low cost and a long shelf life because it does not have any seals that can rupture or degrade over time?
   a. Ampule
   b. Prefilled syringe
   c. Vial
   d. Nebule

9. What is the term used to describe the decrease in desired effect of a drug after it is taken regularly over a period of time?
   a. Tolerance
   b. Cross-tolerance
   c. Habituation
   d. Drug dependency

Critical-Thinking Questions

10. Why do you think extensive burns, rashes, or other skin conditions would be a contraindication to topical or transdermal drug administration?

11. How do the physical and physiologic differences of pediatric and geriatric patients (introduced in Chapter 7) affect the absorption, distribution, effects, and elimination of drugs?

12. A patient is taking the anticoagulant drug warfarin, which binds to albumin in the plasma. He begins taking a second drug, which also binds to albumin. What do you predict will happen with regard to the levels and effects of the drugs?

References

Centers for Disease Control and Prevention. (2011). *National diabetes fact sheet: National estimates and general information on diabetes and prediabetes in the United States, 2011: Centers for Disease Control and Prevention*. Retrieved June 14, 2011, from Centers for Disease Control and Prevention: http://www.cdc.gov/diabetes/pubs/pdf/ndfs_2011.pdf

Sung Sug (Sarah) Yoon, Y. O. (2010, October). *Recent Trends in the Prevalence of High Blood Pressure: Centers for Disease Control and Prevention*. Retrieved June 14, 2011, from Centers for Disease Control and Prevention: http://www.cdc.gov/nchs/data/databriefs/db48.pdf

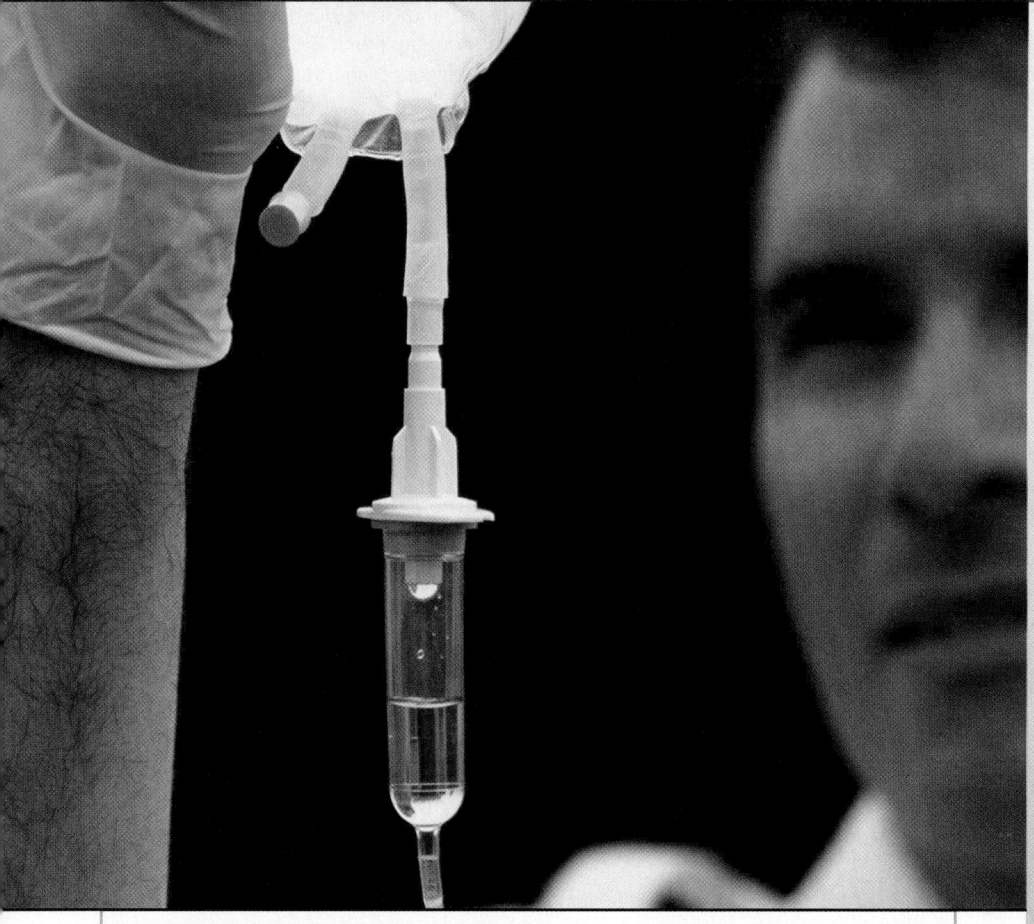

12 Medication Administration

Content Area: Pharmacology

Advanced EMT Education Standard: Applies fundamental knowledge of medications in the Advanced EMT scope of practice to patient assessment and management.

Objectives

After reading this chapter, you should be able to:

12.1   Define key terms introduced in this chapter.

12.2   Explain the medical direction mechanisms by which an Advanced EMT may be authorized to administer a medication.

12.3   Explain Advanced EMT practices that are necessary with regard to medication administration safety.

12.4   Differentiate between enteral and parenteral routes of drug administration.

12.5   Describe each of the following routes of medication administration:

   – Inhaled (gases and nebulized medications)

   – Intramuscular (IM)

   – Intraosseous infusion (pediatric)

(continued)

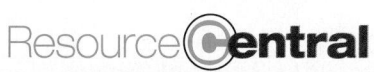

Resource Central

To access Resource Central, follow the directions on the Student Access Card provided with this text. If there is no card, go to www.bradybooks.com and follow the Resource Central link to Buy Access. Under Media Resources, you will find:

• *Alert! Alert!* Read and understand what is meant by high-alert medications.

• *Quiz on!* Learn how to make your very own drug flashcards the easy way.

• *The "Little Stick."* Discover how to troubleshoot common IV complications.

CASE STUDY

"Ambulance Seven, respond to eleven fifteen Trumbull Road for an unresponsive person. That is one-one, one-five Trumbull Road. Law enforcement is en route."

The Advanced EMTs assigned to Ambulance Seven, Loretta Budreau and Grant Hughes, arrive at the address 9 minutes later. Law enforcement is on the scene. Sheriff's deputy Frank Brooks informs the crew that he found drug paraphernalia, including a syringe, inside the residence and that the patient is a 35-year-old woman who is unresponsive. He tells the crew that the caller is no longer on the scene, and he suspects the caller made the 911 call after the patient overdosed and left to avoid being arrested. Deputy Brooks also tells the crew that there is a lot of clutter inside the home and cautions them to be careful.

Once inside the home, Grant sees that the patient appears to be breathing, although slowly and shallowly, and hears faint snoring. The patient is pale with cyanosis of her lips and there are no obvious signs of trauma. Grant confirms that she is unresponsive to painful stimuli and opens the airway with a head-tilt/chin-lift maneuver. He determines that she has a weak radial pulse that he estimates to be between 60 and 70 beats per minute. Taking over airway positioning from Grant, Loretta inserts an oropharyngeal airway and begins assisting the patient's ventilations with a bag-valve mask device and supplemental oxygen.

Grant performs a rapid medical exam and, because he suspects an IV drug overdose, he carefully checks the patient's pupils and looks for needle marks. The patient's pupils are constricted to pinpoint size and he finds fresh needle punctures over veins in the patient's forearms, as well as scarring that indicates a long history of IV drug abuse. Grant consults Loretta about his initial treatment plan. They agree that starting an IV and administering the narcotic antagonist naloxone are immediate priorities in improving the patient's ventilations.

Problem-Solving Questions

1. What equipment does Grant need to start an IV and administer a medication intravenously?
2. How can Grant and Loretta ensure patient safety and minimize the risks of complications from IV therapy and medication administration?
3. What should Grant include in his documentation about the IV and medication administration?

(continued from previous page)

- – Intravenous bolus
- – Intravenous infusion
- – Oral (PO)
- – Subcutaneous (subQ)
- – Sublingual (SL)

12.6	Properly interpret verbal and written drug orders.
12.7	Use proper abbreviations and terminology with respect to drug administration.
12.8	Calculate drug dosages from drug orders, including proper use of the metric system.
12.9	Explain the concept of medical asepsis.
12.10	Demonstrate the following skills under instructor supervision:

- – Administering drugs by small-volume nebulizer
- – Administering nitrous oxide
- – Assisting patient with the use of a metered-dose inhaler
- – Intramuscular injection
- – Intravenous access
- – Intravenous and intraosseous fluid administration
- – Intravenous medication bolus
- – Oral medication administration
- – Pediatric intraosseous access
- – Subcutaneous injection
- – Sublingual medication administration
- – Use of an auto-injector device

Introduction

Medications are some of the most powerful treatments at the Advanced EMT's disposal. Administered correctly, medications can be lifesaving. Administered incorrectly, medications can cause harm and even death. Always maintain awareness of the principles of medication administration, as well as other information about drugs, when contemplating the use of medication in patient care. Unfortunately, medication errors are common, but are preventable.

Proper medication administration begins with recognizing the indications and contraindications of a drug, and knowing other aspects of the drug profile. (See Chapter 13.) You also must know how to interpret standing medication orders and individual patient medication orders, and how to receive verbal medication orders from medical direction. You must understand the advantages and disadvantages of various routes of medication administration, and use the proper techniques and equipment for each route of administration. You must be able to calculate drug dosages, select the correct medication, select and properly prepare the medication, and adhere to principles of safe medication administration. In addition, the responsibilities of medication administration include careful documentation of how the medication order was carried out and the patient's response to it.

Principles of Safe Medication Administration

Medication administration does not stand alone as a skill. In each situation, you must use your knowledge of anatomy, physiology, pathophysiology, and pharmacology, as well as your skills in history taking, assessment, and clinical reasoning to determine whether or not it is in a patient's best interests to administer a drug. Failure to consider all factors in the situation can lead to patient harm. Drug packaging, labeling, and safety policies contribute to patient safety, as well.

The most common type of medication administration error resulting in death is giving the wrong dosage of the drug, which accounts for over 40 percent of all medication administration error–related deaths (Hughes & Blegen, 2008). Giving the wrong drug and administering drugs by the incorrect route also contribute to significant numbers of deaths related to medication administration errors. Some phases of the medication administration process are particularly error prone, including:

- Giving the drug order
- Transcribing (interpreting) the order
- Administering the drug (including dosage and route of administration errors)
- Patient monitoring
- Documentation

There are principles you must always keep in mind when contemplating drug administration.

Six Rights of Medication Administration

Several principles of medication safety are remembered as the *Six Rights of Medication Administration*, described as follows:

- *The right patient.* In the prehospital setting, you usually care for only one patient at a time, particularly in medical emergencies that require medication administration, so that matching the right drug to the right patient is not a common concern. However, if you work in an emergency department or other setting, there are usually multiple patients being cared for at one time. In such cases, the employer generally has policies in place for correctly identifying the patient. For example, you may be required to ask the patient his full name and date of birth, so that you can match the information against his chart, or you may be required to match the patient's identification or medical record number on his wrist band to the chart.

- *The right medication.* Confirm the medication order to ensure that you know what medication is to be given. Be aware that many medication containers look alike, and many medication names sound alike and are spelled similarly. Carefully check the name of the medication on each layer of packaging. For example, if a vial is contained within a box, check the label on both the box and the vial. Some medications come in more than one concentration, such as epinephrine 1:1,000 and epinephrine 1:10,000. Read and check the label three times for name and concentration of the medication as follows:
  - When you first select the medication
  - As you prepare the medication for administration
  - Just before giving the patient the medication

  A good practice is to have a second health care provider who can administer the same medication check the medication before you administer it. Also ensure that the medication is not expired, the packaging is undamaged, and the medication appears as it is supposed to (for example, it does not contain particulates and is not discolored).

Advanced EMT Herb Barker: I was nervous the first time I administered a medication, even though I had practiced the skills and had a preceptor supervising me. I knew that 50 percent dextrose would raise the blood glucose level and quickly improve the patient's level of responsiveness, but I had never seen it work before. I prepared the medication and expelled air from the syringe. My preceptor double-checked the medication. I cleaned the injection port in the IV line with alcohol and attached the syringe. I clamped the tubing and slowly injected the medication. Fifty percent dextrose is thick and sticky and a lot harder to push than I thought. After the medication had been injected, I flushed the IV tubing and readjusted the drip rate. The patient suddenly cried out, "My head, oh, my head! It's killing me!" I was startled. I wondered if I had done something wrong, but I couldn't think of anything. My preceptor was startled, too, but recovered quickly. He must have anticipated my feeling that I had done something wrong, and reassured me that I hadn't.

Before we could assess the patient to see what the problem was, she became alert and oriented and knew right away that she had suffered a hypoglycemic episode. When I asked her if her head hurt, she said that it didn't. We continued our assessment, including rechecking her blood glucose level, which was normal. At the hospital emergency department, I included the reaction in my report to the triage nurse. She said she had seen similar reactions a few times, but that it wasn't common. Memorizing the drug profile is one thing, but seeing what the drug actually does is another!

■ *The right dose.* Carefully calculate drug dosages and double-check them. If possible, have a second provider verify your calculation. Standardized dosing tables are a good reference for verifying your dosage.

■ *The right route.* You must know the routes by which medications can be administered and ensure that you give medications only by those routes. For example, 50 percent dextrose solution can be lifesaving when administered intravenously, as intended. However, the highly osmotic solution causes tissue necrosis if administered intramuscularly.

■ *The right time.* Most often, you will give drugs immediately upon receiving the order or recognizing the need according to standing orders. Many drugs that you give will be administered only once, while others, such as nitroglycerin, may be repeated at intervals. When giving intravenous infusions, you must calculate the drip rate that delivers the order as intended. Some intravenous injections are given rapidly, while others are pushed slowly. You must know which intravenous injections are given slowly and which are given rapidly.

■ *The right documentation.* You must document all relevant drug administration information for medical and legal reasons. To plan further treatment without harming the patient, other health care providers must know what medications you gave the patient, in what dosages they were given, by what routes, and when they were given.

Additional Medication Safety Considerations

Increased attention to patient safety has led to many changes in the way drugs are packaged, labeled, stored, dispensed, and administered. For example, the drug lidocaine, used as an antidysrhythmic and local anesthetic, comes in many different concentrations. In the past, a concentrated solution of the drug was supplied in a syringe for the purpose of health care providers mixing solutions for intravenous infusions. The prefilled syringes contained 2 grams (2,000 mg) of lidocaine, whereas the usual dose for IV injection is 50 to 100 mg. This resulted in some cases where the highly concentrated solution, intended to be diluted in 500 mL of intravenous fluid, was administered by IV injection, resulting in patient death. It is now rare that the 2-gram syringe would be found in a patient care area. Instead, the drug is supplied premixed for intravenous infusion by the manufacturer, or mixed and labeled in a hospital pharmacy.

Medications stored in patient care areas are frequently packaged in individual containers holding approximately the amount given in a single dose to reduce the chances of medication dosage errors. Whenever you calculate a drug dosage, be suspicious of an error if results call for more than one container (vial, ampule, or prefilled syringe) or only a small fraction of the amount of a single-dose container.

Routes of Drug Administration

A route of drug administration is the way in which the drug gains access to the body. The two broad categories of routes are enteral and parenteral. **Enteral** routes are those that allow access through the vasculature of the gastrointestinal system, where drugs enter the portal vein circulation. Drugs for enteral administration are generally liquid, solid, or semisolid. **Parenteral** routes are those that bypass the gastrointestinal tract. Drugs for parenteral administration are usually in liquid, gas, or semisolid forms. Some routes of parenteral drug administration are percutaneous. **Percutaneous** routes are those that require injection through the skin. There are advantages and disadvantages to each type of route (Table 12-1).

Enteral routes include giving medications by mouth to be swallowed, called *per os,* and abbreviated *PO.* Advanced EMTs commonly give aspirin to patients with chest pain by this route for its platelet aggregation–inhibiting effects. Although it is not in the Advanced EMT scope of practice, rectal administration (per rectum, or *PR*) is also an enteral route.

Many texts classify the sublingual (SL) route as an enteral route. However, the capillaries of the sublingual plexus allow absorption directly into the systemic circulation, bypassing the hepatic portal system. Drugs that can readily be absorbed through the mucous membranes under the tongue, such as nitroglycerin, can be given sublingually. Oral glucose paste is absorbed through the mucous membrane of the buccal surface (inner cheek), also bypassing the hepatic portal circulation.

Enterally administered drugs travel through the hepatic portal system to the liver before entering the systemic circulation, although sublingual and rectal routes also allow some direct systemic absorption. The liver changes many drugs in first-pass metabolism before they enter the systemic circulation, where they can have their effect on target tissues. Some drugs, such as benzodiazepines (for example, Valium) are given in an inactive form that is activated upon first-pass metabolism. Other drugs are extensively broken down by first-pass metabolism and cannot be given enterally.

The onset of action of drugs given by the sublingual and rectal routes is relatively quick. However, orally administered drugs are largely absorbed through the duodenum, rather than the stomach. The onset of action depends on the amount of food in the stomach and the rate of gastric emptying. In addition, some drugs, such as insulin, are broken down into inactive components by the pepsin and hydrochloric acid in the stomach, and must be given parenterally.

Parenteral routes of drug administration in the Advanced EMT scope of practice include inhalation, subcutaneous injection, intramuscular injection, intravenous **bolus**, intravenous infusion, and in pediatric patients, intraosseous administration. The time to onset of action of parenterally

TABLE 12-1	**Advanced EMT Routes of Medication Administration**	
	Route	**Description**
Enteral routes	Oral (PO)	Liquid, solid, or semisolid drugs are placed in the mouth and swallowed. The speed of onset is slow and depends on the drug form, nature of the drug, stomach contents, and rate of gastric emptying. The route is contraindicated in patients who are restricted from oral intake. This route is generally safe and drug forms for oral administration are often less expensive than other forms. The skills required to administer drugs orally are relatively simple and the route is well-accepted by most patients.
Parenteral routes: Sublingual	Sublingual (SL)	Many textbooks consider the sublingual route an enteral route, but drugs given this way are absorbed directly into the systemic circulation, bypassing the hepatic portal circulation. The thin, moist mucous membrane beneath the tongue allows rapid absorption of drugs into the dense network of capillaries beneath the tongue, allowing for a rapid onset of action. Few drugs are available for administration by this route.
Parenteral routes: Percutaneous All percutaneous routes require specialized skills and equipment. These routes of administration may cause pain, fear, and infection. In general, the onset of action is rapid.	Subcutaneous (subQ or subcut)	A short, fine needle is used to inject 1 mL or less of fluid into the subcutaneous tissue. This route is slower than IM and IV routes and the predictability of absorption is affected by peripheral circulatory status.
	Intramuscular (IM)	A needle is used to inject up to 5 mL of fluid (depending on the site selected) into skeletal muscle tissue. Greater circulation in the skeletal muscle, as compared to the subcutaneous tissues, results in a more rapid onset of action, but absorption is affected by peripheral circulation.
	Intravenous (IV)	Drugs are administered directly into the peripheral circulation by intravenous injection or infusion (drip). The onset of action is nearly immediate.
Parenteral routes: Inhalation	Inhalation	Gases, microdroplets, and fine powders are absorbed quickly across the large surface area of the respiratory membrane. Onset of action is rapid. Drug administration is impaired in patients with inadequate ventilation.

administered drugs depends on the length of time it takes the medication to enter the circulation.

The slowest of the routes is the subcutaneous route, abbreviated *subQ* or *subcut*. Subcutaneous medications are in liquid form and are injected beneath the dermis, into the subcutaneous tissue (Figure 12-1). Medications are absorbed relatively slowly, but steadily, when circulation to the skin is normal. However, in patients with poor peripheral circulation, such as those in shock, absorption is too slow and unpredictable. For anaphylaxis, 1:1,000 epinephrine is sometimes given by the subcutaneous route, but the intramuscular route is preferred, because absorption is faster and more predictable.

Intramuscular drugs are liquids injected into large skeletal muscle masses, such as the deltoid or gluteus muscles (Figure 12-2). Increased circulation in the muscle, as compared to subcutaneous tissues, allows a slightly more rapid onset of action. Drugs commonly given by this route in the prehospital setting include 1:1,000 epinephrine for anaphylaxis, and glucagon for hypoglycemia, when intravenous access is not available.

Intravenous (IV) drugs are liquids injected (by syringe) or infused (dripped from a bag of IV fluid) directly into the venous system. To give drugs by either method, an IV catheter is placed through the skin and into a superficial vein and secured in place. Either a short piece of tubing filled with saline (a saline lock) (Figure 12-3) or tubing connected to a bag of IV fluid is connected to the catheter. An injection port in the saline lock or IV tubing allows medications to be injected into the circulatory system. When IV fluid, with or without medication added, is allowed to flow from an IV bag through the tubing and into the vein, it is called an *IV infusion*.

Drugs administered by the IV route have a rapid onset of action. Accordingly, this route is preferred for most drugs given in an emergency situation. Advanced EMTs may give dextrose solutions (such as 25 percent or 50 percent dextrose) and naloxone (a narcotic antagonist) by IV injection, and may infuse unmedicated IV fluids.

The intraosseous (IO) route involves placing a hollow needle into the medullary cavity of a bone, where medication is rapidly absorbed through the medullary vasculature (Figure 12-4). The proximal tibia is the preferred site for IO access in pediatric patients. A saline lock or IV tubing is attached to the IO needle, similar to the technique for intravenous access. The same drugs and IV fluids that are given by the IV route may be administered by injection or infusion by the IO route.

Drugs for inhalation are generally gases, such as oxygen and nitrous oxide, or aerosolized liquids or powders, such as albuterol and ipratropium bromide for asthma and COPD. Gases and aerosolized medications are absorbed quickly across the respiratory membrane.

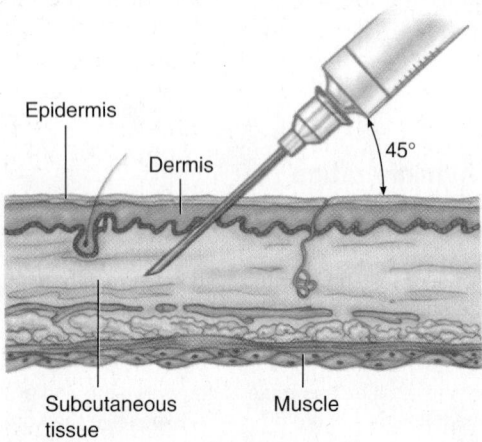

FIGURE 12-1

Needle placement for subcutaneous injection.

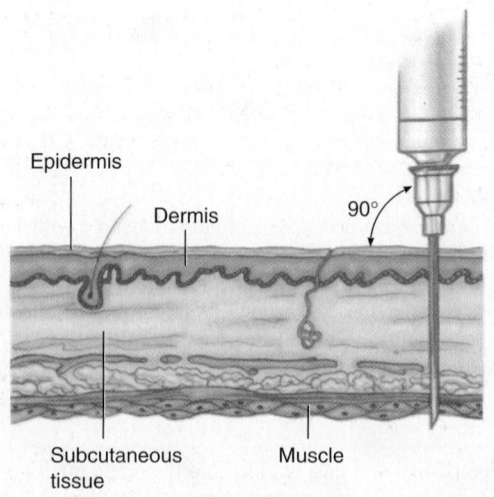

FIGURE 12-2

Needle placement for intramuscular injection.

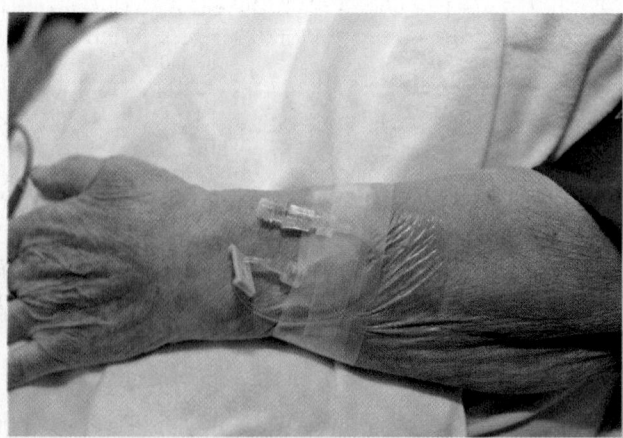

FIGURE 12-3

A saline lock.

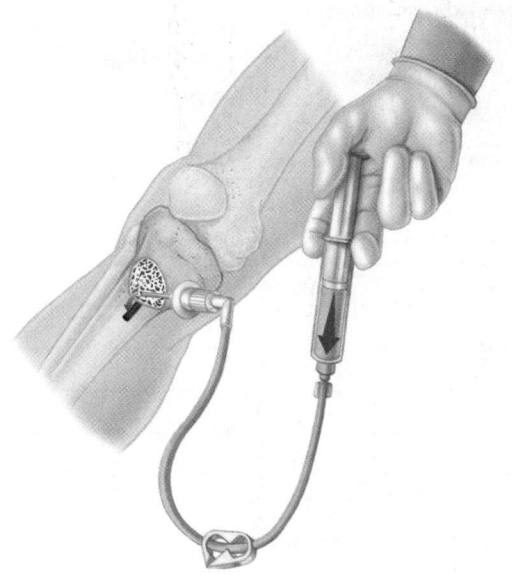

FIGURE 12-4

Needle placement for intraosseous infusion.

Drug Orders

Advanced EMTs may only administer drugs on the order of a licensed physician providing EMS medical direction. Those orders may be written in the form of standing orders, written orders (hard copy or electronic) for individual patients, or verbal orders received from the physician in person or over the radio or telephone.

A standing order gives you the ability to administer a drug to a patient under specific circumstances without first making contact with medical direction. Standing orders are written and signed by the EMS service physician medical director. They are used when delaying medication to consult with medical direction could result in jeopardy to the patient. For example, the administration of 1:1,000 epinephrine for anaphylactic shock is a common standing order. Standing orders also may be used when the EMS service medical director is confident that all personnel are able to accurately recognize indications and contraindications for the drug and give it safely without consultation. The use of oxygen is the most common example of that.

You will most likely rely on written orders for individual patients if you work in an emergency department or other hospital or clinic setting. In those cases, the physician caring for the patient either writes the order on the patient's paper chart, or enters the orders for the patient electronically. Written orders use abbreviations and symbols and follow certain conventions for writing dosages. You must know those abbreviations, symbols, and conventions, and must use them in your documentation. Written orders are preferred to verbal orders, because the document serves as verification of the physician's order.

You may receive verbal orders over the radio or phone in an emergency. To make a decision about the order, the physician relies on you to paint an accurate but concise picture of the relevant information. *Once you receive the order, you must always repeat it back to the physician, word for word, to verify understanding.*

If you believe the order to be erroneous or unsafe, tactfully question the order by repeating it back. If the physician corrects the order, repeat the correct order back to verify. If he verifies the order you believe to be in error, request further clarification. Never carry out a medication order you believe to be dangerous or in error. The conversation should go something like this:

Advanced EMT: "This is ambulance 21, Advanced EMT Keller. We are on the scene of a 54-year-old male who is alert and oriented to person, place, and time, and complaining of retrosternal chest discomfort. The pain began 30 minutes ago while he was sitting at his desk at work, and nothing makes the pain better or worse. He took three nitroglycerin tablets sublingually without relief and he states that the bottle is approximately four years old. He describes the discomfort as a heavy pressure and rates it a 7 on a scale from 1 to 10. The pain does not radiate. He has a past history of myocardial infarction six years ago. The patient has no medication allergies and does not regularly take any medications. He has not taken any medications today except nitroglycerin. His last oral intake was breakfast, about 2 hours ago. His skin color is normal, and the skin is warm and moist to the touch. Breath sounds are clear and equal bilaterally, and there is no peripheral edema or jugular venous distention. Vital signs: blood pressure 162/90; pulse 84, strong at the radial artery with occasional irregular beats; respirations 16; and SpO_2 was 96 percent on room air. The patient is on 4 L/min of oxygen by nasal cannula, which increased the SpO_2 to 99 percent. We have administered 162 mg aspirin PO, and established an IV of normal saline with an 18-gauge catheter in the left forearm. Due to the age of the patient's nitroglycerin tablets and their lack of effect, we are requesting an order for additional sublingual nitroglycerin. We have an ETA of 20 minutes."

Physician: "This is Dr. Marley. Give up to three 0.4 doses of sublingual nitroglycerin spray, 5 minutes apart, as long as the patient's systolic blood pressure is above 90 mmHg and he continues to have chest pain or discomfort."

Advanced EMT: "Clear, Dr. Marley. We will give up to three 0.4 mg doses of sublingual nitroglycerin spray, 5 minutes apart, as long as the patient's systolic blood pressure is above 90 mmHg and he continues to have chest pain or discomfort."

Physician: "Affirmative, Ambulance 21. Notify us of any changes. We will see you in about 20 minutes."

Face-to-face verbal orders may be given in an emergency situation in the hospital, such as during cardiac arrest resuscitation attempts, or in other situations with critical patients. Follow the same procedure for verification as you would for a radio or telephone order. In such cases, there is usually one health care provider assigned to be a scribe. The scribe records notes on all of the activity of the resuscitation. Once you have given the medication, state it aloud for the scribe to record. For example, "25 grams of 50 percent dextrose given IV push through the right antecubital IV line at 2150 hours."

No matter how the order is received, you must document all pertinent information about how you carried out the order, any complications, and the patient's response to the medication. If you gave medication on a standing order or verbal order, it is usually required that you have the ordering physician sign or otherwise acknowledge that he gave or approved the order. Each EMS service has procedures for physician acknowledgement of orders.

Ethically, you are obligated to report any medication error that occurs, whether or not it results in patient harm. The exact procedures for reporting errors, and to whom they are reported, are dictated by the policies of your employer. However, you must immediately report the error to the physician caring for the patient so that any needed measures can be taken and to prevent other treatments, which now may be contraindicated, from being carried out. Interestingly, though it may seem counterintuitive, there is no evidence that patients are more likely to sue when medication errors are reported to them, if a sincere apology is made.

Interpreting Drug Orders

A complete drug order consists of the following information:

- Drug name
- Drug concentration, if applicable
- Drug dosage
- Route of administration
- Rate or frequency of repetition, if applicable

The following orders appear as they may be written in standing orders:

- Aspirin 325 mg PO
- Nitroglycerin (NTG) 0.4 mg SL, every 5 minutes, up to three doses
- Naloxone 2 mg IV push

A number of abbreviations are used in giving and documenting drug orders (Table 12-2). In recent years, some abbreviations have fallen out of favor because they led to confusion and medication errors. It is critical that standard abbreviations are used to avoid confusion. You must clearly understand commonly used standard abbreviations and must seek clarification from the physician giving the order if you are not sure about the order as it is written.

TABLE 12-2 Selected Abbreviations Used in Medication Administration

Abbreviation	Meaning
$\bar{a}$	before
admin	administer
amp	ampule
ASA	aspirin
$\bar{c}$	with
d/c	discontinue
et	and
g	gram
gtt/gtts	drop/drops
HHN	handheld nebulizer
IM	intramuscular
IO	intraosseous
IV	intravenous
IVP	intravenous push (injection)
kg	kilogram
KO	keep open (IV infusion)
KVO	keep vein open (IV infusion)
L	liter
max	maximum
MDI	metered-dose inhaler
mcg	microgram
mg	milligram
min	minute
mL	milliliter
NKA	no known allergies
NKDA	no known drug allergies
NTG	nitroglycerin
$\bar{p}$	after
po	by mouth
prn	as necessary
q	every
Rx	treatment
$\bar{s}$	without
subQ, subcut	subcutaneous
stat	immediately
SVN	small-volume nebulizer
TKO	to keep vein open (intravenous infusion)

Conventions of drug orders include always placing a leading zero before dosages of less than one unit. For example, the dosage of nitroglycerin is always written *0.4 mg*, not .4 mg. Without the leading zero, .4 can easily be misinterpreted as 4, resulting in a tenfold increase of the intended dose. Zeros are not used with whole numbers. For example, you would document *25 g dextrose, slow IV push*, not 25.0 g.

Drug Dosage Calculation

Mathematical operations are required to convert drug orders to the units in which the drug will be administered. You must understand how to systematically perform the operations for various types of drug orders, including giving tablets, injections, and intravenous infusions. Drug dosages are given in metric units, necessitating understanding of the metric system.

Review of the Metric System

The metric system is a base-10 system used in science and medicine. Base units of measurement for weight, length, and volume are converted to larger and smaller units using multiples and submultiples of ten (Table 12-3). Standard prefixes are used for multiples and submultiples. Whole numbers are placed to the left of a decimal and fractions are represented by place values to the right of a decimal. For example, 2.25 is equal to 2 and 25/100. Common weights used in pharmacology are kilograms (kg) (for patients' weights), grams (g), milligrams (mg), and micrograms (mcg). Common volumes used in pharmacology are liters (L) and milliliters (mL). In some cases, it is helpful to be able to convert between the system of household measures used in the United States and metric units (Table 12-4). For example, you may receive an order to administer an IV fluid bolus of 30 milliliters per kilogram of body weight (30 mL/kg). To carry out the order, you will most likely have to convert the patient's weight in pounds to kilograms.

In most cases, the general rule for rounding decimals applies: Round up to the next highest whole number for five-tenths and above, and round down to the whole number for four-tenths and lower. However, in some cases, greater precision is needed. In general, the smaller the patient, the more precision you should use.

Translating the Order to Units to Administer

As an Advanced EMT, the two most common types of calculations you are called upon to perform are basic drug dosage calculations and IV drip rate calculations. In some cases, the calculation must consider another factor: the patient's weight.

This text presents simple, straightforward steps for drug calculations. Instructors and practicing EMS providers may provide other methods of calculating drug dosages. It is best to first learn the basic method, rather than trying to learn multiple ways of doing calculations at the same time. Once you have mastered the basic calculations, you can use other methods of setting up and solving the problems, such as dimensional analysis, if you find they make more sense to you.

TABLE 12-4	Common U.S. Customary Metric Equivalents
U.S. Customary Unit	**Metric Equivalent**
1 teaspoon	5 mL
1 tablespoon	15 mL
1 fluid ounce	30 mL
1 quart	950 mL
1 gallon	3.8 L
1 inch	2.54 cm
1 pound	0.45 kg (1 kg = 2.2 lb)

TABLE 12-3 Metric System Bases and Multiples Commonly Used in Pharmacology

Property	Base Unit	Abbreviation	1/1,000,000 (10^{-6} or 0.000.001)	1/1,000 (10^{-3} or 0.001)	1/100 (10^{-2} or 0.01)	1,000 (10^3)
Mass (weight)	gram	g	microgram (mcg)	milligram (mg)		kilogram (kg)
Volume	liter	L		milliliter (mL)		
Length	meter	m		millimeter (mm)	centimeter (cm)	

Basic Calculations

A basic drug calculation is finding the amount of drug to administer when given a physician's order and the concentration of drug available. For example, you receive an order to give 0.3 mg of epinephrine, 1:1,000, IM. You have available a vial of the drug containing 1 mg/mL (1 milligram per 1 milliliter). Here is what you know:

The order: 0.3 mg of epinephrine, 1:1,000, IM

The concentration on hand: 1 mg/mL

The information that is not explicit in the facts you have is the volume of the drug to give. However, from the information you have, you can determine it. In this case, you will find the volume in milliliters. The easiest way to do this is to set up the problem using fractions and solve for the unknown information. Remember, in this example, you are solving for the unknown number of milliliters.

Begin with what you know: the concentration of the drug on hand, which is 1 mg/mL. Write it as a fraction:

$$\frac{1\ mg}{1\ mL}$$

Compare what you know with what you need to find out, using x to represent the unknown:

$$\frac{1\ mg}{1\ mL} = \frac{0.3\ mg}{x\ mL}$$

Solve the equation by cross-multiplying. Multiply each numerator (top number) by the denominator (bottom number) of the other fraction. Multiply 1 mg by x mL (represented as $1x$), and place it on the left side of a new equation, and multiply 0.3 mg by 1 mL, and place it on the right side of the equation, as follows:

$$1x = 0.3 \times 1$$

Simplified, the equation is:

$$1x = 0.3$$

The equation is solved by isolating x on one side of the equation. To do that, move the 1 on the left side of the equation to the right side, where it becomes the denominator in a new fraction, remembering the units you are solving for (milliliters):

$$x = \frac{0.3}{1}\ mL$$

IN THE FIELD

Although most high-stakes tests prohibit the use of calculators in order to test the accuracy of your math skills in drug dosage calculation, always use a calculator when possible to calculate drug dosages.

Finally, simplify the fraction by dividing the numerator by the denominator (0.3 divided by 1):

$$x = 0.3\ mL$$

You will administer 0.3 mL of epinephrine, 1:1,000, IM. In this case, you might have surmised the solution, because the ratio of milligrams to milliliters was one-to-one (1 mg per 1 mL). However, drug concentrations vary, as illustrated by the next example:

You receive an order to give 2 mg of naloxone IV. You have on hand 10-mL vials of naloxone with a concentration of 0.4 mg/mL. You must find out the volume of drug to give in milliliters. Set up and solve the problem using the steps from the previous problem:

Set up the equation:

$$\frac{0.4\ mg}{1\ mL} = \frac{2\ mg}{x\ mL}$$

Cross-multiply:

$$0.4x = 2 \times 1$$

Simplify:

$$0.4x = 2$$

Solve for x:

$$x = \frac{2}{0.4}\ mL$$

Simplify:

$$x = 5\ mL$$

Some drug concentrations are given as a percent. Keep in mind that *percent* means *per hundred*. In this case, percent means per 100 mL. Unless otherwise noted, the weight of the drug is in grams. For example, 50 percent dextrose means that the concentration is 50 grams per 100 mL.

You receive an order for 25 grams dextrose given by IV push (25 g dextrose IVP). The drug is supplied in a 50-mL syringe in which the concentration of the drug is 50 percent, called D_{50}. You can solve the problem—to find the volume to be administered—as in the previous examples:

Set up the equation:

$$\frac{50\ g}{100\ mL} = \frac{25\ g}{x\ mL}$$

Cross-multiply:

$$50x = 100 \times 25$$

Simplify:

$$50x = 2,500$$

Solve for x:

$$x = \frac{2,500}{50} \text{ mL}$$

Simplify:

$$x = 50 \text{ mL}$$

The previous examples used liquid drugs given by injection, but the formula holds true for other drug forms as well. For example:

You receive an order to give 162 mg of aspirin by mouth. You have on hand a bottle of 81-mg tablets of chewable aspirin.

Set up the equation:

$$\frac{81 \text{ mg}}{1 \text{ tablet}} = \frac{162 \text{ mg}}{x \text{ tablets}}$$

Cross-multiply:

$$81x = 1 \times 162$$

Simplify:

$$81x = 162$$

Solve for x:

$$x = \frac{162}{81} \text{ tablets}$$

Simplify:

$$x = 2 \text{ tablets}$$

Weight-Based Dosage Calculations

Many drugs have a relatively wide margin of safety, allowing a standard dosage to be administered to most adult patients. However, in pediatric patients and with drugs that require a very precise dosage, the dosage is calculated based on the patient's body weight. When weight-based dosages are given, they are usually given based on the patient's weight in kilograms. Few people in the United States routinely use kilograms, meaning you will need to convert the patient's weight in pounds to kilograms. To do that, divide the patient's weight in pounds by 2.2. It is not acceptable to estimate by dividing the patient's weight in pounds by two; the reason a weight-based dosage is given is because a precise dosage is needed.

Studies have shown that health care providers are not very accurate when estimating a patient's weight. Always determine as accurately as you can the patient's weight. If possible, ask the adult patient his weight. You can use a length-based resuscitation tape, such as a Broslow tape, for pediatric patients. Lay the tape next to the patient. The drug dosage recommendations are listed according to the patient's length.

You are given an order to administer 0.01 mg/kg of epinephrine, 1:1,000, IM to a 45-pound pediatric patient. Epinephrine 1:1,000 is supplied in a concentration of 1 mg/mL. Before using the steps described for basic dosage calculations, you must find the amount of the drug to be given in milligrams.

Find the patient's weight in kilograms:

$$\frac{45 \text{ lb}}{2.2} = 20.45 \text{ kg}$$

Find the dosage in milligrams:

$$20.45 \text{ kg} \times 0.01 \text{ mg/kg} = 0.2045, \text{ which can now be rounded to } 0.2 \text{ mg}$$

Set up the equation:

$$\frac{1 \text{ mg}}{1 \text{ mL}} = \frac{0.2 \text{ mg}}{x \text{ mL}}$$

Cross-multiply:

$$1x = 0.2 \times 1$$

Simplify:

$$1x = 0.2$$

Solve for x:

$$x = \frac{0.2}{1} \text{ mL}$$

Simplify:

$$x = 0.2 \text{ mL}$$

IV Drip Rate Calculations

IV drip rates are calculated using a formula that includes the **drip factor** of the IV tubing set. The drip factor is the number of drops needed to infuse 1 mL of IV fluid. The smaller the drop, the more drops that are needed to equal 1 mL. When greater precision is needed, such as with patients who could be easily overloaded with fluids and when medications are added to an IV infusion, a 60-drop set (sometimes called a *microdrip set*) is used. That means that it takes 60 drops (gtts) to infuse 1 mL of fluid.

When a faster infusion of fluid is needed, an IV tubing set that delivers larger drops is used. The drip factors of those sets may be 10 gtts/mL, 15 gtts/mL, or 20 gtts/mL. Those sets are sometimes called *macrodrip sets*, but because there are various tubing drip factors that could be considered macrodrip, it is best to specify the exact drip factor, rather than using the term *macrodrip*.

Always check the IV tubing package for the drip factor. In addition, a 60-gtts/mL set has a small, needlelike metal tube that you can see in the drip chamber of the tubing (Figure 12-5).

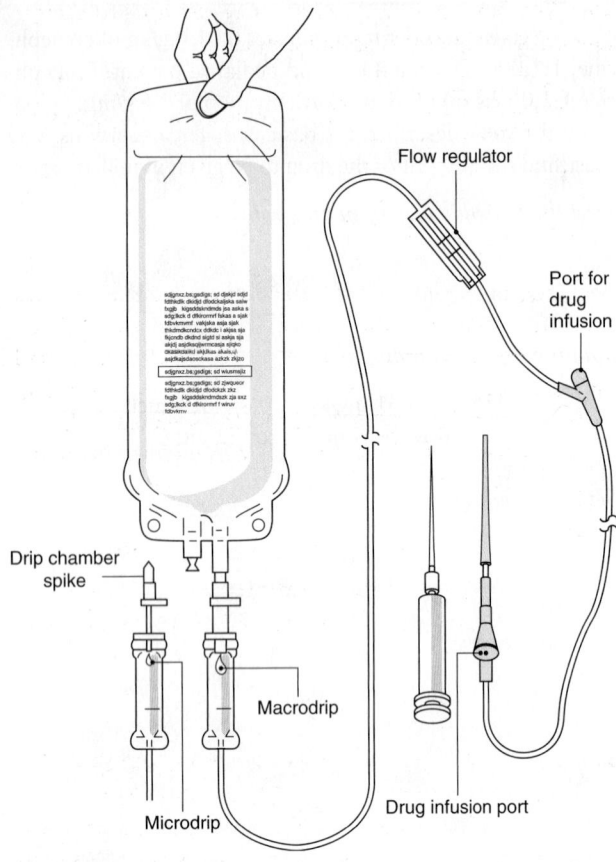

FIGURE 12-5

Parts of an IV administration set.

A standard IV infusion order is usually given as a volume of fluid to be infused over a given amount of time, often in milliliters per hour. However, the order also may be given in liters over a period of several hours. A standard formula is used to determine the number of drops per minute needed to deliver the amount given in the order:

$$\frac{\text{amount to be infused in milliters} \times \text{tubing drip factor}}{\text{time in minutes}} = \text{gtts/min}$$

For example, you receive an order to infuse lactated Ringer's solution (a common isotonic IV fluid) at a rate of 200 mL/hour. Because you are giving fluids at a relatively fast rate, you will use a tubing set that delivers larger drops. Your service uses 15-gtts/mL sets for this purpose. Here is what you know:

- The amount to be infused in milliliters is 200.
- The tubing drip factor is 15.
- The time in minutes is 60.

Set up the formula:

$$\frac{200 \times 15}{60} = x \text{ gtts/min}$$

Simplify the terms. In this case, because 15 goes into 60 four times, the formula is simplified as follows:

$$\frac{200 \times 1}{4} = x \text{ gtts/min}$$

Simplify further and solve the equation:

$$\frac{200}{4} = 50 \text{ gtts/min}$$

You will adjust the drip rate to 50 drops per minute.

In another order, you are given an order to give 30 mL/hour of normal saline. Such a small dosage is best administered using a 60-gtts/mL tubing set.

Set up the formula:

$$\frac{30 \times 60}{60} = x \text{ gtts/mL}$$

Simplify the terms. In this case, because the drip rate and minute terms are both 60, they cancel each other out. In other words, 60 goes into 60 one time, so each term of 60 becomes 1. The formula is simplified as follows:

$$\frac{30 \times 1}{1} = x \text{ gtts/min}$$

Simplify further and solve the equation:

$$\frac{30}{1} = 30 \text{ gtts/min}$$

You will adjust the drip rate to 30 drops per minute.

It is not coincidence that, in the previous example using 60-gtts/mL tubing, the number of milliliters in the order is equal to the number of drops per minute needed to achieve the dosage. All of the drip factors used (60, 20, 15, and 10) are multiples of 60, allowing simplification of the terms whenever the order is given for 1 hour (60 minutes). When the order is given in milliliters per hour, simply divide the milliliters to be given per hour as follows:

- For 60-gtts/mL tubing, divide by 1.
- For 20-gtts/mL tubing, divide by 3.
- For 15-gtts/mL tubing, divide by 4.
- For 10-gtts/mL tubing, divide by 6.

Always make sure you check the time over which the volume is to be infused before calculating the drip. Although IV infusion orders are often given in milliliters per hour, this is not always the case. Particularly when medications are involved, the dosage is given in milligrams or micrograms per minute, an order that requires a complex calculation. It is typically not within the Advanced EMT scope of practice to administer intravenous infusions of medications, but this information is covered in Appendix 4. In other cases, such as in severely dehydrated or burned patients, you may be given an order for intravenous fluids in terms of liters per hour, or per several hours. An example:

You receive an order to give 3 L of normal saline over 8 hours. For this purpose, you will use 15 gtts/mL. First, find the amount of fluid to give in 1 hour by setting up an equation to solve for the unknown volume.

Set up the equation:

$$\frac{3 \text{ L}}{8 \text{ hr}} = \frac{x \text{ L}}{1 \text{ hr}}$$

Cross-multiply. (Note that the same method as described previously is used to solve the equation, even though x is on the right side of the equation in this example):

$$(3 \times 1) = 8x$$

Solve for x to find the volume to be given in 1 hour:

$$\frac{3}{8} = x \text{ L} = 0.375 \text{ L/hr}$$

Now, convert liters to milliliters, remembering that there are 1,000 mL in a liter. Moving the decimal point three places to the right is the same as multiplying 0.375 by 1,000:

$$0.375 \text{ L} = 375 \text{ mL (to be given in 1 hr)}$$

Set up and solve the problem following the standard formula for drip rate problems:

$$\frac{375 \text{ mL} \times 15 \text{ gtts/mL}}{60 \text{ min}}$$

$$= 93.75 \text{ (rounded to 94) drops per minute}$$

Often, you will be asked to set an IV infusion to a "keep-open" rate, abbreviated TKO (to keep open) or KVO (keep vein open). A standard TKO or KVO rate is 30 mL/hour.

Weight-Based IV Drip Rate Calculations

In some cases, you are given weight-based IV infusion orders. Before proceeding with the standard formula, you must first obtain the patient's weight and, if necessary, convert the weight in pounds to kilograms. For example:

You are given an order to infuse normal saline at a rate of 2 mL/kg/hour. The patient weighs 90 pounds. You will use 15 gtts/mL tubing. First, convert the weight in pounds to kilograms by dividing 90 by 2.2:

$$\frac{90 \text{ lb}}{2.2} = 40.9 \text{ (rounded to 41 kg)}$$

Next, find the total amount of fluid to be administered each hour by multiplying 2 mL by 41 kg:

$$2 \times 41 = 82 \text{ mL}$$

Now, you have all of the information you need to use the standard drip rate calculation formula:

$$\frac{82 \text{ mL} \times 15 \text{ gtts/mL}}{60 \text{ min}} = 20.5 \text{ (rounded to 21) gtts/min}$$

Setting the Drip Rate

Once you have determined how many drops per minute of IV fluid must be administered to deliver the ordered amount, you must adjust the flow rate to the calculated number of drops. Observe the drops dripping into the drip chamber and adjust the roller clamp (flow regulator) to increase or decrease the flow rate. Determine the timing of the drops as follows.

EXAMPLE 1: You must deliver 60 gtts/minute. This example is easy. Because there are 60 seconds in 1 minute, you will time the drops to be delivered one every second.

EXAMPLE 2: You must deliver 40 gtts/minute. By estimation, you can determine that, because fewer drops will be given than there are seconds in a minute, that drops will be more than 1 second apart. In such cases, the easiest way to adjust the flow rate is to determine how many drops should be given in a fraction of a minute, such as 15 seconds. That way, you can use the second hand on your watch or on a wall clock to count the number of drops in a 15-second period. To find the number of drops in 15 seconds, divide 40 (the number of drops to be given in 1 minute) by 4 (the number of times 15 seconds goes into 1 minute):

$$\frac{40}{4} = 10 \text{ gtts every 15 sec}$$

EXAMPLE 3: You have calculated a drip rate of 80 drops per minute: In this case, you can estimate that you will be giving more than one drop per second. Use the method above to determine how to adjust the flow rate:

$$\frac{80}{4} = 20 \text{ gtts every 15 sec}$$

In the hospital setting, and sometimes in the prehospital setting, IV infusion pumps are used to calculate and adjust the IV infusion rate (Figure 12-6). Some devices are very simple and use a dial to set the infusion at a given number of milliliters per hour, while others are digital and the information used to calculate the drip rate is programmed into the pump. Most IV infusion pumps use special tubing, which you must carry if your service uses IV infusion pumps.

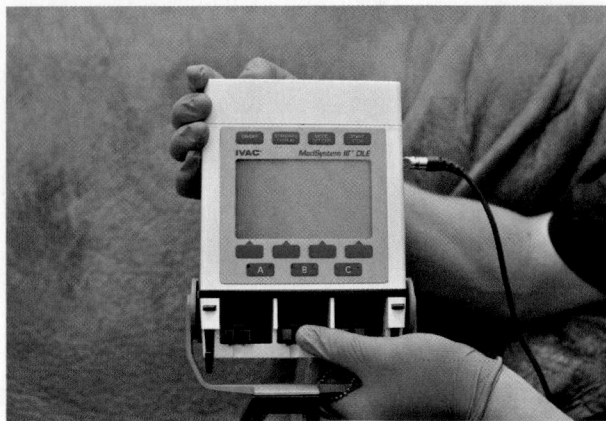

FIGURE 12-6

An IV infusion pump.

Techniques of Medication Administration

Before giving any medication, you must perform a history and assessment to determine that the medication is indicated, and that it is not contraindicated. That includes asking about medications the patient currently takes, about drug allergies, and about conditions that could contraindicate a particular drug. For example, the use of a drug for erectile dysfunction within the past 24 to 48 hours is a contraindication to administering nitroglycerin, because a dangerous drop in blood pressure can occur.

Ask specifically about allergies to the drug you plan to give. A patient who is experiencing stress because he is having chest pain may not think to tell you that he is allergic to aspirin when you ask about medication allergies in general. However, if you specifically ask, "Are you allergic to aspirin?" he may give you a different answer.

Obtain a complete set of baseline vital signs before administering medications. Without them, you may miss a contraindication for the medication you are going to give. You also will not know if the patient's vital signs are a result of his condition or a result of the medication. One possible exception is with a known asthmatic patient who is wheezing and has a significant respiratory distress; you may administer an inhaled beta$_2$ agonist before obtaining a blood pressure. Even in that situation, ideally, your partner or another provider would obtain a blood pressure as you are setting up the equipment to administer the medication.

Medication administration is not complete until you have documented the procedure. Make sure that your documentation contains the findings that made it clear the medication was indicated and **pertinent negatives** that make it clear there were no contraindications. Document the authorization to administer the medication, such as the name of the medical direction physician who gave the order over the radio or that the medication was given according to standing order. Document the name of the medication, the amount given, and the route by which it was given. If appropriate, such as with percutaneous medications, document the site of administration. Document the time the medication was given, and any complications that occurred.

After giving medications, you must reassess the patient at appropriate intervals and document the findings. The frequency of reassessment depends on the medication and the patient's condition.

Ask the patient if he has experienced a change in the symptoms for which the medication was administered and if he has any new symptoms. It is important to note whether the medications are having the desired effects in reducing the severity of the patient's symptoms. Failure of the medication to reduce symptoms may mean that the condition is refractory (resistant) to treatment. You should also reconsider your original field impression. It is possible that the medication did not have the desired effect because the problem is different than you initially thought. New symptoms may indicate worsening of the patient's condition, drug side effects, or that the patient's condition is something other than your original field impression.

Reassess pertinent signs and compare subsequent sets of vital signs to their baseline values. Analyze the possible meanings of your reassessment to determine the effectiveness of treatment, as well as whether you should reconsider your original field impression.

Aseptic Technique

Infection is a risk from any percutaneous (through the skin) route of medication administration. Strict adherence to **aseptic** technique helps minimize the risk of infection. Use aseptic technique for intramuscular and subcutaneous injection and for intravenous access and intravenous injection through a medication administration port on intravenous tubing. For those procedures, the minimum aseptic technique is the application of friction with an isopropyl alcohol wipe (Figure 12-7). You can use povidone iodine (Betadine) solution swabs, as well. Keep in mind that neither of those solutions sterilizes the skin, and that the use of friction, particularly with alcohol, is an important part of cleaning and disinfecting the skin. Follow the guidelines below when preparing the skin for percutaneous medication administration:

- Identify the site where you will puncture the skin and use the swab in a circular motion, creating increasingly larger concentric circles. The key is to move from "clean" to "dirty." The area that must be cleanest is the point of insertion of the needle. Debris and pathogens are dragged outward, away from the site by using concentric circles. Do not go back over an area you have already cleaned with the swab.

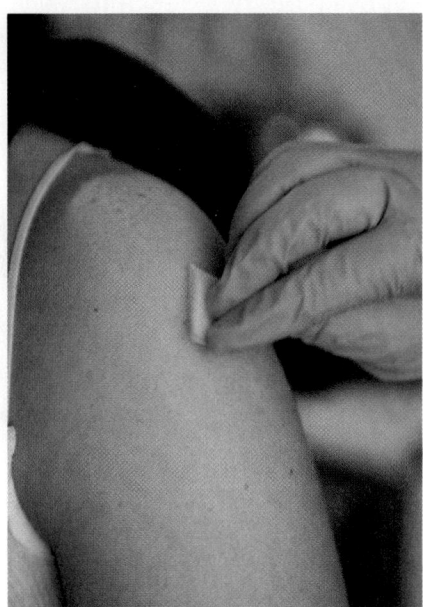

FIGURE 12-7

Use an alcohol wipe (shown) or povidone iodine swab to disinfect the skin prior to percutaneous injection.

■ Once you have disinfected the area, do not touch it.

■ Allow the skin to dry completely to complete the disinfection process. Do not blow on or fan the area to speed drying, as both practices reintroduce pathogens to the area. Puncturing the skin through wet alcohol or povidone iodine can also increase pain.

■ If the disinfected area becomes contaminated before the injection is performed, start the disinfection process over again.

■ Before giving an intravenous injection through a medication port on IV tubing, cleanse the port with an alcohol swab.

Do not allow any equipment or solution that will enter the body to become contaminated. This includes avoiding contact between those items and nonsterile surfaces or items. Needles, IV catheters, infusion straws, and IV tubing connections all must be kept sterile. Good hand washing and cleaning and disinfection of equipment and surfaces are also important measures in infection control.

EMS Provider Safety

Always use Standard Precautions for percutaneous procedures. (See Chapter 3.) Gloves are required for IV catheterization. Although gloves are not a requirement of Standard Precautions for intramuscular and subcutaneous injections, your employer's policy may require them and some health care providers prefer to wear them for those procedures.

Never recap contaminated needles. Use needleless systems and devices with needle guards when possible. Dispose of needles in an approved biohazard container. Make it a

habit to include disposal of sharps as a step continuous with the procedure, rather than laying them aside for later disposal. Never stick needles into the stretcher mattress or seat cushions. Do not leave sharps at the scene of a call. Whenever possible, avoid performing percutaneous procedures in a moving ambulance. Either perform the task before you leave the scene, or have the driver stop for a moment so you can safely perform the task.

Oral Medication Administration

The most common medication administered orally by Advanced EMTs is aspirin. Aspirin is given to patients with signs and symptoms of acute coronary syndrome (ACS) to prevent further aggregation (clumping) of platelets in the narrowed coronary arteries. To shorten the time to onset of action, it is preferred that non–enteric-coated, chewable tablets are given. Because oral medications are given to patients who are alert, your primary tasks are selecting the proper number of tablets and handing them to the patient with instructions to chew and swallow them. If available, a small plastic medication cup reduces the likelihood that either you or the patient will drop the tablets.

An example of documentation is as follows:

162 mg chewable aspirin administered PO, according to standing orders, at 0412 hours.

Sublingual Medication Administration

The most common medication administered sublingually by Advanced EMTs is nitroglycerin (NTG), which comes in tablet and metered-dose spray forms. Nitroglycerin is given to patients with suspected ACS to dilate the coronary arteries through smooth muscle relaxation, allowing increased blood flow through the coronary arteries. The sublingual route allows rapid onset of action. Nitroglycerin has several side effects for which you must monitor the patient.

To administer a tablet sublingually, tell the patient that you are going to place a tablet under his tongue, and that he should allow it to dissolve there, rather than swallowing the tablet. Ask the patient to lift up his tongue, and then place the tablet beneath it (Figure 12-8). Wear gloves when handling nitroglycerin tablets. Moisture on your hands can allow the tablet to begin to dissolve and be absorbed through your skin.

To administer nitroglycerin spray, explain to the patient that you are going to spray the medication under his tongue. Ask him to lift up his tongue, then, holding the spray canister just outside the patient's mouth with the spray directed toward the sublingual space, depress the spray button on the top of the canister.

An example of documentation is as follows:

Per radio order from Dr. Blume at Channing Hospital, 0.4 mg NTG administered by sublingual tablet at 0731 hours.

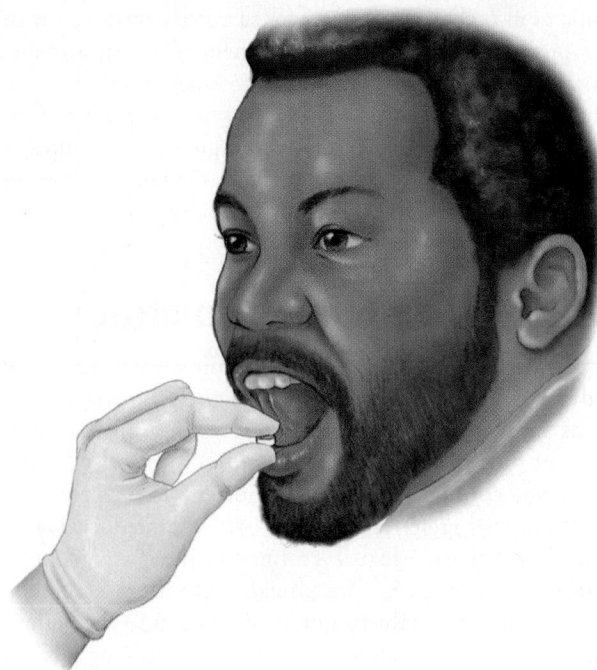

FIGURE 12-8

Sublingual medication administration.

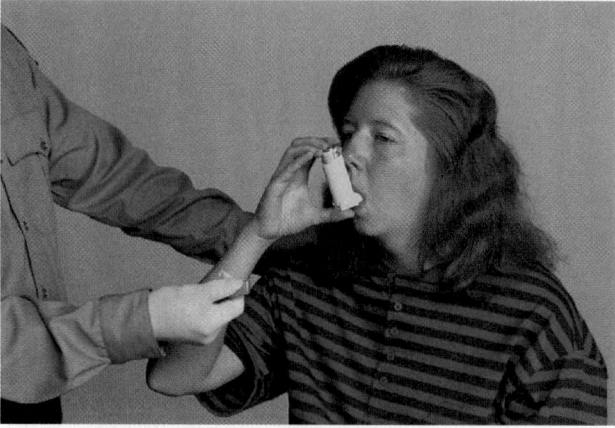

FIGURE 12-9

Assisting a patient with metered-dose inhaler administration.

Nebulized Medication Administration

Beta$_2$ agonists such as albuterol and levalbuterol, and anticholinergics such as ipatropium bromide (alone or in combination with beta$_2$ agonists) are supplied as liquids that are nebulized, or turned into a fine mist, by compressed air or pressurized oxygen flowing through the liquid. The mist is inhaled, and the droplets come in contact with the respiratory membrane. A small-volume nebulizer (SVN) consists of tubing that connects the oxygen or air source to a small cup that holds the medication and either a mouthpiece or facemask. The patient must hold the mouthpiece, while the mask is placed in the same way as an oxygen mask. (See Scan 12-1.)

An example of documentation is as follows:

2.5 mg albuterol in 1.5 mL normal saline administered by SVN at 1513 hours per standing order.

Medication Administration by Metered-Dose Inhaler

Many patients who require administration of medication by metered-dose inhaler (MDI) are familiar with the use of the device, because they are often prescribed a similar device for use at home (Figure 12-9). Nonetheless, you cannot be sure that the patient uses the device correctly at home, and you must still provide instruction. For patients unfamiliar with the use of the device, you may need to assist them in

depressing the canister as you instruct them to inhale. MDIs must be shaken prior to use. The patient places the mouthpiece in his mouth and seals his lips around it. Just as he begins a deep inhalation, the canister is depressed to dispense the medication as the patient continues to inhale and then hold his breath briefly before exhaling.

An example of documentation is as follows:

Two 90-mcg sprays of albuterol administered by MDI at 2310 hours on the order of Dr. Boggs at Brown County Hospital.

Nitrous Oxide Administration

Nitrous oxide is a self-administered analgesic gas that is a 50:50 mix of oxygen and nitrogen (Figure 12-10). Nitrous oxide systems may consist of two tanks or a single tank. You must follow the manufacturer's directions for the use of any particular system. The patient holds a mask against his face and is instructed to breathe normally. One of the effects of the drug is to alter the mental status. The patient will no longer be able to hold the mask against the face when that occurs. Never hold the mask against the patient's face for him. Nitrous oxide must be used only in well-ventilated areas. Because of the risk of complications, pregnant dental technicians do not administer nitrous oxide, even in settings in which scavenging systems are in place to limit their exposure.

Equipment Used for Injections

You will need some special equipment to prepare and administer a subcutaneous, intramuscular, or intravenous injection, as follows:

- Gloves for Standard Precautions.
- Alcohol or povidone iodine swabs to prepare the site of injection, and if applicable, the membrane of medication vials.

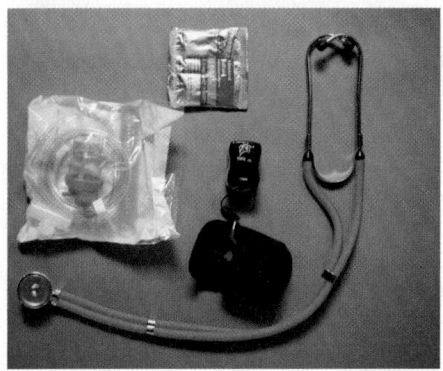

1. Assemble all of the equipment needed for the procedure.

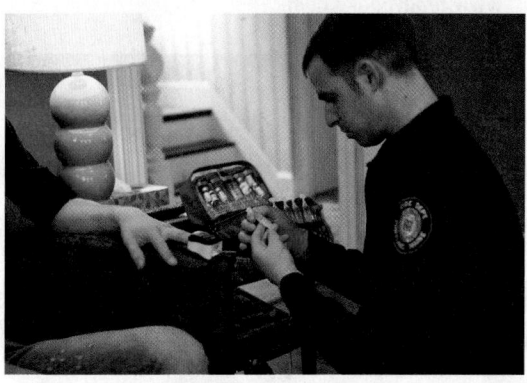

2. Select and check the medication.

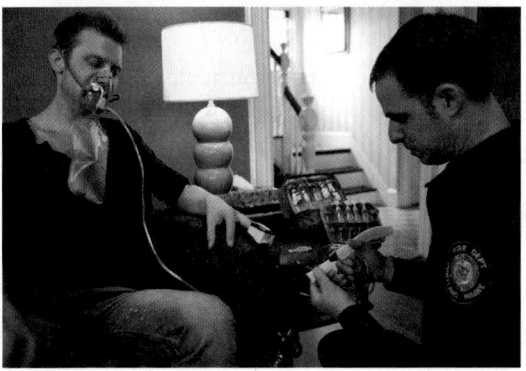

3. Assemble the nebulizer by connecting the mouthpiece to the "T" connector atop the medication cup.

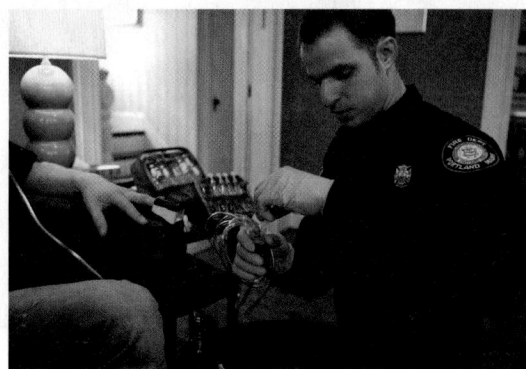

4. Unscrew the cap of the medication cup. Place the medication in the medication cup of the small volume nebulizer.

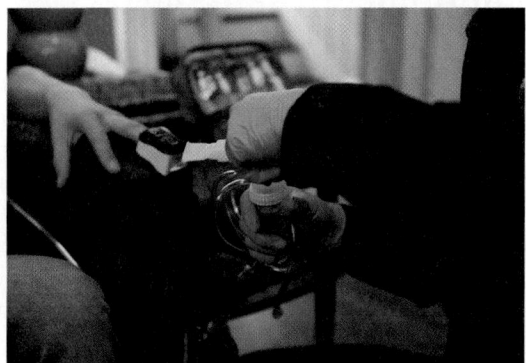

5. Replace the cap on the nebulizer.

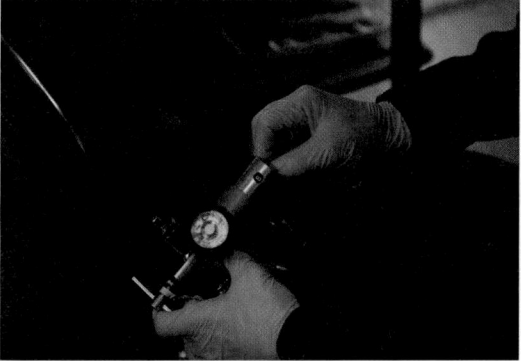

6. Connect the tubing from the nebulizer to oxygen and adjust the oxygen flow rate to 8 L/min.

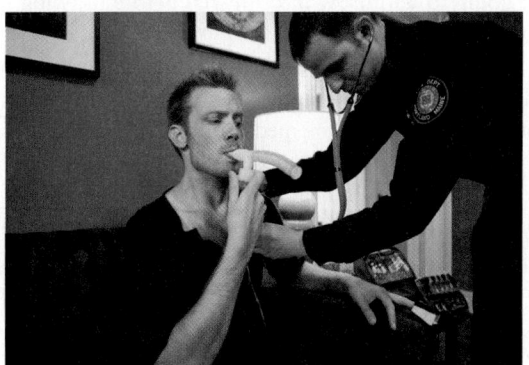

7. Instruct the patient to place the mouthpiece in his mouth and breathe in the medication and breathe it out. Reassess the patient.

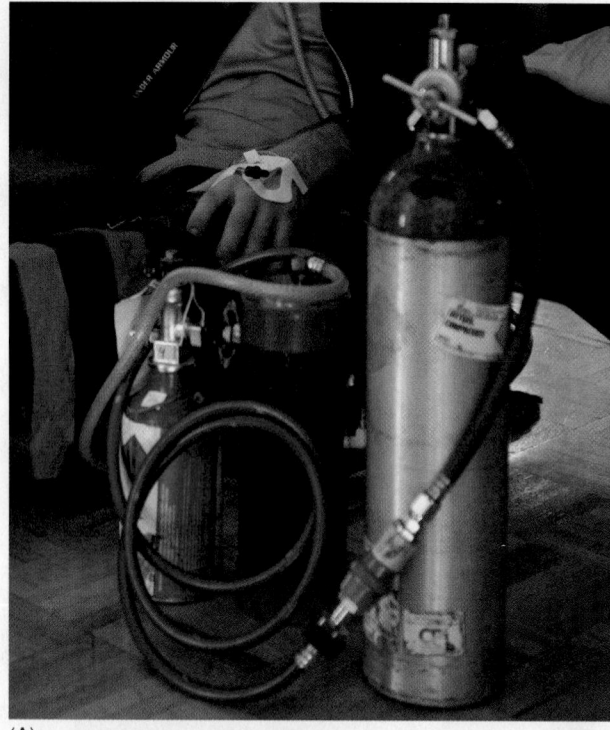

(A)

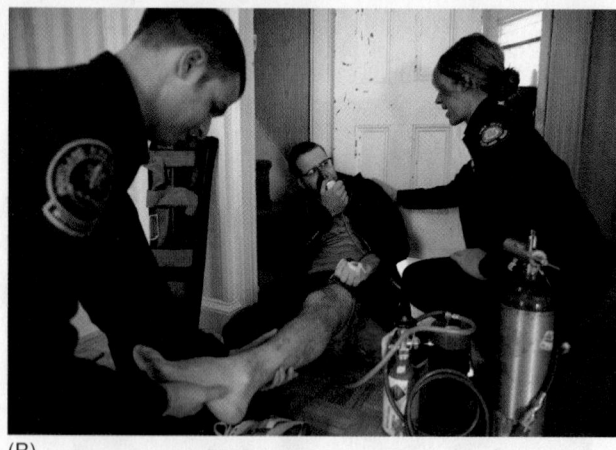

(B)

FIGURE 12-10

(A) Nitrous oxide administration set. (B) A patient self-administering nitrous oxide.

- Syringe of the proper size and with the proper graduations for the precision of the dosage to be administered. Typical syringe sizes are 1 mL, 3 mL, 5 mL, and 10 mL. Prefilled syringes containing medications to be administered intravenously may contain larger volumes of medication. Use the syringe volume that most closely matches the volume of medication to be administered. The degree of precision decreases slightly as the syringe volume increases. That is not consequential when using a 10-mL syringe to administer 5 mL of medication. However, it may be substantial when using a 3-mL syringe to administer

0.3 mL of medication. When giving 1 mL or less of medication, always use a 1-mL syringe.

- Needles or filter straws for drawing up and administering the medication. Hollow needles for medication administration come in various gauges and lengths. *Gauge* refers to the diameter of the needle. The smaller the number of the gauge, the larger the diameter of the needle. An 18-gauge needle is fairly large in diameter, and is used to draw up medications, but not to administer them subcutaneously or intravenously. Smaller diameter 21-gauge and 23-gauge needles are used for intramuscular injections. 25-gauge needles are used for subcutaneous injection. A longer needle, 1 to 1½ inches, is used for intramuscular injections in adults. A shorter needle, ½ to ⅝ inches, is used for subcutaneous injections.

- Small gauze square to apply pressure if minor bleeding occurs after injection.

- Small adhesive bandage to cover the puncture site.

- Vial, ampule, or prefilled syringe of medication to be administered.

- Sharps disposal container.

Drawing Medication from Ampules and Vials

Many medications administered by percutaneous routes are supplied in vials and ampules, and must be drawn into a syringe in preparation for administration. The technique is slightly different for ampules (Scan 12-2) than it is for vials (shown in Scan 12-4 for IM injection). When drawing a medication from an ampule, first hold it upright between your thumb and fingers and shake it downward to ensure all medication is below the neck of the ampule. Do not draw air into the syringe or inject air into the ampule before drawing up the medication.

When drawing up medication from a vial, you must inject a volume of air equal to the volume of medication you are going to withdraw into the vial before drawing up the medication.

When drawing up medications from an ampule or vial, it is common to use a larger needle, usually 18 gauge, than you will use to inject the medication. The use of a fill needle or filter straw (needleless mechanism) makes drawing up the medication easier. If a fill needle or filter straw is used, you must discard it after the syringe contains the proper amount of medication and replace it with the proper gauge (diameter) and length of needle for the route of administration.

When filling a syringe with medication from an ampule or vial, always make sure that the bevel of the needle is fully covered by liquid to avoid drawing air into the syringe (Figure 12-11). Draw a volume of medication slightly more than the amount needed. Remove the needle from the ampule or vial and hold the syringe with the needle pointing upward. Flick or tap the barrel of the syringe to dislodge air

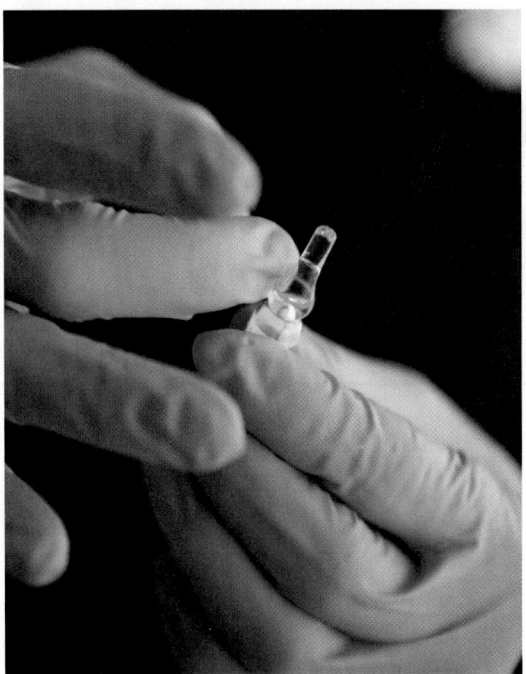

1. Hold the ampule upright and gently tap the top until all medication has moved into the bottom chamber of the ampule.

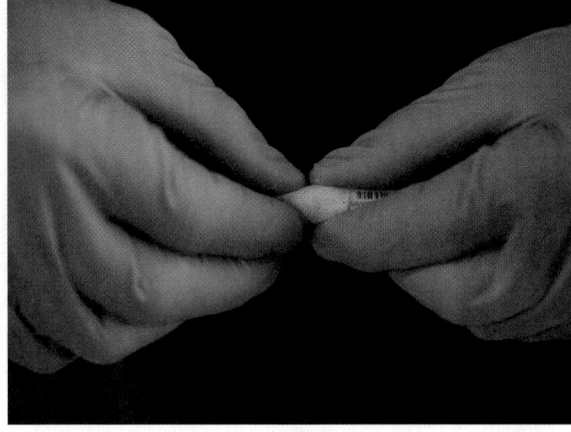

2. Grasp the top of the ampule with a piece of gauze or alcohol swab.

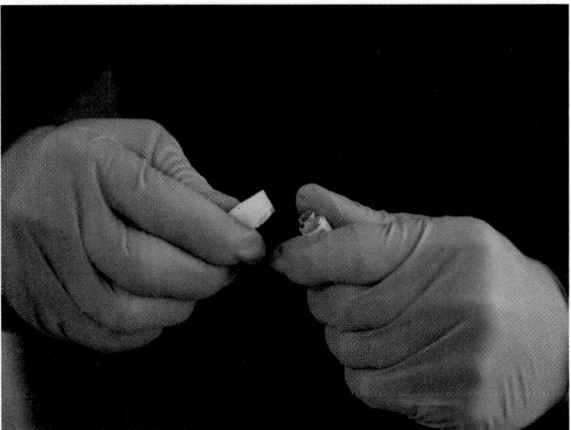

3. Snap off the top of the ampule, taking care not to spill any medication.

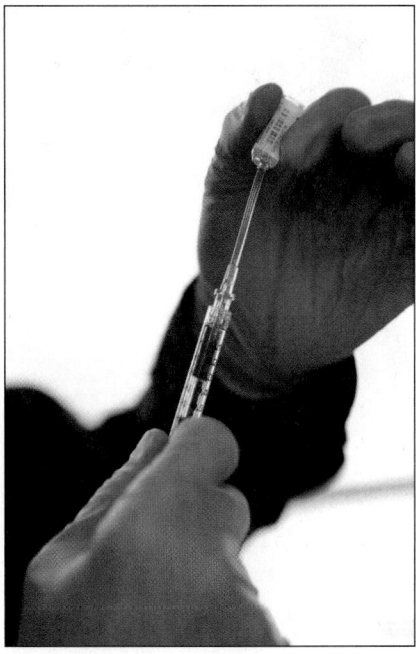

4. Draw the medication from the ampule.

bubbles, and allow them to migrate upward. Slightly and carefully depress the syringe plunger until the top edge of the black disk at the top of it, called the *meniscus,* is at the line on the syringe barrel that indicates the proper volume for administration. When checking the amount of medication in the syringe, hold the syringe at eye level to ensure accurate measurement.

If necessary, remove the fill needle or filter straw and replace it with the appropriately sized needle for medication administration.

Subcutaneous Injection

In some cases, you may give epinephrine, 1:1,000 subcutaneously, for patients in anaphylaxis. Several sites are acceptable for subcutaneous injection (Figure 12-12). In the prehospital setting, the upper arm is usually the most convenient site. To ensure the medication is injected into the subcutaneous tissue and not into the dermis or muscle, pinch a 1-inch fold of skin between your thumb and forefinger (Scan 12-3). You can inject a maximum of 1 mL of

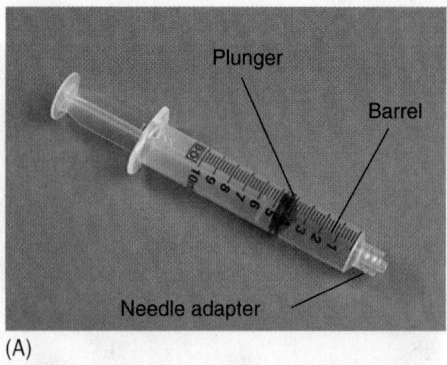
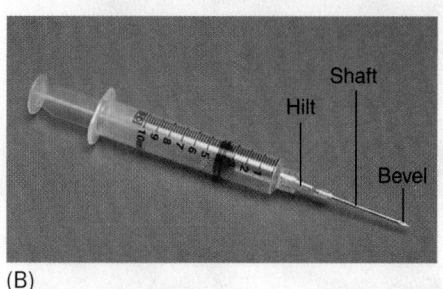

(A)   (B)

FIGURE 12-11

(A) Parts of a syringe. (B) Parts of a percutaneous needle.

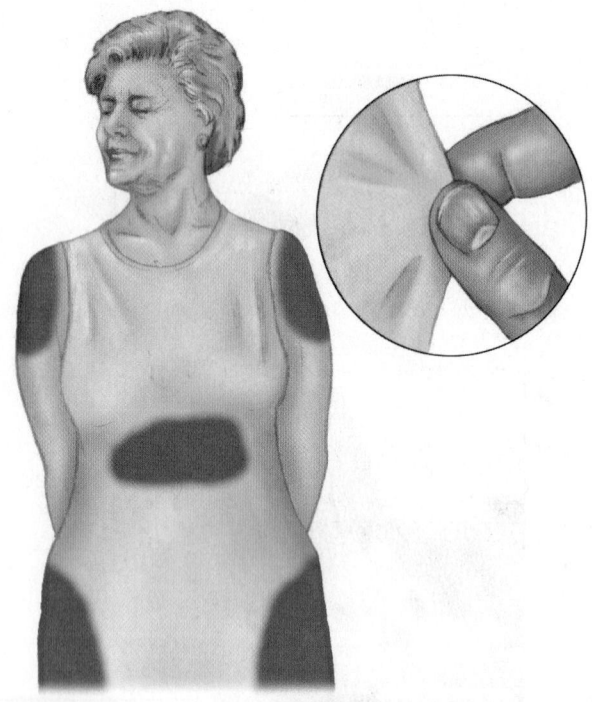

FIGURE 12-12

Sites for subcutaneous injection.

Pediatric Care

Percutaneous needles of shorter lengths and smaller gauges are used for pediatric patients. In smaller pediatric patients, the muscles of the thigh are preferred over the deltoid muscle for IM injection.

use the deltoid muscle in the upper arm for its convenience and because the volume of medication to be injected is usually 1 mL or less. To ensure medication is injected into the muscle, use a 21-gauge or 23-gauge needle (23 or 25 gauge in pediatric patients). A needle length of ¾ inch is suitable for most pediatric patients. A needle length of ¾ to 1 inch is suitable for most adults, but a 1½-inch needle is used for deep IM injection in the gluteal muscle, and may be required in very obese patients. You can inject a maximum of 1 mL of medication into the deltoid muscle, while you can inject 2 mL into the muscles of the thigh. Though you can inject 5 mL into the gluteal muscles, it is generally advisable to divide such a large volume of medication into two smaller doses. (See Scan 12-4.)

An example of documentation is as follows:

1 mg glucagon administered IM in the right deltoid at 1015 hours by radio order of Dr. Taylor, Baptist Emergency Department.

Intravenous Injection

Advanced EMTs can administer dextrose solutions to hypoglycemic patients, such as 50 percent dextrose for adults and 25 percent dextrose for pediatric patients (except neonates), and naloxone for suspected narcotic overdose, by intravenous injection. Intravenous injections may either be given through an intravenous line or a saline lock (both discussed in a later section). Always know the drug profile of

medication subcutaneously. Use a 25-gauge needle, ½ to ⁵/₈ inches long, for subcutaneous injection.

An example of documentation is as follows:

0.5 mg epinephrine 1:1,000 given subQ in the left upper arm at 1400 hours per standing orders.

Intramuscular Injection

Two drugs you may give intramuscularly are epinephrine 1:1,000 and glucagon, which is given for hypoglycemia when an IV cannot be established. Several sites are acceptable for IM injection (Figure 12-13). In most cases, Advanced EMTs

(*Text continued on page 306*)

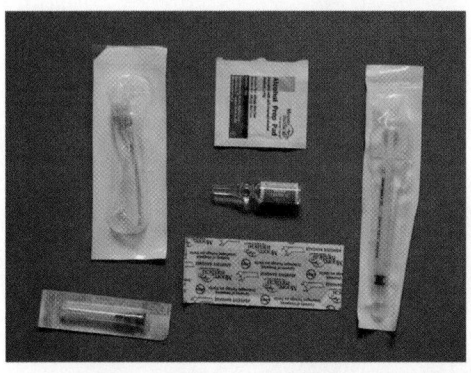

1. Assemble all of the equipment needed for the procedure.

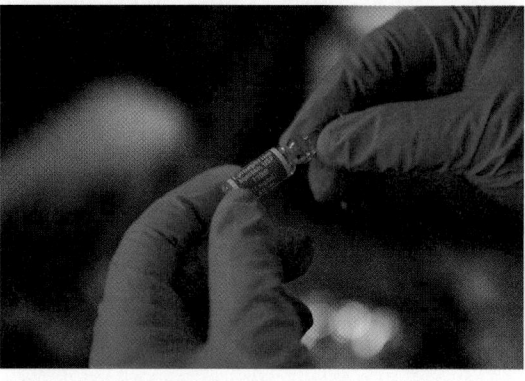

2. Verify the medication.

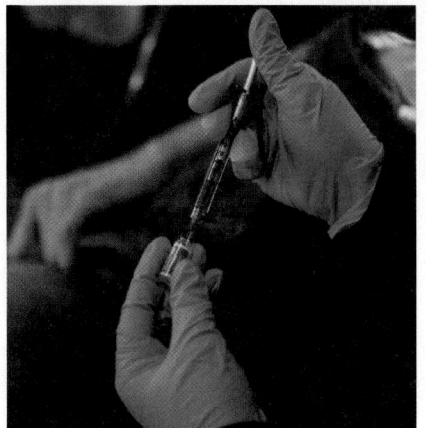

3. Draw up the medication into a syringe.

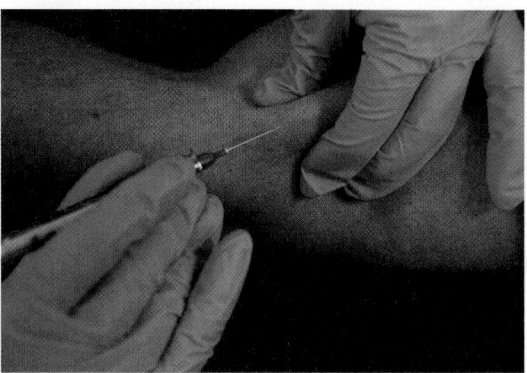

4. After disinfecting the skin, pinch up fold of skin and position the needle at a 45-degree angle to the skin.

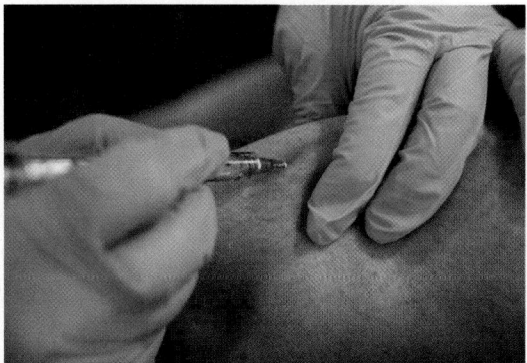

5. Insert the needle into the skin and inject the medication.

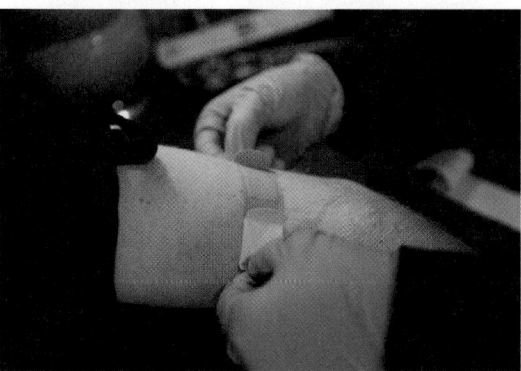

6. Place an adhesive bandage over the injection site.

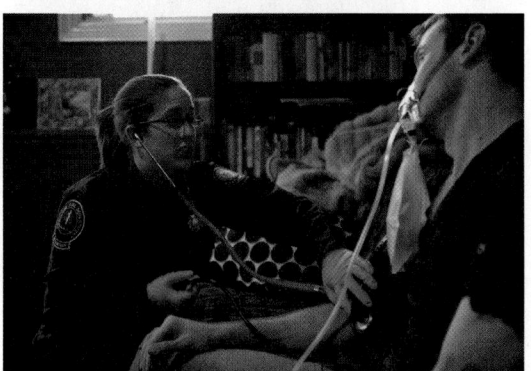

7. Reassess the patient.

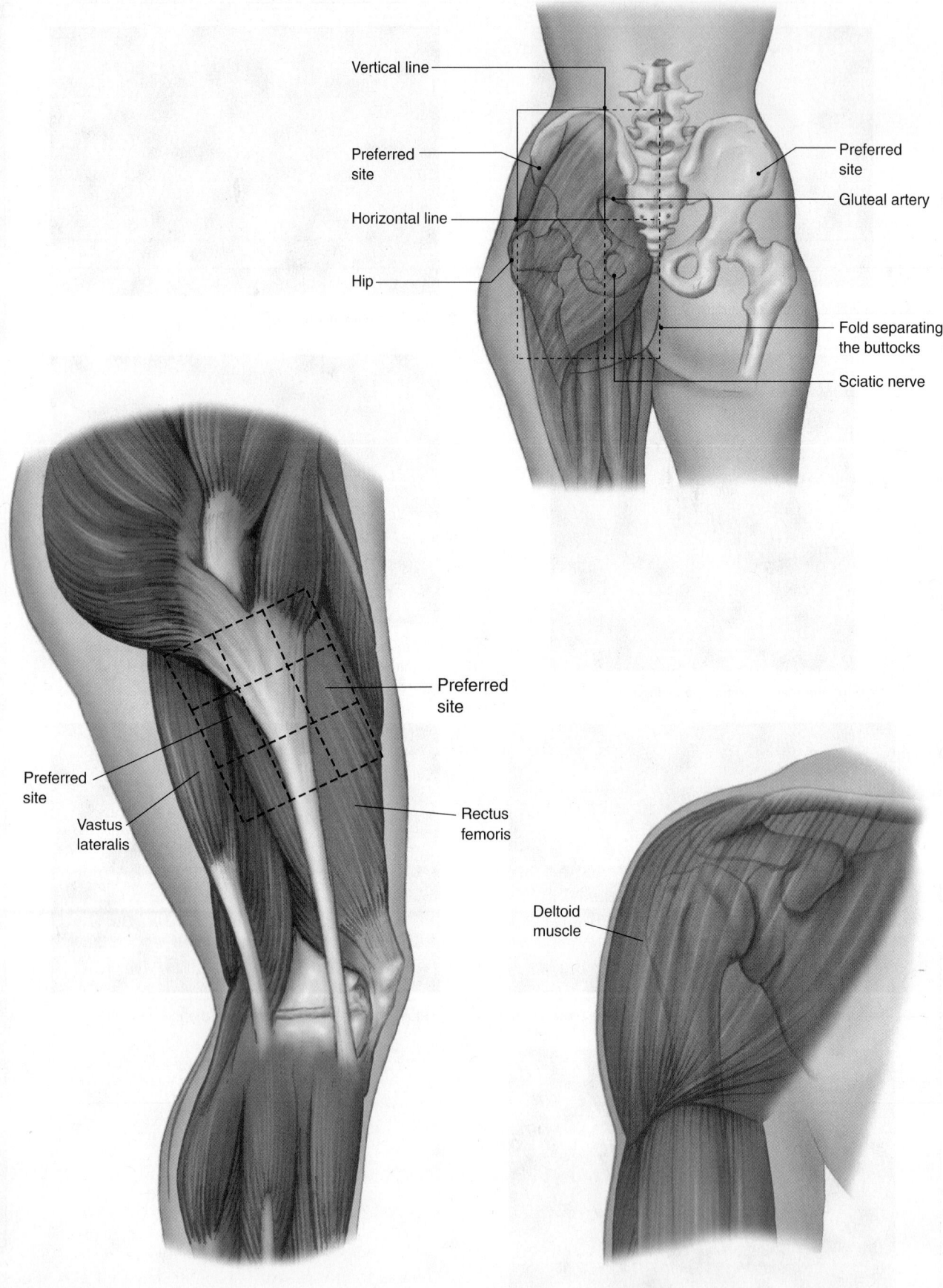

FIGURE 12-13

Sites for intramuscular injection.

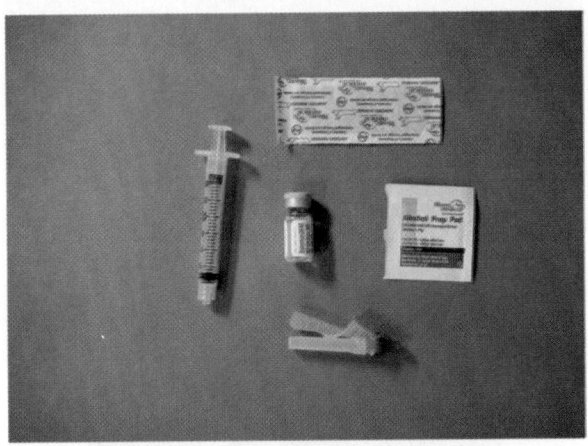

1. Assemble all of the equipment needed for the procedure.

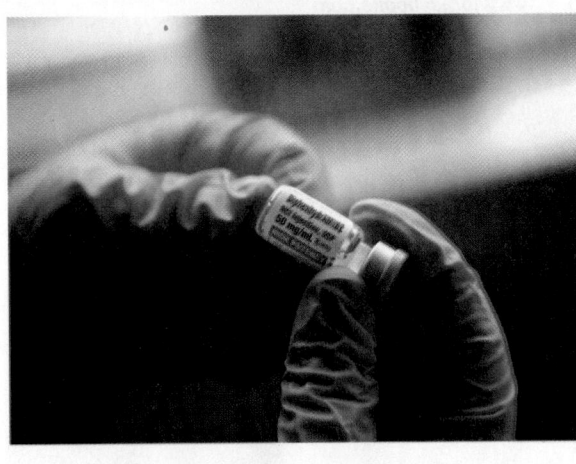

2. Select and verify the medication.

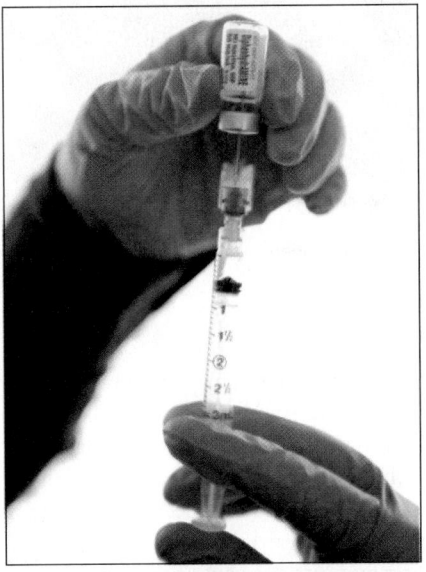

3. Inject a volume of air slightly greater than the volume of medication to be withdrawn and draw the medication from the vial.

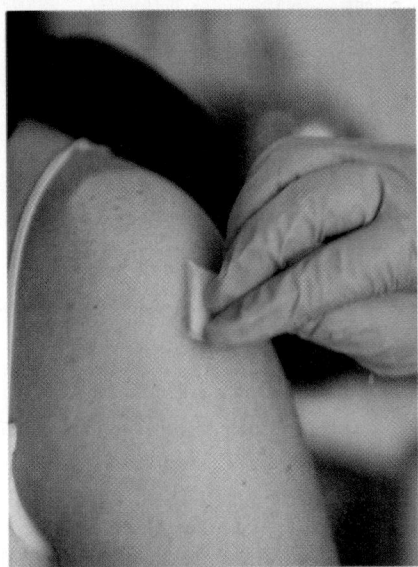

4. Disinfect the skin at the injection site.

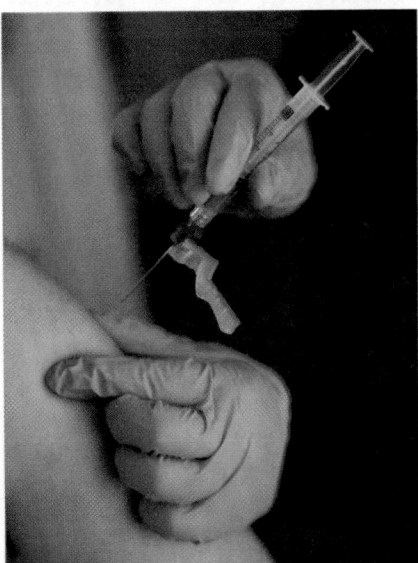

5. Stabilize the skin over the site and place the needle at a 90-degree angle to the skin.

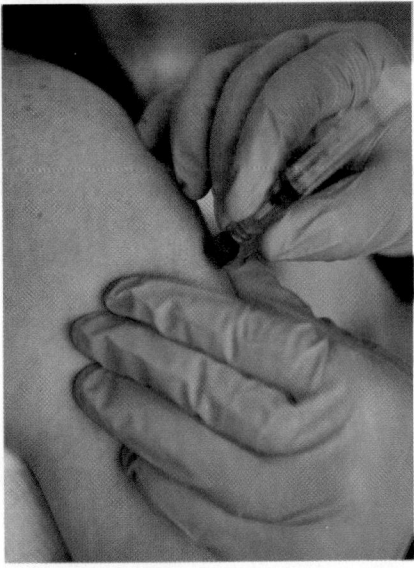

6. Insert the needle and inject the medication. Draw back on the syringe plunger slightly. You should not be able to aspirate blood. If blood is aspirated, do not inject the medication. Remove the needle from the skin and start over in another site.

(continued)

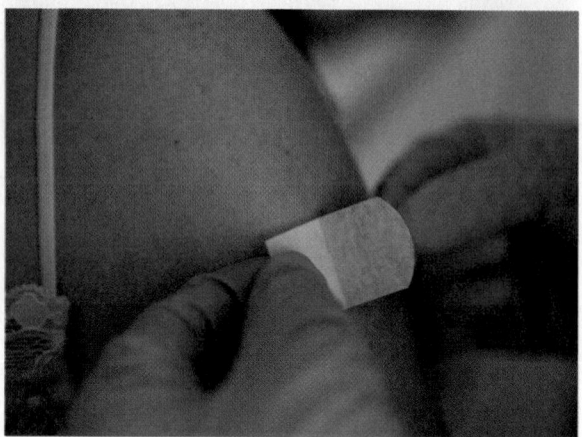

7. Place an adhesive bandage over the site.

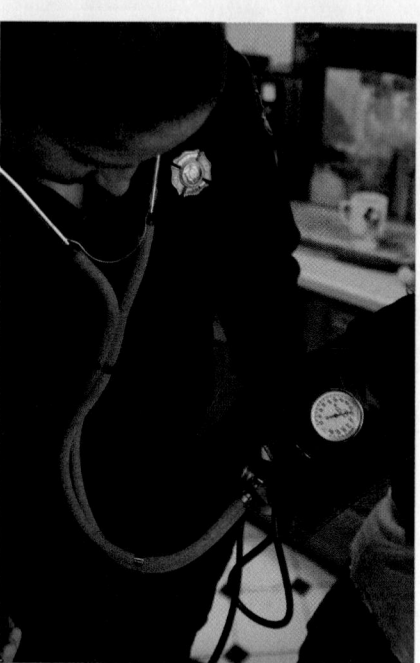

8. Reassess the patient.

the medication you are giving, including whether it should be given by slow IV push or by rapid IV push or bolus.

Before giving any intravenous medication, check to make sure the IV or saline lock is patent (flows freely or can be easily flushed with saline from a syringe) and is not infiltrated (fluid is not leaking from the vein into the surrounding tissue). Attempting to administer a drug through an IV that is not patent or that is infiltrated can cause phlebitis and tissue damage.

Preferably, a needleless system is used to administer intravenous injections, but you may use syringes with needles, as well. The procedure for administering a medication through an IV line varies slightly from the procedure for administering a medication through a saline lock. Whereas you can flush a medication administered through an IV line through the catheter by briefly opening up the roller clamp on the tubing and allowing IV fluid to flow through the tubing before readjusting the drip rate, you must flush a medication

administered through a saline lock through the catheter with a syringe full of sterile normal saline, called a *saline flush*.

To administer an injection through an IV line, you must pinch off or clamp the tubing above the injection port in the tubing to prevent the medication being injected from flowing upward toward the IV bag, rather than through the IV catheter and into the vein. (See Scan 12-5.)

Establishing a Peripheral Intravenous Line

Peripheral intravenous access is indicated for any patient in whom fluid administration or a means for giving emergency medicines is required or anticipated. Intravenous access is obtained by using a catheter that surrounds a hollow needle (Figure 12-14). The needle is used to puncture the skin and

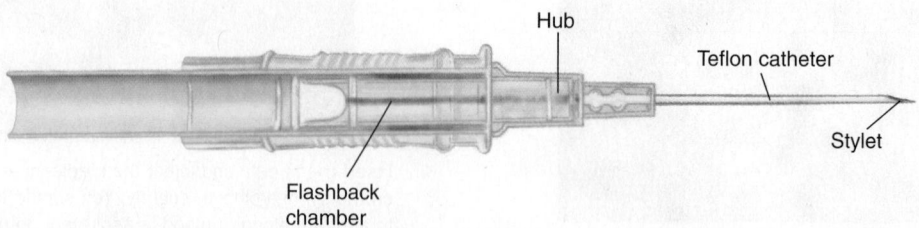

FIGURE 12-14

Parts of a catheter-over-needle device for intravenous access.

SCAN 12-5 Intravenous Injection

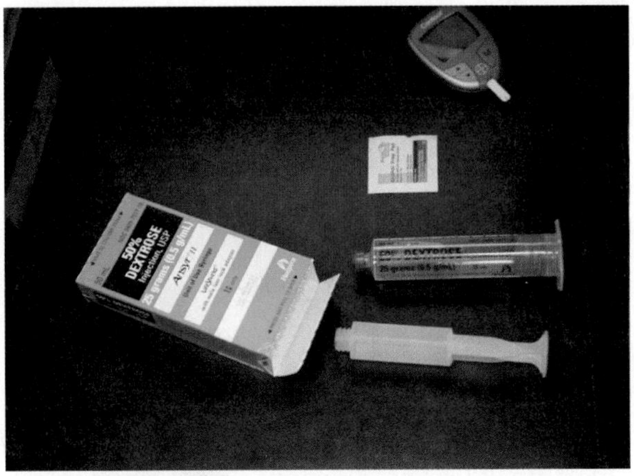

1. Assemble all of the equipment needed for the procedure.

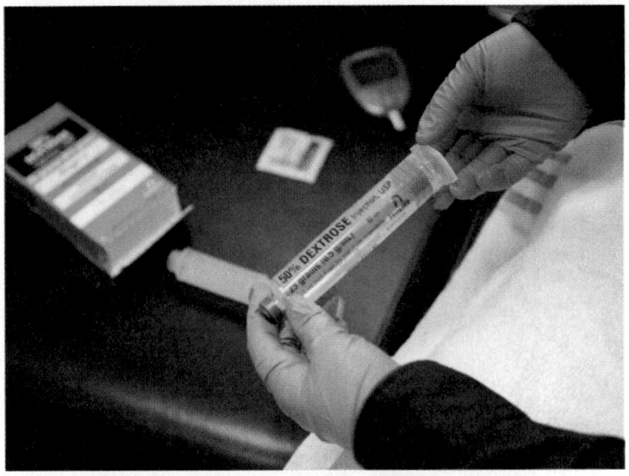

2. Verify the medication.

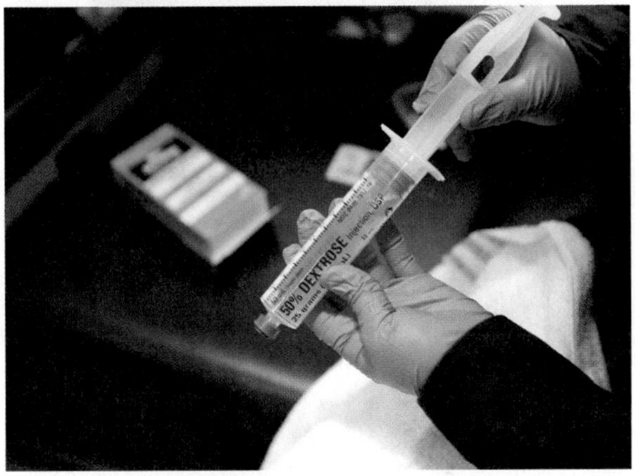

3. Prepare the medication syringe.

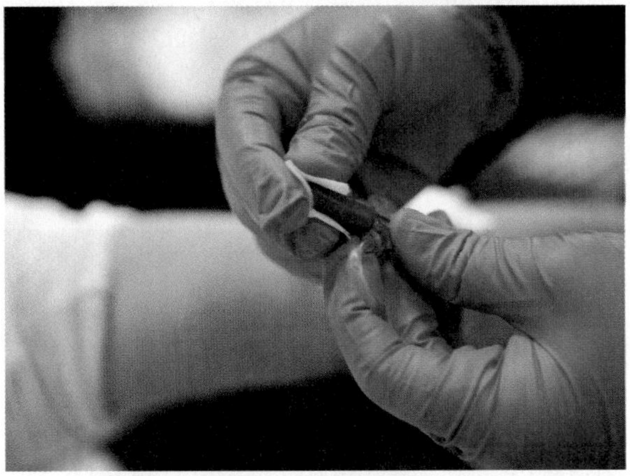

4. Clean the IV injection port with an alcohol swab.

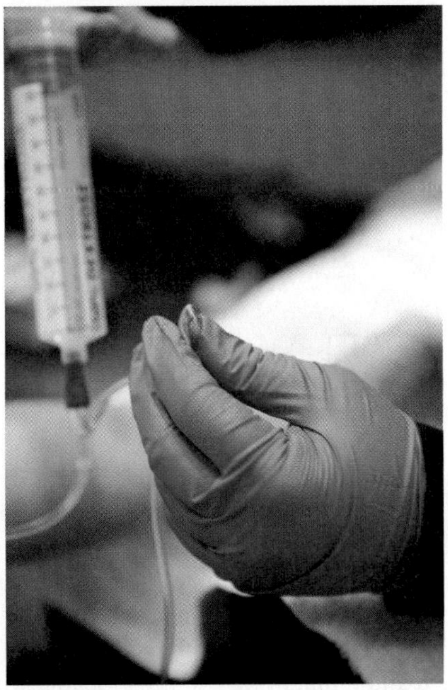

5. Attach the syringe to the injection port and crimp the IV tubing above the site of administration.

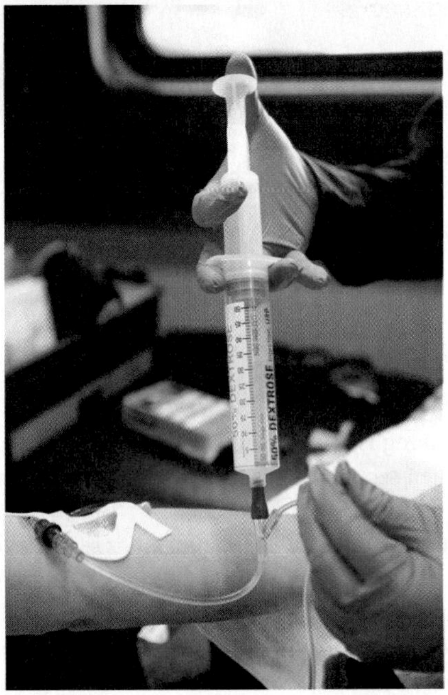

6. Inject the medication at the proper rate.

(continued)

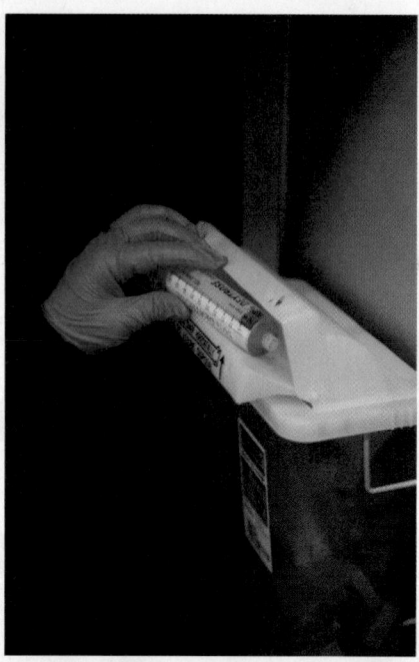

7. Discard the syringe in a sharps disposal container.

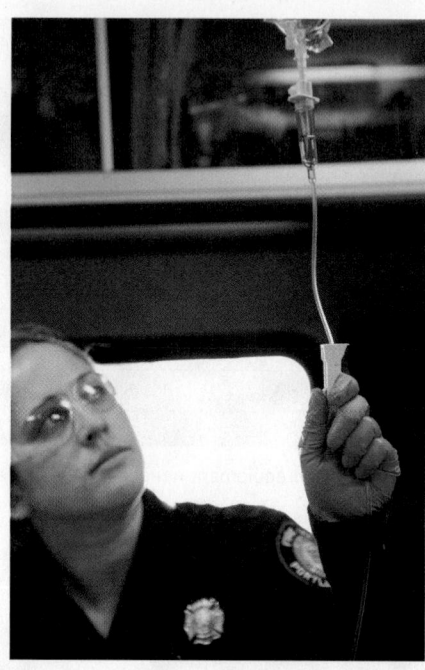

8. Flush the IV tubing and readjust the drip rate.

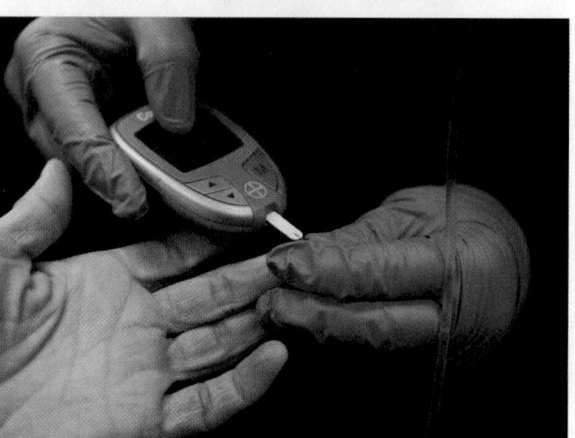

9. Reassess the patient.

wall of the vein and serves as a guide over which the flexible catheter is threaded into the vein. Once the catheter is positioned in the vein, the needle is removed and a saline lock or IV tubing is attached to the hub of the catheter. The catheter is then secured in place, allowing fluid infusion and medication administration as needed.

Whether a saline lock or IV infusion is selected depends on the patient's fluid needs. A saline lock is a convenient way to obtain access without administering fluids. If an IV infusion is selected, the type of fluid depends on the patients needs. Some EMS services carry only normal saline as an all-purpose fluid, while some may also carry lactated Ringer's solution and 5 percent dextrose solution. Follow your protocols regarding the selection of fluids.

Equipment for Establishing IV Access

As with any procedure, collect and organize the needed equipment before beginning the task of starting an IV. An IV tray or pack that contains all needed equipment and that is checked and restocked frequently makes preparing for the task much more efficient. In addition, commercially prepared IV start kits often contain all of the items needed except the IV needle/catheter combination and the saline lock or IV fluid and tubing. You will need the following:

- Gloves for Standard Precautions
- Venous constricting band

- Alcohol or povodine iodine swab
- Saline lock and saline flush or IV fluid bag and IV tubing
- Catheter-over-needle IV access device, such as an Angiocath
- Small gauze squares to control minor bleeding
- Commercial IV dressing (preferred) or 2 strips each ½ inch wide of adhesive tape and sterile gauze for dressing
- Adhesive tape (½- to 1-inch width torn into three or four 2- to 3-inch long pieces) to secure the IV tubing
- Antibiotic ointment
- Tincture of benzoin, which is helpful for securing IVs to diaphoretic skin

Catheter Size

IV needle/catheter combinations come in a variety of diameters and lengths. The catheter gauge is an even number, while its slightly smaller needle is an odd number. For example, a 14-gauge catheter is inserted over a 15-gauge needle. When documenting the IV initiation, always use the catheter size, including the gauge and length. IV catheters may be as small as 24 gauge, ¾ inch, or as large as 14 gauge. For 20-gauge and larger catheters, the 1¼-inch length should be used for IV access. Although 2-inch catheters are available, they create increased resistance to fluid flow. The 20- and 18-gauge catheters are suitable for routine IV access in adults. When medications will be given, use at least an 18-gauge catheter. When rapid infusion of fluids is required, use a 16-gauge or 14-gauge catheter. The 22-gauge and 24-gauge catheters should be reserved for patients who have extremely small diameter or fragile veins, making access with a larger catheter difficult.

Setting Up the IV Fluid and Tubing

Remember: IV fluids are medications. You must carefully check the IV fluid bag, just as you would a vial, ampule, prefilled syringe, or other medication container. Check the name of the fluid, check the expiration date, inspect the bag for damage or leakage, and observe the fluid for clarity, color, and any visible contaminants.

Open the packaging that contains the IV tubing and ensure that the roller clamp is turned off (rolled downward to crimp the tubing). Remove the seal from the port on the IV fluid bag, taking care that nothing comes in contact with the exposed port. Remove the cover from the spike on the IV tubing, making sure that nothing comes into contact with the exposed spike. Use a slight twisting motion to insert the spike into the port on the IV bag.

Squeeze the clear drip chamber on the IV tubing to fill it one-third to one-half full with IV fluid. Then, open the roller clamp to flush the IV tubing of air and fill it with fluid. If fluid does not flow, you may need to loosen the cap that covers the end of the tubing that connects to the IV catheter. However, do not allow the sterile portion of the tubing to come into contact with anything. Place the end of the tubing where it will be within your reach after you perform the **venipuncture.**

Selecting a Suitable Vein

Learning how to identify a suitable vein for IV access takes practice. Suitable veins for prehospital access are those in the back of the hand and forearm and in the **antecubital fossa** of the anterior elbow (Figure 12-15). Some EMS systems may allow Advanced EMTs to start IVs in the lower extremities (dorsum of the foot or ankle) or in the external jugular vein in the neck (a tourniquet is not used in this case). There is a higher rate of complication for lower extremity IVs and they should not be used if another site for venous access is available. If you are permitted to start external jugular IVs, you must be specifically trained in the procedure, because there are some special considerations.

A venous tourniquet is used to restrict venous return and engorge the veins to make them easier to find by both visualization and palpation (feeling the vein with your fingertips). Although the term *tourniquet* is frequently used, it is a misnomer. You should think of it as a venous constricting band. A common mistake in starting an IV is placing the constricting band too tightly. When the constricting band is too tight, it restricts arterial flow into the distal area, which, in turn, reduces the amount of blood that returns to the veins. A tight constricting band is unnecessarily painful for the patient and counterproductive to your goal of distending the veins.

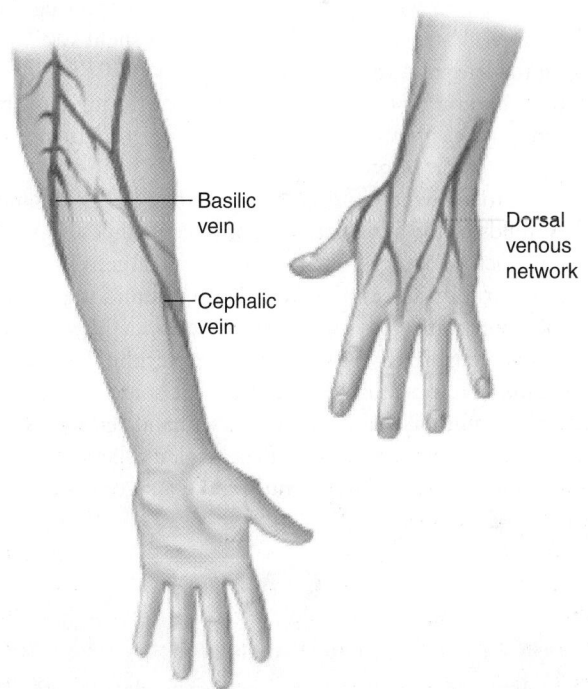

Basilic vein

Cephalic vein

Dorsal venous network

FIGURE 12-15

Sites for peripheral venous access.

Geriatric Care

With age, superficial veins often become more mobile as the surrounding connective tissue thins. Be sure to stabilize the vein above and below the puncture site to minimize movement of the vein when starting an IV.

You can use prominent, more superficial veins that are readily visible and deeper veins that may not be readily visible. Superficial veins, though easily seen, are more mobile and can move away as the tip of the needle makes contact with them. This can often be prevented by stabilizing the vein both above and below the site by placing the middle finger of your nondominant hand above the contemplated puncture site and your thumb below it. Superficial veins also tend to be more stable at the point of bifurcation, making bifurcations an option for IV placement.

Whether visible or only palpable deeper in the tissues, a suitable vein has a spongy, springy feeling on palpation. However, if the vessel you are palpating has a pulse (meaning you are palpating an artery, not a vein) or there is a pulse very close to it, you must not insert the needle at that location. The anatomical location of arteries is more predictable than that of veins. Knowledge of the anatomical location of superficial arteries, such as the radial and brachial arteries, helps you avoid inadvertent arterial puncture. Also keep in mind that arteries are deeper in the tissues, so keep the needle at a lower angle (less than 45 degrees) when inserting it to avoid arterial puncture.

Remember that veins have valves to prevent retrograde blood flow. Valves can sometimes be seen as slight swellings along the length of the vein. Avoid starting an IV too close to the valve on its distal side; the IV catheter may not be able to pass easily through the valve when you attempt to thread the catheter into the vein.

In patients who require or may require larger volumes of IV fluids or the administration of large volumes of medication (such as 50 percent dextrose), use a larger vein, such as a forearm or antecubital vein. Keep in mind that an IV in the antecubital fossa may become occluded by the patient's movement. If you must use an antecubital vein and occlusion becomes a problem, use a short board splint (arm board) to immobilize the elbow. Dorsal hand veins are suitable IV sites for many patients. In general, it is better to start the IV more distally. If you must make a second attempt,

Pediatric Care

Antecubital veins are often the most suitable for IV placement in pediatric patients, but an arm board will be required to immobilize the elbow.

you can do so more proximally so that IV fluid will not flow through the site of venous injury.

Performing the Venipuncture

After disinfecting the site, hold the IV needle at a 45-degree angle or less to the skin with the bevel up. Another common mistake when starting an IV is to hold the IV needle at too steep an angle to the skin. A 30-degree angle allows a better chance of entering the vein without skimming along the top of it, yet decreases the chances that the needle will pierce both sides of the vein. Line up the direction of the needle with the direction of the vein. (See Scan 12-6.)

The tip of the needle is very sharp, requiring only gentle force to puncture the skin and underlying tissue. As you enter the lumen of the vein, you may feel a sudden decrease in resistance. When the tip of the needle enters the vein, blood flows through the needle and into a small, clear chamber at the back of the needle. This is called "getting a flash."

Once you see blood in the flash chamber, lower the angle of the needle until it is almost flush with the skin and advance the needle and catheter as a single unit about 1 to 2 mm further into the vein to ensure that the end of the catheter is within the lumen of the vein. Then, hold the needle in place and slide the catheter over it into the vein. Advance the catheter until its hub rests against the skin.

Never pull the catheter back over the needle or advance the needle through the catheter. Those actions can cause the sharp tip of the needle to shear off the flexible catheter, creating an embolus that can travel through the venous system. If you cannot thread the catheter completely into the vein, do not force it. In such cases you must withdraw both the catheter and needle and discontinue the IV attempt at that site. Release the tourniquet, hold a gauze square over the entry site, pull out the catheter and needle as a single unit, and apply pressure to the site. Dispose of the IV needle in a sharps collection container.

Once you have completely threaded the catheter into the vein, immediately release the constricting band. Use a fingertip to apply pressure to the vein proximal to the end of the catheter to occlude blood flow, then withdraw the needle and dispose of it in a sharps disposal container.

Keeping your fingertip on the vein to occlude it, use your other hand to connect the saline lock or IV tubing. Remove your fingertip from the vein and flush the saline lock or IV tubing to clear the catheter of blood and to check the patency of the IV. Observe for tissue swelling, which indicates **infiltration** of the tissues with intravenous fluid. If the IV is patent, secure it and, if you have connected an IV line, adjust the drip rate. If the IV fluid does not flow freely, check for infiltration and make sure you have removed the constricting band. Also make sure that all clamps on the tubing are open, that the patient's arm or hand position is not occluding the flow, and that the IV bag is above the level of the patient's heart. If the IV is infiltrated, discontinue the IV immediately.

If blood backs up into the tubing rapidly, suspect that you may have inadvertently **cannulated** an artery.

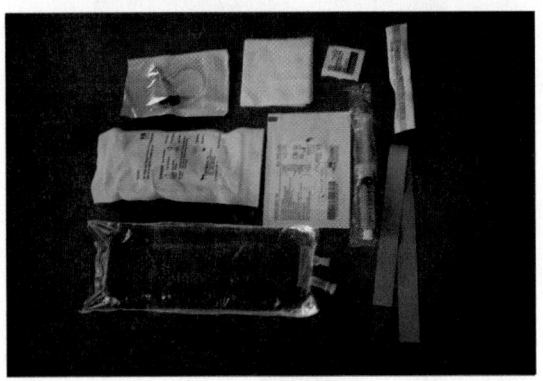

1. Prepare all of the necessary equipment before beginning the procedure.

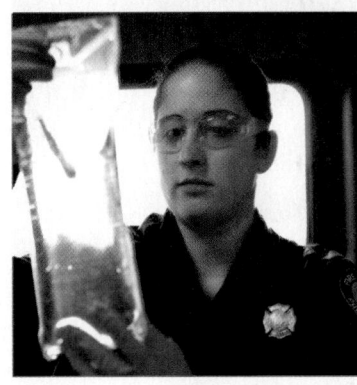

2. Check the name of the fluid, inspect it for clarity, and ensure that it is not expired.

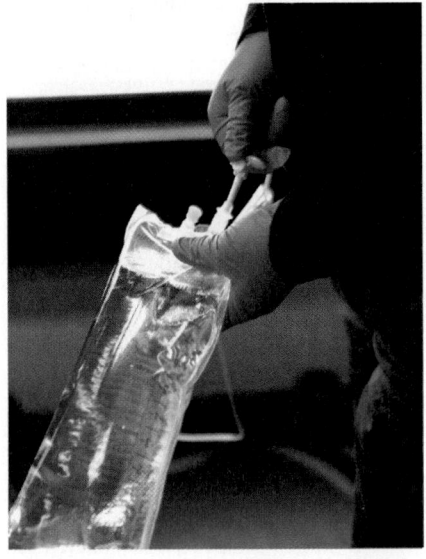

3. Insert the spike of the IV tubing into the fluid bag and squeeze the drip chamber, then allow it to fill about one third of the way.

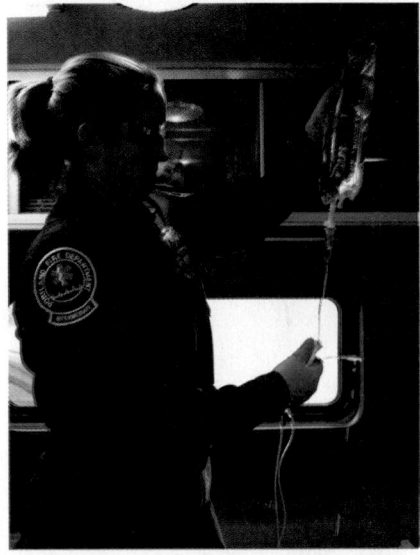

4. Open the roller clamp and allow the fluid to fill the tubing, ensuring that all air bubbles are expelled from the tubing.

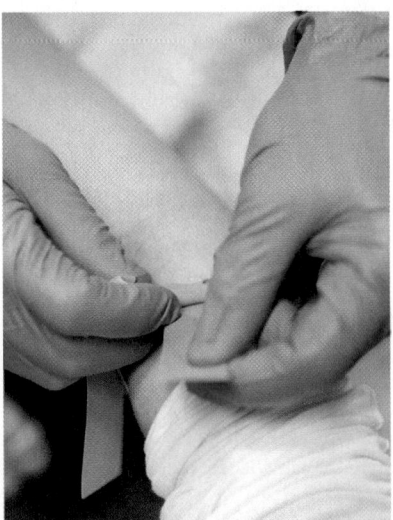

5. Apply a venous constricting band above the venipuncture site.

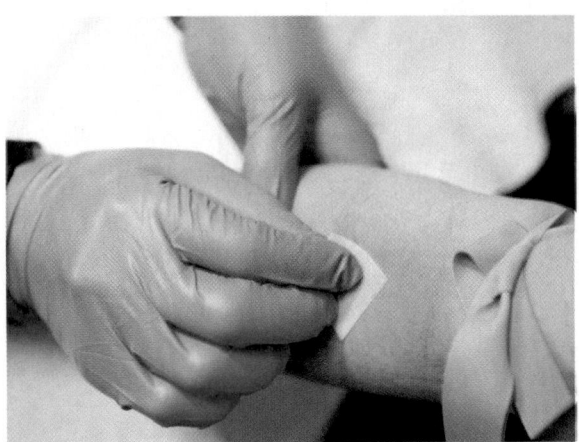

6. Disinfect the venipuncture site using aseptic technique.

(continued)

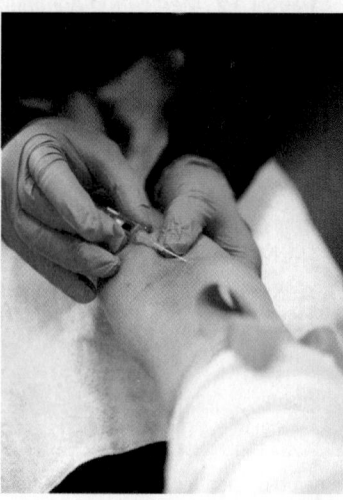

7. Stabilize the skin. Holding the IV access device bevel up at no higher than a 45-degree angle, insert the tip of the needle into the vein and advance it until blood is seen in the flash chamber.

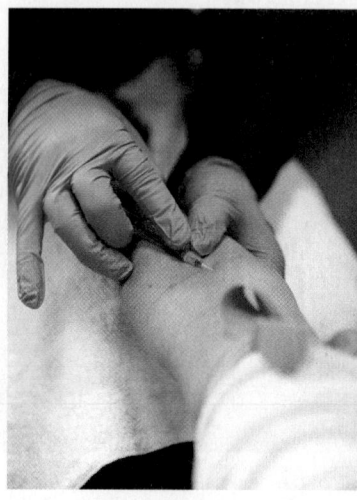

8. When flashback occurs, advance the device 1 to 2 mL further. Stop advancing the needle and push the catheter over the needle until the hub is in contact with the patient's skin.

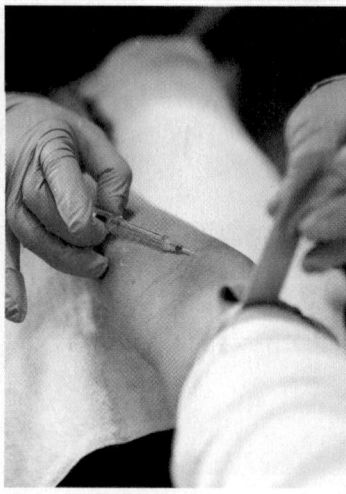

9. Release the constricting band.

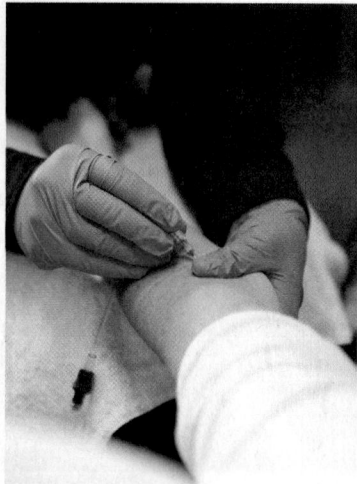

10. Occlude the vein above the end of the catheter. Withdraw the needle and discard it in a sharps disposal container. Connect the IV tubing to the catheter hub. Wipe any blood from the site using a gauze square.

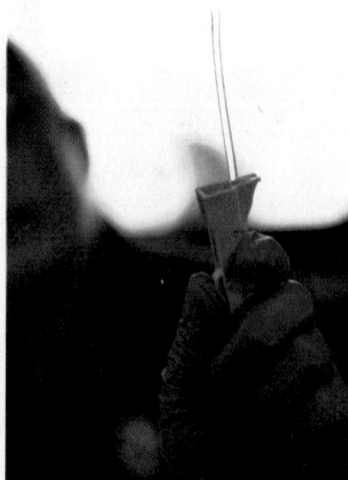

11. Flush the tubing, check the site for infiltration, and adjust the flow of fluid to the desired rate.

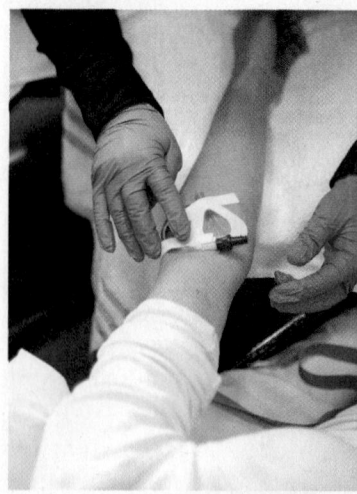

12. Use a commercial dressing to protect the site and secure the tubing in place with tape.

Discontinue the IV immediately and apply pressure to the site to control bleeding. If smaller amounts of dark red blood are seen in the IV tubing, ensure the IV bag is above the level of the patient's heart and open up the roller clamp to flush the blood through the line.

Unsuccessful IV Attempts and Discontinuing IV Therapy

In some cases, an IV attempt will not be successful. This may happen if the vein moves away from the needle, or the needle punctures both sides of the vein, the catheter meets resistance from a valve, or the angle of insertion is wrong. If you make an unsuccessful IV attempt, you must remove the IV needle/catheter combination and dispose of it safely and apply pressure to the site.

If the vein moves or the angle or insertion is wrong, you may pull the needle/catheter combination back slightly as a unit, keeping the tip of the needle in the skin, and redirect the tip of the needle. Keep in mind that attempts to reposition the needle are painful for the patient and increase tissue damage. Do not make repeated attempts to reposition the needle. In such cases, it is better to abandon the attempt and start over. If you pull the tip of the needle out of the skin, do not reinsert it through the skin. Discard the device and start over.

In a patient with fragile veins or blood clotting disorders, in patients taking anticoagulants, or when the venous tourniquet is too tight, blood may escape rapidly under the skin when the vein is punctured by the needle, causing a hematoma. The IV usually is not patent in such cases. Remove the needle/catheter combination as a unit, apply pressure to the site, and start over.

If an IV must be discontinued after the tubing is connected, always begin by closing the roller clamp or clamp on a saline lock to prevent leakage of contaminated fluid when the catheter is removed. Do not disconnect the tubing from the IV, because this will cause blood to flow out of the catheter. Remove the IV dressing and tape on the tubing. Place a small gauze square over the insertion site and grasp the catheter by the hub. Smoothly pull the catheter out of the skin and apply pressure with the gauze square. When bleeding has stopped, apply an adhesive bandage. Discard the contaminated catheter and tubing in a biohazard collection bag.

Changing an IV Bag

When large volumes of fluid are administered or when transport times are long, you may need to replace the original bag of IV fluid with a fresh one as the amount gets low. It is preferable to change the bag when a few milliliters of fluid are left in the bag, rather than allowing it to empty completely, which allows the residual air in the bag to enter the IV tubing. Although pressure from the venous system keeps the fluid in the tubing from emptying into the vein,

when a new bag of fluid is placed, the residual air will flow through the tubing as fluid from the bag begins to move through it.

When the first IV bag is nearly empty, close the roller clamp to prevent further fluid from entering the tubing and to prevent air from entering the tubing when you remove the spike from the IV bag. Have the new bag of fluid ready, because you will need to hold the tubing in one hand, making it difficult to prepare the new bag after you remove the old one from the tubing. Hold the empty bag upside down. Pull on the tubing just above the drip chamber to remove the spike from the bag. Spike the new bag and make sure the drip chamber is one-third to one-half full. Readjust the flow rate.

Complications of IV Therapy

There are several potential complications of intravenous access and fluid administration. They include infection, infiltration, air or catheter embolism, bruising or hematoma, thrombosis, phlebitis, **pyrogenic reaction**, and fluid overload.

Infection is a risk of any percutaneous procedure. Sick and injured patients are more susceptible to infection than healthy individuals and can develop phlebitis and sepsis from IV catheter–associated infections. If the infectious organism is antibiotic resistant, it is very difficult to treat. You can reduce the risk of infection by doing the following:

- Using proper aseptic technique to disinfect the IV puncture site
- Ensuring that your hands are clean and that you are wearing clean gloves
- Not touching the puncture site after disinfecting it or after completing the procedure
- Applying antibiotic ointment
- Using a transparent commercial IV dressing
- Preventing sterile portions of equipment (IV needle and catheter, IV tubing spike and connection, IV bag port) from being contaminated during the procedure, and replacing any equipment that becomes contaminated
- Carefully checking the expiration date of the IV fluid and checking for indications of contamination of the fluid

Infiltration occurs when the vein is injured, allowing IV fluid to leak from the vein and into the surrounding tissues. Infiltration causes pain and swelling of the tissue, and the IV will not flow freely. The affected area is firm and cool to the touch. Extravasated hypertonic IV fluids and some medications (such as 50 percent dextrose and vasopressors) can cause tissue necrosis. If signs of infiltration are present, discontinue the IV.

Air embolism may occur if there are large amounts of air in the IV tubing. When setting up the IV, always flush the IV tubing with fluid. It is not possible to remove all tiny bubbles from the tubing, but they are not harmful. Catheter shear may result in a piece of the intravenous catheter entering the circulation. Once you have advanced the catheter over the needle, never pull the catheter back over the needle or insert the needle back through the catheter.

Bruising and hematoma occur more easily in patients with fragile veins (such as the elderly), patients taking corticosteroids (such as prednisone) or anticoagulants (such as warfarin [Coumadin]), and those with blood clotting disorders (such as liver disease and hemophilia). However, a traumatic IV attempt can result in bruising or hematoma in any patient. Apply pressure to stop bleeding.

Phlebitis is an inflammation of the vein, which can be caused by infection or from the administration of irritating IV fluids or medications. Thrombophlebitis occurs when the clotting cascade is activated by the inflammatory process, resulting in occlusion of the vein. The area will be painful, tender, red, and warm to the touch. The IV should be discontinued.

Pyrogens are any foreign proteins capable of causing fever, and can be found in contaminated IV fluid or equipment. A pyrogenic reaction produces a sudden fever, chills, backache, headache, nausea, and vomiting. Shock also can occur. Discontinue the IV if a pyrogenic reaction occurs. Start another IV, preferably with equipment and fluid from a different lot number than those originally used.

Fluid overload is a potential complication in any patient receiving IV fluids. Some patients, such as those with heart failure, the elderly, and pediatric patients, are at greater risk. Always calculate the infusion rate accurately and monitor the rate of the IV infusion carefully to prevent fluid overload. Check for signs of fluid overload in your reassessment. Shortness of breath and the presence of crackles (rales) on auscultation of the lung sounds indicate significant fluid load.

Pediatric Intraosseous Access

Intravenous access can be difficult in some patients, especially those who are critically ill or injured. If a patient requires immediate access to the circulatory system, but an IV cannot be obtained, intraosseous (IO) access is an alternative. Your standing orders likely specify the maximum number (usually two in pediatric patients) of IV attempts allowed in critical patients before IO access should be considered. Pediatric IO access is in the Advanced EMT Scope of Practice Model. In some services, you also may be permitted to perform adult IO access. (See Appendix 3.)

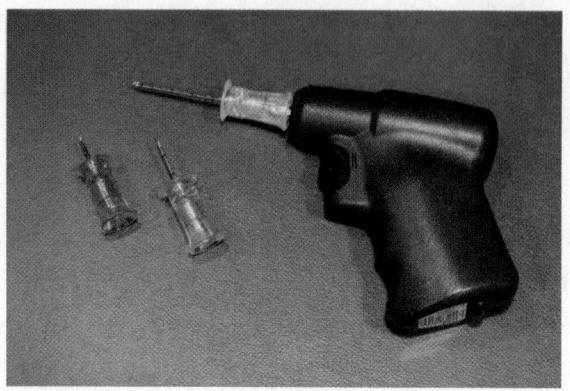

FIGURE 12-16

EZ IO device. Different sized needles are available for some devices. Shown here is a bariatric needle (yellow), a standard adult needle (blue), and a pediatric needle (red).

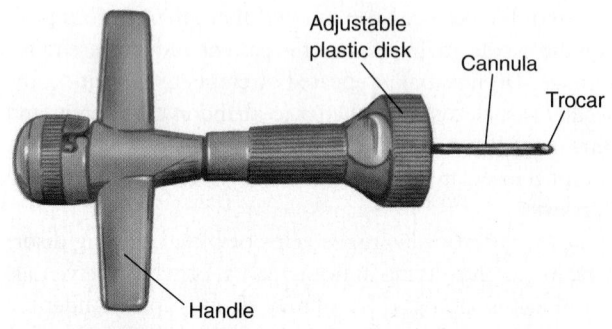

Adjustable plastic disk

Cannula

Trocar

Handle

FIGURE 12-17

A manual intraosseous needle.

The easiest way to obtain IO access is with a commercial device that uses battery power or a spring-loaded mechanism. Two devices approved for pediatric use are the EZ IO (Vidacare) device (shown in Scan 12-7) and the Bone Injection Gun, or BIG (WaisMed) device (Figure 12-16). Manual access is possible, but difficult (Figure 12-17). The proximal tibia is the preferred site of access for pediatric IO infusion. The distal tibia may be used in older children.

Conditions that contraindicate IO infusion include fracture of the extremity, previous IO attempt or placement in the same bone, and the bone disease *osteogenesis imperfecta* (a congenital bone disease that occurs in about 1 of 20,000 live births), osteoporosis, and infection over the site of insertion. Do not place an IO device through burned tissue unless

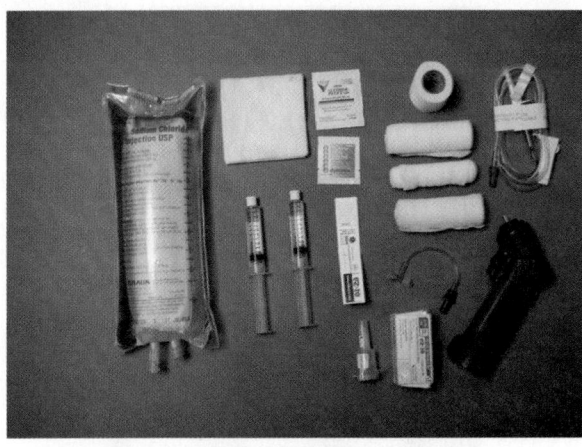

1. Assemble all needed equipment. Set up an IV line and prefill the extension tubing provided with the saline. Leave the syringe attached to the tubing.

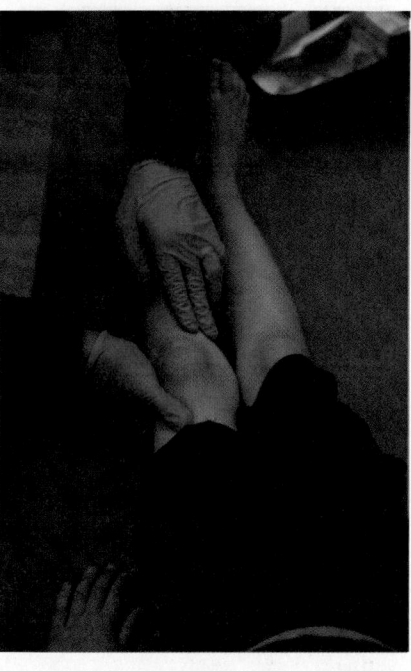

2. Find the proper insertion site, two fingerbreadths below the tibial tuberosity along the anteriomedial surface.

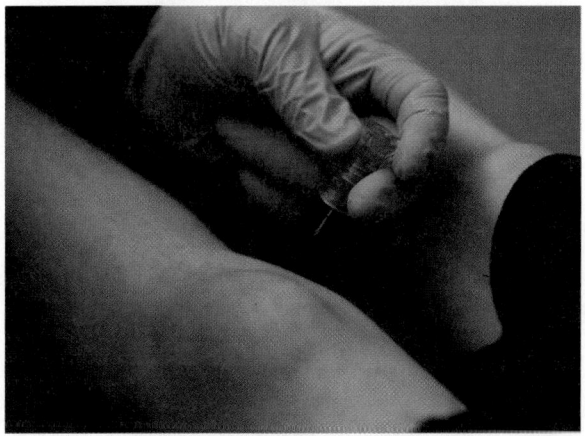

3. Ensure the correct needle length for the size of the patient.

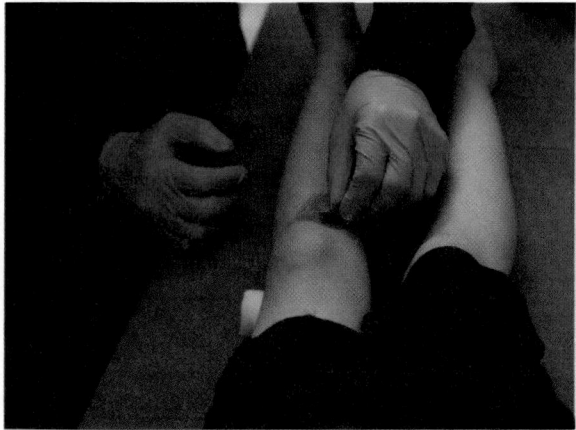

4. Prepare the site with a povidone iodine swab.

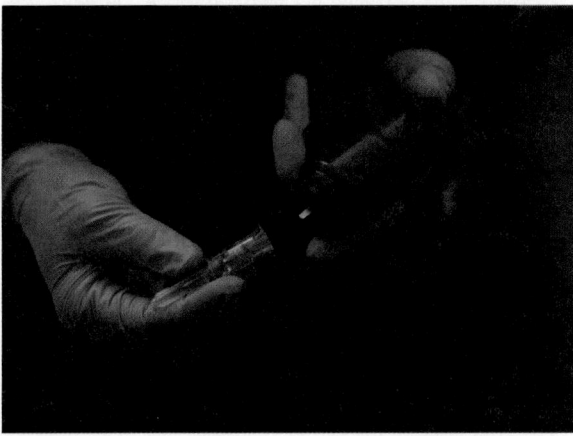

5. Place the needle on the driver.

(continued)

Pediatric Intraosseous Access Using the EZ IO Device (continued)

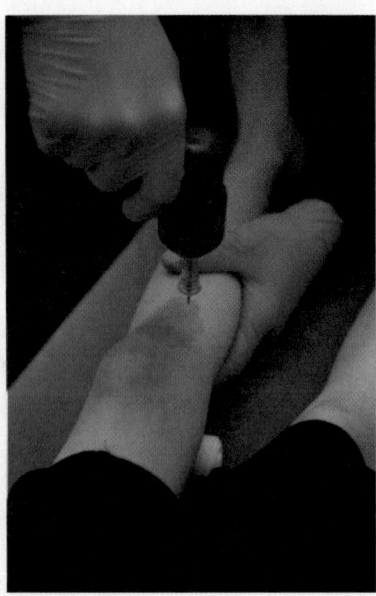

6. Hold the driver at a 90-degree angle to the leg and drill the needle into the bone.

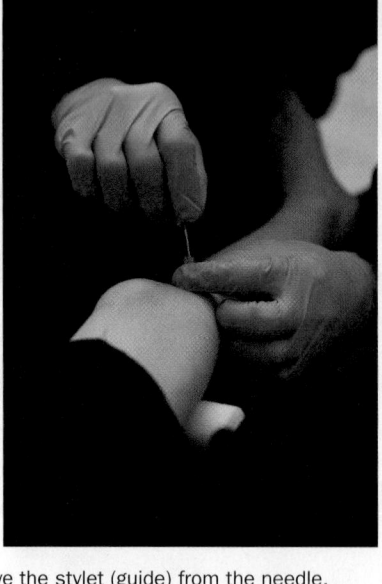

7. Remove the stylet (guide) from the needle.

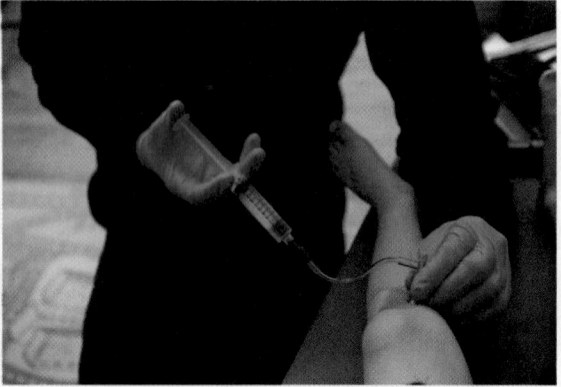

8. Attach the tubing prefilled with normal saline and flush the needle. Observe for free flow of fluid and absence of infiltration into the soft tissues.

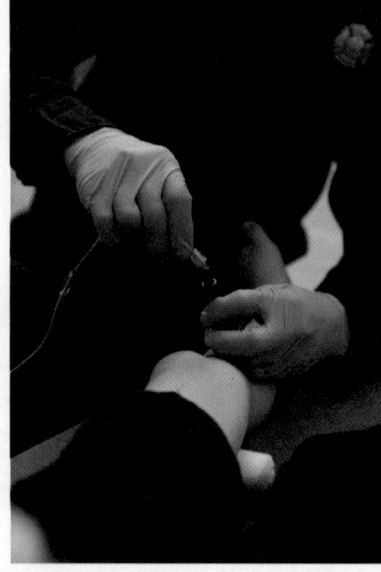

9. Attach the IV tubing to the extension tubing and adjust the flow rate.

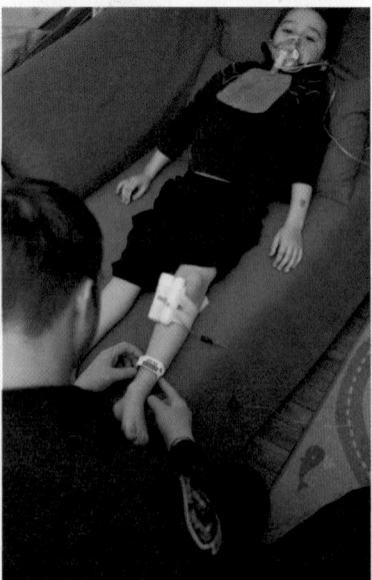

10. Secure the needle and tubing and attach the information band to the extremity.

there are no other options. Do not attempt to place an IO device if you cannot locate the anatomical landmarks. Complications of IO attempts and IO access include the following:

- Incorrect placement due to incorrect identification of landmarks

- Obstruction of the needle with bone marrow, a blood clot, or bone fragments

- Fracture, from excessive force or bone disorders

- Infection of the superficial tissues (cellulitis) or bone (osteomyelitis)

- Compartment syndrome (accumulation of fluid in the muscle compartment caused by infusion of fluid into a damaged bone)

- Possible fat embolus

Begin the procedure by collecting and organizing all needed equipment and setting up an intravenous line. You will need a manual IO needle, or the needle supplied with a commercial insertion device. You also need a saline lock, or similar piece of equipment supplied with the IO device. An empty syringe is used to aspirate bone marrow to check for correct placement, although it is common that no marrow can be aspirated, even when placement is correct. A syringe filled with sterile saline is used to flush the needle after placement.

You also will need gloves for Standard Precautions, an antiseptic to disinfect the skin, gauze squares to stabilize the needle in place, scissors, and tape.

To locate the anatomical landmarks for proximal tibial insertion, the patient's knee should be slightly flexed. Use one hand to stabilize the lower leg. Locate the tibial tuberosity, the prominence on the anterior tibia just below the knee (Figure 12-18). The insertion site is two fingerbreadths (one fingerbreadth in infants) below the tibial tuberosity on the anteromedial aspect of the tibia. Use povidone iodine to disinfect the skin (Scan 12-7).

The needle is then inserted manually or with a commercial device, following the manufacturer's directions. Once you have confirmed placement and you have flushed the needle and begun the infusion, stabilize the needle in place with gauze squares and tape. You can administer medications in the same manner as for IV injection.

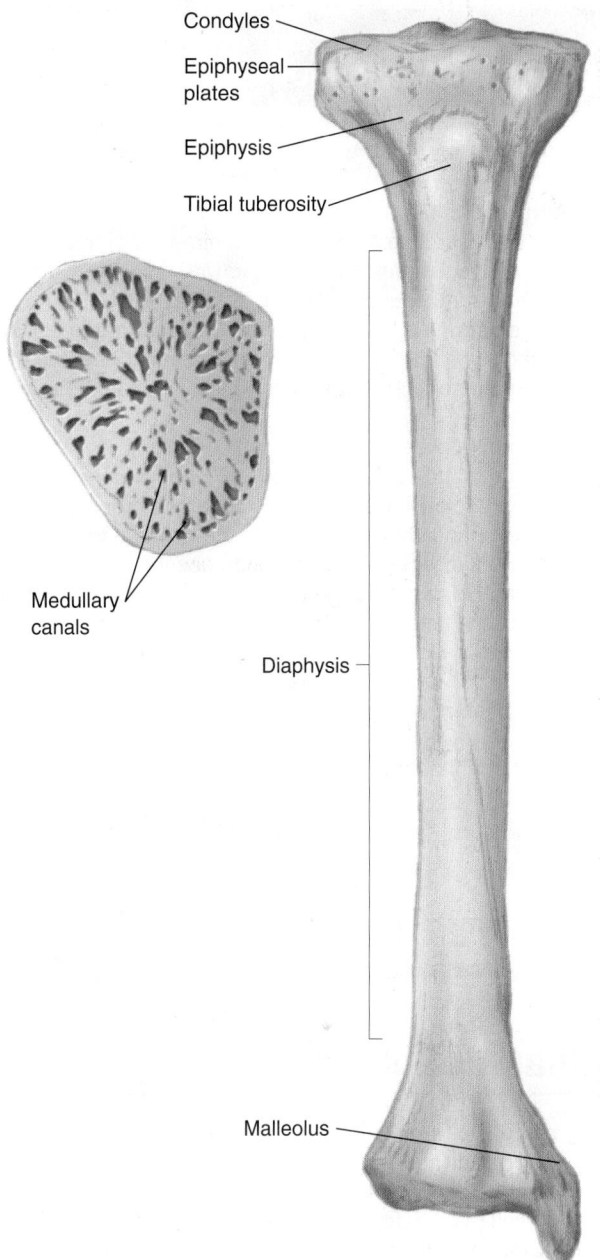

FIGURE 12-18

Anatomy of the tibia.

CASE STUDY WRAP-UP

Clinical-Reasoning Process

Advanced EMTs Loretta and Grant are at the scene of an unresponsive female whom they suspect is suffering from a narcotic overdose. According to their standing orders, they can administer 2 mg of naloxone intravenously for patients with suspected narcotic overdose with respiratory depression.

Grant anticipates potential difficulty in starting an IV because of the patient's scarring from past IV drug abuse. As he sets up his equipment, he decides to use a 16-gauge, 1¼-inch catheter because the sturdier needle is better suited to penetrate scar tissue. The patient needs a route for medication administration, but has no immediate needs for fluids, so he decides to use a saline lock, rather than an IV fluid infusion. He collects, organizes, and prepares his equipment.

Grant applies a venous constricting band just above the patient's elbow and begins searching for a suitable vein. He realizes that the patient has mostly used superficial veins for injection, so he palpates to feel for deeper veins. He finds one just below the antecubital fossa and prepares the site with povidone iodine. As the site dries, he selects a vial of naloxone and checks it carefully. He hands it to Loretta so she can confirm the medication.

After successfully placing and securing the saline lock, Grant calculates the medication dosage and verifies it with Loretta. He draws up the naloxone in a syringe administers it by slow IV push using a needleless system. He makes a note of the time of administration and begins monitoring the patient for the effect of the drug as he and Loretta prepare her for transportation to the closest emergency department.

After the call, Grant carefully documents his assessment and treatment, including the details of the IV and medication administration and his reassessment findings.

CHAPTER REVIEW

Chapter Summary

Advanced EMTs can administer several beneficial, potentially lifesaving medications under medical direction. Administering medications comes with tremendous responsibility for patient safety. Following safety principles, including the Six Rights of Medication Administration, is a professional obligation you have to your patients. You must ensure that the medication is indicated for the patient and that it is not contraindicated and that you are giving the right medication to the right patient. Carefully calculate and verify drug dosages and select the proper route of administration. Administer medications at the right time and rate and document the details of medication administration in your patient care report. If required, obtain the physician's signature for drug orders.

You can take many other steps to improve patient safety. Use aseptic technique to minimize the risk of infection when performing percutaneous procedures. Select the proper equipment and techniques for medication administration tasks. Know how to troubleshoot problems and actively look for signs of complications during reassessment.

By upholding professional standards for medication administration, you provide patients with the best chances for recovery with the least risk of complications and errors.

Review Questions

Multiple-Choice Questions

1. Which one of the following is an enteral route of medication administration?

   a. Intraosseous
   b. Inhalation
   c. Oral
   d. Intramuscular

2. You receive an order to give a medication PO. How should you administer the medication?

   a. By mouth
   b. Under the tongue
   c. Through a needle in the bone
   d. By applying it topically

3. Of the following routes of medication administration, which one allows the fastest onset of action?
   a. Sublingual
   b. Subcutaneous
   c. Intramuscular
   d. Intravenous

4. One liter is equal to _____ milliliters.
   a. 10
   b. 100
   c. 1,000
   d. 10,000

5. A patient weighs 185 pounds. This means he weighs _____ kilograms.
   a. 84
   b. 93
   c. 125
   d. 370

6. You receive an order to give 0.5 mg of epinephrine 1:1,000 intramuscularly. The drug is supplied in 1-mL ampules in a concentration of 1 mg/mL. You should give _____ mL of the drug.
   a. 0.05
   b. 0.5
   c. 5
   d. 50

7. What is the amount of drug contained in 5 mL of a 10-percent solution?
   a. 100 milligrams
   b. 500 milligrams
   c. 1 gram
   d. 5 grams

8. Standing orders allow you to give 0.01 mg/kg of epinephrine 1:1,000 for pediatric patients with anaphylaxis. How much drug should be given to a 60-pound patient?
   a. 2.7 mg
   b. 0.27 mg
   c. 1.3 mg
   d. 0.13 mg

9. You are going to start an IV and administer lactated Ringer's solution at a rate of 75 mL/hour using a 20-gtts/mL tubing set. What is the drip rate in gtts/minute?
   a. 25
   b. 50
   c. 75
   d. 100

10. You receive an order to give 2 L of normal saline over 3 hours. What is the drip rate using 10-gtts/mL tubing?
    a. 333
    b. 167
    c. 111
    d. 56

11. You have calculated a drip rate of 45 gtts/minute. How many drops should be counted in 15 seconds?
    a. 6
    b. 11
    c. 23
    d. 30

12. Which one of the following needles are most appropriate for a subcutaneous injection?
    a. 18 gauge, 1½ inches
    b. 21 gauge, 1¼ inches
    c. 23 gauge, 1 inch
    d. 25 gauge, ¾ inch

13. You have just started an IV. The IV fluid will drip and the area around the insertion site is swollen, firm, and cool to the touch. There is no discoloration. The findings described are most consistent with:
    a. pyrogenic reaction.
    b. hematoma.
    c. phlebitis.
    d. infiltration.

14. A patient needs a rapid infusion of 500 mL of fluid. Of the following, which IV catheter is best suited for this purpose?
    a. 20 gauge, 1¼ inches
    b. 20 gauge, 2 inches
    c. 16 gauge, 1¼ inches
    d. 16 gauge, 2 inches

15. The preferred site of intraosseous placement in pediatric patients is the:
    a. proximal tibia.
    b. distal tibia.
    c. proximal humerus.
    d. distal humerus.

Critical-Thinking Questions

16. Explain how the medication safety principle of "right patient" applies in prehospital care.

17. You received an order to give 12.5 grams of 50 percent dextrose intravenously, but inadvertently gave 25 grams.

You immediately realize you have made an error. What should you do?

18. You have started an IV but the IV fluid will not drip. Explain your process of troubleshooting the problem.

References

Hughes, R. G., & Blegen, M. A. (2008). Medication administration safety. In R. G. Hughes (Ed.), Patient safety and quality: An evidence-based handbook for nurses (pp. 2-397–2-457). Rockville, MD: Agency for Healthcare Research and Quality.

Additional Reading

Bledsoe, B. E., Porter, R. S., & Cherry, R. A. (2009). *Paramedic care: Principles and practice* (3rd ed., Vol. 1). Upper Saddle River, NJ: Pearson.

Franscone, R. J., Jensen, J., Wewerka, S. S., & Salzman, J. G. (2009). Use of the pediatric EZ-IO needle by emergency medical services providers. *Pediatric Emergency Care 25*(5), 329–332.

13 Medications

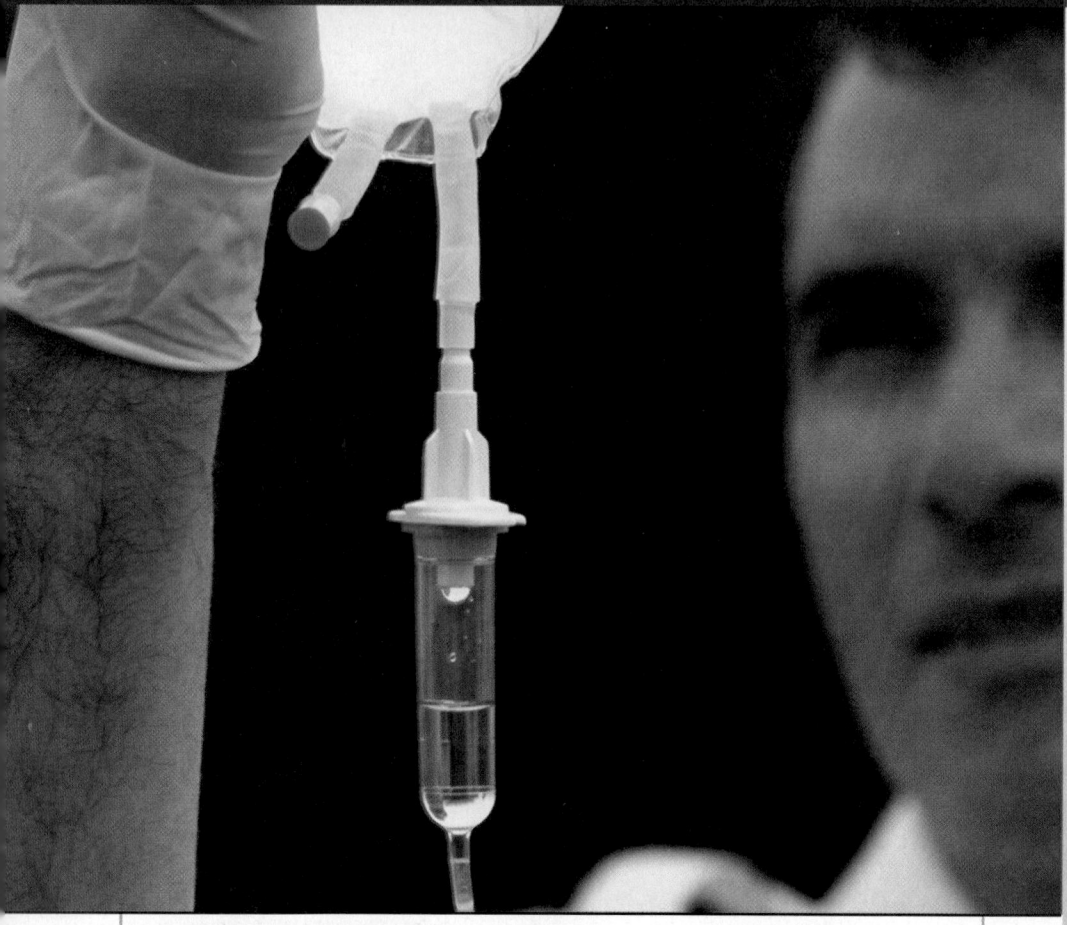

Content Area: Pharmacology

Advanced EMT Education Standard: Applies fundamental knowledge of medications in the Advanced EMT scope of practice to patient assessment and management.

Objectives

After reading this chapter, you should be able to:

13.1   Define key terms introduced in this chapter.

13.2   Describe the drug profiles for each of the following medications:

- acetaminophen
- activated charcoal
- aspirin
- dextrose 50 percent, 25 percent, and 10 percent for treating hypoglycemia, and 5 percent in water for intravenous infusion
- epinephrine, 1:1,000
- glucagon
- ibuprofen

(continued)

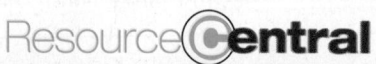

Resource**Central**

CASE STUDY

Advanced EMTs David Babin and Christy Trammel are in the ambulance bay at Mercy Hospital getting their ambulance ready for their next call when dispatch calls. "Unit 3, respond to 2410 University Blvd. for an unconscious person," says the dispatcher. After verifying the location of the call, David jumps in the driver's seat as Christy finds the address on a map.

They arrive at the location, a residence in an affluent part of town. As Christy tells dispatch they have arrived on scene, David grabs their gear and starts toward the house with Christy following. As they reach the front porch, a woman meets them and says, "I just came home from work and I can't wake up my son."

A male patient about 20 years old is lying prone on the couch. Christy asks the patient's mother if he has any medical conditions or takes prescription medications. She tells Christy that her son does not have any medical conditions and has not taken any prescriptions that she knows of since he had the flu six months ago.

After placing the patient in a supine position and using a head-tilt/chin-lift maneuver to open the airway, David continues the assessment. He points out to Christy that the patient's pupils are constricted. The patient responds to a painful stimulus by groaning. The patient's vital signs are as follows: blood pressure 94/64; heart rate 70, slightly weak, but regular; respiration 10, shallow, nonlabored; SpO_2 94 percent on room air.

Problem-Solving Questions

1. What are some initial hypotheses about causes of the patient's condition?
2. What additional information would assist David and Christy in determining the cause of the patient's condition?
3. What treatments should David and Christy implement as they continue their assessment?

(continued from previous page)

- inhaled beta$_2$ agonists
- lactated Ringer's solution for intravenous infusion
- naloxone
- nitroglycerin tablets and spray
- nitrous oxide
- oral glucose
- other isotonic intravenous solutions as allowed by medical direction
- oxygen
- sodium chloride solution 0.9 percent for intravenous infusion

Introduction

Advanced EMTs administer a limited number of medications to patients, but those medications are potent and must be administered only for the purposes intended and by the appropriate route. Safe medication administration includes knowing key information about each drug you administer. That key information is organized into a drug profile. However, a drug profile does not contain all of the information that is known about a drug. Therefore, do not hesitate to contact medical direction for guidance when needed. The drugs in the profiles in this chapter are commonly carried by EMS agencies for use by Advanced EMTs, but you must only administer medications approved by your medical director. Individual states, municipalities, and agencies may allow Advanced EMTs to use medications not included here.

Medications in Patient Care

Medications are part of your supplies and equipment for patient care and they must be inventoried at the beginning of each shift. During this process, you will account for each medication listed in your inventory and ensure that all medications are available in the required amounts and that they are not expired.

Before you can safely administer any medication, you must know the indications, contraindications, mechanism of action, correct dose, expected effects, side effects, and any special considerations applicable to the medication. You will use some medications more frequently than others and will therefore remain more familiar with them. Others will not be used as frequently and you might become less familiar with them over time. To remain knowledgeable about every medication that you are allowed to administer, you must review medication information from time to time.

Always perform a patient assessment and take a history to determine whether a drug is indicated and whether there are any contraindications to administering the drug. A known drug allergy to the intended drug is always a contraindication.

Once a medication is administered, you cannot take it back! Always calculate and prepare the dosage carefully. Follow the proper procedure for administering medications in order to prevent errors that could be detrimental to your patient's condition.

IV Solutions

Intravenous fluids are medications that have indications, contraindications, and side effects, as well as other properties and effects of which you must be aware. The two general indications for obtaining IV access in the prehospital setting are to replace lost circulatory volume from blood loss, burns, and dehydration and to establish a route for administration of medications. In patients who require access for medication administration but who do not require intravenous fluids, you can use a saline lock. If you administer IV fluids, the type of fluid selected depends on the patient's condition. In many cases, 0.9 percent sodium chloride solution (normal saline) is satisfactory for short-term use in the prehospital setting. In fact, many EMS protocols specify normal saline except in special circumstances.

Normal saline is a crystalloid solution. A **crystalloid** solution contains water and electrolytes, and in some cases, dextrose. Crystalloid solutions may be **hypotonic, isotonic,** or **hypertonic** with respect to body fluids. Isotonic fluids, given in therapeutic amounts, do not cause significant fluid or electrolyte shifts in patients with normal fluid status. However, in patients with blood loss, only about one third of the fluid is still in the vascular space 1 hour after it is administered. Isotonic crystalloid solutions are preferred for fluid replacement in the prehospital setting. The volume of fluid infused is guided by the patient's condition and current evidence about the role of fluid replacement for various conditions. For patients with blood loss, remember that IV fluids do not correct the oxygen-carrying deficit caused by the loss of red blood cells.

Hypertonic fluids cause water to leave the cells and enter the vascular space. The increased osmotic pressure of hypertonic crystalloid solutions can increase the circulating volume by more than the volume of intravenous fluid administered. Hypotonic fluids cause a shift of fluid from the intravascular space to the intracellular space. The sugar in dextrose solutions may make them isotonic or even hypertonic, but the dextrose is metabolized quickly upon administration, rendering the solution hypotonic.

IV fluids that contain proteins or large starch molecules are known as **colloids**. The large protein and starch molecules do not easily leave the intravascular space, allowing them to exert substantial osmotic pressure (in the form of colloid oncotic pressure). Relatively small amounts of colloid solutions increase the circulating volume by attracting interstitial fluid into the vascular space. However, colloid solutions are expensive and have several other drawbacks.

In addition to the active solutes they contain, IV fluids also contain preservatives and additives to adjust their pH.

The following are the most common IV fluids used in EMS:

- Normal saline (0.9 percent sodium chloride solution)
- Dextrose, 5 percent in water
- Lactated Ringer's solution

Normal Saline

Normal saline, or 0.9 percent saline solution, is sterile water with sodium chloride (NaCl) added to equal the amount found in the human body. Keep in mind, though, that plasma contains many solutes in addition to sodium and chloride. However, normal saline is useful for rehydration, vascular volume replacement, and diluting medications for intravenous infusion. Saline solutions also come in other concentrations, both hypotonic and hypertonic.

D$_5$W

Five percent dextrose in water (D$_5$W) is a solution of sterile water containing 5 percent dextrose. That is, there are 5 grams of dextrose in every 100 mL of water. Dextrose solution also is available in 10 percent solution (10 grams of dextrose per 100 mL) and in combination with other IV fluids, such as normal saline or lactated Ringer's solution. Dextrose solutions are used when the patient can benefit from intravenous carbohydrates, such as patients who cannot have anything by mouth for a period of time. D$_5$W also is useful for a keep-open IV in patients who are prone to fluid overload because it does not remain in the vascular space.

Lactated Ringer's Solution

Lactated Ringer's (LR) solution is an isotonic crystalloid that contains sodium, chloride, potassium, calcium, and lactate. Because lactate is involved in the blood buffer system, it can be useful in patients with acidosis, such as those with hypovolemic shock or diabetic ketoacidosis. The addition of potassium makes lactated Ringer's solution useful in patients with suspected hypokalemia, but potentially dangerous in patients with hyperkalemia, such as patients with crush syndrome.

IV Fluids

Normal Saline (0.9 Percent Sodium Chloride Solution) for Intravenous Infusion

Normal saline is the most commonly used IV solution in EMS care. It is routinely used safely and effectively to replace lost circulatory volume. The following is key information about normal saline:

- *Class:* Isotonic crystalloid.
- *Description:* Clear liquid containing water, 154 mEq per liter sodium, and approximately 154 mEq per liter of chloride to match the concentration found in the human body.
- *Mechanism of action:* Used to temporarily expand the vascular volume by replacing water and electrolytes.
- *Indications:* Hypovolemia, heat exhaustion, heat stroke, and diabetic ketoacidosis.
- *Contraindications:* Should not be given to patients with heart failure, because fluid overload may occur.
- *Precautions:* Patients receiving large volumes of normal saline should be carefully monitored for fluid overload. In patients who have lost significant amounts of electrolytes, it may be more appropriate to use lactated Ringer's solution or an alternative IV fluid containing electrolyte replacement.
- *Side effects:* Administration of large amounts of normal saline may result in hemodilution and electrolyte imbalance.
- *Dosage:* Depends on the condition for which normal saline is being administered. Follow your protocols. A keep-open rate is 30 mL/hour.
- *Route:* Intravenous infusion.
- *How supplied:* Normal saline is commonly supplied in 250-, 500-, and 1,000-mL bags designed to be used with an IV drip set. To avoid inadvertent fluid overload, select a container volume appropriate to the patient's condition.

5 Percent Dextrose in Water for Intravenous Infusion

D_5W can be used for a keep-open IV because the danger of fluid overload is reduced. However, a saline lock is also useful for that purpose and does not require additional storage space for bags of IV fluid. Therefore, not all EMS

Pediatric Care

You can use IV administration sets with a flexible graduated cylinder between the IV fluid bag and infusion tubing to precisely measure the maximum amount of IV fluid to be administered. The maximum volume of the cylinder is 150 mL. The device is sometimes called a burette, Buretrol, or Volutrol.

services carry D_5W. The following is key information about D_5W:

- *Class:* Hypotonic carbohydrate-containing solution.
- *Description:* Sterile water containing 5 percent dextrose (5 g/100 mL).
- *Mechanism of action:* D_5W combines dextrose and water in a hypotonic concentration that will not remain in the vascular space, reducing the danger of fluid overload.
- *Indications:* D_5W is used for prophylactic IV access or to dilute concentrated drugs for IV infusion.
- *Contraindications:* D_5W should not be used for patients who require IV fluid replacement or in patients who are hyperglycemic. Do not use in patients with traumatic brain injury or stroke.
- *Precautions:* D_5W may be more irritating to the tissues than normal saline, so the IV site should be closely monitored for irritation, swelling, or redness.
- *Side effects:* Rare when given in therapeutic doses.
- *Interactions:* D_5W should not be used for blood product infusion.
- *Dosage:* Usually administered at a keep-open rate (30 mL/hour).
- *Route:* IV infusion.
- *How supplied:* D_5W is most commonly supplied in 250-mL or 500-mL bags.

Lactated Ringer's Solution

The following is key information about lactated Ringer's solution:

- *Class:* Isotonic crystalloid solution.
- *Description:* Sterile water containing the following electrolytes:
  - Sodium, 130 mEq/L
  - Potassium, 4 mEq/L
  - Calcium, 30 mEq/L
  - Chloride, 109 mEq/L
  - Lactate, 28 mEq/L
- *Mechanism of action:* Lactated Ringer's solution is used to replace fluid and electrolytes.
- *Indications:* Significant burns and hypovolemia.

- *Contraindications:* Do not use in patients with heart failure, renal failure, or suspected hyperkalemia.
- *Precautions:* Monitor closely for signs of circulatory overload.
- *Side effects:* Rare in therapeutic dosages.
- *Interactions:* Do not use with blood product infusion.
- *Dosage:* Depends on the condition for which lactated Ringer's solution is being administered. Follow your protocols. A keep-open rate is 30 mL/hour.
- *Route:* IV infusion.
- *How supplied:* Lactated Ringer's solution is commonly supplied in 1,000-mL bags.

Medications

Albuterol Sulfate

The Advanced EMT Scope of Practice Model includes the administration of inhaled bronchodilators to patients with wheezing due to asthma and COPD. Albuterol is a prototypical bronchodilator drug used for that purpose. The following is key information about albuterol:

- *Class:* Beta$_2$-selective sympathomimetic; bronchodilator.
- *Description:* Albuterol sulfate (Proventil, Ventolin) is a sympathetic beta$_s$ agonist used to reverse bronchiolar smooth muscle constriction in patients with asthma and chronic obstructive pulmonary disease.
- *Mechanism of action:* Acts on beta$_2$ sympathetic receptors in bronchiolar smooth muscle to cause bronchodilation.
- *Indications:* Wheezing caused by asthma, and COPD, and some other conditions.

IN THE FIELD

Levalbuterol (Xopenex) is a beta$_2$ selective bronchodilator used in place of albuterol in some EMS systems. In addition, some EMS systems allow ipratropium bromide (Atrovent), an anticholinergic drug, to be given in conjunction with an inhaled beta$_2$ agonist.

- *Contraindications:* Hypersensitivity and symptomatic tachycardia.
- *Precautions:* Albuterol has minimal beta$_1$-adrenergic effects, but may increase heart rate and myocardial oxygen demand. Use with caution in patients with heart disease.
- *Side effects:* Anxiety, palpitations, chest discomfort, headache, and perspiration.
- *Interactions:* Other beta agonists should not be administered concurrently with albuterol.
- *Dosage:* Metered-dose inhaler: one or two 90-mcg sprays. The use of a spacer device is preferred when administering albuterol by metered-dose inhaler, especially in pediatric patients. Small-volume nebulizer: 2.5 mg diluted in 2.5 mL over 5 to 15 minutes; pediatric dosage, 0.15 mg/kg diluted in 2.5 mL normal saline.
- *Route:* Inhalation.
- *How supplied:* Metered-dose inhaler or 2.5 mg/0.5 mL nebule.

Aspirin

Aspirin (acetylsalicylic acid [ASA]) is one of the most important medications in the treatment of acute myocardial infarction. No other medication has been shown to be as effective for so little cost. Aspirin inhibits platelet aggregation to reduce additional blood clotting. The following is key information about aspirin:

- *Class:* Platelet aggregation inhibitor; nonsteroidal anti-inflammatory; analgesic.
- *Description:* Aspirin is a salicylate that reduces platelet aggregation by inhibiting the release of a prostaglandin called thromboxane A$_2$.
- *Mechanism of action:* Aspirin blocks part of the chemical reaction responsible for activating platelets.
- *Indications:* In the prehospital setting, acute coronary syndrome and stroke.
- *Contraindications:* Hypersensitivity; not given to children or adolescents with suspected viral illnesses because it is associated with an increased risk of Reye's syndrome.
- *Precautions:* Administer with caution in patients with asthma or seasonal allergies, stomach ulcers, liver disease, alcohol abuse, kidney disease, or coagulopathies.

PERSONAL PERSPECTIVE

Advanced EMT Jill Bailey: It is amazing to see the effects of medications on patients. With some drugs, like aspirin, you can't see the effects immediately. But when you give albuterol to an asthmatic, or nitroglycerin to a patient with chest pain, or 50 percent dextrose to a hypoglycemic patient, or naloxone to a patient who isn't breathing so well from a narcotic overdose, the effects are fast and dramatic. Having those drugs available as tools to help patients is very satisfying, but it is still a big responsibility that can never be taken lightly.

- *Side effects:* GI upset, bleeding, nausea, vomiting, and wheezing.
- *Interactions:* Few interactions for a single dose in the prehospital setting.
- *Dosage:* The American Heart Association currently recommends 160 to ~~325~~ mg of chewable aspirin. **324 or** Children's aspirin is preferred because it is chewable, **die!** which increases the rate of absorption, and does not require water to assist swallowing (American Heart Association, 2010).
- *Route:* Oral.
- *How supplied:* Chewable tablets containing 81 mg/tablet.

50 Percent Dextrose

Dextrose is used to supply sugar to patients with acute hypoglycemia who have a decreased level of responsiveness and cannot receive oral glucose. It is a concentrated solution that contains 500 mg of dextrose per 1 mL. There are some risks to the administration of hypertonic dextrose solutions. They can cause local irritation of the vein and, if accidentally introduced into the tissues through an infiltrated IV line, it can cause tissue necrosis. Only administer 50 percent dextrose through a patent, free-flowing IV line. Push the medication slowly to avoid injuring the vein and causing infiltration of the tissues. The following is key information about dextrose 50 percent:

- *Class:* Carbohydrate.
- *Description:* High concentration (50 g/100 mL) of dextrose in sterile water for IV administration.
- *Mechanism of action:* Increases glucose concentration in the blood for the reversal of acute hypoglycemia.
- *Indications:* Hypoglycemia in adult patients.
- *Contraindications:* Intracranial hemorrhage (traumatic brain injury, stroke) and hyperglycemia.
- *Precautions:* Check the blood glucose level prior to administration. A solution of 50 percent dextrose is hypertonic and will cause severe tissue necrosis if infiltration occurs.
- *Side effects:* Localized irritation of the vein.
- *Interactions:* There are no significant interactions in emergency situations.
- *Dosage:* 25 g slow IV push; may be repeated in 10 to 15 minutes if blood glucose level (BGL) remains below

70 mL/dL. Pediatric dosage: 0.5 g/kg (500 mg kg) of a 25 percent solution (25 g/100 mL) of dextrose; 10 percent (10 g/100 mL) for neonates.
- *Route:* Slow IV push through at least an 18-gauge IV catheter in a large vein. Monitor the IV site for infiltration during administration.
- *How supplied:* Prefilled syringe containing 25 grams of dextrose in 50 mL.

Epinephrine 1:1,000

Epinephrine is commonly available for injection in two concentrations, 1:10,000 (1 g/10,000 mL) and 1:1,000 (1 g/1000 mL). The 1:10,000 solution is administered by intravenous injection in cardiac arrest and severe, refractory anaphylaxis by paramedics and hospital personnel. Advanced EMTs can give 1:1,000 epinephrine to patients with anaphylaxis, either by assisting a patient with his epinephrine autoinjector (such as an EpiPen) or by drawing up the medication in a syringe and giving it by subcutaneous or intramuscular injection. The following is key information about epinephrine 1:1,000:

- *Class:* Sympathomimetic.
- *Description:* Epinephrine is a naturally occurring hormone (adrenalin) secreted by the adrenal glands in response to sympathetic nervous system stimulation. Epinephrine binds to $alpha_1$ $beta_1$, and $beta_2$-adrenergic receptor sites, causing vasoconstriction, increased heart rate and force of contraction, and bronchiolar smooth muscle relaxation.
- *Mechanism of action:* Epinephrine, 1:1,000 is administered in anaphylaxis to cause vasoconstriction and relax bronchiolar smooth muscle.
- *Indications:* Acute anaphylaxis.
- *Contraindications:* Use with caution in patients with significant cardiovascular disease or hypertension.
- *Precautions:* Epinephrine is inactivated by exposure to sunlight or when given with an alkaline solution. Because epinephrine causes a strong sympathetic stimulus, patients may experience chest pain, palpitations, anxiety, nausea, or headache. Monitor the patient's heart rate and blood pressure.
- *Side effects:* Palpitations, tachycardia, anxiety, headache, dizziness, nausea, and vomiting are common side effects. Patients with underlying cardiac disease also may experience chest pain and acute myocardial infarction.
- *Interactions:* The effects of epinephrine can be intensified in patients taking some antidepressants.
- *Dosage:* 0.3 to 0.5 mg subcutaneously or intramuscularly every 15 minutes as needed; pediatric dose, 0.01 mg/kg.
- *Route:* Subcutaneous or intramuscular injection.
- *How supplied:* 1 mg/1 mL in vials, ampules, or prefilled autoinjector devices.

Pediatric Care

Use 25 percent dextrose to treat hypoglycemia in pediatric patients. If a prefilled syringe of 25 percent solution for pediatric administration is not available, dilute 50 percent dextrose 1:1 with sterile water or normal saline.

Glucagon

Glucagon is a naturally occurring hormone that promotes the breakdown of glycogen in the liver to glucose to increase blood glucose levels. Intramuscular glucagon is indicated for emergency treatment of severe hypoglycemia when it is not possible to establish an IV line to administer dextrose. Patients who have inadequate liver glycogen stores, such as those with severe liver disease or malnutrition, will not respond to glucagon. The following is key information about glucagon:

- *Class:* Hormone with antihypoglycemic action.
- *Description:* Glucagon is a pancreatic hormone that affects the blood glucose level by promoting glycogenolysis and gluconeogenesis and inhibiting glycogenesis.
- *Mechanism of action:* Glucagon causes a release of stored glycogen and its conversion to glucose when released into the circulation. When administered, it causes an increase in blood glucose levels if the patient has adequate stores of glycogen for conversion to glucose.
- *Indications:* Inability to establish intravenous access in patients with significant hypoglycemia.
- *Contraindications:* Hypersensitivity.
- *Precautions:* Glucagon will not be effective if the patient has already depleted glycogen stores.
- *Side effects:* Side effects are rare, but hypotension, dizziness, headache, nausea, and vomiting may occur.
- *Interactions:* Few interactions when given in an emergency situation in therapeutic doses.
- *Dosage:* 1 mg.
- *Route:* Intramuscular injection.
- *How supplied:* Glucagon a supplied as a kit containing the powdered medication and solvent that must be combined before administration.

Glucose

Glucose is administered orally or applied to the buccal mucosa in hypoglycemic patients who are awake and are not at risk of aspiration. The following is key information about glucose:

- *Class:* Carbohydrate.
- *Description:* Glucose is a simple carbohydrate that can be absorbed across the buccal mucosa or through the gastrointestinal tract.

- *Mechanism of action:* Increases blood glucose levels.
- *Indications:* Acute hypoglycemia in a patient who is awake and can protect his own airway.
- *Contraindications:* Inability to maintain a patent airway.
- *Precautions:* Carefully monitor the patient for the potential of aspiration.
- *Side effects:* Nausea and vomiting.
- *Interactions:* None.
- *Dosage:* 15 grams by mouth or applied to the buccal mucosa.
- *Route:* Oral or buccal.
- *How supplied:* Single-dose 1.3 oz (37.5 g) sealed tube containing 15 g d-glucose (40 percent glucose) tube with a twist-off cap.

Naloxone (Narcan)

Naloxone (Narcan) is a narcotic antagonist used to reverse respiratory depression associated with narcotic overdose. Naloxone has a greater affinity for narcotic receptor sites than opiates, thereby displacing them from the receptor. Because it has a shorter duration of effects than most narcotics, the narcotic can reoccupy the receptor sites when naloxone's half-life is exceeded, necessitating further naloxone administration to maintain adequate respirations.

Naloxone should not be used indiscriminately as a diagnostic tool to determine if narcotic overdose is the cause of respiratory depression. Many EMS systems recommend that administration be started at the low end of the dosage range and titrated to the minimum needed to maintain the patient's respiratory rate instead of improving level of responsiveness. The following is key information about naloxone:

- *Class:* Narcotic antagonist.
- *Description:* Medication used to reverse respiratory depression associated with narcotic overdose.
- *Mechanism of action:* Naloxone has a higher affinity for narcotic receptor sites and when administered, displaces the narcotic, blocking its effects.
- *Indications:* Naloxone is indicated to reverse the respiratory depression associated with narcotic overdose.
- *Contraindications:* Known hypersensitivity.
- *Precautions:* Rapid administration and large doses may cause withdrawal in narcotic-addicted patients. Many EMS systems titrate the dosage to the minimum amount needed to ensure adequate breathing rather than complete reversal of the narcotic.
- *Side effects:* These are rare, but hypotension, hypertension, nausea, vomiting, and cardiac arrhythmias may occur.

- *Interactions:* May cause withdrawal symptoms in patients addicted to narcotics.
- *Dosage:* 1 to 2 mg slow IV push titrated to restore respiratory rate. If no effect, may be repeated at 5-minute intervals. An intranasal formulation is also available.
- *Route:* Slow IV push.
- *How supplied:* Prefilled syringe, vial, or ampule.

Nitroglycerin—Sublingual Tablets and Spray

Nitroglycerin (NTG) is used in the treatment of patients with acute coronary syndrome (ACS). It causes vascular smooth muscle relaxation, resulting in dilation of the coronary arteries and systemic vasculature to increase myocardial perfusion and reduce the myocardial workload. Nitrates can cause a significant drop in blood pressure, even when used carefully. Nitroglycerin must not be administered to patients with a systolic blood pressure lower than 90 mmHg. The following is key information about nitroglycerin:

- *Class:* Nitrate; vasodilator.
- *Description:* Supplied as tablets or a metered-dose spray for sublingual administration in the treatment of acute coronary syndrome.
- *Mechanism of action:* Nitrates are potent vasodilators that increase blood flow to the coronary arteries and decrease cardiac workload by dilating the peripheral vasculature and reducing preload.
- *Indications:* Chest pain associated with acute coronary syndrome.
- *Contraindications:* Hypotension, increased intracranial pressure, and use of erectile dysfunction medications within 24 to 36 hours.
- *Precautions:* NTG deteriorates rapidly when exposed to light or air. Monitor blood pressure closely and discontinue administration if the systolic blood pressure falls below 90 mmHg.
- *Side effects:* NTG is a potent vasodilator and commonly causes an immediate headache. May cause dizziness, weakness, tachycardia, hypotension, dry mouth, nausea, and vomiting. The spray or tablets may cause a burning sensation on administration.
- *Interactions:* Effects may be accentuated by alcohol use, erectile dysfunction medications, and beta blockers.
- *Dosage:* Administer 0.4 mg sublingually. If chest pain persists and the systolic blood pressure remains at least 90 mmHg, the dose may be repeated every 5 minutes to a total of three doses.
- *Route:* Sublingual.
- *How supplied:* Calibrated spray delivering 0.4 mg/spray or as a small tablet containing 0.4 mg/tablet.

Nitrous Oxide (Nitronox)

Nitrous oxide is used as an inhaled anesthetic or analgesic in the presence of severe pain due to musculoskeletal injury or acute MI. Because it is inhaled, the onset is extremely rapid but the effects subside quickly when administration is discontinued. In the prehospital setting, the patient self–administers the drug by holding the mask to the face and breathing in the gas. If the patient administers too much, he will no longer be able to keep the mask against his face and will discontinue the drug. The system consists of two pressurized gas cylinders, one filled with oxygen and the other with nitrous oxide. Some systems (Entonox) use a single cylinder. The following is key information about nitrous oxide:

- *Class:* Analgesic and anesthetic.
- *Description:* A 50/50 mix of oxygen and nitrous oxide delivered to a modified-demand valve and mask that the patient self-administers by holding the mask and inhaling.
- *Mechanism of action:* CNS depressant.
- *Indications:* Severe musculoskeletal pain, and chest pain associated with acute coronary syndrome and not relieved by nitroglycerin.
- *Contraindications:* Decreased level of responsiveness, inability to follow instructions, traumatic brain injury, COPD, suspected pneumothorax, abdominal pain, and suspected bowel obstruction.
- *Precautions:* Only use in well-ventilated area to prevent sedation of the medical staff. Teratogenic; should not be used by or around pregnant patients or health care providers.
- *Side effects:* Dizziness, decreased mental status, hallucinations, nausea, and vomiting.
- *Interactions:* Do not use with sedative–hypnotic medications, narcotics, or alcohol.
- *Dosage:* Self-administered mixture of 50 percent nitrous oxide and 50 percent oxygen.
- *Route:* Inhalation.
- *How supplied:* Modified-demand valve with mixer to combine 50 percent of each gas for inhalation.

Oxygen

The following is key information about oxygen:

- *Class:* Gas.
- *Description:* Colorless, odorless, tasteless gas.
- *Mechanism of action:* Oxygen is necessary for cellular energy production. When inhaled, oxygen molecules cross the respiratory membrane to attach to hemoglobin in red blood cells for transport to the tissues.
- *Indications:* Dyspnea, hypoxia; SpO_2 <95 percent.
- *Contraindications:* There are no absolute contraindications to the use of oxygen. however, there are

complications associated with hyperoxemia, particularly in neonates and patients resuscitated from cardiac arrest.

- *Precautions:* Patients with chronic obstructive pulmonary disease who depend on hypoxic drive for respiratory drive may experience respiratory depression if high concentrations of oxygen are administered for a prolonged period of time. Oxygen is a vasoactive drug that causes cerebral and coronary artery vasoconstriction. Oxygen is not recommended for routine use in uncomplicated acute coronary syndrome. Oxygen administration should be titrated to maintain an SpO_2 of 95 percent or higher. Do not use near an open flame or sources of combustion. Compressed gas cylinders may become projectile hazards if knocked over and damaged. Always leave the bottle on its side and use a protective guard over the flow meter to prevent damage.

- *Side effects:* There are few side effects associated with short-term administration of therapeutic amounts of oxygen. If used for prolonged periods of time without a humidifier, it may cause drying of the mucous membranes and nose bleeds.

- *Interactions:* None.

- *Dosage:* Oxygen administration should be titrated to maintain a SpO_2 of 95 percent or higher. High oxygen concentrations for prolonged periods of time can cause oxygen toxicity. Therefore, ventilator patients are often kept below 50 percent oxygen when possible.

- *Route:* Inhalation via nasal cannula, face mask, nonrebreather mask, or bag-valve-mask device.

- *How supplied:* Oxygen is supplied as a compressed gas in a high-pressure cylinder.

Activated Charcoal (Actidose)

While not commonly used, activated charcoal may still be used as an absorbent for ingested toxins. The following is key information about activated charcoal:

- *Class:* Absorbent.

- *Description:* Finely powdered charcoal activated with oxygen, commonly diluted in water for oral administration.

- *Mechanism of action:* Binds with ingested toxins in the GI tract to prevent absorption.

- *Indications:* Oral ingestion of toxins.

- *Contraindications:* Decreased level of responsiveness or increased risk of aspiration; or ingestion of corrosives, caustics, or petroleum distillates.

- *Precautions:* Activated charcoal will inactivate other oral medications.

- *Side effects:* Black, tarry stools, and constipation.

- *Interactions:* None.

- *Dosage:* 1 g/kg orally (adults and pediatric patients).

- *Route:* Oral.

- *How supplied:* Premixed slurry of 50 grams/250 mL.

Acetaminophen (Tylenol)

Acetaminophen is a nonprescription analgesic and anti-pyretic that, while not carried by most EMS systems, may be administered by the Advanced EMT in some situations. The following is key information about acetaminophen:

- *Class:* Analgesic, antipyretic (fever reducer).

- *Description:* Nonprescription medication used for the relief of mild to moderate pain and as a fever reducer.

- *Mechanism of action:* The mechanism of action is not completely understood, but acetaminophen increases the pain threshold by blocking prostaglandin synthesis and inhibits the effect of pyrogens in the central nervous system.

- *Indications:* Mild to moderate pain and fever.

- *Contraindications:* Hypersensitivity.

- *Precautions:* Acetaminophen is hepatotoxic in high doses and should be used with caution in patients with known liver disease.

- *Side effects:* Acetaminophen is generally well-tolerated and there are no significant side effects in therapeutic doses. In large doses, the medication can be hepatotoxic.

- *Interactions:* Alcohol increases liver toxicity.

- *Dosage:* Adults 650 to 1,000 mg every 4 to 6 hours, 4-gram maximum per 24 hours; pediatric dosage, 10 to 15 mg/kg every 4 to 6 hours, 40 mg/kg maximum per 24 hours.

- *Route:* Oral.

- *How supplied:* Capsules, tablets, chewable tablets, suspension, elixir, and suppositories (for rectal administration).

Ibuprofen (Motrin)

Commonly known as Motrin, ibuprofen is a nonsteroidal anti-inflammatory or NSAID. While not commonly carried by EMS units, the Advanced EMT may administer ibuprofen in some situations. The following is key information about ibuprofen:

- *Class:* Nonsteroidal anti-inflammatory (NSAID) (analgesic and antipyretic).

- *Description:* Nonprescription medication used for the relief of mild to moderate pain and to reduce fever.

- *Mechanism of action:* Inhibits inflammatory response by blocking formation of cyclo-oxygenase (COX-2), a chemical mediator of inflammatory chemicals such as prostaglandins.

- *Indications:* Mild to moderate pain and fever.

- *Contraindications:* Known allergy to ibuprofen or other NSAIDs.
- *Precautions:* High-dose ibuprofen is known to cause significant gastrointestinal irritation and increases the risk of gastrointestinal bleeding.
- *Side effects:* Gastric irritation.
- *Interactions:* Do not give with aspirin or other NSAIDs.
- *Dosage:* 200 to 400 mg every 6 to 8 hours; pediatric dosage, 5 to 10 mg/kg every 6 to 8 hours.
- *Route:* Oral.
- *How supplied:* Coated tablets, chewable tablets, capsules, suspension, and elixir.

Nerve Agent Antidote Kits

Many EMS agencies are now carrying nerve agent antidote kits as part of homeland security precautions. The kits consist of prefilled injectors of atropine (2 mg) and pralidoxime chloride (600 mg). The medications are antidotes for organophosphate nerve agents, such as tabun, sarin, and VX. They reduce parasympathetic nervous system stimulation by blocking the production and uptake of acetylcholine. The kits are not intended for the public, but rather for the EMS crew on the ambulance if they are exposed to a suspected nerve agent. You can use the auto injectors to inject the medication subcutaneously in either the gluteus or the vastus lateralis muscles.

CASE STUDY WRAP-UP

Clinical-Reasoning Process

Advanced EMTs Christy and David are on the scene of a 20-year-old man who responds only to painful stimulus and who has depressed respirations and constricted pupils. David has ensured an open airway with a head-tilt/chin-lift maneuver. He places the patient on 15 L/min of oxygen by nonrebreather mask. He recognizes the patient's shallow respirations at 10 per minute, resulting in a SpO_2 of 94 percent, as a developing problem that must be corrected. Considering the patient's reaction to pain and current respiratory status, David decides that assisting the patient's ventilations is not warranted at the moment. He searches for an immediately correctable cause of the problem. However, he knows he must continually monitor the patient's airway, breathing, and oxygenation.

David's assessment reveals no signs of injury or other clues to the nature of the underlying problem. As David obtains the patient's blood glucose level (BGL), which is within normal limits, he asks the patient's mother additional questions to get a better idea of what may be going on with the patient. The mother states that she spoke to the patient about 3 hours before coming home to find him this way. She says that "this has never happened before" and she doesn't know "what is going on."

The patient's altered mental status, depressed respirations, vital signs, and constricted pupils make David think of narcotic overdose. He asks the patient's mother if anyone in the household has a prescription for pain medication. It turns out that the patient's father had a prescription for Lortab, which David recognizes as a narcotic. "Would you mind checking to see if they are missing?" asks David.

When the mother returns, she says, "They were in the medicine cabinet yesterday, but they are not there now."

David recognizes the indications for naloxone: suspected narcotic overdose with respiratory depression. Improving the patient's respiratory status is a high priority, so as Christy retrieves the stretcher, David starts an IV of normal saline in the patient's forearm, using an 18-gauge catheter. David selects a prefilled syringe of naloxone and confirms the medication. He administers 1 mg of the drug slowly by IV push and rechecks the patient's ventilations. The patient's ventilations are now 12 per minute, and his SpO_2 is 99 percent with oxygen by nonrebreather mask.

David and Christy place the patient on the stretcher and load the stretcher into the ambulance for the 10-minute ride to the emergency department. Later that day, they follow up with the emergency department physician and learn that the patient's toxicology screen was positive for the narcotic drug.

CHAPTER REVIEW

Chapter Summary

EMS is a field that demands continuing education in order to provide appropriate treatment to patients. As an Advanced EMT, you will be responsible for not only knowing which medication is indicated for use in a particular patient but also what that medication will do to, and for, the patient. It is up to you to maintain a good working knowledge of the medications discussed in this chapter as well as any new medications that are introduced into your protocols for the remainder of your career.

Review Questions

Multiple-Choice Questions

1. Which one of the following medications is indicated for the treatment of chest pain associated with acute coronary syndrome?
   a. 50 percent dextrose
   b. Naloxone
   c. Nitroglycerin
   d. Epinephrine

2. Which one of the following is a contraindication to administering nitroglycerin?
   a. Chest pain
   b. Systolic blood pressure less than 90 mmHg
   c. Hyperglycemia
   d. SpO_2 below 95 percent

3. Which one of the following IV fluids is the best choice for a patient with a history of heart failure?
   a. Normal saline
   b. Lactated Ringer's
   c. 5 percent dextrose in water
   d. 2 percent sodium chloride

4. Which one of the following is an analgesic?
   a. Naloxone
   b. Oxygen
   c. Glucagon
   d. Nitrous oxide

5. Which one of the following medications can be administered by Advanced EMTs in the treatment of wheezing due to asthma?
   a. Epinephrine
   b. Albuterol
   c. Aspirin
   d. Nitrous oxide

6. Which one of the following IV fluids has the advantage of providing a treatment for metabolic acidosis?
   a. Lactated Ringer's
   b. Normal saline
   c. 5 percent dextrose in water
   d. 0.45 percent sodium chloride

7. You are caring for a 40-year-old diabetic patient who is unresponsive and severely hypoglycemic (BGL = 20 mg/dL). You are unable to obtain an IV. Which one of the following is the best course of action?
   a. 50 percent dextrose, IM
   b. 2 mg naloxone, IM
   c. 0.5 mg epinephrine, 1:1,000 IM
   d. 1 mg glucagon IM

8. Which one of the following is the reason aspirin is given to patients with suspected acute coronary syndrome?
   a. It is an analgesic.
   b. It inhibits platelet aggregation.
   c. It dilates the coronary arteries and decreases preload.
   d. It breaks down fibrin clots.

9. Albuterol is classified as a(n):
   a. antiadrenergic.
   b. cholinergic.
   c. anticholinergic.
   d. sympathomimetic.

10. The pediatric dosage of epinephrine, 1:1,000 is:
    a. 0.3 to 0.5 mg.
    b. 0.3 to 0.5 mg/kg.
    c. 0.1 mg/kg.
    d. 0.01 mg/kg.

Critical-Thinking Questions

11. Explain the differences in hypotonic, hypertonic, and isotonic solutions.

12. Explain why glucagon may not be effective in the treatment of hypoglycemia in an alcoholic patient.

References

American Heart Association. (2010). Part 10: Acute coronary syndromes: 2010 American Heart Association guidelines for cardiopulmonary resuscitation and emergency cardiovascular care. *Circulation, 122,* S787–S817.

Additional Reading

Bledsoe, B. E., Porter, R. S., & Cherry, R. A. (2009). *Paramedic care: Principles and practice* (3rd ed., Vol. 1). Upper Saddle River, NJ: Pearson.

Camargo, C. A. (2006). A model protocol for emergency medical services management of asthma exacerbations. *Prehospital Emergency Care, 10*(4), 418–29.

SECTION 4

Assessment and Initial Management

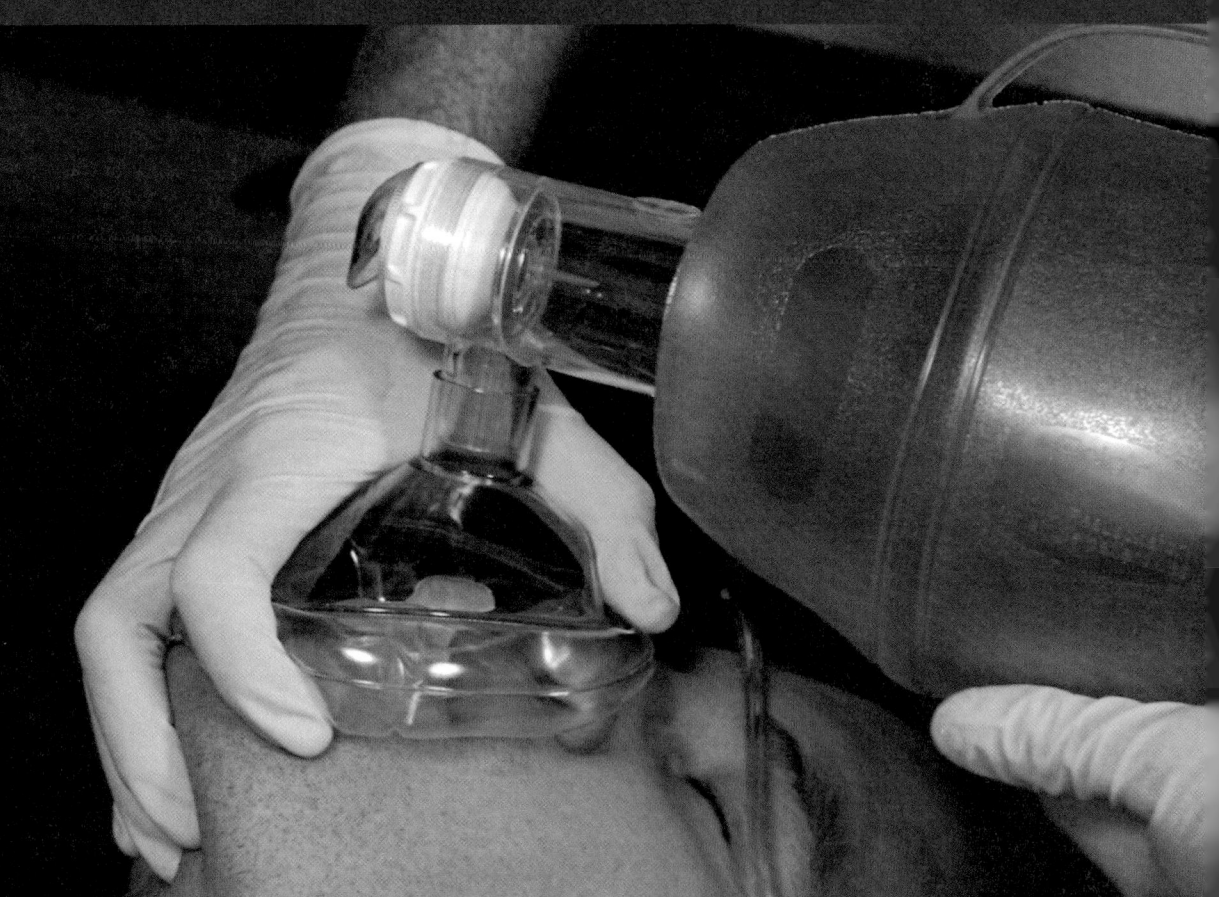

14 General Approach to Patient Assessment and Clinical Reasoning

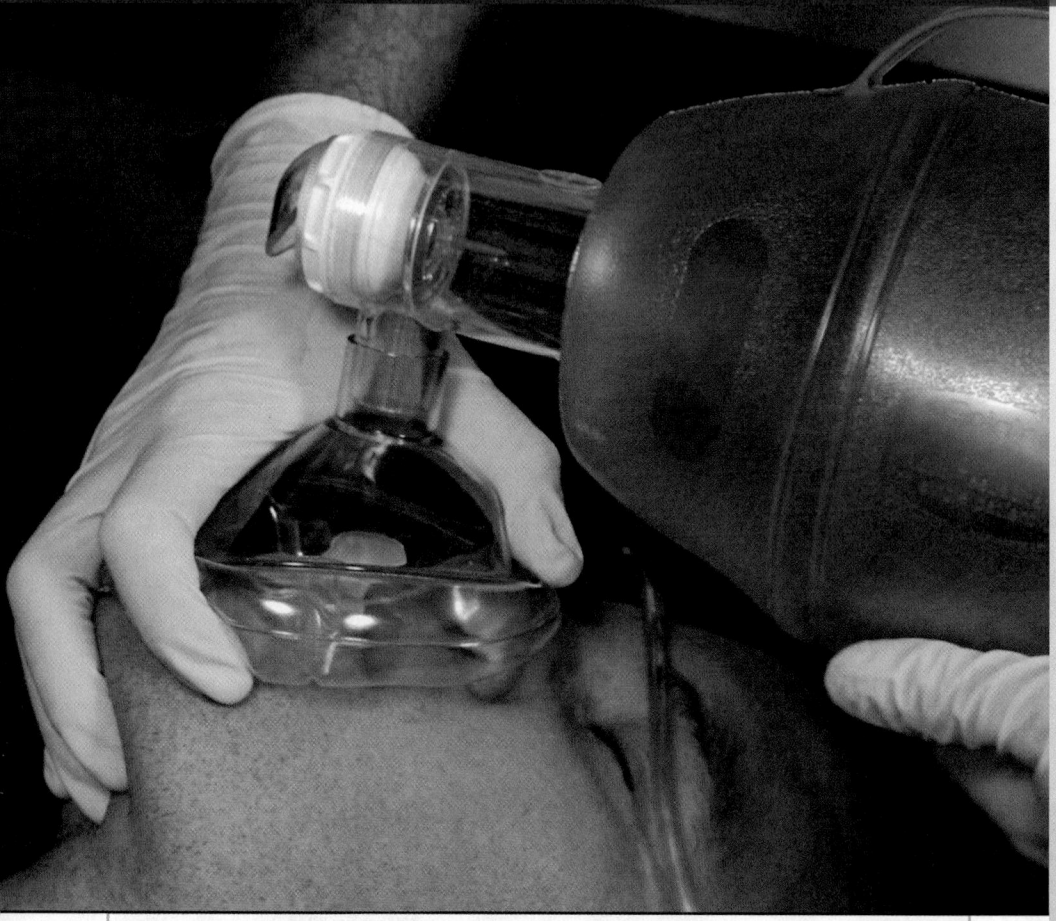

Content Area: Assessment

Advanced EMT Education Standard: Applies scene information and patient assessment findings (scene size-up, primary and secondary assessment, patient history, and reassessment) to guide emergency management.

Objectives

After reading this chapter, you should be able to:

14.1   Define key terms introduced in this chapter.

14.2   Describe the purpose and goals of patient assessment.

14.3   Describe the components of the patient assessment process.

14.4   Discuss the decisions that must be made during the patient assessment process.

14.5   Explain the importance of both a systematic approach and adaptability in patient assessment.

14.6   Explain the importance of various decision-making and problem-solving approaches in the patient assessment and patient care processes.

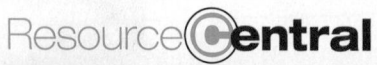
Resource **C**entral

To access Resource Central, follow the directions on the Student Access Card provided with this text. If there is no card, go to www.bradybooks.com and follow the Resource Central link to Buy Access. Under Media Resources, you will find:

• *Mechanism of Injury.* Watch how EMS professionals use clues at the scene to determine the MOI.

• *Patient Assessment Facts.* Learn how to stay focused for an effective patient assessment.

• *First Things First!* Learn more about the importance of the primary assessment and the interventions that may be used.

Advanced EMTs Julia Payne and Beth Mercer arrive in the 6500 block of East Grant Street where law enforcement has requested a "check out" of a person in custody. The patient is a disheveled man in his 30s with his hands cuffed behind his back. He is struggling with two police officers, cursing, thrashing about, and yelling, "Let me go!"

One of the officers, Lieutenant Avila, tells Julia and Beth that the patient's supervisor called 911 when the patient became unruly at work. The patient, Brian Nelson, began work only a week ago and the supervisor knows little about him beyond the information from his employment application. Lieutenant Avila called for EMS because she couldn't find an explanation for the patient's sudden change in behavior, and wants to have the patient "checked out" by EMS before transporting him to the detention center.

Problem-Solving Questions

1. What can Julia and Beth determine about the patient's condition with the information they have so far?
2. What information do they need to determine the nature of the patient's problem?
3. In what order should they collect this information?

Introduction

At its most basic level, the **patient assessment** process involves continually asking, "In what ways does this patient's presentation differ from a healthy state of functioning?" To answer this question, an Advanced EMT must systematically and thoroughly collect relevant information about the patient and the situation. He must then compare those findings to what healthy functioning looks like.

An overview of what normal functioning looks like appears in Chapters 8 and 9. Pathophysiology was introduced in Chapter 10. However, a great deal of study, classroom time, lab practice, and clinical experience are still needed. Each will help you gain confidence in your ability to recognize the many variations of both normal and abnormal patient presentations.

This chapter offers an overview of the patient assessment process, or a "big picture" perspective. Subsequent chapters will provide detailed information on each of the components of the patient assessment process.

Purpose and Goals of Patient Assessment

Patient assessment is a process that begins with information about the call, most often through the dispatch center. The patient assessment process continues throughout the call until patient care has been transferred to other health care personnel.

The term **assessment-based management** underscores the use of information collected and analyzed during the patient assessment process to make patient care decisions. For example, as an Advanced EMT, you must immediately treat the assessment finding of difficulty breathing by providing supplemental oxygen. But that is not enough. You also must engage in a process of **clinical problem solving** to search for treatable underlying causes of the problem. You must understand the significance of a collection of findings. You must understand in what way abnormal findings are a threat to the patient's health. Based on that understanding, you can decide what specific interventions are needed.

By systematically collecting and analyzing information, comparing it to your knowledge of various causes of difficulty breathing, for example, you can determine if more specific treatment is needed. For example, a **field impression** of bee sting anaphylaxis will lead you to one treatment. A field impression of an asthma attack will lead you to a different treatment.

Frequently, other EMS providers and hospital personnel rely on your assessments for information they might not otherwise have. You are in a unique position. You can collect information about the patient's environment and the **mechanism of injury** because you are there, at the scene. For example, the potential severity of injuries to a patient involved in a motor vehicle collision (MVC) may not be apparent to the emergency department physician or trauma surgeon. Your description of the damage to the vehicle, the position in which the patient was found, how long it took to extricate him from the vehicle, and whether or not he was wearing his seatbelt are vital (Figure 14-1).

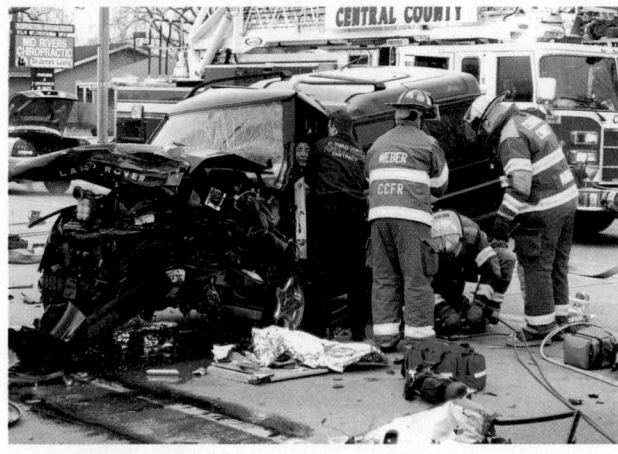

FIGURE 14-1

EMS providers are in a unique position to observe the mechanism of injury and the patient's surroundings.
(© Ray Kemp/Triple Zilch Productions)

In the patient assessment process, the goals include efficiently determining the answers to the following questions:

- Is it safe to approach the patient and begin care in the patient's current location? If not, what must you do to solve this problem?

- What is the nature of the patient's problem?

- How sick is the patient?

- Which interventions, resources, and actions are required immediately?

- Which health care facility can best meet the patient's immediate needs?

- How should the patient be transported to receive that care?

- What do you need to do to support the patient's vital functions from the time you arrive at the scene to the time you transfer patient care to other health care personnel?

- Is the patient's condition stable, improving, or worsening?

The answers to the questions are determined by using an approach that incorporates both structure and flexibility. You must perform the major steps of patient assessment for every patient. However, the way in which you determine the information at each step can vary based on the patient's condition.

General Approach to Patient Assessment

An overall systematic approach to patient assessment that has been learned well and practiced will allow you to be efficient. It also minimizes chances that you will overlook an important clue to a patient's problem. Such an assessment could allow you to collect hundreds of pieces of information. But that would be neither efficient nor useful. Instead, you must use the preliminary information you obtain to direct the rest of your assessment.

As you move through this text, you will learn what information is most useful when assessing patients with particular presentations and complaints. You also will learn to tailor the focus of your assessment and history-taking approach to the needs of the patient.

Components of the Patient Assessment Process

Successful patient assessment requires that you first establish trust and rapport with the patient. The process of therapeutic communication, described in Chapter 6, is critical to quickly establish a professional relationship with a patient in a stressful situation. The patient's trust in you will increase greatly by professionalism in dress, demeanor, and an organized, confident approach.

Patient assessment consists of the following four essential components (Figure 14-2; Scan 14-1):

- *Scene size-up.* During **scene size-up**, you determine the safety of the scene and formulate a general impression of the nature of the situation.

- *Primary assessment.* During the **primary assessment,** you look for and manage any immediate threats to the patient's life and establish priorities for treatment and transport.

- *Secondary assessment.* During the **secondary assessment,** you collect vital signs, obtain a medical history, and look for additional signs of injury and illness.

- *Reassessment.* During **reassessment,** you monitor the patient's condition for changes, assess the effects of treatment, and make adjustments in treatment as needed.

By necessity, any narrative description of the patient assessment process is linear and step-wise in nature. This can be deceiving. Although EMS personnel might speak of performing each component of assessment in turn, in reality, they are gathering a wealth of information while they are performing many different components of the assessment simultaneously. For example, as you approach an injured gymnast, you can see that she is sitting on the floor at the end of the balance beam, holding her deformed right forearm against her body with her left hand, and tearfully telling her coach that it hurts. That observation has simultaneously given you information that is pertinent to the scene size-up, primary assessment, and secondary assessment.

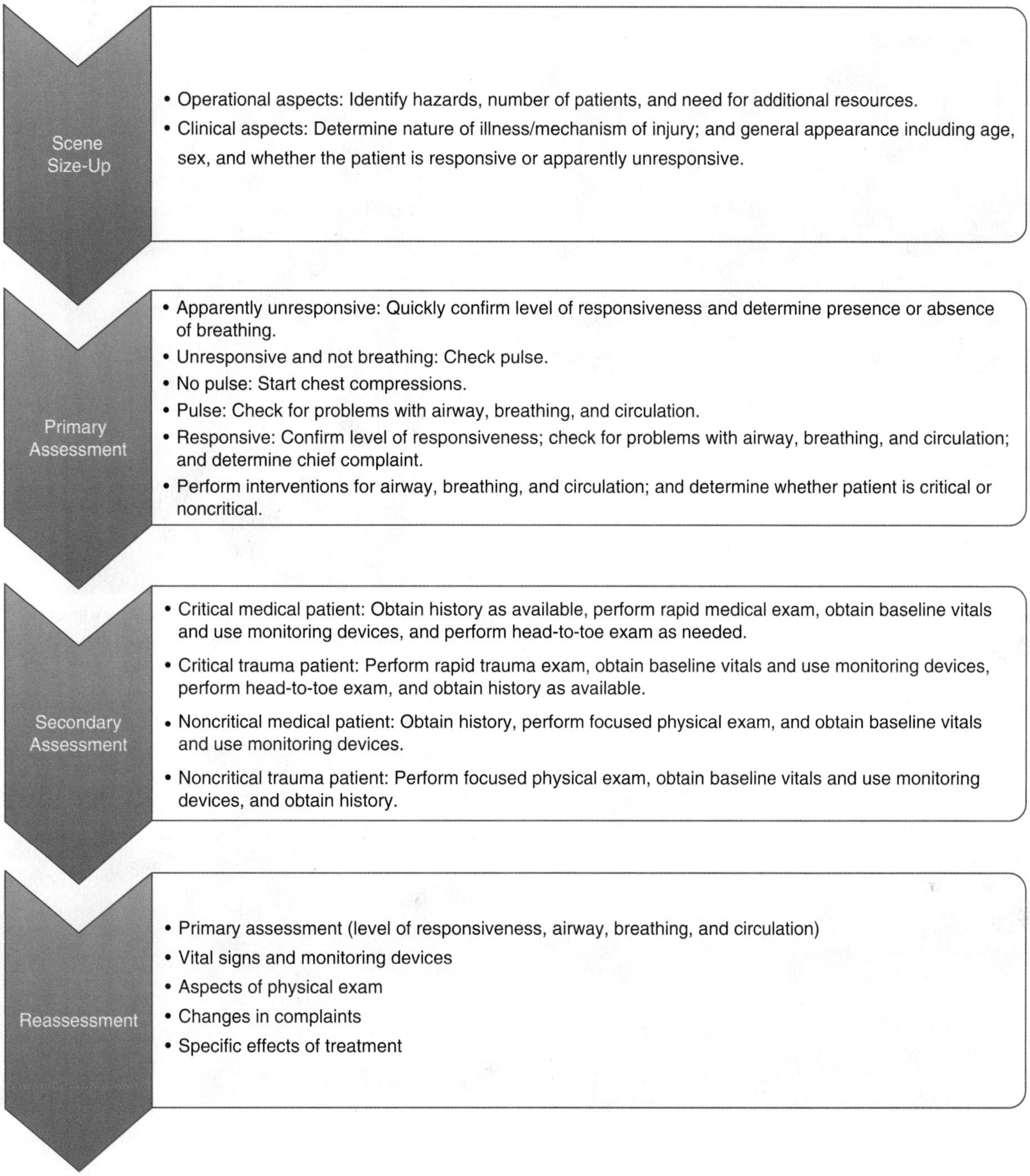

| Scene Size-Up | • Operational aspects: Identify hazards, number of patients, and need for additional resources. |
| | • Clinical aspects: Determine nature of illness/mechanism of injury; and general appearance including age, sex, and whether the patient is responsive or apparently unresponsive. |

Primary Assessment	• Apparently unresponsive: Quickly confirm level of responsiveness and determine presence or absence of breathing.
	• Unresponsive and not breathing: Check pulse.
	• No pulse: Start chest compressions.
	• Pulse: Check for problems with airway, breathing, and circulation.
	• Responsive: Confirm level of responsiveness; check for problems with airway, breathing, and circulation; and determine chief complaint.
	• Perform interventions for airway, breathing, and circulation; and determine whether patient is critical or noncritical.

Secondary Assessment	• Critical medical patient: Obtain history as available, perform rapid medical exam, obtain baseline vitals and use monitoring devices, and perform head-to-toe exam as needed.
	• Critical trauma patient: Perform rapid trauma exam, obtain baseline vitals and use monitoring devices, perform head-to-toe exam, and obtain history as available.
	• Noncritical medical patient: Obtain history, perform focused physical exam, and obtain baseline vitals and use monitoring devices.
	• Noncritical trauma patient: Perform focused physical exam, obtain baseline vitals and use monitoring devices, and obtain history.

Reassessment	• Primary assessment (level of responsiveness, airway, breathing, and circulation)
	• Vital signs and monitoring devices
	• Aspects of physical exam
	• Changes in complaints
	• Specific effects of treatment

FIGURE 14-2

An overview of the patient assessment process.

IN THE FIELD

Establishing a safe scene, identifying the number of patients, and determining the need for additional resources are all critical components of the scene size-up. (See Chapter 5 to review its operational aspects.)

Scene Size-Up

The scene size-up begins as you arrive at the scene. Its purpose is twofold. First, from an operational standpoint, you are concerned with determining whether or not the scene is safe, if you have more than one patient to care for, and if additional resources are needed. From a **clinical** standpoint, you are simultaneously collecting information about

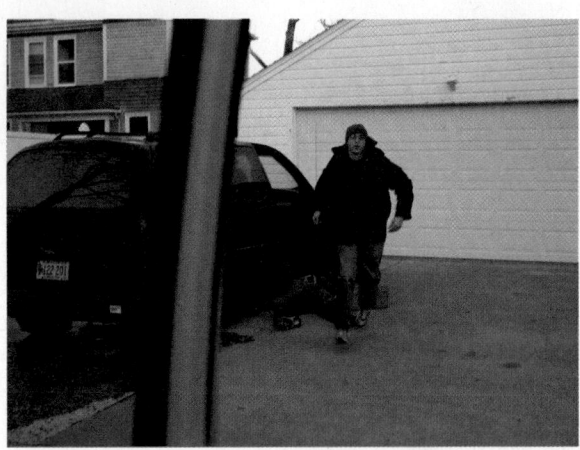

1. Perform a scene size-up to determine scene safety, the nature of the situation, the number of patients, and the need for additional resources.

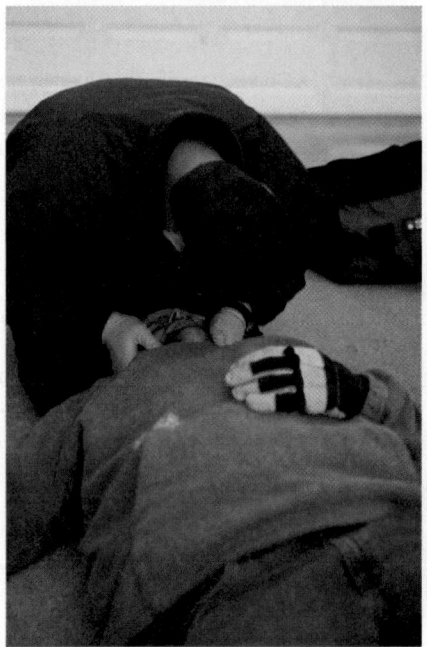

2. Perform a primary assessment for immediately life-threatening problems with the airway, breathing, and circulation.

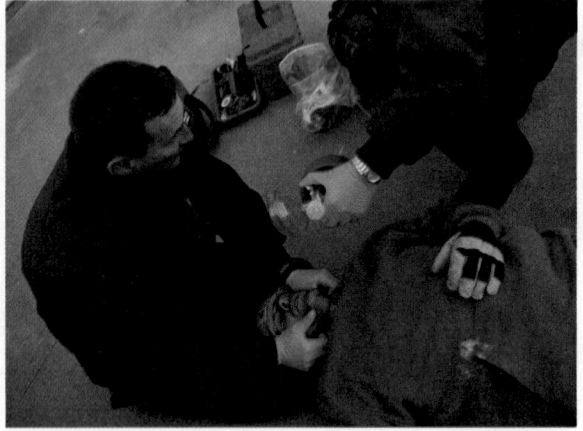

3. Correct immediate threats to life before proceeding with additional assessment.

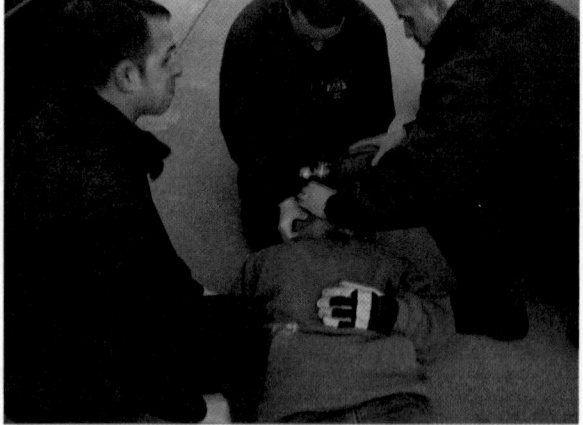

4. Make a decision about the patient's priority for transport.

(continued)

the patient and his or her situation. This information allows you to form an initial general impression of the patient's problem. The general impression determines how you will approach the primary assessment.

Mechanism of Injury and Nature of Illness

One of your first clinical goals of patient assessment is to determine if the patient's problem is due to an injury or a medical problem. If the patient has been injured, you will assess the mechanism of injury. If the patient is complaining of a medical problem, you will seek additional information to establish the nature of the illness.

Some of the information you collect about the safety of the scene also will give you information about the patient. For example, if the scene is unsafe because a vehicle was discovered with the engine running in an enclosed garage, you must consider exposure to carbon monoxide gas a potential problem for any occupants of the vehicle, garage, and house.

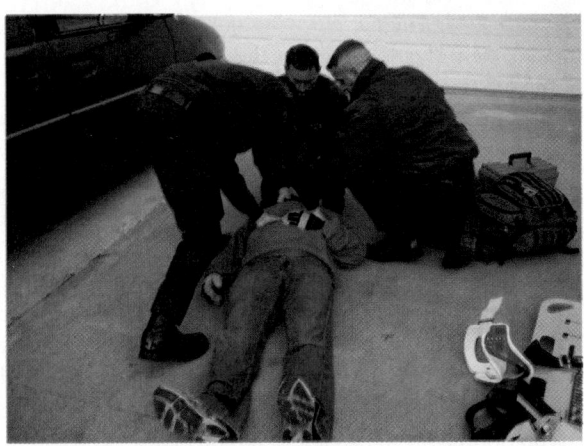

5. Decide how to approach the secondary assessment. For a critical patient such as this, perform a rapid physical exam, begin transport, and then complete the secondary assessment.

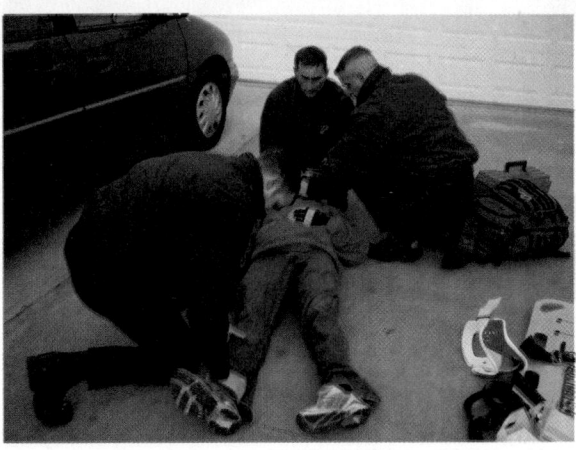

6. The secondary assessment includes a physical examination, vital signs, and medical history.

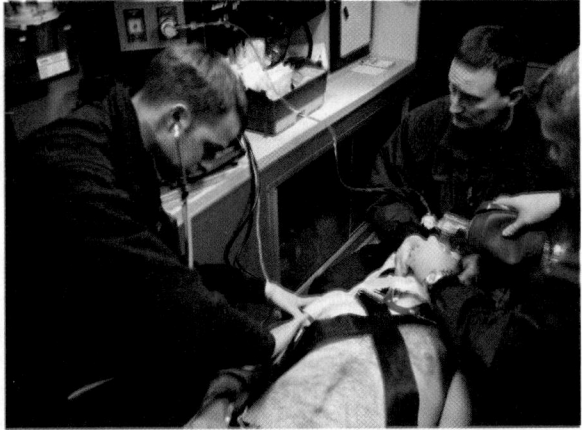

7. Critical patients are reassessed every 5 minutes and noncritical patients are assessed every 15 minutes to detect changes in condition and the effects of treatment.

General Impression

Your initial general impression of the patient will help you determine the urgency of the situation. For example, you will take a much more relaxed approach to the 11-year-old girl sitting on the sidewalk with one rollerblade off, holding her swollen ankle in her hands, than you would to the 65-year-old woman sitting on a chair, gasping for breath with a distressed look on her face. You will take still a different approach to the patient who appears to be unresponsive and cyanotic.

One of the key determinations in the initial general impression is whether the patient is obviously responsive or appears to be unresponsive. The differentiation between responsive and apparently unresponsive determines how you approach the primary assessment. A patient whom you confirm to be unresponsive may be in cardiac arrest. If the patient is unresponsive and his breathing is absent or abnormal, the next step is to quickly check a carotid pulse. If the patient is in cardiac arrest, you must immediately start chest compressions to circulate blood to his vital organs and attach him to an automatic external defibrillator.

If the patient is awake, responds to your voice or to a painful stimulus, or is unresponsive but breathing, you will assess the quality of his airway, breathing, and circulation by performing a systematic primary assessment to determine the patient's level of distress.

Primary Assessment

During the primary assessment, you will further develop the general impression of the nature and seriousness of the patient's problem that you began formulating in the scene size-up. You will confirm the **level of responsiveness**, look for and correct any immediate threats to life, and establish the priorities for patient care and transport.

The mnemonic *ABCD* represents the components of the primary assessment for all patients. *ABCD* makes sense alphabetically and helps remember what the components of the primary assessment are, but it is not necessarily the sequence in which the components are addressed. In the mnemonic, disability (D) refers specifically to checking for any alteration in the patient's level of responsiveness (neurologic disability). You have made an initial determination of the patient's disability by the time you form an initial general impression in the scene size-up. In fact, you will often have simultaneously collected information about the patient's airway, breathing, and circulation (ABC). But at the general

impression stage, your information is presumptive and must be confirmed. The patient who appears unresponsive may, indeed, be unresponsive, but he also may be sleeping or **obtunded** (Figure 14-3).

With the 11-year-old patient mentioned earlier, you can quickly determine that she is alert, her airway is open, she is breathing adequately, and her circulation is adequate. You will most likely begin by introducing yourself, asking the patient's name, and asking her what happened. So, your primary assessment was nearly effortless, and you are quickly able to move on to the secondary assessment. In contrast, you will look more closely and deliberately at the 65-year-old patient to determine the patient's level of consciousness and the quality of her airway, breathing, and circulation. Your approach to a patient who appears unresponsive and is cyanotic differs, as well.

Disability: Level of Responsiveness

An alteration in a patient's level of responsiveness (ability to respond to the environment, also called *level of consciousness*), or other aspects of the **mental status** (such as clarity of thinking and appropriate behavior), means there is a potential for life-threatening problems. While it will likely require more information to determine the underlying cause of the alteration in level of responsiveness, you will use your initial determination of the level of responsiveness to help determine the seriousness of the situation.

At this early stage of assessment, you are simply determining whether the patient is alert, responds to voice, responds only to painful stimuli, or is completely unresponsive. You can remember this assessment using the mnemonic *AVPU* to determine the patient's best response to stimuli. If the patient is awake and completely aware of his surroundings, he is alert (A). If the patient is not alert, check

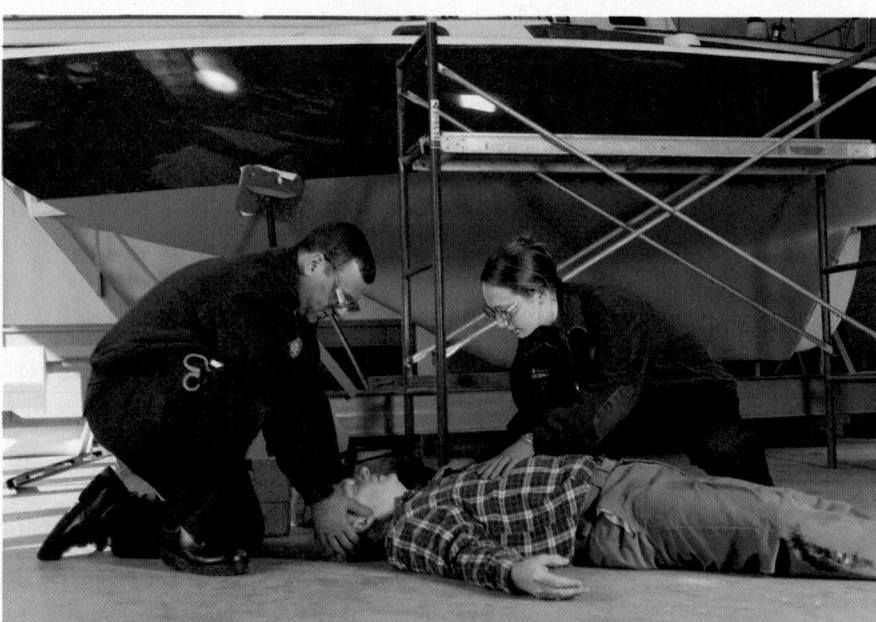

FIGURE 14-3

During the primary assessment, Advanced EMTs confirm the level of responsiveness and check for and correct immediately life-threatening problems involving the airway, breathing, and circulation.

to see if he responds to verbal stimuli (V). If the patient does not respond to your voice, check to see if he responds to painful stimuli (P). Finally, the patient may be completely unresponsive to all stimuli (U).

Airway, Breathing, and Circulation

Immediate threats to life include any problem with the patient's airway, breathing, or circulation—the ABCs. You have already learned that checking for the absence of breathing and circulation is your highest priority in an unresponsive patient. In a patient who is not in cardiac arrest, an obstructed airway prevents oxygenated air from reaching the lungs to oxygenate red blood cells. No oxygen will be delivered to the cells, and the patient will quickly asphyxiate and die. In this case, an obstructed airway must be managed immediately.

A patient whose airway is open, but who is breathing inadequately to ventilate the lungs, will quickly become hypoxic. Inadequate breathing, too, must be corrected immediately (Figure 14-4). (Chapter 16 will provide the details of how to intervene to correct an obstructed airway, maintain an open airway, and provide artificial ventilation and oxygen.)

There are two considerations in assessing circulation. First, you are concerned with the overall quality of the patient's perfusion. If the patient is pulseless and meets criteria to begin resuscitation, you will begin CPR. Beyond the presence of the pulse, you are concerned with whether the pulse rate is within normal range, and the strength and regularity of the pulse. The other consideration in addressing circulation is to control ongoing hemorrhage. Uncontrolled hemorrhage will lead to shock and death. Patients with poor perfusion and significant bleeding are critical and require rapid intervention and transport without delay.

Establishing Priorities

As an EMS provider, you naturally are concerned about what interventions your patients need. However, do not forget that a major intervention is getting your patient to the hospital. All other tasks are planned around that need. The primary assessment helps to establish your priorities for treatment and transportation. At that point, your general impression of the patient's condition can tell you if the patient is best served by taking a few more minutes at the scene to gather more information or by preparing for transport immediately. That decision is based on your categorization of the patient as critical or noncritical.

Critical patients are those who need, or are on the verge of needing, emergent interventions. Quickly implementing interventions aimed at supporting the airway, breathing, and circulation, and getting critical patients to the hospital without undue delay best serve them. You will continue your assessment and treatment en route to the hospital. Ideally, your partner or other EMS providers at the scene are making transport preparations while you are conducting your primary assessment and making initial interventions. Teamwork and communication are essential in making things work smoothly in time-critical situations.

Critical patients include those in cardiac arrest, with difficulty breathing, cardiac chest pain, signs and symptoms of stroke, and those with a significant mechanism of injury (Table 14-1). Patients with cardiac chest pain, for example, are at risk of cardiac arrest and other life-threatening complications that are best managed in the hospital. Those patients need quick intervention to prevent further damage to the heart. Critical trauma patients may have uncontrolled internal hemorrhage that requires prompt surgical intervention. Delay at the scene serves only to delay the definitive interventions that such patients need.

Noncritical patients are those who need to be evaluated and treated at the hospital, but whose conditions do not require immediate intervention. They include the following types of patient:

- Patients with no immediate concern for airway, breathing, or circulation

- Patients with a mental status that is not altered

- Patients with no life-threatening medical conditions or mechanisms of injury

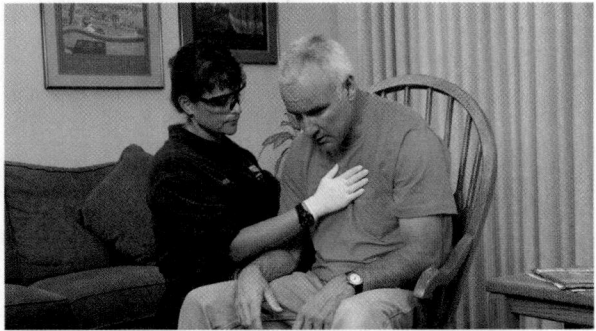
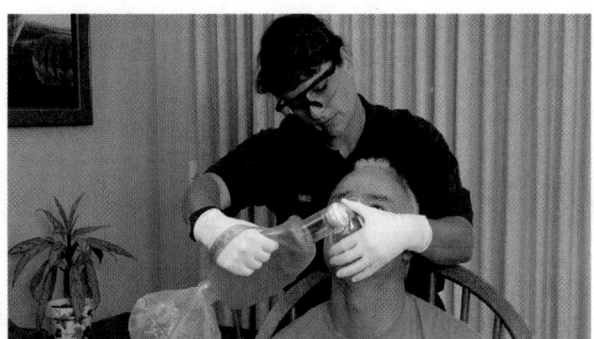

FIGURE 14-4

Hypoxia and inadequate breathing must be corrected during the primary assessment, before moving on to a more detailed assessment.

TABLE 14-1   National Trauma Triage Protocol

VITAL SIGNS AND LEVEL OF RESPONSIVENESS
- Glasgow Coma Scale < 14
- Systolic blood pressure < 90 mmHg
- Respiratory rate < 10 or > 20 breaths per minute (< 20 in infant < 1 year old)

ANATOMY OF INJURY
- All penetrating injuries to head, neck, torso, and extremities proximal to elbow and knee
- Flail chest
- Two or more proximal long-bone fractures
- Crushed, degloved, or mangled extremity
- Amputation proximal to wrist or ankle
- Pelvic fracture
- Open or depressed skull fracture
- Paralysis

MECHANISM OF INJURY AND EVIDENCE OF HIGH-ENERGY IMPACT
- Falls
  - Adults > 20 ft (1 story = 10 ft)
  - Children >10 ft or two to three times patient's height
- High-risk auto crash
  - Intrusion > 12 in. occupant site; > 18 in. any site
  - Ejection (partial or complete) from automobile
  - Death in same passenger compartment
  - Vehicle telemetry data consistent with high risk of injury
- Auto versus pedestrian/bicyclist thrown, run over or with > 20 mph impact
- Motorcycle crash > 20 mph

SPECIAL PATIENT OR SYSTEM CONSIDERATIONS
- Age
  - Risk of injury death increases after age 55 years.
  - Children should be preferentially triaged to pediatric-capable trauma centers.
- Anticoagulation and bleeding disorders
- Burns
  - Without other trauma: Triage to burn facility
  - With trauma mechanism: Triage to trauma center
- Time-sensitive extremity injury
- End-stage renal disease requiring dialysis
- Pregnancy > 20 weeks
- EMS provider judgment

Source: Data from Centers for Disease Control. (2006). *Field triage decision scheme: The national trauma triage protocol.* Retrieved November 20, 2010, from http://www.cdc.gov/fieldtriage/index.html

analgesic prior to transport. Similarly, taking time to splint an isolated forearm fracture will make transportation much more comfortable for the patient. It also can minimize further injury induced by unnecessary movement of the injured extremity (Figure 14-5).

Unfortunately, it may not always be as easy as it sounds to make a determination of how sick a patient is. When in doubt, do not delay unnecessarily at the scene. Manage problems with the airway, breathing, and circulation; initiate transport; and continue your assessment and management en route.

It also is not as easy as it sounds to make clean distinctions between either performing or not performing the secondary assessment and additional management at the scene. For example, unresponsive patients have threatened airways. The airway is a primary assessment concern. Unresponsive patients are at risk for airway obstruction by the tongue and for aspiration of blood or vomit into the lungs. Even our best methods for managing the patient's airway are not as good as the patient's own ability to manage his airway if he is responsive. As an Advanced EMT, you will have the ability to treat select causes of unresponsiveness in a manner that quickly improves the patient's level of responsiveness and ability to manage his airway. In such cases, you may be warranted in providing treatment while on the scene, rather than delaying it to prepare the patient for transport.

Imagine, for example, that you and you partner are on the scene of an unresponsive diabetic patient and there are no additional providers available to respond. You have completed the primary assessment, including airway management and oxygen, and you have performed a rapid head-to-toe exam. Because you have determined the patient is a diabetic, you suspect his unresponsiveness may be the result of a blood glucose level that is too low. In this case, it may be best to test his blood glucose level before preparing him for transport. If needed, you can start an IV at the scene, and administer a 50 percent dextrose solution. Within a few minutes, you may have a responsive patient who can manage his own airway.

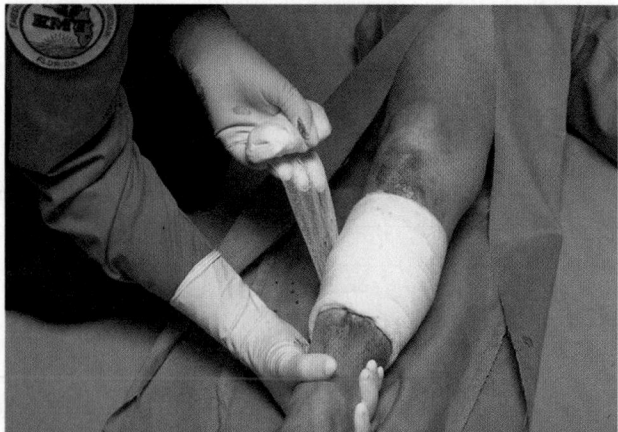

FIGURE 14-5

Many patients benefit from simple treatments prior to being transported.

For example, the chef who splashed boiling water on his hand and forearm is in pain and certainly needs medical attention for his injury. But you can provide temporary management of the wound during transport. If allowed by protocol, you also can treat the patient's pain with an

On the other hand, for a patient without a history of diabetes, the best choice may be to defer the blood glucose test until you are en route to the hospital, because chances are much less that the patient has a low blood glucose level. For this patient, it is more likely that you cannot treat the underlying problem in the prehospital setting. The patient is better served by being transported without delay to the hospital.

The thought of making such decisions may be overwhelming at the moment. Learning to make them is a long process. You will develop critical thinking skills and judgment as you progress throughout your training program, and you will develop a better sense of the types of things you should consider to make good decisions.

Secondary Assessment

After you have identified threats to the patient's ABCs, a secondary assessment is performed to collect additional information. This new information helps you determine what the patient's problem is and how it should be managed. Your approach to the secondary assessment depends on whether the patient's problem is medical or traumatic. It also depends on the severity of the patient's condition. With critically ill patients, a **rapid physical exam** may be performed while preparing for transport, but a complete secondary assessment may be best performed during transport to the hospital. For most patients, though, you will perform a complete secondary assessment.

The secondary assessment consists of the following steps:

- Obtaining a medical history from the patient
- Measuring **baseline vital signs**
- Conducting a physical examination

A rapid physical exam may be performed prior to transport for critical medical patients (**rapid medical exam**) and must be performed for all critical trauma patients (**rapid trauma exam**). The rapid physical exam procedure is essentially the same for medical and trauma patients, but different findings are anticipated. A rapid physical exam for both medical and trauma patients is used to quickly check the head, neck, torso, and proximal extremities for any life-threatening conditions that were not found in the primary assessment. The rapid physical exam does not replace a complete secondary assessment en route to the hospital. Vital signs, medical history, and a more detailed physical exam must still be performed en route.

The order in which to perform each task depends on the nature and severity of the patient's condition and the resources available. For example, in general, the history will receive more emphasis than the physical exam for a medical patient. If there are plenty of EMS providers on scene and just one patient, providers could team up to perform two or more tasks at once (Figure 14-6). Or it may be best to wait until the patient is in the ambulance, away from bystanders, to ask history questions.

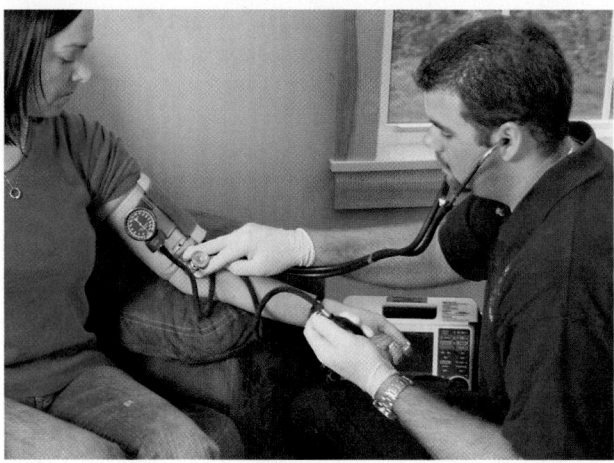

FIGURE 14-6

With teamwork, many components of the patient assessment process can proceed simultaneously.

Secondary Assessment of Medical Patients

The secondary assessment of patients with medical complaints depends on whether the patient is critical or noncritical. An unresponsive patient should always be considered critical. A responsive patient may be either critical or noncritical.

For a patient who is responsive (that is, a patient who is alert and can answer your questions), start the secondary assessment by obtaining a medical history. Focus it on the patient's **chief complaint**. Obtain baseline vital signs, and then focus your physical exam on those aspects that can give you relevant information about the patient's condition. This is called a **focused physical exam**.

For an unresponsive medical patient (one who is not alert and who cannot answer your questions), perform a rapid physical exam to detect any serious problems that were not found in the primary assessment. Baseline vital signs will give you more information about the severity of the patient's condition. Meanwhile, another EMS provider can question family, friends, or bystanders to get as much information about the patient and the event as possible. If you have not determined a cause of the patient's condition from the rapid physical exam, vital signs, and available history, a complete **head-to-toe exam** performed en route to the hospital may provide more information.

Secondary Assessment of Trauma Patients

The approach to the secondary assessment of a trauma patient depends on the severity of the patient's condition. You will judge severity based on the mechanism of injury and primary assessment findings.

Some EMS providers describe severity in terms of a "critical" versus a "stable" patient. However, only the terms "critical" and "noncritical" are used to categorize trauma patients for the purposes of directing the secondary assessment. A critical adult patient meets one or more of the criteria for trauma triage to a specialized trauma center. Noncritical patients are those who have non–life-threatening and non–limb-threatening isolated injuries, or who do not have a mechanism of injury anticipated to produce life- or limb-threatening injuries.

For a critical trauma patient, time is of the essence in stabilizing immediate life threats. It also is important to perform a rapid trauma exam while preparing the patient for transport (Figure 14-7). The purpose of such an assessment is to further check vital areas of the body for indications of potentially life-threatening injuries.

You can remember the link between the primary assessment and secondary assessment by the mnemonic *ABCDE*. You check the airway, breathing, circulation, and disability as described for the primary assessment. The "E" indicates that you will quickly expose (E) and check vital areas of the patient's body. This is a quick head-to-toe exam meant to find any indications of significant injury, such as open wounds, bruises, and deformities. Once en route to the hospital, if the patient's condition and the available resources allow, you will perform a complete head-to-toe physical exam (sometimes called a detailed physical exam), obtain baseline vital signs, and then gather a medical history. Note that assessments, treatments, and preparations for transport must proceed simultaneously. This need for multitasking is one of the great challenges of EMS.

The approach to secondary assessment of noncritical trauma patients contains the same components as for critical patients. However, the physical exam is modified so that it focuses on the isolated injury (focused physical exam). You obtain baseline vital signs, and then gather a

medical history to complete the secondary assessment. For example, imagine you have responded to the stockroom of a large department store for a patient who cut his hand with a box cutter while opening a box. It is not necessary to perform a head-to-toe exam on this patient. You will examine the injury, control bleeding, and check circulation, motor function, and sensation distal to the injury. You will then take vital signs and a patient history. You will manage the patient's injury, and then transport him for further evaluation and care.

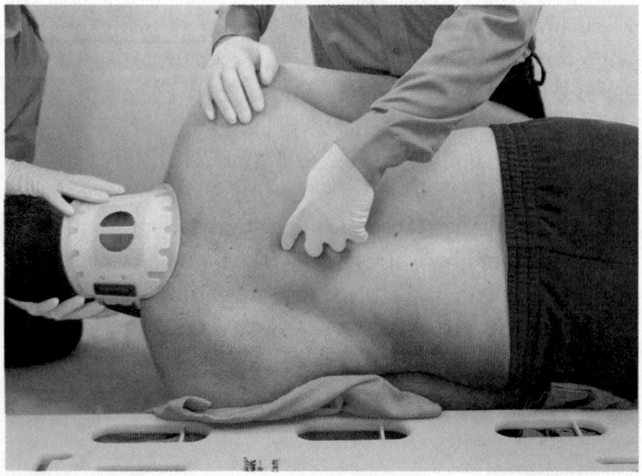

Reassessment

Patient assessment continues throughout the call. You begin collecting information, forming impressions, and making decisions as soon as you see the patient. Information gathering and analysis continue through the primary and secondary assessments. Although the technical term is *reassessment*, think of it as an ongoing assessment during which you continue to make observations about the patient while preparing him for transport and initiating treatment. However, you also will periodically and systematically reassess specific information based on the patient's initial complaints and condition, and the interventions you performed.

For a critically ill or injured patient, you will reassess every 5 minutes or sooner. You will reassess a noncritical patient every 15 minutes, or at least once during transport. You also will reassess a patient any time there is a change in his condition. For example, if a patient you are transporting for difficulty breathing suddenly complains of chest pain, you will immediately reassess him based on both his original and new complaints.

Clinical Reasoning and Problem Solving

Patient assessment is more than just a process of collecting information. You must analyze the information and use it to direct decision making. You also must determine what additional information is relevant or not relevant to the current problem. You must determine the nature of the patient's problem and decide what interventions are needed. You must continue to collect and further analyze information to check for the accuracy of our initial impression, the effects of treatments, and identify trends in the patient's condition.

Finding the answers to the questions listed in Table 14-2 requires a process of problem solving that is called *clinical problem solving* or *clinical reasoning*. Patient safety depends on all health care providers having excellent problem-solving skills. Many errors in medicine, including EMS, are made because of faulty clinical reasoning processes.

Advanced EMTs do not make definitive diagnoses of patients' problems. However, you do use the information

FIGURE 14-7

For critical trauma patients, a rapid trauma exam is performed before packaging and transporting the patient, but a detailed head-to-toe exam is deferred until you are en route to the hospital.

TABLE 14-2	Questions Guiding the Patient Assessment Process

- Is it safe to approach the patient and begin care in the patient's current location? If not, what must you do to solve this problem?
- What is the nature of the patient's problem?
- How sick is the patient?
- Which interventions, resources, and actions are required immediately?
- Which health care facility can best meet the patient's immediate needs?
- How should the patient be transported to receive this care?
- What do you need to do to support the patient's vital functions from the time you arrive at the scene to the time you transfer care to other health care personnel?
- Is the patient's condition stable, improving, or worsening?

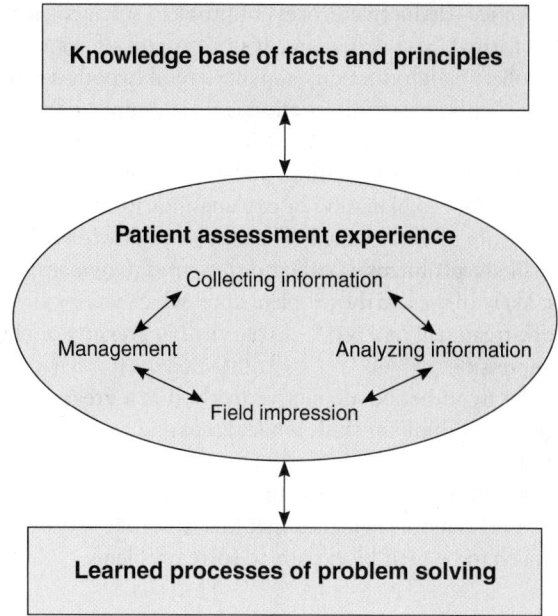

FIGURE 14-8

Model of Clinical Problem Solving. In clinical problem solving, there is a relationship between experience, knowledge base, and learned processes for clinical problem solving.

obtained from the assessment to understand the patient's immediate problems. That is, you formulate field impressions to determine what actions to take. Sometimes your field impression may be general, as with the patient who has no history of respiratory problems and a sudden onset of difficulty breathing. For such a patient, your clinical impression may be "respiratory distress." You will treat the patient with oxygen and, if needed, assist with ventilations. Other times, your clinical impression may be more specific. For example, it is often possible to be reasonably certain that a specific patient is experiencing acute coronary syndrome. Specificity is important in this case, because you will give medications intended to treat some of the specific concerns with myocardial infarction, in addition to providing more general supportive treatment.

As allowed by protocol, Advanced EMTs may give medications for hypoglycemia, acute coronary syndrome, asthma, anaphylaxis, and narcotic overdose. In each of those cases, you must have a reasonable degree of certainty about your field impression.

Readiness for Problem Solving

Accurate problem solving requires an adequate knowledge base of the facts and principles of anatomy and physiology, pathophysiology, pharmacology, and other information you will learn in your training program. Accurate and efficient problem solving is also a function of your learned methods for solving problems. Like all skills, problem-solving ability is improved with practice.

Consciously thinking about your approach to clinical problems and getting feedback from your instructors will help you develop problem-solving skills. You will be expected to "think about your thinking" as you proceed through your training program. Be sure to reflect on your performance in case studies, lab scenarios, and clinical experiences.

The Model of Clinical Problem Solving (Figure 14-8) represents the relationship among experience, knowledge base, and learned processes for clinical problem solving. There are many approaches to clinical problem solving, and many pitfalls, too. The goal of this section is to introduce to you some concepts in problem solving.

The Hypothetico–Deductive Approach to Problem Solving

Much is made of the need for critical thinking skills in EMS. Indeed, it plays an important role. But there are other considerations as well. Usually, when we talk about critical thinking, we are referring to the hypothetico–deductive approach to solving problems, which is often held up as the ideal approach to problem solving. However, it offers both advantages and disadvantages. At times, other approaches to problem solving can serve us better.

If you have ever watched the television series *House*, you have seen a version of the hypothetico–deductive approach to clinical problem solving at work. The hypothetico–deductive process of problem solving is structured, formal, and deliberate. It is a process of systematically collecting information, forming several hypotheses, and then collecting more information in an attempt to "prove" or "disprove" each hypothesis. It is a repetitive process of forming, refining, eliminating, and adding hypotheses until the most likely explanation or explanations for the patient's problem are all that remain. The narrowed-down list of the most likely problems is called *differential diagnoses*. The most likely of these is the problem upon which you base your specific treatment and is called your *field impression* or clinical impression.

The hypothetico–deductive method is a great way to learn critical thinking skills while discussing case studies or scenarios, but it requires the luxuries of time and information that are not always available in the prehospital setting. There is also ample evidence that this is not the most likely approach to be used by experts to solve problems.

Pattern Recognition

Experts often use a problem-solving process called *pattern recognition*. The expert immediately recognizes problems based on their similarity to previously encountered problems. In order to develop and store these patterns (called *illness scripts*) in long-term memory, you must have a substantial amount of experience. Without experience with a

---

IN THE FIELD

EMS personnel cannot collect the type of information needed to "prove" or "disprove" hypotheses, or to "rule in" or "rule out" hypotheses. Instead, you must rank hypotheses in terms of what is more or less likely, and then act on the most likely hypothesis.

---

variety of patient presentations and feedback to check the accuracy of your impressions, your illness scripts may be inaccurate or insufficient to serve you (or your patients) well. Those immediate impressions are based on typical experiences. The narrower your range of experience, the more likely you will lack a script that matches a given patient's presentation. The usefulness of pattern recognition is developed with experience and feedback over time. This method of problem solving can be quite useful. When a problem is accurately identified, the associated script also contains other information about the problem, such as what treatment is indicated. Pattern recognition can be prone to what is called *premature diagnostic closure*, meaning that there is inadequate consideration given to other possibilities. Whenever a pattern is recognized, you must still search for information that can both corroborate and refute the initial impression.

Heuristics: Rules of Thumb

Another approach to clinical problem solving is the use of *heuristics*, or rules of thumb. Some heuristics in medicine are formal, and some are developed by individuals based on their experiences. An example of a heuristic often used in medicine is, "When you hear hoof beats, think horses, not zebras." Simply put, this means that the most common cause (the "horse") of a collection of signs and symptoms (the "hoof beats") is a more likely conclusion than the uncommon cause (the "zebra"). As an example, the most common cause of shock in a trauma patient is hypovolemia. You should assume that shock in a trauma patient is due to hypovolemia, and treat accordingly, until there is evidence to the contrary. You should not initially assume less likely causes of shock, such as cardiogenic or neurogenic shock.

Heuristics are used because, by and large, they are useful. But heuristics, too, can be prone to error. Notice that,

---

PERSONAL PERSPECTIVE

Advanced EMT Student Evan Gregory: "I was pretty confident in what I had learned in class about patient assessment, and thought I'd done pretty well in practice scenarios. But on my first emergency department clinical shift, I felt tongue-tied when I followed my preceptor in to talk to a 49-year-old male patient complaining of back pain. The patient was pacing around and refused to lie down, despite the fact that he said his back was killing him. My preceptor asked the patient to show her where his back hurt. When he put his hand over the lower ribs on his right side, my preceptor asked the patient if he'd ever had a kidney stone before. That threw me for a loop! I wondered where she came up with that question, but I was even more surprised when the patient

answered that he had had a kidney stone before. Afterward, I asked my preceptor, Barb, what made her ask that question. She told me that the patient fit a pattern she recognized after working as a nurse in the ED for three years. "Middle-aged male, good vital signs on his triage note, complaining of flank pain on one side, pacing about and looking extremely uncomfortable. One of the first things you think of is kidney stone," she told me. I learned from Barb that many problems present with what she called classic findings. "Classic findings are useful," she told me. "They help us recognize the way some problems typically present. Just make sure you follow through with your history and assessment to make sure there isn't something else going on.""

while initial treatment of the trauma patient in shock is based on the heuristic, you also must consider the possibility of other causes, even though they are less common.

Pitfalls in Clinical Reasoning

One way to reduce errors in clinical reasoning is to be aware of some common pitfalls. Many of those pitfalls occur because human beings have predispositions to respond to information in certain ways. In fact, those pitfalls are not unique to thinking about clinical problems. In fact, errors in thinking often are made in everyday life.

Search Satisficing

Consider the pitfall of search **satisficing**. Imagine you are shopping for a gift for a family member. You are pressed for time and a few dollars' variation in price is not a concern for you. The mall is crowded and traffic is a mess. If you are like most people, you will be tempted to settle for the first satisfactory item, even if it is not the perfect gift. The biggest risk here is that your gift may get a lukewarm reception. Unfortunately, search satisficing is much riskier in medicine. Imagine you are assessing a patient who has fallen from a second-story rooftop. He is complaining of pain in his arm and you find that his right arm is deformed above the elbow. Assuming that this is the patient's biggest or only problem is an example of search satisficing. As soon as something was found, the search for anything else stopped when, in fact, the patient might have much more significant injuries.

Fundamental Attribution Error

Fundamental attribution error occurs when you wrongly attribute a person's behavior to his personality or disposition, rather than to circumstances. If you walked into the emergency department and encountered a visitor arguing with the staff, your assumption might be that the visitor is a troublemaker. Could there be another explanation? Imagine the patient who is being dismissive of his potential for injuries and walking away from you each time you try to get information and ask him a few questions. It would be easy to attribute the patient's behavior to his personality, but a number of medical issues can cause illogical or even hostile behavior. The patient may have a traumatic brain injury and be confused or combative. He may be a diabetic with hypoglycemia or he may have had a stroke or may be hypoxic.

Closely related to fundamental attribution error is a pitfall called "psych out" error. In this case, there is a failure to pay sufficient attention to the possibility that a patient has a medical problem because he has a history of psychiatric illness. Instead, the assumption is that his complaints or behaviors are related to his psychiatric diagnosis.

Commission Bias

A particularly notable error in EMS is called *commission bias.* This means that EMS providers can sometimes have a hard time *not* initiating treatment. It is difficult to realize that sometimes the less one does, the better. Providers often have a tendency to overtreat patients because it makes them feel better to do something for a patient. Remember, there must be a clear indication for any test or treatment that is provided to a patient. You must be able to defend everything you do on medical grounds.

Narcotic antagonists, such as naloxone, which is a drug that may be given by Advanced EMTs, provides a prime example of commission error. Naloxone is indicated for patients with suspected narcotic overdose who have respiratory depression. However, many EMS providers feel relatively helpless when faced with an unresponsive patient and give naloxone, even when respirations are not depressed or when the likelihood of narcotic overdose is remote, believing that doing anything is better than doing nothing.

Less likely, but also possible, is the opposite, an *omission error.* Omission error occurs when something should be done, but the provider hesitates to do it. It may be daunting to consider placing a mask over the face of a conscious patient in severe respiratory distress, and providers may hesitate to do it. However, it is the treatment the patient requires and you must not hesitate to intervene when it is needed.

Anchoring

Anchoring is a pitfall that occurs when a piece of information revealed early in the assessment process is seized upon and made to be more significant than it really is. It is essentially an error made by jumping to conclusions. Imagine a patient tells you that she has a headache. Because she told you very early in the process that she is a diabetic, there is a tendency to anchor on that information, attributing the headache to diabetes, perhaps assuming that she is hypoglycemic. But what if diabetes is not the cause of the patient's problems today? What if she is having a stroke or has some other cause of headache? Of course, you should consider the possibility that diabetes is involved, but you must not dismiss other causes of the problem, either.

Avoiding Pitfalls

There are literally dozens of pitfalls in both everyday thinking and in clinical reasoning, and those are but a few common examples. Reflect on your thinking processes for each call. Share your thought processes with your partner, a preceptor, or mentor. Get feedback on your patients' outcomes to determine if your thinking was accurate. Read case studies, review text material from time to time, and read journal articles. The more practice you get using information and solving problems, provided you get feedback on your accuracy, the better you become at solving problems.

Clinical-Reasoning Process

Advanced EMTs Julia Payne and Beth Mercer are on the scene of a disheveled man in his 30s with his hands cuffed behind his back, struggling with two police officers. The patient is cursing, thrashing about, and yelling, "Let me go!" The patient's supervisor called 911 when the patient, Brian Nelson, became unruly at work. The supervisor knows little about him beyond the information from his employment application.

The patient's ability to speak without difficulty indicates to Julia and Beth that his airway is open, he is breathing, and has adequate circulation. But the patient's behavior indicates that he has an altered mental status. While law enforcement and the supervisor are leaning toward thinking this is some sort of drug-induced or psychiatric problem, Beth and Julia know that a number of serious medical problems might account for the patient's behavior.

Following their customary way of approaching similar calls, Beth talks with the supervisor to get as much information as she can, including an emergency contact number for Brian. Meanwhile, Julia observes that Brian's general appearance is pale and he is sweating profusely. As an Advanced EMT for four years, Julia has seen a number of similar cases where the cause of the patient's behavior is hypoglycemia. She recognizes this pattern almost immediately.

She knows that there are other potential causes of the patient's presentation, but she wants to check her suspicion about diabetes first, for a couple of reasons. First, it is a very likely explanation for the patient's presentation. And if confirmed, it can easily be treated in the field. The patient's age makes other problems, such as a cardiac event or pulmonary embolism, less likely. Second, untreated hypoglycemia will progress, and the patient's condition may worsen.

Julia asks Beth to see if she can find out if the patient has a history of diabetes, along with any other medical history she can get. Julia then asks the police officers if they can help hold Brian still long enough for her to check his blood glucose level. Beth reports back that the patient is a diabetic, and the blood glucose level of 40 mg/dL confirms that he is hypoglycemic. Meanwhile, Brian is still uncooperative, but is becoming more confused and lethargic. With the assistance of law enforcement officers, Julia and Beth place Brian on their stretcher and load him into the ambulance.

While Beth prepares to administer oxygen by nasal cannula, Julia starts an IV of normal saline in Brian's left forearm with an 18-gauge catheter, and begins administering 25 grams of 50 percent dextrose by slow IV push. As Julia pushes in the last of the D_{50}, Brian becomes more alert and says, "My sugar got low, didn't it?"

"It sure did," answers Julia. "We got 40 on our blood glucose meter and we've given you some sugar through an IV. I'm glad you're feeling better. What hospital do you want to go to, Brian?"

"Mercy, I guess, if I have to go."

"Well, Brian, I think it is best if you go and get your blood sugar stabilized and see if adjustments should be made to your medications or diet. We'll have you there in about 15 minutes. In the meantime, I'd like to ask you some questions and take your vital signs, if that's okay."

"Okay, I guess that's best. Can you call my wife and let her know?"

"I will," says Beth. "I just spoke to her a few minutes ago. I'll let her know we're on our way to Mercy."

CHAPTER REVIEW

Chapter Summary

Now that you have an overview of the patient assessment and clinical decision-making processes, you have a framework for learning the information in subsequent chapters. In practice, many components of assessment, treatment, and preparation for transportation must occur simultaneously. Knowing each component well and engaging in teamwork with good communication will help you with the required multitasking. With so much going on at once,

you must remember your priorities. Always prioritize scene safety, airway management, management of ventilation and oxygenation, and maintaining the patient's circulation. Developing your assessment and problem-solving skills takes background knowledge and experience. Take every opportunity you can to improve your knowledge base and to practice—and get feedback on—your patient assessment and decision-making skills.

Review Questions

Multiple-Choice Questions

1. The status of a patient's airway should be checked in the:

a. scene size-up.
b. primary assessment.
c. secondary assessment.
d. baseline vital signs.

2. Which one of the following factors, on its own, should be considered in making a determination that a patient is critical?

a. Patient complains of severe pain in his fractured ankle.
b. Patient states he has vomited four times this morning.
c. Patient responds only to a painful stimulus, such as pinching his shoulder.
d. Patient tells you he has a history of diabetes.

3. You have performed a scene size-up and primary assessment, and have determined that you have a critical trauma patient. Your next step should be to:

a. immediately load the patient for transport.
b. conduct a rapid trauma assessment.
c. get baseline vital signs.
d. find out the patient's medical history.

4. For most medical patients, you will get the most useful information, and will therefore emphasize, which one of the following components of the secondary assessment?

a. The medical history
b. The rapid medical assessment
c. The name of the patient's personal physician
d. The blood glucose level

5. Which one of the following best describes the process by which experts typically identify a patient's problem?

a. Long, complicated chains of hypothetico–deductive reasoning
b. Testing for every possible problem the patient could have
c. Assuming that each patient has the worst possible problem he could have, based on his signs and symptoms
d. Recognizing patterns of patient presentations made familiar through experience

Critical-Thinking Questions

6. Explain the purpose of obtaining baseline vital signs.

7. How is the mnemonic *ABCD* applied in the primary assessment?

8. For each of the following items, indicate when it is performed. Write "P" for the primary assessment, "S" for the secondary assessment, or "R" for reassessment. NOTE: Some items may be performed in more than one part of the patient assessment process.

a. Checking the airway _____
b. Taking baseline vital signs _____
c. Taking the patient's history _____
d. Assessing the effects of treatment _____
e. Performing a focused physical examination _____

References

Centers for Disease Control. (2006). *Field triage decision scheme: The national trauma triage protocol.* Retrieved November 20, 2010, from http://www.cdc.gov/fieldtriage/index.html

Additional Reading

Alexander, M. (2009). *Reasoning processes used by paramedics to solve clinical problems* (Unpublished doctoral dissertation). The George Washington University, Washington, DC.

American Heart Association. (2010). *2010 American Heart Association guidelines for cardiopulmonary resuscitation and emergency cardiovascular care. Circulation, 122.*

15

Scene Size-Up and Primary Assessment

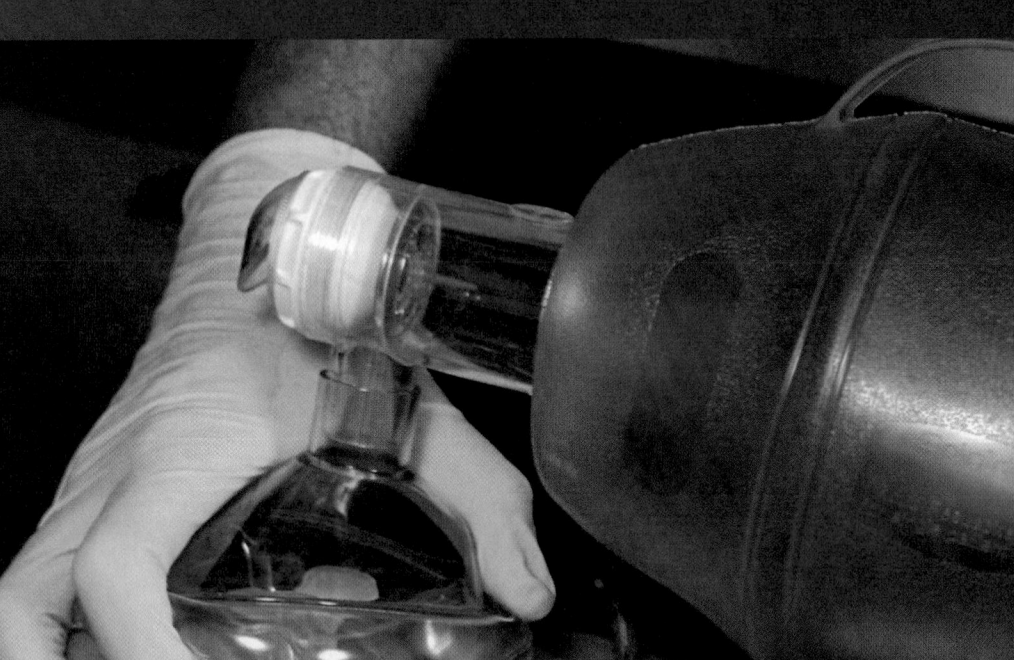

Content Area: Assessment

Advanced EMT Education Standard: Applies scene information and patient assessment findings (scene size-up, primary and secondary assessment, patient history, and reassessment) to guide emergency management.

Objectives

After reading this chapter, you should be able to:

15.1	Define key terms introduced in this chapter.
15.2	Use information from the scene size-up and initial approach to the patient to formulate a general impression of the nature and seriousness of the patient's condition.
15.3	Use the primary assessment findings to identify immediate threats to life.
15.4	Accurately assess a patient's level of responsiveness using the AVPU approach.
15.5	Determine whether a patient's airway is patent.
15.6	Differentiate between adequate and inadequate breathing.
15.7	Determine whether a patient has adequate circulation.

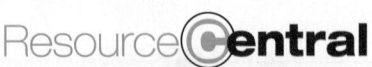

Resource **Central**

CASE STUDY

Advanced EMTs Kyle Davis and Eric Chen have just been dispatched to a motor vehicle collision (MVC) involving a motorcycle on a rural highway about 15 minutes from their station. While they are en route, dispatch informs them that the sheriff's deputy on scene is reporting two patients, one conscious and one unconscious. Dispatch sends a BLS ambulance for backup, with an ETA several minutes after Kyle and Eric will arrive.

As their vehicle approaches the scene, Eric and Kyle can see that the crash is in a sharp curve in the road. Additional law enforcement officers have arrived and stopped traffic in both directions. A state police officer motions Kyle to drive past the barricade.

Through the windshield, Kyle and Eric see a badly damaged motorcycle several yards from a dented and scuffed guardrail. Skid marks and the damage to the motorcycle and guardrail suggest that the motorcycle entered the curve too fast and lost control, striking the guardrail. Law enforcement officers have used absorbent material to manage the small amount of fluid leaking from the motorcycle. There are no downed power lines or damaged objects that could pose a danger to the crew.

A figure is lying motionless on the far side of the guardrail, with a sheriff's deputy manually stabilizing his cervical spine. About 6 feet away, a female with an obviously deformed left thigh is struggling to sit up. The deputy with her is trying to calm her and get her to lie still.

As they get out of the ambulance with reflective vests in place, Eric says to Kyle, "I'll take the patient who's not moving. You check on the other one." He approaches the motionless patient, a male with a bloody face and gurgling respirations. He asks the deputy, "Are there any other patients?"

Problem-Solving Questions

1. What is the next thing Eric should do?
2. What should Kyle look for as he approaches his patient?
3. What equipment must each have to provide patient care in the next few minutes?
4. What decisions must they make within the first few minutes?

15.8 Integrate the use of manual airway maneuvers, simple airway adjuncts, bag-valve-mask ventilations, supplemental oxygen, CPR, defibrillation, and bleeding control into the primary assessment.

15.9 Use the primary assessment findings to re-evaluate the general impression and determine the priority for patient transport.

15.10 Use primary assessment findings to make a decision about the next step in the assessment and management of the patient.

15.11 Describe the processes of gaining and maintaining control of the scene, teamwork, and reducing the patient's anxiety in preparation for obtaining the history and assessing the patient.

Introduction

Advanced EMTs take in and analyze a wealth of information in the first moments after they arrive at the scene. The information collected guides decisions about scene management and immediate patient care. The two phases of patient assessment that provide this initial information are the scene size-up and primary assessment.

Collecting information in a meaningful way requires that you build a mental framework for patient assessment. You must actively look for particular things, determine what they mean, and decide what to do about them. The scene size-up and primary assessment are not just checklists of steps to be completed mindlessly by rote. They are deliberate processes of collecting information that inform decisions about further assessment and treatment.

In the scene size-up, look for indications of scene safety, the number of patients involved, and the general nature of the incident. This information guides operational decisions about safety precautions and additional resources needed. It also gives you an indication of how to initially approach your patient for the primary assessment.

The primary assessment involves collecting and acting on information about immediate threats to the patient's

---

life. You collect information through the senses of sight, hearing, smell, and touch. Rapid analysis of this information tells you whether you must take immediate action to manage the patient's airway, breathing, or circulation. The patient's chief complaint, combined with his general appearance, level of responsiveness, and other primary assessment findings, gives you a preliminary impression of how sick the patient is, what actions you must take immediately, and how quickly the patient must be prepared for transport.

Information from the scene size-up and primary assessment allows you to care for patients in the first few moments of an emergency call. Despite the several pages of text required to discuss the details of the primary assessment, it is a process that should be completed within 30 seconds, with many observations made simultaneously. In this chapter you learn what information to collect from the scene size-up and primary assessment, how to collect it, and how to analyze it. You also gain knowledge of decisions that must be made and actions that must be taken before proceeding with the rest of the patient assessment.

Scene Size-Up

Advanced EMTs start collecting information in the scene size-up, well before making initial contact with their patients. You learned in Chapters 5 and 14 that the scene size-up has an operational aspect and a patient care aspect. The operational aspect includes assessing scene safety and identifying the number of patients. This information informs decisions about additional resources that may be needed to manage the scene.

One of the decisions to think about in your initial approach to the scene is what personal protective equipment (PPE) you will need. If you will be inside a heavily damaged vehicle to care for a patient during extrication, you will need a protective helmet, eyewear, and turnout gear, including heavy gloves. If you see that a patient is bleeding as you make your initial approach, you will decide whether PPE, in addition to latex or vinyl gloves, is needed. (See Chapter 3 for a review of Standard Precautions and PPE.)

The focus in this chapter is on the patient assessment aspect of scene size-up. This aspect focuses on determining the mechanism of injury (MOI) or nature of the illness. Sometimes, obtaining this information is relatively straightforward. Other times, determining the MOI or nature of the illness merges with the primary assessment. You may not know what the nature of the problem is until you make contact with the patient, noting his general appearance and chief complaint.

MOI refers to the types and amounts of energy that a patient was subjected to, resulting in injury (Figure 15-1). Types of energy that can result in injury to human body tissues include the energy of objects in motion (**kinetic energy**), heat (thermal energy), electricity, radiation, and chemical energy.

Kinetic energy can produce blunt or penetrating injuries. Impact with an object that has high surface area and relatively low velocity (speed) does not penetrate the body.

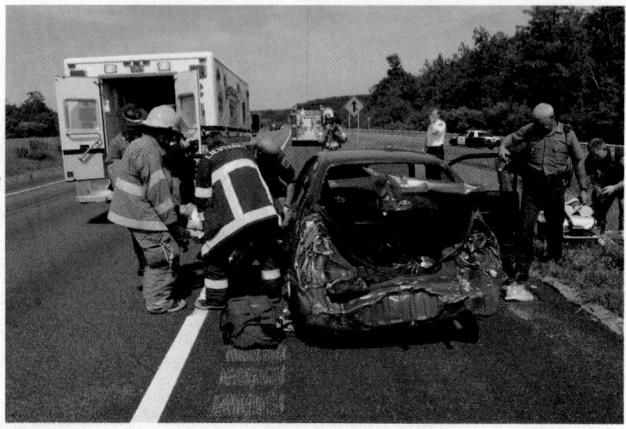

FIGURE 15-1

Observe the scene to determine the mechanism of injury.
(© Mark C. Ide)

This is called **blunt force injury**. Examples of blunt force injury include being struck with a baseball bat, falls, and forces applied in MVCs. Blunt force trauma can result in open injuries when the force is great enough. For example, an elderly patient slips on a throw rug and falls backward, striking her head on a tile floor. This mechanism is blunt, but frequently results in a laceration (cut or tear in the skin).

Penetrating trauma occurs when an object impacting the body has a small surface area. When the surface area is small, a low velocity impact can result in penetration. For example, very little force is needed for the sharp edge of a knife to penetrate the tissues. A bullet usually has a relatively blunt tip, and therefore a greater surface area than the edge of a knife. Much greater velocity is required for the bullet to penetrate the tissues. Some MOIs transfer enough energy to the body that the patient is considered at high risk, even if he does not seem to be seriously injured (Table 15-1).

TABLE 15-1   Critical Mechanisms of Injury

- Complete or partial ejection in a motor vehicle collision (MVC)
- MVC that causes death to another occupant of the same vehicle
- Rollover mechanism MVC
- High-speed MVC
- Intrusion (damage) of > 12 inches into the passenger compartment of a vehicle, or vehicle crush of > 18 inches at any point on the vehicle
- Pedestrian or bicyclist struck by a motor vehicle
- Motorcyclist involved in collision at > 20 mph
- Fall from a height > 20 feet
- Blast (explosion) trauma
- Penetrating trauma except distal to the elbow or knee
- Amputation or near-amputation proximal to the fingers or toes
- Trauma with burns

TABLE 15-2 Indications of Cervical-Spine Injury

- Penetrating injury to the head, neck, or torso
- Shallow-water diving injuries
- Pedestrian–vehicle injuries
- Motor vehicle collisions
- Motorcycle collisions
- Contact sport injuries
- Recreational vehicle (personal watercraft, all-terrain vehicle) injuries
- Hanging
- Falls from a height
- Electrical (including lightning) injuries
- Unresponsive trauma patient

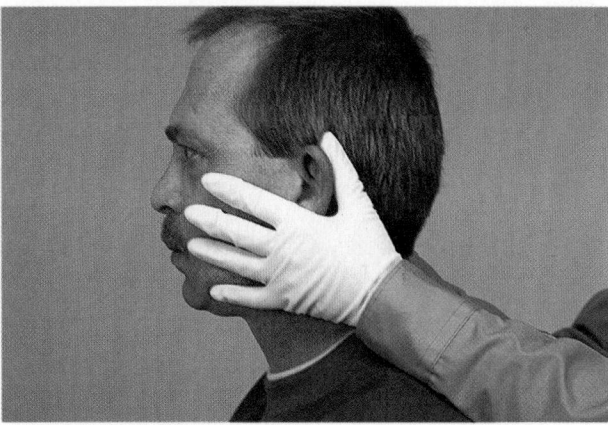

(A)

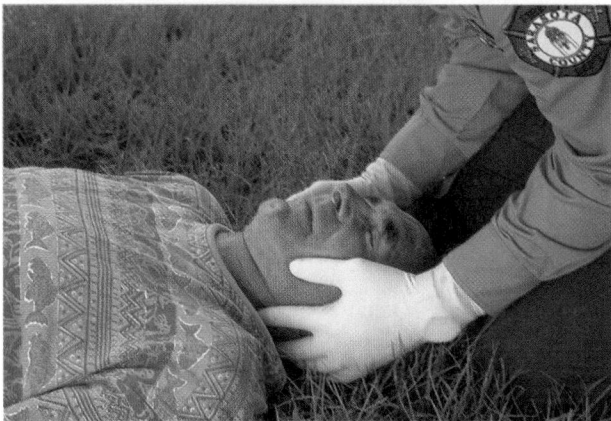

(B)

FIGURE 15-2

When the mechanism of injury is consistent with the possibility of cervical-spine injury, provide in-line manual stabilization of the head and neck as soon as you are at the patient's side. (A) Place your hands on either side of the patient's head to keep the head and neck in a neutral position and prevent movement. (B) Maintain manual stabilization until the patient is fully immobilized to a long backboard with a cervical immobilization collar in place.

(See Chapter 34 for an in-depth discussion of mechanisms of injury.)

Assessment of MOI is used to determine if in-line **manual stabilization** of the cervical spine should be taken upon contact with the patient. Whenever there is an MOI that might have produced injury to the cervical spine, you must take or direct another EMS provider to take **cervical-spine precautions** (Table 15-2).

If the patient is conscious, explain that you are placing your hands on his head to prevent him from moving his head and neck in case he has neck injuries (Figure 15-2). If the patient is unresponsive, first check the carotid pulse. If a pulse is present, open the airway with a **modified jaw-thrust maneuver**, rather than a **head-tilt/chin-lift maneuver** (Figure 15-3). If a carotid pulse is not detected within 10 seconds, follow your protocols for initiating resuscitation in pulseless trauma patients. The head-tilt/chin-lift maneuver is an effective way of opening the airway, but requires hyperextension of the neck, which may aggravate an existing cervical-spine injury. The modified jaw-thrust maneuver (jaw thrust without head extension) is more difficult, particularly when only one provider is available to manage airway and ventilation, but opens the airway without hyperextension of the neck. (See Chapter 16.)

Fortunately, injuries to the cervical spine occur infrequently, even with significant trauma (Hackl, Hausberger, Sailer, Ulmer, & Gassner, 2001; Mithani et al., 2009). If you are unable to maintain an airway with a modified jaw-thrust maneuver, use a head-tilt/chin-lift. The patient must have an open airway to survive, and the risk of causing paralysis of a trauma patient through airway management procedures is much lower than it is often presumed to be. Nonetheless, there is no reason to be careless with the cervical spine of a patient with significant trauma and a modified jaw-thrust maneuver should be used if it effectively maintains the patient's airway.

Information about the nature of the illness is typically very general during the scene size-up (Figure 15-4). You may hear a patient with a wet cough as you approach or you may see a patient holding a hand over his chest. The patient may appear very sick, or may seem to be in little distress. He may be alert, notice your arrival, and make eye contact, or he may have a decreased level of responsiveness and not be aware of your approach. In some cases, a family member or coworker will meet you outside and tell you what kind of problem the patient is experiencing. In each of these cases, your observations contribute to forming a general impression of the situation. The general impression gives you an indication of how to approach the primary assessment.

Imagine that you were dispatched for an MVC. When you size up the scene through the windshield of the ambulance, you see two badly damaged vehicles in the intersection. One vehicle has front-end damage and the other has

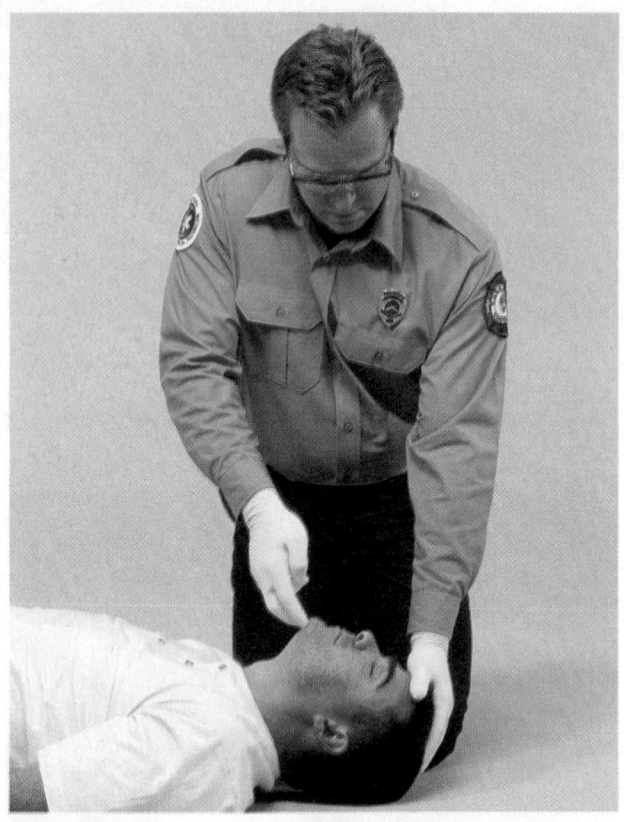

(A)

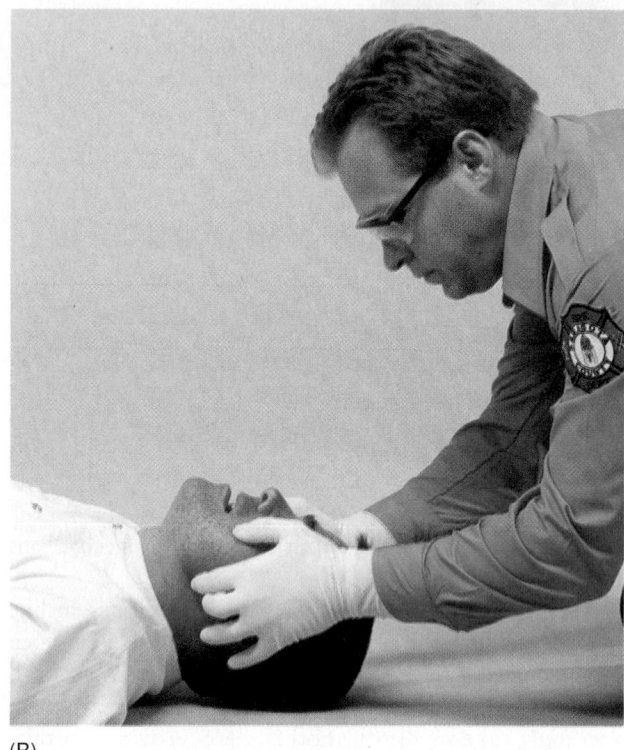

(B)

FIGURE 15-3

Manual maneuvers to open the airway: (A) a head-tilt/chin-lift maneuver; (B) a modified jaw-thrust maneuver.

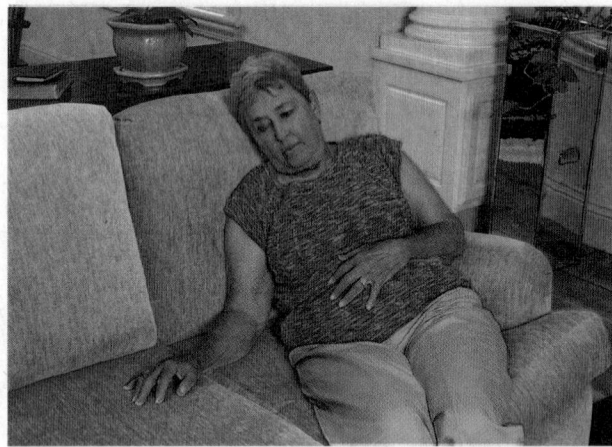

FIGURE 15-4

In the scene size-up, determine the general nature of the illness.

damage to the driver's side, focused at the front door. This would seem to confirm the MOI.

However, imagine you arrive on the scene to find a single vehicle that has struck a light pole in a parking lot. The vehicle has moderate damage. Approaching the driver's side window, you notice that the patient's injuries seem more severe than the mechanism indicates. His shirt is blood soaked and there are three gunshot wounds in his chest.

Or picture yourself walking up to a vehicle that went through a red light without slowing down. The car was struck a glancing blow by a vehicle in cross-traffic and is resting atop a broken fire hydrant. The patient is unresponsive, pale, and sweaty, but there are no obvious signs of injuries. Pulling his necklace out of the collar of his shirt, you see a medical information tag imprinted with the word "Diabetic."

Patient assessment information gained in the scene size-up gives you a good starting point. All the patients just mentioned had an obvious MOI that required investigation. For two of the patients, however, the scene size-up alone did not tell the entire story of the MOI and nature of the illness. The moral of these stories is, "Don't assume." You must ask yourself questions even when the appearance of the scene seems to present an obvious scenario.

Say you approach an apparently unresponsive patient lying about 10 feet from the base of a ladder propped against a two-story house. Ask yourself, "Did the patient fall from the ladder?" "Was he stung by a bee as he approached the ladder, collapsing in anaphylactic shock?" "Was he on the ladder when he suffered a medical problem, such as a seizure or syncopal (fainting) episode?"

IN THE FIELD

Scene size-up and primary assessment are the first considerations in patient assessment, but they are not complete at the beginning of a call. Scene size-up continues until you leave the scene. Primary assessment continues until you turn over patient care to another health care provider.

On another call you see a sign on the door of a residence that says, "No smoking. Oxygen in use." Your patient may have a chronic respiratory or cardiac problem that requires him to be on oxygen—but maybe today his problem is that his speech suddenly became slurred. The oxygen may be an important part of his history, but may not be an indication of the problem the patient is having *today*. Possibly, the oxygen belongs to another person living in the home, and is not even the patient's at all.

Do not think of the scene size-up as a step of the assessment that is complete at the beginning of the call. Clues about your patient's condition may not all present themselves at the beginning of the call. Your thinking about scene size-up will continue alongside your thoughts about primary and secondary assessment and patient treatment. Perhaps on the scene of an elderly woman with abdominal pain, you ask if you can check her nightstand for medications as your partner takes her blood pressure. Or you find a container holding bloody vomit, though the patient had denied nausea or vomiting.

As you size up the scene and approach the patient, you must not only *look* for clues about the scene and patient, but you also must listen for any sounds that concern you, detect any odors that might give clues, and use your sense of touch. For example, do you hear the engine of a crashed vehicle still running? Do you hear screams, yelling, or other noises? You also must talk and listen to first responders, law enforcement officers, family members, bystanders, and others with information. Do you smell natural gas, smoke, or chemical smells? Does the environment feel unusually hot or cold? Those clues not only give you information about possible hazards, but also can give you information about the patient. As you make your initial approach, be cautious but confident. You must bring and maintain order at a scene that may be mildly stressful or wildly chaotic.

The scene size-up begins as you approach the scene. It provides valuable information about the presence of hazards, the number of patients, and additional resources needed. The scene size-up also provides information about the nature of the illness or MOI. The information you obtain is important. You must follow up on it. However, you must never assume that the scene size-up tells the entire story about the nature of the illness or the mechanism of injury. Scene size-up continues alongside patient assessment and management, and does not end until you leave the scene.

Primary Assessment

The purpose of the primary assessment is to immediately identify and correct conditions that can cause the patient's death if not remedied at once. Conditions that will rapidly result in death or irreversible harm if not corrected are conditions that interfere with perfusion, the delivery of oxygenated blood to the cellular level. Without adequate perfusion, cell damage and death begin within minutes. The highest priority in patient care is to recognize and correct those problems.

The actions of the primary assessment are represented by *ABCD*, which stand for airway, breathing, circulation, and disability. (Disability refers to neurologic disability as determined by the patient's level of responsiveness.) While the mnemonic *ABCD* is useful for remembering the components of primary assessment, the order in which they are followed actually begins with *D*. The next decisions you make are determined by whether the patient is responsive or apparently unresponsive.

If the patient is alert or responds to either verbal or painful stimuli, or if the patient is apparently unresponsive but breathing normally, it means that there is some degree of cellular perfusion taking place. In this case the priority is determining the status of the patient's airway, breathing, and circulation, in that order: A, B, C.

In patients who appear to be unresponsive and not breathing or breathing ineffectively, you must check a carotid pulse *before* opening the airway. The order is circulation, airway, and breathing: C, A, B (American Heart Association, 2010). When the primary cause of cardiac arrest is sudden cardiac death, residual air in the lungs contains some oxygen. However, the problem is that no blood is circulating through the lungs to pick up the oxygen and deliver it to the tissues. The most important step in resuscitation of patients in cardiac arrest is restoring circulation. When only a single rescuer is present, chest compressions and defibrillation take higher priority than opening the airway and providing ventilation. (See Chapter 17.) When more than one rescuer is present, you can manage airway and ventilation in conjunction with chest compressions and defibrillation.

You must ensure that some specialized equipment and supplies are available during the primary assessment. You must take this equipment to the patient's side and make the equipment immediately accessible. Essential equipment and supplies for patient care are generally carried from the ambulance to the patient's location in one or two bags specially designed to organize EMS equipment. Ensure that the following minimum equipment is immediately available to perform the primary assessment:

- Personal protective equipment
- Portable suction unit
- Simple airway adjuncts (oropharyngeal and nasopharyngeal airways)

- Additional airway devices in the scope of practice (for example: King LTD, CombiTube)
- Bag-valve-mask device or pocket face mask
- Oxygen cylinder
- Oxygen delivery devices (for example: nasal cannula, nonrebreather mask)
- Automatic external defibrillator
- Bandage shears
- Absorbent dressings and bandages
- Tourniquet

Assessing the General Appearance

The primary assessment begins by looking at the patient's general appearance and determining the age and sex of the patient (Figure 15-5). One of the first things you notice about the patient is whether he appears to be responsive or unresponsive. If the patient is responsive, you have some idea of his *ABCD*. A patient who is walking around his crashed car and looking at the amount of damage, for instance, is alert and his airway, breathing, and circulation are not immediate cause for concern.

Note the patient's skin color. If he is pale, this indicates that perfusion of the skin is decreased, perhaps from shock. **Cyanosis**, a bluish or purple discoloration, indicates hypoxia (Figure 15-6). Cyanosis may be generalized, or may be present in areas such as the ears, lips, or nail beds. A patient who is flushed in appearance may have a fever. **Jaundice**, a yellowing of the skin, indicates severe liver disease (Figure 15-7).

Assess the patient's general level of distress. Is he smiling, or grimacing in pain? Is he pacing about, holding his hands on his back as if in pain? Or is he lying very still with his legs drawn up, avoiding any movement? If your impression "from the doorway" is that the patient appears sick, is in distress, or has a decreased level of responsiveness, primary assessment requires a more detailed process.

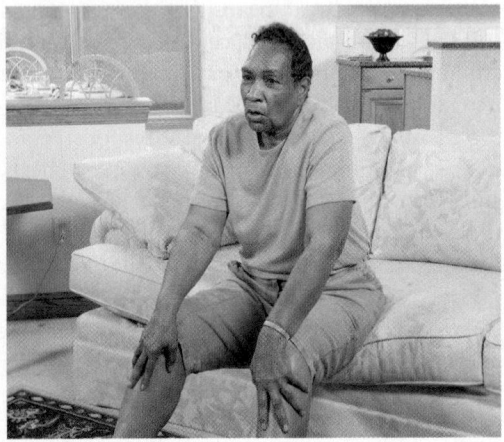

FIGURE 15-5

Begin the primary assessment by observing the patient's general appearance.

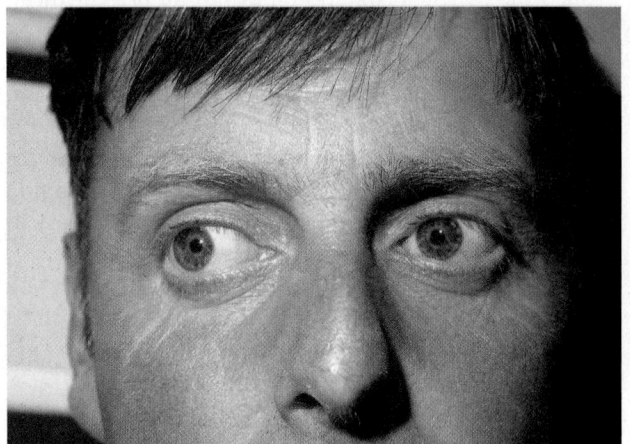

FIGURE 15-7

Jaundice. (© John Callan/Shout Picture Library)

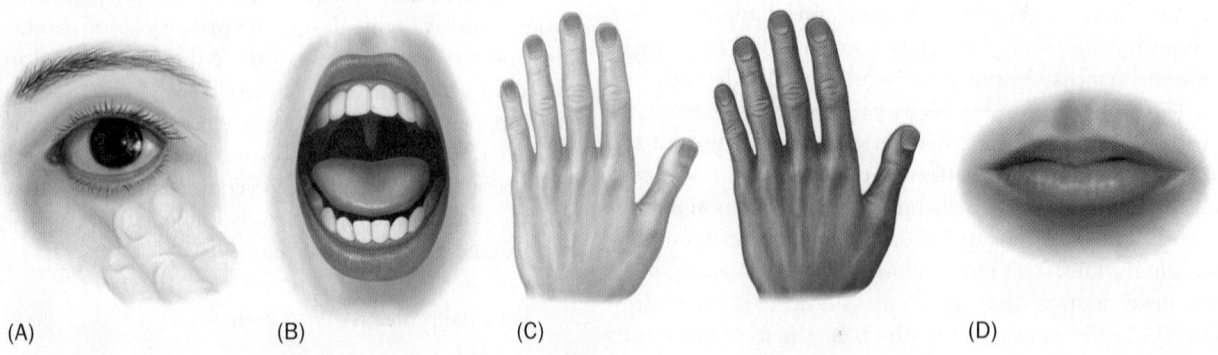

(A)   (B)   (C)   (D)

FIGURE 15-6

Cyanosis in the (A) conjunctiva, (B) mucosa, (C) fingernail beds, (D) circumoral area.

Assessing Level of Responsiveness

Although *D* appears in alphabetical order to make *ABCD* easy to remember, the patient's level of responsiveness (potential disability) is assessed first. A patient who is merely sleeping may not react well to having a stranger grasp his head in order to open his airway to relieve snoring.

The mnemonic *AVPU* is used to initially assess the level of responsiveness. Patients are categorized as alert, responsive to verbal stimuli, responsive to painful stimuli, or unresponsive to all stimuli. The **Glasgow Coma Scale (GCS)** is a more specific way of assessing the level of responsiveness.

Assessing AVPU

A patient whose eyes are purposefully open and is aware of the environment around him, including your approach, is alert. If the patient's eyes are closed or he seems unaware of your presence, check to see if he responds to verbal stimuli. Speak to the patient by asking if he can hear you. If he

reacts to your voice by opening his eyes, he is responsive to verbal stimuli.

If he does not respond, check for response to painful stimuli. The use of the term "painful stimuli" is a bit misleading. For a patient whose eyes are not spontaneously open and who has not responded to your voice, your first approach is to gently but firmly shake his shoulder. If he does not respond, there are a few generally acceptable ways to check for response to pain (Figure 15-8). For example, you may pinch the trapezius muscle of the shoulder, ensuring that you are applying pressure to the muscle, and not just the overlying skin and fatty tissue. Another way to check for response to pain is to apply pressure on the supraorbital ridge. Firmly pressing your knuckles over the patient's sternum and rubbing it also produces pain.

It has been suggested that a patient attempting to withdraw from those types of stimuli may move his shoulders, neck, or head. Therefore, in some systems, the use of those stimuli is discouraged in patients who may have a cervical-spine injury. Follow your system's protocols in the use of these techniques.

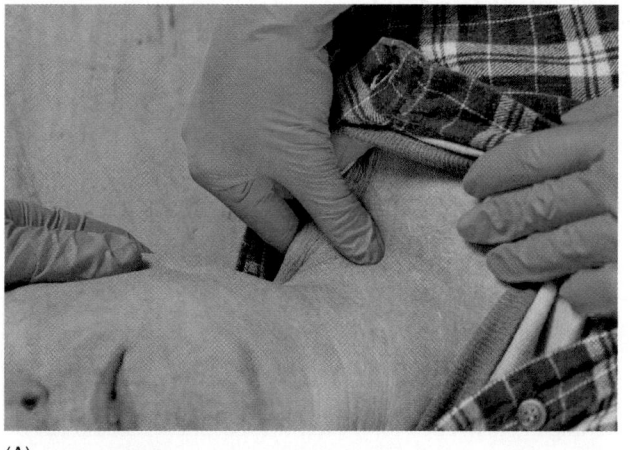
(A)

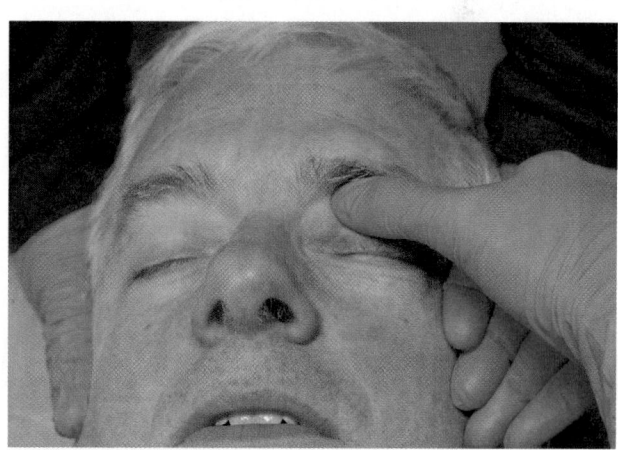
(B)

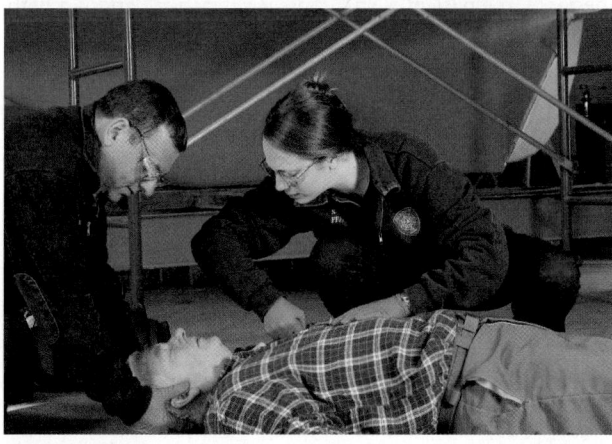
(C)

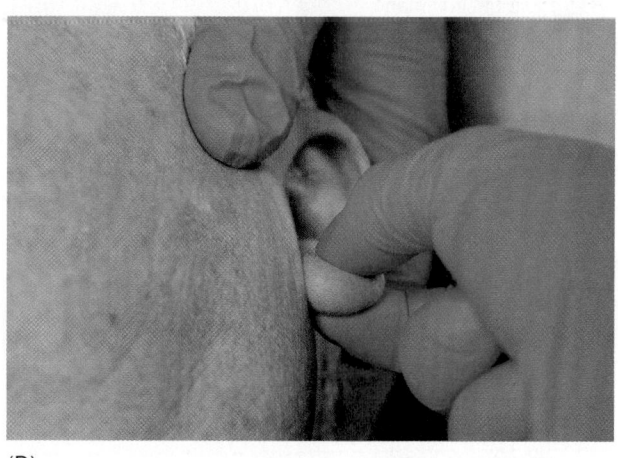
(D)

FIGURE 15-8

Methods of checking for response to painful stimuli include (A) a trapezius pinch, (B) supraorbital pressure, (C) a sternal rub, and (D) an earlobe pinch.

Another acceptable way to apply a painful stimulus is through interdigital pressure (inter = between; digital = pertaining to the finger). Place an object, such as a pen, between the patient's index and middle fingers and squeeze the fingers together. You also can apply pressure to the nail bed, using the side of a pen or similar object to produce pain.

Assessing the GCS Score

The Glasgow Coma Scale (GCS) score (Table 15-3) should be determined for every patient, although you should not delay any part of the primary assessment to do so. It takes experience using the GCS with a variety of patients before you will be able to calculate it automatically, without referring to a pocket card or wall chart. In fact, using the pocket card or wall chart will ensure accuracy, regardless of your experience level. A GCS wall chart is posted in most trauma resuscitation rooms for reference, and may also be posted in the patient compartment of the ambulance.

TABLE 15-3   Glasgow Coma Scale

BEST EYE OPENING RESPONSE	
Spontaneous	4
To verbal command	3
To pain	2
No response	1
BEST VERBAL RESPONSE	
Oriented and converses	5
Disoriented and converses	4
Inappropriate words	3
Incomprehensible sounds	2
No response	1
BEST MOTOR RESPONSE	
Obeys verbal commands	6
Localizes pain	5
Withdraws from pain (flexion)	4
Abnormal flexion in response to pain (decorticate posturing)	3
Abnormal extension in response to pain (decerebrate posturing)	2
No response	1

As a matter of practicality, the GCS is often calculated later in the assessment, using the information gained in the primary assessment. All the information needed to determine the GCS is available from the AVPU assessment. AVPU is a quick way to determine the level of responsiveness for initial decision making. The GCS is more precise. Its scores are used to predict the severity of the patient's condition and his likely outcome, particularly in trauma.

The GCS is calculated on a scale from 3 to 15. Up to 6 points are given for the patient's eye-opening response, up to 5 points for the patient's verbal response, and up to 4 points for the patient's motor (movement) response. Note that complete unresponsiveness is awarded a GCS of 3, not zero.

Keep in mind that neither AVPU nor the GCS is a complete assessment of the patient's **mental status**. Mental status goes beyond level of responsiveness and includes assessment of higher **cognitive functions**, such as memory, understanding, and reasoning. Assessment of mental status is part of the secondary assessment, and is particularly important in patients suspected of having a traumatic brain injury, stroke, or behavioral emergency.

Decision Making

When a patient's level of responsiveness is less than alert (using the AVPU scale) or less than 14 (using the GCS), he has a decreased level of responsiveness. A patient who has a GCS score of 3 or who does not respond to either verbal or painful stimuli is unresponsive. The initial impression for these patients is that they are critical, or potentially critical, and a high priority for transport.

Decreased responsiveness is an indication that the brain is deprived of oxygen, circulation, or glucose, or that there is an injury to the brain. Other causes of decreased level of responsiveness include drug overdose, toxic exposure, environmental extremes, infection, and endocrine or metabolic derangements. Therefore, even if subsequent assessment of the airway, breathing, and circulation reveals that they are adequate, the patient is still considered critical, and is a high priority for transport.

Also keep in mind, though, that there are two underlying causes of decreased responsiveness and unresponsiveness that Advanced EMTs may be able to correct prior to transport. If the patient's history and the information from the scene size-up are highly consistent with hypoglycemia, a diabetic emergency, check the blood glucose level and administer 50 percent dextrose or glucagon according to protocol or on-line medical direction. If the patient's respirations are depressed and the situation is highly consistent with narcotic overdose, consider administering naloxone before inserting an airway other than a nasopharyngeal or oropharyngeal airway.

In both situations, you must use excellent clinical reasoning. If the cause of unresponsiveness is not immediately correctable, you must not delay inserting an appropriate airway, performing ventilation, and transporting the patient. However, if you can improve the patient's condition so that he can manage his own airway and ventilation, that situation is preferable to using **airway adjuncts** and artificial ventilation.

Additionally, prolonged hypoglycemia is detrimental to brain cells, and must be corrected as quickly as possible. In addition to delaying treatment for hypoglycemia, using airway devices other than a nasopharyngeal or oropharyngeal airway in a patient who is likely to regain consciousness will result in complications. If the patient situation is consistent with hypoglycemia, use less invasive airway adjuncts while checking the blood glucose level. Placing a CombiTube, King LTD airway, or similar airway device in the pharynx, and then "waking up" the patient by administering 50 percent dextrose can result in vomiting, aspiration, soft-tissue damage to the airway, and extreme stress for the patient.

Responsive Versus Unresponsive Patients

The next steps in primary assessment proceed differently, based on the patient's level of responsiveness. You can assess patients who are fully responsive more rapidly than those whose level of responsiveness is decreased. Airway, breathing, and circulation are required (at least to some degree) to perfuse the cerebrum well enough to support responsiveness. Therefore, you have an initial impression of the responsive patient's airway, breathing, and circulation.

Introduce yourself to the patient and determine his chief complaint. The chief complaint is the reason the patient states, in his own words, that he needs medical assistance. Do not assume that you know what the patient's chief complaint is. A patient may seem obviously short of breath, but his chief complaint may be chest pain. The initial exchange with a responsive patient may go something like this:

EXAMPLE 1:

You: "Hi, I'm John. I'm an Advanced EMT with the fire department. This is my partner, Tabby. What's your name, sir?"

Patient: "I'm Fred. Fred Wyant."

You: "It's nice to meet you, Mr. Wyant. How can we help you today?"

Patient: "I'm feeling so weak I can hardly get out of this chair today."

EXAMPLE 2:

You: "Good morning, Mrs. DeBaca, I'm Deb with the ambulance service. Your daughter called the ambulance because she was concerned about you. How are you feeling?"

Patient: "My heart is racing. I can feel it beating in my chest. My chest is starting to feel heavy and I'm having trouble breathing."

You: "Which of these things is bothering you the most?"

Patient: "It's the sensation in my chest."

You: "Do you mean the sensation of your heart racing, or the heaviness?"

Patient: "The heaviness. I can't say it hurts. It just feels heavy."

EXAMPLE 3:

You: "Hi, sir. My name is Ben and this is my partner, Leo. It looks like you crashed your bicycle. Do you hurt anywhere?"

Patient: "Just my pride and my skinned-up hands."

You: "Let me have a look at your hands. Do you hurt anywhere else?"

As you talk to responsive patients, you will continue to observe them for any evidence that their airway, breathing, or circulation is compromised. You will also use the chief complaint and information from the scene size-up to evaluate the possibility of life-threatening conditions.

Regardless of other primary assessment findings, some chief complaints make patients a higher priority for transport (Table 15-4).

For patients who have a decreased level of responsiveness, you will take a more active approach to assessing and managing the airway, breathing, and circulation. For apparently unresponsive patients who do not appear to be breathing normally, the order of primary assessment changes to *CAB* (circulation, airway, and breathing). An unresponsive patient without circulation, as determined by the absence

TABLE 15-4	Selected High-Priority Chief Complaints and Presenting Problems

- Abdominal pain
- Acute nonmusculoskeletal back/flank pain in a patient > 60 years old
- Indications of GI bleeding (blood in vomit or stool)
- Other indications of internal bleeding (profuse hematuria or hemoptysis)
- Chest pain or discomfort in a patient > 35 years old
- Difficulty breathing/shortness of breath
- Dizziness in a patient > 65 years old
- Acute, severe headache
- Acute onset of neurologic deficit (slurred speech, facial droop, weakness, paralysis)
- Seizures
- Immersion/submersion incident (drowning)
- Electrocution or lightning strike
- Poisoning/overdose
- Syncope
- Abdominal pain

of a carotid pulse, is in cardiac arrest. If the patient's pulse is absent, begin resuscitation by immediately starting chest compressions and applying the **automatic external defibrillator (AED)**. For unresponsive patients who have a pulse, proceed to assessing the airway.

Assessing the Airway

For air to move in and out of the lungs for the exchange of gases, the passageway between the lungs and the environment must be open. This is sometimes referred to as having a "patent" airway. You must check the patency of the upper airway (Figure 15-9) in the primary assessment. Without an open airway, the patient's life is in immediate jeopardy from hypoxia.

Immediately correct any condition that partially or completely obstructs the airway. In many cases, correction is not difficult, despite the critical nature of the task. Often,

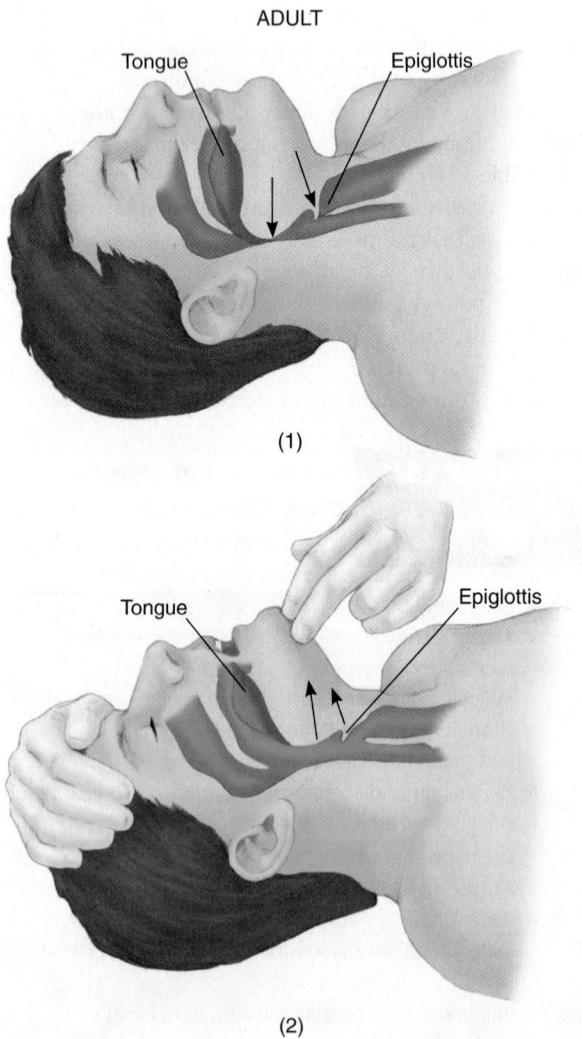

ADULT

Tongue

Epiglottis

(1)

Tongue

Epiglottis

(2)

FIGURE 15-9

The airway passage must be open to allow air movement in and out of the lungs. The tongue is the most common cause of airway obstruction.

manual positioning and simple airway adjuncts, such as a **nasopharyngeal airway** or **oropharyngeal airway**, will provide an open airway.

Patients whose airway is currently open but at risk for airway compromise must be managed, as well. (Chapter 16 provides the details of the airway management and ventilation equipment and techniques that are introduced in this chapter.)

There are several conditions that pose an immediate risk to a patient's airway. Any patient who has a decreased level of responsiveness is at risk of airway obstruction for two reasons. First, in unresponsive patients, the muscles that normally hold the jaw and tongue anteriorly and elevate the epiglottis relax. The epiglottis closes over the glottis and the tongue falls back into the posterior pharynx, obstructing it. In fact, relaxation of those muscles is the most common cause of airway obstruction.

When the obstruction is partial, such as when someone is deeply asleep, snoring occurs as air being forced through the restricted opening of the pharynx vibrates the soft tissues. Snoring is a sign of partial airway obstruction, and when it occurs in a patient, you must correct it by manually positioning the airway.

The second reason that the airway of a patient with a decreased level of responsiveness is at risk is that there may be no gag reflex. The gag reflex normally keeps us from aspirating food and fluids into the airway. Many conditions that result in a decreased level of responsiveness also increase the risk of vomiting. A patient whose gag reflex is impaired may aspirate blood, vomit, gum, tobacco, or other foreign substances in the mouth or pharynx.

Patients who have had a stroke may have impaired ability to swallow and are at risk for aspiration. Patients who are vomiting or at risk for vomiting must be positioned to maintain a clear airway. Suction must be immediately available to assist the patient in clearing the airway, if necessary. Bleeding from the nose (epistaxis) or injuries to the head or face also can lead to aspiration. Other causes of airway obstruction include soft-tissue swelling, such as from injuries, anaphylactic (severe allergic) reactions, airway burns, and foreign bodies (food, or small toys or objects).

Most patients you encounter will be alert and obviously have an open airway. An adequate airway will be evident in the patient's general appearance through the level of responsiveness, skin color, and ease of speaking and breathing. Your primary assessment of those patients is essentially completed by the time you reach the patient's side.

For patients who present with a general impression that is poor or causes concern, assess the airway by deliberately looking, listening, and feeling to check for air movement through the airway. An obvious and immediate sign of airway obstruction is abnormal breathing sounds. Snoring, stridor, gurgling, and coughing all indicate partial upper airway obstruction.

- *Snoring.* This sound is caused by obstruction of the pharynx by the tongue, and is relieved by manually positioning the head and jaw to move the tongue.

- *Stridor.* A high-pitched whistling sound, **stridor** is heard primarily during inspiration, that results from turbulent airflow through the trachea or larynx. Stridor is an indication of partial upper airway obstruction from a foreign body or swelling of the airway. In small children, stridor can be an indication of **epiglottitis**, which can quickly lead to airway obstruction. These conditions require rapid advanced interventions.

- *Gurgling.* This sound indicates fluid in the upper airway, which must be removed by suctioning. Proper positioning can prevent the accumulation of additional fluids in some patients. A patient who is unresponsive but has adequate breathing and no indications of cervical-spine trauma is placed on his left side, in the **recovery position**, to aid in drainage of fluids from the mouth.

- *Coughing.* Coughing can occur because of problems in the upper or lower airways, including partial upper airway obstruction by fluids or foreign bodies.

If the patient has a decreased level of responsiveness, begin by manually positioning the airway. If there is no risk of cervical-spine injury, use a head-tilt/chin-lift maneuver. If there is a possibility of cervical-spine injury, use a modified jaw-thrust maneuver.

Next, look toward the patient's chest, with the side of your face several inches above the patient's nose and mouth. By doing this, you can simultaneously look for the rise and fall of the patient's chest, listen for air movement from the mouth and nose, and feel for the movement of air from the nose and mouth (Figure 15-10).

Air movement confirms that the airway is open. Decreased air movement means one of two things: Either the airway is partially obstructed, or the airway is open but the patient is not breathing adequately. If there is inadequate air movement, attempt to ventilate the patient using a **bag-valve-mask device**. If you are able to ventilate without difficulty, the

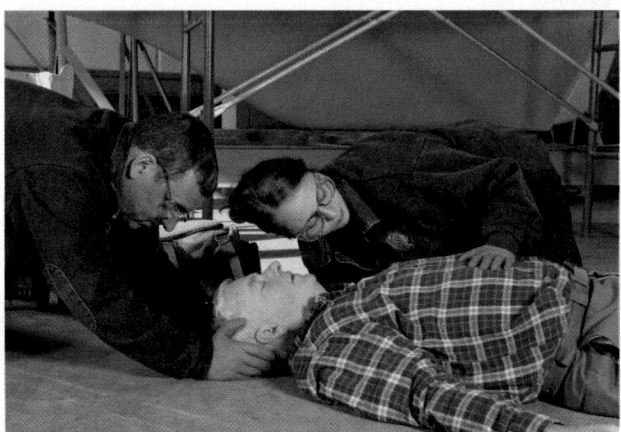

FIGURE 15-10

Assess the airway by looking for chest rise and fall, listening for air movement at the mouth and nose, and feeling for air movement from the mouth and nose.

Pediatric Care

Anatomical differences in infants and small children require modification of airway assessment and management and ventilation techniques and devices. Those differences are covered in detail in Chapters 9 and 44.

airway is open. If ventilation is difficult or impossible, check that you have positioned the head and neck properly to open the airway and attempt again to ventilate. If you are still not able to ventilate, manage the patient for an obstructed airway. Continue ventilating the patient whose airway is open but who is either not breathing or is not breathing adequately.

Assessing Breathing

Once you have determined that the airway is open, the next step is to determine the adequacy of breathing. Your initial general impression of the patient may already have given you information about his breathing status. The patient's level of responsiveness, skin color, and general level of distress are indications of breathing status. You also may have heard **wheezing** or **crackles** (**rales**) as you approached the patient, which are indications of respiratory distress.

You must not miss signs of inadequate breathing (Table 15-5). Patients with **respiratory distress, respiratory failure,** and **respiratory arrest** need immediate intervention. The same "look, listen, and feel" techniques that you used to assess the airway also will have given you some information about the patient's breathing.

Normal breathing is effortless and quiet. Patients who must work to breathe are suffering from respiratory distress. Patients with significant respiratory distress cannot even complete a sentence without pausing to take a breath. The more severe the **dyspnea**, the fewer words the patient can speak between breaths. With severe dyspnea, patients will use **accessory muscles of breathing** to assist the normally effortless process (Figure 15-11).

TABLE 15-5 Signs of Inadequate Breathing

- Increased work of breathing/use of accessory muscles
- Noisy breathing (stridor, snoring, gurgling, wheezing, crackles)
- Decreased or absent air movement or breath sounds
- Apnea/respiratory arrest
- Ventilatory rate < 8 or > 30 per minute in an adult
- Irregular breathing
- Cyanosis

PERSONAL PERSPECTIVE

Advanced EMT Janice Kelso: I was walking to class on campus about a year ago when I saw a cluster of people in an intersection, just in front of a car with a dent on the hood. I walked over and discovered that the car had struck a young man as he crossed the street. He was lying on his back, and I saw immediately that his face and upper body were purple. A lady was holding his head still, but the guy wasn't breathing at all.

I stepped forward and knelt down beside the patient's head and said, "I'm an EMT. Let me help you." I checked the patient's carotid pulse and found that it was strong and regular, so I said, "Let's get his airway open." The lady said, "You can't move him. His neck might be broken!" I replied that a broken neck was a possibility, but the patient would die in the next few minutes without an airway. "I'll be careful of his neck," I said, and opened his airway with a modified jaw-thrust maneuver. He still wasn't breathing.

Some of my friends have called me a geek for carrying around a pocket mask, but I was glad I had it. I had a bystander pull it out of my backpack. I heard ambulance sirens approaching in the distance as I carefully placed the mask on the patient's face and gave a breath. Just as I prepared to give a second breath, the patient took in a deep breath on his own, and his color started to improve almost immediately. I recognized one of the Advanced EMTs on the ambulance and gave him a quick report.

I saw on the local news that night the patient had been treated in the hospital emergency department and released. I called the Advanced EMT on the run and asked if I'd heard right. "He had a slight concussion, but his airway became obstructed from the position he was in while he was unconscious. Other than that, all he had was a laceration on his backside, but he probably wouldn't be going home tonight if you hadn't opened his airway."

Patients whose ventilation and oxygenation are poor, even with increased work of breathing, are in respiratory failure. As oxygenation decreases, despite the need for more oxygen to fuel the increased work of breathing, the patient becomes more and more hypoxic and acidotic. The work of breathing may decrease, air movement may decrease, and the patient may become sleepy and less responsive.

Respiratory arrest is the absence of breathing, or **apnea**. Once respiratory arrest occurs, cardiac arrest will follow quickly if it is not corrected. Some patients in respiratory arrest have a period of slow, shallow, gasping, ineffective respirations called **agonal** (dying) **respirations**.

Assess the rate, depth, rhythm, and effort of the patient's breathing, and listen for any abnormal breathing noises that indicate respiratory distress. Healthy adult patients breathe regularly at a rate of 12 to 20 times per minute. Consider whether the amount of air being moved in and out of the lungs with each breath is adequate. Normal **tidal volume** for the average adult is about 500 mL. Because 150 mL of this air remains in the conducting airways, unavailable for gas exchange, only a small decrease in tidal volume is tolerated, even with a compensatory increase in ventilatory rate.

Wheezing, which can sometimes be heard without a stethoscope, indicates constriction of the bronchioles. Bronchiolar constriction interferes with movement of air into and out of the alveoli. Crackles (rales), which also can sometimes be heard without a stethoscope, indicate the presence of fluid in the alveoli. The presence of fluid interferes with gas exchange. Finally, the presence of cyanosis, which may have been noted in the patient's general appearance, indicates that the patient's hemoglobin is not carrying an adequate amount of oxygen.

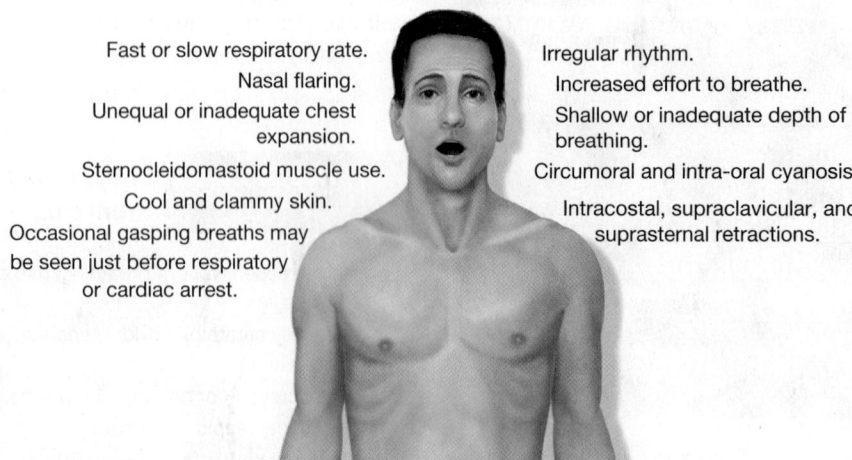

Fast or slow respiratory rate.
Nasal flaring.
Unequal or inadequate chest expansion.
Sternocleidomastoid muscle use.
Cool and clammy skin.
Occasional gasping breaths may be seen just before respiratory or cardiac arrest.

Irregular rhythm.
Increased effort to breathe.
Shallow or inadequate depth of breathing.
Circumoral and intra-oral cyanosis.
Intracostal, supraclavicular, and suprasternal retractions.

FIGURE 15-11

Look for indications of respiratory distress.

TABLE 15-6	Indications for Administration of Oxygen

- Cardiac or respiratory arrest
- Respiratory distress or respiratory failure
- Any patient requiring assisted ventilations
- SpO_2 less than 95 percent
- Inadequate tidal volume
- Respiratory rate < 8 or > 30
- Patient has an altered mental status/decreased level of responsiveness
- Patient complains of difficulty breathing/shortness of breath
- Patient complains of chest pain
- Other medical conditions that can cause hypoxia, such as seizures, stroke, overdose, toxic inhalation, and wheezing
- Signs and symptoms of shock or severe internal or external bleeding
- Major or multiple trauma

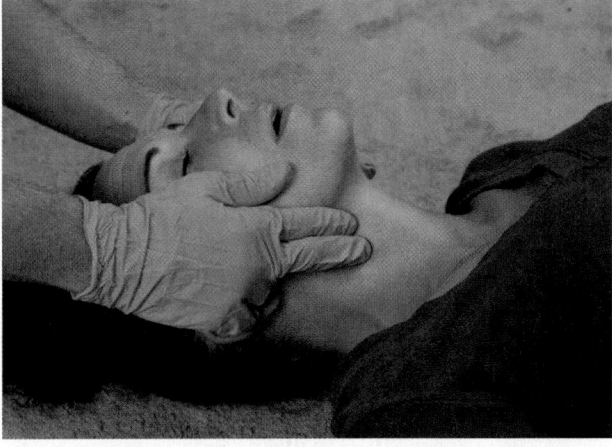

(A)

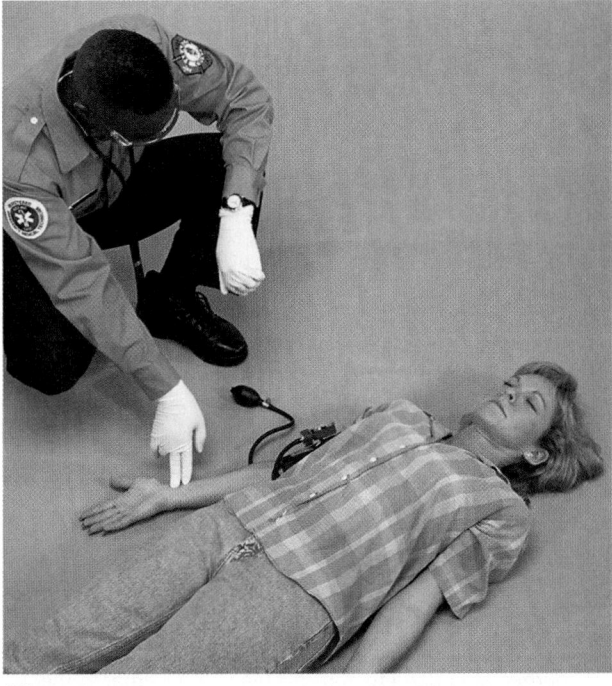

(B)

FIGURE 15-12

(A) Assess the carotid pulse in unresponsive patients, and (B) the radial pulse in responsive patients.

Based on the assessment of breathing, you will decide on necessary interventions. The patient may require oxygen by nonrebreather mask or nasal cannula (Table 15-6). Patients with inadequate or absent breathing will need assistance with ventilation. For some patients, **continuous positive airway pressure (CPAP)** may be appropriate. Others must have their ventilations assisted with a bag-valve-mask device; those in respiratory arrest must have artificial ventilation by bag-valve-mask.

Assessing Circulation

Once the airway is open and air is flowing in and out of the lungs, the oxygen must be circulated to the cells. For this to happen, there must be enough blood in the circulatory system, and the heart must be pumping it adequately throughout the body. Therefore, the next steps in the primary assessment are to check the pulse and control bleeding.

Again, with most patients, these steps are straightforward and you will accomplish them as you approach the patient. A patient who is alert, has good skin color, and has no significant ongoing bleeding has adequate circulation for the purposes of the primary assessment.

For unresponsive patients, check the carotid pulse before opening the airway (Figure 15-12). For both responsive

Pediatric Care

The brachial pulse along the medial aspect of the humerus is checked in infants (age 1 month to 1 year). The normal respiratory and heart rates for pediatric patients are provided in Chapters 9, 18, and 44.

patients and unresponsive patients with a carotid pulse, check the radial pulse in the wrist at the base of the thumb. (See Chapter 18.) The average healthy adult has a strong radial pulse at a regular rate of 60 to 100 times per minute. Good perfusion is also indicated by dry, warm skin without **pallor** (paleness).

Search for and control significant external bleeding with **direct pressure** (Figure 15-13). When direct pressure is inadequate to control bleeding from the extremities proximal to the elbow or knee, you can use a **tourniquet,** according to your protocol (Figure 15-14). The loss of red blood cells means a loss of oxygen-carrying capability. This results in tissue hypoxia when a critical amount of red blood cells has been lost.

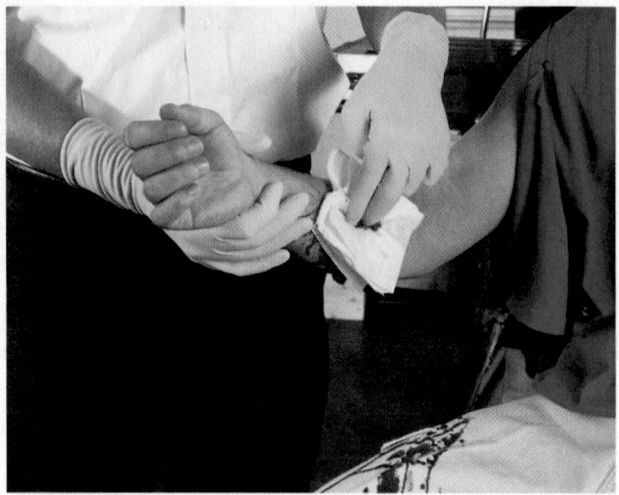

FIGURE 15-13

Use direct pressure to control bleeding.

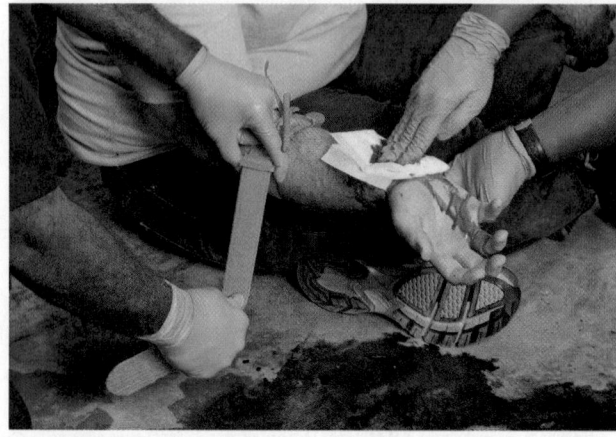

FIGURE 15-14

A tourniquet is used to control bleeding proximal to the knee or elbow when direct pressure cannot control it.

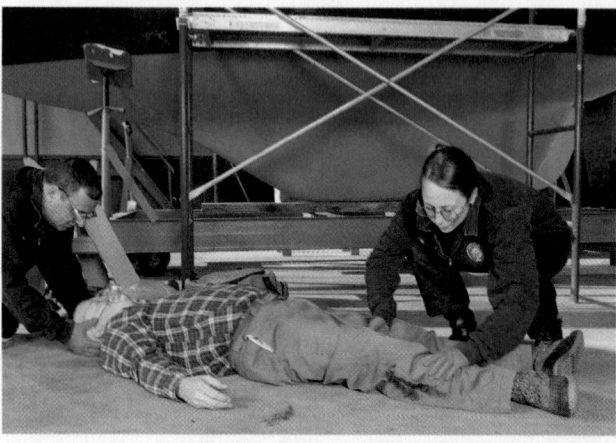

(A)

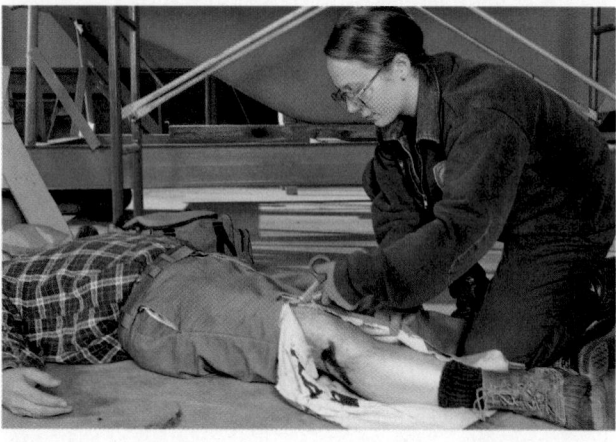

(B)

FIGURE 15-15

Expose trauma patients to ensure you have identified all significant external bleeding. (A) Check for major bleeding. (B) Cut away blood-soaked clothing to expose potentially life-threatening bleeding.

Assessing a conscious bleeding patient with an isolated injury is generally straightforward in daylight. However, imagine that you have responded to a motor vehicle collision (MVC) at night. You find your unresponsive patient with his head down on the floorboard, underneath the dash. You can tell, when you reach in to stabilize his spine and open his airway, that there is a lot of blood coming from somewhere, but the darkness and the amount of blood make it difficult to see. Because the patient was not restrained, it is difficult to picture the exact trajectory he took on impact to end up in the position he is in. It is difficult to imagine what he came in contact with, and where his injuries may be. This situation is challenging, but you must look for and control bleeding. You need light and assistance getting the patient out of the vehicle so you can expose and inspect him to be sure that you have located and controlled

all ongoing external bleeding (Figure 15-15). Adding an *E* to *ABCD*, creating the mnemonic *ABCDE*, serves as a reminder to expose (E) patients with significant trauma to check for bleeding.

Patient Care Decisions

Once you are managing immediate life threats, use information from the scene size-up and primary assessment to make decisions about further assessment, further treatment, and transport. You will come to one of several conclusions, based on your analysis of the information and the guidance provided by your protocols and standing orders:

- The patient is deceased and is not a candidate for resuscitation, either because of presumptive signs of death, or the presence of a do-not-resuscitate order. (See Table 15-7 and Chapter 4.)

CASE STUDY (continued)

Advanced EMTs Kyle Davis and Eric Chen have arrived on the scene of a motorcycle collision involving two patients. Eric approaches an unresponsive male patient with a bloody face and gurgling respirations, as Kyle makes his way to an alert female patient with a deformed thigh.

Eric ensures that the deputy maintaining cervical-spine stabilization is correctly performing a modified jaw-thrust maneuver to open the patient's airway. He pulls a portable suction unit from the airway bag to remove the bloody fluid from the patient's airway. The patient's respirations are irregular, with periods of apnea, so Eric inserts an oropharyngeal airway and begins bag-valve-mask ventilations with supplemental oxygen. The patient has a weak radial pulse at 92 per minute.

While maintaining ventilations, Eric looks for ongoing bleeding and finds that the major source is a large scalp laceration. Eric directs the deputy to apply direct pressure to the laceration with an absorbent dressing. Eric continues to monitor the patient's airway, the effectiveness of the ventilations he is providing, and the patient's circulation as he waits for the backup unit to arrive.

Meanwhile, Kyle notes that his patient is pale, with cool, sweaty skin, with indications of shock. Her airway is open, and she is breathing 24 times per minute. She does not have indications of difficulty breathing, but her radial pulse is weak and rapid. The patient has many abrasions and minor lacerations, but no significant ongoing external bleeding. Kyle convinces the patient to lie down and provides her with 15 L/min of oxygen by nonrebreather mask.

Problem-Solving Questions

1. Are either of these patients in critical condition?
2. What evidence from the scenario supports your answer?
3. What are the next decisions that Eric and Kyle should make?

TABLE 15-7	Signs of Presumptive Death

- Decapitation or midsection transection of the body
- Decomposition
- Dependent lividity (discoloration of the body as blood pools from the effects of gravity)
- Severe charring of the body
- Rigor mortis (rigidity of muscles)

TABLE 15-8	High-Priority Findings in the Primary Assessment

- Poor general impression (cyanosis, pallor, obvious major bleeding or injuries, obvious respiratory distress, diaphoresis, or other indications of serious illness or injury)
- Cardiac or respiratory arrest
- Decreased level of responsiveness/altered mental status
- Compromised or obstructed airway
- Inadequate breathing
- Signs of inadequate perfusion (absent or weak pulse; bradycardia or tachycardia; pale, cool, diaphoretic skin)
- Significant external bleeding or suspected internal bleeding

- The patient is not critical (he is alert and does not have immediate problems with airway, breathing, or circulation), but needs additional assessment and treatment. For example, the patient has an isolated ankle injury that should be splinted before he is moved.

- The patient is critical (Table 15-8), but immediate intervention may improve the situation. For example, if the patient is in cardiac arrest, you will follow through with the initial sequence of resuscitation without interruption to prepare for transport. (See Chapter 17.) You also may need to start an albuterol treatment for an asthmatic patient, or to start an IV and give 50 percent dextrose to a diabetic patient with hypoglycemia.

- The patient is critical and must be packaged and transported without delay on the scene for further assessment and interventions. Some patients may have hypovolemic shock, traumatic brain injury, suspected abdominal aortic aneurysm, or other conditions that cannot be improved in the field. These patients require emergent intervention in a medical facility capable of providing the specific services that the patient's condition requires.

Primary Assessments Compared

You cannot overlook any part of the scene size-up or primary assessment, but the way the steps play out varies, depending on the situation. You must use a balance of the prescribed approach (Figure 15-16; Scans 15-1 and 15-2), common sense, flexibility, and concern for the patient's best interests. Common sense tells you that the patient who got up to answer the door in response to your knock does not have immediately life-threatening problems with airway, breathing, or circulation. This does not mean that the patient is not sick. It simply means he is not dying before your eyes from an obstructed airway, inadequate breathing, or compromised circulation. He may, in fact, end up complaining of shortness of breath and have some signs and symptoms of respiratory distress, but he is not immediately categorized as a critical patient.

Scene Size-Up
- Operational aspects: Identify hazards, number of patients, and need for additional resources.
- Clinical aspects: Determine nature of illness/mechanism of injury; and general appearance including age, sex, responsive or apparently unresponsive.

Primary Assessment
- Apparently unresponsive: Quickly confirm level of responsiveness and determine presence or absence of breathing.
- For unresponsive patients, the pulse should be checked prior to checking breathing.
- No pulse: Start chest compressions.
- Pulse present: Check for problems with airway, breathing, and circulation.
- Responsive: Confirm level of responsiveness; check for problems with airway, breathing, and circulation; and determine chief complaint.
- Perform interventions for airway, breathing, and circulation; and determine whether patient is critical or noncritical.

Secondary Assessment
- Critical medical patient: Obtain history as available, perform rapid medical exam, obtain baseline vitals and use monitoring devices, and perform head-to-toe exam as needed.
- Critical trauma patient: Perform rapid trauma exam, obtain baseline vitals and use monitoring devices, perform head-to-toe exam, and obtain history as available.
- Noncritical medical patient: Obtain history, perform focused physical exam, and obtain baseline vitals and use monitoring devices.
- Noncritical trauma patient: Perform focused physical exam, obtain baseline vitals and use monitoring devices, and obtain history.

Reassessment
- Primary assessment (level of responsiveness, airway, breathing, and circulation)
- Vital signs and monitoring devices
- Aspects of physical exam
- Changes in complaints
- Specific effects of treatment

FIGURE 15-16

The patient assessment flowchart.

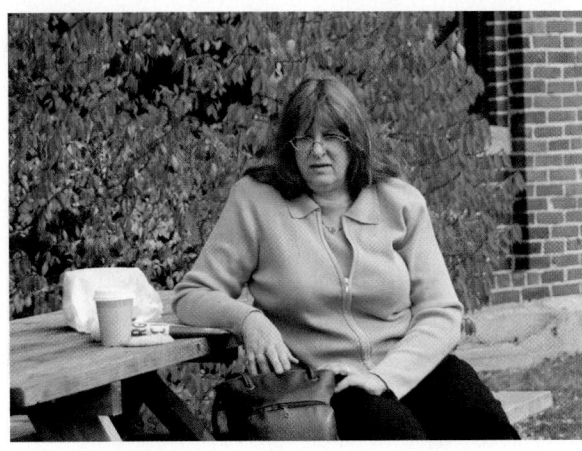

1. Perform a scene size-up to determine scene safety, the nature of the situation, the number of patients, and the need for additional resources.

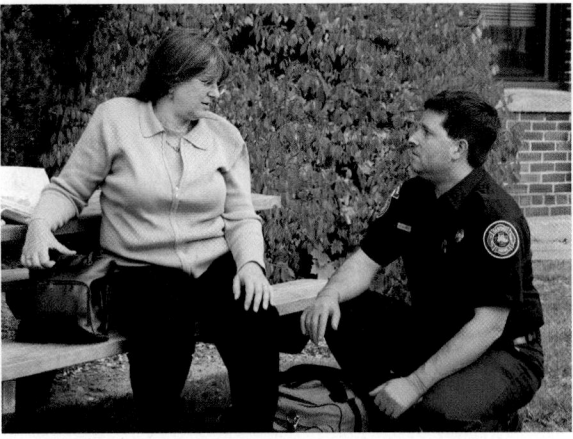

2. Note the patient's general appearance, such as skin color, obvious injuries, level of distress, and level of responsiveness.

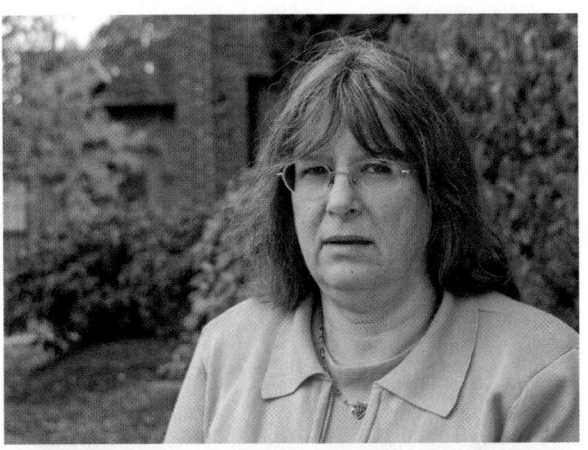

3. Look and listen for evidence of airway problems, such as struggling to breathe, noisy breathing, and cyanosis.

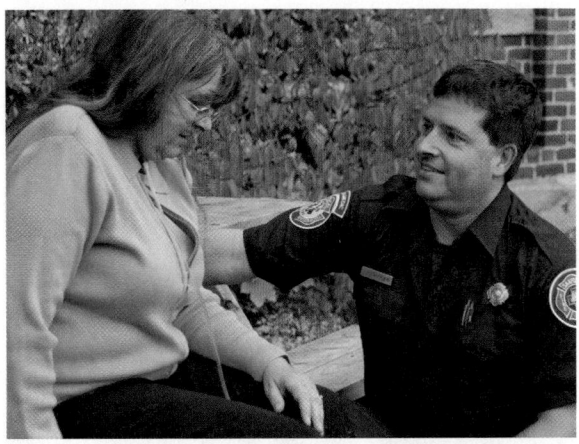

4. Assess the patient's breathing, looking and listening for signs of difficulty breathing.

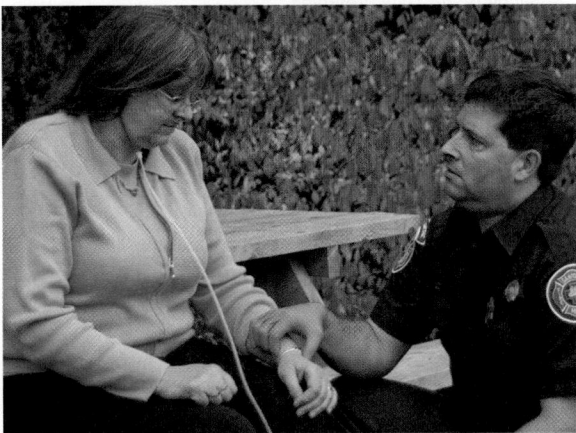

5. Check the patient's circulation.

Primary Assessment—Unresponsive Patient with a Pulse

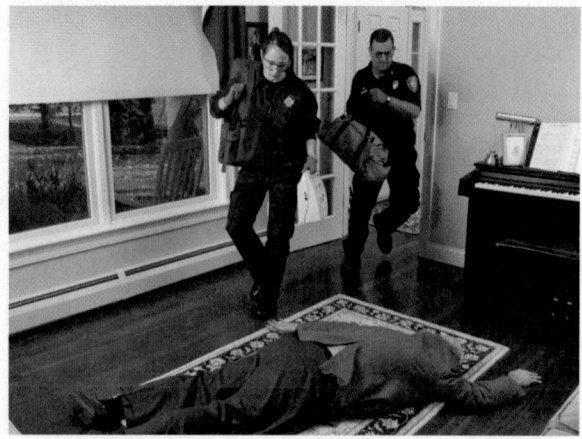

1. Perform a scene size-up to determine scene safety, the nature of the situation, the number of patients, and the need for additional resources.

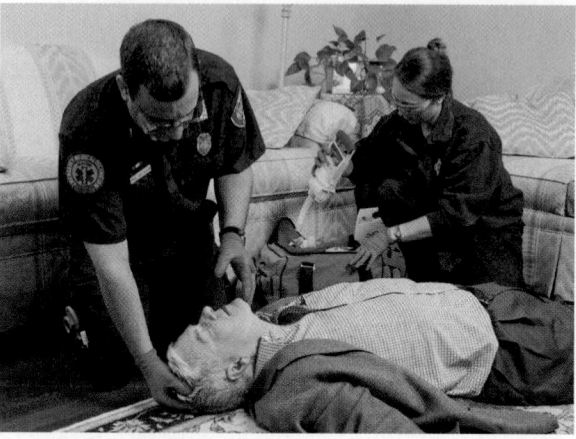

2. If spine injury is suspected, manually stabilize the head and neck during initial contact with the patient. Note the patient's general appearance, such as skin color, obvious injuries, and level of distress. Check the patient's level of responsiveness.

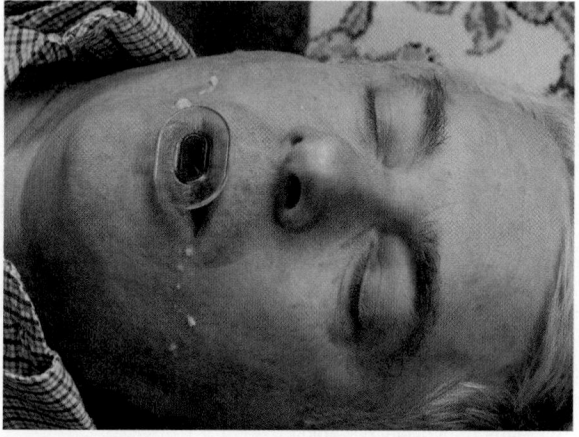

3. Position the patient and check the airway. Use a head-tilt/chin-lift maneuver for patients without suspected spine injury. Use a modified jaw-thrust maneuver to open the airway if spine injury is suspected. If needed, use suction and a basic airway adjunct to maintain an open airway.

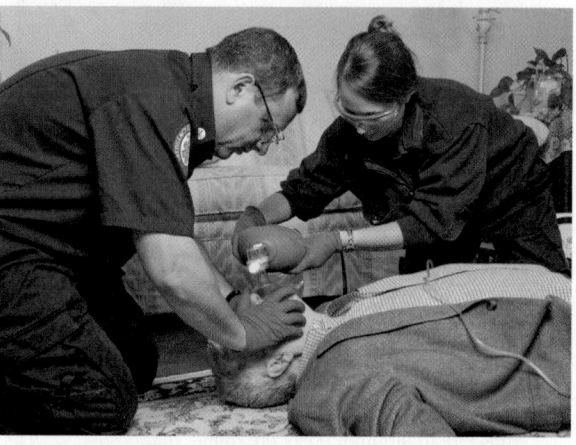

4. Assess the patient's breathing by looking and listening for signs of difficulty breathing.

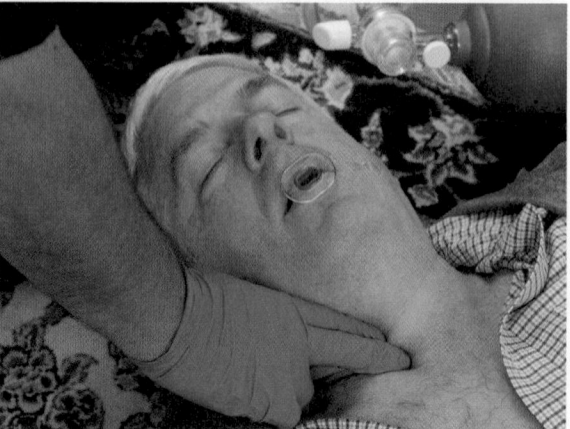

5. Check the rate and quality of the pulse. Control obvious hemorrhage.

In another situation, a distraught man might meet you at the door and tell you that his brother collapsed and he cannot wake him. The patient is lying motionless on the floor, cyanotic. You know immediately that this is a critical patient. Double-check to make sure the scene is safe. Is he unresponsive and cyanotic because of a gas leak? Does it look like there may have been a struggle with an assailant? Is there a distraught family member who may pose a danger? Quickly go to the patient's side. His cyanosis tells you that he has a problem with perfusion. Quickly check the carotid pulse. If the patient is pulseless, immediately begin chest compressions and apply the AED (for consistency with AHA guidelines), depending on whether or not his collapse was witnessed. If the patient has a pulse, or as soon as feasible during cardiac resuscitation, open the airway, insert an airway adjunct, begin ventilations, and provide supplemental oxygen. Work with your partner to request additional resources, prepare needed equipment and supplies, get a history from the family, and prepare the patient for transport.

Other times, the critical/not critical decision is not as easy. For example, on a call for a "sick person," you might enter a residence to find a young adult female patient lying on a sofa. Her eyes are closed and something about her appearance tells you she is sick, but you can see her breathing. She is not cyanotic, and there is no blood or emesis around the patient. You call out to her and place your hand on her shoulder, and she opens her eyes. You ask what her name is, but she mumbles something incomprehensible. At this point, because she has an altered mental status, you decide that she is a critical patient. Her airway is open, and she is breathing, but you notice that her breathing is deep and rapid. You then check her radial pulse. It is weak and rapid, but her skin is dry and flushed. Her abnormal breathing and pulse confirm to you that she is a critical patient. Apply oxygen to maintain an SpO$_2$ of 95 percent or higher by nonrebreather and collect a medical history from the family while your partner prepares for transport.

In yet another case, you respond to a call for a "sick person," and find a young adult female patient lying on a sofa with her eyes closed. When you call out to her and put your hand on her shoulder, she opens her eyes and says, "I don't feel well." Her skin is warm, moist, and slightly pale. She answers all of your questions appropriately. Her breathing is effortless, and she has a strong, regular radial pulse of 88 per minute. The patient's illness may or may not be serious, but there are no immediate threats to her airway, breathing, or circulation. More information is needed to determine her priority for transport.

Reassessment and Documentation

Primary assessment findings can change. You will not be aware of changes in the patient's general appearance, level of responsiveness, airway, breathing, or circulation unless you actively look for them. The initial findings serve as a baseline from which to track improvement or deterioration in the patient's condition.

Document the patient's initial condition, the interventions you implemented, and the effects of the interventions. Keep in mind, as well, that your verbal communication and documentation of scene size-up and primary assessment findings provide information that hospital staff otherwise might not have. Consider the narrative information in the following examples, noting that complete narrative documentation includes additional information about the secondary assessment and other treatments:

EXAMPLE 1: The pt is a 38 y/o male who was the unrestrained driver of a vehicle that left the highway at a high rate of speed and rolled over multiple times. The pt was ejected into an open field and was found prone approximately 25 feet from the vehicle.

Primary assessment: The pt was unresponsive to painful stimuli. He had shallow, irregular, gurgling respirations at a rate of 6 per minute. The radial pulse was strong and regular at 58 per minute. The pt was log-rolled onto a long backboard with manual stabilization of the cervical spine. The airway was opened with a modified jaw-thrust maneuver, and 60 mL of bloody fluid was suctioned from the mouth. The pt tolerated an oropharyngeal airway without a gag reflex. Bag-valve-mask ventilations were initiated at a rate of 10 per minute with 15 L/min of supplemental oxygen. The pt required frequent suctioning to remove bloody fluid from his mouth.

EXAMPLE 2: The pt is a 16 y/o female found sitting on a barstool at home, alert, with a chief complaint, "I can't breathe."

Primary assessment: The patient was leaning forward, using accessory muscles to breathe, and able to speak only three to four words at a time without pausing to breathe. The respiratory rate was 24 times per minute. Wheezing was heard without a stethoscope. The patient's skin was warm and moist without cyanosis, and the radial pulse was strong with a rate of 116 per minute. An albuterol treatment of 2.5 mg in 3 mL of normal saline was nebulized with 8 L/min of oxygen.

(Following other information): After the albuterol treatment, she stated she had less difficulty breathing. The respiratory rate decreased to 20 times per minute and no wheezing was heard on auscultation of the lungs. The radial pulse remained strong at 116 per minute.

CASE STUDY WRAP-UP

Clinical-Reasoning Process

Advanced EMTs Kyle Davis and Eric Chen are on the scene of two patients from a motorcycle collision. Both patients are critical, but the unresponsive male has the most immediately life-threatening conditions. Both patients have a mechanism of injury that requires transport to a trauma center. The male patient is unresponsive with impaired airway and breathing, along with significant bleeding. The female is alert and has little evidence of external bleeding, but her pulse is weak and rapid. Along with her pale, sweaty skin and obvious injuries, the findings make her a critical patient as well. Kyle and Eric realize both patients could deteriorate rapidly.

While waiting for the second ambulance to arrive, Kyle contacts the trauma center and tells them they will arrive in 30 to 35 minutes with two critical trauma patients from a motorcycle collision. He gives a brief initial report on both patients. When the backup ambulance crew arrives, they help package and load Eric's patient first, and then Kyle's.

Both ambulances depart for the trauma center. Kyle is able to perform a full secondary assessment and splint the patient's injured extremity. Eric's attention remains on his patient's airway and breathing. He is able to complete a rapid trauma assessment, determining that the patient has multiple fractures and likely chest and abdominal injuries in addition to his head injuries.

CHAPTER REVIEW

Chapter Summary

A scene size-up and primary assessment are performed on every patient to identify the general nature of the problem and immediately detect and correct problems with the airway, breathing, or circulation.

In the scene size-up, determine the mechanism of injury or nature of the illness. Begin to form an impression of the patient's general appearance. Note whether he appears to be responsive or unresponsive. Also note his skin color (pale, cyanotic, flushed, jaundiced), obvious injuries or problems, and general level of distress. Overlooking any aspect of the primary assessment can result in patient harm, or even death. The patient must have an open airway, be adequately ventilated, and have adequate circulation before other assessments or interventions are begun.

Assess the patient's level of responsiveness to determine whether he is alert, responsive to verbal stimuli, responsive to painful stimuli, or unresponsive. Noting how the patient responds to verbal and painful stimuli gives additional information that is used to calculate a GCS score.

If the patient is unresponsive, immediately check the carotid pulse. If he is pulseless, begin chest compressions. If a pulse is present, proceed with assessing the airway and breathing.

Observe responsive patients for indications of problems with the airway, breathing, or circulation, and obtain the chief complaint. Apply oxygen to any patient whose breathing is adequate, but who is at risk for hypoxia.

For patients with a decreased level of responsiveness, begin by ensuring that the airway is open, which may require manual maneuvers and simple airway adjuncts. Assess the adequacy of the patient's breathing, and use a bag-valve-mask device with supplemental oxygen to assist any patient with inadequate or absent breathing.

Assess the patient's pulse, and check for significant external bleeding. Control bleeding with direct pressure. If necessary, use a tourniquet for uncontrollable bleeding proximal to the knee or elbow. Expose the patient if indicated to ensure that you have located all ongoing bleeding.

Use the information from the scene size-up and primary assessment to determine the patient's priority for transportation, how you will approach the secondary assessment, and what additional initial interventions are necessary. Reassess the primary assessment findings. Document both initial and subsequent assessment findings.

Review Questions

Multiple-Choice Questions

1. At what point should you make an initial decision about what type of PPE you should use for a particular patient?
   a. When you have decided the patient's transport priority
   b. After the primary assessment
   c. In the scene size-up
   d. After checking the airway

2. Which one of the following is an example of a mechanism of injury?
   a. Exposure to fire
   b. A broken leg
   c. Chest pain
   d. Unresponsiveness

3. Which one of the following decisions is based on assessment of the mechanism of injury?
   a. Whether to transport the patient to the hospital
   b. What specific organs were injured
   c. What type of airway adjunct to insert
   d. Whether to use manual stabilization of the cervical spine

4. If you believe a patient may have suffered an injury to his cervical spine, you should use a _____ maneuver to open the airway.
   a. head-tilt/chin-lift
   b. tongue/jaw pull
   c. modified jaw-thrust
   d. neck-flex

5. Which one of the following best describes the purpose of the primary assessment?
   a. To identify all injuries and problems
   b. To find and treat all immediately life-threatening problems
   c. To decide whether to transport the patient
   d. To make a diagnosis of the patient's problem

6. A numeric score can be assigned to the level of responsiveness using the:
   a. level of responsiveness.
   b. AVPU scale.
   c. Glasgow Coma Scale.
   d. ABCD mnemonic.

7. Which one of the following is an acceptable method of checking for response to painful stimuli?
   a. Needle stick
   b. Interdigital pressure
   c. Pinching the skin
   d. Thumping the chest

8. A bluish-purple discoloration of the skin indicates:
   a. hypoxia.
   b. liver disease.
   c. fever.
   d. shock.

9. Snoring is an indication of airway obstruction caused by:
   a. swelling of the trachea or larynx.
   b. fluids in the airway.
   c. the tongue.
   d. a foreign body in lower airway.

10. Which one of the following chief complaints makes a patient the highest priority for transport?
    a. Sore throat
    b. Difficulty breathing
    c. Low back pain
    d. Fever

Critical-Thinking Questions

11. You have determined that an adult patient who is responsive only to pain is breathing 8 times per minute. Explain what steps you will take next.

12. Why are patients with decreased levels of responsiveness at risk for airway compromise?

13. Why must a primary assessment be performed on every patient?

14. How is the concept of tidal volume used in the primary assessment?

15. What are some causes of airway obstruction? How is each managed?

References

American Heart Association. (2010). 2010 American Heart Association guidelines for cardiopulmonary resuscitation and emergency cardiovascular care. *Circulation.* Retrieved October 18, 2010, from http://circ.ahajournals.org/cgi/content/full/122/18_suppl_3/

Hackl, W., Hausberger, K., Sailer, R., Ulmer, H., & Gassner, R. (2001). Prevalence of cervical spine injuries in patients with facial trauma. *Oral Surgery, Oral Medicine, Oral Pathology, Oral Radiology, and Endodontology, 92,* 370–376.

Mithani, S. K., St. Hilaire, H., Brooke, B. S., Smith, I. M., Bluebond-Langer, R. & Rodriguez, E. D. (2009). Predictable patterns of intracranial and cervical spine injury in craniomaxillofacial trauma: Analysis of 4786 patients. *Plastic and Reconstructive Surgery, 123,* 1293–1301.

16 Airway Management, Ventilation, and Oxygenation

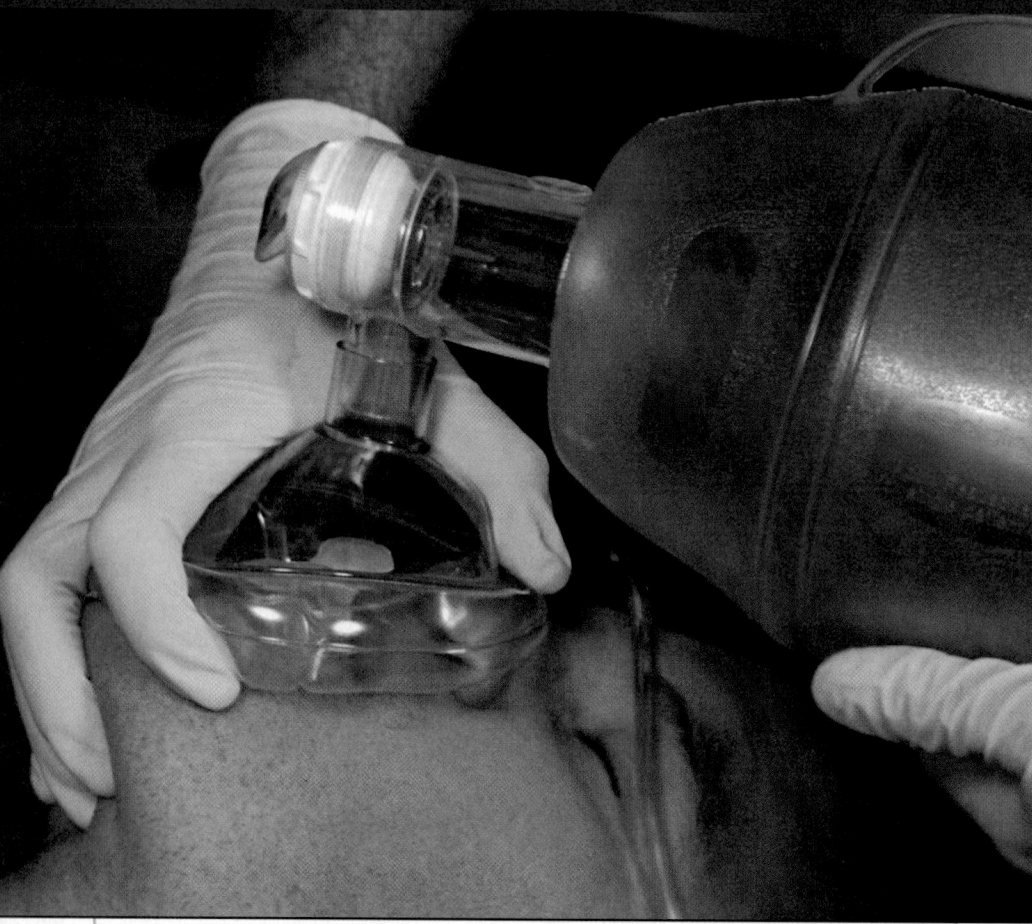

Content Area: Airway Management; Respiration; and Artificial Ventilation

Advanced EMT Education Standard: Applies knowledge of upper airway anatomy and physiology to patient assessment and management in order to ensure a patent airway, adequate mechanical ventilation, and respiration for patients of all ages.

Objectives

After reading this chapter, you should be able to:

16.1   Define the key terms introduced in this chapter.

16.2   Relate the anatomy and physiology of the respiratory system to oxygenation, perfusion, and removal of carbon dioxide.

16.3   Give examples of complaints and conditions that are associated with risk of hypoxia and hypoventilation.

16.4   Relate findings from the assessment of the airway and ventilation to the patient's need for interventions in airway, oxygenation, and ventilation.

16.5   Recognize signs and symptoms of mild, moderate, and severe hypoxia.

16.6   Distinguish between adequate and inadequate breathing.

16.7   Measure oxygenation by pulse oximetry.

KEY TERMS (continued)

tracheostomy *(p. 393)*

trauma chin lift *(p. 380)*

tripod position *(p. 380)*

ventilation *(p. 372)*

ventilation–perfusion (VQ) mismatch *(p. 377)*

Yankauer *(p. 393)*

CASE STUDY

It is 0600 and Advanced EMTs Brian Calley and Tiffany Bombard are checking their ambulance as they begin their shift. The tone goes off and they are dispatched to 240 Butternut Street for a 70-year-old patient with difficulty breathing. They stop what they are doing and immediately notify dispatch that they have begun their response.

After acknowledging that the ambulance is responding, the dispatcher notifies Brian and Tiffany that the patient has had shortness of breath since last night and that the caller indicated the patient is "not doing well at all."

Brian turns to Tiffany and says, "I have a bad feeling about this one," and the partners begin to formulate a plan of action. They discuss what equipment they will bring into the house and what roles they each will play. Tiffany points out that the patient's shortness of breath seems to have been going on for several hours and suggests a few possible etiologies.

They arrive at a small home in a residential neighborhood. A woman in a housecoat is in the doorway waving the ambulance in. Brian and Tiffany grab their gear and quickly look around for any possible safety hazards. Seeing none, they approach the house. The woman is very upset. As the providers approach, she says, "Please hurry, I don't think he is going to make it." She directs them to the back bedroom and rushes down the hall. The house is stuffy and oxygen tubing crisscrosses the floor.

Brian and Tiffany find the patient seated on the edge of the bed. He is in tripod position and is rocking back and forth slightly as he breathes. His color is dusky with cyanosis of his mouth, ears, and nail beds. He is wearing a nasal cannula and he seems disoriented, showing no indication that he is aware of the Advanced EMTs.

Problem-Solving Questions

1. How would you describe your general impression of the patient? What evidence supports your description?
2. What does the evidence indicate should be Brian and Tiffany's first action?
3. What additional information do you need about this patient?
4. How will Brian and Tiffany integrate the need to collect further information with the need to treat and transport the patient?

16.8   Measure exhaled carbon dioxide by colorimetric capnometry or wave-form capnography.

16.9   Incorporate the values of pulse oximetry and capnometry into decisions regarding management of airway, breathing, and oxygenation.

16.10   Demonstrate the proper technique of auscultating breath sounds.

16.11   Describe the causes of abnormal breathing sounds, including:
   – Decreased and absent breath sounds
   – Gurgling
   – Crackles (rales)
   – Rhonchi
   – Snoring
   – Stridor
   – Wheezing

(continued)

(continued from previous page)

16.12   Identify the different presentations and needs of pediatric and geriatric patients with regard to airway, ventilation, and oxygenation.

16.13   Take immediate action to correct impaired airway, breathing, or oxygenation.

16.14   Utilize manual positioning and suction (portable and fixed devices) to keep the airway clear.

16.15   Given a variety of scenarios, select and insert an oropharyngeal or nasopharyngeal airway.

16.16   Given a variety of scenarios, select and insert an appropriate advanced airway device (Combitube or supraglottic airway).

16.17   Administer supplemental oxygen via devices suited to individual patients' needs, including:
  – Nasal cannula
  – Nonrebreather mask
  – Partial rebreather mask
  – Simple face mask
  – Tracheostomy mask
  – Venturi mask

16.18   Describe the concept of positive end-expiratory pressure (PEEP).

16.19   Ventilate or assist the ventilations of patients using the following devices, as appropriate to various situations:
  – Automatic transport ventilators
  – Bag-valve-mask device
  – Combitube
  – Continuous positive airway pressure (CPAP)
  – Laryngeal mask airway (LMA)
  – Manually triggered ventilation devices
  – Mouth-to-mask
  – Supraglottic airway devices, such as the King LTD or Cobra

16.20   Employ appropriate safety precautions when handling, transporting, and administering oxygen.

16.21   Properly utilize oxygen cylinders and regulators to ensure adequate patient oxygenation.

16.22   Modify techniques of managing airway, ventilation, and oxygenation for the following situations:
  – Patients with abnormal facial structure and dental appliances
  – Patients with facial trauma
  – Patients with foreign body airway obstruction
  – Patients with potential cervical-spine injuries
  – Patients with stomas and tracheostomies
  – Pediatric and geriatric patients

16.23   Discuss the physiologic differences, including potential complications, of artificial ventilation.

16.24   Suction the airway of an intubated patient.

Introduction

The function of the respiratory system is to obtain oxygen needed for cell metabolism and to eliminate carbon dioxide produced by cell metabolism. Without the support for cell metabolism provided by the respiratory system, death occurs quickly. Respiratory support for metabolism requires the mechanical process of **ventilation** and the process of gas exchange, called *respiration*. Ventilation relies on an open airway and basic principles of physics to create the conditions for air to flow in and out of the lungs. Respiration relies on the microscopic anatomy of the alveoli and capillaries, as well as the principle of gradients, which are differences in the concentrations of gases from one area to another. A problem with any aspect of ventilation or respiration can quickly result in death. The body has sophisticated compensatory mechanisms, but unless the underlying problem is corrected, these mechanisms become overwhelmed.

Restoring function in patients who have problems with ventilation and respiration requires that Advanced EMTs are skilled in a variety of techniques, ranging from simple and noninvasive to more complex. But this process is not primarily about tools and gadgets. It is about assessment and decision making. Although it is important to be skilled in the use of devices and techniques, it is far more important to understand when and why to utilize those skills. Airway and ventilatory management requires providers to use clinical judgment and critical thinking to determine the most appropriate intervention given the situation at hand.

In all cases, the best way to manage a patient's airway is whatever technique ensures adequate oxygenation and ventilation for that particular patient with minimal complications. Making the right decisions first requires the ability to quickly recognize problems with airway, ventilation, and respiration. You must know what options are available to you for managing the situation and must carefully but quickly weigh the utility and potential drawbacks of each option. In doing this, you must take into consideration the patient's condition, the amount and type of help available to you, any factors that may complicate the situation, and the amount of time for which your chosen option must work for the patient.

The primary focus of this chapter is adult airway and ventilatory management. Infant and pediatric airway and ventilatory management considerations are given additional attention in Chapters 43 and 44.

Anatomy and Physiology Review

The process of moving air in and out the lungs is a mechanical process called *ventilation* (Figure 16-1). Once air enters the lungs, oxygen and carbon dioxide are exchanged across the respiratory membrane composed of the alveolar and pulmonary capillary walls in a process called *external respiration*. The exchange of oxygen and

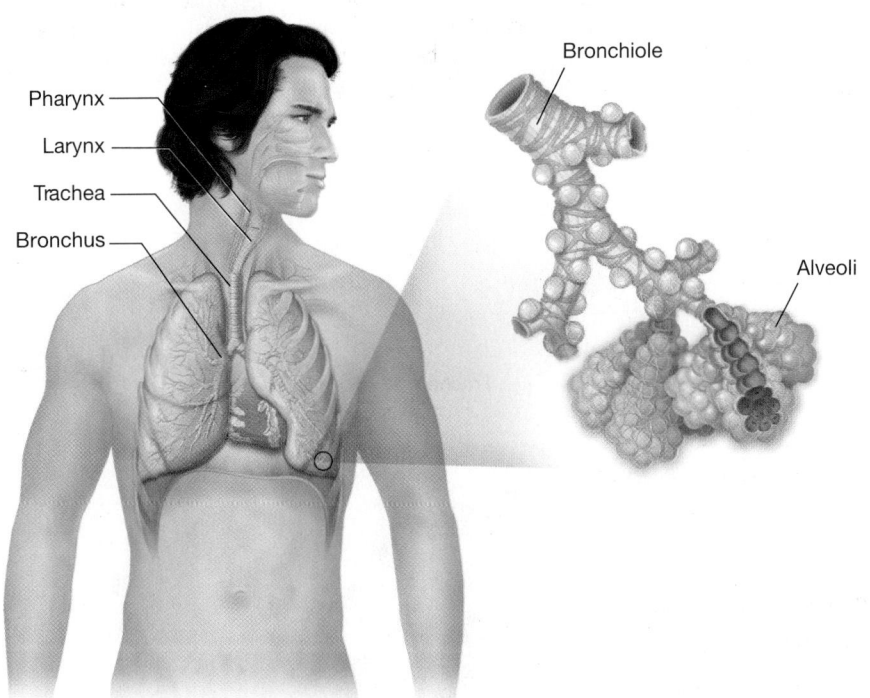

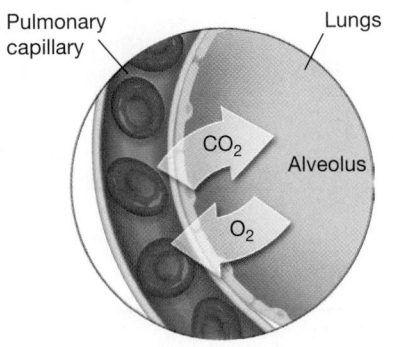

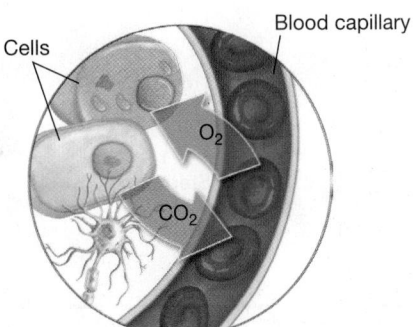

FIGURE 16-1

Ventilation is required for external and internal respiration.

carbon dioxide between the blood and the cells of the body is called *internal respiration*. Ventilation relies on basic principles of physics to create the conditions for air to flow in and out of the lungs. Respiration relies on the microscopic anatomy of the alveoli and capillaries, as well as the principle of gradients—differences in the concentrations of gases from one area to another.

Physiology of Air Movement

Ventilation is controlled by the levels of carbon dioxide (CO_2) and oxygen (O_2) in the blood and cerebrospinal fluid (CSF). Chemoreceptors in the aortic arch, carotid arteries, and central nervous system signal the inspiratory center in the medulla oblingata of the brain stem when carbon dioxide levels increase or oxygen levels decrease. In turn, signals from the inspiratory center stimulate contraction of the diaphragm and intercostal muscles, which increases the volume of the thoracic cavity and lungs (Figure 16-2). As the volume increases, the pressure of the gas within the cavity decreases with respect to atmospheric pressure (Boyle's law). Provided that the upper and lower airways are unobstructed, air flows from the higher atmospheric pressure to the lower intrapulmonary pressure.

Stretch receptors in the lungs send signals that terminate inspiration and the diaphragm and intercostal

IN THE FIELD

The decrease in intrathoracic pressure during inspiration also assists with return of blood to the heart, allowing an increase in cardiac output. If intrathoracic pressure is abnormally increased, such as occurs with aggressive artificial ventilation, cardiac output is decreased.

IN THE FIELD

Compression and release of the chest wall, such as occurs during chest compressions in CPR, causes changes in the size of the thoracic cavity and in intrathoracic pressure. When the chest is compressed, the increase in intrathoracic pressure forces blood out of the heart. However, unless the chest wall is allowed to completely recoil between compressions, the increased intrathoracic pressure impedes return of blood to the heart. Therefore, it is extremely important to allow the chest wall to recoil completely between compressions. The same decrease in intrathoracic pressure that allows blood to return to the heart may also allow some passive movement of air into the lungs, while the increase in intrathoracic pressure accompanying chest compression will move air out of the lungs.

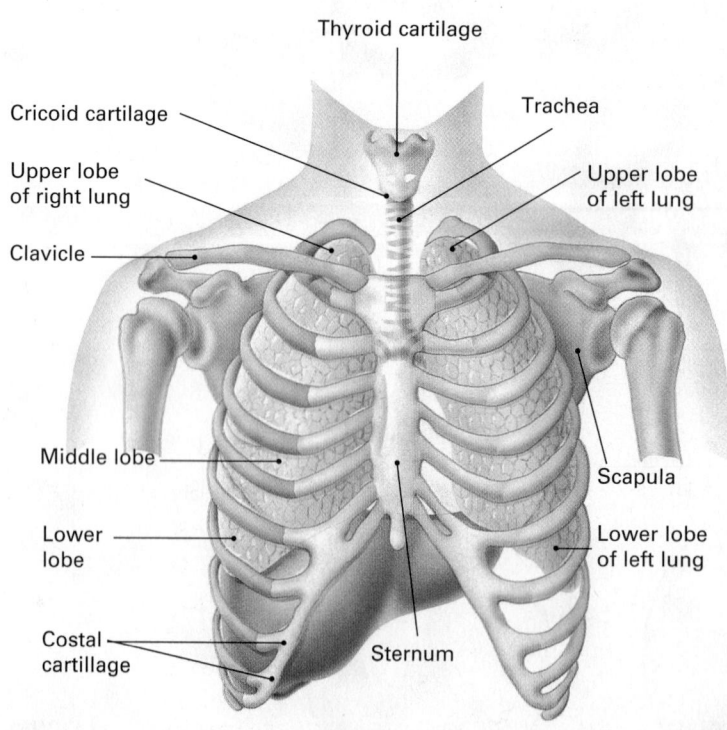

FIGURE 16-2

The thoracic cavity.

muscles relax (Hering–Breuer reflex). As the muscles relax, the intrathoracic and intrapulmonary volumes decrease, causing an increase in pressure. Provided that there are no obstructions in the airway, air flows from the higher intrapulmonary pressure to the relatively lower atmospheric pressure.

Upper Airway

The upper airway consists of the structures above the glottis. Air enters the body through the mouth and nose (Figure 16-3). In the nose, air is filtered, humidified, and warmed as it winds its way through the folds of the nasal turbinates. Air from the nose enters the posterior pharynx at an area called the *nasopharynx*. When air enters through the mouth, the important functions of the nasal turbinates are bypassed. The roof of the oral cavity anteriorly is composed of the hard palate, which transitions to the soft palate in the posterior oral cavity. The uvula is a fleshy protuberance from the soft palate that hangs inferiorly into the oropharynx. The tongue arises from the floor of the oral cavity posteriorly. Small masses of lymphoepithelial tissue are found at the lateral aspects of both the oropharynx and the nasopharynx. In the oropharynx, these are called *tonsils* and in the nasopharynx, they are called *adenoids*. Both tonsils and adenoids can become inflamed and swollen due to infection, and also are highly vascular.

The hypopharynx, also known as the *laryngopharynx*, is the most inferior area of the throat and is just superior to the openings of the trachea and esophagus. The oral cavity, oropharynx, and hypopharynx provide a common passageway for both the digestive and respiratory systems.

This arrangement necessitates protective mechanisms to prevent food and liquids intended for the digestive system from entering the respiratory system. During swallowing, a leaf-shaped flap of tissue called the *epiglottis* closes over the glottis, which is the opening of the larynx and lies between the vocal cords. Reflex elevation of the soft palate prevents foods and fluids from traveling upward into the nasopharynx. The gag reflex is an involuntary elevation of the palate and contraction of pharyngeal muscles in response to stimulation of the posterior pharynx and soft palate, which prevents foreign material from entering the hypopharynx. In some individuals, a larger area of the brainstem appears to be stimulated by the gag reflex, which can result in vomiting. One of the cranial nerves responsible for the gag reflex, the vagus nerve (CN X), also has branches that inhibit the rate of the sinoatrial node of the heart. When the vagus nerve is stimulated by way of the gag reflex, bradycardia can sometimes occur.

The cough reflex occurs when inflammation or irritants, such as aspirated food or liquid, or toxic gases stimulate sensory receptors in the lining of the airways. The result is inspiration of air followed by closing of the glottis and contraction of the abdominal muscles, diaphragm, and intercostal muscles. Muscular contraction decreases the volume of the thorax, but the closed glottis prevents expiration, resulting in increasing intrapulmonary pressure. When the glottis suddenly opens, air is forcefully propelled out through the airways, hopefully removing the irritant with it. The vocal cords themselves provide some protection to the lower airway when they are closed. In the presence of irritation, the vocal cords can spasm, closing the glottic opening. This is known as **laryngospasm**.

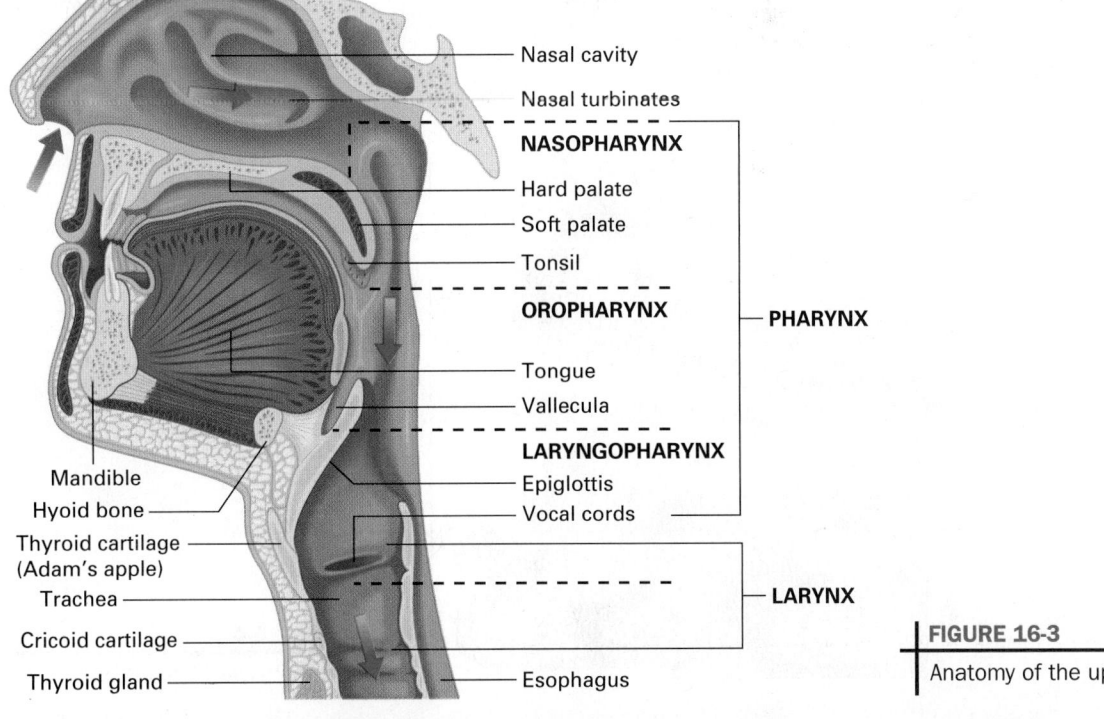

Nasal cavity
Nasal turbinates
NASOPHARYNX
Hard palate
Soft palate
Tonsil
OROPHARYNX
Tongue
Vallecula
LARYNGOPHARYNX
Epiglottis
Vocal cords
PHARYNX

Mandible
Hyoid bone
Thyroid cartilage (Adam's apple)
Trachea
Cricoid cartilage
Thyroid gland
Esophagus
LARYNX

FIGURE 16-3

Anatomy of the upper airway.

A certain degree of muscle tone is required to keep the tongue from relaxing and falling posteriorly into the pharynx, where it can obstruct airflow. Some degree of muscle tone is maintained even during sleep in normal circumstances. Yet, laxity of the tongue is reflected in snoring, caused by partial airway obstruction. The obstruction increases the turbulence of airflow and vibrates the soft tissues of the pharynx. Always remember that snoring is an indication of partial airway obstruction. In patients with a decreased level of responsiveness, laxity of the tongue can result in partial or complete airway obstruction. In fact, the tongue is the most common cause of airway obstruction.

Manually positioning the head and neck elevates the mandible, thus lifting the tongue to relieve upper airway obstruction. While basic airway adjuncts, such as an **oropharyngeal airway** and a **nasopharyngeal airway** can displace the soft tissue of the tongue, they do not replace the need for manual positioning of the head and neck. In trauma patients suspected of a cervical-spine injury, manual airway maneuvers are modified to prevent hyperextension of the neck. (See Chapter 14 for indications of cervical-spine injury.)

Lower Airway

The lower airway begins at the glottic opening and proceeds into the trachea (Figure 16-5). The trachea is formed by up to 20 rings of cartilage beginning with the cricoid ring. The cricoid ring is the only true ring. The others are "C" shaped and connected in back by a strip of smooth muscle. This posterior smooth muscle connection allows for the movement of food through the esophagus, which lies against the posterior aspect of the trachea.

As it proceeds into the chest, the trachea bifurcates into the right and left mainstem bronchi at the carina, which lies roughly at the level of the fourth thoracic vertebra and angle of Louis (angle formed by the junction of the manubrium and body of the sternum). The left mainstem bronchus angles more sharply, while the right mainstem bronchus takes a straighter path from the carina. As a result, aspirated foreign bodies tend to lodge in the right mainstem bronchus. An endotracheal tube (advanced airway device placed for positive pressure ventilation) and suction catheter inserted too deeply also tend to end up in the right mainstem bronchus.

Smaller bronchi branch from the left and right bronchi, serving each of the three lobes of the right lung and both

(P) Pediatric Care

Pediatric patients have a proportionally larger tongue and epiglottis than adults (Figure 16-4). This can mean increased vulnerability to obstruction due to decreased muscle tone. The laryngopharynx is also more anterior and superior than that of an adult. In an adult, the narrowest point in the airway is the glottic opening. In small children and infants, the narrowest point is just below the glottic opening at the level of the cricoid ring. This causes the airway to be somewhat funnel shaped and prone to the dangers of obstruction and subglottic edema in infection.

IN THE FIELD

In the past, the application of pressure to the cricoid ring, also called *Sellick's maneuver,* was employed in cardiac arrest management to press the cricoid ring posteriorly against the esophagus. The idea was that this might prevent regurgitation of stomach contents past this point to protect against aspiration and prevent air from entering the stomach during bag-valve-mask ventilations. However, studies have not supported the use of cricoid pressure and indicate that its application may delay other, more critical airway procedures. The 2010 American Heart Association Emergency Cardiac Care Guidelines no longer recommend the routine use of this procedure.

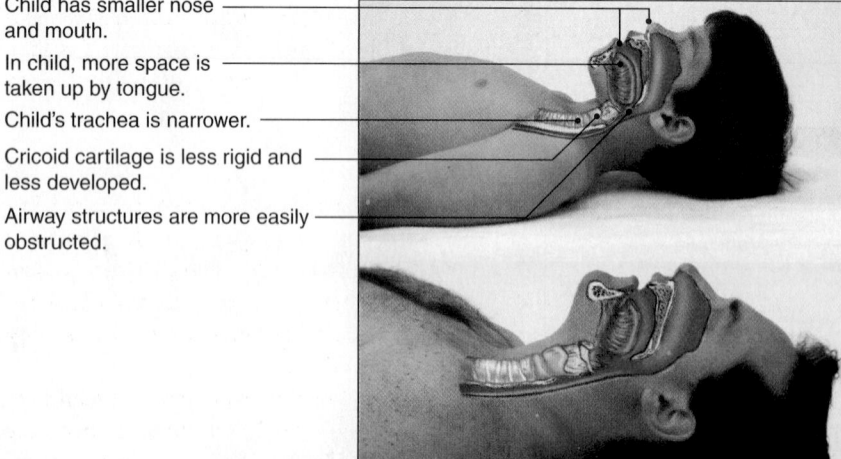

Child has smaller nose and mouth.

In child, more space is taken up by tongue.

Child's trachea is narrower.

Cricoid cartilage is less rigid and less developed.

Airway structures are more easily obstructed.

FIGURE 16-4
Pediatric airway differences.

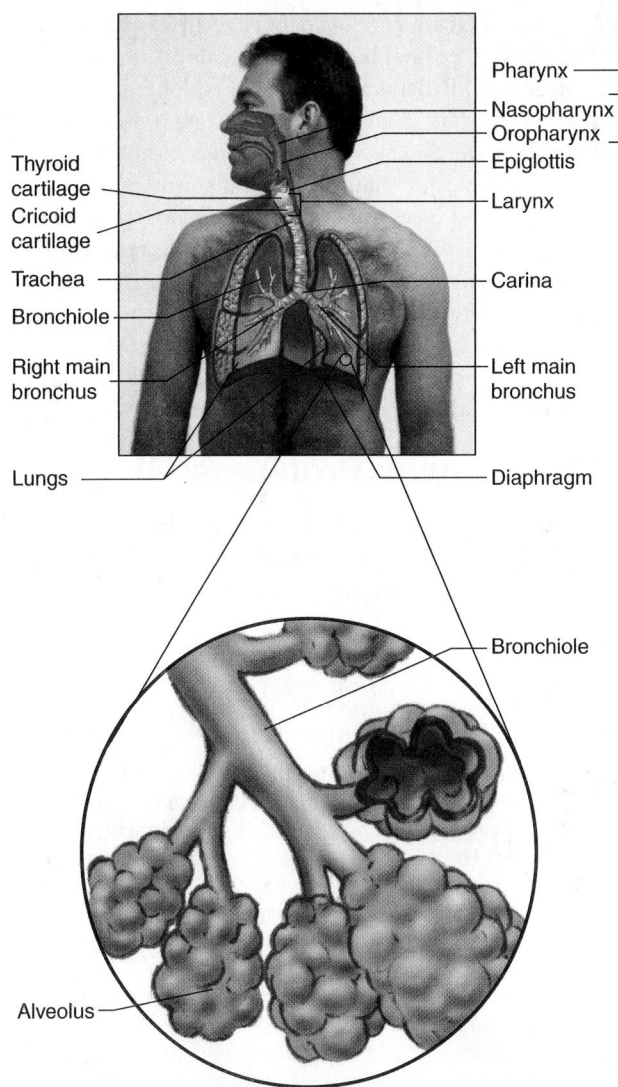

Pharynx
Nasopharynx
Oropharynx
Epiglottis
Larynx
Carina
Left main bronchus
Diaphragm

Thyroid cartilage
Cricoid cartilage
Trachea
Bronchiole
Right main bronchus
Lungs

Bronchiole
Alveolus

FIGURE 16-5

Anatomy of the lower airway.

lobes of the left lung. These bronchi continue dividing into smaller and smaller and smaller branches until they become terminal bronchioles leading into clusters of alveoli. The bronchi and bronchioles are lined with specialized endothelial tissue. The bronchioles have a layer of smooth muscle, the cells of which have sympathetic beta$_2$ receptor sites that respond to epinephrine from sympathetic nervous system stimulation and beta$_2$ agonist drugs. When the beta$_2$ receptors are stimulated, smooth muscle relaxes, increasing the diameter of the bronchioles to allow greater airflow.

Gas Exchange

Alveoli are tiny air sacs surrounded by pulmonary capillaries. It is here that the process of diffusion allows oxygen from inhaled air to move into the bloodstream and carbon dioxide from the bloodstream to move into the alveoli for expiration in the process of external respiration. Effective external respiration requires a match between the amount of

lung ventilated and the amount of lung perfused. Anything that interferes with ventilation to a lung or any portion of it or anything that interferes with distribution of blood through the pulmonary circulation results in what is called a **ventilation–perfusion (VQ) mismatch**. External respiration is affected by any process that increases the distance across which gases must diffuse. An example is increased interstitial fluid at the alveolar–capillary interface, such as occurs with **pulmonary edema.**

Internal respiration occurs when oxygen is delivered to the cellular level by the hemoglobin in red blood cells, and carbon dioxide from cellular metabolism diffuses into the blood. This process can be affected by metabolic changes and toxins, such as carbon monoxide and cyanide.

Ventilation

Alveolar ventilation is the volume of air that reaches the alveoli each minute. It is a function of both respiratory rate and tidal volume. Tidal volume is the volume of air inhaled and exhaled in a single breath. Tidal volumes can vary depending on the size and respiratory pattern of the patient, but are approximately 5 to 7 mL per kilogram of body weight. For purposes of discussion, normal tidal volume for an average-size person is about 500 mL. **Minute volume** combines tidal volume and respiratory rate to measure the volume of air breathed each minute. But measurement of minute volume does not ensure that air has reached the alveoli. Of a 500 mL tidal volume, typically only 350 mL reach the alveoli. The remaining 150 mL of air occupies space in the trachea and large bronchial tubes and never reaches the alveoli. This nonalveolar air is called *dead space air*. When the tidal volume decreases, the volume of dead space remains constant at the expense of alveolar ventilation.

Pathophysiology of the Airway, Ventilation, and Oxygenation

The goal of providing oxygen to the cells and eliminating carbon dioxide can be disrupted at any point from the upper airway to the cellular level. Problems are generally classified as either upper airway problems or lower airway problems.

Upper Airway Problems

Upper airway problems can occur by a variety of mechanisms. A common cause of upper airway obstruction is poor muscle tone due to decreased level of responsiveness (Figure 16-6). Fourteen different muscle groups control airway patency. Loss of tone in one of those groups can lead to partial or complete obstruction.

When a patient's level of responsiveness is diminished, the muscles of the pharynx relax. In the supine patient, the tongue falls back, which obstructs the oropharynx and impedes airflow through the trachea. When the obstruction is

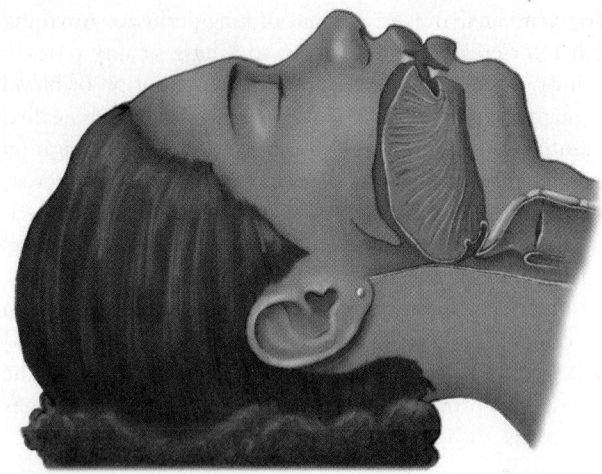

FIGURE 16-6

In patients with decreased muscle tone, the tongue and epiglottis can obstruct the upper airway.

partial, a snoring noise indicates turbulent airflow vibrating the soft tissues of the palate and pharynx (Table 16-1). The airway may also be obstructed in the patient who develops a decreased level of responsiveness in a sitting position. When the neck flexes forward, the trachea can be obstructed. Partial and complete airway obstruction in patients with decreased responsiveness is typically easily relieved by manually positioning the head and neck.

Foreign bodies are also a cause of upper airway obstruction. Any matter that obstructs airflow can be involved. Sometimes, the reason EMS is requested is that a patient is choking on food or another object. A patient who is unresponsive because of a stroke, drug overdose, or trauma may vomit and stomach contents may be aspirated into the airway. Not only does this result in immediate airway problems, but it also leads to subsequent pneumonitis and

pneumonia. Trauma patients may have airway obstruction due to active bleeding, blood clots, or direct injury to airway structures. Patients who are choking on a solid object require maneuvers to clear the obstruction, while patients with fluids in the airway require suction to clear the airway.

The airway is of relatively small diameter and can easily be obstructed by edema. Causes of upper airway edema include trauma, burns, anaphylaxis, and infection. Patients with airway edema require advanced life support procedures. When you encounter a patient with airway edema, request advanced life support response if available, or prepare for transport without delay to the closest emergency facility capable of managing the airway problem.

Lower Airway Problems

The lower airway involves all structures below the glottic opening. By far the most common cause of widespread obstruction to airflow in the lower airway is

Pediatric Care

Epiglottitis is a bacterial infection that can obstruct the airway. It was formerly more common in children, but widespread vaccination against the causative bacteria has decreased its incidence in children. Always ask about a child's immunization against Hib (haemophilus influenza B) when airway obstruction is suspected. The patient generally has a sore throat and fever. Epiglottitis also can occur in adults. Drooling occurs because of the pain involved in swallowing. If the airway is jeopardized, the patient will often present in tripod position and exhibit stridor with inspiration. Do not attempt to inspect the airway or insert anything in the mouth when epiglottitis is suspected because additional inflammation can convert a partial airway obstruction to a complete airway obstruction.

TABLE 16-1	**Abnormal Respiratory Sounds**	
Sound	**Description**	**Significance**
Snoring	Harsh, vibrating, rattling sound that may be soft or loud	Partial obstruction of the upper airway by the tongue
Gurgling	Liquid, bubbling sound	Fluid in the upper airway
Stridor	Harsh inspiratory sound	Partial upper airway obstruction; may indicate laryngeal edema, foreign body airway obstruction, or epiglottitis
Coughing	Spasmodic forceful air expulsion that may sound "dry" or "wet"	Irritation of the respiratory mucosa from infection or irritants
Wheezing	Whistling, musical sound of the lower airways, often heard on expiration but can be heard on inspiration	Narrowing of the bronchioles from edema or bronchoconstriction
Crackles (rales)	Fine bubbling, crackling sounds heard in the lower airways	Fluid in the alveoli and lower airways
Rhonchi	Coarse, liquid, lower airway sound	Secretions in the bronchi

bronchoconstriction affecting the smaller airways, the bronchioles. The decreased diameter of the bronchioles can result from inflammation, smooth muscle contraction (bronchospasm), or a combination of both. Obstruction to airflow occurs during both inspiration and expiration. However, because the bronchioles expand slightly on inspiration and inspiration is an active process, the patient initially may have more obstruction to expiration than to inspiration. The result is that patients with **bronchoconstriction** often have wheezing on expiration. As bronchoconstriction progresses and deoxygenated gases accumulate in the alveoli, the respiratory rate may be fast, but oxygenated air is not reaching the alveoli.

Bronchoconstriction can be caused by a variety of problems. Asthma is a common problem in patients of all ages. Respiratory syncytial virus (RSV) can lead to severe lower airway obstruction in infants and small children, and the chronic obstructive pulmonary diseases (COPD), emphysema and chronic bronchitis, affect middle-aged and older patients. Allergic reactions, toxic inhalation, and other respiratory diseases also cause bronchoconstriction. In addition to the narrowing of the bronchioles from inflammation and bronchospasm, many of these conditions are exacerbated by increased mucus secretion, resulting in plugging of the bronchioles.

Gas exchange can also be impaired by accumulation of fluid or pus in the alveoli and smaller bronchioles, such as occurs in pulmonary edema or pneumonia. In acute pulmonary edema, air reaches the alveoli only to find it filled with fluid or deflated under the weight of interstitial fluid (atelectasis). When air does reach the alveoli, the distance across which gases must diffuse is increased by an increase in interstitial fluid in the respiratory membrane.

Ventilation Problems

Any trauma or medical problem that interferes with the ability to move the chest wall or diaphragm and generate negative intrathoracic and intrapulmonary pressures impairs ventilation. Underlying problems include paralysis of the respiratory muscles due to degenerative neurologic diseases, stroke, or spinal cord trauma; or trauma that disrupts the integrity of the chest wall, trachea, bronchi, or lung parenchyma. Drug overdoses and neurologic trauma and diseases can depress the respiratory center in the medulla, resulting in hypoventilation.

Assessment of the Airway, Ventilation, and Oxygenation

Every patient receives an evaluation of airway, ventilation, and oxygenation in the scene size-up and primary assessment. The goal of this assessment is to rapidly identify anything that presents an immediately life-threatening problem to the patient's airway, ventilation, or respiration. When you

identify an immediate threat to life, correct it. A relatively small and simple, yet critically important, set of skills is used in this initial intervention, regardless of the underlying cause of the problem. You will obtain additional information about breathing in the secondary assessment and history. The additional information helps you determine whether more specific treatments aimed at the underlying problem are indicated. In your continued interaction with the patient you will reassess his airway, ventilation, and oxygenation status. Your problem-solving process will continue throughout the call as you assess the effects of your interventions and decide what additional actions to take.

Scene Size-Up

While you will be alert to the many clues that are provided by the environment before you reach the patient, you will form a general impression based on your first glimpse of him. One of the first things to notice is whether the patient is obviously responsive or unresponsive (Figure 16-7). If he is unresponsive, there is a high probability that there also

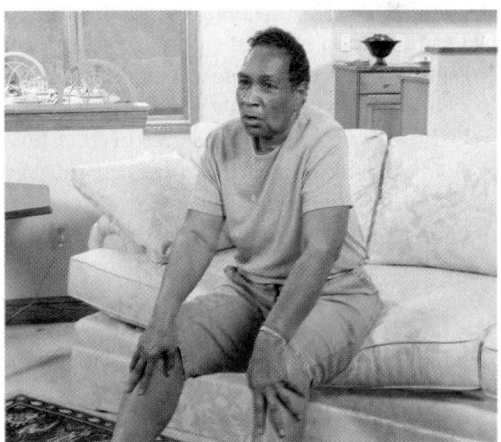
(A)

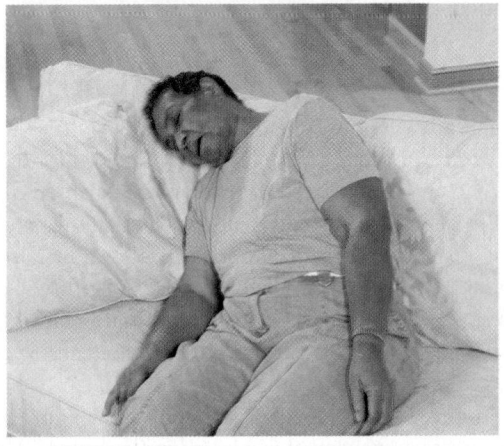
(B)

FIGURE 16-7

Form a general impression of the patient's level of responsiveness and degree of distress. (A) A responsive patient. (B) An apparently unresponsive patient.

may be an associated airway problem. Quickly note the position he is in and any indications of injury or distress, such as bleeding, pale skin, or an active seizure.

As you gain clinical experience, you will quickly learn to recognize patients in respiratory and cardiac arrest. Typically, severe respiratory distress is obvious. Indications include the use of increased effort to breathe, the use of the accessory muscles of breathing, abnormal breathing sounds, sitting in the **tripod position,** and cyanosis. Any one of those findings should focus your attention on the patient's airway and breathing.

The goal of the clinical aspects of the scene size-up is to develop a general impression of the problem, including a sense of the urgency with which you must perform your next tasks. The approach to the remainder of the scene size-up and primary assessment depends on whether the patient is apparently unresponsive or responsive, and if responsive, the apparent level of distress. For unresponsive patients, you must obtain information from other sources about the nature of the illness or mechanism of injury.

For responsive patients, the scene size-up concludes as you determine the patient's chief complaint and form a general impression of the seriousness of his condition. As the patient tells you his chief complaint, you will begin to obtain additional information about the primary assessment. His ability to speak in complete sentences can demonstrate not only an open airway, but also how severe any dyspnea might be. Consider the quality of the patient's speech. A hoarse or scratchy voice can indicate a partially obstructed airway. Can the patient speak more than a single word without taking a breath? If not, it is unlikely that air movement is sufficient.

Primary Assessment

Any airway and breathing problems must be identified in the primary assessment. Findings from your general impression may guide you, but in the primary assessment, evaluation of the level of responsiveness, airway, breathing, and circulation must be definitive.

Apparently Unresponsive Patient

It is generally obvious when an unresponsive patient is in cardiac or respiratory arrest. He is cyanotic or mottled and has either no respiratory effort, or what is called *agonal breathing.* Agonal breathing is ineffective, shallow, irregular gasping respiratory effort that continues for a brief period following respiratory or cardiac arrest. When the patient is unresponsive and has absent or abnormal breathing, the next step is to check his carotid pulse. If you cannot detect a carotid pulse in 10 seconds, the patient is in cardiac arrest and you must begin chest compressions. (The approach to cardiac arrest management is detailed in Chapter 17.)

Not all patients who appear unresponsive are actually unresponsive. Patients who are sleeping, intoxicated, or suffering from other medical or traumatic problems may respond to a loud voice command or painful stimulus, such as a sternal rub or pinch of the trapezius muscle. If the patient awakens to verbal or painful stimuli, approach the assessment as you would for other responsive patients. If you have confirmed that a patient is unresponsive to stimuli, or responds in any way other than becoming alert, take steps to open and assess the airway and evaluate breathing and circulation.

Open the Airway

For patients in whom cervical-spine injury is not suspected, use a **head-tilt/chin-lift maneuver** to open the airway (Figure 16-8). This maneuver elevates the tongue to prevent it from obstructing the airway. Use a **modified jaw-thrust maneuver** (also called a *trauma jaw thrust*) for patients in whom you suspect cervical-spine injury, such as those who have fallen from a height, been involved in a significant motor vehicle collision, or undergone another significant mechanism of injury (Figure 16-9) (McSwain, Salomone & Pons, 2007). The modified jaw-thrust maneuver displaces the mandible forward without hyperextending the neck. However, it is somewhat less effective than a head-tilt/chin-lift maneuver because some of the airway muscles remain lax. The steps of the manual maneuvers are detailed in an upcoming section.

A head-tilt/chin-lift maneuver is **relatively contraindicated** in patients with suspected cervical-spine injury, but the airways of some trauma patients can be extremely difficult to manage and a modified jaw-thrust maneuver may be inadequate. What you must remember in such cases is that, even with significant head and face trauma, the incidence of cervical-spine injury is still fairly low. However, if your patient does not have a patent airway, he will die within minutes. If you must choose between some movement of the spine to establish an airway and not being able to establish an airway, always choose to establish an airway.

An additional airway maneuver that can assist in difficult situations is the triple airway maneuver, which combines a head-tilt/chin-lift with a jaw-thrust. If you are performing a potentially risky maneuver, take a moment to observe whether there is movement in all extremities prior to the procedure.

A final manual maneuver to open the airway of a trauma patient is the **trauma chin lift.** To perform this maneuver, grasp the patient's mandible by inserting the thumb of a gloved hand in the patient's mouth behind his lower incisors and placing the index finger under the chin. Then pull the mandible forward. Disadvantages to this maneuver include placing your thumb in the patient's mouth and the inability to apply an oxygen mask or use a bag-valve-mask device with a provider's hand in this position.

If the patient's airway contains fluid, such as blood or vomit, suction the airway to clear it. The aspiration of fluid from the airway into the lungs results in pneumonitis or pneumonia, which can be fatal for the patient. A basic airway adjunct, either an oropharyngeal or nasopharyngeal airway, can be inserted at this point, if the patient is deeply unresponsive. However, do not delay assessment of

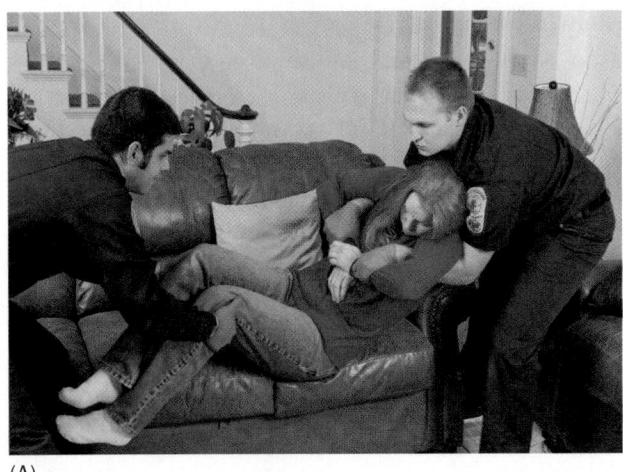
(A)

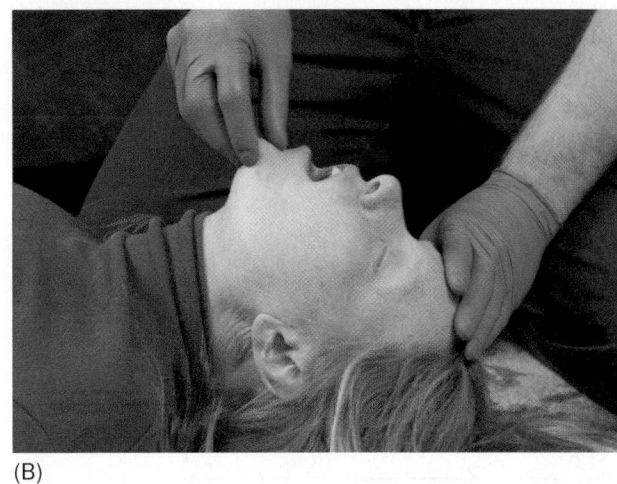
(B)

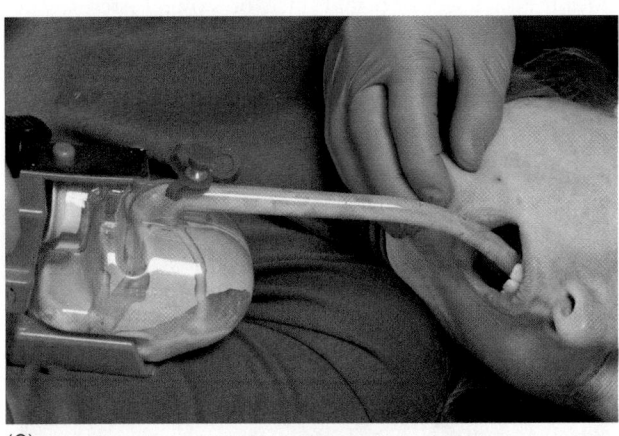
(C)

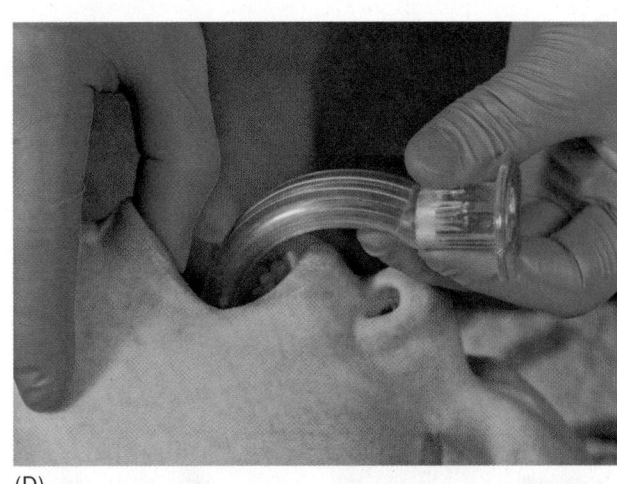
(D)

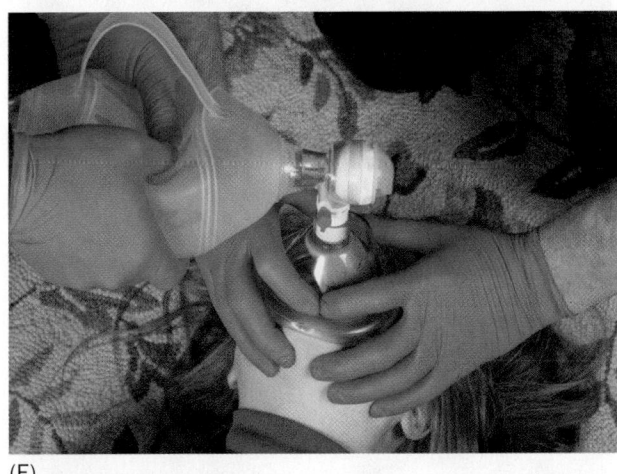
(E)

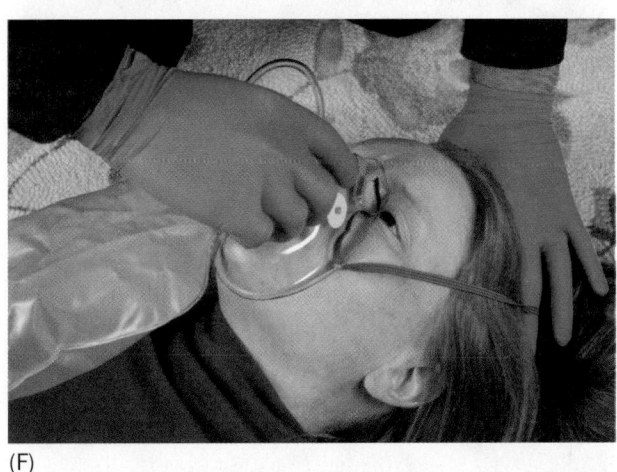
(F)

FIGURE 16-8

Assessing and managing the airway of an unresponsive patient.
(A) Move the patient to the floor.
(B) Open the airway.
(C) Suction if necessary.
(D) Insert an oral airway if the patient is responsive without a gag reflex.
(E) Ventilate the patient if he or she is not breathing or is breathing inadequately.
(F) Administer oxygen if the patient is breathing adequately.

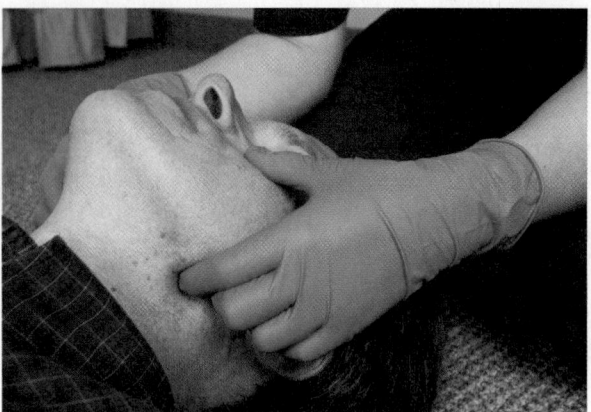

FIGURE 16-9

A modified jaw-thrust maneuver. (© Daniel Limmer)

breathing and implementation of ventilations. Also keep in mind that neither a nasopharyngeal nor oropharyngeal airway can keep the airway open on its own. Their use must always be accompanied by an appropriate manual maneuver.

Assess Breathing

As you form a general impression of your patient, note whether he is breathing. This is just a quick determination to guide your next step. For patients who are not breathing or who do not have normal breathing, you must check the pulse. If the pulse is absent, begin chest compressions. However, if the patient's pulse is present, open the airway. Once the airway is open, assess breathing.

To assess breathing, use the techniques of looking, listening, and feeling (Figure 16-10). This is best accomplished by kneeling next to the patient's head, turning your head to the side to observe the patient's chest and abdomen, and placing your ear above the patient's mouth and nose. Look at the chest: Does the movement indicate adequate tidal volume or decreased tidal volume? Do both sides of the chest move symmetrically? If you are not sure, place your hands on the chest wall to feel for movement. Does the rate seem normal, fast, or slow? Listen for air movement at the mouth and nose and determine the volume of airflow. You may quickly use your stethoscope to listen for the presence of breath sounds. Simply listen for

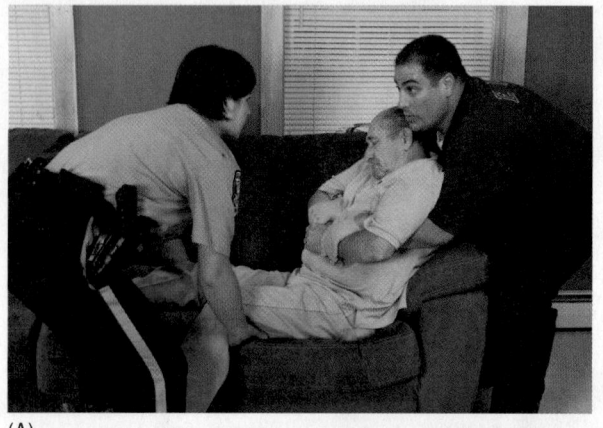
(A)

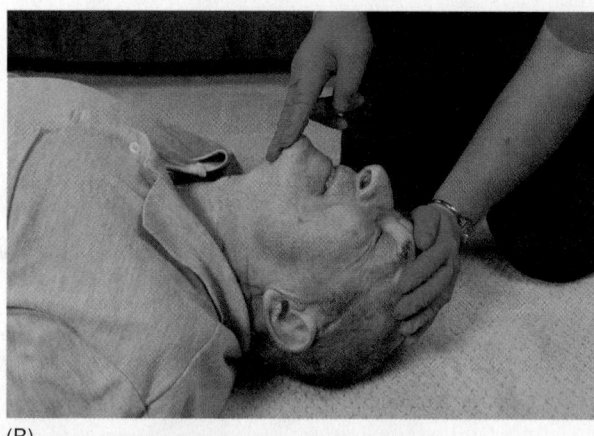
(B)

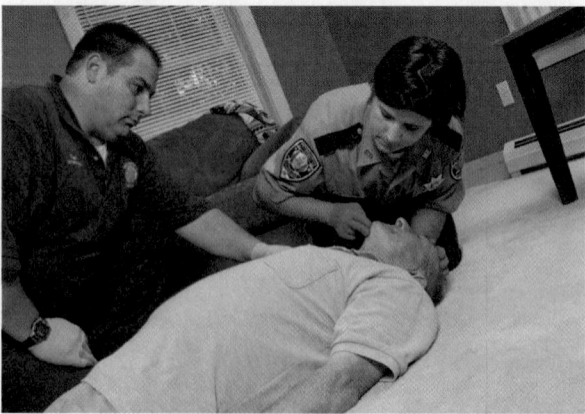
(C)

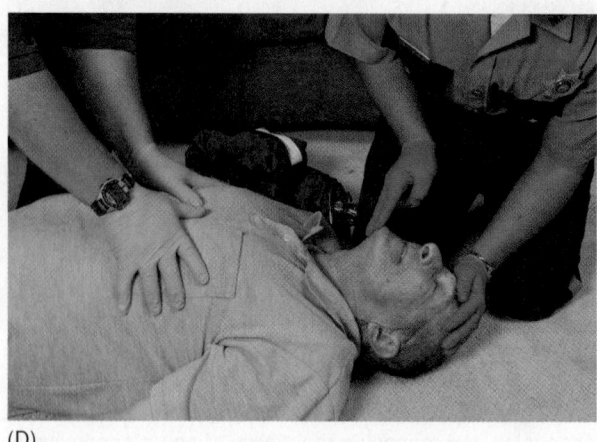
(D)

FIGURE 16-10

Assessing the airway and breathing of an unresponsive patient with a pulse. (A) Move the unresponsive patient to the floor or another firm surface. Maintain neutral alignment of the head and neck if trauma is suspected. (B) Open the airway with a head-tilt/chin-lift maneuver. Use a modified jaw-thrust maneuver if trauma is suspected. (C) Observe the patient's rate of breathing. (D) Place a hand over each side of the patient's chest to feel for adequate/equal expansion.

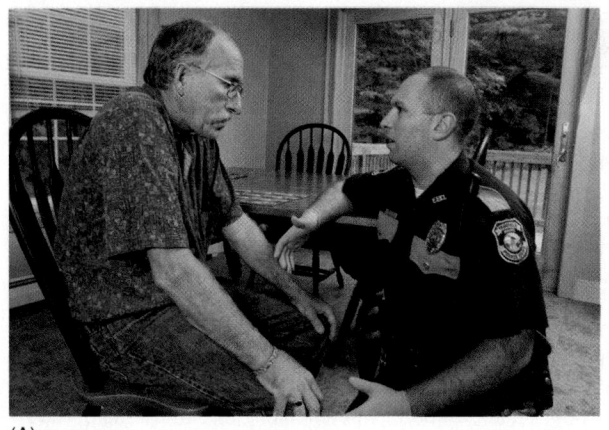 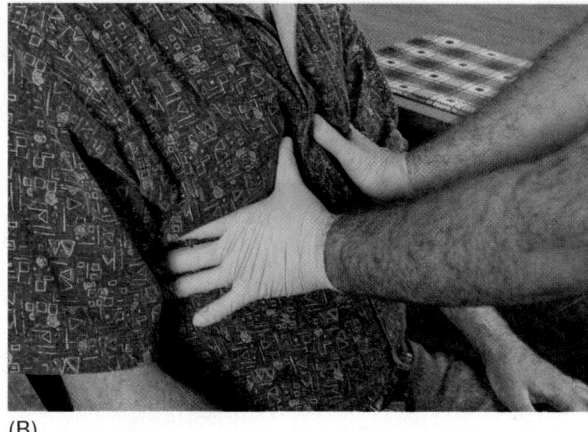

(A) (B)

FIGURE 16-11

Assessing the airway and breathing of a responsive patient. (A) Observe the patient's general appearance. Note signs of distress or anxiety. Observe skin color and accessory muscle use. (B) Spread your fingers over the patient's ribs with thumbs near the sternum. Assess rate and depth of respirations. Feel for equal and adequate chest expansion.

one inspiration and expiration at one location on the anterior of each side of the chest.

If breathing is inadequate or absent, use a **bag-valve-mask device** to assist the patient's ventilations or to provide artificial ventilation. If ventilations are obstructed and repositioning the airway does not help, suspect a foreign body airway obstruction.

Assess Circulation

While forming a general impression, determine that the patient has a pulse. During the primary assessment, check the patient's carotid pulse to determine the strength, rhythm, and whether the rate is slow, normal, or fast. Ensure that you have located and controlled significant bleeding.

Responsive Patients

With responsive patients for whom you have already determined that the patient has an airway, is breathing, and has a pulse, determine whether there is an immediate problem with the quality of the airway, breathing, or circulation (Figure 16-11). Looking and listening techniques are used to assess the patient's airway and breathing. A significant sign of **hypoxia** is a decreasing level of responsiveness. Although the patient may initially have been responsive, this can change quickly. Look at the chest to determine if rise and fall are adequate. Look for indications of respiratory distress, such as accessory muscle use, tripod position, and cyanosis. In the patient who is responsive, abnormal sounds are an important way of determining the status of the airway (Table 16-2). Indications of airway obstruction include stridor, coughing, gurgling, and wheezing. Sounds also provide information about breathing. Severe wheezing and crackles (rales) can sometimes be heard without the use of a stethoscope. If in doubt about air movement, quickly auscultate both sides of the chest with your stethoscope (Figure 16-12).

Clinical Decision Making

The goal of the primary assessment is to identify and intervene in any situations that pose an immediate threat to

TABLE 16-2 Findings That Indicate Inadequate Breathing

SIGNS OF INADEQUATE BREATHING
- Increased work of breathing/use of accessory muscles
- Noisy breathing (stridor, snoring, gurgling, wheezing, crackles [rales])
- Decreased or absent air movement or breath sounds
- Apnea/respiratory arrest
- Ventilatory rate < 8 or > 30 per minute in an adult
- An SpO_2 of less than 95 percent
- Irregular breathing
- Cyanosis

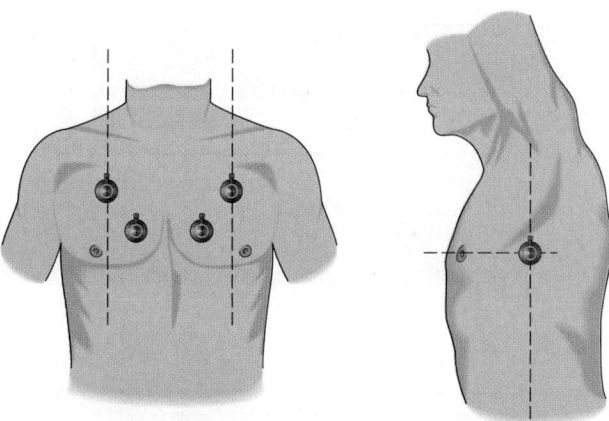

FIGURE 16-12

Quickly auscultate the lungs in the primary assessment to assess breathing.

PERSONAL PERSPECTIVE

Advanced EMT Nicole Sutton: At my old service I worked with a paramedic partner whom I wish had heard my current medical director's airway management motto: Ego eats brain. My old partner and I responded to a motor vehicle collision involving five teenagers who were seriously injured. We were assigned a 15-year-old girl with an altered mental status, facial trauma, and some long-bone fractures. She was responsive to painful stimuli but gave inappropriate answers to questions. She was able to maintain her airway, so I'm not sure what my partner's thinking was when she tried to insert an oropharyngeal airway. The patient gagged on the oral airway, so my partner decided to sedate her and intubate. She couldn't get the tube, but she wouldn't stop to ventilate the patient. I told my partner that the patient's SpO_2 was dropping, but she kept insisting that she "almost had it." I told her we needed to use a backup airway, a Combitube or a King LTD. She said she couldn't bring the patient in not

intubated now that she had sedated her. It seemed like the more trouble she had intubating, the more determined she was to get the tube in. By that time, the patient had blood in her airway from the trauma of the ongoing futile intubation attempt. I had suction ready, but my partner just kept trying to pass the tube. The patient's SpO_2 was in the 60s and her heart rate was starting to drop. I got on the radio and notified the ED that our patient had been sedated and had a difficult airway, and that we were going to need some help on arrival. Dr. Simpson heard the report and gave an order to use a Combitube. Finally, my partner seemed to get it. When she backed away from the patient's airway, I quickly suctioned the blood and started bagging the patient. Once her oxygen sats came up, I slipped in the Combitube. It was a really close call. The patient's injuries were serious, but not life threatening, yet she almost died from hypoxia. Not because of her injuries, but because of poor decision making.

life (Figure 16-13). If the patient is in cardiac arrest, start CPR. If the patient has a pulse, deliberately assess airway and breathing and check for and control significant bleeding. In its entirety, the primary assessment should take only 30 to 60 seconds to accomplish and for the most part, problems will be fairly obvious. When problems are found in the primary assessment, they are cues to provide immediate intervention. For any patient in whom you had to correct a problem during the primary assessment, then who needs

additional interventions, consider this patient critical and prepare him for transport without delay.

The best approach to managing a patient's airway is moving from simple to complex instead of jumping ahead to the most advanced technique at your disposal. When simple interventions provide an open airway, it may not be necessary to move on to more advanced techniques. It is equally as important to recognize when simple interventions are not sufficient to maintain an airway. Being an excellent EMS provider is not

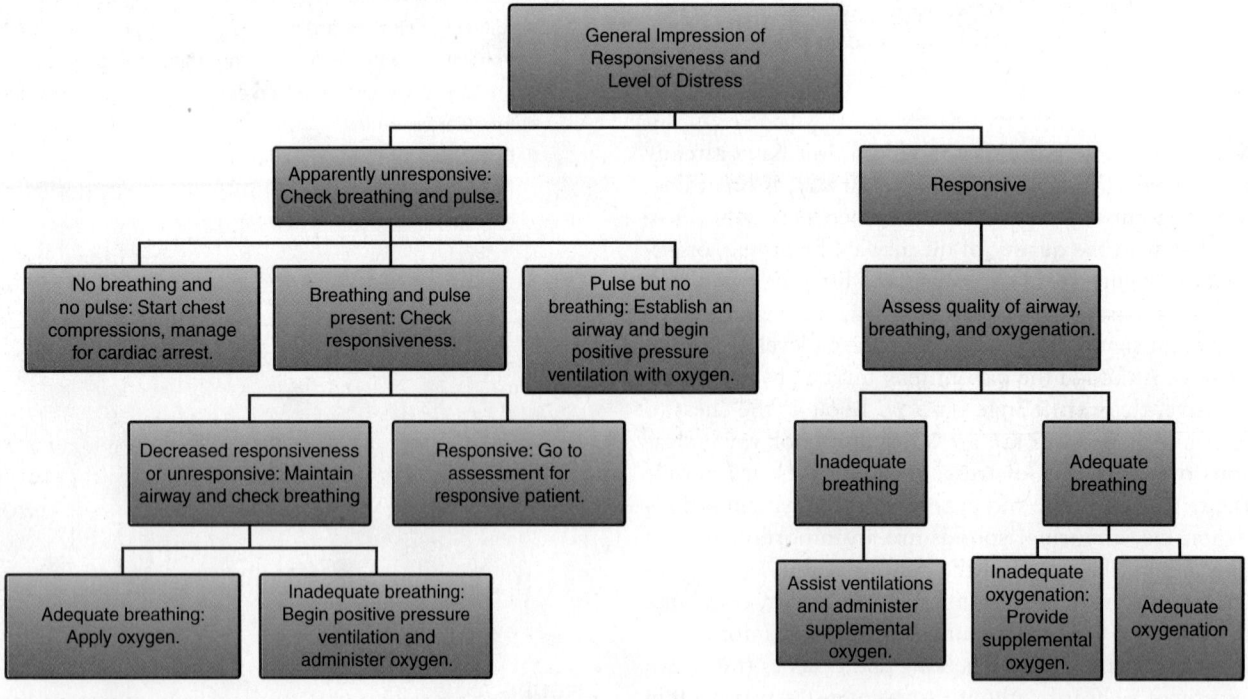

FIGURE 16-13

Clinical decision making in airway and ventilation management.

about how aggressive you are with interventions. It is about the level of sophistication with which you make decisions.

If simple airway management techniques to provide an airway are working, you still must ask some additional questions. Based on the patient's condition and the situation, are those techniques anticipated to remain sufficient? What are the risks and benefits of additional actions being considered? What are the consequences of maintaining the current approach versus taking additional actions? When simple techniques do not provide an adequate airway, you must recognize the situation and rapidly select a more advanced approach.

In all cases, the best approach to airway management is the one that will provide an adequate airway with the least risk for the patient. Sometimes that approach will not go beyond a manual maneuver. Sometimes, you will use a simple adjunct. Other times, you will use a more advanced adjunct. Less frequently, none of the tools you have available to you will provide a satisfactory airway. In this case, you must recognize the limitations of the tools at your disposal and get more advanced care to the patient, or get the patient to more advanced care while managing him to the best degree possible. Often, there is no simple answer. In each case, the situation must be assessed and critical thinking used to make the most appropriate decisions.

All patients with a complaint of dyspnea or any indications of impaired ventilation and oxygenation must receive supplemental oxygen. In the patient whose ventilations are being provided or assisted by a bag-valve-mask device, supplemental oxygen is always provided by connecting the oxygen tubing from the bag to an oxygen source. In patients with adequate spontaneous ventilation, oxygen is provided in varying concentrations by a nasal cannula or one of several types of oxygen masks.

One of your determinations in the primary assessment is whether the patient is in, or at risk for, respiratory distress or respiratory failure. Beyond your initial interventions, you must make decisions about continued management of the patient's airway, ventilation, and oxygenation. In some cases, you will have enough information to begin decision making at the end of the primary assessment. Consider the case of an unresponsive patient with significant head trauma who is vomiting and has irregular respirations. It is obvious that you will need to aggressively manage the airway with a more advanced adjunct and that you will need to continue assisting with ventilations. Respiratory failure requires immediate action. The patient's own efforts are not adequate to meet the metabolic demands of his body. If you do not intervene, respiratory failure will progress to respiratory arrest.

If the patient is not in respiratory failure, then you must consider how to best support the patient's respiratory efforts. This may include looking for correctable causes and administering supplemental oxygen and medications. Since the patient is not in respiratory failure, you have more time to complete a differential diagnosis. The information provided by secondary assessment helps you select the treatment likely to have the best effect. For example, you will need some history and additional assessment findings to determine if the patient requires a nebulized beta$_2$ agonist for asthma or COPD, or whether a patient with an anaphylactic (severe allergic) reaction requires an injection of epinephrine. The diabetic patient to whom you will give dextrose or glucagon will be unhappy, to say the least, if he regains consciousness with an advanced airway device in his hypopharynx, as will the narcotic overdose patient who may awaken with the administration of naloxone.

In yet other cases, you will recognize that immediate intervention is not required, but you must carefully monitor the patient for anticipated changes. Once you have ensured that an airway is present, ask yourself if it is likely that the airway will remain open. In some cases, the answer has a great deal to do with the etiology of the problem. Problems such as airway burns and neck trauma have a likelihood of developing obstruction due to laryngeal swelling. If you identify such a problem, it is reasonable to anticipate airway difficulties.

Signs of a potentially problematic airway include hoarse speech or changing speech quality; difficulty swallowing or drooling; and the high-pitched, upper airway sound of stridor. Ongoing bleeding and failure to control secretions also can potentially impact the flow of air. Never forget that a decreasing level of responsiveness is a serious threat to the patency of an airway. Patients with changing levels of responsiveness are at a high risk for losing an otherwise patent airway.

Secondary Assessment and Reassessment

The primary assessment is a brief evaluation of immediate life threats and may not be thorough enough to identify subtle indicators of impending problems. After completing the primary assessment, take a closer look at the airway, ventilation, and oxygenation. You have several skills at your disposal to assist in this process. (Also see Chapters 15 and 18.)

Respiratory Rate and Pattern

The primary assessment provides a gross indication of the presence and adequacy of breathing. The secondary assessment provides a specific respiratory rate and allows for detection of specific respiratory patterns. The respiratory rate is determined by counting the number of complete respirations (one inspiration plus one expiration) in 30 seconds

---

IN THE FIELD

It may be difficult to decide to intervene when a patient is responsive and breathing on his own. However, you must recognize when what the patient is doing on his own is not enough. Do not talk yourself out of necessary interventions.

TABLE 16-3   Normal and Abnormal Respiratory Patterns

	Condition	Description	Causes
	Eupnea	Normal breathing rate and pattern	
	Tachypnea	Increased respiratory rate	Fever, anxiety, exercise, shock
	Bradypnea	Decreased respiratory rate	Sleep, drugs, metabolic disorder, head injury, stroke
	Apnea	Absence of breathing	Deceased patient, head injury, stroke
	Hyperpnea	Normal rate, but deep respirations	Emotional stress, diabetic ketoacidosis
	Cheyne-Stokes respirations	Gradual increases and decreases in respirations with periods of apnea	Increasing intracranial pressure, brainstem injury
	Biot's respirations	Rapid, deep respirations (gasps) with short pauses between sets	Spinal meningitis, many CNS causes, head injury
	Kussmaul's respirations	Tachypnea and hyperpnea	Renal failure, metabolic acidosis, diabetic ketoacidosis
	Apneustic respirations	Prolonged inspiratory phase with shortened expiratory phase	Lesion in brainstem

Source: Bledsoe, Bryan E.; Porter, Robert S.; Cherry, Richard A., Intermediate Emergency Care: Principles and Practice, 1st Edition, © 2004. Reprinted with permission of Pearson Education, Inc., Upper Saddle River, NJ.

and multiplying by 2. Although you can count the number of respirations in 15 seconds and multiply by 4, the slower rate of respirations (as compared to the pulse) makes this approach slightly more prone to error. The normal adult respiratory rate is 12 to 20 per minute. Abnormal respiratory patterns are associated with a number of neurologic and metabolic problems (Table 16-3). Also, reassess the depth of breathing to evaluate tidal volume.

Auscultation of Breath Sounds

Although you may have initially auscultated the lungs quickly to determine the presence and equality of breath sounds and any gross abnormalities, a more detailed assessment of breath sounds is performed in the secondary assessment (Figure 16-14). The patient's clothing will obscure lung sounds, so remove or loosen as many layers as possible given your circumstances. In doing so, do not neglect the patient's modesty or warmth. Listen first to one side and then move your stethoscope to the opposite side. (See Chapter 18.) Breath sounds should be equally present at each level on both sides. Remember that lung fields reach as high as the shoulders and can reach as low as the level of the umbilicus. Auscultation usually begins high in the chest or back and works its way down to the low bases. Normal breathing should be quiet and free of unusual sounds.

Pulse Oximetry

Pulse oximetry uses infrared technology to assess the oxygen saturation of hemoglobin in the peripheral tissues. This is accomplished by attaching a noninvasive probe to the end of a finger, toe, or earlobe (Figure 16-15). The probe passes a light beam through peripheral capillaries. The different light wavelengths are absorbed by oxygen-saturated hemoglobin, which is a brighter red color, and unsaturated hemoglobin, which is a darker red color. The device then calculates saturation by measuring the amount of light that was absorbed. The reading represents a percentage of hemoglobin saturated by oxygen.

A normal pulse oximetry reading is between 95 and 100 percent at lower geographic elevations and 90 to 100 percent at higher altitudes. At lower elevations, readings of 91 to 94 percent indicate mild hypoxia, readings of 86 to 90 percent indicate moderate hypoxia, and readings 85 percent or less indicate severe hypoxia. The patient care goal is to maintain an SpO_2 of 95 percent or higher by administering oxygen and, if needed, assisting with ventilations.

Hemoglobin saturation, abbreviated SpO_2 when measured by pulse oximetry, is a useful tool in assessing the oxygenation status in your patient, but should be used only as an adjunct to a good patient assessment. Because the majority of the oxygen in the blood is attached to hemoglobin, pulse oximetry correlates with the partial pressure of oxygen in arterial blood. However, this correlation is not exact and must be taken in context. Pulse oximetry measures saturation of hemoglobin, but does not measure the amount of hemoglobin present. In general, technology should confirm your assessment, not replace it. Pulse oximeters are very reliable, but their accuracy can be affected by ambient light sources, nail polish and nail accessories, and by low perfusion states such as shock and hypothermia. Furthermore, other molecules, such as carbon monoxide, can bind with hemoglobin, resulting in a falsely high reading.

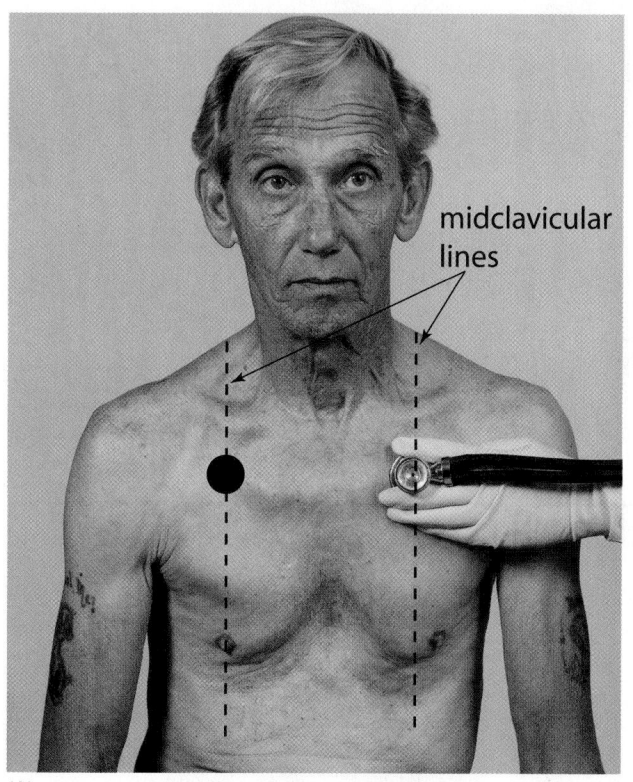

(A)

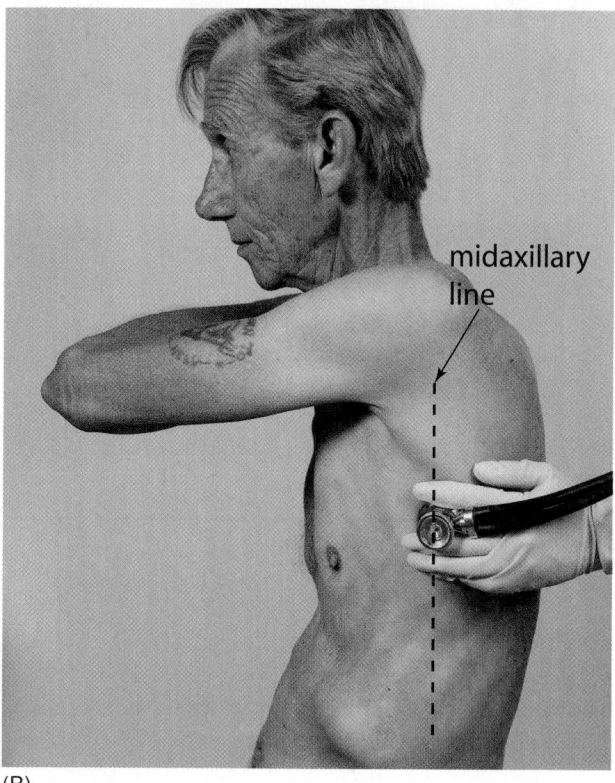

(B)

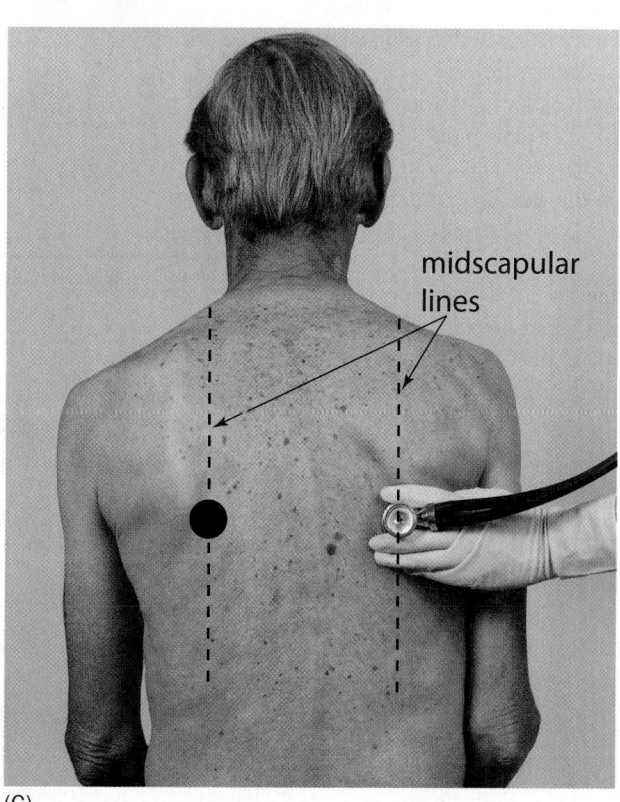

(C)

FIGURE 16-14

Locations for auscultating breath sounds. (A) Auscultate the anterior chest at the second intercostal space at each midclavicular line. (B) Auscultate the lateral chest at the fourth to fifth intercostal space at each midaxillary line. (C) Auscultate the posterior chest below the tip of the scapula on each midscapular line.

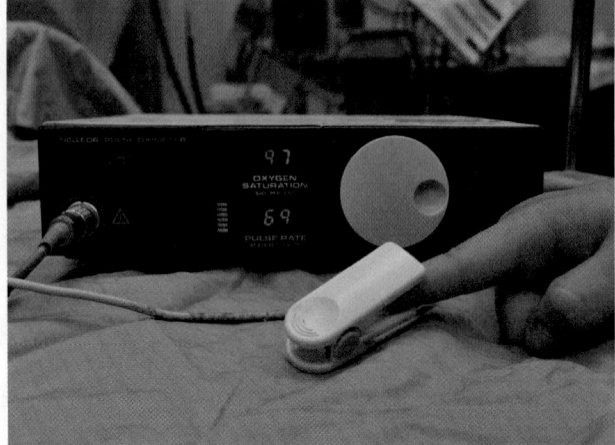

FIGURE 16-15

A pulse oximeter. (© Edward T. Dickinson, MD)

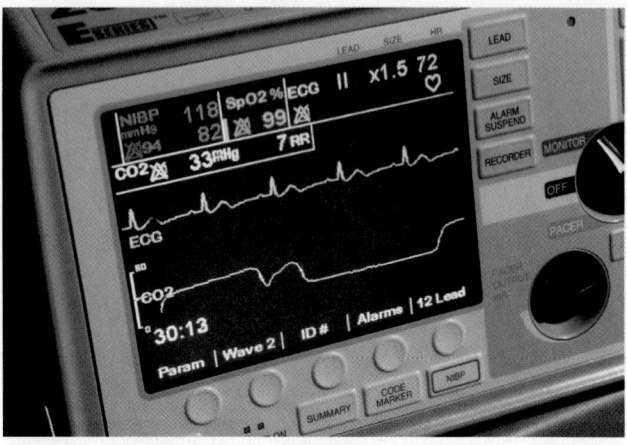

FIGURE 16-16

An electronic capnography device.

Capnometry

Capnometry is the measurement of carbon dioxide in exhaled air. **Capnography,** or waveform carbon dioxide monitoring, not only provides a numeric measurement, but also a waveform of the changes in the levels of carbon dioxide the patient is expiring over the course of each expiration (Figure 16-16). Colorimetric devices are simpler and essentially only provide a yes or no answer as to whether exhaled air contains carbon dioxide. Colorimetric devices are used to confirm placement of endotracheal tubes in patients with spontaneous circulation (Figure 16-17). (Inadequate cellular perfusion in cardiac arrest means that the aerobic metabolism required to produce carbon dioxide is minimal.) As with pulse oximetry, carbon dioxide monitoring is an adjunct to excellent assessment skills.

Exhaled carbon dioxide is measured by a sensor in a special mask or nasal cannula, or placed on the end of an airway device such as a laryngeal mask airway (LMA) or endotracheal tube (Figure 16-18). As the sample is processed, the monitor assesses the level of exhaled carbon dioxide. A normal capnometry value is 35 to 45 mmHg. Higher levels indicate **hypercapnia,** which is often due to inadequate ventilation. Low levels of carbon dioxide, known as **hypocapnia,** can mean that the body has eliminated an excess amount of carbon dioxide, as can sometimes happen in hyperventilation syndrome. Although this measurement often correlates well to blood levels of carbon dioxide, this correlation is not guaranteed. Consider the following examples:

■ *A severely bronchoconstricted patient.* Here, the airways are tightened to the point that air is moving only minimally. The sample examined outside the patient's mouth and nose likely only contains tracheal air and does not represent air trapped at the alveolar level. If measured, this sample will likely contain only minimal carbon dioxide despite high levels of carbon dioxide present in the bloodstream and at the alveolar level.

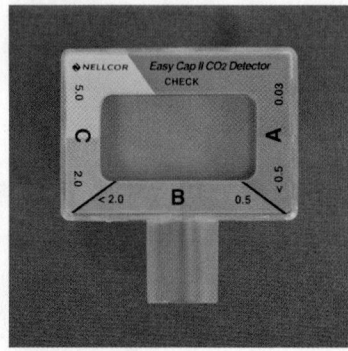

FIGURE 16-17

Colorimetric capnometry device. (© Edward T. Dickinson, MD)

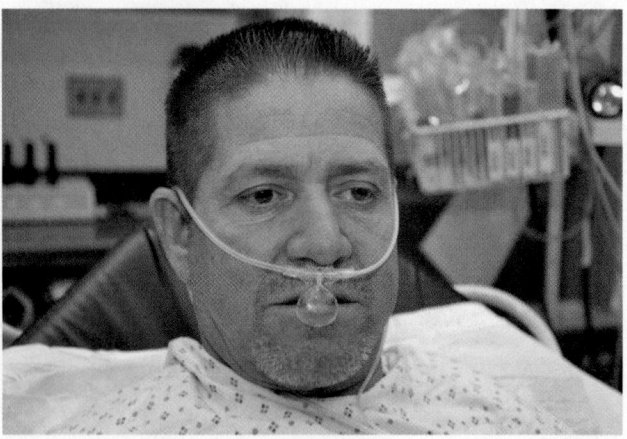

FIGURE 16-18

Capnometry sensor. (© Edward T. Dickinson, MD)

Brian and Tiffany are on the scene of a 70-year-old male, Pete Campbell, who is working hard to breathe and has indications of hypoxia. Mrs. Campbell has informed the Advanced EMTs that her husband has COPD. As Brian opens the airway and oxygen bag, Tiffany introduces herself but Mr. Campbell does not respond. Tiffany notices cyanosis around his lips and accessory muscle use. She quickly auscultates the patient's chest, hearing minimal air movement and pronounced expiratory wheezes.

Problem-Solving Questions

1. What is the best approach to correcting the patient's hypoxia?
2. What are the pros and cons of different options available for treating the patient?
3. How should Tiffany and Brian prioritize the various actions needed?

- *A patient in cardiac arrest.* Although an airway device may be properly placed and the patient is being ventilated, the reduced perfusion occurring during CPR permits minimal aerobic metabolism and therefore produces minimal carbon dioxide.

As with any technology, you must rely upon a thorough patient assessment and good clinical judgment to assess the value of the information provided by capnometry.

Peak Expiratory Flow Rate

The **peak expiratory flow rate (PEFR)** is a measurement of the maximal flow rate of air during expiration. Patients with asthma or COPD may use a **peak flow meter (PFM)** at home. A decrease in PEFR can signify the onset of an asthma attack or decompensation in COPD. PFMs are relatively inexpensive and easy to use, and may be used in some EMS systems to obtain a baseline reading before treatment and a comparison reading after treatment. PFMs determine the flow of air in liters per minute (L/min) during a forced expiration that follows a maximal inspiration. Three measurements are obtained and the best of the three is used as a baseline. If used in your system, follow protocol and never delay treatment of a patient in severe respiratory distress or respiratory failure to obtain this reading. If your system uses PEFR measurements, the device will most likely be accompanied by a table of predicted PEFR values based on the patient's age, gender, and size. **Spirometry** is a broader term that includes several measurements of pulmonary function. It uses more sophisticated equipment and can be performed in a hospital or doctor's office.

Reassessment

Without intervention, respiratory distress can rapidly progress to respiratory failure. Remember that compensation requires oxygen and energy and the patient already has deficits in both these areas. Hypoxia and fatigue can rapidly overwhelm your patient's ability to compensate. You

must be ever vigilant and watchful for these changes. Constant and regular reassessment is the key. Compare ongoing findings to the baseline values obtained in your primary and secondary assessments. Changes in skin color and condition, mental status, respiratory rate, respiratory effort, breath sounds, and pulse oximetry and capnometry values are all important indicators of improvement or deterioration in your patient's condition.

Airway Management

Airway management, ventilatory support, control of bleeding, chest compressions, and other actions are best carried out simultaneously through teamwork. For the sake of organization, airway management is traditionally discussed first, because in the patient with a pulse, the airway must be open in order for ventilation to occur. Initial airway management focuses on the upper airway, but the lower airway must be open as well to allow air to reach the alveoli. In patients who are not able to maintain their own airways due to altered mental status, trauma, bleeding, or vomiting, interventions range from positioning the patient, to manual airway maneuvers, suction, and simple airway adjuncts to more advanced airway adjuncts.

IN THE FIELD

Airway management requires you to put yourself in close proximity to the patient's respiratory tract. As air is expired or forcefully expelled through coughing, you may be exposed to the patient's body fluids including saliva, sputum, and blood. When managing an airway, always wear gloves and eye protection at a minimum. Consider additional personal protective equipment if the situation presents a higher risk.

Positioning and Manual Maneuvers

Often, ensuring an open airway is as simple as making sure the patient is positioned to be able to maintain his own airway. Responsive patients who are vomiting, who may vomit, or who have epistaxis (nosebleed) or other bleeding that can compromise the airway should be placed in a sitting or lateral recumbent position to prevent aspiration (Figure 16-19). Positioning may be effective, as well, for stroke patients with impaired swallowing and those with an airway narrowed by epiglottitis or other causes of airway edema. Keep suction immediately available to assist the patient and be prepared to intervene further if the patient's ability to maintain his own airway diminishes.

Manual airway maneuvers take advantage of the attachments of the tongue to indirectly reposition it to relieve or prevent airway obstruction. When the neck is hyperextended or the mandible is displaced anteriorly, the tongue is pulled away from the posterior pharynx.

Head-Tilt/Chin-Lift Maneuver

The head-tilt/chin-lift maneuver adjusts the head to a position that naturally moves the mandible anteriorly (Figure 16-20). This head position lines up the internal structures of the airway and prevents obstruction of the glottic opening. Because the head-tilt/chin-lift maneuver hyperextends the neck, do not use it in a patient with suspected spine injury unless a modified jaw-thrust maneuver does not provide an adequate airway.

Use the following steps to perform the head-tilt/chin-lift maneuver:

1. Move the patient to a supine position.
2. Place one hand on the patient's forehead and the other hand beneath the bony prominence of the patient's mandible.
3. Gently tilt the head by applying pressure to the patient's forehead.
4. Simultaneously lift the mandible, taking care not to put pressure on the soft tissue beneath the lower jaw because this can obstruct the airway.

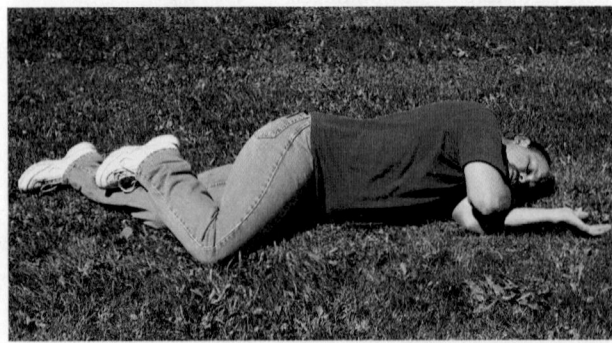

FIGURE 16-19
Left lateral recumbent (recovery) position.

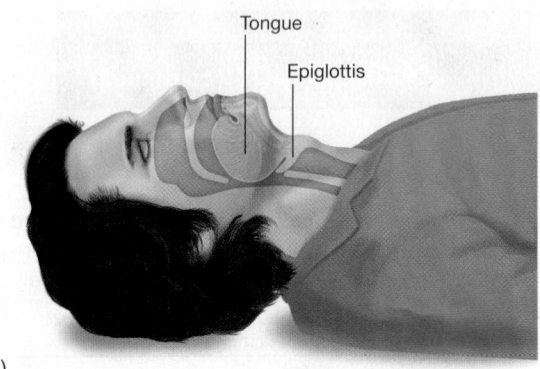
(A)

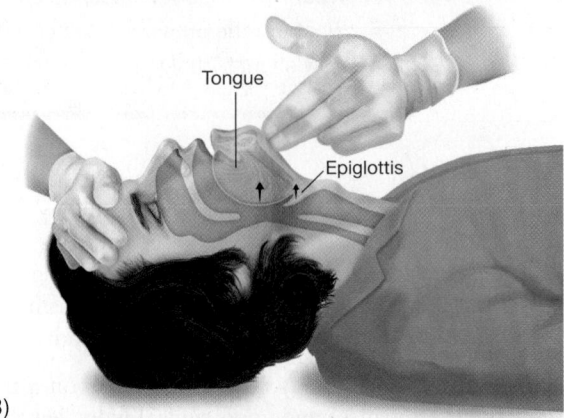
(B)

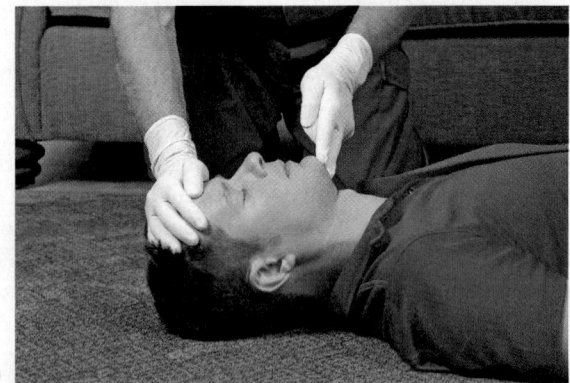
(C)

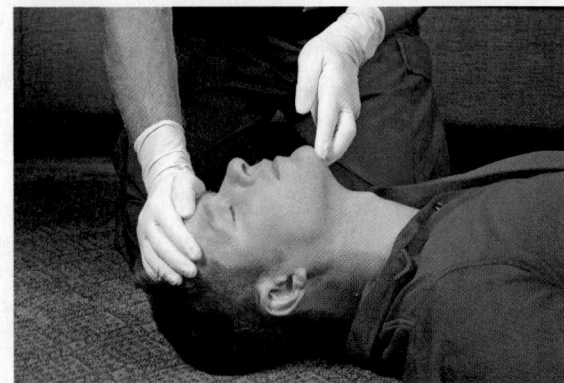
(D)

FIGURE 16-20
Head-tilt/chin-lift maneuver. (A) The supine adult. (B) The head-tilt/chin-lift maneuver in the adult. (C) Head-tilt/chin-lift maneuver in the adult in a neutral starting position. (D) Head-tilt/chin-lift maneuver in the adult in final tilting position.

Once a head-tilt/chin-lift maneuver has been accomplished, you must maintain the position to keep the airway open. Assess breathing and determine whether an airway adjunct and artificial ventilation are required.

Modified Jaw-Thrust Maneuver

The modified jaw-thrust maneuver is used to open the airway in patients with suspected spine injury because it causes less movement of the cervical spine than a head-tilt/chin-lift maneuver (Figure 16-21). However, it also may be somewhat less effective than a head-tilt/chin-lift maneuver in relieving airway obstruction. Do not assume that you have opened the airway with any manual maneuver. After employing the manual maneuver, you must confirm that the airway is open.

Use the following steps to accomplish the modified jaw-thrust maneuver:

1. Ensure that the patient is in a supine position and that manual cervical-spine immobilization has been accomplished.
2. Place your fingers on the posterior angles on each side of the patient's mandible, just below the ears.
3. Displace the mandible anteriorly without moving the head itself.

Again, you must maintain this position in order to keep the airway open. Assess breathing and consider the need for an airway adjunct. If a modified jaw thrust maneuver does not provide an adequate airway, use a head-tilt/chin-lift maneuver to establish an airway.

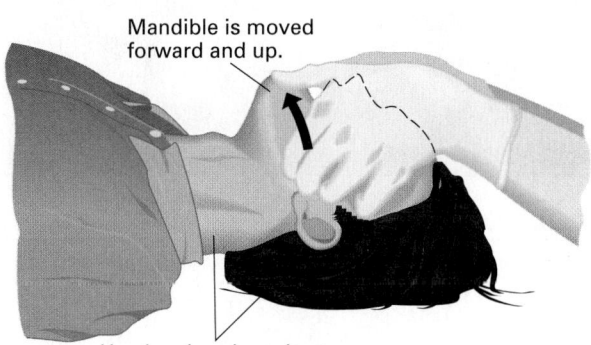

Mandible is moved forward and up.

Head and neck are kept in neutral in-line position.

(A)

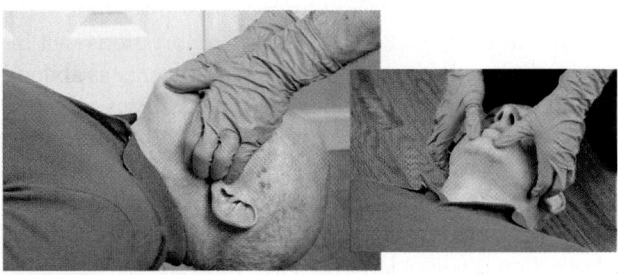

(B)

FIGURE 16-21

Modified jaw-thrust maneuver. (A) Procedure. (B) Two views.

As mentioned earlier in the chapter, the trauma chin lift and triple airway maneuvers may be considered in patients in whom the head-tilt/chin-lift and modified jaw-thrust maneuvers are ineffective.

Removing Foreign Bodies and Fluids from the Airway

Fluids and foreign bodies can obstruct the flow of air and must be removed before initiating **positive pressure ventilation** (**PPV**). Blood, vomit, secretions, broken teeth, food, gum, chewing tobacco, and other objects can completely or partially obstruct the airway. Patients with complete airway obstruction will not be able to move any air and may be severely hypoxic, unresponsive, and approaching or in cardiac arrest by the time you arrive. Bystanders may give a history consistent with foreign body airway obstruction, such as the patient suddenly choking during a meal, or you may not find the obstruction until you unsuccessfully attempt to ventilate the patient.

Patients with partial airway obstruction may have either adequate or inadequate air movement. A foreign body or fluids that require removal may cause airway obstruction, but obstruction also may be caused by edema. Obtaining a history of the event is critical in determining the course of action to take. Noisy breathing can indicate partial airway obstruction as air is forced through the narrowed airway or through fluid in the airway. The harsh, crowing sound of stridor is an indication of upper airway obstruction, while localized wheezing in one lung indicates an area of partial airway obstruction in a bronchus. Bubbling or gurgling noises indicate fluid in the airway.

Positioning the patient on his side and using a gloved hand to sweep matter out of the airway may be the best way to quickly and effectively remove large amounts of debris in the airway. If cervical-spine injury is suspected, use manual stabilization of the cervical spine while positioning

---

IN THE FIELD

You must clear the airway of debris and fluid before attempting ventilation. While it is true that the patient must be ventilated and oxygenated, forcing debris and fluid deeper into the airway will further impair ventilation and oxygenation.

Pediatric Care

Never perform a blind finger sweep in a pediatric patient. You could push a foreign object deeper in the airway, worsening the obstruction.

Geriatric Care

It is often best to leave dentures and dental appliances in place. However, remove them if they interfere with airway management and ventilation.

the patient. In such cases, suctioning will not be effective to quickly remove large amounts of fluid or particles that are too large for the bore of the suction tubing. Suctioning may help after large debris and copious amounts of fluid are removed manually.

Foreign Body Airway Obstruction

Foreign body airway obstruction (FBAO) may result in either mild or severe airway blockage. A partial obstruction allows some air to pass around it, but a complete obstruction prevents air movement altogether. The distinction between mild and severe FBAO is an important one to make, because the treatment pathways are very different. A patient with a mild FBAO may be coughing, but will have air movement. Signs of severe airway obstruction include poor air exchange (such as a silent, ineffective cough), cyanosis, and inability to speak or breathe. Occasionally, the patient will clutch his neck, the universal sign of choking.

FBAO can be obvious, as in a conscious person choking; or, it may be unknown, as in a person found unresponsive. You must be prepared to initiate FBAO procedures any time you are unable to ventilate a patient and you suspect that the difficulty may be due to an obstruction.

Mild Obstruction

Do not interfere with the coughing and breathing efforts of a patient with only a mild FBAO. Allow the person to continue to attempt to expel the obstruction on his own. Because an oxygen mask could interfere with the patient's efforts to expel the obstruction, administer oxygen by nasal cannula, if needed. Monitor the patient carefully, because he can become fatigued and progress to severe FBAO. Always transport the patient, even if he clears the obstruction. Occasionally, a FBAO can cause swelling in the hypopharynx even hours after the incident.

Severe Obstruction

For a conscious patient with a severe FBAO, use repeated abdominal thrusts to clear the obstruction (Figure 16-22). To deliver an abdominal thrust, stand behind the patient and place your fist just below his diaphragm on or around his navel. Use your other hand to quickly and firmly pull your fist toward you and into the patient's abdomen. Repeat this step until the obstruction is relieved or the patient becomes unconscious. If you are unable to encircle your arms around the abdomen, as with a late-stage pregnant patient or an extremely obese one, consider positioning your

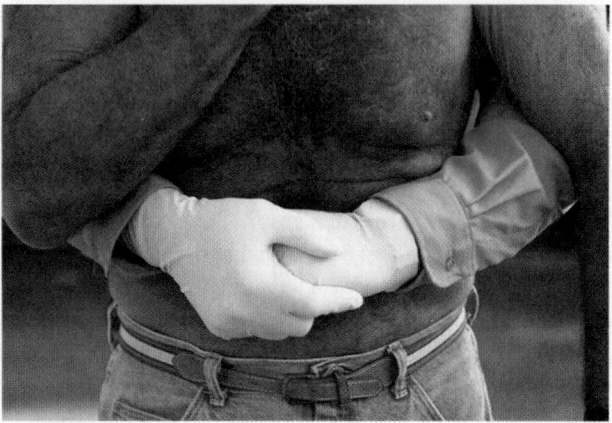

FIGURE 16-22

Use a series of abdominal thrusts for a conscious adult with foreign body airway obstruction.

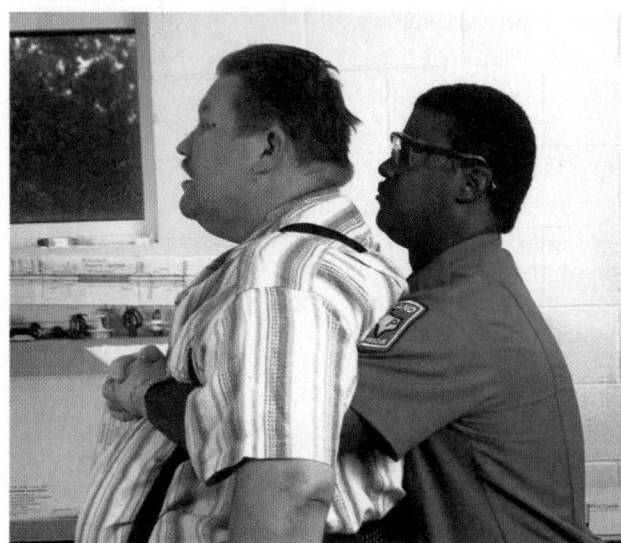

FIGURE 16-23

Chest thrusts can be used in place of abdominal thrusts in obese or pregnant patients.

hands around the patient's chest and performing a chest thrust instead (Figure 16-23).

If the patient becomes unresponsive, lower him to the ground and begin CPR. (The chest compressions will increase pressure in the airway in the same manner as abdominal thrusts to help expel the object and will ensure blood circulation.) Attempt to complete cycles of 30 compressions and 2 positive pressure ventilations. Each time you open the airway and attempt to ventilate, inspect the airway and remove any objects you see. Continue these cycles until the obstruction is relieved.

Pediatric Airway Obstruction

In much the same way as with an adult, if the FBAO is mild, do not interfere. Allow the pediatric patient to clear his own

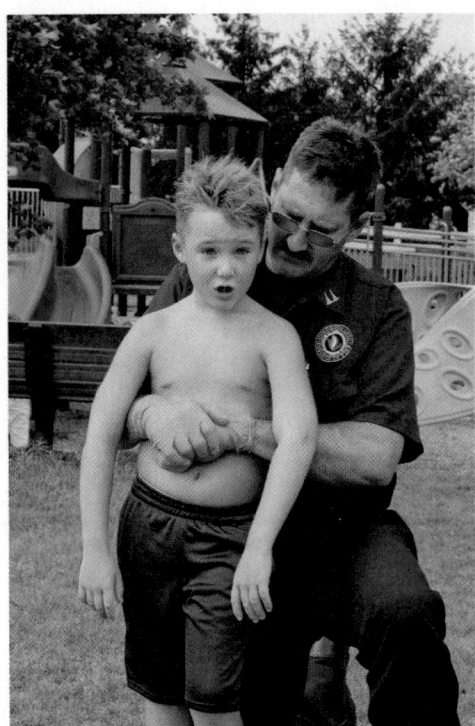

FIGURE 16-24

Abdominal thrusts in a pediatric patient.

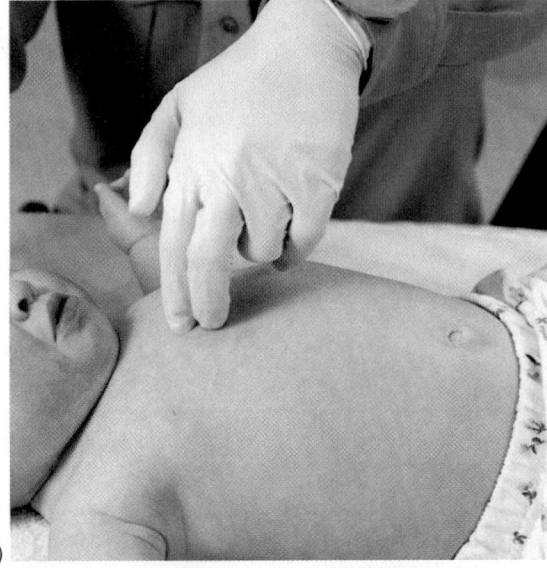

(A)

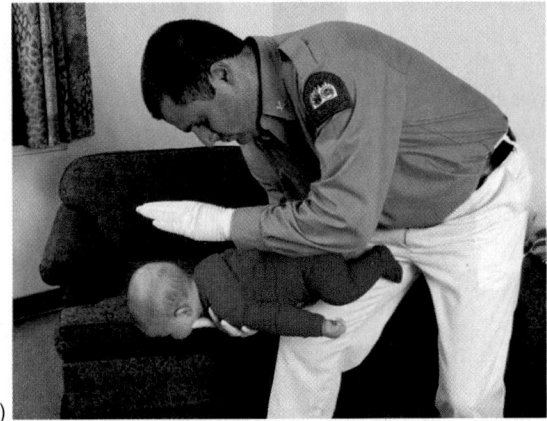

(B)

FIGURE 16-25

Foreign body airway obstruction relief in an infant:
(A) chest thrusts and (B) back blows.

airway by coughing while you continue to reassess for signs of severe FBAO. For a conscious child with a severe (complete) FBAO, perform subdiaphragmatic abdominal thrusts in the same manner as you would on an adult (Figure 16-24). Continue abdominal thrusts until the object is expelled or the patient becomes unresponsive.

If the child becomes unresponsive, initiate 30 chest compressions. (Do not perform a pulse check.) After completing 30 compressions, open the airway using a head-tilt/chin-lift maneuver or a modified jaw-thrust maneuver. Attempt to visualize the airway. If you see a foreign body, remove it but do not perform blind finger sweeps because a child's airway is funnel shaped and a blind finger sweep might actually push the object further into the airway. Attempt to deliver 2 positive pressure ventilations, and then continue with cycles of 30 chest compressions and 2 ventilations until the object is expelled.

Infant Airway Obstruction

For a conscious infant, use a combination of back blows (Figure 16-25) and chest thrusts. Hold the infant prone along your forearm with his head in a slightly dependent position. Use your hand to deliver five blows to the center of his back, then turn the patient over and deliver five chest compressions just as if you were doing CPR. Continue alternating five back blows and five chest thrusts until the object is expelled or the patient becomes unresponsive. Do not use abdominal thrusts on an infant.

If the infant is found or becomes unconscious, use the same procedure as for an unconscious child with severe FBAO.

Suction

Suction is the use of negative pressure (vacuum) to remove liquids from the upper airway and from the lower airway of patients with an endotracheal or **tracheostomy** tube in place (Figure 16-26). Suction units can be either portable or fixed in position in the ambulance or to the wall in the hospital setting. A properly functioning suction device must have an air flow rate of least 30 L/min and generate a vacuum of no less than 300 mmHg when the suction tube is clamped.

Suction typically uses a wide lumen, noncollapsible tube to collect liquids into a disposable collection basin. One of two types of suction catheters is attached to the end of the suction tubing. Rigid suction catheters, otherwise known as **Yankauer** or tonsil-tip catheters, are used to

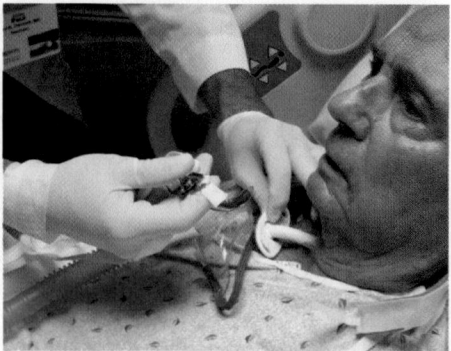

FIGURE 16-26

Tracheostomy. (© B. Slaven, MD/Custom Medical Stock Photo)

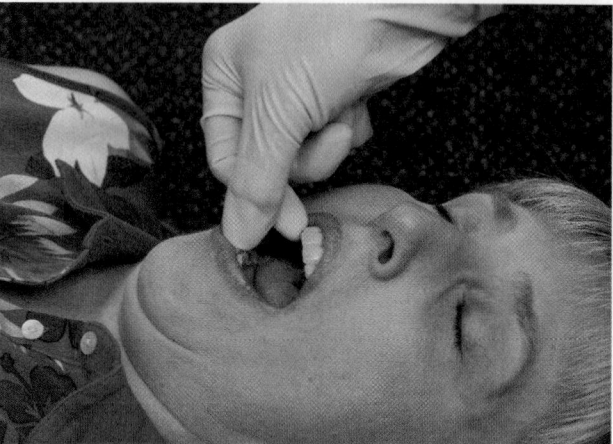

FIGURE 16-27

Cross-finger technique of opening the mouth.

suction the oropharynx. They are not flexible, which allows greater control over their position, and they have a larger lumen than soft catheters.

Soft catheters are used for suctioning the trachea of patients with an endotracheal tube in place. They are directed through the endotracheal tube to the level of the carina to remove bronchial secretions, because the intubated patient cannot cough to remove his own secretions. Soft catheters come in various diameters, using **French units (Fr.)** of sizing. The larger the French size, the larger the diameter of the suction catheter. One Fr. unit is equal to 0.33 mm. Therefore, a size 16 Fr. catheter is 5.3 mm in diameter and an 18 Fr. catheter is 6 mm in diameter. A 14 Fr. catheter is the typical size used for endotracheal suctioning of an average-size adult patient.

When suctioning is not emergent, such as in routine suctioning of an intubated patient, the patient is preoxygenated prior to suctioning, because suction removes oxygen from the airway and interrupts ventilations. However, in a patient who is in immediate jeopardy of aspirating fluids into the airway, do not delay suctioning. When suctioning is not emergent, perform it for no more than 10 seconds at a time. If additional suctioning is needed, ventilate the patient again and preoxygenate the patient before suctioning. But when a patient's airway is full of blood or vomit, clear the airway before ventilating the patient, keeping in mind that you must accomplish this quickly. You must not allow or cause the patient to aspirate fluids into the lungs by failing to clear the airway of fluids.

Suction is an essential, potentially lifesaving skill. But it is not without risks to the patient. Those risks include causing or worsening hypoxia, trauma to the oropharynx, stimulating a gag reflex (resulting in vomiting), and inducing bradycardia through stimulation of the hypopharynx. Suction also presents a risk to you by potentially exposing you to the patient's blood or body fluids. As with any airway management procedure, use gloves and eye protection as minimum PPE.

Suctioning the Oropharynx

Begin by ensuring the proper catheter is connected to the suction unit and switching on the unit (Scan 16-1). Ideally,

you should measure the Yankauer tip prior to insertion by placing the tip of the catheter at the corner of the patient's mouth and measuring to the earlobe.

Open the patient's mouth using a cross-finger technique (Figure 16-27). While facing the patient, place your gloved hand at the level of the patient's teeth. Place your thumb on the bottom edge of the upper teeth and your middle or index finger on the top edge of the bottom teeth. Simultaneously push upward with your thumb and downward with your finger to open the patient's mouth.

While inserting the catheter, do not cover the side port of the suction catheter. This prevents a vacuum at the tip of the catheter, because suction is only applied as the catheter is withdrawn. If measuring the insertion depth prior to insertion is not possible, insert the tip of the catheter only as far as you can see. In other words, you should be able to see the tip of the catheter at all times. This helps avoid stimulation of the gag reflex and the vagus nerve and reduces the potential for soft-tissue trauma. If the patient begins to gag, pull the catheter away from the posterior pharynx.

Cover the side port on the suction catheter and apply suction as you withdraw it. Remember, the patient is becoming hypoxic as you suction. So, ideally, you should apply suction for no longer than 10 seconds. Also keep in mind that the airway must be clear of fluids before beginning or resuming bag-valve-mask ventilations.

Pediatric Care

Pediatric patients are especially prone to hypoxia, to which they respond with bradycardia. Keep suctioning as brief as possible in pediatric patients.

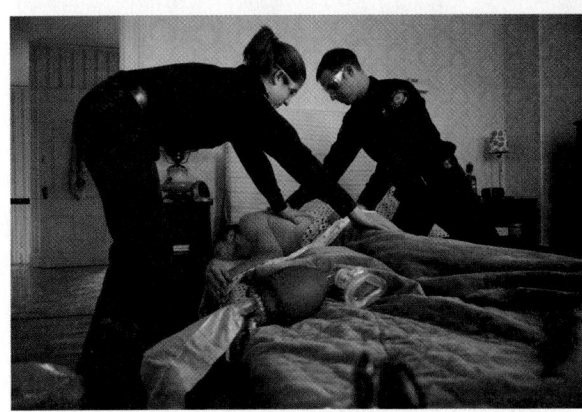

1. Move the patient to the left lateral recumbent position.

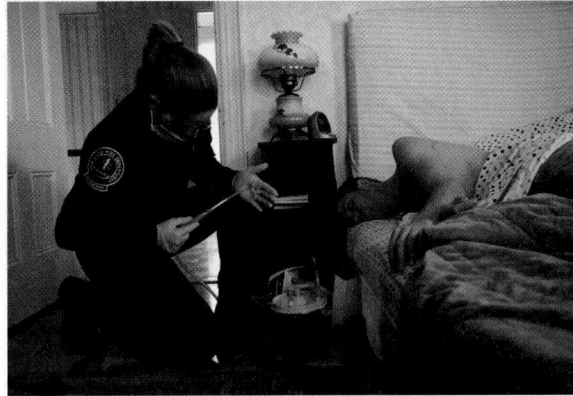

2. Make sure the suction unit is properly assembled.

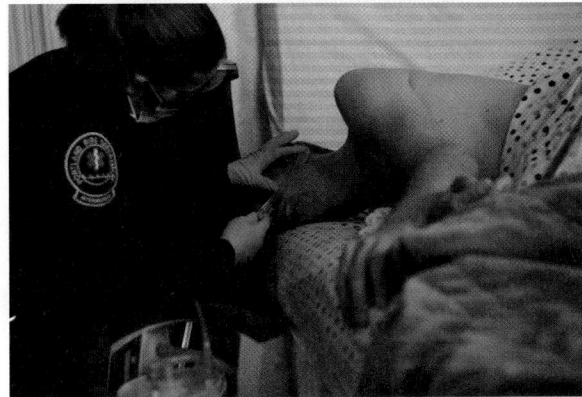

3. Measure the catheter from the corner of the patient's mouth to the earlobe.

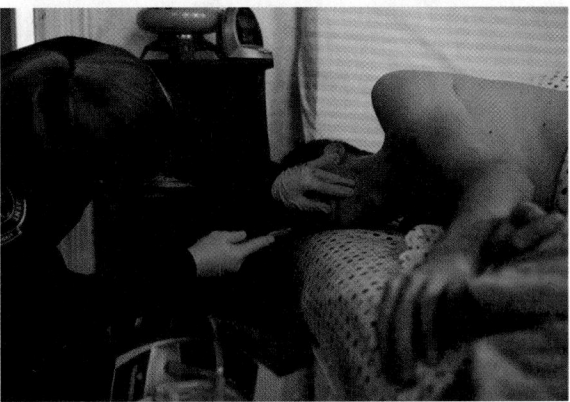

4. Open the patient's mouth and insert the catheter.

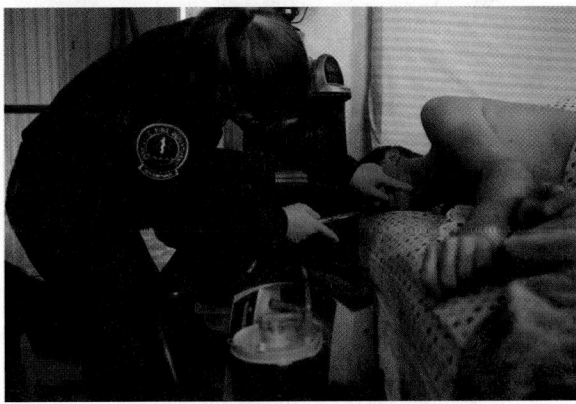

5. Apply suction as you withdraw the catheter.

After withdrawing the suction catheter, insert the tip into a container of sterile water and suction some water through the tubing to clear it. For especially viscous fluid, removing the Yankauer tip and using the end of the suction tubing itself may better achieve suction. Suctioning may be a one-time event for a particular patient, or it may require frequent repetition. Each situation is different and requires critical thinking to develop an effective strategy to accomplish the overall goal of clearing the airway.

Suctioning the Lower Airway

Patients who have an endotracheal tube or tracheostomy tube occasionally require suction to clear the trachea of secretions (Scan 16-2). A soft suction catheter is used, and because it is introduced into the lower airway, you must use sterile equipment and sterile technique. In the adult patient, you will typically use a 14 Fr. suction catheter. For pediatric patients it is best to have a reference guide readily available.

Tracheal Suctioning of an Intubated Patient

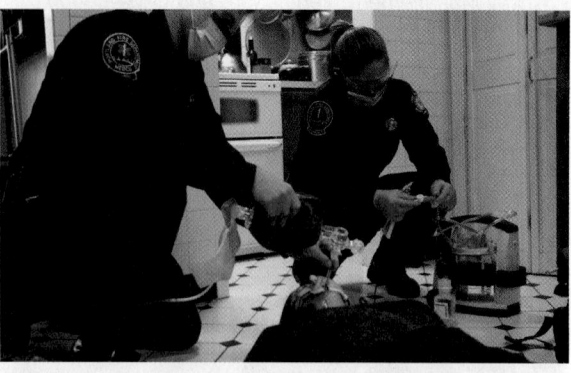

1. If possible, preoxygenate the patient prior to suctioning. If copious secretions are preventing ventilation and oxygenation, suction them immediately.

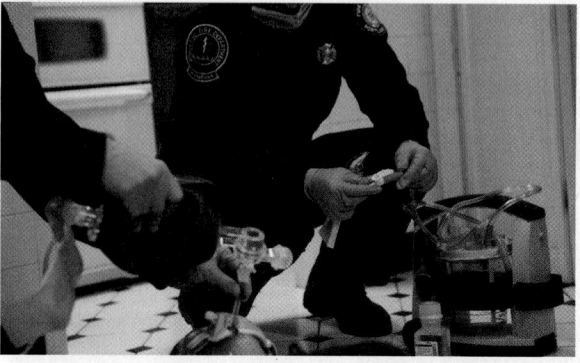

2. Assemble and check the suction equipment. Maintain sterility of the flexible suction catheter by keeping it covered with the packaging.

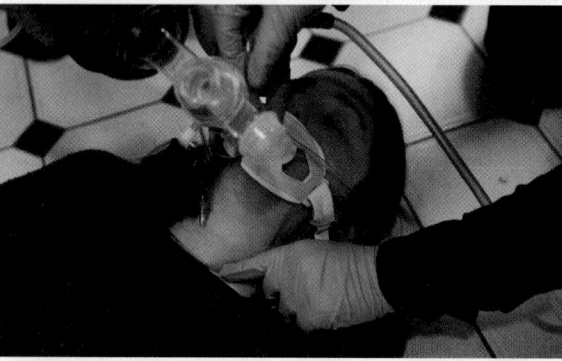

3. Maintaining the sterility of the suction catheter, measure the suction catheter from the earlobe, around the top of the ear, and down the neck to the sternal notch.

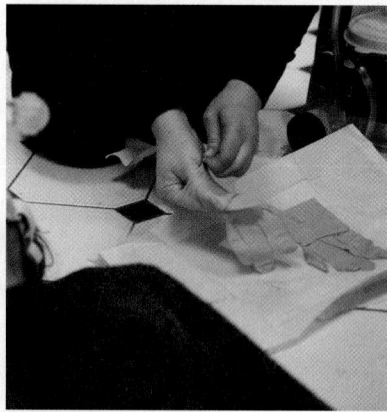

4. Use a sterile glove to handle the suction catheter.

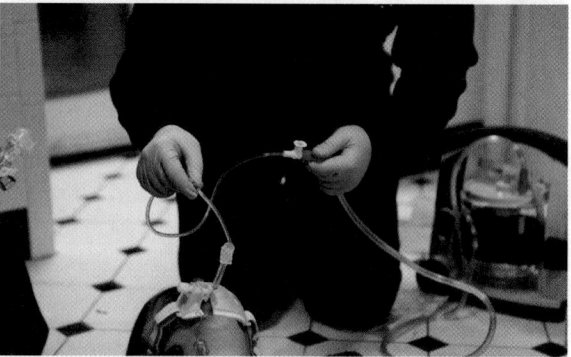

5. Insert the suction catheter into the endotracheal tube to the measured depth without applying suction.

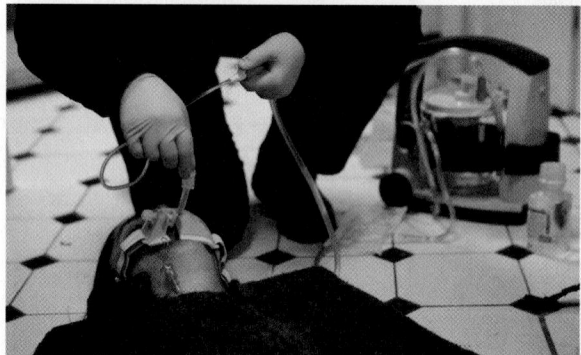

6. Cover the side port and apply suction as you slowly withdraw the catheter using a twisting motion. Monitor SpO$_2$ and cardiac rhythm while suctioning.

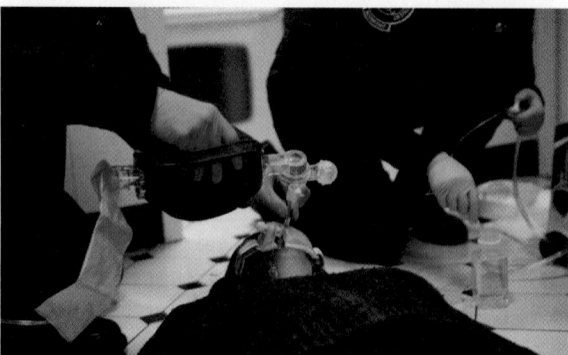

7. Limit suctioning to 10 seconds. Ventilate the patient before suctioning again. If suctioning is to be repeated, suction sterile water through the catheter to clear it.

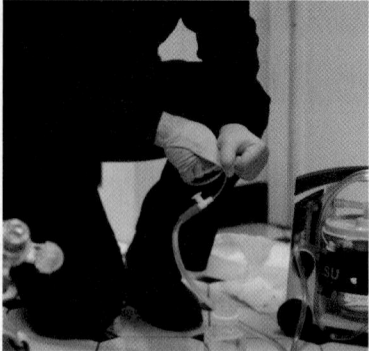

8. Dispose of the used suction catheter by wrapping it around your gloved hand. Turn the glove inside out as you remove it. Dispose of the glove and catheter in a biohazardous waste bag.

If a guide is not readily available, use a suction catheter that is approximately half the diameter of the internal diameter of the endotracheal tube.

While the suction catheter is in its unopened sterile packaging, measure it from the tip of the endotracheal tube or stoma to the level of the carina, which lies at approximately the sternal notch. To account for the curvature of the upper airway, when measuring from the tip of an endotracheal tube, run the suction catheter from tip of the tube to the corner of the mouth, around the ear, and then down to the sternal notch.

In patients with thick secretions, it is helpful to instill 5 mL of sterile saline from a sealed, premeasured plastic ampule into the trachea just prior to suctioning. The saline will help loosen the secretions, making them easier to remove. A prepackaged sterile kit for endotracheal suctioning includes sterile gloves and a sterile suction catheter. Handle the suction catheter only with sterile gloves and do not allow either the gloves or catheter to touch any surface. For most patients who require endotracheal or tracheostomy tube suctioning, preoxygenation is feasible and should be performed. Monitor the patient's SpO_2 and heart rate during the procedure.

Advance the suction catheter into the tube to the premeasured point without applying suction. Once you reach the proper depth, cover the side port with your thumb to generate suction at the catheter tip. Slowly withdraw the catheter with a slight swirling or rotating motion. Limit each suction attempt to 10 seconds. Clear the catheter and tubing with sterile water. If you will suction the patient again immediately, keep the catheter sterile while you reoxygenate the patient. If additional suctioning is not immediately required, discard the used catheter and your gloves in a biohazard disposal container.

Airway Adjuncts

Once you have manually opened and cleared the airway, you must ensure that the airway remains open. In some cases, you simply need to monitor the patient vigilantly

and if possible, treat the underlying cause of airway impairment, such as unresponsiveness due to hypoglycemia or narcotic overdose. A patient who is responsive can protect his airway more effectively than EMS providers can protect it by using airway adjuncts. In other cases, a simple or more advanced airway adjunct is required. In most cases, the tools at your disposal as an Advanced EMT are sufficient. In some cases, such as severe airway obstruction due to edema (for example from anaphylaxis or burns) or trauma, an endotracheal tube or cricothyrotomy (surgical incision into the cricoid membrane) is required to establish an airway. You must provide the best airway possible and determine whether it is more feasible to request ALS response (by ground or air) or to transport the patient to the nearest facility capable of managing the problem.

Remember that the most effective method of airway management is whatever method gets air into your patient with the fewest complications. That method may very well be the most basic approach.

Oropharyngeal Airways

An oropharyngeal (oral) airway is a curved device used to displace the soft tissue of the tongue to provide a channel for air to flow through the oropharynx (Figure 16-28). Because the tip of an oropharyngeal airway reaches the hypopharynx, it stimulates a gag reflex and must only be used in patients who are unresponsive and do not have a gag reflex. Oropharyngeal airways do not stand alone as an airway management device. They are an adjunct to the use of a manual airway maneuver.

Proper oropharyngeal airway size is essential to its effectiveness. A device that is too small will not displace the tongue effectively. A device that is too large may obstruct the airway and may cause trauma to the soft tissues. Measure the length from the corner of the patient's mouth to the angle of the jaw, just below the earlobe (Scan 16-3). If a patient measures between two sizes, select the airway that

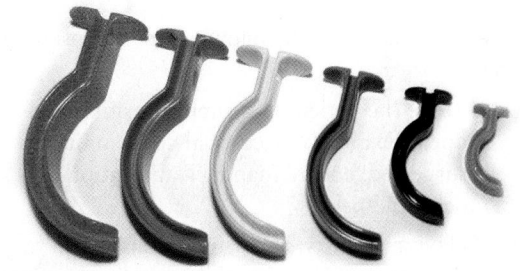

FIGURE 16-28

Oropharyngeal airways come in a variety of sizes, from neonatal to large adult. (© Edward T. Dickinson, MD)

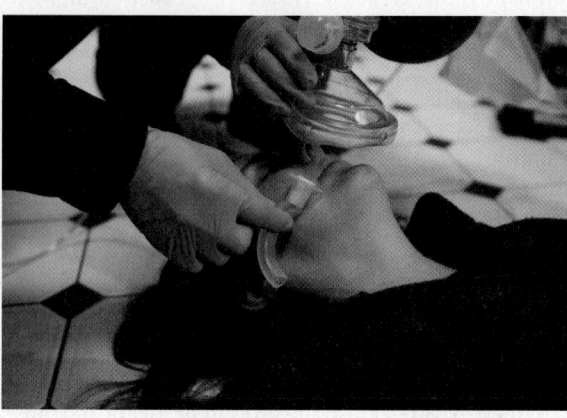

1. Measure to ensure the correct size.

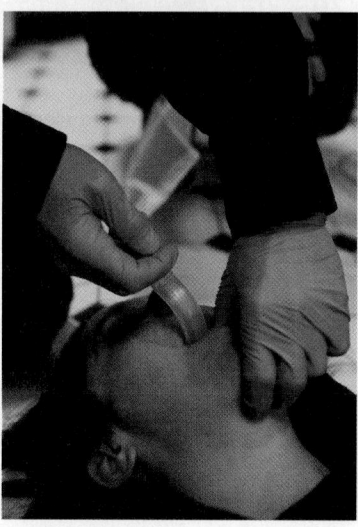

2. Insert with tip pointing up toward roof of mouth.

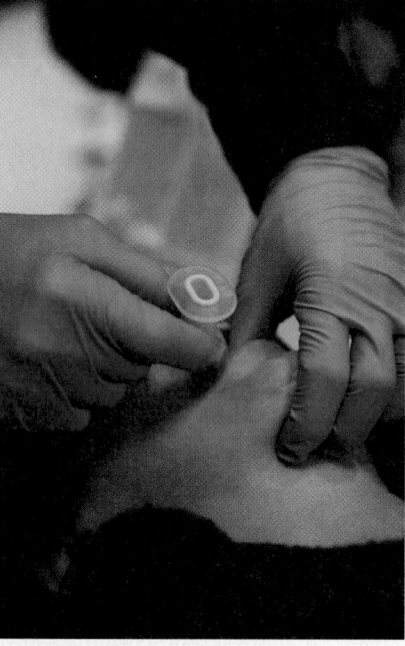

3. Advance while rotating 180 degrees.

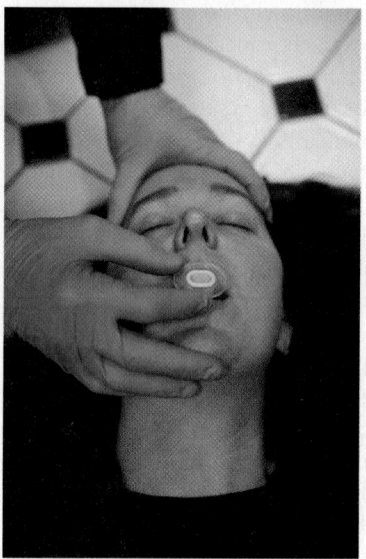

4. Continue until flange rests on the teeth.

best fits the patient. Use the following steps to insert an oropharyngeal airway:

1. Move the patient to a supine position and open the airway. If cervical-spine injury is suspected, ensure manual stabilization of head and neck.

2. Have suction available in case the patient has a gag reflex and vomits while attempting to insert the airway. Be prepared to turn the patient to the side and suction.

3. Wearing appropriate PPE, open the patient's mouth using the cross-finger technique described previously.

4. Insert the airway with the tip curved upward toward the patient's hard palate. Alternatively, you can use a tongue blade to depress the tongue, which will allow you to insert the device with the tip curved downward as you visualize it.

5. As you insert the device, gently rotate it 180 degrees so that that tip follows the curvature of the airway. If the patient gags, remove the device.

6. When properly positioned, the flange (collar) of the device should rest against the patient's lips.

7. Maintain the use of a manual maneuver in addition to the oropharyngeal airway.

8. Frequently reassess airway patency.

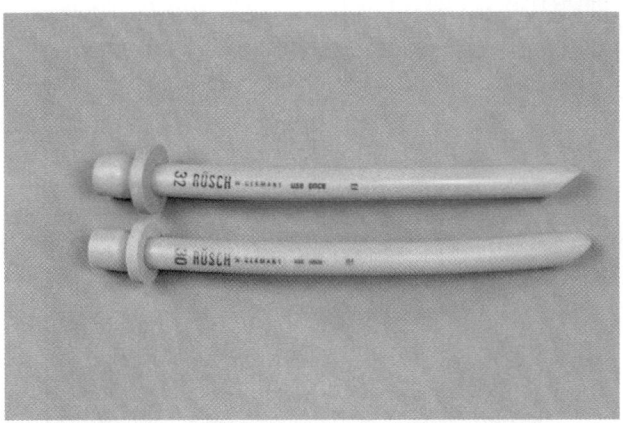

FIGURE 16-29

Nasopharyngeal airways.

Nasopharyngeal Airways

Nasopharyngeal (nasal) airways can be used in patients when access to the oropharynx is impossible (Figure 16-29). Some patients with a gag reflex who cannot tolerate an oropharyngeal airway may be able to tolerate a nasopharyngeal airway.

A nasopharyngeal airway is a flexible tube inserted through the nose and into the hypopharynx. When properly placed, the device provides a channel for air to move past the tongue. Sizing is essential and a nasopharyngeal airway does not replace the need for manual airway positioning. A nasopharyngeal airway is measured from the tip of the patient's nose to the angle of the mandible, just below the earlobe.

Nasopharyngeal airways have some disadvantages and contraindications. The nasal mucosa has a rich blood supply and is easily traumatized. Epistaxis often occurs as a result of attempting to pass a nasopharyngeal airway. The airway is then jeopardized by blood flowing into the pharynx, particularly in a patient taking a medication that impairs hemostasis. For this reason, you should always lubricate a nasopharyngeal airway with a water-soluble lubricant prior to insertion and insert it gently.

You must understand the anatomy of the nose in relation to the pharynx to properly direct the device and avoid trauma to the nasal turbinates. In addition, the device must not be forced past a point of resistance. Some patients may have a deviated nasal septum or other anatomic variations that make insertion of a nasopharyngeal airway difficult. By convention, the right naris is often chosen as the side into which nasopharyngeal airway insertion is first attempted. However, it can be inserted on either side as long as the bevel is oriented toward the septum.

While the risk is largely theoretical and minimal if the device is oriented properly during insertion, a nasopharyngeal airway could potentially enter the cranial vault in a patient with a basilar skull fracture. Bacteria from the nasal cavity can be introduced into the cranial vault when this occurs. You should avoid inserting a nasopharyngeal airway in patients with severe head or midface trauma or other indications of a basilar skull fracture, such as leakage of CSF from the nose (CSF rhinorrhea), with or without blood.

To insert a nasopharyngeal airway, use the following steps (Scan 16-4):

1. Position the patient in a supine position and open the airway with a manual maneuver. If cervical-spine trauma is suspected, ensure manual stabilization of the head and neck.

2. Have suction available. While vomiting is less likely, the risk of bleeding into the pharynx is increased with use of a nasopharyngeal airway. Be prepared to turn the patient to the side and suction.

3. Measure the device from the tip of the nose to the angle of the mandible and ensure the external diameter is compatible with the size of the patient's external nares.

4. Lubricate the last 1 to 2 inches of the outside of the tube with a water-based lubricant.

5. By convention, the right naris is often chosen, but if there is obvious obstruction, begin with the left. Align the bevel (angled portion at the tip) toward the septum.

6. Insert the airway into the patient's nostril and advance posteriorly (not at an upward angle) until the flange is seated against the patient's nostril. If minor resistance is met, slightly rotating the device from side to side by rolling it between your fingers may help. However, *never force insertion of a nasopharyngeal airway*.

7. If insertion on the first side attempted is unsuccessful, you may attempt insertion on the other side. Remove the airway and attempt insertion in the other nostril.

Just as with an oropharyngeal airway, maintain head position to help ensure airway patency. A head-tilt/chin-lift maneuver or modified jaw-thrust maneuver may still be necessary.

Combitube and Supraglottic Airway Devices

In many cases, you can effectively and safely maintain a patient's airway by using manual airway maneuvers and a simple airway adjunct. In such cases, this is often the best way to manage the patient's airway until arrival at the hospital. One of the limitations of these methods, though, is that they cannot protect the patient from aspirating fluids into the trachea and lungs. When patients are at high risk for aspiration (for example, a patient who is bleeding into the airway or vomiting) or when simpler methods are not effective in providing an airway that can be ventilated, you must consider the use of a more advanced airway adjunct.

As an Advanced EMT, you have two types of more advanced airway devices available to you. Neither type

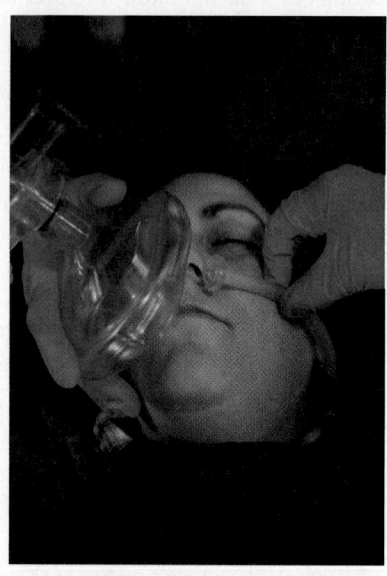

1.   Measure the nasopharyngeal airway.

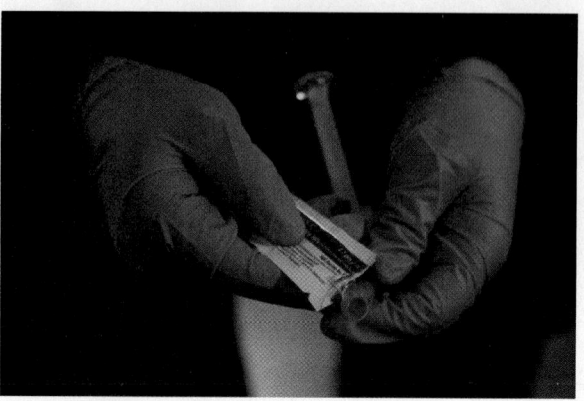

2.   Lubricate it with water-soluble lubricant.

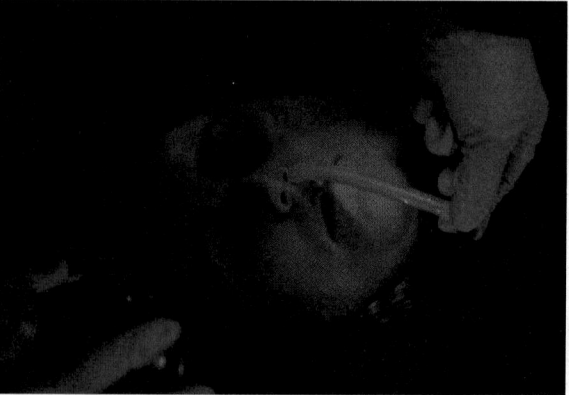

3.   Insert the airway with the bevel toward the septum or base of the tonsil.

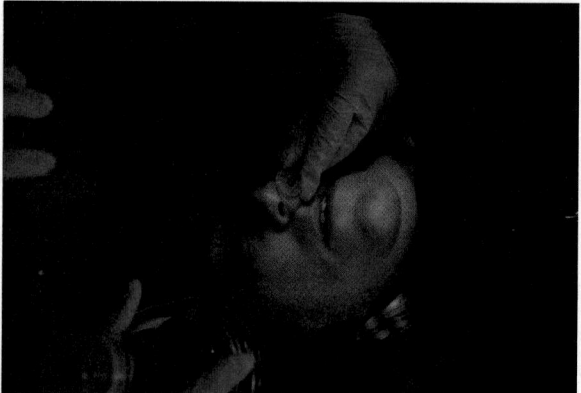

4.   Advance the airway until the flange is seated against the patient's nostril. Advance the airway until the flange is seated against the patient's nostril.

requires direct visualization of the glottic opening as insertion of an endotracheal tube does. This is an advantage in that visualization is often the most difficult and time-consuming part of endotracheally intubating a patient, especially when the patient's head cannot be hyperextended out of concern for cervical-spine trauma. Because visualization of the glottis is not required, those devices are called *nonvisualized airways* or, sometimes, *blind insertion devices*. The devices offer at least minimal protection of the glottis against aspiration and a more defined pathway. But, they do not isolate the trachea and are not effective in patients with subglottic edema. The devices are, however, relatively easy to use and can be inserted quickly.

The number of nonvisualized airway devices and variations on each of them has increased in the past few years, providing a variety options. The specific devices allowed in the Advanced EMT scope of practice vary by state and by EMS medical director. General information about nonvisualized airway devices is presented in this chapter. You must follow manufacturer directions and your protocols for proper insertion and use procedures for the airway devices used in your EMS service.

The first type of device is the esophageal tracheal Combitube (usually called a *Combitube*), which is designed to function when placed in the esophagus by obstructing the esophagus and pharynx so that, by default, air enters the trachea (Figure 16-30). However, the dual-lumen design of the Combitube allows it to function if it inadvertently enters the trachea. Patients must meet certain criteria in order for the Combitube to be used (Table 16-4).

The second type of device is a supraglottic device (also called an *extraglottic device*) because it sits in the hypopharynx, just above the glottic opening. Laryngeal mask airways (LMA), King LTD, and Cobra devices are

protection to the glottic opening for as long as the seal is maintained, and the glottic opening is reasonably protected from secretions and foreign matter. Movement of the patient can frequently dislodge this type of airway.

Ventilation

Once you have secured the airway, you will evaluate the patient's breathing (although it may already be obvious that the patient's breathing is absent or inadequate) and assess the need for artificial ventilation. In some cases, the need for positive pressure ventilation is obvious. In the patient in respiratory arrest, the need for positive pressure ventilations is clear. In other cases, the need for ventilatory assistance may not be as clear. Consider the asthma patient with respiratory distress. Your assessment may initially reveal that he requires supplemental oxygen and a nebulized bronchodilator. In contrast, if he shows signs of respiratory failure, such as altered mental status, cyanosis, and ineffective breathing, you must assist his ventilations. (It is possible to use a nebulizer in conjunction with a bag-valve-mask device if your service carries a T-connector that allows the nebulizer chamber to be placed in line with the bag-valve-mask.)

Unfortunately, it is not always so clear-cut. In the past, there was little that could be done for patients who were not compensating well, but were not quite in respiratory failure. In recent years, **continuous positive airway pressure (CPAP)** devices have become widely available in the prehospital setting (Figure 16-32). CPAP assists the patient approaching respiratory failure and may improve oxygenation enough that he can avoid being intubated and being placed on a ventilator in the hospital (which carries a high risk of infection and other complications).

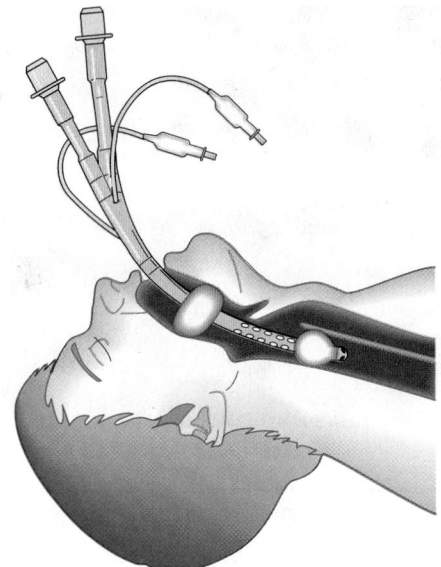

FIGURE 16-30

An esophageal tracheal Combitube®.

examples of supraglottic devices (Figure 16-31). As with the Combitube, patients must meet certain criteria for insertion of a supraglottic airway device. Improvements are constantly being made to existing devices and new devices are continuously under development. You must follow the manufacturer's directions and your protocols for using any airway device.

Supraglottic devices are inserted into the hypopharynx and create a seal around the glottic opening. A cuff is inflated to create the seal and then positive pressure is applied to force air into the trachea. This seal also adds a level of

TABLE 16-4 **Indications and Contraindications for Advanced EMT Airway Devices**

COMBITUBE		LARYNGEAL MASK AIRWAY		KING LTD	
Indications	Contraindications	Indications	Contraindications	Indications	Contraindciations
Patient is unresponsive without a gag reflex and requires a more secure airway and route of ventilation than can be provided by more basic means.	Patient under 5 feet tall (a small adult size exists and can be used in patients between 4½–5 feet tall). Patient under 16 years old. Presence of esophageal disease or trauma. Laryngectomy with stoma.	Patient is unresponsive without a gag reflex and requires a more secure airway and route of ventilation than can be provided by more basic means.	No contraindications for use as a rescue airway in patients who are completely unresponsive and do not have gag reflex (Laryngeal Mask Airway Company, 2010). Laryngectomy with stoma.	Patient is unresponsive without a gag reflex and requires a more secure airway and route of ventilation than can be provided by more basic means.	Patient under 4 feet tall. Laryngectomy with stoma.

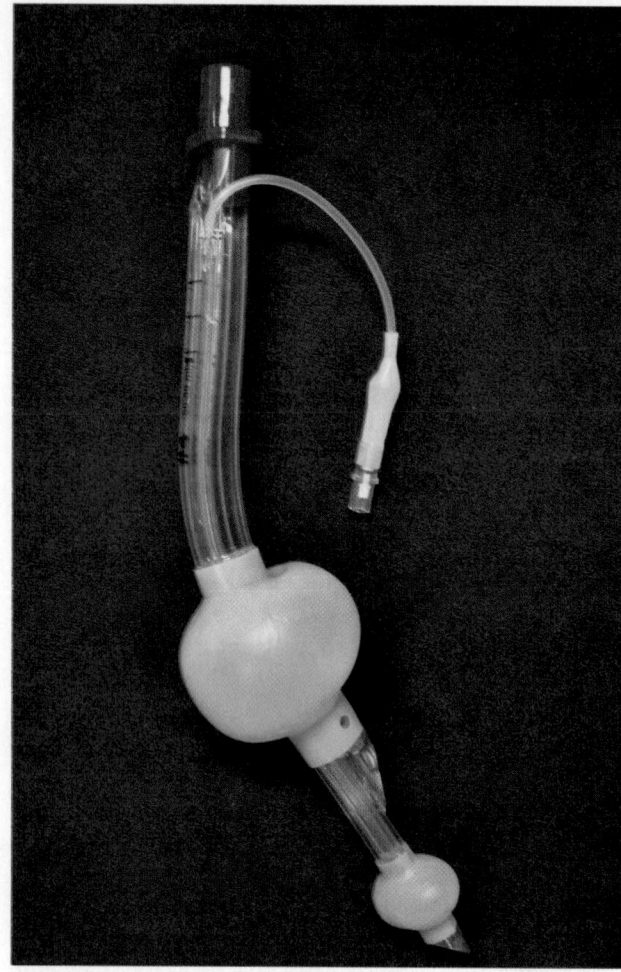

FIGURE 16-31

King LTD airway. (© Edward T. Dickinson, MD)

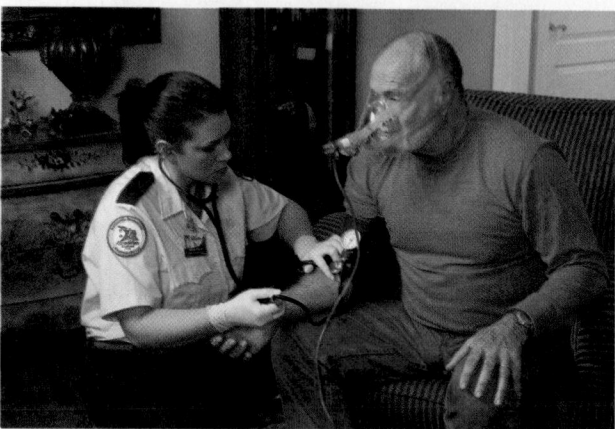

FIGURE 16-32

Continuous positive airway pressure (CPAP) device.

During respiratory distress, the patient has a respiratory problem for which his body is attempting to compensate with a greater or lesser degree of success. When the body's compensatory mechanisms cannot result in adequate tissue oxygenation, the patient is in respiratory failure. In respiratory distress, the patient will likely have an increased respiratory rate, may be seated in a tripod position, and may be using accessory muscles. When compensatory mechanisms are meeting the metabolic needs of the body, the patient's mental status is normal (although he is likely to be anxious) and there are no signs of hypoxia. These patients require supplemental oxygen administration and treatment of the underlying cause of respiratory distress. In severe respiratory distress, respiratory failure, and respiratory arrest, you must either supplement the patient's spontaneous respiratory effort, or provide him with artificial ventilation using positive pressure ventilation.

Positive Pressure Ventilation

In normal breathing, air movement on inspiration is generated by negative intrathoracic pressure. The use of artificial ventilation devices moves air into the lungs because it is being forced in under increased pressure, and is therefore called *positive pressure ventilation*. There are four options available for assisting or providing ventilations in the prehospital setting. They are CPAP, bag-valve-mask devices with supplemental oxygen, manually triggered ventilation devices, and automatic transport ventilators. The use of each can result in complications due to reliance on positive pressure.

Recall that the negative intrathoracic pressure generated on inspiration contributes to preload and thus cardiac output. The use of positive pressure impairs cardiac output, especially when excessive pressures are used and intrathoracic pressure is increased above normal. In a low perfusion state, such as shock or during CPR, any decrease in cardiac output is a serious problem.

With negative pressure ventilations, the opening of the esophagus is pulled into a closed position. With positive pressure, the esophagus is forced open, leading to air entry into the stomach. Air in the stomach in a limited quantity is not a significant problem, but as the volume increases, vomiting is likely and gastric distention is possible. In gastric distention, the air-filled stomach limits the excursion of the diaphragm and thus decreases the total capacity of the lungs.

Also keep in mind that the airway is designed for low pressures. Under increased pressure, trauma to the trachea, bronchi, and lung parenchyma can occur. This risk is increased when excessive pressures are used, the patient has pre-existing lung disease (such as COPD), and in pediatric patients.

Although positive pressure ventilation may be associated with complications, apnea and respiratory failure quickly result in death. When you determine that a patient requires positive pressure ventilations, you can limit complications through the use of good technique and by fully understanding how poor technique harms the patient.

Bag-Valve-Mask Ventilations

Providing bag-valve-mask ventilations is a relatively simple skill, but it requires finesse. Your technique can either cause or minimize the unintended consequences of positive pressure ventilation. A bag-valve-mask device consists of a self-inflating bag attached to a mask that creates a seal around the patient's mouth and nose and has a reservoir for collecting oxygen (Figure 16-33). With the mask tightly sealed, air is expelled from the bag when it is squeezed by hand. If the mask is not sealed, this air under pressure will leak out of the sides of the mask instead of entering the airway. Bag-valve-mask devices are available in adult, pediatric, infant, and neonatal sizes. With the use

of a reservoir and 15 L/min of oxygen flow, bag-valve-mask devices can deliver a concentration of oxygen approaching 100 percent.

Using a bag-valve-mask device requires that the patient's airway is open. You must coordinate sealing the mask to the face, maintaining the head and jaw in proper position, and squeezing the bag to deliver ventilations. It is preferred that two providers work together to manage the airway and ventilation. However, you can achieve good ventilation by yourself if you must, although it is challenging. When a patient has a more advanced airway in place, such as an endotracheal tube, Combitube, or supraglottic airway, you should detach the mask and fit the standard 15-mm adapter on the bag to the airway device to deliver ventilations more directly to the lower airway.

Achieve a Good Mask Seal

Choose an appropriately sized mask. Face masks come in a variety of shapes and sizes. The mask should cover the face from the bridge of the nose to the depression between the lower lip and tip of the chin with sufficient coverage of the mouth (Figure 16-34). The mask should be soft enough to create a seal when pressed against the soft tissue of the face. If you are managing airway and ventilation alone,

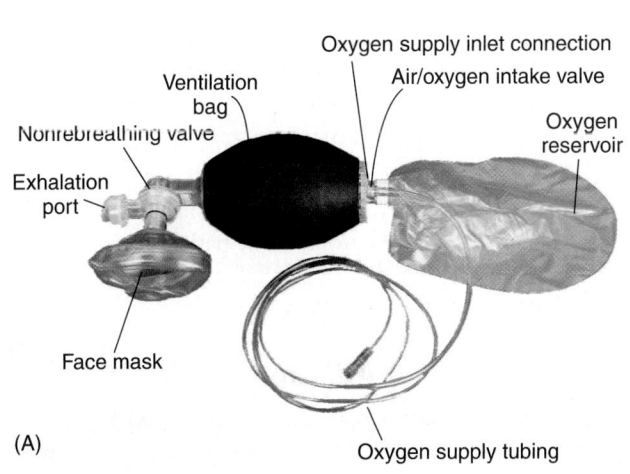

Ventilation bag

Oxygen supply inlet connection

Air/oxygen intake valve

Nonrebreathing valve

Oxygen reservoir

Exhalation port

Face mask

(A)

Oxygen supply tubing

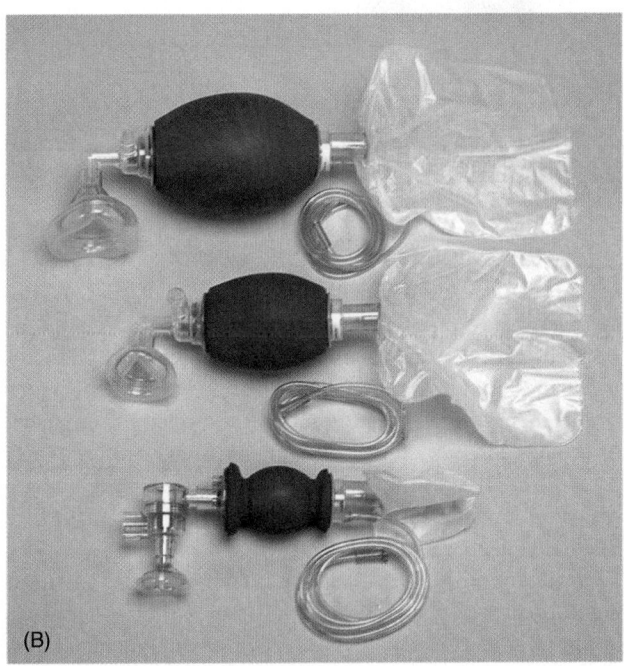

(B)

FIGURE 16-33

(A) Bag-valve-mask device with oxygen bag reservoir. Tubing-type reservoirs are also available.
(B) Adult, child, and infant bag-valve-mask devices.

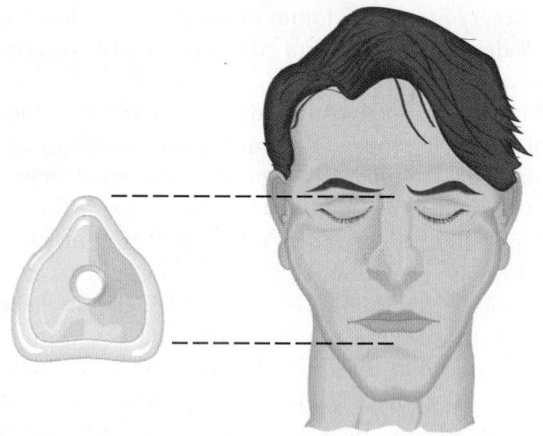

FIGURE 16-34

Use a mask that fits the patient properly.

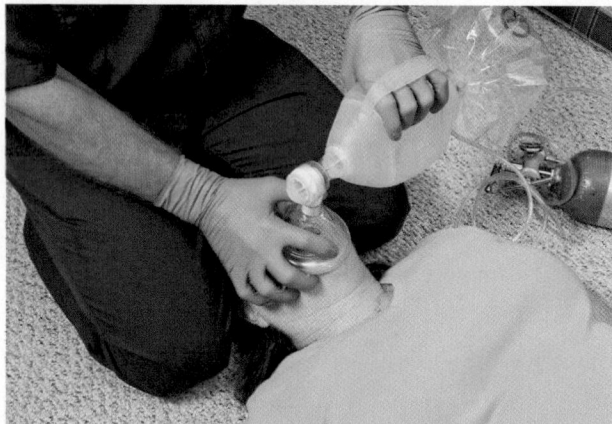

FIGURE 16-35

Obtain a mask seal and maintain proper airway position when using a single-provider bag-valve-mask technique by using an "E-C" grip.

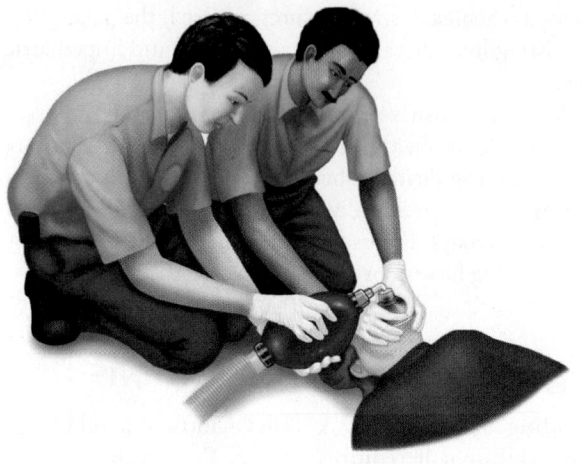

FIGURE 16-36

Two-provider bag-valve-mask ventilation technique.

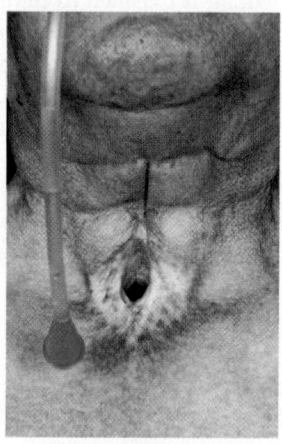

FIGURE 16-37

To ventilate a patient with a stoma, place the BVM mask over the stoma. (© Biophoto Associates/Photo Researchers, Inc.)

use an "E-C technique" to form a seal (Figure 16-35). Use the thumb and index finger of one hand to hold the mask (forming a C). At the same time, apply downward pressure to the mask to seal it on the face. Place the middle, ring, and small fingers of the same hand on the boney prominence of the patient's mandible (forming an E) and pull the jaw toward the mask. In a patient with suspected spine injury, avoid unnecessary movement of the head. Use your other hand to squeeze the bag.

With two providers, one can use both hands to obtain a good seal with the mask and the other can provide ventilation (Figure 16-36). The two-person technique facilitates the ability to perform a modified jaw-thrust maneuver in combination with securing the mask. If you are delivering mouth-to-mask ventilations, you can use either of the techniques to obtain a good seal. In this case, the positive pressure comes from your lungs instead of from a bag-valve-mask device.

You can ventilate patients with a tracheostomy by attaching the 15-mm adapter of the ventilation bag to the tracheal tube or by placing a mask over the stoma (Figure 16-37). Usually, a pediatric-size face mask will allow a better seal over the stoma if the patient does not have a tracheal tube (in which case you will attach the ventilation bag directly to the tracheal tube).

Ventilate at the Appropriate Depth

To minimize the complications associated with positive pressure ventilations, use just the volume necessary to provide adequate tidal volume. Normal tidal volume is 5 to 7 mL/kg of body weight. However, it is difficult to gauge the volume of air that is being squeezed from the bag. To approximate appropriate tidal volume, gently squeeze the bag over 1 to 1½ seconds, until the chest just begins to rise. Any additional pressure is unneeded and leads to gastric distention and decreased venous return to the heart. This rule of thumb is true regardless of the size of the patient. Watch for chest rise and stop ventilation upon moving the chest wall.

Ventilate at the Appropriate Rate

Just as more is not better in terms of ventilatory volume, it is not better in terms of ventilatory rate. Hyperventilation is harmful. Adult patients are ventilated 10 to 12 times per minute except in select cases of severe traumatic brain injury. This means that a single ventilation is delivered once every 5 to 6 seconds. During CPR, the delivery of ventilations follows American Heart Association (AHA) guidelines, which may differ from the ventilatory rates provided for patients with a pulse. Always follow your protocol and the most up-to-date AHA guidelines.

Ventilating at a rate faster than normal leads to gastric distention and allows for elimination of an increased amount of carbon dioxide. Both excessively high PaO_2 and low $PaCO_2$ result in cerebral vasoconstriction, thereby reducing blood flow to the brain. Both low PaO_2 and high $PaCO_2$, however, lead to cerebral vasodilation. While this may not seem harmful on the surface, it is in fact quite harmful to patients with cerebral edema. Patients who require ventilation often have conditions, such as stroke or traumatic brain injury, that are a primary cause of cerebral edema. Hypoxia from any cause can also lead to cerebral edema. Your technique of ventilation must be refined to avoid unnecessary changes in pH and blood gases. The use of both pulse oximetry and capnometry can provide feedback about your ventilations.

While ventilating a patient, be alert to any indication that ventilations are either ineffective or excessive (Table 16-5). Pay attention to the patient's skin color and condition, breath sounds, and vital signs. Increased resistance to bagging can mean that the airway has become occluded, there is air trapping in the lungs due to

Pediatric Care

Positive pressure ventilation in children requires the use of pediatric-size equipment, including airway adjuncts, mask, and bag. Excessive ventilatory volume in children can result in gastric distention, reduced ventilation, hypoxia, bradycardia, and vomiting.

overventilation, there is gastric distention, or a tension pneumothorax is developing as a result of lung injury.

Maintaining the proper rate of ventilations can be made more difficult by anxiety, multitasking, and simply failing to accurately time ventilations. Overventilation and underventilation have significant negative consequences. Concentrate carefully on the rate and depth of positive pressure ventilations. Failure to do so can result in a poor patient outcome.

In some cases, positive pressure ventilation is used to assist a patient who is breathing, but breathing inadequately (Figure 16-38). The goals of positive pressure ventilation in these patients are to increase oxygen delivery, reduce fatigue, and improve tidal volume. Inadequate breathing may occur with either fast or slow respiratory rates. As the rate increases beyond a certain point, tidal volume decreases. For these patients, you can use positive pressure ventilation to increase tidal volume, although you will not assist every breath the patient is taking. You will assist the adult patient at a rate of 10 to 12 per minute, aiming for an adequate tidal volume.

Positive pressure ventilation is also required for patients becoming fatigued from severe respiratory distress and the increased work of breathing. In such cases, determine to what degree the patient needs assistance with ventilatory rate and ventilatory volume. Positive pressure ventilation on

TABLE 16-5 Indications of Effective and Ineffective Positive Pressure Ventilation	
Adequate Ventilation	**Inadequate Ventilation**
Good seal of mask to face, mask covers mouth and nose.	Air leaks around face mask during ventilation.
Tidal volume is appropriate to patient; each ventilation delivered over about 1½ seconds until patient's chest just begins to rise.	There is excessive chest rise, no chest rise, or abdominal distention.
Ventilation rate is appropriate to patient's age: 10–12 per minute for adults, 12–20 per minute for pediatric patients, >20 per minute for infants.	Ventilation rate is too fast or too slow for the patient's age.
Air flows into the lungs with slight resistance.	There is no resistance to airflow (check connections and seals) or significant/increasing resistance to airflow (check for airway position and gastric distention; check breath sounds).
Patient's condition stabilizes or improves.	Patient's condition fails to improve or deteriorates (check mental status, skin color, breath sounds, vital signs, and SpO_2 and CO_2 levels).

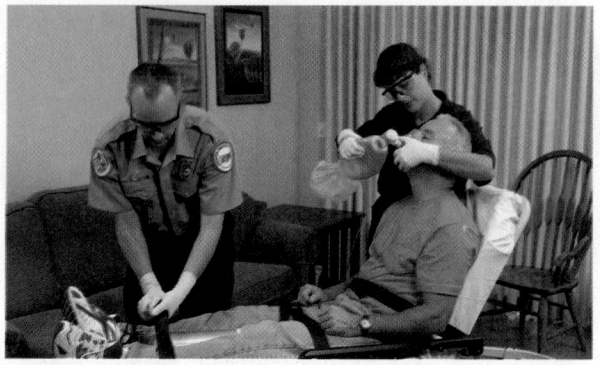

FIGURE 16-38

Using a bag-valve-mask device to assist a patient in severe respiratory distress or respiratory failure.

a breathing patient is not an easy skill. It requires careful timing and communication with the patient. In some cases, you may find that the patient will not tolerate mask intervention. This can be a sign of improvement, but it also may be a sign that further interventions are needed. Similarly, the patient who stops resisting assistance may either be tolerating the mask, or may be deteriorating and unable to resist.

Complications of delivering positive pressure ventilations to a conscious person include gastric distention and intolerance of the procedure. If the timing is not correct, air can be swallowed and enter the stomach. In this case, vomiting is a significant hazard.

Manually Triggered Ventilation Devices and Automatic Transport Ventilators

The manually triggered ventilation device and the **automatic transport ventilator (ATV)** deliver positive pressure without the provider needing to squeeze a bag or blow air into a mask. The advantages of the devices include reducing rescuer fatigue involved with manual resuscitative efforts. ATVs allow the operator to set the rate and volume of ventilations, thereby reducing errors from over- and under-ventilation. While ATVs have alarms that indicate excessive airway pressures, manually triggered devices operate under higher pressure and do not allow the provider to detect the sensation of increased resistance to ventilation. Both of the devices require specialized training. ATV operation varies by manufacturer and medical director. You must receive training specific to any device used in your system and have your medical director's approval to use it.

Flow-Restricted Oxygen-Powered Ventilation Device

A manually triggered ventilation device, also known as a **flow-restricted oxygen-powered ventilation device (FROPVD)**, uses the power of compressed oxygen to deliver

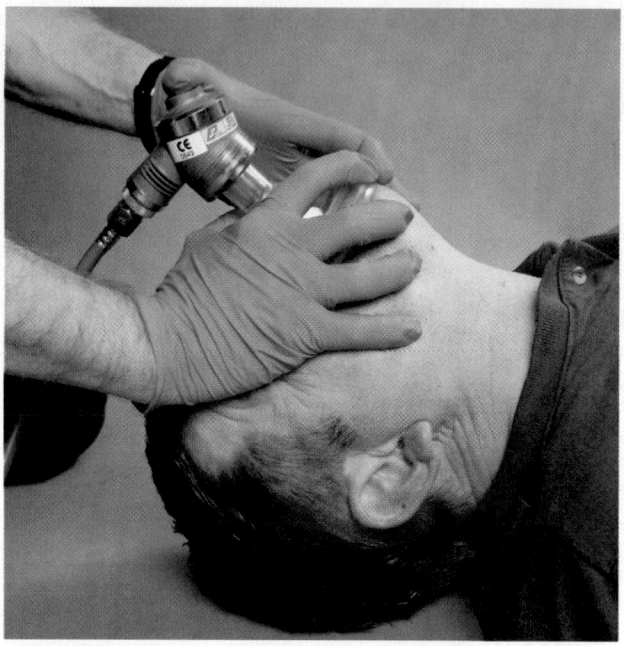

FIGURE 16-39

A flow-restricted oxygen-powered ventilation device (FROPVD).

ventilations (Figure 16-39). Oxygen is delivered with positive pressure through either a face mask or an advanced airway, The provider uses a trigger device to deliver ventilations. Commonly, the devices can deliver between 90 and 100 percent oxygen at up to 40 L/min. Typically, they also are regulated with a pressure relief valve that opens at approximately 60 cm H_2O. Use of the devices is very similar to bag-valve-mask ventilation. You must maintain an open airway and appropriate mask seal (if a mask is used instead of a Combitube or supraglottic device). Ventilate patients with only enough volume to cause chest rise and at a rate of 10 to 12 breaths per minute. Take special care taken when ventilating patients with chest trauma because it will be difficult to judge compliance when delivering ventilations. Use only enough pressure to obtain chest rise and be wary of the creation of a pneumothorax.

Standard manually triggered ventilation devices are designed for adult use only. Pediatric specific models do exist, but will require specialized training.

Automatic Transport Ventilators

Automatic transport ventilators can be used for any patient requiring bag-valve-mask ventilation (Figure 16-40). They are often used in the interfacilty transport of patients requiring ongoing positive pressure ventilation, but can be used during any prolonged transport situation in which the patient has a need for positive pressure ventilation. The advantage of an automatic transport device is that it allows the rate and depth of ventilation to be set by the provider and then delivered by the device in a hands-free operation. Because the rate and depth are mechanically delivered, you

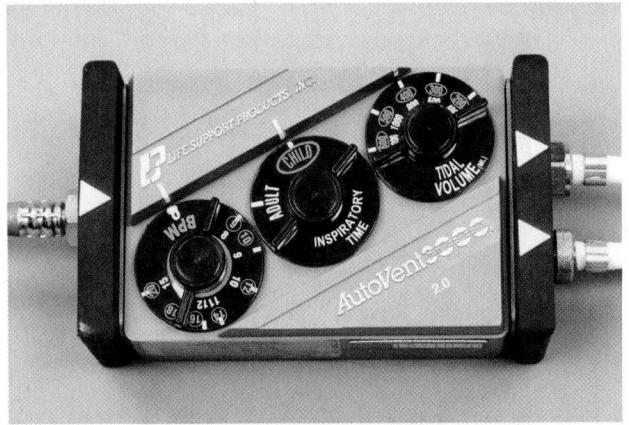

FIGURE 16-40

An automatic transport ventilator.

must ensure proper settings initially and reassess the settings to ensure they are safe and adequate for the patient. Pneumothorax and diving-related lung injuries are contraindications to the use of an ATV. If you are using a face mask in conjunction with the ATV, maintain proper airway position, use an airway adjunct, and ensure the mask has a good seal to the face.

Continuous Positive Airway Pressure

Continuous positive airway pressure (CPAP) devices use positive pressure to improve air flow in spontaneously breathing patients. In fact, CPAP and bilevel positive airway pressure (BiPAP) devices are used at home by many patients with respiratory disease and sleep apnea. A mask is sealed over the patient's mouth and nose and airflow is generated to provide pressure against which the patient can breathe. This is known as **positive end-expiratory pressure (PEEP)** and it creates a higher pressure within the entire airway tract from upper airway to alveoli. PEEP is valuable because it "pneumatically splints" the airways and keeps them from collapsing. In many cases, this pressure will prevent atelectasis and improve the surface area for oxygen exchange.

Although CPAP uses positive pressure, it is not mechanical ventilation. It is not a ventilator. The pressures utilized, typically around 10 cm H_2O, are not sufficient to ventilate a nonbreathing patient. CPAP is used to improve the ventilations that are already taking place. CPAP is used only in patients who are responsive and able to follow commands. It is not used in patients who cannot follow commands.

CPAP is particularly useful in patients suffering from acute pulmonary edema. The PEEP generated from CPAP can splint open the otherwise collapsing alveoli and sustain oxygen-exchanging capacity. The pressure from CPAP also helps prevent the influx of fluid into the alveoli. CPAP can cause many of the same complications as positive pressure ventilation. Because it causes increased pressure within the chest, it can drop cardiac output and cause a decrease in blood pressure. As such, use CPAP with caution in patients with lower than normal blood pressures.

CPAP can be delivered using room air or oxygen. When used in most EMS settings, CPAP combines oxygen and room air to create high levels of airflow at the CPAP mask. This combination makes CPAP a highly effective supplemental oxygen delivery system in addition to the benefits gained by creating PEEP.

Oxygenation

All patients with complaints of dyspnea or who are in respiratory distress, respiratory failure, or respiratory arrest should receive supplemental oxygen (Scan 16-5). Supplemental oxygen is beneficial to patients with an SpO_2 of less than 95%. (See Table 16-6.)

Oxygen as a Medication

In its concentrated form, oxygen is a medication. Like all medications, oxygen must be administered according to its indications by acceptable routes in approved dosages. Although most side effects associated with oxygen require long-term administration of high concentrations, you still must remember to use supplemental oxygen critically, and not just because it is an available tool. It has specific effects and mechanisms of actions and is not a cure-all. Recent studies have identified hyperoxia as a factor that increases morbidity and mortality in patients resuscitated from cardiac arrest. As a vasoactive drug, oxygen causes vasoconstriction and can actually decrease perfusion to ischemic tissues.

PERSONAL PERSPECTIVE

Mrs. Bertha Johnson: "When I had my heart attack, I just couldn't breathe. All of a sudden I just couldn't catch my breath. I thought I was going to die. When the ambulance folks got there, they put a mask over my face and began to breathe for me. It was terrifying. I couldn't breathe and now these people were pressing a mask over my face. At first I struggled. I couldn't help it. But as the man holding the mask on my face talked to me, I calmed down. Soon, by communicating we were able to time the breathing and I actually began to feel better. It was still scary, but soon the mask was actually helping me. It wasn't easy, but I think it saved my life."

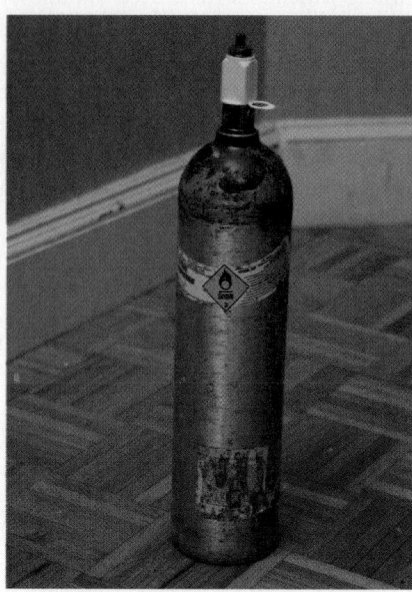

1. Select the desired cylinder. Check for label "Oxygen U.S.P."

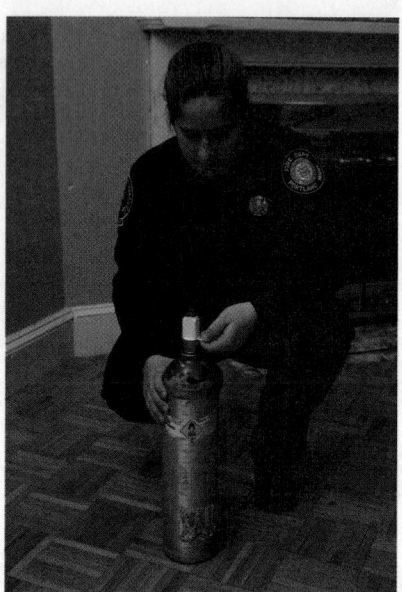

2. Place the cylinder in an upright position and stand to one side.

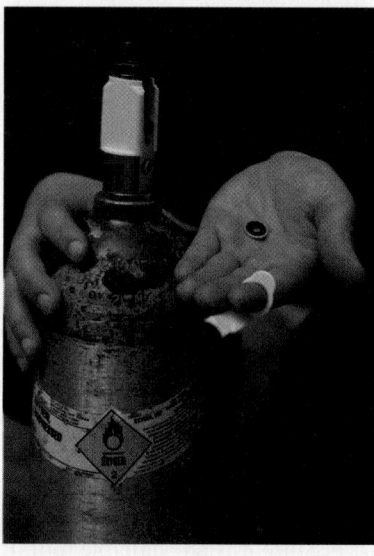

3. Remove the plastic wrapper or cap protecting the cylinder outlet. Keep the plastic washer (some setups).

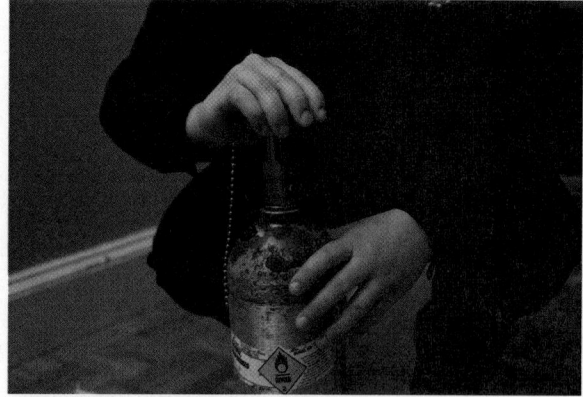

4. "Crack" the main valve for 1 second.

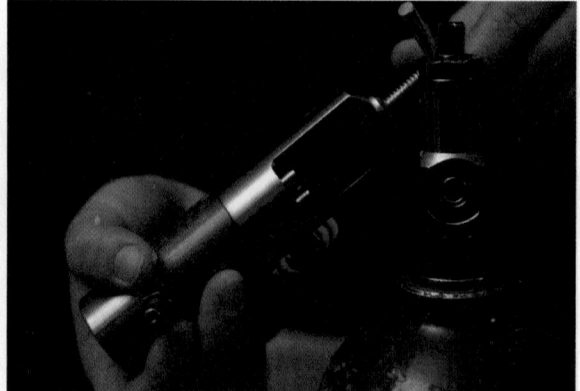

5. Select the correct pressure regulator and flow meter. A pin yoke for portable tanks is shown.

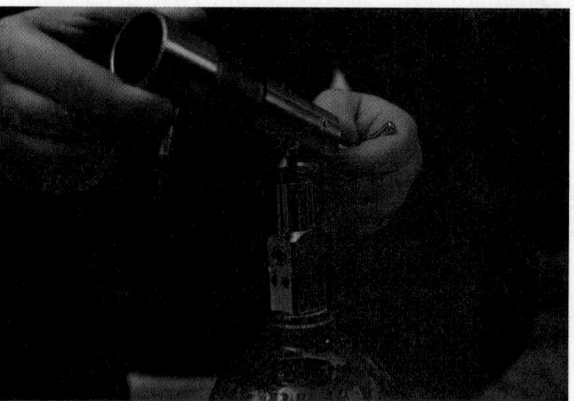

6. Align the pins.

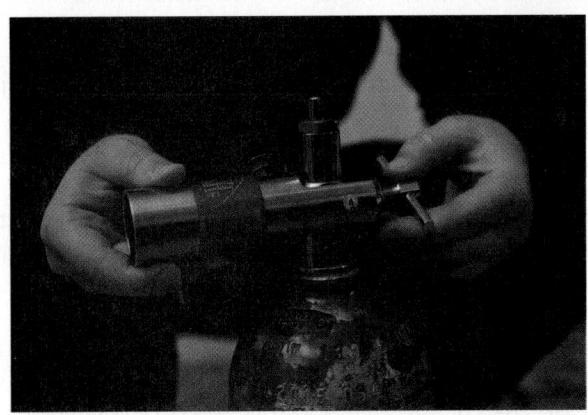

7. Tighten the T-screw for the pin yoke.

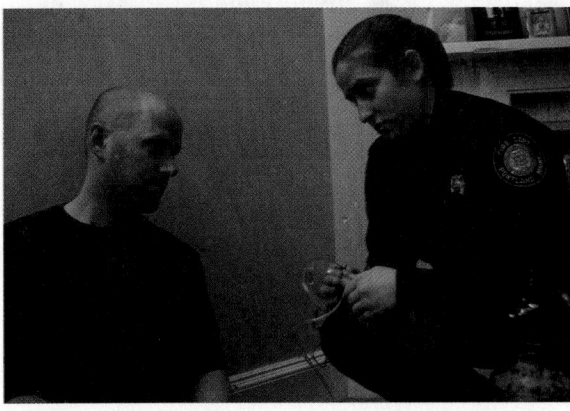

8. Explain to the patient the need for oxygen.

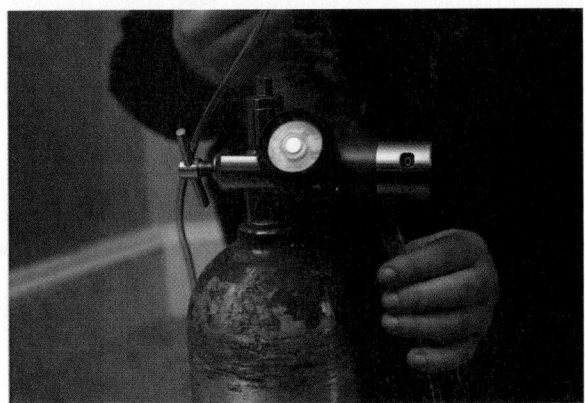

9. Attach the tubing and delivery device.

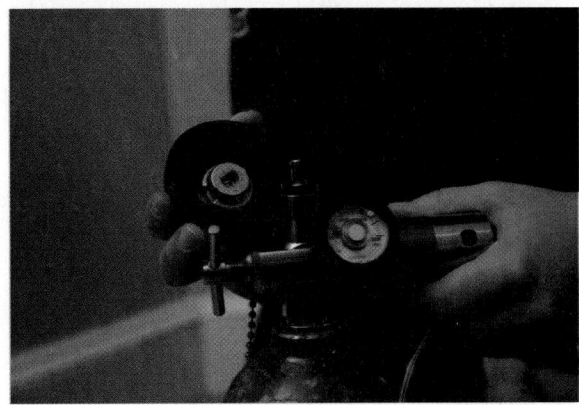

10. Open the main valve.

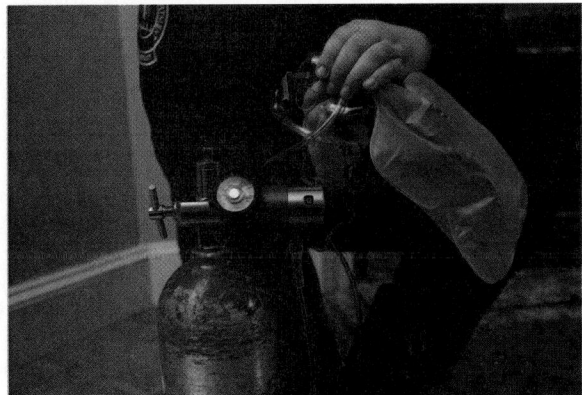

11. Adjust the flow meter.

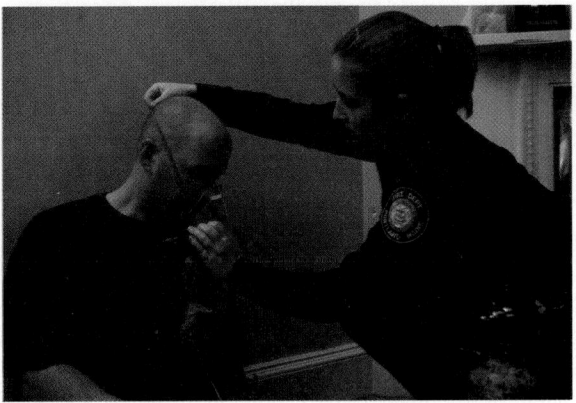

12. Place an oxygen delivery device on the patient.

Among the less serious side effects of oxygen administration is drying and irritation of the mucous membranes. Oxygen directly from the cylinder is not humidified and can dry the respiratory passages. Humidifiers exist for fixed oxygen delivery systems, such as the one in the ambulance, but must be meticulously maintained to prevent them from becoming reservoirs for bacteria. Because prehospital oxygen administration is usually of short duration, humidifiers are not usually used.

Some patients with COPD become accustomed to increased levels of carbon dioxide and thus rely on their secondary stimulus to breathe: decreased oxygen. In some cases, oxygen administration can subsequently decrease the patient's respiratory drive. However, never withhold oxygen from a patient who needs it. It is uncommon that the hypoxic drive would be suppressed in the prehospital setting and if the patient's respirations diminish, the solution is to assist the patient's ventilations, not decrease the oxygen his tissues need.

TABLE 16-6	Indications for Administration of Oxygen

Indications for Administration of Oxygen

- Cardiac or respiratory arrest.
- Respiratory distress or respiratory failure.
- Any patient requiring assisted ventilations.
- Inadequate tidal volume.
- Respiratory rate < 8 or > 30.
- SpO_2 less than 95 percent.
- Patient has an altered mental status/decreased level of responsiveness.
- Patient complains of difficulty breathing/shortness or breath.
- Patient complains of chest pain.
- Other medical conditions that can cause hypoxia, such as seizures, stroke, overdose, toxic inhalation, and wheezing.
- Signs and symptoms of shock or severe internal or external bleeding.
- Major or multiple trauma.

IN THE FIELD

Your decision to administer oxygen should not rely solely on an adequate SpO_2 value. While a low value should be interpreted as hypoxia, a high value does not necessarily mean the tissues are receiving oxygen. In low perfusion states, there is no guarantee that the oxygen on the hemoglobin is reaching the peripheral tissue, and pulse oximetry does not measure the amount of hemoglobin present. Maximizing the concentration of oxygen in the blood may help in this situation.

Oxygen Equipment

In the prehospital setting, oxygen is supplied in small portable tanks called *cylinders* and large tanks in vehicles and in buildings. A cylinder has a pressure regulator that reduces the pressure to a level that is medically safe. A cylinder also has a flow meter that allows the amount of oxygen being delivered to be adjusted to the individual patient's needs.

Oxygen cylinders are typically filled to pressures equal to 2,000 pounds per square inch (psi). Your EMS service may have a specific minimum pressure level at which you must change or refill the cylinder, but in general, the minimum safe residual level is 200 psi. Oxygen cylinders should never be allowed to empty below this level. For long-distance interfacility transports, always calculate the amount of oxygen required for the duration of the trip and ensure you have an adequate supply.

Pressurized oxygen first passes through a regulator and then into an oxygen delivery device. The pressure regulator adjusts the 2,000 psi pressure of the cylinder down to a lower pressure that can be used to administer oxygen to the

patient. Typically, pressure is regulated down to 30 to 70 psi. On portable tanks (E size or smaller), the pressure regulator is connected directly to the tank. An oxygen-specific fitting consisting of two pins on the regulator ensures that medical-grade oxygen is being used. A plastic washer or gasket is inserted between the oxygen cylinder stem and the regulator to ensure a seal between them to prevent a high-pressure oxygen leak. Larger tanks utilize valves connected directly to the tank. When attaching any regulator, the tank should be briefly opened prior to fitting the regulator to clear any debris from the point of connection.

A flow meter is connected to the regulator to allow for the adjustment of oxygen flow to the patient. There are two basic types of flow meters. One consists of a graduated tube in which a metal ball is elevated by the flow of oxygen to indicate the rate. Because the readings are affected by gravity, you are more likely to see this type of regulator in the hospital, where it is fixed to the wall, than in the prehospital setting. In the prehospital setting, the flow meter/regulator combination consists of a gauge that displays the amount of oxygen in the tank in psi and a second gauge or dial that shows the liter flow per minute. Most flow meters used in prehospital care allow delivery of up to 25 L/min. However, in most instances, a flow rate of 15 L/min provides concentrations of oxygen approaching 100 percent, depending on the delivery device. Oxygen masks and cannulas and ventilation devices are connected to the low-pressure outlet on the oxygen regulator. Some regulators also have a high-pressure outlet.

A number of pressurized medical gases are used in health care settings. Always ensure the gas you are administering is, in fact, oxygen. There are several ways to confirm this. An oxygen cylinder is green or silver with a green band, is labeled that it contains oxygen, and accepts only an oxygen regulator.

Oxygen Safety

Safety is a prime consideration when administering oxygen. Always take into account the following safety considerations:

- *Oxygen enhances combustion when exposed to fire.* Avoid open flame or sparks when administering oxygen. Never allow smoking near an oxygen cylinder and avoid metal tools that might produce a spark. Take care to avoid leaks that might lead to high oxygen concentrations in an enclosed space because this can be a serious a fire hazard. Make sure connections are tight and that disposable gaskets have been replaced with each cylinder change. Turn off the main cylinder valve when the cylinder is not in use.

- *Oxygen is a pressurized gas.* A crack or break in a pressurized metal cylinder can cause the cylinder to become a deadly missile. Secure oxygen cylinders appropriately. Never stand a cylinder upright without a proper securing device and never drop or drag a tank. Your service or oxygen supplier must follow manufacturer's recommendations and regularly conduct hydrostatic testing on oxygen cylinders to ensure tank integrity.

- *Petroleum products can react with oxygen.* Avoid using grease or adhesive tape on oxygen cylinders or regulators.

Oxygen Delivery Devices

Aside from administering supplemental oxygen during positive pressure ventilation, you can administer oxygen to spontaneously breathing patients using either a nasal cannula or a variety of face masks (Table 16-7). The most common type of face mask used in the prehospital setting is a nonrebreather mask, although a simple face mask or Venturi mask may be used on occasion.

Nonrebreather Mask

A nonrebreather mask allows delivery of high concentrations of oxygen because of its oxygen reservoir bag and simple flaps that act as one-way valves to direct both oxygen flow and the patient's exhaled air (Figure 16-41). A nonrebreather mask connected to 15 L/min of oxygen can provide concentrations of oxygen approaching 100 percent.

Because a one-way valve on the front of the mask allows only a minimal amount of ambient air to enter the mask, the plastic bag that acts as an oxygen reservoir for the mask must always be inflated before the mask is placed on the patient's face. During use, carefully monitor the reservoir to ensure that in remains inflated. An empty oxygen tank can lead to asphyxia in a patient wearing a nonrebreather mask. A flow rate of 12 to 15 L/min is required to keep the oxygen reservoir full as the patient inhales from it. When the patient exhales, the one-way valve on the front of the mask allows expired air to exit the mask but prevents ambient air from being pulled in during inspiration. A one-way valve between the mask and the oxygen reservoir allows oxygen to enter the mask, but does not allow expired air to enter the reservoir.

TABLE 16-7	**Comparison of Oxygen Delivery Devices**	
Device	**Flow Rate (in L/min)**	**Oxygen Concentration Delivered**
Nasal cannula	1–6 (rates over 4 L/min are irritating to nasal mucosa; usual prehospital flow rate is 2 to 4 L/min)	24–44 percent
Simple face mask	6–10	35–60 percent
Venturi mask	4–8	25–60 percent
Partial rebreather mask	5–10	40–60 percent
Nonrebreather mask	10–12 (flow rate must be adequate to keep reservoir bag inflated)	95 percent
Bag-valve-mask device	12–15	>95 percent

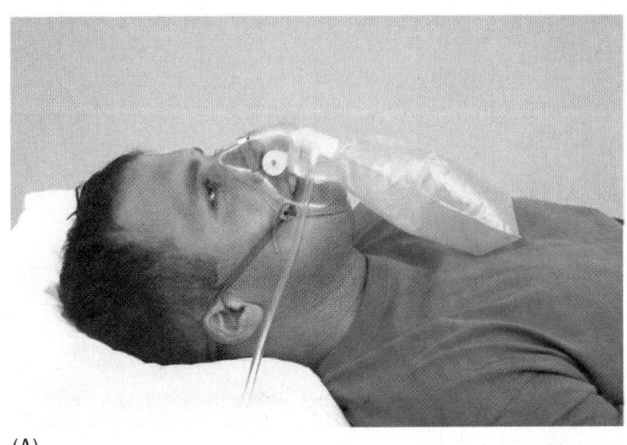

(A)

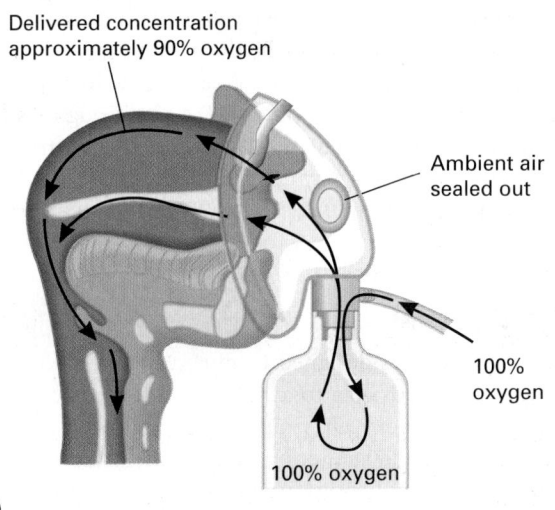

Delivered concentration approximately 90% oxygen

Ambient air sealed out

100% oxygen

100% oxygen

(B)

FIGURE 16-41

(A) A nonrebreather mask. (B) Cutaway view of a nonrebreather mask.

A nonrebreather mask is a good choice for patients who have adequate ventilations but who need a high concentration of supplemental oxygen. A nonrebreather mask must never be used on a patient with inadequate ventilation; use a bag-valve-mask device to assist ventilations and deliver oxygen. Patients having significant respiratory distress, who are in shock, or who otherwise are suspected of having general hypoxia or localized ischemia should generally receive oxygen by nonrebreather mask.

Past practice included providing oxygen by nonrebreather mask to patients with suspected acute coronary syndrome (ACS). The American Heart Association 2010 guidelines cite inadequate evidence to support the routine use of oxygen for patients with uncomplicated ACS whose SpO_2 is 94 percent or higher (American Heart Association, 2010). As mentioned, oxygen is a vasoconstrictor and can potentially decrease perfusion to ischemic tissues in high concentrations. However, you must follow your protocols for treatment.

A potential downside to a nonrebreather mask is that some patients feel suffocated by having something placed over the mouth and nose. Reassurance can often calm the patient and allow him to accept the mask. However, if the patient is made agitated or anxious by the mask, a nasal cannula should be used.

A partial rebreather mask is similar to a nonrebreather mask but has no one-way valve in the opening to the reservoir bag. It can deliver 40 to 60 percent oxygen at a flow rate of 6 to 10 L/min. Because there is no one-way valve, the patient will rebreathe some of his exhaled air.

Nasal Cannula

A nasal cannula consists of a length of oxygen tubing that resembles a lasso and has two short prongs that are placed in nares to deliver oxygen (Figure 16-42). It is a low-flow device that provides oxygen concentrations between 24 and 44 percent at flow rates between 4 and 6 L/min. In order to successfully deliver oxygen by nasal cannula, the patient must be able to breathe through his nose. For example, a nasal cannula would not be effective for a patient with a broken nose who cannot move air through his nasal passages. Nasal cannulas are a good choice for patients who complain of mild dyspnea and who have no more than mild hypoxia (SpO_2 between 90 and 95 percent) on room air.

Venturi Mask

A Venturi mask is designed to mix specific amounts of ambient air and oxygen to achieve specific, relatively low concentrations of oxygen (Figure 16-43). Venturi masks are typically used for longer-term oxygen administration in patients with COPD. Venturi masks either have an adjustable port or interchangeable fittings designed to deliver different oxygen concentrations.

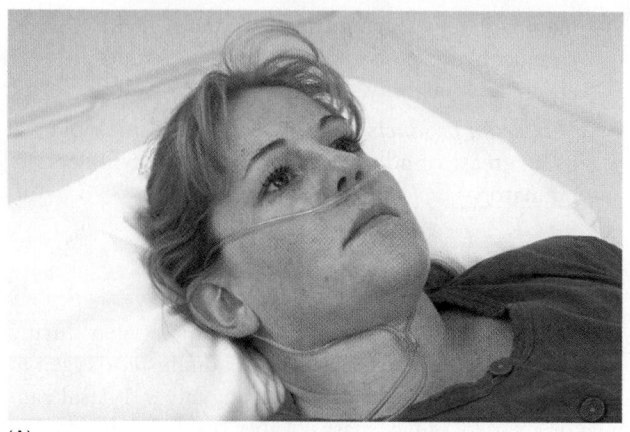
(A)

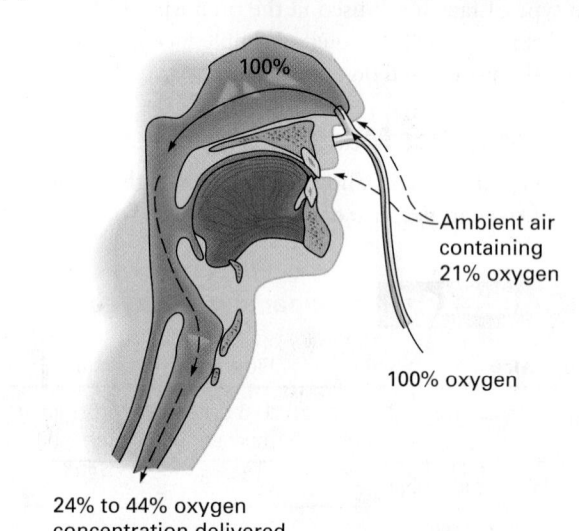
(B)

FIGURE 16-42

(A) A nasal cannula. (B) Cutaway view of a nasal cannula.

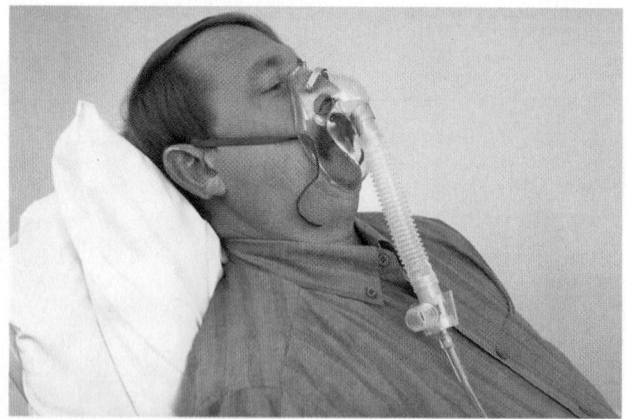

FIGURE 16-43

A Venturi mask.

Simple Face Mask

A simple face mask does not have one-way valves or a reservoir bag. This mask delivers lower concentrations of oxygen at a flow rate of 6 to 10 L/min. Actual concentrations of oxygen delivered vary greatly depending on respiratory rate, mask fit, and the amount of room air mixed with ventilations.

Tracheostomy Mask

A tracheostomy mask is used to provide supplemental oxygen to patients who have a tracheostomy tube or stoma and who do not require positive ventilation (Figure 16-44). The mask is a small cuplike device that is placed over the tracheostomy tube or stoma. An amount of 8 to 10 L/min of oxygen provides adequate oxygenation using these masks.

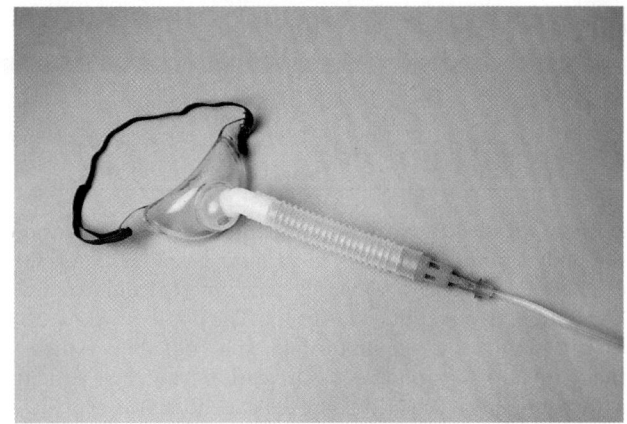

FIGURE 16-44

A tracheostomy mask. (© Carl Leet)

CASE STUDY WRAP-UP

Clinical-Reasoning Process

Brian and Tiffany recognize immediately that Mr. Campbell is in respiratory failure. Their general impression is that he is exhausted with an altered mental status and other signs of hypoxia. They recognize that, although the patient's airway is open, ventilation and oxygenation are inadequate to meet the patient's metabolic needs. Without immediate intervention, the patient will continue to deteriorate. Brian calls for additional manpower so he and Tiffany can devote their full attention to Mr. Campbell's treatment.

Because Mr. Campbell is severely hypoxic and unable to follow commands, he is not a candidate for CPAP. Brian hands Tiffany a bag-valve-mask device as he connects it to the oxygen cylinder. Tiffany positions herself behind Mr. Campbell and quickly explains to him that she is going to place a mask on his face to help him breathe. She seals the mask against his face and begins delivering positive pressure ventilations, synchronizing her ventilations with the patient's to provide better tidal volume than the patient can obtain himself.

Tiffany and Brian realize that bagging will be minimally effective because of bronchoconstriction indicated by wheezing breathing sounds. However, they also realize that they cannot stop assisting the patient's ventilations to administer an albuterol treatment. Fortunately, their service carries a small-volume nebulizer that they can use in conjunction with a bag-valve-mask device. As Tiffany continues bagging the patient, Brian sets up the device and obtains a baseline set of vital signs. As anticipated, the patient's SpO_2 remains low despite bagging with supplemental oxygen and administering the bronchodilator. "He is satting at 79 percent," Brian tells Tiffany, referring to the patient's SpO_2.

When the engine company arrives, Brian works with his colleagues to ready the stretcher for immediate transport. As Mr. Campbell is being loaded into the ambulance, Brian stays behind to talk briefly to Mrs. Campbell. As soon as Brian returns with additional patient history, a member of the engine company begins driving the ambulance toward the closest emergency department. En route, Brian inserts an IV and completes a secondary assessment of the patient. After speaking to the medical director, the EMTs prepare an albuterol treatment to be connected to the bag-valve-mask device.

The transport is short and the patient's status does not change significantly. Both Brian and Tiffany anticipate the need for further ventilatory support and expect that the ED physician will intubate the patient when they arrive. They continuously monitor the patient closely, knowing that respiratory and cardiac arrest are very real possibilities.

At the hospital, Tiffany delivers an oral report while Brian assists in transferring the patient over to the trauma room bed.

Care for this patient was limited. After identifying a primary assessment problem, the crew took immediate action to control the patient's airway, assist ventilations, and provide supplemental oxygen. The secondary assessment and patient history was not ignored. It was addressed after the primary issues were taken care of. Brian and Tiffany identified the underlying cause of respiratory failure as an exacerbation of the patient's COPD and implemented a beta$_2$ agonist to promote bronchodilation and improve alveolar ventilation. The crew's quick and accurate problem solving and interventions prevented the patient from deteriorating further during transport.

CHAPTER REVIEW

Chapter Summary

Without an adequate airway, ventilations, and oxygenation, the body cannot perform even its most basic task: normal cellular metabolism. Without adequate internal and external respiration, hypoxia quickly ensues. The body can compensate only for a short time through anaerobic metabolism. In a patient with spontaneous circulation, your first patient care priorities are ensuring that the patient has an open airway, adequate ventilation, and adequate oxygenation. You have a variety of skills and tools available to help you assess the patient's oxygenation status and to provide interventions when needed.

You must be able to quickly determine, through the scene size-up and primary assessment, whether the patient has adequate or inadequate breathing. Immediate problems with the patient's airway and breathing are addressed in the primary assessment. You may use a variety of manual airway maneuvers and basic airway adjuncts, FBAO maneuvers, suction, oxygen, and a bag-valve-mask device at the point to restore and maintain the patient's airway, ventilation, and oxygenation. In some patients, a more definitive airway and method of ventilation are required. You may use a Combitube, supraglottic airway, FROPVD, CPAP, or ATV to assist in airway management and ventilation.

The secondary assessment provides additional information about the quality of the patient's airway, breathing, and oxygenation. Finding a correctable underlying cause for the patient's impaired airway and breathing, such as unresponsiveness due to hypoglycemia or narcotic overdose, or impaired ventilation due to bronchospasm, are preferable to continued airway management. An alert patient can protect his airway better than you can protect it with mechanical devices. Artificial ventilations are not successful when the airways are so constricted that air cannot move in and out of the lungs.

Airway management techniques, positive pressure ventilation, and oxygen administration are not without undesired consequences. Although each of those methods and devices must be used when indicated, you also must ensure that you are applying them correctly to minimize complications. Being more aggressive than indicated can have a negative impact on patient outcomes. The goal of airway management, positive pressure ventilation, and oxygen administration is to prevent hypoxia. There are a variety of different strategies to achieve this goal. Always use the findings of your patient assessment and good clinical judgment to select the most appropriate therapy for each patient.

Review Questions

Multiple-Choice Questions

1. Which one of the following findings would differentiate respiratory distress from respiratory failure?

   a. Increased respiratory rate
   b. Accessory muscle use
   c. Altered mental status
   d. Wheezes on auscultation

2. A low level of oxygen in the body tissues is known as:

   a. hypoxia.
   b. dyspnea.
   c. hypocapnia.
   d. apnea.

3. Pulse oximetry measures the amount of:

   a. hemoglobin.
   b. oxygen dissolved in the blood.
   c. oxygen bound to hemoglobin.
   d. carbon dioxide bound to hemoglobin.

4. Which one of the following is a common complication of positive pressure ventilation?

   a. Hypertension
   b. Increased preload to the heart
   c. Gastric distention
   d. Hypercapnia

5. When compared to an adult, the larynx of a child is:

   a. more superior.
   b. more inferior.
   c. wider below the glottic opening.
   d. more rigidly held in place.

6. Normal capnometry values range from _____ mmHg.

   a. 20 to 40
   b. 35 to 45
   c. 65 to 80
   d. 90 to 100

7. Of the 500 mL average tidal volume, about _____ mL remains in the anatomic dead space.

   a. 75
   b. 150
   c. 275
   d. 350

8. Which one of the following best describes how far to insert a rigid suction tip?

   a. To the level of the carina
   b. Only as far as you can see
   c. Until the flange rests on the patient's lips
   d. Until a gag reflex is stimulated

9. When using positive pressure to ventilate an apneic adult patient with a pulse, you should ventilate once every _____ seconds.
   a. 5 to 6
   b. 6 to 10
   c. 10 to 12
   d. 12 to 20

10. Which one of the following is the most appropriate way to achieve the desired tidal volume when using a bag-valve-mask device on an infant?
    a. Use an infant-size bag.
    b. Use an adult-size bag but ventilate only until you see the chest begin to rise.
    c. Ventilate at a rate of 60 per minute.
    d. Do not exceed a volume of 100 mL/kg.

11. Which one of the following oxygen delivery devices provides the highest concentration of oxygen?
    a. Simple face mask
    b. Partial rebreather
    c. Venturi mask
    d. Nonrebreather mask

12. Which one of the following abnormal airway sounds indicates partial upper airway obstruction?
    a. Stridor
    b. Wheezing
    c. Crackles (rales)
    d. Rhonchi

13. For a conscious adult patient with a mild foreign body airway obstruction, the preferred method of management is:
    a. a blind finger sweep to remove the object.
    b. suction with a wide-bore catheter.
    c. to allow him to expel it on his own.
    d. a series of abdominal thrusts.

14. Which one of the following describes preferred management of an unresponsive infant with a foreign body airway obstruction?
    a. Chest thrusts
    b. Back blows and chest thrusts
    c. Abdominal thrusts
    d. Blind finger sweep

15. When your medical director says you should use a supraglottic airway device, you should select a(n):
    a. oropharyngeal airway.
    b. Combitube.
    c. laryngeal mask airway.
    d. endotracheal tube.

Critical-Thinking Questions

16. What should you look for to determine if a patient is likely to be hypoxic?

17. What signs should you look for to determine if a patient with spontaneous breathing requires assistance with a bag-valve-mask device?

18. How would you determine if a patient is a candidate for continuous positive airway pressure (CPAP)?

19. What will you look for to determine if your positive pressure ventilations are effective?

20. How would you troubleshoot to find the cause of poor positive pressure ventilations?

21. What are some considerations in deciding whether you should use a nasal cannula or a nonrebreather mask to deliver oxygen to a patient?

22. What are the consequences of allowing your oxygen cylinder to be completely emptied while you have a patient on a nonrebreather mask?

23. Explain how aggressive positive pressure ventilation can be detrimental to a patient.

References

American Heart Association. (2010). 2010 American Heart Association guidelines for cardiopulmonary resuscitation and emergency cardiovascular care. *Circulation, 122,* S640–S861.

Laryngeal Mask Airway Company. (2010). *Instruction manual.* Retrieved November 19, 2010, at http://www.lmaco.com/unique.php

McSwain, N. E., Salomone, J. P., & Pons. P. T. (Eds.). (2007). *Prehospital trauma life support* (6th ed.). St. Louis, MO: Elsevier.

17

Resuscitation: Managing Shock and Cardiac Arrest

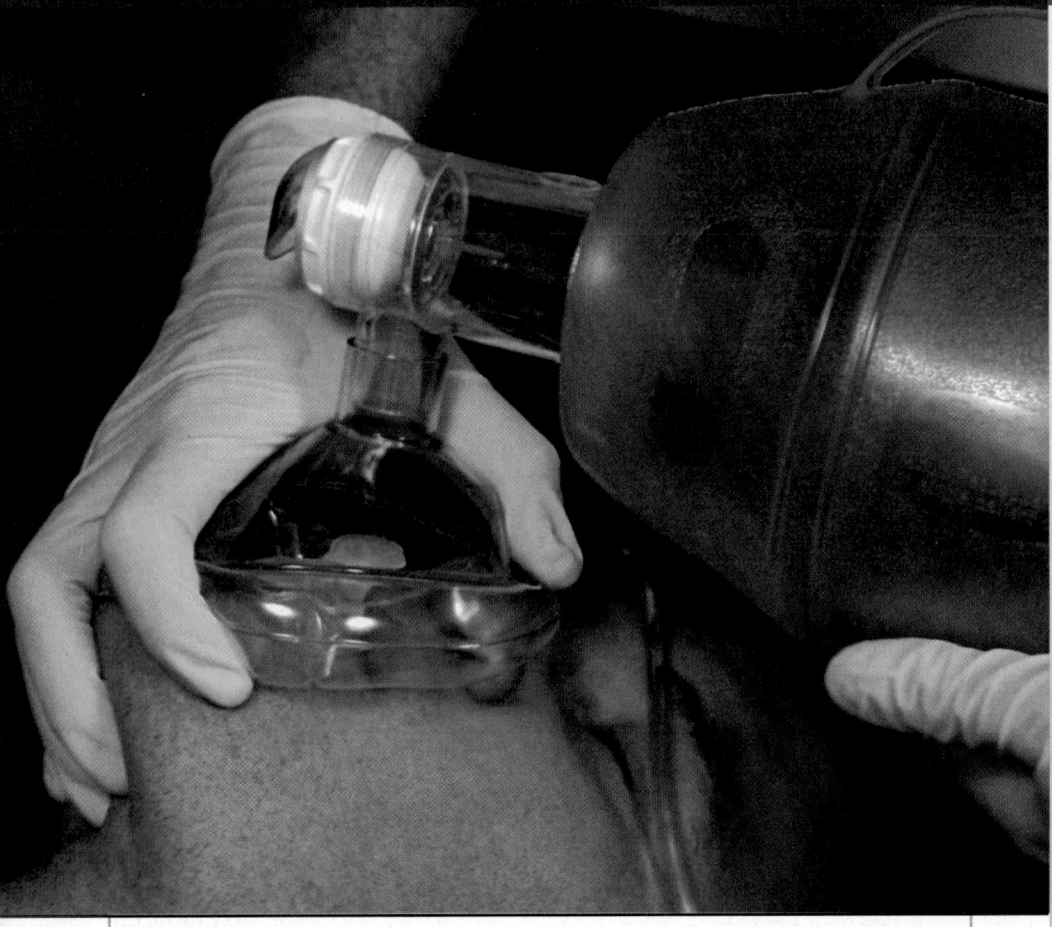

Content Area: Assessment

Advanced EMT Education Standard: Applies fundamental knowledge of the causes, pathophysiology, and management of shock, respiratory failure or arrest, cardiac failure or arrest, and postresuscitation management.

Objectives

After reading this chapter, you should be able to:

17.1 Define key terms introduced in this chapter.

17.2 Identify situations in which you should withhold resuscitative attempts.

17.3 Explain each of the links in the Chain of Survival of cardiac arrest.

17.4 Explain the importance of early defibrillation in cardiac arrest.

17.5 Explain the rationale for the "push hard and push fast" approach to CPR.

17.6 Describe the features, functions, advantages, disadvantages, use, and precautions in the use of automatic external defibrillators (AEDs).

17.7 Compare and contrast ventricular fibrillation, ventricular tachycardia, asystole, and pulseless electrical activity.

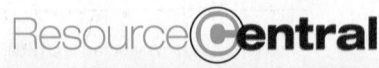

Resource **Central**

To access Resource Central, follow the directions on the Student Access Card provided with this text. If there is no card, go to www.bradybooks.com and follow the Resource Central link to Buy Access. Under Media Resources, you will find:

• *Cardiac Arrest.* See common causes and how to quickly recognize the signs of cardiac arrest.

• *Shock.* Learn the most common causes of shock.

• *Shock Management.* Review the signs and symptoms of hemorrhage and techniques to help you manage it.

CASE STUDY

Advanced EMTs Mary Campbell and Grace Gene are cleaning and restocking their ambulance when they hear the dispatcher request their unit. "Unit 144, respond to 1854 County Road 375 East, the Fitness-Pro Gym, for a 45-year-old man in cardiac arrest. CPR is in progress." Acknowledging that they are en route, Mary and Grace depart for the scene.

Problem-Solving Questions

1. What should Mary and Grace anticipate as possible causes of cardiac arrest?
2. How should they prioritize their interventions once they arrive at the scene?
3. What factors are likely to affect the patient's outcome? What can Mary and Grace do to influence those factors?

17.8   Describe the safety precautions to be taken to protect yourself, other EMS providers, the patient, and bystanders in resuscitation situations.

17.9   Given a series of cardiac arrest scenarios involving infants, children, and adults, demonstrate appropriate assessment and resuscitative techniques, including the integrated use of CPR, AEDs, airway management, and ventilation.

17.10   Explain the purpose and procedure for reassessing patients in shock and cardiac arrest.

17.11   Given a cardiac arrest scenario, make decisions regarding transport and requesting advanced life support (ALS) backup.

17.12   Demonstrate assessment and management of a postcardiac arrest patient with return of spontaneous circulation (ROSC).

17.13   Explain the importance of AED maintenance, EMS provider training and skills maintenance, medical direction, and continuous quality improvement in the Chain of Survival of cardiac arrest.

17.14   Discuss special considerations in the use of an AED in patients with cardiac pacemakers and implanted cardioverter–defibrillators.

17.15   Discuss the use of mechanical CPR devices.

17.16   Demonstrate effective mechanisms for controlling external hemorrhage.

17.17   Discuss the indications, contraindications, complications, and administration of fluids to patients in cardiac arrest and hemorrhagic shock.

17.18   Discuss the use of the pneumatic antishock garment (PASG) in patients with hemorrhagic shock.

17.19   Discuss current trends and research in resuscitation and shock management.

Introduction

Shock, respiratory failure and arrest, and cardiac failure and arrest all result in the final common pathway of inadequate perfusion to maintain cellular metabolism. There are many underlying causes of those conditions, but they share the same initial prehospital care priority: restoring the conditions for aerobic cellular metabolism. The series of interventions used to manage those patients is called **resuscitation.**

When resuscitation is required, it means a patient's life hangs in the balance. Resuscitation scenes necessitate quick action and are often stressful. The keys to success are to understand resuscitation priorities, maintain focus on the priorities of the situation, have well-practiced skills, and apply your skills critically to meet the patient's immediate needs. Algorithms can provide direction for care, but cannot account for the unique aspects of each situation. Resuscitation requires teamwork. Establishing a team leader is important, but no one's ego must get in the way of ensuring the patient's best chances of survival. Everyone must be able to make suggestions without fear of reprisal and everyone must be willing to listen to suggestions. Everyone must review each resuscitation situation to assess opportunities for learning and improved patient care.

Pathophysiology of Shock

Shock is sometimes described as a momentary pause in the act of dying. It is the result of a physiologic insult that poses a threat to cellular perfusion. The body has remarkable compensatory mechanisms, but they are not unlimited. When the underlying problem, such as blood loss or damage to the myocardium, is too severe, the body's compensatory mechanisms are inadequate to maintain cellular perfusion. Without medical intervention to restore perfusion, the patient will die.

Ideally, intervention occurs before cellular death begins. In some cases, resuscitation restores perfusion in the short term, but cellular death leads to organ failure and death within days. Sometimes, despite immediate access to the best medical care, the patient cannot survive the underlying problem. It is not possible to know in the prehospital setting the point at which cellular death begins or the point at which irreversible organ damage has occurred. You must provide the highest quality care to every patient in shock.

Hypoperfusion

Perfusion is adequate when each cell in the body receives the blood supply it needs to provide oxygen and nutrients for metabolism and to remove metabolic wastes. At its most basic level, perfusion requires three conditions, as follows:

- Adequate onloading of oxygen to the hemoglobin in red blood cells
- Adequate transportation of the oxygen-carrying red blood cells to the tissues
- Adequate offloading of oxygen for use at the cellular level

In order for the cardiovascular system to provide the three conditions needed for perfusion, the heart must be functioning as a pump, the blood vessels must provide peripheral vascular resistance by maintaining a certain degree vasoconstriction, and there must be a sufficient volume of blood with adequate oxygen-carrying capacity.

Shock is a state of hypoperfusion that occurs when any condition interferes with delivery of oxygen to the cellular level. In the initial stages of shock, the signs and symptoms reflect the body's attempts at compensation. The body's ability to compensate for challenges to the cardiovascular system is remarkable, but in the end it is temporary at best. In later stages, signs and symptoms reflect the consequences of inadequate tissue perfusion.

Mechanisms of Shock

The mechanisms that lead to shock are categorized as hypovolemic, distributive (vasogenic), cardiogenic, obstructive, and respiratory/metabolic. Within each of the categories, there are specific causes of shock (Figure 17-1, Table 17-1). The recognition and management of respiratory failure/metabolic shock was discussed in Chapter 16.

Hypovolemic Shock

A sufficient volume of blood is required to maintain pressure within the vascular system to permit perfusion. Blood also is the transport medium for oxygen, nutrients, chemical messengers, drugs, and wastes. *Hypovolemia* results from an absolute decrease in vascular volume from any cause, and is a common cause of shock in the prehospital setting. Hypovolemia can result from either medical problems or trauma.

Significant blood loss results in both overall volume loss and loss of oxygen-carrying capacity. Specifically, this is called *hemorrhagic shock*. Hemorrhagic shock can occur from medical causes, such as gastrointestinal tract bleeding, or from traumatic injury (Figure 17-2).

Hypovolemia also occurs when body fluids are lost from excessive vomiting or diarrhea, inadequate fluid intake, or extensive burns. It also can occur due to loss of fluid into the interstitial spaces, which can occur when there is increased vascular permeability, as in anaphylaxis or overwhelming infection (sepsis). In those cases, although hypovolemia contributes to shock, the primary mechanism is vasodilation.

Progression of Hemorrhagic Shock

A description of the progression of hemorrhagic shock presents an overall pattern of the homeostatic response to shock in general, in which the failing component of perfusion results in compensation by the functioning components of perfusion (Figure 17-3). When blood volume decreases, cardiac preload decreases, resulting in decreased cardiac output. The decreased cardiac output translates to a decrease in blood pressure. The decreased blood pressure is detected by baroreceptors in the carotid arteries. As a result, the sympathetic nervous system and the renin–angiotensin system are activated.

When the sympathetic nervous system is activated, two adrenal medullary hormones—epinephrine and norepinephrine—are secreted. Cells with $alpha_1$, $beta_1$, and $beta_2$ receptors respond to epinephrine resulting in a fight-or-flight response, then norepinephrine provides additional $alpha_1$ stimulation and a lesser amount of $beta_1$ stimulation. Blood vessels constrict and the heart rate and force of contraction increase to maintain blood pressure. The respiratory rate increases slightly to increase oxygenation.

The effects of the renin–angiotensin system are less immediate than those of the sympathetic nervous system. Overall, the complex mechanism of the renin–angiotensin system prevents further fluid loss and causes vasoconstriction. (See Chapter 8 for a review.)

The early signs of shock represent the body's attempt to compensate for blood loss. Sympathetic nervous system stimulation results in diaphoresis and anxiety. Peripheral vasoconstriction decreases circulation to the skin, resulting in pale, cool skin and thready peripheral pulses, yet the blood pressure remains normal as long as significant fluid loss is not ongoing. As fluid loss continues, the body can no longer compensate and blood pressure, as well as perfusion to the vital organs, decreases.

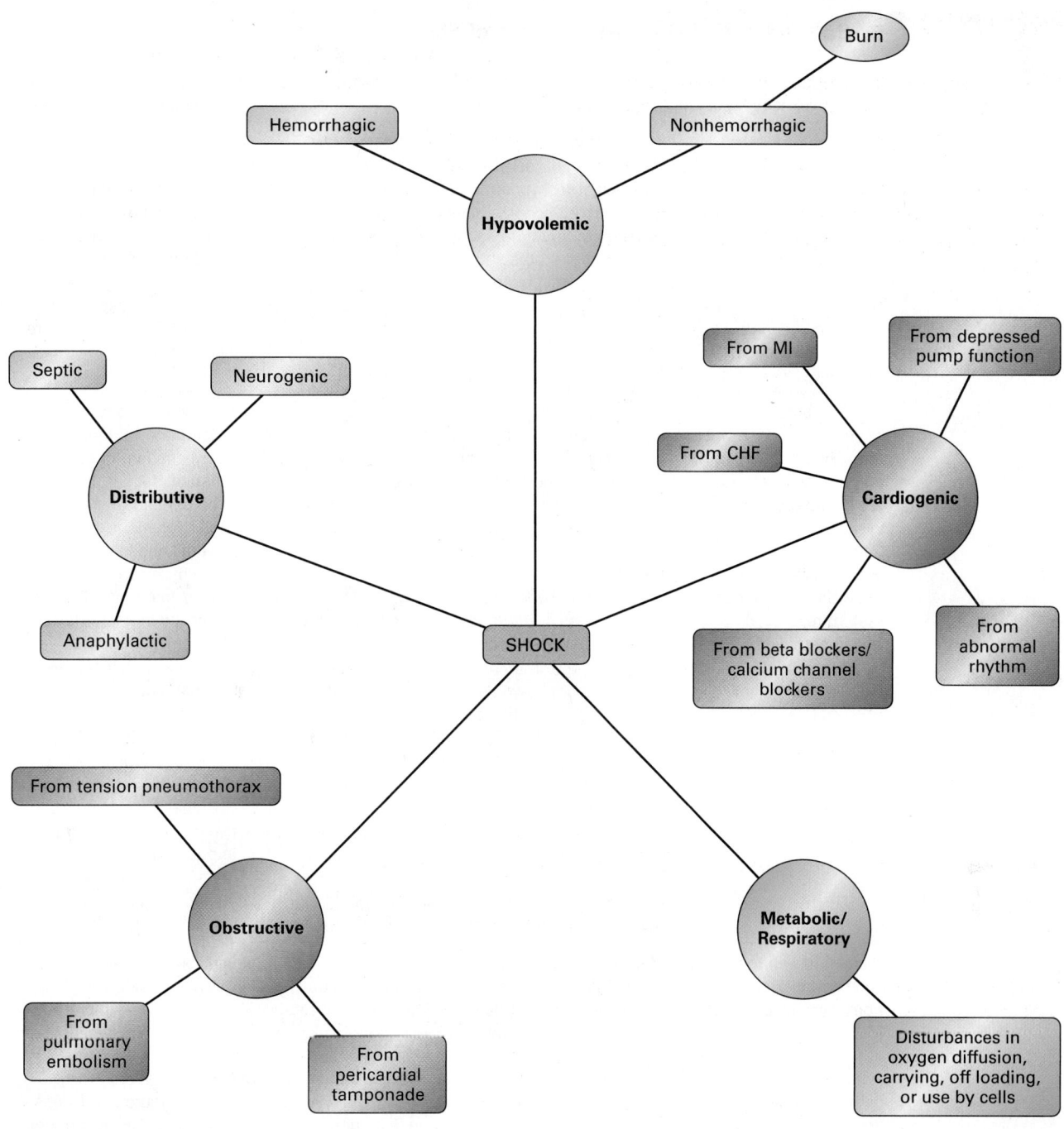

FIGURE 17-1

Mechanisms of shock.

Stages of Blood Loss and Phases of Shock

Hemorrhagic shock is classified into four stages by the signs and symptoms that occur at given percentages of volume loss (Table 17-2). Physiologically, shock can also be classified as compensated, decompensated, and irreversible (Table 17-3). At the tissue level, shock occurs in three phases: ischemic, stagnant (correlates with irreversible shock), and washout (Table 17-4).

In the initial stages of blood loss, both the precapillary and postcapillary sphincters—the smooth muscle at each

IN THE FIELD

Shock does not begin with hypotension. Hypotension means the patient has transitioned from compensated shock to decompensated shock. You must know in what circumstances to anticipate shock and actively search for its early signs and symptoms. Pregnant women can be in shock with few signs because placental circulation is compromised to maintain the mother's perfusion, despite significant blood loss.

TABLE 17-1   Comparing and Contrasting Types of Shock

Type of Shock	Description and Pathophysiology	Signs and Symptoms	Management
Hypovolemic	Fluid loss from dehydration, burns, or blood loss results in decreased vascular volume. The body attempts to maintain cardiac output and perfusion by increasing the heart rate and peripheral vascular resistance.	Early signs and symptoms include thirst; anxiety; slight tachycardia; cool, pale skin; and slight tachypnea. As shock progresses, the patient becomes diaphoretic, hypotension occurs, tachycardia and tachypnea increase, and mental status changes (confusion, agitation, decreased responsiveness).	Ensure an open airway, adequate ventilation, and oxygenation. For hemorrhagic shock, control external bleeding. Consider the need for fluid replacement in the prehospital setting. Transport to the nearest hospital capable of providing the care the patient needs.
Distributive	Blood volume is normal but cannot be distributed throughout the body for perfusion because the capacity of the vasculature is increased. Causes include sepsis, anaphylaxis, and loss of sympathetic nervous system regulation of vasoconstriction.	Anaphylactic shock: There may be a history of exposure to an antigen (bee sting, medications, etc.), or the patient may have edema, dyspnea, hives, vomiting, abdominal cramps, or diarrhea. The airway may be obstructed by edema, and wheezing may be present. The patient is tachycardic and hypotensive. Mental status decreases in response to hypoxia and hypoperfusion. The skin may be mottled, rather than pale, and the patient may be diaphoretic. Septic shock: The patient may have a history of infection or have risk factors for infection, such as a Foley catheter or intravenous access. The patient is hypotensive and usually tachycardic, with altered mental status. The skin may be cool and mottled, and the patient may be hypothermic. Neurogenic shock: Occurs in the context of high spinal-cord injury. The patient is hypotensive, but the skin is warm and dry and the heart rate is normal. Mental status may be impaired, but often, perfusion is not profoundly impacted.	Ensure an open airway and adequate ventilation and oxygenation. In the prehospital setting, fluids may be beneficial to increase vascular volume. However, the overall need is to return the size of the vascular container to normal. This can be achieved in anaphylaxis by the administration of epinephrine, which causes vasoconstriction. In neurogenic shock, assess for accompanying hemorrhagic shock, based on the mechanism of injury. With spinal-cord injury above C5, the diaphragm is impaired and the patient may require positive pressure ventilation.
Cardiogenic	A problem with the heart, such as muscle death from myocardial infarction (death of 40 percent or more of the left ventricle), heart failure, or an abnormal heart rate decreases cardiac output.	May have signs and symptoms of ACS (chest pain or discomfort, dyspnea, nausea, vomiting), signs of pulmonary edema (crackles [rales], dyspnea), pale, cool, diaphoretic skin, altered mental status (confusion, syncope, decreased responsiveness), systolic blood pressure < 90 mmHg, varied heart rate depending on underlying cause, jugular venous distention, or cardiac dysrhythmia.	In addition to managing the airway and providing oxygen, ventilation may be improved in patients with pulmonary edema through the use of CPAP. Assist or provide positive pressure ventilations if necessary. IV fluids may help increase preload and increase cardiac output, but may also be poorly tolerated by patients with heart failure. Consult with medical direction concerning fluid administration.
Obstructive	There is a mechanical obstruction to blood flow, such as a pulmonary embolism, tension pneumothorax, or cardiac tamponade, that decreases venous return to the heart (preload).	The onset of signs and symptoms may be abrupt, and may include severe dyspnea, altered mental status, hypotension, tachycardia, and jugular venous distension. In tension pneumothorax, breath sounds will be decreased or absent, initially on the injured side, but later on both sides.	Manage the airway, ventilation, and oxygenation. IV fluids may temporarily increase preload, but the underlying cause must be corrected.

end of a capillary bed—constrict (Figure 17-4). Blood is shunted away from peripheral capillary beds. This is the ischemic phase of shock, in which the peripheral tissues do not receive adequate perfusion. The cells of these tissues cannot participate in aerobic metabolism. Energy production is reduced and lactic acid accumulates in the tissues. However,

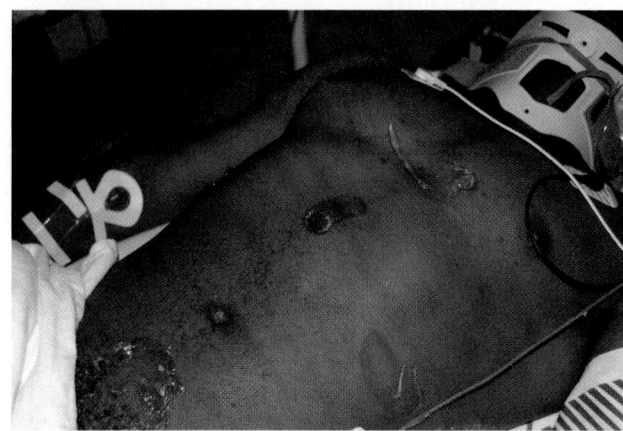

FIGURE 17-2

A patient with penetrating trauma and probable internal bleeding. (© Edward T. Dickinson, MD)

TABLE 17-2	**Classification of Hemorrhage**

CLASSIFICATION OF HEMORRHAGE

Class	Blood Volume Loss in a 70-kg Adult	Signs
Class I Hemorrhage	Up to 15 percent (750 mL)	Usually well tolerated; can lead to mild tachycardia
Class II Hemorrhage	15–30 percent (750–1,500 mL)	Moderate tachycardia, pale skin, delayed capillary refill
Class III Hemorrhage	30–40 percent (1,500–2,000 mL)	Tachycardia Failure of compensation Hypotension
Class IV Hemorrhage	40–50 percent (2,000–2,500 mL)	Profound hypotension End-organ failure (e.g., bradycardia, anuria) Death

CYCLE OF HEMORRHAGIC SHOCK

TRAUMA

Loss of blood volume from the vascular space decreases cardiac output and pressure in the aorta, carotid, and peripheral arteries.

Decrease in the delivery of oxygen and glucose to cells and the removal of carbon dioxide.

Baroreceptors trigger hormone release and sympathetic nervous system stimulation to increase cardiac output, blood pressure, and perfusion.

Further decrease in blood volume, perfusion, and blood pressure leads to brain tissue death, multiple organ failure, and eventual patient death.

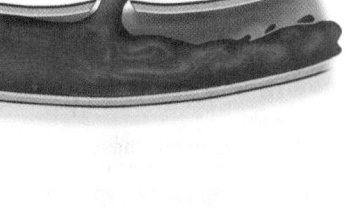

Heart rate and contractility increase, vessels constrict, respiratory rate increases, and urine output decreases in an attempt to compensate and increase cardiac output, blood pressure, and perfusion.

Patient becomes unresponsive, heart rate severely increases and then drops dramatically, blood pressure decreases significantly and may not be obtainable, respirations decrease and become inadequate.

Brain becomes ischemic and medulla fails, causing a severe drop in perfusion and blood pressure.

Continued volume loss overwhelms compensatory mechanisms and blood pressure falls, tachycardia and tachypnea further increase, peripheral pulses are extremely weak or absent, mental status deteriorates.

Patient exhibits tachycardia, weak peripheral pulses, decreased mental status, tachypnea, and pale, cool and clammy skin.

FIGURE 17-3

The cycle of hemorrhagic shock.

TABLE 17-3	Compensated and Decompensated Shock

COMPENSATED SHOCK	
Sign	**Physiologic Explanation**
Anxiety	Response to epinephrine from sympathetic nervous system response (fight-or-flight reaction).
Normal blood pressure	Peripheral vasoconstriction shunts blood away from capillary beds and increases peripheral vascular resistance; heart rate increases to maintain cardiac output.
Tachycardia (100–120 per minute)	Decreased stimulation of baroreceptors results in increased heart rate via sympathetic nervous system stimulation of the SA node.
Pulse quality	Thready in extremities, becoming weak.
Slight to moderate tachypnea (20–30/min)	Increased stimulation of respiratory center in medulla in response to increased $PaCO_2$ and decreased PaO_2.
Pale, cool skin; skin is moist	Vasoconstriction in response to epinephrine and norepinephrine from sympathetic nervous system to divert remaining volume from nonvital to vital areas of the body.
DECOMPENSATED SHOCK	
Sign	**Physiologic Explanation**
Altered mental status (agitation, confusion, decreased responsiveness)	Cerebral hypoperfusion.
Hypotension	Blood loss exceeds ability of compensatory mechanisms (>30 percent blood volume loss); failure of compensatory mechanisms due to hypoxia and acidosis.
Marked tachycardia (>120; at 140 and above, patient's circumstance is dire); may progress to bradycardia	Continued response to hypotension; bradycardia as heart becomes hypoperfused and fails.
Pulse quality	Weak, becoming absent.
Air hunger (tachypnea [>30/minute]/ hyperpnea); progresses to respiratory failure	Acidosis, hypoxia.
Skin	White, waxy, cold.

TABLE 17-4	Ischemic, Stagnant, and Washout Phases of Shock

Ischemic Phase	Stagnant Phase	Washout Phase
Selective vasoconstriction shunts blood flow away from capillary beds, causing tissues served by those capillary beds to become ischemic. The precapillary sphincter of the arteriole leading into the capillary bed and the postcapillary sphincter of the venule leaving the capillary bed are both constricted. The affected tissues must use anaerobic metabolism, resulting in acidosis.	Progressing hypoxia and acidosis result in failure of the precapillary sphincters. Blood enters the capillary bed, but the postcapillary sphincter remains constricted. Blood stagnates in the capillary beds. Shock is considered irreversible at this point (McSwain, Salomone & Pons, 2007).	Further hypoxia and acidosis cause the postcapillary sphincters to fail. Accumulated acids and microemboli formed in the capillary beds are now released into the circulation, worsening acidosis.

Source: This article was published in Publication, Prehospital Trauma Life Support, 6ed, Salomone, J.P., Pons, P.T.; Copyright Elsevier.

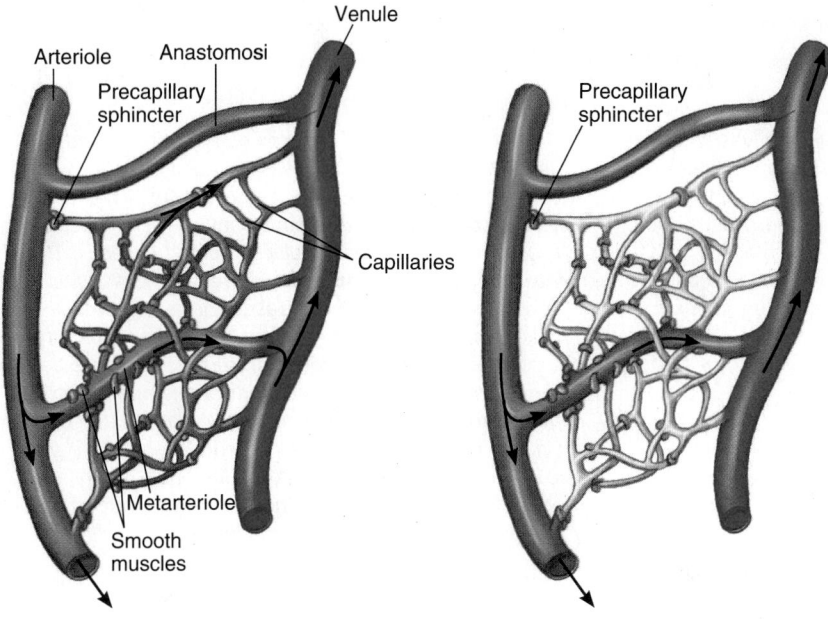

(A) Blood directed to the tissue.

(B) Blood bypassing the tissue.

FIGURE 17-4

(A) Normal microvascular perfusion. (B) Peripheral capillary beds are bypassed in response to sympathetic nervous system stimulation.

it is vasoconstriction, in part, that allows the body to compensate for shock.

Different tissues of the body have different levels of ischemic sensitivity. Skeletal muscle may survive a few hours with inadequate perfusion, while the brain and heart cannot survive more than several minutes without adequate perfusion. The body's compensatory mechanisms are aimed at shunting blood away from tissues with less sensitivity to **ischemia** while maximizing perfusion of tissues with greater ischemic sensitivity. If perfusion is restored quickly, shock is reversible at this stage.

As blood loss continues, the body's compensatory mechanisms are no longer sufficient to provide perfusion to organs with greater ischemic sensitivity. Despite increased heart rate, blood volume is inadequate to maintain blood pressure. If shock is not corrected, lack of energy and decreased pH lead the precapillary sphincters to fail. Blood then enters the capillary bed, but cannot flow through because the postcapillary sphincter is still constricted. This is the stagnant phase of shock. As a result of stagnation, blood cells clump together.

As tissue hypoxia and acidosis progress, the postcapillary sphincter fails. In the washout phase, the accumulated wastes and microemboli (formed during stagnation) are flushed from the capillary beds and into the circulation. The results are devastating, leading to additional tissue and organ damage.

In the presence of continued hypoxia and acidosis, the cellular sodium/potassium pump fails. The accumulation of sodium within cells results in movement of water into the cell, causing the cell membrane to rupture. As cells die, their lysosomes release potent lysozymes, which are destructive enzymes. Lysozymes break down adjacent cell membranes, causing further tissue injury and death. Once a critical number of the cells of any organ die, the organ fails and the patient enters irreversible shock. In some cases, death occurs immediately. In other cases, the patient is resuscitated to the point of immediate survival, but dies hours to days later from complications, such as **acute respiratory distress syndrome (ARDS)**, **multiple organ dysfunction syndrome (MODS)**, or **disseminated intravascular coagulation (DIC)**.

IN THE FIELD

The speed at which shock progresses depends upon the rate of blood loss and the patient's ability to compensate. The body of a patient with massive bleeding from a lacerated aorta will not have time to even try to compensate before death occurs from exsanguination. Patients with such severe injuries die immediately, or within the first few minutes, prior to EMS arrival. Unfortunately, such severe injuries are not survivable. Even if the injury occurred in a hospital surgical suite, the patient would die.

Patients with significant bleeding may have lost a large volume of blood prior to your arrival, presenting in decompensated shock with unresponsiveness, hypotension, and a barely present carotid pulse. Yet, immediate intervention and quick access to surgical facilities might allow the patient to survive. Other patients may have only subtle signs of compensatory shock, which could be mistaken for activation of the fight-or-flight response from fear. If the mechanism of injury or nature of the illness warrants it, patients must be suspected of being in, or at high risk for developing shock.

Pediatric Care

Pediatric patients initially compensate well for a loss in volume and can maintain normal blood pressure despite significant blood loss. The increased energy required to fuel compensatory mechanisms is soon depleted, though, because children have less stored glycogen than adults. Decompensation occurs quickly. Suspicion of shock and early recognition are vital to the pediatric shock patient's survival.

Distributive Shock

Under normal conditions, both the sympathetic and parasympathetic nervous systems exert control over the diameter of blood vessels. When more vasoconstriction is required to maintain blood pressure, the sympathetic nervous system dominates. When a greater degree of vasodilation is needed to maintain normal blood pressure, the parasympathetic nervous system dominates. When vasoconstriction occurs, the vascular container gets smaller. Given the same amount of fluid, an increase in blood pressure occurs.

As you just learned, the body compensates for decreased vascular volume through vasoconstriction to maintain blood pressure. Conversely, when vasodilation occurs the vascular container gets larger, yet holds the same amount of fluid, leading to a decrease in blood pressure. Usually, this is a normal homeostatic mechanism, which allows the body to regulate the blood pressure according to its needs at any given time. When a pathologic state results in excessive vasodilation, the blood pressure decreases below normal, resulting in hypoperfusion. The amount of blood is the same, but it cannot be distributed adequately to the tissues, thus leading to distributive shock (Figure 17-5).

Among the mechanisms that can lead to *distributive shock* are anaphylaxis, sepsis, and loss of sympathetic nervous system control over the vascular system.

Anaphylactic Shock

In *anaphylaxis* (severe allergic reaction), substances that cause tissue inflammation are released from basophils in the bloodstream and mast cells in the tissue. (See Chapter 8 for a review of the immune response.) Among the substances released is *histamine*, which causes vasodilation. The chemical mediators of anaphylaxis also can lead to airway edema and obstruction, vomiting, and diarrhea. Normally, vasodilation is a functional part of the body's inflammatory response. However, vasodilation is limited to the area of injury in order to increase blood flow to the area and promote healing. In anaphylaxis there is widespread, systemic vasodilation that substantially increases the size of the vascular container. Increased permeability of the capillaries to fluid accompanies vasodilation. The resulting loss of fluid into the interstitial spaces reduces vascular volume, compounding the effects of vasodilation.

Geriatric Care

Both the effects of aging on organ systems and medications taken for cardiovascular disease can impair compensatory mechanisms of older adults. A diseased or aged cardiovascular system cannot efficiently respond to the increased demands placed upon it in shock. The maximum heart rate, strength of contraction, and ability to vasoconstrict are all decreased. Beta blockers, ACE inhibitors, and other medications can further impair the response of the cardiovascular system. Therefore, elderly patients and patients on these medications may not exhibit tachycardia as an early sign of shock, nor the expected pale, cool, diaphoretic skin. Patients over the age of 55 years are at greater risk for death due to injury and shock. Accordingly, the threshold for transportation to a trauma center is lower.

Septic Shock

Septic shock occurs due to the combined effects of the body's aggressive response to massive infection and effects of the pathogen itself. In some cases, bacterial pathogens release toxins that result in vasodilation and increased capillary permeability. As with anaphylactic shock, the widespread vasodilation accompanying septic shock is largely a result of an exaggeration of the body's normal immune response.

Neurogenic Shock

Neurogenic shock is a result of impaired sympathetic nervous system function. The sympathetic nerves that control blood vessel diameter exit from the cervical and thoracic spinal cord. With high spinal-cord injury, the pathway between the spinal cord and the peripheral vascular system is severed. The effects of the parasympathetic nervous system dominate, resulting in unopposed vasodilation.

IN THE FIELD

Septic shock is often missed in the prehospital setting and its diagnosis and treatment can be delayed in the hospital emergency department. Septic shock has a high mortality rate, and recent research has highlighted the need for rapid recognition and management of septic shock. One reason for failing to recognize septic shock in the prehospital setting is that, unlike other patients with infectious illnesses, patients with sepsis may not have a fever. In fact, heat loss from massive vasodilation and impairment of heat regulating mechanisms can leave these patients hypothermic. It is possible to measure blood lactate levels as an indication of septic shock. Although it is not yet a widespread practice, it is possible to measure lactate in the prehospital setting for early identification of septic shock. A pitfall is that lactate may also be elevated after a seizure, but an early lactate level can be a helpful clue in the ongoing assessment and care of the patient.

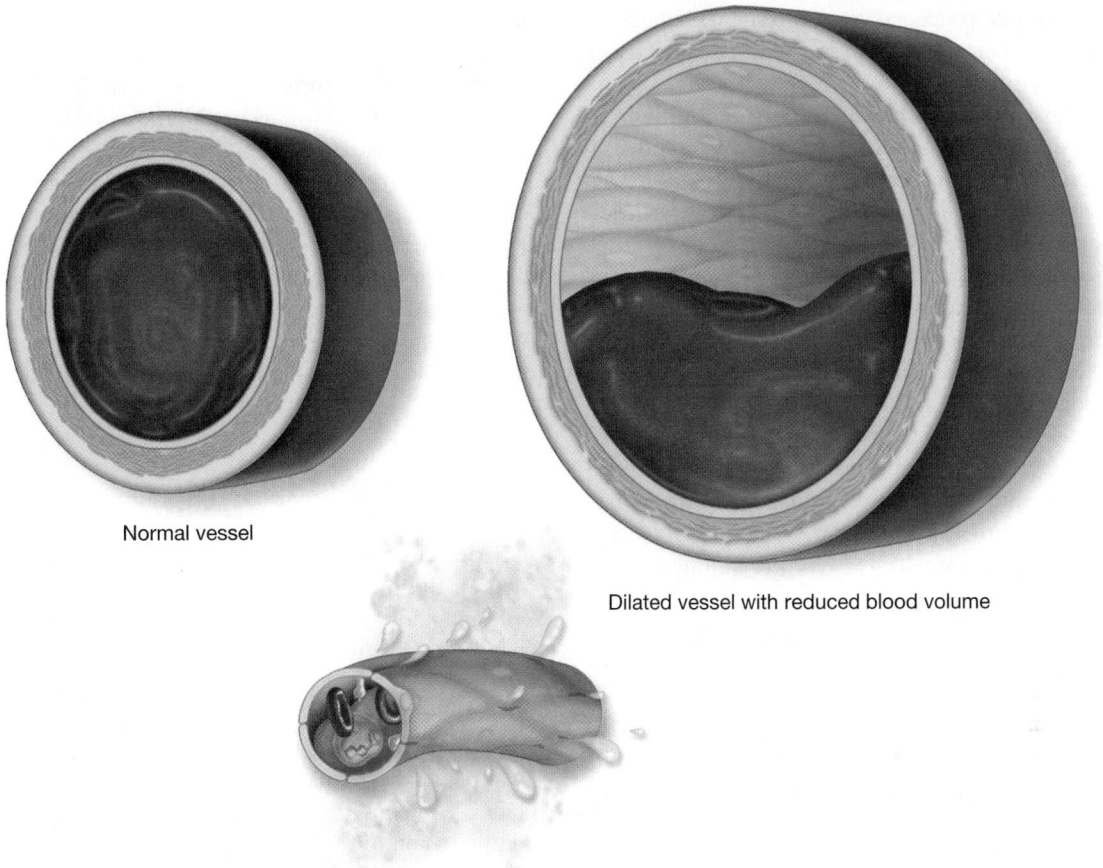

Normal vessel

Dilated vessel with reduced blood volume

Permeable capillaries

FIGURE 17-5

Distributive shock is caused by vasodilation and increased capillary permeability.

Distributive Shock Signs

The mechanisms that cause distributive shock prevent one of the body's primary compensatory mechanisms for shock: vasoconstriction. In septic and anaphylactic shock, other sympathetic nervous responses, primarily increased heart rate, are intact. Therefore, patients with those types of shock typically have tachycardia and may be diaphoretic. In neurogenic shock, the cardioaccelerator nerves, which arise from the thoracic spinal cord, cannot stimulate the SA node to increase the heart rate, which means that the body cannot compensate for decreased blood pressure by increasing cardiac output.

Because of the poor distribution of blood caused by vasodilation, patients can present with blotchy and mottled skin, in contrast to hypovolemic shock in which blood is shunted away from the surface, causing pale skin. Patients with neurogenic shock may present with warm, dry skin and a normal heart rate despite hypotension.

Cardiogenic Shock

When the heart's failure as a pump is the reason for inadequate perfusion, the patient is in *cardiogenic shock* (Figure 17-6). The ability of the heart to provide adequate output depends upon its rate and force of contraction. (Remember: CO = HR × SV.)

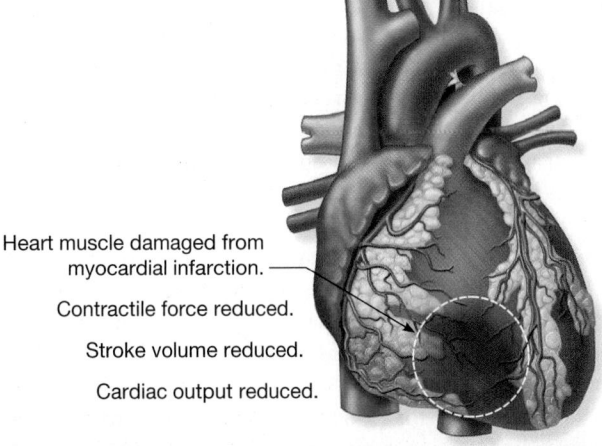

Heart muscle damaged from myocardial infarction.

Contractile force reduced.

Stroke volume reduced.

Cardiac output reduced.

FIGURE 17-6

Cardiogenic shock from myocardial infarction.

Physical damage of the myocardium, such as occurs in heart failure or acute myocardial infarction, can reduce the ability of the heart to contract and eject an adequate amount of blood with each contraction. The body's normal compensatory responses—increased peripheral vascular resistance (afterload) and increased heart rate—both increase the workload of the already impaired heart.

Although patients with heart failure can initially be hypertensive, the body cannot maintain this compensatory mechanism. The function of the heart becomes further impaired and hypotension ensues. When the left ventricle fails, it cannot accept the volume of blood being returned to the left side of the heart from the pulmonary vasculature. The pulmonary vasculature becomes congested and fluid is forced out of the capillaries under the increased hydrostatic pressure, resulting in pulmonary edema.

Cardiogenic shock also may occur when the electrical conduction system of the heart functions abnormally. Bradycardia can result in a decrease in blood pressure because the heart simply does not contract frequently enough to maintain pressure in the vascular system. Hypotension may occur when the rate drops to 60 per minute and the incidence of hypotension increases when the rate drops below 50 per minute. When bradycardia is due to increased parasympathetic nervous system stimulation by way of the vagus nerve, vasodilation may further impair perfusion.

In tachycardia, primarily at rates greater than 150 beats per minute, there is not sufficient time for ventricular filling between ventricular systoles. The stroke volume decreases, thereby decreasing cardiac output. A further increase in the heart rate will only decrease cardiac output more. Because the coronary arteries are only perfused during left ventricular diastole, the myocardium becomes ischemic at a time when its workload, and thus oxygen demand, is already increased.

Obstructive Shock

Obstructive shock occurs when there is some mechanism that mechanically creates an obstruction to blood flow to such a degree that cardiac output is significantly diminished. Among the causes of obstructive shock are pulmonary embolism, **cardiac tamponade**, and tension pneumothorax. When a massive pulmonary embolism (blood clot in the pulmonary arterial system) occurs, blood cannot flow through the pulmonary vasculature beyond that point. The more proximal the obstruction is to the right heart, the larger the size of the artery affected, and the more pulmonary circulation is impaired. In some cases, not one embolus, but multiple smaller emboli affect multiple branches within the pulmonary system.

The inability for blood to flow past the obstruction has two immediate consequences. First, gas exchange cannot occur in the affected areas of the lung, producing hypoxia and hypercarbia. Second, because blood cannot get past the arterial obstruction to the pulmonary venous circulation, blood does not return to the left side of the heart. Preload is decreased, thereby decreasing cardiac output.

In the case of cardiac tamponade, accumulation of fluid or blood within the pericardial sac compresses the volume of the heart chambers. Less blood can enter the heart,

decreasing cardiac output. Tension pneumothorax occurs when an injury to the lung allows a large amount of air to accumulate under pressure within the thoracic cavity. Initially, the alveoli of the lung on the affected side collapse and are unable to participate in ventilation and gas exchange. However, a large enough defect in the lung, such as a lacerated bronchus, allows more air to enter with each inspiration. As intrathoracic pressure increases, the low pressure of blood in the vena cava is unable to overcome the resistance and preload and cardiac output decrease. As structures in the mediastinum are shifted, both the vena cava and aorta may become obstructed, further decreasing cardiac output.

Assessing for Shock

A patient in shock always has signs and symptoms, but early in the process signs and symptoms may be subtle. They may not "jump out" at you. Instead, you must know when to anticipate shock and actively look for other indications of shock.

In all cases, there is some indication of hypoperfusion. Early in shock, some of the indications are indirect. For example, an increased heart rate is an indication that the body is compensating to maintain adequate blood pressure and perfusion of the brain and other vital organs. Yet, peripheral tissues are being hypoperfused. You must consider shock in the differential diagnosis of patients with tachycardia and look at other indications.

Scene Size-Up

Even before arrival at the scene, preliminary information from dispatch may lead you to anticipate a patient in shock (Figure 17-7). Upon arriving at the scene, as you look for hazards, assess the need for additional resources, and determine the number of patients, you will also get a general idea of the mechanism of injury. Gunshot and stab wounds, assaults, falls from a height, motor vehicle collisions, industrial incidents, and power tool injuries are some examples of mechanisms that increase suspicion of shock.

With medical patients, the nature of the illness begins to unfold as with clues at the scene and information from the patient and others. You may see or smell evidence of gastrointestinal bleeding, or the patient or family may offer a glimpse of the patient's history as you make initial contact. A history of heart failure, a sudden onset of difficulty breathing, or other information can provide immediate clues.

Obvious significant bleeding, pale or mottled skin, decreased level of responsiveness, and respiratory distress all contribute to a general impression of a patient in shock. Determine if the mechanism of injury is consistent with the potential for cervical spine injury. If it is, prepare to provide manual stabilization of the head and neck as you approach the patient. Double-check to ensure that your PPE is adequate to the situation.

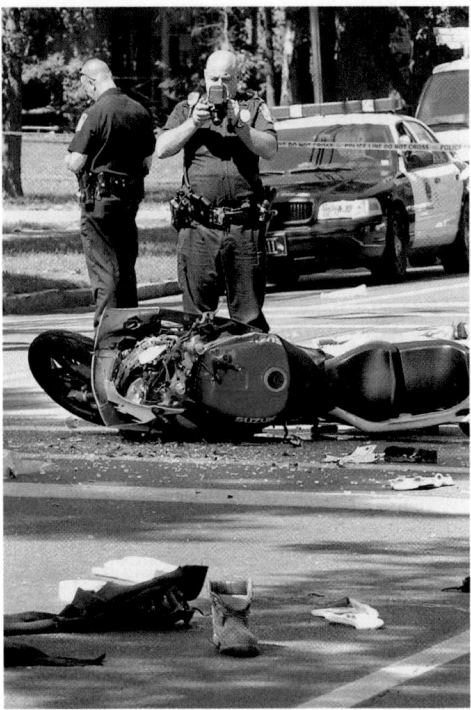

FIGURE 17-7

Look for indications of shock in the scene size-up.

(© CW McKean/Syracuse Newspapers/The Image Works)

Primary Assessment

Deliberately make note of the responsive patient's airway, breathing, and circulation. Does the patient have facial injuries that can jeopardize the airway? Is there blood in the airway? Is there swelling of the face or neck? Is the patient's voice hoarse? Does he appear dyspneic?

Intervene as needed to ensure an open airway and adequate ventilation and oxygenation. Anticipate vomiting. Position the patient to protect his airway and have suction available. Control significant external bleeding with direct pressure. In the occasional event that direct pressure is not effective, you must use additional methods to control significant, ongoing external bleeding.

For the patient who appears unresponsive, quickly confirm the level of responsiveness and determine if breathing is present. If breathing is absent, check the patient's carotid pulse. For the patient who is breathing, or who is not breathing but has a pulse, systematically assess and manage the patient's airway, breathing, and circulation. Use manual maneuvers, suction, and airway adjuncts as indicated to maintain the airway. Provide bag-valve-mask ventilations for the patient with inadequate ventilations, and give supplemental oxygen to all patients in, or at risk for, shock. For patients without a pulse, begin chest compressions and apply an AED.

Confirm your initial impression of the patient and establish priorities for treatment and transport. Patients in shock are critical and require hospital treatment without delay. However, appropriate steps to restore or maintain tissue perfusion must be carried out during preparation for transport.

Secondary Assessment

Follow the guidelines previously presented for determining the approach to secondary assessment. Patients in shock, whether from medical or traumatic causes, receive a rapid physical examination. Assess baseline vital signs, apply monitoring devices, and obtain a medical history. When indicated, such as in a patient with the potential for multisystems trauma, perform a head-to-toe physical exam.

Clinical Reasoning

You must engage in a process of clinical reasoning to determine the most likely underlying cause of shock and determine treatment beyond that initiated in the primary assessment. Physical exam clues are important. For instance, in hemorrhagic shock lung sounds are normal, but in heart failure they sound like wet crackles (rales).

The goal of treatment is to interrupt the progression toward decompensation and irreversible shock. Selecting the wrong treatment or inappropriate prioritization of treatment and transport can be detrimental to the patient. A patient with fluid loss from vomiting and diarrhea requires volume replacement with intravenous fluids. The same amount of fluid can be detrimental to the patient in hemorrhagic shock from a lacerated liver, or to the patient with heart failure.

Advanced interventions, such as starting an IV, are often best carried out during transport to prevent delays in reaching definitive care. But, in some cases, additional treatment may be warranted during preparation for transport. A case in which this might be considered is severe anaphylaxis, in which giving an initial dose of epinephrine can have an immediate impact on the patient's condition. In contrast, the patient in hemorrhagic shock or with a pulmonary embolism requires immediate hospital care.

Reassessment

Patients with conditions leading to shock can deteriorate rapidly. Vigilantly reassess the patient's level of responsiveness, airway, breathing, oxygenation, and circulation, and the effects of interventions. Use the information from reassessment to determine the overall trend in the patient's condition and make decisions about treatment.

Managing Bleeding and Shock

Untreated shock inevitably leads to death. Shock is a negative downward spiral that is not reversed on its own and requires intervention (McSwain, Salomone & Pons, 2007). The best treatment for shock is to prevent it. In the case of blood loss, simple interventions may be quite effective in preventing shock. In other cases, early recognition and interventions to restore and maintain tissue perfusion are fundamental to improving the patient's chances of survival.

Bleeding Control

In the patient with significant bleeding, the priorities are, after airway and breathing, stopping further loss of oxygen-carrying red blood cells, enhancing perfusion, and transporting the patient to the best available source of definitive care. Internal bleeding control requires medical or surgical treatment in the hospital. In most cases, external bleeding can be controlled by direct pressure in the prehospital setting. Occasionally, bleeding is too severe to be controlled with direct pressure, or the number of critically injured patients may require that bleeding is controlled by other means.

Do not neglect any external source of bleeding. In a multisystems trauma patient, a laceration to the arm may represent only small amount of the total bleeding. By itself, the bleeding from the laceration may not be enough to cause shock. But combined with bleeding from an injured liver or spleen, or from a long-bone fracture, this seemingly small amount of blood contributes to the total amount of blood loss. Blood cells from the same cardiovascular system are being lost regardless if they are flowing out of the patient's liver or out of his arm. By stopping bleeding from the arm, you keep more blood in the patient even though that bleeding is less severe than the bleeding in his liver.

Hemostasis

The body has an amazing and intricate process for responding to injury and stopping bleeding. The process of **hemostasis** occurs in three phases (Figure 17-8). In the vascular phase, the smooth muscle coat of the vessel constricts, narrowing the lumen of the vessel and reducing blood flow through it. In the next phase, platelets activated by exposure to tissue collagen from the injured vessel are attracted to the injured area and are able to adhere together to form a platelet plug. Finally, the coagulation cascade, which requires a

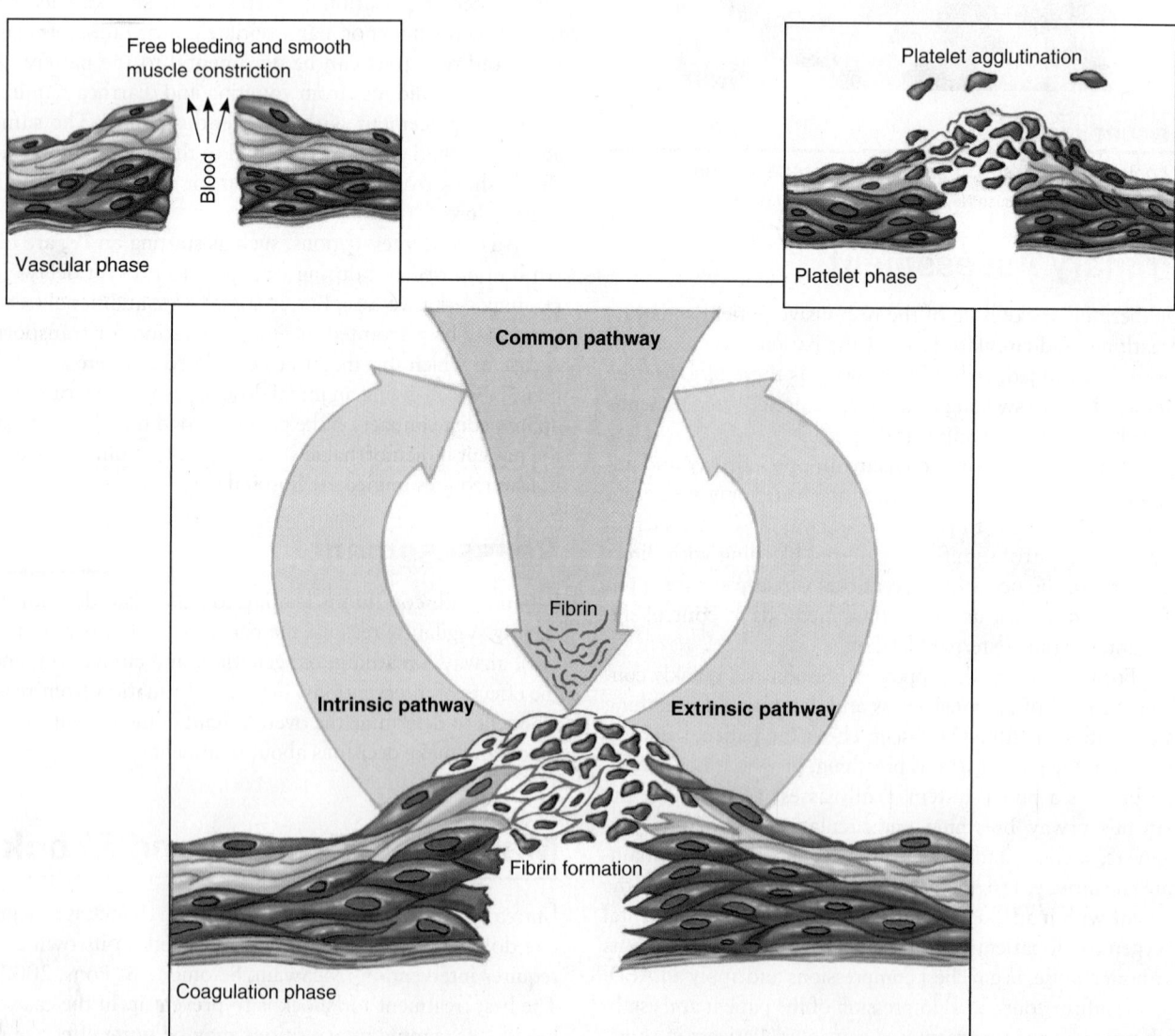

FIGURE 17-8

Steps of hemostasis.

number of circulating clotting factors, transforms the platelet plug into a stable fibrin clot.

In some cases, the body's hemostatic mechanisms are overwhelmed by the magnitude of the injury or impaired by drugs, illness, or other factors. The higher pressure of blood in the arterial system can interfere with formation of a platelet plug and clotting (Figure 17-9). Bleeding from injuries that cleanly cut across a vessel is more likely to respond to the body's hemostatic response (Figure 17-10). When the vessels are torn or crushed, their ability to constrict is impaired. Despite the lower pressure of blood in the venous system, blood loss from larger veins can be severe, because the large size makes formation of a platelet plug difficult.

A number of medications and dietary supplements can impair blood clotting (Table 17-5). In patients who are at risk of clot formation, this action is desirable, but it does place the patient at risk of bleeding that is difficult to control.

Direct Pressure

Direct pressure is best applied by placing a sterile, absorbent dressing over the wound and applying firm pressure using a gloved hand until bleeding is controlled (Figure 17-11). You should then secure the dressing in place using a pressure dressing. (See Chapter 35.) If the initial dressing becomes saturated with blood, place an additional dressing over the top of it. Removing the dressing in contact with the wound may disrupt blood clots that have begun to form. You can apply additional dressings, but too many dressings can decrease the amount pressure transmitted through them to the

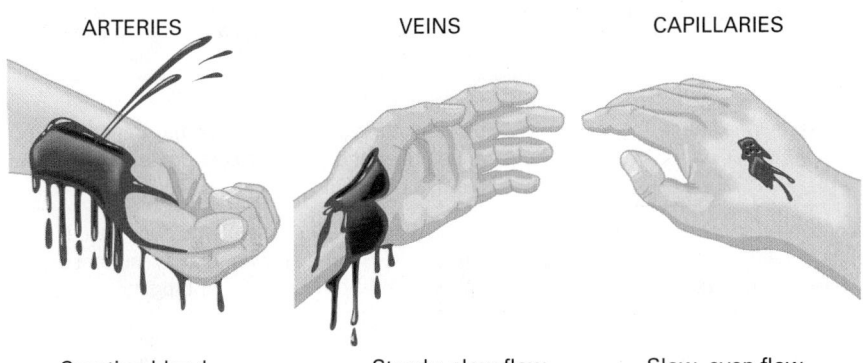

ARTERIES

Spurting blood.
Pulsating flow.
Bright red color.

VEINS

Steady, slow flow.
Dark red color.

CAPILLARIES

Slow, even flow.

FIGURE 17-9

Types of bleeding.

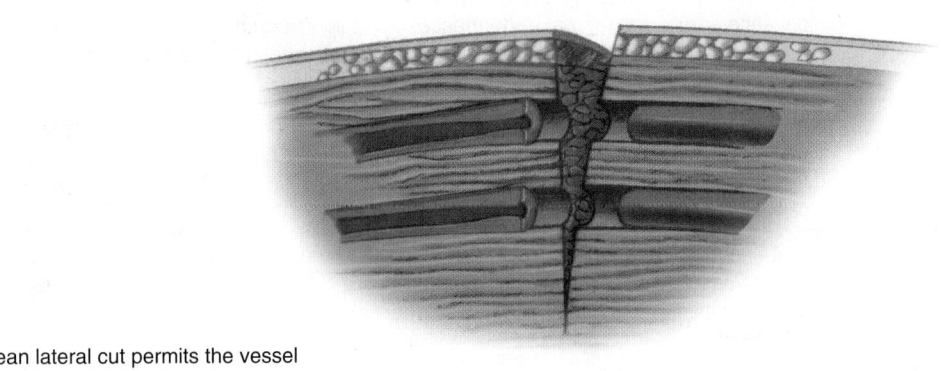

A clean lateral cut permits the vessel to retract and thicken its wall.

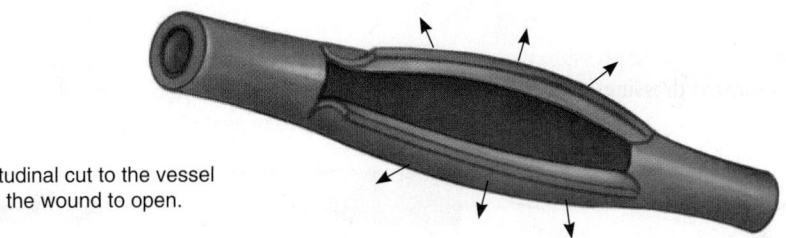

A longitudinal cut to the vessel causes the wound to open.

FIGURE 17-10

The type of injury to a vessel affects its ability to contract and slow bleeding.

TABLE 17-5	Medications and Supplements That May Affect Blood Clotting	
Medication/Supplement	**Use**	**Effects on Hemostasis**
aspirin	Over-the-counter analgesic and anti-inflammatory; used to inhibit platelet aggregation in patients at risk for ACS.	Reduces ability of platelets to clump together and form a platelet plug.
clopidogrel (Plavix)	Prescription platelet aggregation inhibitor.	Reduces ability of platelets to clump together and form a platelet plug.
dipyridamole (Persantine)	Prescription platelet aggregation inhibitor.	Reduces ability of platelets to clump together and form a platelet plug.
dong quai	Herbal supplement taken for many conditions, including menopausal symptoms.	Herbal and dietary supplements can reduce blood clotting on their own, or may interact with antiplatelet and anticoagulant drugs to increase the risk of bleeding.
feverfew	Taken for migraine headaches.	Herbal and dietary supplements can reduce blood clotting on their own, or may interact with antiplatelet and anticoagulant drugs to increase the risk of bleeding.
fish oil	Taken for omega-3 fatty acids to reduce the risk of cardiovascular disease.	Herbal and dietary supplements can reduce blood clotting on their own, or may interact with antiplatelet and anticoagulant drugs to increase the risk of bleeding.
garlic	Taken in concentrated form (oil, extract, capsules) for anti-inflammatory, effects on immune system, and to reduce the risk of cardiovascular disease.	Herbal and dietary supplements can reduce blood clotting on their own, or may interact with antiplatelet and anticoagulant drugs to increase the risk of bleeding.
gingko biloba	Taken to improve memory and concentration.	Herbal and dietary supplements can reduce blood clotting on their own, or may interact with antiplatelet and anticoagulant drugs to increase the risk of bleeding.
ginseng	Taken to relieve fatigue and stress and to enhance sexual and mental performance.	Herbal and dietary supplements can reduce blood clotting on their own, or may interact with antiplatelet and anticoagulant drugs to increase the risk of bleeding.
heparin	An injectable anticoagulant that interferes with the blood clotting cascade. Prescribed for a variety of conditions in which blood clotting may be increased.	Formation of fibrin clots is impaired.
warfarin (Coumadin)	Oral anticoagulant that interferes with the clotting cascade. Prescribed for a number of conditions in which blood clotting may be increased.	Formation of fibrin clots is impaired.

wound. If you are unable to maintain adequate pressure on the wound, remove some of the saturated dressings (not the one in contact with the wound).

Topical Hemostatic Agents

A variety of chemical and physical hemostatic agents are available to surgeons and have been used for many years in the surgical setting (Figure 17-12). The use of topical hemostatic agents is more recent in the prehospital setting

and there are few studies either supporting or refuting their effectiveness, safety, and feasibility in the prehospital setting. Therefore, availability and protocols for use vary from

IN THE FIELD

Direct pressure is the best way to control most bleeding in the prehospital setting.

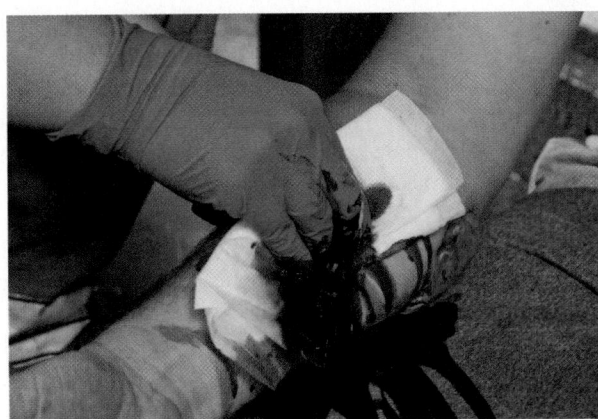

FIGURE 17-11

Direct pressure controls most external bleeding.

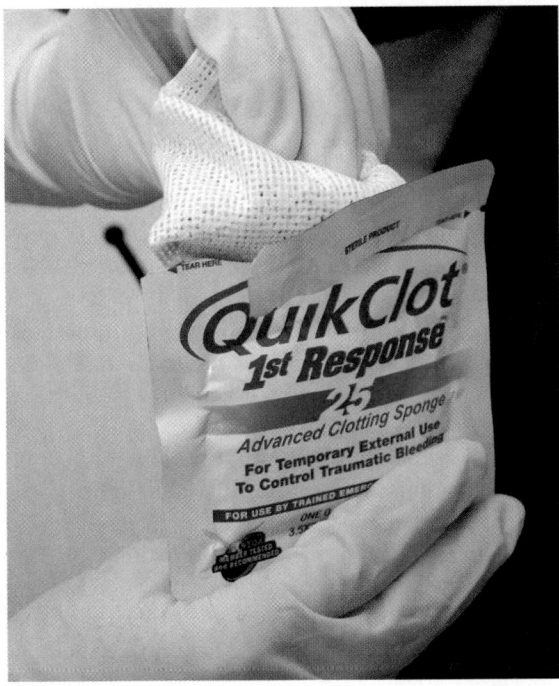

FIGURE 17-12

A topical hemostatic agent.

system to system. When used, topical hemostatic agents are an adjunct to direct pressure in the control of severe, ongoing external bleeding. There are three kinds of topical hemostatic agents available for use in the prehospital setting. HemCon is a dressing made with chitosan, a protein derived from shrimp shells. There has been some successful experience with HemCon on the battlefields of Iraq and Afghanistan. In addition to its hemostatic properties, HemCon has some antibacterial action. Although shellfish allergy is a contraindication to the use of chitosan, there have been no reports of cross-sensitivity to chitosan in patients with shellfish allergies to date (Achneck et al., 2010; McSwain, Salomone & Pons, 2007).

QuikClot is a mineral zeolite dressing derived from volcanic rock. The dressing absorbs water from blood, concentrating the elements needed for clotting. Earlier versions generated a significant amount of heat on application, although newer versions have been modified to avoid this complication. There have been mixed results in research of plant-based starch hemostatic agents, such as TraumaDex, and much of the research relies on animal studies (Gegel et al., 2010).

If protocols allow, you may apply the agents directly to the wound to help control bleeding. Improper use yields topical hemostatics ineffective. You must follow manufacturer's instructions for use of specific agents. The typical steps for application include wiping away pools of blood first, applying the dressing or other form of the agent to the wound, then continuing direct pressure.

Tourniquets

When bleeding is severe and ongoing despite direct pressure, a tourniquet can save the patient's life. A tourniquet is a wide band applied to constrict both venous and arterial blood flow (Figure 17-13). Tourniquets are used to control bleeding from extremity wounds by placing the tourniquet between the wound and the heart. Therefore, they are not appropriate to all sources of life-threatening bleeding. Tourniquets are applied as close to the wound as possible to limit the amount of tissue ischemia. You can use tourniquets for life-threatening hemorrhage either proximal or distal to the elbow or knee. Some sources have suggested that tourniquets should not be applied distal to the elbow or knee. However, the further the distance between the wound and the tourniquet, the greater the area of ischemic tissue and potential tissue damage (McSwain, Salomone & Pons, 2007).

There are a variety of commercially available tourniquets. However, in one recent study, none was found to be superior to an improvised tourniquet using a cloth (similar to a triangular bandage) with a windlass (Swan, Wright, Barbagiovanni, Swan, & Swan, 2009). When using a commercial tourniquet, follow the manufacturer's instructions.

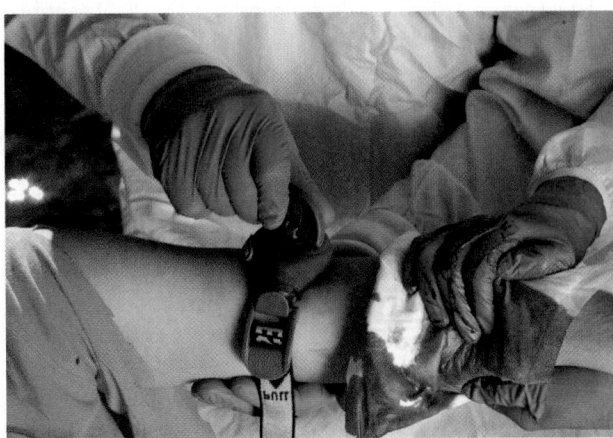

FIGURE 17-13

A commercial tourniquet.

The ideal material for a tourniquet is a wide material (approximately 1 to 4 inches) that will not cut into the patient's skin. For example, rope, twine, and wire are not appropriate materials. A folded cloth is an ideal material, but a belt can also work. A material that is too stretchy may not allow sufficient tightening of the tourniquet.

A windlass is a device that uses a handle to transfer mechanical energy to create leverage. In the case of a tourniquet, the cloth is wrapped around the extremity twice and tied with a half knot. An improvised handle, such as a sturdy stick about 6 to 8 inches long, is then placed on top of the knot. The ends of the cloth are then tied into a knot over the top of the stick. The handle is then twisted (like turning on a faucet) until the tourniquet is tight enough to control bleeding. Once bleeding has stopped, the handle must be secured in place to prevent the tourniquet from loosening.

It is often suggested that a blood pressure cuff can serve as an improvised tourniquet. You must be certain that there are no leaks in the tubing that would allow an air leak that allows pressure to decrease in the cuff over time. You must ensure that the valve on the cuff is securely closed and that the Velcro on the cuff overlaps sufficiently and is not worn, which would allow the cuff to suddenly release. In addition, most blood pressure cuffs are not large enough for use on the thigh or in patients with large extremities.

The larger the extremity, the greater the pressure you must apply to control bleeding. Tighten the tourniquet until bleeding stops and secure it. Attach a label (such as a piece of tape) on the tourniquet and write "TK" followed by the time the tourniquet was applied. Do not cover the tourniquet with bandages or clothing. It must be clearly visible upon arrival at the hospital. Frequently check to ensure that the tourniquet continues to control hemorrhage. Tourniquets have been left in place for up to 2 to 2½ hours without significant tissue damage (McSwain, Salomone & Pons, 2007). However, even with prolonged transport times, you must realize that saving the patient's life takes precedence over potential damage to the limb.

The application of a tourniquet can be painful for a patient who is alert, and analgesia should be considered for patients who are not in decompensated shock. If feasible, you should transport patients who have had a tourniquet applied to the highest level trauma center available.

Extremity Elevation and Arterial Pressure Points

Up until the past few years, extremity elevation and compression of proximal arterial pulse points were mainstays in teaching about bleeding control. Recently, both of the techniques have come into question because of lack of evidence for their effectiveness. Swan et al. (2009) found that, while enough pressure could be applied to the brachial artery at the medial arm and the femoral artery, blood flow quickly returned to distal areas. The brachial artery at the elbow and the popliteal artery were less accessible and more difficult to compress. Neither the Prehospital Trauma Life Support Committee (McSwain, Salomone & Pons, 2007) nor the **American Heart Association (AHA)** (2010) recommend the use of pressure points as a way of controlling bleeding.

Theoretically, elevating a distal extremity above the level of the heart while applying direct pressure should slow bleeding due to the effect of gravity. While there is no evidence showing that extremity elevation actually does contribute to bleeding control, this is not the same as saying that studies have shown it to be ineffective. However, keep in mind that bleeding from an extremity may be accompanied by an extremity fracture. Elevating an extremity with an unsplinted extremity can aggravate the injury and lead to increased bleeding. In addition, elevation may detract from the application of other, more important measures in the management of the patient with significant bleeding. The AHA (2010) no longer recommends the use of elevation as a method of bleeding control in its first aid guidelines. However, as an Advanced EMT, you must follow your protocols.

Intravenous Access and Fluid Administration

In a patient in shock, the first treatment priorities are managing problems with the airway, ventilation, and oxygenation, controlling bleeding, and preparing the patient for transport without delay to the most appropriate facility to manage his problems. Intravenous access is important for the in-hospital management of the patient, and sensible use of intravenous fluids may be of benefit to some patients during transport (Figure 17-14).

To understand why you must carefully consider intravenous fluid administration for the patient in hemorrhagic shock, recall that the blood must maintain specific concentrations of plasma and formed elements to do its job. Plasma is not simply water. While water is its major constituent, it contains vital electrolytes, proteins, chemical messengers, and other substances. When blood is lost, those substances

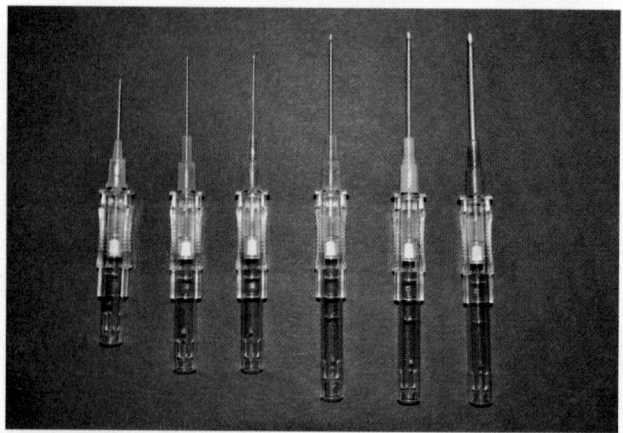

FIGURE 17-14

The greater the diameter of an intravenous catheter, the greater the rate of flow it can provide. (© Edward T. Dickinson, MD)

are lost, as well, and prehospital intravenous fluids cannot replace them. Among the proteins lost are blood-clotting factors and albumin. When intravenous fluid is added, the remaining blood is diluted. This means that blood loses oncotic pressure and cannot effectively maintain intravascular volume. (See Chapter 8.) Intravenous fluids will quickly leave the vascular space and enter the interstitial space. The clotting factors needed to stop ongoing bleeding are diluted in concentration, as well.

In the same manner, the concentration of red blood cells is decreased. The overall oxygen-carrying capacity is reduced and can only be replaced by the infusion of whole blood or packed red blood cells. Therefore, intravenous fluids may raise the blood pressure, but cannot solve the underlying problem of cellular ischemia and acidosis. The increase in blood pressure, along with the accompanying dilution of clotting factors and platelets, can increase bleeding.

The patient is already hypothermic and the addition of large volumes of intravenous fluids lowers his body temperature and taxes his metabolism even more. Even seemingly warm intravenous fluids still take heat from the body to raise their temperature to body temperature. Taking a further toll, the body's blood clotting mechanisms are impaired in the presence of hypothermia. The patient who has lost blood has lost heat. He can generate very little heat in the presence of anaerobic metabolism, and does so at the cost of acidosis.

The administration of intravenous fluids for patients in hemorrhagic shock (and for all patients) is guided by your protocols. In general, the current practice is to differentiate between patients in whom hemorrhage is ongoing and those in whom hemorrhage has been controlled. Only external hemorrhage can be controlled in the prehospital setting. Therefore, any patient with internal bleeding in the prehospital setting has uncontrollable bleeding. In patients with externally accessible bleeding, you can infuse intravenous fluids to increase the blood pressure to normal and maintain it. This does not mean administration of large amounts of fluid. You must monitor the intravenous infusions to avoid giving more than the amount needed to maintain the patient's blood pressure.

In patients with ongoing bleeding, intravenous fluids are administered with a goal of **permissive hypotension**. This means that you are trying to strike a balance between maintaining a level of perfusion without worsening the patient's situation through excessive fluid administration. A typical target systolic blood pressure in the patient in shock with ongoing bleeding is 80 to 90 mmHg. This is often

Pediatric Care

As a rule of thumb, pediatric patients are given 20 mL of intravenous fluid for each kilogram of body weight. If an adequate response is not achieved, a second bolus may be considered in consultation with medical direction.

Geriatric Care

Geriatric patients can easily be overloaded with intravenous fluids. Carefully monitor for signs of fluid overload, including assessing breath sounds for indications of pulmonary edema.

achieved by administering an initial bolus of 500 mL of isotonic crystalloid fluid (normal saline or lactated Ringer's solution). If the target blood pressure is not reached, an additional bolus of 500 mL is given.

In the patient with hemorrhagic shock and traumatic brain injury with suspected increased intracranial pressure, the mean arterial pressure must exceed the intracranial pressure sufficiently to allow cerebral perfusion. In those cases, the target systolic blood pressure is slightly higher: 90 to 100 mmHg (McSwain, Salomone & Pons, 2007).

Fluid Resuscitation in Nonhemorrhagic Shock

Shock is always best treated by reversing the underlying cause. The pathophysiology of various types of shock helps you understand the benefits and limitations of fluids in their treatment. That knowledge also helps you understand your protocols and anticipate orders from medical direction.

Patients in septic and anaphylactic shock have both distributive and hypovolemic components. Even in the hypovolemic component, the problem is not necessarily an overall loss of fluid, but movement from the vascular space to the interstitial space. In anaphylaxis, the administration of epinephrine causes vasoconstriction to reduce the vascular container size and reduce the increased permeability of capillaries that is allowing fluid to leak into the interstitial spaces. In this case, fluids are an adjunct to treatment with epinephrine.

Patients in septic shock may be dehydrated from the underlying infection, in addition to third-spacing of fluid and vasodilation. They can require large amounts of fluid administration, but the amount that should be delivered in the prehospital setting is not agreed upon. In contrast, the patient in cardiogenic shock may not be able to handle additional fluid load without developing pulmonary edema. If hypotension is caused by a slow heart rate, the

IN THE FIELD

You must never delay on the scene to establish intravenous access in a patient with hemorrhagic shock.

CASE STUDY (continued)

Advanced EMTs Mary and Grace arrive at FitnessPro Gym, where a 45-year-old man is reported to be in cardiac arrest with CPR in progress. A gym employee meets Mary and Grace at the door and leads them to the cardiovascular training area. On the way, she provides some initial information.

The patient, Frank Cutler, just joined the gym a few weeks ago to train for an upcoming marathon. He has not worked out regularly for several years and is obese. Despite being cautioned by his assigned personal trainer, he has been working out too hard for his current fitness level. Today, after about 10 minutes on the treadmill, he suddenly collapsed. Another gym member called out for help and found that Mr. Cutler was unresponsive and was making gasping attempts at breathing. Two gym employees arrived within seconds with an AED, while another called 911.

Problem-Solving Questions

1. What additional information do Mary and Grace need from the two employees who responded with the AED?
2. As the team leader, what does Grace need to communicate to her team, and how should she communicate it?
3. How does the information provided about the history of the present illness affect your ideas about the underlying cause of cardiac arrest and the patient's chances for survival?

administration of large amounts of fluid can, paradoxically, slow the heart even more. By increasing blood pressure, the carotid baroreceptors stimulate the cardiovascular center in the brain to slow the heart rate.

In obstructive shock, fluids can increase preload and temporarily increase cardiac output and blood pressure. But fluids do not treat the underlying problem and as the underlying problems advance, fluid administration will not be sufficient to overcome the problem. Neurogenic shock is temporary, though the spinal-cord injury may be permanent. Despite hypotension, perfusion may not be severely impaired.

Pneumatic Anti-Shock Garments

Pneumatic antishock garments (PASGs) are trousers with inflatable compartments (Figure 17-15). The device was originally thought to work by forcing blood from the legs and pelvis to the upper body, resulting in an autotransfusion of blood. Although most providers who used PASG

IN THE FIELD

Fluid overload can be detrimental to patients in shock. Consequences include worsening of heart failure, pulmonary edema, increased bleeding and impaired clotting in hemorrhagic shock, and electrolyte imbalances.

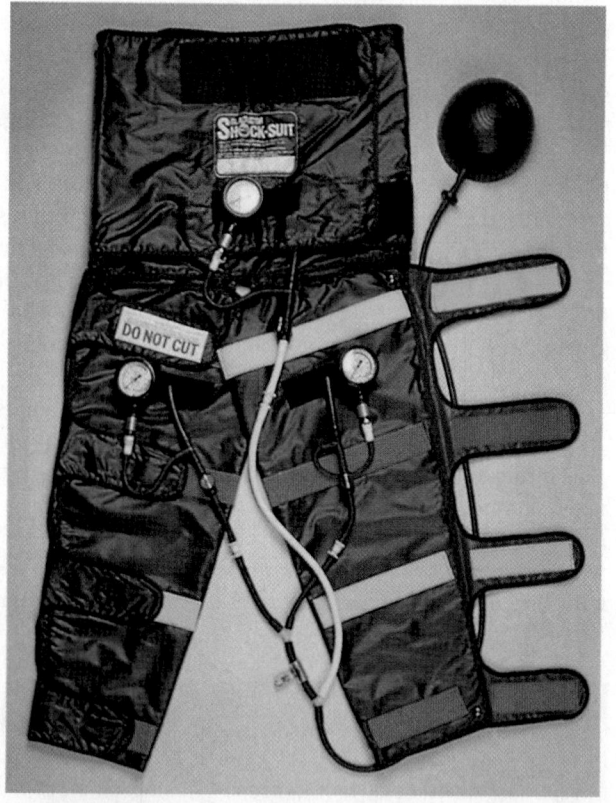

FIGURE 17-15

Pneumatic antishock garment (PASG).

saw an initial increase in the patient's blood pressure, research indicated that they do not improve survival. Their use may complicate some conditions and their application can interfere with treatments that should have a higher priority in the management of shock. As a result, the use of PASG has largely fallen out of favor. In some cases, they remain in EMS system protocols as a means of stabilizing pelvic fractures. (See Chapter 36.) However, other devices are available to stabilize a fractured pelvis.

Cardiac Arrest

In adults, **sudden cardiac arrest (SCA)** is most likely to occur due to a primary cardiac cause, such as acute coronary syndrome (ACS) or another cause of sudden cardiac **dysrhythmia**. Genetic abnormalities of the ion channels in the cardiac conduction system have been implicated in some cases of sudden cardiac arrest, including cardiac arrest in young athletes. Cardiac arrest is more rare in children. When cardiac arrest occurs in children, it is most often a result of respiratory failure. Other causes of cardiac arrest include trauma, hypothermia, drug overdoses, electrolyte imbalances, toxins, stroke, and pulmonary embolism.

Sudden cardiac arrest occurs when the heart develops a dysrhythmia that does not produce mechanical contraction sufficient to generate cardiac output. As a result, perfusion ceases and the patient becomes pulseless, unresponsive, and apneic (or has ineffective gasping respirations). Once perfusion ceases, tissues become ischemic. In some cases, if you can restore a perfusing rhythm before extensive cellular damage occurs, the patient can survive.

About 25 percent of the time, the initial rhythm in adult sudden cardiac arrest is a pulseless ventricular rhythm, either *ventricular fibrillation* or *ventricular tachycardia* (Figure 17-16). Other pulseless dysrhythmias include *asystole* and *pulseless electrical activity (PEA)*. Cardiac arrest is also caused by respiratory arrest, hypoxia, acidosis, and other problems. In those cases, the patient first develops an underlying problem that leads to cardiac arrest if not corrected and is not classified as sudden cardiac arrest. Whether sudden or not, the same initial interventions are used in treatment. After initial treatment is begun, developing hypotheses about correctable underlying conditions allows specific corrective interventions. For example, you may not be able to resuscitate a patient who is hypothermic until the body temperature is raised to near-normal.

Body tissues and organ systems are rapidly damaged by this lack of perfusion. The brain and heart are extremely sensitive to ischemia. Cellular death can begin in 4 to 6 minutes and if perfusion is not restored, death is likely in 8 to 10 minutes.

The Chain of Survival

The key to treating cardiac arrest is restoring perfusion and stopping the progression of cellular damage. In order for this to occur, a series of events called the *Chain of Survival*

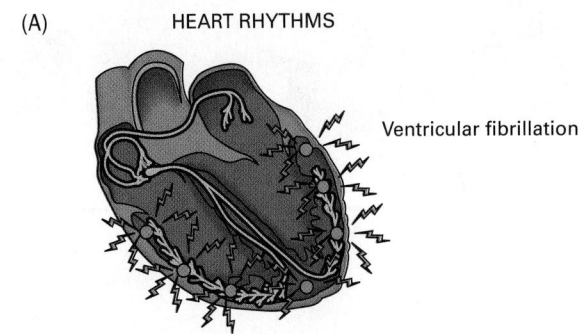

HEART RHYTHMS

Ventricular fibrillation

Chaotic electrical discharge (ventricular fibrillation) as seen on an ECG tracing

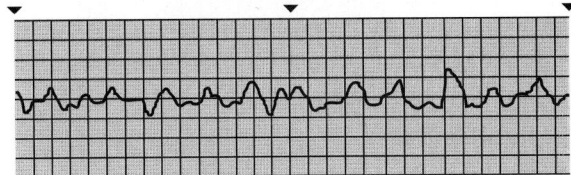

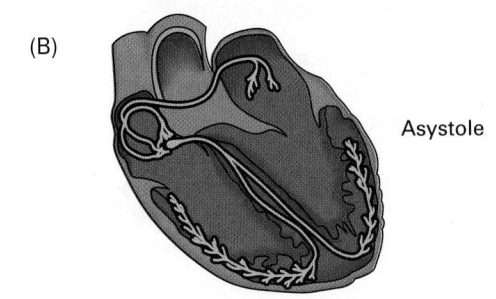

(B) Asystole

ECG tracing of asystole

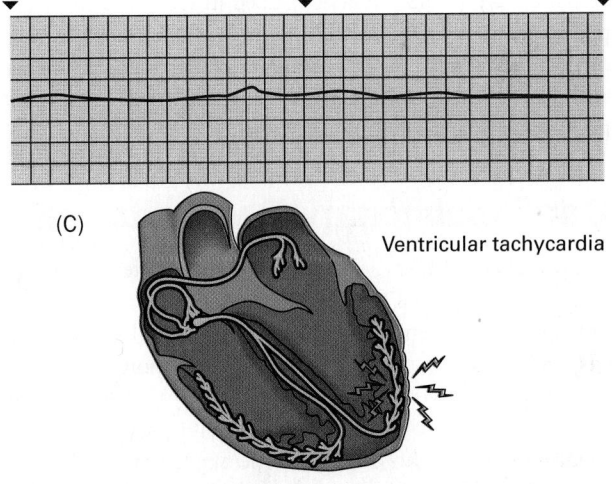

(C) Ventricular tachycardia

ECG tracing of ventricular tachycardia

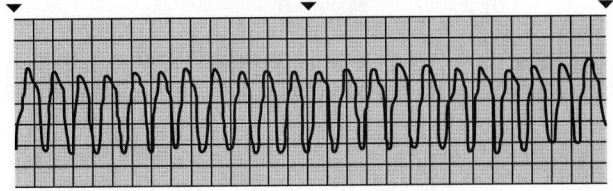

FIGURE 17-16

Lethal cardiac arrest dysrhythmias: (A) Ventricular fibrillation, (B) Asystole, (C) Ventricular tachycardia.

FIGURE 17-17

The Chain of Survival.

is required (Figure 17-17)(AHA, 2010). The links in the Chain of Survival are as follows:

- Immediate recognition of cardiac arrest by bystanders and activation of the emergency response system
- Early CPR with emphasis on chest compressions
- Rapid **defibrillation**
- Early advanced life support
- Integrated post–cardiac arrest care

As with all chains, if any of the links are weak or missing, the other links are rendered ineffective. The best EMS system cannot save a patient in whom cardiac arrest recognition and EMS notification were delayed.

Resuscitation from cardiac arrest is most likely to be successful if defibrillation is performed in the first 5 minutes after collapse (for patients in whom the initial dysrhythmia is ventricular fibrillation or ventricular tachycardia). Because the interval from collapse to arrival of EMS is typically longer than 5 minutes, the potential for survival is highest when the public is trained in CPR and there are **public access defibrillation** (PAD) programs. The placement of EMS providers in the community makes them ideal candidates for teaching CPR and leading efforts to implement public access defibrillation programs.

Cardiopulmonary Resuscitation

As an Advanced EMT, you have a slightly different threshold for initiating CPR. Lay rescuers are taught that any unresponsive patient with absent or abnormal (ineffective, gasping) breathing requires immediate initiation of 30 chest compressions. Recent research has found that laypersons are often unable to distinguish between a patient who has a pulse and one who does not. The approach to CPR has changed to reflect this. Learning to detect the presence or absence of a pulse takes practice with both patients who

have a pulse and those who do not. That type of practice is not typically available to lay rescuers. Therefore, lay rescuers should not delay chest compressions to check for a pulse.

Health Care Provider CPR

Your approach is similar to that of the lay responder, but you will also quickly check the patient's carotid pulse (Table 17-6). Some research has also found that health care providers cannot always reliably determine the presence or absence of a pulse in an unresponsive patient. As a result, the pulse check has been de-emphasized in health care provider CPR. If a pulse is not detected within 10 seconds, begin chest compressions (Figure 17-18).

Unlike lay rescuers, EMS providers give the patient the advantage by responding in teams. That allows you the advantage of responding in teams OR an advantage by responding in teams. As one provider begins chest compressions, another prepares the AED. With additional responders, you can make preparations for airway management and transportation. Throughout the remainder of this chapter, keep in mind that you can simultaneously accomplish many of the tasks discussed in a stepwise manner through teamwork.

Scene Size-Up and Primary Assessment

There are cases in which you will be dispatched to a known cardiac arrest. Emergency medical dispatchers are trained to recognize the need for CPR and give prearrival instructions to bystanders before crews arrive. When this occurs, you will be dispatched for a cardiac arrest or advised that CPR is in progress. In other cases, the information that the patient is in cardiac arrest may not have been relayed to the dispatcher, but another bystander may arrive in the meantime and be performing CPR when you arrive on the scene.

Sometimes bystanders are present but are not performing CPR. In those cases, you will have an apparently unresponsive patient whom you must quickly assess for cardiac arrest. Although not every apparently unresponsive person is in cardiac arrest, you must immediately determine if this is the case (Figure 17-19). At times, the general impression of an unresponsive patient (including cyanotic or mottled skin) tells you there is an immediate need to resuscitate. In patients in whom cardiac arrest is not immediately apparent in the general impression, quickly check for responsiveness, breathing, and a pulse.

As you approach an apparently unresponsive patient, first use a loud voice to assess the level of consciousness. "Mrs. Johnson, are you awake? Are you alright?" If the patient does not respond to your voice, approach carefully and use your hand to gently shake the patient's shoulder. Take care to remain just out of the patient's reach in case the patient reacts violently to being startled awake. As you take the initial steps to determine the level of responsiveness, also

| **TABLE 17-6** | **Approach to CPR in Adults, Children, and Infants** | | | | |

CPR is indicated in patients who are unresponsive and who are not breathing or who have agonal breathing. EMS providers should check the patient's pulse.

	Pulse	Overview (EMS teams should perform steps simultaneously)	Hand Placement	Compressions	Ratio of Chest Compressions to Ventilations
Adult 8 years and older	No carotid pulse detected within 10 seconds	Call EMS, begin chest compressions	Both hands over lower half of the sternum	Compress 2 inches at a rate of at least 100 per minute	30-to-2
Child 1 to 8 years	Pulse <60 and poor perfusion	2 minutes of chest compressions, call EMS	1 or both hands over lower half of the sternum	Compress 2 inches at a rate of at least 100 per minute	30-to-2 for 1 rescuer; 15:2 for 2 rescuers
Infant less than 1 year	Pulse <60 and poor perfusion	2 minutes of chest compressions, call EMS	2 fingers over the sternum just below the nipple-line	1.5 inches at a rate of at least 100 per minute	30-to-2 for 1 rescuer; 15:2 for 2 rescuers

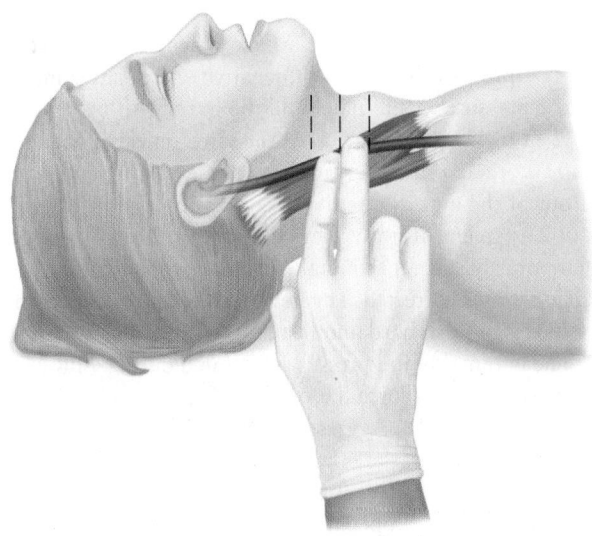
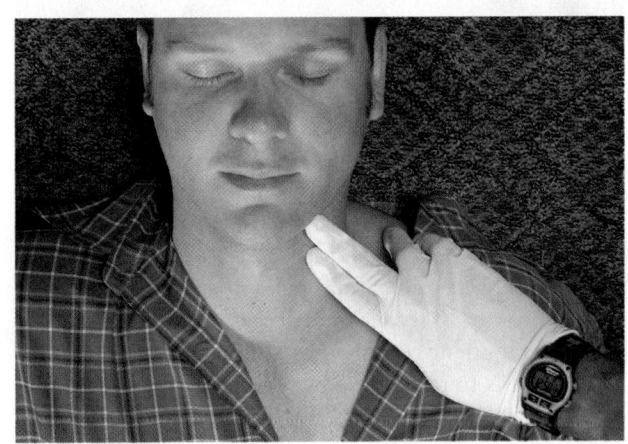

FIGURE 17-18

If a carotid pulse is not detected in 10 seconds, begin chest compressions.

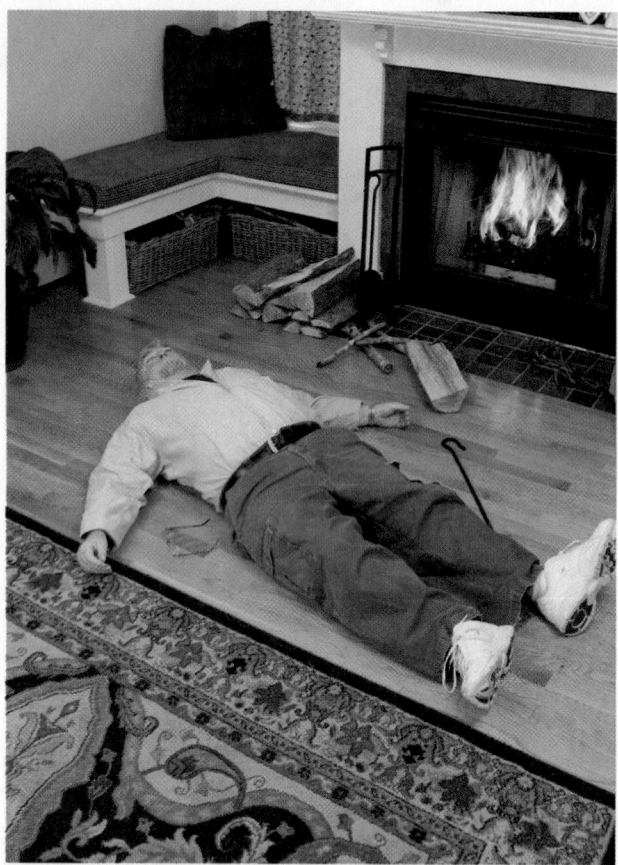

FIGURE 17-19

Quickly assess for cardiac arrest in apparently unresponsive patients.

quickly check to see whether the patient is breathing. If the patient is unresponsive and has apnea or agonal respirations, quickly check a carotid pulse. If you do not detect a carotid pulse in 10 seconds, begin chest compressions.

If the patient responds to your voice or to painful stimuli, or is unresponsive but breathing (except agonal respirations), continue with the primary assessment as you normally would. Keep in mind that patients in whom you identify a problem in the primary assessment are critical and may deteriorate to cardiac arrest. Frequent reassessment is required.

Chest Compressions

The most important element of cardiac arrest treatment is the rapid initiation of chest compressions. Once the arrest is recognized, compressions must be started. This idea may initially seem at odds with the usual airway, breathing, circulation (ABC) approach to patient assessment and care. The pathophysiology of sudden cardiac arrest requires a different approach to restore perfusion. The sequence of patient care, once cardiac arrest has been identified, is circulation, airway, and breathing: CAB.

Rationale for Compressions First

When sudden cardiac arrest occurs, a certain amount of oxygen is in the blood and in the lungs. When deoxygenated blood reaches the pulmonary system, it is not *unoxygenated*. It still has a PaO$_2$ of about 40 mmHg. After a normal exhalation, the lungs still contain about 2,200 mL of air that can continue to exchange oxygen with the blood. Although the amount of oxygen available is not ideal, the patient's immediate problem is that the available oxygen is not being circulated at all.

In addition to the revised perspective on the pathophysiology of cardiac arrest, studies evaluated by the AHA (2010) indicated that one of the obstacles to lay rescuers performing CPR was hesitation to provide mouth-to-mouth or mouth-to-mask ventilations. Rather than have a lay rescuer avoid CPR, it is better to do chest compressions only. There also are reasons health care provider CPR initially focuses on chest compressions, as well. As stated, there is some oxygen in the blood, but it is not being circulated in cardiac arrest. The time taken to assess and establish an airway and begin bag-valve-mask ventilations delays the circulation of this blood.

There is yet another reason chest compressions are performed first in sudden cardiac arrest. When done correctly, chest compressions create both negative and positive intrathoracic pressure to alternately fill the heart with blood and squeeze it out into circulation. At the same time, the changes in intrathoracic pressure can allow some air movement in and out of the airway. Artificial circulation produces only about 21 percent of normal circulation, but that is enough to temporarily sustain minimal perfusion while the cause of cardiac arrest is corrected. The key to delivering quality compressions is to push hard and fast and to limit interruptions.

The minimal blood pressure generated during CPR also underscores the importance of one of the principles presented in Chapter 16. Aggressive ventilation and overinflation of the chest interferes with the return of blood to the heart. With only 21 percent of normal cardiac output being produced, increased impedance to blood returning the heart will reduce this amount even more.

Compression Technique

During an EMS response, one provider begins chest compressions while another prepares the defibrillator. If you are alone and a defibrillator is not immediately

IN THE FIELD

Teamwork and communication are required to perform procedures, prepare the cardiac arrest patient for transport, and transfer to the ambulance with minimal interruption in chest compressions.

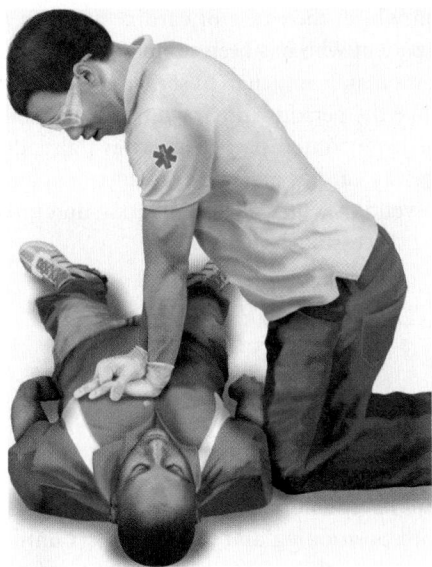

FIGURE 17-20

Hand placement for adult chest compressions.

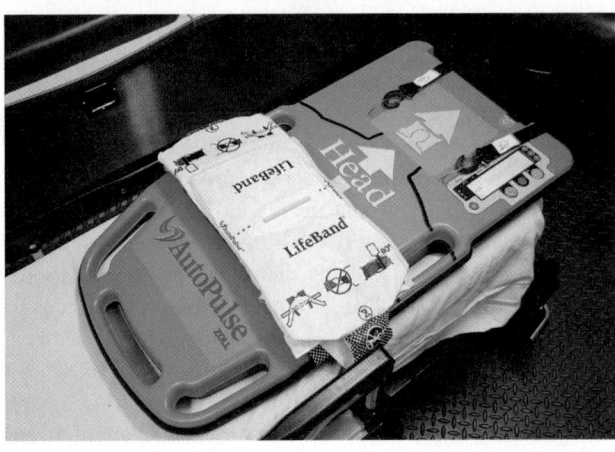

(A)

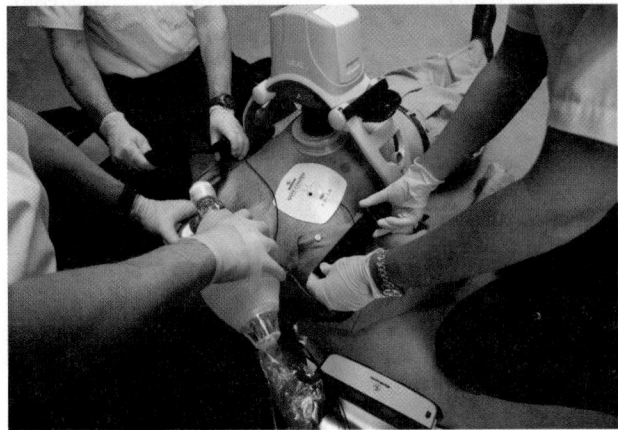

(B)

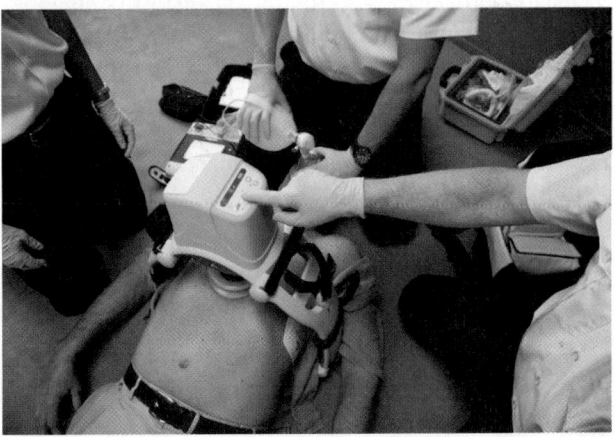

(C)

available, perform chest compressions until another provider arrives. For an adult patient, position your hands over the lower half of the sternum with the heel of one hand in the center of the patient's chest and the second hand on top of the first (Figure 17-20). Compress to a depth of 2 inches and then allow the chest to fully recoil. Adequate compression followed by complete recoil maximizes pressure changes within the chest to provide for the movement of blood.

Common pitfalls include compressions that are too shallow (commonly due to provider fatigue) or keeping constant pressure on the chest and not allowing full recoil. It is appropriate to leave your hands in place, but be sure they are not impeding recoil.

Compress at a rate of at least 100 compressions per minute in a pattern of 30 compressions followed by 2 ventilations until an advanced airway is placed. This rate allows a buildup of pressure within the cardiovascular system to allow perfusion. Minimize interruptions. Each time compressions are interrupted, blood pressure falls and perfusion is decreased.

After initiating resuscitation, you will deliver 30 chest compressions before moving on to the airway.

Mechanical CPR Devices

Mechanical CPR devices can be a useful tool in the case of prolonged CPR or in situations where manpower is scarce (Figure 17-21). The efficacy of CPR delivered by the devices seems to be equivalent to that of manual compressions, but the research is still limited. If using those devices, follow the manufacturer's instructions and adhere to your protocols.

FIGURE 17-21

Mechanical CPR devices.
(A) The AutoPulse, a load-distributing band CPR device, compresses the thorax.
(B) The Lucas (Jolife) device actively compresses and decompresses the thorax. (Courtesy of PhysioControl, Inc.)
(C) The Lucas (Jolife) device applied to a patient. (Courtesy of PhysioControl, Inc.)

Airway and Ventilations

Unlike lay rescuers, who perform compression-only CPR, health care providers follow each set of 30 chest compressions by opening the airway with a head-tilt/chin-lift or modified jaw-thrust maneuver and deliver 2 ventilations by bag-valve mask-device or mouth-to-barrier mask (Figure 17-22). Deliver each ventilation over 1 second using just enough volume to obtain visible chest rise. After delivering the 2 ventilations, resume compressions. The ratio of 30 chest compressions to 2 ventilations continues until a defibrillator is available or an advanced airway is placed.

If you cannot deliver an attempted ventilation, check that you have effectively opened the airway and attempt ventilation again. If air does not enter despite ensuring proper airway position, suspect foreign body airway obstruction (FBAO). Essentially, the treatment for FBAO is chest compressions, although you must also periodically check to see if the object has been dislodged. (See Chapter 16 for FBAO management.)

Cardiac arrest can be accompanied by vomiting or regurgitation of stomach contents. You must ensure that suction is immediately available to clear the airway.

After an advanced airway device (for example, LMA, KingLTD, Combitube, or endotracheal tube) is placed, ventilations are delivered every 6 to 8 seconds without interrupting chest compressions. Once an advanced airway is in place, chest compressions are delivered continuously at a rate of at least 100 per minute.

If enough personnel are available, frequently rotate the provider performing chest compressions. The quality of compressions including rate, depth, and recoil are affected as a provider begins to tire. The quality of compressions can diminish within just a few minutes, even when the provider does not feel tired. Ideally, you should rotate roles every 2 minutes.

The AHA expects that trained health care providers will exercise good clinical judgment. For example, in

patients in whom the cause of cardiac arrest is asphyxia, such as a patient who has been submerged in a body of water, ventilation and oxygenation should receive a higher priority. Unlike the person who has suffered a sudden cardiac arrest, the asphyxiated patient will have already become hypoxic before cardiac arrest occurs. Hypoxia may prevent other interventions, such as defibrillation and medications, from being successful.

Integrating Advanced Airway Devices

There are several advantages to using a Combitube or supraglottic airway, such as the King LTD, as discussed in Chapter 16. A disadvantage, though, is that they can delay or interrupt chest compressions. It is better to maintain an airway with positioning and basic adjuncts until there are sufficient personnel to assist with insertion of a more advanced device. In the case of endotracheal intubation, it provides a means of measuring carbon dioxide, which can provide important information, but often requires an interruption in chest compressions. However, once an advanced airway device is in place, you can perform chest compressions continuously, without interruption for ventilation. Remember the importance of minimizing interruptions in chest compressions when making decisions about advanced airway devices.

Defibrillation

Early defibrillation is critical for patients presenting in a pulseless ventricular rhythm. Patients presenting with those rhythms have a higher probability of survival than patients presenting in asystole or PEA. However, the window of opportunity closes quickly. The greater the interval between arrest and beginning rescuscitation, the poorer the patient's chances of survival. Aside from time, one of the factors that influences the success of defibrillation is the effectiveness of chest compressions. To maximize the chances that defibrillation is successful, keep chest compression interruptions to a minimum.

Ventricular Fibrillation

Ventricular fibrillation occurs when thousands of electrical foci in the heart depolarize independently. The appearance of the electrical activity on the cardiac monitor is chaotic. The myocardium quivers in response to the chaotic electrical activity, but cannot respond normally by contracting to eject blood. Unlike ventricular fibrillation, ventricular tachycardia appears to be organized on the cardiac monitor. It sometimes produces a pulse, and sometimes does not. Pulseless ventricular tachycardia is treated identically to ventricular fibrillation. Inadvertent defibrillation of a patient in ventricular tachycardia with a pulse is avoided by following a simple rule of AED use: Never apply an AED to a patient with a pulse.

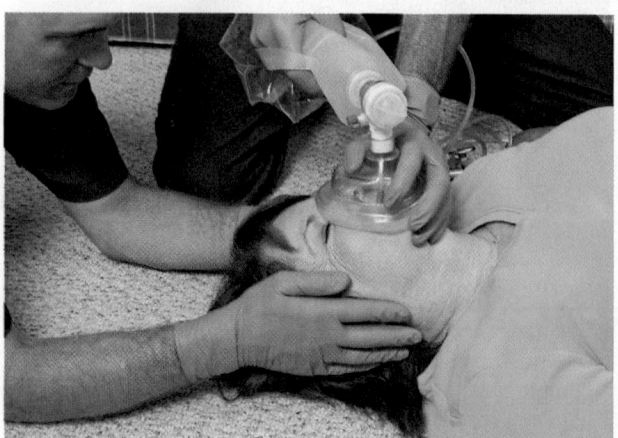

FIGURE 17-22

Open the airway and begin ventilations after 30 chest compressions.

Physiology of Defibrillation

Immediate bystander CPR significantly improves the response to defibrillation, but does not terminate a lethal dysrhythmia. Defibrillation does not, as urban legend would have us believe, re-start the heart. During defibrillation, an electrical current is passed through the heart in order to depolarize the cardiac electrical cells uniformly to stop them from working independently of the cardiac conduction system. Defibrillation actually stops the heart momentarily. The myocardium and conduction system can then repolarize uniformly, with the intent of the sinoatrial (SA) node regaining control of the heart.

Automatic External Defibrillation

Defibrillators used in the prehospital setting come in three operational designs. Manual defibrillation requires significant training in the recognition of dysrhythmias and allows the operator complete control over the timing and energy levels used in defibrillation. Semiautomatic external defibrillators (SAEDs) and automatic external defibrillators (AEDs) are often lumped together in the same category and referred to simply as *AEDs* (Figure 17-23). However, there is a critical difference you must be aware of.

Once the pads of an AED are applied and it is powered on, no additional input is required from the provider. The AED analyzes the cardiac rhythm, determines whether the pattern meets the criteria for defibrillation, and delivers the shock. This type of device is most commonly seen in public places as part of a public access defibrillation program.

An SAED analyzes the rhythm in the same way, but instead of delivering shock, it advises the user that a shock is indicated. The user must then push a button to deliver the shock. While paramedics use a manual defibrillator, similar to the ones used in the hospital, Advanced EMTs, EMTs, and EMRs use either SAEDs or AEDs. As an Advanced EMT, it is more likely that you will use an SAED. For simplicity, except when explaining device operation, the term *AED* will be used in this text to mean both fully automatic and semiautomatic defibrillators.

Using an AED

Correct use of an AED begins before the call. All AEDs require preventive maintenance to ensure readiness. Always follow the maintenance plan specified by the AED manufacturer and adhere to your employer's policies regarding AED maintenance. You must check AEDs regularly and replace batteries at specified intervals. The defibrillation pads used with an AED also expire and you must replace them before expiration.

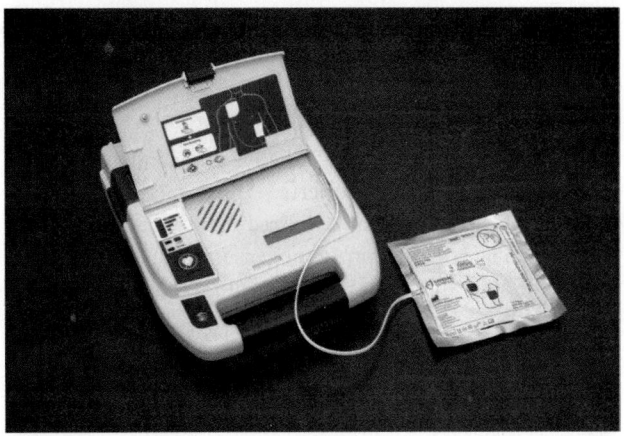

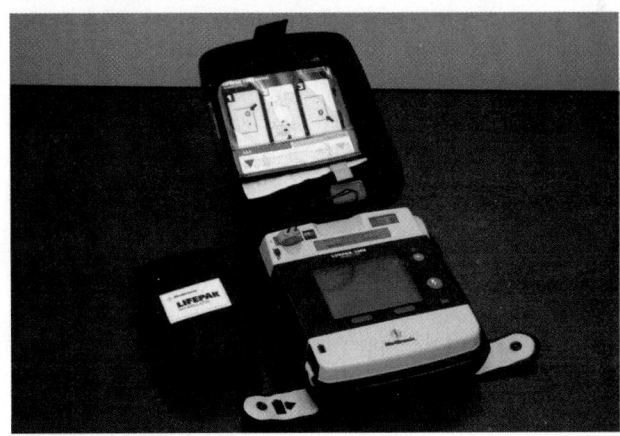

FIGURE 17-23

Automatic external defibrillators.

An AED is applied only to a patient in cardiac arrest. That is, a patient who is unresponsive, apneic, and pulseless. Never apply an AED to a patient with a pulse. AEDs are incredibly reliable in differentiating dysrhythmia that require defibrillation from those that do not, but the potential still exists for inadvertent defibrillation of a patient with an organized cardiac rhythm.

If a defibrillator is immediately available upon a patient's collapse, apply it and use it as quickly as possible, but with as little interruption in chest compressions as possible. When bystanders do not initiate CPR, especially if the collapse is not witnessed, it has been suggested that 1½ to 3 minutes of CPR prior to defibrillation may improve patient outcome. However, evidence supporting this is conflicting. You must follow your protocols to determine in which instances CPR is started or continued by EMS personnel prior to defibrillation, and in which cases defibrillation is performed immediately. However, in practice, with more than one EMS provider, CPR can be performed while the defibrillator is prepared, without delaying defibrillation.

Defibrillator Pad Placement

Defibrillator pads have both adhesive and conductive properties. The conductive properties allow the rhythm to be detected and energy to be delivered through the defibrillator leads. The adhesive properties ensure proper contact between the skin and conductive medium to ensure electricity is delivered efficiently.

Connect defibrillator pads to the AED leads and apply them to the patient's bare chest, following the manufacturer's recommendations for placement. If placement recommendations are not given, one pad is placed on the upper right chest, beneath the right clavicle, and the other is placed on the left lateral chest wall near the apex of the heart (Figure 17-24). Make sure the pad is placed under the breast tissue. If the patient is wet, wipe the chest dry before applying the pads. If necessary and possible, use a safety razor to shave excessive chest hair before placing pads (keep a safety razor with the AED and defibrillator pads). Do not place pads over jewelry or medication patches. Remove such items prior to attaching the pads.

Do not place pads directly over internally implanted pacemakers or defibrillators. They are identified as a bulge under the skin of the upper left chest (Figure 17-25). If you encounter such a device, offset the pad slightly or adjust to an anterior–posterior placement. On occasion, a pacemaker can interfere with AED detection of ventricular fibrillation. In patients with implanted defibrillators, the device detects ventricular fibrillation and delivers a cycle of low-energy shock directly to the heart. This cycle should be completed by the time you arrive. If it is not (as indicated by twitching of the patient's muscles), allow 30 to 60 seconds for the implanted device to complete its cycle.

Defibrillation Energy Levels

AEDs are preprogrammed to deliver shocks at a given level, but it is important to understand how defibrillation energy levels are determined. Newer AEDs and manual defibrillators deliver biphasic energy. Older models that deliver monophasic energy may still be in use. In *monophasic*

defibrillation, the electrical energy is delivered in only one direction between the defibrillation pads. In *biphasic defibrillation*, the energy is delivered in one direction for half of the duration of the shock and in the opposite direction for the second half (Bocka, 2009).

Biphasic defibrillators can terminate ventricular fibrillation at lower energy levels of 120 to 200 joules (J), but studies have not determined the optimum energy level for either initial or subsequent shocks. Monophasic defibrillators should generally be set to deliver 360 J.

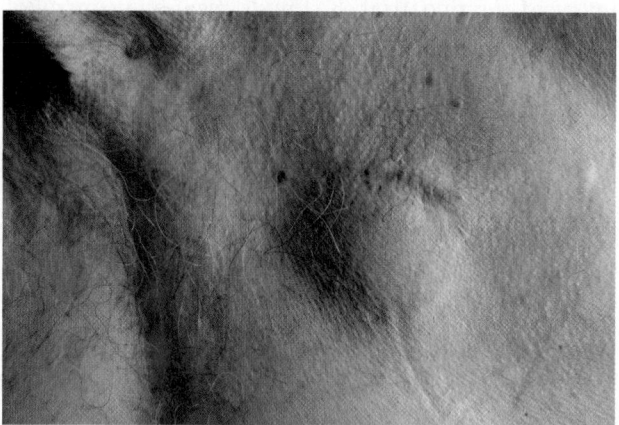
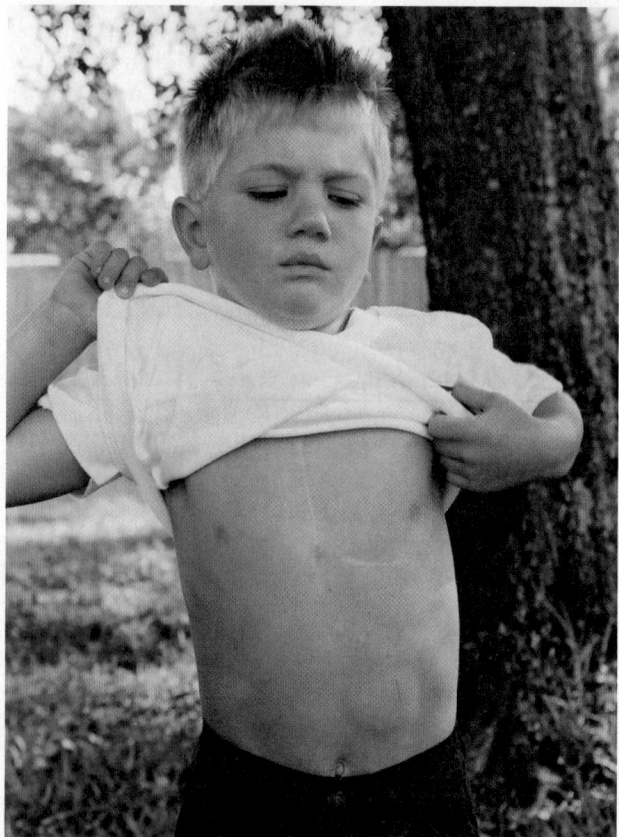

FIGURE 17-25

Examples of implanted pacemakers. Adjust AED pad placement so that they are not placed over an implanted device. (Both Photos: © Michal Heron)

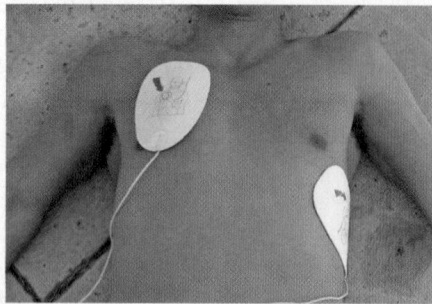

FIGURE 17-24

Typical defibrillator pad placement.

Analyzing the Rhythm and Delivering a Shock

Position the AED next to the patient and turn it on (Scan 17–1). Chest compressions should continue as you ready the device. If the device you are using gives voice prompts, follow the prompts. Attach pads to the AED and apply them to the patient's chest. You must stop chest compressions and clear all personnel from the patient to allow the machine to detect and analyze the patient's cardiac rhythm. Rhythm analysis may proceed automatically, or you may have to initiate rhythm analysis by pushing the appropriate button on the machine. Rhythm analysis may take several seconds.

If a shock is advised, the AED will alert the operator and indicate that the patient should be "cleared" in preparation for delivering a shock. Clearing the patient means that no one is in direct or indirect (such as by ventilating through an advanced airway device) contact with the patient. Remember: A fully automated defibrillator will charge and deliver a shock once ventricular fibrillation or ventricular tachycardia is detected. You must remain clear of the patient while the machine delivers the shock.

With an SAED, ensure that no one is in contact with the patient before delivering the shock. Usually, the device automatically charges in preparation to shock once a "shockable" rhythm is detected. However, with some devices you will need to push a button to manually charge the device. Once the device is charged, the machine will alert you that the shock may be delivered.

As soon as the shock is delivered, resume CPR. If defibrillation was successful, cardiac output remains diminished in the first moments and CPR can be beneficial. The time taken to check a pulse or cardiac rhythm delays the resumption of CPR, whether or not the shock was successful. After about five cycles or 2 minutes of CPR, ending with 30 compressions, reanalyze the rhythm. If shock is advised, deliver the shock as quickly as possible. The less time between the last compression of a CPR cycle and defibrillation, the better. If a shock is not advised, resume CPR.

Checking for Return of Spontaneous Circulation

You must monitor the patient for signs of the return of spontaneous circulation (ROSC) with minimal interruption of chest compressions. Obvious signs of ROSC include resumption of spontaneous breathing and response to stimuli. However, these occur rarely. The most useful tool for the Advanced EMT, in most cases, is detection of a carotid pulse during a pause in chest compressions. However, you should check the pulse infrequently to minimize interruptions in CPR and do not assess the pulse for more than 10 seconds. If a definite pulse is not detected within 10 seconds, you must resume CPR.

End-tidal carbon dioxide monitoring is useful in intubated patients in detecting ROSC, but its use in patients with a supraglottic airway has not been adequately studied.

During CPR, carbon dioxide is produced, but it is not circulated to the lungs in normal amounts. Therefore $ETCO_2$ is low in patients in cardiac arrest, despite chest compressions and ventilation. When spontaneous circulation returns, carbon dioxide delivery to the lungs is increased. A sudden and sustained increase in $ETCO_2$ in intubated patients is, therefore, an indicator of ROSC.

If your particular scope of practice includes cardiac monitoring, the presence of an organized rhythm when a shock is not indicated is a prompt to check the pulse. Do not rely solely on the presence of an organized rhythm to establish ROSC. It is quite possible for the heart to generate electrical activity that does not produce mechanical contraction of the heart. This condition is called *pulseless electrical activity (PEA)*.

If ROSC is detected, the patient requires ongoing care, detailed later in this chapter.

AED Safety

The energy used for defibrillation can be up to 360 J. The function of defibrillation pads is to direct as much of this energy as possible through the heart. However, some structures of the body are good conductors of electricity and some electricity is conducted throughout the body when the shock is delivered. If another person is contact with the patient, directly or indirectly, electricity can be conducted to them, as well. That is why you must always clearly instruct all personnel (and bystanders) to clear the patient and look to make sure they are not in contact with the patient when you deliver a shock. Each EMS system may use slightly different phrases, but those are generally some variation of "Everybody clear," or "Everybody off."

Defibrillation in a moving ambulance is an unsafe practice. In addition, ambulance movement may interfere with the AED's rhythm analysis. You should not analyze or defibrillate a patient while the ambulance is moving.

It is possible for defibrillation to create a spark, although this is not likely. Because oxygen supports combustion, a spark could cause a fire in an oxygen-enriched atmosphere. Even though you may be administering oxygen to your patient during defibrillation, this does not enrich the atmosphere. However, a faulty oxygen system in an enclosed space, such as the back of the ambulance, could potentially result in an oxygen-enriched atmosphere. Ensuring that defibrillation pads are securely adhered to the patient minimizes the likelihood of a spark. However, it is not

IN THE FIELD

While it was once believed that CPR on a patient with a spontaneous pulse could cause a dysrhythmia, there is inadequate evidence to establish this as a significant concern. In a patient whose cardiac output is inadequate to produce clear signs of spontaneous circulation, chest compressions are continued.

Initial Cardiac Arrest Management for Adult Patients

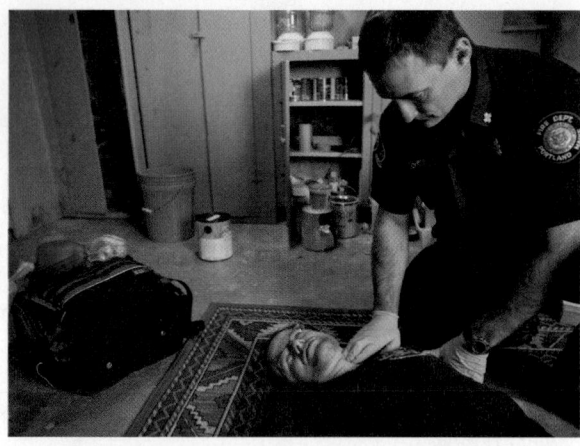

1. If a patient is apparently unresponsive and not breathing normally, check the carotid pulse for no more than 10 seconds.

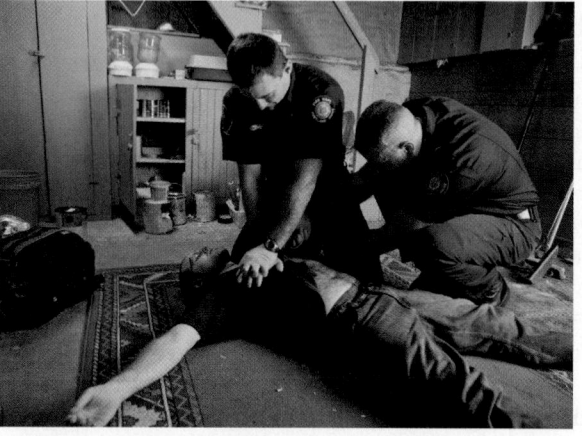

2. If you do not detect a carotid pulse in 10 seconds, begin chest compressions. A second EMS provider should prepare to apply an AED while chest compressions are performed at a ratio of 30 compressions to 2 ventilations.

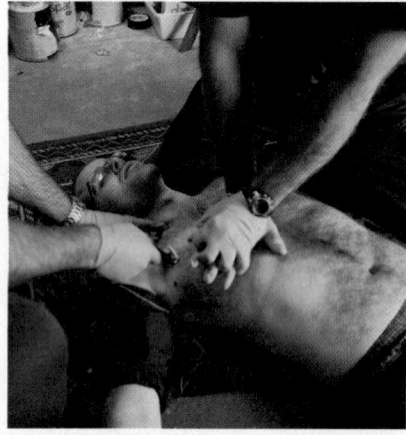

3. Shave excess hair from the patient's chest to ensure good contact between the AED pads and the skin.

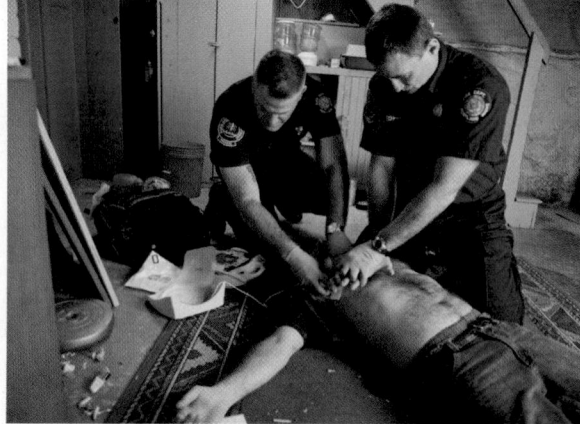

4. Apply the pads as directed by the manufacturer. The default position is to place the first pad on the upper right chest, just below the clavicle and to the right of the sternal border.

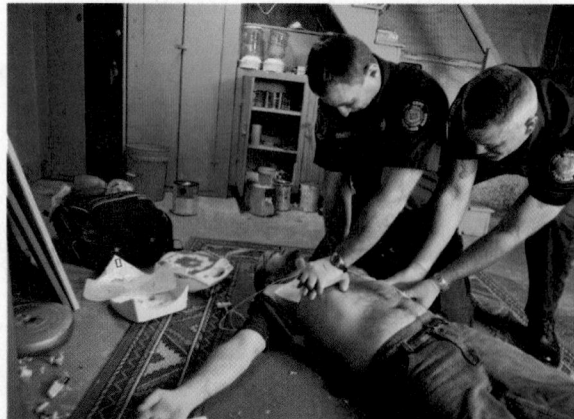

5. The default position for the second pad is the lower left lateral chest.

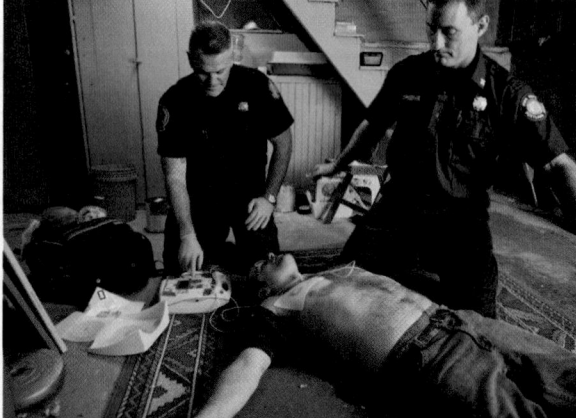

6. When the defibrillator has been powered on (either before or after applying the pads, according to the manufacturer's directions), stop CPR, ensure everyone is completely clear of the patient, and press the designated button to analyze the rhythm (or allow the AED to analyze the rhythm automatically, depending on the configuration). Allow the machine to shock, or press to deliver a shock when prompted. Resume CPR.

advisable to defibrillate in any environment you believe to be enriched with a combustible substance.

Because water is an excellent conductor of electricity, do not defibrillate in wet conditions. Quickly move the patient out of wet conditions and dry his chest before applying defibrillation pads.

Intravenous Access and Medications

CPR, defibrillation, establishing an airway, and providing ventilations all take precedence over starting IVs and administering medications. Even in Advanced Cardiac Life Support (ACLS), administered by paramedics and in-hospital personnel, the role of medications during cardiac arrest has been de-emphasized. Therefore, IVs are established by Advanced EMTs only when sufficient personnel are present to allow it without interrupting or delaying more critical procedures. This may mean that an IV is not established until you are en route to the hospital, or it may not be established at all, depending on resources available.

Intravenous fluids have not been shown to improve cardiac arrest outcomes and are generally not required. The only time you should administer significant amounts of fluid is if hypovolemia is the cause of, or a contributing factor to, cardiac arrest.

Resuscitation Outcomes and Postresuscitation Care

Successful resuscitation means, in the short term, that the patient has ROSC. Ultimately, though, it means discharge from the hospital neurologically intact. For a variety of reasons, most out-of-hospital resuscitation attempts are, unfortunately, not successful. However, according to the AHA (2010), with all links of the Chain of Survival in place and functioning well, up to 50 percent of witnessed out-of-hospital cardiac arrest patients with an initial rhythm of ventricular fibrillation could be resuscitated.

Every community should have a continuous quality improvement program that sets benchmarks for resuscitation attempts and measures them. Measurement must be accompanied by changes in practice as indicated. EMS providers can assist greatly in data collection with thorough documentation, including whether the cardiac arrest was witnessed, whether bystander CPR was initiated, and the interval to defibrillation.

CPR in Infants and Children

In the adult population, cardiac arrest is often caused by a primary cardiac problem. In contrast, pediatric patients do not have coronary artery disease, which is a common reason for adult cardiac arrest. Pediatric patients are far more likely to experience cardiac arrest as a secondary event from hypoxia. The most frequent cause of cardiac arrest in pediatric patients is a problem with the airway or breathing. The

Pediatric Care

Pediatric patients present special resuscitation challenges. Pediatric cardiac arrest situations can be emotionally charged and difficult to manage. When possible, give immediate consideration to the well-being of family members. In most cases, family members are encouraged to remain with the patient during resuscitation. However, if their presence interferes with resuscitation efforts, a bystander, law enforcement officer, or an extra EMS provider should move them away from the patient and stay with them.

precipitating event could be FBAO, asthma, respiratory infection, drowning, electrocution, overdose, or trauma. Early intervention in pediatric airway and breathing problems to prevent progression to cardiac arrest is essential.

As with adults, survival rates are improved by bystander CPR and when ventricular fibrillation occurs, prompt defibrillation. For health care providers as well as lay rescuers, the sequence of resuscitation events once cardiac arrest is detected begins with chest compressions. A lone rescuer applies chest compressions at a ratio of 30:2, while two rescuers use a ratio of 15:2 in recognition of the likelihood of asphyxial cardiac arrest. In both cases, the compression rate is at least 100 per minute. In all cases of cardiac arrest, it is desirable for lay rescuers to begin chest compressions while someone simultaneously calls 911. In adults, when this is not possible, the lay rescuer requests EMS first, then begins chest compressions so that the patient can be defibrillated as quickly as possible. In children, lay rescuers first provide about 2 minutes (5 cycles) of CPR to immediately restore perfusion, then request EMS.

For the purposes of CPR, an infant is under one year old and a child is from one year old until there are signs of puberty (beginning of breast development in girls and the presence of axillary hair in boys). Adolescents with signs of puberty are managed according to adult CPR guidelines.

Infant CPR

In infants, the brachial pulse along the medial arm is checked. (Figure 17-26). Compressions are performed either by using two fingers placed over the sternum just below an imaginary line between the patient's nipples (recommended for lone rescuers) or by encircling the chest with your hands and using your thumbs to compress the lower third of the sternum (recommended for two rescuers).

The depth of compression is approximately 1½ inches, or one third of the anterior–posterior dimension of the chest. Perform compressions at a rate of at least 100 per minute, using a 30:2 ratio for a single rescuer and a 15:2 ratio for two rescuers. As with adults, once an advanced airway is in place, do not interrupt chest compressions for ventilation. Provide ventilations once every 6 to 8 seconds, taking care to avoid overventilation.

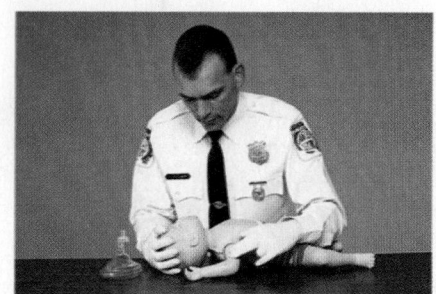

(A)

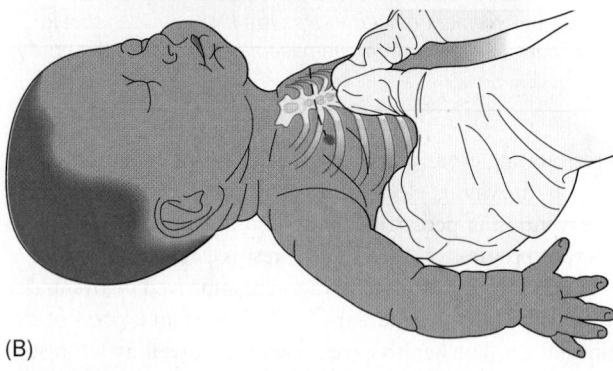

(B)

FIGURE 17-26

(A) Check the brachial pulse in infants.
(B) With two providers, encircle the infant's chest with your hands and place your thumbs over the sternum to provide chest compressions.

It is preferred that pediatric defibrillation pads are used as well as an AED in which the amount of energy delivered can be decreased. However, if these features are not available, you can still use an AED. This is a better alternative than not promptly defibrillating ventricular fibrillation.

Gastric distention from ventilation is more likely in children than in adults when you have not placed an advanced airway. Gastric distention decreases the quality of CPR and ventilation. Although routine use of cricoid pressure to limit gastric distention was recommended in the past, it has not been shown to be effective in most circumstances, and may interfere with ventilation. Nonetheless, cricoid pressure may be beneficial in some circumstances. If allowed in your protocols, locate the cricoid cartilage, just below the thyroid cartilage and press posteriorly so that the firmer cartilage of the airway occludes the esophagus. Be aware that application of excess pressure will obstruct the trachea.

A final difference in infant (and child) CPR is that chest compressions are used when the heart rate is less than 60 per minute with signs of poor perfusion.

Child CPR

In children, the carotid pulse is checked for no more than 10 seconds, as with adults. With the exception of hand placement and depth of chest compressions, CPR is performed as it is for infants. Depending on the size of the child, use one or two hands (as for adults) over

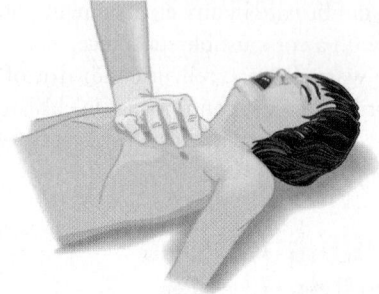

FIGURE 17-27

Hand placement for child CPR.

the lower half of the sternum (Figure 17-27). Compress the chest 2 inches, or one third of the anterior–posterior dimension of the chest. For larger children, you may need to use two-handed compressions similar to the adult technique in order to achieve the appropriate compression depth.

As with adults, if you suspect FBAO, continue chest compressions, but periodically check the airway for the presence of the foreign body. (Chapter 16 covers FBAO management.)

Secondary Assessment and History Taking in Resuscitation

Rapid intervention is required for patients in cardiac arrest, but it is also necessary to perform a rapid medical assessment and obtain a history from family or bystanders before you leave the scene. The immediate goal of the rapid medical assessment and patient history is to find potentially correctable causes of cardiac arrest. The AHA uses the six Hs and five Ts as a mnemonic to remember potentially correctable causes of cardiac arrest (Table 17-7).

As an Advanced EMT, you may not be able to address each of these issues, but a good assessment and history may help the next link in the Chain of Survival to address them. There are, however, critical interventions that are within your scope of practice. Checking a blood glucose level is a fast and easy test for a condition for which you have an immediate intervention, if necessary. Obtain a history of the present illness. Knowing the events that preceded cardiac arrest can help identify toxins, trauma, and other potentially correctable conditions.

Ethical and Legal Considerations

There are many situations where death is obvious and resuscitative efforts would be futile. You must follow your protocols for when resuscitation is and is not indicated. But, generally, you should not initiate resuscitative efforts on patients who have rigor mortis, dependent lividity, obvious decomposition, or other injuries incompatible with life (such as decapitation or transection of the torso). The

TABLE 17-7	Additional Steps in Resuscitation	
Situation	**Potential Causes**	**Actions**
Pediatric patient	Hypoxia is the most common cause of cardiac arrest in pediatric patients.	Ensure an open airway and adequate ventilations and provide supplemental oxygen.
Environmental temperature or impaired temperature regulation	Hyperthermia, hypothermia; dehydration, electrolyte imbalance	Passive rewarming for hypothermia; cooling for hyperthermia
Trauma	Tension pneumothorax, cardiac tamponade, hypovolemia	Immediate ALS or surgical interventions required. Follow protocols for fluid resuscitation in traumatic arrest.
Hemorrhage (internal or external)	Hypovolemia	Immediate surgical intervention required. Follow protocols for fluid resuscitation.
Diabetic	Hypoglycemia, acidosis, potassium imbalance	Check the blood glucose level and correct hypoglycemia
Kidney Disease or Dialysis	Electrolyte imbalance	Requires immediate laboratory testing and correction
Quality of resuscitation	Uncorrected hypoxia or acidosis	Ensure high-quality CPR with adequate depth and rate of chest compressions. Ensure an open airway and adequate ventilations with supplemental oxygen.
Sudden collapse	Stroke, cardiac arrhythmia, pulmonary embolism	May benefit from interventional procedure
Potential for or evidence of overdose or exposure to toxin	Opiates, other CNS depressants, bites or stings, toxic inhalation	May benefit from treatment for specific overdose or toxin

survival rate from traumatic cardiac arrest is extremely low and many systems discourage beginning CPR in trauma patients found without a pulse, particularly in blunt trauma.

Terminally ill patients may have do not resuscitate (DNR) or do not attempt resuscitation (DNAR) orders in place, indicating their wishes, and their physicians' agreement, that resuscitative measures not be implemented in the event of cardiac arrest. Your protocols specify requirements for determining the validity of DNRs (or DNARs). These situations often require consultation with medical direction or your supervisor.

Cardiac arrest is a dramatic event. In most cases, it means the loss of a loved one to family members present. Although this may be a clinical event for you, be sure to delegate appropriate resources to look after the well-being of bystanders and family members.

Return of Spontaneous Circulation

Resuscitation of cardiac arrest is most frequently unsuccessful. However, in some cases, patients have ROSC. You must be prepared to manage these patients. Prehospital treatment can rarely address the underlying cause of cardiac arrest, which means that patients with ROSC are at high risk for a second cardiac arrest. Once you detect ROSC, you must continuously monitor the patient for subsequent deterioration and cardiac arrest.

Patients with ROSC rarely regain responsiveness in the prehospital setting, although it is possible. Usually, the hypoxic insult to the brain results in unresponsiveness. In some cases, aggressive management can allow the brain time to heal and the patient may recover neurologically intact. Unfortunately, this is not always the case and permanent neurologic deficit is common among those with ROSC.

Manage the airway and breathing. Consider placing an advanced airway if one is not already in place. Use positive pressure ventilation, but remember that aggressive ventilation decreases venous return to the heart and impairs cardiac output. It is likely you will need to deliver shocks again, so keep defibrillation pads in place. Unless there is a protocol in place to induce **therapeutic hypothermia** following ROSC, take steps to maintain the patient's body temperature. If the patient is hypotensive, consult medical direction about administering a bolus of IV fluid.

Obtain vital signs and, if possible, complete a head-to-toe exam and continuously reassess the patient. Use other monitoring devices, such as pulse oximetry and capnometry, and obtain a blood glucose level if not already done.

Therapeutic Hypothermia

Recent research has demonstrated improved outcomes for patients with ROSC following ventricular fibrillation and ventricular tachycardia arrest when therapeutic hypothermia was induced. Therapeutic hypothermia involves reducing the patient's core temperature, typically by the administration of chilled IV fluid. The best results have been obtained by cooling the patient following resuscitation and maintaining hypothermia over a prolonged period.

CASE STUDY WRAP-UP

Clinical-Reasoning Process

Having anticipated cardiac arrest, Mary and Grace brought their airway and equipment bags and their AED to the patient's side, along with the stretcher and a long backboard. When Mary and Grace arrive at the patient's side, they notice that his face is cyanotic, providing initial confirmation that the patient is in cardiac arrest. One of the gym employees is performing chest compressions using good technique and AED pads have been applied to the patient's chest. In response to Grace's questions, the second gym employee states that the machine has delivered one shock and that the current cycle of CPR is nearly complete. Grace responds to the employees, "Please complete the cycle of CPR, then switch places while I analyze the rhythm." To Mary she says, "Get ready to manage the airway and ventilate."

Mary pulls the bag-valve-mask device from the airway bag and positions herself at the patient's head. As the current cycle of CPR is completed, Grace checks for a pulse for 10 seconds, but no pulse is present. She clears everyone from the patient and uses the gym's AED to analyze the patient's rhythm. The AED indicates and delivers a shock. The second gym employee, at Grace's request, begins chest compressions. At that moment, the EMT crew arrives and Grace directs them to prepare to place the patient on the backboard. By coordinating efforts, they are able to do so with minimal interruption of chest compressions.

The team coordinates replacing the gym's AED with their own and places the patient on the stretcher with the backboard beneath him and secures him with the straps. The two gym employees assist with CPR while the crew moves the stretcher toward the ambulance. They coordinate a brief interruption in CPR to load the stretcher. Grace quickly thanks the gym employees as they close the ambulance doors. After completing a cycle of chest compressions, she again analyzes the patient's rhythm. She delivers the indicated shock and one of the EMTs resumes chest compressions. Mary inserts a supraglottic airway so that chest compressions can continue without interruption, and attaches a capnometry sensor.

En route, a sudden increase in the patient's $ETCO_2$ prompts Grace to check a pulse at the conclusion of the current cycle of CPR. A carotid pulse is present and the patient's color is improving. Grace notifies the hospital emergency department of this latest development and continues to monitor the patient's condition. She inserts an IV just as they arrive at the hospital. Mary and Grace later learn that the patient was admitted to the critical care unit, but his neurologic outcome is uncertain at the present time.

CHAPTER REVIEW

Chapter Summary

Advanced EMTs must rapidly identify patients in shock and cardiac arrest and take immediate action to improve the patient's chances of survival. In both cases, the goal is to quickly restore tissue perfusion. The interventions and priorities for shock and cardiac arrest differ. In shock, the patient has some degree of cardiac output, although it may be significantly impaired. The priorities are to establish an airway and ensure that the patient is adequately ventilated and oxygenated, and that external bleeding, if any, is controlled.

In cardiac arrest, chest compressions are the highest priority in order to re-establish circulation in both adults and pediatric patients. Prompt defibrillation is required for patients in ventricular fibrillation and pulseless ventricular tachycardia. The need to establish an airway and provide ventilation is still critical, but must be done with minimal interruption of chest compressions.

In both cardiac arrest and shock, resuscitation requires teamwork, communication, and searching for an underlying cause. Basic resuscitation measures can sustain a minimal amount of perfusion for a brief period of time, but rarely correct the underlying problem. Identifying an underlying cause may allow more specific treatment, such as providing epinephrine to a patient in anaphylactic shock or treating hypoglycemia in a diabetic patient in cardiac arrest. For all critically ill patients, you must apply clinical reasoning to determine when additional interventions are required and how they should be prioritized with the need to transport the patient for definitive care.

Therapies for shock and cardiac arrest continue to be researched to find the best methods for prehospital treatment. To continue to provide patients with the best opportunity for survival, maintain awareness of the most current research and anticipate changes in protocols.

Review Questions

Multiple-Choice Questions

1. Which one of the following is most likely to lead to obstructive shock?

   a. Pulmonary embolism
   b. Myocardial infarction
   c. Massive infection
   d. Spinal-cord injury

2. Your patient is a female in her 70s who collapsed while walking with a friend. She is unresponsive, cyanotic, and not breathing. Which one of the following should you do first?

   a. Open the airway with a head-tilt/chin-lift maneuver.
   b. Obtain a past medical history.
   c. Quickly check for a pulse.
   d. Defibrillate three times in quick succession.

3. Which one of the following statements best describes the rationale for allowing full recoil of the chest wall during CPR?

   a. It permits venous return to the heart before the next compression.
   b. It prevents gastric distention and regurgitation.
   c. It allows the rescuer time to check a pulse between compressions.
   d. It can spontaneously terminate ventricular fibrillation.

4. Your patient is a seven-year-old child who suddenly collapsed whole playing soccer. Your AED is not equipped to decrease the amount of energy delivered from the amount for adult patients. Which one of the following is the best solution?

   a. Apply the defibrillation pads further apart than you normally would, placing one on the upper right chest and the other on the left thigh.
   b. Omit defibrillation as part of the treatment and perform CPR only.
   c. Delay defibrillation as long as possible in the hopes that CPR will result in ROSC.
   d. Apply and use the defibrillator, using the preset energy levels for adult patients.

5. Which one of the following best explains the pathophysiology of septic shock?

   a. Inability of the heart to maintain adequate forward flow of blood
   b. Loss of sympathetic nervous system influence on the vascular system
   c. Vasodilation and increased capillary permeability
   d. Increased resistance to venous blood return to the heart

6. When two health care providers are performing CPR on a five-year-old child, the ratio of chest compressions to ventilations is:

   a. 15:1.
   b. 15:2.
   c. 30:2.
   d. 30:4.

7. When performing CPR for an adult, the rate of compressions is at least _____ per minute.

   a. 50
   b. 80
   c. 100
   d. 150

8. In which one of the situations below is it recommended that chest compressions be performed by encircling the patient's chest with your hands and placing your thumbs over the lower sternum?

   a. Two-year-old child, when there are two health care providers present
   b. Two-year-old child when there is one health care provider present
   c. Three-month-old child when there are two health care providers present
   d. Three-month-old child when there is one health care provider present

9. You have just entered a scene where a 14-year-old child was found unresponsive by his parents. He is not breathing and does not have a pulse. Which one of the following should you do first?

   a. Deliver 30 chest compressions.
   b. Open the airway with a head-tilt/chin-lift maneuver.
   c. Determine if the parents want you to attempt resuscitation.
   d. Apply an AED.

10. Your patient is a 50-year-old female who was shot in the thigh in a hunting incident. She is awake, but pale and diaphoretic with a significant amount of bleeding from the wound. You should first attempt to control bleeding by applying:

    a. a topical hemostatic agent.
    b. a tourniquet.
    c. a PASG.
    d. direct pressure.

11. Your patient is a 27-year-old male who fell from a one-story roof and was impaled in the right flank by a screwdriver that was in his tool belt. He is confused, with pale, cold, diaphoretic skin and a very weak radial pulse. There is little external bleeding from the wound. After initial management of his airway and breathing and applying oxygen by nonrebreather mask, you determine that he has a systolic blood pressure of 70 mmHg. You do not suspect that he has a significant traumatic brain injury. After establishing two 14-gauge IVs of normal saline, which one of the following is the best approach to intravenous fluid administration in this patient?

    a. Administer an initial bolus of 2 L.
    b. Give a 500-mL bolus, and check to see if the systolic blood pressure is between 80 and 90 mmHg.
    c. Maintain both IVs at a keep-open rate.
    d. Infuse as much fluid as needed to achieve and maintain a systolic blood pressure of at least 120 mmHg.

12. In which one of the following situations may therapeutic hypothermia be useful?

    a. In cardiac arrest when ROSC cannot be obtained
    b. In cardiac arrest after ROSC occurs
    c. In decompensated hemorrhagic shock
    d. In patients with hemorrhagic shock and traumatic brain injury

Critical-Thinking Questions

13. A 19-year-old female has multiple stab wounds to her torso. She is unresponsive, with pale, cold, diaphoretic skin. Her radial pulse is absent and her carotid pulse is weak and rapid. What is happening in the body that explains the findings?

14. You are working with a veteran partner who proclaims that he disagrees with the CAB approach to cardiac arrest. How can you explain to him the rationale that supports this approach?

15. Your patient is a 60-year-old male who is unresponsive, but who has warm, dry skin. His radial pulse is weak, but present at a rate of 38 beats per minute. Is this patient in shock? What is the rationale for your answer?

16. The survival rate from out-of-hospital cardiac arrest in your community is lower than average. What are some possible explanations? What are some ways to improve survival rates?

References

Achneck, H. E., Sileshi, B., Jamiolkowski, R. M., Albala, D. M., Shapiro, M. L., & Lawson, J. H. (2010). A comprehensive review of topical hemostatic agents: Efficacy and recommendations for use. *Annals of Surgery, 251*, 217–228.

American Heart Association. (2010). Part 5: Adult Basic Life Support: 2010 Guidelines for Cardiopulmonary Resuscitation and Emergency Cardiac Care. *Circulation, 122* S685-705 DOI: 10.1161/CIRCULATIONAHA.110.970939

Bocka, J. L. (2009). Automatic defibrillation. *eMedicine*. Retrieved November 28, 2010, from http://emedicine.medscape.com/article/780533-overview

Gegel, B., Burgert, J., Cooley, B., MacGregor, J., Myers, J., Calder, S., Johnson, D. (2010). The effects of Bleed Arrest, Celox, and TraumaDex on hemorrhage control in a porcine model. *Journal of Surgical Research, 164*, e125–e129.

McSwain, N.E., Salomone, J., & Pons, P. T. (Eds.). (2007). *Prehospital trauma life support* (6th ed.). St. Louis, MO: Elsevier.

Swan, K. G. Jr., Wright, D. S., Barbagiovanni, S. S., Swan, B. C., & Swan, K. G. (2009). Tourniquets revisited. *Journal of Trauma Injury, Infection, and Critical Care, 66*, 672–675.

18

Vital Signs and Monitoring Devices

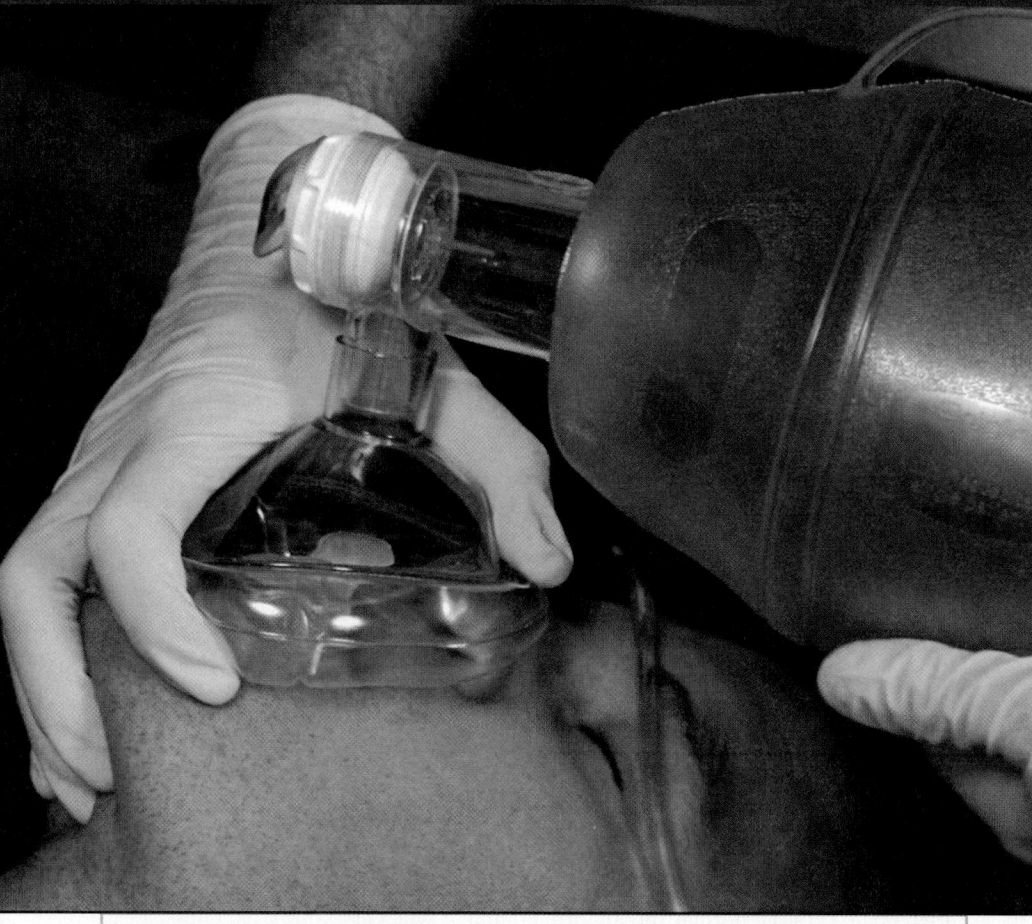

Content Area: Assessment

Advanced EMT Education Standard: Applies scene information and patient assessment findings (scene size-up, primary and secondary assessments, patient history, and reassessment) to guide emergency management.

Objectives

After reading this chapter, you should be able to:

18.1   Define key terms introduced in this chapter.

18.2   Discuss the importance of accurate assessment and documentation of vital signs over the course of contact with the patient to identify problems and changes in the patient's condition.

18.3   Perform the steps required to assess the patient's breathing, pulse, skin, pupils, blood pressure, and oxygen saturation.

18.4   Consider a patient's overall presentation when interpreting the meaning of vital sign findings.

(continued)

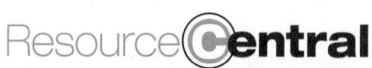

To access Resource Central, follow the directions on the Student Access Card provided with this text. If there is no card, go to www.bradybooks.com and follow the Resource Central link to Buy Access. Under Media Resources, you will find:

• *Heath & Physical Assessment.* Watch how to effectively perform a health assessment.

• *Riding the Wave.* Learn about the types of end-tidal CO_2 monitoring devices.

• *Blood Glucose Monitoring.* Review the steps for measuring blood glucose.

KEY TERMS (continued)

pyrexia *(p. 465)*

rhonchi *(p. 464)*

sphygmomanometer *(p. 454)*

static ECG *(p. 471)*

systolic blood pressure
(p. 458)

tachycardia *(p. 456)*

turgor *(p. 466)*

tympanic temperature *(p. 465)*

vital signs *(p. 454)*

CASE STUDY

Advanced EMTs Matt Brewer and Marcie Pickett have just entered the office of Denny Haines. Mr. Haines is awake and alert, though he appears to be in pain, and is squinting and rubbing the back of his head. Mr. Haines is a 42-year-old man with a busy, active schedule who just told Matt and Marcie that he had a sudden headache that started in the back of his head. He describes it as the worst headache he's ever had—a 10 on a scale of 10. He says he was sitting at his desk when "it felt like a miniature grenade went off inside my head."

Matt and Marcie have determined that Mr. Haines' airway is not in immediate jeopardy, his breathing is adequate, and so is his perfusion. They recognize, though, that this is a serious chief complaint, requiring prompt transport to the hospital.

Problem-Solving Questions

1. How should Marcie and Matt go about getting vital signs for this patient while considering the patient's priority for transport?
2. How will they know if the patient's vital signs are normal or abnormal?
3. What other types of information should they obtain from special monitoring devices?

(continued from previous page)

18.5 Differentiate between normal and abnormal findings when assessing a patient's breathing to include the respiratory rate, depth of respirations, rhythm of respiration, and signs that indicate respiratory distress or respiratory failure.

18.6 Differentiate between normal respiratory rates for adults, children, infants, and newborns.

18.7 Evaluate the need to administer treatment based on assessment of a patient's breathing.

18.8 Auscultate breath sounds to determine the presence of breath sounds, equality of breath sounds, and the presence of abnormal breath sounds.

18.9 Identify abnormal sounds associated with breathing with the likely underlying cause, including snoring, gurgling, stridor, wheezing, crackles (rales), and rhonchi.

18.10 Assess the pulse at each of the following pulse points: carotid, femoral, radial, brachial, popliteal, posterior tibial, and dorsalis pedis.

18.11 Consider the patient's age and level of responsiveness when selecting a site to palpate the pulse.

18.12 Differentiate between normal and abnormal findings when assessing a patient's pulse to include the pulse rate, quality of the pulse, and rhythm of the pulse.

18.13 Differentiate between normal heart rates for adults, children, infants, and newborns.

18.14 Associate abnormalities in the assessment of pulses with possible underlying causes.

18.15 Describe pulsus alternans and pulsus paradoxus.

18.16 Recognize normal and abnormal findings in the assessment of skin and mucous membrane color, skin temperature and condition, and capillary refill time.

18.17 Associate abnormal findings in skin color, temperature, and condition with potential underlying causes.

18.18 Explain factors that can affect capillary refill time.

18.19 Differentiate among normal, dilated, and constricted pupils.

18.20 Recognize anisocoria (inequality of pupils) greater than 2 mm.

18.21 Assess the pupils for size, equality, and reactivity to light.

18.22 Associate abnormal pupil findings with potential underlying causes.

18.23 Explain the underlying physiologic processes being evaluated by measuring systolic and diastolic blood pressure.

18.24 Demonstrate the proper techniques of obtaining blood pressure by auscultation, palpation, and noninvasive blood pressure monitoring.

18.25 Relate the methods, techniques, and equipment for obtaining a blood pressure measurement to differences in findings and potential errors in blood pressure measurement.

18.26 Determine whether a blood pressure value is consistent with expected values for the patient's age and gender.

18.27 Use the blood pressure value to find the patient's pulse pressure and mean arterial pressure (MAP).

18.28 List potential causes of abnormal findings or changes in blood pressure and pulse pressure.

18.29 Explain the concept of orthostatic (postural) hypotension.

18.30 Given a patient scenario, determine the frequency with which vital signs should be reassessed.

18.31 Explain what is being measured when pulse oximetry is used.

18.32 Describe factors and limitations that should be taken into consideration when interpreting the meaning of pulse oximetry findings.

18.33 Explain what is being measured when capnography is used.

18.34 Describe factors and limitations that should be taken into consideration when interpreting the meaning of capnography findings.

18.35 Explain what is being measured when a glucometer is used.

18.36 Use glucometry values as an adjunct in determining the need for supplemental glucose/dextrose administration.

18.37 Describe factors and limitations that should be taken into consideration when interpreting the meaning of glucometry findings.

18.38 Describe the value of continuous ECG monitoring.

18.39 Obtain a Lead II ECG recording.

Introduction

Vital signs, assessment of the skin and pupils, and information from a variety of patient monitoring devices are obtained during the secondary assessment. Those observations provide a wealth of information to assist with further patient assessment and decision making. You must know what information to collect, how and when to collect it, and what it means to each particular patient's condition.

Vital signs include pulse rate, blood pressure, respiratory rate, and temperature. Making observations about the patient's skin and pupils also gives initial information about the patient's general condition. Monitoring devices that may be used by Advanced EMTs include electronic vital sign monitoring, pulse oximetry, capnography, electrocardiogram (ECG) monitoring, and blood glucose level determination.

The information available from vital signs, assessment of the skin and pupils, and monitoring devices is useful only if it is relevant and integrated into an overall impression of the patient's condition. A single finding in isolation from the patient's other signs and symptoms is not useful, and may result in misguided patient care decisions. In this chapter, you will learn how to assess vital signs, the skin and pupils, and how to use monitoring devices. Your understanding of when to use these skills and how to interpret the results will continue to develop through subsequent chapters and through experience.

Integrating Vital Signs and Monitoring Devices into the Assessment Process

Smoothly integrating assessment of **vital signs** and the use of monitoring devices into the patient care process requires teamwork, as well as your general impression of the patient from the primary assessment. A full set of baseline vital signs should be obtained as soon as possible for all patients. For a critical *trauma* patient, this may mean that you obtain the vital signs after the patient is packaged and loaded into the ambulance for transport. For a critical *medical* patient, this may mean your partner gets vital signs while you start an IV at the scene. For a noncritical patient, take vital signs while your partner takes a history, writes down a list of medications, or talks to a family member. Note that some patients require blood glucose testing, and some do not, and some patients need a pulse oximetry reading sooner than others.

The key is that you must properly prioritize these tasks in relation to the patient's condition, anticipated treatment, and other tasks that you must complete. You also must consider the amount of help you have available at the scene and during transport. Communicate with your team members as needed to ensure that tasks are properly prioritized.

The frequency with which vital signs and information from monitoring devices is reassessed depends on your determination of how critical the patient is and the treatments you are providing. Assess critical patients' vital signs every 5 minutes, or sooner. Assess noncritical patients' vital signs every 15 minutes, or at least once after obtaining the baseline. If you work in an area where some transports are only 5 to 10 minutes long, it may be sufficient to obtain baseline vital signs and one additional set of vital signs, based on your protocols.

Assess vital signs before and after giving medications. Reassess vital signs if the patient offers additional complaints, has increased distress, or you suspect the patient's condition is worsening. For example, pulse oximetry devices and ECG monitors allow continuous monitoring of the heart rate. A sudden unexplained change in heart rate should prompt reassessment of the primary assessment and vital signs.

Vital Signs

The four vital signs are pulse, respirations, blood pressure, and temperature. You must obtain pulse and respirations on all patients. Blood pressure is measured on all patients over the age of three years. To evaluate perfusion in patients who are younger than three, **capillary refill time** is used in conjunction with the other vital signs and the patient's general appearance.

A temperature is not routinely obtained in the prehospital setting. In some cases, however, it is important. For

example, if you suspect fever or a heat-related or cold-related emergency, it is important to assess the body temperature with a thermometer. Body temperature changes relatively slowly. Unless transport time is prolonged, the temperature is usually not taken a second time.

Some simple equipment is needed to obtain a set of vital signs. You will need the following:

- Watch or clock with a second hand (you can use a digital watch with a stopwatch feature)
- Stethoscope
- **Sphygmomanometer** (blood pressure cuff)
- Thermometer
- Penlight (for assessment of the pupils)

Assessing the Pulse

The pulse is the intermittent wave of pressure felt in arteries as a result of left ventricular systole (contraction). Each time the left ventricle ejects blood into the aorta, there is a brief increase in blood pressure. This expands the arteries as the pressure wave passes through them. You can feel (**palpate**) the pulsation of each pressure wave in superficial arteries that pass over firmer underlying tissues (Figure 18-1). Assessing the pulse gives information about cardiac function and tissue perfusion. The pulse is assessed as an indication of both systemic circulation and circulation to individual extremities.

In general, the greater the blood pressure, the further away from the heart you can feel a pulse. **Peripheral pulses** are assessed in responsive patients. **Central pulses** are assessed in unresponsive patients. In responsive adults, the radial pulse in the wrist is assessed. In unresponsive adult patients, the carotid pulse in the neck is palpated. During

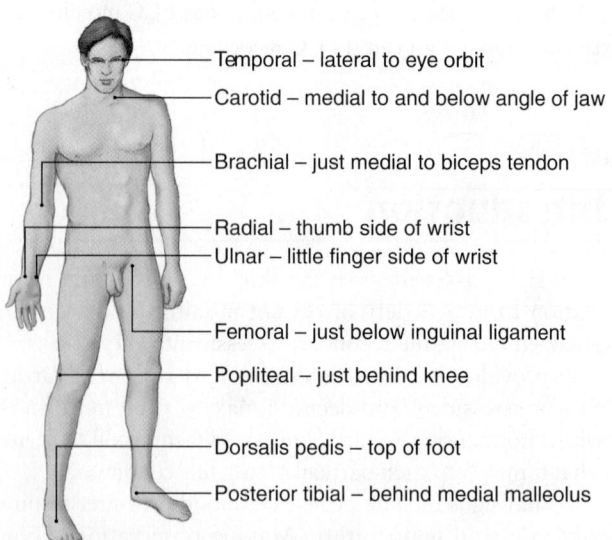

FIGURE 18-1

Pulse locations.

resuscitation efforts and in critical unresponsive patients without a radial pulse, you can assess the femoral pulse. It is sometimes difficult to find the radial pulse in small children. In that case, you can palpate the brachial pulse in the **antecubital fossa** (Figure 18-2). In infants, the brachial pulse along the medial humerus is palpated.

The pulse is assessed for rate, rhythm, volume, and strength. The sensation of a normal pulse is learned through experience. Take every opportunity to practice assessing pulses. You will soon learn what is within the normal range. Being familiar with "normal" allows you to quickly recognize when a patient's pulse is not normal.

Press lightly with the tips of your index and middle fingers over the location of the artery to find the pulse (Figure 18-3). Do not use your thumb, because it has a pulse of its own that you could confuse with the patient's pulse. If your pressure is too light, you will not be able to feel the pulsations. If your pressure is too firm, you can occlude the artery, and you will not feel the pulse. While maintaining your fingertips on the pulse, look at a clock or watch with a second hand. Count the number of pulsations in 15 seconds. Multiply by 4 to obtain the number of pulsations in 1 minute.

The normal heart rate in adults is from 60 to 100 beats per minute. Normal heart rates for infants and children vary with age (Table 18-1). While counting, pay attention to the strength and volume of the pulse, as well as its rhythm. The

IN THE FIELD

Because you can occlude the pulse with fingertip pressure, you should never check the carotid pulse on both sides at the same time.

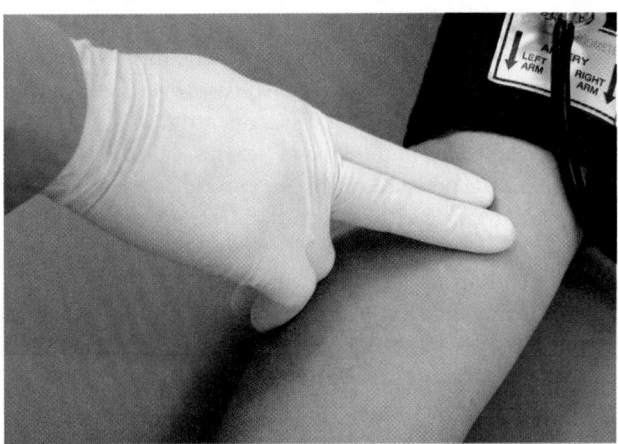

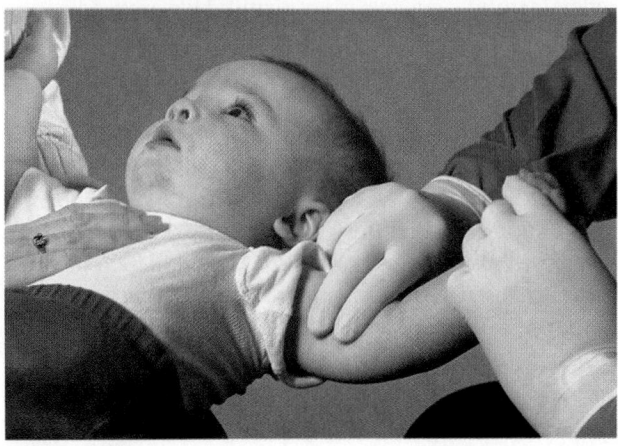

FIGURE 18-2

The brachial pulse is palpated in the antecubital fossa in adults, and along the medial humerus in infants. (Bottom photo: © Daniel Limmer)

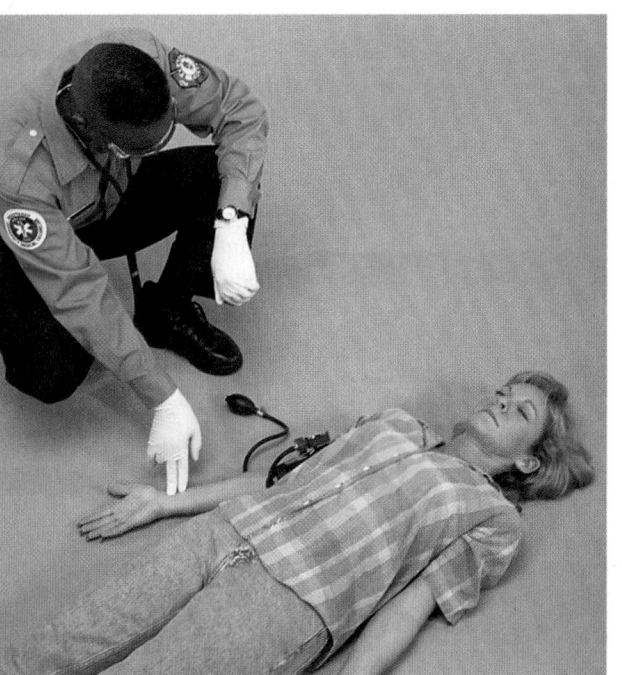

FIGURE 18-3

Palpate the radial pulse by counting the number of beats in 15 seconds and multiplying by 4.

TABLE 18-1	**Normal Pediatric Vital Signs**		
Age Group	Respiratory Rate	Heart Rate	Systolic Blood Pressure
Newborn	30–60	100–180	70–90
Infant	25–40	100–160	70–90
Toddler	24–30	80–130	72–100
Preschooler	22–34	80–120	78–104
School age	18–30	70–110	80–115
Adolescent	12–20	60–105	88–120

pulse should be regular, strong, and full. Count an irregular, abnormally fast, or abnormally slow pulse for a full minute to obtain an accurate rate.

Heart Rate

A heart rate that is faster than normal (>100 per minute in an adult) is called **tachycardia**. Tachycardia can be caused by anxiety, fear, pain, blood loss, dehydration, fever, hypoxia, heart failure, caffeine or other stimulants, or by cardiac dysrhythmia. Attribute tachycardia to anxiety or fear only after investigating for potentially life-threatening causes. Even then, remember that your patient is just that—a patient. There is some mechanism of injury or illness present that prompted a call for EMS.

Maintain an appropriate index of suspicion for a pathologic cause of tachycardia. An acute stress response presents with similar signs and symptoms, whether the cause is a perceived threat or actual physical harm. The signs and symptoms of stress, including an increased heart rate, involve the body's response to the release of adrenalin (epinephrine). A patient who has just crashed his car is very likely to be upset. The adrenalin released in the stress response will increase his heart rate. However, if the patient is bleeding from internal injuries sustained in the collision, the heart rate will increase to compensate for the decrease in blood volume—also in response to adrenalin.

You must consider the causes of tachycardia, but you must also consider its consequences. A heart that is working faster requires more oxygen, and therefore more perfusion of oxygenated blood to each cell in the heart. If the blood volume remains normal, the heart can maintain adequate cardiac output up to a rate of 150 per minute or so. Beyond this point, there is not enough time between each contraction of the ventricles for them to fill sufficiently with blood. Therefore, each contraction of the ventricles delivers a volume of blood that is less than adequate. The blood pressure may drop and the tissues, including the heart itself, will not be adequately perfused.

At very high heart rates, the heart requires more oxygenated blood than normal, but receives less oxygenated blood than normal because the diastolic time, during which the myocardium is perfused by the coronary arteries, is greatly reduced. The result is myocardial ischemia. The risk of ischemia is even greater in patients who have pre-existing coronary artery disease. The decrease in perfusion to the

brain may result in confusion or decreased level of responsiveness, as well as other signs of shock. (See Chapter 10.)

Bradycardia is a slower-than-normal (<60 per minute in an adult) heart rate. In some well-conditioned athletes, the heart may be so efficient that the "normal" heart rate for these individuals would be considered bradycardic for most people. As always, consider the heart rate in the context of the patient's complaint, history, and overall condition. Bradycardia can occur in response to a problem with the cardiac conduction system, excessive stimulation of the vagus nerve, or as a reflex response to hypertension, including hypertension caused by increased intracranial pressure.

The vagus nerve, the tenth pair of cranial nerves that exit from the brainstem, serves many organs of the body, including the sinoatrial node of the heart, and organs of the gastrointestinal system. The vagus nerve is part of the parasympathetic nervous system. The overall responsibilities of the parasympathetic nervous system include digestion and other routine body functions. When the vagus nerve is stimulated, its effect is to inhibit the sinoatrial node of the heart. Inhibition of the heart's normal pacemaker can result in a heart rate of less than 60. Occasionally, stimulation of the vagus nerve by way of the digestive system can result in vagal stimulation of the sinoatrial node. Vomiting, a distended stomach, or straining to have a bowel movement have been known to result in bradycardia. Typically, this type of bradycardia is temporary, and is called *vasovagal bradycardia*, which may result in vasovagal syncope.

Special nerves in the carotid arteries, called *baroreceptors*, detect the pressure within the carotid arteries and send feedback to the heart by way of the nervous system. When the pressure detected is low, the sympathetic nervous system responds by increasing the heart rate to increase cardiac output. This would occur, for example, when blood volume is lost because of hemorrhage. When the pressure detected is high, the parasympathetic nervous system responds by inhibiting the sinoatrial node, decreasing the heart rate.

Some individuals have a very sensitive carotid sinus reflex (carotid sinus hypersensitivity). Hyperextending the neck to look upward, or even wearing a tight shirt collar, can place pressure on the nerves in the carotid arteries, resulting in reflex bradycardia. In such cases, the temporary decrease in cardiac output interrupts blood flow to the cerebrum sufficiently to cause a temporary loss of consciousness, called a *syncopal (fainting) episode*. When the pressure inside the cranium (intracranial pressure, or ICP) increases, such as when the brain swells in response to injury, blood pressure must increase to overcome the resistance. This increase in blood pressure can result in a reflex slowing of the heart rate.

Geriatric Care

As body systems age, they become less able to respond in ways that maintain homeostasis. A normal response to significant bleeding is for the heart rate to increase. The heart rate of an elderly person may not increase as much as expected. Diseases of the cardiac conduction system and some medications, such as beta blockers, also can keep the heart rate from increasing to meet the body's needs.

Pediatric Care

Bradycardia in pediatric patients is an indication of hypoxia. Reassess the patient's airway, breathing, and oxygenation.

This combination of **hypertension** and bradycardia in a patient with a brain injury is known as **Cushing's reflex**.

Normally, there is a balance between the sympathetic and parasympathetic nervous systems, so the heart rate is fine-tuned to exactly meet the body's demands on a moment-to-moment basis. In some patients with high blood pressure or certain cardiac dysrhythmias, though, it is desirable to decrease the effects of the sympathetic nervous system. Beta blockers are a class of medications that inhibit functions of the sympathetic nervous system. An overdose—either accidental or intentional—can result in bradycardia that is extremely difficult to treat. Overdose of calcium channel blocker medications also causes bradycardia. (See Chapter 21 for additional information.)

Bradycardia can lead to a decrease in cardiac output that is sufficient to cause hypoperfusion. In the case of a syncopal episode, the hypoperfusion is temporary. It is corrected by gravity when the patient falls (the heart does not have to pump against gravity) or when the heart rate returns to normal. In other cases, such as a problem with the cardiac conduction system, bradycardia is not as easily corrected. Intravenous medications or a temporary or permanent pacemaker may be required in such cases.

Heart Rhythm

A regular pulse means that there is the same amount of time between all heartbeats. In some individuals, the heart speeds up slightly with each inspiration and slows slightly with each expiration. This is a normal phenomenon. In some patients, you will detect irregularity in the pulse. You may note beats that come earlier than expected, or longer-than-expected pauses between beats in an otherwise regular rhythm. In some patients, there is no regularity to the rhythm at all.

A regular pulse does not necessarily mean that all is well with the patient, and an irregular pulse does not necessarily indicate an immediately life-threatening condition. As with all findings, you must interpret the regularity of the pulse in the context of the patient's complaint, medical history, and overall presentation.

Under the right conditions, anyone can experience a few irregular heartbeats without clinical significance. In a patient complaining of chest pain, though, an irregular pulse can mean that the patient is at risk for a lethal dysrhythmia. Some patients have a chronically irregular heart rhythm called **atrial fibrillation** (Figure 18-4). If it has previously been diagnosed, the patient may be able to tell you when you gather his history. Risk factors for atrial fibrillation include age, heart failure, and chronic lung disease. Many patients with atrial fibrillation take medications to control the heart rate (keeping it under 100 per minute), but the irregularity persists. In some cases, an irregular heartbeat can result in decreased cardiac output, with associated signs of poor perfusion.

Pulse Volume and Strength

Pulse volume is a reflection of arterial diameter, whereas pulse strength is an indication of blood pressure. Normally, the volume of the pulse is "full," but this is not often noted in prehospital documentation. When there is significant vasoconstriction, such as in shock, the pulse may feel "thready." You should document this finding.

Under normal conditions, the pulse is strong. When blood pressure is increased, the pulse may be even stronger, a feeling described as "bounding." When blood pressure is low, the pulse may feel weak.

Assessing Blood Pressure

Blood pressure is the amount of force exerted against the walls of the arteries by the blood flowing through them. In medicine, this pressure is measured in units of millimeters of mercury (mmHg). A certain amount of pressure is necessary for blood to circulate from the heart, through the miles of blood vessels in the body, and back to the heart again. Without adequate pressure, oxygenated blood cannot circulate through the capillary beds to deliver oxygen, nutrients, and other substances to the tissues and carry away waste products of metabolism. Adequate blood pressure is required for tissue perfusion. When disease processes result

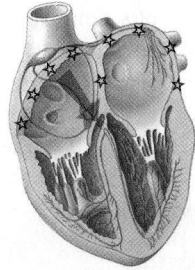

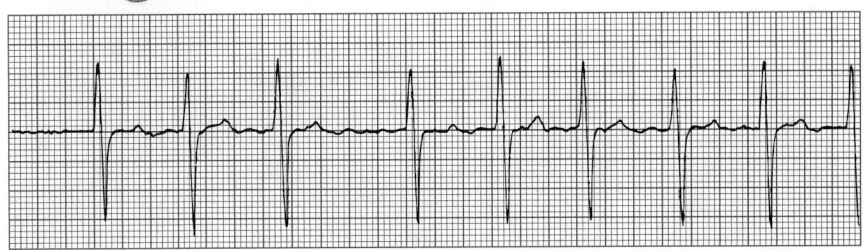

FIGURE 18-4

Atrial fibrillation is a cardiac dysrhythmia that produces an irregular pulse.

in chronic high blood pressure, tissue and organ damage occur. Very high blood pressure, even in the short term, can cause organ damage as well. It is important to take a blood pressure measurement for all patients.

Blood pressure depends on the volume of blood available, the effectiveness of the heart as a pump, and the capacity of the vascular system at any given moment. To understand the concept of blood pressure, you must understand stroke volume (SV), cardiac output (CO), and systemic vascular resistance (SVR). Blood pressure, represented by the **mean arterial pressure (MAP)**, is represented by the following formula:

$$MAP = CO \times SVR$$

Cardiac output is the volume of blood that leaves the left ventricle every minute, measured in liters per minute. It is determined by multiplying the amount of blood that leaves the left ventricle with each contraction (SV) by the number of times the heart contracts each minute (HR). Cardiac output is represented as the following formula:

$$CO = SV \times HR$$

A person with a stroke volume of 70 mL and a heart rate of 75 beats per minute has cardiac output of 5,250 mL/min, or 5.25 L/min.

The relationship between stroke volume and heart rate means that if one of those components decreases, cardiac output can be maintained by an increase in the other component. For example, if the stroke volume decreases to 50 mL, cardiac output can be maintained if the heart rate increases to 105 per minute. However, this ability to compensate has limits. Recall from the previous discussion on the pulse rate, that the ventricles do not have time to adequately fill when the heart rate is very rapid.

Systemic vascular resistance is based on the diameter of the blood vessels at any given time. The more constricted the blood vessels are, the smaller their diameter. The smaller their diameter, the more resistance there is to blood flow. The more resistance provided by the vascular system, the higher the pressure is within the vessels. Conversely, the more relaxed and dilated the vascular system, the lower the blood pressure will be, unless the heart rate goes up to compensate by increasing cardiac output.

As in the relationship between heart rate and stroke volume, a decrease in one component of the blood pressure equation can be compensated for by an increase in the other—to a degree. For example, if a loss of blood volume causes a decrease in stroke volume, you can expect to see increases in both heart rate and systemic vascular resistance to maintain blood pressure. This explains why in early hypovolemic shock, a patient's blood pressure may be normal, but the heart rate is increased and the skin is pale and cool because the peripheral blood vessels are constricted.

During each cardiac cycle, blood pressure is highest during ventricular systole. With each contraction, blood is ejected from the left ventricle and pushed through the arterial system. Each contraction of the heart causes an increase in pressure above the pressure in the arteries between contractions. The higher pressure associated with ventricular contraction is the **systolic blood pressure**. The lower blood pressure present during ventricular relaxation, or diastole, is the **diastolic blood pressure**.

The blood pressure is recorded as the systolic pressure "over" the diastolic pressure. A systolic pressure of 110 with a diastolic pressure of 70 is recorded as 110/70 mmHg. The typical range of adult systolic blood pressure is from 100 to 140 mmHg and the typical range of adult diastolic blood pressure is 60 to 90 mmHg. However, the National Heart Lung and Blood Institute (NHLBI) of the National Institutes of Health (NIH) considers a systolic blood pressure of less than 120 mmHg and a diastolic pressure of less than 80 mmHg healthy in adults (NHLBI, 2010). Blood pressures that are consistently above those levels are classified as follows:

- Systolic blood pressure of 120 to 139 mmHg or diastolic blood pressure of 80 to 89 mmHg is prehypertensive.
- Systolic blood pressure from 140 to 159 mmHg or diastolic blood pressure from 90 to 99 mmHg is stage I hypertension (high blood pressure).
- Systolic blood pressure 160 mmHg or above or diastolic blood pressure 100 mmHg or above is stage II hypertension.

Chronic hypertension is not diagnosed based on the blood pressure readings taken on a single occasion, particularly under stressful conditions, such as those that require EMS. However, hypertension is a common, serious, often "silent" disease that increases the risk of heart attack and stroke. **Hypotension** (low blood pressure) is also of concern in the prehospital setting.

Some healthy young adults, particularly females, may normally have a systolic blood pressure that is slightly below 100 mmHg. This underscores the importance of looking at vital signs in context and taking multiple sets of vital signs to detect trends. Children's blood pressures increase with age (Table 18-1). You must be familiar with the expected blood pressure measurements in patients of all ages.

By measuring the systolic and diastolic blood pressure, it is possible to calculate two other measurements that can be helpful. Although these readings are not typically recorded on the prehospital care report, they can provide useful information about critically ill and injured patients. Pulse pressure is the difference between the systolic and diastolic blood pressures, represented by the following formula:

$$systolic - diastolic = pulse\ pressure$$

Pulse pressures may get progressively narrower or wider over multiple readings in some conditions. For example, in patients with increased ICP, the pulse pressure may get progressively wider as the systolic blood pressure increases more than the diastolic blood pressure.

The mean arterial pressure (MAP) is the "average" amount of pressure in the arterial system. A MAP of at least 60 mmHg is required to adequately perfuse the brain, coronary arteries, and kidneys. A common way of estimating MAP is to add one third of the pulse pressure to the diastolic pressure. A person with a blood pressure of 110/80 mmHg has a pulse pressure of 30 mmHg. One third of the pulse pressure is 10 mmHg. By adding the diastolic pressure of 80 to one third of the pulse pressure, you obtain a MAP of 90 mmHg (MAP = 1/3 [110 − 80] = 90 mmHg).

Pulsus paradoxus is a drop in the systolic blood pressure of greater than 10 mmHg during inspiration. Normally, there is a slight drop in systolic pressure during inspiration, because the increased pressure within the chest cavity decreases cardiac output slightly. In some conditions, such as cardiac tamponade (accumulation of fluid or blood in the pericardial sac around the heart), there is a greater drop in systolic pressure during inspiration. Because the pulse is associated with the systolic blood pressure, pulsus paradoxus can be reflected by a pulse that gets weaker during inspiration. **Pulsus alternans** is an alternating pulse specifically due to left ventricular failure and is not related to breathing.

A stethoscope and a sphygmomanometer are used to measure blood pressure (Figure 18-5). You can obtain automated blood pressure readings by machine (Figure 18-6), but you should obtain a manual reading first as a baseline. Whether manual or automatic, you must calibrate all equipment, and ensure that it is in proper working order and is the proper size for the patient. A blood pressure cuff that is too narrow will result in an artificially high blood pressure reading, and one that is too wide will result in an artificially low reading. The width of the blood pressure cuff should be about 40 percent of the circumference of the patient's arm.

A blood pressure cuff consists of an inflatable bladder with a fabric or vinyl cover that has Velcro to secure it around the arm. The bladder has two tubes attached to it. One of the tubes is attached to a bulb that is squeezed to inflate the bladder. There is a valve at the junction of the tubing and bulb that is rolled open and closed, allowing the cuff to be inflated and deflated. The other tube is attached to a gauge that measures pressure in increments of 2 mmHg from 0 to 300. Because the markings on the gauge are in

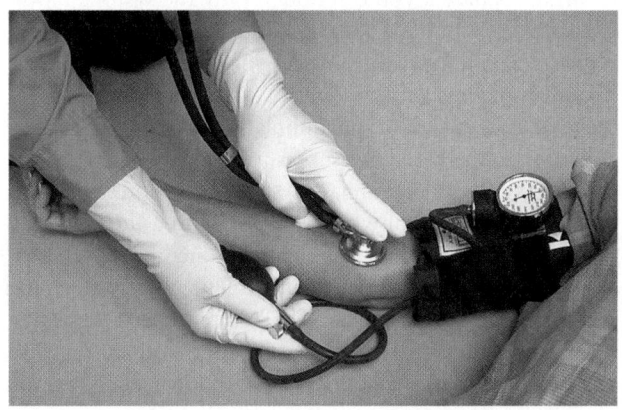

FIGURE 18-5

A blood pressure cuff and stethoscope are used to auscultate the blood pressure.

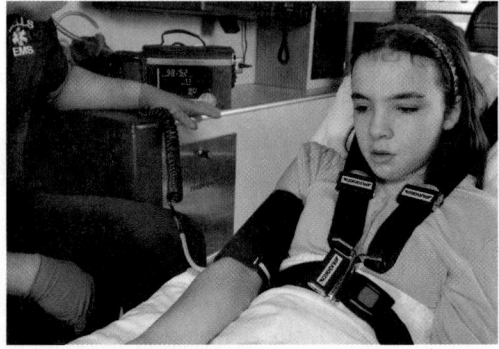

FIGURE 18-6

An automated blood pressure cuff.

increments of 2 mmHg, blood pressures taken manually are always recorded using only even numbers.

Blood pressure cuffs have a mark that is lined up with the brachial artery in the antecubital fossa. When a blood pressure cuff is positioned properly over the brachial artery, inflating the bladder occludes blood flow through this artery. As the blood pressure cuff is slowly deflated, the point at which the pressure in the brachial artery exceeds the pressure in the bladder is noted. You can do this by **auscultation** (listening) or palpation (feeling) over the brachial artery.

You can hear the force of the first pulsations of blood that exceed the pressure in the cuff with a stethoscope. These sounds, called **Korotkoff sounds**, are used to determine the systolic and diastolic blood pressure. Systolic blood pressure is determined by noting the position of the needle in the blood pressure gauge at the time the first sound is heard. The sounds are at first sharp, tapping sounds, but become muffled and then disappear. The sounds continue until the pressure in the cuff is equal to the diastolic blood pressure. Diastolic blood pressure is determined by noting the position of the needle in the gauge at the time of the last sound.

When palpating the blood pressure, the pulse in the radial artery is palpated as the cuff is deflated. The point at which the first pulsation is felt is the systolic blood pressure. Because the pulse will continue to be felt as the cuff is further deflated, you can obtain only the systolic blood pressure by palpation. Therefore, it is always preferable to obtain a blood pressure by auscultation, rather than by palpation. Sometimes, the amount of background noise at the scene or in the back of the ambulance interferes with auscultation, so the blood pressure is palpated.

Another way to estimate systolic blood pressure is to apply a waveform pulse oximetry probe to a finger on the same extremity in which you will be taking the blood pressure. Inflate the blood pressure cuff until the waveform on the pulse oximeter is obliterated. The point at which the waveform is obliterated is recorded as the systolic blood pressure (Mohler & Hart, 1994). In patients with low blood pressure, the Korotkoff sounds may be difficult to hear. You can sometimes palpate a blood pressure even though you cannot hear it.

When you inflate the blood pressure cuff, it is important that you do not overinflate it. Overinflating the cuff can artificially increase the blood pressure reading and is uncomfortable for the patient. Underinflating the cuff can result in missing the first Korotkoff sounds. To reach the proper inflation point, palpate the radial artery as you inflate the cuff. When the radial pulse disappears, inflate the cuff only about 20 mmHg more. For example, as you inflate the cuff, if you last feel the pulse at 140 mmHg, you should inflate the cuff only to 160 mmHg.

The steps of auscultating a blood pressure are as follows (Scan 18-1):

1. Tell the patient what you are going to do.
2. Remove heavy clothing from the arm (taking the blood pressure over heavy clothing, such as a sweater or jacket, artificially raises the reading; a thin shirt sleeve is okay).
3. Position the blood pressure cuff as follows:
   - Place the blood pressure cuff around the patient's arm, with its bottom edge about 1 inch above the crease in the elbow.
   - Ensure that the cuff is snug, and the marker on the cuff is in line with the brachial artery.
   - Palpate the brachial artery to ensure the cuff is placed properly. Note the location of the brachial artery, because this is where you will place the stethoscope.
   - Make sure you have a clear view of the dial on the gauge.
4. Support the patient's arm at the level of his heart.
5. Close the clamp on the inflation bulb.
6. Place the earpieces of the stethoscope in your ears.
7. Locate the radial pulse and continue to palpate it.
8. Inflate the cuff as follows:
   - Squeeze the inflation bulb several times quickly and firmly while palpating the radial pulse and watching the needle on the gauge.
   - Inflate the bulb 20 mmHg past the point at which the radial pulse disappears.
   - Close the valve on the inflation bulb.
9. Place the diaphragm of the stethoscope over the brachial pulse with light pressure.
10. Deflate the cuff and listen for the blood pressure as follows:
    - Watch the needle on the gauge.
    - Slowly and steadily open the valve to allow air to gradually escape from the bladder in the cuff. (Deflate at a rate of about 5 to 10 mmHg/second.)
    - Listen for Korotkoff sounds.
    - Note the pressure in the gauge at the time you hear the first sound. This is the systolic blood pressure.
    - Note the pressure in the gauge at the time of the last sound. This is the diastolic pressure.
    - Quickly release the remaining air from the cuff.
11. Take the earpieces of the stethoscope from your ears and remove the cuff from the patient's arm (unless the patient is critical and requires frequent blood pressure measurement).

IN THE FIELD

Some hypertensive patients have an ausculatory gap in the Korotkoff sounds. This means that there is an initial single tapping sound, followed by a pause, before you hear steady sounds. If you miss the initial sound and pick up only on the steady sounds, you will significantly underestimate the blood pressure.

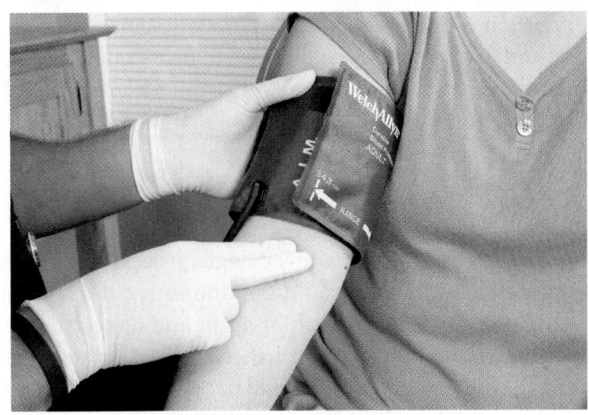

1. Tell the patient what you are going to do. Position the blood pressure cuff around the patient's arm with its bottom edge 1 inch above the crease of the elbow. The cuff should be snug and the marker on the cuff should be in line with the brachial artery.

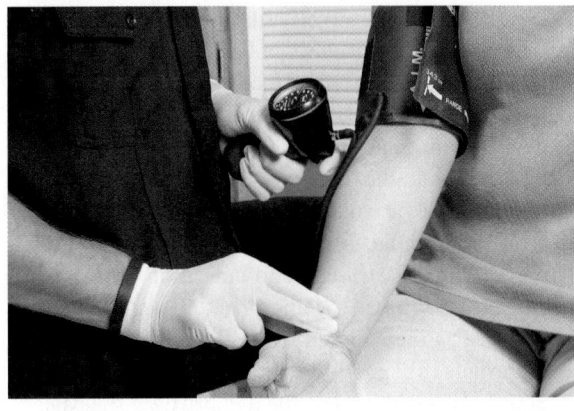

2. Locate the radial pulse and keep your fingers on it. Close the valve on the inflation bulb. Inflate the cuff by squeezing the bulb several times quickly and firmly while watching the needle on the gauge. Inflate the cuff 20 mmHg past the point where the radial pulse disappears.

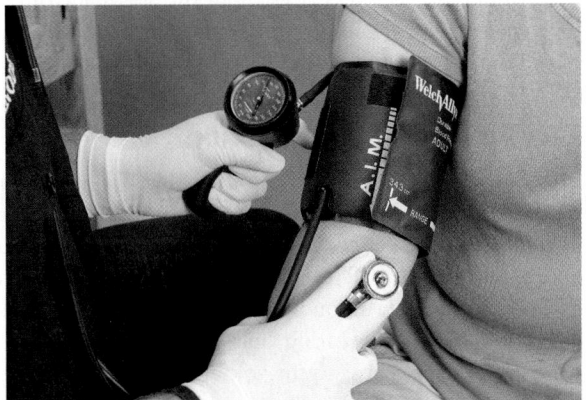

3. With the earpieces of the stethoscope in your ears, place the diaphragm of the stethoscope over the patient's brachial artery.

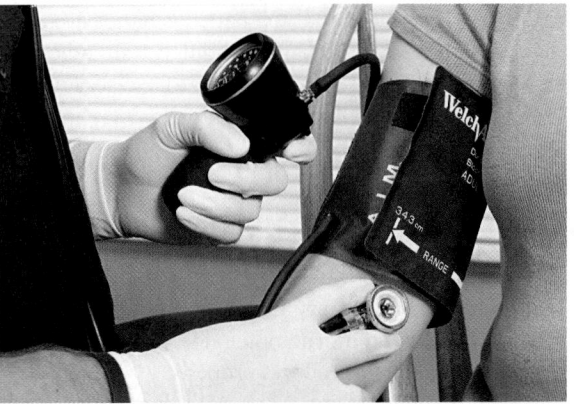

4. Listen and watch the gauge while slowly opening the valve on the inflation valve to deflate the cuff at a rate of 5 to 10 mmHg per second. Listen for the Korotkoff sounds. The position of the gauge when you hear the first sound is the systolic blood pressure. The position of the gauge when you hear the last sound is the diastolic blood pressure. Quickly release the remaining air from the cuff.

12. Determine what the patient's blood pressure reading means.

13. Record the reading as the systolic number over the diastolic number. For example: 122/74 mmHg.

To palpate a blood pressure, modify your technique as follows:

1. Instead of using the stethoscope to listen, keep your fingers on the point where you last felt the radial pulse when you inflated the cuff.

2. Continue to feel for the pulse as you slowly deflate the cuff, watching the needle on the gauge.

3. The point at which you first feel the radial pulse reappear is the systolic blood pressure.

4. Record the blood pressure as the systolic number over "palp" or "P." For example, 98/P mmHg.

IN THE FIELD

Never take a blood pressure in an arm with a hemodialysis access site (shunt or fistula). Do not take a blood pressure in the arm on the same side on which a woman has had a mastectomy that involved the removal of lymph nodes. Patients are educated to avoid procedures such as blood draws and blood pressure measurement on the affected side.

The cuff of an automated blood pressure device is positioned in the same way as if you are measuring the blood pressure manually. However, the tubes that emerge from the bladder are connected to the automated device. The device is powered on before the cuff is placed. Once the machine is ready, you can either push a button to take a blood pressure on demand or set a program to take the blood pressure at prescribed intervals. Automated devices give a digital readout of the patient's pulse and blood pressure. Most devices also calculate mean arterial pressure (MAP). Many automated blood pressure devices are part of monitoring devices with other functions, such as a thermometer, cardiac monitor, and the pulse oximeter.

Blood pressures are not routinely obtained on children under three years of age in the prehospital setting. Instead, capillary refill time is assessed as an indication of peripheral perfusion status. Squeeze the end of the patient's finger to apply pressure to the nail bed, then release. Squeezing the nail bed prevents capillary blood flow from reaching it. You can notice the lack of blood as the nail briefly turns pale, or blanches. The nail bed will turn pink again as blood flow is restored. This should occur in less than 2 seconds (about the time it takes for you to say, "capillary refill," to yourself).

A delay in capillary refill is an indication of poor perfusion to the peripheral tissues. This can be an indication of shock, but also can mean that the patient's hands are cold. Capillary refill time is less reliable in adults as an indication of perfusion status. Pre-existing circulatory disease, cigarette smoking, and other factors can cause a delay in capillary refill in adults.

Orthostatic Vital Signs

Taking orthostatic vital signs can provide useful information, but it is time consuming. Therefore, you should weigh the possible benefits of information gained against the time needed to perform the procedures properly.

Orthostatic hypotension or **postural hypotension** can occur in some individuals when they change from a prone to a standing position. From 300 to 800 mL of blood can move into the lower extremities when an individual moves from a supine (or prone) position to a standing position, because of the effects of gravity. Under normal circumstances, muscle contraction in the lower extremities and constriction of the blood vessels returns the blood into the circulation within a minute or two. When something interferes with the ability to compensate and return circulation to normal, the blood pressure remains low. This can cause a feeling of lightheadedness, or even syncope. Factors that can interfere with returning the circulation to normal include medications that prevent vasoconstriction or increase in heart rate, dehydration, and blood loss.

Orthostatic vital signs (pulse and blood pressure) can be useful when you suspect that a medical (not trauma) patient may be suffering from dehydration or blood loss, but there is not clear evidence that this is the case. If there is already clear evidence of those conditions, it is not necessary to take orthostatic vital signs in the prehospital setting. In fact, doing so could result in syncope and patient injury.

To take orthostatic vital signs, the patient must lie in a supine position for at least 3 minutes first. After you take the patient's blood pressure and heart rate, leave the cuff in place and have the patient stand for 3 minutes. Then, retake

the blood pressure and heart rate. Orthostatic (postural) hypotension is defined as a drop in systolic blood pressure of 20 mmHg or more, or an increase in heart rate of 20 beats per minute or more, 3 minutes after the patient assumes an upright position.

Assessing Respirations

Respiration is a complex physiologic process that requires ventilation, external respiration, and internal respiration. Ventilation is the movement of air in and out of the lungs. External respiration is the exchange of gases between the alveoli in the lungs and the blood in the capillary networks surrounding the alveoli. Internal respiration is the exchange of gases between the blood in the tissue capillaries and the cells.

Assessment of the respiratory rate is really an assessment of the ventilatory rate. Adequate ventilations are required for respiration, but ventilations alone cannot tell you everything you need to know about the adequacy of tissue oxygenation and the removal of carbon dioxide (CO_2) produced during cellular metabolism.

The Process of Ventilation

Effective ventilation requires a functioning brainstem, functioning nerve pathways, integrity of the chest wall and diaphragm, contact between the visceral and parietal pleura, and an open airway. The stimulus that starts a respiratory cycle is an increased amount of carbon dioxide in the blood. The movement of air during ventilation is based on the inverse relationship between the volume and pressure of a gas, and the fact that air moves from an area of higher pressure to an area of lower pressure.

The amount of carbon dioxide is detected by specialized receptors in the lining of the arch of the aorta, called *chemoreceptors*. When the level of carbon dioxide increases, the chemoreceptors, as well as an increased level of carbon dioxide in the cerebrospinal fluid (CSF), stimulate the respiratory center in the medulla oblongata of the brainstem. The medulla sends nerve impulses to the diaphragm and intercostal (between the ribs) muscles. When the diaphragm contracts, it moves downward and flattens, increasing the size of the chest cavity. When the intercostal muscles contract, they lift the ribs upward and outward, also increasing the size of the chest cavity. The potential space between the parietal pleura covering the lungs and the visceral pleura of the chest wall is occupied only by a thin layer of pleural fluid. As the chest wall moves, a pressure gradient is created between the layers so that the lungs are expanded as well.

The increased volume of the chest cavity and lungs results in lower air pressure within the chest and lungs. Air moves from the higher pressure of the atmosphere to the lower pressure within the lungs. When the lungs have expanded to a certain degree, stretch receptors in the lungs signal the brainstem to stop signaling the respiratory muscles to contract. This is called the *Hering–Breuer reflex*. When the diaphragm relaxes and moves upward, and the intercostal muscles relax, allowing the ribs to resume their resting position, the volume of the chest cavity becomes smaller. The smaller volume results in higher air pressure within the chest. Air moves from the higher pressure within the chest to the atmosphere. Movement of air out of the lungs is exhalation. Inhalation is the active phase of ventilation, and exhalation is normally passive. Ventilation is controlled by the autonomic nervous system, but can be temporarily altered by conscious effort.

Rate, Depth, Effort, and Regularity of Ventilations

Although you are, more accurately, assessing the patient's ventilations, this vital sign has been traditionally called the *respiratory rate (RR)*. Ventilations are assessed for rate, depth, effort, and regularity. The normal adult respiratory rate is from 12 to 20 breaths per minute at rest, regular in rhythm, and effortless. (See Table 18-1 for pediatric respiratory rates.) The amount of air that is inhaled and then exhaled in a normal breath is the tidal volume (TV). The average adult has a TV of 5 to 10 mL/kg of body weight (about 500 mL). Although it is not feasible to measure TV in the prehospital setting, it is important to understand the concept, and to get a sense of what normal TV "looks like." Just as you will learn through experience what a normal pulse feels like, you will learn what normal tidal volume looks like. Both TV and respiratory rate must be adequate to maintain an adequate minute volume of respiration.

Minute volume is calculated as TV × RR. A person with a respiratory rate (RR) of 16 and tidal volume (TV)

of 500 mL has a minute volume of 8,000 mL (8 L). If the tidal volume decreases, as in a patient whose chest muscles are paralyzed, the respiratory rate will increase to compensate. This compensatory mechanism is limited, though. Of the 500 mL of tidal volume, 350 mL reaches the alveoli and bronchioles, but 150 mL remain in the upper airway and bronchi, unavailable for gas exchange. The amount of air available for gas exchange is 5,600 mL (5.6 L) per minute. The 150 mL in the upper airways and bronchi is called *dead space air*. The amount of dead space does not decrease as tidal volume decreases. If tidal volume decreases to 300 mL, 150 mL remains unavailable for gas exchange, and the amount of air reaching the alveoli is reduced to 150 mL. So, although the minute volume is 4,800 mL (4.8 L), only 2,400 mL (2.4 L) is available for gas exchange.

Evaluation of ventilations begins in the primary assessment. You note if the patient is using accessory muscles, "tripoding" (leaning forward on the arms), exhibiting abnormal noises with ventilation, or has other signs of respiratory distress, such as cyanosis or altered mental status (Figure 18-7). Further assessment of ventilation includes obtaining a respiratory rate and carefully observing the depth and rhythm of ventilations (Table 18-2).

A patient's awareness that you are assessing his ventilations can make him feel conscious of the ventilations, which may alter them. It is preferred to observe the patient's ventilations unobtrusively. Keep your fingers on the radial pulse after you have calculated the heart rate so the patient is not aware that you have finished checking his pulse. Observe the patient's chest rise and fall. Each cycle of inspiration and expiration is one ventilation (one inspiration + one

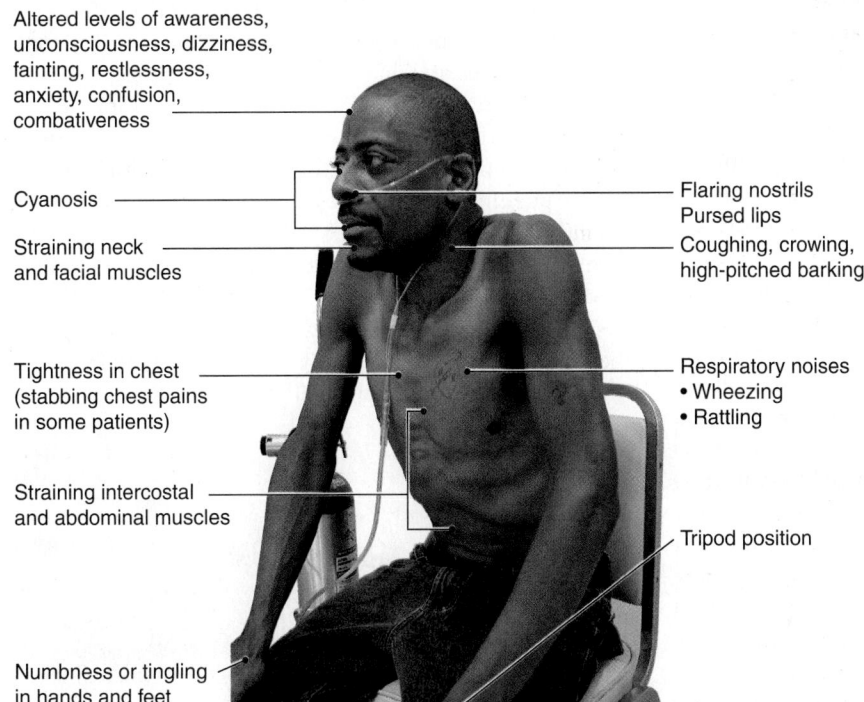

Altered levels of awareness, unconsciousness, dizziness, fainting, restlessness, anxiety, confusion, combativeness

Cyanosis

Straining neck and facial muscles

Tightness in chest (stabbing chest pains in some patients)

Straining intercostal and abdominal muscles

Numbness or tingling in hands and feet

Flaring nostrils
Pursed lips

Coughing, crowing, high-pitched barking

Respiratory noises
• Wheezing
• Rattling

Tripod position

FIGURE 18-7

Signs and symptoms of difficulty breathing. (© Ray Kemp/Triple Zilch Productions)

TABLE 18-2 Breathing Patterns

Condition	Description	Causes
Eupnea	Normal breathing rate and pattern	
Tachypnea	Increased respiratory rate	Fever, anxiety, exercise, shock
Bradypnea	Decreased respiratory rate	Sleep, drugs, metabolic disorder, head injury, stroke
Apnea	Absence of breathing	Deceased patient, head injury, stroke
Hyperpnea	Normal rate, but deep respirations	Emotional stress, diabetic ketoacidosis
Cheyne-Stokes respirations	Gradual increases and decreases in respirations with periods of apnea	Increasing intracranial pressure, brainstem injury
Biot's respirations	Rapid, deep respirations (gasps) with short pauses between sets	Spinal meningitis, many central nervous system causes, head injury
Kussmaul's respirations	Tachypnea and hyperpnea	Renal failure, metabolic acidosis, diabetic ketoacidosis
Apneustic	Prolonged inspiratory phase with shortened expiratory phase	Lesion in brainstem

expiration = one ventilation). Count the ventilations for 15 seconds and multiply by 4 to obtain the ventilatory rate. If you count three ventilations in 15 seconds, the patient's ventilatory rate is 12 per minute; four ventilations in 15 seconds means a ventilatory rate of 16, and so forth. Document your findings in the patient care report (PCR).

Assessing Breath Sounds

A complete assessment of ventilations includes assessing breath sounds. You should have noted and addressed abnormal upper airway sounds in the primary assessment (Chapter 15), but those sounds may develop later and you must address them as soon as you note them.

Abnormal upper airway sounds include snoring, gurgling, and stridor. Snoring is caused by partial occlusion of the upper airway by the tongue, and is corrected by manual positioning and, if indicated, an oropharyngeal or nasopharyngeal airway. Gurgling is an indication of fluid (for example, blood or vomit) in the airway. You must clear the airway of fluids to prevent aspiration and keep the airway open. Use suction to remove fluids. If not contraindicated, the recovery position can help prevent aspiration.

Stridor is a high-pitched sound that is an indication of partial obstruction of the larynx or trachea, such as by edema or a foreign body. If initial measures are ineffective in correcting upper airway problems, you may need to use more advanced airway adjuncts. (See Chapter 16.)

Lung sounds are auscultated using a stethoscope to listen for normal air movement and for extra, abnormal sounds (adventitious sounds). Place the diaphragm of the stethoscope directly on the chest wall with gentle pressure.

Friction of the diaphragm over clothing will cause noise that interferes with listening to breath sounds.

Abnormal breath sounds include crackles (rales), **rhonchi**, and wheezes. Crackles (rales) indicate fluid in the terminal bronchioles and alveoli. Crackles are a fine, popping, crackling sound, sometimes compared to the initial "fizzing" sounds after a can of soda is opened. Crackles typically are heard during inspiration. Crackles that disappear after a deep breath may be caused by collapsed alveoli opening up. You will hear crackles associated with heart failure and pulmonary edema first in the lowest areas of the lungs, but the level becomes higher as the condition progresses.

Rhonchi are lower-pitched, coarser rumbling sounds associated with secretions in the larger airways. Rhonchi are heard mostly on expiration in patients with bronchitis or pneumonia. Wheezes are high-pitched whistling sounds heard during exhalation. Wheezes are caused by constriction of the bronchioles, such as occurs in asthma and COPD.

When documenting lung sounds, note whether you heard breaths sounds bilaterally (on both sides) and whether they were clear, or if abnormal sounds were present. Also

Pediatric Care

Bronchiolitis and asthma can present similarly in infants. However, in bronchiolitis, it is more typical to hear fine rales, rather than wheezes, when auscultating the lung sounds. Bronchiolitis is associated with respiratory syncytial virus (RSV) and is common in the winter months.

note the location in which you heard any abnormal sounds. Examples include the following:

- Breath sounds were clear and equal bilaterally.
- Wheezes were heard in all lung fields on expiration.
- Rhonchi were heard in the left lower lung.
- Crackles were heard in the lower lungs bilaterally.

Assessing Body Temperature

Checking a patient's skin temperature gives a general indication of body temperature, but sometimes an exact temperature reading is desired. In some systems with longer transport times, Advanced EMTs may be able to give acetaminophen or ibuprofen to children with fevers, but you will need to measure the temperature first, using a thermometer. Other instances in which it is useful for you to know a patient's body temperature include heat-related and cold-related emergencies.

The average normal body temperature taken orally is 37 degrees Celsius (C), or about 98.6 degrees Fahrenheit (F). The temperature fluctuates over the course of the day and may be as low as 35.8°C or 96.4°F, or as high as 37.3°C or 99.1°F. Temperatures taken rectally are about 0.5°C or 1°F higher than oral temperatures, and **tympanic temperatures** may be up to 0.8°C or 1.4°F higher than oral temperatures. If you must take an axillary (under the arm) temperature, keep in mind that it is a less accurate method, takes longer to register, and is about 0.5°C or 1°F lower than an oral temperature.

Fever, or **pyrexia**, is an elevation of the body temperature above normal. Fever is often caused by infection, but also can be caused by blood transfusion reactions, medication reactions, and hyperthyroidism. The term *hyperthermia* is used to refer to an increase in body temperature because of the environment. **Hypothermia** is a lower-than-normal body temperature, and may be caused by environmental exposure, impaired vasoconstriction (as in patients with septic shock), or hypothyroidism.

A fever is not considered medically significant unless it is above 38°C or 100.4°F. However, you do not necessarily need to treat low-grade fever unless the patient is uncomfortable. You must treat fever that is above 40°C or 104°F. **Hyperpyrexia** is an extreme elevation in body temperature, above 40.1°C or 106°F.

A variety of types of thermometers are marketed, and there has been some debate about the accuracy of the different types. Older thermometers consisted of a closed glass tube containing mercury. Most thermometers used today give a digital reading of the temperature in degrees Celsius, degrees Fahrenheit, or both. Most people in the United States are more familiar with degrees Fahrenheit, so it is useful to be able to convert a temperature reading obtained in degrees Celsius to the Fahrenheit scale (Table 18-3). A pocket reference guide that contains a conversion scale is very useful.

Advanced EMTs will most often use an oral or tympanic (ear) thermometer, but may occasionally need to take a rectal or axillary temperature. Forehead thermometer strips have recently become available, but their accuracy is questionable. Before using any oral, tympanic, or rectal thermometer to take a patient's temperature, you must cover the tip of the thermometer or thermometer probe with a disposable cover.

Place the tip of an oral thermometer under the tongue and you must keep the mouth closed to obtain an accurate reading (Figure 18-8). A digital thermometer generally gives

TABLE 18-3	Celsius–Fahrenheit Conversion Table
Degrees Celsius	**Degrees Fahrenheit**
35	95
36	96.8
37	98.6
38	100.4
38.6	101.4
39	102.2
39.6	103.2
40	104

To convert Celsius to Fahrenheit, multiply by 9/5 and add 32. To convert Fahrenheit to Celsius, subtract 32 and multiply by 5/9.

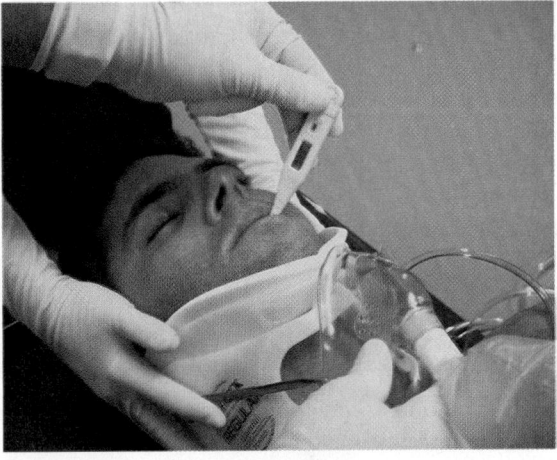

FIGURE 18-8

Taking an oral temperature.

Geriatric Care

The elderly are less likely than younger patients to exhibit fever in response to infection. An elderly patient may have a serious infection without a fever. Elderly patients are also more prone to hypothermia, with or without an infection.

CASE STUDY (continued)

Advanced EMTs Matt and Marcie are on the scene with Mr. Haines, a 42-year-old man complaining of a sudden headache. "Sounds like the squad just pulled up," says Matt.

"Okay," says Marcie. "I got a pulse of 72, regular and strong. The respirations are 12, and depth is good. I'll help them get ready to transport while you get a quick BP and pulse ox."

Already wrapping the blood pressure cuff around Mr. Haines' left arm, Matt asks, "Do you have a history of diabetes, Mr. Haines?"

"Yeah, I'm a diabetic. I just checked my glucose though. It was 91. This sure doesn't feel like a problem with my sugar."

"We'll wait until we're in the ambulance," says Matt, but we'll double-check your glucose level, just to be sure."

Problem-Solving Questions

1. What other signs should Matt check for at the scene?
2. Why do you think Matt chose to delay blood glucose testing until they were in the ambulance?

---

a readout in about 10 seconds. This method is not acceptable for small children (under about three years old) who cannot follow instructions or who might bite the thermometer, or for any patient who is unresponsive, cannot close the mouth, or cannot follow instructions. Oral temperatures can be inaccurate if the patient has had something to eat or drink or has smoked within the past 10 to 15 minutes.

Tympanic thermometers use an infrared light to detect the temperature at the tympanic membrane (eardrum). A tympanic thermometer can be quick and accurate. However, if it is not aligned correctly in the ear canal (the light should be directed at the tympanic membrane), or if there is a large amount of cerumen (earwax), then readings can be inaccurate.

Rectal thermometers resemble oral thermometers, but the tip may be shorter. On electronic devices that have a probe for oral use and a probe for rectal use, the oral probe is blue and the rectal probe is red. You must lubricate the tip of the rectal thermometer, preferably with a water-soluble lubricant, before inserting it into the rectum. Injury can occur if the tip of the thermometer is inserted too far. In infants, the tip is inserted about 1.0 inch, and in adults, about 1.5 inches. You can take an axillary temperature by placing the (covered) tip of the thermometer in the axilla (armpit) and having the patient keep his arm at his side.

Assessing the Skin

A patient's skin can give important information about his condition. You should check the skin for color, moisture, temperature, mobility, and **turgor** (Figure 18-9). Also check for a change in color, such as pallor (paleness), redness, cyanosis, and jaundice. Changes in skin color may be

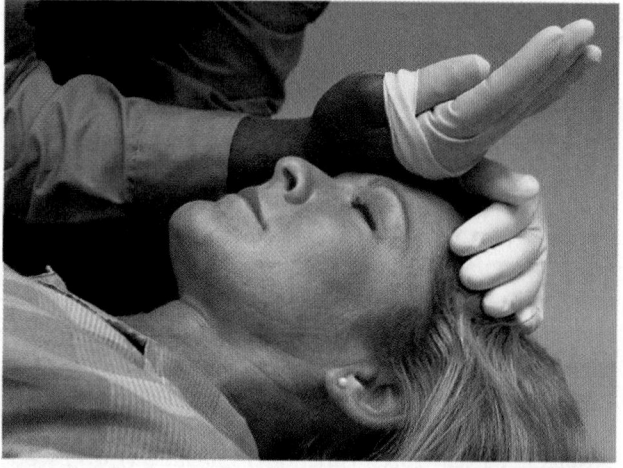

FIGURE 18-9

Check the patient's skin temperature with the back of your hand.

generalized and easily noted, or may be noted in specific areas. Pallor may be best noted by checking the mucous membranes of the mouth and inner lining of the lower eyelid. Cyanosis may be present in the lips, ears, or nail beds. You may first see jaundice, a yellowing of the tissues that occurs in liver disease, in the sclera (white part) of the eye. This is called **icterus**. Redness may be generalized, such as from a hot environment, exertion, or fever, or it may be localized to an area of inflammation. Table 18-4 provides information on possible causes of changes in the color of the skin and mucous membranes.

Check the patient's skin for excessive dryness or sweating. Excessive dryness can have several contributing causes, including dehydration. Sweating is expected in

TABLE 18-4	Skin Assessment Findings and Possible Significance
Skin Finding	**Possible Significance**
Pink	Normal skin color in lighter-skinned individuals; normal color of mucous membranes in all individuals
Pale	Peripheral blood vessel constriction; may indicate shock or fright
Cyanosis	Hypoxia resulting from inadequate ventilation, oxygenation, circulation
Flushed	Fever, exertion, hyperthermia, excitement, embarrassment
Jaundice	Liver disease
Mottled	Exposure to cold, shock
Cold	Hypothermia, poor circulation
Cool	Shock, fright, anxiety
Warm	Normal
Hot	Fever, hyperthermia
Dry	Normal
Excessive dryness	Dehydration, hypothyroidism
Moist/wet	Fever, exertion, hyperthermia, shock, fear, anxiety
Poor mobility (skin is "tight")	Edema
Poor turgor (skin lacks elasticity)	Dehydration

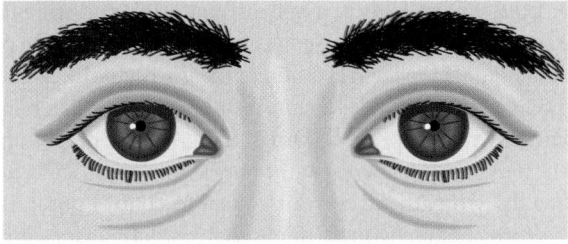

Constricted pupils

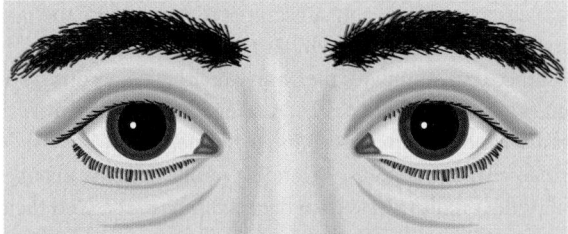

Dilated pupils

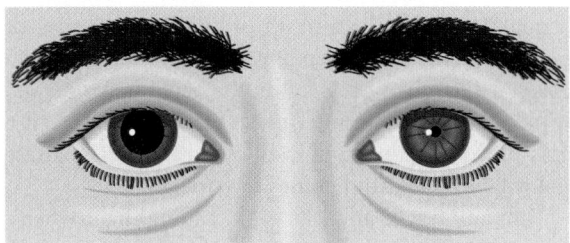

Unequal pupils

FIGURE 18-10

Check for pupil size, equality, and reaction to light.

Assessing the Pupils

The pupil is the opening in the center of the ring-shaped muscle of the eye, the iris. The iris adjusts the size of the pupil, dilating it to let more light reach the inside of the eye, and constricting it to limit the amount of light that enters. The size of the pupil is controlled by the oculomotor nerve (cranial nerve III) and by sympathetic nerve fibers. Parasympathetic stimulation causes the pupils to constrict, and sympathetic stimulation causes the pupils to dilate.

Pupil size is determined by a balance of sympathetic input and parasympathetic input (from the oculomotor nerve). The size of the pupils, their ability to react to light, and whether they are equal tell us something about the presence of various stimuli. Under normal circumstances, the pupils are larger (more dilated) in dim light, and smaller (more constricted) in bright light (Figure 18-10). When you shine a light into the eye, the pupil constricts. The pupils react consensually, which means that when you shine a light into one eye, both pupils constrict at the same time. The pupils are normally round and equal in size. Size ranges from 2 to 8 mm in diameter.

warm conditions or during exertion. Excessive sweating in the absence of these conditions, however, is known as *diaphoresis*, and is an indication of increased sympathetic nervous system activity. Diaphoresis may be present in shock, myocardial infarction (heart attack), and other serious conditions.

To check mobility and turgor, gently pinch and lift up a fold of the patient's skin, such as the skin on the back of the hand, and then release it. Mobility is the ease with which the fold of skin can be lifted. It can be decreased in edema. Turgor is the speed with which the fold of skin returns to its original position. A delay in returning to the original position is called *poor skin turgor*, and is an indication of dehydration. If the skin remains raised, it is described as "tenting" of the skin.

Fear, anxiety, shock, dim light, and drugs that stimulate the sympathetic nervous system (such as cocaine) result in pupil dilation. Complete relaxation of the iris occurs in cerebral hypoxia and death, resulting in the pupils being dilated and nonreactive to light (fixed). Drugs that block the parasympathetic nervous system prevent the pupils from constricting and allow the sympathetic nervous system to control pupil size. Eye drops containing medications that block the parasympathetic nervous system are used to dilate the pupils to allow examination of the retina in the back of the eye. Bright light, some narcotic drugs, and substances that stimulate the parasympathetic nervous system cause pupil constriction. One substance that stimulates the parasympathetic nervous system is an organophosphate pesticide, which is also a potential terrorist weapon. Epinephrine and atropine, two drugs used in cardiac resuscitation, also dilate the pupils, making examination of the pupils useless in patients who have received them.

Anisocoria (slightly unequal pupils) is normal in a small number of people. Typically, though, the pupils should be equal in size. Anisocoria of 2 mm or greater is of concern. Unequal pupils can be a result of injury to one eye, or a sign of increased ICP. When pressure inside the cranium increases, it can cause pressure on the oculomotor nerve on one side. The pressure interferes with the function of the nerve, preventing the pupil from constricting. The affected pupil will be dilated and nonreactive to light.

Dim any bright ambient (surrounding) light when assessing the pupils. Note the size of the pupils, and whether they are equal. Many penlights have a reference guide along the side to determine the size of the pupils in millimeters. Briefly shine your penlight into one eye (Figure 18-11). Both pupils should constrict together, then return to their original size when the light is removed. This response should occur quickly, which is often described as a "brisk" response. Repeat the procedure for the other eye. Normal pupil reaction is documented as "pupils equal [and] react to light." This is abbreviated as *PERL* or *PEARL*.

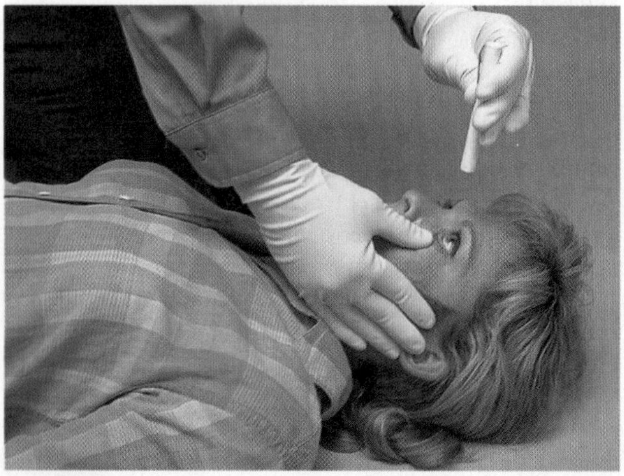

Monitoring Devices

A variety of electronic monitoring devices can provide additional information about patients' conditions. Pulse oximeters indicate the percentage of hemoglobin saturation with oxygen. Capnography is used to measure the carbon dioxide in exhaled air. A glucometer can measure the amount of glucose in a drop of blood. A cardiac monitor can provide a visual representation of the electrical activity of the heart.

Pulse Oximetry

A certain amount of dissolved oxygen must be present in the arterial blood in order for oxygen to bind with hemoglobin for transportation to the cells. The amount of oxygen in arterial blood is measured by obtaining a sample of arterial blood to measure the partial pressure of oxygen in the blood (PaO_2). Measuring PaO_2 is invasive and requires laboratory facilities for analysis. Pulse oximetry is a noninvasive method that gives slightly different information about oxygenation (Figure 18-12).

Pulse oximetry uses light to measure how saturated with oxygen the hemoglobin in red blood cells is. This is possible because different colors absorb different wavelengths of light. Saturated hemoglobin turns blood a bright red color, and desaturated hemoglobin results in a darker red color. The more hemoglobin molecules that are saturated, the brighter red the blood. The light sources of the pulse oximeter are placed on one side of a capillary bed, such as a finger or earlobe, and the sensors are placed on the other side. The more of a specific wavelength of light emitted by the pulse oximeter that is absorbed by either saturated or desaturated hemoglobin, the less of that specific wavelength of light that reaches the sensor on the other side.

FIGURE 18-11

Use a penlight to check pupils' reactivity to light.

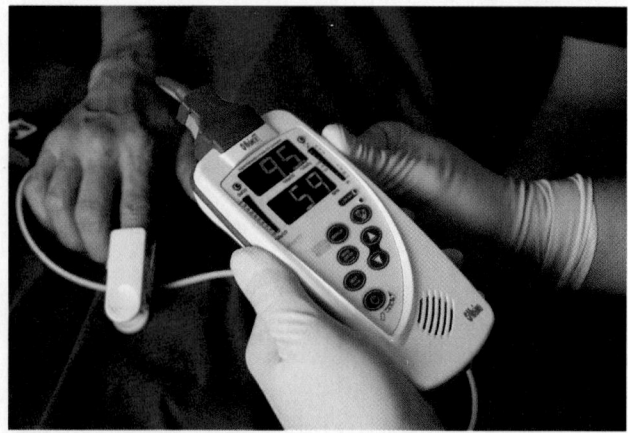

FIGURE 18-12

Pulse oximetry uses different wavelengths of light to measure the saturation of hemoglobin with oxygen.

Pulse oximetry gives the saturation percentage of oxygen (SpO₂) and displays the pulse rate. A normal pulse oximetry reading is between 95 and 99 percent at lower geographic elevations, readings of 91 to 94 percent indicate mild hypoxia, readings of 86 to 90 percent indicate moderate hypoxia, and readings 85 percent or less indicate severe hypoxia. The patient care goal is to maintain an SpO₂ of 95 percent or higher by administering and, if needed, assisting with ventilations.

In most cases, oxygen molecules binding with hemoglobin cause the hemoglobin to be saturated. However, carbon monoxide (CO) also binds to hemoglobin. A pulse oximeter cannot tell what is causing the hemoglobin to be saturated. It can determine only how saturated it is. Patients with carbon monoxide poisoning can have a high SpO₂. Therefore, it is critical to remember your clinical reasoning skills. Pulse oximetry contributes a piece of information, but does not tell the whole story. Pulse oximetry also cannot tell how much hemoglobin is present. It can tell only how saturated the hemoglobin is. Therefore, a patient with a low red blood cell count, such as an anemic patient, may have a high SpO₂, yet the tissues may not be getting an adequate amount of oxygen.

Pulse oximetry readings also can be affected by high-intensity ambient lighting, poor circulation in the capillary bed, and anything that interferes with the light source passing through the tissue to the sensor. Pulse oximetry can be very useful in determining changes in a patient's condition. After obtaining a baseline reading, you can monitor the effects of oxygen administration and medication administration.

End-Tidal Carbon Dioxide Monitoring

Exhaled carbon dioxide monitoring, or capnometry, measures the amount of carbon dioxide in exhaled air (Figure 18-13). Capnography is a display of the measurements of exhaled

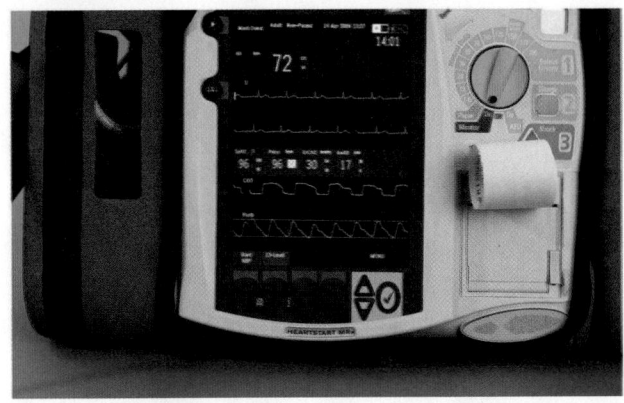

FIGURE 18-13

An end-tidal carbon dioxide detector integrated into a cardiac monitor.

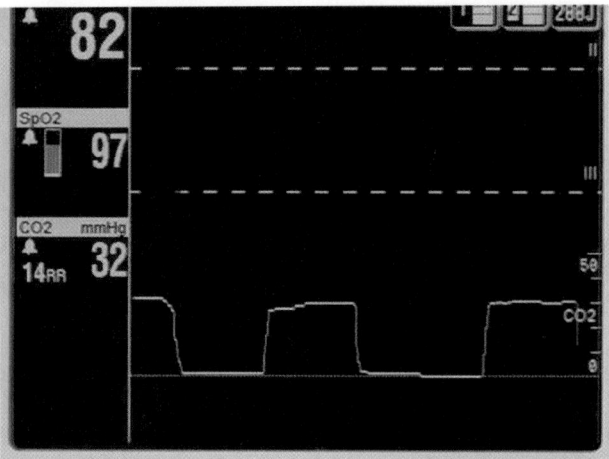

FIGURE 18-14

A capnogram displayed in continuous waveform capnography.

carbon dioxide monitoring. A capnogram is a display of a waveform that represents the amount of exhaled carbon dioxide (Figure 18-14). Capnometry measures the percentage of carbon dioxide in exhaled air and uses it to calculate the pCO₂. Carbon dioxide is an end product of normal aerobic metabolism. Oxygen combines with the hydrogen ions (H⁺) contained in the acidic products that result from the earlier stages of energy metabolism. When oxygen is inadequate, those acids cannot be broken down, resulting in acidosis. Oxygen accepts the H⁺ from the acids, resulting in carbon dioxide and water (H₂O). The carbon dioxide in the blood is then eliminated through the lungs.

The traditional way of measuring the amount of carbon dioxide remaining in arterial blood after exhalation is to obtain an arterial blood sample. However, this is not feasible in the prehospital setting. Exhaled carbon dioxide is a way to noninvasively monitor the amount of carbon dioxide being eliminated from the body. Exhaled carbon dioxide is measured by sensors that you can use either in patients

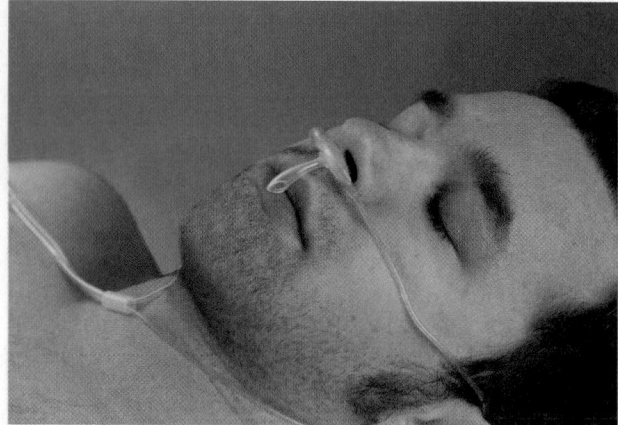

FIGURE 18-15

End-tidal carbon dioxide detection in a spontaneously breathing patient.

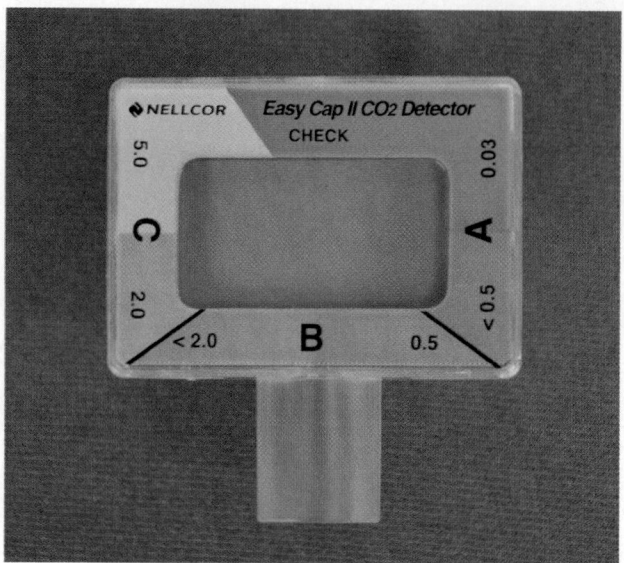

FIGURE 18-16

A colorimetric end-tidal carbon dioxide detection device.
(© Edward T. Dickinson, MD)

who are being artificially ventilated or in those who are breathing spontaneously (Figure 18-15). The normal range of **end-tidal carbon dioxide** (ETCO$_2$) in exhaled air is 35 to 45 mmHg, which correlates to a pCO$_2$ in the arterial blood of 38 to 45 mmHg. The amount of carbon dioxide exhaled is not consistent throughout exhalation. This amount can be represented on a graphic readout to show the how the level of carbon dioxide changes throughout exhalation. This is useful in more advanced assessment to identify specific respiratory problems.

Exhaled carbon dioxide monitoring in the prehospital setting is useful for patients with respiratory complaints and in critically ill patients, but is particularly useful as a method for confirming and monitoring endotracheal tube placement. The carbon dioxide in exhaled air from the lungs is detected if the endotracheal tube is properly placed in the trachea, which contains carbon dioxide. If the tube is in the esophagus, there is no carbon dioxide to be detected. A low carbon dioxide reading in an intubated patient should trigger investigation of tube placement.

Circulation is required for the metabolism that produces carbon dioxide. Therefore, a low carbon dioxide reading is also an indication of inadequate circulation. Increased carbon dioxide readings can indicate hypoventilation.

IN THE FIELD

A recently consumed carbonated beverage can result in inaccurate carbon dioxide measurement, because the gas may be contained within the stomach, rather than being produced by metabolism. You must always use more than one method of assessing adequate ventilation and circulation. Like all tools, carbon dioxide monitoring is an adjunct to, not a replacement for, clinical skills and judgment.

Colorimetric devices are a less sophisticated way to measure exhaled carbon dioxide (Figure 18-16). The device is placed over the end of the airway device, such as an endotracheal tube. A special paper filter in the device changes color from purple to yellow in the presence of carbon dioxide.

Blood Glucose Level

Glucose is an essential source of energy for cellular metabolism. Very little glucose can enter cells without the help of insulin. Brain cells do not require insulin to use glucose, but they also are not able to use fats or proteins as energy sources. Therefore, for the brain to function, a constant adequate supply of glucose is required. Type 1 diabetics do not produce insulin, while Type 2 diabetics either produce inadequate insulin or their cells are resistant to insulin. With no or inadequate insulin, very little glucose in the blood can enter cells. The **blood glucose level** (BGL) gets very high, but the cells are starved for a source of energy. Type 1 diabetics require daily administration of insulin (often several times a day). Type 2 diabetics usually take medications that stimulate the pancreas to produce insulin or decrease cellular resistance to insulin.

With the right amount of insulin, glucose enters the cells in the amount needed over time. However, with too much insulin, or inadequate food intake for the amount of insulin present, the available glucose quickly enters the cells. This leaves an inadequate amount of glucose in the blood to meet cells' ongoing needs. Type 1 diabetics are most prone to **hypoglycemia** (low blood glucose), but this emergency can occur in Type 2 diabetics as well.

When brain cells do not have an adequate amount of glucose, they begin to malfunction, starting with the highest functions of the brain. The patient may become confused, exhibit bizarre behavior, or become unresponsive. Advanced EMTs can treat hypoglycemia either by administering glucose, or administering the medication glucagon, a hormone that breaks down stored glycogen in the liver into glucose.

When the amount of insulin available is inadequate, the blood glucose level can become very high. Over a period of hours to days, the hyperglycemic diabetic can become quite ill. One of the complications of **hyperglycemia** is dehydration, which Advanced EMTs can treat with IV fluids.

You should measure the blood glucose level in all diabetic patients, especially when their signs and symptoms suggest that hypoglycemia or hyperglycemia is present. Hypoglycemia and hyperglycemia are not common in patients without diabetes, but you should check the blood glucose level in all medical patients with altered mental status or a neurologic deficit. A patient with undiagnosed diabetes may first present in the prehospital setting, not knowing that undiagnosed diabetes is the cause of his signs and symptoms. A complete history may not be available in patients with an altered mental status, so do not rule out diabetes. Checking the blood glucose level is a quick, simple test, and unrecognized severe hypoglycemia can be life threatening.

Glucose is measured in milligrams per deciliter (100 mL) of blood. However, the concentration of glucose is the same in each drop of blood. Therefore, you can use the amount of glucose in a single drop of blood to determine how much glucose is present in 100 mL. The normal BGL is 70 to 110 mg/dL. This level can be slightly higher in healthy individuals immediately following a meal. A variety of small, handheld blood glucose monitors are available; you must follow the manufacturer's instructions for each device (Figure 18-17). A drop of blood is placed on a test strip in the device for analysis, giving a digital readout of the BGL.

Only a small drop of blood is required for analysis (Scan 18-2). The sample is obtained from the pad of one of the fingers. If the patient is conscious, he may have a preference as to which finger to use. Otherwise, the middle or ring finger is used. Clean the pad of the finger with an alcohol wipe and let it dry completely. Use a new, sterile, single-use lancet to pierce the skin with a quick motion. A great deal of force is not required. Avoid an approach that is too tentative so you will not have to puncture the skin a second time to obtain an adequate sample.

Allow the blood drop to fall on the indicated spot on the test strip in the device. Do not squeeze or "milk" the finger to obtain the sample. Use a small gauze pad to stop any bleeding that continues after you obtain the sample. Compare the reading to normal values and follow your protocols for treatment.

Cardiac Monitoring

The electrical activity of the heart is assessed by obtaining an **electrocardiogram** (ECG). Advanced EMTs can assist paramedics, nurses, and physicians in connecting a patient to an ECG monitor and obtaining a rhythm strip. In some locations, Advanced EMTs may be expected to recognize a limited number of cardiac dysrhythmias on the ECG. A brief overview of cardiac monitoring is provided in this chapter. The topic is covered in detail in Chapter 21 and Appendix 2.

ECG monitors use electrodes placed on the skin to detect the minute amount of electricity from cardiac impulses that travels to the skin (Figure 18-18). The electrodes conduct the electricity through wires to the ECG monitor. The ECG monitor provides a continuous display of real-time electrical activity on a screen. This is called a **dynamic ECG.** You can record short periods of the electrical activity onto graph paper for documentation and later reference. This is a **static ECG.**

Cardiac monitoring detects and displays a representation of electrical activity as it flows between a positive electrode and a negative electrode. The typical monitoring lead is called **Lead II.** Lead II "looks" at the electrical activity

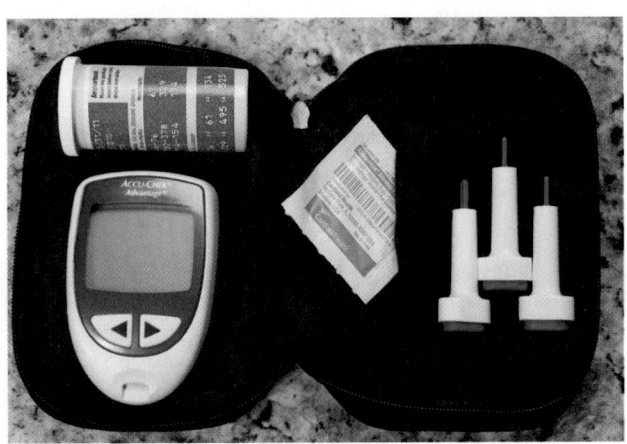

FIGURE 18-17

A glucometer uses a drop of blood on a test strip to measure the blood glucose level.

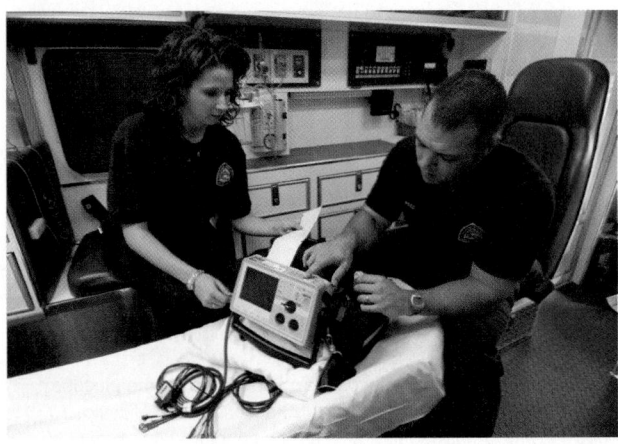

FIGURE 18-18

A portable cardiac monitor–defibrillator.

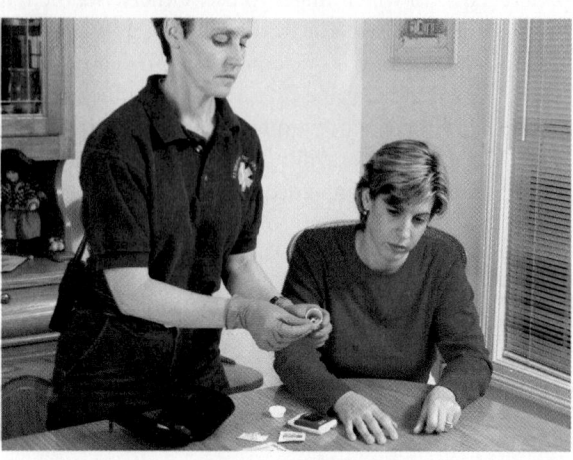

1. Prepare the blood glucose meter, including a test strip and a lancet.

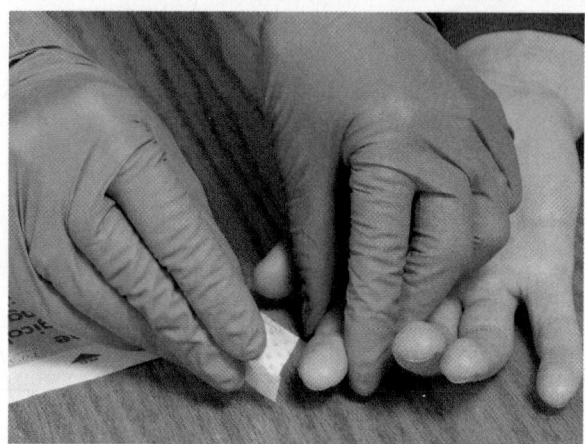

2. Cleanse the skin with an alcohol preparation. Allow the alcohol to dry before performing the finger stick.

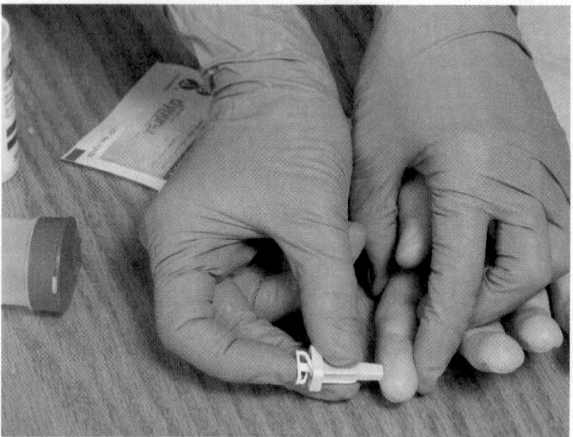

3. Use the lancet to perform a finger stick. Wipe away the first drop of blood that appears. Squeeze the finger if necessary to get a second drop of blood.

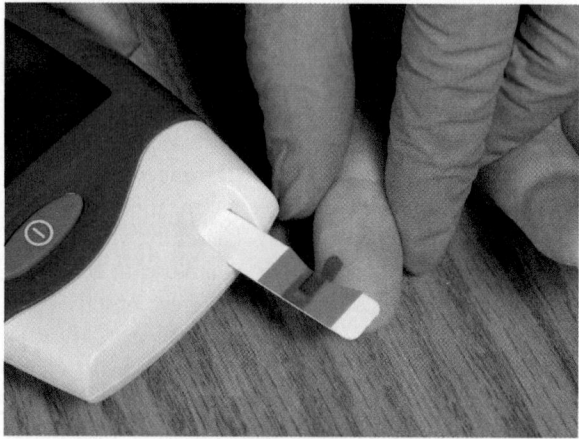

4. Apply the blood to the test strip. You may do this by holding the strip to the finger to draw the blood into the strip.

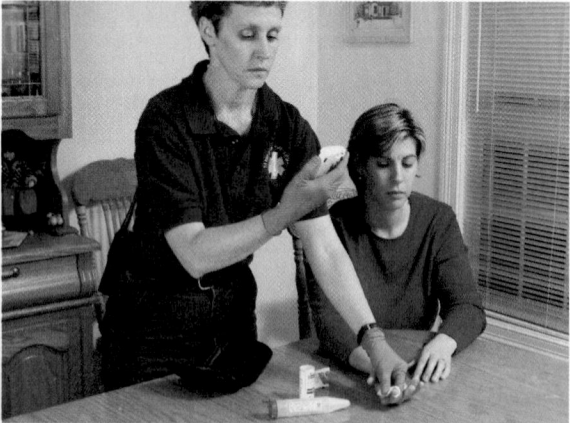

5. Read the blood glucose level displayed on the glucose meter. (It may take 15 to 60 seconds for the device to provide a reading.) Assess the puncture site and apply direct pressure or a bandage to the site if bleeding continues.

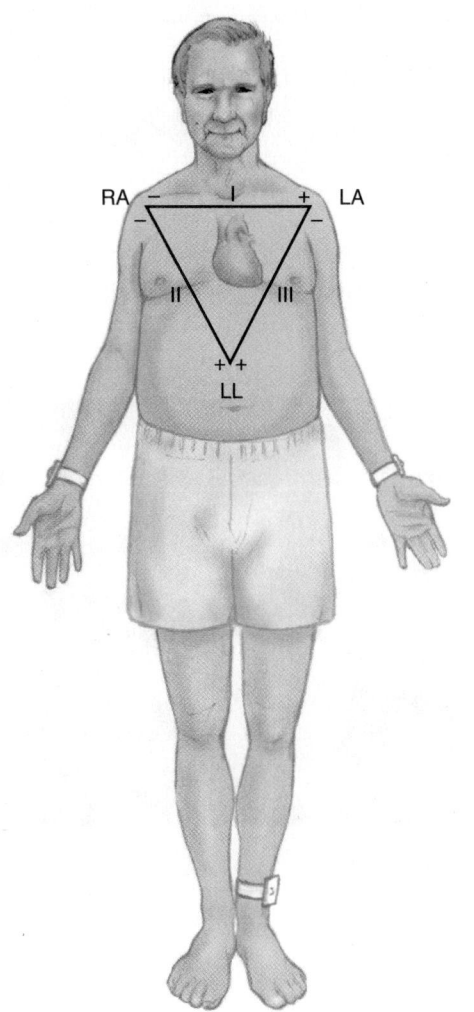

FIGURE 18-19

Einthoven's triangle forms cardiac monitoring leads I, II, and III.

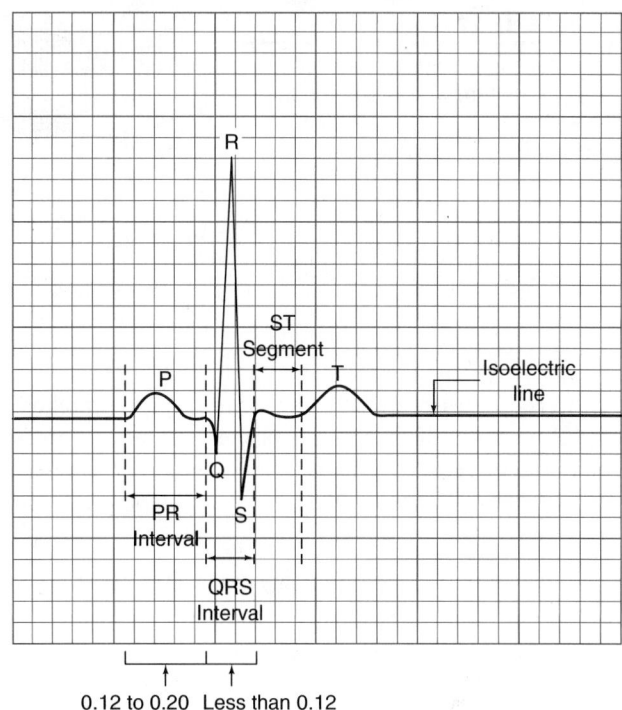

FIGURE 18-20

The waveforms of an ECG.

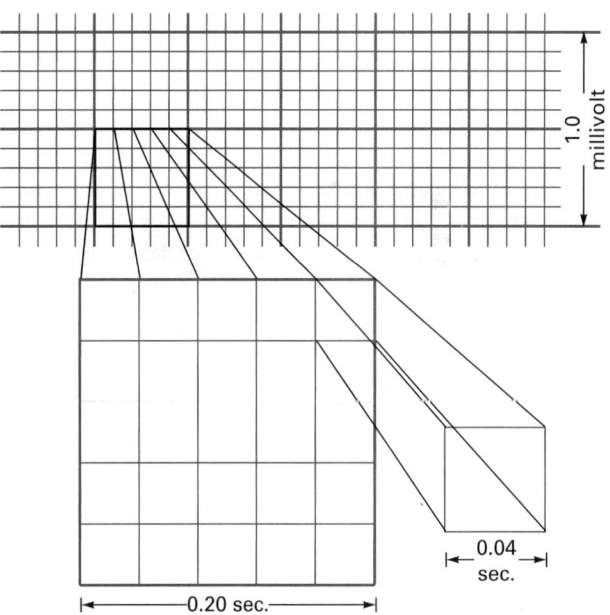

FIGURE 18-21

ECG paper.

between a positive electrode on the patient's right shoulder and a negative electrode placed on the skin below the apex of the heart, usually on the lower left chest (Figure 18-19). Looking at electrical activity in a single lead allows you to determine the heart rate, rhythm, pacemaker site, and the presence of delays or blocks in electrical conduction. A 12-lead (or 15-lead) ECG is used to look at multiple views of the heart to give information about the presence and location of myocardial ischemia and infarction, and changes in the size and position of the heart.

The waveforms of the ECG show the amount and direction of electricity being conducted through the heart as waves of different sizes, durations, and directions. The waves are assigned letters and represent specific parts of the cardiac electrical cycle (Figure 18-20). Graph paper with a grid of 1-mm squares moves through the ECG machine at a standard rate of 25 mm/second (Figure 18-21). This allows the grid to serve as a basis for measuring the amount of electricity conducted on the vertical axis, and the time it

takes electricity to travel through the heart on the horizontal axis. When the heart rate and each of those measurements are within normal limits, the rhythm is called **normal sinus rhythm (NSR)** (Figure 18-22). NSR originates in the normal pacemaker of the heart, the sinoatrial node. This is the expected cardiac rhythm, and the rules that it follows serve as the basis of comparison for cardiac dysrhythmia.

FIGURE 18-22

Normal sinus rhythm produces a regular rhythm with characteristic waveforms, at a rate between 60 and 100 per minute.

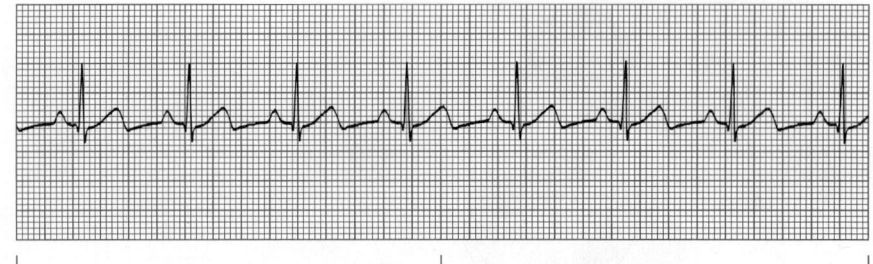

Certain measurements are important in the prehospital setting. On the horizontal axis, each 1-mm square is equal to 0.04 seconds. Heavier lines every 5 mm represent 0.20 seconds. The waves analyzed in ECG monitoring are as follows:

- *P wave*, representing electricity moving through the atria
- *PR interval (PRI)*, representing the length of time for a cardiac impulse to travel through the atria and atrioventricular (AV) node
- *QRS complex*, representing movement of electricity through the ventricles
- *T wave*, representing the flow of electricity as the cells in the ventricles resume their electrical charge

When using an ECG monitor, you must remember that it gives information only about the electrical activity of the heart. It does not give information about the mechanical function of the heart. It is quite possible for the heart to have electrical activity that, for a variety of reasons, does not result in mechanical contraction of the heart. You must always base your assessment of perfusion on primary assessment findings and vital signs, not on the cardiac monitor.

ECG monitors in the prehospital setting are combined monitor–defibrillators with multiple functions. The steps here apply only to ECG monitoring. The basic functions of each machine are the same, but their configurations and some features differ. Refer to the manufacturer's instructions for the location of the power button and monitor controls.

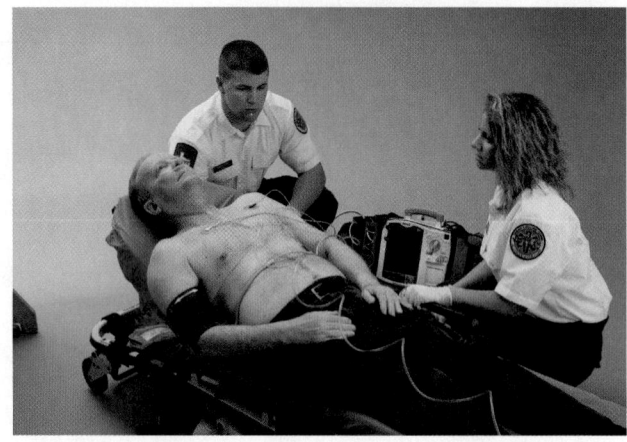

FIGURE 18-23

ECG monitoring in the prehospital setting.

To monitor the ECG (Figure 18-23):

- Explain to the patient what you are going to do.
- Power on the cardiac monitor.
- Ensure that the monitor is set to Lead II.
- Attach monitoring electrodes to each of the monitoring lead wires.
- Ensure that the patient's skin is clean and dry. If needed, you can use an alcohol pad to remove oils, dirt, blood, and so on.

The lead wires are typically labeled for placement, as follows:

- *Right arm (RA)* is on the anterior chest, just below the right clavicle
- *Left arm (LA)* is on the anterior chest, just below the left clavicle
- *Left leg (LL)* is on the lower left anterior chest wall, below the apex of the heart
- *Right leg (RL, if present)* is on the lower right anterior chest wall

Check the quality of the ECG waveforms displayed. Poor electrode adhesion or patient movement can cause interference. Press or tap the "print" button or icon to obtain a static ECG.

IN THE FIELD

An easy way to determine the heart rate from a monitor strip is to count the number of large (5-mm) boxes between QRS complexes and apply the following rule that relates to the number of large boxes to the heart rate: 1 large box = HR 300, 2 large boxes = HR 150, 3 large boxes = HR 100, 4 large boxes = HR 75, 5 large boxes = HR 60, and 6 large boxes = HR 50.

CASE STUDY WRAP-UP

Clinical-Reasoning Process

Advanced EMTs Matt Brewer and Marcie Pickett are taking care of Mr. Denny Haines, a 42-year-old patient who had a sudden onset of a severe headache. Mr. Haines' blood pressure is 168/72 mmHg. This concerns Matt, given Mr. Haines' complaint. He considers the possibility of a stroke. Matt wants to transport without further delay. Mr. Haines' level of responsiveness indicates that his blood glucose level measurement can wait, but if he is having a stroke, his condition could quickly worsen.

While taking Mr. Haines' blood pressure, Matt notices that his skin is slightly moist, with normal color. Mr. Haines' SpO_2 is 99 percent with the nasal cannula in place. Just before placing Mr. Haines on the stretcher, Matt checks his pupils. "So far, so good," he thinks, noting that the pupils are equal and reactive to light. He makes a plan to include rechecking the pupils in his reassessment plan.

En route to the emergency department, Matt starts an IV of normal saline at a keep-open rate and determines that Mr. Haines's BGL is 100 mg/dL. Mr. Haines continues to complain of a severe headache without relief. A second set of vital signs is obtained, with a blood pressure of 172/78, heart rate 68, and respiration 12. The SpO_2 is stable at 99 percent. Matt recognizes the possibility of increasing intracranial pressure.

As Matt prepares to recheck the pupils, he notices that Mr. Haines is having difficulty speaking. The left pupil is now 2 mm larger than the right, and sluggish to respond to light. Matt's suspicion of a hemorrhagic stroke with increasing intracranial pressure is increased. Recognizing his patient's rapid deterioration, he includes the new findings in an update to the emergency department. "Clear, Ambulance 12. We will see you in 2 to 3 minutes in resuscitation room 2."

CHAPTER REVIEW

Chapter Summary

Vital signs provide essential information about a patient's baseline condition and how his condition changes over time. As part of the secondary assessment, vital signs and monitoring devices are integrated into the priorities established for each patient, based on his condition and the amount of help you have available.

The pulse and blood pressure provide information about the function of the cardiovascular system and adequacy of perfusion. The pulse is assessed for rate, rhythm, strength, and volume. The blood pressure provides information about cardiac output and peripheral vascular resistance. The depth, rate, and volume of ventilations, along with the presence of an abnormal upper airway or lung sounds, provide information about the adequacy of ventilation. Using a thermometer to measure the body temperature is important when fever, hyperthermia, or hypothermia are suspected.

The color, temperature, moisture, mobility, and turgor of the skin give a wealth of information about perfusion, hydration, and underlying disease processes. Examination of the skin can reveal signs of shock, hypoxia, fever, and liver disease. Examining the pupils provides information about the central nervous system. It also can provide clues about drugs or toxins patients may have been exposed to.

A variety of monitoring devices give additional information to guide patient care. Pulse oximetry measures the degree to which hemoglobin is saturated with oxygen. This gives additional information about respiration that goes beyond what you can obtain by assessing ventilations. Capnometry measures the amount of carbon dioxide being exhaled, providing information about perfusion and ventilation. Blood glucose measurement is important in diabetics and patients with altered mental status or neurologic deficit. As an Advanced EMT, you may assist in obtaining ECGs and you may be expected to recognize selected cardiac dysrhythmias. Continuous ECG monitoring provides real-time information about the electrical function of the heart.

You must analyze all the information obtained by measuring vital signs, examining the skin and pupils, and using monitoring devices in the context of the whole patient. Patient care decisions made on a single piece of information taken out of context can lead to unnecessary or inappropriate treatment, or can let serious conditions to go undetected. Vital signs and monitoring devices are invaluable, but provide only part of the information needed to engage in sound clinical reasoning.

Review Questions

Multiple-Choice Questions

1. Which one of the following is a vital sign?
   a. Blood pressure
   b. Pulse oximetry
   c. Blood glucose level
   d. End-tidal carbon dioxide

2. The heart rate is recorded as the number of beats in _____ seconds.
   a. 10
   b. 15
   c. 30
   d. 60

3. Which one of the following heart rates represents tachycardia in an adult?
   a. 50
   b. 75
   c. 90
   d. 105

4. Systolic blood pressure is best described as the pressure in the:
   a. venous system.
   b. arteries when the heart contracts.
   c. arteries when the heart relaxes.
   d. veins and arteries on average.

5. A healthy systolic blood pressure in adults is _____ mmHg or less.
   a. 90
   b. 100
   c. 120
   d. 140

6. Pulse pressure is calculated as:
   a. diastolic pressure plus one third of the systolic pressure.
   b. systolic pressure minus mean arterial pressure.
   c. diastolic pressure plus systolic pressure.
   d. systolic pressure minus diastolic pressure.

7. Which one of the following is a normal respiratory rate for an adult?
   a. 8
   b. 16
   c. 22
   d. 28

8. Which one of the following sounds indicates upper airway obstruction?
   a. Rhonchi
   b. Rales
   c. Stridor
   d. Wheezing

9. Normal body temperature in degrees C is:
   a. 34.
   b. 35.
   c. 36.
   d. 37.

10. A fever is considered medically significant when it is above _____ degrees F.
    a. 99.0
    b. 100.4
    c. 101.1
    d. 104.0

11. Which one of the following pupil findings is abnormal?
    a. When a light is shined into one eye, both pupils constrict.
    b. The right pupil is 4 mm in diameter and the left is 5 mm.
    c. Both pupils are 2 mm in diameter in a dimly lit room.
    d. Both pupils are 6 mm in diameter.

12. A blue or purple discoloration of the skin or mucous membranes is an indication of:
    a. liver disease.
    b. fever.
    c. blood loss.
    d. inadequate ventilation.

13. Your partner says a patient has jaundice. You will agree with him if the patient's skin appears:
    a. pale.
    b. yellow.
    c. mottled.
    d. red.

14. Poor skin mobility is a sign of:
    a. edema.
    b. dehydration.
    c. fever.
    d. hypoxia.

15. Which one of the following best describes the measurement obtained by pulse oximetry?
    a. PaO_2
    b. Percent of hemoglobin carrying oxygen
    c. Amount of carbon dioxide bound to hemoglobin
    d. Amount of oxygen in exhaled air

16. Pulse oximetry may be inaccurate in which one of the following situations?
    a. Hypoxia
    b. Anemia
    c. Hypercarbia
    d. Carbon monoxide poisoning

17. Capnometry in the prehospital setting measures:
 a. oxygen in the blood.
 b. oxygen in exhaled air.
 c. carbon dioxide in the blood.
 d. carbon dioxide in exhaled air.

18. Which one of the following is a normal blood glucose level?
 a. 55
 b. 102
 c. 135
 d. 154

19. Cardiac monitoring gives information about:
 a. heart rate.
 b. pulse strength.
 c. perfusion.
 d. blood pressure.

20. The term *hyperpyrexia* refers to a high:
 a. blood glucose level.
 b. blood pressure.
 c. level of carbon dioxide.
 d. body temperature.

Critical-Thinking Questions

21. What factors should you consider when determining at what point you will take a particular patient's vital signs?

22. When you arrive at the scene of a four-year-old patient at a daycare center, the director tells you she measured the child's temperature with a forehead strip. What is the usefulness of this information?

23. Your patient is located in a noisy factory and there is too much background noise to auscultate a blood pressure. What other options do you have? What are the limitations of those methods?

24. Your 23-year-old patient has a heart rate of 124. What are some underlying causes you should consider?

25. In what types of patients should you obtain a blood glucose level?

26. How often should you reassess vital signs?

27. Your patient has a low exhaled carbon dioxide reading. What possible causes should you look for?

28. How should you use SpO_2 readings to determine a patient's oxygenation status?

29. What information can assessment of the pupils provide?

References

Mohler, J., & Hart, S. C. (1994). Use of a pulse oximeter for determination of systolic blood pressure in a helicopter air ambulance. *Air Medical Journal, 13*(11–12), 479–482.

National Heart, Lung, and Blood Institute. (2010). *Reference card from the seventh report on the Joint National Committee for the Prevention, Detection, Evaluation, and Treatment of High Blood Pressure.* Retrieved July 22, 2010, from http://www.nhlbi.nih.gov

Additional Reading

Bickley, L. S. (2003). *Bates' guide to physical examination and history-taking* (8th ed.). Philadelphia, PA: Lippincott Williams & Wilkins.

19 History Taking, Secondary Assessment, and Reassessment

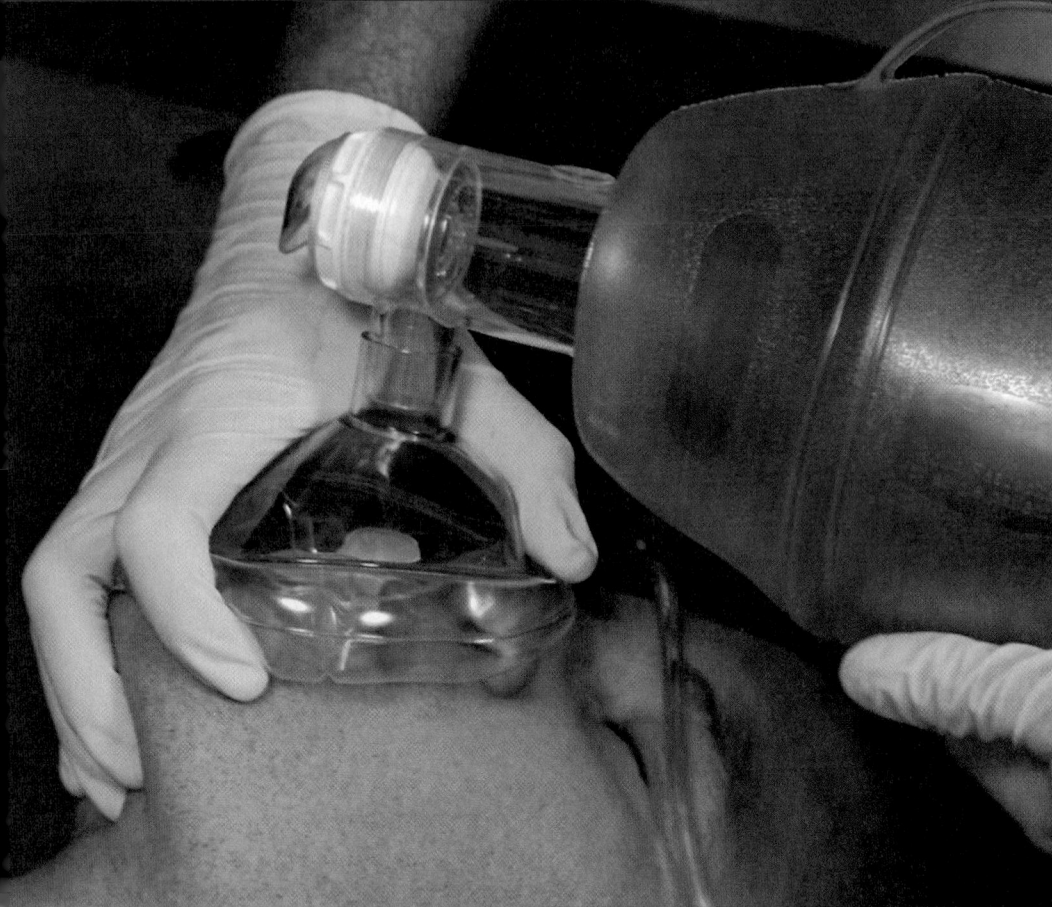

Content Area: Assessment

Advanced EMT Education Standard: Applies scene information and patient assessment findings (scene size-up, primary and secondary assessment, patient history, and reassessment) to guide emergency management.

Objectives

After reading this chapter, you should be able to:

19.1   Define key terms introduced in this chapter.

19.2   Determine a patient's chief complaint.

19.3   Given a scenario, efficiently elicit an adequate patient history using both closed and open-ended questions, as well as active listening techniques.

19.4   Use the mnemonics SAMPLE and OPQRST to ensure that a complete prehospital patient history has been obtained.

19.5   React appropriately when confronted with the need to ask questions about sensitive topics or when caring for patients who present special challenges to the history-taking and assessment processes.

Resource Central

To access Resource Central, follow the directions on the Student Access Card provided with this text. If there is no card, go to www.bradybooks.com and follow the Resource Central link to Buy Access. Under Media Resources, you will find:

• *The Assessment.* Watch a patient assessment.

• *Taking a History.* Learn some effective interviewing techniques.

• *The Reassessment.* View a short video to see the importance of reassessment.

CASE STUDY

Advanced EMTs Lindsay Peoples and Teresa Stewart have responded to a dispatch for a patient with abdominal pain. They have sized up the scene and determined there is nothing that appears to pose a hazard. A man in his 60s met them at the door and informed them that his sister was in a bedroom down the hallway, complaining of "terrible stomach pain."

Lindsay makes a note of the patient's general appearance from the doorway of the bedroom. The patient appears to be in her late 60s. She is awake, but is lying still. She is positioned on her right side with her knees drawn up. She is pale, but her skin is dry and there is no obvious cyanosis. The patient's facial expression indicates that she does not feel well. Lindsay steps next to the bed and bends down on one knee to be at eye level with the patient. "Good morning, ma'am. My name is Lindsay and this is my partner, Teresa. What is your name?"

"I'm Gretchen Snyder. I'd say I'm pleased to meet you, but I wish it was under different circumstances," she says softly.

Reaching over to check Ms. Snyder's radial pulse, Lindsay says, "I'm sorry to hear you're not feeling well. What seems to be the problem?"

"I've got a pretty bad pain in my belly. I think I need to go to the hospital."

Problem-Solving Questions

1. Based on the primary assessment, what priority should Lindsay and Teresa give Ms. Snyder for transport?
2. What is Ms. Snyder's chief complaint?
3. What information about the patient's history will Lindsay and Teresa use to decide how to treat the patient?
4. What should Lindsay and Teresa look for in their physical examination of the patient?

19.6	Differentiate between relevant and less relevant patient history questions in the prehospital setting.
19.7	Given a variety of patient scenarios, adapt your approach to the secondary assessment to meet the demands of the situation.
19.8	Given a variety of patient scenarios, differentiate between normal and abnormal findings in the secondary assessment.
19.9	Provide possible explanations for abnormal secondary assessment findings.
19.10	Recognize critical findings in the secondary assessments of medical and trauma patients.
19.11	Explain the anatomical and body system approaches to secondary assessment.
19.12	Compare and contrast the approaches to the secondary assessment in medical and trauma patients.
19.13	Compare primary and secondary assessment findings with reassessment findings to identify changes in the patient's condition.
19.14	Integrate history taking into the patient assessment process.
19.15	Integrate findings of the scene size-up, primary and secondary assessments, and patient history to formulate an overall impression of the patient's condition and make transport decisions.
19.16	Communicate pertinent patient assessment findings to other health care providers orally and in writing.

Introduction

Advanced EMTs identify patients' problems by taking medical histories and performing physical examinations. Combined with their knowledge of pathophysiology, Advanced EMTs use this information to anticipate associated complaints and problems and ask about them. Secondary assessment allows you to gather additional information about patients after you have sized up the scene and performed a primary assessment. (To review the patient assessment process, see Figure 19-1.)

All patients receive a secondary assessment, but the approach, timing, and level of detail differ. The approach to the secondary assessment depends on whether the patient has a medical problem or traumatic injury, what his chief complaint is, whether he is a critical or noncritical patient, and the circumstances at the scene. Circumstances at the scene include safety, the presence of bystanders and

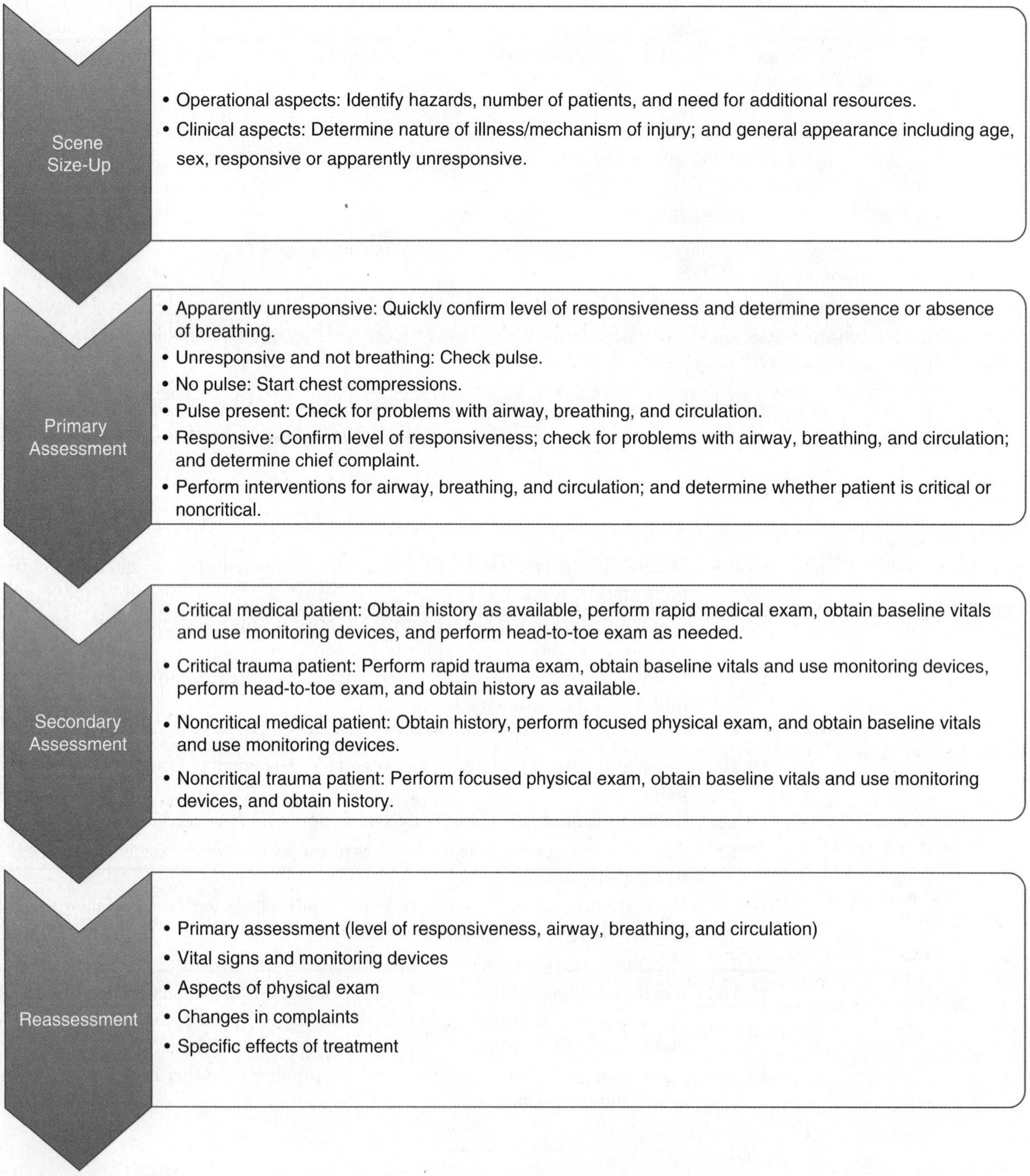

Scene Size-Up
- Operational aspects: Identify hazards, number of patients, and need for additional resources.
- Clinical aspects: Determine nature of illness/mechanism of injury; and general appearance including age, sex, responsive or apparently unresponsive.

Primary Assessment
- Apparently unresponsive: Quickly confirm level of responsiveness and determine presence or absence of breathing.
- Unresponsive and not breathing: Check pulse.
- No pulse: Start chest compressions.
- Pulse present: Check for problems with airway, breathing, and circulation.
- Responsive: Confirm level of responsiveness; check for problems with airway, breathing, and circulation; and determine chief complaint.
- Perform interventions for airway, breathing, and circulation; and determine whether patient is critical or noncritical.

Secondary Assessment
- Critical medical patient: Obtain history as available, perform rapid medical exam, obtain baseline vitals and use monitoring devices, and perform head-to-toe exam as needed.
- Critical trauma patient: Perform rapid trauma exam, obtain baseline vitals and use monitoring devices, perform head-to-toe exam, and obtain history as available.
- Noncritical medical patient: Obtain history, perform focused physical exam, and obtain baseline vitals and use monitoring devices.
- Noncritical trauma patient: Perform focused physical exam, obtain baseline vitals and use monitoring devices, and obtain history.

Reassessment
- Primary assessment (level of responsiveness, airway, breathing, and circulation)
- Vital signs and monitoring devices
- Aspects of physical exam
- Changes in complaints
- Specific effects of treatment

FIGURE 19-1

Overview of the patient assessment process.

family members, whether there is enough light and space to properly perform an exam, and how much help is available.

Secondary assessment of critical patients begins immediately after the primary assessment with either a rapid trauma exam or rapid medical exam. Secondary assessment further consists of obtaining vital signs, using monitoring devices as indicated, and performing either a focused or head-to-toe (detailed) physical examination. Aspects of the secondary assessment are reassessed based on the patient and situation.

Obtaining a relevant and adequate patient history requires effective therapeutic communication (Chapter 6), knowledge of anatomy and physiology (Chapter 8) and pathophysiology (Chapter 10), and clinical reasoning skills (Chapter 14) to adapt your approach as information emerges.

The history consists of the history of the present illness and a relevant past medical history. Mnemonics help the Advanced EMT remember all of the key information in the history, but they are not a substitute for truly understanding what information is important in particular situations. This chapter introduces you to a clinical reasoning approach to secondary assessment, history taking, and reassessment. The chapter presents the techniques of physical examination and discusses considerations in how to apply them.

General Approaches to the Secondary Assessment and History Taking

Information from the scene size-up and primary assessment help you form an initial impression of the nature of the illness or MOI, and whether the patient is critical or noncritical. The goal is to transport critical patients sooner. This does not mean that the approach is rushed and haphazard. In fact, you must be calm and organized to prevent undue delays at the scene. Even for critical patients, you must perform some treatments at the scene without delay. Defibrillation of a patient in cardiac arrest is one example.

Complete secondary assessment of critical patients is usually deferred until you are en route to the hospital, but a rapid medical exam or rapid trauma exam is performed as the patient is prepared for transport. Some aspects of the history, such as eyewitness accounts of the mechanism of injury, may not be available once you leave the scene and you should obtain this information before transport.

Remember, many of the tasks of patient assessment, packaging, and transport may proceed simultaneously, depending on the situation. Your partner may take vital signs while you take a medical history. Additional personnel may carry the stretcher up the porch steps as you and your partner work with the patient, or they may obtain information from a family member.

Medical Patients

Noncritical Medical Patients

A medical patient is noncritical if there are no threats to airway, breathing, or circulation, the patient is responsive, and the patient does not have a chief complaint that indicates an immediately life-threatening medical condition. Noncritical patients must be evaluated and treated at the hospital, but their conditions are not as time-sensitive as those of critical patients. An example of a noncritical patient is a 30-year-old man who is sitting up on the edge of his hotel bed, alert and complaining of several episodes of vomiting and diarrhea. An alert four-year-old child complaining of an earache is also likely to be noncritical. Take some time in such cases to gather additional information before deciding on treatment and preparing for transport (Figure 19-2). If available information is ambiguous, it is better to transport without delay and obtain more history and secondary assessment information en route.

The medical history provides a substantial amount of the information you need to form a **field impression** for medical patients. It also provides information that will guide you in the physical examination.

Begin by obtaining a medical history based on the patient's chief complaint. Different chief complaints are associated with different concerns; thus, there are questions that are relevant to some chief complaints but not others. For example, you will not ask the date of the last menstrual period in the history of a 65-year-old woman complaining of difficulty breathing. But this information is extremely relevant for an 18-year-old woman complaining of lower abdominal pain and vaginal bleeding.

Obtain vital signs, and then perform a focused physical exam based on the patient's complaint, history, and vital signs. Tailor the physical exam to give you relevant information about the patient's condition. You will not likely gain useful information from palpating the abdomen of an asthma patient who began wheezing on a hiking trail. Listening to his breath sounds, though, will provide information you can use. You will learn more about what is relevant for specific complaints as you progress in your Advanced EMT training.

To form a field impression, apply your knowledge of pathophysiology to all the information you have collected. Revise your general impression and the priority for transport if you discover that the patient's condition is more serious than you originally thought, or if the patient's condition is deteriorating. Implement treatment that is indicated. Reassess noncritical patients every 15 minutes, or more frequently if indicated.

Critical Medical Patients

To prepare to transport a critical medical patient, you must simultaneously obtain key pieces of information and begin treatments that cannot be delayed. Therefore, effective assessment and management of critical patients cannot take

Scene size-up	Primary assessment	Secondary assessment	Reassessment
Goals Determine nature of the incident and need for additional resources Determine scene safety	**Goals** Formulate a general impression of the problem Find and correct immediate threats to life Determine priority for transport	**Goals** Determine problem Plan treatment Reevaluate priority decision	**Goals** Detect trends in patient condition Detect new complaints, signs, symptoms Determine effects of treatment Evaluate treatment plan and patient priority
• Nature of incident: medical • Single patient; assess need for additional resources • No hazards/hazards controlled • Nature of illness/general appearance: **Noncritical medical patient**	• Patient is alert AND • Has good general appearance AND • No impairment of airway, breathing, or circulation AND • Chief complaint is not concerning for life-threatening illness • Confirm general impression: **Noncritical medical patient; transport may be delayed for further assessment and treatment**	• Take history based on chief complaint or presenting problem • Take vital signs and use monitoring devices • Perform focused secondary assessment based on chief complaint and patient priority • Formulate field impression • Plan treatment and transport • Reevaluate priority for transport • Communicate with medical direction and receiving facility as needed	• Reassess every 15 minutes or more frequently as indicated • Perform primary assessment • Take vital signs and use monitoring devices • Perform aspects of secondary assessment • Make changes in treatment as needed • Reevaluate patient priority • Communicate changes as needed

FIGURE 19-2

Assessment of a noncritical medical patient.

place without teamwork. The need for swift action and decision making does not mean that you should hurry to the point of being disorganized and omitting critical steps. You must be calm and deliberate.

For example, if you are on a call with a patient complaining of chest pain, you cannot jump to a field impression of acute coronary syndrome (ACS) without additional information. To be efficient, though, you must carefully choose the questions you ask and the examinations you perform on the scene. In this case, the OPQRST of the chest pain is critical to your field impression. Whether the patient has a family history of coronary artery disease is important, but will not change your immediate actions because you cannot use this information to rule out ACS. You can defer the question until you are en route.

Collect key information from the SAMPLE history, obtain baseline vital signs, use relevant monitoring devices, and perform a physical exam (Figure 19-3). If the problem is clear, the physical exam is focused by the chief complaint. If the problem is not clear, perform a **rapid medical exam**. For example, you would perform a rapid medical exam for an unresponsive patient for whom no cause could be identified in the primary assessment or from the initial information available. The rapid medical exam is similar to the **rapid trauma exam**. It is a quick check of vital areas to see if there are any potentially life-threatening problems that were not apparent from the primary assessment.

The initial information you obtain, in addition to the chief complaint, is used to make treatment decisions. Taking an in-depth history, performing a head-to-toe exam, or moving the patient from his location to the ambulance should not delay some types of treatment. However, you should not unduly delay transport by performing tasks at the scene that you could more efficiently perform en route to the hospital.

The lack of a definitive answer about exactly what to do in every situation can be frustrating. There are principles

IN THE FIELD

You must make decisions about the timing of treatment and transport on a case-by-case basis. A textbook is only one source of information that helps inform your decisions. You also need medical direction, experience, and knowledge of particular EMS systems to guide you. Among the questions you should ask yourself are these: How long will it take to move the patient from his current location to the ambulance? How much help do you have? What are the consequences of delaying medication administration for a certain patient? Will medication be delayed for 1 minute or 5 minutes, based on how difficult it is to package and move the patient? How do the consequences of delaying transportation for 2 minutes to give a medication compare to delaying the medication for 5 minutes to prepare for transport?

Scene size-up	Primary assessment	Secondary assessment	Reassessment
Goals	**Goals**	**Goals**	**Goals**
Determine nature of the incident and need for additional resources	Formulate a general impression of the problem	Determine problem	Detect trends in patient condition
Determine scene safety	Find and correct immediate threats to life	Plan treatment	Detect new complaints, signs, symptoms
	Determine priority for transport	Reevaluate priority decision	Determine effects of treatment
			Evaluate treatment plan and patient priority

• Nature of incident: medical	• Patient has decreased level of responsiveness OR	• Take history based on chief complaint or presenting problem	• Reassess every 5 minutes or more frequently as indicated
• Single patient; assess need for additional resources	• Poor general appearance OR	• Take vital signs and use monitoring devices	• Perform primary assessment
• No hazards/hazards controlled	• Impaired airway, breathing, or circulation OR	• Perform focused secondary assessment based on chief complaint and patient priority	• Take vital signs and use monitoring devices
• Nature of illness/general appearance: **Critical medical patient**	• Chief complaint is concerning for life-threatening illness	• If problem is not clear perform rapid medical assessment	• Perform aspects of secondary assessment
	• Begin interventions for ABCs	• If problem remains unclear, perform head-to-toe exam	• Make changes in treatment as needed
	• Confirm general impression: **Critical medical patient; immediate priority for transport**	• Formulate field impression	• Reevaluate patient priority
		• Plan treatment (on scene vs. en route)	• Communicate changes as needed
		• Reevaluate priority for transport	
		• Communicate with medical direction and receiving facility	

FIGURE 19-3

Assessment of a critical medical patient.

and guidelines, but each situation has its own specific needs. You must continually analyze your decisions throughout the call. That is the basis of professional insight and judgment.

Trauma Patients

Noncritical Trauma Patients

Noncritical trauma patients are those who have non–life-threatening and non–limb-threatening isolated injuries, and who do not have a mechanism of injury anticipated to produce life- or limb-threatening injuries. An example is the patient who cut his hand with a kitchen knife or one who fell while roller-skating at low speed, injuring his forearm. A focused physical exam gives the most relevant and useful information in this case (Figure 19-4). Also take baseline vital signs and a SAMPLE history. The history can reveal, for example, that a patient is taking antiplatelet or anticoagulant medications that impair blood clotting. This is important information in the management of any patient. Manage the isolated injury and transport.

Critical Trauma Patients

Trauma patients who have serious mechanisms of injury; who have problems with airway, breathing, or circulation; or who have an altered mental status are critical (Table 19-1). Time is of the essence in stabilizing immediate life threats, immobilizing the spine if indicated, and preparing for transportation to the most appropriate facility (Figure 19-5). While preparing the patient for transport, perform a rapid trauma exam to check vital areas of the body for potentially life-threatening injuries.

You can remember the link between the primary assessment and secondary assessment by using the mnemonic *ABCDE*. Perform ABCD in the primary assessment. The "E" is a reminder to quickly expose the patient to perform a rapid trauma exam. You must not omit this step. However, take care to preserve the patient's privacy and prevent hypothermia.

The rapid trauma exam is a quick, systematic head-to-toe exam. It is performed to look for signs of significant injury, such as open wounds, bruises, and deformities. Obtain

Scene size-up	Primary assessment	Secondary assessment	Reassessment
Goals	**Goals**	**Goals**	**Goals**
Determine nature of the incident and need for additional resources Determine scene safety	Formulate a general impression of the problem Find and correct immediate threats to life Determine priority for transport	Determine problem Plan treatment Reevaluate priority decision	Detect trends in patient condition Detect new complaints, signs, symptoms Determine effects of treatment Evaluate treatment plan and patient priority
• Nature of incident: trauma • Single patient; assess need for additional resources • No hazards/hazards controlled • Mechanism of Injury/general appearance: **Noncritical trauma patient**	• Patient is alert AND • Has good general appearance AND • No impairment of airway, breathing, or circulation AND • Chief complaint/MOI is not concerning for life-threatening injury • Confirm general impression: **Noncritical trauma patient; transport may be delayed for further assessment and treatment**	• Perform a focused exam based on chief complaint or presenting problem • Take vital signs and use monitoring devices • Gather a medical history • Formulate field impression • Plan treatment and transport • Reevaluate priority for transport • Communicate with medical direction and receiving facility as needed	• Reassess every 15 minutes or more frequently as indicated • Perform primary assessment • Take vital signs and use monitoring devices • Perform aspects of secondary assessment • Make changes in treatment as needed • Reevaluate patient priority • Communicate changes as needed

FIGURE 19-4

Assessment of a noncritical trauma patient.

Scene size-up	Primary assessment	Secondary assessment	Reassessment
Goals	**Goals**	**Goals**	**Goals**
Determine nature of the incident and need for additional resources Determine scene safety	Formulate a general impression of the problem Find and correct immediate threats to life Determine priority for transport	Determine problem Plan treatment Reevaluate priority decision	Detect trends in patient condition Detect new complaints, signs, symptoms Determine effects of treatment Evaluate treatment plan and patient priority
• Nature of incident: trauma • Single patient; assess need for additional resources • Hazards controlled • Mechanism of Injury/general appearance: **Critical trauma patient** • Determine need for manual stabilization of cervical spine	• Patient has decreased level of responsiveness OR • Poor general appearance OR • Is alert but has impaired airway, breathing, or circulation OR • Chief complaint/MOI is concerning for life-threatening injury • Begin interventions for ABCs • Confirm general impression: **Critical trauma patient; immediate priority for transport**	• Perform rapid trauma exam • Take vital signs and use monitoring devices • Gather a medical history • Formulate field impression • Plan treatment (on scene vs. en route) • Perform a head-to-toe exam • Reevaluate priority for transport • Communicate with medical direction and receiving facility	• Reassess every 5 minutes or more frequently as indicated • Perform primary assessment • Take vital signs and use monitoring devices • Perform aspects of secondary assessment • Make changes in treatment as needed • Reevaluate patient priority • Communicate changes as needed

FIGURE 19-5

Assessment of a critical trauma patient.

TABLE 19-1	Criteria for Critical Trauma Patients

CRITICAL MECHANISMS OF INJURY

- Complete or partial ejection in a motor vehicle collision (MVC)
- MVC that causes death to another occupant of the same vehicle
- Rollover mechanism MVC
- High-speed MVC
- Intrusion (damage) of > 12 inches into the passenger compartment of a vehicle, or vehicle crush of > 18 inches at any point on the vehicle
- Pedestrian or bicyclist struck by a motor vehicle
- Motorcyclist involved in collision at > 20 mph
- Fall from a height > 20 feet
- Blast (explosion) trauma
- Penetrating trauma except distal to the elbow or knee
- Amputation or near-amputation proximal to the fingers or toes
- Trauma with burns

PATIENT CHARACTERISTICS

- Obstructed, inadequate, or threatened airway
- Impaired ventilation
- Significant hemorrhage (external or suspected internal)
- Altered mental status or neurologic deficit
- Presence of serious medical conditions (e.g., bleeding disorder, taking anticoagulants, heart disease, lung disease)
- Age > 55 years
- Hypothermia
- Pregnancy

TABLE 19-2	Questions Guiding the Patient Assessment Process

- Is it safe to approach the patient and begin care in the patient's current location? If not, what must you do to solve this problem?
- What is the nature of the patient's problem?
- How sick is the patient?
- Which interventions, resources, and actions are required immediately?
- Which health care facility can best meet the patient's immediate needs?
- How should the patient be transported to receive this care?
- What do you need to do to support the patient's vital functions from the time you arrive at the scene to the time you transfer care of the patient to hospital personnel?
- Is the patient's condition stable, improving, or worsening?

a set of baseline vital signs and measure the SpO_2. If the patient's condition and available resources allow, perform a head-to-toe exam en route to the hospital. Obtain as much relevant medical history as possible. At times, there may be little information available about unresponsive patients until they have arrived at the hospital and family members have been contacted.

Field Impression

The information you have collected through the scene size-up, primary assessment, secondary assessment, and medical history is used to form a field impression of the patient's problem. Ask yourself the questions introduced in Chapter 14 to guide your reasoning through the patient assessment process (Table 19-2). The clinical reasoning process may confirm an early hypothesis, or the information may change your initial impression of the problem. Be aware of the clinical reasoning process and its pitfalls (Chapter 14).

A field impression is not a definitive diagnosis of the patient's problem. It is an understanding of the patient's

immediate problems. Beyond the immediate actions taken in the primary assessment, your field impression provides the basis of management decisions.

Reassessment

Reassessment is a process of comparing later findings to baseline patient assessment findings. Reassess to track changes in a patient's condition and evaluate the effects of treatment. Use reassessment information to determine if changes in patient care are needed. Picture a patient whose initial SpO_2 before oxygen administration was 92 percent. Because the patient was mildly hypoxic, you began administering 4 L/min of oxygen by nasal cannula. Five minutes later, the patient's SpO_2 is 94 percent. The patient's SpO_2 has improved, but the goal is to achieve and maintain an SpO_2 of 95 percent or higher. If the patient originally was wheezing and you also started an albuterol treatment, you might decide to wait until he finishes the treatment and reassess. If the patient's original problem did not indicate an albuterol treatment, you may decide to increase the amount of oxygen being administered and switch the patient to a simple face mask.

Critical patients are reassessed every 5 minutes, or more frequently. Noncritical patients are reassessed every 15 minutes. Reassess the patient's chief complaint and associated complaints, the primary assessment findings, and vital signs. Other aspects of reassessment depend on the results from monitoring devices and the type of secondary assessment you performed. If a patient has an isolated ankle injury, you will reassess the injured extremity. If a patient was hypoglycemic and you administered dextrose, you will recheck his blood glucose level (BGL).

For a critical trauma patient, re-examine problems you found in the secondary assessment, and repeat the rapid trauma assessment to detect any emerging problems. Whenever a patient has an additional complaint, or his initial complaints worsen, you should reassess him. If you notice a change in the patient's condition between planned reassessments, reassess him. For example, if the patient becomes confused, his heart rate changes significantly, or his SpO₂ drops, perform a reassessment. Sometimes a change can be explained by something as simple as the pulse oximeter clip becoming dislodged from the patient's finger. However, sometimes the patient has taken a sudden change for the worse and you must be ready to intervene immediately.

Documentation

Mentally organize assessment information in preparation for giving a radio report/or a handoff report that concisely conveys key pieces of information. You also must document assessment findings in the PCR (Chapter 6). Document results of the scene size-up, primary assessment, secondary assessment, and patient history. Document the treatment performed, the results of reassessment, and any changes made in treatment.

You must document both positive findings and **pertinent negatives** from the secondary assessment and history. They will, of course, depend on the situation. For example, it is important to document that a patient with an isolated leg injury had a strong pedal (dorsalis pedis) pulse. It is not important to document that the patient denied a history of measles as a child. Your judgment about what is pertinent will develop over time. Feedback on your documentation from your medical director and experienced EMS providers will help you refine your documentation skills.

Taking a Medical History

Establish rapport with your patient to ensure effective therapeutic communication. Begin by introducing yourself and your partner and letting the patient know you are there to help. If you must address sensitive topics, wait until you are in the privacy of the ambulance, overcome special challenges to communication, and make other adaptations to your approach as needed.

Keep in mind the principles and techniques of interviewing and therapeutic communication covered in Chapter 6. Your next questions are guided by obtaining the patient's chief complaint. The following exchange illustrates how you might begin:

Advanced EMT: "Hi. My name is Owen Griego. This is my partner, France Morgan. What is your name, sir?"

Patient: "Hi. I'm Derrick Wolfe."

Advanced EMT: "How can we help you today, Mr. Wolfe?"

Patient: "I was bitten by a stray cat I tried to pick up and I think it's getting infected."

Advanced EMT: "Where did it bite you?"

Patient: "Right here, on my right hand [showing hand]."

Advanced EMT: "I see it. How does it feel?"

Patient: "It hurts like heck! See how it's swelling up? It feels tight and I'm having trouble bending my fingers."

Advanced EMT: "Which of those symptoms is bothering you the most?"

Patient: "It's the pain. That's why I thought it was getting infected, and then it started to swell."

In this exchange, the cat bite is the mechanism of injury, and right-hand pain is the chief complaint. It also is correct to say the patient's chief complaint is "right-hand pain and swelling," because the pain and swelling together made the patient concerned about infection, prompting his call for the ambulance. The patient expressed possible infection as a concern, but his concern was based on his symptoms: pain and swelling.

The SAMPLE History

The mnemonic *SAMPLE* is used to ensure all aspects of the history of the present illness and past medical history are obtained. The letters in SAMPLE stand for the following:

S – Symptoms
A – Allergies
M – Medications
P – Past medical history
L – Last oral intake
E – Events leading to the problem

SAMPLE serves as a useful checklist to make sure you have completed the history, but the information does not always emerge in SAMPLE order. After all, SAMPLE and other mnemonics are *your* tools, not the patient's.

Make sure you are listening to everything the patient says, even if it does not fit the SAMPLE sequence. If necessary, confirm any information that is not clear, or ask the patient to elaborate on something mentioned previously. It is detrimental to therapeutic communication to ask questions to which the patient already clearly gave you answers. However, if you forget the answer the patient gave you, simply say, "I'm sorry. I know you told me the answer to this, but I don't recall what you said," and then repeat your question. Do not let pride or embarrassment keep you from obtaining critical information.

Symptoms

Symptoms are a patient's subjective complaints of perceived changes in the body. Patients may complain of symptoms such as leg pain, dizziness, muscle aches, difficulty breathing, inability to urinate, coughing, and many other things. Health care personnel cannot directly perceive most symptoms but some, such as coughing, can be observed.

Symptoms, including the chief complaint, are best elicited by asking open-ended questions. For example, "What is bothering you today, Ms. Griffin?" A follow-up question might be, "In addition to the stomach pain, are you having any other problems or concerns?" You may need to follow up again by asking, "Anything else?" Patients tend not to mention things they think might not be related to the problem, things that might be embarrassing, or things that are not bothering them at the moment.

Ask specifically about symptoms the patient has not mentioned that are commonly associated with the chief complaint. For example, because you have likely had a cold or the flu, you are familiar with their collection of symptoms. So, if a patient complains of a cough, ask about difficulty breathing, fever, muscle aches, headache, and other associated symptoms. If the patient states that he has one or more of them, include them in your oral and written reports.

If the patient states that he does *not* have a symptom that is typically associated with the chief complaint, this is called a *pertinent negative*. Pertinent negatives also are included in your reports. This is usually recorded in the form of "The patient denies [specific symptoms]."

The **history of the present illness** elaborates on the story of the patient's symptoms. Note that some of the information obtained early in the patient interview will actually fall under the category of *events leading up to the problem*.

A useful mnemonic for exploring the history of the present illness is *OPQRST*. The letters stand for the following:

O – Onset of the symptoms
P – factors that Provoke or Palliate (**relieve**) the symptoms
Q – subjective Quality of the symptoms
R – Radiation of pain or discomfort
S – Severity of the symptoms
T – Time or duration of the symptoms

Pain is a symptom, and a frequent complaint. It is useful to be able to anticipate some of the ways patients describe it (Table 19-3).

To determine the onset of symptoms, ask the patient what he was doing at the time the symptoms occurred, or how it was that he became aware of the symptoms. This works best for symptoms of relatively short duration. When patients offer a long-standing complaint, ask what changed to make the patient more concerned than usual.

You may notice that this information can overlap with the "E" in SAMPLE. This is not a problem. It serves as a double-check that you have all information. Ask the patient if anything makes the symptoms better or worse. Anything that makes the symptoms better is a *palliating* factor. Anything that makes them worse is a *provoking* factor.

TABLE 19-3 Pain Descriptions

Type of Pain	Description
Visceral pain	Pain arising from the organs. Usually experienced as vague and diffuse. May be described as "dull" pain.
Somatic pain	Pain arising from inflammation of the lining of body cavities, such as the peritoneum. Usually well-localized, intense, and tender to palpation. May be described as a "sharp" pain.
Neuropathic pain	Pain arising from nerves, such as in sciatica. May be described as shooting, stinging, or burning and can be accompanied by numbness and tingling sensations.
Colic (colicky pain)	Arises from spasm of hollow organs, such as the intestines and ureters. Tends to occur in waves.
Referred pain	Pain that is felt in another part of the body than the organ that is producing. For example, pain from an injured spleen may be referred to the left shoulder.
Radiating pain	Pain that originates in one place but is also experienced in other locations. For example, chest pain from acute coronary syndrome may also be experienced in the neck, jaw, or arm.
Throbbing pain	Associated with inflammation or increased circulation. May occur in some headaches and localized injuries.

Determine the subjective quality of the complaint by asking the patient to describe it in his own words. Start with an open-ended question, such as "Describe the exact sensation you are feeling in your lower back." If the patient cannot describe the quality of pain, you will have to ask more focused questions. Ask if the pain is sharp or dull and whether it is constant or comes and goes. Other questions about the quality of symptoms will depend on the particular complaint.

Sometimes patients experience pain that starts in a primary location but then extends to other locations. This is called **radiation**, which you should not confuse with *referred* pain. A patient with a kidney stone (renal calculus) may complain of pain in the side or back (flank) that radiates to his groin. The patient is not likely to use the term "radiate." More likely he will say something like, "The pain starts at the right side of my back and moves down into my groin." Patients having ACS may have chest pain or discomfort that radiates to the shoulder, jaw, back, or other locations. **Referred pain** is pain that is experienced in a location in the

Pediatric Care

For small children who might not understand a numerical scale for assessing the level of pain, a visual scale with cartoon faces that range from happy to very distressed is useful.

Geriatric Care

Severity of pain can diminish with age. The elderly may feel a lesser amount of pain than expected for their condition. Do not underestimate the severity of the elderly patient's condition because he does not describe the pain as severe.

body that is *not* the actual site of the problem. A patient with ACS who complains of pain in his left arm *instead of* chest pain or discomfort is experiencing referred pain.

As with all symptoms, the experience of pain is subjective. You cannot see or objectively measure the severity of a patient's pain. Nonetheless, the patient's subjective experience of the pain is important, even if he is not experiencing it the way another person might.

Assessing and managing pain have become very important issues in health care. Establishing the patient's baseline level of pain allows you to track response to treatment or worsening of the situation. Pain is assessed using a scale from 1 to 10, with 1 being the least amount of pain (0 is no pain) and 10 being the worst pain the patient has ever experienced.

Using OPQRST, the "T" for time refers to the duration of the symptoms. The symptoms may have started suddenly, prompting the call for EMS, or may have gradually increased over a period of hours, or even days. Even though a patient has had the pain for a long period of time, it does not mean that the situation is not serious. A patient may delay getting help for a number of reasons, during which time his condition can become worse. In such patients, there is increased urgency in getting him to definitive care, because some treatments, such as fibrinolytic therapy, must be given within a narrow window of opportunity.

Allergies

Ask the patient specifically about the allergies he may have. In particular, ask about drug allergies, but allergies to foods and other substances are important, too. Common medication allergies include those to aspirin, codeine, penicillin, and sulfa and other antibiotics.

Some patients confuse medication allergies with any adverse reaction to a medication. When a patient states he has an allergy, it is helpful to ask, "What happens when you take [the medication]?" Common signs and symptoms of allergic reactions include swelling, hives, itching, and difficulty breathing. Ask specifically about allergies to any medications that you may administer to the patient.

Medications

Find out what medications the patient is taking. This includes all prescription and over-the-counter medications, vitamins, herbal supplements, and homeopathic medications. A helpful question is, "Have you tried anything to treat this problem?" The answer may or may not involve a medication, but can provide information that you might not otherwise get.

A patient's medications can give you information about his medical conditions that he might not think to include when you ask about his past medical history. If a medication has several uses or you are not sure what it is for, ask the patient for the reason he is taking it. Ask to see the medication containers, if possible (Figure 19-6). The names of many medications sound alike, so it is important to write down the exact name of the medication, as well as the dosage. Also ask if the patient is taking medications as prescribed. Information that a patient is taking more or less of a medication than prescribed could help explain the patient's condition.

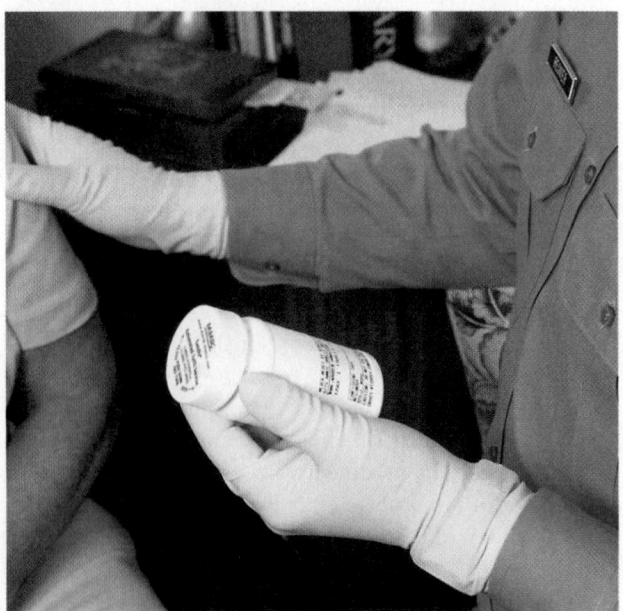

FIGURE 19-6

Record the names of all medications exactly as they appear on the label.

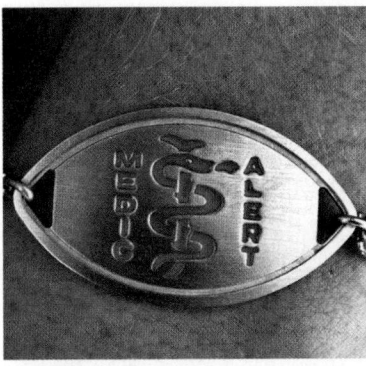

(A)

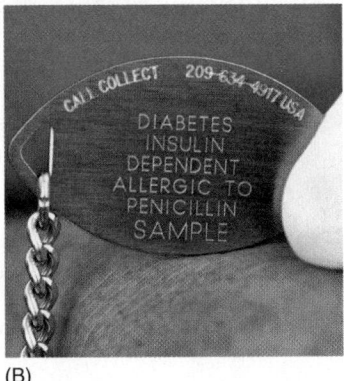

(B)

FIGURE 19-7

Medical identification jewelry. (A) Front. (B) Back.

Ask about over-the-counter medications, supplements, herbs, and alternative therapies, because these all can impact a patient's health and medical care.

Past Medical History

A pertinent **past medical history** includes ongoing chronic illnesses, serious past illnesses, and significant surgeries, injuries, and hospitalizations. It is important to know about heart disease, high blood pressure, breathing problems, diabetes, kidney disease, seizures, liver disease, and other serious illnesses, even if the current problem does not seem to be related to them (Figure 19-7). Those diseases can affect the patient's ability to compensate for other problems and the treatment he may need.

Other aspects of the past medical history depend on the current situation. For medical complaints, ask the patient if he has had the same problem in the past. Also consider the nature of the situation when deciding what questions to ask. For example, in prehospital care it is usually not important to ask a woman about any past pregnancies. However, if the patient is presenting with an obstetric (pregnancy-related) or gynecologic (reproductive system) complaint, this information is important.

Last Oral Intake

Ask the patient when the last time was that he had anything to eat or drink. Sometimes this is relevant to the chief complaint itself, such as when a patient has vomiting, diarrhea, stomach cramps, or an allergic reaction to a food. The last time a patient ate or drank is important in assessing diabetics, and in patients who are possibly dehydrated or malnourished. This information also can help you anticipate if the patient has a full stomach and could vomit in response to pain, injury, or medications. It also is important if the patient will require anesthesia or conscious sedation for a surgical procedure in the hospital.

Events Leading to the Problem

Make sure you completely understand the patient's story of the events that led to the call for EMS. In most cases, the information should come from the patient. If the patient is confused or uncooperative, supplement his information with information from family, bystanders, or caregivers. If the patient is unresponsive, you will have to rely solely on the information provided by others.

When you have obtained all the information required for a SAMPLE history, summarize your understanding of the pertinent parts of the history to the patient and ask if you have understood correctly. Follow up by asking if there is anything else the patient wants to tell you that could be helpful in understanding the problem. If you have forgotten to ask something, or another question occurs to you later on, be sure to ask about it.

Working from the Presenting Problem or Chief Complaint

Patients do not present a field impression up front. They present with complaints and **presenting problems**. You must manage some presenting problems, such as cardiac arrest, immediately. Even then, because there are different causes of cardiac arrest, you still must collect information to determine the presence of any other problems in order to form a field impression. You must work *from* the scene size-up, primary assessment, and chief complaint *to* a field impression. Because they are life threatening, you will treat some problems, such as problems with airway, breathing, and circulation, along the way.

You should know how to obtain the history from, and how to examine patients with, the complaints and presenting problems listed in Table 19-4. By the end of your Advanced EMT program, you should be able to provide prehospital emergency care and transportation for patients with each of those complaints and problems. The details of assessing and managing those patients are covered in upcoming chapters.

Patient complaints and problems are not limited to those listed, of course. Patients will present with other complaints and problems, including those in Table 19-5.

CASE STUDY (continued)

Advanced EMTs Lindsay and Teresa are at the home of Ms. Gretchen Snyder, who is complaining of severe abdominal pain. She told the Advanced EMTs, "I've got a pretty bad pain in my belly."

"When did the pain start?" asks Lindsay.

"It woke me up during the night, about 2:00 AM, I think. I didn't sleep much after that," Ms. Snyder replies.

"Have you ever had pain like this before?"

"Nothing like this. No."

"Have you been able to do anything that makes the pain better?" Lindsay asks.

"As long as I lie still, curled up like this, it's not as bad. If I stretch out or move, though, it hurts a lot worse."

"Can you describe what the pain feels like?"

"I can't really pinpoint what hurts. It hurts all around the middle of my stomach. It started out kind of dull, but it feels a little sharper now."

"On a scale from 1 being the least pain to 10 being the worst pain," says Lindsay, "where would you rate this pain?"

"A seven, I'd say."

"Are you having pain anywhere else?"

"No, just my stomach."

"Can you point to where the pain is?"

"Here," Ms. Snyder replies, drawing an imaginary circle around her umbilicus.

"Teresa is going to check your blood pressure while I ask you a few more questions. Okay, Ms. Snyder?"

Problem-Solving Questions

1. What do Lindsay and Teresa know about the SAMPLE history, so far?
2. What are the next questions Lindsay and Teresa should ask?
3. At what point should Lindsay and Teresa perform a physical exam?
4. What should Lindsay and Teresa assess during the physical exam?

TABLE 19-4   Selected Chief Complaints

■ Abdominal pain	■ Chest pain	■ Gastrointestinal bleeding	■ Poisoning
■ Abuse/neglect	■ Constipation	■ Headache	■ Rash
■ Altered mental status/decreased level of responsiveness	■ Cyanosis	■ Hematuria	■ Rectal pain
	■ Dehydration	■ Hemoptysis	■ Shock
■ Anxiety	■ Diarrhea	■ Hypertension	■ Sore throat
■ Apnea	■ Dizziness/vertigo	■ Hypotension	■ Stridor/drooling
■ Ataxia	■ Dysphasia	■ Joint pain/swelling	■ Syncope
■ Back pain	■ Dyspnea	■ Multiple trauma	■ Urinary retention
■ Behavioral emergency	■ Edema	■ Nausea/vomiting	■ Visual disturbances
■ Bleeding	■ Eye pain	■ Pain	■ Weakness
■ Cardiac arrest	■ Fatigue	■ Paralysis	■ Wheezing
■ Cardiac rhythm disturbances	■ Fever	■ Pediatric crying/fussiness	

Some complaints are more common than others, and some complaints indicate more urgent problems than others. You must know how to obtain history and physical exam information from patients with each of these complaints.

TABLE 19-5	Additional Patient Complaints

In addition to the complaints and problems mentioned specifically in the Advanced EMT Education Standards, patients present with other complaints with which you should be familiar. They include:

- Ascites
- Congestion
- Cough/hiccups
- Dental pain
- Dysmenorrhea
- Dysuria
- Ear pain
- Feeding problems
- Hearing disturbance
- Incontinence
- Jaundice
- Malaise
- Pruritus
- Red eye/pink eye
- Tinnitus

Overview of the Physical Examination

In the prehospital setting, there are two complementary approaches to the physical examination in the secondary assessment: the anatomical approach and the body systems approach. The anatomical approach systematically assesses the body from head to toe. It is used in the rapid trauma exam, rapid medical exam, and head-to-toe exam. A more thorough, detailed, head-to-toe exam is performed on critical and potentially critical trauma patients. A detailed head-to-toe exam is less often performed on medical patients. It is most helpful with an unresponsive medical patient in whom the primary assessment, SAMPLE history, and rapid medical exam have not allowed you to determine the nature of the problem. With isolated injuries, the anatomical approach is used to perform an exam that is focused on the area of complaint (focused exam).

The body systems approach is used in both trauma and medical patients. In medical patients, this approach receives more emphasis than the anatomical one, based on the chief complaint. The major body systems assessed are the respiratory, cardiovascular, neurologic, and musculoskeletal systems.

The complementary nature of the anatomical and body systems approaches is illustrated by the following example: Imagine you are conducting a head-to-toe exam on a trauma patient and palpate a hematoma on the back

of his head. After finishing your head-to-toe exam (the anatomical approach), you then focus on collecting additional information about neurologic function (the body systems approach).

The techniques of inspection, palpation, and auscultation are used in the physical examination, as well as in specific tests or exams (Table 19-6). The mnemonic *DCAP-BTLS* is one way of remembering the signs you may find during examination (Table 19-7). *Inspection* is a visual examination of the body during which you look for signs of illness or injury. You may see a rash or variety of other skin lesions, deformity, swelling, open or closed soft-tissue injuries, burns, skin discoloration, cerebrospinal fluid leaking from the ears or nose, and other signs (Figure 19-8). Also take note of any unusual odors on the patient. Certain breath odors can indicate the presence of specific toxins, diabetic ketoacidosis, alcohol intoxication, or poor oral hygiene (Table 19-8). An odor of urine on the body and clothing can indicate urinary **incontinence** or renal failure. Other odors can give clues to a patient's recent activities, which may help in determining the nature of the problem.

Palpation is used to feel for abnormalities (Figure 19-9). You may feel a lump that represents a hematoma, deformity, swelling, **crepitus**, or a mass within the abdomen, or guarding. Guarding is voluntary or involuntary abdominal muscle contraction in response to painful abdominal conditions. In voluntary guarding, the patient can relax the abdominal muscles when instructed to do so, although he may be reluctant. A patient with involuntary guarding cannot relax the muscles. When a patient complains of pain in response to palpation, this is called *tenderness*.

Auscultation is listening to sounds within the body (Figure 19-10). It is useful to listen to breath sounds—and in some cases, heart sounds—in the prehospital setting. Although you can auscultate the abdomen to assess bowel sounds, the information provided is not immediately useful in prehospital care. When you perform abdominal auscultation, you should do it prior to palpation.

In specific cases, it is useful to perform physical exam tests that give information about particular conditions. One such example is checking for signs of meningeal irritation in a patient whose history and physical exam findings suggest a hypothesis of meningitis. When a supine patient flexes his hips and knees in response to flexion of the neck, this is a positive Brudzinski's sign, which is an indication of inflammation of the meninges (Figure 19-11). Specific tests are discussed in later chapters.

Some findings are *pathognomonic*. This means that a sign or symptom is so distinctive to a particular disease that a diagnosis can be made from the finding. An example is the characteristic "slapped cheek" appearance of a child with fifth disease (a common childhood viral illness) (Figure 19-12). Unfortunately, there are few such findings that assist in forming a field impression. You must make the field impression based on a collection of findings that may or may not be an exact match to a "classic" presentation.

TABLE 19-6   Selected Physical Exam Tests

Test	Indication	Technique	Results
Cincinnati prehospital stroke scale	History, symptoms, or signs of a possible stroke	Ask patient to smile and show you his teeth.	Patient's facial expression should be symmetrical. Asymmetry or drooping can be caused by stroke.
		Ask the patient to hold his arms out in front of him, palms up.	Drifting or pronation of one arm indicates weakness, which can be due to a stroke.
		Ask the patient to repeat, "You can't teach an old dog new tricks."	Any difficulty or confusion in repeating back the phrase may be the result of a stroke.
Heel-Drop test (Markle test)	Abdominal pain that suggests inflammation of the peritoneum	Have patient stand on balls of the feet and suddenly drop down on the heels.	Resulting pain in the abdomen is a sign of peritonitis.
Homan's sign	Pain or swelling in the leg that may be caused by deep vein thrombosis	Support the patient's leg and dorsiflex his foot.	Pain caused by dorsiflexion is a sign of deep vein thrombosis.
Percussion	To detect an abnormal collection of air or fluid, or a tumor	Place the fingers of one hand flat against the part to be percussed (abdomen or chest). Strike the middle finger of the hand with the tip of the opposite middle finger to elicit sound.	Hollow, air-filled structures have a resonant sound. Solid or fluid-filled structures have a dull percussion note.
Murphy's sign	Possible liver or gallbladder problem	As you palpate the abdomen, gently "hook" your fingers around the inferior border of the right costal margin while asking the patient to inhale.	Increased pain indicates involvement of the liver or gallbladder.
Orthostatic vital signs	Dehydration or occult bleeding without obvious signs of shock	Measure blood pressure and pulse while patient is supine. Have patient then stand for 3 minutes, and repeat measurements.	An increase in pulse of 10 beats per minute or more, or a decrease in systolic blood pressure of 10 mmHg or more, indicates orthostatic hypotension.
Range of motion	Possible joint injury without obvious signs	Have the patient move the joint in all directions to check for mobility and pain.	Pain and limited motion are indications of joint injury.
Visual acuity	Complaints of sudden changes in or loss of vision; eye injury	In the prehospital setting, you can examine vision grossly by holding up your fingers and having the patient tell you how many fingers he can see.	Depends on patient's baseline visual acuity.

At a minimum, you need the following equipment to complete the secondary assessment, including vital signs:

- Exam gloves
- Other personal protective equipment (PPE) as appropriate to the situation
- Large bandage or "trauma" shears
- Stethoscope
- Blood pressure cuff
- Penlight
- Pulse oximeter and other monitoring devices as indicated

If the patient is responsive, explain what you are going to do before you do it. Talk to the patient during the exam to keep him informed about what you are doing, and to determine whether your examination is causing discomfort.

As much as possible, protect the patient's privacy and modesty. Conduct the exam away from bystanders. If you expose an area, cover it again when you have finished examining that area. If you must cut the patient's clothing to conduct the exam, have a sheet available to cover the patient, for both warmth and modesty.

Anatomical Approach to Secondary Assessment

The anatomical approach for the rapid examination of trauma and medical patients is a quick, focused version of the more detailed head-to-toe exam. The techniques are the

TABLE 19-7   DCAP–BTLS Mnemonic

D – Deformities

C – Contusions

A – Abrasions

P – Punctures, penetrations

B – Burns

T – Tenderness

L – Lacerations

S – Swelling

The mnemonic DCAP–BTLS is one way of remembering signs of injury.

TABLE 19-8   Body Odors That May Be Noted on Physical Examination

Odor	Possible Significance
Fruity, acetone odor on breath	Diabetic ketoacidosis
Alcohol	Ingestion of alcoholic beverage
Urine/ammonia	Urinary incontinence/kidney failure
Bitter-almond breath odor	Cyanide poisoning
Sweet, putrid	Infection, gangrene
Fecal odor	Bowel incontinence, bowel obstruction (fecal odor on breath)
Musty	Liver disease

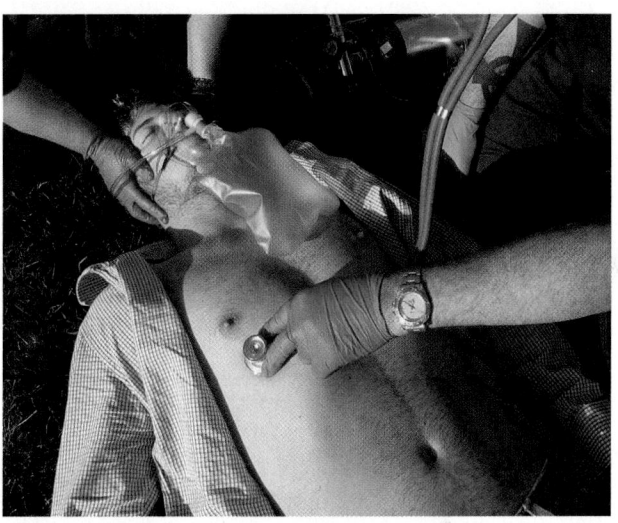

FIGURE 19-9

Use palpation to feel for deformity, swelling, crepitus, and other signs of injury and illness.

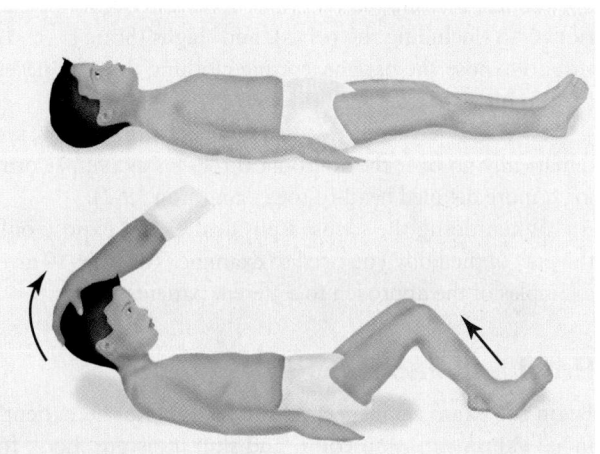

FIGURE 19-10

Auscultate the patient's breath sounds. (© Daniel Limmer)

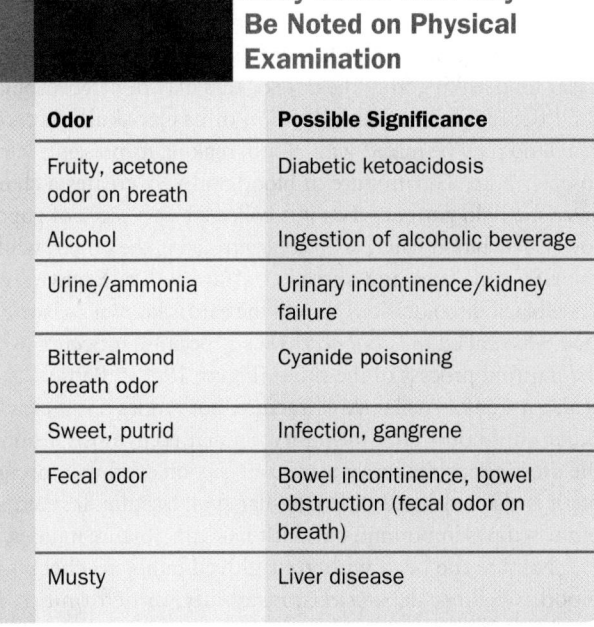

FIGURE 19-8

Use inspection to visually examine the body for signs of injury and illness.

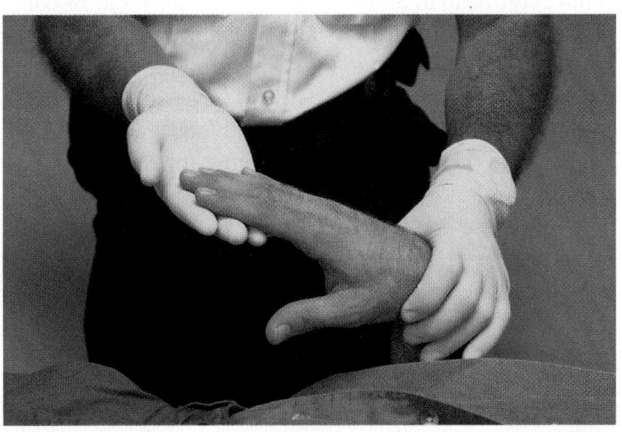

FIGURE 19-11

Brudzinki's sign is an indication of irritation of the meninges.

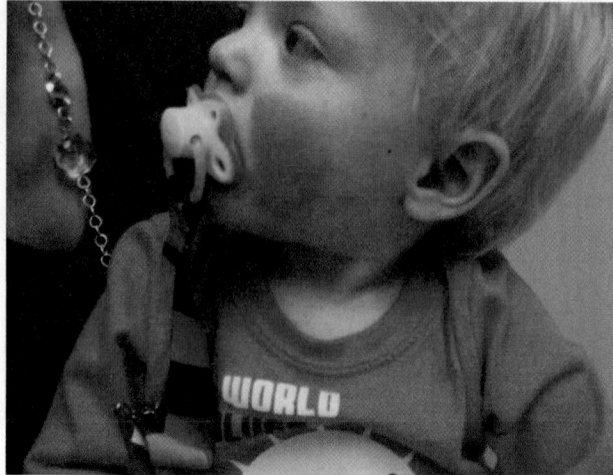

FIGURE 19-12

Fifth disease has a pathognomonic rash. (© Melissa Alexander)

Geriatric Care

Elderly patients, and sometimes homeless and mentally ill patients, wear many layers of clothing, even in warm weather. Those many layers can make examination difficult. Homeless and poor patients may be very concerned about not having replacement clothing. Find out how the hospitals you transport to handle this. Many hospitals provide donated clothing to patients who do not have another set of clothing to wear.

same, but you are to look only for life-threatening conditions that you must treat immediately (Table 19-9).

The anatomical approach is systematic, using the same general format in all cases so no components are omitted. You should complete the rapid trauma exam in about 30 seconds, focusing on the head, neck, anterior and posterior torso (including the pelvis), and thighs (Scan 19-1). Be sure to expose the patient, cutting clothing away as necessary, in order to examine his body.

After you have addressed all immediate life threats, systematically go over the anatomical regions again, performing a more detailed head-to-toe exam (Scan 19-2).

When doing the focused physical exam, expose only the part of the body you need to examine. Table 19-10 gives examples of the approach to different patients.

Head and Face

Begin the exam by inspecting the face. Note the patient's facial expression, skin color, and skin moisture. Look for symmetry of the facial features, open wounds, deformities, contusions, hematomas, and other injuries and abnormalities. Use your penlight to check the pupils and the inside of the mouth. Check inside the mouth for injuries, bleeding,

IN THE FIELD

There are special considerations in the examination of some patient populations, such as those who are technology dependent, have sensory impairments, or have other special needs. Differences in physical examination of these patients are discussed in Chapter 46.

Pediatric Care

The approach to the physical exam in small children differs in important ways. Modifications for examination of pediatric patients are presented in Chapters 43 and 44.

and foreign objects that may obstruct the airway, such as broken teeth or dentures, gum, food, or tobacco.

Take note of any bleeding or fluid from the nose and ears. Clear fluid leaking from the nose or ears may be cerebrospinal fluid (CSF), which is an indication of basilar skull fracture. The fluid may be mixed with blood, making its presence hard to determine. The mixture of blood and CSF creates a characteristic halo pattern when it is collected on a piece of paper towel. The blood will remain concentrated in the center, while the CSF separates and spreads out around it. **Ecchymosis** (blue/black discoloration) behind the ears is known as *Battle's sign* (also called *mastoid ecchymosis,* because it occurs over the mastoid process of the skull) (Figure 19-13). Battle's sign is also a sign of basilar skull fracture, but it does not typically occur until hours after the injury. Similar ecchymosis around the eyes (periorbital ecchymosis or raccoon eyes) may occur, but it is also a delayed sign of basilar skull fracture. Inspection of the scalp is important, but thick hair can obscure injuries.

Palpate the head with your gloved hands to check for blood, swelling, depressions, instability, or deformities. If cervical-spine injury is suspected, gently slide your hands beneath the head to prevent movement of the neck. Bleeding may not be immediately obvious in the primary assessment if the blood is soaking into the carpet, ground, or something else beneath the head. After palpating the back of the head, check your gloves for the presence of blood.

Palpate the facial bones, checking for tenderness, instability, and other signs of injury. Instability of the facial bones can lead to airway compromise. Signs of soft-tissue or bony injuries to the head and face should increase your index of suspicion for underlying traumatic brain injury.

Neck

In trauma patients, you must assess the neck before you apply a cervical collar. Inspect and palpate the neck for signs of injury, keeping in mind that it contains vital structures of the airway, major arteries and veins, and the cervical spinal cord.

TABLE 19-9	Significant Findings in Rapid Secondary Exam	
Body Region	**Finding**	**Possible Significance**
Head	**TRAUMA PATIENT**	
	Trauma to the head or face	Traumatic brain injury
	Unequal or nonreactive pupils	Traumatic brain injury
	Cerebrospinal fluid from nose or ears	Traumatic brain injury
	MEDICAL PATIENT	
	Unequal, nonreactive, or constricted pupils	Stroke
	Constricted pupils	Narcotic overdose, toxic exposure
	Dilated pupils	Overdose, toxic exposure, hypoxia
	Facial drooping	Stroke
Neck	**TRAUMA PATIENT**	
	Swelling, crepitus	Hematoma, tracheal injury
	Tracheal deviation	Tension pneumothorax
	Jugular venous distention (JVD)	Pericardial tamponade, tension pneumothorax
	Tenderness or deformity of cervical spine	Spinal-column injury, possible spinal-cord injury
	MEDICAL PATIENT	
	Swelling	Severe allergic reaction
	Jugular venous distention (JVD)	Right-sided heart failure, pericardial tamponade
Thorax	**TRAUMA PATIENT**	
	Unequal breath sounds	Pneumothorax, hemothorax, tension pneumothorax
	Tenderness, contusions, crepitus, instability, open injuries	Thoracic wall injuries, underlying lung injuries
	MEDICAL PATIENT	
	Unequal breath sounds	Pneumonia, pneumothorax
	Wheezing	Asthma, chronic obstructive pulmonary disease, allergic reaction
	Crackles	Pulmonary edema
	Rhonchi	Bronchitis
Abdomen	**TRAUMA PATIENT**	
	Contusions, tenderness, guarding, wounds	Internal bleeding or peritonitis from organ injury
	MEDICAL PATIENT	
	Discoloration, guarding, tenderness, distention	Peritonitis, hemorrhage, fluid (ascites), liver disease
Pelvis	**TRAUMA PATIENT**	
	Instability, tenderness, crepitus	Pelvic fracture
Extremities	**TRAUMA PATIENT**	
	Swelling, deformity, crepitus, tenderness, numbness, contusions, hematomas, wounds	Fractures, soft-tissue injuries
	Paralysis (bilateral)	Spinal-cord injury
	MEDICAL PATIENT	
	Swelling (bilateral)	Right-sided heart failure
	Swelling (one extremity)	Venous thrombosis (obstructed venous flow)
	Paralysis or weakness (unilateral)	Stroke

Observe for use of the sternocleidomastoid muscle during breathing as an indication of respiratory distress. Check the trachea to see if it is in the midline, and look for jugular venous distention (JVD). Tracheal deviation is not often seen, but is very significant when present, because it is a sign of tension pneumothorax.

The external jugular veins usually are visible when the patient is supine or reclining at less than a 45-degree angle. In patients positioned at greater than a 45-degree angle, the effects of gravity make the jugular veins less prominent. JVD in patients positioned at an angle that is greater than 45 degrees suggests that blood return through the superior vena cava

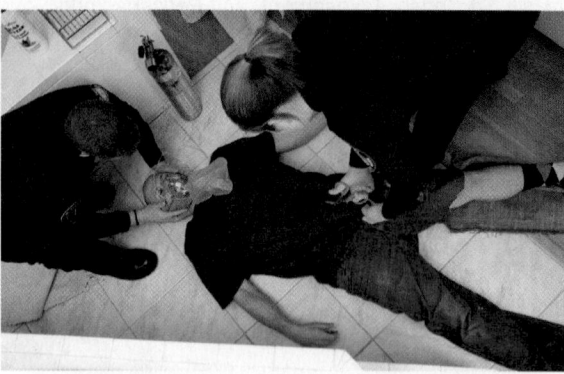

1. Expose critical trauma and medical patients to perform a rapid physical examination after the primary assessment.

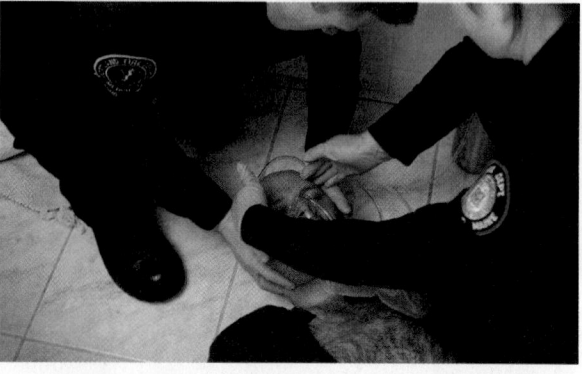

2. Inspect and palpate the patient's head and face.

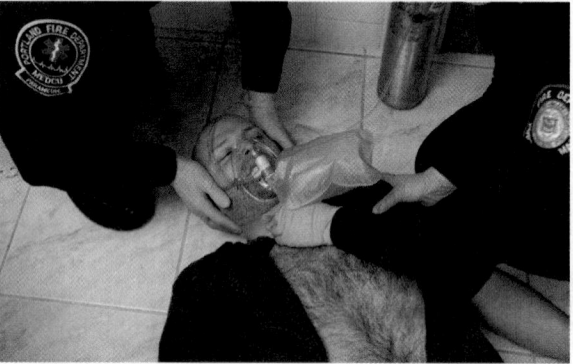

3. Inspect and palpate the patient's neck.

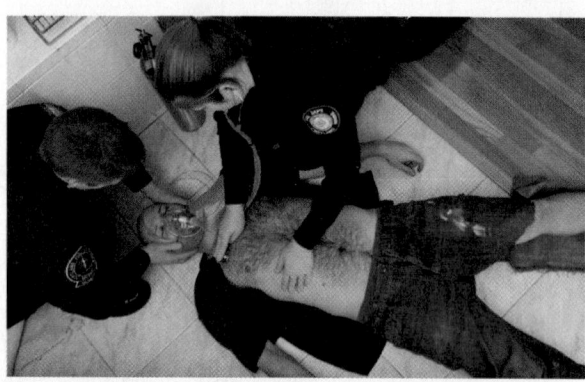

4. Inspect, palpate, and auscultate the chest.

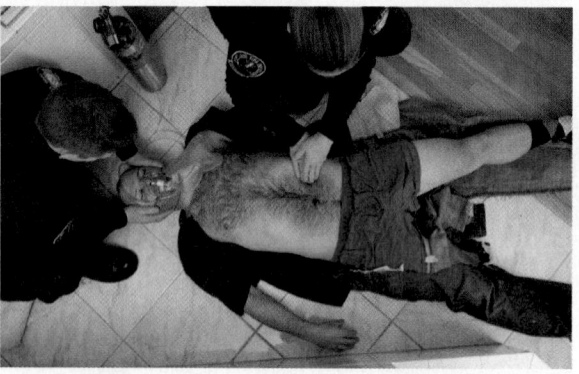

5. Inspect and palpate the abdomen.

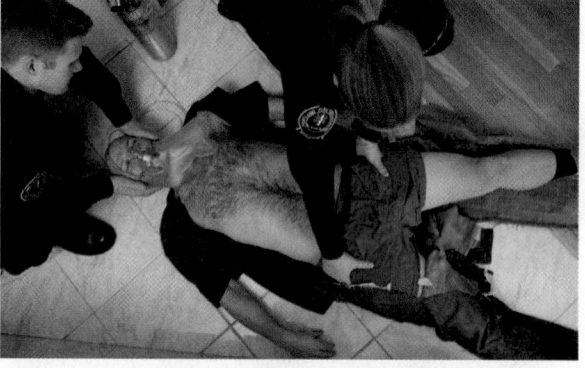

6. Compress the pelvis to check for stability. Inspect for signs of trauma.

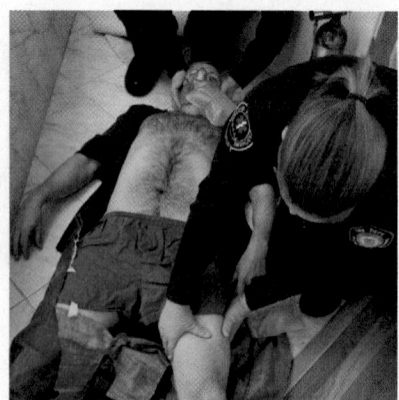

7. Quickly palpate and inspect the lower extremities.

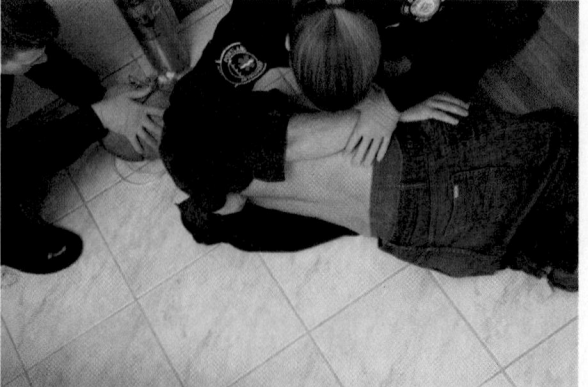

8. Log-roll the patient and check the posterior aspect of the body.

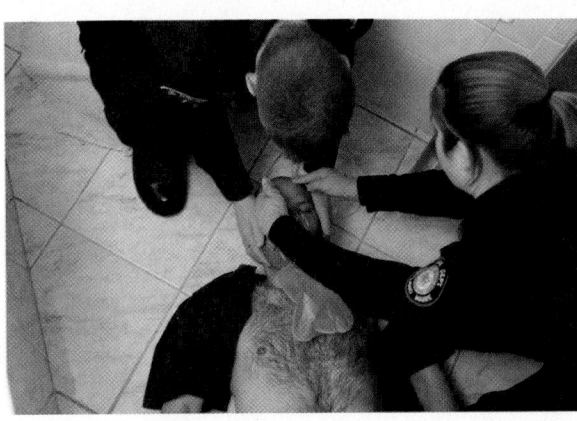

1. Inspect and palpate the patient's head. Hair can obscure injuries. Feel carefully for deformities, crepitus, instability, and lacerations. After palpation, check your gloves for blood.

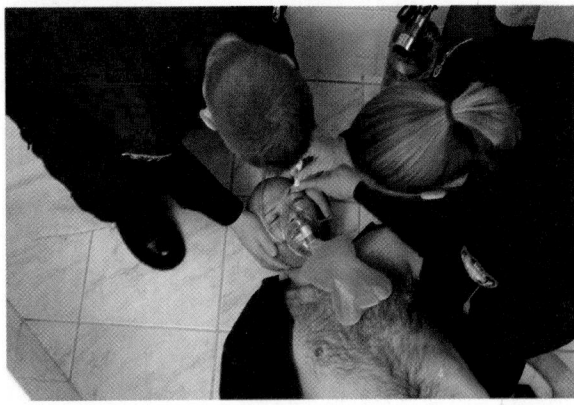

2. Inspect and palpate the patient's face. Use a penlight to check the eyes for injury and pupil response.

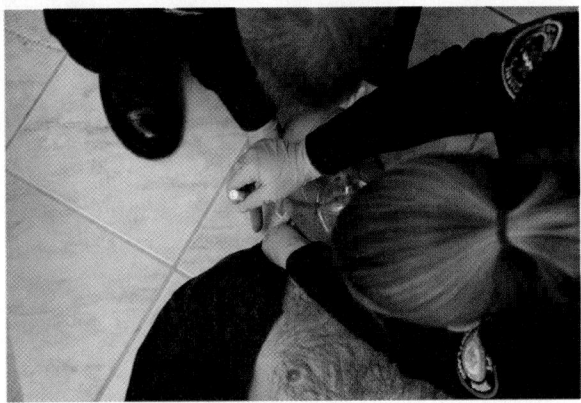

3. Check the ears for draining blood or fluid.

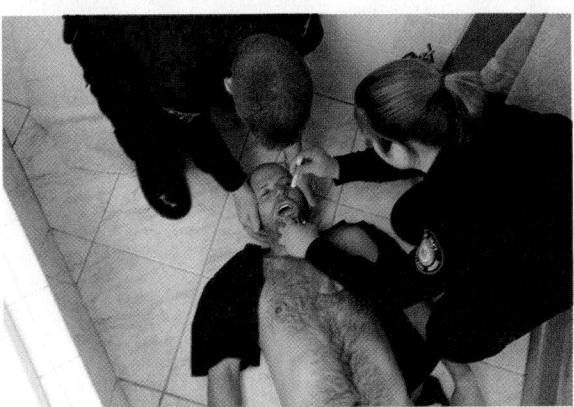

4. Check the mouth for loose or broken teeth, foreign bodies, swelling, and lacerations. Manage any situations that threaten the airway.

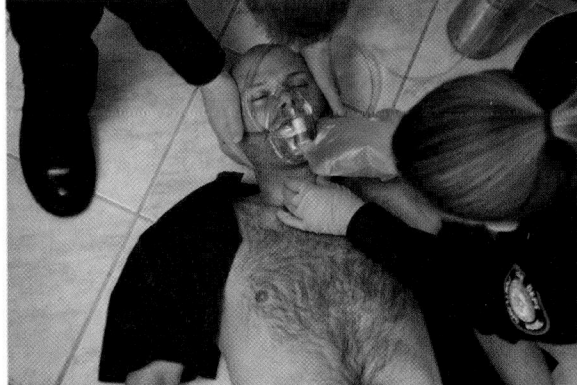

5. Check the neck for jugular venous distention, swelling, discoloration, wounds, crepitus, and tracheal deviation.

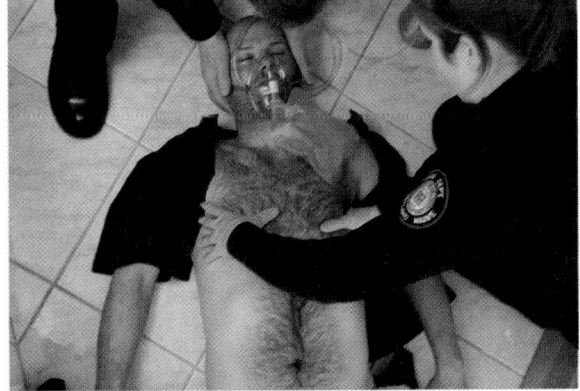

6. Inspect and palpate the chest, checking wounds, crepitus, and symmetry of chest wall movement.

(continued)

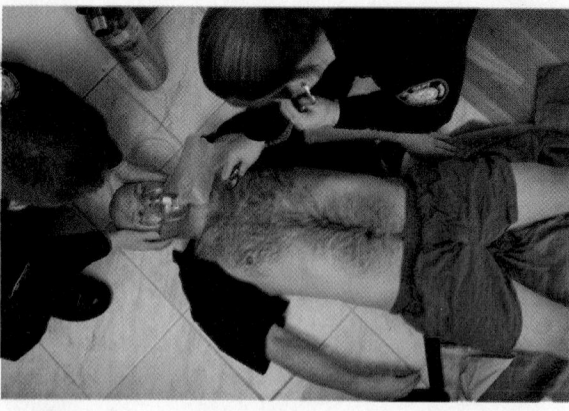

7. Auscultate the breath sounds for presence, equality, and abnormal breathing sounds.

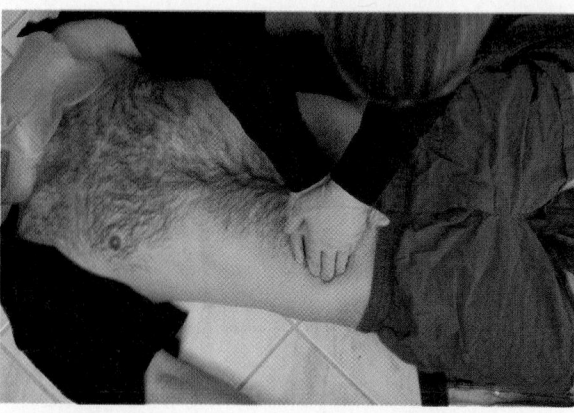

8. Inspect and palpate the abdomen. Check for distention, guarding, tenderness, discoloration, and wounds.

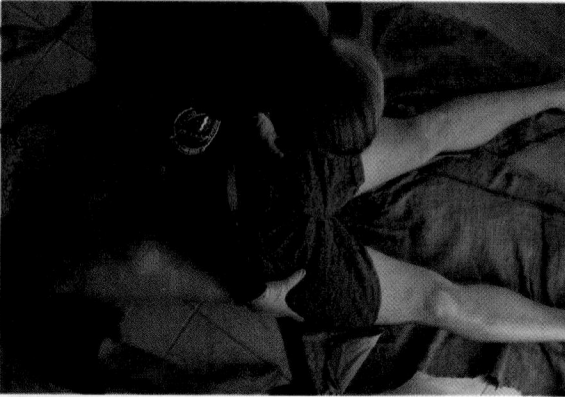

9. Gently compress the pelvis to check for tenderness, instability, and crepitus. Inspect for bleeding and incontinence. Also check the posterior body by placing your hands beneath the patient's back.

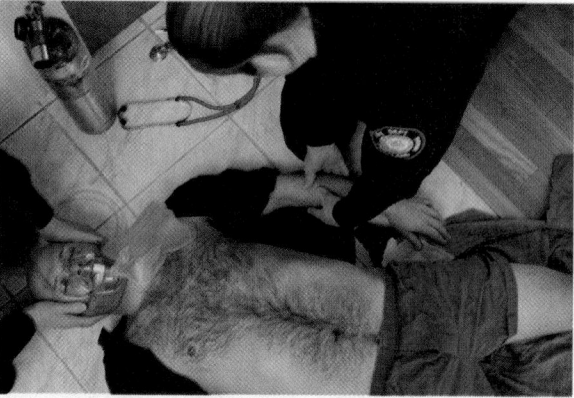

10. Inspect and palpate the upper extremities from shoulder to fingertips. Assess for pulse, motor function, and sensation.

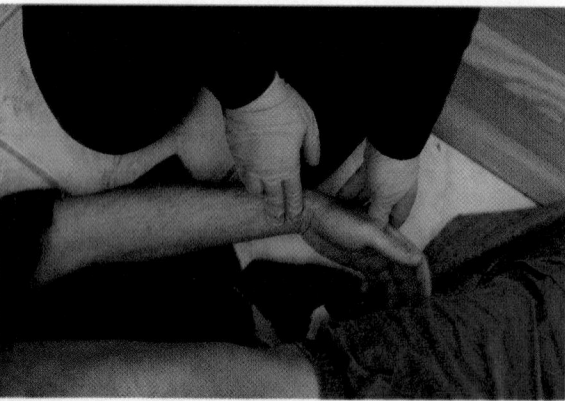

11. Assess the upper extremities for pulse, motor function, and sensation.

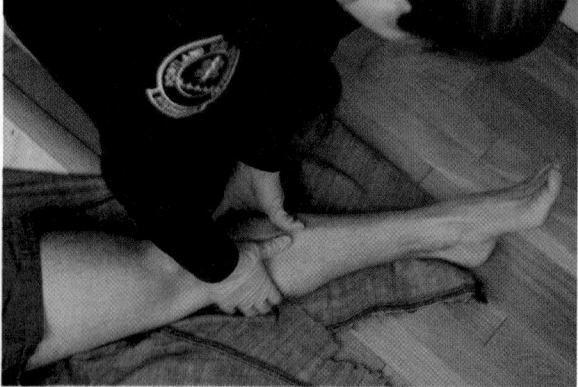

12. Inspect and palpate the lower extremities. Also assess for pulse, motor function, and sensation.

TABLE 19-10	Examples of Approaches to Secondary Assessment

Patient	Scene Size-Up	Primary Assessment	Impression	Secondary Assessment	Reassessment
• 13-year-old-male fell onto outstretched arm while skateboarding. • Chief complaint is right forearm pain.	• No indications of danger. • There is one patient. • No additional resources are needed. • Patient is sitting up, awake, holding arm; good general appearance.	• Patient is alert. • Airway is open. • Breathing is adequate. • Circulation is adequate.	• Noncritical trauma patient	• SAMPLE history • Vital signs • Focused anatomical exam of injury	• Vital signs • Focused anatomical exam of injury • Effects of interventions
• 49-year-old male patient, unrestrained driver of a vehicle that left the road at about 50 mph and rolled over several times. • Fire department personnel report that the patient is unresponsive.	• Fire department is stabilizing the vehicle and applying absorbent to leaking fluids; no downed power lines or indications of fire. • There is one patient. • Consider the need for and availability of ALS or air medical transportation. • Patient has a poor general appearance.	• Patient is unresponsive to painful stimuli. • Use manual maneuver for stabilization of cervical spine. Patient has gurgling with respirations—use suction and insert a basic airway adjunct. • Breathing is irregular and shallow—use a bag-valve-mask device with supplemental oxygen. • Radial pulse is present at 70 beats per minute; control bleeding from lacerations.	• Critical trauma patient	• Rapid trauma exam while preparing for transport • Vital signs en route to hospital • Monitoring devices: pulse oximetry, $ETCO_2$, cardiac monitor, blood glucose level • Head-to-toe exam en route to hospital • SAMPLE history if available	• Primary assessment • Rapid trauma exam • Vital signs and monitoring devices • Reassessment of specific injuries and treatments
• 10-year-old female stung on the hand by fire ant; no history of allergy to bites or stings. • Chief complaint is burning pain in the left hand.	• Patient has been moved inside—no indications of danger. • There is one patient. • No additional resources are needed. • Patient is sitting up, awake, holding a wet paper towel around her hand. Patient has a good general appearance.	• Patient is alert. • Airway is open. • Breathing is adequate. • Circulation is adequate.	• Noncritical medical patient	• SAMPLE history • Vital signs • Focused examination of hand	• Vital signs • Focused examination of hand • Effects of interventions

(continued)

TABLE 19-10   Examples of Approaches to Secondary Assessment—continued

Patient	Scene Size-Up	Primary Assessment	Impression	Secondary Assessment	Reassessment
■ 55-year-old female complaining of severe shortness of breath.	■ There are no indications of danger. ■ There is one patient. ■ Consider the need for ALS. ■ Patient is cyanotic, sweating profusely, and has signs of respiratory distress. The patient has a poor general appearance.	■ Patient is awake but sleepy and slow to respond. ■ Airway is open. ■ Breathing is rapid, shallow, and ineffective. Assist ventilations with bag-valve-mask device and supplemental oxygen. ■ Patient has a rapid radial pulse.	■ Critical medical patient	■ SAMPLE history ■ Vital signs ■ Monitoring devices: pulse oximetry, ETCO$_2$, cardiac monitor ■ Body systems assessment: cardiovascular and respiratory systems	■ Primary assessment ■ Vital signs and monitoring devices ■ Cardiovascular and respiratory systems ■ Effects of interventions

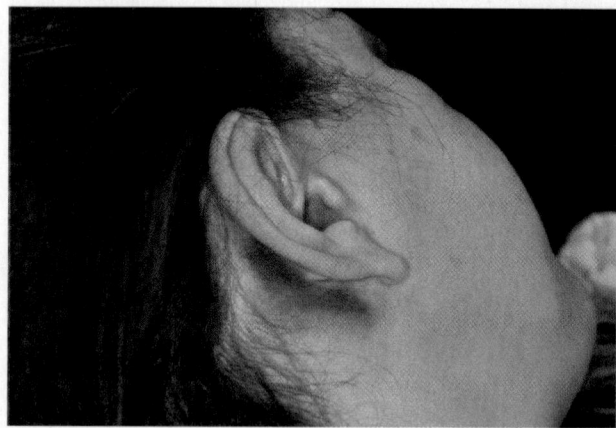

FIGURE 19-13

Battle's sign. (© Edward T. Dickinson, MD)

to the heart is obstructed to some degree. Right-sided heart failure is a cause of JVD in medical patients. Suspect tension pneumothorax or pericardial tamponade in trauma patients.

Edema or hematomas in the soft tissues of the neck can lead to airway obstruction, which you must monitor. Check the neck for the presence of subcutaneous air. Air escaping from an injured trachea or bronchus can accumulate beneath the skin, causing swelling. Palpation of areas of subcutaneous air can reveal crepitus.

Cover open wounds to the neck with an occlusive dressing. In trauma patients, also palpate the posterior neck for indications of injury. Note any tenderness or swelling. The spinous processes of the vertebrae should be in alignment. Although it is very unusual to find palpable displacement of the vertebrae, it is a critical finding that indicates injury to the spinal column with the potential for spinal-cord injury.

Torso

You must examine the torso, including the chest, abdomen, and pelvis, both anteriorly and posteriorly. Vital organs of the respiratory and cardiovascular systems are located in the thorax. Injuries of the abdomen and pelvis can result in life-threatening hemorrhage. Abdominal pain in medical patients can result from a number of serious problems. It is usually easiest to assess the entire anterior torso, and then assess the posterior torso as the patient is rolled to one side. For critical trauma patients, it is efficient to examine the posterior torso when the patient is log-rolled onto a long backboard.

Inspect the thorax for any indications of respiratory distress. Look for accessory muscle use and retraction of the tissues above the clavicles or between the ribs. Observe the chest for symmetrical movement and areas of **paradoxical movement**, and look for signs of injury. Paradoxical movement is an indication of flail chest, in which two or more adjacent ribs are each fractured in two or more places. Place your hands on both sides of the thoracic cage for a complete inspiration and expiration to feel for symmetry in chest movement. Palpate the chest wall, including over the sternum, for tenderness, instability, and crepitus. Crepitus may indicate a rib fracture, or may be a sign of subcutaneous air from a lung injury. Cover any open wounds with an occlusive dressing. Auscultate the breath sounds to determine their presence and equality, and to check for the presence of abnormal breath sounds.

Inspect the abdomen for injuries, distention, and areas of discoloration. Ecchymosis around the umbilicus is Cullen's sign and ecchymosis of the flanks is Grey-Turner's sign. Both are indications of internal hemorrhage—in particular, retroperitoneal bleeding. These signs may be seen in ruptured ectopic pregnancy or acute pancreatitis, but are not diagnostic of either condition. Neither Cullen's sign nor Grey-Turner's sign is commonly seen, especially in the first 24 hours.

Distention may be caused by fluid, air within the abdomen, intestinal gas, or intestinal obstruction. A tremendous volume of blood is required to cause distention or rigidity of the abdomen. Therefore, absence of distention or rigidity of the abdominal wall does not rule out the presence of serious injury with potentially life-threatening bleeding. Patients who have lost the amount of blood necessary to cause distention or rigidity of the abdomen are in life-threatening hypovolemic shock.

You must palpate the abdomen to check for areas of tenderness, the degree of relaxation of the abdominal wall, and abnormal masses. However, if the patient is complaining of abdominal pain, ask him to point to the area where he is experiencing it. Palpate that area *last*. If the patient experiences increased pain when you palpate that area, his abdominal muscles are likely to tense and he will have difficulty relaxing them. This is known as *voluntary guarding*. The tense muscles will affect the rest of your abdominal exam. For the same reason, make sure your hands are warm and tell the patient what you are going to do before you do it.

A technique for palpating the abdomen begins by placing the fingertips of one hand over the back of the fingers of your other hand. Gently press down on the abdomen with the top hand, creating a rolling motion. Palpate over each of the four quadrants of the abdomen. Practice abdominal palpation when possible so that you will be able to differentiate between normal abdominal findings and abnormal ones. Normally, the abdominal muscles are relaxed, making the abdomen soft. A tense or rigid abdominal wall that cannot be relaxed is an indication of peritonitis (inflammation of the peritoneum). You must palpate more deeply in patients with a large amount of abdominal fat in order to feel the muscles beneath.

Note the location of tenderness during palpation, as well as **rebound tenderness**. Without practice, it may be difficult to distinguish between the normal sensation of palpating abdominal organs and the presence of a mass. One particularly concerning finding is a large, pulsating mass in the abdomen. This can be an indication of an abdominal aortic aneurysm (AAA) (Chapter 21). However, that sign is not present in all cases of AAA. In addition, in thin individuals, you may be able to feel the normal pulsation of the aorta.

If a pulsating mass is noted, do not palpate the abdomen further. Relate the findings of your assessment to your knowledge of anatomy. Tenderness or bruising over the flanks can indicate a kidney injury, for example, whereas pain in the left upper quadrant may indicate a problem with the stomach or spleen.

The pelvis is part of the lower extremities, but anatomically it makes sense to assess it with the torso. Assessing the pelvis is an important part of the rapid trauma exam, because pelvic fractures can result in massive internal hemorrhage. In trauma patients, check the stability of the pelvic bones. Place your hands on both sides of the pelvis and gently compress it medially. Instability, pain on compression, and crepitus are signs of pelvic fracture. Do not vigorously "rock" the pelvis. If the patient has a pelvic fracture, you will cause additional pain and injury by doing so. In addition, you may aggravate any injury to the spine, because the pelvis is attached to the spine.

In trauma patients, visualize the external genitalia. Pelvic fractures and other injuries can cause swelling of the genitalia or bleeding from the urethra. Severe pelvic fractures can result in tearing of the perineum.

If you find an unstable pelvis, suspect hypovolemic shock. Treat the patient as a critical patient if the decision to do so has not already been made. Priapism, an involuntary erection of the penis, can indicate spinal-cord injury in male patients. In both trauma and medical patients, note whether there are signs of incontinence (loss of bladder or bowel control). (Examination of obstetric and gynecologic patients is covered in Chapters 25 and 43.) Inspect and palpate the patient's posterior torso including the spine and, if possible, auscultate the lungs posteriorly.

Extremities

Inspect the extremities for swelling, symmetry of length and circumference, abnormal internal or external rotation or positioning, discoloration, deformity, and other signs of injury and illness. Palpate the length of each extremity individually, from proximal to distal, feeling for swelling, deformity, crepitus, and tenderness. The clavicles are part of the upper extremities, forming part of the shoulder joint. However, because of their position over the first rib, anteriorly, fractured clavicles can sometimes cause injury to the lungs.

Proper examination of the lower extremities requires that the patient's shoes and socks be removed. This is necessary for critical trauma patients and patients with isolated lower extremity injuries or complaints. For patients wearing specialized athletic gear, ask for assistance from an athletic trainer, if available. If necessary, cut the socks to avoid undue movement of painful lower extremity complaints.

When examining the extremities, distal neurovascular status is assessed to determine the presence of circulation and nerve function. Assessing nervous function includes checking both sensation and movement. Ask the patient if he has any pain or tingling sensations (paresthesia) in each extremity as you begin your assessment of that extremity.

To assess sensory function, instruct the patient not to look at you for a moment and to tell you which finger or toe you are touching. Different sensory nerve tracts carry light touch and pain sensations. Assess for light touch sensation by lightly touching the finger or toe. Check for pain sensation with a firmer pinch. Because different nerves supply medial and lateral sensory function, touch the first and last digits.

In patients suspected of having a stroke, evaluate motor function by testing for **pronator drift**. Ask the patient to close his eyes and hold both arms straight out in front of him with the palms up for 10 seconds. If the patient is unable to hold both arms at the same level, or if one arm turns palm down (pronates), this is an indication of stroke (Figure 19-14).

Test for strength and equality of motor function in the upper extremities by having the patient grasp both your hands with his and squeeze. Test strength and equality of the lower

PERSONAL PERSPECTIVE

Advanced EMT Brian Dillinger: My partner and I responded to a report of shots fired with multiple patients. We were one of four ambulances on the scene, and we were assigned to a young man who was up and walking around, complaining of being shot in his backside. Sure enough, he had a small-caliber wound on his right buttock. He was upset about the shooting, and didn't want to lie down or cooperate with us. He was convinced that he just needed to get the bullet extracted from his buttock, and it was difficult to convince him that we needed to undress and examine him.

I'm glad we were persistent, though. It turns out that the exit wound was in his perineum. There wasn't much blood, so it hadn't soaked through his pants. We would have missed it if we hadn't undressed him. It turns out that the bullet entered his lower abdominal cavity and did some damage to his bowel. The surgeon said that infection was a big risk with this patient. He ended up having surgery and was released several days later. I hate to think what would have happened if he'd left the scene, convinced that he just had a bullet in his buttock.

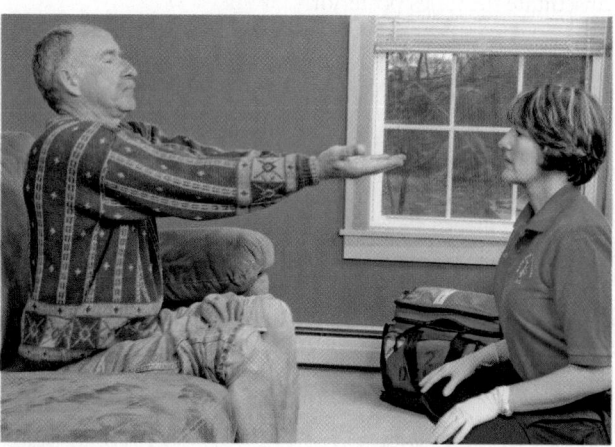

FIGURE 19-14

Check for pronator drift.

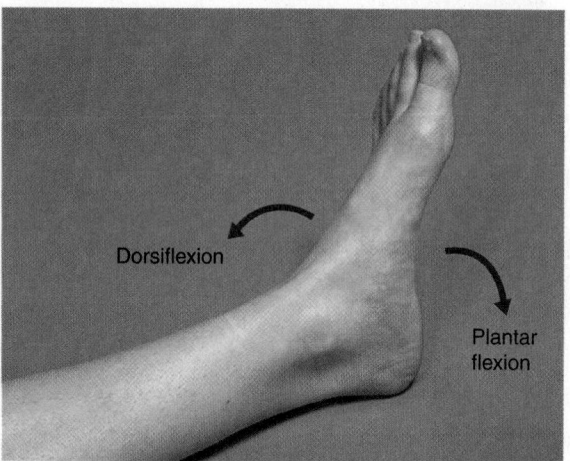

FIGURE 19-15

Dorsiflexion and plantar flexion.

extremities by having the patient first **dorsiflex** the feet against the resistance of your hands, and then **plantar flex** against resistance (Figure 19-15). Pain in the calf of the leg, particularly on one side, during dorsiflexion is called the *Homan's sign,* a sign of deep vein thrombosis (abnormal clot formation in the deep veins of the lower leg). Unequal strength can be a sign of brain or spinal-cord injury, stroke, or injury to one extremity. Bilateral weakness (paresis) or paralysis is an indication of spinal-cord injury. Although they are not sophisticated tests of neurologic function, the prehospital examination is designed to identify **gross** sensory and motor deficits.

Assess circulation in the extremities by noting their color and temperature and by checking distal pulses. A cold, pale, mottled, cyanotic, or pulseless extremity on one side is an indication of arterial occlusion, which is a limb-threatening emergency. A painful swollen extremity on one side can be an indication of venous occlusion, a problem with lymphatic drainage, or an injury.

In the upper extremities, check the radial pulses, and in the lower extremities, check either the dorsalis pedis or posterior tibial pulses. The dorsalis pedis and posterior tibial pulses can be challenging to locate. You must remove the patient's shoes and socks to feel the dorsalis pedis. Take

the opportunity to practice this skill in your labs. The more practice you have, the better you will be at it.

Compartment syndrome is a complication of injury that can jeopardize a limb. Each muscle is contained within a tough, fibrous sheath called *fascia.* The fascia cannot expand to accommodate bleeding or swelling of the muscle within it. If swelling or collection of blood continues, the pressure within the compartment formed by the fascia becomes greater than the pressure of blood within the capillaries. This interferes with tissue perfusion.

Signs and symptoms of compartment syndrome can be remembered as the five Ps: pain, paralysis, pallor, paresthesia, and pulselessness. Pulselessness does not have to occur, though, for the tissues to be jeopardized. The first symptom is often pain that seems out of proportion with the injury sustained.

IN THE FIELD

Do not check for strength or ask patients to move extremities if they have obvious bone or joint injuries.

Body Systems Approach to Secondary Assessment

Each finding noted in an anatomical approach to assessment is related to one or more body systems. Therefore, you must think about what body systems may be involved, as either a cause or a consequence of the finding. For example, a contusion over the right upper quadrant of the abdomen can represent an injury to the liver, which lies beneath it. The liver is a highly vascular organ, and injury to it can result in life-threatening hemorrhage. Therefore, assessment of the cardiovascular system is essential. However, shock also affects the respiratory and nervous systems, so you must assess them, too.

Many of the components of a body systems approach will already have been examined if you performed an anatomical secondary assessment. However, you must put the findings together to understand how each major body system is affected. For example, skin color tells you about the respiratory system and cardiovascular system. You must make the link between cyanotic skin color, use of accessory muscles of the neck, and sluggish pupils to understand that respiratory system may be compromised.

The major body systems assessed in the prehospital setting are the nervous, respiratory, cardiovascular, and musculoskeletal systems. The emphasis each of the examinations receives depends on the nature of the patient's illness or mechanism of injury, chief complaint, and other information. For example, for a young patient with a history of asthma who is complaining of wheezing that came on while he was playing baseball, your focus will be on the respiratory system. For an elderly patient who is complaining of sudden slurred speech and facial drooping, you will focus on the nervous and cardiovascular systems. This is not to say that you are not concerned with the patient's respiratory status, but you will have the essential information you need about the respiratory status from the primary assessment, vital signs (including auscultation of breath sounds), and SpO$_2$ measurement.

Assessment of the Nervous System

In the primary assessment, an exam of the nervous system begins with determining the patient's level of responsiveness using AVPU. The Glasgow Coma Scale (GCS) is used to more accurately describe the patient's level of responsiveness. Examination of the pupils gives additional information about the nervous system. Examination of the extremities can give you information about any focal neurologic deficits, such as weakness of the left arm or impaired sensation in the lower extremities.

You also must be concerned with assessing the patient's mental status. Mental status includes level of responsiveness, but it also includes an assessment of the patient's thought content and process, mood, perceptions, and memory. At the very least, you will determine whether the patient is oriented to person, time, and place.

In addition, note any abnormalities of speech processes (such as slurred speech), or speech content (such as using nonsensical or invented words). Observe for abnormal motor activity, such as weakness, paralysis, tics, spasms, repetitive movements, or tremors. (More in-depth assessment of mental status is considered in Chapter 22.)

There are specific neurologic tests used in the prehospital setting to determine the likelihood that a patient is having a stroke (Chapter 22). The tests are the Cincinnati Prehospital Stroke Scale and the Los Angeles Prehospital Stroke Screen (LAPSS). The Cincinnati Prehospital Stroke Scale consists of three components, as follows:

- Ask the patient to smile (or show you his teeth) while you observe for symmetry of facial movement. Facial droop can indicate stroke (Figure 19-16).
- Check for pronator drift (discussed under assessment of the extremities).
- Ask the patient to repeat the following phrase, "You can't teach an old dog new tricks." Listen for slurred speech or other speech abnormalities. Difficulty speaking is called *dysphasia*. Inability to speak is called *aphasia*.

An abnormal finding in any of the components of the Cincinnati Prehospital Stroke Scale should result in a high index of suspicion for stroke. Because some strokes are treatable within a few hours of their onset, many EMS systems have stroke protocols that include notifying the receiving hospital so that they can prepare to rapidly assess and treat the patient on arrival.

The LAPSS considers additional factors, including the patient's age (greater than 45 years), no prior history of seizures, duration of symptoms (less than 24 hours), patient

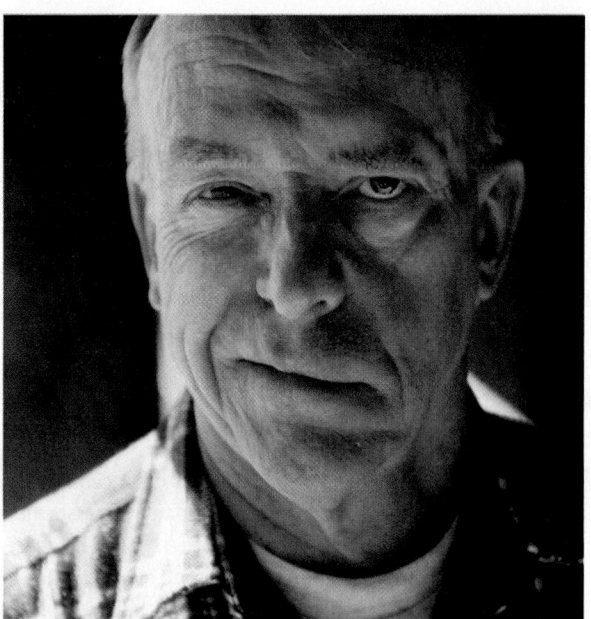

FIGURE 19-16

Ask the patient to smile; check for facial symmetry.
(© Michal Heron Photography)

not confined to bed or a wheelchair, patient has a blood glucose level between 60 and 400 mg/dL, and whether there is asymmetry evidenced as facial droop, arm drift, or grip strength. The purpose of the expanded assessment of the LAPSS is to determine whether there are other possible causes of the patient's signs and symptoms, such as a diabetic emergency or seizure.

Assessment of the Cardiovascular System

The primary assessment, along with assessment of skin color and condition, pulse, and blood pressure, give initial information about the function of the cardiovascular system. You can obtain further information through cardiac rhythm monitoring, when indicated. For patients with complaints that indicate a possible cardiovascular problem, the presence or absence of specific other findings is helpful in determining the seriousness of the situation and refining your field impression.

Crackles, as described in Chapter 18, indicate pulmonary edema, which can be caused by left-sided heart failure. Check the neck for evidence of JVD, which can indicate right-sided heart failure or pericardial tamponade. Ascites (a collection of fluid in the abdomen) and edema, particularly in the sacral area (in supine patients) and lower extremities, also can indicate right heart failure (Figures 19-17 and 19-18). However, ascites and edema have other causes, including liver failure.

A great deal of skill and practice are required to accurately assess heart sounds. Individuals who have the opportunity to practice auscultating heart sounds with feedback from an experienced practitioner can detect abnormalities of the cardiovascular system. The typical sound made by the heart is a "lub-dub" that occurs with the closing and opening of heart valves during each cardiac cycle. Abnormal sounds include extra sounds and murmurs. Heart sounds can be muffled in pericardial tamponade.

Assessment of the Respiratory System

You can first obtain information about the respiratory system from the primary assessment, vital signs, and SpO_2 measurement. In particular, observe carefully for cyanosis, work of breathing, use of accessory muscles, and abnormal breath sounds.

Assessment of the Musculoskeletal System

Assessment of the musculoskeletal system is best accomplished either in the anatomical approach to secondary assessment of critical or potentially critical trauma patients, or in a focused examination of patients with isolated medical or traumatic musculoskeletal complaints. Musculoskeletal injuries are of immediate concern in the prehospital setting when they produce life-threatening hemorrhage, or when the limb is endangered.

Musculoskeletal injuries of particular concern include skull fractures, vertebral column injuries, thoracic cage

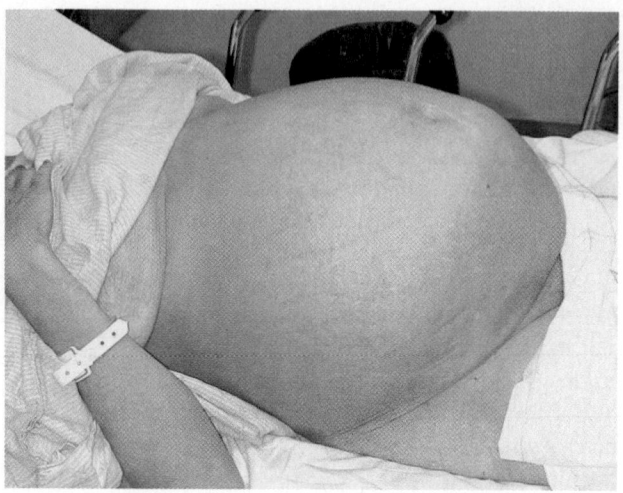

FIGURE 19-17

Ascites is an abnormal collection of fluid within the abdomen. (© Charles Stewart, MD, and Associates)

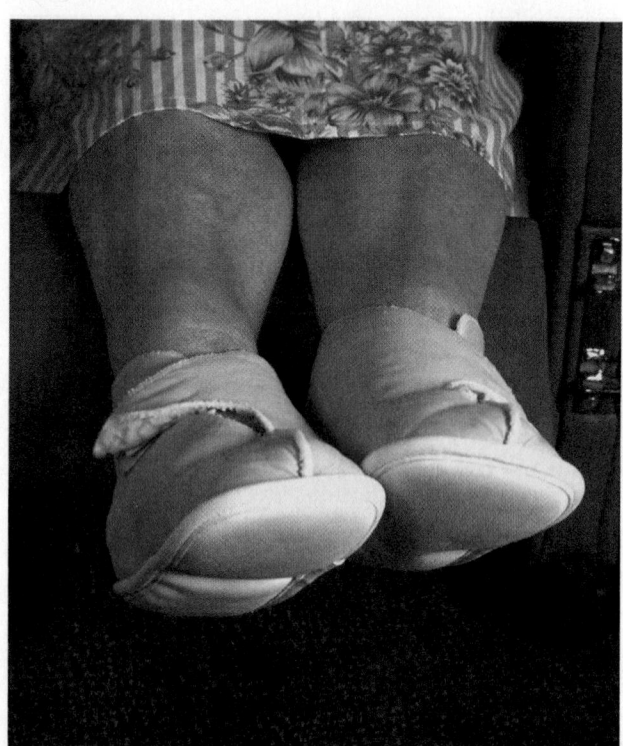

FIGURE 19-18

Edema of both lower extremities is an indication of right-sided heart failure.

injuries, pelvis fractures, and femur fractures. Multiple long-bone fractures that individually would not result in life-threatening hemorrhage can cause significant blood loss. Injuries that result in loss of distal pulses or neurologic function put the limb in jeopardy. Fractures of the scapula and first rib are associated with higher mortality because the mechanisms that result in those injuries are likely to produce life-threatening intrathoracic trauma.

CASE STUDY WRAP-UP

Clinical-Reasoning Process

Advanced EMTs Lindsay and Teresa are assessing Ms. Gretchen Snyder, who is complaining of severe, diffuse periumbilical abdominal pain that woke her from sleep at 2:00 AM. The pain feels better when Ms. Snyder lies still, with her hips flexed, but is worse when she moves or stretches. Lindsay recognizes the signs and symptoms of peritonitis.

While Teresa finishes taking vital signs, Lindsay completes the history and prepares to perform a secondary assessment. "Ms. Snyder, I know it's uncomfortable, but I need you to lie on your back for a moment so I can examine your abdomen. You can keep your knees bent."

When she exposes Ms. Snyder's abdomen, Lindsay can see that the abdomen looks distended, but there is no discoloration. Beginning in the right upper quadrant, Lindsay moves in a clockwise direction, palpating each of the abdominal quadrants. Palpation around the umbilicus produces more pain than palpation of the quadrants, causing Ms. Snyder to tense her abdominal muscles. Lindsay did not palpate any masses, but the abdomen was distended and tender to palpation in all four quadrants, and especially over the umbilical area.

Suspecting possible ischemia of the bowel, Lindsay asks Teresa to administer 4 L/min of oxygen by nasal cannula. Lindsay and Teresa untuck the bedsheet and use it to gently lift Ms. Snyder onto their stretcher, where she prefers to lie on her side, with her legs drawn up. Concerned about dehydration and the seriousness of abdominal pain that has lasted several hours, especially in a patient of Ms. Snyder's age, Lindsay plans to start an IV en route to the hospital.

"We're going to take a nice, easy ride to the hospital, Ms. Snyder," says Teresa. "I'll make it as smooth a ride as possible, and I'll let you know if we are going to go over any bumps." Lindsay takes a second set of vital signs as they depart for the hospital, and checks to see how Ms. Snyder is feeling. She gives a radio report and reassesses the patient frequently en route.

CHAPTER REVIEW

Chapter Summary

Secondary assessment and history taking are used to gather additional information about presenting problems and complaints in order to form a field impression for each patient and to plan specific treatments. A medical history, secondary assessment, and reassessments are performed for every patient. Decisions about how to proceed with the history, secondary assessment, and reassessment depend on the nature and severity of the problem, the circumstances, and the resources you have available.

For critical or potentially critical trauma patients, begin the secondary assessment with a rapid trauma exam. Keep in mind that the goal is to minimize scene time. Baseline vital signs, history, and a head-to-toe exam are usually performed en route to the hospital.

Reassess critical trauma patients at least every 5 minutes, including constant monitoring of the airway, breathing, and circulation, repeat vital signs and the rapid trauma exam, and a check of the effects of interventions. You should perform a focused physical exam of the injury for noncritical trauma patients with isolated non–life-threatening and non–limb-threatening injuries, in addition to assessing vital signs and taking a medical history. Reassess noncritical trauma

patients at least every 15 minutes, including reassessment of the primary assessment, vital signs, focused secondary assessment, and effects of interventions.

For critical medical patients perform a rapid medical exam similar to the rapid trauma exam. However, if the problem is clear after the scene size-up, primary assessment, and rapid medical exam, a detailed head-to-toe exam is not likely to provide additional useful information. Instead, the medical history, vital signs, and a body systems approach to secondary assessment, based on the chief complaint or presenting problem, should yield the most information.

Similar to critical trauma patients, reassess critical medical patients at least every 5 minutes. Constantly monitor airway, breathing, and circulation. Repeat critical aspects of the secondary assessment, reassess vital signs and monitoring devices, and check the effects of interventions. You should perform a focused secondary examination of noncritical medical patients based on the chief complaint and medical history. Take vital signs and use appropriate monitoring devices. Reassess noncritical medical patients at least every 15 minutes, repeating the primary assessment, vital signs, and focused secondary assessment, and checking the effects of interventions.

Review Questions

Multiple-Choice Questions

1. A patient with a chief complaint of stomach pain says that he was working in the garage when he became sweaty and dizzy, and then vomited before the stomach pain began. The sweating, dizziness, and vomiting are part of the:

   a. mechanism of injury (MOI).
   b. focused physical exam.
   c. history of the present illness.
   d. past medical history.

2. Which one of the following patients would be classified as a noncritical medical patient?

   a. 27-year-old with a burn on the palm of her hand
   b. 11-year-old with a cough and fever
   c. 36-year-old diabetic who is unresponsive to painful stimuli
   d. 54-year-old who was the unrestrained driver of a vehicle that hit a tree at about 45 mph

3. Your patient complains of body aches, a fever, and vomiting, but states that he has not had diarrhea. In this case, diarrhea is a:

   a. symptom.
   b. pertinent negative.
   c. chief complaint.
   d. provoking factor.

4. Which one of the following is a sign of illness or injury?

   a. Discoloration around the eyes
   b. Chest pain
   c. Nausea
   d. Painful urination

5. A patient tells you that walking around reduces her abdominal discomfort. In this case, walking around describes:

   a. the onset of the complaint.
   b. radiation of the pain.
   c. a palliating factor.
   d. the quality of the pain.

6. A patient says he has severe lower back pain that shoots down the back of his leg. This describes _____ pain.

   a. radiating
   b. referred
   c. visceral
   d. phantom

7. You feel a grating, crunching sensation under your fingers when you palpate over a patient's neck. This is known as:

   a. ecchymosis.
   b. tenderness.
   c. asymmetry.
   d. crepitus.

8. You feel a large, pulsating mass while palpating a patient's abdomen. You should:

   a. palpate again to make sure you actually felt it.
   b. ask your partner to palpate it.
   c. leave it alone, but include the information in verbal and written reports.
   d. consider it normal.

9. You notice bruising behind the ears of a patient. This indicates:

   a. the patient received a basilar skull fracture within the past few minutes.
   b. a ruptured eardrum.
   c. the patient received a basilar skull fracture hours or days ago.
   d. an ear infection.

10. To assess the circulation of the distal lower extremities, you will palpate the _____ pulses.

    a. dorsalis pedis or posterior tibial
    b. popliteal or brachial
    c. ulnar or radial
    d. femoral or popliteal

Critical-Thinking Questions

11. What is the relationship between mental status and level of responsiveness?

12. A patient who injured his leg a day ago complains of increasingly severe pain in the leg. He says he can no longer move his ankle and toes and that he has some painful "tingling" in his foot. The leg is pale, and the pedal pulse is very weak. How can you use this information in developing a field impression?

13. In your rapid trauma exam of a patient involved in a fall from a height, you notice paradoxical motion of the chest wall. What impact does this have on your field impression?

14. You notice an odor that reminds you of nail polish remover, which you quickly associate with acetone, on the breath of an unresponsive patient you are assessing. What is the significance of the odor?

Additional Reading

Bickley, L. S. (Ed). (2003). *Bates' guide to physical examination and history-taking* (8th ed.). Philadelphia, PA: Lippincott Williams & Wilkins.

Bledsoe, B. E., Porter, R. S., & Cherry, R. A. (2009). *Paramedic care: Principles and practice* (3rd ed., Vol. 2). Upper Saddle River, NJ: Pearson.

SECTION 5

Medical Emergencies

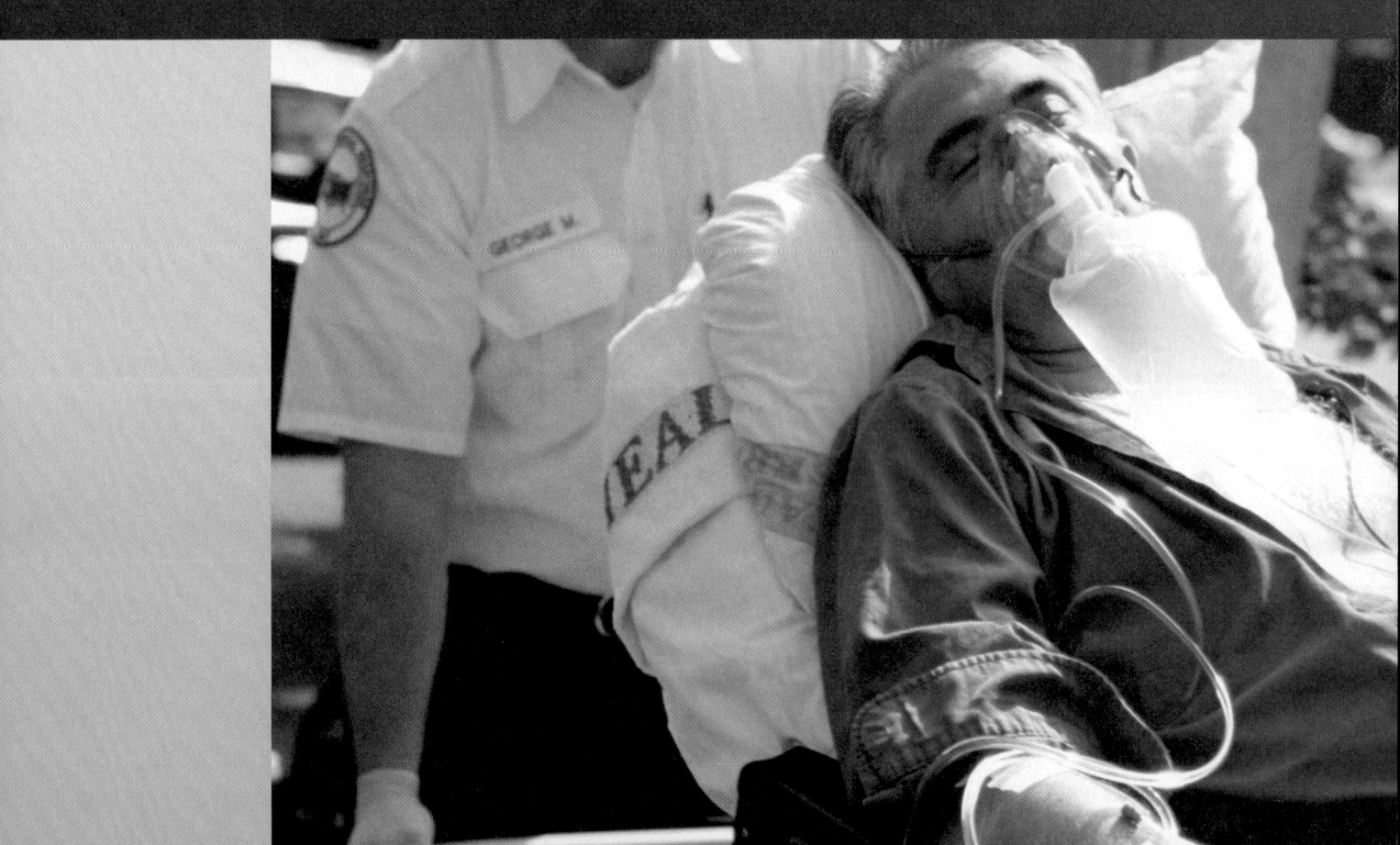

20

Respiratory Disorders

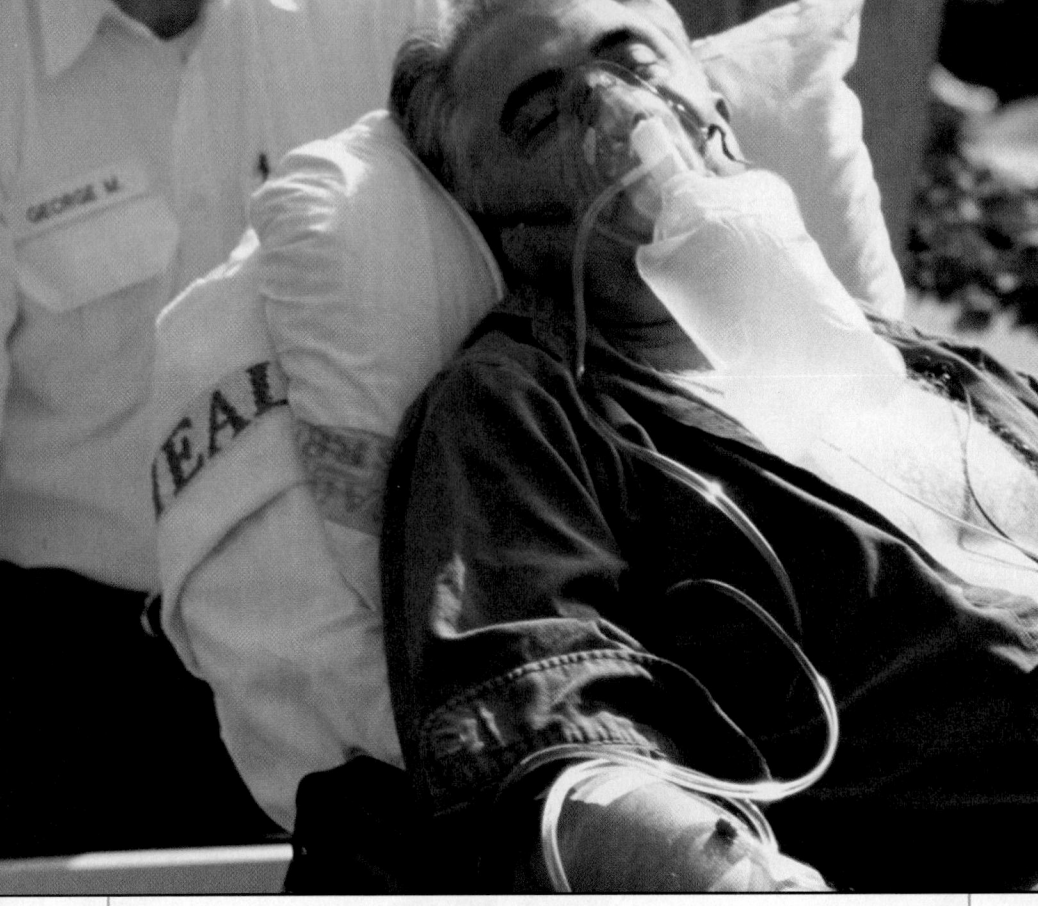

Content Area: Medicine

Advanced EMT Education Standard: Applies fundamental knowledge to provide basic and selected advanced emergency care and transportation based on assessment findings for an acutely ill patient.

Objectives

After reading this chapter, you should be able to:

20.1 Define key terms introduced in this chapter.

20.2 Explain the importance of being able to quickly recognize and treat patients with respiratory emergencies.

20.3 Obtain an appropriate history for a patient with a respiratory problem.

20.4 Conduct an appropriate examination for a patient with a respiratory problem.

20.5 Explain the relationship between dyspnea and hypoxia.

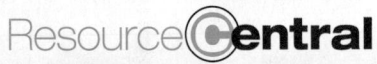

Resource **C**entral

To access Resource Central, follow the directions on the Student Access Card provided with this text. If there is no card, go to www.bradybooks.com and follow the Resource Central link to Buy Access. Under Media Resources, you will find:

- *Chronic Obstructive Pulmonary Disease. See* the causes and treatment of COPD.

- *Understanding Respiratory Failure.* Learn about V-Q mismatch, shunting, and pulse oximetry monitoring.

- *The Spontaneous Pneumothorax.* View its signs, symptoms, and prehospital management.

CASE STUDY

Advanced EMTs Toby Marshall and Brent Croft are responding to a call for difficulty breathing. They have responded to this address before and know that the patient is a 60-year-old man with a history of COPD.

Today, when they enter the home, they see that Mr. Emerson seems especially short of breath. He is wearing his nasal cannula and sitting on the edge of a sofa with his hands placed on his thighs to support himself. He is working hard to breathe and barely acknowledges the presence of the Advanced EMTs. His ears and lips are a dusky blue color and he is using the muscles in his neck to assist with breathing.

Just as Toby and Brent reach his side, Mr. Emerson coughs some rusty-colored sputum into a tissue. Placing his hand on Mr. Emerson's shoulder, Toby notices that his skin is hot and moist. Toby asks Mr. Emerson, "How are you doing today?"

Mr. Emerson is barely able to get out a response, "Can't seem . . . to get . . . a breath," he gasps.

Mr. Emerson's son, Peter, tells the crew that his father's bronchitis had been "acting up" since the previous night. He started having increased difficulty breathing, with chills and a fever, earlier this morning. He initially refused to let Peter take him to the doctor, but Peter called 911 when Mr. Emerson became confused and more short of breath.

Mr. Emerson is an obese man with bilateral edema of his ankles and feet. His breath sounds have rhonchi and wheezing scattered throughout his lungs, and there are crackles in the lung bases bilaterally. His respirations are 30 per minute and labored, his pulse is 124 and irregular, his blood pressure is 164/102, and his SpO_2 is 82 percent with the 3 liters of oxygen he is receiving from his nasal cannula.

Problem-Solving Questions

1. What are your hypotheses about Mr. Emerson's problem?
2. What additional information should you obtain to help you arrive at a clinical impression?
3. What treatments should you begin prior to transport?

20.6　Describe the pathophysiology by which each of the following conditions leads to inadequate oxygenation:
- Asthma
- Cystic fibrosis
- Hyperventilation syndrome
- Lung cancer
- Obstructive pulmonary diseases (emphysema and chronic bronchitis)
- Pneumonia
- Poisonous/toxic exposures
- Pulmonary edema
- Pulmonary embolism
- Spontaneous pneumothorax
- Viral respiratory infections

20.7　Use patient histories and clinical presentations to differentiate among causes of respiratory emergencies.

20.8　Engage in effective clinical reasoning in order to recognize indications for the following interventions in patients with respiratory complaints/emergencies:
- Establishing an airway
- Administering oxygen

(continued)

(continued from previous page)

- Positive pressure ventilation
- Administering/assisting with self-administration of an inhaled beta$_2$ agonist
- Expediting transport
- ALS backup

20.9 Given a list of patient medications, recognize medications that are associated with respiratory disease.

20.10 Differentiate between short-acting beta$_2$ agonists appropriate for prehospital use and respiratory medications that are not intended for emergency use.

20.11 Use reassessment to identify responses to treatment and changes in the conditions of patients presenting with respiratory complaints and emergencies.

Introduction

Patients who present in respiratory distress can deteriorate rapidly into respiratory failure and respiratory arrest. No matter what the underlying cause, death follows quickly unless measures are taken to restore ventilation and oxygenation.

A number of problems arising in the respiratory system can interfere with delivery of oxygen to the tissues. The oxygen deficit is exacerbated by two factors that increase oxygen demand when its supply is already jeopardized. First, the sensation of not being able to breathe is terrifying; and the associated stress response increases the demand for oxygen. Second, increased use of respiratory muscles creates an even higher need for cellular oxygen in the face of the decreased supply. Cellular metabolism with inadequate oxygen results in inefficient energy production and respiratory acidosis. The combination of the uncorrected underlying problem, exhaustion, and acidosis can overwhelm the body's attempts to compensate and restore homeostasis.

As an Advanced EMT, you must be able to quickly recognize patients with difficulty breathing and intervene. You must ensure an open airway, adequate ventilation, and circulation of oxygenated blood to the tissues. In some cases, you will implement specific treatment measures for the underlying cause of respiratory distress. In other cases, the best prehospital treatment for the patient is to continue to ensure an open airway and provide support for ventilation and oxygenation while transporting the patient without delay for definitive care.

Understanding the anatomy and physiology of ventilation and respiration, and the pathophysiology of respiratory problems assists you in giving the best care possible to patients with difficulty breathing. There are treatments within the Advanced EMT scope of practice that you can use to treat patients with specific causes of respiratory distress. You must understand when specific medications should be considered, as well as when IV fluids may help and when they may result in harm.

Anatomy and Physiology Review

Cellular energy production, and thus life itself, depends on oxygen from the atmosphere reaching each individual cell. Oxygen from the air that enters the lungs is carried through the blood. It then moves into cells from the network of capillaries that provide circulation to body tissues. This process is more complex than it seems on the surface. It depends on the particular way that the organs of the respiratory and circulatory system are structured and the precise way in which they work together.

For oxygen to reach the microscopic alveoli of the lungs, where gases are exchanged with the circulatory system, there must be an adequate amount of oxygen in the atmosphere. The upper and lower portions of the airway must be open to allow that air to reach the alveoli. Each alveolus must be in close contact with a network of capillaries so that oxygen and carbon dioxide can be exchanged between the lungs and the blood (Figure 20-1).

The red blood cells must contain an adequate amount of hemoglobin to carry oxygen to the cells. The body's temperature, acid–base balance, and other factors must be in the proper ranges for hemoglobin to accept oxygen from the lungs (external respiration) and release it to the cells (internal respiration).

The right side of the heart must be able to receive deoxygenated blood that is high in carbon dioxide and pump it through the pulmonary artery and into the lungs. The left side of the heart must be able to receive oxygenated blood that is low in carbon dioxide and pump it through the arterial and capillary systems to the cellular level.

Anything that interferes with this complex set of conditions can lead to hypoxia, cell dysfunction, and death.

The Need for Oxygen

Cells must produce energy to carry out their functions. The functions of brain cells, muscle cells, and liver, kidney,

Respiratory System

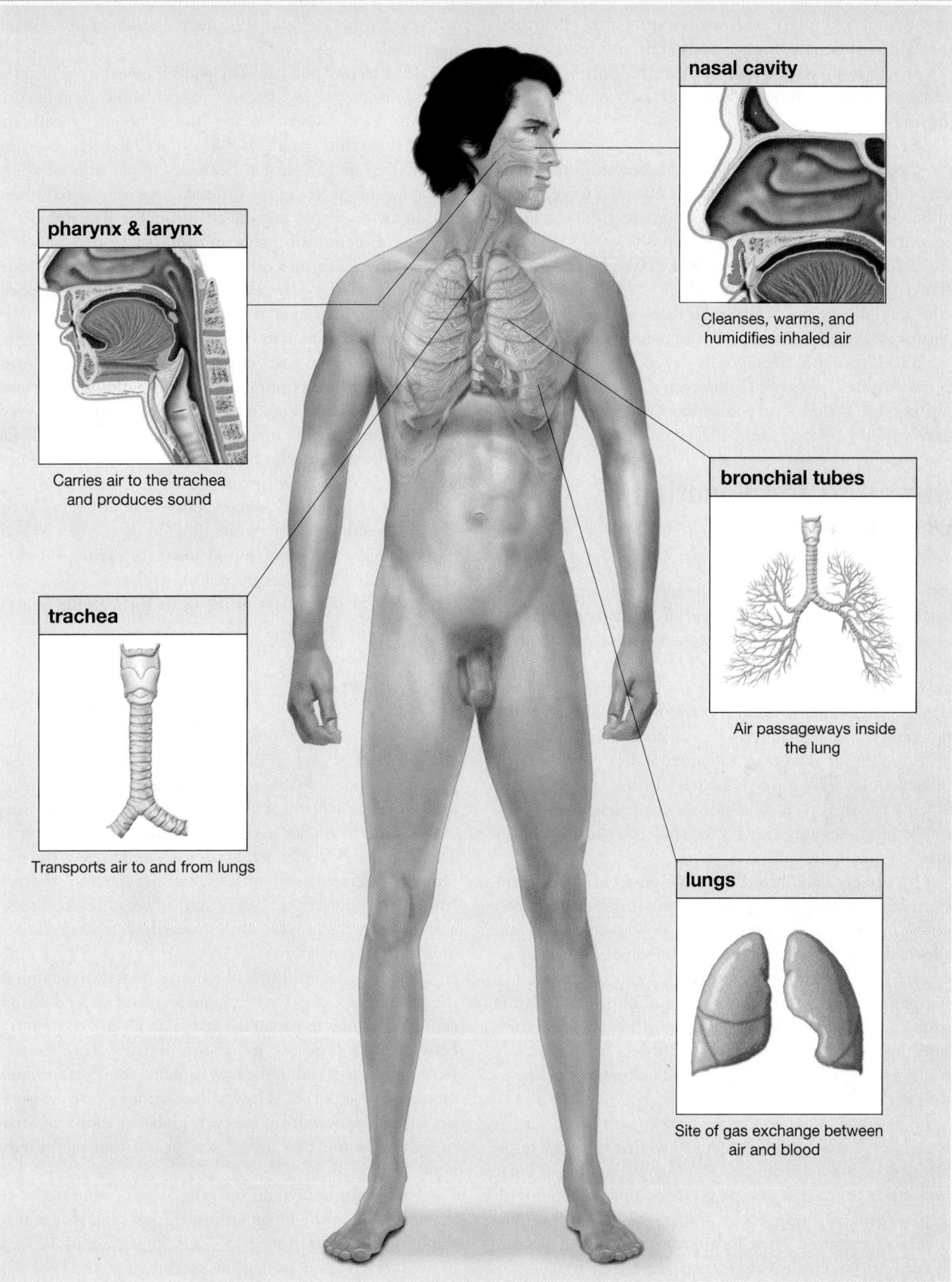

nasal cavity

Cleanses, warms, and humidifies inhaled air

pharynx & larynx

Carries air to the trachea and produces sound

trachea

Transports air to and from lungs

bronchial tubes

Air passageways inside the lung

lungs

Site of gas exchange between air and blood

FIGURE 20-1

Components of the respiratory system.

and cardiac cells all include maintaining their own cell membranes and internal structures and performing their specialized functions for the body. Energy production in the presence of oxygen (aerobic metabolism) is efficient and results in byproducts that are easily eliminated by the body.

In the process of producing energy, hydrogen ions (H^+) are produced. An increase in H^+ concentration decreases the body's pH, leading to acidosis. Cells need oxygen (O_2) to bind to the hydrogen ions (H^+) that are produced in energy metabolism. By doing so, two products, water (H_2O) and carbon dioxide (CO_2), are formed, which can be easily eliminated.

Without oxygen, in anaerobic metabolism, energy production is severely limited and H^+ accumulates in the form of lactic acid. Anaerobic metabolism is a compensatory mechanism when the body's need for oxygen is greater than its supply, but it is a short-term compensatory mechanism. Unless oxygenation is restored, death will occur.

Structure and Function of the Lungs

The lungs are spongy tissues with millions of microscopic air sacs, called *alveoli*, which allow the exchange of gases between the internal environment of the body and the atmosphere. Air enters the lung through the nose or mouth in the upper airway, travels through the pharynx, and moves into the larynx and trachea. The trachea divides at the carina into right and left main-stem bronchi, which enter the right and left lungs, respectively, at their hilum.

Once inside the lungs, the bronchi divide into smaller branches that serve the two lobes of the left lung and three lobes of the right lung. The bronchi divide into smaller and smaller branches until they become microscopic bronchioles that enter each alveolus.

The trachea and bronchi are composed of sturdy cartilage rings that keep them from collapsing. The bronchioles, however, have a substantial amount of smooth muscle that allows their diameter to change in response to the amount of alveolar ventilation required. The smooth muscle has **sympathetic beta₂ receptors** that respond to epinephrine from the body, as well as to drugs with beta₂ properties. The effect of beta₂ receptor stimulation is smooth muscle relaxation, which increases bronchodilation (an increase of the diameter of the bronchioles).

The lining of the respiratory tract contains cells that secrete mucus, which traps contaminants that enter the respiratory system along with air. Microscopic, hairlike cellular projections called *cilia* sweep the mucus upward, along with trapped contaminant particles, so they can be expelled (mucociliary clearance). The cilia are paralyzed by the nicotine in cigarette smoke, leaving the smoker unable to clear the lungs of toxins.

The walls of the distal (terminal) bronchioles and alveoli are a single cell-layer thick. A network of capillaries, which also are a single cell-layer thick, surrounds each alveolus. The alveoli and capillaries are in close contact with each other, separated by a small amount of extracellular fluid.

The alveolar and capillary walls together are called the *respiratory membrane*. Because oxygen and carbon dioxide can diffuse only short distances, this respiratory membrane must remain thin. An increase in extracellular fluid between the capillary and alveolar walls, for example, or fluid or pus in the alveoli, increase the distance between the red blood cells in the capillaries and the air within the alveoli.

The direction of diffusion of gases depends on their relative concentrations on each side of the cell membrane. Gases diffuse from where they are higher in concentration to where they are lower in concentration.

For gas exchange to occur, deoxygenated blood from the right side of the heart must reach the lungs. Blood from the right ventricle is pumped into the pulmonary artery, which divides into right and left branches to deliver deoxygenated blood to both lungs. The pulmonary arteries divide into smaller and smaller branches until they form the network of capillaries that surround each alveolus.

At the arterial end of the capillary bed, blood is lower in oxygen and higher in carbon dioxide. At the venous end, blood is higher in oxygen and lower in carbon dioxide. Oxygenated blood enters the pulmonary venous system and returns to the left atrium of the heart through the pulmonary vein (Figure 20-2).

Ventilation

Chemically, ventilation is stimulated primarily by an increased level of carbon dioxide in the blood and in cerebrospinal fluid. A secondary stimulus is a decreased level of oxygen. Those chemical changes stimulate the inspiratory center of the brain, located in the medulla of the brainstem. The inspiratory center sends nervous impulses to the diaphragm and intercostal muscles, causing them to contract. Muscular contraction flattens and lowers the diaphragm and lifts the ribs upward and outward, increasing the volume of the thoracic cavity.

The increase in thoracic volume creates a vacuum in the potential space between the parietal and visceral pleura, causing the lungs to expand. There is an inverse relationship between the volume of a gas and its pressure. The increased intrapulmonary (within the lung) volume results in intrapulmonary pressure that is lower than atmospheric pressure. Because air moves from areas of higher pressure to areas of lower pressure, air moves from the environment into the lungs (Figure 20-3).

Under normal conditions, the average amount of air that moves into the lungs on inspiration (and then out of the lungs on expiration) is 5–7 mL/kg, or about 500 mL in an average-sized adult. This is known as the tidal volume. Of this 500 mL, 150 mL remains in the conduction portion of the airway (trachea and bronchi), unavailable for gas exchange. This is known as anatomical dead space air. The amount of air available for alveolar ventilation is

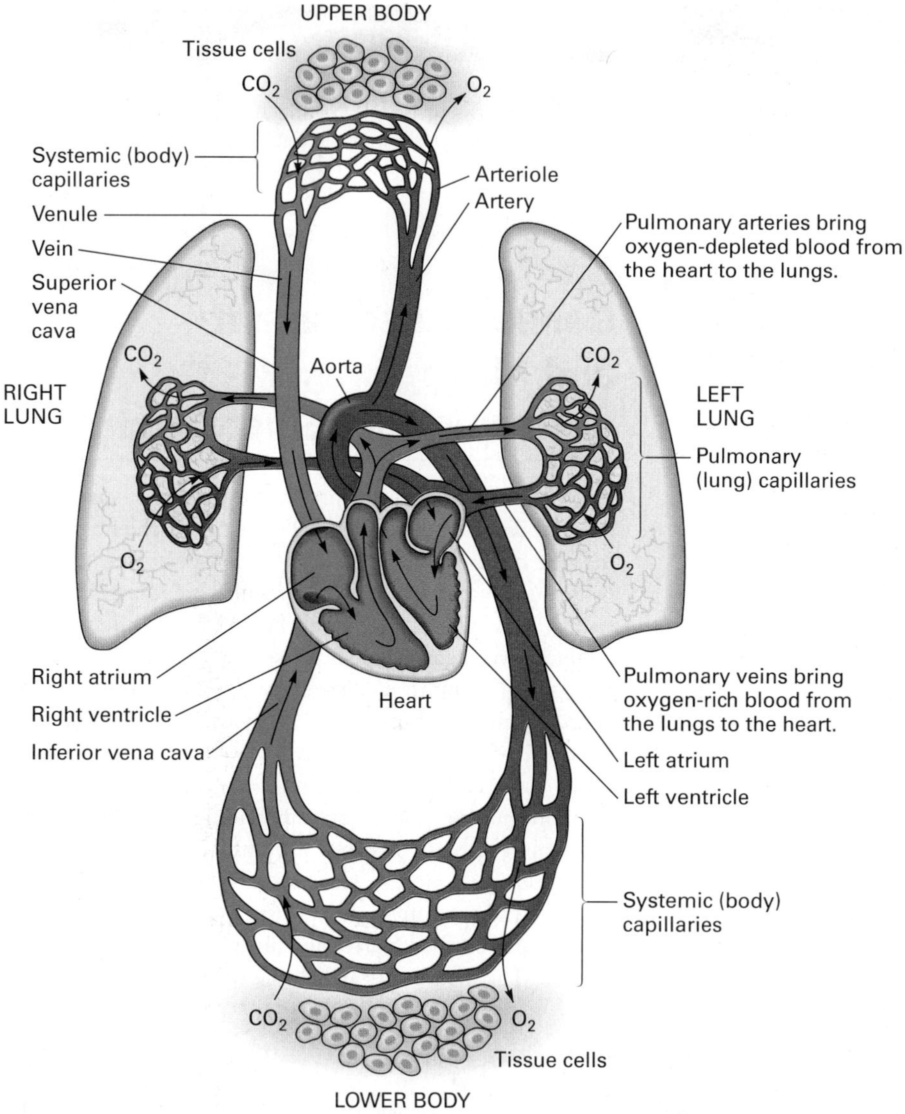

FIGURE 20-2

Relationship between pulmonary and systemic circulation.

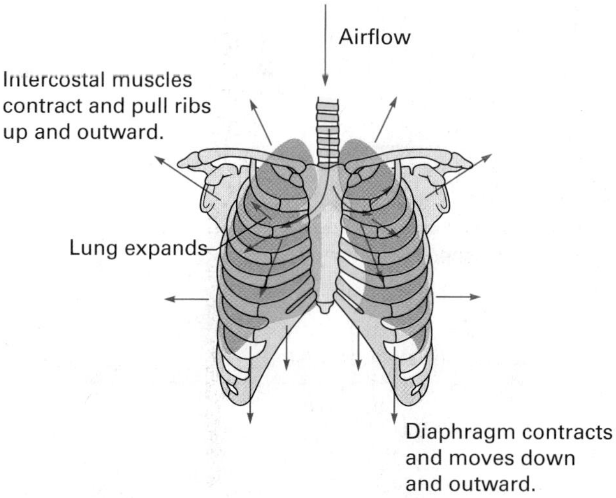

UPPER BODY

Tissue cells
CO_2 O_2

Systemic (body) capillaries

Arteriole
Artery

Pulmonary arteries bring oxygen-depleted blood from the heart to the lungs.

Venule
Vein
Superior vena cava

CO_2 Aorta CO_2

RIGHT LUNG

LEFT LUNG

Pulmonary (lung) capillaries

O_2 O_2

Right atrium
Right ventricle
Inferior vena cava

Heart

Pulmonary veins bring oxygen-rich blood from the lungs to the heart.

Left atrium
Left ventricle

Systemic (body) capillaries

CO_2 O_2
Tissue cells

LOWER BODY

Airflow

Intercostal muscles contract and pull ribs up and outward.

Lung expands

Diaphragm contracts and moves down and outward.

FIGURE 20-3

The diaphragm and intercostal muscles contract, increasing the volume of the thoracic cavity, which lowers intrathoracic (and intrapulmonary) pressure, allowing inspiration.

350 mL. The volume of anatomical dead space does not change. If tidal volume decreases to 300 mL, 150 mL remains in the dead space and alveolar ventilation is decreased to 150 mL.

Expiration is stimulated by the Hering–Breuer reflex. When stretch receptors in the lungs are activated, nervous signals stimulate the expiratory center and inhibit the inspiratory center in the brainstem. As the diaphragm and intercostal muscles relax, the volume of the thoracic cavity, and therefore the lungs, decreases. This results in higher intrapulmonary pressure with respect to the environment, so air flows out of the lungs (Figure 20-4).

IN THE FIELD

Anything that decreases tidal volume decreases alveolar ventilation. Shallow breathing means that the amount of oxygen delivered to the cells is decreased.

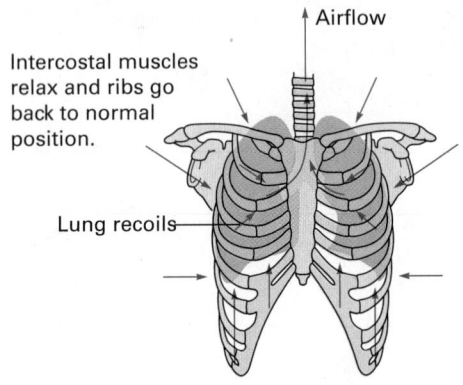

Airflow

Intercostal muscles relax and ribs go back to normal position.

Lung recoils

Diaphragm relaxes and moves upward.

FIGURE 20-4

The diaphragm and intercostal muscles relax, which reduces the volume of the thoracic cavity and increases intrathoracic (and intrapulmonary) pressure, allowing expiration.

When the level of carbon dioxide rises, another respiratory cycle begins. When more carbon dioxide is produced and more oxygen is required, the respiratory rate is faster and the depth is increased.

General Assessment and Management of Respiratory Emergencies

Patients with respiratory problems present in varying degrees of distress (Table 20-1). The patient's chief complaint may be mild dyspnea, which is often described as being "short of breath" or "having difficulty breathing." Patients with severe dyspnea may barely be able to offer a chief complaint between gasps for air. Dyspnea may be accompanied by signs of respiratory distress, such as tripoding, wheezing, coughing, and use of accessory muscles of respiration (Figure 20-5). Signs of hypoxia and exhaustion such as cyanosis, altered mental status, and weak respiratory effort indicate respiratory failure and impending respiratory arrest. Patients in respiratory arrest present with ineffective respiratory effort, or apnea. Cardiac arrest will follow quickly without intervention (Figure 20-6).

All patients with dyspnea must receive supplemental oxygen. The method for delivering oxygen and the amount

TABLE 20-1	Signs of Respiratory Distress, Respiratory Failure, and Respiratory Arrest			
	Normal Breathing	**Respiratory Distress**	**Respiratory Failure**	**Respiratory Arrest**
Respiratory rate	12–20 per minute	May be normal, but likely slightly outside normal range	8 or less, or 30 or greater	Agonal or absent
Tidal volume	Free movement of air, adequate depth	May be increased or decreased	Inadequate	Minimal to absent
Breath sounds	No abnormal sounds, breaths sounds present and equal in all lung fields	May have stridor, wheezing, rhonchi, crackles (rales); breath sounds may be diminished or unequal	May have stridor, wheezing, rhonchi, crackles (rales); breath sounds may be diminished, reflecting inadequate air movement	Absent
Work of breathing	Normal	Slightly to moderately increased	Increased, but patient may be showing signs of fatigue	Minimal to absent
Patient appearance	Good skin color	Anxious	Anxious, may have cyanosis, level of responsiveness may begin to decrease, patient may be confused	Decreased responsiveness, cyanotic
Necessary interventions	Oxygen by nasal cannula if indicated by complaints, history, clinical findings	Oxygen by nonrebreather	Assist ventilations with CPAP, bag-valve-mask device, or FROPVD	Provide ventilations using bag-valve-mask device, FROPVD, or ATV

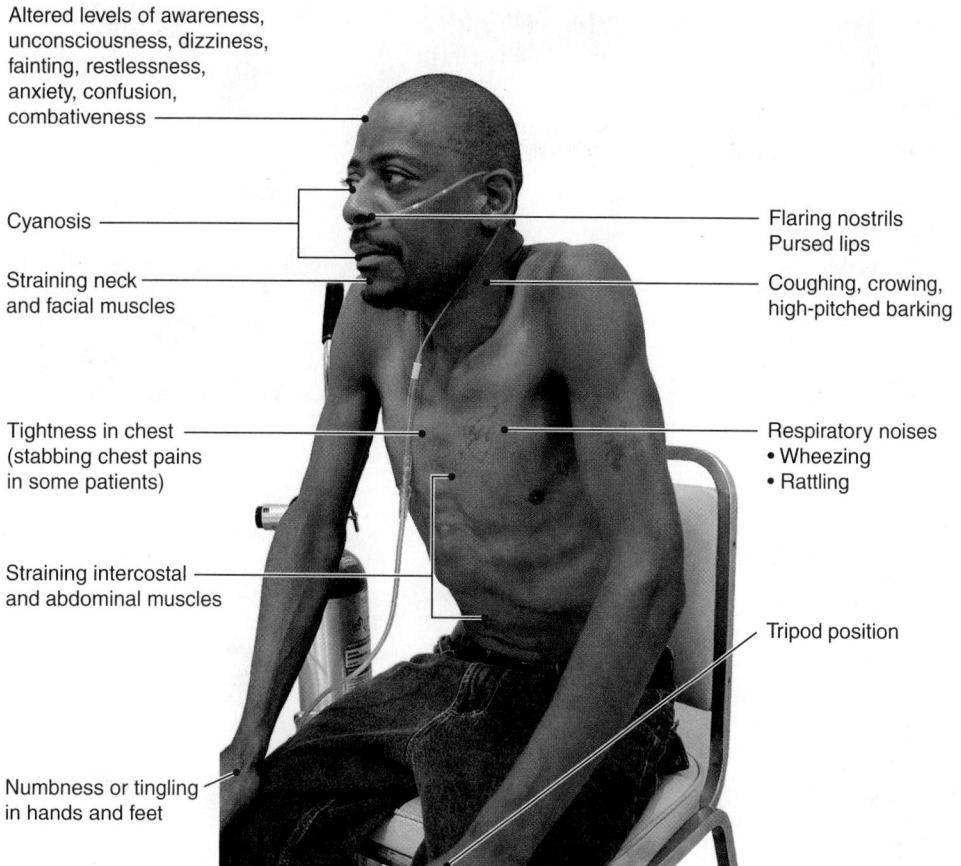

Altered levels of awareness, unconsciousness, dizziness, fainting, restlessness, anxiety, confusion, combativeness

Cyanosis

Straining neck and facial muscles

Tightness in chest (stabbing chest pains in some patients)

Straining intercostal and abdominal muscles

Numbness or tingling in hands and feet

Flaring nostrils
Pursed lips

Coughing, crowing, high-pitched barking

Respiratory noises
• Wheezing
• Rattling

Tripod position

FIGURE 20-5

Signs of respiratory distress. (© Ray Kemp/Triple Zilch Productions)

provided depends on the patient's degree of distress, adequacy of ventilation, pulse oximetry value, and suspected underlying condition. Patients with **chronic obstructive pulmonary disease (COPD)** who present with a mild increase in dyspnea and few signs of respiratory distress may do well with oxygen by nasal cannula. Patients with severe dyspnea but adequate ventilation require oxygen by nonrebreather mask to maintain an SpO_2 of 95 percent or higher. Other supportive measures include allowing the patient to assume a position of comfort. For most patients, sitting upright and perhaps leaning forward will provide the greatest level of comfort, as long as other conditions (decreased level of responsiveness or hypotension, for instance) do not contraindicate it. Reassure the patient by telling him that you are there to help.

All patients with inadequate ventilation require supplemental oxygen and assistance with ventilation by bag-valve-mask device. None of the general signs and symptoms described earlier gives information about the specific underlying cause of the problem. Maintaining the patient's airway, breathing, oxygenation, and circulation are critical, but those measures are not directed at reversing the underlying cause of the problem. Unless the underlying problem is corrected, the supportive measures only buy a little time. They do not provide a solution. The patient's history is often the key to determining the underlying cause of the problem.

Scene Size-Up

Begin, as always, with a scene size-up. Occasionally, a respiratory emergency may not be obvious. Hypoxic patients can behave irrationally because of cerebral dysfunction. Even as you must always ensure your own safety, always consider that there may be a medical cause of the patient's behavior.

Next, form a general impression before deciding how to proceed with the primary assessment. Respiratory failure and respiratory arrest may present as a decreased level of responsiveness. In this case, respiratory effort may be decreased or absent. For these patients, once you have assessed scene safety, take immediate steps to establish the level of responsiveness and check a carotid pulse. If the pulse is absent after checking for 10 seconds, begin chest compressions and prepare to apply an AED. If the carotid pulse is present, ensure an open airway, and provide or assist ventilations with a bag-valve-mask device and supplemental oxygen.

In more responsive patients, the presence of respiratory distress or failure may be obvious from your first glimpse of the patient. Note the patient's position. Often, patients with respiratory distress are sitting upright and may be leaning forward, supporting themselves with their arms (tripod position). You may see exaggerated chest and abdominal movement and use of accessory muscles, indicating labored breathing. The patient may appear drowsy or confused. You

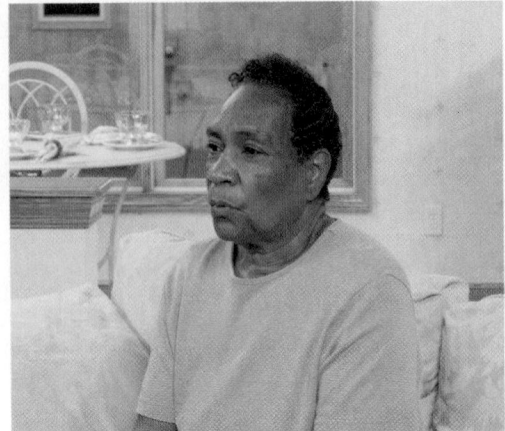

(A)

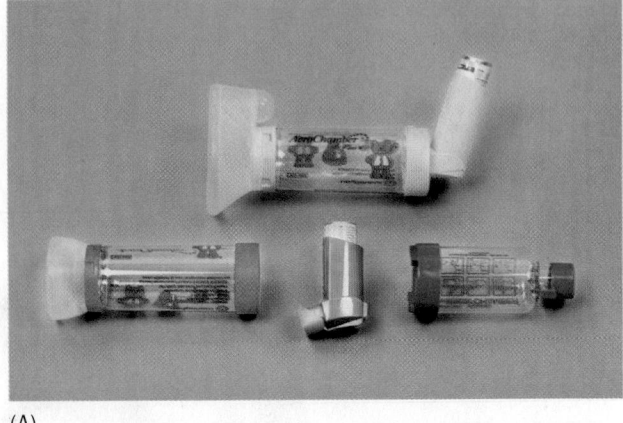

(A)

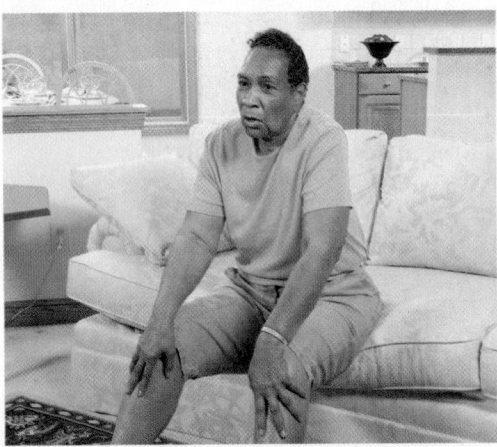

(B)

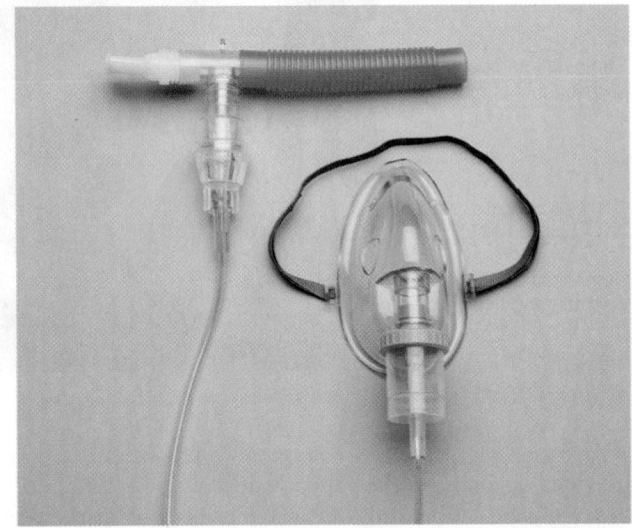

(B)

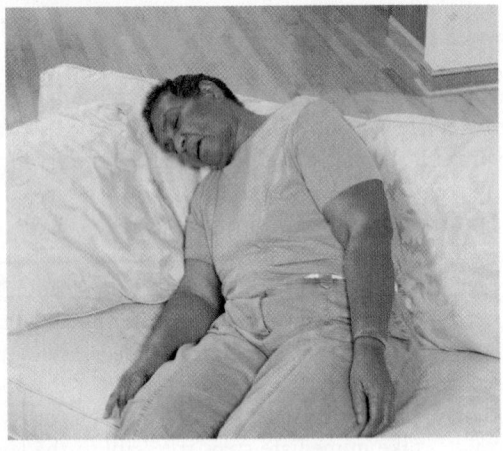

(C)

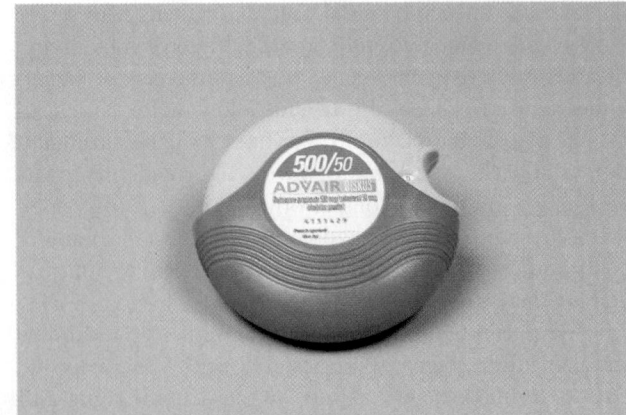

(C)

FIGURE 20-6

(A) Progression from respiratory distress
(B) to respiratory failure (C) and respiratory arrest.

FIGURE 20-7

A patient's medications, including inhalers and nebulizers, can provide an important clue to a history of respiratory problems. (A) Metered-dose inhaler with spacer devices. (B) Small-volume nebulizer. (C) Advair Diskus. (All photos: © Carl Leet)

may see cyanosis, especially of the lips, ears, and nail beds. You may hear wheezing, coughing, crackles (rales), stridor, or coughing.

If the patient is on oxygen, you will have an immediate indication that the patient has a serious chronic illness. The presence of a nebulizer and a metered-dose inhaler (MDI) also provides a clue that the patient has a respiratory illness (Figure 20-7).

Pediatric Care

Pediatric patients often exhibit bradycardia, rather than tachycardia, in response to hypoxia.

Geriatric Care

Elderly patients may not exhibit an increase in heart rate in response to hypoxia.

As you introduce yourself and ask about the patient's problem, listen for the ease with which he is able to speak. Can he speak an entire sentence without taking a breath? Or must he take a breath after two or three words?

Primary Assessment

In the primary assessment, ensure that the patient has an open airway. Use manual positioning, suction, and basic adjuncts as needed. Assess the adequacy of breathing, checking for adequate air movement. Decreased tidal volume means decreased alveolar ventilation. An increase in respiratory rate can only compensate for this decrease to a certain point. Assist ventilations by bag-valve-mask device with supplemental oxygen if the patient's breathing is inadequate (Figure 20-8). For patients with adequate ventilation, begin treatment with oxygen. Select the administration device according to the patient's degree of distress. The goal is to maintain an SpO_2 of 95 percent or higher. Assess the patient's pulse. Tachycardia is an indication of hypoxia.

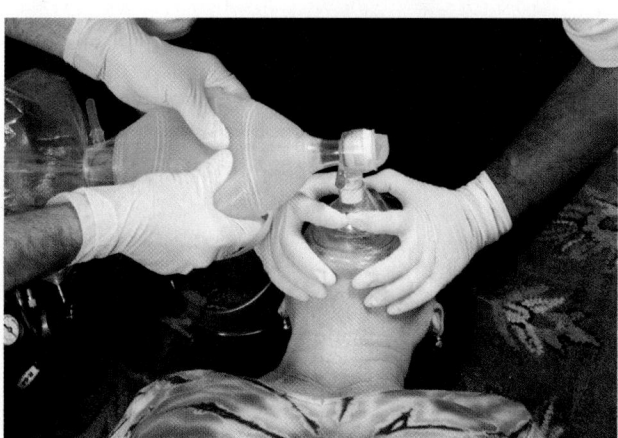

FIGURE 20-8

Use a bag-valve-mask device to assist with or provide ventilations for any patient with inadequate or absent breathing.

Make an initial determination of the patient's priority for transport. Because dyspnea is an indication of a problem with breathing, patients with this complaint are a high priority for transport.

Respiratory distress can quickly progress to respiratory failure and respiratory arrest. However, effective prehospital treatment can substantially improve the patient's condition. Be prepared to change the patient's priority based on reassessment findings. Consider early communication with the receiving hospital, if it appears that the patient will need endotracheal intubation.

Secondary Assessment

In the secondary assessment, focus on things that will provide you with the most relevant information first. That includes auscultation of breath sounds, vital signs, pulse oximetry, capnometry and cardiac monitoring if available, and the patient's medical history.

The history may prompt you to check for additional signs and symptoms, such as edema in the lower extremities. The patient's medications and history yield important clues (Table 20-2). Whether or not the patient has a history of respiratory disease, heart disease, allergic reactions, recent surgery, or other medical problems plays a crucial role in clinical reasoning.

Clinical-Reasoning Process

Understanding the pathophysiology of various causes of difficulty breathing will help you know what questions to ask as you begin to develop and test hypotheses about the underlying cause of a respiratory emergency. A history of emphysema, for example, tells you not only that the patient has a chronic respiratory disease, but also that he is at risk of heart failure, cardiac dysrhythmia, and complications related to long-term corticosteroid use. On the other hand, sudden respiratory distress in a patient with no history of respiratory disease should lead you to think of acute emergencies, such as pulmonary embolism or spontaneous pneumothorax.

Treatment

In addition to basic treatment aimed at maintaining the patient's airway, breathing, oxygenation, and circulation, other treatments may be indicated. Patients who are unresponsive and without a gag reflex may require the use of a Combitube or supraglottic airway device. Continuous positive airway pressure (CPAP) may be indicated to provide ventilatory support for patients with pulmonary edema (Figure 20-9).

IV fluids are important in patients with asthma and pneumonia, and bronchodilators can assist patients with asthma or COPD. If protocols allow, patients with pulmonary edema from heart failure can benefit from

Auscultate the breath sounds for changes and communicate with the patient to determine whether treatment has relieved his symptoms. Recheck the vital signs and SpO_2. If cardiac monitoring and capnometry have been implemented, reassess their results frequently, as well. Be prepared to change treatment, if needed, based on the results of reassessment.

Chronic Obstructive Pulmonary Disease

Chronic obstructive pulmonary disease (COPD) includes both **emphysema** and **chronic bronchitis**, and is the fourth leading cause of death in the United States (American Lung Association, 2010b). Emphysema and chronic bronchitis typically occur in middle age and are almost exclusively caused by cigarette smoking. Smoking causes 85–90 percent of COPD deaths; most other cases can be attributed to secondhand smoke exposure, occupational exposure, and air pollution. Rarely (2–3 percent of cases), emphysema is caused by a genetic disorder in which there is a deficiency of a lung-protective protein.

Although emphysema and chronic bronchitis have some different features, most patients with COPD have some degree of both diseases, with the features of one or the other predominating. Difficulty breathing is caused by progressive destruction of lung tissue with one or more of the following: decreased diameter of the small airways, loss of elasticity of the airways, obstruction because of inflammation and increased mucus production, and decreased alveolar surface area for gas exchange (National Heart, Blood, and Lung Institute, 2010a).

Increased resistance to blood flow through the pulmonary vasculature means that the right ventricle of the heart must work harder to circulate blood through the lungs. This can result in enlargement of the right ventricle and **right-sided heart failure**, as well as pulmonary artery hypertension. Damage to the right side of the heart can lead to the cardiac dysrhythmia atrial fibrillation, which is common in patients with COPD. Atrial fibrillation is an irregular heart rhythm and it is not unusual to detect an irregular pulse in patients with a history of COPD. Right-sided heart failure results in edema, particularly of the lower extremities and

within the abdomen. Right-sided heart failure caused by pulmonary disease is called **cor pulmonale** (Figure 20-10).

Chronic hypoxia leads to a condition called *clubbing of the fingers* (Figure 20-11). Some patients with COPD become accustomed to having an increased level of carbon dioxide, making their primary respiratory drive a low oxygen level (hypoxic drive) instead of a high carbon dioxide level.

Chronic Bronchitis

In patients with chronic bronchitis, the mucus-producing cells in the bronchi are increased in size and produce more mucus than normal, resulting in a persistent "smoker's cough." Destruction of the cilia that line the airway makes it more difficult to rid the airway of the mucus, which allows bacteria to become trapped in the lungs (Figure 20-12). The patient is stable for periods of time but has episodes of decompensation called *acute exacerbation*, often caused by infection.

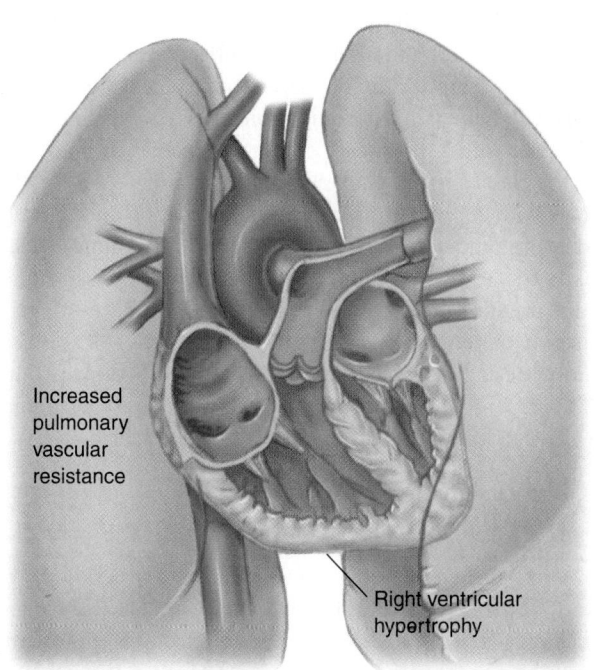

Increased pulmonary vascular resistance

Right ventricular hypertrophy

FIGURE 20-10

Cor pulmonale is right-sided heart failure that occurs because of increased resistance in the pulmonary vasculature.

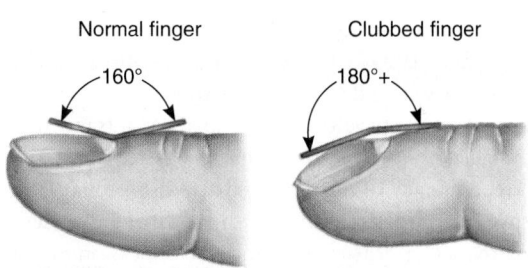

Normal finger 160°   Clubbed finger 180°+

FIGURE 20-11

Patients with COPD can exhibit "clubbing" of the fingers.

IN THE FIELD

Hypoxic drive, the reliance on decreased oxygen levels as the stimulus to breathe, may occur in some COPD patients. In such cases, prolonged administration of high levels of oxygen may result in respiratory depression. However, you must never withhold oxygen from a patient who needs it. Monitor the patient's ventilations and provide assistance by bag-valve-mask device if respiratory effort becomes inadequate.

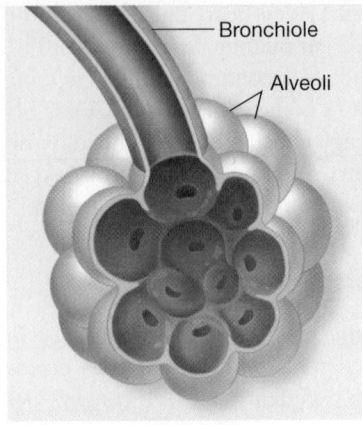
Normal

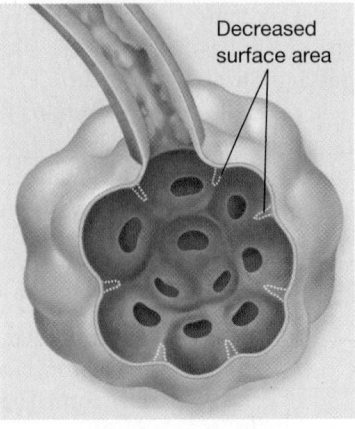
Emphysema

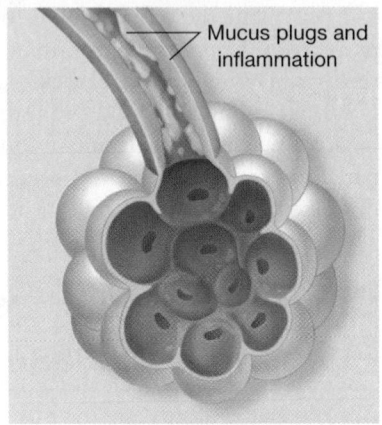
Chronic Bronchitis

FIGURE 20-12

Pathophysiology of chronic bronchitis and emphysema.

Chronic bronchitis is characterized by a cough that produces sputum for a total of three months during two consecutive years (Fayyaz, Hmidi, Nascimento, Olade, & Lessnau, 2010). Patients with chronic bronchitis are typically over 50 years old. As the disease progresses, the patient may take on the classic appearance referred to as a *blue bloater*. Patients with chronic bronchitis become cyanotic during exacerbations, and are prone to right-sided heart failure, which leads to peripheral edema. During acute exacerbations, the patient's cough may be more frequent and more productive, there may be a change in the character of sputum, and wheezing may occur as a result of bronchoconstriction. Patients with chronic bronchitis are prone to hypercapnia, which can lead to confusion, drowsiness, and headache.

Emphysema

Patients with emphysema have extensive destruction of the walls of the alveoli, resulting in reduced surface area for gas exchange (Figure 20-12). Because of chronic hypoxia, the body compensates by increasing production of red blood cells to carry oxygen. The increased red blood cell level allows the patient to have good skin color, despite being short of breath. The classic presentation of a patient with emphysema is thus called the *pink puffer*.

Patients with emphysema also are prone to acute exacerbations, which may be triggered by exposure to smoke, cold air, or other irritants. The level of respiratory distress increases, and narrowed airways result in wheezing. Patients with emphysema tend to be thin, with well-developed accessory muscles of respiration (Figure 20-13). Air trapped within the damaged alveoli leads to a "barrel-chested" appearance.

The tendency of the damaged alveoli to collapse causes patients to compensate by breathing through pursed lips. This provides increased resistance to expiration and keeps pressure in the lungs higher. This reflex results in conditions similar to positive end-expiratory pressure (PEEP) ventilation used in automatic ventilator settings.

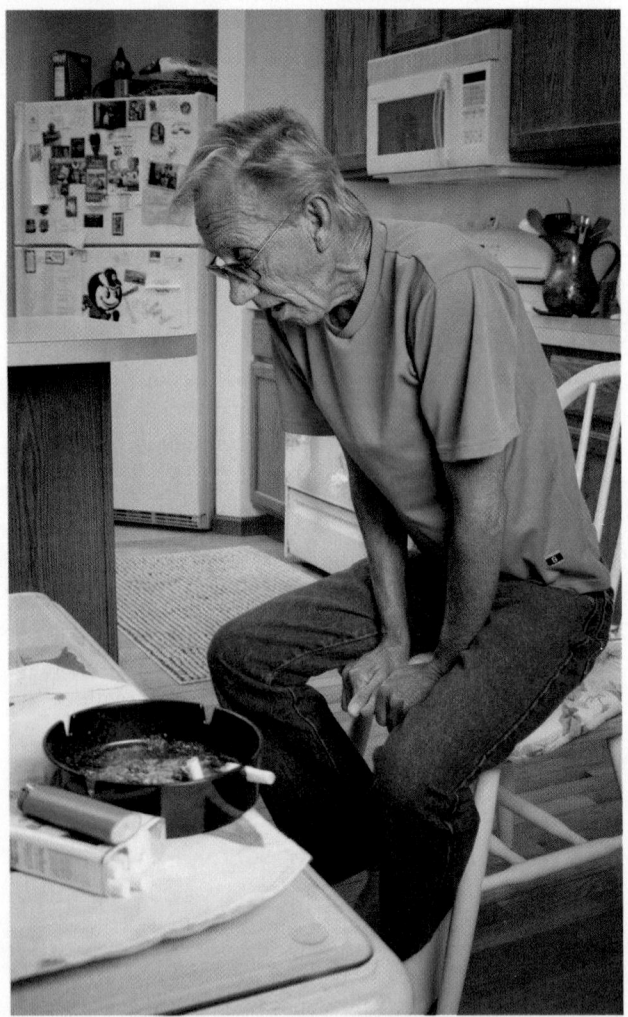

FIGURE 20-13

Classic appearance of a patient with emphysema.

COPD Management

In both types of disease—chronic bronchitis and emphysema—patients' quality of life can be severely affected. Both diseases are progressive and cannot be reversed. However, stopping smoking is an important step in slowing the progress of the disease.

In mild cases, patients suffer from dyspnea on exertion. As the disease progresses, dyspnea is more frequent and more severe.

Pneumonia and spontaneous pneumothorax are complications of COPD. Patients are typically treated with corticosteroids or other anti-inflammatory drugs to reduce inflammation. However, the drugs have significant side effects, including increased risk of infection. Long-acting bronchodilators are used to prevent bronchoconstriction, and short-acting bronchodilators (sometimes called *rescue inhalers*) are used to treat episodes of increased dyspnea.

Bronchodilators include beta$_2$ agonists and parasympatholytic (anticholinergic) drugs. Acute exacerbations of chronic bronchitis are often treated with antibiotics. As the disease progresses, patients may rely on supplemental oxygen part or all of the time.

Despite some differences in the diseases, the goals of prehospital treatment are the same: to improve ventilation and oxygenation. In addition to providing supplemental oxygen and (if needed) assisted ventilation, sympathetic beta$_2$ agonists (albuterol, for example) can be used to treat bronchoconstriction in patients who are wheezing. In some EMS systems, a combined beta$_2$ agonist/parasympatholytic agent, such as ipratropium (Atrovent), is preferred.

Thick, dehydrated mucus in the lungs can lead to obstruction of the bronchi. Hydration decreases mucus plugging. Keep in mind, though, that patients with COPD are prone to heart failure, and fluid overload can be detrimental. Follow protocols for IV fluid administration, and check with medical direction if you have questions about the rate of fluids for specific patients.

Check lung sounds frequently for both improvement in wheezing and development of crackles (rales). The saline used to nebulize bronchodilators will help with **expectoration**, and humidified oxygen should be used if available.

If transport times are long or for interfacility transport, the physician may order a Venturi mask at a specific oxygen setting. CPAP is used with caution because the increased pulmonary pressures in the weakened lung tissues can lead to pneumothorax.

Asthma

Twenty-three million people in the United States suffer from asthma, a chronic inflammation of the airways with reversible episodes of obstruction (American Lung Association, 2010a). Asthma affects people of all ages, and untreated asthma can lead to death.

Asthma is thought to have a significant genetic component, but can be caused by certain respiratory illnesses in childhood and early exposure to certain viruses and environmental contaminants when the immune system is developing.

Asthma rates are higher in children in urban areas. One reason is thought to be the increased exposure to antigens from cockroaches and other urban contaminants (National Heart, Lung, and Blood Institute, 2010b). Asthma triggers include cigarette smoke, pet dander, pollutants, exercise, respiratory infections, and other irritants.

Asthma Pathophysiology

There are two components to asthma. Patients have chronic inflammation of the bronchioles, which can be exacerbated, causing an "asthma attack." During an asthma attack, the airways narrow because of smooth muscle constriction, and the underlying inflammation increases (Figure 20-14).

One of the body's normal responses to lung irritants is constriction of the bronchioles to limit exposure. This response is exaggerated in asthmatics, leading to significant constriction of the bronchioles. The reaction is especially pronounced on expiration, because the bronchioles normally dilate on inspiration and constrict on expiration (Martini, Bartholomew, & Bledsoe, 2008). The result is expiratory wheezing and overinflation of the alveoli (air trapping) (Table 20-3).

Even when bronchiolar smooth muscle constriction is treated by beta$_2$ agonists, the underlying increase in inflammation may just be starting. The increased inflammation leads to swelling of the bronchioles and increased mucus production. Additional medications are needed to treat the inflammatory component.

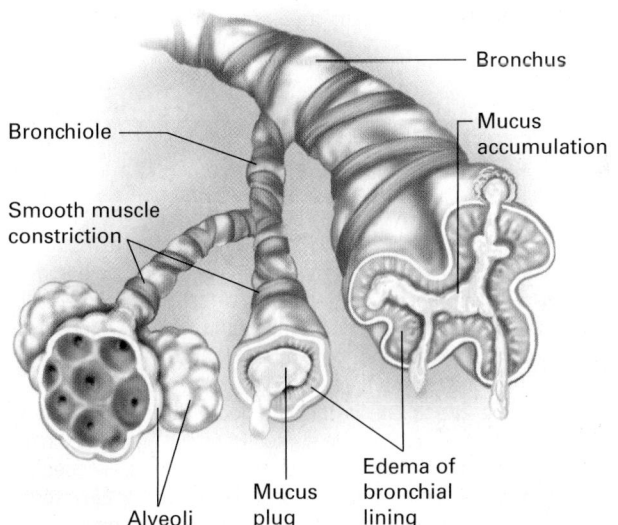

FIGURE 20-14

Asthma has inflammatory and bronchoconstrictive components.

TABLE 20-3 Signs and Symptoms of an Asthma Attack

SIGNS AND SYMPTOMS OF A MILDER ASTHMA ATTACK

- Nonproductive cough (may be worse at night, causing inability to sleep, or may be worse in early morning)
- Wheezing (may be induced by exercise, infection, or exposure to triggers; usually expiratory)
- Chest tightness
- Shortness of breath
- Tachypnea
- Tachycardia (below 150 beats/min.)
- Anxiety
- $SpO_2 > 95$ percent before oxygen

SIGNS AND SYMPTOMS OF SEVERE ASTHMA ATTACK

- Fatigue, exhaustion
- Inability to speak
- Confusion or drowsiness
- Cyanosis
- Diminished or absent breath sounds
- Tachycardia or bradycardia
- Tachypnea (>30 beats/min.)
- Diaphoresis
- $SpO_2 < 90$ percent with oxygen

Asthma Management

Two types of medications are used to treat asthma. Anti-inflammatory agents such as corticosteroids, cromolyn sodium, and **leukotriene inhibitors** are used to decrease inflammation and prevent asthma attacks. Bronchodilators, usually beta$_2$ agonists and anticholinergics, are used to prevent asthma attacks and to relax bronchiolar smooth muscle to treat acute attacks. In severe asthma attacks that do not respond well to the short-acting beta$_2$ agonists, additional anti-inflammatory medication may be needed.

Often, an asthma patient or those around him will call 911 after his attempts to reverse an attack with a rescue inhaler have failed. A patient may successfully use his rescue inhaler to treat the initial bronchoconstriction that occurs after exposure to a trigger, but the inflammatory phase that develops hours after exposure to the trigger will cause recurrence of symptoms that cannot be treated by beta$_2$ agonists. **Status asthmaticus** is a severe, prolonged, life-threatening asthma attack that does not respond to treatment with bronchodilators. The patient may be approaching or in respiratory failure by the time the ambulance arrives.

Prehospital treatment of asthma patients begins with an assessment of the patient's level of responsiveness, airway, breathing, oxygenation, and circulation. Altered mental status and signs of exhaustion, cyanosis, and diminished air movement are signs that the patient's condition is immediately life threatening.

Immediately establish an airway, assist with ventilation, and provide supplemental oxygen. The patient must be transported without delay with an IV established en route. Contact the receiving facility for notification and consult with medical direction about the possibility of using SubQ or IM epinephrine to treat status asthmaticus.

For asthma patients who are awake and breathing adequately, begin oxygen administration as you complete your assessment and obtain a history. Base oxygen administration on the patient's level of distress, vital signs, and SpO_2. Obtain as much information as possible about what the patient has done to treat the asthma attack. Patients may already have used more than the recommended amount of their rescue inhaler without significant relief. They may be experiencing side effects associated with the medications, including increased anxiety, palpitations, and tachycardia. If this is case, consult with medical direction before

PERSONAL PERSPECTIVE

Advanced EMT Raleigh Fisher: I never took asthma that seriously—until the night I saw a teenage boy die from it. I was working the overnight shift as a tech in the emergency department when a guy came running in from the ambulance bay yelling for someone to help him. His 15-year-old son was in the car, and he was unresponsive. The dad said his son had an asthma attack late in the afternoon, but he was able to control it with his inhaler. He started wheezing again later in the evening, but his inhaler didn't seem to be working. He used the inhaler several times, but the wheezing just kept getting worse.

The boy was very agitated, his dad said, but he suddenly seemed to relax. The father's relief lasted only seconds. He realized that he was exhausted and barely moving air. He put his son into the car and sped to the ED. The drive took only two to three minutes, but by the time we got to the boy, he was in respiratory arrest.

I started bagging him immediately, but his lungs were so "tight" I couldn't really get any air in. We got him into the resuscitation room. The ED doc intubated him, but his heart rate dropped quickly from 130 into the 60s, then 50s, and then cardiac arrest. We did CPR, started IVs, and gave medications, but it was futile.

I was shocked and saddened. I knew intellectually that asthma could be lethal, but I had just seen it happen to a 15-year-old kid right before my eyes. From that point forward, I've never taken an asthma patient lightly, even when his distress seems to be mild. I always look to see how tired he is and how much air he is moving.

administering additional beta₂ agonists. Otherwise, follow your protocol in administering a beta₂ agonist or combined beta₂ agonist/anticholinergic by small-volume nebulizer.

Patients with asthma benefit from hydration with IV fluids. Follow protocols in the amount of fluids to administer. Frequently reassess the asthma patient, including mental status, airway, breathing, vital signs, breath sounds, level of distress, and SpO₂. Keep in mind the possibility of deterioration and be prepared to provide an airway and start ventilations by bag-valve-mask device.

Pulmonary Embolism

Pulmonary embolism (PE) is a condition in which there is an obstruction to blood flow in the pulmonary arterial system by a blood clot (embolus). This means that part of the lung is not able to participate in gas exchange. Early in the process, air enters the alveoli of the affected part of the lung, but the absence of circulation in the surrounding capillaries means that oxygen does not enter the blood. This imbalance in ventilation and perfusion in the lung is called a **ventilation–perfusion (VQ) mismatch**.

Because part of the lung is not available for gas exchange, hypoxia can result. The degree of distress suffered by the patient depends on the degree to which lung perfusion is affected. A small embolus affecting circulation to a relatively small number of alveoli may cause mild shortness of breath.

It is not uncommon for patients to present with vague signs and symptoms up to a week before being diagnosed with PE. However, many pulmonary emboli are larger, obstructing large areas of blood flow.

In some cases, a number of smaller emboli may obstruct many different branches of pulmonary circulation. In such cases, patients generally experience a sudden onset of severe dyspnea. This may be accompanied by hypotension and signs of severe respiratory distress and hypoxia. In some cases, the patient will also complain of a sudden onset of sharp chest pain (Table 20-4).

Patients with significant PE can deteriorate quickly, getting worse despite all attempts to oxygenate and ventilate him and increase the blood pressure through fluid

TABLE 20-4	Signs and Symptoms of Pulmonary Embolism

- Unexplained shortness of breath
- Tachypnea
- Tachycardia
- Hypotension
- Feeling of dread, anxiety
- Syncope
- Diaphoresis
- Chest pain (pleuritic)
- Coughing, hemoptysis
- New cardiac dysrhythmia
- Swollen, tender lower extremity (calf)

administration. Definitive treatment requires anticoagulation to prevent further embolus formation, fibrinolytic therapy to breakdown the existing clot, or less frequently, embolectomy by surgery or catheterization.

Patients at greatest risk for a pulmonary embolism usually have existing medical conditions that predispose them to abnormal blood clot formation. A common source of the embolus is deep vein thrombosis (DVT) of the pelvis or lower extremities.

Although blood clots are the most common cause of pulmonary embolism, air, fat, bone marrow, and amniotic fluid in the circulation also can cause it. Some risk factors include recent surgery, cancer, immobilization (from a fracture, major injury, illness, or obesity), estrogen use (hormone replacement or contraceptives), pregnancy (all trimesters and up to 6–12 weeks postpartum), and older age.

Suspect pulmonary embolism in patients with otherwise unexplained dyspnea and hypoxia (SpO₂ < 95 percent) (Sutherland, 2010). Early in the process, breath sounds are clear and equal, although the nonperfused portion of the lung will undergo **atelectasis** 24–72 hours after the onset.

The patient's history may reveal risk factors that increase your suspicion for pulmonary embolism. Other signs and symptoms may exist, but their absence cannot rule it out. Additional signs and symptoms include chest, back, shoulder, or upper abdominal pain. Chest pain may be **pleuritic**. The patient may experience syncope (fainting), and may have hypotension, tachycardia, **hemoptysis**, or swelling of one leg. Severely hypoxic patients may present with cyanosis or mottling; cool, diaphoretic skin; altered mental status; respiratory failure; or respiratory arrest.

Treat patients with suspected pulmonary embolism with oxygen by nonrebreather mask, if ventilations are adequate, or bag-valve-mask device if ventilations are inadequate. Start an IV. If the patient is hypotensive, administer fluids. Patients with pulmonary embolism who have hypotension are likely to be severely hypoxic and acidotic. Be prepared for respiratory and cardiac arrest. As with any critical patient, notify the receiving facility and if questions about treatment arise, consult with medical direction.

IN THE FIELD

Although wheezing is a common sign of an asthma attack, keep two things in mind. First, all that wheezes is not asthma. Other conditions, which may require different treatment, also cause wheezing. Second, wheezing can occur only if a certain amount of air is moving through the bronchioles. In a severe asthma attack, little air is moving and wheezing may not be heard. Silence is an ominous sign when auscultating the chest of a patient with respiratory distress.

Pulmonary Edema

Pulmonary edema occurs when there is an increase in interstitial fluid that increases the distance of gas diffusion between the alveoli and pulmonary capillaries. Pulmonary edema is classified as cardiogenic or noncardiogenic.

Cardiogenic Pulmonary Edema

In cardiogenic pulmonary edema, congestion of the pulmonary capillaries from left-sided heart failure can force fluid into the alveoli, where it mixes with air, producing crackles (rales) on auscultation and frothy sputum (Figure 20-15). (See Chapter 21 for the pathophysiology of heart failure.)

Because cardiogenic pulmonary edema is caused by increased afterload (amount of resistance the heart has to overcome to eject blood from the ventricles) and pulmonary vascular congestion, medications that cause vasodilation are important in its treatment. One such medication carried by Advanced EMTs is nitroglycerin. Nitroglycerin may be administered sublingually, according to your protocol or in consultation with medical direction.

Noncardiogenic Pulmonary Edema

Noncardiogenic causes of pulmonary edema include **acute respiratory distress syndrome (ARDS)** and delayed toxin-induced lung injury (McSwain, Salomone, & Pons, 2007).

ARDS is a complication of severe illnesses and is rarely seen in the prehospital setting. Some factors that can directly or indirectly injure the lungs and result in ARDS are shock, sepsis, drug overdose, severe pneumonia, severe trauma or illness, aspiration of stomach contents, and exposure to inhaled toxins. ARDS carries a high mortality rate.

There are measures that you can take to decrease a patient's risk of developing ARDS. They include recognizing and managing shock by controlling bleeding and ensuring adequate oxygenation, and preventing aspiration of stomach contents through proper airway management, including positioning the patient and having suction readily available.

A number of toxic substances that reach the lungs either by inhalation or blood circulation can lead to noncardiogenic pulmonary edema and other damage to the lungs that may not be evident immediately after exposure. This is sometimes referred to as *delayed toxin-induced lung injury* (McSwain, Salomone, & Pons, 2007). You should maintain a high index of suspicion for later complications in patients who have a history of exposure to toxins, even when they appear noncritical immediately following the incident.

Toxic causes of noncardiogenic pulmonary edema by inhalation of fumes include smoke produced by fires, chlorine gas, anhydrous ammonia, acid fumes or vapors (such as hydrogen fluoride or sulfur dioxide), hydrogen sulfide (from sewage treatment or farming operations), phosgene, and others (Mullen, 2007).

Toxins introduced to the circulation through injection or oral administration include heroin, methadone, and other opioid drugs; narcotic antagonists such as naloxone (rarely);

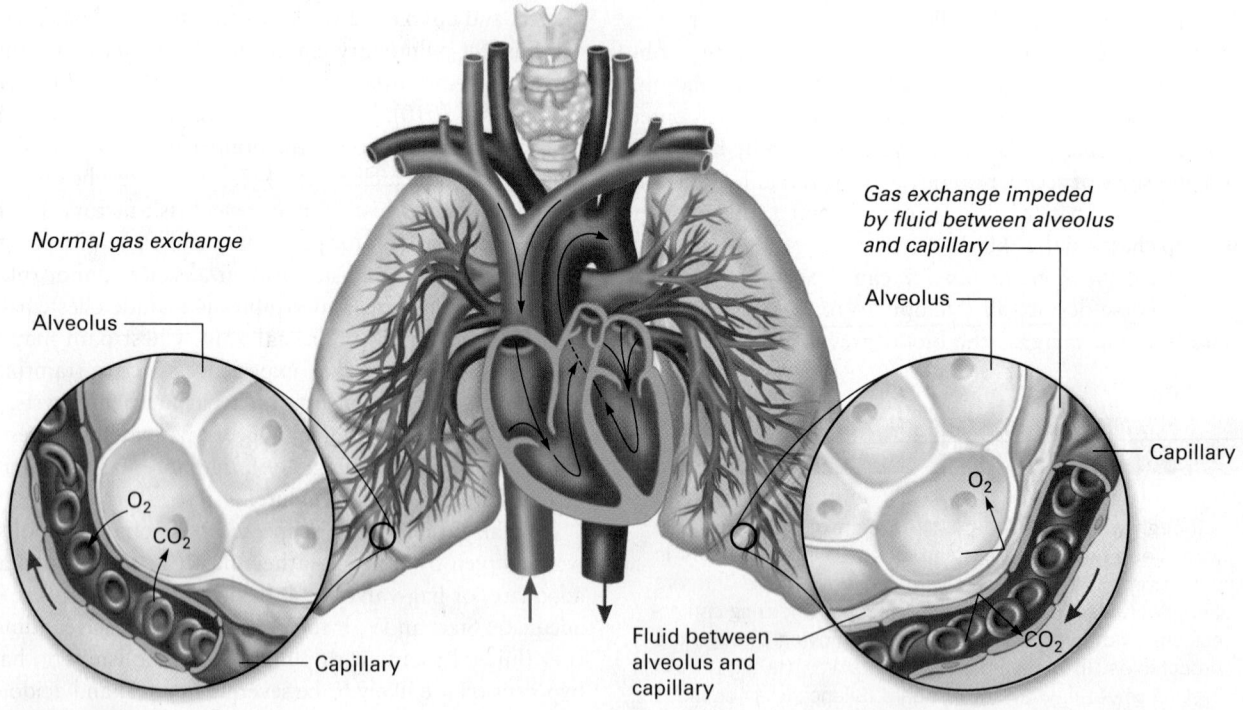

Normal gas exchange

Alveolus

O_2
CO_2

Capillary

Gas exchange impeded by fluid between alveolus and capillary

Alveolus

Capillary

O_2

CO_2

Fluid between alveolus and capillary

FIGURE 20-15

Pathophysiology of cardiogenic pulmonary edema.

aspirin overdose; calcium channel blocker overdose; some herbal remedies; and scorpion envenomation. In those cases, obtaining and communicating a complete history, including that of herbal medications, occupational exposure to substances, and illicit drug use is critical. Prehospital treatment includes management of ventilation and oxygenation.

Spontaneous Pneumothorax

Pneumothorax is a condition in which air has accumulated within the pleural cavity, outside the lung, interfering with the ability of the lung to expand during inspiration (Figure 20-16). In lay terms, this is referred to as a *collapsed lung*. The degree of impaired ventilation and hypoxia depend on how much air has accumulated within the pleural space.

Although pneumothorax is often the result of trauma, medical patients can have risk factors for pneumothorax. When pneumothorax occurs without trauma, it is referred to as a **spontaneous pneumothorax**. Lung diseases, such as lung cancer and COPD, result in weakened areas of the lung that can rupture spontaneously or in response to coughing. Some otherwise healthy individuals are at higher risk of spontaneous pneumothorax, possibly due to an inherent weakness in the connective tissues of the lung. Those individuals are likely to be young, tall, thin males. In addition to coughing, any other activity that leads to an increase in intrapulmonary pressure, such as exhaling against a closed glottis when lifting something heavy, may result in pneumothorax in these individuals.

Simple Pneumothorax

When an area of the lung ruptures, air leaks out and accumulates in the pleural space. In most cases, the defect in the lung is small and self-sealing. This limits the amount of air that escapes from the lung. This condition is called *simple pneumothorax*. The term "simple" can be deceiving, because the amount of air in the pleural cavity on the affected side can be substantial, leading to respiratory distress and hypoxia.

Spontaneous pneumothorax may present with pain, and patients often present with a sudden onset of dyspnea, which may have been preceded by coughing or an activity that would increase intrapulmonary pressure. The amount of dyspnea varies from mild to severe, and may be stable or increasing (Table 20-5).

Lung sounds will often will be absent in the affected area, but this can be difficult to detect unless the pneumothorax is large. Breath sounds from the functioning area of the lung can be transmitted to the chest wall over the nonfunctioning portion. You may detect this as diminished, rather than absent, breath sounds. Further complicating assessment of breath sounds, the accumulation of air in the pleural cavity will collect at the top of the pleural cavity. The aspect of the chest that is "at the top" depends on the patient's position.

Other indications of simple spontaneous pneumothorax depend on the severity of the pneumothorax. The patient may have tachypnea, tachycardia, and a decreased SpO_2. Your suspicion should increase in patients with a history that includes risk factors for spontaneous pneumothorax.

Provide the patient with oxygen. His level of distress and SpO_2 guide dosage and administration. Allow the

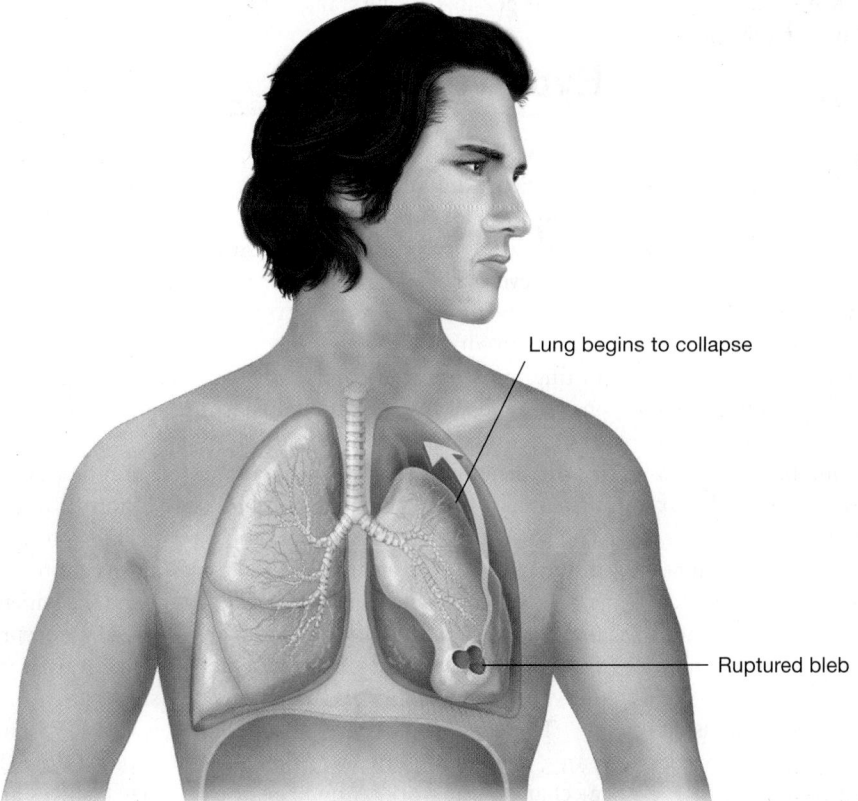

Lung begins to collapse

Ruptured bleb

TABLE 20-5   Signs and Symptoms of Simple and Tension Pneumothorax

Feature	Simple Pneumothorax	Tension Pneumothorax
Dyspnea	Mild to severe	Increasingly severe, progressing to respiratory failure
Hypoxia	Mild to severe	Increasingly severe
Lung sounds (sounds from the unaffected lung may be transmitted to the affected side)	Decreased on affected side	Decreased first on affected side, later on both sides
Chest pain	May be present	Present in 90 percent of cases
Circulation	May have tachycardia related to anxiety and dyspnea	Hypotension, tachycardia, impaired return of blood to heart results in jugular venous distension; if untreated, cardiac arrest with pulseless electrical activity or asystole
Other possible physical findings (these signs may rarely be seen and may be subtle; be aware of their meaning, but do not rely on their presence to identify tension pneumothorax)		Pulsus paradoxus, tracheal deviation away from affected side, hyperexpansion of the chest, hyperresonance of the chest to percussion

patient to assume a position of comfort, which will often be sitting up. Provide reassurance.

If ventilations are inadequate, assist using a bag-valve-mask device. Be aware that positive pressure ventilation from a bag-valve mask can increase the leakage of air from the affected lung. Use the minimum amount of force needed to achieve adequate ventilation. If resistance to bagging increases, suspect tension pneumothorax, described in the next section. *Never use CPAP or administer nitrous oxide to a patient with a suspected pneumothorax.*

Use judgment in starting an IV. A patient in mild distress whose condition is stable may not require an IV in the prehospital setting. A patient in moderate to severe distress should have an IV. Reassess the patient frequently, monitoring mental status, breathing, lung sounds, oxygenation, and vital signs.

Tension Pneumothorax

In some cases, the defect in the lung is large and cannot seal itself. This may occur when the rupture of the lung includes a larger bronchus. Air continues to accumulate and cannot escape. Pressure increases within the thorax, first compressing the lung on the affected side, then pushing the structures in the mediastinum toward the other lung, and finally collapsing the opposite lung. This is called a **tension pneumothorax**. It is a critical, life-threatening emergency.

In addition to signs and symptoms of simple pneumothorax, indications of tension pneumothorax include increasingly severe dyspnea, respiratory failure, cyanosis, distended neck veins, and hypotension. Very late in the condition, the trachea may be deviated away from the affected side. The poor outcome associated with tension pneumothorax is due to obstructive shock. The high intrathoracic pressure impedes blood return to the heart, reducing cardiac output.

Paramedics can perform a life-saving procedure called *needle thoracostomy* (needle chest decompression) to decompress the chest. If you suspect tension pneumothorax, request ALS. If ALS is not available, transport the patient as quickly as possible while assisting with ventilation. Be aware, however, that ventilation can increase the amount of air escaping from the damaged lung. Use the least amount of pressure needed to ventilate the patient. Start an IV and infuse fluids for hypotension. Notify the receiving facility as early as possible during transport.

Hyperventilation Syndrome

Hyperventilation syndrome (HVS) is a condition in which the patient's minute ventilation exceeds his metabolic demands (Kern & Rosh, 2009). When this occurs, the patient's arterial pCO_2 may drop, although in some cases the patient's pCO_2 level is not low enough to explain the signs and symptoms. Patients with HVS may present with dyspnea, anxiety, chest pain, dizziness, near-syncope, weakness, **paresthesia** (a tingling sensation, particularly around the mouth and in the hands), and **carpopedal spasm** (contraction of the muscles of the hands and feet).

Patients often have a feeling of suffocation despite an increased respiratory rate and volume and a normal SpO_2. The patient may report mental changes, such as a feeling of unreality. Often, an emotionally distressing event preceding the onset of symptoms can be identified, and the patient may have a past history of similar episodes. HVS occurs more frequently in females, and usually occurs in patients between the ages of 15 and 55 (Kern & Rosh, 2009).

There is a high degree of overlap between HVS and panic disorder. However, there are still physiological mechanisms at work. A number of electrolyte changes are induced by hypocapnia, and the resulting symptoms are very real. Therefore, you should recognize that the patient cannot simply "calm down."

It is thought that increased levels of lactate or carbon dioxide can induce hyperventilation in some patients, especially those with panic disorder. Other theories are that patients with panic disorder–induced HVS have an exaggerated fight or flight response.

Do not assume that a patient with increased ventilation has HVS. Hypoxia also causes increased ventilation and anxiety. Death from HVS is rare, but death from hypoxia can occur quickly if not corrected. Consider spontaneous pneumothorax and pulmonary embolism as differential diagnoses.

Although chest pain associated with HVS is usually sharp in nature, it can present similarly to the chest pain of acute coronary syndrome (ACS). HVS also induces ECG changes that can appear similar to those of ACS. If in doubt, older patients should be treated for ACS, but nitroglycerin will not relieve chest pain from HVS. However, hypocapnia from HVS can result in coronary vasospasm, which would be expected to respond to nitroglycerin. Death can occur in severe HVS as a result of vasospasm induced by low carbon dioxide levels and impaired dissociation of oxygen from hemoglobin at the cellular level.

Although you may suspect HVS in the field, it cannot be diagnosed in the field. Conditions leading to serious hypoxia may be present, and HVS itself can have significant complications. Do not take the condition lightly. Supplemental oxygen will not harm, and may help, the patient. Reassurance is important, but do not become frustrated if it seems to have minimal effect. Coaching the patient to use "diaphragmatic" breathing may help. Instruct the patient to focus on using his abdominal muscles to breathe.

Infectious Respiratory Diseases

Viruses, fungi, and bacteria can all cause infection of the upper or lower respiratory system. An **upper respiratory infection (URI)** may be **sinusitis** (sinus infection), **pharyngitis** (sore throat), and rhinovirus infection—the common cold. URIs are rarely life threatening. One exception is epiglottitis, a bacterial infection that causes swelling of the epiglottis, which can lead to airway obstruction. Fortunately, widespread vaccination against *Haemophilis influenza* has all but eradicated this disease, which now is mostly seen in unvaccinated adults. **Laryngitis** can occasionally result in respiratory distress as evidenced by stridor. **Laryngotracheobronchitis**, or **croup**, produces stridor and a characteristic "seal bark" cough. Both

epiglottitis and croup are primarily seen in children and are discussed in Chapter 44.

Lower respiratory infections can lead to impairments of oxygenation and become life-threatening. Pneumonia, influenza, and acute bronchitis are most common and occur in patients of all ages. Respiratory syncytial virus (RSV), which causes inflammation of the bronchioles (bronchiolitis), is most often seen in children and can require hospitalization. (See Chapter 44.) Metapneumovirus is the second most common cause of bronchiolitis.

Two less common but very serious conditions are severe acute respiratory syndrome (SARS), caused by a corona virus, and **hantavirus pulmonary syndrome (HPS)**, which is spread by deer mice and is typically concentrated in the Four Corners region of the United States (Arizona, Colorado, New Mexico, Utah). Pertussis (whooping cough), which was once under control due to widespread vaccination, is now on the increase and is of particular concern in infants and small children. (See Chapters 28 and 44.)

Pneumonia

Pneumonia is an infectious disease that results in inflammation of the lungs. The causative agent and the products of the body's inflammatory response to the infection infiltrate the tissues. Pneumonia may be community-acquired or hospital-acquired (nosocomial). Pneumonia can be fatal in individuals with weakened immune systems, including the elderly. Patients with asthma, COPD, heart failure, and other medical problems, as well as smokers, are at increased risk of pneumonia, which exacerbates underlying respiratory conditions.

Pneumonia is quite common in patients who are immobile (for example, because of stroke, surgery, or other problems) or who reside in extended-care facilities. Pneumonia also occurs as a complication of other lower respiratory infections, such as influenza.

Patients with pneumonia can be quite ill, presenting with a cough, difficulty breathing, shaking chills, fever, and malaise. In the elderly, in whom the immune response is diminished, fever may or may not be a prominent sign. Elderly patients may present with altered mental status, such as confusion, because of infection and associated hypoxia.

Dyspnea and respiratory distress range from mild to severe. The patient's cough is usually productive and the sputum may be yellow or tinged with a rust color.

Pneumonia occurs in one or more lobes of the lung. Breath sounds will be diminished in the affected areas on auscultation. Pneumonia presents a VQ mismatch, in which part of the lung is not ventilated. The blood circulating around the affected alveoli is therefore not oxygenated before circulating back to the tissues.

Differentiating between pneumonia and pulmonary edema can be difficult (Table 20-6). Basic treatment of hypoxia and impaired ventilation is the same. However, some treatments indicated for one condition are not appropriate for the other. Both patients require administration of supplemental oxygen, often by nonrebreather mask.

TABLE 20-6	Comparing and Contrasting Cardiogenic Pulmonary Edema and Pneumonia	
Feature	**Pulmonary Edema**	**Pneumonia**
Cause	Left-sided heart failure	Bacterial, viral, or fungal infection
Risk factors	Known heart failure or heart disease, acute myocardial infarction (AMI), history of hypertension	Smoking, COPD, asthma, influenza, immunocompromise
Pathophysiology	Increased hydrostatic pressure in pulmonary capillaries results in increased interstitial fluid between capillaries and alveoli; fluid may enter alveoli Affects both lungs	Alveoli filled with fluid and pus; often localized to a single lobe of one lung, but may be bilateral
Onset	Often occurs at night when the patient lies down, but can occur at any time Onset is often sudden	May be a history of recent respiratory infection (influenza, bronchitis) Chills and fever may occur suddenly Dyspnea tends to be progressive
Signs and symptoms	Orthopnea (needs to sit up to breathe) History of dyspnea on exertion Paroxysmal nocturnal dyspnea (PND) Altered mental status Jugular venous distention (JVD) Pink, frothy sputum Peripheral edema Decreased SpO_2 Hypertension or hypotension Crackles (rales) may be heard without a stethoscope, or may require auscultation of the lungs; may be present in both lungs, beginning at the bases Some wheezing may be heard	Malaise Loss of appetite Fever (may not always occur) Chills Dyspnea Cough (productive or nonproductive) Green, yellow, or rust-colored sputum Altered mental status (especially in the elderly) Tachypnea Decreased SpO_2 Localized crackles (rales) Wheezing and rhonchi in affected lung Decreased lung sounds over affected area May complain of pleuritic chest pain Diaphoresis and cyanosis may occur
Management	Oxygen, assist ventilations if needed, CPAP may be useful Start IV at a keep-open rate Nitroglycerin may be ordered by medical direction Medical direction may order a nebulized bronchodilator if wheezing is significant	Oxygen Assist ventilations if needed IV fluids for dehydration Medical direction may order a nebulized bronchodilator for significant wheezing

Patients with pneumonia tend to be dehydrated and need fluids, whereas patients with pulmonary edema have fluid overload (actually, redistribution of fluids to the lungs), which will be aggravated by aggressive fluid resuscitation.

IN THE FIELD

Patients sometimes complain to EMS providers that their physician refused to prescribe antibiotics for them or for their children for earaches, sore throats, or respiratory infections. Although antibiotics used to be prescribed indiscriminately for such complaints, this is no longer considered acceptable medical practice. Antibiotics are ineffective against the viruses that cause so many upper and lower respiratory infections and their associated complaints. Widespread use of antibiotics (medically and agriculturally) has led to antibiotic-resistant strains of a number of bacterial infections.

In both cases, your protocol may allow you to treat wheezing caused by bronchospasm with an inhaled beta$_2$ agonist. However, by failing to identify cardiogenic pulmonary edema, the patient may not receive the benefit of treatment with nitroglycerin in the field. Nitroglycerin, however, may cause hypotension in the fluid-depleted patient with pneumonia.

Acute Bronchitis

Acute bronchitis causes inflammation of the bronchi, with increased mucus production. The presence of mucus in the larger airways produces the rhonchi characteristically heard on auscultation of the lungs. Although anyone can get bronchitis, smokers and patients with lung disease are at increased risk. Acute bronchitis can be caused by viruses (including influenza), bacteria, and irritants.

Patients with acute bronchitis may experience wheezing, coughing, shortness of breath, fever, chills, and malaise.

The cough is typically productive and sputum may be yellow, green, or streaked with blood.

Provide oxygen to treat dyspnea and hypoxia. Patients who are wheezing may benefit from a nebulized bronchodilator, as allowed by protocol or in consultation with medical direction. IV fluids may be beneficial for patients who are dehydrated due to fever or decreased fluid intake.

Viral Respiratory Diseases

Influenza, SARS, and HPS (Table 20-7) are all viral diseases that can lead to death from hypoxia. In most people, most strains of influenza are unpleasant, but not life threatening. However, influenza can be fatal in susceptible patients.

Widespread influenza vaccination is important not only for preventing influenza in individuals, but also for producing herd immunity. Herd immunity means that if the majority of people are vaccinated, the chances of an infected person and an unimmunized person coming into contact with each other are greatly reduced.

Influenza vaccinations are different each year, based on the three strains of influenza predicted to be most prevalent in a given year. Immunization begins in September and it is recommended that individuals be vaccinated as early as possible. However, even as late as February, vaccination can still be beneficial.

Lung Cancer

Lung cancer is a common and deadly disease, with 222,520 new cases and 157,300 deaths predicted in 2010 (National Cancer Institute, 2010). The primary cause of lung cancer is smoking, although some types of lung cancer are a result of occupational exposure to asbestos and some have an underlying genetic predisposition. Exposure to radon gas and air pollution also can play a role. Radon gas is produced from the natural decay of uranium in the soil. It seeps into homes through cracks in the foundation and can accumulate. Inexpensive radon detection kits are available, and vent pipe systems can be installed to reduce radon levels.

Lung cancer is often not diagnosed early enough for a cure. The five-year survival rate after diagnosis is just 15.8 percent, in part due to the presence of few signs and symptoms until the disease has progressed.

There are two types of lung cancer: small cell and non-small cell. Small cell lung cancer is less common (13 percent of cases) but spreads very quickly. Non-small-cell lung cancer accounts for the remaining 87 percent of cases.

A patient may inform you of what stage his cancer is in. Staging is based on the degree to which the cancer has metastasized. Stages of lung cancer range from stage 0, in which the cancerous cells are localized to the innermost

TABLE 20-7 Influenza, SARS, and HPS

Feature	Influenza	SARS	HPS
Cause	Any one of several influenza viruses	A corona virus	Hantavirus
Description	Common and seasonal, may affect anyone but the very young, elderly, pregnant women, immunocompromised, and health care providers are at increased risk Can be prevented through immunization	An outbreak that likely originated in China resulted in an outbreak in North America (Toronto) in 2002–2003 but no community-acquired cases have been reported since However, during that time there were 8,000 cases with an approximately 10 percent mortality rate Not known if another outbreak could occur Most patients have a known history of contact with a SARS-infected individual	Also called *sin nombre* (no name) virus Virus contracted through airborne dust-containing rodent saliva or dropping particles Rare Most cases have occurred in the Four Corners region of the United States, with a mortality rate of 37 percent
Signs and symptoms	Usually mild, but can be severe, leading to pneumonia in some cases Malaise, fever, muscle and joint pain, cough	Fever and pneumonia	Signs and symptoms occur in two stages Early-stage symptoms are difficult to distinguish from those of influenza In second stage, the cardiopulmonary stage, pulmonary edema (ARDS), shock, and multiple organ failure may occur
Treatment	Oxygen and assisted ventilation if indicated IV fluids for dehydration	Use respiratory droplet precautions when dealing with suspected cases Treat hypoxia and respiratory distress IV fluids for dehydration	Patient may require aggressive respiratory resuscitation

lining of the lung and have not spread, to stage IV, in which the cancer has metastasized to distant organs. Lung cancer most often spreads to the lymph nodes, brain, adrenal glands, liver, and bones.

You may be involved in transporting a cancer patient for chemotherapy or radiation treatments, or you may respond to an emergency involving dyspnea or another aspect of the disease. Dyspnea may be caused by the obstruction of bronchi and destruction of lung tissue associated with tumors of the lung. However, a sudden increase in dyspnea may be the result of a pneumothorax. Often, but not always, this sudden increase in dyspnea follows an episode of coughing. Pulmonary effusion (collection of fluid in the thoracic cavity) also causes dyspnea, and lung cancer increases the risk of pulmonary embolism.

Patients may have respiratory depression and hypotension caused by high doses of potent narcotic medications. Cancer patients also may suffer a variety of other problems related to the progression of the disease. Behavioral changes may be due to brain metastasis, hypoxia, or side effects of medications. Pathological fractures may occur as a result of bone metastasis. Cancer results in hypercoagulability, which increases the risk for pulmonary embolism. Patients undergoing chemotherapy often experience severe nausea and vomiting and may become dehydrated. Patients with cancer are often thin and frail, and must be handled gently.

You will often be dealing with issues of death and dying involving lung cancer patients and their families. The patient and family members may be in different stages of the grieving process, ranging from denial to bargaining, to anger to depression, and acceptance. (See Chapter 9.) Patients may be receiving hospice care at home and may have a do-not-resuscitate (DNR) order. (Review Chapter 4.)

Cystic Fibrosis

Cystic fibrosis (CF) is a relatively rare (affecting 30,000 people in the United States) genetic disease of the secretory glands (Cystic Fibrosis Foundation, 2009). Many organs are affected, including the lungs and digestive tract. The presence of two defective genes, one inherited from each parent, results in the production of extremely viscous mucus. In the respiratory tract, the thick secretions can obstruct the airways and lead to life-threatening infection. In the pancreas, mucus blocks the ducts of the exocrine glands that secrete digestive enzymes into the digestive tract.

Until recent years, patients with CF died as children or very early in adulthood. Advances in treatment are allowing CF patients to live into middle age, meaning it is no longer a disease that affects only children. The median life expectancy for patients with CF is in the mid-30s (Cystic Fibrosis Foundation, 2009). Some patients now survive into their 40s and 50s.

You are most likely to encounter CF patients with an acute respiratory emergency, but they are also prone to electrolyte disturbances, bowel obstruction, pancreatitis, dehydration, osteoporosis, and diabetes.

Treat the patient for his signs and symptoms. Administering oxygen without humidification may aggravate the tenacious mucus in the lungs, making it harder to expectorate. However, do not withhold oxygen. IV fluids may assist in hydrating the mucus. Consult with medical direction for the type of fluid and rate of administration. CPAP may be useful for patients with impending respiratory failure (Leder & Dorkin, 2010). Administer a nebulized bronchodilator for wheezing, if allowed by medical direction.

CASE STUDY WRAP-UP

Clinical-Reasoning Process

Advanced EMTs Toby Marshall and Brent Croft are providing care for Mr. Emerson, a 60-year-old with a history of COPD who presents today with respiratory distress, fever, confusion, and a productive cough. Mr. Emerson is severely hypoxic; his breath sounds include wheezes, rhonchi, and crackles (rales); and he has bilateral pedal edema.

Toby and Brent realize that they must immediately begin to correct Mr. Emerson's hypoxia. They administer oxygen by nonrebreather mask, with plans to start an albuterol treatment for the bronchospasm indicated by wheezing.

Toby knows that he must carefully observe Mr. Emerson for signs of respiratory failure and be ready to intervene. En route to the hospital, while Mr. Emerson is receiving an albuterol treatment by small-volume nebulizer, Toby starts an IV of normal saline at 30 mL/hour.

Once the albuterol treatment is finished, Mr. Emerson's wheezing is reduced, but he remains short of breath with rhonchi and crackles (rales). Despite oxygen and the albuterol treatment, his SpO$_2$ is 87 percent, and he is becoming more exhausted. Toby begins treatment with CPAP and notifies the hospital emergency department of Mr. Emerson's condition. He continues to reassess Mr. Emerson's condition en route.

CHAPTER REVIEW

Chapter Summary

Acute and chronic respiratory problems can be life threatening because of impaired ventilation and oxygenation. Respiratory distress can quickly progress to respiratory failure and respiratory arrest as the underlying problem progresses and the patient becomes exhausted, hypoxic, and acidotic.

Problems include COPD and lung cancer, which are highly associated with smoking, as well as asthma, pulmonary edema, hyperventilation syndrome, infectious diseases, and cystic fibrosis.

Your ability to recognize signs and symptoms, obtain a relevant history, and develop a clinical impression of the problem are important in deciding how to best manage the patient. Quick recognition of the patient's level of distress and intervention to restore and maintain ventilation and oxygenation can be life saving.

In some cases, you will administer specific treatments, such as bronchodilators, aimed at treating the underlying cause of respiratory distress. In all cases, your ability to empathize and calmly interact with the patient is critical.

Review Questions

Multiple-Choice Questions

1. The reason sympathetic beta$_2$ agonists are indicated in asthma is because they:
   a. reduce inflammation.
   b. increase expectoration.
   c. relax bronchiolar smooth muscle.
   d. stimulate respiratory drive.

2. An average-size adult who has taken a narcotic overdose has a tidal volume of 250 mL. The amount of air reaching the alveoli for gas exchange is about _____ mL.
   a. 250
   b. 200
   c. 150
   d. 100

3. The primary chemical stimulus to breathe is a(n) _____ level.
   a. increased carbon dioxide
   b. decreased carbon dioxide
   c. increased carbon dioxide
   d. decreased oxygen

4. The most important medication for any patient with respiratory distress is:
   a. albuterol.
   b. ipatroprium.
   c. oxygen.
   d. epinephrine.

5. COPD includes which one of the following conditions?
   a. Emphysema, chronic bronchitis
   b. Acute bronchitis, chronic bronchitis
   c. Emphysema, cystic fibrosis
   d. Asthma, cystic fibrosis

6. The two components of asthma are:
   a. infection and inflammation.
   b. infection and bronchospasm.
   c. inflammation and bronchospasm.
   d. loss of alveolar surface area and bronchospasm.

7. Which one of the following best describes the underlying problem in cystic fibrosis?
   a. Secretion of thick, sticky mucus
   b. Smooth muscle spasms
   c. Abnormal cell growth
   d. Exposure to toxins

8. Which one of the following would you expect in the early stages of a pulmonary embolism?
   a. Absent breath sounds on the affected side
   b. Fever
   c. Sudden onset of dyspnea
   d. Rhonchi

9. The primary cause of lung cancer is:
   a. asbestos exposure.
   b. smoking.
   c. genetic.
   d. radon gas.

10. Which one of the following is contraindicated in suspected pneumothorax?
    a. Oxygen by nonrebreather mask
    b. Nitrous oxide
    c. IV fluids
    d. Bag-valve-mask device

Critical-Thinking Questions

11. How would you recognize a patient with a tension pneumothorax?

12. What are some risk factors for pulmonary embolism?

13. What are some circumstances in which you would suspect noncardiogenic pulmonary edema?

14. Compare and contrast expected findings in cardiogenic pulmonary edema and pneumonia.

References

American Lung Association. (2010a). *Asthma*. Retrieved September 28, 2010, from http//www.lungusa.org/lung-disease/asthma/resources/facts-and-figures/asthma-children-fact-sheet.html

American Lung Association. (2010b). *COPD*. Retrieved September 28, 2010, from http//www.lungusa.org/lung-disease/copd/resources/facts-figures/COPD-Fact-Sheet.html

Cystic Fibrosis Foundation. (2009). *About CR*. Retrieved October 7, 2010 from http://www.cff.org/AboutCF/

Fayyaz, J., Hmidi, A., Nascimento, J., Olade, R. B., & Lessnau, K. D. (2010). *Bronchitis*. Retrieved September 28, 2010, from http://emedicine.medscape.com/article/297108-overview Bronchitis

Kern, B., & Rosh, A. J. (2009). Hyperventilation syndrome. *e-medicine*. Retrieved September 27, 2010, from http://emedicine.medscape.com/article/807277-overview

Leder, E., & Dorkin, H. (2010). Chapter 99: Emergencies in cystic fibrosis. In G.R. Fleisher & S. Ludwig (Eds.), *Textbook of pediatric emergency medicine* (6th ed.). Philadelphia: Lippincott, Williams, & Wilkins.

Martini, F. H., Bartholomew, E. F., & Bledsoe, B. E. (2008). *Anatomy and physiology for emergency care* (2nd ed.). Upper Saddle River, NJ: Pearson.

McSwain, N.E., Salomone, J., & Pons, P. T. (Eds.). (2007). *Prehospital trauma life support* (6th ed.). St. Louis, MO: Elsevier.

Mullen, W. H. (2007). Toxin-related non-cardiogenic pulmonary edema. *American College of Chest Physicians*. Retrieved September 29, 2010, from http://www.chestnet.org/accp/pccsu/toxin-related-noncardiogenic-pulmonary-edema?page=0,3

National Cancer Institute. (2010). *Lung cancer*. Retrieved October 7, 2010, from http://www.cancer.gov/cancertopics/wyntk/lung/

National Heart, Lung, and Blood Institute. (2010a). *COPD*. Retrieved September 29, 2010, from http://www.nhlbi.nih.gov/health/dci/Diseases/Copd/Copd_WhatIs.html

National Heart, Lung, and Blood Institute. (2010b). *Asthma*. Retrieved September 29, 2010, from http://www.nhlbi.nih.gov/health/dci/Diseases/Asthma/Asthma_Causes.html

Sutherland, S.F. (2010). Pulmonary embolism. *Medscape Reference*. Retrieved September 29, 2010, from http://emedicine.medscape.com/article/759765-overview

21

Cardiovascular Disorders

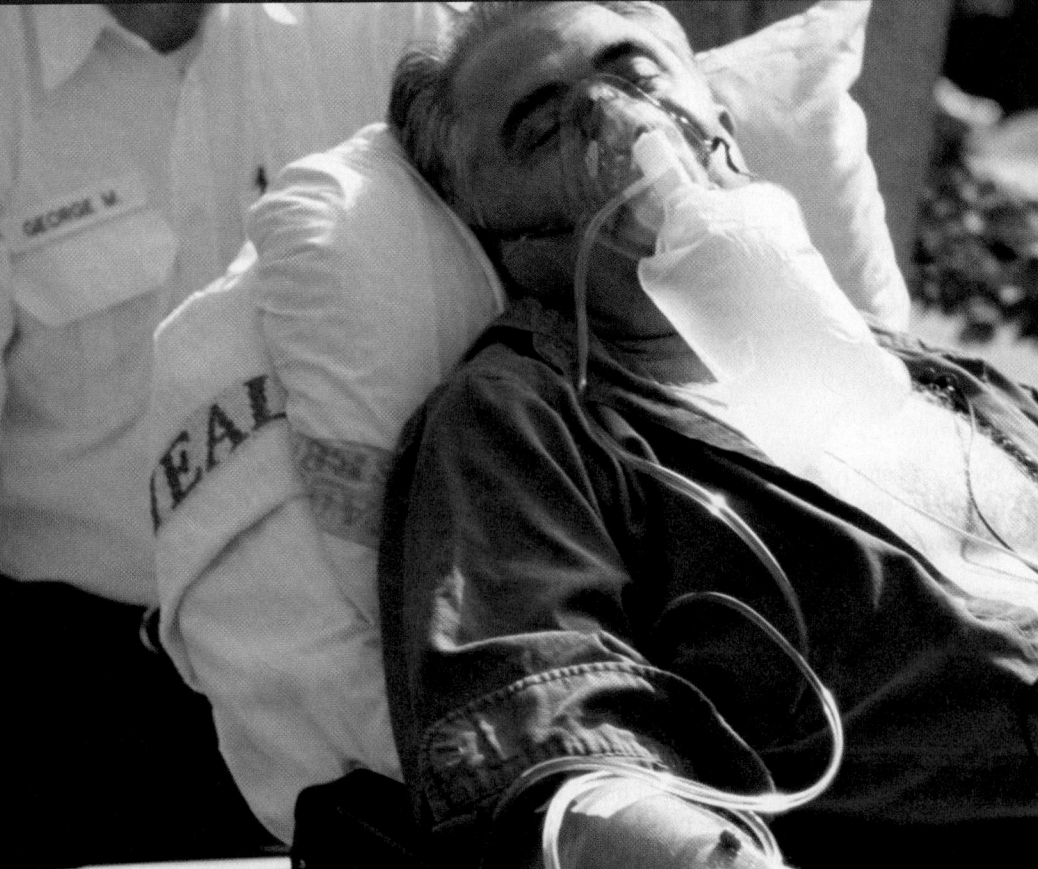

Content Area: Medicine

Advanced EMT Education Standard: Applies fundamental knowledge to provide basic and selected advanced emergency care and transportation based on assessment findings for an acutely ill patient.

Objectives

After reading this chapter, you should be able to:

21.1 Define key terms introduced in this chapter.

21.2 Explain the relationship between electrical and mechanical events in the heart.

21.3 Describe the processes of depolarization, repolarization, and the flow of electricity through the cardiac conduction system.

21.4 Relate the waves and intervals of a normal Lead II ECG to the physiologic events they represent.

21.5 Discuss the relationship between hypoxia, damage to the cardiac conduction system, premature ventricular contractions, ventricular tachycardia, and ventricular fibrillation.

(continued)

Resource**Central**

To access Resource Central, follow the directions on the Student Access Card provided with this text. If there is no card, go to www.bradybooks.com and follow the Resource Central link to Buy Access. Under Media Resources, you will find:

- *Ischemic Heart Disease.* Learn about it and how to reduce your risk.

- *American Heart Association (AHA).* Discover the AHA's role in the prevention, treatment, and education of patients, families, and health care professionals.

- *The 12-Lead ECG.* Understand the importance of prehospital 12-lead ECGs.

CASE STUDY

Rusty Kypers is sitting in his favorite recliner searching for an early morning program on his television to watch while he enjoys the sausage and pancakes his wife makes every Sunday. As he decides on a recap of the week's hockey, he has a sudden jolt of pain in his jaw. He opens wide, as though giving half a yawn, to stretch the muscle, with no relief. He then feels as though a pickup truck hit him head-on and pinned him against a wall. As he tries to breathe, he drops his plate to the ground and clutches his chest. He starts thinking about the first time he held his newborn daughter in the hospital. He wonders if he will die as he yells for his wife. "Laura, help me," he calls, as he plunges to the floor, unable to catch himself.

Laura rushes in from the kitchen. "Rusty, what's happening?"

"Call 911," he says, "I think I'm dying."

Within minutes, the emergency response team arrives at the door. Advanced EMTs Will Rose and Justin Dobbs hear Laura's calls and enter the house. Making their way to the living room, they find Rusty lying on his back with his neck propped against a recliner. Rusty watches them approach and they hear him utter, "Help me, I'm having a heart attack."

"We're here to help you," says Will. "What happened?" he asks, as Justin opens his supply bag to get a pulse oximeter.

Problem-Solving Questions

1. What specific questions should Will and Justin ask to determine the problem?
2. What treatments should the patient receive in the prehospital setting?
3. What are the considerations in deciding how to transport the patient, and to what hospital?

(continued from previous page)

21.6   Describe the roles of the heart and blood vessels in maintaining normal blood pressure, including the concepts of cardiac output and systemic vascular resistance.

21.7   Explain the importance of early recognition of signs and symptoms, and early treatment of patients with cardiac emergencies.

21.8   Explain the pathophysiology of the following:
   - Acute coronary syndrome, including classic and unstable angina pectoris and myocardial infarction
   - Aortic aneurysm and dissection
   - Atherosclerosis
   - Cardiac arrest
   - Hypertension
   - Left- and right-sided heart failure
   - Cardiogenic shock

21.9   Recognize cardiac emergency patients with both typical and atypical presentations.

21.10   Differentiate between patients with adequate perfusion and patients with inadequate perfusion.

21.11   Explain the importance of managing the airway, breathing, and circulation in patients with cardiac problems.

21.12   Explain the indications, contraindications, mechanism of action, side effects, dosage, and administration of the following in the context of a cardiac emergency:
   - Aspirin
   - Nitroglycerin
   - Nitrous oxide
   - Oxygen

21.13 Given a series of scenarios, demonstrate the management of a variety of patients with cardiovascular emergencies, including the following:
- Angina pectoris
- Aortic aneurysm or dissection
- Cardiac arrest (including CPR and AED use)
- Cardiogenic shock
- Congestive heart failure
- Hypertensive emergencies
- Myocardial infarction

21.14 Discuss the purpose of fibrinolytic therapy and percutaneous coronary interventions (PCIs) in patients with cardiac emergencies.

21.15 Discuss considerations in requesting advanced life support personnel to transport patients with cardiovascular emergencies.

21.16 Describe the purpose of using CPAP in patients with pulmonary edema.

Introduction

The cardiovascular system transports oxygen, chemical messages, nutrients, and other important substances throughout the body, and transports waste products to the organs designed to eliminate them. The heart is a strong and resilient muscle, capable of carrying out tremendous work, but also is prone to life-threatening diseases. The heart pumps blood, a complex liquid transportation medium, through a series of blood vessels to the lungs and tissues of the body, and back to the heart. Anything that interferes with the ability of the heart and blood vessels to transport blood to and from the tissues compromises the ability of the body to function.

Advanced EMTs can make a significant difference for patients with cardiovascular emergencies by quickly recognizing signs and symptoms of cardiovascular emergencies and providing prompt treatment. Treatment of those emergencies includes administering medications, and transporting the patient to a hospital equipped to provide definite cardiac care.

Understanding the anatomy and physiology of the heart and the pathophysiology of cardiovascular diseases is essential to identifying and managing patients with cardiovascular emergencies. This chapter begins by reviewing the anatomy and physiology of the cardiovascular system and introducing cardiac electrophysiology. Explanation of the pathophysiology, assessment, and management of cardiovascular emergencies follows the anatomy review.

Anatomy and Physiology Review

The heart lies in the mediastinum, in the center of the chest. Its apex (lowest end) is tilted toward the left, and the right side is rotated slightly anteriorly (Figure 21-1). The heart is

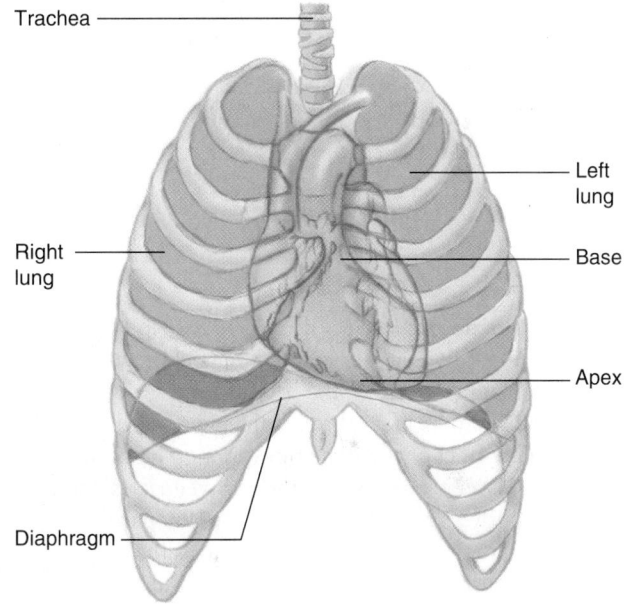

Trachea
Right lung
Left lung
Base
Apex
Diaphragm

FIGURE 21-1

Position of the heart in the chest.

a hollow, muscular organ with four chambers (Figure 21-2). The two upper chambers are called *atria* (singular, *atrium*) and the two lower chambers are called the *ventricles*.

The specialized muscle is called *myocardium*. The electrical properties of myocardium allow the heart to beat on its own. A smooth layer called *endocardium* lines the chambers of the heart, allowing blood to flow smoothly through it.

A double-walled sac surrounds the heart. The inner layer of the sac, which adheres to the myocardium, is called the *epicardium* (or visceral pericardium). The outer, fibrous layer is the *pericardium*. Normally, about 15 to 50 mL of pericardial fluid is present within the pericardial sac to allow frictionless movement of the heart with each heartbeat.

FIGURE 21-2

Cross section of the heart.

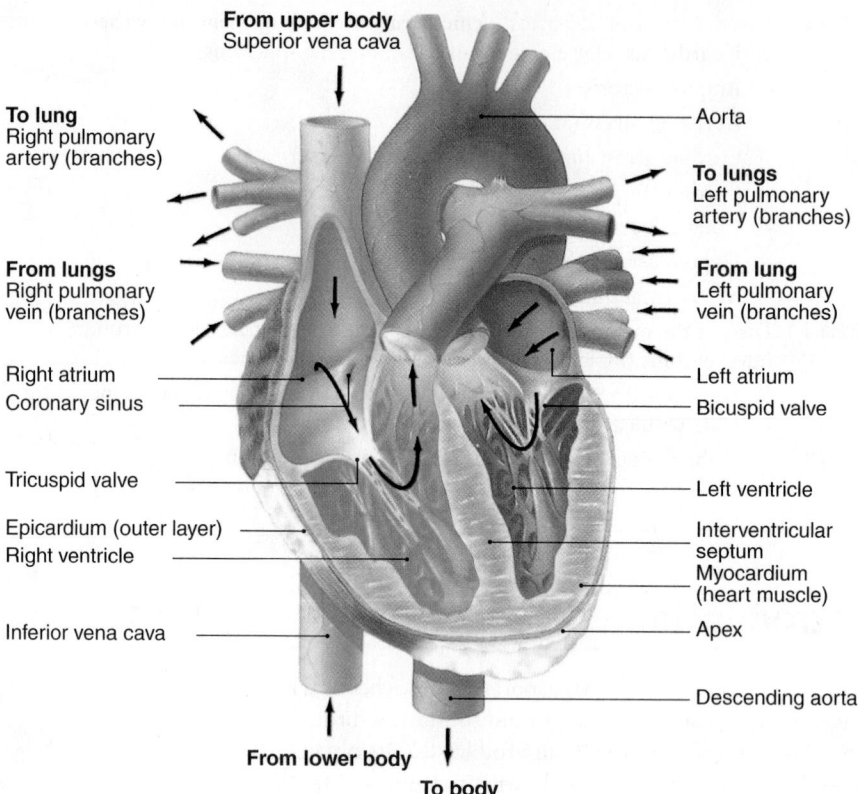

The right atrium receives deoxygenated blood from the systemic circulation via the superior vena cava and inferior vena cava. Simultaneously, the left atrium receives oxygenated blood from the lungs through the pulmonary vein. The two atria contract at the same time, forcing blood into the ventricles. After a brief pause, the two ventricles contract simultaneously, forcing blood into the pulmonary and systemic circulation. Oxygenated blood leaves the more muscular left ventricle through the aorta, and deoxygenated blood from the right ventricle enters the pulmonary artery and travels to the lungs.

Four valves work to maintain forward flow of blood through the heart: the aortic semilunar valve, the pulmonary semilunar valve, the bicuspid (mitral) valve, and the tricuspid valve. The aortic semilunar valve is situated in the left ventricle at the entrance to the aorta. It closes immediately after blood is ejected from the ventricle to prevent it from flowing back into the heart. Though the aortic valve is open as the ventricle contracts (systole), its flaps cover the entrance of the coronary arteries. When the aortic valve closes during ventricular relaxation (diastole), blood from the aorta flows into the coronary arteries to perfuse them.

The pulmonary semilunar valve is at the junction of the right ventricle and pulmonary artery, where it prevents backflow of blood following right ventricular systole.

The bicuspid, or mitral, valve sits between the left atrium and ventricle. It is open during diastole to allow passive filling of the ventricle as blood enters the atrium. The valve remains open as the atria contract to complete ventricular filling. The valve then closes so that blood is not forced backward into the atrium (retrograde blood flow) when the left ventricle contracts.

The tricuspid valve is situated between the right atrium and ventricle. Its role is very similar to that of the bicuspid valve, preventing retrograde bloodflow into the right atrium during right ventricular systole. Improperly functioning valves impair *cardiac output*. A valve that does not open properly narrows the pathway for bloodflow (stenosis), which restricts the forward flow of blood through the heart. A valve that does not close properly allows regurgitation (backflow) of blood.

Coronary Circulation

The heart muscle requires a constant supply of oxygenated blood to do its work. Even though the heart chambers fill with blood, none of this blood reaches the heart muscle itself. Instead, two coronary arteries immediately branch from the aorta as it leaves the left ventricle, and extend along the surface of the heart. They are the right and left coronary arteries (Figure 21-3). Those two arteries branch many times to supply the myocardium with oxygenated blood. When the aortic valve opens during ventricular systole (contraction), its cusps (flaps) cover the opening of the coronary arteries. During diastole (relaxation), the aortic valve closes, allowing blood from the aorta to enter the

FIGURE 21-3

The coronary arteries.

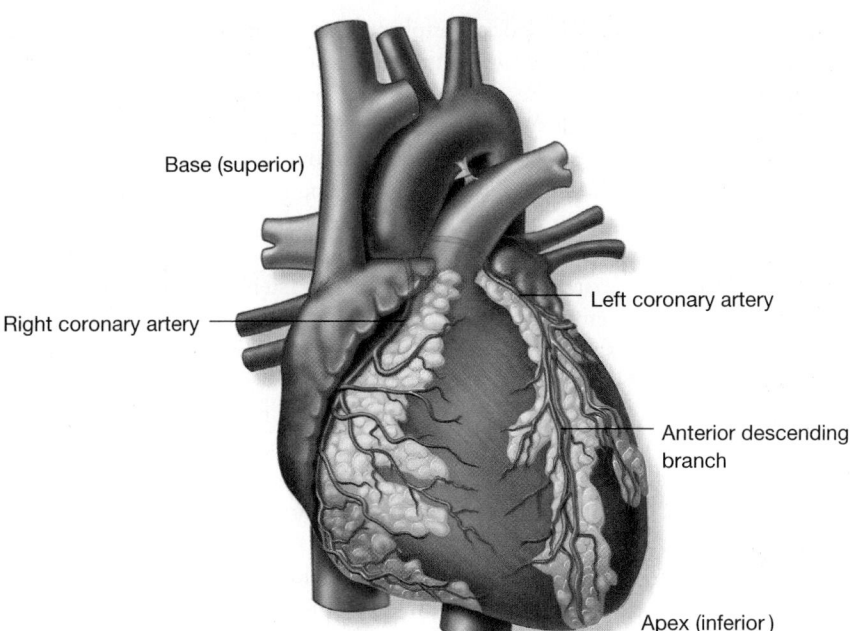

coronary arteries. After circulating through capillaries at the cellular level of the myocardium, blood flows through the coronary veins and empties into the right atrium through an expanded portion of vein, the coronary sinus.

Any obstruction to coronary blood flow deprives the affected area of oxygen, resulting in *ischemia*. Ischemia impairs the function of the heart and typically causes pain. If not quickly relieved, ischemia leads to injury of the myocardial cells. If perfusion to the cardiac tissue is not restored, infarction, or death, of that portion of the myocardium occurs. The degree to which overall heart function is affected depends on the location and extent of the myocardial infarction.

The Vascular System and Blood

The blood vessels are collectively known as the *vasculature*. The vascular system is comprised of three types of vessels: arteries, veins, and capillaries (Figure 21-4). Arteries are thick-walled vessels designed to carry the higher-pressure blood leaving the heart. They consist of three layers, or coats. There is a smooth inner lining of endothelium (tunica intima), a middle layer of smooth muscle (tunica media), and an outer layer of fibrous and elastic tissue (tunica externa, or tunica adventitia). A thin membrane, the elastic lamina, lies between the endothelial cells and the smooth muscle layer. Arteries have varying relative amounts of

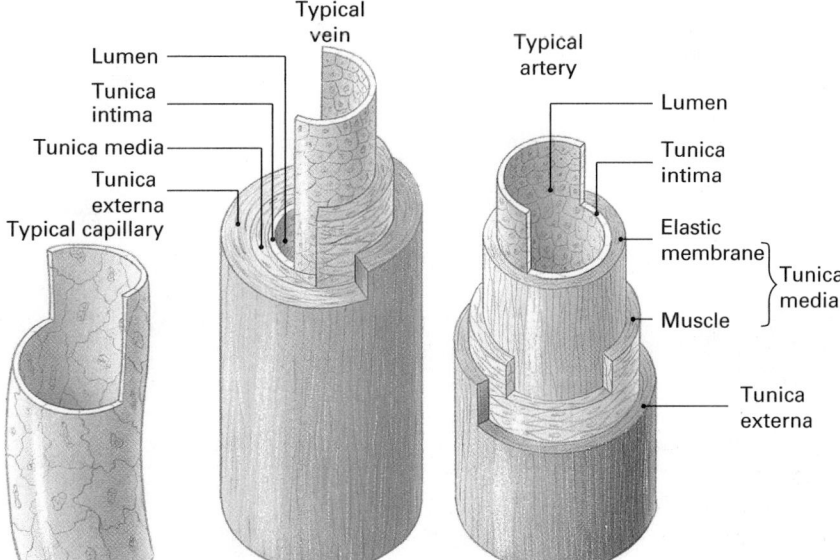

FIGURE 21-4

Layers of the blood vessels.

elastic and smooth muscle tissue. For example, the largest artery, the aorta, is elastic, but has little ability to constrict.

Arterioles, the smallest arteries, have more smooth muscle tissue, allowing them to constrict and dilate. The ability of arterioles to constrict and dilate is key in the control of blood pressure and tissue perfusion.

The aorta, which receives oxygenated blood from the left ventricle of the heart, has major branches supplying the upper body, thoracic and abdominal organs, and lower extremities. Each of the branches divides into smaller and smaller branches. The smallest branches, the arterioles, enter capillary networks, or beds.

Capillaries are microscopic blood vessels that are a single cell-layer thick, with a diameter just wide enough to admit red blood cells in single file. Each cell of the body must be in close enough proximity to a capillary to receive the oxygen that diffuses from red blood cells, through the thin capillary wall, and into the interstitial fluid surrounding the cell. Carbon dioxide and other cellular wastes diffuse in the opposite direction, out of the cell, into the interstitial fluid, and into the capillaries.

Capillary beds converge to form tiny veins, called *venules.* Venules converge into veins, which merge into larger and larger veins. The largest veins, the inferior and superior vena cavae, empty back into the right atrium. Veins also have three layers, but are thinner-walled overall. Because blood in the veins is under low pressure, and mostly traveling against gravity, veins contain valves that prevent backflow of blood. Contraction of skeletal muscle also increases venous return.

Circulation through the aorta to the body, and back to the heart through the vena cavae, is called the *systemic circulation.* The part of the systemic circulation closer to the surface of the body, such as blood vessels in the skin, fatty tissue, and skeletal muscles, is called *peripheral circulation.* Blood in the large arteries and the supply of blood to the internal organs is called *central circulation.*

In shock, peripheral circulation is sacrificed to redirect blood to the central circulation. Reduced peripheral perfusion is responsible for the pale, cool skin associated with shock. Within the systemic circulation, veins of the gastrointestinal system enter the hepatic portal vein and travel through the liver before being returned to the general systemic venous system. The hepatic portal system allows the liver to process nutrients and drugs from the digestive system before they enter the systemic circulation. The systemic circulation also includes the bronchial arteries, which supply oxygen and nutrients to the lungs. A special type of circulation occurs between the mother and her developing fetus, which delivers oxygen and nutrients from the mother through the placenta. (See Chapter 43.)

The pulmonary circulation leaves the right side of the heart through the pulmonary artery and returns through the pulmonary veins. In the lungs, carbon dioxide is removed and oxygen is added to this blood. The pulmonary artery is the only artery in the body that carries unoxygenated blood away from the heart. The pulmonary veins are the only veins in the body that carry oxygenated blood to the heart.

Blood is a tissue that consists of a fluid medium called *plasma,* and three types of cells: red blood cells, white blood cells, and platelets (Figure 21-5). Plasma contains proteins, such as albumin and antibodies, and serves as a transportation medium for electrolytes, hormones, drugs, wastes, nutrients, and other substances. Unlike other cells, mature red blood cells do not have nuclei. The cells are flattened and indented on both sides.

Red blood cells contain *hemoglobin,* which is a molecule that consists of protein and iron. The configuration of hemoglobin allows it to bind to oxygen under the conditions in the pulmonary circulation, and to release oxygen under the conditions of the systemic capillary beds. Hemoglobin also carries some of the carbon dioxide released by tissue cells back to the lungs for elimination.

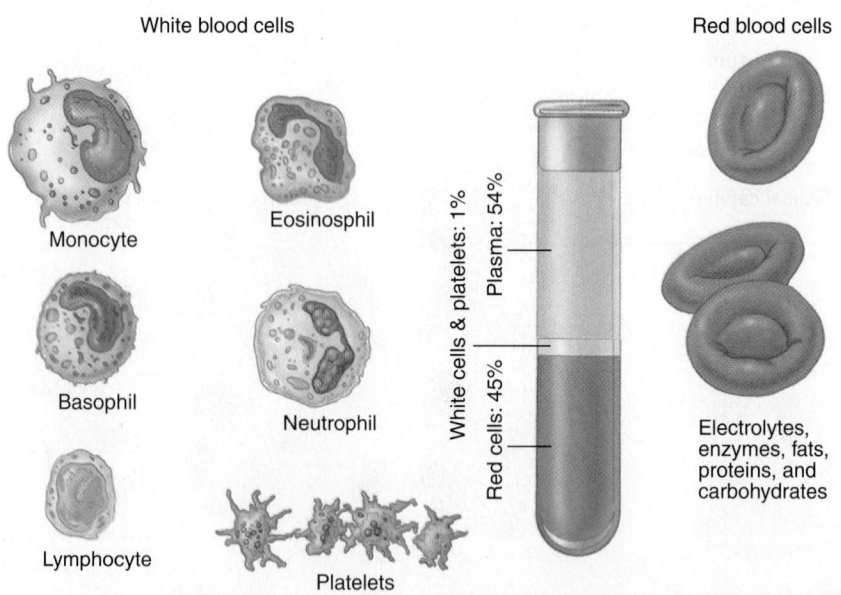

FIGURE 21-5

Components of the blood.

The several types of white blood cells are part of the immune system, functioning in various ways to protect the body from illness.

Platelets are a first line of defense in blood clotting. Under normal conditions, they simply move through the circulatory system. When a blood vessel is disrupted, chemical messages from the injured tissue cause a number of events that result in a clot being formed. One of the results is that platelets are activated. When activated, platelets are attracted to the injured area and secrete a substance that makes them "sticky." The activated platelets aggregate, or clump together, at the site of injury to form a temporary plug until a blood clot is formed.

Perfusion, Cardiac Output, and Blood Pressure

Perfusion, the circulation of oxygenated blood to the cells of the body (Figure 21-6), depends on adequate blood pressure (BP). Adequate blood pressure, in turn, depends on the volume of blood available, the output of blood from the heart, and the capacity of the blood vessels. There are four concepts that are important to understanding blood pressure, as follows:

- Mean arterial pressure (MAP)
- Stroke volume (SV)
- Cardiac output (CO)
- Systemic vascular resistance (SVR)

Mean arterial pressure (MAP) is a way of defining the overall average blood pressure at a given time. It is represented by diastolic blood pressure (DBP) + one third of the pulse pressure, which is the systolic blood pressure (SBP) − DBP, represented by the following equation:

$$MAP = 1/3 \ (SBP - DBP)$$

Blood pressure, represented by MAP, is calculated by the following equation:

$$MAP = CO \times SVP$$

Cardiac output (CO) is the volume of blood leaving the heart every minute, measured in liters per minute. It is determined by multiplying the volume of blood that leaves the heart with each contraction (SV) by the number of times the heart contracts each minute (HR). Cardiac output is represented by the following equation:

$$CO = SV \times HR$$

Stroke volume (SV) is determined by subtracting the amount of blood left in the left ventricle after contraction (end-systolic volume, or ESV), from the amount of blood that was in the left ventricle just before contraction (end-diastolic volume, or EDV). EDV is also called **preload**. Stroke volume is represented as follows:

$$SV = EDV - ESV$$

A measure of heart function is the **ejection fraction**, which is the SV expressed as a percentage of EDV. Even in healthy

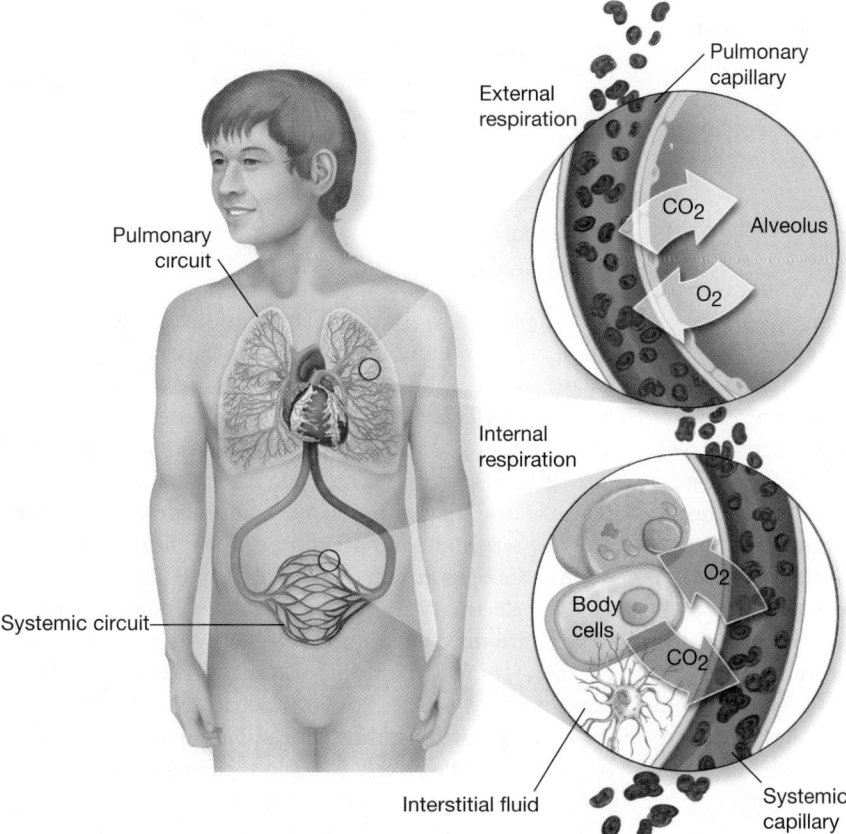

External respiration

Pulmonary capillary

Pulmonary circuit

CO_2

Alveolus

O_2

Internal respiration

Systemic circuit

Body cells

O_2

CO_2

Interstitial fluid

Systemic capillary

FIGURE 21-6

Overview of tissue perfusion.

hearts, not all of the EDV is ejected. Ejection fraction is typically 55 to 70 percent. Ejection fraction can be substantially reduced following myocardial infarction or in heart failure.

Systemic vascular resistance (SVR) is based on the diameter of small blood vessels at any given time. The more constricted the blood vessels, the smaller their diameter. The smaller the diameter, the more resistance there is to blood flow. The greater the resistance to blood flow, the higher the pressure within the vessels. The greater the pressure in the arterial system (afterload), the harder the heart must contract to force more blood into the system.

The exact measurement of blood pressure can only be done invasively, by placing a special catheter in an artery. Except in critical care settings, this is not feasible and the risk is not acceptable. Instead, an approximate measure of blood pressure is obtained using a sphygmomanometer and stethoscope, as discussed in Chapter 18. However, the concepts behind blood pressure are important to understanding what happens when we lose blood, the heart muscle is weak, the heart rate is too slow or too fast, or the diameter of blood vessels changes.

A healthy adult heart has an average stroke volume of 70 mL and a rate of 75 beats per minute. This means the cardiac output is 5,250 mL (5.25 L) per minute. Cardiac output can increase to almost 30 L/min in a trained athlete to perfuse the continually contracting muscles.

In a patient who is losing blood from a gunshot wound to the abdomen, there is less blood returning to the heart with each contraction. The preload drops in proportion to the amount of blood lost from the wound. If preload is decreased, then stroke volume is decreased, lowering cardiac output and blood pressure. To compensate, the nervous system responds by increasing the heart rate, which increases cardiac output, and by increasing systemic vascular resistance through vasoconstriction, which increases blood pressure. However, the compensatory mechanisms are limited.

During an **acute myocardial infarction (AMI)**, the ventricles may not contract properly. Stroke volume can decrease due to incomplete emptying of the ventricles. The effect can be profound enough to result in tachycardia and hypotension, called *cardiogenic shock.* It is often assumed that tachycardia in a patient with chest pain is the result of pain or anxiety. Keep in mind that tachycardia may be a physiologic response to reduced heart function.

A blood pressure measurement consists of the amount of pressure exerted against arterial walls at two different times. Systolic blood pressure is the pressure in the arteries at the time of cardiac contraction and *diastolic blood pressure* is the pressure that remains within the arteries after the heart has relaxed. The normal range for systolic blood pressure is 100 to 140 and for diastolic blood pressure it is 60 to 90.

When blood pressure is above the normal range, it is called *hypertension.* Sustained hypertension over time carries many health risks. The heart must work harder, causing the overworked ventricles to enlarge and weaken over time. The blood vessels are damaged from the increased pressure against the lining. Those changes can lead to kidney, heart, and peripheral vascular disease, as well as stroke. Low blood pressure is called *hypotension,* and can result in hypoperfusion of the tissues, or shock.

Cardiac Electrophysiology

The electrical activity of cardiac cells is designed to lead to mechanical contraction of the cardiac muscle, much as a power tool requires electricity for mechanical movement of its parts. The relatively small amount of electricity generated by the human body is measured in millivolts (mV). The electrical activity of the heart is conducted to the surface of the skin, where it is detected by electrodes and is represented on an ECG as a series of waves.

ECG tracings provide important information to health care providers about the function of the heart. Even when using an AED, it is the computerized analysis of the ECG that determines whether a shock is advised, even though the ECG tracing might not be displayed on a screen or printout that the provider can see.

There are three types of cardiac cells, as follows:

- Pacemaker cells
- Conductive cells
- Contractile cells

Those cells work together to produce each heartbeat. An electrical stimulus is generated in a pacemaker cell. Pacemaker cells have a property known as *automaticity,* meaning that they can generate electrical impulses on their own. The impulses generated by pacemaker cells are transmitted throughout the heart via the conductive cells to the contractile cells, resulting in mechanical contraction of the heart. The electrical stimulus normally begins at the **sinoatrial (SA) node** in the right atrium (Figure 21-7).

For electricity to move, or flow, from one cell to the next, there must be a difference between their electrical charges. The electrical impulse that travels through the heart is based on the flow of electrically charged chemical particles, or ions, through channels in cell membranes (Figure 21-8). Positively charged ions involved in cardiac function are sodium (Na^+), potassium (K^+), and calcium (Ca^{++}). The negatively charged ion is chloride (Cl^-). Cell

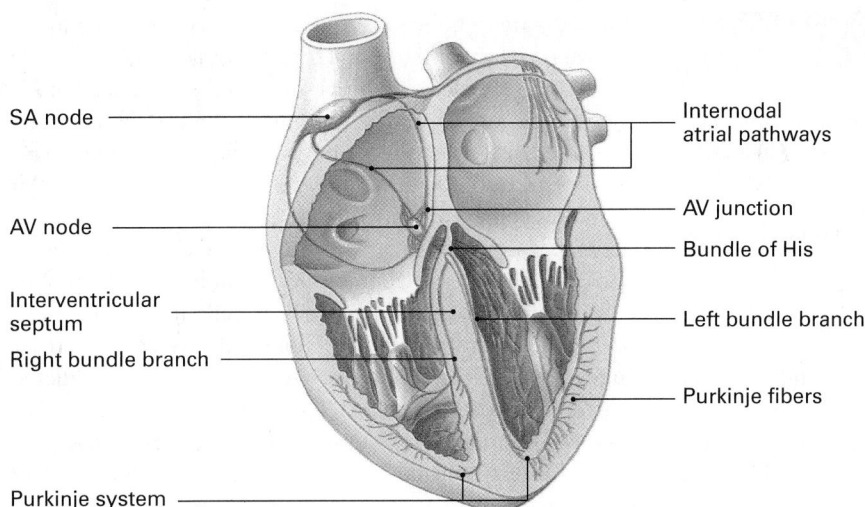

FIGURE 21-7

The cardiac conduction system.

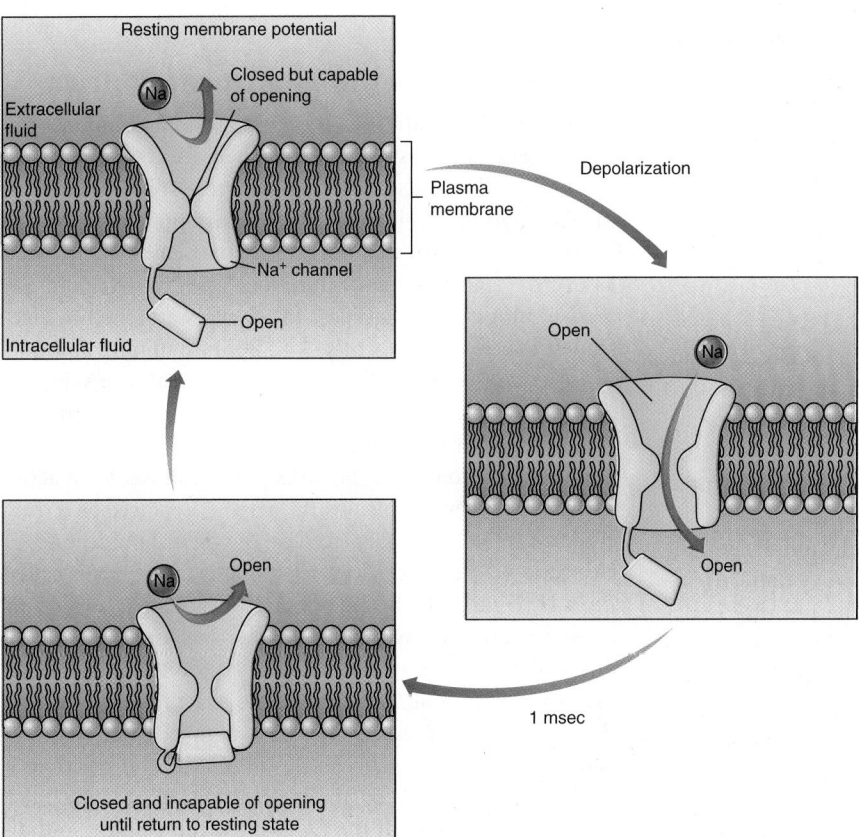

FIGURE 21-8

Cell membrane channels.

membrane channels open and close selectively to the ions at different times.

Electricity normally flows from areas in which the net (overall) charge is positive to areas where the net charge is negative, in an attempt to neutralize the difference, much like the concepts of fluid and solute movement discussed in Chapter 8. A difference in electrical charge on each side of a cell membrane is called *polarity*. When the cell membrane is polarized, there is a potential for electricity to flow across the membrane.

Action Potentials: The Electrical Cycle of the Heart

A repetitive cycle of electrical events is required to generate each heartbeat. The electrical cycle of the heart consists of depolarization and repolarization. Depolarization occurs when positively charged ions flow to a less-positively charged area until the electrical difference between the two areas becomes zero. In repolarization, the difference in charges is restored. Because ions must move against the typical direction of electrical flow, active cellular mechanisms (the sodium/potassium pump) that use energy in the form of ATP are required for repolarization and to maintain the polarized state (the resting potential) until the next depolarization. The waves of an ECG represent the flow of electricity in depolarization and repolarization.

Ca^{++} is required for muscle contraction. Its presence activates the contractile fiber system of cardiac cells, transforming the electrical activity of the heart into mechanical activity. When the contractile system is activated, the muscle fibers contract, and shorten. This action occurs simultaneously in a group of cells, causing them to contract as a unit. This allows the two atria to contract simultaneously, and the two ventricles to contract simultaneously.

Cardiac Pacemakers and Impulse Conduction

The SA node sets the normal, regular rate of electrical activity for the heart. It generates impulses, or "fires," 60 to 100 times per minute. This is its *intrinsic rate*. The rate can slow if the parasympathetic nervous system is stimulated, or it can speed up under the influence of the sympathetic nervous system.

Impulses from the SA node are conducted to the cells of the atria and to the **atrioventricular (AV) node**, at the junction of the atria and ventricles. The impulse is delayed slightly at the AV node to allow the atria time to contract and finish filling the ventricles before the ventricles are stimulated to contract. If the AV node is diseased, impulses may be delayed or blocked from being conducted to the ventricles. From the AV node, impulses are conducted through a pathway (the His–Purkinje system) that travels to the apex of the heart before transferring the impulse to the myocardial cells of the ventricles. This allows the ventricles to contract from the bottom (apex) of the heart up toward the aortic and pulmonic valves, directing blood flow into the aorta and pulmonary artery and aorta.

The AV node, and some cells in the ventricles, also display the property of automaticity. Because the intrinsic rate of the SA node is faster than the intrinsic rate of the "lower" pacemakers, they are normally kept from generating impulses. If the SA node is damaged or under excessive parasympathetic nervous system control via the vagus nerve, it may not generate impulses, or may generate them at a much slower rate. The lower pacemakers act as a backup or "escape" mechanism, but their rates are slower.

In the absence of an impulse from the SA node, the AV node has a rate of 40 to 60 per minute. In the absence of an impulse from either the SA or AV node, the ventricles have a rate of 20 to 40 per minute. Because AV and ventricular impulses come from different locations in the heart's electrical system, their configurations on the ECG are different.

Under some circumstances, such as ischemia or the influence of stimulants, other cells in the heart can demonstrate automaticity. Those cells are called **ectopic pacemakers**. Their impulses spread and are conducted through the rest of the cardiac conduction system. The ectopic impulse shows up as extra electrical activity on the ECG. Its unusual appearance indicates which part of the heart it came from. Ectopic impulses generally result in mechanical contraction of the heart. An individual may experience this as **palpitations**, a sensation of abnormal heartbeats in the chest.

Introduction to the Electrocardiogram

An electrocardiogram (ECG) is an important component of cardiac patient assessment. Although an ECG uses 12 leads, a subset of the leads is used in the prehospital setting for cardiac rhythm monitoring. The primary prehospital use of 12-lead ECGs is for diagnosis of cardiac emergencies such as myocardial ischemia, infarction, and dysrhythmias. A cardiac monitor uses at least three wires attached to electrodes placed on a patient's skin. Because minute amounts of electricity from cardiac impulses travel to the skin, the electrodes can capture and conduct the impulses to the cardiac monitor or ECG machine.

Cardiac monitoring involves looking at electrical activity from one view. Typically, the activity is viewed as it travels between an electrode placed on the right shoulder and an electrode placed on the lower left chest. This view is called *Lead II* (Figure 21-9). The primary purpose is to determine the heart rate and rhythm, pacemaker site, and the presence of any delay in conduction. A 12-lead (or 15-lead) ECG is used to look at multiple views of the heart to give information about the presence and location of myocardial ischemia and infarction, as well as changes in the size and position of the heart.

The waveforms of the ECG show the amount and direction of electricity being conducted through the heart as waves of different sizes, durations, and directions. The

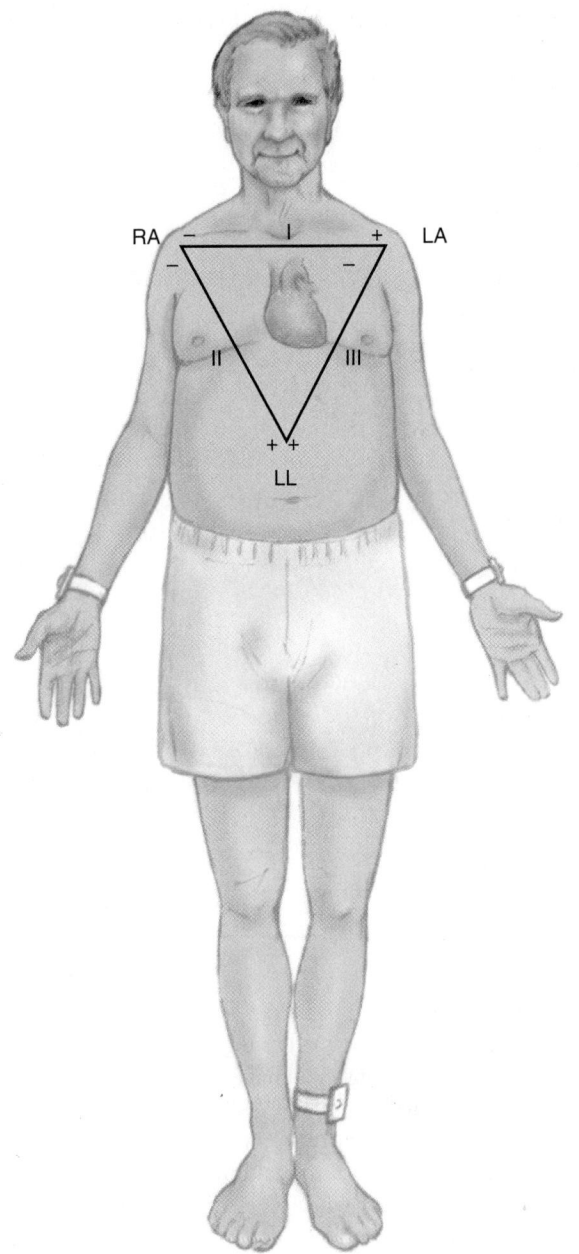

IN THE FIELD

Another way of determining the heart rate is by counting the number of 5-mm boxes between the same point on two consecutive ECG heartbeats. The rates for a distance of 1, 2, 3, 4, 5, and 6 boxes are 300, 150, 100, 75, 60, and 50, respectively.

IN THE FIELD

The electrical activity of the heart does not give information about the strength of cardiac contractions. Despite critical decreases in cardiac output—in some cases to zero—organized electrical activity can appear on the ECG. The ECG tells only part of the story. You must assess the mechanical activity of the heart by checking pulses, measuring blood pressure, and assessing other indications of perfusion.

FIGURE 21-9

The triangle formed by the three ECG monitoring leads is called *Einthoven's triangle.* Most prehospital ECG monitoring uses Lead II.

waves are assigned letters, and represent specific parts of the cardiac electrical cycle (Figure 21-10). Graph paper with a grid of 1-mm squares moves through the ECG machine at a standard rate of 25 mm/second. This allows the grid to serve as a basis for measuring the amount of electricity conducted (on the vertical axis) and the time it takes the impulse to travel through the heart (on the horizontal axis).

Certain measurements are helpful in the prehospital setting (Figure 21-11). On the horizontal axis, each 1-mm square is equal to 0.04 seconds. Heavier lines every 5 mm

are 0.20 seconds apart. Measurements that are helpful in understanding how the ECG relates to the cardiac cycle are as follows:

- *P wave:* Atrial depolarization.
- *P–R interval (PRI):* Length of time for the depolarization wave to travel through the atria and AV node, normally 0.12 to 0.20 seconds (three to five small boxes).
- *QRS complex:* Ventricular depolarization, normally less than 0.12 seconds (less than three small boxes).
- *T wave:* Ventricular repolarization (the small amount of energy involved in atrial repolarization is covered up by ventricular depolarization).

The expected rhythm of the heart is the normal sinus rhythm (NSR). Dysrhythmias are diagnosed by comparing their characteristics, or rules, to the rules of NSR. Figures 21-12, 21-13, and 21-14 provide the rules for NSR, and show sinus tachycardia and sinus bradycardia for comparison. Appendix 2 provides information on recognizing additional dysrhythmias.

General Assessment of Cardiovascular Complaints

Patients present with complaints, not diagnoses. It is important that you not jump immediately from the patient's complaint or initial presentation to a field impression. You must engage in clinical reasoning to develop a list of differential diagnoses and your ultimate field impression.

FIGURE 21-10

Relationship of cardiac electrical activity and ECG waves.

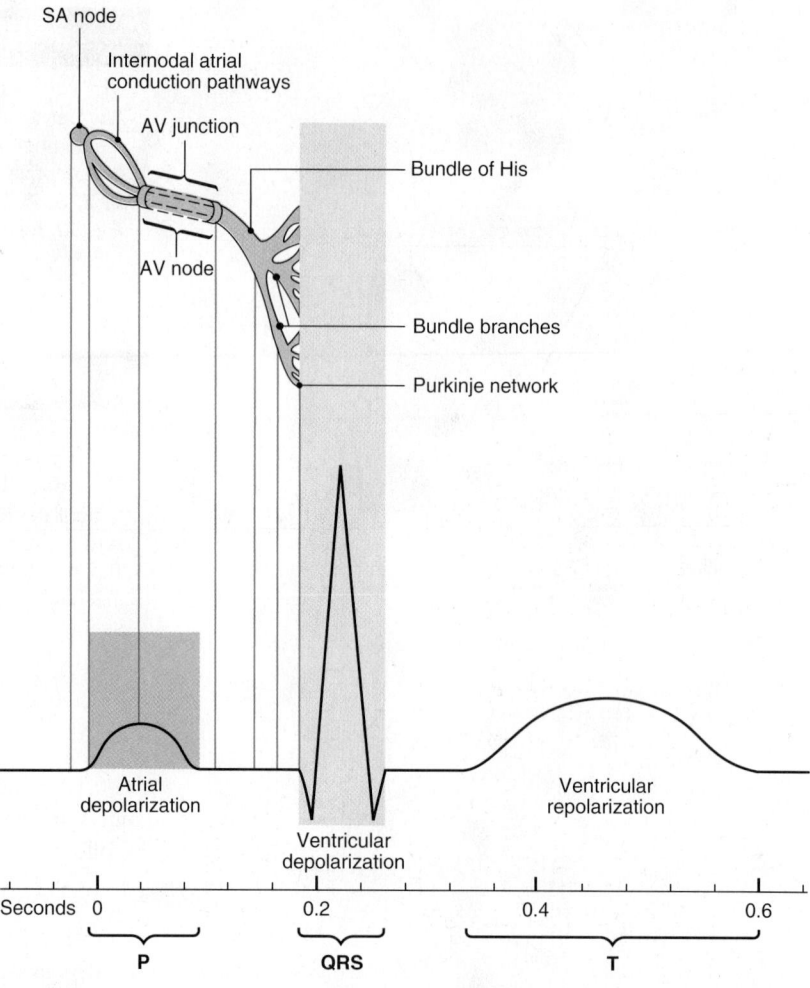

FIGURE 21-11

The waves, segments, and intervals used to interpret the ECG.

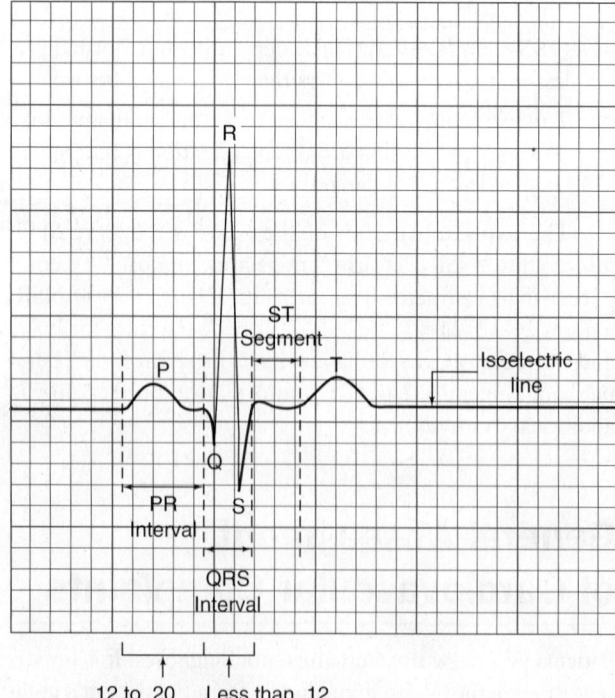

You will not know whether the patient is having a cardiovascular problem until you have collected more information about the chief complaint, as well as obtain a history and vital signs and perform a physical exam. The way in which you collect this additional information will be based on your knowledge of what types of problems are associated with different complaints. Most complaints are associated with more than one kind of problem.

General treatment begins even before forming a field impression, as part of the initial general impression obtained in the primary assessment. The approach to a responsive medical patient differs from the approach to an unresponsive medical patient. In either case, assess the airway and the need for assisted ventilation and oxygen. Get an idea of the adequacy of perfusion through the patient's general appearance and assessment of the pulse.

If an unresponsive patient is pulseless, begin resuscitation by applying the AED and performing CPR as indicated. A responsive patient with signs of hypoxia or poor perfusion needs oxygen, no matter what the chief complaint or underlying cause.

During the primary assessment of a responsive patient, you also will determine the chief complaint. However, jumping to conclusions about the underlying cause will likely lead to the wrong field impression, and incorrect further

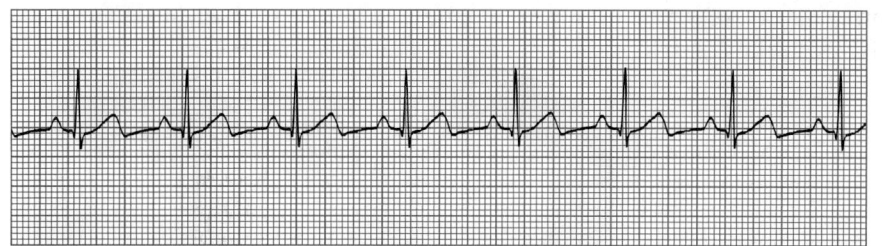

FIGURE 21-12

Normal sinus rhythm originates in the SA node. It is regular at a rate of 60 to 100 per minute. The P wave is upright, with a P–R interval of 0.12 to 0.20 seconds. There is the same number of P waves as QRS complexes. The QRS wave is less than 0.12 seconds.

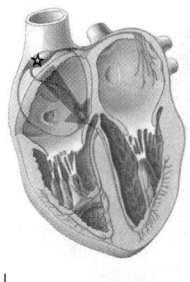

FIGURE 21-13

Sinus tachycardia originates in the SA node. It is regular at a rate of 100 to 150 per minute. The P wave is upright, with a P–R interval of 0.12 to 0.20 seconds. There is the same number of P waves as QRS complexes. The QRS wave is less than 0.12 seconds.

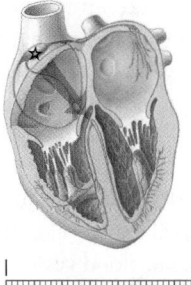

FIGURE 21-14

Sinus bradycardia originates in the SA node. It is regular at a rate of less than 60 per minute. The P wave is upright, with a P–R interval of 0.12 to 0.20 seconds. There is the same number of P waves as QRS complexes. The QRS wave is less than 0.12 seconds.

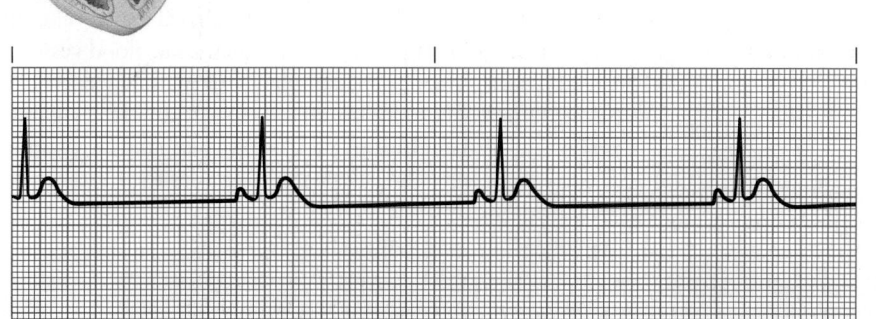

treatment. A reasonably accurate field impression is necessary before deciding if specific medications are warranted. For example, if dyspnea is caused by chronic obstructive pulmonary disease (COPD), albuterol may be indicated. If dyspnea is related to left-sided heart failure, albuterol is not given in most cases, but other medications are. An incorrect assumption that the patient's difficulty is caused by COPD not only means that he gets the wrong treatment, but also means that he will not get the right treatment.

The history and further assessment are guided by the question, "What are the possible causes of the patient's complaint?" Following the preceding example, the two causes of dyspnea that are of immediate concern are cardio-vascular problems and respiratory problems. Initial questioning will attempt to identify which system is involved. A reasonable place to start is to ask, "Has this ever happened before?" Find out if previous events were diagnosed. Determine what other signs and symptoms are present. Consider the past medical history and current medications.

As you proceed, continually compare the emerging collection of information to your mental scripts for respiratory problems and cardiovascular problems, revising your approach to the history and assessment as you go.

Patients with cardiovascular disorders may present with complaints of chest pain or discomfort; pain or discomfort in the arms, shoulders, neck, or jaw; difficulty breathing; weakness; palpitations; **syncope**; altered mental status; nausea; vomiting; or cardiac arrest. Patients presenting with abdominal or back pain may have an abdominal **aortic aneurysm**. Patients with headache or visual disturbances may be acutely hypertensive.

A script consisting of an understanding of the pathophysiology and signs and symptoms of various cardiovascular disorders will help you determine whether the patient's complaint relates to a cardiovascular problem.

Acute Coronary Syndromes

There is a range of disorders under the umbrella term **acute coronary syndrome (ACS)**. All share the common pathophysiology of insufficient oxygen supply to meet the heart's need for oxygen. With an insufficient oxygen supply, the myocardium becomes ischemic. The most common cause of ischemia is **coronary artery disease (CAD)**, caused by a buildup of fatty tissue in the coronary arteries, called **atherosclerosis**. This fatty tissue, or **plaque**, decreases the amount of blood that can reach the myocardium. ACS includes **unstable angina**, acute myocardial infarction, and sudden cardiac arrest.

Atherosclerosis

For more than a century, it was thought that a high-cholesterol diet was the only culprit in atherosclerosis development. Recent research, however, shows that genetics, inflammatory response, smoking, diabetes, and hypertension all contribute to the disease.

The first event in atherosclerosis development is disruption of the endothelium of the tunica intima (Figure 21-15). Injury and inflammation prevent the intima from acting as a barrier between blood components and the elastic lamina and tunica media beneath it. Causes of injury and inflammation include cigarette smoking, elevated blood glucose levels, increased blood lipid (fat) levels, and hypertension.

In the second step of atherosclerosis development, the damaged endothelial layer allows lipids from the bloodstream to enter and accumulate in the tissues beneath the

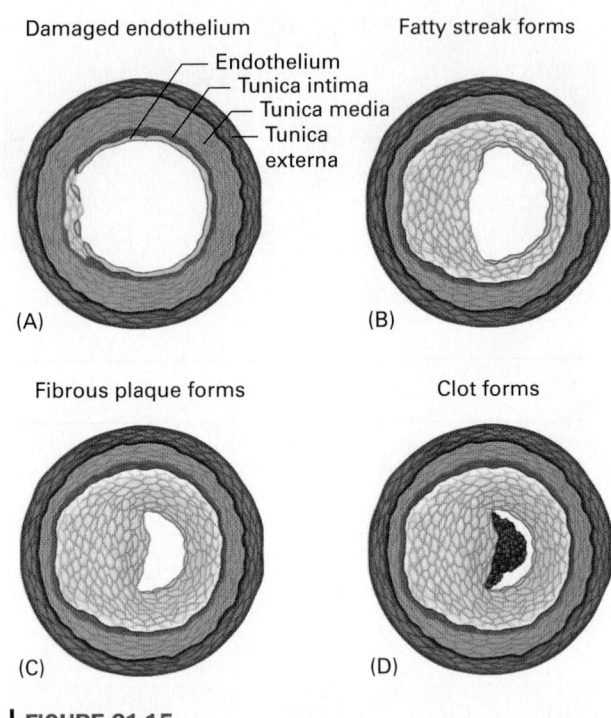

FIGURE 21-15

Development of atherosclerosis. (A) Damage to the endothelium of the tunica intima. (B) Formation of a fatty streak. (C) Development of plaque with a fibrous cap narrows the artery lumen. (D) Rupture of the plaque and platelet aggregation occlude the artery.

intima. Because the lipids are deposited in tissues where they normally would not be, they are seen as "foreign invaders" by the immune system. White blood cells take up the fat, and die, but remain in the tissue as foam cells. The changes initially appear as a fatty streak when the vessel is dissected at autopsy. Fatty streak formation is present in most people in developed countries by the age of 20.

After decades of foam cell buildup, smooth muscle cells begin to migrate from the tunica media into the tissues just beneath the intima. The smooth muscle cells also take up lipids. This expanding mass in the wall of the blood vessel is called *plaque*. The presence of plaque narrows the coronary artery lumen. The smooth muscle cells begin secreting material that forms a **fibrous cap** over the expanding plaque. Foam cells secrete an enzyme that degrades the fibrous cap, which may cause the plaque to rupture. Rupture of the plaque is the event that leads to AMI.

Angina Pectoris

As the buildup of foam cells and weakening of the fibrous cap continues, the lumen of the artery is continuously narrowed, decreasing the amount of blood that can pass through it. At rest, myocardial blood flow may be sufficient. When the heart must work harder, though, such as during exercise or stress, it cannot receive enough oxygenated blood.

EARLY SIGNS OF ACUTE CORONARY SYNDROME (HEART ATTACK)

FIGURE 21-16

Chest pain or discomfort from ACS may be experienced in, or radiate to, those areas.

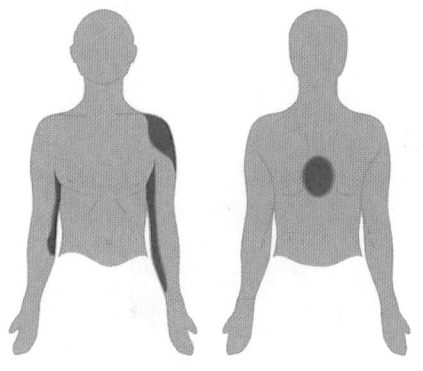

Just under sternum, midchest, or the entire upper chest.

Midchest, neck, and jaw.

Midchest and the shoulder and inside arms (more frequently the left).

Upper abdomen, often mistaken for indigestion.

Larger area of the chest, plus neck, jaw, and inside arms.

Jaw from ear to ear, in both sides of upper neck, and in lower center neck.

Shoulder (usually left) and inside arm to the waist, plus opposite arm, inside to the elbow.

Between the shoulder blades.

Angina pectoris is chest pain that occurs when the myocardial oxygen demand is higher than the amount of oxygen that diseased coronary arteries can supply. The pain is usually retrosternal and described as "pressure" or "tightening." The pain can radiate to the neck, jaw, or left arm (Figure 21-16). Nausea, vomiting, pallor, diaphoresis, and dyspnea sometimes occur with angina.

Angina typically occurs during physical activity or stress and is relieved by rest. Nitroglycerin may be prescribed to patients with angina. When chest pain does not go away with rest, the patient takes nitroglycerin to relax the smooth muscle of the coronary arteries. This allows vasodilation and improved blood flow.

Recurrent chest pain that comes on only during exercise or stress and resolves with rest or nitroglycerin is called **stable angina**, and is usually due to an increase in oxygen demand. Unstable angina occurs at rest, occurs more frequently than usual, hurts or radiates more than usual, and is not relieved by rest within 20 minutes or three doses of nitroglycerin. Unstable angina is usually due to a decrease in oxygen supply. Without prompt treatment, this will progress to an acute myocardial infarction.

Acute Myocardial Infarction

When the fibrous plaque of coronary artery disease ruptures, the damaged blood vessel initiates the body's clotting cascade (Figure 21-17). This further narrows or completely obstructs the artery, and myocardial cells deprived of oxygen begin to die (Figure 21-18). This is an *acute myocardial infarction (AMI)*.

An AMI very often is not triggered by stress or activity. It usually occurs at rest. The pain is similar to that of angina pectoris. It is often retrosternal and may radiate to the shoulder, neck, or jaw. If the patient has a history of angina, AMI pain is typically more intense, lasts more than 20 minutes, and has little or no relief with rest and nitroglycerin.

Signs and Symptoms of ACS

The classic response to myocardial ischemia, whatever the cause, is chest pain (Figure 21-19). Often, the "pain" is not described as pain, but as a discomfort, ache, or pressure. It is a good practice to ask a patient if he is having chest *discomfort,* as opposed to pain, or simply "How does your chest feel?" The pain is usually retrosternal, but can be left

FIGURE 21-17

Pathophysiology of acute coronary syndromes.

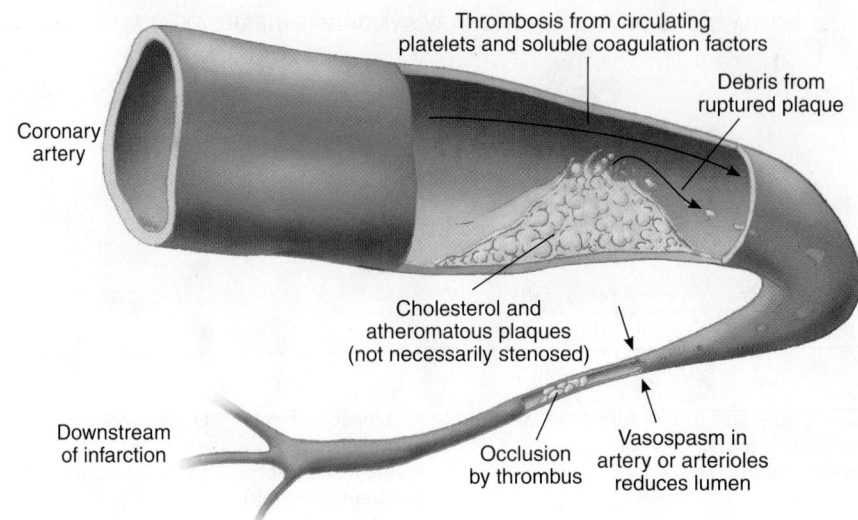

Thrombosis from circulating platelets and soluble coagulation factors

Debris from ruptured plaque

Coronary artery

Cholesterol and atheromatous plaques (not necessarily stenosed)

Downstream of infarction

Occlusion by thrombus

Vasospasm in artery or arterioles reduces lumen

FIGURE 21-18

Myocardial infarction results in death of the affected heart muscle.

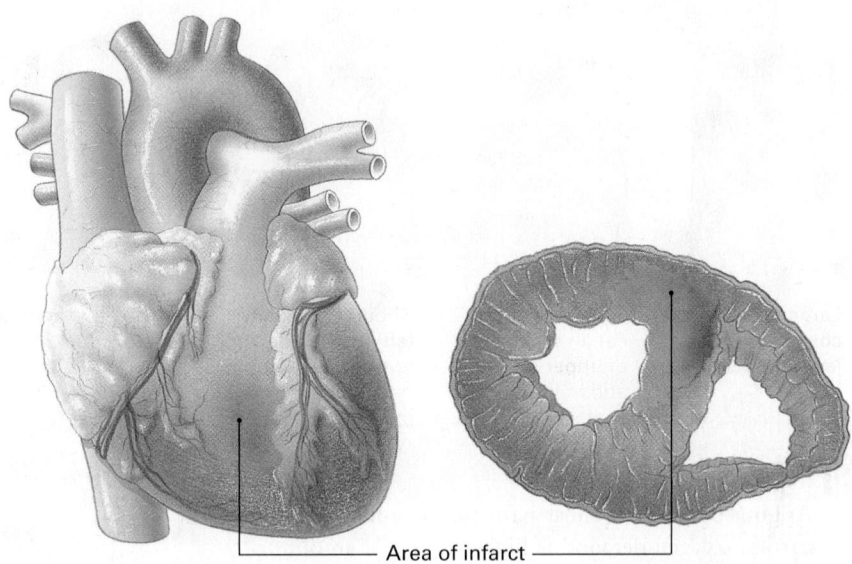

Area of infarct

or right sided, diffuse throughout the chest, or in the back, flank, or upper abdomen. Keep in mind that some ACS patients present atypically, and do not experience pain. The ability to reproduce the pain by palpating the area cannot "rule out" ACS as the cause of pain.

Other signs and symptoms may or may not be present. Only a few, or perhaps no, other signs and symptoms will be present in any given patient. Approximately 25 percent of myocardial infarctions are **silent MIs**, in which an AMI occurs without symptoms and is found on an ECG at a later time. Signs and symptoms other than those in the following list may also be present. Some typical signs and symptoms of ACS include the following:

- Cool, clammy skin
- Pale or ashen appearance
- Diaphoresis
- Nausea

- Vomiting
- Lightheadedness or weakness
- Dyspnea
- Anxiety or sense of impending doom
- Arm, shoulder, back, neck, or jaw discomfort
- Lung sounds that are often clear, but auscultation may indicate pulmonary edema from acute heart failure
- ECG tracing may be normal or abnormal

Atypical Presentations of ACS

Individuals in some groups often present with different symptoms from the "classic" symptoms described earlier. When a patient whose heart is clearly deprived of oxygen experiences signs and symptoms other than typical chest pain, those signs and symptoms are called **anginal equivalents**.

COMPARING ANGINA PECTORIS AND MYOCARDIAL INFARCTION

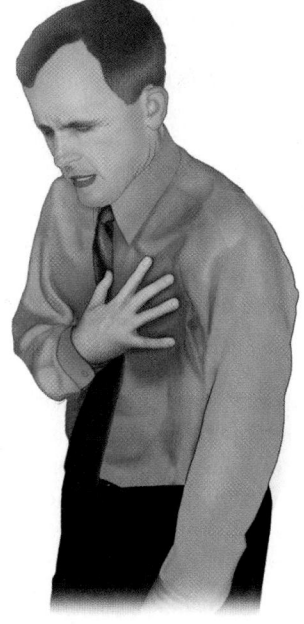

	Angina Pectoris	Myocardial Infarction
Location of Discomfort	Substernal or across chest	Same
Radiation of Discomfort	Neck, jaw, arms, back, shoulders	Same
Nature of Discomfort	Dull or heavy discomfort with a pressure or squeezing sensation	Same, but maybe more intense
Duration	Usually 2 to 15 minutes, subsides after activity stops	Lasts longer than 10 minutes
Other Symptoms	Usually none	Perspiration, pale gray color, nausea, weakness, dizziness, lightheadedness
Precipitating Factors	Extremes in weather, exertion, stress, meals	Often none
Factors Giving Relief	Stopping physical activity, reducing stress, nitroglycerin	Nitroglycerin may give incomplete or no relief

FIGURE 21-19

The signs and symptoms of angina pectoris and AMI are similar. Differentiating between them in the prehospital setting is difficult, but both the pain of angina and of AMI are treated the same way.

PERSONAL PERSPECTIVE

It's kind of funny, you know? I had chest pains a few years ago every time my grandkids came over and as if I were like Superman, would have me pick them up and hold them. I thought it was muscle aches at first, then age. My wife saw me grab my chest one time and panicked. She told me, "You need to see Dr. Abelman." ["You think he listens to me?," his wife yells from the kitchen. "Of course he didn't. He never does."] I had the appointment and missed it because I forgot I had tickets to the Cubs game. But the pain started coming more often and once I even had pain just walking up the steps from the garage. Then, I was at the pub with the guys from work just watching the Cubs losing. This was about a year ago. I was sitting there, I just finished a meatball sandwich and I couldn't breathe! It was like a car ran off a bridge and landed on my chest. I guess it was like the pain I'd had before, but this time it was terrible. I'd never felt anything like it before. I could feel it all the way into my teeth, like I was biting down on a hot coal. Anyway, my buddies were asking, "You okay? You okay?" I couldn't even talk. I was clutching my chest and trying to breathe. It was like breathing underwater. It took everything I had. And it was cold! I couldn't tell, but I'm sure I looked like a glass of milk on a hot day, completely white and covered in sweat. I wanted to wipe the sweat out of my eyes and tell them it was okay, but I fell to the floor. Somebody called 911, but I don't remember. All I was thinking about was my wife and how I never saw the Cubs win the Series. [Don't tell my wife I said that. She hates baseball.]

So I was on the floor thinking I was dead. This firefighter walks over to me and starts asking those around me questions. Then he looks at me and smiles, says his name is Frank. I don't remember his first couple of questions, but I remember he gave me some little aspirins and some oxygen and I started feeling a little better. As they wheeled me to the ambulance, he told me they were going to take good care of me. All I could do was believe the guy, and I did. It felt better than the morphine they gave me later in the hospital, knowing I would see my family again, you know?

Frank was a great guy. He told me he was an Advanced EMT. He did so much to help me that I think he brought me back from the edge of death. He saved my life. I know the doctor who did my bypass fixed me, but without Frank, I never would have made it that far. My wife made his station some pies and cookies. Did I tell you she makes the best pies? ["Oh honey, you can be so sweet when you want to be," she yells from the kitchen.] Anyway, Frank and I still talk sometimes. I saw him at the Fourth of July parade one time and we got a picture together with my grandkids. There should be more people like him, you know? Well, since then I've changed a lot. I quit smoking and only eat brats at Wrigley. My wife learned to cook "heart healthy," whatever that means. But I feel better, younger. I get to see my grandkids graduate, and I wouldn't have, if he hadn't been there to help me.

Geriatric Care

Many geriatric and diabetic patients may complain not of chest pain, but only of dyspnea, weakness, nausea, or vomiting. Maintain a high index of suspicion for ACS when older women, diabetics, and elderly patients present with those symptoms.

Anginal equivalents include atypical chest pain, such as pain that is sharp in character; pain in the back, arms, or jaw; abdominal discomfort or a sensation of indigestion; and weakness, nausea and vomiting, faintness or fainting, or general weakness.

Acute coronary syndromes (ACSs) can present with less-specific signs and symptoms in women, the elderly, and diabetics. The prevalence of ACS in women was once underestimated. In fact, older women with ACS are more likely to die from the event than are men. Symptoms in women may also differ from those in men; chest pain may be a minor complaint secondary to pain elsewhere, such as the back or shoulder.

Assessment and Management of ACS

The signs and symptoms of stable and unstable angina and AMI overlap considerably. It can be difficult to differentiate between them, even with sophisticated in-hospital diagnostic tests. As a general rule, *suspect that any patient with chest pain or chest discomfort is having a cardiac emergency.*

Dispatch Information and Scene Size-Up

Remember, the goals of the scene size-up are to determine the nature of the incident, the need for additional resources, and scene safety. Dispatch information may or may not be accurate, because dispatchers rely on the person making the call to relate the nature of the problem. Nearly any type of dispatch could result in a patient with a cardiovascular emergency.

Do not assume the scene is safe based on the nature of the dispatch. The situation may be something other than that described by the caller, or a family member or even the patient himself may be a danger to you.

Do not let a dispatch for chest pain limit your thinking about problems other than ACS. Experienced EMS providers can often describe having seen patients whom they immediately recognized as having an AMI. Their immediate general impression is most likely that of a very sick, anxious patient with pale, cool, diaphoretic skin.

Your first impression of the patient's degree of distress is important. The size and location of the patient, the presence of bystanders, and other factors may necessitate requesting additional resources.

Primary Assessment

Make note of the patient's general appearance and age to help guide your clinical reasoning. Obtain the chief complaint and determine if there are any immediate threats to life. Often the patient's chief complaint will be chest pain or chest discomfort. Sometimes, the sensation of pressure may make the patient think he is suffering from "indigestion." The chief complaint also may be pain in the arm, shoulder, neck, or jaw.

Keep in mind that the chief complaint may not be pain at all, especially in women, diabetics, and the elderly. Patients may complain of weakness, nausea, vomiting, or shortness of breath.

Most patients with ACS are alert and able to maintain an airway. However, patients with compromised perfusion may have an altered mental status. If your general impression does not provide you with a clear assessment of the patient's airway, carefully assess the airway and take initial measures to maintain it.

If breathing is inadequate, assist the patient's ventilations with a bag-valve-mask device. While previous practice has been to apply oxygen by nonrebreather mask to all patients with suspected ACS, there is insufficient evidence to support the practice in stable patients with uncomplicated ACS (American Heart Association [AHA], 2010). In patients with suspected ACS who have dyspnea, indications of heart failure, or signs of hypoxia, administer oxygen to maintain a SpO_2 of 95 percent or greater. Follow your protocols for oxygen administration to patients with suspected ACS.

If the patient is alert, assess the radial pulse, checking for rate, strength, and regularity. Patients with ACS are at risk of dysrhythmia and decreased perfusion. Check the carotid pulse if the patient's level of responsiveness is decreased. Patients with myocardial ischemia are at increased risk of cardiac arrest. An AED must be present and ready for operation at all times. The patient's mental status may be affected in ACS. Many patients are anxious. If cerebral perfusion is impaired, patients can be confused or combative, or have a decreased level of responsiveness.

At this point, communicate with your team about the next steps to take, based on your determination of the patient's priority for transport. Quickly decide how you will integrate further assessment, treatment, and preparation for transport. Even for patients whom you want to transport quickly, you should carry out some treatments and assessments while transport preparations are made.

Secondary Assessment

A focused history, vital signs, and focused assessment form the secondary assessment. Ideally, your partner can obtain vital signs while you ask questions based on the chief complaint. You can integrate parts of the focused physical exam and treatment with the history.

If the patient's chief complaint is pain, use the mnemonic *OPQRST* to get additional information. Compare the information with your knowledge of the nature of pain associated with ACS. Keep in mind that the severity of the pain need not be a 9 or 10 on a scale from 1 to 10 to be consistent with ACS. In fact, many patients will attempt to minimize the severity of their pain in their description.

The initial pain scale rating will provide a point of comparison for ongoing assessment. You should be especially concerned about unstable angina and AMI if the pain came on at rest, is not relieved by rest or nitroglycerin, and has persisted for more than 20 minutes.

Some typical characteristics of cardiac chest pain are that the pain or discomfort may be described as "dull," "heavy," "aching," "squeezing," "pressure," or "tightness." The pain or discomfort is often felt beneath the sternum. It may originate in the chest, but radiate to one or both arms or shoulders, the neck, jaw, or back.

Check for associated symptoms and pertinent negatives. Dyspnea, nausea, vomiting, anxiety, or weakness may accompany ACS. For some patients, one or more of the symptoms may be the chief complaint.

Ask the patient about his past medical history, including the components of the SAMPLE history. Ask about any additional symptoms. Check for allergies, medications, pertinent past medical history, last oral intake, and events leading up to the onset of the problem.

You may have covered some of those points, such as symptoms and events, in your exploration of the chief complaint. Some aspects of the past medical history will increase your suspicion that the patient is experiencing ACS. Risk factors for ACS include hypertension, diabetes, high lipid levels, obesity, smoking, a previous history of CAD, and a family history of CAD. The absence of risk factors does not rule out ACS, however. Base your suspicion primarily on the patient's current signs and symptoms.

Vital signs and monitoring should include blood pressure, heart and respiration rates, and pulse oximetry. A systolic blood pressure of at least 90 mmHg is required in order to administer nitroglycerin. A systolic blood pressure of less than 90 mmHg is typically inadequate for perfusion, and is treated by intravenous fluid boluses, if allowed by protocol.

Cardiac patients may experience dysrhythmia, which may be noted by bradycardia, tachycardia, or an irregular pulse. If cardiac monitoring is within your scope of practice, it provides additional information about the cardiac rhythm. Cardiac patients can deteriorate quickly, so you must monitor vital signs frequently.

Assess the patient's breath sounds. The presence of crackles (rales) in the lungs is an indication of in acute heart failure with pulmonary edema. This is a result of extensive damage to the left ventricle, which impairs cardiac output. Patients with heart failure may have edema of the lower extremities, although this takes time to develop. They should not receive additional fluid boluses.

At this point, you should make a decision about your field impression in order to plan further treatment and reassess transport plans. If the patient's condition is consistent with ACS, transport the patient without undue delay to a hospital that can provide definitive interventions for ACS.

Definitive interventions are aimed at reopening the blocked artery. This can be accomplished either by administering **fibrinolytic** medications or by percutaneous coronary intervention (PCI), also called *percutaneous coronary angioplasty (PCA)*. Cardiac catheterization is a diagnostic procedure in which the coronary arteries are examined for blockage. If there is blockage, PCI can be performed. If the affected portion of myocardium can be reperfused, injured cells that otherwise might have died may be saved, minimizing damage to the heart. The interventions can succeed only if initiated within a narrow window of opportunity. If transport time is long, consider air medical or ground ALS transport according to your protocols.

ACS Treatment

In addition to administering oxygen as indicated by the patient's degree of distress and oxygen saturation, typical management of the alert ACS patient includes administering aspirin, starting an IV, and giving nitroglycerin. In some cases, you also may give an analgesic, such as nitrous oxide. If you work with a paramedic, you can anticipate that the patient will receive a narcotic analgesic, such as fentanyl or morphine.

Immediate administration of aspirin can reduce the morbidity and mortality of ACS. The therapeutic effect of aspirin in ACS is that it reduces platelet aggregation, which helps prevent further clotting at the site of the plaque rupture (Table 21-1). Specifically ask about an allergy to aspirin and follow your protocol in administering 160 to 325 mg of chewable aspirin.

Nitroglycerin is important in ACS, but can cause a drop in blood pressure. Usually this occurs in patients who have never received nitroglycerin before or who have had a hypotensive response to it in the past. For that reason, most protocols encourage having an IV in place prior to administering nitroglycerin. For patients who are normotensive, an IV at a keep open TKO rate is indicated. Protocols may direct you to administer a fluid bolus to ACS patients with a systolic blood pressure less than 90 mmHg.

It is essential that you listen to the patient's lung sounds before administering a fluid bolus. Additional fluids are contraindicated for patients with pulmonary edema. Normal saline is an acceptable IV fluid. The potassium in lactated Ringer's solution makes it undesirable for ACS.

Nitroglycerin may be administered if systolic blood pressure is greater than 90 mmHg and the patient meets other criteria. You can administer up to three 0.4-mg dosages of nitroglycerin spaced 3 to 5 minutes apart sublingually, either by a tablet that dissolves quickly under the tongue, or by metered-dose spray.

Assess the patient's blood pressure and pain level before and after each dose of nitroglycerin. Nitroglycerin not only dilates coronary arteries to improve myocardial

TABLE 21-1	Emergency Medications for Acute Coronary Syndromes			
Medication	**Indications**	**Contraindications**	**Dose**	**Side Effects**
Aspirin	Chest pain of suspected cardiac cause (angina, acute MI)	Patient unable to chew, swallow, or protect airway; gastric ulcers, allergy to aspirin; asthmatic patient	81 to 325 mg (chewable tablets)	Usually none with a single dose; some patients may complain of stomach upset or pain
Nitroglycerin	Chest pain of suspected cardiac cause (angina, acute MI); left-sided heart failure with pulmonary edema	Systolic BP <90 to 100 mmHg; heart rate less than 50 or greater than 100, patient has already taken 3 doses of drug or has recently used a drug for erectile dysfunction	0.4 mg tablet or spray administered sublingually every 5 minutes, up to a total of 3 doses.	May cause hypotension. Check BP before each dose. May cause headache and flushed skin.
Nitrous oxide	Chest pain	Patients who cannot follow instructions or who are intoxicated	Self-administered; sedating effects limit dosage	Sedation
Oxygen	SpO$_2$ <95%	Generally none in an emergency setting, but only administer if indicated	2 to 15 L/min. by a variety of administration devices	Usually none in an emergency setting. May cause dryness of mucosa

perfusion, but also relaxes all vascular smooth muscle, which can lead to hypotension. If hypotension occurs, administer IV fluids to increase the systolic blood pressure to above 90 mmHg again. Consult with medical direction before administering additional nitroglycerin following an episode of hypotension.

Reassessment

Monitor the ACS patient closely for changes. Re-evaluate the status of the patient's airway, breathing, and oxygenation. Check the pulse for changes in rate, rhythm, or strength. Continue to assess vital signs. In particular, the patient's blood pressure may drop as a side effect of nitroglycerin, or an indication of cardiogenic shock. Reassess the patient's level of pain in response to treatment, using a scale from 1 to 10.

Alter your treatment plan as necessary, paying attention to the need for IV fluids and pain management. Early notification of the receiving hospital can allow preparation for the patient's arrival in the emergency department, and if available, preparation of the cardiac catheterization lab.

The single most important field management of a patient suspected of having an acute MI is obtaining an ECG and communicating the results to the emergency department. In this way, they can be prepared for an acute MI in advance. In some systems, a patient with a positive ECG for AMI in the field may go directly to a catheterization lab, bypassing the emergency department entirely.

Sudden Cardiac Death and Cardiac Arrest

Lethal cardiac dysrhythmias can occur as an individual's first indication of CAD in 10 percent of cases, or as a complication shortly following the onset of ACS symptoms. Ventricular fibrillation is the most common initial dysrhythmia in cardiac arrest, but ventricular tachycardia also may occur.

In the ischemic heart, cells in the ventricles can become irritable and may depolarize at random. When one or a few of the ectopic pacemakers fires occasionally, it is called a **premature ventricular contraction (PVC)** (Figure 21-20). (The term "contraction" is misleading, though, because PVC refers to the electrical activity, not mechanical activity.) Sometimes one or more ectopic ventricular pacemakers will fire in rapid succession in a dysrhythmia called *ventricular tachycardia* (Figure 21-21). Ventricular tachycardia may

occur with or without a pulse. When multiple—perhaps hundreds—of cells in the ventricles become ectopic pacemakers, the result is chaotic electrical activity that cannot produce effective contraction of the heart. The heart muscle quivers, or fibrillates. This is called *ventricular fibrillation*. There are no definable P, QRS, or T waves on the ECG (Figure 21-22). There is no cardiac output. The patient is unresponsive and pulseless. The only way to reverse ventricular fibrillation and pulseless ventricular tachycardia is immediate electrical defibrillation.

Automated external defibrillators (AEDs) are applied only to patients who are unresponsive and pulseless, because the AED detects ventricular tachycardia as well as ventricular fibrillation. Defibrillating the patient who is in ventricular tachycardia with a pulse may result in ventricular fibrillation. Subsequent defibrillation may be unsuccessful in reversing the resulting ventricular fibrillation.

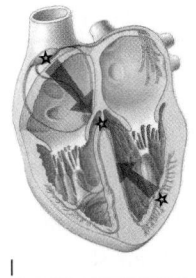
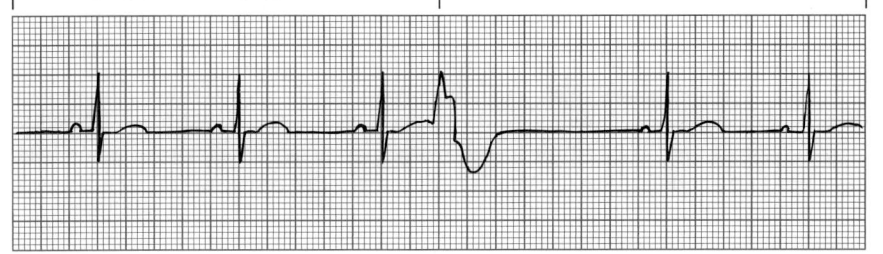

FIGURE 21-20

A premature ventricular complex (PVC) is an abnormal ECG complex that arises from an ectopic pacemaker in the ventricles, causing a bizarre-looking complex earlier than the next expected complex.

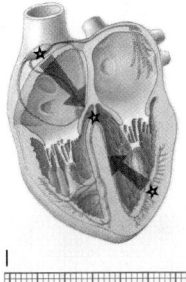
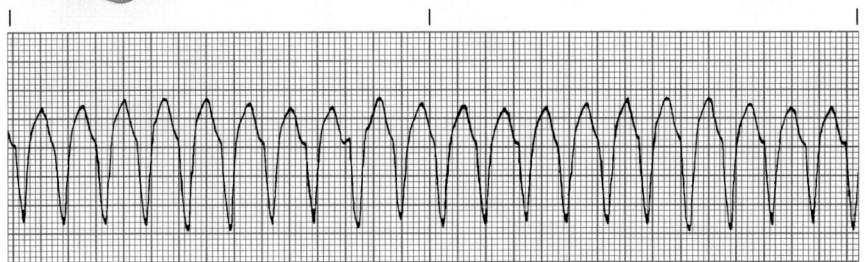

FIGURE 21-21

Ventricular tachycardia (VT) arises from a rapidly firing ectopic pacemaker in the ventricles. The complexes are wide, with no P wave visible. The rate is typically between 100 and 250 per minute, and may occur with or without a pulse. VT is recognized and defibrillated by the AED; therefore, the AED is never placed on a patient with a pulse.

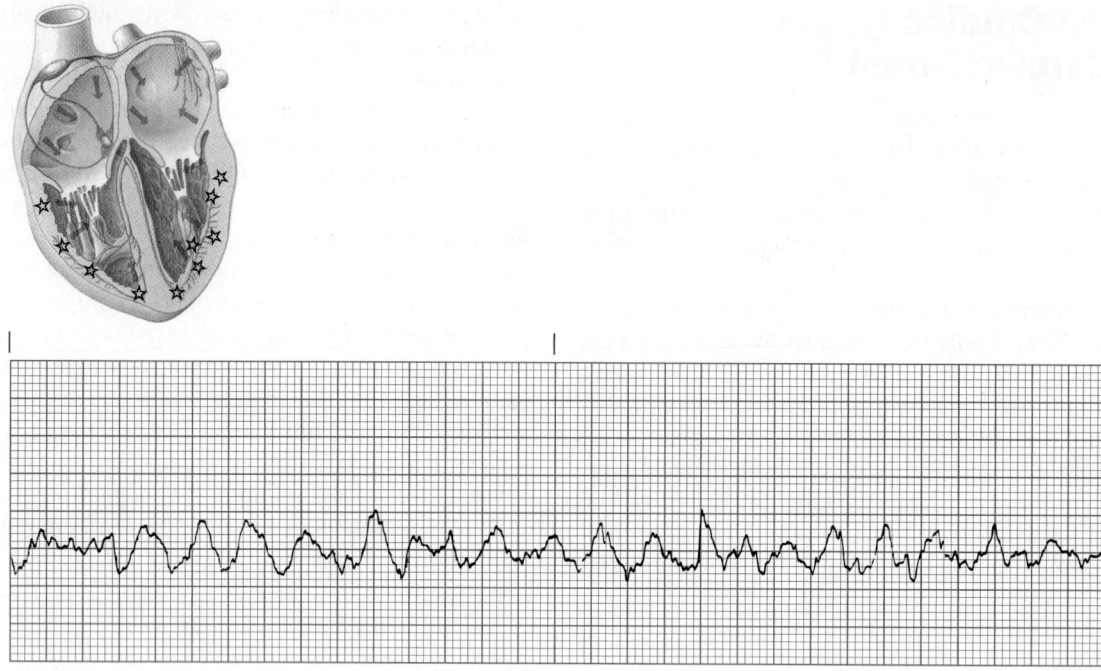

FIGURE 21-22

Ventricular fibrillation (VF) is a chaotic, disorganized electrical activity resulting from multiple, rapidly firing ectopic pacemakers in the ventricles. Electrical activity is not conducted normally, and there is no cardiac output. VF is recognized and defibrillated by the AED.

If ventricular tachycardia is seen on the cardiac monitor in a patient who has a pulse, advanced life support treatment includes synchronized cardioversion and medications that are typically not in the Advanced EMT's scope of practice.

Asystole is a complete absence of cardiac electrical activity, resulting in cardiac arrest (Figure 21-23). Asystole is not typically the initial rhythm in cardiac arrest, but untreated dysrhythmia and other underlying problems can lead to asystole. The chances of survival from asystole are slim.

ACS is not the only cause of cardiac arrest. Trauma, stroke, toxins, environmental exposure, and metabolic imbalances are all causes of cardiac arrest (Table 21-2). In those cases, the underlying problem must be addressed in addition to following emergency cardiac care guidelines. (See Chapter 17 for a review of resuscitation techniques.)

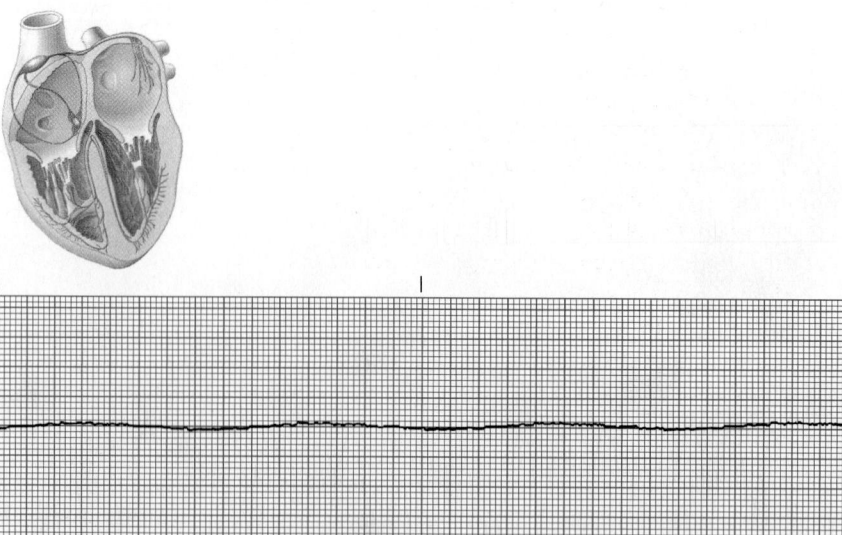

FIGURE 21-23

Asystole is an absence of cardiac electrical activity, resulting in cardiac standstill.

TABLE 21-2	Possible Causes of Cardiac Arrest

- Hypoxia
- Hypovolemia
- Hydrogen ion (acidosis/alkalosis)
- Hypo/hyperkalemia (potassium)
- Hypoglycemia
- Hypothermia
- Toxins
- Tension pneumothorax
- Tamponade (cardiac tamponade)
- Thrombosis (coronary, pulmonary, cerebral)
- Trauma

Heart Failure

Heart failure occurs when the heart cannot pump enough blood to meet the metabolic demands of the body or when it can do so only if venous pressure is unusually high. Heart failure can be the most severe and terminal representation of many cardiac diseases, including coronary artery disease and myocardial infarction. Heart failure affects 5 million people in the United States. More than half a million cases are diagnosed each year. The five-year survival rate following heart failure diagnosis is 50 percent, which is less than that of most cancers.

Pathophysiology of Heart Failure

To maintain blood pressure and perfusion, the heart must contract with enough force to eject blood against the pressure in the arterial system. The pressure within the arterial system that must be overcome by the left ventricle is called **afterload**. Anything that impairs ventricular contraction to the point at which it cannot pump out the amount of blood that is being returned to it results in a backup of blood behind the affected ventricle.

The ventricle may sustain enough damage from an AMI that its function is immediately impaired, or when infarcted myocardium is replaced with fibrous tissue that does not contract. When the ventricle must work harder than normal over time to overcome increased resistance, the muscle enlarges and becomes less effective at contraction. This condition is called *myocardial hypertrophy*. Left ventricular hypertrophy may occur in response to long-standing hypertension.

The most common cause of right-sided heart failure is left-sided heart failure. As the pulmonary vasculature becomes congested from left-sided heart failure, it becomes harder for the right ventricle to pump blood into the pulmonary vasculature. The right ventricle may also have difficulty overcoming resistance in the lungs from COPD or pulmonary embolism. Right-sided heart failure that occurs from increased resistance in the lungs is called *cor pulmonale*.

When cardiac output is reduced in heart failure, the kidneys become hypoperfused. Because hypoperfusion often occurs in response to a loss of circulating volume, the kidneys attempt to compensate by secreting substances that result in water retention and other mechanisms to increase blood pressure.

The increased volume of blood returned to the heart stretches the cardiac muscle fibers. According to a physiologic principle called *Frank–Starling's law of the heart*, the greater the stretch on myocardial contractile fibers, the greater the force with which they will contract. However, as with all compensatory mechanisms, this works only to a certain point. If the volume increases too greatly, contractility does not compensate and venous congestion ensues.

Other mechanisms of compensation are chronic vasoconstriction and tachycardia. Those mechanisms work well initially to compensate, but ultimately lead to worsened heart failure and further reduction in cardiac output.

As blood backs up into either the systemic or pulmonary capillaries, the increased pressure in the vascular system forces fluid out of the capillaries and into the interstitial spaces. The result is edema. When the left ventricle fails, pulmonary edema interferes with the ability of oxygen and carbon dioxide to diffuse between the capillaries and alveoli (Figure 21-24). As the pressure increases and more fluid accumulates, the alveoli can fill with fluid, resulting in wet lung sounds and production of frothy sputum.

Systemic edema typically is affected by gravity; thus, failure of the right ventricle is often evident from swelling of the feet and ankles (Figure 21-25). Patients with right-sided heart failure also often have jugular venous distention (JVD), congestion of peripheral veins, and fluid in the abdominal cavity (ascites).

Assessment and Management of Heart Failure

Most people who have heart failure are aware of it and may provide that information early in the encounter. The signs and symptoms vary, depending on the severity of the heart failure and whether it is left or right sided.

Dispatch Information and Scene Size-Up

Often calls for heart failure are dispatched as calls for difficulty breathing, and it is not uncommon to receive them during the nighttime hours. Patients with heart failure may be on oxygen at home. The presence of oxygen may be an indication of the severity of the patient's illness. As with all patients, assess scene safety and determine the need for additional resources.

FIGURE 21-24

Left-sided heart failure.

LEFT-HEART FAILURE

Signs
- Cyanosis
- Tachycardia
- Noisy labored breathing
- Rales
- Coughing
- Blood-tinged sputum
- Gallop rhythm of the heart

Symptom
- Dyspnea

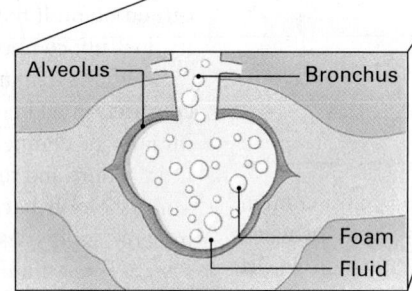

FIGURE 21-25

Right-sided heart failure.

RIGHT-HEART FAILURE

Signs

- Tachycardia
- Neck veins engorging and pulsating
- Edema of body and lower extremities
- Engorged liver and spleen
- Abdominal distention (ascites)

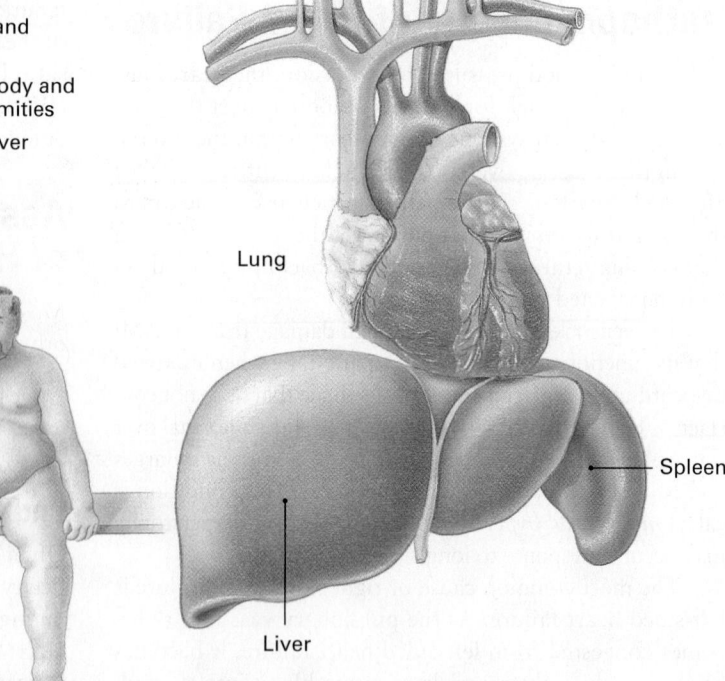

Primary Assessment

Your initial glimpse of the patient may reveal the nature and severity of the problem. A patient with severe pulmonary edema is frequently sitting up and struggling to breathe. The skin is often wet, with poor color. You may hear bubbling crackles as you approach the patient, and the patient may have foamy, pink-tinged sputum.

The patient may be anxious and exhausted from the effort of breathing. Poor cerebral perfusion and hypoxia may result in confusion, agitation, or decreased level of responsiveness. Such patients need immediate attention to airway, breathing, and oxygenation. Other patients may present less dramatically, and need further evaluation to determine the nature of the problem.

Assisting with airway and breathing can be a challenge in pulmonary edema. Unless they are in complete respiratory failure, most patients with pulmonary edema will not tolerate a position other than sitting up. It may be necessary to assist ventilations with the patient in a sitting position.

Patients may be in dire need of airway and ventilation management, yet be too responsive to tolerate airway devices. Continuous positive airway pressure (CPAP) can play an important role in improving ventilation and oxygenation in patients with pulmonary edema. The positive end-expiratory pressure provided by CPAP can reduce the amount of fluid that can cross into the alveoli. Typical CPAP pressures used in pulmonary edema are from 2.5 to 5 cmH$_2$O.

Increased oxygen in the alveoli will help improve diffusion of oxygen across the edematous respiratory membrane. Depending on the patient's level of responsiveness and degree of distress, interventions may include oxygen by nonrebreather mask, CPAP, assisted ventilations with a bag-valve-mask device, insertion of airway adjuncts, and artificial ventilation. If you are working with a paramedic and the patient has been intubated, you may perform endotracheal suctioning to remove fluid from the lower airway.

Check the patient's pulse. The pulse is likely to be rapid as the body attempts to improve cardiac output. Bradycardia may be a sign of respiratory failure and impending cardiac arrest. The pulse is often bounding as a result of hypertension. A weak pulse may indicate cardiogenic shock as cardiac output continues to fall. Patients with respiratory failure are in acidosis and may deteriorate to cardiac arrest. Be prepared to apply the AED and perform CPR.

For patients who are able to speak, determine the chief complaint. Often, the chief complaint is difficulty breathing, but patients may also offer a chief complaint of chest pain or weakness. Determine the patient's priority for transport. Communicate with your team about the priorities for further assessment, treatment, and transportation.

Secondary Assessment

Determine the OPQRST of the patient's chief complaint. Often, patients with heart failure wake up at night, while lying supine or semireclined, in acute respiratory distress.

Sometimes, after resuming an upright position, the distress is resolved. This is called **paroxysmal nocturnal dyspnea (PND)** and is quite common in heart failure patients.

Of particular note in the SAMPLE history, the patient may often have a history of heart failure, hypertension, and other cardiovascular problems. Medications may include **angiotensin-converting enzyme (ACE) inhibitors, diuretics,** and **beta blockers.**

Assess the vital signs, determine oxygen saturation, and perform a focused physical examination. Patients with heart failure frequently have a chronic cardiac dysrhythmia called **atrial fibrillation.** The heartbeat is irregular, resulting in an irregular pulse. Often, the patient is hypertensive.

As noted, hypotension is an indication of cardiogenic shock. Respirations are likely to be increased in response to hypoxia. Slow or irregular respirations indicate respiratory failure. Oxygen saturation may be low; the goal is to maintain the SpO$_2$ at 95 percent or higher.

The focused physical examination includes auscultation of the lungs and assessing for edema. Fluid backup from the right ventricle can cause swelling of the liver, inducing tenderness and pain in the right upper quadrant of the abdomen. Fluid overload may fill the abdominal cavity and distend the abdomen. The lower extremities may be swollen as well. Use the results of the secondary assessment to plan specific treatment and re-evaluate the patient's priority for transport.

Prehospital Management of Heart Failure

Pay close attention to managing the patient's airway, breathing, and oxygenation. Ideally, oxygen is administered by nonrebreather mask. However, patients with respiratory distress can panic if something is placed over the nose and mouth. Reassure the patient that the mask delivers high levels of oxygen.

If the patient cannot tolerate a facemask, the anxiety he is experiencing may increase his demand for oxygen and place even more stress on the heart. If necessary, use a nasal cannula instead.

Place the patient in a position of comfort, which is usually sitting upright. Follow protocols for specific indications for continuous positive airway pressure (CPAP). Take a good history to ensure that the patient does not have conditions that contraindicate the use of CPAP. (See Chapter 16 for a review of CPAP.) Ventilatory assistance with a bag-valve-mask device is indicated if the patient shows signs of inadequate respirations or decreasing mental status.

If chest pain or discomfort is present, administration of aspirin is indicated. Starting an IV may be difficult because of significant swelling of the extremities. You should maintain IV fluids at a TKO rate.

Nitroglycerin is beneficial by reducing pulmonary edema through vasodilation and reducing myocardial workload. Protocols may allow up to three 0.4-mg doses of nitroglycerin, based on the patient's blood pressure and use of nitroglycerin before your arrival. Be prepared for respiratory or cardiac arrest, especially in patients with decreasing mental status or hypotension.

Advanced (paramedic-level) prehospital management of acute pulmonary edema may include diuretics, such as furosemide and morphine. Furosemide initially causes vasodilation, and ultimately results in removal of excess fluid through urination. Morphine also causes vasodilation and can reduce the patient's anxiety. If needed to manage airway and ventilation, paramedics may intubate the patient in the prehospital setting.

You must take care to ensure that the patient is not a COPD exacerbation, which appears much the same as acute heart failure. No history of heart failure or a history of COPD may help make this distinction. Lung sounds can sometimes be deceiving because they are so noisy in both conditions. Use of diuretics in COPD and the use of albuterol in heart failure can worsen the situation, so the correct assessment is critical.

Reassessment

Continuously re-evaluate the components of the primary assessment. Altered mental status—including confusion, agitation, and decreased level of responsiveness—are an indication of progressively poor perfusion and cerebral hypoxia. A decreasing level of responsiveness or increasing secretions may jeopardize the patient's airway status. Use suction as needed to keep the airway clear.

Respiratory distress can quickly progress to respiratory failure and respiratory arrest. Monitor the need to use airway adjuncts, assist ventilations, and use CPAP. If you have already implemented those interventions, monitor their effectiveness.

Cardiac arrest may occur. Be ready to initiate CPR and use the AED. Reassess vital signs and oxygenation, noting the effects of interventions and trends in the patient's condition.

Cardiogenic Shock

Under conditions of significantly low cardiac output and hypotension (less than 90 mmHg) resulting from left ventricular dysfunction, the heart cannot provide enough blood flow to perfuse the tissues of the body. This is called *cardiogenic shock*. Cardiogenic shock can be caused by MI in which more than 40 percent of the left ventricle is affected, or by heart failure or other cardiac problems. Cardiogenic shock can be a downward spiral. Once hypotension develops, coronary artery perfusion decreases, leading to more myocardial damage. The mortality from cardiogenic shock is more than 70 percent.

The body's early attempts to compensate for decreased cardiac output from left ventricular damage result in tachycardia, pallor, cool skin, and diaphoresis. Hypotension, the distinctive sign of cardiogenic shock, follows.

Hypoperfusion of the brain leads to altered mental status, anxiety, or unresponsiveness. Patients may have signs of heart failure, such as pulmonary edema, JVD, and dyspnea.

Airway management is the first priority. You should anticipate the insertion of at least a basic adjunct, followed by positive pressure ventilations with a bag-valve-mask device and 100 percent oxygen. If the airway is patent, you can administer oxygen to maintain the patient's oxygen saturation at 95 percent or higher.

Managing patients with cardiogenic shock can present a paradox because of coexisting hypotension and pulmonary edema. If the patient can tolerate it, the supine position is preferred to enhance brain and coronary perfusion. You should obtain large-bore intravenous access.

In the absence of pulmonary edema, a bolus of intravenous fluid may help increase preload and cardiac output. You must accompany administration of fluid with ongoing assessment of the lungs for signs of pulmonary edema. Additional fluids will worsen existing pulmonary edema, decreasing gas exchange.

Hypotension is a critical condition. Do not delay transport. If transport time is long, consider air medical or ground ALS transport. Transport to a facility with surgical and intensive care capabilities is preferred for invasive hemodynamic monitoring and definitive treatment.

Paramedic and initial emergency department management typically include medications such as dobutamine or dopamine to increase the contractility of the heart to improve cardiac output, blood pressure, and tissue perfusion.

Once hospitalized, the patient may be implanted with an intra-aortic balloon pump, a mechanical device that improves tissue perfusion while decreasing myocardial oxygen demand. This and similar devices may be in place during interfacility transport, requiring monitoring by EMS personnel.

Hypertension

Hypertension is a complex and poorly understood disease. At least 25 percent of the people of the United States are affected by the disease. Patients diagnosed with "hypertension" have what is called *primary* or *essential hypertension*. This is a syndrome with many contributing factors that is diagnosed once other causes of hypertension (secondary hypertension), such as renal diseases or **aortic dissection**, are ruled out. An exact cause of hypertension has not been identified, but genetic factors that affect vascular tone and diuresis appear to be involved.

Hypertension is defined as systolic blood pressure greater than or equal to 140 mmHg and/or diastolic blood pressure greater than or equal to 90 mmHg. Primary treatment is aimed at reducing blood pressure below those levels (Table 21-3). Treatment is important in reducing complications of hypertension, which include left ventricular

TABLE 21-3 Drugs Commonly Prescribed for Patients with Cardiovascular Disease

Drug	Classification	Use
doxazosin (Cardura), prazosin (Minipress)	Alpha-receptor blockers, which block alpha effects of sympathetic nervous system	Hypertension
atenolol (Tenormin), metoprolol (Lopressor), propranolol (Inderal)	Beta-receptor blockers, which block the beta effects of the sympathetic nervous system	Angina, tachycardia, hypertension
labetalol (Normodyne, Trandate)	Combined alpha- and beta-blocker, which blocks both alpha and beta sympathetic nervous system effects	Hypertension
lisinopril (Zestril), enalapril (Vasotec), captopril (Capoten)	Angiotensin-converting enzyme (ACE) inhibitors, which prevent production of angiotensin II, a hormone that causes vasoconstriction	Hypertension, heart failure
amiodarone (Cordarone), digoxin (Lanoxin), procainamide (Pronestyl)	Antidysrhythmics	Cardiac dysrhythmia suppression; digoxin also used in heart failure
aspirin, dipyridamole (Permole), clopidogrel (Plavix)	Antiplatelet drugs	Platelet aggregation prevention, AMI and stroke risk reduction
warfarin (Coumadin)	Anticoagulant	Blood clotting prevention
diltiazem (Cardizem), nifedipine (Procardia), verapamil (Covera)	Calcium channel blocker, which reduces muscle contraction to cause vasodilation	Angina, hypertension, and dysrhythmia
atorvastatin (Lipitor), lovastatin (Mevacor), simvastatin (Zocor)	Statins, which reduce cholesterol	High blood lipid levels for AMI risk reduction
hydrochlorothiazide (HydroDiuril), bemetanide (Bumex), furosemide (Lasix)	Diuretics, which reduce excess fluid volume	Hypertension and heart failure
nitroglycerin	Vasodilator	Angina

hypertrophy, heart failure, myocardial ischemia, stroke, aortic aneurysm or dissection, and renal failure.

Hypertensive emergency or crisis is defined as a rapid, symptomatic increase in blood pressure with a systolic pressure greater than 160 mmHg and/or diastolic blood pressure greater than 94 mmHg. The systolic blood pressure can go above 250 mmHg.

It is usually the onset of other signs and symptoms, not the blood pressure itself, that causes the patient to seek medical care. Patients may present with acute renal failure or **hypertensive encephalopathy.** Hypertensive encephalopathy results when the elevated blood pressure causes cerebral edema and increased intracranial pressure. Patients may present with severe headache and possibly neurologic deficits, such as visual disturbances or altered mental status. Other conditions that present with hypertension include myocardial infarction, intracranial hemorrhage, aortic dissection, and hypertensive disorders of pregnancy.

Symptoms of hypertensive emergencies include hematuria (blood in the urine), chest pain, blurred vision, headache, neurologic changes, pulmonary edema, bounding pulse, nausea, vomiting, seizures, oliguria (very low urine output), and epistaxis (nosebleed).

Aortic Aneurysm and Dissection

The aorta is the largest blood vessel in the body. The amount of resistance it provides is responsible for a large amount of mechanical stress that occurs with each cardiac contraction. Like the other arteries of the body, it contains three layers. Collagen fibers provide strength and support, and elastic fibers (elastin) allow the tissue to stretch in response to the blood pumped into it with every heartbeat.

Over time, elastin begins to break down and collagen replaces it within the arterial wall. This causes the aorta to become stiff and narrow. The reduced ability to stretch causes an increase in systolic blood pressure.

Aortic Aneurysm

As the support proteins for the aorta degrade and disappear in all three layers, the pressure within the aorta can cause the weakened area to dilate (Figure 21-26). When the diameter of the aorta increases 50 percent or more from its original size, by definition, an aortic aneurysm has developed. The normal diameter of the aorta is 2 to 2.5 cm. An aneurysm is a focal widening greater than 3 to 4 cm. It can be found in the ascending, descending, abdominal aorta, or all three.

The abdominal aortic aneurysm (AAA) is the most common location, accounting for more than 90 percent of cases. As the aneurysm enlarges and the wall becomes thinner, the risk of rupture increases. Once the aneurysm ruptures, survival is unlikely, even if it occurs while the patient is in the emergency department or operating room. Rapid bleeding into the abdominal cavity is the most common cause of death.

Risk factors for aortic aneurysm include genetic disposition, male gender, old age, bacterial infection, and atherosclerosis and its risk factors: smoking, hypertension, inflammation, and lipid disease. In its early stages, aortic aneurysms are usually asymptomatic. The aneurysm is usually found on accident or during a routine physical exam. Ultrasound or CT scan confirms the physical findings. As the aneurysm enlarges, a pulsating mass may be felt on palpation of the abdomen. The patient may complain of abdominal "fullness," abdominal pain, back pain, or vague gastrointestinal symptoms. The most common complaints for which emergency response is initiated are abdominal pain, back pain, syncope, or cardiac arrest.

The presence of pain or hypotension usually indicates that the aneurysm is rupturing, in which case the prognosis is poor. Physical examination of the abdomen may reveal a pulsating mass, but this finding is not always present.

Advanced EMT management for a patient with aortic aneurysm is rapid transport to a surgical facility. You should administer oxygen, and initiate at least one IV with a large-bore catheter and blood tubing, if available. Follow protocols for fluid resuscitation.

Aortic Dissection

Aortic dissection occurs when there is a tear in the tunica intima of the arterial wall. Blood enters the tear and is forced between the tunica media and tunica externa, creating a false lumen (Figure 21-27). The mechanisms and risk factors for aortic dissection are similar to those that result in aneurysms. An injury in which there was sudden deceleration of the body, such as a high-speed motor vehicle collision (MVC) or fall from a height, can stretch and tear the tunica intima, as well, resulting in dissection.

Dissection most commonly occurs in the ascending thoracic aorta, followed in incidence by the descending thoracic aorta, aortic arch, and abdominal aorta. Complications are often fatal and need to be diagnosed rapidly. Complications include obstruction of arteries branching from the aorta, which can lead to stroke, myocardial infarction, renal failure, and pulseless extremities. Massive hemorrhage may occur if the tunica externa ruptures. The aortic valve may rupture,

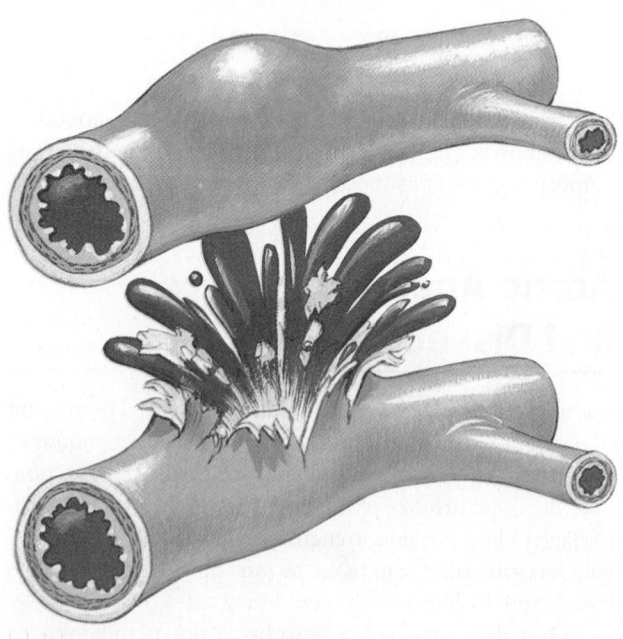

FIGURE 21-26

Aortic aneurysm and aortic rupture.

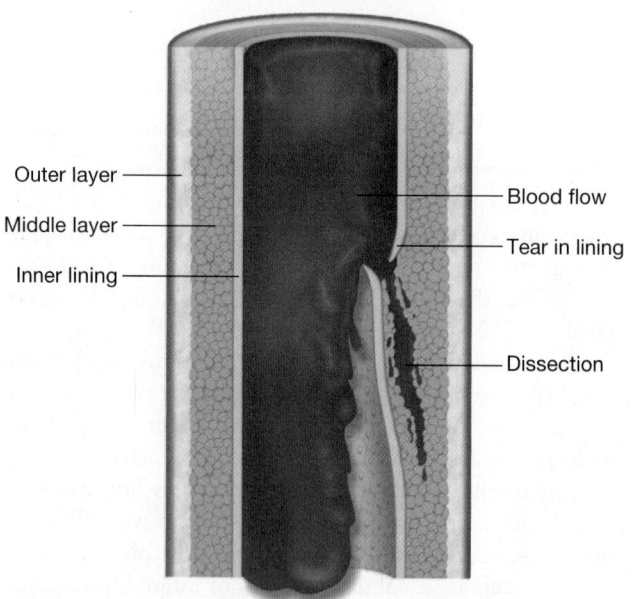

Outer layer

Middle layer

Inner lining

Blood flow

Tear in lining

Dissection

FIGURE 21-27

Aortic dissection. A tear in the tunica intima allows blood to be forced between the layers of the aorta.

leading to heart failure, and blood may leak into the pericardial sac, resulting in **cardiac tamponade**. Diagnosis may be difficult because of the similarity to other cardiac emergencies.

The most common complaint during dissection is tremendous pain in the chest, with a "tearing" or "ripping" sensation. The pain also may be felt in the back, especially when the dissection is present in the descending aorta. Pain may not be present, although this is rare. If dissection extends to one of the subclavian arteries, blood pressure may differ significantly between one arm and the other.

If you suspect aortic dissection, ensure a patent airway with adequate ventilation and administer high-flow oxygen. During transport to a surgical facility, start at least one large-bore IV at a TKO rate. Unless hypotension is present, do not administer fluids, because even a slight increase in blood pressure can extend the dissection or cause it to rupture. If hypotension is present, rupture of the adventitia has likely occurred. Administer fluids according to protocol.

Heart Rate Disturbances

The normal adult heart rate ranges from 60 to 100 beats per minute. A healthy individual can compensate for slight increases or decreases for short periods of time, but both tachycardia and bradycardia can lead to hypotension, chest pain, and altered mental status.

Bradycardia

Although some athletes have a normal resting heart rate of less than 60 beats per minute, bradycardia often leads to an emergency. Bradycardia may be due to abnormal stimulation of the vagus nerve, or due to abnormalities in the cardiac conduction system called *heart blocks*. In some cases, bradycardia is due to intentional or accidental drug overdose, such as with cardiac medications. A bradycardic heart rhythm may be regular or irregular.

When bradycardia is noted, it is classified as either symptomatic or asymptomatic. Asymptomatic patients should receive basic supportive treatments, such as oxygen and an IV, along with transport to a receiving facility with cardiac care capabilities. A patient who has signs or symptoms as a result of the bradycardia, such as chest pain, dyspnea, syncope or near-syncope, confusion, a decreased level of responsiveness, hypotension, or other signs of poor perfusion requires emergency treatment. If available, request ALS. Paramedics can give medications to increase the heart rate and can perform transcutaneous pacing to increase the heart rate.

Ensure the patient has an open airway, using positioning, adjuncts, and suction as necessary. Assist ventilations if they are inadequate, and provide high-flow supplemental oxygen. The patient needs IV access and should be transported without delay. Contact the receiving hospital of the patient's condition, including any indication that the underlying problem may be a drug overdose. If the patient is hypotensive, consult with medical direction about administering a fluid bolus.

Tachycardia

A variety of conditions can lead to an increase in heart rate. The heart rate is expected to increase in response to exertion, anxiety, blood or fluid loss, fever, and some drug overdoses. In those cases, the heart rate is typically less than 150 beats per minute and the treatment is aimed at correcting the underlying cause. Certain cardiac abnormalities can cause rapid heart rates, often at greater than 150 beats per minute.

Paroxysmal supraventricular tachycardia (PSVT) is a dysrhythmia in which the heart beats very rapidly (between 150 and 250 times per minute). This dysrhythmia can occur at any age, and in individuals without known underlying heart disease. In some individuals, there is a defect in the cardiac conduction system that leads to the dysrhythmia, but in others it may be induced by caffeine, smoking, or overexertion. The patient may complain of palpitations, lightheadedness, shortness of breath, or chest pain. The primary problems in PSVT are increased myocardial oxygen consumption and reduced cardiac output.

In PSVT, the heart may beat so rapidly that there is not adequate time between cardiac contractions for the ventricles to fill before contracting again. The stroke volume drops, and may result in hypotension. In some cases, the hypotension is severe enough to impair cerebral perfusion, resulting in altered mental status.

The rapid contraction of the heart increases its need for oxygen, but the decreased stroke volume and cardiac output mean that the coronary arteries are not adequately perfused. Therefore, patients may experience chest pain. Young, healthy individuals may be able to tolerate short periods of PSVT without harm, but untreated, PSVT can lead to congestive heart failure.

Suspect PSVT in a patient who complains of palpitations, perhaps with chest pain or shortness of breath. Often, such patients have a history of similar episodes. You may feel a radial pulse if cardiac output is not severely reduced, but it can be too rapid to get an accurate count. You may only be able to palpate the carotid pulse. If applying a cardiac monitor is within your scope of practice, you will see a regular rhythm with narrow QRS complexes at a rate between 150 and 250 per minute. If cardiac output is severely reduced, the patient may be pale, diaphoretic, and have altered mental status.

Patients with PSVT require high-flow oxygen and should have an IV in place. Treatments for PSVT are typically not within the Advanced EMT's scope of practice. However, if transport time is long, medical direction may instruct you to have the patient perform a Valsalva maneuver: The patient holds his breath and bears down as if to have a bowel movement. This stimulates the vagus nerve, which in turn, may decrease the heart rate. At the paramedic level and in the hospital emergency department, PSVT is treated with medications and synchronized cardioversion.

It is important to note that chest pain from PSVT does not have the same underlying mechanism as ACS, so you should not use nitroglycerin.

Clinical-Reasoning Process

Advanced EMTs Justin and Will are at the residence of Rusty Kypers, who suffered a sudden onset of chest pain at rest. In response to Will's question, Rusty describes his chest pain as a 10 on a scale from 1 to 10. Justin obtains vital signs. Rusty's pulse is 90, strong, and irregular at the radial artery. His blood pressure is 152/94 mmHg, his SpO$_2$ is 97 percent on room air, and his respirations are 22 breaths per minute, with increased respiratory effort. Justin places a nasal cannula on Mr. Kypers with an oxygen flow rate of 4 L/min. Will has determined that Rusty has a medical history of hypertension and high cholesterol.

Laura, Rusty's wife, collects Rusty's medications, which include lisinopril, lovastatin, nitroglycerin, and children's aspirin. Rusty says he hasn't taken his medications in a few days because of his busy work schedule and trying to finish shopping for their wedding anniversary.

After Rusty says he has no allergies, Will hands him two chewable aspirin to prevent further platelet aggregation in the coronary arteries, and Rusty chews them while rubbing his jaw. Even though Rusty's oxygen saturation is normal, the increased respiratory effort concerns Will, so he administers 2 L/min of oxygen by nasal cannula. Justin has prepped an intravenous line of normal saline and tells Rusty, "I'm going to start an IV before we can give you another medication to help with your chest pain." The needle stick barely distracts Rusty from his pain.

As the IV is secured, Laura asks, "Is he going to be okay?"

Will lays a hand on her shoulder and says, "We're doing everything we can and your husband is in good hands, but we need to get him to the hospital as soon as possible."

Justin tells Will the IV is flowing well and pulls out a spray bottle of nitroglycerin from the medication box. Instructing Rusty to open his mouth and lift his tongue, Justin gives a single spray sublingually. En route to the hospital, Rusty receives two more doses of nitroglycerin, which reduce his pain to 4 on a scale of 10 and his blood pressure to 110/64.

At the hospital, a 12-lead ECG is acquired, showing an AMI, and a cardiologist is called to prepare the cath lab. The cardiologist places a stent, opening the artery and relieving some of Rusty's pain. Rusty is discharged from the hospital after several days of anticoagulant therapy and IV nitroglycerin. He begins to exercise more and starts eating cereal on Sunday mornings.

CHAPTER REVIEW

Chapter Summary

The ability to survive depends on the heart's continuous work of effectively pumping blood throughout the body to perfuse cells with oxygen and nutrients and to remove wastes. The cardiovascular system is prone to disease processes that can make the heart less effective as a pump, damage the blood vessels, or even cause sudden death. Acute coronary syndromes result from atherosclerosis, which limits, or even stops altogether, the flow of oxygenated blood to the myocardium. Ischemia and infarction of the myocardium ensue.

You can play a critical role in improving survival from cardiovascular emergencies. Advanced EMTs have the ability to administer some of the most important and therapeutic medications given at any level of licensure, in the initial treatment of ACS.

When the heart is damaged by AMI, long-standing hard work against high blood pressure, or other mechanisms, it can fail as a pump. Two resulting presentations are heart failure and cardiogenic shock. You must recognize the presentations of those emergencies, provide initial treatment, and transport the patient to the hospital emergency department for definitive management. Other cardiovascular emergencies that Advanced EMTs must recognize and be prepared to manage include aortic aneurysm and dissection, hypertensive emergencies, and sudden cardiac death.

Review Questions

Multiple-Choice Questions

1. Blood enters the coronary arteries, allowing perfusion of the myocardium, during:
   a. atrial systole.
   b. atrial diastole.
   c. ventricular systole.
   d. ventricular diastole.

2. Which cardiac electrical event below is represented by the interval on the ECG from the beginning of the QRS complex to the end of the T wave (QT interval)?
   a. Complete cardiac electrical cycle
   b. Ventricular systole and diastole
   c. Ventricular depolarization and repolarization
   d. Atrial depolarization and repolarization

3. A 55-year-old male patient complains of chest pain and dizziness while at rest. Initial vital signs are: heart rate 55, blood pressure 86/52, respiratory rate 22, SpO$_2$ 92 percent on room air. You have initiated oxygen by nonrebreather mask at 15 L/min, given the patient 162 mg chewable aspirin, and started a large-bore IV of normal saline. The next thing you should do is:

   a. administer 0.4 mg SL nitroglycerin.
   b. administer 4 mg morphine, IVP.
   c. contact medical direction concerning a possible fluid bolus.
   d. give a second dose of aspirin, 81 mg PO.

4. In what way do white blood cells play a role in athero-sclerosis?

   a. By sticking together, providing the basis for a blood clot in the artery
   b. By causing initial damage to the intimal layer of the vessel
   c. By forming a fibrous cap over the plaque
   d. By ingesting cholesterol and becoming foam cells in the plaque

5. Which one of the following patients is most likely to present with atypical signs and symptoms of ACS?

   a. 60-year-old woman with diabetes
   b. An otherwise healthy 52-year-old man
   c. 35-year-old man with high blood lipid levels
   d. Any patient who is overweight

6. Which one of the following cardiac dysrhythmias may be present either with or without a pulse?

   a. Normal sinus rhythm
   b. Ventricular fibrillation
   c. Ventricular tachycardia
   d. Asystole

7. Which one of the following would make a patient a poor choice for fibrinolytic therapy?

   a. Takes aspirin every day
   b. Recently had surgery
   c. Has a history of coronary artery disease
   d. Has a family history of stroke

8. Which one of the following most commonly places a patient at highest risk for hypertensive encephalopathy?

   a. Failing to take prescribed medicines for high blood pressure
   b. Regular exercise
   c. Taking antidepressant medication
   d. Acute myocardial infarction

9. Which one of the following best describes the pathophys-iology of aortic dissection?

   a. A weakened area of arterial wall balloons out.
   b. A tear in the lining of the aorta allows blood to seep between the layers, creating a false lumen.
   c. An undetected aneurysm ruptures, causing massive hemorrhage.
   d. A large blood clot forms at the point at which the aorta branches into the lower extremities.

10. Which one of the following is a contraindication for giv-ing nitroglycerin in the prehospital setting?

   a. Systolic blood pressure is less than 120 mmHg.
   b. Patient rates the chest pain as a 5 or less on a scale from 1 to 10.
   c. Patient describes a sensation of heaviness or tight-ness, rather than pain.
   d. Patient states he took three doses of nitroglycerin before you arrived.

Critical-Thinking Questions

11. In what way(s) can the body maintain cardiac output if the blood volume decreases?

12. Describe what your concerns should be if a patient with signs and symptoms of ACS presents with tachycardia.

13. Why are early recognition and treatment important for patients with ACS?

14. How can CPAP help the patient with pulmonary edema resulting from heart failure?

15. How are left-sided and right-sided heart failure the same and how are they different?

Reference

American Heart Association. (2010). Part 10: Acute coronary syndromes: 2010 American Heart Association Guidelines for Cardiopulmonary Resuscitation and Emergency Cardiovascular Care. *Circulation, 122,* S787–S817.

Additional Reading

Field, J. M. (Ed.). (2006). *Advanced cardiovascular life support provider manual.* Dallas, TX: American Heart Association.
Libby, P. (Ed.) (2008). *Braunwald's heart disease: A textbook of cardiovascular medicine* (8th ed.). Philadelphia, PA: Saunders Elsevier.
Lilly, L. S. (Ed.). (2007). *Pathophysiology of heart disease* (4th ed.). Baltimore, MD: Lippincott Williams & Wilkins.
Mistovich, J., & Karren, K. (2010). *Prehospital emergency care* (9th ed.). Upper Saddle River, NJ: Brady Pearson.

22

Neurologic Disorders

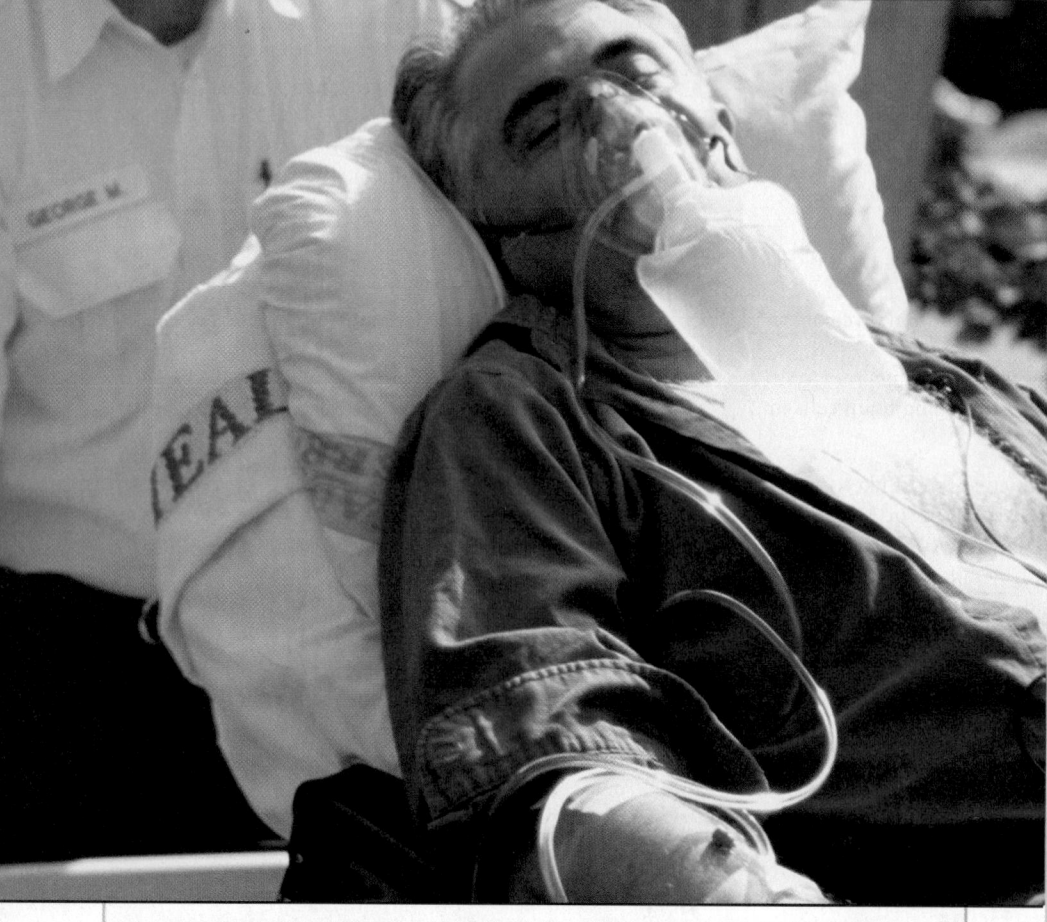

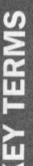
Content Area: Medicine

Advanced EMT Education Standard: Applies fundamental knowledge to provide basic and selected advanced emergency care and transportation based on assessment findings for an acutely ill patient.

Objectives

After reading this chapter, you should be able to:

22.1 Define key terms introduced in this chapter.

22.2 Recognize complaints that may indicate a neurologic problem.

22.3 List possible underlying causes of altered mental status, neurologic deficit, headache, seizures, and syncope.

22.4 Explain the importance of airway assessment and management in patients with altered mental status and neurologic deficit.

22.5 Obtain information in the patient history that is focused on the evaluation of altered mental status, neurologic deficit, headache, seizure, or syncope.

22.6 Given a scenario with a patient with altered mental status, neurologic deficit, headache, seizure, or syncope, perform a physical examination that is focused on relevant findings and anticipated consequences.

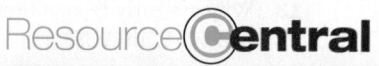
Resource Central

CASE STUDY

Advanced EMTs Anna Chu and Brian Davis are at 542 Walker Avenue for a report of a patient with a headache. A girl of about seven years old opens the door, telling the crew that her mother has a really bad headache and needs your help. The patient, 44-year-old Regina Lear, is lying on her left side on a sofa, holding a small pillow over her eyes. Brian introduces himself and Anna to the patient and asks, "How can we help you today, Ms. Lear? You look as if you're not feeling well."

"It's my head," replies Ms. Lear. "It's killing me."

Problem-Solving Questions

1. What are some potential causes of the patient's headache?
2. What level of concern should Anna and Brian have for a chief complaint of severe head pain?
3. What is the best way to approach the gathering of this patient's history?
4. What aspects of the examination will provide the most important information in this case?

22.7   Integrate scene size-up information, the patient's history, vital signs, and physical exam findings with knowledge of anatomy and physiology and pathophysiology to identify more likely causes of the patient's condition.

22.8   Determine the need for the following interventions in patients with a neurologic emergency:

- Interventions to open and maintain the airway
- Manual spinal stabilization
- Oxygenation
- Ventilation

22.9   Identify the signs and symptoms of stroke.

22.10   Describe the pathophysiology of stroke.

22.11   Explain the importance of early recognition of stroke signs and symptoms by patients, family or bystanders, and EMS personnel.

22.12   Describe the relationship between stroke and transient ischemic attack.

22.13   Assess the patient with possible stroke for neurologic deficits, including use of a stroke scale:

- Cincinnati Prehospital Stroke Scale
- Los Angeles Prehospital Stroke Scale

22.14   Discuss the role of blood glucose determination in the assessment of patients with altered mental status, neurologic deficits, and seizures.

22.15   Describe ways of communicating with patients who have difficulty speaking.

22.16   Recognize indications that a headache may have a potentially life-threatening underlying cause, such as toxic exposure, hypertension, infectious disease, or hemorrhagic stroke.

22.17   Describe measures that you can take to improve the comfort level of the patient suffering from a headache.

22.18   Explain the importance of reassessment of the patient with altered mental status, neurologic deficit, headache, seizure, or syncope.

22.19   Describe the various ways that seizures can present.

22.20   Discuss possible underlying causes of seizures.

22.21   Explain the concerns associated with prolonged or successive seizures.

22.22   Describe the assessment and emergency medical care of patients with tonic–clonic, simple partial, complex partial, febrile, and absence seizures, and patients in a postictal state.

(continued)

(continued from previous page)

22.23 Anticipate bystander reactions to patients having seizures and measures needed to stop any unnecessary or inappropriate interventions.

22.24 Compare and contrast features of dementia and delirium.

22.25 Describe basic information about various neurologic disorders, such as Bell's palsy, vertigo, Parkinson's disease, Wernicke-Korsakoff syndrome, multiple sclerosis, normal pressure hydrocephalus, and others that may affect the assessment and management of patients.

Introduction

Neurologic disorders can arise in either the central or peripheral divisions of the nervous system. Typically, those that are most serious arise in the central nervous system, although peripheral nervous disorders can be painful and debilitating. Altered mental status, behavioral changes, and neurologic deficits are common manifestations of nervous system disorders, but have other causes, too. Some of those underlying problems can be corrected or improved by measures in the Advanced EMT's scope of practice. In other cases, understanding the pathophysiology of disease processes helps you understand the importance of your actions in improving the patient's potential for recovery by preventing secondary brain injury. In the case of stroke, recognition of signs and symptoms and prompt transport to a specialized stroke center, if available, can limit the amount of damage and, in some cases, restore lost neurologic function.

This chapter covers the assessment and management of patients with altered mental status and pathophysiology, assessment, and management of patients with specific neurologic disorders. Topics include stroke, seizures, headaches, dementia, delirium, selected chronic and degenerative neurologic diseases, infectious neurologic disorders, and nontraumatic back pain.

Anatomy and Physiology Review

The nervous system is one of the two major control systems of the body. Compared to the endocrine system, the nervous system responds more quickly to stimuli in order to maintain homeostasis. The nervous system is divided anatomically into the central nervous system (CNS), consisting of the brain and spinal cord; and peripheral nervous system, which consists of all neural tissue outside the brain and spinal cord (Figure 22-1). Functionally, the nervous system is divided into the somatic (voluntary) and

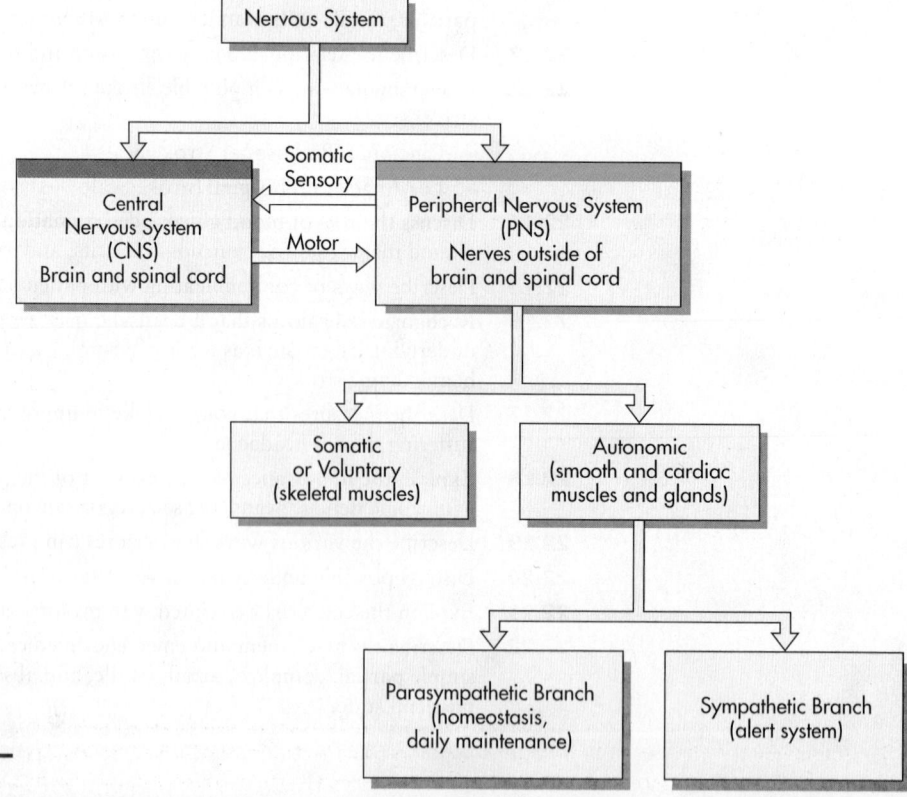

FIGURE 22-1

Divisions of the nervous system.

TABLE 22-1	Functions of the Sympathetic and Parasympathetic Divisions of the Autonomic Nervous System			
	SYMPATHETIC			**PARASYMPATHETIC**
Alpha$_1$ Receptors	**Beta$_1$ Receptors**	**Beta$_2$ Receptors**		
Constriction of arterioles and veins Pupil dilation	Increased heart rate, strength of contraction, automaticity, and conduction	Bronchodilation Dilation of arterioles Inhibition of uterine contractions Skeletal muscle tremors		Pupil constriction Decreases heart rate, strength of contraction, and blood pressure Bronchoconstriction Increases gastrointestinal tract activity

autonomic (involuntary) divisions. The autonomic division is further divided into the parasympathetic division, responsible for vegetative functions and reproduction, and the sympathetic division, responsible for the response to stressors (Table 22-1). The sympathetic and parasympathetic divisions work together to meet the demands on the body, with each exerting a greater or lesser degree of control as needed.

The overall function of the nervous system is to monitor input from the body's internal and external environments,

integrate the sensory input from the environment, and coordinate both voluntary and involuntary responses to the input. Input is received from the external environment from somatic sensory receptors, such as those involved in vision and hearing; and from the internal environment by visceral receptors, such as the baroreceptors that monitor blood pressure and the chemoreceptors that monitor carbon dioxide and oxygen levels in the blood. Input travels by way of afferent nerve fibers to the central nervous system where it is integrated and a response is coordinated (Figure 22-2).

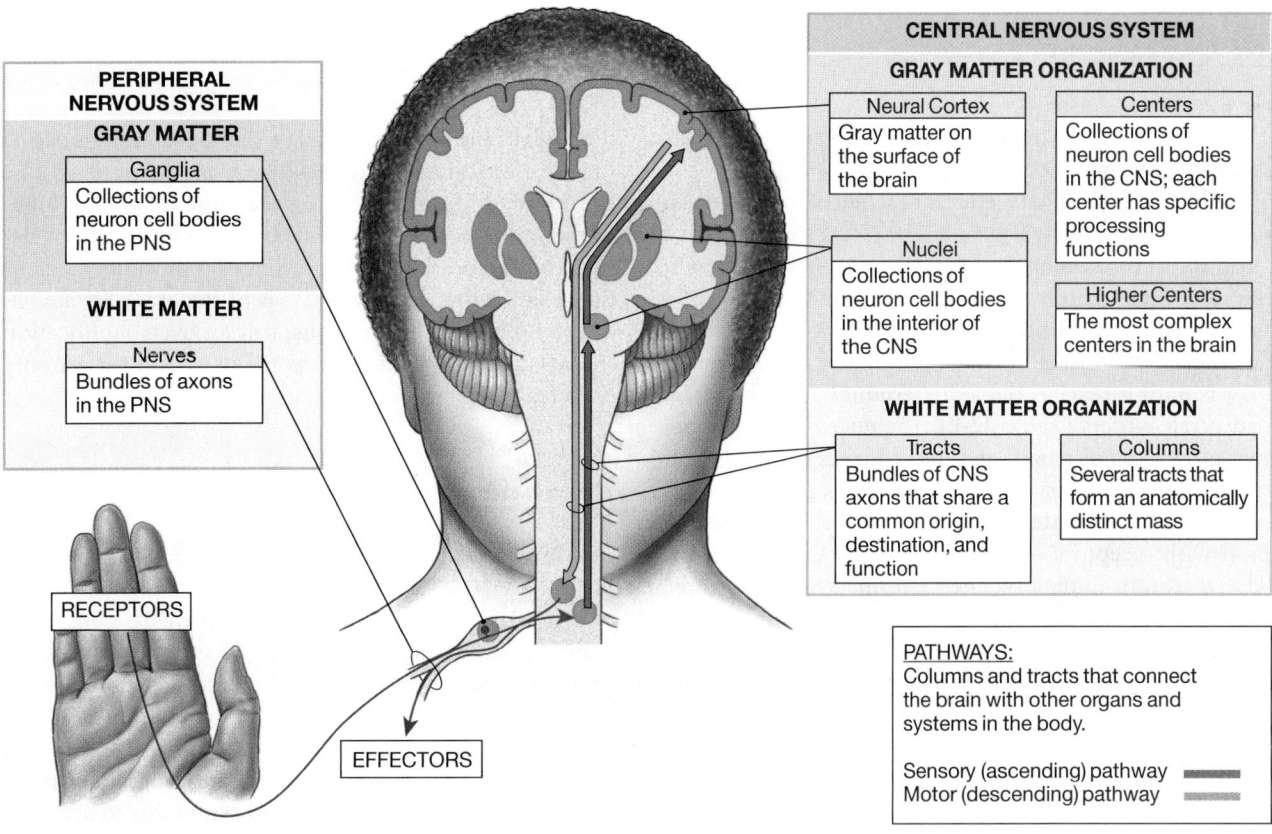

FIGURE 22-2

Communication in the nervous system. (Bledsoe, Bryan E.; Martini, Frederic H.; Bartholomew, Edwin F.; Ober, William C.; Garrison, Claire W.; Anatomy & Physiology for Emergency Care, 2nd Edition, © 2008. Reprinted with permission of Pearson Education, Inc., Upper Saddle River, NJ)

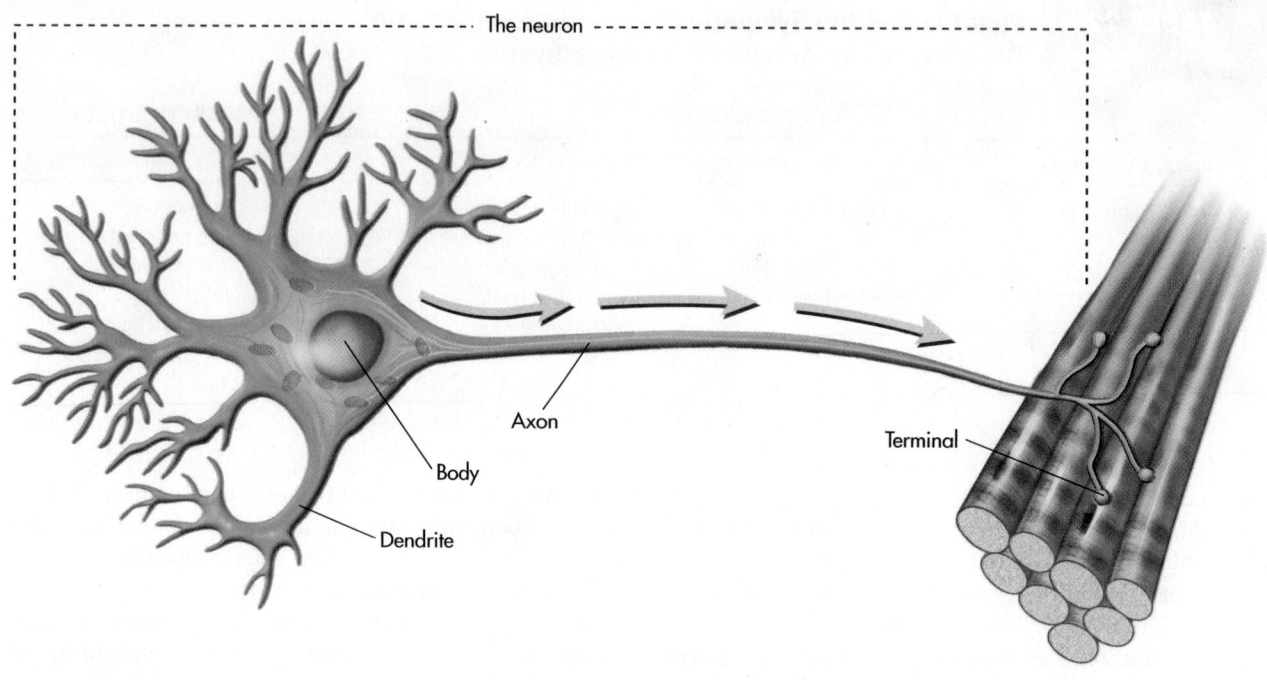

```
                                    The neuron
```

Axon

Body

Terminal

Dendrite

FIGURE 22-3

A representative neuron.

The response stimuli travel by way of efferent nerve fibers to target effector tissues.

The basic unit of structure of the nervous system is a *neuron*, or nerve cell (Figure 22-3). Nerve cells can take various forms based on their function, but have basic similarities. Each neuron consists of a cell body, or soma; a projection with dendrites, which receive input; and a projection called an *axon* through which a nervous impulse travels until it reaches the axon terminals, which secrete neurotransmitters (Table 22-2). The microscopic gap between the axon terminals and the dendrites of an adjacent neuron or the effector tissue is called a *synapse*. Molecules of the neurotransmitter are secreted into the synapse and bind with receptors on the dendrites of effector tissue. The neurotransmitters secreted into the synapse must be broken down to prevent continuous nervous stimulation (Figure 22-4).

The human brain consists of six major parts: the cerebrum, diencephalon, midbrain, pons, medulla oblongata, and cerebellum (Figure 22-5). The cerebrum is the uppermost portion of the brain, responsible for higher brain functions (Figure 22-6). The cerebral cortex is the outermost portion of the cerebrum. The cerebrum is divided by the longitudinal fissure into right and left hemispheres. Each hemisphere is composed of the frontal, temporal, parietal, and occipital lobes, corresponding to the areas of

the skull of the same names. The central sulcus (groove or furrow) separates the frontal lobe from the parietal lobe behind it. Additional sulci separate the remaining lobes of the brain from each other. Higher brain functions depend on integration and coordination of many areas of the brain. Although certain areas of the brain are associated with particular functions, it is an oversimplification to view any brain function as being dependent on only one area of the brain (Table 22-3).

Assessment of Neurologic Complaints

You must work from the patient's presentation, complaints, and history to determine if the problem is due to neurologic causes or something else. The patient may present with altered mental status, behavioral changes, sensory impairment, headache, weakness, paralysis, or other complaints. You must use knowledge of various causes of the presenting signs and symptoms to arrive at a field impression. Knowledge of the pathophysiology of common neurologic problems is an important part of being able to develop and test hypotheses in your clinical reasoning process.

TABLE 22-2	Selected Neurotransmitters
Neurotransmitter	**Function**
Acetylcholine	The preganglionic neurotransmitter of the sympathetic nervous system and the pre- and postganglionic neurotransmitter of the parasympathetic nervous system. Also acts at the neuromuscular junction.
Dopamine	In the brain, affects areas of the brain responsible for movement, emotions, and the ability to experience pleasure. Dopamine regulation may play a role in addictions. Death of dopamine-producing cells in a specific area of the brain results in Parkinson's disease. Some antipsychotics are used to decrease dopamine activity on certain dopamine receptors in the brain to treat schizophrenia. Some older antidepressants work by blocking the enzyme that breaks down dopamine, thus increasing dopamine's action in the brain.
GABA (gamma-aminobutyric acid)	Inhibits central nervous system activity. Deficiency can play a role in anxiety and insomnia. Benzodiazepines, such as Valium and Xanax, work to decrease anxiety by stimulating GABA receptors.
Glutamate	Plays a role in learning and memory; may be deficient (or certain receptors for it may be damaged) in Alzheimer's disease and alcoholic brain damage.
Norepinephrine	Helps regulate the reticular activating system. Excess in the amygdala and forebrain can produce anxiety. Reduced norepinephrine activity may play a role in depression. Some types of antidepressants prevent reuptake of norepinephrine.
Serotonin	In the brain, regulates mood, emotion, appetite, and sleep. Responsible for general feelings of well-being. Lack of serotonin in the brain may lead to depression. Many currently used antidepressants block the reuptake of serotonin in brain synapses (selective serotonin reuptake inhibitors or SSRIs).

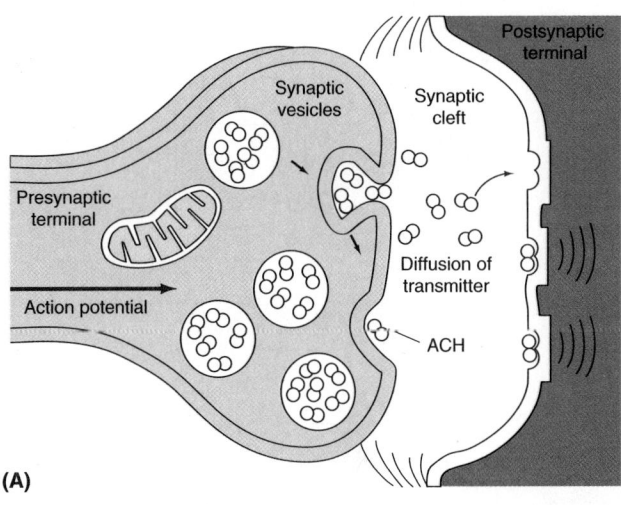
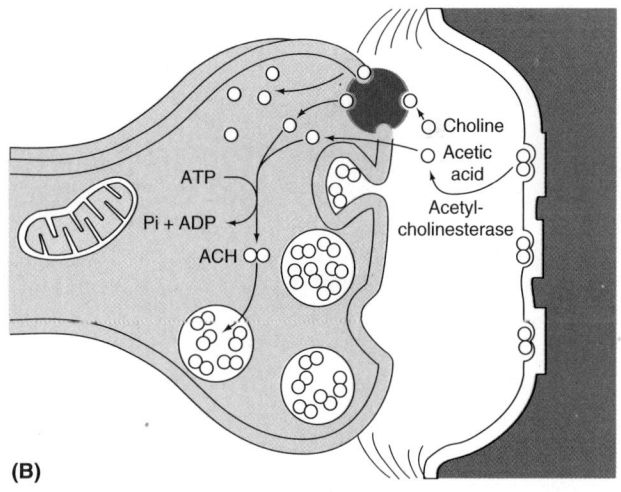

(A)   **(B)**

FIGURE 22-4

Neurotransmitter action at a synapse. (A) Acetylcholine is released into the synapse and binds with receptors. (B) Acetylcholine is broken down by acetylcholinesterase and its components are reused to make additional acetylcholine.

Scene Size-Up

Because you do not know the exact nature of the problem at the beginning, your scene size-up incorporates standard operational and patient care aspects. Before you can further assess the patient and provide care, you must ensure your safety and the patient's. You may note some early

IN THE FIELD

If your scene size-up shows that there are multiple patients with altered mental status, suspect exposure to a toxin and do not enter the area. Notify dispatch of a possible hazardous materials situation.

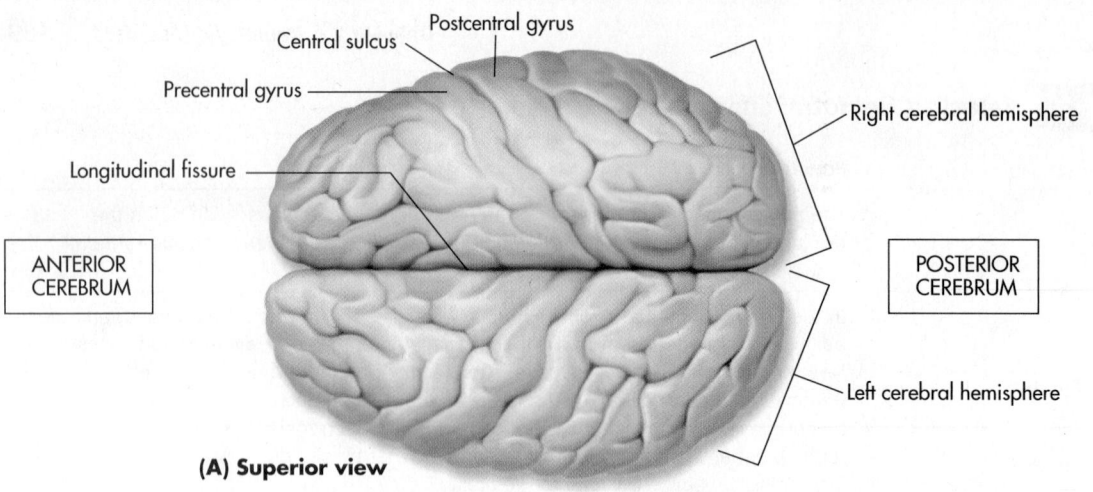

(A) Superior view

Central sulcus
Postcentral gyrus
Precentral gyrus
Longitudinal fissure
Right cerebral hemisphere
Left cerebral hemisphere

ANTERIOR CEREBRUM

POSTERIOR CEREBRUM

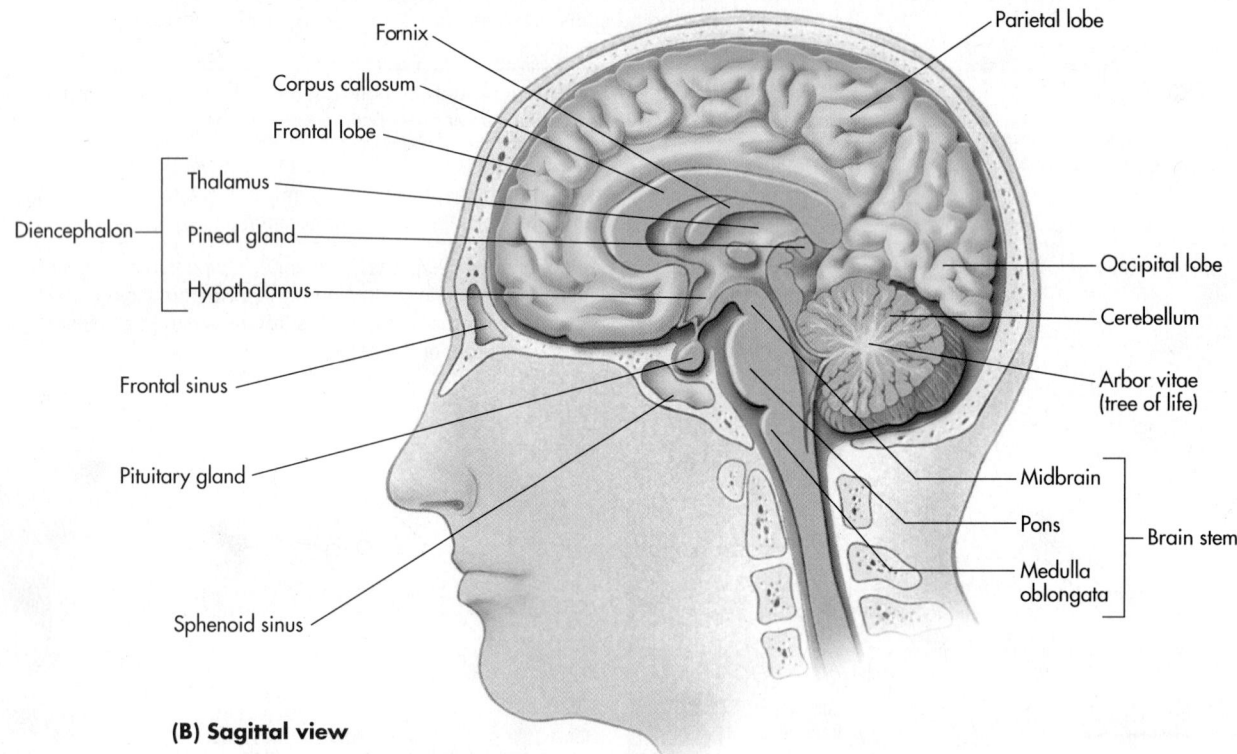

Fornix
Corpus callosum
Frontal lobe
Thalamus
Pineal gland
Hypothalamus
Diencephalon
Frontal sinus
Pituitary gland
Sphenoid sinus
Parietal lobe
Occipital lobe
Cerebellum
Arbor vitae (tree of life)
Midbrain
Pons
Medulla oblongata
Brain stem

(B) Sagittal view

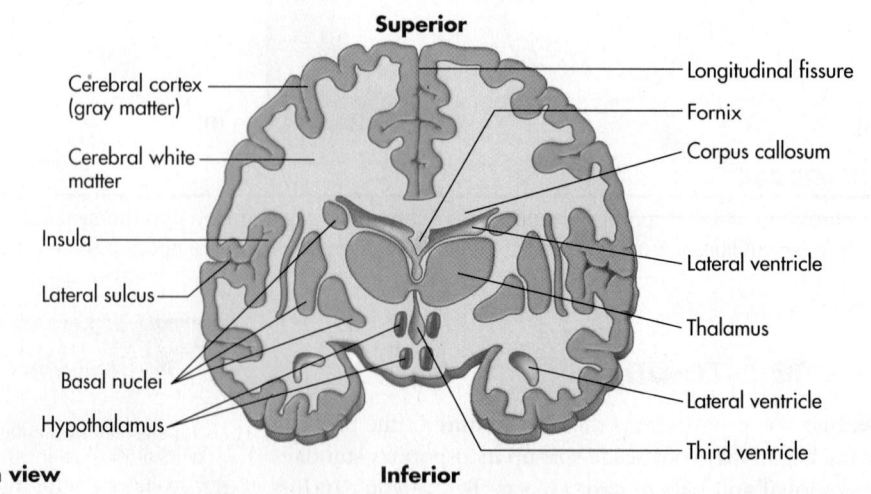

Superior

Cerebral cortex (gray matter)
Cerebral white matter
Insula
Lateral sulcus
Basal nuclei
Hypothalamus
Longitudinal fissure
Fornix
Corpus callosum
Lateral ventricle
Thalamus
Lateral ventricle
Third ventricle

(C) Frontal section view

Inferior

FIGURE 22-5

Structure of the brain. (A) Superior view. (B) Sagittal view. (C) Frontal section view.

TABLE 22-5	Stroke Assessment	
Sign of Stroke	**Patient Activity**	**Interpretation**
Unilateral or bilateral facial droop	Have the patient look directly at you and smile or show their teeth	Normal: symmetrical movement to both sides Abnormal: one side does not move or neither side moves
Arm drift	Have the patient extend their arms outward and hold them there for several seconds while their eyes are closed	Normal: the arms do not drift downward Abnormal: one arm drifts downward while the other remains extended
Abnormal speech	Have the patient repeat a sentence to you	Normal: the patient correctly repeats the sentence to you Abnormal: the patient speaks with slurred words, cannot speak, or uses incorrect words

TABLE 22-6	Stroke Screening Tool			
Criteria		**Yes**	**No**	**Unknown**
Greater than 45 years of age				
Seizure activity prior to symptom onset				
Blood glucose between 60 and 400 mg/dL				
Abnormal findings during stroke assessment				

Reasoning and Decision Making

Recognizing signs and symptoms of neurologic problems requires inductive reasoning from the collection of signs and symptoms to their potential causes. To do this effectively, you must understand the basic functions of the nervous system and causes of neurologic signs and symptoms. Altered mental status, behavioral emergencies, headache, slurred speech, and other indications of neurologic emergencies have several underlying causes. You can remember those causes by the mnemonic AEIOU-TIPS (Table 22-8).

Some causes are extracranial, caused by conditions arising elsewhere in the body that affect brain functioning, such as infection, metabolic problems (hypoglycemia, hyperglycemia), hypoxia, hypoperfusion, toxins, environmental conditions, and overdoses. Some of those causes can be addressed in the prehospital setting and must be identified immediately. Correcting problems with the airway, breathing, and oxygenation may improve mental status. Patients who are hypoglycemic will improve with an increase in blood glucose level, and patients with narcotic overdoses may improve with naloxone administration. Other causes

TABLE 22-7   Glasgow Coma Scale

EYE OPENING	
Spontaneous	4
To verbal command	3
To pain	2
No response	1
VERBAL RESPONSE	
Oriented and converses	5
Disoriented and converses	4
Inappropriate words	3
Incomprehensible sounds	2
No response	1
MOTOR RESPONSE	
Obeys verbal commands	6
Localizes pain	5
Withdraws from pain (flexion)	4
Abnormal flexion in response to pain (decorticate rigidity)	3
Extension in response to pain (decerebrate rigidity)	2
No response	1

TABLE 22-8   Mnemonic AEIOU-TIPS for Causes of Altered Mental Status

A	–	Alcohol, anoxia
E	–	Environment, epilepsy
I	–	Insulin (diabetes and other endocrine disorders)
O	–	Overdose
U	–	Uremia (renal failure)
T	–	Trauma (shock, traumatic brain injury)
I	–	Infection
P	–	Psychosis, poisoning
S	–	Stroke

may not be immediately correctable in the prehospital setting, but the care you provide can improve the patient's outcome, and the history you collect can be instrumental in guiding the emergency department care of the patient.

Intracranial causes of neurologic emergencies include traumatic brain injury, stroke, and epilepsy. Although you cannot address those underlying problem, there is much you can do to improve the patient's outcome. The management of airway, ventilation, and oxygenation is critical. Controlling bleeding and maintaining blood pressure in the trauma patient with a brain injury helps maintain brain perfusion, preventing secondary brain injury. Transporting the stroke or traumatic brain injury patient to the right facility for care can make a tremendous difference in the patient's outcome.

Reassessment

Patients with neurologic emergencies can be critically ill. Reassess critical patients every 5 minutes, including the primary assessment, vital signs, complaints, and relevant aspects of the secondary assessment. Perform reassessment more frequently, if warranted. Include serial assessments of the patient's mental status, pupil response, and other aspects of neurologic examination. Reassess noncritical patients every 15 minutes. The interventions you provide will depend on the nature of the problem, but you must check their effectiveness.

Altered Mental Status

Altered mental status (AMS) is not a disease in itself, but an indication of an underlying problem that is affecting brain function. There are many causes of AMS, some of which you can immediately correct or improve in the prehospital setting. Regardless of the underlying cause, patients with AMS are vulnerable. They cannot protect themselves from the environment and may have lost their gag and cough reflexes, putting them at risk for aspiration. Muscle tone may be impaired, leading to airway obstruction by the epiglottis and tongue, and respirations may be depressed. Patients with involvement of the hypothalamus and brainstem may lose the ability to control body temperature, blood pressure, heart rate, and respirations. Many of the conditions leading to AMS also can place the patient at risk for seizures.

Treatment of patients with AMS includes managing the airway, breathing, and circulation, and searching for potentially correctable underlying causes. If you believe the patient's AMS may be due to hypoglycemia or narcotic overdose, defer insertion of oropharyngeal and advanced airway devices until you have treated the patient for those conditions. This does not mean that you should not appropriately manage the patient's airway and ventilations. It means instead that you should use manual maneuvers and potentially a nasopharyngeal airway to prevent the patient with an immediately correctable cause of AMS from waking up with a device in his airway that could cause him to panic and lead to injury. A patient who is conscious can protect his airway and adjust his ventilations better than EMS providers can.

Syncope

Syncope is a temporary loss of consciousness caused by inadequate brain perfusion. Common causes of syncope and near-syncope include transient cardiac dysrhythmia, volume depletion (especially when the patient changes from a supine or sitting position to standing), medications that prevent an increase in heart rate or vasoconstriction when the patient changes from a supine or sitting position to standing, and a vasovagal response (stimulation of the parasympathetic nervous system temporarily over-rides the sympathetic nervous system mechanisms that allow an increase in heart rate and vasoconstriction). Note that the underlying cause of syncope in most cases is cardiovascular, not neurologic.

The vasovagal response may occur in patients who have a highly sensitive carotid sinus or in response to stimuli such as the sight of blood or needles. Witnesses usually report that the patient became pale and may have exhibited some shaking of the extremities that may be described as a "seizure." The patient often describes a narrowing of the field of vision (tunnel vision), loss of vision, "seeing stars," or roaring in the ears just prior to loss of consciousness.

By definition, syncope is transient. If the patient remains unresponsive on your arrival, the problem is not syncope, but something else. Although syncope can be benign, there are also potentially life-threatening causes. In addition, it is possible for a patient to sustain injury if he falls during the syncopal episode. All patients who have experienced syncope or a near-syncopal episode must be thoroughly evaluated and encouraged to be transported to the hospital. Depending upon the patient's history (age, medications, other complaints), cardiac monitoring and checking orthostatic vital signs may be indicated.

Stroke

Stroke is a leading cause of death and disability, with 795,000 cases of new or repeat strokes annually (American Heart Association [AHA], 2010). Stroke occurs when an area of the brain is deprived of circulation, and thus of oxygen and glucose. The two mechanisms of stroke are ischemic and hemorrhagic (Figure 22-7). **Ischemic stroke** occurs when a blood clot blocks arterial blood flow to a

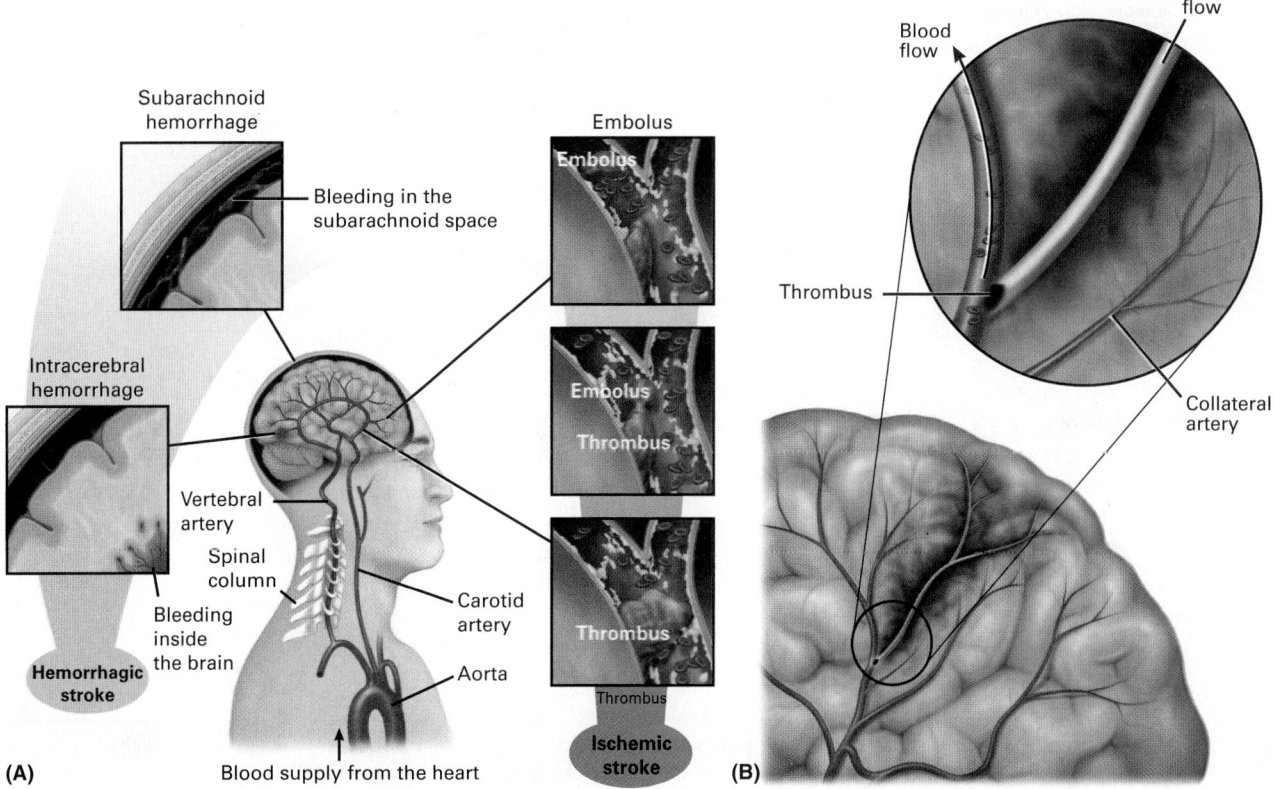

FIGURE 22-7

Causes of stroke. (A) Blood is carried from the heart to the brain by way of the carotid and vertebral arteries, which form a ring and branches within the brain. A hemorrhagic stroke occurs when a cerebral artery ruptures and bleeds into the brain (examples shown: subarachnoid bleeding on the surface of the brain; intracerebral bleeding within the brain). An ischemic stroke occurs when a thrombus is formed on the wall of an artery or when an embolus travels from another area until it lodges in and blocks an arterial branch. (B) Brain tissues distal to a rupture, thrombus, or embolus receive little or no perfusion and become ischemic (starved of oxygen) and eventually infarcted (dead). When a thrombus grows slowly enough, collateral arteries may form parallel to the blocked artery to perfuse or partially perfuse the oxygen-starved area of the brain.

portion of the brain. Ischemic stroke most commonly occurs from thrombus formation, but also can occur from an embolus. Hemorrhagic stroke occurs when there is a rupture of a blood vessel within the cranium. An intracerebral hemorrhage occurs when an aneurysm or **arteriovenous malformation** (AVM) ruptures within the brain itself, while a **subarachnoid hemorrhage** occurs when a weakened vessel bleeds into the subarachnoid space between the brain and arachnoid layer of the meninges.

Stroke Pathophysiology

Ischemic stroke is often a result of atherosclerosis of cerebral arteries, or of the internal carotid arteries that supply blood to the brain. The risk factors for atherosclerosis are the same as those for cardiovascular disease (Table 22-9).

TABLE 22-9 Stroke Risk Factors

- Hypertension
- Diabetes
- Cardiovascular disease
- Prior stroke
- Transient ischemic attack
- Hypercholesterolemia
- Age > 55 years
- Gender (male)
- Ethnicity (African Americans and Hispanics have twice the risk as the population as a whole)
- Family history
- Hypercoagulative states (pregnancy, sickle cell disease, cancer)
- Smoking
- Obesity
- Atrial fibrillation
- Inactivity
- Cocaine, IV drug abuse
- Excessive alcohol use
- Hormonal contraceptives
- History of migraine headaches with an aura

A blood clot or plaque from the internal carotid arteries can also break loose, forming an embolism that travels into the brain circulation until it reaches a point where it becomes lodged and obstructs blood flow. The cardiac dysrhythmia atrial fibrillation can lead to the formation of blood clots in the atria, which can then be ejected into the systemic circulation and travel to the brain. Hemorrhagic strokes can occur due to rupture of an aneurysm in the brain, or from an AVM, an abnormal connection between arterial and venous circulation in the brain. Hypertension and atherosclerosis are risk factors for hemorrhagic stroke, but patients also may have a congenital abnormality that leads to hemorrhage.

The high demand of the brain for both oxygen and glucose means that dysfunction of the affected areas occurs immediately and neurologic damage and death can begin to occur within 4 minutes. Depending on the artery affected, there can be collateral circulation that provides some perfusion to the affected area, increasing the amount of time before irreversible damage is done. If perfusion is restored, injury can be reduced, or even reversed. The initial signs and symptoms of stroke reflect the area of the brain deprived of perfusion (Table 22-10). In severe stroke, secondary brain injury and edema can lead to worsening of signs and symptoms and progress to altered mental status and impaired breathing. Common warning signs of stroke include the following:

- Sudden numbness or weakness of the face, arm, or leg, especially on one side of the body
- Sudden confusion or difficulty speaking or understanding (aphasia)
- Sudden difficulty with vision in one or both eyes
- Sudden loss of coordination, difficulty walking, dizziness, or loss of balance
- Sudden, severe headache with no other known explanation

Other stroke signs and symptoms include sudden onset of inappropriate display of emotions (inappropriate laughing or crying), or inability to control emotions. A common difference in the onset of ischemic and hemorrhagic stroke is

TABLE 22-10 Stroke Terminology

Term	Definition
Aphasia	Difficulty with or loss of language skills; may be receptive (difficulty understanding) or expressive (difficulty expressing oneself); can include spoken or written language
Ataxia	Lack of coordination
Dysarthria	Difficulty speaking due to weakness or paralysis of muscles involved in speech
Hemianopsia	Loss of half the visual field
Hemiparesis	Weakness on one side of the body
Hemiplegia	Paralysis on one side of the body

that hemorrhagic strokes often begin with a sudden, severe headache unlike other headaches the patient has experienced, followed by progressively worsening signs and symptoms. The brain itself does not have pain sensors, meaning that ischemic stroke is not initially painful. However, the meninges do have pain sensors. Blood within the cranial cavity is irritating to the meninges, causing pain. Depending on the speed and amount of bleeding, mental status may decrease rapidly and intracranial pressure may increase. In ischemic stroke, there often is no headache and signs and symptoms are their worst at or near the time of onset (Figure 22-8).

Patients also can present with signs and symptoms of stroke that resolve, usually within 1 to 2 hours, without cerebral infarction (Easton et al., 2009). This is called a **transient ischemic attack (TIA)**, in which there is a temporary interruption in perfusion (usually from atherosclerotic disease or emboli). Signs and symptoms can sometimes last up to 24 hours, but you must never take a "wait and see" approach to the patient who has signs and symptoms of stroke. The diagnosis of TIA is ultimately based on whether or not there is permanent neurologic deficit, not on the duration of the signs and symptoms. The patient who has experienced a TIA is at high risk for subsequent stroke and must be transported for further evaluation, even if the signs and symptoms have resolved.

Stroke Treatment

There is a stroke chain of survival, very much like the chain of survival for cardiac arrest. One of the weakest links in this chain often is the patient's or bystanders' ability to recognize signs and symptoms of stroke. This often leads to a delay in seeking care. Public education and advances in stroke treatment have led to better outcomes for stroke, but as many as half of all stroke patients arrive at the emergency department by means other than ambulance. The steps of

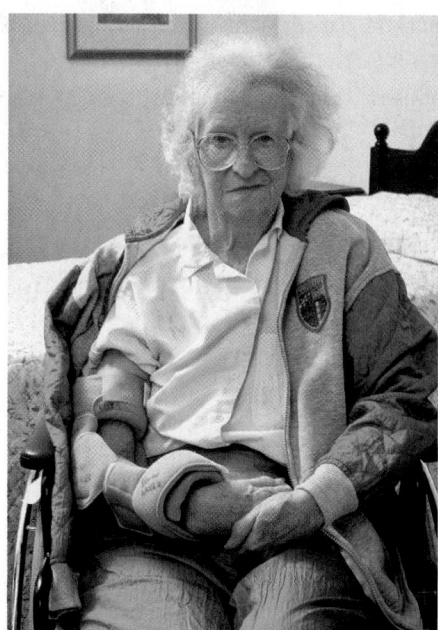

FIGURE 22-8

Stroke can result in paralysis affecting one side of the body.

appropriate stroke care are detailed below (Table 22-11). Currently there is emphasis on the development of community stroke centers that specialize in prompt diagnosis and treatment of stroke.

The role of EMS providers is to quickly recognize the possibility of stroke, provide immediate treatment, and transport the patient without delay to the most appropriate facility. Key EMS provider actions include the following:

- Recognize signs and symptoms that may indicate stroke.
- Use a prehospital stroke screening tool to identify stroke patients.

TABLE 22-11	**Keys to appropriate stroke care**
Early recognition of stroke	Bystanders must be able to recognize signs and symptoms of stroke. This is done through public education and awareness campaigns.
Timely activation and dispatch of EMS	Once stroke is identified bystanders must activate 911 in a timely manner to initiate EMS response.
Timely EMS assessment, recognition, and transport to an appropriate facility	EMS must complete an assessment, recognize stroke, and initiate transport to a facility capable of providing definitive care to the patient.
Timely triage, evaluation, and management in the emergency department	Upon arrival at the emergency department staff must identify stroke in a timely manner and activate the appropriate resources needed to manage the patient.
Appropriate therapy initiation	Specialists, usually stroke neurologists, must select the appropriate treatment using information gathered from bystanders, EMS, emergency department staff, and their own assessment.
Timely admission to stroke unit	Once treatment is initiated the patient should be admitted to a stroke unit for further treatment and monitoring.

- Support the patient's airway, breathing, and circulation.

- Administer oxygen to patients with an SpO_2 less than 95 percent.

- Manage hypotension (systolic blood pressure of less than 90 mmHg).

- Establish the time of onset of signs and symptoms.

- Select the most appropriate receiving facility, preferably a stroke center.

- Transport without delay.

- Be prepared to manage seizures.

- Notify the receiving facility so they can prepare for the patient.

- Check the patient's blood glucose level.

- In some EMS systems, EMS personal perform an initial screening to determine the patient's eligibility for fibrinolytic therapy.

As with all patients, care of the patient with a stroke begins in the primary assessment. Patients with stroke are at risk for upper airway obstruction and aspiration due to vomiting and impaired swallowing. Use positioning, manual maneuvers, and suction to open the airway and help the patient manage secretions. If the patient's level of responsiveness is impaired, use basic and more definitive airway adjuncts as needed. If the patient's ventilations are inadequate, assist them using a bag-valve-mask device. Although it has long a been a practice to administer high-flow oxygen to all patients suspected of having a stroke, be aware that an elevated PaO_2 can cause vasoconstriction, further impairing perfusion of the ischemic brain. Treat hypoxia, but do not over administer oxygen.

Patients with stroke may be hypertensive, but it is currently not recommended that you treat high blood pressure in the prehospital setting. Lowering the mean arterial pressure will lower the cerebral perfusion pressure. If the cerebral perfusion pressure is decreased too much, the ischemic brain will not be adequately perfused, leading to additional damage. A stroke patient who is hypotensive, with a systolic blood pressure less than 90 mmHg, also is at risk of having an inadequate cerebral perfusion pressure. Follow your protocols or consult with on-line medical direction regarding intravenous fluid administration in hypotensive stroke patients.

Once you are managing the patient's airway, breathing, and circulation, determine the time of onset of signs and symptoms as exactly as possible (if you have not already obtained this information). If the patient awoke from sleep with signs and symptoms, determine the last time the patient was seen without signs and symptoms. For fibrinolytic treatment to be effective, if the patient is a candidate, it must be initiated within 3 to 4½ hours from the onset of signs and symptoms. However, the more quickly it is administered, the less brain cell death will occur. It is estimated that for each minute without adequate perfusion, a pea-sized portion of brain tissue dies, including 1.9 million neurons and 14 billion synapses. In some cases, it may be desirable to transport a family member who is knowledgeable about the patient's medical history to the hospital with him. Several very specific questions must be answered to determine if the patient is a candidate for fibrinolytic therapy (Table 22-12).

It is critical to transport the patient without delay to the most appropriate facility in order to maximize the patient's chances for improvement in neurologic status. Stroke centers are available regionally in most areas, although air

---

TABLE 22-12   Criteria for fibrinolytic treatment of stroke

Inclusionary criteria	Exclusionary criteria
Stroke identified with neurologic deficit not resolving	Traumatic head trauma or stroke in the past 3 months
Symptoms onset <3 hours (may vary depending upon facility treatment guidelines)	Confirmed intracranial hemorrhage
18 years of age or older	Arterial cannulation within the past 7 days
	Hypertension
	Any active bleeding
	Blood glucose <50 mg/dL
	Resolving neurologic deficits
	Seizure activity at onset of symptoms
	Surgery or traumatic injury in the past 2 weeks
	Myocardial infarction in past 3 months

transport may be required to reach the facility in a timely manner if you are in a rural area. Several factors determine the advisability of air transport. Always follow your protocols and policies regarding the preferred destination and mode of transport for stroke patients.

Your protocol may include starting at least one, and possibly more, IVs on stroke patients in preparation for medication administration upon arrival at the hospital. You should also obtain a blood glucose level on patients suspected of having a stroke. Only administer glucose in consultation with medical direction. Hypoglycemia worsens neurologic outcome, but hyperglycemia does as well. Glucose enters brain cells readily, and an excessive glucose level in cells can cause water to enter the cell osmotically, producing edema.

Advise the receiving facility that you are transporting a patient with signs and symptoms of stroke. The time of onset, the patient's neurologic status, the results of stroke screening instruments, vital signs, blood glucose level, and the patient's medical history are all critical aspects of the report.

Seizures

A seizure is an abnormal discharge and spread of neuronal activity through the cerebral cortex, which interferes with neurologic functioning. In some cases, the abnormal brain stimulation results in abnormal generalized motor activity, while in other cases the motor activity is localized, or the seizure manifests as behavioral change. Seizures have many underlying causes, but the cause of many seizures is idiopathic and diagnosed as **epilepsy**. Toxins, drugs, metabolic disturbances, trauma, stroke, tumors, and fever may all cause seizures. Febrile seizures can occur in pediatric patients. (See Chapter 44.) A key piece of information is whether or not the patient has a history of seizures. A physician must attempt to establish the cause of a new onset of seizures to determine whether or not there may be a life-threatening cause, such as cerebral hemorrhage or brain tumor.

Seizures have two major classifications, each with subtypes. **Generalized seizures** include tonic–clonic and absence seizures. **Tonic–clonic seizures** are motor seizures involving the entire body (Figure 22-9). They begin with a hypertonic

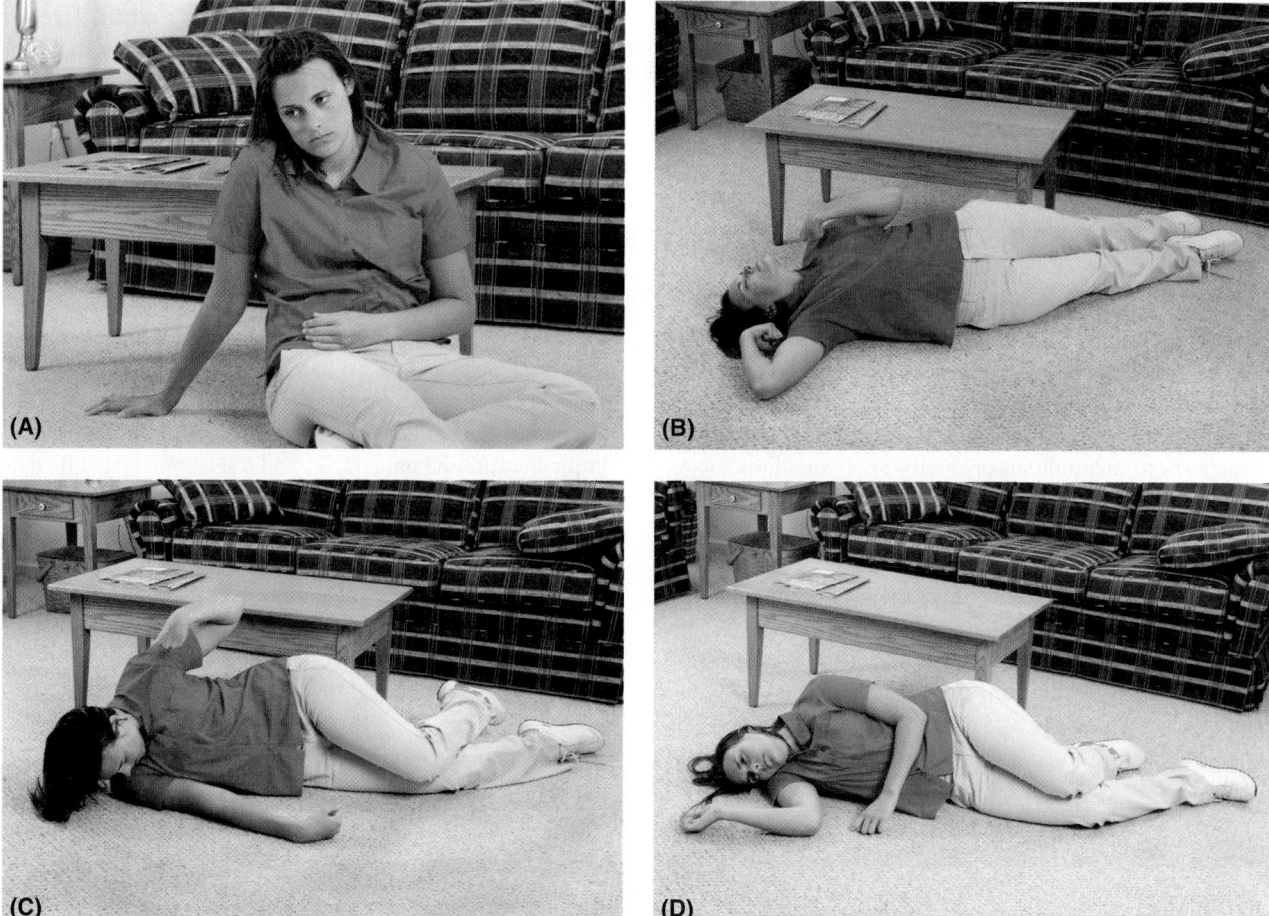

(A)

(B)

(C)

(D)

FIGURE 22-9

A generalized tonic–clonic, or grand mal, seizure is a sign of abnormal release of electrical impulses in the brain: (A) aura, (B) loss of consciousness followed by tonic phase, (C) clonic phase, and (D) postictal phase.

state of the muscles, in which the body becomes rigid, followed by a clonic phase in which there are rapid, rhythmic contractions of the muscles. Tonic–clonic seizures are typically followed by a **postictal** state, in which the brain is recovering from the massive neuronal discharge. Absence seizures are most common in children and involve a loss of awareness, but no change in muscle tone or activity. A brief absence seizure may appear to the observer as the patient simply staring off into space or daydreaming.

Partial seizures are focal, or localized to one area of the brain, as opposed to being generalized. Partial seizures may either be simple or complex. Simple partial seizures can include motor, sensory, psychic, or autonomic phenomena. The patient maintains consciousness unless there is secondary generalization of the seizure activity in the brain. Complex partial seizures may be accompanied by an **aura** and involve impairment of awareness associated with stereotyped movements, such as stair-stepping. They also are accompanied by a postictal period. Complex partial seizures may be dispatched as a behavioral emergencies.

Tonic–clonic seizures are the most common type EMS providers respond to. While they are usually uncomplicated, life-threatening complications are possible. Patients may be injured during the seizure, become hypoxic or acidotic during the seizure, or suffer airway obstruction during the postictal period.

Usually, you will arrive to find a patient who is no longer having an active seizure, but who is in a postictal state. Patients in a postictal state have some impairment of mental status, from unresponsive to awake but confused and slow to respond to questions. Patients may continue to be sleepy for several hours following the seizure.

In the immediate postictal period, patients have copious oral secretions and often require positioning (recovery position) and suctioning to clear the airway. The secretions may contain blood if the patient bit his tongue or soft tissues of the mouth during the seizure. Use manual airway maneuvers to maintain an open airway. If an adjunct is required, the patient may more easily tolerate a nasopharyngeal airway. If you suspect that there was trauma involved with the seizure, for example if the patient fell from a height at the onset of the seizure, consider the need for manual stabilization of the cervical spine.

Postictal patients often have slightly increased ventilations, but if ventilations are inadequate, assist with a bag-valve-mask device attached to supplemental oxygen. Administer oxygen in the immediate postictal period, because ventilations can be impaired during a seizure. Control any major bleeding noted.

Assess the patient for injuries and indications of other abnormalities and obtain as much information as possible from any witnesses or family members, including a description of the seizure activity and how long it lasted. Obtain vital signs and a blood glucose level. Hypoglycemia is one cause of seizures. Glucose may become depleted in prolonged seizures, especially in children. Determine if the patient has a history of seizures, recent trauma, or medical problems, and any medications the patient is taking. Do not forget to check for medical identification jewelry that can provide you with information about the patient's history. Your protocols may require that you start an IV in patients who have suffered a seizure. If a subsequent seizure occurs, the IV provides a route for medication administration.

The postictal period can last up to 30 minutes before the patient is able to answer questions appropriately. In many patients this time period is shorter, and patients who have had a seizure, particularly those with a history of seizures, sometimes refuse transport to the hospital. This presents a dilemma. Often, the reason for a seizure in a patient with a known history of seizures is that the level of anticonvulsant medication in the blood is below the level needed to prevent seizures. The most common cause of the life-threatening condition status epilepticus is an inadequate level of anticonvulsant medication in a patient with a history of seizures. However, even in patients who take their medication as directed, seizures occasionally happen. Usually, they occur without consequence and the patient may not seek medical assistance. If a seizure occurs in the presence of someone not familiar with the patient and his seizures, the dramatic appearance of the seizure often prompts a call for EMS.

As with any patient who refuses treatment and transport, assess the patient's competence to make decisions. But, simply because the patient has had a seizure is not sufficient reason to assume that the patient is unable to make decisions. Attempt to understand the reason for his reluctance. Inform the patient of the potential risks of refusal and, if at all possible, ensure that the patient is not left alone. Follow your protocol for contacting medical direction and obtaining a refusal of care.

IN THE FIELD

Oxygen can correct hypoxia in a postictal patient, but does not speed resolution of the postictal state. The patient's altered mental status is a result of the massive, abnormal neuronal discharge he has just experienced.

IN THE FIELD

Benzodiazepines, such as lorazepam (Ativan), and diazepam (Valium), and sometimes midazolam (Versed), are administered in the hospital emergency department and by paramedics in the prehospital setting to terminate active tonic–clonic seizures. Lorazepam is used in the emergency department to reduce the recurrence of alcoholic seizures.

Advanced EMTs Brian Davis and Anna Chu are caring for patient Regina Lear, who has just offered a chief complaint of severe head pain. While Anna takes a set of vital signs, Brian begins taking a history from Ms. Lear, observing her speech and mental status as well as contemplating her answers. "Have you ever had a headache like this before?" he asks.

"I have a history of migraines, but this headache just hit me all of the sudden, with no warning."

Brian detects a hint of slurring to the patient's speech, and notices that the right side of her face might be weak. "What were you doing when the headache came on?" he asks.

"I was playing a board game with my daughter."

"I see you were holding a pillow over your eyes when we came in. Does that help with the pain?"

"The tiniest bit of light really hurts my eyes. I'm just trying to block out the light, but the pillow doesn't help my headache at all."

Meanwhile, Anna has completed an initial set of vital signs. The heart rate is 72 with a strong, regular radial pulse, the blood pressure is 138/84, respirations are regular at 12 per minute, and the patient's SpO$_2$ is 99 percent on room air.

Problem-Solving Questions

1. What have the findings so far suggested about causes that should be higher on Brian and Anna's list of possible differential diagnoses?
2. What line of questioning should Brian pursue next?
3. How should Brian and Anna approach treatment and transport decisions for this patient?

Status Epilepticus

Status epilepticus is a tonic–clonic seizure lasting more than 5 minutes, or consecutive seizures without an intervening period of consciousness. Status epilepticus is a life-threatening emergency. Request advanced life support, if available, or transport without delay to the closest emergency department. Manage the patient's airway and ventilation. It may be difficult to insert an oropharyngeal airway or advanced airway because of the seizure activity. If it is not possible to insert an advanced airway, use a nasopharyngeal airway and a bag-valve-mask device to manage the airway. Start an IV and check the patient's blood glucose level. Consult with medical direction about fluid administration because rhabdomyolysis (skeletal muscle breakdown) can occur in status epilepticus, so IV fluid infusion may be beneficial. Do not use a bite-block or insert anything between the patient's teeth to attempt to prevent him from biting his tongue. Move objects away from the patient to prevent injury, and place padding, such as a folded blanket, beneath the head to protect it from hard surfaces.

Sudden Unexpected Death in Epilepsy

Sudden unexpected death in epilepsy (SUDEP) is the cause of 8 to 17 percent of deaths in patients with epilepsy (Nouri & Balish, 2009). This phenomenon does not occur during a seizure, but may occur shortly afterward, or may be unwitnessed. Autopsy findings associated with SUDEP include cerebral edema, hypoxia in the area of the hippocampus, sclerosis of the amygdala, neurogenic pulmonary edema, fibrosis of the cardiac conduction system, and liver congestion. Obstructive apnea and cardiac dysrhythmias, particularly bradydysrhythmias, may be implicated.

Headache

Headaches result in millions of emergency department visits each year and can sometimes have life-threatening underlying causes. The key to differentiating between non–life-threatening and life-threatening causes of headache is the history. Explore the chief complaint of headache using the OPQRST mnemonic. Determine if there is a change in pattern from the patient's other headaches. Also identify any other associated signs and symptoms. There are two classifications of headaches: primary headache syndromes and secondary headache syndromes. In both cases, it is not the brain itself that hurts, because brain tissue is insensitive to pain. Rather, it is pressure or tension on pain-sensitive structures surrounding the brain, or of the muscles of the scalp and neck. Pain in the sinuses, teeth, or jaw also can result in a sensation of headache. Another cause of headaches is abnormal nerve transmission, or neuralgia. Primary headache syndromes include migraines, cluster headaches, and tension headaches. Secondary headache syndromes are caused by other problems, some of which can be life threatening.

Primary Headache Syndromes

Migraine headaches result from abnormal nervous system pain transmission and are thought to be neurochemical in origin, with similarities to epilepsy. There is a familial tendency, with migraines occurring more frequently in females than in males. Onset of migraines typically occurs at a younger age. Migraines last from minutes to hours, with a gradual onset of intense, throbbing pain that is usually unilateral. The patient may experience an aura prior to the onset of the headache, such as flashing lights in the visual field. There may be a known trigger for particular patients, such as alcohol, foods, or medications. Often the pain is accompanied by photosensitivity (sensitivity to light), nausea, and vomiting. However, nearly any neurologic sign or symptom is possible, and there are several variants of the typical migraine experience. Patients with a history of migraine have an increased risk of ischemic stroke. Migraines also are associated with depression and epilepsy.

Noise, light, movement, and other stimulation exacerbate migraines. Provide a dark, quiet environment for the patient. A damp, cool cloth on the forehead or over the eyes may provide a measure of relief. Consult with medical direction about the use of antiemetics (if in your scope of practice) and analgesics.

Cluster headaches are uncommon and occur more frequently in males. They consist of a sudden onset of a series of severe headaches of short duration. They are unilateral, generally in the temporal region or around the eye. Unlike other headaches, there is some indication that high-flow oxygen may be useful in relieving pain from cluster headaches.

Tension headaches are experienced by patients of all ages and are associated with dull, nagging pain that may extend from the shoulders and neck to the scalp. The patient may experience muscle soreness or a feeling of muscle tightness with the headache. Tension headaches may be associated with abnormal serotonin or other neurotransmitter activity, and selective serotonin reuptake inhibitors (SSRIs) such as duloxetine (Cymbalta) may be prescribed for frequent tension headaches.

Secondary Headache Syndromes

Secondary headache syndromes have a variety of underlying causes, including vascular problems, CNS or non-CNS infections, glaucoma, hypoxia, toxins, high altitude, tumors, and hypertension. Vascular causes include intracranial hemorrhage, dissection of the internal carotid or vertebral arteries that supply the brain, and inflammation or spasm of the temporal artery. Hypoglycemia, carbon monoxide exposure, fever, dental problems, pre-eclampsia, and hypertension are causes, and headache may occur following a lumbar puncture.

A subarachnoid hemorrhage occurs when there is bleeding that accumulates between the brain and the arachnoid layer of the meninges. There is typically a sudden onset of a severe headache, unlike any other headache experienced by the patient. The pain may be diffuse or located in the occipital region and may include neck pain. Nausea, vomiting, and altered mental status may occur, along with various neurologic deficits. The patient may have **meningismus**, neck stiffness, and **photophobia** accompanying the headache. Subarachnoid hemorrhage may be precipitated by an activity that raises the blood pressure, such as coughing, defecation, or exertion, or may occur spontaneously. Although there are classic signs and symptoms of subarachnoid hemorrhage, be aware that up to 50 percent of patients have normal vital signs, a normal level of responsiveness, and no neck pain or stiffness. Nonetheless, subarachnoid hemorrhage may result in death or disability.

Dementia and Delirium

Dementia is a progressive condition in which intellectual function is severely impaired, and which may be accompanied by emotional and behavioral changes. Intellectual components include impaired memory, reasoning, and problem-solving, language, and other cognitive skills. The incidence of dementia increases with age, but is not a normal consequence of aging. There are several pathologic causes of dementia, including Alzheimer's disease, multi-infarct dementia, and frontotemporal dementia.

Alzheimer's disease is characterized by the presence of amyloid (a specific type of protein) deposits in the brain and degeneration of the microtubules of cerebral neurons. Alzheimer's disease is not completely understood, but there is a genetic abnormality in some cases in which either too much amyloid protein is produced or it is not removed normally by the brain. Multi-infarct dementia occurs as a result of multiple, small strokes that result in accumulated damage over time. Frontotemporal dementia has a strong familial component and manifests as either loss of inhibitions or severe language deficits.

HIV-associated neurologic disease can result in dementia and other neurologic signs and symptoms, including forgetfulness and memory problems, confusion, changes in behavior, severe headaches, progressive weakness of the extremities, and peripheral neuropathy.

Geriatric Care

A screening mental status exam can give an indication of cognitive impairment. Table 22-13 lists some elements used to screen for cognitive impairment.

TABLE 22-13 **Assessment of Mental State**

Cognitive Function	Assessment
Orientation to time and place	Ask the patient the year, month, and date. Ask the patient the state, city, and specific current location (e.g., home, name of hospital)
Concentration and computational ability	Ask the patient to count backwards from 100 by 7s (stop the patient when they have given 5 numbers); ask the patient to spell the word "world" backwards.
Short-term memory registration and recall	Name 3 unrelated items (e.g., phone, banana, cat) and ask the patient to repeat all three. At the end of the exam ask the patient to repeat the items again.
Language	Point to two common items (one at a time) and ask the patient to name them.

Advanced EMT Al Colbert: Over the years I've taken care of a lot of patients with dementia, but I never really understood its impact on the patient or the family members until my dad developed Alzheimer's disease a few years ago. He started off forgetting small things, which we all attributed to "senior moments." Then it began getting worse. He couldn't remember the names of the grandkids or of the neighbors he'd had for 15 years. It was upsetting to him. He knew there was a problem worse than occasional forgetfulness. His doctor diagnosed him with Alzheimer's and started him on some medication. It seemed to help a little for a while, and maybe, in the end, it gave him and my mom a few more months together at home than they would have had.

He started having trouble understanding how his debit card worked with his checking account, and got confused about how much things cost when he was shopping. One day, he took off in my mom's car and disappeared. We looked all over town, and called everyone we could think of. By evening, we were worried sick and called the police for help. We didn't find him for two days. Police from a city about 150 miles away called. They had pulled him over for erratic driving and found him to be confused and disoriented. He continued to get worse. His personality changed. He became irritable, easily enraged, and cried for no reason. He often thought he was back in the Army, and called my brothers and me by the names of some of the guys he'd served with. I know it was the disease, but sometimes it seemed like he just wasn't concentrating and it was hard not to get annoyed.

My mom had more and more difficulty dealing with him. She couldn't sleep well at night because my dad would get up at all hours during the night and wander around. She contemplated putting him in a care facility, but it made her feel so guilty. Eventually, he wouldn't eat and my mom couldn't manage him. We had to put him in a facility. We all knew it was for the best, but we still felt terrible about it. I hate that it happened, but I learned to be more compassionate with dementia patients and their families.

When managing a patient with dementia, you must be calm and tolerant and realize that the world can be a frightening place for him. Such patients can be agitated and combative, but you must understand that the behavior arises from confusion. Nonetheless, take care that the patient does not injure himself or others. When assessing mental status, ask caregivers if there has been a sudden change from the patient's baseline mental status.

Unlike dementia, which is progressive, delirium is an acute state of confusion that occurs from an underlying problem, such as infection, metabolic disturbances, toxins, or medications. It is more prevalent in elderly patients with renal failure, heart failure, and other chronic illness. Delirium tends to affect the patient less in the morning, worsening in the evening. The patient may have delusions and hallucinations and may be frightened. In addition to protecting the patient from harm and reassuring him, you must transport him for evaluation to find the underlying cause.

Excited delirium is a state of delirium accompanied by agitated, combative behavior, often prompting the involvement of law enforcement. **Excited delirium syndrome (ExDS)** is associated with cocaine and methamphetamine use, as well as the use of other drugs. Other factors are not well understood, but ExDS has been implicated in several deaths of persons in the custody of law enforcement. It is hypothesized that ExDS involves dysregulation of the dopamine transport system in the brain, resulting in excess dopamine activity. Patients may exhibit unusual pain tolerance, tachypnea, sweating, unusual strength, and lack of tiring (Hoffman, 2009). Sudden death can occur and is more often associated with asystole than ventricular fibrillation.

The underlying lesson is that, even though ExDS may initially present as a law enforcement issue, it is, in fact a medical emergency. The possibility of being harmed by a patient with ExDS is significant; however, these patients can be extremely difficult to restrain. If chemical agents (oleoresin capsaicin or pepper spray), a Taser, or other weapons have been used by law enforcement, the patient may require treatment for associated injuries. In any patient who is being combative with law enforcement, be alert to the possibility of ExDS and sudden death.

Vertigo

Vertigo is a subjective sensation of movement when there is none, often described by patients as dizziness. However, patients often confuse dizziness and lightheadedness, so it is important to verify whether the patient is experiencing a sensation of spinning or other movement—either of himself or the environment—or he is feeling like he may faint (lightheadedness). When a patient complains of dizziness, ask him to describe the sensation he is experiencing. Vertigo can be accompanied by nausea, vomiting, and abnormal eye movements (nystagmus), and may be precipitated by sudden movement of the head. Vertigo can be caused by problems with the structures of the inner ear, the eighth cranial nerve (auditory or vestibulocochlear nerve), or a problem with the brainstem, including insufficient blood supply or stroke. Patients may have a history of vertigo from benign paroxysmal positional vertigo (BPPV) or Ménière disease. Be aware that movement may worsen vertigo and the patient is prone to falling and being injured.

Nontraumatic Back and Neck Pain

Back and neck pain can occur from impingement of spinal nerves, often due to herniation or rupture of an intervertebral disc. In addition to pain, the patient may experience weakness, numbness, tingling, or pain along the distribution of the nerve. In the absence of acute trauma, spinal immobilization may increase the patient's pain and should be done according to protocol. The pain, whether neurologic or musculoskeletal in origin, may be severe enough to warrant providing analgesia or sedation prior to moving the patient. If moving the patient will significantly increase pain, check with medical direction about the use of analgesia.

A key responsibility when assessing the patient with back pain is to consider serious medical conditions and potentially life-threatening causes of back pain, of which the most immediately life threatening is abdominal aortic aneurysm. (See Chapter 21.) Other serious medical conditions include pyelonephritis, peptic ulcer, pancreatitis, diverticulitis, and pelvic inflammatory disease (PID).

Geriatric Care

A common cause of severe back pain on one side, particularly in older and immunosuppressed patients, is herpes zoster (shingles), which is a re-emergence of the virus that causes chicken pox. After a bout with chicken pox, the virus lies dormant in a spinal nerve root for many years and emerges when there is a decline in immune system function. Zoster may be accompanied by a large vesicular (blistered) rash along the dermatome supplied by the nerve.

Central Nervous System Infections

Encephalitis, meningitis, and brain abscess can all produce neurologic signs and symptoms. Encephalitis is an inflammation of the brain by a viral infection, such as the West Nile Virus, herpes simplex, or others. Common signs and symptoms of encephalitis include a new onset of psychiatric symptoms, cognitive deficits, confusion, headache, movement disorders, photophobia, and fever.

Meningitis can be either viral or bacterial. Bacterial meningitis can present with a gradual onset or fulminant (sudden, severe, aggressive) presentation. There occasionally are concerns about outbreaks of bacterial meningitis among school-age and college-age populations. Signs and symptoms include photophobia, stiff neck, headache, fever, and altered mental status, and occasionally seizures. Acute meningococcal meningitis can be accompanied by a hemorrhagic skin rash (purpura) and patients may present in shock. A classic sign of meningitis is Brudzinski's sign: When the patient's neck is flexed by moving the chin toward the chest, the knees flex in response. In addition to providing any supportive treatment that the patient's condition indicates, remember that bacterial meningitis can be spread through droplet spray and you should wear a face mask in addition to other indicated Standard Precautions.

A brain abscess is a focal, or localized, bacterial or fungal infection in the brain. An abscess can occur from extension of an ear, sinus, tooth infection, or from pathogens introduced into the blood, for example, from intravenous drug abuse or an infection elsewhere in the body. Patients who are immunocompromised are at greater risk. The most common presenting signs and symptoms are headache, seizure, and fever.

Other Neurologic Disorders

You may care for patients with a variety of other neurologic disorders in the course of interfacility transports or emergencies related to complications of the underlying disease. It is important, as a health care provider, that you are familiar with some of the more common neurologic diagnoses. You can find information about them and many other neurologic problems through the National Institute of Neurologic Disorders and Stroke (NINDS) of the National Institutes of Health.

Bell's Palsy

Bell's palsy is a temporary weakness or paralysis of the facial nerve (cranial nerve VII). There are several factors that may predispose an individual to inflammation of the facial nerve, and it is thought that herpes simplex virus may play a role. Exposure of the face to cold air, pregnancy, and diabetes can increase the risk of Bell's palsy. The signs and symptoms often have onset during the night and the patient awakens with them. In addition to weakness of the facial muscles causing drooping of the affected side, patients may also drool, lose the sense of taste, have numbness on the affected side, and either have a dry eye or excessive tearing.

A distinction between a stroke in the facial nerve distribution and Bell's palsy is that the forehead is generally involved only in Bell's palsy, leaving the patient unable to raise one eyebrow. Although Bell's palsy appears to be a stroke, it is not. Bell's palsy patients may be extremely fearful of having had a stroke, so careful reassurance is important until the diagnosis is made with certainty. The majority of Bell's palsy cases resolve completely in several weeks, although some patients may have ongoing effects.

Normal Pressure Hydrocephalus

Normal pressure hydrocephalus (NPH) is somewhat of a misnomer, because the intracranial pressure can be increased in these patients. However, unlike patients with congenital causes of hydrocephalus, the collection of cere-brospinal fluid (CSF) that causes the increased pressure is more gradual and the pressure is not as high. NPH occurs when the CSF produced within the ventricles of the brain cannot be properly reabsorbed or drained, allowing it to collect in abnormal amounts. The condition occurs most commonly in patients over the age of 55 and there often is a history of subarachnoid hemorrhage, traumatic brain injury, infection, or a tumor. The early symptoms overlap with the cognitive impairment of Alzheimer's disease and the motor impairment of Parkinson's disease, and the diagnosis may be missed or delayed. NPH is characterized by a symptom triad of **ataxia** (loss of coordination, often presenting as dif-ficulty walking), dementia, and urinary incontinence.

Once the problem is diagnosed, a shunt may be placed to drain the excess fluid. The shunt is a piece of tubing with a valve that is placed with one end in the ventricle of the brain and the other end passed through a tunnel in the skin into another area of the body (usually the abdominal cavity) to allow the fluid to drain. A problem with the shunt may cause obstruction and an increase in ICP.

Parkinson's Disease

Parkinson's disease typically occurs in patients over the age of 50, but can occur earlier. The mechanism is a loss of dopamine-producing cells in the brain, resulting in move-ment disorder. The early signs and symptoms are subtle and have a gradual onset. Signs and symptoms include muscle tremors, muscle rigidity, slowed movements, and prob-lems with balance and coordination. Eventually, the signs and symptoms impair daily activities, and depression, sleep disruption, eating problems, and difficulty speaking may occur. The disease is progressive, but medications can help with the signs and symptoms.

Multiple Sclerosis

It is believed that multiple sclerosis is an autoimmune dis-ease in which the myelin sheath of nerves is destroyed, re-sulting in problems with nerve conduction. The onset of the disease is generally first noticed between the ages of 20 and 40 and the initial symptoms may include difficulty with vi-sion. Other signs and symptoms include muscle weakness, which may progress to paralysis, tingling sensations and fre-quently, cognitive symptoms such as depression, inability to concentrate, and poor memory.

Myasthenia Gravis

Myasthenia gravis is an autoimmune condition in which the acetylcholine receptors in the skeletal system are blocked or destroyed, preventing the action of acetylcholine at the neuromuscular junction. Typically, muscle weakness oc-curs during activity and improves with rest. The facial mus-cles are often affected, but the respiratory muscles can be

affected and patients may require assisted ventilation. Medi-cations can decrease the severity of signs and symptoms.

Two emergencies associated with myasthenia gravis are myasthenic crisis and cholinergic crisis (Goldenberg & Sinert, 2010). Myasthenic crisis occurs when the patient does not re-ceive an adequate amount of medication. The presentation includes muscle weakness or paralysis, wheezing, increased bronchial secretions, respiratory failure, and diaphoresis. Cholinergic crisis occurs when the patient is overmedicated. The presentation resembles the presentation of organophos-phate poisoning. The associated muscle weakness or paralysis makes distinguishing myasthenic crisis from cholinergic crisis difficult. Patients with cholinergic crisis also may have pupil-lary constriction and can present with the SLUDGE signs that occur in organophosphate poisoning (salivation, lacrimation [tears], urinary incontinence, diarrhea, gastric distress, emesis [vomiting]), but those signs are not reliably present.

Peripheral Neuropathy

Peripheral neuropathies are disorders of the nerves of the peripheral nervous system, which result in sensory, and sometimes, motor signs and symptoms. Patients with dia-betes are especially prone to peripheral neuropathy. They may experience decreased sensation of the lower extremi-ties, resulting in unnoticed injuries. Because healing is poor and infections common in diabetics, the wounds can lead to serious illness. In other cases, neuropathies may be autoim-mune, a result of injury, or due to toxins, infection, mal-nutrition, and numerous other causes. Signs and symptoms can include pain, burning sensations, numbness, tingling weakness, and wasting of affected muscle groups.

Tardive Dyskinesia and Acute Dystonic Reaction

Tardive dyskinesia is a permanent side effect of taking cer-tain classes of medications, often medications used as an-tipsychotics. However, medications used as antipsychotics have other uses, including use as antiemetics. Patients with tardive dyskinesia suffer from repetitive, involuntary, pur-poseless movements. This can include grimacing, blinking the eyes, tongue protrusion, and smacking or puckering the lips. Patients sometimes exhibit stereotyped behaviors such as appearing to play an imaginary piano or guitar.

An acute dystonic reaction is a temporary side effect of taking the types of medications implicated in tardive dys-kinesia. Acute dystonic reaction is seen often in patients who have purchased illegal drugs that they did not know were from that class of medications. The onset may oc-cur within hours or days after a patient receives medica-tions that act on certain types of dopamine receptors in the brain. The patient experiences a sudden onset of sustained or intermittent involuntary muscle contractions, which can affect skeletal muscle in any part of the body. Often, the face and neck muscles are involved. The reaction itself is not life threatening, but if spasm of the pharyngeal or laryngeal muscles occurs, the airway can be compromised. The reaction is usually frightening and confusing for the patient. Particular reactions include oculogyric crisis, in which the eyes involuntarily move in all directions, protrusion of the tongue, spasm of the jaw preventing mouth opening (trismus), and torticollis—a spasm of the neck muscles that causes the head to be held in an awkward position. Fortunately, a common, inexpensive medication—diphenhydramine (Benadryl)—usually quickly relieves the symptoms.

Wernicke-Korsakoff Syndrome

Wernicke-Korsakoff syndrome is a spectrum of degenerative neurologic disorders that includes Wernicke's encephalopathy and Korsakoff's amnesic syndrome. Both are caused by thiamine (vitamin B_1) deficiency, which is common in alcoholics, those with eating disorders, and patients who are malnourished. Wernicke's encephalopathy is the acute phase of the disorder, which can be treated with the administration of thiamine. Signs and symptoms include vision impairment, confusion, decreased level of responsiveness, hypothermia, hypotension, and ataxia. Some prehospital protocols include the administration of thiamine, along with 50 percent dextrose, in the treatment of some hypoglycemic patients with risk factors for thiamine deficiency. This is critical, because thiamine is needed to metabolize glucose. Korsakoff's amnesic syndrome includes difficulty retaining new information and retrieving stored memories, and represents permanent damage to the areas of the brain involved.

CASE STUDY WRAP-UP

Clinical-Reasoning Process

Brian continues to question Ms. Lear as Anna applies oxygen by nasal cannula at 4 L/min. In addition to her history of migraine headaches, the patient has a history of depression. She takes butybarbitol with aspirin and caffeine (Butalbitol) for her headaches and duloxetine (Cymbalta) for her depression. She also takes zolpidem (Ambien) on occasion for insomnia. Ms. Lear also takes an herb (feverfew) for migraine prevention. She is not allergic to any medications and Brian learns that her last oral intake was a cup of tea and some cookies about 90 minutes ago.

She tells Brian that her head hurts mostly in the back, rates the headache pain a 10/10 and states that her neck is beginning to hurt. She is unable to differentiate whether she is feeling a sharp pain or a dull pain, she says it just hurts. Brian decides to come back to that question later. He establishes that the onset of pain was about 15 minutes ago, that exposure to light makes it worse, and nothing makes it better.

Brian has observed that the patient is alert and oriented to person, place, and time. Other than a slight slurring to her speech, the patient's speech and language are otherwise normal, within the limits of the prehospital examination. Brian continues the neurologic exam as Anna lowers the stretcher next to her. He asks the patient to give him a smile that shows her teeth, and he notices that there is weakness on the right side of the face, but that it does not include the forehead. She has normal strength and sensation in all of her extremities, and there is no arm drift when Brian applies the Cincinnati Prehospital Stroke Scale. "I know your eyes are sensitive to light, Ms. Lear, but I need to check your pupils with my penlight. I'll make it as quick as possible." Her pupils are equal and both respond to light.

Considering the patient's presentation and history, Brian believes she may have a subarachnoid hemorrhage. The patient's headache differs from her usual migraines in severity, suddenness of onset, location in the occipital area, and presence of associated slurred speech and unilateral facial weakness. He realizes that the patient may be experiencing an atypical migraine headache, but maintains a higher suspicion that the patient is having a stroke caused by a subarachnoid hemorrhage.

Currently, there are no clear indications of increased ICP, but Brian realizes the importance of reassessing vital signs and neurologic findings. He will be especially alert to changes in level of responsiveness and other aspects of mental status, pupil reaction, blood pressure, pulse, and respiratory patterns. En route Brian obtains a blood glucose level. He realizes there is no history of diabetes, but he knows that blood glucose management is an important part of preventing secondary brain injury in stroke. In the unlikely event that the patient's signs and symptoms are due to hypoglycemia, the prehospital treatment is simple. He starts an IV on the patient, knowing that a subarachnoid hemorrhage could lead the patient to have a seizure, and that the patient will need IV access for treatment in the hospital.

Thanks to Brian notifying the emergency department, a physician is awaiting their arrival and quickly assesses the patient. Labs are drawn and a second IV is started while the patient is prepared for a CT scan. The CT scan shows a small subarachnoid hemorrhage, but subsequent testing does not find a source of the bleeding. The neurologist informs Ms. Lear that it is actually good news that an aneurysm or AVM was not found. She is admitted to the intensive care unit, where her blood pressure is monitored and she is treated for pain and anxiety to minimize additional bleeding. The neurologic symptoms resolve over time, and Ms. Lear has a complete recovery.

CHAPTER REVIEW

Chapter Summary

Patients with neurologic emergencies can present with a variety of signs and symptoms. Signs and symptoms can be general, such as altered mental status, weakness, or fatigue. Always keep in mind that the complaints and signs that can indicate a neurologic problem may be caused by other problems. The patient's presentation, medical history, and a list of the patient's medications help you begin to focus your investigation of signs and symptoms. Knowledge of the function of the nervous system and the pathophysiology of specific neurologic disorders further help in your clinical reasoning process. This knowledge contributes to your ability to consider a variety of explanations for the patient's presentation and anticipate additional problems.

The goals for managing patients with suspected neurologic problems include managing the airway, breathing, and circulation, and looking for immediately correctable causes of the problem. As an Advanced EMT, you have many tools to treat patients who present with neurologic signs and symptoms. Airway management and ventilation can be impaired by a number of disorders. Ensure an open airway and adequate ventilation and oxygenation. Perfusion of the brain may be affected by dehydration, impairment of fluid regulation, decreased metabolism, and cardiac dysrhythmia. Administer fluids as needed to maintain adequate perfusion. Patients with hypoglycemia require oral or IV administration of glucose, or IM administration of glucagon. If you suspect altered mental status, it may be due to a narcotic overdose. So if the patient has decreased respirations, consider administering naloxone. Finally, remember that neurologic problems can be frightening and frustrating for patients and their families. Be empathetic and provide reassurance.

Review Questions

Multiple-Choice Questions

1. When blood flow to part of the brain is obstructed by a blood clot, resulting in death of neurons, this type of stroke is known as a(n) _____ stroke.
   a. microvascular
   b. ischemic
   c. idiopathic
   d. hemorrhagic

2. An abnormal formation of blood vessels, which can rupture and cause intracerebral hemorrhage, is called a(n):
   a. embolus.
   b. neoplasm.
   c. arteriovenous malformation.
   d. aneurysm.

3. Which one of the following best describes a transient ischemic attack?
   a. Temporary obstruction to blood flow to a portion of the brain, resulting in neurologic deficits lasting less than one day
   b. Temporary loss of consciousness due to hypoperfusion of the brain
   c. A paroxysmal episode in which the patient experiences a sensation of whirling or spinning despite being stationary
   d. Sudden onset of weakness or paralysis of the face on one side, which resolves on its own in several weeks

4. You are transporting a patient with signs and symptoms consistent with a stroke. The patient's vital signs and testing results are: blood pressure 180/102, heart rate 68, SpO_2 100 percent on room air, blood glucose level 74 mg/dL. Which one of the following actions is most beneficial for this patient?
   a. Transport without delay to a stroke center.
   b. Administer oxygen, 15 L/min by nonrebreather mask.
   c. Administer 0.4 mg nitroglycerin, sublingually.
   d. Administer 25 g of 50 percent dextrose intravenously.

5. Which one of the following best describes a seizure?
   a. Abnormal electrical activity in the brain
   b. Rhythmic muscle contractions
   c. Sensation of smelling or tasting something in the absence of actual stimuli
   d. The period of altered mental status that follows a convulsion

6. A tonic–clonic seizure lasting more than 5 minutes, or a series of tonic–clonic seizures without an intervening period of consciousness, is known as:
   a. a postictal state.
   b. SUDEP.
   c. a complex partial seizure.
   d. status epilepticus.

7. Which one of the following patients is most likely to experience symptomatic relief from the administration of high-flow oxygen?
   a. Patient with cluster headaches
   b. Patient having an ischemic stroke
   c. Patient with vertigo
   d. Postictal patient

8. Which one of the following is a cause of a primary headache syndrome?
   a. Dissection of a vertebral artery
   b. Brain tumor
   c. Migraine
   d. Subarachnoid hemorrhage

9. Which one of the following terms is used to describe a problem with language, either receptive or expressive, associated with stroke?
   a. Ataxia
   b. Dysarthria
   c. Dyskinesia
   d. Aphasia

10. Alzheimer's disease is a type of:

    a. delirium.

    b. dementia.

    c. movement disorder.

    d. dopamine disorder.

11. Of the following, which one should be your primary concern when caring for a patient with excited delirium syndrome?

    a. Sedating him with an antipsychotic drug

    b. Anticipating sudden death

    c. Administering thiamine

    d. Restraining the patient in a prone position

12. Your patient is a 19-year-old college freshman who lives in a dormitory. She presents with a fever, headache, photophobia, stiff neck, malaise, and blotchy, reddish-purple discoloration of the skin. This is most characteristic of:

    a. bacterial meningitis.

    b. subarachnoid hemorrhage.

    c. normal pressure hydrocephalus.

    d. acute dystonic reaction.

13. Your patient is a 70-year-old man who had a stroke six months ago. He now has a shunt in place to drain cerebrospinal fluid into his abdominal cavity. This is most consistent with a history of:

    a. normal pressure hydrocephalus.

    b. myasthenia gravis.

    c. Parkinson's disease.

    d. tardive dyskinesia.

14. Your patient has just returned from the emergency department, where she received an intravenous medication for nausea and vomiting. She now is presenting with a rigid spasm of her neck muscles. She has no chronic health conditions and otherwise takes no medications. Her condition is most consistent with:

    a. myasthenia gravis.   c. tardive dyskinesia.

    b. acute dystonic reaction.   d. simple partial seizure.

15. Wernicke-Korsakoff syndrome is a result of:

    a. long-term use of antipsychotic medications.

    b. vitamin B_1 deficiency.

    c. lack of dopamine in the brain.

    d. autoimmune destruction of acetylcholine receptors.

Critical-Thinking Questions

16. Your patient is a 32-year-old man who is unresponsive. Describe the considerations in selecting an appropriate airway management technique for this patient.

17. Your patient is a 60-year-old man who is complaining of severe back pain. What are some initial hypotheses you should consider?

18. Your patient states she suddenly became dizzy when she got out of her car. What are some important questions to ask this patient?

19. What is the importance of having a basic understanding of common neurologic disorders such as Parkinson's disease, multiple sclerosis, and myasthenia gravis?

References

American Heart Association (2010). Guidelines for cardiopulmonary resuscitation and emergency cardiac care. *Circulation, 122* (Supplement). Retrieved October 18, 2010, from http://circ.ahajournals.org/cgi/content/full/122/

Easton, J. D., Saver, J. L., Albers, G. W., Alberts, M. J., Chaturvedi, S., Feldmann, & Sacco, R. L. (2009). Definition and evaluation of transient ischemic attack: A scientific statement for healthcare professionals from the American Heart Association/American Stroke Association Stroke Council; Council on Cardiovascular Surgery and Anesthesia; Council on Cardiovascular Radiology and Intervention; Council on Cardiovascular Nursing; and the Interdisciplinary Council on Peripheral Vascular Disease. *Stroke, 40,* 2276–2293. Retrieved March 7, 2011, from http://stroke.ahajournals.org

Goldenberg, W. D., & Sinert, R. H. (2010). Myasthenia gravis in emergency medicine. *eMedicine.* Retrieved March 7, 2011, from http://emedicine.medscape.com/article/793136-overview

Hoffman, L. (2009). ACEP recognizes excited delirium syndrome. *Emergency Medicine News, Scientific Assembly Edition.*

Nouri, S., & Balish, M. (2009). Sudden unexpected death in epilepsy. *eMedicine.* Retrieved December 30, 2010, from http://emedicine.medscape.com/article/1187111-overview

Rovner, B. W., & Folstein, M. F. (1987). Mini-mental state exam in clinical practice. *Hospital Practice, 22*(1A), 99, 103, 106, 110.

Shah, M. N., Jones, C. M., Richardson, T. M., Conwell, Y., Katz, P., & Schneider, S. M. (2011). Prevalence of depression and cognitive impairment in older adult emergency medical services patients. *Prehospital Emergency Care, 15*(1), 4–11.

Additional Reading

Bledsoe, B. E., Porter, R. S., & Cherry, R. A. (2009). *Paramedic care: Principles & practice, vol. 3* (3rd ed.). Upper Saddle River, NJ: Pearson/Prentice Hall.

Martini, F. H., Bartholomew, E. F., & Bledsoe, B. E. (2008). *Anatomy & physiology for emergency care* (2nd ed.). Upper Saddle River, NJ: Pearson/Prentice Hall.

National Institute of Neurologic Disorders and Stroke (2010). http://www.ninds.nih.gov/disorders

23

Endocrine Disorders

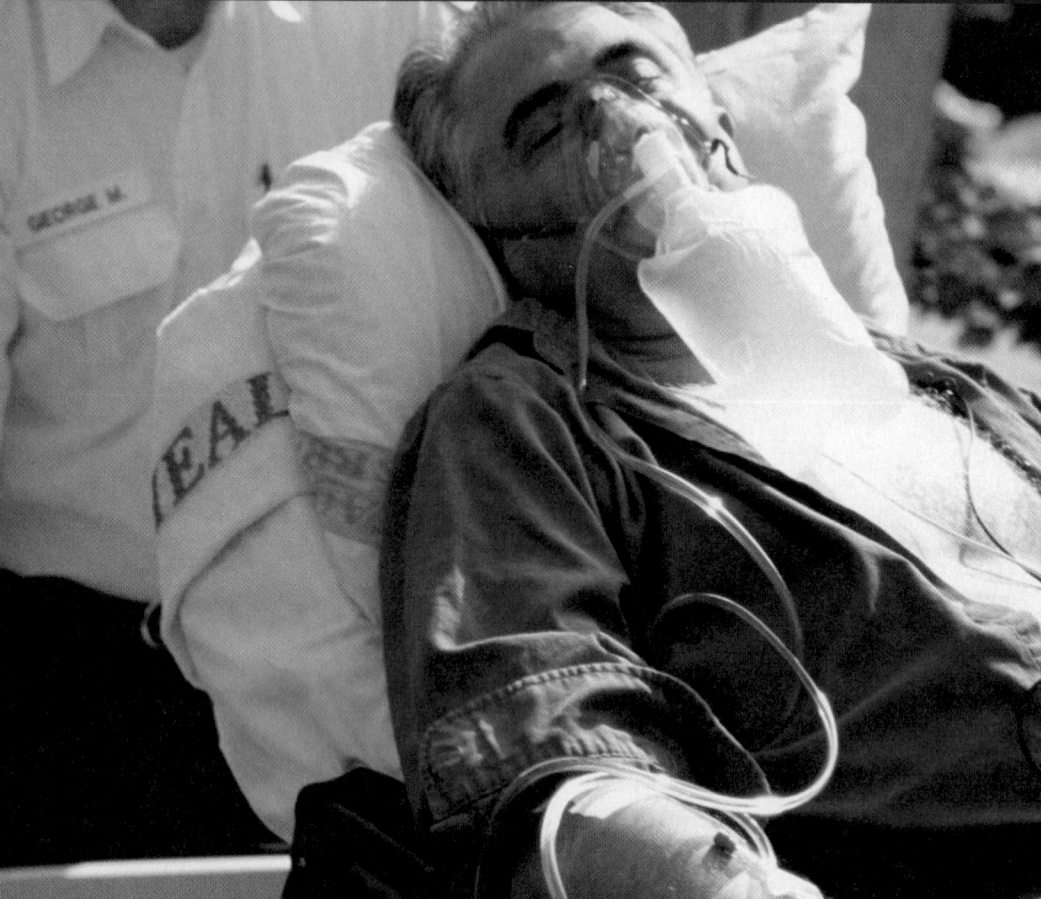

Content Area: Medicine

Advanced EMT Education Standard: Applies fundamental knowledge to provide basic and selected advanced emergency care and transportation based on assessment findings for an acutely ill patient.

Objectives

After reading this chapter, you should be able to:

23.1   Define key terms introduced in this chapter.

23.2   Describe the pathophysiology of diabetes mellitus to include:

- Differences from normal glucose metabolism
- Roles of insulin and glucagon
- Consequences to cellular metabolism and water balance of insufficient insulin
- Similarities and differences between type 1 and type 2 diabetes mellitus
- Mechanisms by which the classic signs and symptoms of untreated diabetes mellitus are produced
- Events leading to hypoglycemia

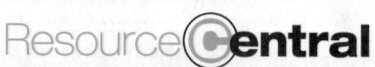

CASE STUDY

Advanced EMTs Will Hoover and Mia Bartlett are en route to a call for an unresponsive person in a downtown office building. During the 4-minute response, Will and Mia review possible causes of unresponsiveness with each other. Keeping in mind that some causes of unresponsiveness, such as exposure to toxins, could be a risk to them, they also plan their approach to the scene size-up.

After finding a suitable place to park the ambulance, they approach the building, maintaining awareness of potential hazards. They take the elevator to the ninth floor, the reported location of the patient. Will and Mia's cautious approach reveals a crowd of seven or eight coworkers surrounding a woman in her 30s who appears to be unresponsive.

"Hurry," urges a portly middle-aged man. "She's a diabetic. I think she needs sugar."

Problem-Solving Questions

1. What are the next steps Will and Mia should take?
2. How can they determine whether the patient's coworker is right about her condition?
3. If the patient's blood sugar is low, what are the steps in treating the condition?

23.3	Given a patient's blood glucose level, determine whether it is within normal limits.
23.4	Recognize the brain's particular sensitivity to decreased blood glucose levels.
23.5	Predict the consequences of insufficient glycogen stores.
23.6	Compare and contrast the speed of onset and signs and symptoms of hypoglycemia and hyperglycemia.
23.7	Compare and contrast diabetic ketoacidosis (DKA) and nonketotic hyperosmolar coma (NKHC).
23.8	Describe how to conduct direct history taking and assessment to obtain information relevant to the patient with a diabetic emergency.
23.9	List common complications of diabetes.
23.10	Given a scenario with a patient suffering a diabetic emergency, provide emergency medical care for the patient.
23.11	Identify indications and contraindications to the administration of oral glucose, intravenous dextrose, and intramuscular glucagon.
23.12	Describe the reassessment of a patient with a diabetic emergency.
23.13	Document the assessment and management of a patient with a diabetic emergency.
23.14	Give a brief overview of the pathophysiology and the signs and symptoms of hyperthyroidism and hypothyroidism.
23.15	Give a brief overview of the pathophysiology and the signs and symptoms of disorders of the adrenal glands, including Cushing's syndrome and Addison disease.

Introduction

The endocrine system consists of glands that secrete chemical messengers called *hormones*. Hormones affect individual body cells to regulate body functions, including energy metabolism, response to stressors, thirst, reproduction, and many others. When endocrine functions are disrupted to a significant degree, life-threatening complications can occur.

The complex function of the endocrine system can lead patients with endocrine emergencies to present with a variety of signs and symptoms. The patient who presents with abdominal pain, nausea and vomiting, cardiac dysrhythmia, altered mental status, dehydration, fatigue, or weakness may have an underlying endocrine problem. In addition, patients with endocrine disorders are at higher risk for other diseases, such as cardiovascular disease and stroke.

Even when the presenting problem is not an immediate endocrine emergency, you must recognize that endocrine disorders contribute to other health problems. Because the endocrine system plays such a crucial role in maintaining homeostasis, patients with endocrine disorders cannot respond well to stressors, such as injury, illness, and surgery. They can exacerbate the underlying endocrine problem, resulting in an endocrine emergency.

Because endocrine problems can be life threatening, your ability to identify and manage problems with the patient's airway, ventilation, oxygenation, and circulation are critical in supporting vital functions. There are other specific interventions you can perform that can improve the condition of patients with endocrine emergencies as well. A basic understanding of hormones and the relationship between the nervous and endocrine systems will help you associate patients' complaints with endocrine emergencies, anticipate complications, and develop effective treatment plans.

As an Advanced EMT, the most urgent endocrine problems you are likely to see are those related to the dysfunction of the pancreas and of the thyroid and adrenal glands. Diabetes mellitus is a disease of the pancreas in which the regulation of the blood glucose level (BGL) is impaired. Both high and low blood glucose levels can be life threatening. It is within the Advanced EMT's scope of practice to assess BGLs and to manage patients with both high and low BGLs. You also can play a role in the stabilization of patients with emergencies related to hyperthyroidism and hypothyroidism, as well as those suffering from deficiencies or excess of hormones secreted by the adrenal cortex.

Anatomy and Physiology Review

The endocrine system is a collection of ductless glands in the body that secrete chemical messenger molecules, which interact with specific cellular receptors in or on target cells (Figure 23-1). Hormones can circulate throughout the blood, having their actions on target cells distant from the gland that secreted them, or can act locally on adjacent cells.

Many circulating hormones are active for only a short time. Hormone molecules that do not quickly bind with target cell receptors or proteins in the blood are broken down in the body. This allows precise regulation of hormonal effects.

Understanding certain terminology makes remembering the actions of hormones easier. The suffix –*tropic* (or –*tropin*) means *to stimulate*. For example, adrenocorticotropic hormone (ACTH) stimulates the adrenal cortex to secrete its hormones. Some hormones are named more simply, such as thyroid-stimulating hormone (TSH), which acts on the thyroid gland, stimulating it to secrete thyroid hormones. *Releasing hormones* act on other endocrine glands, causing them to release their hormones. *Inhibiting hormones* act to decrease action. Somatostatin, or growth hormone-inhibiting hormone (GHIH), for example, reduces the secretion of growth hormone.

Only cells with a receptor for specific hormone molecules are affected by the presence of the hormone. Think of hormones as keys that can unlock only the doors they

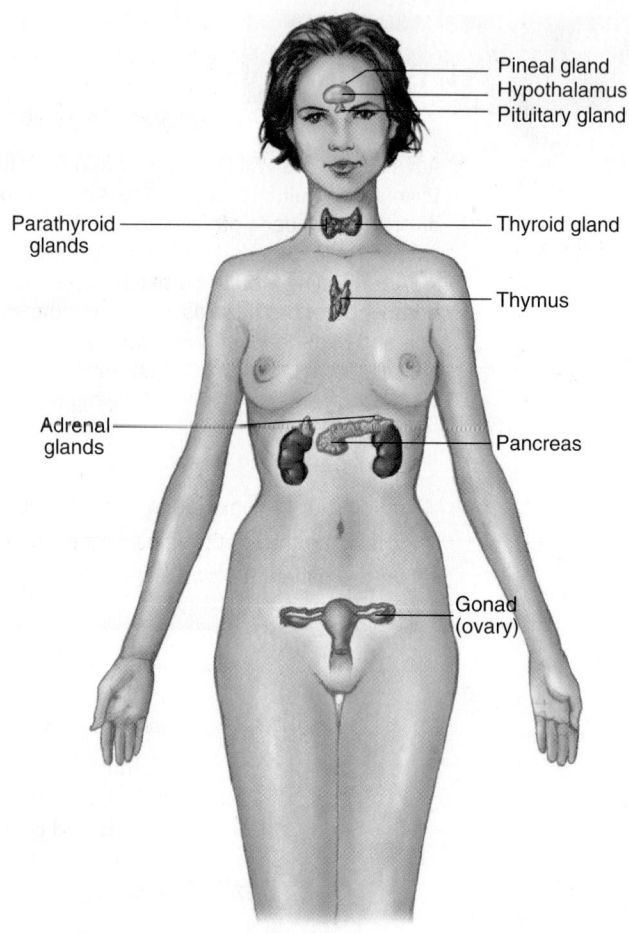

FIGURE 23-1

Structures of the endocrine system.

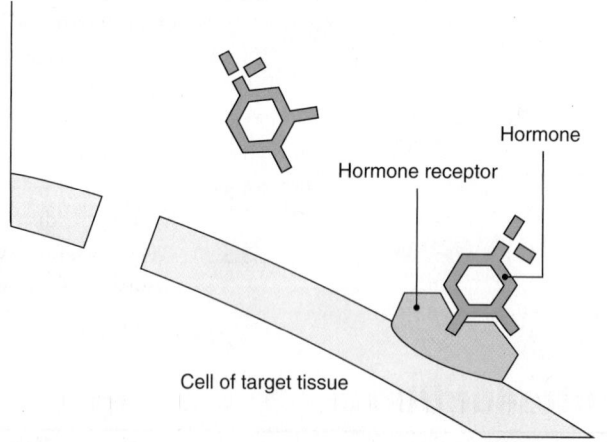

FIGURE 23-2

Hormones act only on cells that have specific receptors for them. Some hormones bind to receptor sites on the cell membrane, whereas others cross the cell membrane to bind with receptors inside the cell.

are specifically made to open (Figure 23-2). Some hormones cannot cross the cell membrane, so they bind with a receptor on the membrane of target cells. Activation of the receptor triggers a second messenger inside the cell.

The second messenger then causes a change in cellular activity. Other hormones, such as steroid hormones (for example, estrogen and testosterone) can cross target cell membranes and bind with receptors inside it. The resulting hormone–receptor complex activates changes in the cell's function.

Hormonal secretion is regulated by negative feedback (Figure 23-3). Negative feedback works in the same way as a thermostat regulates a heating system. When a thermostat detects a low level of heat, it sends a message to the heating system to increase heat production. The thermostat monitors heat production; when the heat level is high enough, the thermostat tells the heating system to shut down heat production.

The body regulates hormone levels as a thermostat regulates heat levels. When the body detects an abnormal condition, such as low blood glucose or high blood glucose, it stimulates a series of events to restore conditions to normal.

When the blood glucose level (BGL) is low, certain cells in the pancreas secrete **glucagon**, a hormone that increases the glucose level. When the glucose level is high, glucagon levels drop and other pancreas cells secrete **insulin**, a different hormone. Insulin decreases the BGL back to the normal range. In fact, many hormones such as insulin and glucagon work in pairs with opposite actions. Endocrine regulation involves more steps than in this example, but negative feedback is the basic mechanism at work in maintaining homeostasis.

There are three ways in which an endocrine gland can receive messages to either increase or decrease hormone secretion (Martini, Bartholomew, & Bledsoe, 2008). Some endocrine glands are stimulated or inhibited directly by the composition of the extracellular fluid that surrounds them (for example, the amount of glucose). Other endocrine glands are stimulated or inhibited by hormones from other endocrine glands. Finally, some endocrine glands are controlled by the release of neurotransmitters from neurons in contact with them.

Endocrine control is often the result of a cascade of events that begin with stimulation of the hypothalamus and pituitary gland (hypophysis). The hypothalamus is the connection between the nervous system and endocrine system. The three main endocrine functions of the hypothalamus are (1) controlling the pituitary gland through the secretion of releasing and inhibiting hormones, (2) making two hormones that are released by the posterior pituitary gland, and (3) nervous stimulation of the medullae of the adrenal glands.

The pituitary gland has two parts: the anterior pituitary gland and the posterior pituitary gland. The anterior pituitary gland is surrounded by a network of capillaries. This network allows hormones to be absorbed and distributed throughout the body.

Specific releasing and inhibiting hormones secreted by the hypothalamus affect different types of cells in the anterior pituitary. Many hormones secreted by the cells of the anterior pituitary are **tropic hormones** that affect other endocrine glands (Table 23-1). For example, thyrotropin-releasing hormone (TRH) from the hypothalamus stimulates the anterior pituitary gland to secrete thyroid-stimulating hormone (TSH), also called *thyrotropin*. TSH then acts on the thyroid gland, which secretes two forms of thyroid hormone, T_3 and T_4.

The posterior pituitary gland hormones are antidiuretic hormone (ADH), also called **vasopressin** (it decreases the amount of water lost through the kidneys and causes vasoconstriction) and oxytocin. Sensitivity of uterine smooth muscle to oxytocin increases late in pregnancy, inducing uterine contractions. Oxytocin also plays roles in the release of milk during breastfeeding and in male and female sexual response.

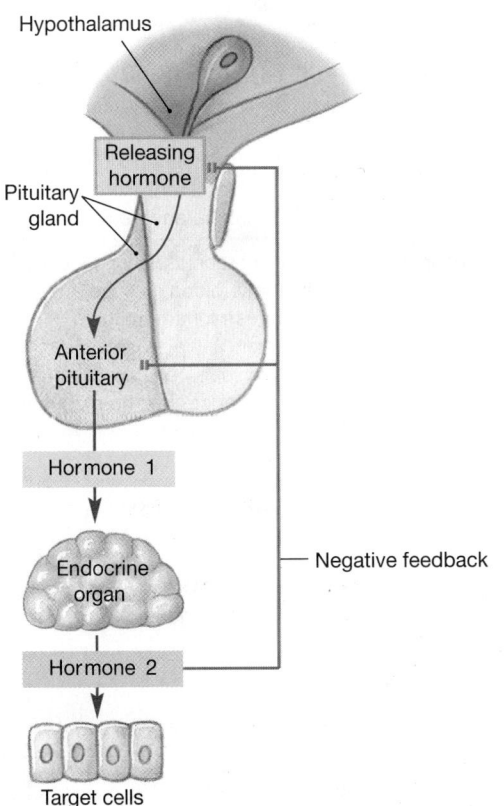

FIGURE 23-3

The vast majority of hormones are regulated by negative feedback. (Bledsoe, Bryan E.; Martini, Frederic H.; Bartholomew, Edwin F.; Ober, William C.; Garrison, Claire W.; Anatomy & Physiology for Emergency Care, 2nd Edition, © 2008. Reprinted with permission of Pearson Education, Inc., Upper Saddle River, NJ)

The Pancreas and Blood Glucose Level

Glucose is a simple carbohydrate molecule, or sugar, that is the preferred source of energy for cells. Normal cell metabolism requires a steady source of glucose. Simple carbohydrates such as glucose are rapidly absorbed from the digestive tract to provide a source of fuel.

TABLE 23-1   Overview of Selected Endocrine Functions

Gland	Stimulated By	Hormones Released	Hormone Targets and Effects
Hypothalamus	Autonomic nervous system	Releasing and inhibiting hormones, including growth hormone-releasing hormone (GHRH), somatostatin (growth hormone-inhibiting hormone [GHIH]), corticotropin-releasing hormone (CRH), thyrotropin-releasing hormone (TRH), gonadatropic-releasing hormone (GnRH), and prolactin-releasing and inhibiting hormones (PRH, PIH)	Anterior pituitary gland; stimulation and inhibition of anterior pituitary hormone secretion.
Anterior pituitary gland	Hypothalamic hormones, levels of various hormones	Growth hormone (GH), adrenocorticotropic hormone (ACTH), thyroid-stimulating hormone (TSH), follicle-stimulating hormone (FSH), luteinizing hormone (LH), prolactin (PRL)	GH affects all cells, ACTH affects adrenal cortices, TSH acts on the thyroid gland, FSH and LH act on the ovaries and testes, and PRL acts on the mammary glands.
Posterior pituitary gland	Hypothalamus	Antidiuretic hormone (ADH, vasopressin), oxytocin	ADH acts on the kidneys to prevent water loss, and oxytocin acts on uterine and mammary gland smooth muscle tissue.
Thyroid gland	TSH, calcium level	T_3 and T_4; calcitonin	T_3 and T_4 affect all cells, increasing cellular metabolism. Calcitonin stimulates bone to increase calcium uptake.
Pancreas	Levels of glucose and amino acids	Glucagon (alpha cells), insulin (beta cells), somatostatin (delta cells)	Glucagon promotes an increase in glucose level through glycogenolysis in the liver; insulin affects all cells, promoting glucose uptake and protein, glycogen, and fat synthesis; and somatostatin acts locally to inhibit alpha and beta cells.
Adrenal cortex	ACTH	Glucocorticoids, mineralocorticoids, small amounts of sex hormones (estrogen, testosterone, progesterone)	Glucocorticoids, such as cortisol, increase blood glucose and suppress inflammation and immune reaction. Mineralocorticoids, such as aldosterone, regulate electrolyte and fluid balance. Sex hormones have effects on most cells in males and females.
Adrenal medulla	Sympathetic nervous system, via the hypothalamus	Epinephrine, norepinephrine	Epinephrine acts on the muscle, liver, and cardiovascular system to stimulate the fight-or-flight response. Norepinephrine causes vasoconstriction.

Glucose that is not used right away is converted to a more complex molecule, glycogen, through a process called *glycogenesis*. The primary storage reservoir for glycogen is the liver. As glucose levels start to decrease, glycogen is broken down again into glucose in a process called *glycogenolysis*. To supplement the glucose obtained this way, the body can create glucose from amino acids and fatty acids using a process called *gluconeogenesis*.

Without glucose, many types of cells begin to use fats for energy. However, the brain cannot quickly convert to using fats. Without a constant supply of glucose, brain cells cannot function. This is why hypoglycemia is a life-threatening emergency. Unless glucose levels are quickly restored, brain cells will suffer damage and die. Although other types of cells can use fat as a source of energy, fats are an inefficient and dirty fuel. When fat is burned at an excessive rate, toxic byproducts accumulate in the blood.

The use and storage of glucose is regulated by secretion of hormones from the pancreas, which lies in the retroperitoneal space behind the stomach. The pancreas is both an endocrine organ and an exocrine organ. The exocrine function of the pancreas is controlled by the vagus nerve. It secretes digestive enzymes and bicarbonate into the digestive tract. In acute pancreatitis it is the action of these powerful digestive enzymes that causes pancreatic tissue destruction with associated severe pain.

The endocrine function of the pancreas takes place in clumps of tissue called the *islets of Langerhans* (Figure 23-4). The islets of Langerhans consist of different types of cells. Alpha cells secrete glucagon, beta cells secrete insulin, and delta cells secrete somatostatin, which acts locally to decrease the action of adjacent alpha and beta cells. The levels of glucagon and insulin must be in balance to meet the metabolic needs of the body (Table 23-2).

The relative amount of each hormone at any given time depends on blood glucose and amino acid levels, input from the sympathetic and parasympathetic nervous systems, and the levels of other hormones, such as GH and ACTH.

Glucagon

Glucagon is secreted when the BGL is low. It acts on the liver to accelerate glycogenolysis, stimulate gluconeogenesis, and enhance glucose release into the blood. Under stress, cortisol from the adrenal glands stimulates an increase in glucagon, and thus an increase in BGL, to provide energy. When the BGL increases, secretion of somatostatin from the delta cells inhibits production of glucagon by the alpha cells.

TABLE 23-2	Hormonal Effects of Insulin and Glucagon	
Insulin		**Glucagon**
Dominant hormone when blood glucose level is high		Dominant hormone when blood glucose level is low
MAJOR EFFECTS ON TARGET TISSUES All cells: uptake glucose		**MAJOR EFFECTS ON TARGET TISSUES**
Liver: ↑ production of glycogen, protein, fat		Liver: ↑ glycogenolysis → glucose
Liver, fat: ↑ production of fats		Liver: ↑ gluconeogenesis (protein, fat → glucose)

Insulin

Insulin is secreted when the BGL rises. It acts on cells to increase the amount of glucose that can enter them. Although cortisol increases glucagon secretion to increase blood glucose levels, it also stimulates insulin secretion so that the glucose created can enter the cells.

IN THE FIELD

Brain cells require a constant supply of glucose, but do not require insulin for glucose to cross the cell membrane. However, brain cells cannot quickly switch to another source of energy when blood glucose is low. Without a constant supply of glucose, brain cells cannot function. Dysfunction begins in the higher levels of the brain, causing personality changes, bizarre behavior, and confusion. With prolonged, severe hypoglycemia, dysfunction progresses to lower areas of the brain responsible for controlling vital functions. Permanent cell damage and death can occur.

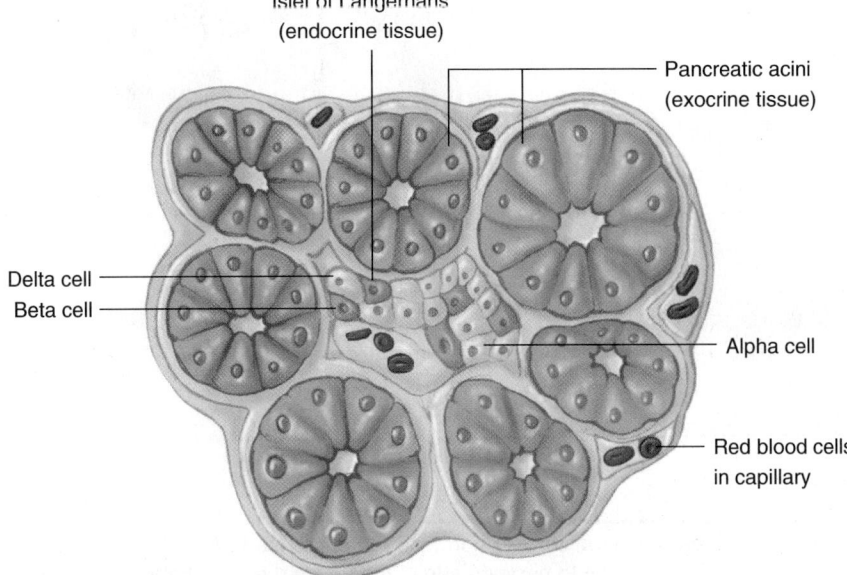

Islet of Langerhans (endocrine tissue)

Pancreatic acini (exocrine tissue)

Delta cell
Beta cell

Alpha cell

Red blood cells in capillary

FIGURE 23-4

The blood glucose level is regulated by the hormones glucagon and insulin. Glucagon raises glucose levels, whereas insulin lowers glucose levels.

Insulin is inhibited by the release of somatostatin from delta cells adjacent to the insulin-secreting beta cells. Insulin is also secreted in response to increased amino acids to promote protein synthesis, and increases storage of fats.

The Thyroid Gland and Metabolism

Thyroid gland hormones control the rate of energy metabolism by cells. T_3 and T_4 affect the mitochondria of cells, accelerating the production of ATP. Overproduction and underproduction of thyroid hormones have serious metabolic effects.

The Adrenal Glands

The adrenal glands, which sit atop each kidney, consist of an outer cortex and an inner adrenal medulla (Figure 23-5). The adrenal medullary hormones are epinephrine and norepinephrine, which are secreted in response to sympathetic nervous system stimulation (from neurons arising in the hypothalamus). Their effects are to increase the heart rate and blood pressure, accelerate glycogen breakdown, and increase glucose and fat breakdown.

A rare condition of the adrenal medulla, but one that you will see listed as a contraindication to drugs that affect the sympathetic nervous system, is pheochromocytoma. This is a tumor that secretes epinephrine when pressure is applied to it, such as when the patient moves, causing anxiety, increased heart rate, and increased blood pressure.

Most adrenal gland disorders are disorders of the adrenal cortex, which produces several corticosteroid hormones that are divided into three classes. The mineralocorticoids control electrolyte balance. A key mineralocorticoid is aldosterone, which promotes sodium and water retention and potassium excretion. Glucocorticoids (such as cortisol, cortisone, and corticosterone) affect glucose metabolism and have anti-inflammatory effects. Excess glucocorticoids result in immunosuppression and delayed wound healing. Androgens, such as testosterone, are secreted from the adrenal cortex in small amounts in both sexes. The exact role of androgens excreted by the adrenal cortex is not clear.

Assessment of Endocrine-Related Complaints

As all patients, endocrine patients present with complaints, not diagnoses. You must work from the patient's complaints, history, and presentation to determine whether the problem is endocrine or something else.

The patient may present with altered mental status, weakness, fatigue, palpitations, fever, abdominal pain, or other complaints. He may tell you that he thinks his symptoms are caused by a known endocrine problem. This history is important, but you still must evaluate all the available information to avoid jumping to conclusions.

You must use knowledge of various causes of the presenting signs and symptoms to arrive at a field impression. Knowledge of the pathophysiology of common endocrine

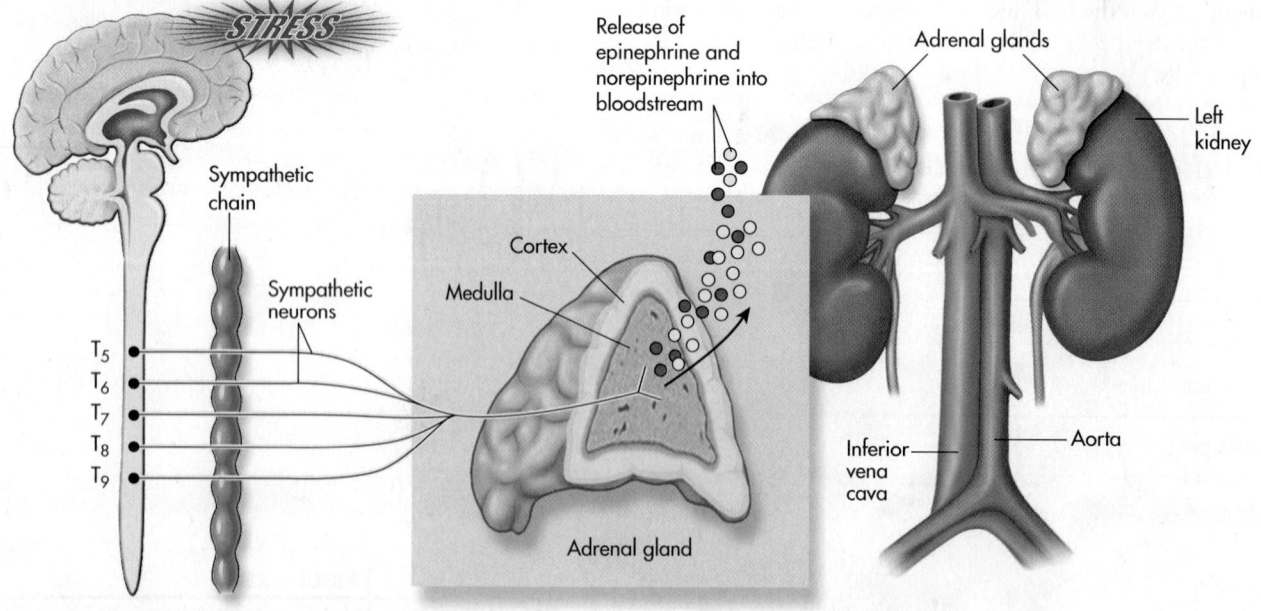

FIGURE 23-5

The adrenal glands consist of an outer cortex that secretes adrenal cortical hormones in response to ACTH and an inner medulla that secretes epinephrine and norepinephrine in response to nervous stimulation from the hypothalamus.

problems is an important part of being able to develop and test hypotheses in your clinical-reasoning process.

Scene Size-Up

Because you do not know the exact nature of the problem at the beginning, your scene size-up incorporates standard operational and patient care aspects.

You may note some early indications that the problem may be endocrine related. Patients with hypoglycemia can be agitated, confused, and combative. Before you can further assess the patient and provide care, you must ensure your safety and the patient's. Other clues to the problem may be evident, as well. For example, a hypoglycemic patient may have been in the process of trying to unwrap a candy bar or buy a soda.

Additional clues may not make sense until you start to form an initial hypothesis. Hyperthyroid patients, for example, are excessively hot, even in a cool environment. You may not initially attribute much significance to the presence of a fan in a cool home, but it may start to make sense in context. Note the patient's general appearance and, if his mental status allows, obtain his chief complaint.

Primary Assessment

In the primary assessment, determine the level of responsiveness using AVPU. Many patients with endocrine (and other) emergencies are awake, but may be confused (Table 23-3). A more in-depth assessment of mental status is required. (See Chapter 22.) Patients with endocrine

TABLE 23-3 Causes of Altered Mental Status

Endocrine emergencies can result in altered mental status. You can remember causes of altered mental status by using the mnemonic AEIOU TIPS.

A – Acidosis (including diabetic ketoacidosis), alcohol
E – Epilepsy (hypoglycemia may result in seizures)
I – Infection (diabetics and patients with adrenal disease are prone to infection)
O – Overdose (may include overdose of insulin or antihyperglycemic agents)
U – Uremia, kidney failure (diabetics are prone to kidney failure)
T – Trauma, tumor, toxin
I – Insulin (too much or too little)
P – Psychosis, poison
S – Stroke, shock, seizures (diabetics are at higher risk for stroke)

Source: Bledsoe, B. E., Porter, R. S., & Cherry, R. A. (2009). *Paramedic care: Principles & practice, Vol. 3* (3rd ed.). Upper Saddle River, NJ: Pearson/Prentice Hall.

IN THE FIELD

Although patients who have an altered mental status are a high priority for transport, suspicion of a diabetic emergency (history from bystanders, presence of medical identification jewelry, clues from the scene size-up, or other indications) should prompt you to check the blood glucose level early in your assessment, after assessing and managing airway, breathing, and circulation. Hypoglycemic patients do not have a source of fuel that allows brain cells to maintain normal function. Prolonged hypoglycemia can lead to permanent cell damage and death. Every second counts in identifying and reversing hypoglycemia.

problems can be deeply unresponsive, leading to airway obstruction and decreased ventilation.

Determine the adequacy of the patient's airway, breathing, and circulation. Intervene as needed to ensure that the patient's airway is not jeopardized and that he is adequately ventilated and oxygenated. If the patient does not have a pulse, move to the resuscitation algorithm. (See Chapter 17.) However, keep in mind that the underlying cause of cardiac arrest may be an endocrine problem.

A history of an endocrine problem can be key in determining and correcting the underlying problem. Recall that hypoglycemia and acidosis, both complications of endocrine problems, are causes of cardiac arrest. Any patient who has an altered mental status or whose airway, breathing, or circulation is compromised is a critical patient and a high priority for transport.

Secondary Assessment

Once the primary assessment is completed and initial interventions are begun, obtain information about the patient's medical history. If the patient is awake and able to offer a chief complaint, tailor your questions to follow up on it. If the patient is not able to offer a chief complaint or provide a history, obtain as much information as possible from family, bystanders, and the scene.

Many patients with endocrine disorders have already been diagnosed. This information will be helpful in determining the current problem. Occasionally, the emergency will be due to a new onset of an endocrine problem. Medications can provide vital clues to the underlying problem (Table 23-4).

Obtain vital signs, pulse oximetry, and if the patient has an altered mental status or history of diabetes, a blood glucose level (BGL). Perform a rapid physical examination for critical patients, and a focused physical examination for noncritical patients.

A detailed, head-to-toe physical examination must be considered for critical patients for whom you cannot determine the problem. Knowledge of the pathophysiology of endocrine (and other) disorders allows you to look purposefully for specific signs in the secondary assessment process.

TABLE 23-4 Medications That May Indicate an Endocrine Emergency

Medication	Condition
levothyroxine (Synthroid), thyroid hormone	Treats hypothyroidism; overdose may cause signs and symptoms of hyperthyroidism.
methimazole (Tapazole)	Treats hyperthyroidism by blocking thyroid hormone synthesis. May indicate Graves' disease.
steroids (prednisone, prednisolone, dexamethasone, cortisone, hydrocortisone, methylprednisolone, others)	Corticosteroids are used to treat inflammatory conditions and replace adrenal cortical hormones. Many have mineralocorticoid effects in addition to the desired glucocorticoid effects. May result in signs and symptoms of Cushing's syndrome. Sudden withdrawal can result in adrenal insufficiency.
insulin (Humulin, Lispro, others) (various forms with different durations of action, including regular, NPH, Lente, Semi-lente, and Ultralente)	Increases cellular uptake of glucose; overdose may result in hypoglycemia.
drugs for type 2 diabetes: Oral antihyperglycemics include tolbutamide (Orinase), chlorpropramide (Diabinese), metformin (Glucophage), glyburide (Micronase), glipizide (Glucotrol), rosiglitazone (Avandia), sitagliptin (Januvia). Injectable drugs include exenatide (Byetta).	Various mechanisms of action to increase insulin production or enhance insulin use.

Reasoning and Decision Making

Recognizing signs and symptoms of endocrine disorders when the history is unknown requires a process of inductive reasoning, from the collection of signs and symptoms to their potential causes. To do this effectively, you must understand the basic functions of the glands most often involved in endocrine emergencies.

A patient's immediate problem may be caused by an excess or insufficient amount of one or more hormones. Signs and symptoms are related to an increase or decrease in the functions controlled by those hormones. Endocrine disorders increase the risk of many other illnesses, such as cardiovascular disease and stroke, so be alert to the possibilities in patients with a history of endocrine problems.

Patients with endocrine disorders have an impaired ability to respond to surgery, infection, trauma, and other stressors. A stressor may exacerbate the endocrine problem, and the endocrine problem may worsen the effects of the stressor. Some endocrine disorders are the result of autoimmune disease, putting patients at risk for other endocrine disorders.

Reassessment

Patients with endocrine emergencies can be critically ill. Reassess critical patients every 5 minutes, including the primary assessment, vital signs, complaints, and relevant aspects of the secondary assessment. Perform reassessment more frequently, if warranted. Reassess noncritical patients every 15 minutes.

The interventions you provide will depend on the nature of the problem, but you must check their effectiveness. If you have given oral glucose, 50 percent dextrose, or glucagon to treat hypoglycemia, you must re-evaluate the patient's blood glucose level.

Diabetes and Diabetic Emergencies

Diabetes mellitus is a disease of glucose regulation that takes two forms (Table 23-5). In **type 1 diabetes,** destruction of the beta cells of the pancreas results in insufficient insulin production. Type 1 diabetes generally has its onset in childhood, adolescence, or young adulthood. It is sometimes called *insulin-dependent diabetes mellitus (IDDM)* because patients must receive regular injections of insulin to control their blood glucose levels. However, patients with **type 2 diabetes** may progress to the point at which insulin injections are required as well.

The term *juvenile diabetes* is sometimes used to describe type 1 diabetes, but the growing rate of obesity in the United States has resulted in children suffering from type 2 diabetes as well. Using the terms *type 1* and *type 2* makes the nature of the patient's problem clearer.

Type 2 diabetes typically occurs in middle-aged, obese individuals and is more likely to be controlled by medications other than insulin, including oral **antihyperglycemic agents.** For those reasons, you may hear type 2 diabetes referred to as *adult-onset* or *non–insulin-dependent diabetes* (NIDDM). Type 2 diabetes occurs when there is both a decrease in the

TABLE 23-5	Comparing and Contrasting Type 1 and Type 2 Diabetes Mellitus	
Feature	**Type 1 Diabetes**	**Type 2 Diabetes**
Other names	Insulin-dependent diabetes mellitus (IDDM), juvenile-onset diabetes.	Non–insulin-dependent diabetes mellitus (NIDDM), adult-onset diabetes.
Cause	Autoimmune destruction of pancreatic beta cells leading to insulin deficiency, resulting in starvation metabolism and hyperglycemia.	Reduced amount of insulin produced by pancreas and increased resistance of cells to insulin, resulting in hyperglycemia.
Risk factors	Genetic factors.	Genetic factors, obesity.
Hypoglycemia	May occur when the amount of insulin administered is too great for the amount of calories ingested.	May occur when the dose of antihyperglycemic medications is too great for the amount of calories ingested.
Hyperglycemic emergencies	Diabetic ketoacidosis (DKA) occurs in undiagnosed or poorly controlled diabetes or in response to increased glucose levels produced by the stress response as a complication of surgery, infection, major illness, or trauma.	Nonketotic hyperosmolar coma (NKHC) may occur in poorly controlled diabetes or in response to increased glucose levels produced by the stress response as a complication of surgery, infection, major illness, or trauma.
Complications	Blindness, cardiovascular disease, stroke, kidney failure, amputation, peripheral neuropathy, peripheral vascular disease, nonhealing wounds, gangrene.	Blindness, cardiovascular disease, stroke, kidney failure, amputation, peripheral neuropathy, peripheral vascular disease, nonhealing wounds, gangrene.
Management	Diabetic diet, careful monitoring of blood glucose level (BGL), insulin.	Weight loss through diet and exercise, diabetic diet, careful monitoring of BGL, medications for type 2 diabetes, insulin in severe cases.

PERSONAL PERSPECTIVE

Advanced EMT Charla Mirabal: I wasn't surprised when I was diagnosed with type 2 diabetes. As a Latina, I know I had about a one in four chance of having diabetes. There are a lot of diabetics in my family, both on my mom's side and my dad's. I worry about the complications. My aunt is diabetic and has kidney failure and is blind. My cousin had his lower leg amputated because of poor circulation and a sore on his foot that got infected. My doctor told me that my chances of complications are lower if I take good care of myself. It's hard to make some of the changes I have to make, but it is important to me and I'm trying.

amount of insulin produced and a decrease in cellular response to insulin (insulin resistance). A third type of diabetes, gestational diabetes, occurs only during pregnancy.

Diabetes as a Chronic Illness

Diabetes is a serious chronic illness that results in a number of complications. Chances of complications decrease with early detection and proper management, but diabetes is a significant cause of death and disability. Complications include cardiovascular disease, stroke, blindness, amputations, nonhealing wounds, peripheral neuropathy, peripheral vascular disease, and kidney failure. Therefore, you will care for patients whose immediate problem is not a diabetic emergency, but a condition related to a complication of diabetes.

Not only are diabetics at higher risk for acute myocardial infarction (AMI), but they also often present atypically.

The history of diabetes is a crucial part of analyzing the patient's presentation, anticipating problems, and developing differential diagnoses.

The management of medical and trauma emergencies in diabetic patients is complicated by impaired glucose homeostasis. In healthy individuals, the pancreas responds to changes in the need for insulin. When stress results in increased production of cortisol and increased blood glucose, the beta cells respond by producing more insulin. In diabetics, the pancreas cannot fine-tune insulin secretion to control blood glucose. Do not forget that insulin has other actions in addition to facilitating entry of glucose into cells, and that these actions are also impaired.

Both type 1 and type 2 diabetics must be followed closely by their physicians, monitor their blood glucose levels, be compliant with medications, and adopt and maintain lifestyle changes (such as diet and exercise) to control their disease.

When taking a history from a diabetic patient, he may mention his "A1c" levels (you may have heard this term in television commercials, too). Hemoglobin A1c (HbA1c) is glycated (or glycosylated) hemoglobin. This is hemoglobin to which glucose has bound. The more glucose there is in the blood, the more glycated hemoglobin there will be.

When a patient takes blood glucose readings, he just gets a snapshot of what his level is at that moment. But levels fluctuate according to meals, insulin or oral diabetic medications, and other factors. HbA1c levels correlate to the average glucose level over the past three months. Therefore, it gives an indication of how well controlled the blood glucose level really is. The American Diabetes Association recommends that a diabetic's HbA1c levels be 6.5 percent or less.

Diabetic Emergencies

Acute diabetic emergencies occur when the BGL is either dangerously low (**hypoglycemia**) or dangerously high (**hyperglycemia**). Normal BGLs are between 70 and 110 mg/dL. Hypoglycemic patients require treatment when their BGL is less than 60 mg/dL. Hyperglycemia exists when the BGL is greater than 140 mg/dL (Martini et al., 2008).

Hyperglycemia

Technically, a BGL above normal is hyperglycemia. Clinically, there are additional factors that determine whether hyperglycemia constitutes an emergency. The BGL in hyperglycemic emergencies is at least 250 mg/dL, but may reach 300 to 500 mg/dL in **diabetic ketoacidosis (DKA)**, and even higher levels, up to 1,000 mg/dL, in **nonketotic hyperosmolar coma (NKHC)** (Kefer, 2004).

Hyperglycemia is at the root of problems suffered by undiagnosed diabetics. In diagnosed diabetics, hyperglycemia occurs whenever the amount of insulin present is insufficient for the amount of glucose present. This may occur because the medication dose needs to be adjusted, the patient is noncompliant with medications, consumes excess calories, or the body is responding to a stressor such as surgery, infection, or myocardial infarction (MI).

Hyperglycemia occurs in both type 1 and type 2 diabetics. However, because type 2 diabetics produce some insulin, the consequences associated with hyperglycemia are somewhat different (Table 23-6). Type 1 diabetes is associated with diabetic ketoacidosis (DKA). Type 2 diabetes is associated with nonketotic hyperosmolar coma (NKHC).

Diabetic Ketoacidosis

Without insulin, metabolism is like that of a starving person. Although there is an abundance of glucose in diabetes,

TABLE 23-6 Comparing and Contrasting DKA and NKHC

Feature	Diabetic Ketoacidosis (DKA)	Nonketotic Hyperosmolar Coma (NKHC)
Patients typically affected	Type 1 diabetics.	Type 2 diabetics.
Cause	Inadequate insulin to allow glucose to enter cells for metabolism, resulting in hyperglycemia and use of fats for energy.	Decreased amount of insulin allows some glucose into cells for metabolism, but cannot lower BGL to normal.
Consequences	Hyperglycemia leads to dehydration through osmotic diuresis. Electrolytes are lost through the large amounts of urine. Use of fats for energy results in ketone production, lowering the blood pH. Dehydration, acidosis, and electrolyte abnormalities lead to altered mental status and increase the risk of cardiac dysrhythmias. Kussmaul's respirations are an attempt to compensate for metabolic acidosis.	Hyperglycemia leads to dehydration through osmotic diuresis. Electrolytes are lost through the large amounts of urine. Dehydration and electrolyte abnormalities lead to altered mental status and increase the risk of cardiac dysrhythmias.
Onset	Hours to days. May be preceded by surgery, trauma, infection, or illness.	Several days. May be preceded by surgery, trauma, infection, or illness.
Signs and symptoms	Gradual onset of altered mental status; warm, dry skin; poor skin turgor, orthostatic hypotension; tachycardia; history of polyuria, polydipsia, and polyphagia; Kussmaul's respirations; acetone odor on breath; abdominal pain; nausea, vomiting. BGL may be 300–500 mg/dL.	Gradual onset of altered mental status; warm, dry skin; poor skin turgor, orthostatic hypotension; tachycardia; history of polyuria, polydipsia, and polyphagia. BGL may reach 1,000 mg/dL.
Prehospital management	Management of airway, breathing, and oxygenation; IV rehydration.	Management of airway, breathing, and oxygenation; IV rehydration.

there is no insulin to facilitate its entry into cells. Therefore, blood glucose levels are very high, but little glucose enters cells for energy metabolism. Cells (except neurons and red blood cells, which do not require insulin to use glucose) begin using fatty acids to create ATP. That creates the conditions for the three hallmark signs of untreated or inadequately controlled diabetes: polyphagia, polyuria, and polydipsia.

- *Polyphagia.* Polyphagia, or excessive hunger, results from cellular starvation, and is more likely in diabetic ketoacidosis (DKA) than in nonketotic hyperosmolar coma (NKHC). The glucose and amino acids consumed in foods cannot be efficiently used, nor can fats be stored. Classically, an undiagnosed or poorly controlled type 1 diabetic is thin and malnourished.

- *Polyuria.* This results from excess glucose molecules in kidney filtrate (fluid in the kidneys that is being processed into urine). The higher concentration of glucose molecules in the filtrate causes the movement of more water into the filtrate (osmosis). The result is both glucose in the urine and osmotic diuresis, the loss of large amounts of urine.

- *Polydipsia.* The loss of excess water leads to dehydration, which leads to polydipsia, excessive thirst. In DKA, the patient's fluid deficit may be 5 to 10 L (Kefer, 2004). Normally, glucose is not excreted in the urine. Cells in the kidneys are able to reabsorb glucose that enters the filtrate that later becomes urine, preventing glucose from leaving the body in urine. When blood glucose reaches a high enough level (usually greater than 180 mg/dL), this mechanism breaks down and the excess glucose in the filtrate cannot be reabsorbed.

The state of high blood glucose levels and loss of water leads to a hyperosmolar state and significant dehydration. The patient will likely exhibit poor skin turgor and warm, dry skin. Hot skin should lead you to suspect fever, which may mean that an infection is the underlying cause of DKA.

When the body uses fatty acids for energy, it does so at a cost. Fatty acids are inefficient fuels that produce less energy and more waste. The byproducts of fat metabolism, **ketones**, accumulate, decreasing the blood pH. Thus, this creates diabetic *ketoacidosis.*

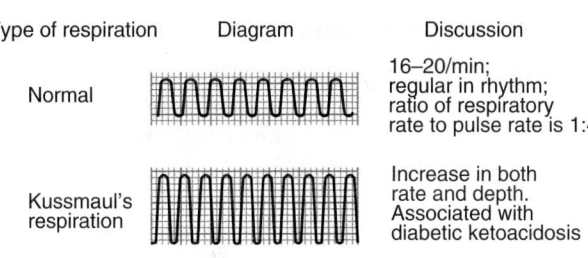

Type of respiration	Diagram	Discussion
Normal		16–20/min; regular in rhythm; ratio of respiratory rate to pulse rate is 1:4
Kussmaul's respiration		Increase in both rate and depth. Associated with diabetic ketoacidosis

FIGURE 23-6

Kussmaul's respirations are rapid, deep respirations that occur to compensate for metabolic acidosis in diabetic ketoacidosis (DKA).

The body attempts to compensate for acidosis by increasing carbon dioxide elimination through fast, deep breathing called **Kussmaul's respirations** (Figure 23-6). Some of the ketones may be eliminated through the lungs, giving the breath the sweet, fruity odor of acetone. Diuresis and acidosis lead to electrolyte abnormalities, such as low potassium (hypokalemia) and decreased bicarbonate ions. The patient may experience altered mental status and cardiac dysrhythmia, and, ultimately, DKA may result in death.

Patients with DKA are weak and lethargic, with varying degrees of decreased responsiveness. Dehydration may lead to hypotension and tachycardia. Vomiting may contribute to dehydration and electrolyte imbalance. An additional symptom of DKA is abdominal pain, particularly in children.

The signs and symptoms of DKA have a relatively slow onset, compared with those of hypoglycemia. Signs and symptoms usually develop over a period hours to days.

Diabetic Ketoacidosis Management

Prehospital management of patients with DKA includes general supportive measures, such as ensuring an open airway and adequate ventilation and oxygenation.

A specific Advanced EMT treatment for DKA is to administer large volumes of isotonic crystalloid IV fluids to begin treatment of dehydration. Start one or two IVs, preferably with at least 18-gauge catheters and administer fluids at the rate prescribed by your medical director, or in consultation with on-line medical direction. Generally, a bolus of fluid (1 to 2 L) is followed by an infusion at a prescribed rate.

Even though the patient is dehydrated, check lung sounds during your reassessment to evaluate for fluid overload. Diabetics may suffer from kidney failure and rapid or excessive fluid administration may be detrimental. Patients in DKA are critically ill and must be evaluated by a physician upon their arrival at the hospital emergency department. Notify the emergency department of your patient's condition and your estimated time of arrival (ETA) in advance.

Nonketotic Hyperosmolar Coma

The primary differences between DKA and NKHC result from the fact that type 2 diabetics continue to use glucose in their cellular metabolism, although all the glucose present in the blood cannot be used. High blood glucose levels lead to loss of glucose and water through the kidneys, resulting in dehydration and thirst. The patient is, therefore, hyperosmolar, leading to osmotic diuresis and both polyuria and polydipsia. However, because fatty acids are not being used as the primary source of cellular fuel, ketones are not produced—the patient is nonketotic. Nonetheless, NKHC is very serious and carries a high mortality rate (40 to 70 percent) (Martini et al., 2008).

The patient's ability to use glucose makes the onset of NKHC slower than that of DKA, perhaps taking several days. The patient may not recognize the seriousness of his illness until he has become quite ill.

Signs and symptoms of DKA and NKHC are similar. However, you will not see Kussmaul's respirations in NKHC because the patient is not ketotic. The prehospital management of both conditions is identical: supporting vital functions and beginning rehydration through isotonic intravenous fluids.

Hypoglycemia

A diabetic's blood glucose level may drop below normal if he has taken too much insulin or other medications to reduce blood glucose levels in relation to the amount of calories he has consumed. An increase above normal physical activity may deplete glucose as well. Hypoglycemia rarely occurs in nondiabetic adult patients.

Glucose levels drop quickly in response to insulin. Therefore, the onset of hypoglycemia is sudden. The brain is particularly sensitive to hypoglycemia, because it needs a constant supply of glucose and cannot readily use other sources of energy. Hypoglycemia can lead to damage and death of brain cells and must be detected and treated immediately.

Of the several signs and symptoms of hypoglycemia (Table 23-7), altered mental status is the most important, because it indicates an insufficient supply of glucose to brain cells. Altered mental status can range from sudden, unexplained rage, to bizarre behavior and confusion, to unresponsiveness.

TABLE 23-7   Signs and Symptoms of Hypoglycemia

- Sudden onset of altered mental status or bizarre behavior
- Irritability
- Weakness, loss of coordination
- Headache
- Weak, rapid pulse
- Pale, cool, diaphoretic skin

Because the brain is so acutely affected by hypoglycemia, seizures may occur. The suddenness of onset may mean that the patient was engaged in an activity, such as driving, hiking, construction work, sports, and the like, when his blood glucose level dropped. Therefore, check the blood glucose level of any patient with an altered mental status, even when trauma seems to explain the condition. A blood glucose level less than 60 mg/dL requires treatment. Hypoglycemia also leads to shaking, headache, impaired vision, and signs of sympathetic nervous system stimulation, such as pale, cool, diaphoretic skin and increased heart rate.

Epinephrine, the cause of the sympathetic nervous system signs, is released as a homeostatic mechanism, because one of its effects is to raise the blood glucose level in the presence of sufficient glycogen. Therefore, the sympathetic nervous system signs may occur as early indicators of hypoglycemia.

After ensuring an airway, breathing, and circulation, the goal of treating hypoglycemia is to increase the blood glucose level. Offer patients who are awake and able to control their airways a concentrated form of sugar to eat or drink. Sucrose (table sugar), fructose (from fruits and juices and added to many sweets), and dextrose are similar in chemical structure to glucose and can be used by the body for energy.

If you are in a setting where it is available, regular soda (not diet soda) or fruit juice, preferably with a packet or two of sugar added, works well and is well accepted by most patients. You may also administer the oral glucose gel or paste carried in your jump kit. Oral administration of the 50 percent dextrose solution for IV use is not recommended.

Patients with a decreased level of responsiveness must never be given anything by mouth. The most effective way of increasing the BGL in these patients is to start an IV and administer a solution of 50 percent dextrose. If you are dealing with a combative patient who has refused to accept oral glucose, this task can be challenging. You will need assistance in restraining the patient from injuring himself, you or your partner, and others. Request additional personnel if needed.

To administer 50 percent dextrose, choose a strong vein and a large enough catheter through which to push the thick liquid. IV placement in an antecubital vein using at least an 18-gauge catheter is preferred. The typical dosage is 25 grams (50 mL) of 50 percent dextrose. Your protocols may allow lower or higher dosages in some situations. The 50 percent dextrose is pushed at a slow, steady rate to avoid injury to the vein. *Never administer dextrose through an IV that is not flowing freely or that has infiltrated.* The hypertonic solution will lead to tissue necrosis if it is extravasated.

The response to intravenous dextrose is rapid. You should see an improvement in the patient's level of responsiveness in 1 to 2 minutes. If your patient does not respond quickly to IV dextrose, recheck his BGL. In general, administration of 50 percent dextrose increases the BGL above normal. If the BGL remains low, additional dextrose is required. Contact medial direction for consultation. If the BGL is above 60 mg/dL, suspect another problem and reassess the patient.

In situations in which you cannot place an IV in a hypoglycemic patient there is another, although indirect, way to increase the BGL. Recall that the hormone glucagon causes the breakdown of glycogen stored in the liver into glucose. You can administer 1 mg of glucagon IM to adult hypoglycemic patients who have a decreased level of responsiveness, and in whom an IV cannot be established. The onset of action is slower, though, and effectiveness relies on the patient having adequate glycogen stores in the liver.

Diabetics Who Refuse Transport

Occasionally, a hypoglycemic patient refuses transport after his BGL increases and he feels better. Once the patient's mental status is normal, you cannot transport him without his consent. Provide the patient with the information he needs to make an informed decision.

The duration of action of the sugar you provide orally or intravenously is much shorter than the duration of insulin or other medication that caused the hypoglycemia to begin with. Some types of insulin, such as Ultralente, and the **sulfonylurea** class oral antihyperglycemics, such as glipizide (Glucotrol), are very long acting. Unless there is a backup source of energy, the BGL will drop again. Make every effort to persuade patients on these medications to accept transport to the hospital emergency department for further evaluation.

If the patient refuses transport, make sure he consumes a meal or snack with adequate protein (cheeses and meats are good choices) to prevent recurrence of hypoglycemia. Proteins are metabolized slowly to provide a steady source of energy. If possible, assist the patient in making a sandwich or getting a snack and ensure he is eating it before you leave.

It is critical that the patient have someone with him in case his BGL drops again. Enlist the help of a friend, coworker, family member, or neighbor to stay with the patient. Advise the patient that he should call 911 if symptoms of hypoglycemia reappear.

Pediatric Care

Because of the hypertonic nature of 50 percent dextrose and the smaller volume of blood in which to dilute it, less concentrated dextrose solutions are used in pediatric patients. In children 25 percent dextrose is used, and 10 percent dextrose is used in newborns and infants.

Your service should supply dextrose in those concentrations. However, if necessary, you may dilute 50 percent dextrose with sterile water or normal saline to create the appropriate concentration.

For hypoglycemic diabetics who refuse transport after treatment, document all assessment and treatment information, including the patient's mental status and BGL after treatment. Include a description of your attempts to persuade the patient to consent to transport and his responses.

Document attempts to have the patient eat an appropriate meal or snack and who was with the patient when you left the scene. Document that you obtained the other person's agreement to observe the patient and informed the person of signs and symptoms of hypoglycemia. Include that you informed the patient and person with him of the risks of refusing transport and that they can call 911 again at any time.

Thyroid Disorders

As with most endocrine disorders, thyroid disorders arise from secreting either too much or too little hormone; in this case, it is thyroid hormone. **Hyperthyroidism** results in increased metabolism, which leads to weight loss, heat

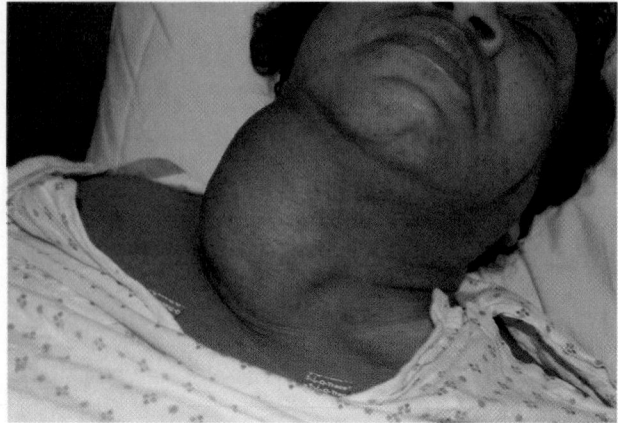

FIGURE 23-7

Goiter results from an enlarged thyroid gland and can be associated with hypothyroidism and hyperthyroidism. (© Edward T. Dickinson, MD)

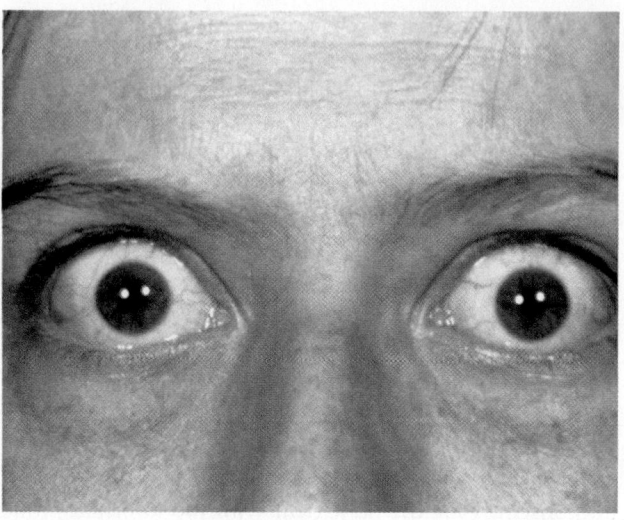

FIGURE 23-8

Exophthalmos, protrusion of the eyes, is a sign of Graves' disease. (© Custom Medical Stock Photo, Inc.)

intolerance, and other problems. **Hypothyroidism** results in weight gain, cold intolerance, and in severe cases, coma.

Goiter is a condition in which the thyroid gland is enlarged, and may be related to either hypothyroidism or hyperthyroidism (Figure 23-7).

Hyperthyroidism

In all forms of hyperthyroidism, signs and symptoms are consequences of increased cellular metabolic activity and increased sympathetic nervous system stimulation (Table 23-8).

Graves' disease is a form of hyperthyroidism that results from an autoimmune disorder that causes increased production of thyroid hormones (Yeung, Habra, & Chiu, 2010). Graves' disease has a characteristic feature called *exophthalmos* that is not seen in hyperthyroidism from other causes (Figure 23-8). Exophthalmos is a condition in which swelling of the tissues behind the eyes causes the eyes to protrude.

In patients with untreated Graves' disease, exposure to a stressor such as infection, surgery, or trauma, can lead to **thyrotoxicosis** (thyroid storm). In thyrotoxicosis, the sympathetic nervous system signs and symptoms of hyperthyroidism increase to a life-threatening level. Prehospital providers cannot treat the underlying cause of thyrotoxicosis, but can manage some of its consequences, such as heart failure.

Hypothyroidism

Hypothyroidism has several causes, including iodine deficiency, surgical removal of the thyroid gland, or damage to the gland from radiation therapy (Schraga, 2010). Mild hypothyroidism is generally caused by autoimmune disease and is treated by supplemental administration of thyroid hormones. Signs and symptoms are consequences of decreased cellular metabolic activity.

TABLE 23-8 Contrasting Hyperthyroidism and Hypothyroidism

Feature	Hyperthyroidism	Hypothyroidism
Cause	Increased thyroid hormone levels	Decreased thyroid hormone levels
Associated conditions	Graves' disease, goiter	Goiter, surgical removal or radiation damage of thyroid gland
Signs and symptoms	Weight loss despite increased appetite, anxiety, intolerance to heat, diarrhea, palpitations, tachycardia, hypertension, nonpitting pretibial edema	Weight gain despite decreased appetite, fatigue and lack of energy, lack of emotion, slowed mental function, intolerance to cold, myxedema in prolonged cases
Emergencies	Thyrotoxicosis (thyroid storm), which may present with heart failure, high fever, vomiting, diarrhea, and psychosis	Myxedema coma, which may be accompanied by bradycardia, hypotension, respiratory depression, elevated capnometry readings, and severe hypothermia

A characteristic sign of severe hypothyroidism is **myxedema**, which is swelling of the skin, particularly in the face. The swelling of myxedema is caused by tissue changes, rather than excess extracellular fluid. Unlike edema from fluid overload, the edema associated with hypothyroidism is nonpitting.

Severe hypothyroidism can progress to a condition called **myxedema coma**. Patients with myxedema coma may present with bradycardia, respiratory depression, and severe hypothermia. Support the patient's airway, breathing, and circulation, and prevent further heat loss. Hypotensive patients may require IV fluids, but be aware that large amounts of IV fluid contribute to hypothermia.

Adrenal Disorders

In **Addison disease**, adrenal cortical hormones are insufficient, whereas in **Cushing's syndrome** (not to be confused with Cushing's triad, the signs of increased intracranial pressure), there is an excess of adrenal cortical hormones. One particular cause of the syndrome is Cushing's disease, in which the cause of adrenal cortical hormone excess is a pituitary tumor that secretes excess ACTH.

Addison Disease

Long-term adrenal insufficiency, or Addison disease, results from damage to the adrenal cortex, which may occur as a result of autoimmune disease, infection, or hypoperfusion. Adrenal insufficiency also may occur because of sudden withdrawal of long-term steroid therapy, so be sure to ask about recent use of steroids. A recent exacerbation of asthma or chronic obstructive pulmonary disease (COPD) or a history of organ or tissue transplant are clues that a patient may have been prescribed long-term steroid therapy. Signs and symptoms arise primarily from decreased amounts of mineralocorticoids, and glucocorticoids (Table 23-9).

Treatment involves replacement of hormones such as cortisone, hydrocortisone, and fludrocortisone. However, the body is unable to adjust to stressors in which there is an increased demand for adrenal cortical hormones, and **adrenal crisis** (Addisonian crisis) may occur. An important example of this would be a patient you might transport who is on adrenal replacement therapy and who has become septic. The patient may have a decreased BGL and electrolyte abnormalities that can result in cardiac dysrhythmia.

Patients in adrenal crisis may present with hypotension that does not respond well to fluid therapy. Be cautious in administering IV fluids, because adrenal crisis is associated with electrolyte imbalance. Hospital treatment includes administration of cortisol.

Cushing's Syndrome

Cushing's syndrome results from long-term overexposure to glucocorticoids. A common cause of Cushing's syndrome is long-term administration of steroids to treat a medical condition such as COPD, asthma, and autoimmune diseases, and to prevent rejection of transplanted organs and tissues. Therefore, a patient with Cushing's syndrome likely will have an underlying chronic disease. In Cushing's disease, a form of Cushing's syndrome, a

TABLE 23-9 Comparing and Contrasting Addison Disease and Cushing's Syndrome

Feature	Cushing's Syndrome	Addison Disease
Cause	Excess adrenal cortical hormones due to glucocorticoid therapy (steroid medications) or pituitary tumor, resulting in increased ACTH.	Insufficient secretion of adrenal cortical hormones due to destruction of adrenal cortex. Adrenal insufficiency may occur as a result of sudden withdrawal of corticosteroid therapy.
Associated conditions	COPD, asthma, cancer, or inflammatory conditions requiring steroid therapy. Diabetes, infection. Increased risk of cardiovascular disease and stroke.	Inability to respond to stressors such as infection, surgery, trauma, or illness.
Signs and symptoms	Weight gain in the trunk, often with thin extremities. "Moon face" appearance, accumulation of fat in the upper back ("buffalo hump"). Thin, easily bruised skin. Delayed wound healing. Development of facial hair in women.	Hyperpigmentation of the skin and gums, fatigue, weakness, weight loss.
Emergencies	Increased risk of MI, stroke, and infection.	Adrenal crisis (Addisonian crisis). May present with hypoglycemia, hypotension, and cardiac rhythm disturbances due to electrolyte abnormalities.

tumor of the anterior pituitary gland causes increased secretion of ACTH, which stimulates the adrenal cortex to secrete excess cortical hormones.

The signs and symptoms of Cushing's syndrome are related to excess levels of glucocorticoids, mineralocorticoids, and androgens. Complications of Cushing's syndrome include osteoporosis (with increased risk of fractures), hypertension, diabetes, muscle wasting, and susceptibility to infection.

In Cushing's syndrome patients the skin is thin and easily injured. Be especially cautious in patient handling and in performing procedures. Patients with Cushing's syndrome may present with a "moon face" appearance, appear obese around the trunk but thin in the extremities, and have an accumulation of excess fat in the upper back ("buffalo hump") (Figure 23-9).

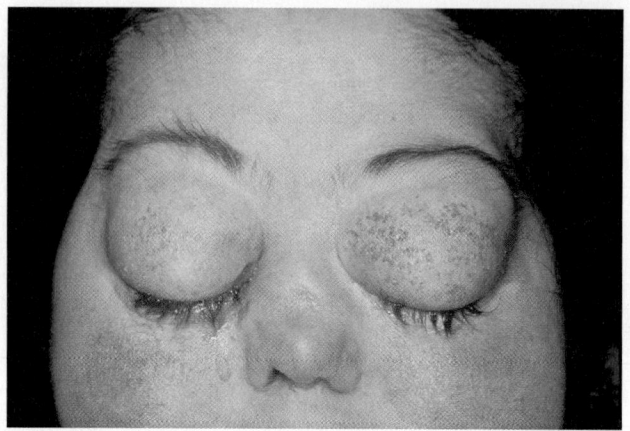

FIGURE 23-9

Characteristic appearance of patients with Cushing's syndrome. (© Biophoto Associates/Photo Researchers, Inc.)

CASE STUDY WRAP-UP

Clinical-Reasoning Process

Advanced EMTs Will Hoover and Mia Bartlett have arrived on the scene of an unresponsive woman in her 30s. Her coworkers have told Mia and Will that the patient is a diabetic. Mia confirms that the patient, Carrie Atkins, is unresponsive. Mia uses a head-tilt/chin-lift maneuver to ensure an open airway and determines that the patient is breathing adequately. Mia notes that the patient's skin is pale, cool, and moist, indicating sympathetic nervous system stimulation. Her radial pulse is thready and rapid.

Meanwhile, having confirmed with coworkers that the patient is a diabetic who takes insulin, Will anticipates hypoglycemia and prepares to check her BGL while starting an IV of normal saline. The patient's BGL is 30 mg/dL. As Will secures the IV, Mia prepares a syringe of 50 percent dextrose. Mia hands the syringe to Will, who confirms the medication again before beginning administration. Will slowly administers 25 grams of dextrose.

Within a few minutes, the patient opens her eyes and is able to answer Will's questions. The patient states that she took her insulin and ate as usual. Unsure of the reason for her low blood sugar level, the patient agrees to transport.

Will obtains a set of vital signs and a complete history en route to the hospital. The patient's BGL just prior to arrival at the ED is 138 mg/dL. She remains alert as Will gives the nurse a report. He and Mia wish the patient well and mark back in service.

CHAPTER REVIEW

Chapter Summary

Patients with endocrine disorders present with a variety of signs and symptoms. Signs and symptoms can be general, such as altered mental status, weakness, or fatigue. In many cases, the patient has a known history of an endocrine disorder. This and a list of the patient's medications help you begin to focus your investigation.

Knowledge of the endocrine system's role in homeostasis and the pathophysiology of specific endocrine disorders further

helps in your clinical-reasoning process. Your knowledge of the complications of endocrine disorders, such as increased risk of silent MI in diabetics, contributes to your ability to consider a variety of explanations for the patient's presentation and to anticipate additional problems. Comparing the patient's symptoms, vital signs, BGL, and physical findings to your knowledge base of medical emergencies, including endocrine disorders, allows you to develop a list of differential diagnoses.

As an Advanced EMT, you have many tools to treat patients with endocrine disorders. Airway management and ventilation can be impaired by a number of disorders. Ensure an open airway and adequate ventilation and oxygenation. Perfusion may be affected by dehydration, impairment of fluid regulation, decreased metabolism, and cardiac dysrhythmia. Administer fluids as needed to maintain adequate perfusion.

Patients with hypoglycemia require oral or IV administration of glucose, or IM administration of glucagon. Patients with thyroid problems may have difficulty with temperature regulation. You must be prepared to treat hyperthermia or hypothermia. Treat underlying problems, such as COPD and chest pain. Perform your treatment keeping in mind that patients with endocrine disorders have impaired regulatory mechanisms and many are especially prone to infection.

Review Questions

Multiple-Choice Questions

1. The structure that links the nervous and endocrine systems is the:
   a. anterior pituitary gland.
   b. pineal gland.
   c. cerebral cortex.
   d. hypothalamus.

2. Addison disease is a condition in which the level of _____ hormones is low.
   a. thyroid
   b. pituitary
   c. adrenal
   d. pancreatic

3. Under which one of the following conditions would you expect the level of insulin to increase?
   a. Immediately after a meal
   b. During sedentary activities
   c. When somatostatin is secreted
   d. When the blood glucose level is low

4. The appropriate concentration of dextrose for treating a four-year-old child with hypoglycemia is:
   a. 5 percent.
   b. 10 percent.
   c. 25 percent.
   d. 50 percent.

5. You have just administered dextrose to increase the blood glucose level of a diabetic who takes a sulfonylurea medication. Which one of the following should you anticipate?
   a. Rebound hyperglycemia
   b. Prolonged risk of another drop in blood glucose level
   c. Increased risk of diabetic ketoacidosis (DKA)
   d. Drug interaction between dextrose and sulfonylureas

6. Your patient presents with a history of type 2 diabetes and a two-day history of progressive fatigue, increased urination, and thirst. He is now responsive to verbal stimuli and has warm, dry skin with poor turgor. These findings are most consistent with:
   a. nonketotic hyperosmolar coma (NKHC).
   b. diabetic ketoacidosis (DKA).
   c. myxedema coma.
   d. hypoglycemia.

7. Which one of the following would you anticipate in a patient with untreated Graves' disease?
   a. Myxedema coma   c. Hyperthermia
   b. Obesity   d. Bradycardia

8. A patient tells you she takes Ultralente insulin. You recognize that the duration of action of this insulin is:
   a. ultra short.   c. intermediate.
   b. short.   d. long.

Critical-Thinking Questions

9. Explain how untreated diabetes leads to the classic signs of polyuria, polydipsia, and polyphagia.

10. Draw an example of a negative feedback loop.

11. What are some common complications of diabetes?

12. Explain why Kussmaul's respirations are seen in DKA but not in NKHC.

References

Bledsoe, B. E., Porter, R. S., & Cherry, R. A. (2009). *Paramedic care: Principles & practice, Vol. 3* (3rd ed.). Upper Saddle River, NJ: Pearson/Prentice Hall.

Kefer, M. P. (2004). Diabetic emergencies. In O. J. Ma, D. M. Cline, J. E. Tintinalli, G. D. Kelen, & J. S. Stapczynski (Eds.), *Emergency medicine manual* (6th ed.). New York, NY: McGraw-Hill.

Martini, F. H., Bartholomew, E. F., & Bledsoe, B. E. (2008). *Anatomy & physiology for emergency care* (2nd ed.). Upper Saddle River, NJ: Pearson/Prentice Hall.

Schraga, E. D. (2010). *Hypothyroidism and myxedema coma: Treatment & medication.* Medscape. Retrieved September 23, 2010, from http://emedicine.medscape.com/article/768053-treatment

Yeung, S. J., Habra, M. A., & Chiu, A. C. (2010). *Graves' disease.* Medscape. Retrieved September 23, 2010, from *http://emedicine.medscape.com/article/120619-overview*

24 Abdominal Pain and Gastrointestinal Disorders

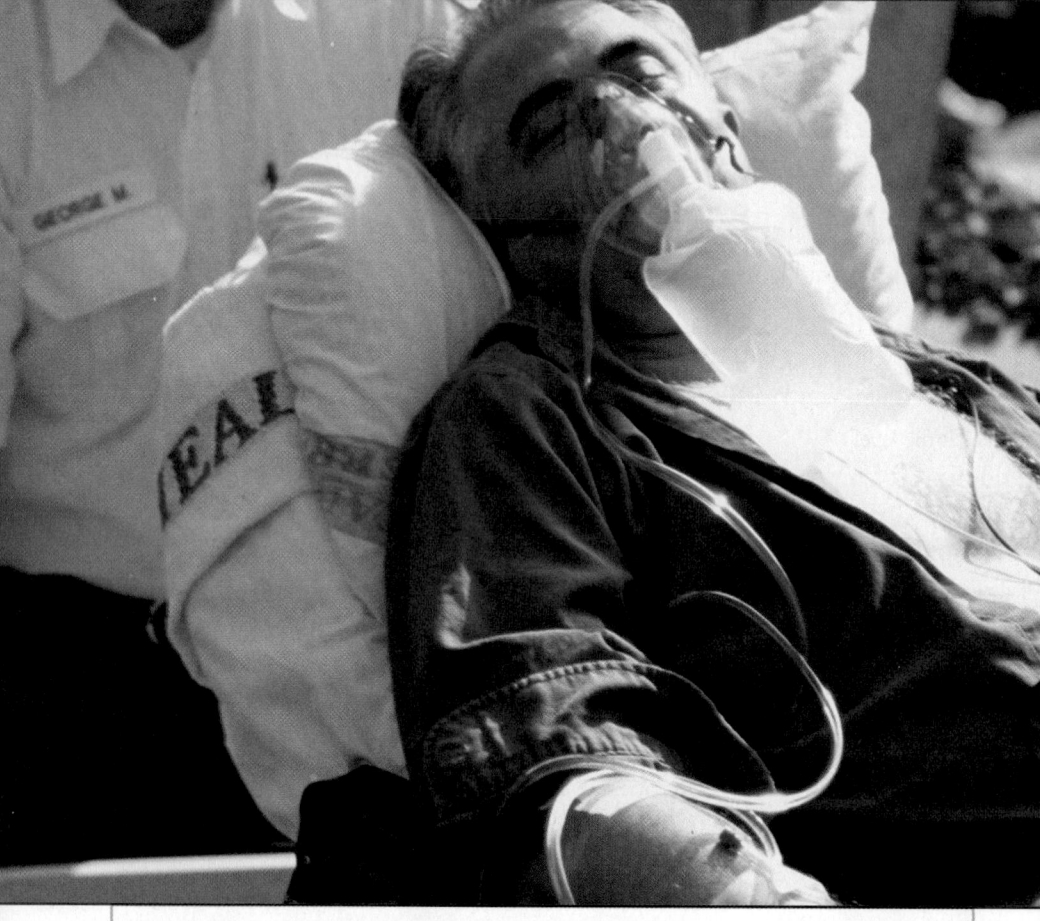

Content Area: Medicine

Advanced EMT Education Standard: Applies fundamental knowledge to provide basic and selected advanced emergency care and transportation based on assessment findings for an acutely ill patient.

Objectives

After reading this chapter, you should be able to:

24.1 Define key terms introduced in this chapter.

24.2 Compare and contrast the general characteristics of hollow and solid abdominal organs.

24.3 List the general mechanisms and types of abdominal pain.

24.4 Describe the pathophysiology, risk factors, assessment, and management of patients with emergencies related to hepatic diseases including viral hepatitis, cirrhosis, and hepatic encephalopathy.

24.5 Explain the pathophysiology, assessment, and management of the following abdominal and gastrointestinal disorders:

- Abdominal aortic aneurysm or dissection
- Appendicitis

(continued)

Resource Central

To access Resource Central, follow the directions on the Student Access Card provided with this text. If there is no card, go to www.bradybooks.com and follow the Resource Central link to Buy Access. Under Media Resources, you will find:

• *Abdominal Aortic Aneurysm (AAA).* Managing AAA in the prehospital setting.

• *My Aching Gut!* Different causes of acute abdominal pain and how to effectively assess the abdomen.

• *Upper & Lower GI Bleeds.* Signs and symptoms, causes, and prehospital management.

Advanced EMTs Elle Hutchings and Becky Weigand have been dispatched to a residence for a patient with abdominal pain. There are no indications of danger outside or inside the residence. An elderly man directs them to a bedroom, where his wife, 82-year-old Thelma Stoker, is lying in a right lateral recumbent position with her hips flexed. She appears pale with dry skin and mucous membranes and her expression indicates she is experiencing discomfort. There is no jaundice or cyanosis. Upon questioning, the patient gives a chief complaint of abdominal pain.

Problem-Solving Questions

1. What are the patient's presenting problems and risk factors that Elle and Becky will use to develop an initial hypotheses on the nature of the illness?
2. What might be Elle and Becky's initial hypotheses about the patient's presenting problem? What systems and processes might be involved?
3. In order to test their hypotheses, what aspects of the history are relevant in determining the underlying problem?

(continued from previous page)

- Bowel obstruction
- Cholecystitis
- Constipation
- Diarrhea
- Esophageal varices
- Gastroenteritis
- Hernia
- Inflammatory disorders of the bowel
- Pancreatitis
- Peritonitis
- Upper and lower gastrointestinal bleeding

24.6 Develop an effective line of questioning for patients presenting with abdominal pain and gastrointestinal complaints.

24.7 Effectively communicate the assessment findings, history, and treatment of patients with gastrointestinal complaints and abdominal pain orally and in writing.

Introduction

Gastrointestinal system disorders often present with abdominal pain, but not all abdominal pain is caused by gastrointestinal disorders. A complaint of abdominal pain may be due to a renal or urinary tract problem, a vascular disorder, gynecologic disorders in women, and even pneumonia or acute myocardial infarction (AMI), as well as gastrointestinal disorders. Many of those problems can be serious, even life threatening, and can cause patients significant discomfort. While it is not possible to make a definitive diagnosis of abdominal pain in the prehospital setting, narrowing the cause down to a set of differential diagnoses helps you develop an appropriate level of concern that the patient's condition could deteriorate. This chapter takes you through the pathophysiology, assessment, and management of patients with abdominal pain and a variety of gastrointestinal disorders.

Anatomy and Physiology Review

The boundaries of the abdominopelvic cavity are the diaphragm superiorly and the floor of the pelvis inferiorly (Figure 24-1a). The organs in the upper quadrants are afforded some degree of protection by the lower ribs. The abdominal and flank muscles and adipose tissue provide protection anteriorly and laterally. Peritoneum is a double layer of serous membrane that adheres to the organs (visceral peritoneum) and the body cavity (parietal peritoneum). The posterior portion of parietal peritoneum separates the abdominal organs from the retroperitoneal organs, which lie between the peritoneum and the posterior body wall. For purposes of physical examination, the abdomen is divided into four quadrants by two imaginary lines that intersect at the umbilicus (Figure 24-1b).

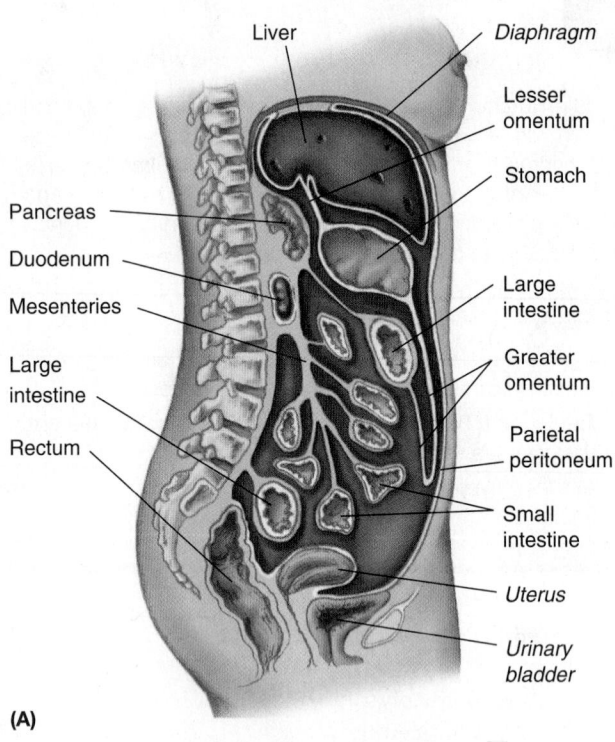

(A)

ABDOMINAL QUADRANTS

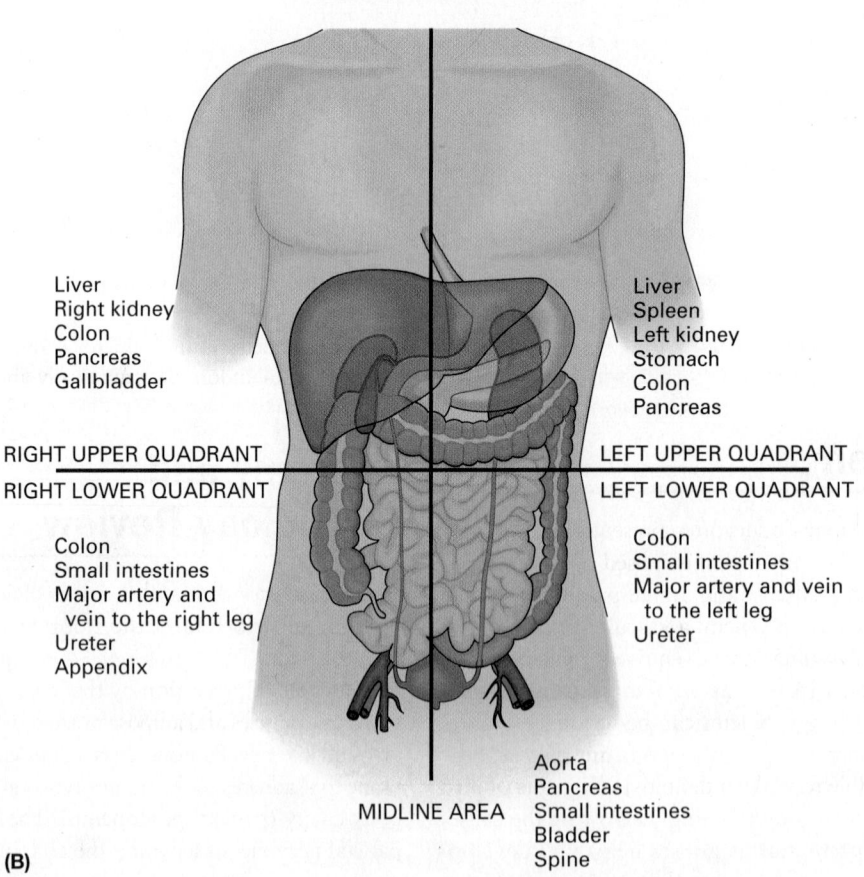

Liver
Right kidney
Colon
Pancreas
Gallbladder

Liver
Spleen
Left kidney
Stomach
Colon
Pancreas

RIGHT UPPER QUADRANT   LEFT UPPER QUADRANT

RIGHT LOWER QUADRANT   LEFT LOWER QUADRANT

Colon
Small intestines
Major artery and
 vein to the right leg
Ureter
Appendix

Colon
Small intestines
Major artery and vein
 to the left leg
Ureter

(B)

MIDLINE AREA

Aorta
Pancreas
Small intestines
Bladder
Spine

FIGURE 24-1

(A) The boundaries of the abdominopelvic cavity. (B) Contents of the abdominopelvic cavity by quadrant.

Abdominal organs are classified as either solid or hollow (Figure 24-2). Solid organs are inelastic and covered by a fibrous capsule. They are dense and highly vascular. Examples of solid organs include the liver, spleen, pancreas, and kidneys (retroperitoneal). Hollow organs are tubelike structures that serve to transport and store substances. Hollow organs have a smooth muscle coat that allows them to contract to propel their contents forward or release them from the body. Examples of hollow organs include the stomach, intestines, gallbladder, ureters, and urinary bladder.

Very large blood vessels course through the abdominal cavity and retroperitoneal space, including the abdominal aorta, vena cava, renal arteries and veins, and the veins of the hepatic portal circulation. Folds of peritoneal tissue called *mesenteries* stabilize the abdominal organs, as well as the blood vessels and nerve supply to the organs. Two mesenteries—the greater omentum and lesser omentum—drape over the abdominal organs to provide protection.

The gastrointestinal (GI) or digestive system consists essentially of a long tube from mouth to anus, and accessory organs (Figure 24-3). The digestive tract begins at the

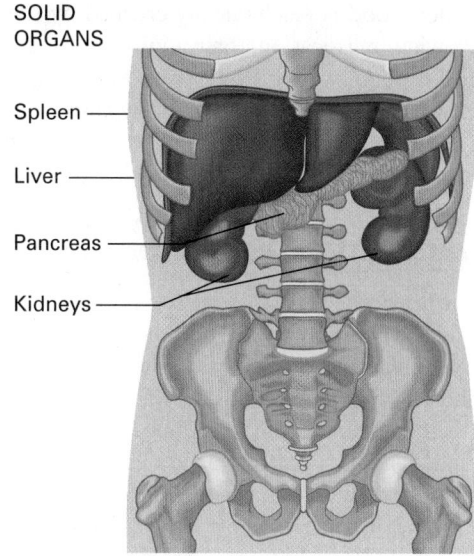

SOLID ORGANS

Spleen
Liver
Pancreas
Kidneys

FIGURE 24-2

Solid abdominal organs.

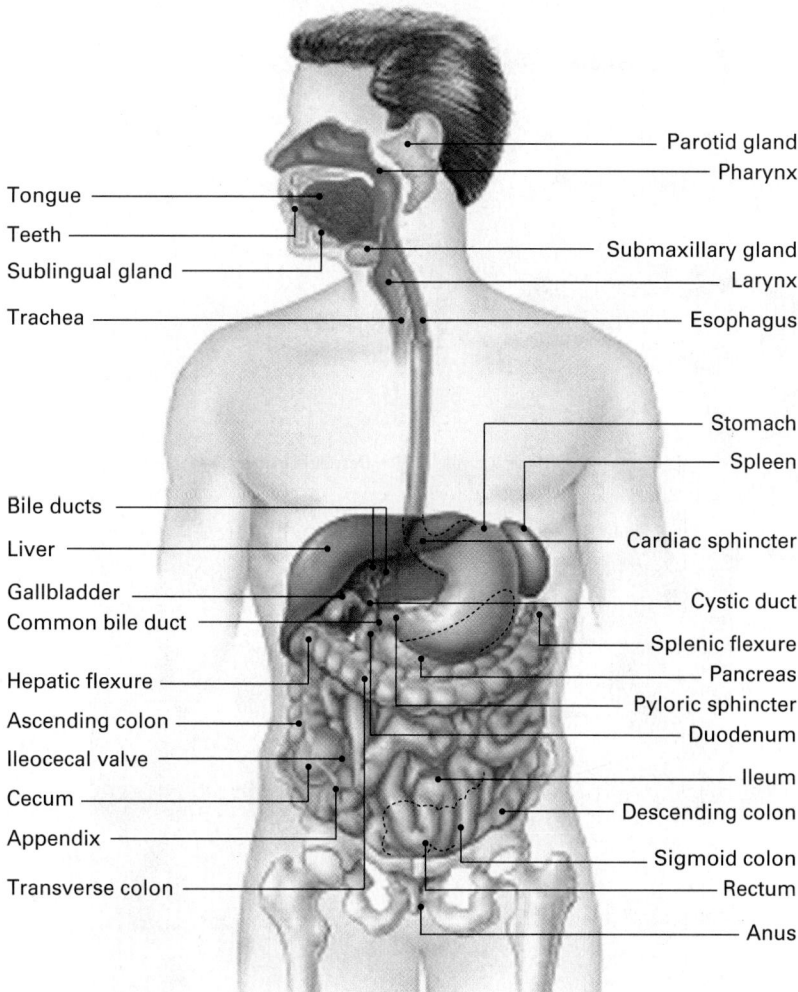

Parotid gland
Pharynx
Tongue
Teeth
Sublingual gland
Submaxillary gland
Larynx
Trachea
Esophagus

Stomach
Spleen

Bile ducts
Liver
Cardiac sphincter

Gallbladder
Common bile duct
Cystic duct

Hepatic flexure
Splenic flexure
Pancreas
Ascending colon
Pyloric sphincter
Duodenum
Ileocecal valve
Ileum
Cecum
Descending colon
Appendix
Sigmoid colon
Transverse colon
Rectum
Anus

FIGURE 24-3

The gastrointestinal system.

mouth, where food is mechanically crushed by the teeth during chewing (mastication). Saliva initiates the chemical breakdown of food, which is then swallowed (deglutition) and propelled through the upper esophageal sphincter and into the esophagus by **peristalsis**. The lower esophageal sphincter opens to admit food into the stomach.

Stomach and Intestines

Food is further broken down in the stomach by the actions of hydrochloric acid and **pepsin**, and the churning motions created by the smooth muscle coats of the stomach. Absorption of nutrients and medications does not take place in the stomach because its thick mucous lining is designed to protect the underlying tissues from the low pH environment of stomach, rather than to absorb nutrients.

The stomach contents, now called **chyme**, enter the first portion of the small intestine, the duodenum. The pH of chyme as it leaves the stomach is between 1.5 and 2.0. Buffers (largely bicarbonate) and digestive enzymes from the pancreas and **bile** from the liver are excreted into the duodenum. The buffers neutralize the chyme, protecting the lining

of the duodenum from the acidic contents entering it from the stomach. Most nutrients are absorbed as the intestinal contents move through the duodenum, and into the second and third portions of the small intestine, the jejunum and ileum.

The intestinal contents then enter the first portion of the large intestine, or colon, at the cecum through the ileocecal valve (Figure 24-4). A blind pouch, the vermiform appendix, projects from the cecum, but its exact functions are not known. From the cecum, the ascending colon travels up the right side of the lower abdomen toward the liver, where it turns and becomes the transverse colon, which crosses from right to left across the abdomen, toward the spleen. The colon then turns inferiorly, becoming the descending colon. The lower portion of the colon is called the *sigmoid colon* for its "S" shape.

Water is absorbed from the large intestine, producing a more solid fecal mass, which is stored in the rectum until there is an urge to defecate. Feces pass through the anus under voluntary control. The anorectal area contains hemorrhoidal cushions, which contribute to sphincter tone and the ability to differentiate between pressure from solids, liquids, and gases. The hemorrhoidal cushions are vascular and can

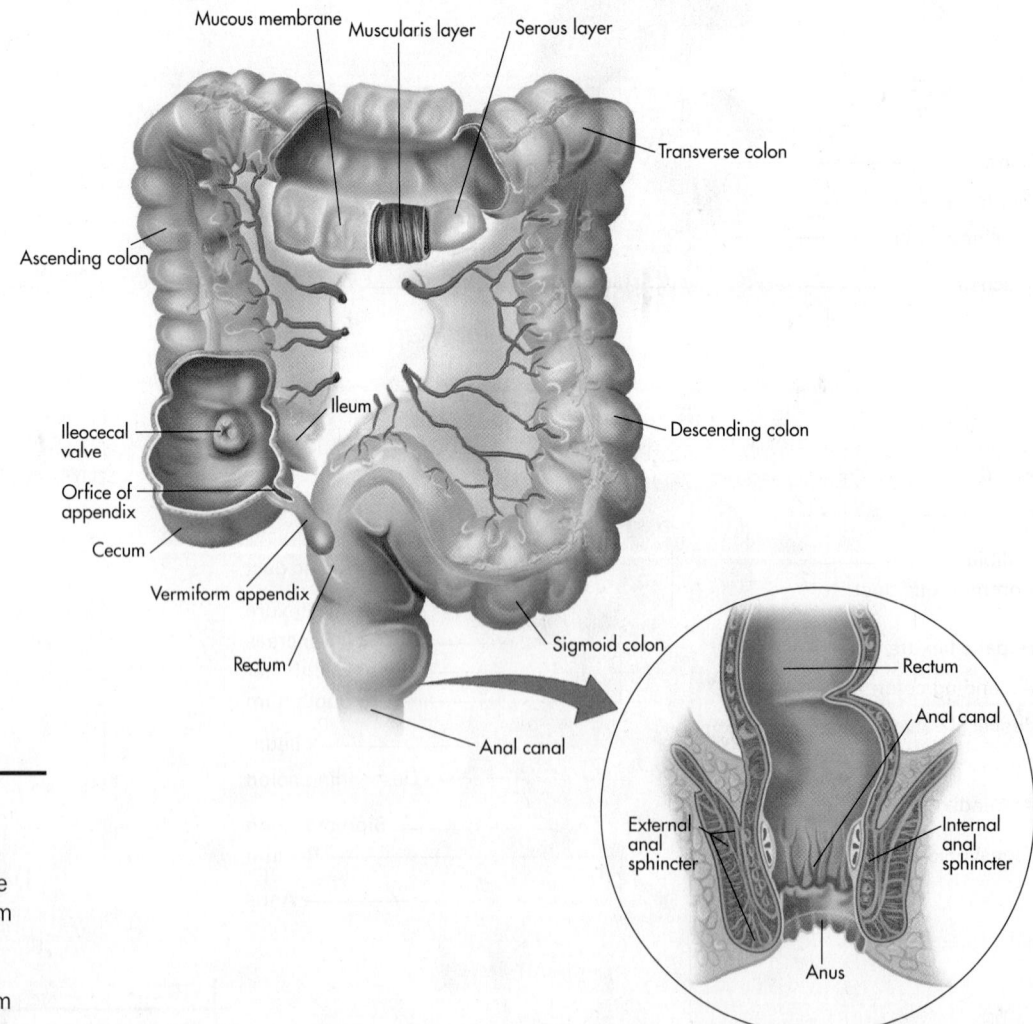

FIGURE 24-4

The colon, or large intestine. The ileum of the small intestine empties into the large intestine at the cecum through the ileocecal valve. The appendix projects inferiorly from the cecum.

become engorged, resulting in protrusion of the tissue from the anus (what most people understand to be hemorrhoids). The tissue can be abraded during bowel movements, resulting in bleeding. The tissue can also become irritated and painful, and can become thrombosed.

Accessory Organs of Digestion

The accessory organs of the digestive system include the salivary glands, the liver, gallbladder, and pancreas. The salivary glands secrete saliva into the oral cavity to moisten food to facilitate its passage through the esophagus. Saliva contains amylase, an enzyme that breaks down complex carbohydrates into simple sugars.

The liver is a complex organ that serves many functions. All venous blood from the digestive tract travels through the liver by way of the hepatic portal circulation prior to returning to the general circulation. The liver processes nutrients and medications absorbed by the GI tract, detoxifies by removing certain substances from the blood, and breaks down, synthesizes, and stores substances. The liver synthesizes albumin, the primary protein that provides the colloid osmotic pressure of the blood, clotting factors, and bile. The characteristic color of bile comes from the pigment bilirubin, a product of the normal breakdown of aged and damaged red blood cells by the liver. The liver is also a major store of glycogen.

Bile produced by the liver can enter the duodenum through the common bile duct (Figure 24-5). Excess bile enters the gallbladder through the cystic duct, where it is stored. The gallbladder is a small sac along the inferior aspect of the liver that stores bile to be secreted into the small intestine, where is serves to emulsify (break up) fats so that they can be absorbed through the intestinal lining.

The pancreas has both endocrine functions and exocrine functions. Its endocrine functions include secretion of insulin and glucagon to regulate blood glucose levels. The pancreas also excretes powerful digestive enzymes and bicarbonate-containing buffer into the gastrointestinal system through the pancreatic duct.

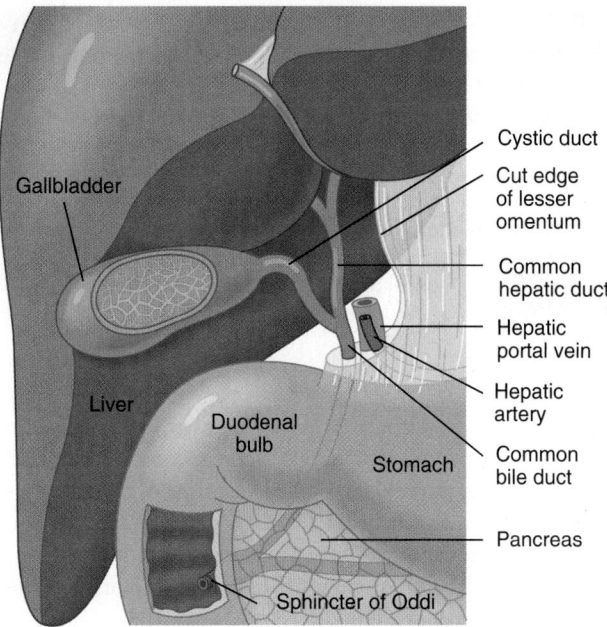

FIGURE 24-5

The liver, gallbladder, and bile ducts. The pancreatic and common bile ducts enter the duodenum through the ampulla of Vater, where their secretions are controlled by the sphincter of Oddi.

General Assessment and Management of Abdominal Complaints

The abdominal cavity houses organs and structures of many body systems. The proximity of organs of different systems can sometimes result in similar signs and symptoms of problems arising from those systems (Table 24-1). In addition to abdominal pain, other complaints and presentations

TABLE 24-1	Possible Sources of Abdominal Pain by Region	
Abdominal Region	**Organs**	**Sources of Referred Pain**
Right upper quadrant	Liver, gallbladder	Pneumonia or pleuritis (right pleural cavity)
Epigastric region	Stomach, pancreas	AMI, appendicitis
Left upper quadrant	Spleen, part of pancreas	Pneumonia or pleuritis (left pleural cavity)
Umbilical and hypogastric	Small intestine, large intestine, aorta, urinary bladder, in females: uterus	Bowel obstruction, appendicitis
Right lower quadrant	Appendix, ascending colon, in females: right ovary and fallopian tube	
Left lower quadrant	Descending colon (diverticula usually are located in the descending colon)	

related to, or potentially related to, gastrointestinal problems include nausea, vomiting, diarrhea, constipation, back pain, bloating, **anorexia**, jaundice, rectal pain, **hematemesis**, **melena**, and **hematochezia**. Patients with abdominal pain and gastrointestinal problems can present in mild discomfort, or with life-threatening **peritonitis** or hemorrhage, dehydration, and electrolyte disorders.

Some of the diseases and problems related to those complaints and presentations include acute and chronic upper and lower gastrointestinal tract bleeding, ulcerative disorders of the intestinal tract, liver disorders such as **cirrhosis** and **hepatitis**, peritonitis, appendicitis, bowel obstruction, gallbladder problems (**cholecystitis**), pancreatitis, hernias, and ingested foreign bodies. Nongastrointestinal disorders can overlap the signs and symptoms of gastrointestinal disorders. Nausea and vomiting, for instance, have numerous causes, such as acute coronary syndrome, diabetic ketoacidosis, and renal colic. Abdominal, back, and flank pain also have nongastrointestinal causes.

While some conditions have so-called classic presentations, keep in mind that patients do not always present with all classic signs and symptoms of disorders, and that there is overlap in the presentations of various disorders (Table 24-2). Therefore, classic presentations give you a starting place for history-taking and assessment, but you still must engage in a thoughtful process of clinical reasoning. Along with knowledge of anatomy, physiology, and pathophysiology, careful assessment is essential in determining the nature of the problem and implementing treatment.

Scene Size-Up

Sometimes, the person who called dispatch may have provided information about the nature of the problem. For example, there may be a report of abdominal pain, or a person vomiting blood. No matter what dispatch information you receive, size up the scene to assess its safety, look for clues to the problem, determine the patient's chief complaint, and obtain an initial impression of the patient. You can get an idea of the patient's degree of distress by noticing his level of responsiveness, facial expression, skin color, and position.

Primary Assessment

Ensure that the patient has an open airway and adequate ventilations, because vomiting is common in patients with gastrointestinal disorders. Provide oxygen as indicated by the patient's complaints and presentation. Assess the adequacy of circulation. Hypotension and tachycardia are signs of shock, which may be due to fluid loss, hemorrhage, or sepsis. Unlike external bleeding, the source of gastrointestinal bleeding is not accessible in the prehospital setting, and the patient requires intervention in the hospital to stop it.

Secondary Assessment

Take a complete set of vital signs to establish a baseline. If dehydration or other volume loss is suspected and the patient's condition allows, check orthostatic vital signs. Examination of the skin can provide clues to anemia from chronic gastrointestinal bleeding or other causes. It also is helpful to check the color of the mucous membranes inside the lower eyelids. *Jaundice* is a clue to liver disease, as is distention of the abdomen with fluid (ascites). Examining the abdomen may reveal distention from gas or fluid, ecchymosis associated with internal bleeding, scars from previous surgery, or an ostomy (surgical opening connecting a portion of the intestine to the abdominal wall, such as **colostomy** or ileostomy). Palpating the abdomen may help localize the area of pain, and can occasionally reveal a pulsating mass associated with abdominal aortic aneurysm. Also note the presence of involuntary or voluntary guarding.

For unresponsive patients, obtain as much history as possible from family, health care providers, or bystanders and perform a rapid secondary assessment. Ensure that all components of the SAMPLE history are included. Patients are often reluctant to discuss bowel habits or problems with medical care providers, especially in the presence of others. It is important that you gain the patient's confidence in order for him to feel as comfortable as possible in sharing the information. In patients who are alert, the focused history and assessment are based on the chief complaint. Determine if there is a history of associated complaints, using your knowledge of disease pathophysiology, which can help you narrow down the cause. Explore the chief complaint, including all components represented by the OPQRST mnemonic.

Ask about nausea, vomiting, pain, lightheadedness, blood in the stools, or dark, tarry stools. Past medical history that may be important in identifying the problem includes known history of ulcers, **diverticulitis**, ulcerative intestinal disorders, cardiovascular disease, diabetes, hypertension, liver failure, cancer, severe endometriosis, and the date of the last menstrual period in menstruating women. Certain medications, such as NSAIDs (for example, aspirin, ibuprofen, naproxen, and some prescription arthritis medications), corticosteroids, some herbal supplements, and excessive alcohol ingestion (either acute or chronic) can increase the risk of gastrointestinal bleeding. Other medications that can

TABLE 24-2	Presentations of Problems Associated with Specific Organs and Problems

Organ or Problem	Common Findings
Liver	■ General: steady, dull pain in right upper quadrant, bleeding tendency, jaundice. ■ Hepatitis: flulike symptoms, enlarged, tender liver. ■ Cirrhosis: ascites; dyspnea from liver enlargement and ascites.
Gallbladder	■ Gallstone obstructing common bile duct: crampy, colicky pain, often 30–60 minutes after eating, especially a high-fat meal. Right upper quadrant pain that may radiate to the right shoulder, scapula, or back. Nausea and vomiting. ■ Cholecystitis: may also have fever, jaundice.
Stomach	■ Gastritis or peptic ulcer disease: steady, burning epigastric pain, possible nausea and vomiting; hematemesis possible. ■ Perforated ulcer: signs of peritoneal irritation.
Acute pancreatitis	■ Sudden onset of constant, severe pain in the epigastric region that may feel as though it is "boring through" to the back; nausea and vomiting, which may be severe.
Spleen	■ Enlarged or irritated: pain in left upper quadrant, pain may be referred to left shoulder and neck. ■ Ruptured spleen: sudden, intense pain subsides and then intensifies and may be accompanied by syncope and orthostatic hypotension.
Large and Small Intestines	■ Gastroenteritis, inflammatory bowel disease, ileitis, colitis: crampy, colicky pain; possible vomiting, diarrhea, and dehydration. ■ Food poisoning: ingestion of contaminated food 2–8 hours before onset of symptoms. Vomiting and diarrhea, dehydration, and electrolyte disturbances are possible. ■ Bowel obstruction: begins with intermittent colicky pain that increases in intensity and becomes constant; pain is poorly localized; shallow respirations due to peritonitis; sepsis may occur. ■ Diverticulitis: signs of peritonitis, fever, diarrhea, lower gastrointestinal bleeding.
Aorta	■ Intense, tearing pain in lower back or abdomen that may radiate down one or both legs, possible vascular and neurologic signs and symptoms in one or both lower extremities, syncope, hypotension, shock, feeling of "impending doom," possible pulsating mass in midline of lower abdomen.
Kidneys and ureters	■ Nephritis: dull, constant flank pain, possible difficulty in urination and hematuria. ■ Kidney stone: sharp, colicky pain that may intensify until the stone is passed, pain may radiate to groin, possible hematuria; patient may be restless, prefer to stand, and be unable to find a comfortable position.
Appendix	■ May begin with poorly localized periumbilical pain, usually localizes to right lower quadrant, may fever. Rupture signified by sudden relief of pain followed by signs of peritonitis.
Ovaries and fallopian tubes	■ Ovarian cyst: dull, constant pain localized to one side in the lower quadrant. ■ Ruptured ovarian cyst: pain may subside briefly followed by signs of peritonitis and pain may radiate to neck or shoulder on affected side. ■ Ectopic pregnancy: crampy, colicky pain that intensifies with rupture, followed by signs of peritonitis, referred pain, orthostatic vital signs, and shock.

indicate a gastrointestinal problem include antacids, H_2 histamine blockers (Tagamet, Zantac), proton pump inhibitors (Prilosec), and laxatives.

Clinical-Reasoning Process

Your primary focus is to ensure an adequate airway, ventilation, oxygenation, and circulation. However, it is also important in the prehospital setting to consider an underlying cause. Be flexible in your history-taking so that you can follow up on the patient's answers. An overly rigid approach

to the history can prevent you from pursuing important lines of questioning. A thorough scene size-up, assessment, and history contribute immeasurably to your ability to anticipate further complications and communicate essential information to receiving facility personnel.

Treatment

Specific things to keep in mind regarding treatment include recognizing that anemia is a frequent complication of chronic **occult** gastrointestinal bleeding. The hemoglobin that is present may be fully saturated with oxygen, resulting in a high SpO_2, but the overall decrease in hemoglobin means that inadequate amounts of oxygen are carried and released to the tissues, resulting in hypoxia at the cellular level. Provide supplemental oxygen, if indicated, to increase the arterial PaO_2. Although it is important to increase perfusion in hypotensive patients, be cautious with the rate of fluid administration in patients who are elderly or who have a history of heart or renal failure. Frequently check the breath sounds for indications of fluid overload.

Anticipate vomiting and the need to provide airway management. Allow the patient to assume a position of comfort unless the need for airway management prevents it. Patients with abdominal pain often are most comfortable lying on their sides with the legs drawn up. Gentle transport is imperative, because each bump can bring excruciating pain to the patient with peritonitis.

The administration of narcotic analgesia does not interfere with diagnosing abdominal pain as once thought. If allowed in your scope of practice, check with medical direction concerning the administration of narcotic analgesia. Nitrous oxide is not contraindicated in abdominal pain in general, but it is contraindicated in patients who may have a bowel obstruction.

Reassessment

Gastrointestinal disorders and other causes of abdominal pain can have life-threatening underlying causes. Patients can be critically ill, and prone to serious complications and rapid decompensation. Establish a baseline of mental status, complaints, vital signs, and physical findings. Reassess critical patients every 5 minutes, or sooner, and noncritical patients every 15 minutes, obtaining at least two complete sets of vital signs.

General Causes and Assessment of Abdominal Pain

The general causes of abdominal pain are inflammation or infection, stretching of tissues from distention or traction, and ischemia. Stretching mechanisms affect the hollow organs and the capsules surrounding solid organs. Rapid distention is especially painful. A crampy or colicky pain is usually caused by distention, infection, obstruction, or inflammation of a hollow organ. Increased peristalsis and pain can occur in gastroenteritis, bowel obstruction with proximal distention of the intestine, intestinal gas, a kidney stone passing through a ureter, and urinary tract infection.

Visceral Pain

Visceral pain arises from the organs in the abdominal cavity and is difficult for the patient to localize. The diffuse nature

of the pain is due to the sparse supply of sensory nerves to the organs. The pain is often experienced in the epigastric and umbilical areas, and is often described as a dull pain. In some conditions, such as appendicitis, pain can begin as a diffuse pain, but as the condition progresses and the peritoneum becomes inflamed, the pain becomes localized.

Somatic Pain

Parietal, or somatic, pain arises from inflammation of the peritoneum that lines the abdominal cavity (parietal peritoneum). The pain is generally intense, constant, and often described as sharp. The pain is well localized, meaning that the patient is able to point to the exact area that hurts.

Referred Pain and Radiating Pain

Referred pain is experienced at a site remote from the affected organ (Figure 24-6). The sensation is often felt in the skin or deeper tissues and is well localized. It arises when the area shares a sensory nerve pathway with the affected organ. Pain from an affected abdominal organ can be referred to the shoulder, back, or leg. Pain in the abdomen can be referred from other sites, such as the myocardium, or pleural cavity in pleuritis or pneumonia.

Radiating pain is pain that is felt in the affected area but which also extends elsewhere. For example, the pain of abdominal aortic aneurysm may be felt in the back and radiate down one or both legs.

Factors Affecting Pain Perception

The experience of pain is affected by age, the presence of other health problems, ingestion of alcohol or other depressant drugs, and the patient's psychological perception of pain and emotional state. Infants and small children are not as well able to localize pain, and are not able to describe the sensation of pain. Confusing the issue, pain is only one of the many causes of infant irritability and crying. The elderly and those with diabetic neuropathy have a decreased sensation of pain and may have serious underlying pathology despite having mild or moderate pain. The way people

IN THE FIELD

The use of nitrous oxide is contraindicated in patients with suspected bowel obstruction, because nitrous oxide diffuses from the blood into air-filled spaces 34 times faster than oxygen. This process can cause further distention of the bowel. Nitrous oxide also should never be used on or around pregnant women.

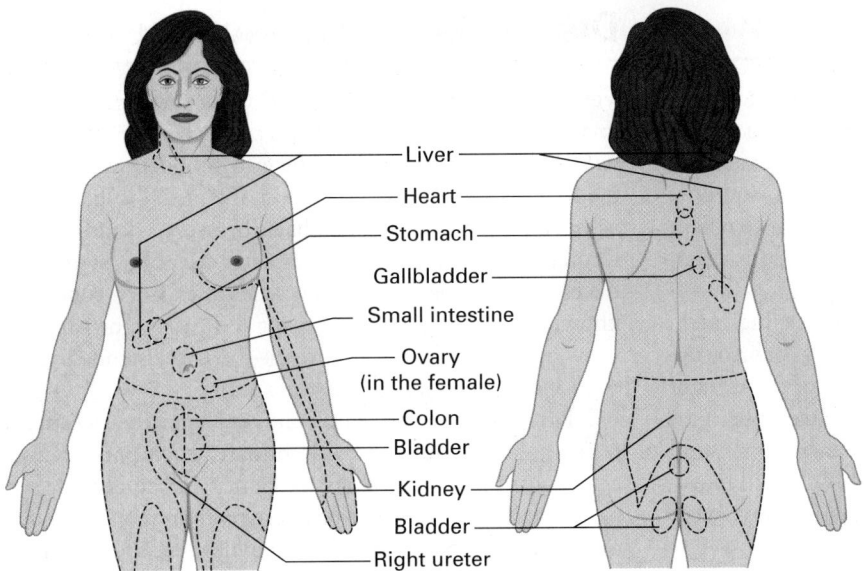

Liver
Heart
Stomach
Gallbladder
Small intestine
Ovary
(in the female)
Colon
Bladder
Kidney
Bladder
Right ureter

FIGURE 24-6

Pain from abdominal problems can be referred to sites other than the location of the problem.

experience and respond to pain varies according to individual and cultural factors.

Ask the patient to compare the current pain to the worst pain he has ever experienced. This is a subjective measure, because the degree of pain suffered in the past is based on individual experience, and different patients perceive pain differently. However, it is the patient's perception of pain that is important to manage, and the initial pain level provides a baseline so you can evaluate whether the patient's pain is increasing or decreasing.

Geriatric Care

Pain sensation can be decreased in the elderly, a population at risk for gastrointestinal disorders. Mild to moderate abdominal pain in an elderly patient does not necessarily mean that the underlying problem is minor. Always consider a serious underlying cause in the elderly patient with abdominal pain.

CASE STUDY (continued)

Mrs. Stoker is alert and oriented to person, place, and time. Her respirations are 24 and shallow. The patient appears anxious, but is lying very still. She is a bit pale and appears uncomfortable. Her pulse is 88 and irregular. Her skin is warm and dry with poor turgor. Her blood pressure is 104/66 and SpO_2 is 95 percent on room air. Mrs. Stoker woke approximately 4 hours ago with intermittent "crampy pain" in the right lower quadrant of her abdomen. The pain has gotten worse, but now is diffuse and she is unable to localize it. She rates the pain as a 6 on a scale of 10. She also complains of nausea, feeling bloated, and being constipated. She denies blood in her stool, dark tarry stools, vomiting, blood in the urine, and difficult or painful urination.

Mrs. Stoker has been generally healthy throughout her life and was only hospitalized when she gave birth to her children. She had an episode of pneumonia about six weeks ago. Severe coughing led her to fracture vertebrae T-8 and T-9, at which time she was diagnosed with osteoporosis, and is being treated with Actonel. The pneumonia was treated with antibiotics, and she was prescribed Tylox for pain due to the fractured vertebrae. Mrs. Stoker is being treated for atrial fibrillation with Cardizem, Tenormin, and Coumadin.

Problem-Solving Questions

1. How might this information help the Advanced EMTs refine their hypotheses?
2. Describe the relevant initial physical examination and interventions needed based on the information so far.

Nausea and Vomiting

Nausea is a sensation that is associated with the anticipation of vomiting. Vomiting is the forcible expulsion of gastrointestinal contents through the mouth. When the involuntary movement of the gastrointestinal system is weak and does not produce **emesis**, it is called *retching*. Just prior to vomiting, there is increased salivation and a sharp, deep involuntary inspiration.

The abdominal muscles contract, increasing intraabdominal pressure. The epiglottis closes to protect the airway, and there are forceful contractions of the inferior portion of the stomach (the pylorus), while the upper part of the stomach (fundus), lower esophageal sphincter, and esophagus all relax. The result is forceful backward movement of stomach contents. But the question remains, what causes vomiting?

Vomiting has several triggers, including sensory nerve stimulation of the pharynx, gastrointestinal tract, heart, and other organs. Local irritation of the stomach activates cells that secrete serotonin. Serotonin acts on specific receptors on afferent vagus nerve (cranial nerve X) fibers, which in turn stimulate the vomiting center in the brain. Endogenous (for example, hormones of pregnancy) and exogenous (opiates, drugs, alcohol, toxins) emetic substances can stimulate the vomiting center, as can increased intracranial pressure and reaction to sensory input (sights, smells, tastes).

The vomiting center in the medulla of the brain receives input from stretch and irritant receptors, conducted by the vagus nerve, mechanical receptors in the throat (gag reflex), the vestibular apparatus of the inner ear (causes vomiting in motion sickness), higher cortical areas of the brain (learned associations), and the chemoreceptor trigger zone (CTZ) in the fourth ventricle of the brain. In this area of the brain, the blood–brain barrier is weak, allowing substances to cross it. The types of receptors involved in the vomiting center allow treatment of vomiting through medications that block the receptors.

Many people describe nausea and vomiting as being the most unpleasant physical sensation they have experienced. This, along with the risks of aspiration, esophageal rupture, dehydration, and electrolyte and pH disturbances make it desirable to treat nausea and vomiting in most cases. A number of EMS services have begun carrying ondansetron (Zofran), an antiemetic drug that blocks certain serotonin receptors.

Pediatric Care

Projectile vomiting in neonates can be an indication of pyloric stenosis, a condition in which the passageway from the stomach into the duodenum is narrowed. The stomach becomes overdistended during feeding and projectile vomiting may occur.

Disorders of the Esophagus

Veins of the esophagus, like other veins of the gastrointestinal tract, empty into the hepatic portal system. In patients with liver disease, the resistance to blood flow through the liver results in back pressure in the portal vein, known as **portal hypertension**. The back pressure is transmitted through the rest of the veins that enter the portal system. In the esophagus, the veins can become distended, a condition known as **esophageal varices** (singular, *varix*), or varicose veins of the esophagus (Figure 24-7). The distended veins can rupture, resulting in massive bleeding.

Patients with bleeding from esophageal varices may aspirate blood and can exsanguinate. Such patients can challenge your clinical skills to the maximum, because supraglottic airways will not be effective in preventing aspiration and will prevent access to the bleeding area. Suction may be inadequate to keep up with the amount of blood in

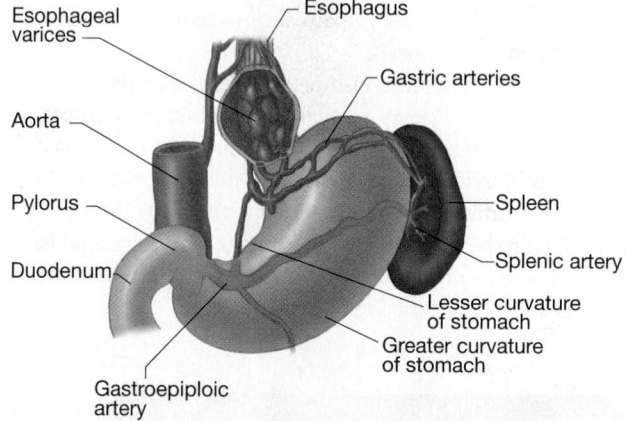

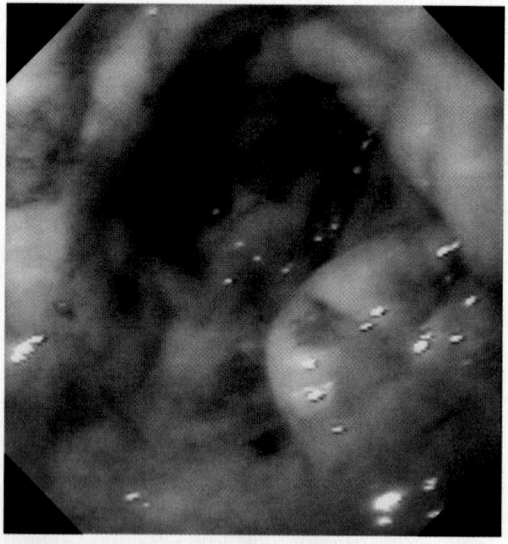

FIGURE 24-7

Esophageal varices. (Bottom photo: David M. Martin, MD/Photo Researchers, Inc.)

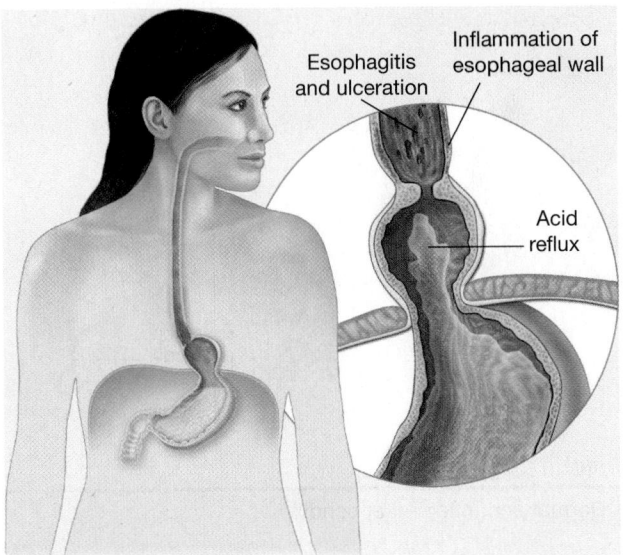
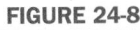
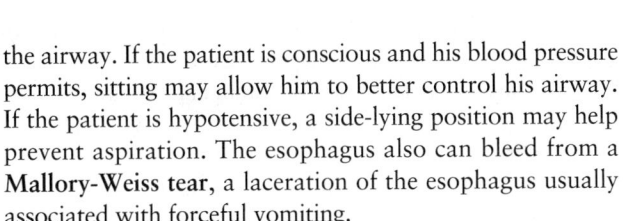

FIGURE 24-8

A hiatal hernia with gastroesophageal reflux.

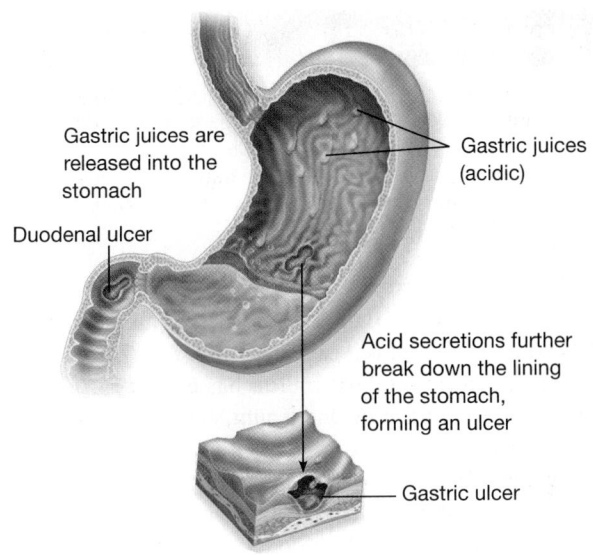

FIGURE 24-9

Peptic ulcers.

the airway. If the patient is conscious and his blood pressure permits, sitting may allow him to better control his airway. If the patient is hypotensive, a side-lying position may help prevent aspiration. The esophagus also can bleed from a **Mallory-Weiss tear**, a laceration of the esophagus usually associated with forceful vomiting.

Esophagitis is an inflammation of the esophagus from the reflux of acidic stomach contents through the lower esophageal sphincter (Figure 24-8). In some patients, the lower esophageal sphincter is weakened, and reflux is a chronic problem (gastroesophageal reflux disease, or GERD). Exposure to stomach contents causes chronic inflammation of the esophageal mucosa and can result in cellular changes (Barrett's esophagus), which can lead to esophageal cancer. Esophagitis is a cause of upper gastrointestinal bleeding. **Hiatal hernia** is a condition in which the stomach slides upward through the opening in the diaphragm through which the esophagus passes. This may result in gastric reflux. In more severe cases, the displaced stomach may cause discomfort by placing pressure on intrathoracic structures.

Disorders of the Stomach and Intestines

Upper gastrointestinal bleeding occurs at any point in the gastrointestinal system from the esophagus to the ligament of Treitz, which supports the small intestine at the junction of the duodenum and jejunum. Lower gastrointestinal bleeding occurs beyond the ligament of Treitz and may be caused by cancer, diverticulitis, or hemorrhoids. Other causes of stomach and intestinal disorders include **peptic**

ulcer disease, gastritis, gastroenteritis, diverticulitis, appendicitis, and bowel obstruction.

Upper Gastrointestinal Bleeding

Upper gastrointestinal bleeding may occur from gastritis, peptic ulcer, or inflammation or ulcers in the duodenum (Figure 24-9). Bleeding from the stomach and duodenum can be accompanied by a burning discomfort in the upper abdominal quadrants, either due to the underlying cause of

IN THE FIELD

Peptic ulcers are erosions of the gastric or duodenal mucosa. Normally, the thick mucosa and mucous secretions of the stomach lining protect it against the hydrochloric acid and pepsin that break down food. Under certain conditions, this protective layer is impaired and the hydrochloric acid and pepsin contact the exposed tissues beneath. One contributing cause is the use of nonsteroidal anti-inflammatory drugs (NSAIDs). NSAIDs inhibit an enzyme that is important in maintaining the protective lining of the stomach. The bacteria *Heliobacter pylori* has been implicated as well. Corticosteroids inhibit tissue repair and can also play a role in the development of ulcers. In the duodenum, if the duct that conducts buffers from the pancreas to the duodenum is blocked, chyme is not neutralized as it enters the duodenum and the lining can be eroded. The relationship between the onset of pain and whether the stomach is empty or full depends on the location of the ulcer. Patients may self-treat recurring discomfort using over-the-counter H_2 antagonists, proton pump inhibitors, and antacids, running the risk of delayed diagnosis of ulcer.

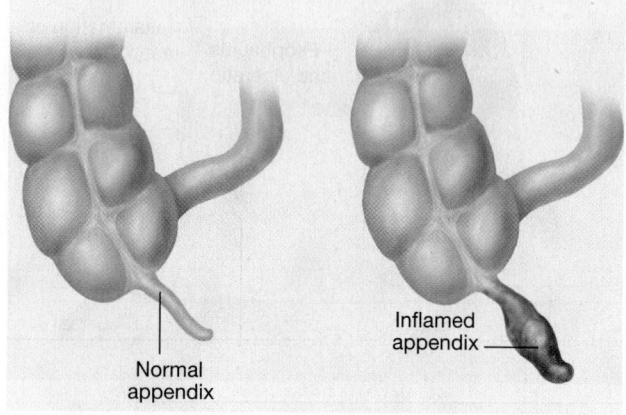

FIGURE 24-10

Normal and inflamed appendix.

inflammation or mucosal erosion (such as an ulcer) or because the blood itself is a gastric irritant. Acute, severe pain can be an indication that an ulcer has eroded through the lining of the stomach or duodenum, causing bleeding into the abdominal cavity.

Patients may vomit fresh blood or the emesis may appear as if it contains coffee grounds when gastric secretions have had time to act on the blood. If a significant amount of blood passes through the gastrointestinal tract, the stool becomes dark and tarry, a condition known as *melena*. When the bleeding is less and is not visible to the eye (occult bleeding), the presence of blood can sometimes be detected by a simple bedside test in which a small amount of stool is placed on a special paper and a chemical reagent that reacts with blood is added.

Acute gastrointestinal bleeding can be massive, leading to shock and death. In some cases, if the bleeding is slower, the patient may present with signs of orthostatic hypotension. Chronic gastrointestinal bleeding can lead to anemia. As with upper gastrointestinal bleeding from the esophagus, airway management can be challenging. Administer oxygen and assist ventilations if needed. For patients with obvious or suspected gastrointestinal bleeding, start an IV and administer intravenous fluids according to protocol.

Gastroenteritis

Gastroenteritis is an inflammation of the stomach and intestines, often due to the presence of a pathogen, which may be viral, bacterial, or parasitic. (See Chapter 28.) Depending on the exact cause and severity, signs and symptoms can include abdominal pain, nausea, bloating, vomiting, diarrhea, and fever. Diarrhea may occur due to inflammation of the intestinal mucosa, causing the intestinal contents to move quickly through the gastrointestinal tract without water being absorbed as it normally would, or pathogenic toxins can poison the sodium pump of intestinal cells, causing massive amounts of sodium and water to enter the lumen of the bowel. Most cases of gastroenteritis are self-limiting, but some can lead to dehydration and electrolyte imbalance.

Appendicitis

Appendicitis in an inflammation of the vermiform appendix, a narrow, blind pouch that projects from the cecum. Inflammation can be caused when the appendix becomes obstructed by stool or foreign body, but in many cases the

cause is unknown (Figure 24-10). The patients most likely to be affected are between 10 and 30 years old, but appendicitis can occur at any age. If untreated, the appendix can rupture, leading to peritonitis.

The abdominal pain associated with acute appendicitis typically comes on suddenly, beginning around the umbilicus but localizing to the right lower quadrant and becoming worse over time. The patient may have a low-grade fever, anorexia, and constipation. Upon palpation of the abdomen, you may notice rebound tenderness in the lower right quadrant. Rebound tenderness is pain that may decrease in intensity when you press down during palpation, but increases in intensity when pressure is released. As with all patients with peritoneal irritation, the patient's pain may increase with movement, especially with jarring movements such as walking.

Diverticulitis

Diverticula are abnormal outpouchings of the wall of the colon that are blind pockets in which fecal material can collect. The condition of having diverticula is called *diverticulosis* (Figure 24-11). Diverticulitis is an infection of a diverticulum that results in signs and symptoms similar to appendicitis. However, most diverticuli are in the distal colon, on the left side of the abdomen. In addition, while appendicitis can occur at any age, it is more common in younger patients, while diverticulitis is more common in patients over the age of 50. The patient presents with abdominal pain, which may localize to the lower left quadrant and fever. The patient may have diarrhea and lower gastrointestinal bleeding. In some cases, a diverticulum ruptures, causing massive lower gastrointestinal bleeding and peritonitis.

Lower Gastrointestinal Bleeding

Lower gastrointestinal bleeding has a number of causes and may be minor or life threatening. Hematochezia may occur with or without abdominal pain. Causes may be relatively

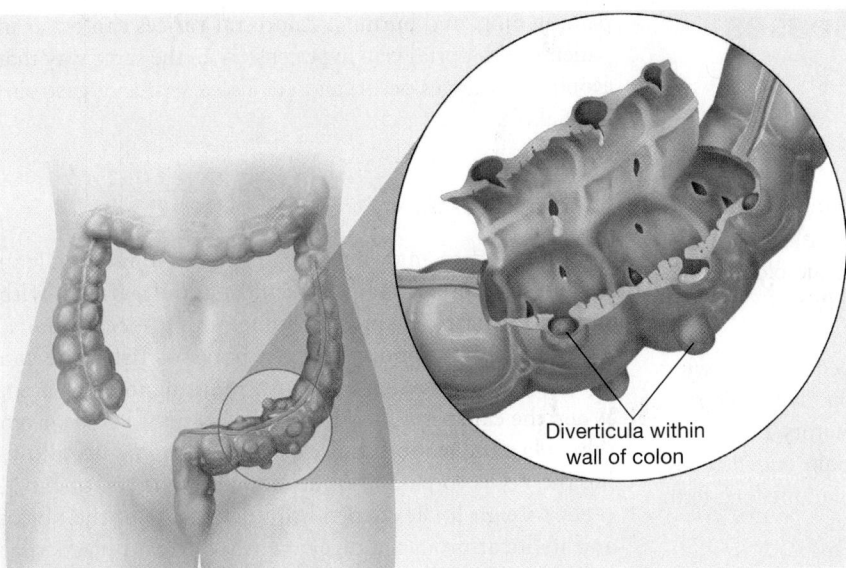

FIGURE 24-11

Diverticula in the colon.

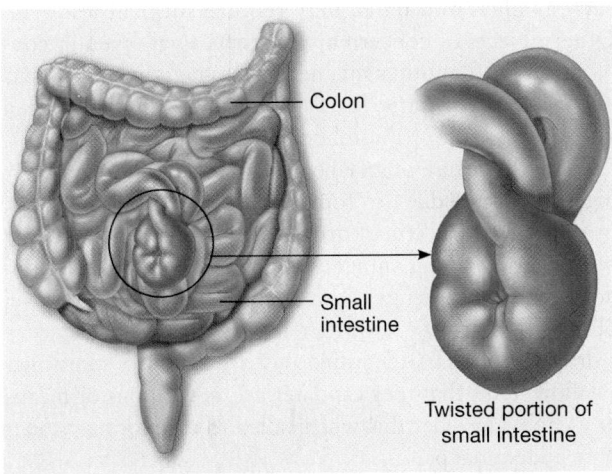

FIGURE 24-12

Volvulus of the small intestine.

benign, such as hemorrhoids or intestinal polyps, or more serious, such as cancers of the colon and rectum and ruptured diverticula. Manage the patient's airway, ventilation, and oxygenation, and administer IV fluids according to protocol.

Bowel Obstruction and Infarction

In adults, bowel obstruction is likely due to fecal impaction, tumor, or bands of adhesions in the abdomen from prior surgery. It also can occur due to **volvulus**, a twisting of the intestine at the cecum or at the sigmoid colon. Paralysis of peristaltic movement, such as may occur after surgery or with a serious intra-abdominal infection, can present like a bowel obstruction (Figure 24-12). Bowel obstruction is more common in the elderly and often begins with an intermittent, colicky, but steadily increasing pain. The pain becomes constant, but may be poorly localized.

Respirations become shallow because movement of the diaphragm further irritates the inflamed peritoneum. As the pressure within the bowel increases, the wall of the intestine can become ischemic, and then necrotic and may rupture, which carries a very high mortality rate. A bowel infarction occurs when a mesenteric artery is obstructed, as may occur in patients with atrial fibrillation. Patients with atrial fibrillation can develop emboli in the improperly contracting left atrium, which can then travel to various parts of the body. The affected portion of bowel becomes ischemic and cannot function. Bacteria that are normally present in the intestine can move through the wall of the intestine, causing sepsis, and the necrotic bowel can rupture.

A hernia is an abnormal opening through which tissue protrudes. In the case of an inguinal hernia or other abdominal wall hernia, a loop of bowel can sometimes become entrapped (incarcerated) and become ischemic. A large hernia may be noted on examination of the stomach, but in other cases, the bowel only protrudes when intra-abdominal pressure increases, such as during coughing.

A patient with a possible bowel obstruction or infarction is a critical patient who requires rapid intervention in the hospital. Administer oxygen if respirations are shallow or the SpO_2 indicates hypoxia, make the patient as comfortable as possible, and start an IV. Administer fluids according to protocol if the patient is hypotensive.

Pediatric Care

Intussusception, *a telescoping of the bowel over itself, is a cause of bowel obstruction in newborns and infants. Bowel obstruction also may occur in those age groups from midgut volvulus or congenital pyloric stenosis, a narrowing of the outlet of the stomach into the duodenum.*

Inflammatory Bowel Diseases

Inflammatory bowel disease (IBD) is a group of disorders that includes ulcerative colitis and Crohn's disease (Figure 24-13). Ulcerative colitis is limited to the colon, but Crohn's disease can affect any part of the gastrointestinal tract. IBD patients have periods of exacerbations and remissions. During exacerbations, or flare-ups, inflammation of the intestinal lining causes abdominal pain and bloody diarrhea. The patient may also have a fever and anorexia. There are several complications of IBD, including rupture of the ulcerations leading to gastrointestinal bleeding, narrowing of the bowel lumen, and bowel obstruction. Irritable bowel syndrome (IBS) is not a form of inflammatory bowel disease. Patients with IBS have abdominal pain but there are no findings on tests of the bowel and none of the long-term problems associated with IBD.

Constipation

Constipation is a condition in which there are infrequent bowel movements with small, hard feces due to excessive water absorption from the colon. It is best to prevent constipation through diet, adequate water intake, and physical activity. Treatments include stool softeners and laxatives.

Hemorrhoids

Hemorrhoids occur when there is congestion of the hemorrhoidal cushions of the anal canal. Bleeding can accompany hemorrhoids and the patient may complain of perianal

pain, itching, and burning. Anorectal varices can occur in patients with portal vein hypertension, in the same way that esophageal varices occur, and are also a source of gastrointestinal bleeding.

Swallowed Foreign Bodies

Foreign bodies may be swallowed accidently or can be ingested intentionally by children and patients with some psychiatric disorders. Sometimes a foreign body, a large bolus of food, a chicken bone, or fish bone can become lodged in the esophagus, resulting in chest pain. When the cause is a food bolus, medications can be given that relax the smooth muscles of the esophagus, allowing the bolus to pass into the stomach. The treatment of other foreign bodies depends on the nature of the object and its location in the digestive tract. Most objects that have passed through the stomach will continue through the digestive tract without a problem. Sharp objects, such as glass and nails, may require surgical removal. Other objects of concern are magnets swallowed in conjunction with another magnet or magnetic metal objects and button-type batteries. Psychiatric patients have been known to swallow a number of bizarre items.

Another cause of an emergency related to foreign body ingestion occurs due to "body packing" by drug smugglers, or swallowed packets of drugs by individuals being taken into custody. Drug smugglers may swallow several condoms filled with drugs. The condoms may result in bowel obstruction, or may rupture, releasing massive amounts of a drug into the gastrointestinal system. Prisoners sometimes swallow items that they can later use as weapons or means of escape. Consider this when called to care for a prisoner with abdominal pain.

Occasionally, patients may seek help for a foreign body in the rectum. The two most common scenarios are objects inserted during erotic activity and objects inserted to avoid detection by law enforcement. Treat the patient with dignity and, as with all patients, keep personal information confidential. Unless bleeding is present, examination usually is not performed in the prehospital setting. Transport the patient for evaluation by a physician.

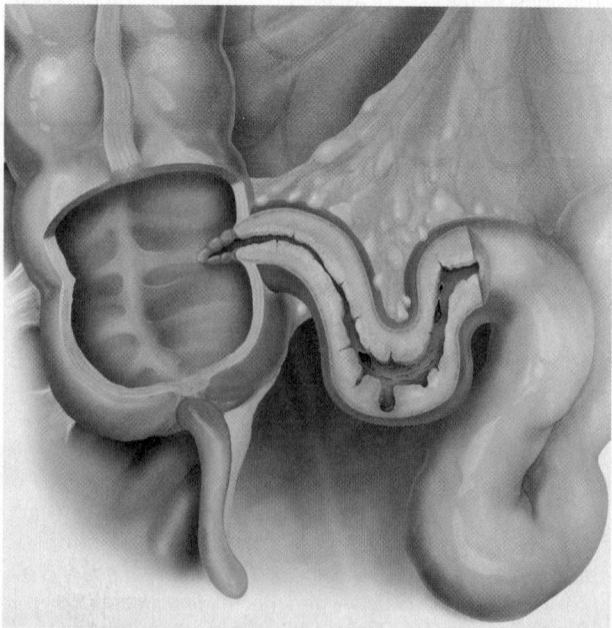

FIGURE 24-13

Crohn's disease.

Pediatric Care

A common household item that is occasionally swallowed by children is a small battery. The environment of the gastrointestinal tract can erode the casing of the battery, allowing the alkaline substance within the battery to come in contact the gastrointestinal tract. This can result in ulceration and even perforation of the affected area. Although physicians may take a "wait and see" approach to many of the foreign bodies swallowed by children, a battery is not one of them.

Pancreatitis

Pancreatitis is an inflammation of the pancreas that results in intense midabdominal pain and a very sick patient (Figure 24-14). The mortality of acute pancreatitis is high because of the risk of sepsis and shock. The most common cause of pancreatitis is alcohol abuse, although there are other causes, such as obstruction of the duct by a gallstone. During acute pancreatitis the digestive enzymes excreted by the exocrine portion of the pancreas come into contact with pancreatic cells, resulting in autodigestion of the pancreatic tissue. There is intense inflammation resulting in pain and edema. In turn, the edema can interfere with tissue perfusion, resulting in ischemia and more edema.

The erosion of the pancreas can include blood vessels resulting in internal hemorrhage. Grey-Turner's sign (ecchymosis of the flanks) and Cullen's sign (periumbilical ecchymosis) are indications of severe pancreatitis. Patients with pancreatitis have intense pain in the epigastric region, which they often describe as boring through to the back. Vomiting may be severe and if there is internal hemorrhage, the patient may be hypotensive.

Liver Disease

Hepatitis has both infectious and noninfectious causes. Most infectious causes are viral. (See Chapter 28.) Noninfectious causes include medications and toxins, such as acetaminophen overdose. Some types of hepatitis are asymptomatic, and some can become chronic, eventually resulting in liver failure. Patients with acute hepatitis can present with pain in the upper right quadrant of the abdomen, nausea, malaise, and fever. Jaundice occurs when the inflamed liver cannot rid the body of bilirubin, which is then deposited in the tissues. Chronic hepatits can lead to liver cancer, cirrhosis, and portal hypertension.

Cirrhosis is a progressive disease caused by chronic inflammation of the liver. As the disease progresses, normal liver tissue is replaced by scar tissue. Common causes of cirrhosis are chronic alcohol abuse, fatty liver, and chronic hepatitis. As normal tissue is lost, the liver cannot metabolize drugs, vitamins, and other substances, rid the body of the pigments from red blood cell breakdown, serve as an effective glycogen store, or produce the albumin, clotting factors, and other substances it normally produces. As a result, levels of

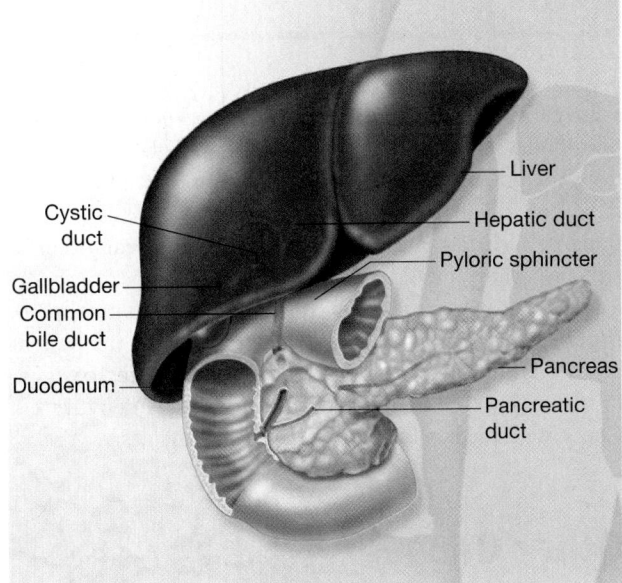

FIGURE 24-14

Accessory organs of digestion. Note the relationship between the liver, gallbladder, and pancreas provided through the cystic and hepatic ducts, common bile duct, and pancreatic duct.

IN THE FIELD

One sign of hepatic encephalopathy is asterixis, a condition in which the patient's hands involuntary "flap" when he holds his hands up with the wrists flexed, such as signaling someone to stop.

PERSONAL PERSPECTIVE

Mr. Charles Flannery: I was at a baseball game last spring, enjoying a picnic and day out with my family when, during the seventh inning of a double-header, I started getting some pain in my upper right stomach and right shoulder. It kept getting worse and I was so nauseated. I wasn't sure what to do, because I didn't feel well enough to walk the half-mile or so to where we had parked. My son-in-law helped me down to the restroom, where I vomited and started feeling even worse. My son-in-law asked a security guard for help. It turns out there was an EMS crew assigned to the stadium.

They got to me in just a few minutes. After they found out what was going on, they alerted the ambulance to come to the closest exit. They started an IV and made me as comfortable as possible, and reassured me that they would get me to the emergency department in just a few minutes. It turns out the problem was my gallbladder. I had surgery that evening and stayed in the hospital for another day. If it hadn't been for the Advanced EMTs, Bob and Shelly, I don't know how I would have gotten out of there and gotten to the hospital. I'm really glad they were there.

As Elle and Becky continue their examination of Mrs. Stoker, they find additional information. Her breath sounds are clear and equal in upper fields, with crackles in the bases bilaterally. The abdomen is distended with diffuse tenderness to palpation and involuntary guarding. There are no scars from a previous surgery. Mrs. Stoker is able to move all of her extremities with intact sensation and peripheral pulses. She has mild edema in both lower extremities. As the Advanced EMTs complete their examination, Mrs. Stoker asks them what they think is wrong with her.

Problem-Solving Questions

1. How might the additional information affect Elle and Becky's hypotheses?
2. Given the patient's age, risk factors, history, and examination findings, what might be Elle and Becky's differential diagnoses?
3. How serious is Mrs. Stoker's condition?
4. How should Elle and Becky respond to Mrs. Stoker's inquiry about what they think the problem is?

ammonia, bilirubin, and other toxins increase, the patient's blood loses oncotic pressure, and blood clotting is impaired.

The resistance to blood flow through the diseased liver results in portal vein hypertension, which can lead to esophageal and anorectal varices. The increased hydrostatic pressure in the portal system, coupled with low albumin result in an accumulation of fluid in the abdomen called *ascites*. Ascites can result in significant abdominal distention and interfere with diaphragmatic movement. When ammonia levels become high from progressive liver failure, hepatic encephalopathy can occur.

Some patients with liver failure are candidates for liver transplantation. Patients who have received a donor liver must take drugs to prevent rejection of the donor tissue. The drugs suppress immune function, making transplant patients prone to infection.

Cholecystitis

Inflammation of the gallbladder commonly occurs from the presence of gallstones. A high proportion of people, though, have asymptomatic gallstones. If a gallstone travels through the common bile duct, it can become lodged, resulting in obstruction. As bile backs up into the gallbladder, it becomes inflamed and distended, resulting in pain. The pain is usually located in the upper right quadrant of the abdomen, and associated irritation of the diaphragm can cause referred pain in the right shoulder. There is often a positive Murphy's sign (tenderness under the right costal margin). Patients with acute cholecystitis are often nauseated and may vomit. In severe cases, the distended gallbladder becomes ischemic and peritonitis can occur.

Factors that may increase your suspicion of acute cholecystitis include a previous history of similar episodes (diagnosed or undiagnosed), onset of pain several hours following a fatty meal (bile is released to emulsify fats in the duodenum), and certain demographic factors. High-risk populations include overweight, Caucasian women with a history of at least one pregnancy ("fat, fair, female, fertile"), Pima Indians, and Hispanics. However, cholecystitis can occur in patients young and old of both genders and any ethnicity.

Manage the patient for vomiting and abdominal pain. If peritonitis results in shallow respirations or the patient has signs and symptoms of shock, administer oxygen. IV fluids may be beneficial if the patient is dehydrated. Check with medical direction concerning analgesia.

Other Causes of Abdominal Pain

While not gastrointestinal in nature, several other causes of abdominal pain must be considered in patients who present with that complaint. Pneumonia can cause referred pain to the upper quadrant of the abdomen on the affected side. Fever, cough, and history of recent respiratory infection should increase your suspicion of pneumonia, and you should listen to the patient's breath sounds.

The pain of myocardial infarction can be experienced in the epigastric region. The patient may experience a sensation of indigestion and have nausea and vomiting. Diabetic ketoacidosis may cause abdominal pain, as can drug withdrawal and sickle cell disease with microinfarction of abdominal organs. In females of reproductive age, consider ovarian cyst, ruptured ovarian cyst, and ectopic pregnancy as potential causes of abdominal pain. (See Chapter 25.)

The spleen, located in the upper left quadrant of the abdomen, has hematologic, immune, and lymphatic functions. It is highly vascular and may rupture if enlarged, resulting in shock from internal hemorrhage. Splenic enlargement can occur in patients with portal hypertension, mononucleosis (an infection caused by the Epstein-Barr virus). Splenic sequestration crisis may occur as a complication of sickle cell disease. (See Chapter 26.) Suspect a splenic problem with left upper quadrant pain, which may radiate to the left shoulder, especially in patients with a recent sore throat and fever or those with a history of liver disease.

Kidney infection and kidney stones may present with flank pain. The pain may radiate to the groin, and the patient may have blood in the urine. Urinary tract infection may include pain over the lower abdomen, as well as pain in the back or flanks.

An abdominal aortic aneurysm results from a weakened area of the aorta that dilates and is prone to rupture. An aortic dissection occurs when a tear in the intimal lining of the aorta allows blood to enter and separate the layers of

the aorta. (See Chapter 21.) The patient may present with intense, tearing pain in the lower back or abdomen and the pain may radiate down one or both legs. The patient may have vascular or neurologic deficits in one or both lower extremities. The patient may have experienced syncope and may be hypotensive and in shock. The patient may have a sense of impending doom (knows something bad is happening, has a feeling he is going to die). In some cases, a pulsating mass can be palpated in the midline of the lower abdomen. In thin individuals the aorta can be palpable in the absence of disease, and a pulsatile mass is not always found on abdominal exam in patients with an abdominal aortic aneurysm. As always, all findings must be placed in context for proper interpretation. An aortic aneurysm or dissection producing signs and symptoms is a critical emergency for which the patient needs immediate in-hospital care.

CASE STUDY WRAP-UP

Clinical-Reasoning Process

Regardless of the underlying cause, Becky and Elle realize that abdominal pain lasting 4 hours is an emergency and that they must make Mrs. Stoker as comfortable as possible, provide oxygen, and treat dehydration. In response to Mrs. Stoker's inquiry about what the problem might be, Becky says, "It is difficult to say without the kinds of tests that can be performed in the hospital. It could be a couple of different things. The doctor will examine you in the emergency department and decide what tests to run. He may order blood tests and X-rays to see what the problem is. If you have any questions about the tests or about what he is thinking, make sure you ask, okay?"

Becky reasons that the underlying cause of abdominal pain in this patient is less likely to be from pneumonia, pancreatitis, gallbladder disease, or liver or renal systems problems. The nature and location of the pain are inconsistent with those problems, and Mrs. Stoker does not have jaundice and has no other symptoms of urinary tract or renal problems. The nature of the pain and other findings also are not consistent with AMI or abdominal aortic aneurysm. Gastrointestinal bleeding, either upper or lower, are not as high on Becky's list of differentials because there is not a history of hematemesis, melena, or hematochezia. The patient's age also makes gynecologic problems less likely.

The differentials highest on Becky's list are bowel obstruction, bowel infarction, diverticulitis, and appendicitis. Appendicitis is less likely in a patient this age, although the pain initially was experienced in the right lower quadrant. Diverticulitis pain is most often on the left side of the abdomen, but cannot be ruled out. Becky thinks there is a high probability of bowel obstruction or, because of the patient's history of atrial fibrillation, bowel infarction. All of the most highly suspected problems are surgical emergencies. Untreated, the patient could experience necrosis and rupture of the affected part of the bowel, leading to severe peritonitis and sepsis.

Elle applies oxygen by nasal cannula at 4 L/min and the Advanced EMTs gently use the draw sheet method to transfer Mrs. Stoker to the stretcher, where they allow her to continue to lie on her side with her hips flexed.

En route to the hospital, Becky starts an IV and administers fluid at 150 mL/hour. The patient is dehydrated, but not hypotensive. Becky suspects the crackles in the lungs may be due to shallow respirations or residual pneumonia, but she cannot be certain that the patient does not have pulmonary edema. At this patient's age, fluid overload could easily occur.

Although Becky would like to administer analgesia to make Mrs. Stoker more comfortable, the substantial possibility of bowel obstruction is a contraindication to nitrous oxide. While Elle takes the smoothest route possible to the hospital, Becky notifies the emergency department that they will be arriving with the patient in 15 to 20 minutes.

Becky and Elle deliver Mrs. Stoker to the emergency department, where Dr. Fields promptly evaluates her and orders an abdominal X-ray and requests a surgical consult. The X-ray suggests cecal volvulus, a twisting of the colon at the cecum. This is confirmed with a barium enema. Although evacuation of the contrast medium can sometimes reduce cecal volvulus, this is not the case with Mrs. Stoker. She undergoes surgery to remove the ischemic portion of the bowel. A temporary colostomy is formed and Mrs. Stoker's postoperative course is uneventful, though healing was prolonged due to her age. Fortunately, her condition was detected and treated prior to the onset of gangrene and perforation of the bowel, which have high mortality.

CHAPTER REVIEW

Chapter Summary

As an Advanced EMT, you will encounter patients with complaints of abdominal pain and other complaints that are associated with gastrointestinal problems. Knowing the anatomy, physiology, and pathophysiology related to the gastrointestinal system and abdomen helps you effectively take the history and perform assessment of the patients, and recognize the significance of their disorders.

Patients may experience abdominal pain that arises from a variety of causes. The life-threatening nature of many of the problems, especially if there is a delay in treatment, requires transportation of patients with abdominal pain for evaluation by a physician.

During transport, make the patient as comfortable as possible, administer oxygen if respirations are shallow or the patient has signs of shock, and consider the need for fluid replacement. Providing analgesia to patients with abdominal pain prior to diagnosis does not interfere with the physician's assessment as it was once thought. Consult with medical direction about the use of analgesia in patients with abdominal pain.

Review Questions

Multiple-Choice Questions

1. The absorption of nutrients from the gastrointestinal tract begins in the:

   a. oral cavity.
   b. esophagus.
   c. stomach.
   d. duodenum.

2. The role of bile is to break down:

   a. proteins.
   b. fats.
   c. carbohydrates.
   d. alcohol.

3. The cecum is located in the _____ quadrant of the abdomen.

   a. right upper
   b. right lower
   c. left upper
   d. left lower

4. The last portion of the colon, just before it becomes the rectum is the _____ colon.

   a. transverse
   b. descending
   c. ascending
   d. sigmoid

5. Which one of the following would be most likely to be associated with a crampy, colicky abdominal pain?

   a. Distention of the bowel
   b. Inflammation of the liver
   c. Pancreatitis
   d. Peritonitis

6. Which one of the following factors in a patient's past medical history would most increase your suspicion of esophageal varices?

   a. He has taken 800 mg ibuprofen three times a day for one month.
   b. He has a history of hepatitis C.
   c. He has a colostomy.
   d. He has a history of renal failure.

7. Your patient gives a history of hiatal hernia. Which one of the following signs or symptoms would most likely be associated with this history?

   a. Bright red bleeding from the rectum
   b. Diarrhea with blood and excessive mucus
   c. An abnormal lump in the lower abdomen during coughing that disappears afterward
   d. Difficulty breathing, especially when lying down

8. Your patient is taking 650 mg of aspirin every 4 to 6 hours for arthritis pain. He complains of burning epigastric pain. Other than arthritis, he has no medical problems. Which one of the following should be highest on your list of hypotheses about the patient's problem?

   a. Gastritis
   b. Diverticulitis
   c. Cholecystitis
   d. Pancreatitis

9. Bile is manufactured by the:

   a. gallbladder.
   b. pancreas.
   c. liver.
   d. small intestine.

10. A patient with a history of peptic ulcers states he has black, tarry stools. You should document this finding as:

 a. melena.
 b. melasma.
 c. hematochezia.
 d. hematemesis.

11. A two-year-old child has swallowed a foreign body. You should be most immediately concerned if the object is a:

 a. marble.
 b. watch battery.
 c. plastic guitar pick.
 d. plastic wheel from a toy car.

Critical-Thinking Questions

12. Create a table to compare and contrast the features of appendicitis and diverticulitis. Use the example shown below.

Feature	Appendicitis	Diverticulitis
Typical age of patients affected		
Character of pain at onset		
Localization of pain		
Associated signs and symptoms		

13. A 17-year-old male patient has had a fever, swollen lymph nodes, and severe sore throat for a week. Today he complains of left upper quadrant abdominal pain and tenderness. Outline the reasoning you would use to develop a clinical impression of the underlying problem.

14. A 74-year-old male patient has a history of type 2 diabetes. He complains of diffuse abdominal pain for several hours, which he rates a 3 on a scale of 10 in severity. How should you interpret the patient's level of pain in relationship to the possible severity of the problem?

Additional Reading

Martini, F. H, Bartholomew, E. F, & Bledsoe, B. E. (2008). *Anatomy and physiology for emergency care* (2nd ed.). Upper Saddle River, NJ: Pearson.

Perry, K. R., & Rosh, A. J. (2009). *Hemorrhoids*. eMedicine. Retrieved January 4, 2011, from http://emedicine.medscape.com/article/775407-overview

25 Renal, Genitourinary, and Gynecologic Disorders

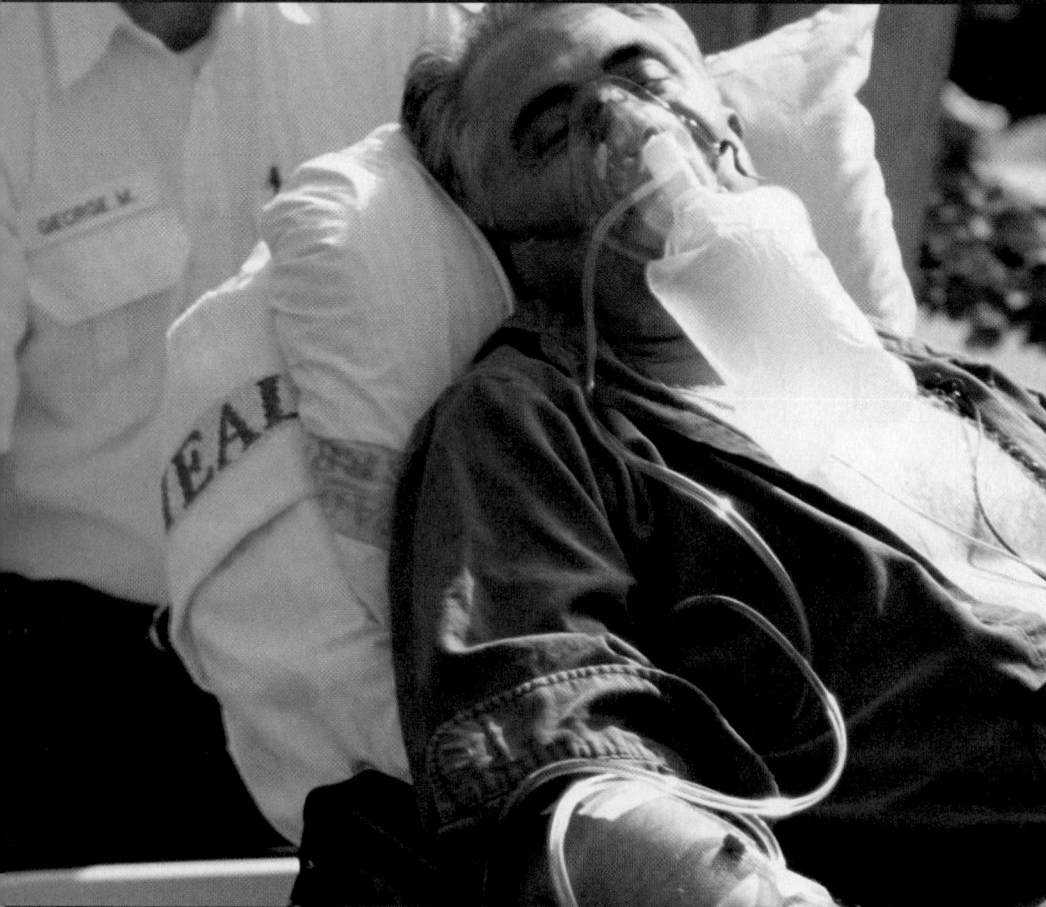

Content Areas: Medicine; Trauma

Advanced EMT Education Standards:
- Applies fundamental knowledge to provide basic and selected advanced emergency care and transportation based on assessment findings for an acutely ill patient.
- Applies fundamental knowledge to provide basic and selected advanced emergency care and transportation based on assessment findings for an acutely injured patient.

Objectives

After reading this chapter, you should be able to:

25.1   Define key terms introduced in this chapter.

25.2   Describe the pathophysiology of acute and chronic renal failure.

25.3   Discuss the complications of end-stage renal disease.

25.4   Explain the assessment and management of patients with emergencies related to renal failure and dialysis.

25.5   Explain the processes of hemodialysis and peritoneal dialysis.

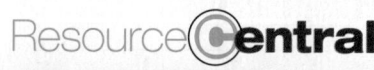

To access Resource Central, follow the directions on the Student Access Card provided with this text. If there is no card, go to www.bradybooks.com and follow the Resource Central link to Buy Access. Under Media Resources, you will find:

- *What Is Dialysis?* Renal failure and the role of dialysis in treating patients with kidney disease.

- *What Is Nephrolithiasis?* Kidney stones, signs and symptoms, and treatment.

- *Sexually Transmitted Diseases (STDs).* Common signs and symptoms and the consequences of untreated STDs.

CASE STUDY

Advanced EMTs John Alcott and Missy Maguire are dispatched for an unresponsive patient at the Methodist Dialysis Center. When they arrive, they are met in the lobby by a dialysis technician named Margo. Margo informs John and Missy that Mr. Thornton, a long-time Monday–Wednesday–Friday dialysis patient, became unresponsive just after being hooked up to the dialysis machine.

Problem-Solving Questions

1. What are the first actions John and Missy should take?
2. What are some initial hypotheses about the cause of unresponsiveness in this patient?
3. What information will help John and Missy determine the cause of the patient's problem?

25.6	Discuss the pathophysiology, assessment, and management of patients with urinary retention.
25.7	Discuss the pathophysiology, assessment, and management of patients with urinary system infections.
25.8	Identify complications associated with catheterization of the urinary bladder.
25.9	Discuss the pathophysiology, assessment, and management of patients with renal calculi.
25.10	Discuss the pathophysiology, assessment, and management of patients with trauma to the male genitourinary system.
25.11	Discuss the pathophysiology, assessment, and management of patients with epididymitis, orchitis, and Fournier gangrene.
25.12	Describe the basic anatomy and physiology of the female reproductive system.
25.13	Obtain a relevant history from patients with a suspected gynecologic problem.
25.14	Describe signs and symptoms associated with common gynecologic and female genitourinary system causes of acute abdominal pain, including:

- Dysmenorrhea
- Endometriosis
- Endometritis
- Ovarian cyst
- Pelvic inflammatory disease
- Sexually transmitted infections
- Urinary tract infection

25.15	Describe special considerations in the assessment and management of patients with:

- Sexual assault
- Vaginal bleeding

25.16	Effectively communicate assessment findings for patients with gynecologic and genitourinary/renal complaints to other health care providers, orally and in writing.

Introduction

Renal disorders are among the most significant negative outcomes of the millions of cases of untreated or poorly treated diabetes and hypertension. The effect on a patient's life resulting from shutdown of the kidneys can be enormous, but is often treatable.

As an Advanced EMT, you may be called on to transport patients with renal emergencies, including emergencies related to dialysis. You also may provide interfacility transportation for patients undergoing hemodialysis (HD). Disorders of the remainder of the urinary system and of the male and female reproductive systems also can lead patients to seek emergency treatment.

In addition to renal failure, this chapter explores kidney stones, urinary tract infections, and medical and traumatic disorders of the male and female reproductive systems.

Anatomy and Physiology Review

The anatomy and physiology of the urinary and reproductive systems overlap to a substantial degree in men, and less so in women. However, the proximity of organs of the urinary tract and reproductive system can sometimes result in similar signs and symptoms of problems arising from those systems.

The Urinary System

Medical care generally divides the urinary system into the upper urinary tract, represented by the kidney, and the lower urinary tract, which is composed of the ureters, bladder, and urethra (Figure 25-1). The renal system refers to the part of the urinary system composed of the kidneys.

Diseases of the kidney are treated by a nephrologist, and generally involve medical, rather than surgical, management. The lower tract, on the other hand, is managed by a urologist. Urologic problems often require surgical management.

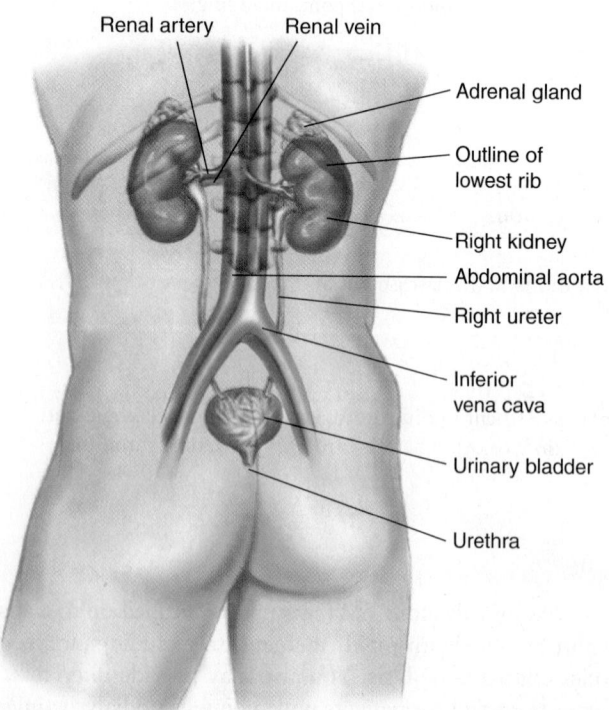

Renal artery   Renal vein

Adrenal gland

Outline of lowest rib

Right kidney

Abdominal aorta

Right ureter

Inferior vena cava

Urinary bladder

Urethra

FIGURE 25-1

The urinary system.

Kidneys

The kidneys lie in the retroperitoneum at their respective costovertebral angles (CVA), which is the point at which the twelfth pair of ribs articulates with T12. Because the kidneys are responsible for filtering the blood and eliminating wastes from it, they receive a large portion of the blood supply from the renal arteries, which branch directly from the aorta.

The arterial blood circulates by way of capillaries through microscopic individual units of the kidney called *nephrons* (Figure 25-2). Each kidney contains about 1 million nephrons. The capillaries take a complex route through the nephron to allow for substances to be filtered from the blood. In the early part of this route, a large amount of water and solutes leave the blood, forming filtrate, and many substances and most of the water are returned to the blood in the later part of the route.

The blood that has circulated through the nephrons returns to the circulation by way of the renal veins, which empty into the inferior vena cava. Meanwhile, the small amount of fluid retained by the nephron, now called *urine*, flows through the collecting tubules of the kidneys and flows through the ureters to the urinary bladder.

The kidney is grossly arranged in two layers, each containing specific microscopic structures (Figure 25-3). The outer layer, the renal cortex, contains the glomerulus and renal tubules. The renal tubules travel toward the inner layer of the kidney, the renal medulla, where they eventually deposit urine in the collecting ducts, which connect to the calyces of the kidney.

This entire entity—from the glomerulus to the collecting duct—is called the *nephron*, the basic functional unit of the kidney. The tissues that occupy the spaces around the tubules and blood vessels are called the *interstitium*. The rate at which filtrate is formed in the kidneys is the *glomerular filtration rate (GFR)*, which is normally about 120 mL/ minute or 7 L/hour. Because most of the filtrate is reabsorbed as it moves through the nephron, the rate of urine production is typically 30 to 40 mL/hour. In kidney failure, the GFR generally is less than 30 mL/minute.

The glomerulus serves three major roles, as follows:

- It filters out the waste products and excess fluid in the blood.

- It begins the process of removing excess electrolytes, such as sodium, potassium, and calcium, to maintain steady levels of the electrolytes in the blood.

- It monitors the pressure in the blood vessels and readjusts the body's blood pressure.

The process of fluid and electrolyte homeostasis continues in the tubules, the interstitium, and the collecting ducts.

After the urine leaves the kidney, it moves into the lower urinary system. Urine leaves the calyces of the kidney and enters the ureters, which course from the retroperitoneal area at the level just inferior to the stomach, down

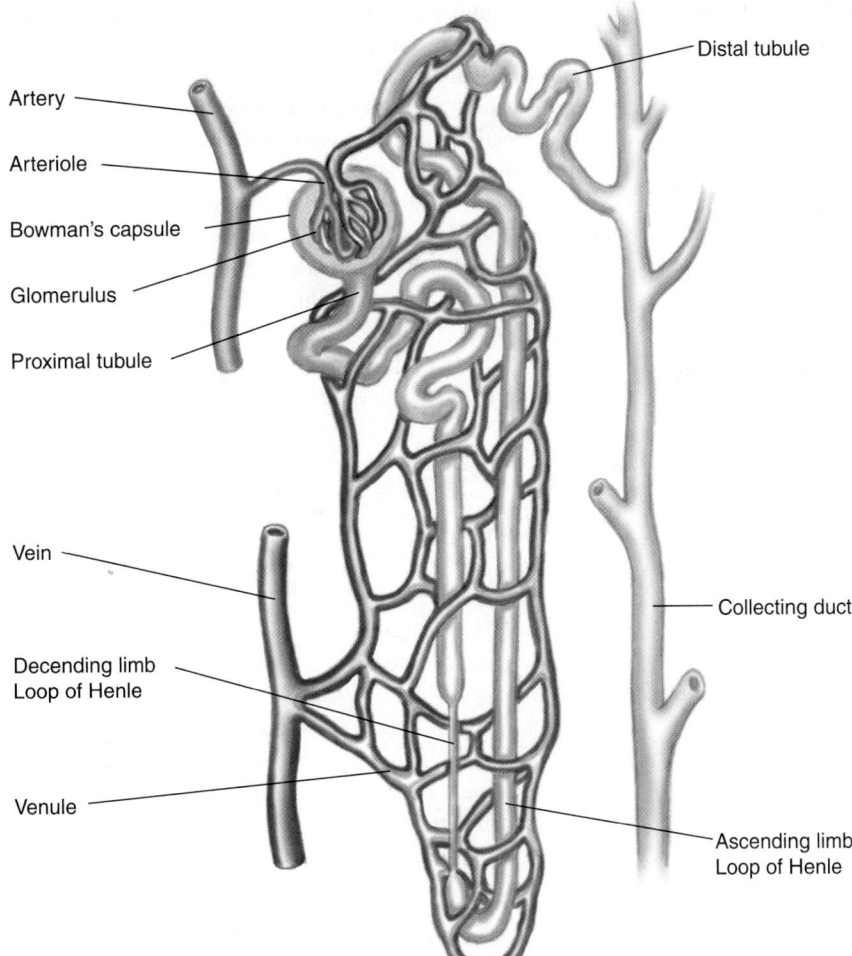

- Distal tubule
- Artery
- Arteriole
- Bowman's capsule
- Glomerulus
- Proximal tubule
- Vein
- Decending limb Loop of Henle
- Venule
- Collecting duct
- Ascending limb Loop of Henle

FIGURE 25-2

Anatomy of the nephron.

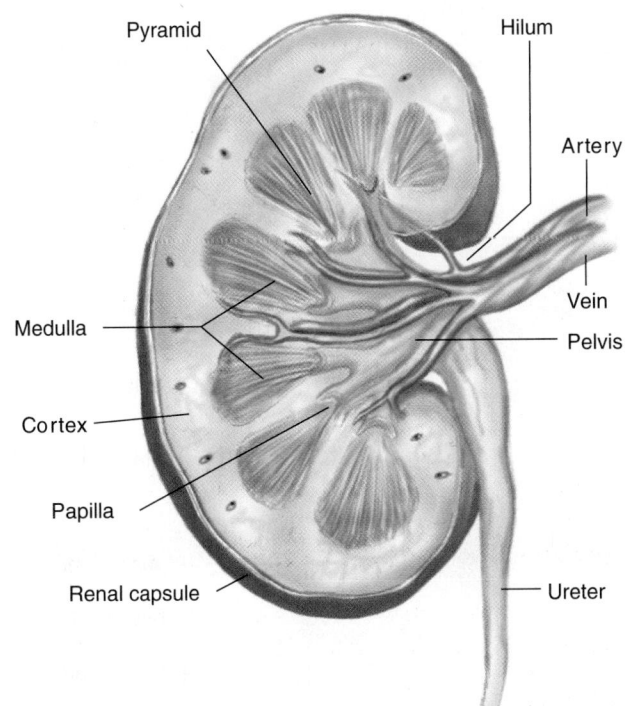

- Pyramid
- Hilum
- Artery
- Vein
- Pelvis
- Medulla
- Cortex
- Papilla
- Renal capsule
- Ureter

FIGURE 25-3

Anatomy of the kidney.

IN THE FIELD

Advanced EMTs may transport or monitor critically ill and injured patients whose fluid intake and output (I&O) must be monitored carefully to assess kidney function. This is accomplished by carefully keeping track of the amount of IV fluids administered and the amount of urine produced.

A lubricated Foley catheter is inserted through the urethral meatus and advanced into the bladder. Once in the bladder, a balloon around the catheter is inflated with water to anchor it in place. The other end of the catheter empties into a collection bag marked with a measuring scale. Patients who are immobile may have a Foley catheter in a home or extended care setting.

the posterior portion of the abdomen, and into the urinary bladder, which is situated anteriorly in the pelvis.

The bladder is a reservoir that can hold a liter or more of urine. Eventually, the feeling of a full bladder leads to the urge to urinate and the urine is released through the urethra. In females, the urethra is a very short tube that follows the anterior wall of the vagina. In males, the urethra is fairly long, coursing through to the end of the penis. This difference in urethral length is the reason that women tend to get more urinary tract infections (UTIs) than men.

Male Reproductive System

The organs of the reproductive system are called *genitals*, or *genitalia*, and are classified as either external or internal genitalia (Figure 25-4). The organs work together, under the influence of the endocrine system, to achieve reproductive functions.

In the male, the urethra is shared by the urinary and reproductive systems, serving as the outlet for both urine and semen. Therefore, problems with the male reproductive system are often handled by a urologist.

The prostate gland is located on the inferior aspect of the male bladder, surrounding the urethra as it leaves the bladder. The portion of the urethra that passes through the prostate is called the *prostatic urethra*. The testicles (or testes), which lie within the scrotum, are connected to the prostate by two structures. The epididymis is located on the posterior portion of the testicle, where it serves as a site for sperm maturation and storage. The vas deferens is a tube that carries testicular secretions from the epididymis to the prostate, where they are deposited in the prostatic urethra.

The external male genitalia consist of the penis and the testicles, which lie within the scrotum. Sperm are produced in the testicle and are transferred to the epididymis for maturation and storage until ejaculation. Just prior to ejaculation, sperm enter the vas deferens, which enter the pelvic cavity through the inguinal canals, and enter the prostate. The combination of prostatic secretions and sperm constitute semen.

Semen continues along the urethra, where it leaves through the urethral meatus. The penis consists of three columns of highly vascular tissues that allow for erection. There are two corpora cavernosa (singular, *corpus cavernosum*) and one corpus spongiosum. Erection occurs when the parasympathetic nervous system causes vasodilation of the penile arterial supply, allowing more blood into the three columns than leaves them.

The foreskin is a double fold of skin and mucous membrane that covers the glans penis (head of the penis) in uncircumcised males. Some males are circumcised (have the foreskin surgically removed) shortly after birth for religious reasons or in compliance with social norms. In uncircumcised males, the foreskin is adherent to the penis until just before puberty, at which time it can be retracted.

Female Reproductive System

The female reproductive system is complex and prone to both medical and surgical problems. Specially trained physicians called *gynecologists* handle those problems. Gynecologists also generally specialize in the management of pregnancy and pregnancy-related disorders, called *obstetrics*.

The female external genitalia consist of the mons pubis, labia majora, labia minora, and clitoris (Figure 25-5). The urethral meatus lies between the clitoris and the introitus, the entrance to the vagina. The vagina is a hollow tubular passageway that connects the external genitalia with the internal genitalia. The vaginal opening is anterior to the anus, separated from it by an area of skin called the *perineum*.

The uterus is a small muscular organ lined with endometrium, tissue that thickens each month during the reproductive years in preparation for the possible implantation of

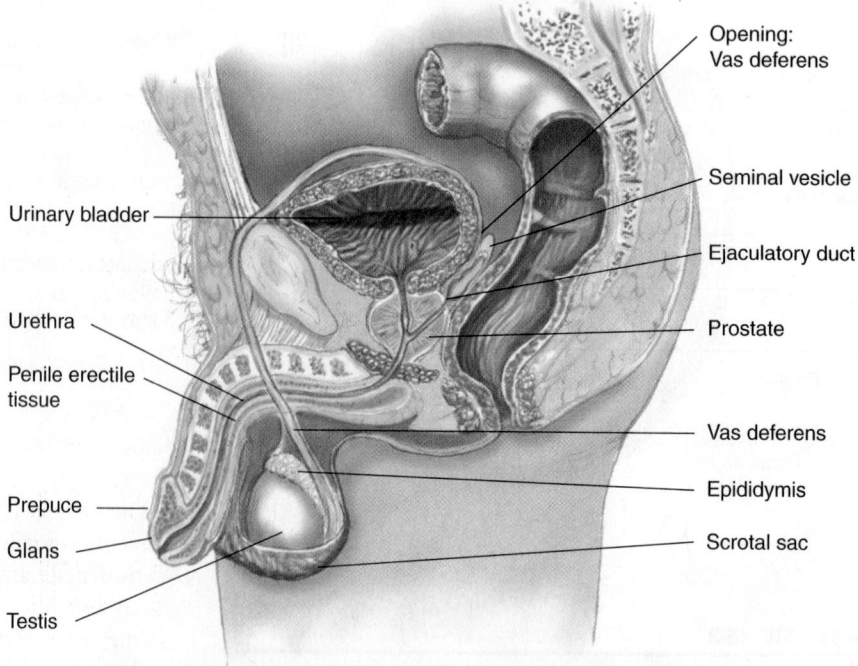

FIGURE 25-4

Anatomy of the male genitourinary system.

Labels: Urinary bladder, Urethra, Penile erectile tissue, Prepuce, Glans, Testis, Opening: Vas deferens, Seminal vesicle, Ejaculatory duct, Prostate, Vas deferens, Epididymis, Scrotal sac

a fertilized ovum (Figure 25-6). The uterus curves around the posterior and superior portions of the female bladder, and lies behind the pubis.

Anatomically, the uterus is divided into three sections, from superior to inferior. The uppermost portion is the fundus and the lowest portion is the cervix, with the body of the uterus lying between. The cervix projects into the upper vagina, where it provides a passageway (os cervix and cervical canal) for sperm to enter the uterus and travel to the fallopian tubes.

Two fallopian tubes, or oviducts, provide a passageway from the interior of the uterus to the area surrounding the left and right ovaries. The outer portion of each fallopian tube drapes around an ovary, providing a passageway for ova to travel toward the uterus. If sperm are present, fertilization normally takes place in the outer third of the fallopian tube. The fertilized ovum continues to travel toward the uterus, where it may be implanted in the endometrium.

The ovaries and endometrium undergo cyclical monthly changes under the influence of the endocrine system, called the *menstrual cycle*. Day 1 of the menstrual cycle is the day that bleeding begins as the endometrium is shed from the uterus in nonpregnant women. The bleeding lasts about five days, but ranges from three to seven days. The total amount of blood lost over this time is about 30 mL.

After the uterine lining is shed, hormonal changes influence it to be rebuilt. Meanwhile, several follicles containing immature ova have already begun developing in the ovaries. In a typical cycle, the development of one of the follicles outpaces that of the others. About 14 days after the first day of menstrual bleeding, the mature follicle ruptures, discharging the ovum into the pelvic cavity near the entrance of the adjacent fallopian tube. This is called *ovulation*. Finger-like projections of the fallopian tube, called *fimbriae*, move in a sweeping motion, which sets up a current that draws the ovum into the tube.

If sperm arrive in the fallopian tube during a short window of time surrounding ovulation, fertilization may occur, resulting in pregnancy. If pregnancy occurs, the rapidly dividing fertilized egg must travel to the uterus, where it will be implanted in the thickened endometrium. Hormones

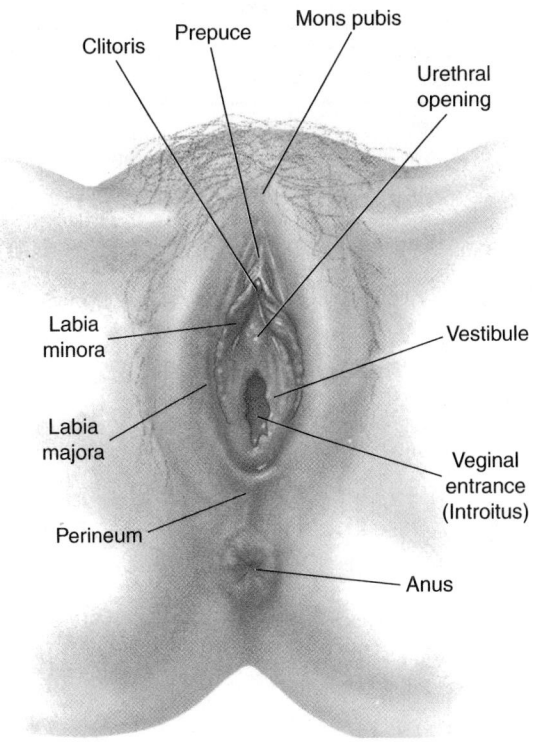

FIGURE 25-5

Female external genitalia.

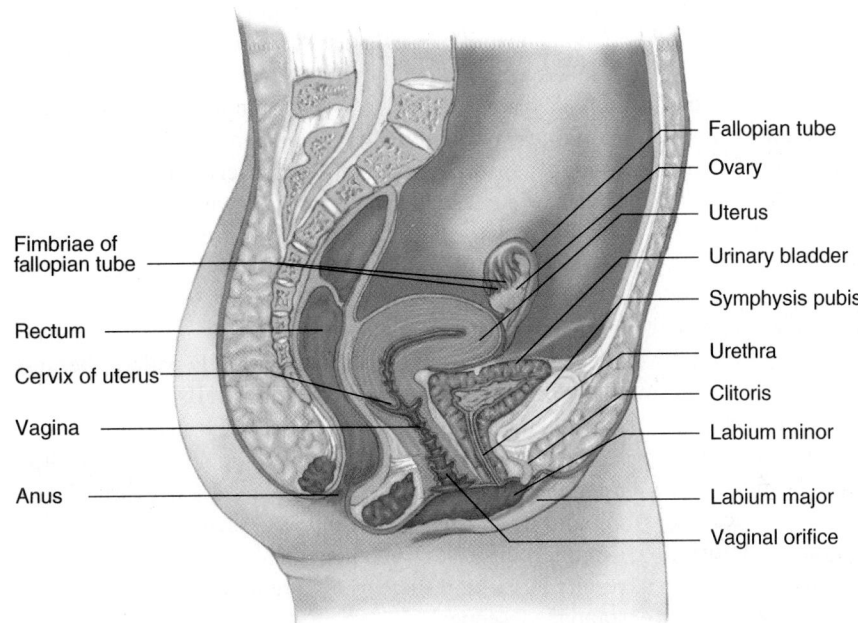

FIGURE 25-6

Female internal genitalia.

released by the developing embryo induce changes that preserve the endometrium and prevent new follicles from beginning to develop.

If fertilization does not occur, hormonal support for the endometrium plummets and the endometrium becomes deprived of blood supply and sloughs, beginning the menstrual cycle over again. On average, the menstrual cycle lasts 28 days, but may vary by a few days. Some women's menstrual periods are very regular, but others are slightly irregular. On the average, menarche, the first menstruation, occurs at about age 12, but may occur as early as age 10, and infrequently, earlier. Menstruation continues until menopause, at an average age of 51.

General Assessment and Management of Urinary System Disorders

Patients with renal disorders present with a variety of complaints and may range in presentation from alert, oriented, and in mild distress to unresponsive with life-threatening hypotension and electrolyte disorders.

Patients with urinary disorders, such as a kidney stone or urinary tract infection, can present with classic signs and symptoms. However, remember that classic signs and symptoms do not occur in all patients, and that there is overlap among the signs and symptoms of different disorders. Therefore, classic presentations give you a starting place for history taking and assessment, but you still must engage in a thoughtful process of clinical reasoning.

A careful assessment, along with knowledge of anatomy, physiology, and pathophysiology, are essential in determining the nature of the problem and implementing treatment.

Scene Size-Up

Often, the general nature of the problem will be known from dispatch. You may be dispatched to a **dialysis** center, or the person who called dispatch may have provided information about the nature of the problem. For example, the patient may have just returned from a hemodialysis (HD) appointment, may have a complication of peritoneal dialysis, or may have a complication related to the HD access site.

No matter what dispatch information you receive, size up the scene for safety, look for clues to the patient's problem, determine the patient's chief complaint, and form an initial impression of the patient.

Clues to a renal disorder include noticing a dialysis access site, peritoneal dialysis equipment, the presence of a **Foley catheter**, or a fishy or ammonia odor indicating renal failure. Complaints and presentations that may indicate a renal problem include decreased urine output, **hematuria**, weakness, dyspnea, flank pain, changes in urination, and altered mental status (Table 25-1).

TABLE 25-1	Signs and Symptoms of Renal Failure
Body System Affected	**Signs/Symptoms**
Fluids and electrolytes	Hypertension, hypotension Peripheral edema Ascites (fluid within the abdomen) Crackles (rales) in the lungs
Cardiovascular/ hematologic	Impaired blood clotting, bruising Anemia
Neuromuscular/ musculoskeletal	Headache Altered mental status/confusion Weakness Muscle cramps and twitching Osteoporosis
Gastrointestinal	Loss of appetite (anorexia) Nausea GI bleeding
Skin	Pruritus, scratches Uremic frost Jaundice Pallor Rash Odor of ammonia
Immune	Immunosuppression, infection
Renal	Decreased urine output

Primary Assessment

Ensure that the patient has an open airway and adequate ventilations. Provide oxygen as indicated by the patient's complaints and presentation. Assess the adequacy of circulation, keeping in mind that hypertension is a leading cause of renal disease, and that hypotension is complication of renal failure and dialysis. Hypotension also may occur as a result of sepsis in patients with an overwhelming UTI, particularly in the elderly and in patients with Foley catheters.

Electrolyte abnormalities—either from dialysis or from missing scheduled dialysis treatment—may result in dysrhythmias and reduced cardiac output, which can lead to cardiac arrest.

Bleeding may be a problem with HD patients because they take anticoagulant medications. HD access sites include both venous and arterial access, which can result in substantial bleeding. Although bleeding must be controlled, use the least amount of pressure necessary to control bleeding and do not use a tourniquet. Vascular access is often extremely difficult to obtain in renal patients. Anything that results in making the current site unusable can have substantial consequences.

Secondary Assessment

Take a complete set of vital signs to establish a baseline. If dehydration or other volume loss is suspected and the patient's condition allows, check orthostatic vital signs. *When determining vital signs in a patient who has an HD access site, avoid taking the blood pressure in that extremity.*

For unresponsive patients, obtain as much history as possible from family, health care providers, or bystanders and perform a rapid secondary assessment. In patients who are alert, the focused history and exam are based on the chief complaint. Because the patient has difficulty with fluid balance, look for signs of dehydration or fluid overload. Listen to breath sounds and heart sounds, check the skin turgor, and look for edema. Check to see if the jugular veins are either distended or flat.

If allowed in your system, cardiac monitoring and an ECG are essential for patients who have renal disease, particularly when they present with weakness, altered mental status, or cardiac complaints. Keep in mind that diabetes is a common cause of renal failure. Check for a history of diabetes and obtain a blood glucose level in diabetic patients and those with altered mental status. Note the patient's skin temperature. Fever may occur with UTI, but its absence does not rule out UTI.

In the history, determine whether or not there have been changes in urination or in the color of the urine. Ask about any difficulty in urinating, inability to urinate, pain with urination, and more frequent urination. Ask about the presence of blood in the urine, dark colored urine, or cloudy or colorless urine.

Past medical history that may be important in recognizing a renal problem includes heart failure, diabetes, hypertension, liver failure, recent infection, prostate enlargement or cancer, lupus, severe **endometriosis**, or cancers of organs in the pelvic cavity. Certain medications, such as diuretics, acetaminophen, and NSAIDs (for example, ibuprofen, naproxen, and some prescription arthritis medications), in conjunction with the rest of the history, may point to a renal disorder. If the patient is on dialysis, it is essential to determine whether or not the patient has kept his scheduled dialysis appointments.

Clinical-Reasoning Process

Patients with renal disorders often have other medical conditions. Do not allow knowledge that the patient has a renal problem keep you from considering other causes of the patient's presentation.

Because of the kidney's role in homeostasis, kidney failure can lead to many complications and can prevent patients from compensating for other illnesses and injuries. If the patient gives a history of kidney transplant or is taking medications to prevent rejection of a transplanted kidney, his immune system is compromised. Keep infection in mind as a differential diagnosis. The presence of a Foley catheter should increase your suspicion of infection.

Your primary focus will be ensuring adequate airway, ventilation, oxygenation, and circulation. However, a thorough scene size-up, assessment, and history can contribute immeasurably to your ability to anticipate further complications and communicate essential information to receiving facility personnel.

Treatment

Specific things to keep in mind regarding treatment include recognizing that anemia is a frequent complication of renal disease and that the kidneys are not able to handle the addition of substantial amounts of fluids.

Patients who are anemic have too little hemoglobin. The hemoglobin that is present may be fully saturated with oxygen, resulting in a high SpO_2. However, the overall decrease in hemoglobin means that inadequate amounts of oxygen are carried and released to the tissues, resulting in hypoxia at the cellular level. Provide supplemental oxygen to increase the arterial PaO_2.

Although it is important to increase perfusion in hypotensive patients, be cautious with the rate of fluid administration. Check the breath sounds for indications of fluid overload frequently. Do not give additional fluids to the renal patient who has crackles (rales) in the lungs.

Reassessment

Patients with renal disorders have impairment in one of the primary homeostatic organs of the body. They are prone to serious complications and may decompensate rapidly. Establish a baseline of mental status, complaints, vital signs, and physical findings. Reassess critical patients every 5 minutes, or sooner, and noncritical patients every 15 minutes, obtaining at least two complete sets of vital signs.

Renal Disorders

Renal disorders are those related to the function of the kidney, and include several forms of renal failure. Many patients have known renal failure as a complication of diabetes or hypertension. Some patients must go to a dialysis center every two or three days to receive HD, some place fluid in their abdomen three times a day to perform peritoneal dialysis, and some undergo renal transplant, one of the most successful transplant surgeries.

Fewer patients encountered by EMS personnel have an acute onset of kidney failure. However, in those cases, the kidney is one of the most remarkable organs in the body in that it has the ability to completely return from renal failure and function reasonably normally. Other kidney disorders, such as **nephritis**, may also result in EMS transport.

The primary diseases of the kidney either cause renal failure, which can be acute or chronic, or can affect the filtering system of the kidney. The causes of acute renal failure

CASE STUDY (continued)

Advanced EMTs John and Missy have responded to a dialysis center for an unresponsive patient, Mr. Thornton. Their scene size-up reveals no obvious problems, such as bleeding from the hemodialysis access site. A technician has already disconnected Mr. Thornton from the dialysis machine.

John's initial impression is that of an African American man in his 50s who appears pale, with his eyes closed, and seems unaware of what is going on around him. A gentle shake of Mr. Thornton's shoulder elicits no response, but he reacts to a sternal rub by mumbling incomprehensible words.

His airway is open and in the process of determining this, John notes that Mr. Thornton's skin is cool and diaphoretic. Respirations are adequate, so John applies the nonrebreather mask that Missy has already connected to the oxygen cylinder. As he applies the mask, he notes that Mr. Thornton has an ammonia-like smell of urine to his breath. John notes a thready, rapid radial pulse in the wrist opposite Mr. Thornton's dialysis access site.

Meanwhile, as Missy prepares the nonrebreather, she obtains some history from Margo, the dialysis tech. Mr. Thornton is 51 years old and an insulin-dependent diabetic with end-stage renal disease. He has hypertension and suffered a mild stroke about a year ago. He is scheduled to receive dialysis three times per week, but missed his last four appointments.

In general, he is poorly compliant with treatment for his diabetes, kidney failure, and hypertension. On today's visit, Mr. Thornton had been hooked to the dialysis machine for about five minutes when a tech noticed that he was unresponsive and requested that someone call 911.

Problem-Solving Questions

1. What additional hypotheses could explain Mr. Thornton's condition? What hypotheses could Missy and John eliminate?
2. What additional information should John and Missy obtain?
3. Are any additional treatments indicated at this point?

IN THE FIELD

Up to 65 percent of all renal failures can be nonoliguric. Thus, you could transport a renal failure patient on dialysis who still urinates regularly and is therefore still susceptible to UTIs.

are further classified by whether the underlying problem occurs outside the urinary system (prerenal causes, such as hypotension); in the kidney, or **intrinsic renal failure** (such as loss of nephrons); or after urine leaves the kidney (postrenal causes, such as obstruction of a ureter).

Renal failure is also categorized by the amount of urine still made by the diseased kidney. This can be oliguria if the kidney is still making urine but less than 400 to 500 mL/24 hours, or less than 16 to 17 mL/hour. When the kidney creates less than 100 mL/24 hours or less than 4 mL/hour, the condition is called *anuria*. On the other extreme, if the kidney is still creating greater than 400 to 500 mL/24 hours (or greater than 20 mL/hour) of urine but there are still indications of renal failure, it is called *nonoliguric renal failure*. If the kidney produces too much urine, it is called *polyuria*.

Acute Renal Failure

Acute renal failure (ARF) is defined as loss of renal function (decreased GFR) over hours to days. It is recognized in the hospital setting by the accumulation of nitrogen-containing wastes in the blood (blood urea nitrogen [BUN] and creatinine [Cr]). When the levels of those substances are increased, it is called *azotemia*. When signs and symptoms of renal failure accompany azotemia, the condition is called **uremia**.

Manifestations of acute renal failure reflect the fact that the kidney cannot remove the following substances from the blood:

- Urea
- Creatinine
- K^+
- H^+
- Na^+, which leads to high blood pressure by increasing the osmotic pressure of the blood
- PO_4^{3-} (phosphate), which leads to a decrease in Ca^{++} in the blood
- Many other toxic substances produced by the body's metabolism that are still not well known or understood
- Medications excreted only by the kidney, such as insulin, leading to accumulation of the drug and toxicity

The pathophysiology of ARF falls into three categories. Cases that are caused by issues or disease elsewhere in the body but that affect the kidney's ability to produce urine are called **prerenal renal failure**, can account for up to 60 percent of cases. Cases caused by diseases in the kidneys, including the glomerulus, tubules, interstitium, and tubules, are called *intrinsic renal failure* and account for up to 40 percent of cases. Cases caused by outflow obstructions that back up the urine into the kidneys are called **postrenal renal failure** and account for up to 5 percent of cases.

Prerenal Acute Renal Failure

The typical presentation of prerenal ARF is that of an elderly patient with a history that suggests decreased blood volume, such as inadequate fluid intake. Additional signs include dry mucous membranes, tenting of the skin, and poor capillary refill and orthostatic vital signs. Decreased effective blood volume can be caused by congestive heart failure, cirrhosis of the liver, and sepsis.

Other prerenal causes of renal failure include severe end-stage liver disease, hypercalcemia, narrowing or blood clots in the renal veins or arteries, and the effect of nonsteroidal drugs such as ibuprofen and naproxen. The typical patient with prerenal renal failure will have some historical evidence of volume loss (for example, diarrhea, acute blood loss) and may show signs of heart or liver disease, evidence of infection, or diuretic use. The patient will usually be thirsty. The best treatment in the field is to correct volume deficits and ensure discontinuation of antagonizing medications such as NSAIDs/COX-2 inhibitors and diuretics.

Postrenal Acute Renal Failure

In cases of postrenal renal failure, the history may include indications of bladder outlet obstruction including urinary frequency, urgency, intermittency, double micturation (the urine stream splits as it leaves the end of the urethra in males), a weak stream, hesitancy, **nocturia**, and incomplete voiding. In addition, the patient may complain of flank pain or hematuria, or have a history of prostate enlargement or cancer, cancer of an organ in the pelvic cavity, or endometriosis.

An obstruction to urine outflow from the bladder results in backflow of urine into the kidney. The backflow results in intratubular pressure increases and changes in the flow of fluid through the kidney, causing the kidney to fail. On physical exam, the patient may have a suprapubic mass, pelvic masses, and adenopathy. When those obstructions are acute, the patient can be in agonizing pain and unable to urinate.

Giving IV fluids to patients with postrenal renal failure will worsen their situation. Allow the patient to find his most comfortable position until he reaches the emergency department, where a Foley catheter will be placed into the bladder to empty it.

Intrinsic Acute Renal Failure

Intrinsic ARF is caused by damage to the kidney itself. Each part of the nephron can be damaged, leading to renal failure. Intrinsic ARF is categorized by whether the glomeruli, tubules, interstitium, or renal blood vessels are the primary involved portion. Other causes of intrinsic disease are autoimmune diseases such as systemic lupus, infections, or no specific attributable cause (idiopathic).

Glomerular Causes

Systemic lupus erythematosus (SLE), or *lupus*, is an autoimmune disease that can profoundly affect kidney function. Patients with lupus nephritis can develop severe damage to the glomeruli of the kidneys, leading to glomerulonephritis.

Although those diseases are relatively rare, one form, which develops as a sequela of strep throat, is more common. Poststrep glomerulonephritis is usually self-limited and does not require significant intervention. An important question in the history is whether the patient had a recent strep throat infection.

Asking about changes in urine color, urinary output, and difficulty in urination is important in evaluating the patient for renal disease.

Tubular Disorders

Tubular disorders are the most common cause of ARF, and are caused by toxins or ischemia. The three major toxins causing tubular damage are radio-contrast dyes (used in CT scans), aminoglycoside antibiotics (such as gentamycin), and toxins produced by muscle breakdown (myoglobin).

Muscle breakdown can occur as a result of crushing trauma, prolonged ischemia of a large muscle mass (such as the alcoholic patient who may lie unconscious on a hard surface for a prolonged period), or excessive exercise, such as running a marathon. Toxins from muscle breakdown—myoglobin, in particular—cause tubular damage. Sloughing of cells from the tubules leads to leakage of the glomerular filtrate through the damaged tubules. A key finding in patients with significant muscle breakdown leading to ARF is dark, tea-colored urine.

Ischemic insults to the kidney occur when blood pressure is lost—for instance, in the patient who is resuscitated from cardiac arrest, a very bad burn, severe blood loss, or an acute myocardial infarction.

The key to managing those patients is to remove the offending toxic agents, if there are any, and maintain good hydration status. These patients can benefit from infusion of fairly large amounts of IV fluids. About 80 percent will have good recovery of renal function.

Interstitial Disorders

Medications are a key cause of interstitial ARF (interstitial nephritis), which affects the renal tissue cells surrounding the nephron and capillaries.

Long-term use of acetaminophen is notorious for affecting the interstitium of the kidney. Keep in mind that acetaminophen can be a "hidden" component of many over-the-counter and prescription drugs. For example, patients often fail to realize that cold and flu preparations, and over-the-counter migraine and menstrual symptom relief products, contain acetaminophen.

Signs and symptoms of renal failure from acetaminophen overuse include fevers and intermittent skin rash, in addition to indications of renal failure. Although acetaminophen is a main cause, other medications such as certain antibiotics (penicillin, cephalosporins, and sulfonamides), phenytoin (used to treat epilepsy), furosemide (a diuretic), and NSAIDs are also implicated.

Vascular Disorders

Vascular renal disorders can be caused by blood clots affecting the blood flow in the kidney. When a clot affects the large vessels near the kidney, you may hear bruits (a "whooshing" noise heard on auscultation) in the abdomen that indicate a narrowing of the renal vessels, which is called *renal artery stenosis (RAS)*. RAS is a potentially reversible cause of hypertension if detected and treated early.

The presence of bruits over the renal arteries (heard in the umbilical region) is an important physical finding in hypertensive patients. The patients also may have physical findings consistent with embolism of other organs, such as stroke or ischemic fingers or toes.

Vascular diseases are the most common cause of renal failure in older adults. Vascular renal disease is also caused by certain food toxins, as illustrated by the recent problem with fresh spinach that caused many stores to pull their spinach from the shelves because of *E. coli* bacterial contamination. Patients with this type of toxic vascular renal disease appear pale, tired, and irritable, may have small, unexplained bruises or bleeding from the nose or mouth and present with high blood pressure and edema. Unlike the vascular disease described earlier, the small-vessel diseases, called **hemolytic uremic syndrome (HUS)**, are the most common cause of short-term renal failure in children.

Acute Renal Failure Management

One of the keys to managing ARF patients is to remove any offending agents and maintain their fluid status as close to normal as possible. Because their kidneys are not functioning well, large fluid boluses, even in the face of hypotension, can be devastating.

A renal failure patient with crackles (rales) in the lungs, indicating fluid overload, should not receive large amounts of saline regardless of blood pressure. Instead, the patient is in need of intravenous medications that raise the blood pressure through vasoconstriction.

Any type of renal failure can leave the patient without functioning kidneys and thus require that he be placed on dialysis. Sometimes renal failure is reversible; sometimes it is not, leading to **chronic renal failure (CRF)**.

Chronic Renal Failure

CRF is defined as irreversible kidney dysfunction with increased urea in the blood for greater than three months. The patient retains products of metabolism, including urea, that were meant to be waste products and that are toxic to the system. The exact nature of all of the toxins is still unknown, but includes small molecules such as urea. Other substances known to build up are serum enzymes and hormones.

To fully understand CRF, it is important to recognize that the kidney has other functions beyond the creation of urine. The first of these is its role in the renin–angiotensin system, which controls blood pressure. Specifically, the kidney produces renin, which affects the peripheral vasculature and blood volume. Additionally, the kidneys activate vitamin D, which plays a key role in calcium and phosphorus management in the blood.

Finally, the kidney produces a hormone called *erythropoietin* that stimulates normal development of red blood cells in the bone marrow. Impairment of those additional functions of the kidney explains the hypertension, low blood calcium levels, and anemia seen in CRF.

Uremia

Uremia is a condition in which urea, a byproduct of protein breakdown in the liver, is not excreted normally by the kidneys. Uremia presents with a constellation of symptoms. Patients may have nausea, vomiting, and diarrhea, and are prone to gastrointestinal bleeding. The breath may smell like ammonia, or be described as "fishy" or "like urine."

The cardiovascular system may be affected, resulting in dyspnea, chest pain, and signs of fluid overload, such as peripheral edema, ascites, and crackles (rales). The patient may be hypotensive and may have cardiac dysrhythmias. Loss of proteins through the damaged kidneys reduces the oncotic pressure of the blood, resulting in edema. Platelet function is impaired, inhibiting blood clot formation, and anemia may be present.

Pericardial tamponade can occur, which may present with the Beck triad: distant heart sounds, hypotension, and jugular venous distension. You may also hear a "rub" on auscultation of the heart, indicative of uremic effects on the pericardial lining.

Neurologic symptoms include restless legs, twitching, and confusion. Ask the patient to extend his arms and hold up his hands as if he is stopping traffic. The hands may "flap," moving forward and backward in a rhythmic motion.

Altered mental status resulting from uremia is called **uremic encephalopathy**. Skin signs include pruritus (itching), bruising, and a rash known as **uremic frost**. Pruritus is associated with the buildup of toxins in the blood. Skin ulcerations may occur as a result of calcium and urea being deposited in the skin. The ulcerations can lead to infections and death, so they are an important finding on the physical exam. The patient also may complain of bone pain and arthritis. All these can be noted on a routine history and exam and may suggest that the patient has developed renal failure.

End-Stage Renal Disease

End-stage renal disease (ESRD) is defined as uremia requiring transplantation or dialysis. There are about 50,000 new cases of CRF in the Unites States each year. The primary causes of ESRD are diabetes and hypertension. Patients with diabetes have 13 times the risk for ESRD, accounting for 30 percent of cases.

Hypertension accounts for about 23 percent of cases. Other causes are glomerulonephritis (acute cases that turn chronic) and **polycystic renal disease**. Polycystic renal disease is one of the most common causes of hereditary renal disease later in life. A family history of renal disease should increase the index of suspicion of renal disease in the presence of other signs and symptoms.

Hemodialysis (HD)

When someone has CRF, he will generally be prepared for long-term HD by having a catheter placed in the subclavian area and an access site, called a **shunt graft**, placed in one arm (Figure 25-7). The subclavian line is used for temporary dialysis access while the graft heals, or "matures." Often this occurs after the patient has been followed for many years and his creatinine level reaches 10 mg/dL (normal being about 1 mg/dL). A shunt graft provides a means by which arterial blood leaves the body to enter tubing that conducts it into the HD machine (Figure 25-8).

In the HD machine, the patient's blood circulates on one side of a synthetic semipermeable membrane while a solution called *dialysate* circulates on the other. The difference in the concentration of substances across the membrane allows wastes to be removed from the blood. The blood then flows from the dialysis machine through tubing that returns it to the venous circulation. To accomplish this task, the graft shunt, which is a small section of tubing, surgically connects an artery and vein.

Although dialysis removes a good deal of the toxins, the removal of the buildup of toxins in the blood is incomplete, which means we do not remove them all and the patient never feels quite normal. Patients are placed on medications to address the body's response to kidney failure: erythropoietin (Epogen) for anemia, vitamin D analogs and phosphate binders for calcium/phosphate balance, and antihypertensives for blood pressure management. Patients with ESRD are at an increased risk of infection and should be vaccinated aggressively.

Complications involving central lines (such as a subclavian catheter) and dialysis shunts may occur. (Central lines are discussed in Chapter 46.) Shunt grafts are a synthetic foreign body, to which the body can react by blood clot formation that prevents flow through them. During your physical exam, lightly touch the graft site. If blood is flowing through it, there will be a "thrill," a light vibration from

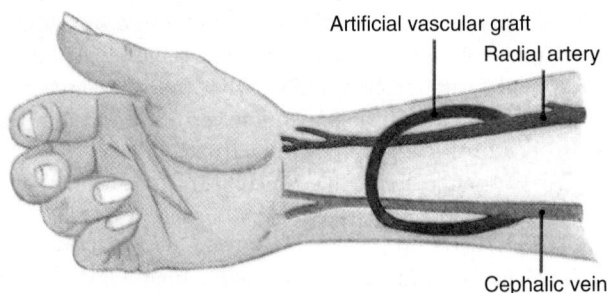

FIGURE 25-7

Vascular access for hemodialysis: a shunt graft.

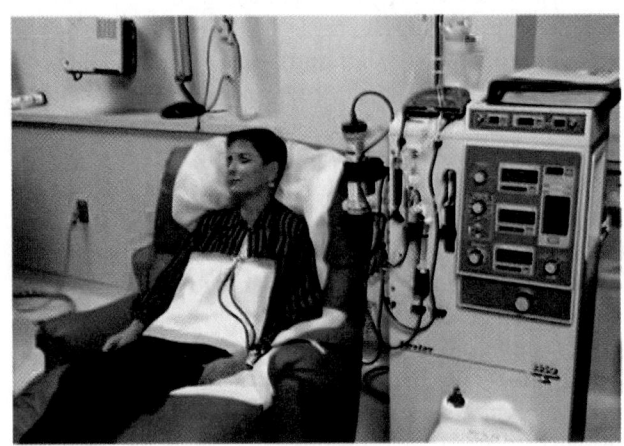

FIGURE 25-8

A patient receiving hemodialysis. (© Michal Heron)

the flow of blood. If the thrill is not there, it may mean the graft has clotted. Determine if the site is warm or tender, suggesting infection, because during every dialysis session it is punctured to connect the patient to the machine. Remember: Do not take the blood pressure, start an IV, or draw blood in the arm containing the shunt graft.

Shunt grafts are susceptible to infection and thrombosis, both of which would require complete graft replacement. The patient would again require placement of a temporary subclavian line, along with its associated risks, followed by weeks of healing for the new graft to mature.

Even without an obvious reason, grafts can develop thrombosis and stenosis, they can get infected, and they can shunt blood from the arterial to the venous blood system. This sets up a "steal" syndrome, in which the heart must pump much harder to keep the blood moving because of the shunting of blood around the capillaries.

You may be called to transport the patient because the graft will not stop bleeding. Remember that CRF patients have poorly functional platelets and are often receiving anticoagulant medications. After the dialysis machine is removed, it may be difficult to stop the graft site from bleeding. The treatment is direct pressure, as always. However, to avoid disrupting normal flow, do not push too hard on the graft.

Patients undergoing HD must receive the procedure three times per week at a special dialysis center, where they are provided with a reclining chair while they are connected to the machine. Dialysis patients never feel "normal." If they forget or skip a day, they feel terrible.

As you can imagine, this attachment to a machine as a lifeline can become a psychological burden. It can lead to medical problems including malnutrition, hypertension, hyperlipidemia, pruritus, and skin rashes. Often, HD patients will call to go to the emergency department for evaluation of other symptoms that may be related to, or worsened by, their underlying renal failure. A key to their care is empathy with how difficult this lifestyle can be.

When you see a dialysis patient, you need to assess how well the patient is doing. Is he making it to his dialysis appointments? What is his nutritional status? Is his blood pressure controlled? Does he have bone disease that requires rehabilitation? What is his level of functioning? These are all important questions in understanding the status of that individual. Some of the information may be available only by assessing the patient's home environment.

A number of complications can occur during the dialysis process, requiring EMS response to a dialysis center. Patients can develop severe hypotension, cramping, nausea, and vomiting. You may be asked to transport the patient to the emergency department for further evaluation, because most dialysis centers do not regularly have a physician available to assess the patient.

Hyperkalemia is a cause of cardiac arrest in patients with renal failure. Cardiac arrest is treated the same in CRF and ARF patients as anyone else. However, prehospital treatment may be ineffective, because the patient requires medications to treat electrolyte abnormalities. Communicate the history of renal failure when notifying the receiving facility that you are transporting a patient in cardiac arrest.

Peritoneal Dialysis

Another group of patients opts to have dialysis done through a catheter placed in the abdomen (Figure 25-9). This is called *peritoneal dialysis (PD)* because it uses the peritoneal membrane of the abdominal cavity to remove wastes from the blood. At varying times during the day, PD patients place large quantities of fluid in their abdomen and wait for the toxins in the blood to equilibrate by osmosis with this fluid before they remove it again. In this manner, they remove many of the toxins without having to be hooked up to an expensive dialysis machine and avoid the required travel to the dialysis center. The machine for peritoneal dialysis is portable and small in comparison to hemodialysis machines.

The advantages of PD are that it does not have a hemodynamic effect, meaning that hypotension is not a side effect. Patients have more freedom and independence, their diets are not as restricted, and they are generally more stable. In addition, if they need antibiotics for a serious

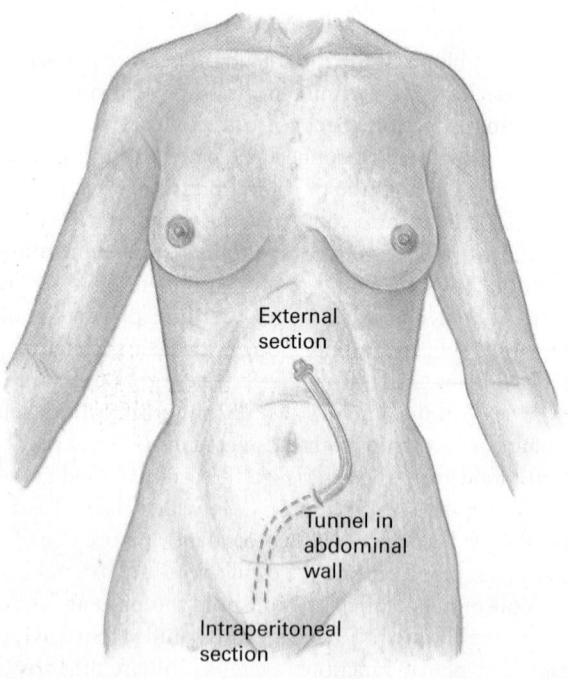

External section

Tunnel in abdominal wall

Intraperitoneal section

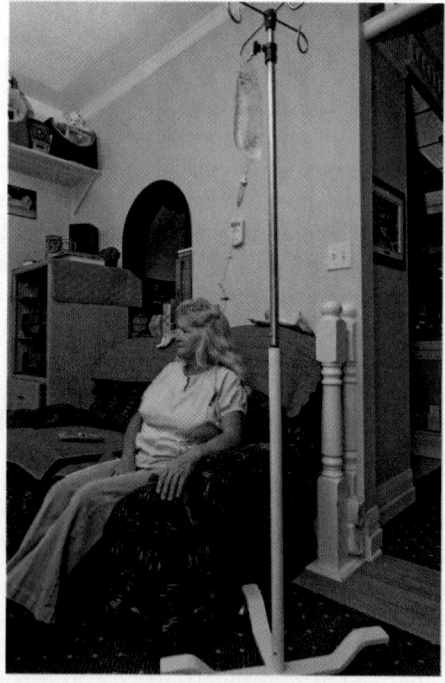

FIGURE 25-9

Peritoneal dialysis uses a catheter surgically implanted in the patient's abdomen to infuse dialysate into the abdominal cavity, where the peritoneal membrane acts as a dialysis filter to remove wastes from the blood. The fluid is then drained from the abdomen. The process is repeated several times a day.

infection, it can be placed in the dialysis fluid and the antibiotic will enter the bloodstream during dialysis.

Unfortunately, although the PD process is gentler, it is less efficient, and may not leave the patient feeling as well as he would after an HD session. PD is time intensive for the patients and can lead to patient burnout. About half the toxins are cleared per week by PD as compared with HD.

Because the catheters are managed by the patient, they can move slightly and lead to catheter malposition or occlusions. If the catheter itself breaks, it can cause a leak of dialysate and may need to be replaced. If the fluid or the entry site becomes contaminated, there is the risk of causing peritonitis, a peritoneal infection, or a tunnel infection along the catheter path into the abdomen.

Careful evaluation of the PD catheter and the entry site is part of a good physical exam of an ESRD patient using PD.

Renal Transplant

Eventually, the patient with end-stage renal disease would like to be free of the dialysis process. This can be accomplished by renal transplantation. The science of transplantation has improved, and our understanding of the immune system and how it rejects a foreign body (which someone else's kidney is) has improved greatly. Today there are better immunosuppressant drugs as well. The patient with a successful renal transplant can actually double his expected five-year survival and, ultimately, his lifespan. The first-year survival currently is around 85 percent.

The demand for the transplants still far outstrips the supply. In 2001, there were 55,000 people on kidney transplant lists and about 16,000 available kidneys. Placing the kidney takes 3 to 4 hours. The kidney is placed in the lower quadrant of the abdomen close to the inguinal ligament and attached to the iliac arteries so the kidney can be felt on abdominal exam.

Post-transplant patients will be on immunosuppressant medications, such as steroids and other medications, including cyclosporin, tacrolimus, alemtuzumab, and mycophenolate. The medications cause adrenal suppression, poor wound healing, osteoporosis, and susceptibility to infection, and they affect the skin, hair, and posture.

Poor bones already weakened by renal failure can be made worse by the medications, leading to easy fracturing and other secondary problems that may be why you are called to evaluate these patients. Most transplant patients die of either cardiac causes or infection. They have an increased risk of skin cancers and lymphomas.

Urologic and Male Genitourinary Disorders

As mentioned previously, from a medical standpoint, the urinary system is split into the kidney and the remainder of the collecting system in the retroperitoneum, the ureters

that connect the kidneys to the bladder, the bladder, and the urethra connecting the bladder to the outside of the body. Problems involving this lower tract portion of the urinary system, as well as emergencies involving the male genitalia, are usually managed by urologists.

Urinary Tract Disorders

Disorders of the urinary tract include acute urinary retention, renal calculi (kidney stones), and urinary tract infections.

Acute Urinary Retention

Urinary retention is often a result of the underlying problem of **benign prostatic hypertrophy (BPH)** that occurs in older men. By the age of 60, most men have developed enlargement of the prostate. Combined with any small insult to the prostate, such as infection, the prostate can enlarge enough to prevent the flow of urine from the bladder. This leads to the backup of urine into the bladder and severe discomfort for the patient.

A physical exam finding in these patients is a large nontympanic (dull to percussion, indicating the presence of fluid) mass in the lower abdomen, which is the enlarged bladder. Urine not only backs up into the bladder, but also through the ureters into the kidney, resulting in ARF.

Spine injuries can disrupt the nervous control over the urethral outflow of urine. Also, it is not unusual to see the development of a bladder obstruction in, for example, a young waitress who cannot reach the bathroom during long shifts.

Relieving the obstruction is done with a Foley catheter in the emergency department. In many cases, the patient requires surgery to prevent future reobstruction. This is a situation in which giving boluses of IV fluids can worsen the patient's condition.

Renal Calculi

Some patients have metabolic problems that result in the production of various small stones in the kidney, usually no bigger than grains of sand. A kidney stone is called a **renal calculus** (Figure 25-10). The composition of the stones varies, but they can pass through the lower urinary tract as long as they are less than 6 mm in size.

Stretching, dilation, and irritation of the affected ureter causes its smooth muscle to spasm. The pain produced by these processes is called **renal colic**. Renal calculi affect men somewhat more often than women, and are most common between the ages of 35 and 45, but can affect both genders at any age.

Patients present with constant, severe flank pain, often radiating to the groin, or lower abdominal pain, tenderness over the costovertebral angle, and nausea. Unlike the pain of appendicitis, when the patient lies as quietly as possible to prevent pain, the renal colic patient will be moving

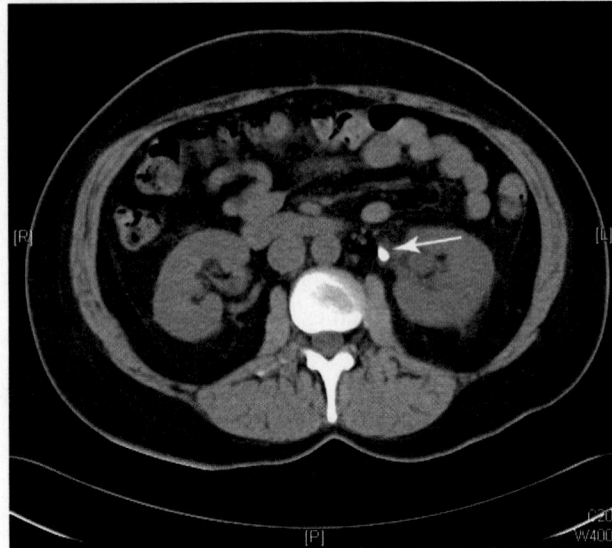

FIGURE 25-10

CT scan showing a kidney stone. (© Edward T. Dickinson, MD)

Geriatric Care

UTIs may initially go unnoticed in the elderly, resulting in severe illness, including vomiting, fever, and sepsis. Always keep UTI among your hypotheses when caring for an elderly patient with nonspecific signs of illness, such as confusion, vomiting, or fever. When responding to a patient who has a Foley catheter in place, always inspect the appearance of the urine in the collection bag. Cloudy or dark urine is an indication of UTI, which is frequent in patients with a Foley catheter.

around the room trying to find a comfortable position. He usually appears pale and diaphoretic. The patient may complain of blood in the urine (hematuria) and have a personal or family history of renal calculi.

The most concerning issue in a patient who you suspect of renal colic, especially if he is elderly, is that it mimics an abdominal aortic aneurysm, which is life threatening. Part of the exam in all renal colic patients should be to determine that there is no pulsating mass in the abdomen, that there is no abdominal bruit, and that the femoral pulses are equal. Abnormalities in any of them would suggest a diagnosis of aortic aneurysm.

Prehospital treatment for renal calculi is to allow the patient to find his most comfortable position. Start an IV, because a bolus of fluid could help flush out the stone and alleviate the pain. The administration of analgesics, in consultation with medical direction, can be helpful.

Urinary Tract Infection

UTIs are more common in females than in males because of their shorter urethra, which allows bacteria to reach the bladder before being eliminated from the urethra during urination. It is also common in patients who have indwelling Foley catheters or who are catheterizing themselves (inserting a catheter to drain the bladder, then removing it) because of inability to control urination, such as patients with spinal-cord diseases or trauma.

Lower-tract urinary infections affect the urethra, the prostate (in males), or the bladder. Those affecting the urethra, commonly called *urethritis*, can be associated with sexually transmitted infections or bacteria from the bowel.

The prostate is like a sponge in consistency, so an infection in the prostate (prostatitis) is very difficult to get rid of. It is often caused by a different group of bacteria than urethritis.

Patients with lower-tract infections may complain of a urethral discharge if they have an infection of the urethra or prostate. If the infection is in the bladder, the usual complaint is painful, frequent, cloudy, and malodorous urine. Infections of the kidney are called *pyelonephritis* and are usually caused by ascending infections from the lower tract. Patients with pyelonephritis may complain of a fever, severe one-sided back pain (unless both kidneys are affected) in the costovertebral angle, and all the same symptoms as in a lower-tract infection.

Field treatment for both lower- and upper-tract infections is to maintain the patient in the best possible position of comfort, start an IV and give a fluid bolus, and consider analgesics. It is important for you to elicit a history of immunosuppression (such as a kidney transplant or steroid use), diabetes, and pregnancy, because they can directly affect the severity of the disease and the hospital management of the patient.

Problems Arising from Foley Catheters

Foley catheters are used in older patients who are confused and cannot control their urination, in patients with BPH prior to surgery to prevent ARF, and in critically ill patients. Occasionally, patients with paralysis due to spinal-cord injuries will have Foley catheters, although most of them catheterize themselves multiple times during the day because this has a lower risk for infection than an indwelling (left in place) Foley catheter.

A Foley catheter is a clear plastic tube with a balloon at one end that is inserted through the urethral meatus and urethra, into the bladder (Figure 25-11). Once in place, the balloon is inflated with water to anchor the catheter in place. The tubing is taped to the leg to prevent tension on the tubing, and a collection bag is placed at a level lower than the bladder to allow the bladder to drain by gravity.

There is a clamp on the tubing that must be released for urine to flow into the collection bag. This clamp should

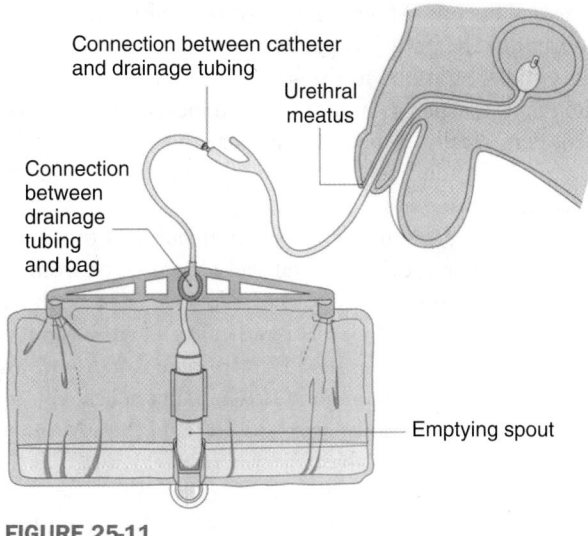

Connection between catheter and drainage tubing

Urethral meatus

Connection between drainage tubing and bag

Emptying spout

FIGURE 25-11

A Foley catheter.

be used when moving a patient if the collection bag must be placed at the level of the patient, to prevent urine from flowing back into the bladder. However, you must then place the bag lower than the bladder and unclamp it to prevent obstruction of urine outflow.

Confused patients may pull on the Foley and in some cases pull it out with the balloon inflated. These patients must be seen in the emergency department and evaluated for possible blood infections and trauma. Remember that Foley catheters can be a source of infection, so when you evaluate the patient, look for signs of infection.

Emergencies Involving the Male Genitalia

There are several emergencies involving the male genitalia. They include Fournier's gangrene, **phimosis** and **paraphimosis**, priapism, testicular torsion, epididymitis/orchitis, and trauma.

Fournier's Gangrene

Fournier's gangrene is a bacterial infection of the skin that affects both the genitals and the perineum, usually developing from a wound or abrasion to the skin. Men are 10 times more likely than women to develop this infection, and it can be fatal.

Often, the appearance on the surface is that of a small scab or lesion, but the infection is so deeply seated in the pelvis that the patients are often rushed to the operating room. Symptoms you might find on exam include crepitus of the area around the scrotum and perineum (a spongy feeling with crackling under the skin), pus weeping from a small gray-colored lesion, a foul odor in the area, severe swelling of the scrotum and penis, and a patient who is lethargic and febrile.

This is a true emergency. Field management is comfort and establishment of an IV for further access in the emergency department. If the patient is hypotensive, fluid replacement is important.

Phimosis and Paraphimosis

Both phimosis and paraphimosis are serious concerns. However, paraphimosis is by far the worse emergency of the two conditions.

A phimosis means that the foreskin cannot be pulled back over the head of the penis. Urine can build up in the area inside the foreskin, causing infections and irritation. Although pediatricians deal with this condition all the time, it is rarely a significant problem that would be addressed by EMS. However, sometimes when the foreskin is pulled down over the shaft of the penis, the small opening can strangle the head of the penis, causing the problem to become a medical emergency. This is called a *paraphimosis*.

Paraphimosis occurs when the foreskin of an uncircumcised male has been retracted and narrows below the glans, constricting the lymphatic drainage and causing the glans to swell. This lack of oxygen from the reduced blood flow can cause tissue death and necrosis. Symptoms include a band of retracted foreskin tissue beneath the glans, necrotic tissue on the glans, inability to urinate, and penile pain, tenderness, redness, and swelling.

Although there are some medications used in the hospital for this condition, about the only assistance that can be given to the patient in the field is an ice pack applied to the area to decrease the swelling, sometimes allowing the foreskin to be "reduced" back over the head of the penis. When using ice, always wrap carefully to prevent skin necrosis due to local freezing. The only real treatment for this emergency is to cut the foreskin, which is performed in the emergency department or the operating room.

Priapism

Priapism is defined as a painful and prolonged erection of the penis usually for more than 4 hours, as has been made famous by television commercials for erectile dysfunction medications.

The penile shaft is composed of a corpus spongiosum, surrounding the urethra, and two corpora cavernosum filling with blood to maintain an erection. Priapism affects the corpora cavernosa without affecting the corpus spongiosum. In priapism, the corpora cavernosa fills with blood for an erection, and then is unable to drain out.

Priapism is a disease of blood buildup. The most common cause of nontraumatic priapism is sickle cell disease, which results in occlusion of the microvasculature. Other medical diseases that cause priapism include leukemia, multiple myeloma, tumors, carbon monoxide poisoning, malaria, black widow spider bites, and certain prescription medications, such as antidepressants. Spine injury is a traumatic cause of priapism. When it is not treated promptly, scarring and permanent inability to achieve an erection (impotence) can result.

Field treatment is similar to that for a paraphimosis. You can apply well-wrapped ice packs to the penis and perineum to reduce swelling. There are some indications that mild exercise, such as walking up a flight of stairs, may help drain the blood.

Testicular Torsion

Testicular torsion is a serious emergency that you may see in the field. If the torsion is not reversed within 6 hours, there is generally death of the testicle. In a torsion, the testicles rotate and twist the spermatic cord, which consists of the vas deferens and the blood supply to and from the testicle. It is much like the supercoiling that occurs with a telephone wire between the base and the receiver. When the spermatic cord is shortened, it supercoils, cutting off the blood supply to the testicle.

Torsion can cause shrinkage (atrophy) and tissue death (necrosis), and may require surgical removal of the testicles (orchiectomy) if not treated within 6 hours. Torsion affects two age groups primarily, infants in the first year of life and adolescent boys aged 12 to 18. It can, however, occur at any age.

The patient may be nauseated and vomiting and complain of hematospermia (blood in the semen), lower abdominal pain, or a lump or swelling in testicle. Often he complains of sudden, severe testicular pain and may have a history of other episodes of the same pain that have occurred intermittently.

Treatment of torsion involves untwisting the testicle. The patient will need an operation, even if the treatment works, to tack down the testicle and prevent rotation in the future.

Epididymitis and Orchitis

Epididymitis is defined as an inflammation of the epididymis at the posterior pole of the testicle. It is a very common finding. It is seen in two separate age groups: young men who have sexually transmitted infections (STIs), and elderly men. The importance of this diagnosis is that it presents much like testicular torsion, a surgical emergency, and therefore is important not to misdiagnose.

Important in the history is whether the patient has a history of STIs and whether the pain has been intermittent and long standing, or if it is really acute and emergent. Ice and elevation of the testicles will help a case of epididymitis, whereas elevation of a torsed testicle will worsen the condition.

Orchitis is inflammation of the testicle itself. On exam, the testicle will be tender, but the epididymis will be normal and nontender. This disease is mostly of historical significance, due to the prevalence of mumps orchitis in the past. However, now that mumps has been virtually eradicated by vaccination, it is very rare.

Trauma to the Male Genitalia

Trauma to the male genitalia may be blunt or penetrating, or may be caused by insertion of a foreign body into the urethra. Trauma may be accidental, self-induced, or a result of sexual assault. Males have most of their genital organs external to the body cavity, which can lead to significant tears and lacerations to the scrotum or penis from straddling injuries (such as may occur on a bicycle or in gymnastics). Periodically, a male will capture the skin of his penis in a zipper, leading to an inability to remove his pants and severe pain at the site.

Other lacerations to the scrotum can lead to the testicle "falling out" of the scrotal sack. It will hang from the vas deferens and must be replaced surgically. The penis can be fractured (actually a soft tissue injury) during vigorous sexual activity. This results in severe pain, often with the penis being bent at an angle. Occasionally, males will present with a foreign body inserted in the urethra. Make no attempt to remove the object.

Injuries to the genitalia are generally quite concerning to patients and may distract both you and the patient from noticing other, potentially life-threatening, injuries. Despite the situation, always conduct a physical examination appropriate to the mechanism of injury and the patient's overall presentation.

Treat problems involving the airway, ventilation, oxygenation, and sources of significant external bleeding first. Cover open wounds with a sterile dressing, apply gentle pressure to control bleeding, and use a wrapped ice pack to reduce swelling. Make the patient as comfortable as possible and transport for further medical care. If injuries are the result of sexual assault, follow the same guidelines discussed later in the chapter for female victims of sexual assault.

Gynecologic Disorders

General Assessment and Management

There are a few special considerations in the assessment and management of patients with suspected gynecologic problems. The history will be helpful in developing differential diagnoses. However, your approach to the history will determine how comfortable the patient feels in sharing information with you. If you appear uncaring, uncomfortable, or unknowledgeable concerning the history or potential problems, the patient is not likely to share information with you.

When a patient complains of abdominal pain, one of the most frequent complaints associated with gynecologic disorders, anticipate the direction your history may take and provide the patient with privacy.

Abdominal pain may be caused by either a gynecologic or an obstetric (pregnancy-related) problem, or may be related to a problem with a different organ system. A second common presentation of gynecologic problems is vaginal bleeding that is abnormal, from either an increased amount of bleeding or unusual timing. The patient may complain of an unusual vaginal discharge, but most often this is not the chief complaint. Instead, it is likely to be associated with a chief complaint of abdominal pain. Both abdominal pain and vaginal discharge may be a result of a sexually transmitted infection. Gynecologic problems also may be related to trauma, including sexual assault.

In addition to information obtained in a routine medical history, specific information is necessary to understand whether a problem may have a gynecologic cause. If you believe a patient's complaint may be caused by a gynecologic problem, questions about her menstrual and reproductive history can add important information to your understanding of her problem. Obtain a history of her menstrual cycles, including whether they are regular, when the last menstrual period (LMP) was, and whether she experiences **dysmenorrhea** (pain) or menorrhagia (particularly heavy bleeding) with them. Ask if she has been pregnant, how many times, and whether the pregnancies have resulted in normal childbirth and healthy, normal children.

Ask about contraceptive methods, because many women do not consider them to be medications and may not volunteer their use unless asked directly. Above all, give the patient the respect she needs by asking questions discreetly, out of the earshot of other people. Also, always consider that a female of reproductive age could be pregnant.

When presenting information about patients with gynecologic complaints to the emergency department, begin with their age and the terms *grava* and *para* to provide her pregnancy history. **Gravidity** (or *grava*) means how many total times the woman has been pregnant (including miscarriage, abortion, stillbirth, and live birth), whereas **parity** (or *para*) means how many successful live births the woman has had. Provide the date of the LMP and any menstrual irregularities. For instance:

"This is a 49 y.o. female grava 4, para 2 with 2 miscarriages. LMP was 6/1, regular in amount and without pain. Today she presents with . . ."

Other useful information may be the age at last period if the patient has stopped menstruating (menopause).

Examination of the genitalia is not performed in the prehospital setting except for the purpose of stopping severe vaginal bleeding from directly observable traumatic lacerations to the external genital area. However, an abdominal examination is part of the focused examination in patients with gynecologic complaints.

Management of gynecologic problems in the prehospital setting is largely supportive. Administer oxygen if needed, and control external bleeding from traumatic injury. Allow the patient to assume a position of comfort and provide empathetic and nonjudgmental care.

Gynecologic Causes of Abdominal Pain

The female patient with abdominal pain is more challenging than the male. In the hospital, males with right lower quadrant pain often go directly to the operating room for appendectomies. Females, however, have too many other possibilities that have to be considered when presenting with pain in the same area.

Causes of abdominal pain include pain with ovulation; ovarian cysts, which can cause pain with and without rupture; endometriosis; endometritis; **ectopic pregnancy**; and pelvic inflammatory disease (PID) or cervicitis, which are usually associated with sexually transmitted infections (STIs).

At the time of ovulation, a small amount of follicular fluid is released along with the ovum, which can cause irritation of the peritoneum and pain, called *mittelschmerz*. Because pain associated with peritoneal irritation tends to be well localized, the patient may be able to pinpoint the painful area.

Ovarian cysts can develop when a follicle continues to develop and fill with fluid instead of degenerating (Figure 25-12). Ovarian cysts usually resolve on their own, but they can become quite large. Although the ovary itself is about 2.5 cm in length, ovarian cysts can grow to be up to 4 cm, or even larger. The cyst may rupture, causing a small amount of bleeding and release of the follicular fluid. This causes irritation of the peritoneum. The cyst may leak, rather than suddenly rupturing, leading to a longer period of peritoneal irritation.

When a cyst is large, it may cause the ovary to twist on its blood supply, similar to testicular torsion in males. This will lead to ischemia of the ovary with accompanying pain. If not corrected, the ovary may become necrotic.

Endometriosis is a condition in which the cells from the endometrium (lining of the uterus) are abnormally implanted outside of the uterus, on the structures within the abdominopelvic cavity. The cells undergo the same hormonally induced cyclical changes as the normal endometrium, resulting in abdominopelvic or lower back pain, which may radiate down the legs. Changes in pain level are often cyclical, accompanying changes in the menstrual cycle.

The abnormally placed (ectopic) tissue can impair the function of other organs and can result in scarring within the abdomen, causing adhesions between the layers of peritoneum. The adhesions can impair organ function and

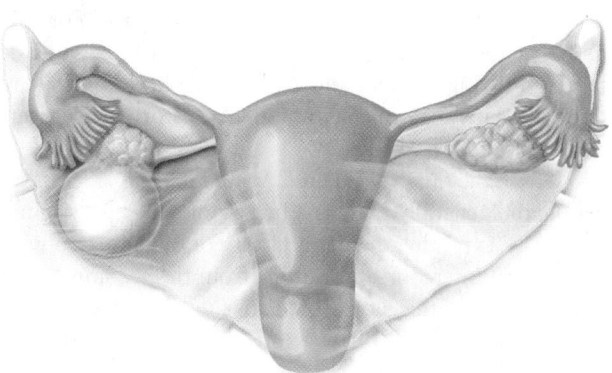

FIGURE 25-12

A cyst on the right ovary.

Gretchen Hendricks: I've never been sick a day in my life and it scared me to death when I got this sudden pain in my left lower abdomen while I was jogging. It wasn't like the usual stitch in your side you get from running. It wouldn't let up and I had to sit down next to the trail.

I must have looked really bad. A woman came over to me and asked if I was all right. I said I didn't know, I thought maybe it was my appendix or something. She waited with me for a few minutes, but the pain just didn't get better. She called 911 and waited with me until the ambulance arrived.

The Advanced EMT, Leah, took my vital signs and asked me a lot of questions. She made sure I was as comfortable as I could be. Her partner was nice, too. He said he'd drive nice and easy to keep from jostling me around too much, and he kept his word.

Leah said my appendix was on the opposite side from the pain, so it didn't seem likely that that was the problem. She reassured me that my vital signs were normal and told me what to expect when I got to the hospital. I ended up in the emergency department for a few hours that morning. It turns out I had a large ovarian cyst that ruptured while I was jogging. I had no idea that could even happen, let alone that it could hurt like that! I ended up taking pain meds for the next week or so, but I was back to jogging a short time later.

cause pain. Often, patients will have a history of ongoing abdominopelvic or lower back pain, which may or may not have been diagnosed as endometriosis.

Ectopic endometrial tissue does not show up well in medical imaging studies and, in the absence of laparoscopy (insertion of a small scope through an abdominal incision to view the organs of the abdominopelvic cavity), it is often a diagnosis of exclusion. Endometriosis is not the same as **uterine fibroids**, or myomas, which are benign tumors of the uterus. Uterine fibroids may become quite large, resulting in abdominal pain.

Endometritis is an infection of the endometrium, most often occurring after childbirth (cesarean or vaginal) or uterine surgery or instrumentation (such as the insertion of an intrauterine device or endometrial biopsy). Therefore, in patients complaining of abdominal pain with fever and abnormal vaginal discharge, it is important to determine whether there is a history of recent childbirth and gynecologic procedures, including abortion and dilation and curettage (D&C).

PID is most frequently a complication of STIs, such as chlamydia or gonorrhea. The infection spreads from the vagina and cervix into the uterus, fallopian tubes, and abdominal cavity, resulting in peritonitis. This inflammation of the peritoneum results in intense pelvic pain. When the patient walks, each heel strike transmits vibration to the peritoneum, resulting in severe pain. For this reason, patients with PID may walk with a shuffling gait to avoid lifting the feet and striking the heel against the floor. Patients may or may not give a history of previous treated or untreated STIs.

Often, the onset of PID follows the patient's menstrual period and generally there is a history of abnormal vaginal discharge. Typically, there is a history of dyspareunia (pain with sexual intercourse), resulting from the accompanying inflammation of the cervix (cervicitis) and movement of the inflamed peritoneum. PID is treated aggressively with antibiotics and may require surgery.

Scarring of the fallopian tubes following PID may narrow the tube so an enlarging fertilized egg cannot pass through it and thus implants in the fallopian tube, resulting in ectopic pregnancy. Although an ectopic pregnancy is any pregnancy in which the fertilized egg is implanted somewhere other than the endometrium, it most frequently occurs in the fallopian tube. As the embryo grows, the tube is stretched, resulting in pain. If not detected and treated, the tube may rupture, resulting in significant bleeding.

Although the patient is pregnant, she may not have a history of a missed menstrual period. Therefore, you cannot rule out ectopic pregnancy even when the patient has no history of a missed period. In other cases, the fallopian tubes are completely blocked by scar tissue, resulting in infertility.

Abnormal Vaginal Bleeding

Causes of vaginal bleeding in the non–trauma patient include pregnancy-associated problems such as spontaneous abortion and placenta previa (see Chapter 43) and particularly heavy periods. In the cases in which trauma is suspected, pursue a history of sexual assault without compromising the patient's privacy or wishes. Other causes include blunt-force injuries to the lower abdomen (for instance, seatbelt injuries in motor vehicle collisions) and foreign bodies in the vagina.

Quantifying the amount of blood loss is difficult for both the patient and medical personnel. A small amount of blood diluted by water in the toilet bowl can seem like a tremendous amount. The best way to give the emergency department an idea of blood loss is to ask the patient how many sanitary pads or tampons are saturated with blood in an hour's time. In the prehospital setting, observe carefully for signs of hypovolemic shock. If you suspect significant loss of blood volume, administer oxygen and start an IV of isotonic crystalloid fluid, according to medical direction.

Female Genital Trauma and Sexual Assault

Small cuts and lacerations commonly occur in the female pediatric population from straddling injuries during gymnastics, from bicycles, and so on. Most of the other female organs are well protected in the pelvis except during pregnancy, which is covered in Chapter 43. Control significant bleeding and if there is significant discomfort or swelling, apply a wrapped ice pack. Consider asking discreet questions regarding the possibility of inappropriate handling or sexual assault.

Males and females of all ages may be victims of sexual assault. Some measures are particularly important in cases where sexual assault is suspected. As always, your concerns begin with scene size-up, primary assessment, secondary assessment, and management of injuries. However, preservation of evidence is a legitimate and significant concern.

Without properly preserved evidence maintained in a documented chain of custody, prosecution of the perpetrator will be extremely difficult, if not impossible. In most cases, the victim desires that the perpetrator be prosecuted, and a few thoughtful actions on your part can contribute to that effort.

Place any garments removed by the patient or by you for medical examination in a paper bag (ideally, individual paper bags) and bring them to the hospital (unless law enforcement is on the scene and assumes custody of evidence). Ensure receipt of the evidence by a specific individual, and document that individual's name in your patient care report.

Discourage the patient from bathing, showering, or otherwise cleaning up prior to transport, because this may remove key evidence in the case. If the patient has cleaned up prior to your arrival, it may still be possible to obtain some evidence in a sexual assault exam at the hospital.

The psychological needs of the patients are critically important, because often he or she may be reluctant to speak with authorities, who can be perceived as being no different than the attacker already encountered. Reassurance is probably the most important intervention that prehospital providers can offer. Do not make statements or ask questions that may imply the victim is somehow at fault for the attack. For example, do not ask, "What were you doing out alone this late?" or "Why didn't you leave when you first became concerned?"

Whenever female EMS providers are available, they should provide care for female sexual assault patients. Do not probe for details of the assault except to ascertain the possibility of serious injury. However, do document anything the patient happens to tell you about the assault. Do not examine the patient unnecessarily, and take care not to unnecessarily remove evidence in your care of the patient. Check your protocols, because each community has specific appropriate facilities where an exam for sexual assault can be done by a qualified team.

Sexually Transmitted Infections (STIs) in Males and Females

STIs are a significant health problem. Except in the case of PID, it is not common that a patient's primary problem in the prehospital setting will be an STI. However, the calls can and do occur, and if you work an emergency department you will be more likely to encounter patients with STIs.

One of the key things to remember is that patients concerned about STIs often feel shame and embarrassment and may delay treatment for their signs and symptoms. Be empathetic and nonjudgmental in your interactions with the patient. Additionally, do not let the patient's age be a determinant of whether or not STIs are part of your differential diagnosis. Recent evidence suggests that the older population of "Baby Boomers" is not only sexually active, but may be taking more risks in sexual behavior than younger populations.

The most common STIs seen are chlamydia, gonorrhea, herpes, and syphilis. Symptoms from STIs may be localized, such as complaints of an ulceration on the genitals, or generalized, such as seen in disseminated gonorrhea.

Chlamydia is the most frequently reported STI in the United States. Patients of either sex may present with a minimal discharge and **dysuria** (burning on urination). However, chlamydia is asymptomatic in 25 percent of men and 75 percent of women. Usually the patient has watery discharge, painful sexual intercourse (dyspareunia), and abdominal pain. Chlamydia is treated with antibiotics such as doxycycline.

Gonorrhea (GC) is the second most frequently reported STI in the United States. The typical presentation is a 20-year-old man with complaints of purulent penile discharge and dysuria. It is a much more difficult disease to determine in women, who are often asymptomatic until two to three weeks later, when they develop a disseminated form of the disease.

The symptoms of disseminated GC include fever, chills, pain in the joints and muscles, and a very characteristic rash. It is usually treated with a cephalosporin antibiotic when it is in either localized or disseminated forms. Hospitalization is necessary, particularly if weight-bearing joints are involved. Gonorrhea is a significant cause of vision loss in newborns when they receive it from the mother during childbirth, and it is the reason that newborns routinely receive eye drops when they are born.

Herpes is a widespread and incurable STI. After a week's incubation of the infection, the patient may complain about the eruption of vesicles on the genitals. Because herpes is never eradicated, the major problems that patients have with herpes is its ongoing reactivation with return of the lesions. Although it is incurable, it can be treated and kept under control with acyclovir.

Syphilis is the oldest documented STI, having been reported since the 1400s. There are three stages to a syphilis infection. Primary syphilis lasts up to six weeks and presents as a painless ulcer on the genitals. Secondary syphilis occurs between the primary and tertiary phases. It includes symptoms such as fever, fatigue, sore throat, hair loss, headache, and muscle pains. Secondary syphilis may present as a rash that has been called the *great imitator* because it appears similar to the rash of many other diseases. A nonpainful, nonitchy rash on the palms of the hands and/or soles of the feet is particularly helpful in diagnosing secondary syphilis.

Tertiary syphilis, the third phase, may return at any time in the future. It affects the brain and spinal cord and causes severe tissue destruction. Often, *latent syphilis* will disappear between the primary and tertiary phases during which the bacteria is quietly spreading throughout the body. Syphilis is one of the treatable causes of congenital diseases in newborns. Treatment is with penicillin.

One other STI you should be aware of is human papilloma virus (HPV). When visible, it presents with pink raised growths often called *genital warts*. However, the virus can be spread by sexual contact even without obvious growths. The reason this disease is so important is that it has been clearly linked to cervical cancer. In recent years, a vaccine has been developed that can prevent the virus that causes the majority of cervical cancer. Because of this, there is a push to vaccinate all young females with Gardasil (recombinant HPV vaccine). Younger individuals, aged 9 to 26 years, are a highly susceptible group who can benefit from vaccination.

CASE STUDY WRAP-UP

Clinical-Reasoning Process

John and Missy are completing their workup of an unresponsive dialysis patient, Mr. Thornton. Missy continues to question the dialysis center staff while John assesses the patient. Mr. Thornton was feeling particularly poorly on arrival today and complained of being very nauseated.

John notes a frosty appearance to the patient's skin in addition to the ammonia-like odor on his breath, both of which he associates with uremia. His blood pressure is 90/70, respirations are 14, heart rate is 120, and SpO_2 is 97 percent just after being placed on a nonrebreather mask at 15 L/min of oxygen. He has jugular venous distention (JVD), crackles (rales) on all lung fields, and very distant heart sounds. He has no abdominal bruits and the hemodialysis graft site in his left antecubital space has a thrill, is oozing blood, and is slightly warm.

John and Missy are looking for an explanation for a sudden loss of consciousness in a diabetic end-stage renal failure patient who had just been hooked up to dialysis. They contemplate several hypotheses: diabetic emergency, uremia, GI bleeding, electrolyte abnormalities, sepsis, and pericardial tamponade. A few of their initial hypotheses are now lower on their list. There are no signs of trauma and bleeding from the shunt graft site is minimal.

Of the hypotheses, immediate information can be obtained about the possibility of a diabetic emergency. John determines that Mr. Thornton's BGL is 100 mg/dL, eliminating hypoglycemia and diabetic ketoacidosis as immediate causes of his altered mental status. John and Missy agree on the following list of differential diagnoses:

- Electrolyte imbalance is likely, due to missing several dialysis appointments and generally poor compliance with treatment. They will not be able to obtain further information about this in the field, but they anticipate that Mr. Thornton will be placed on a cardiac monitor, receive a 12-lead ECG, and have labs drawn when he arrives at the emergency department to check for electrolyte disturbances. However, given this possibility, they realize the patient is at high risk for cardiac arrest.
- Uremia is likely, based on the presence of an ammonia odor to the breath and uremic frost.
- Sepsis is a possibility, based on the warm shunt graft site and increased susceptibility to infection, but would not likely result in sudden loss of consciousness.
- Pericardial tamponade is a possibility, based on findings consistent with Beck's triad: JVD, distant heart sounds, and hypotension.
- GI bleeding is a possibility, because patients with renal failure are at increased risk. There is no evidence of a massive bleed, such as vomiting blood or bloody stools, but a slower ongoing bleed could have aggravated preexisting anemia. The sudden loss of consciousness makes this seem less likely, though.

Mr. Thornton is unresponsive with serious underlying medical problems, making him a critical patient and a high priority for transport. John and Missy note that Mr. Thornton's airway was opened, but he has been able to maintain it without an adjunct. They continue to monitor his airway, realizing this situation could change.

Continuing oxygen therapy, they place Mr. Thornton in a left lateral recumbent position on the stretcher to assist in maintaining his airway. In the back of the ambulance, just prior to initiating transport, John starts an IV. However, because the patient already has signs of fluid overload, he opts for a keep-open rate unless the patient's blood pressure drops further.

En route, John reassesses Mr. Thornton and makes sure that the graft shunt is not obstructed. Mr. Thornton remains in control of his airway and his vital signs are unchanged. John advises the emergency department of the patient's condition and lets them know they will be arriving in 15 minutes.

CHAPTER REVIEW

Chapter Summary

As an Advanced EMT, you will encounter patients with disorders of the kidney, lower urinary tract, and male and female genitalia. To effectively take the history and perform assessment of these patients, and to recognize the significance of their disorders, you must understand the anatomy, physiology, and pathophysiology of the urinary and male and female reproductive systems.

Patients may experience either acute or chronic renal failure that arises from a variety of causes. Impairment of the kidneys' essential role in homeostasis can lead to life-threatening complications. Patients with CRF receive either hemodialysis (HD) or peritoneal dialysis (PD) to remove wastes from the blood. Although HD is more effective than PD, patients are subject to significant complications related to their shunt grafts and the dialysis procedure itself.

The urinary tract may be affected by UTIs, urinary obstruction, and renal calculi, all of which can result in significant discomfort and additional complications. Much of your care of patients with renal and urinary disorders is supportive, but you must understand which patients can benefit from IV fluid boluses, and which patients may be adversely affected by IV fluids.

Renal failure patients in cardiac arrest are managed in the prehospital setting in the same way as other patients in cardiac arrest. However, you must be aware that your interventions may be ineffective until underlying electrolyte abnormalities are corrected in the hospital setting.

Emergencies involving the male genitalia may be either medical or traumatic in origin. They can be emotionally distressing for the patient, can result in permanent loss of function and, in some cases, can be life threatening.

Gynecologic disorders most often present with abdominal pain or vaginal bleeding. Obtaining a pregnancy and menstrual history can be significant in determining the underlying cause.

Both males and females of all ages can be victims of sexual assault. In addition to the care you normally provide, realize the importance of emotional support and preservation of evidence.

Finally, STIs are a significant health problem and patients with an STI may occasionally seek prehospital medical care.

Review Questions

Multiple-Choice Questions

1. You see a patient with severe flank pain that you suspect is renal colic. The most serious diagnosis to consider that would mimic renal colic is:

   a. appendicitis.
   b. pancreatitis.
   c. abdominal aortic aneurysm.
   d. ovarian cyst.

2. The kidney performs all of the following extraurinary functions EXCEPT:

   a. aiding calcium homeostasis.
   b. affecting systemic blood pressure.
   c. increasing bone marrow production of red blood cells (RBCs).
   d. improving digestion of fatty acids.

3. Which one of the following is NOT a difference between epididymitis and testicular torsion?

   a. On raising the testicle, the pain worsens.
   b. The pain is in the scrotal sac.
   c. The patient has a urethral discharge.
   d. The pain has come on gradually over the past month.

4. The parts of the nephron that can become diseased and cause acute renal failure do NOT include:

   a. ureters.
   b. glomerulus.
   c. interstitium of the kidney.
   d. renal tubules.

5. Which one of the following is a normal urine output for a 70-kg man?

   a. 120 mL/hour
   b. 95 mL/hour
   c. 35 mL/hour
   d. 12 mL/hour

6. Which one of the following would be associated with damage to the interstitial tissues of the kidney?

   a. Long-distance runner at the end of the race
   b. Elderly individual who takes acetaminophen for pain four or five times a day
   c. 50-year-old with history of a stroke and three heart attacks
   d. 12-year-old who had strep throat four weeks ago

7. The most significant life-threatening electrolyte abnormality in renal failure is a disorder of which one of the following?

   a. Sodium
   b. Potassium
   c. Calcium
   d. Hematocrit

8. The presence of which one of the following findings indicates a functioning permanent graft for hemodialysis?

   a. Warmth over the graft
   b. A thrill on palpating the graft
   c. A silent graft
   d. Good distal pulses

9. A patient presents with a small scab in the peritoneum, crepitus locally around the area, and a fever. You would be most worried about which one of the following conditions?

   a. Fournier's gangrene
   b. Testicular torsion
   c. Epididymitis
   d. Paraphimosis

10. You transport a 26-year-old woman who tells you that she has had fever plus joint and muscle pains. She had sexual contact with a new partner four weeks ago. You would be most concerned about:

    a. syphilis.
    b. herpes.
    c. chlamydia.
    d. gonorrhea.

11. A female patient has been pregnant four times and has three living children. You would describe her as:

    a. grava 4, para 1.
    b. grava 4, para 3.
    c. grava 3, para 4.
    d. grava 7, para 4.

12. There now is a vaccine that helps to prevent:

    a. syphilis.
    b. cervical cancer.
    c. genital herpes.
    d. chlamydia.

Critical-Thinking Questions

13. What complaints and factors in the patient history would lead you to suspect that a patient has a UTI?

14. What are some of the disorders you should consider in a female patient with abdominal pain?

15. What are the special considerations in managing a sexual assault victim?

Additional Reading

Bledsoe, B. E., Porter, R. S., & Cherry, R. A. (2009). *Intermediate emergency care: Principles & practice*. Upper Saddle River, NJ: Pearson/Prentice Hall.

Brenner, B. M. (2007). *Brenner and Rector's the kidney* (8th ed.). Philadelphia, PA: Saunders Elsevier.

Lameire, N., Biesen, W. V., & Vanholder, R. (2005). Acute renal failure. *Lancet, 365*(9457), 417–430.

Marx, J. A. (2009). *Rosen's emergency medicine* (79th ed.). Philadelphia, PA: Saunders Elsevier.

Wein, A. J. (2007). *Campbell Walsh urology* (9th ed.). Philadelphia, PA: Saunders Elsevier.

Workowski, K. A., & Berman, S. M. (2007). Centers for disease control and prevention sexually transmitted diseases treatment guidelines. *Sexually Transmitted Disease V44* (supplement 3).

26

Hematologic Disorders

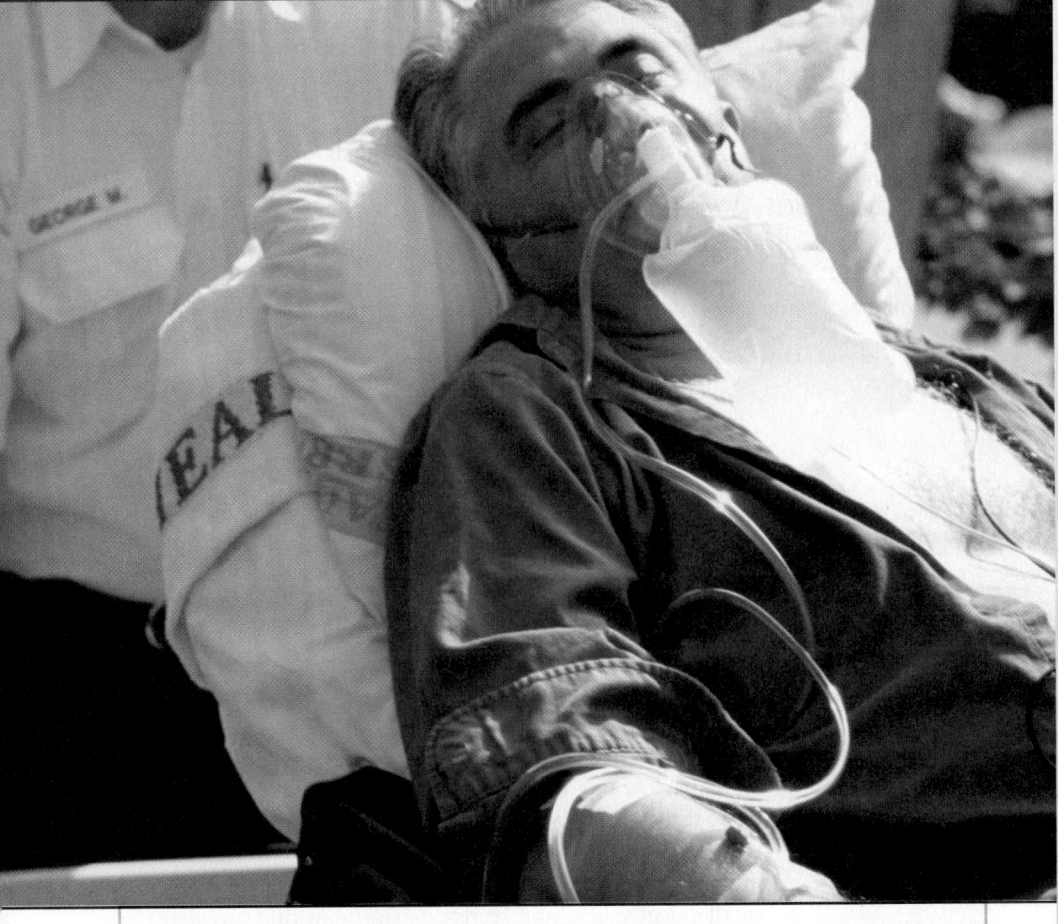

Content Area: Medicine

Advanced EMT Education Standard: Applies fundamental knowledge to provide basic and selected advanced emergency care and transportation based on assessment findings for an acutely ill patient.

Objectives

After reading this chapter, you should be able to:

26.1   Define key terms introduced in this chapter.

26.2   Describe the anatomy and physiology of the hematologic system.

26.3   Describe the pathophysiology and complications of sickle cell disease.

26.4   Recognize the signs and symptoms of vaso-occlusive crisis.

26.5   Describe the etiologies and pathophysiology of anemias.

26.6   Explain the etiology and pathophysiology of diseases of the white blood cells, including leukemias and lymphomas.

26.7   Describe the etiology and pathophysiology of disorders of coagulation and hemostasis, including disseminated intravascular coagulation (DIC) and hemophilia.

(continued)

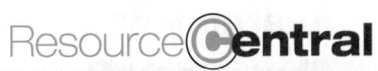

Resource **C**entral

To access Resource Central, follow the directions on the Student Access Card provided with this text. If there is no card, go to www.bradybooks.com and follow the Resource Central link to Buy Access. Under Media Resources, you will find:

• *What Is Sickle Cell Anemia?* Watch and learn about sickle cell anemia and the problems caused by sickled cells.

• *Red Blood Cell Production.* Learn about how red blood cells are manufactured.

• *American Red Cross.* Discover the different blood types and other interesting facts about blood transfusions.

CASE STUDY

Advanced EMTs Cecil Sparks and Eliza Reed are responding to a dispatch for abdominal pain in a child. En route, they discuss some potential causes of abdominal pain in pediatric patients, and how they will go about their assessment and history taking. Their patient is nine-year-old Clancy Heston, who is sitting in a chair with a pained expression on his face. Clancy's mother tells the Advanced EMTs that Clancy has sickle cell disease and began having pain on the left side of abdomen, just under his ribs, about 45 minutes ago, and it has gotten progressively worse.

Problem-Solving Questions

1. How could a history of sickle cell disease relate to a complaint of abdominal pain?
2. What additional information do Cecil and Eliza need to provide the patient with the best care possible?
3. What prehospital interventions should Cecil and Eliza anticipate based on the information so far?

(continued from previous page)

26.8   Discuss the risk factors, signs and symptoms, and consequences of deep vein thrombosis.

26.9   Develop a list of differential diagnoses for patients presenting with signs and symptoms of hematologic disorders.

26.10   Provide prehospital treatment appropriate to the needs of patients with a variety of hematologic disorders.

Introduction

Hematology is the study of the blood and blood-forming (hemopoietic) organs and tissues. Disorders can be related to red blood cells (RBCs), white blood cells (WBCs), platelets, or coagulation. Some of the disorders that you should be familiar with include **hemophilias**, sickle cell disease, **anemias**, cancers of blood-forming tissues, and **coagulopathies**.

Anatomy and Physiology Review

Adults have about 80 to 85 mL/kg of blood volume, giving the average person 5 to 6 liters of blood. Blood consists of a liquid transport medium, plasma, and formed elements with specific functions. The formed elements of the blood are erythrocytes (RBCs), leukocytes (WBCs), and thrombocytes (platelets). Plasma is about 55 percent of the blood volume and contains about 92 percent water, comprising a large proportion of the body's extracellular fluid. Many of the proteins that comprise the remainder of plasma volume, such as albumin and clotting factors, are manufactured in the liver. The formed elements comprise about 45 percent of the blood volume and arise from stem cells in the

bone marrow in adults, and from the bone marrow, spleen, liver, thymus, and lymph nodes during fetal development. The liver, spleen, and bone marrow play roles in eliminating aged and damaged blood cells. The kidneys, and to a smaller degree, the liver, secrete the hormone that stimulates RBC production: **erythropoietin**.

Plasma

In addition to transporting formed elements, plasma contains proteins, such as albumin, clotting factors, and antibodies (globulins). Plasma is also the medium that carries electrolytes, nutrients, medications, hormones, and other substances throughout the body. Albumin is a large protein, which provides blood oncotic pressure (a force that pulls fluid into the blood and out of the tissues) and serves as a medium to which several drugs can bind.

Red Blood Cells

RBCs are flattened disks that are thicker around the edges and thinner in the center, giving them a biconcave structure. This structure provides maximum surface area for gas exchange and allows the cell flexibility enough to squeeze through capillaries. Mature RBCs do not have a nucleus, mitochondria, or ribosomes, and cannot reproduce. They must be manufactured from stem cells in the bone marrow. And they cannot repair themselves when damaged. Without mitochondria, RBCs must engage in anaerobic metabolism. The benefit of this arrangement is that it keeps RBCs from using oxygen, allowing oxygen to be transported to the tissues. Most of the volume of RBCs is occupied by hemoglobin, a protein that has a special pigment (heme) that binds to iron. The iron, in turn, binds with oxygen molecules.

RBCs have a limited life span of approximately 120 days. Damaged and aged RBCs are recognized by macrophages (a type of WBC in the tissues) in the liver, spleen, and bone marrow. Macrophages ingest and break down RBCs, recycling some components for reuse and participating in elimination of others. New RBCs are formed in the red bone marrow under the influence of the hormone erythropoietin. The amount of erythropoietin is adjusted in response to the need for new RBCs (Figure 26-1). For example, emphysema patients with chronic hypoxia have an increased number of RBCs to increase oxygen-carrying capacity, as do individuals who live at high altitudes. Following significant blood loss, erythropoietin increases to stimulate the bone marrow to increase production of RBCs to replace those that were lost.

Hematocrit is the measure of the percentage of blood volume that is composed of formed elements, the majority of which are RBCs. On the average, blood is about 45 percent formed elements, with higher normal levels in

males (40 to 52 percent) and lower normal levels in females (35 to 47 percent). The amount of hemoglobin, the iron-containing protein that carries oxygen and carbon dioxide within RBCs, is important as well (14 to 17.4 g/dL in males and 12.3 to 15.3 g/dL in females). Each hemoglobin molecule has four protein subunits. The iron ion on each hemoglobin subunit can weakly bind with oxygen. The weak bond allows oxygen to be carried, but also to be released at the tissue level. The arrangement allows each hemoglobin molecule to bind with up to four oxygen molecules (one for each protein subunit).

When all four subunits of hemoglobin are bound to oxygen, the molecule is fully saturated with oxygen, giving the molecule a bright red color. Desaturated hemoglobin has a dark red color. The difference in color affects patient's skin and mucous membrane color. When hemoglobin-containing RBCs are decreased in number or diverted away from peripheral tissues, the skin and mucous membranes are pale instead of their normal pink color. When a significant amount of hemoglobin in arterial blood is desaturated, it results in cyanosis. The color difference between saturated and desaturated hemoglobin also serves as the basis of pulse oximetry measurement. (See Chapters 16 and 19.)

White Blood Cells

Although WBCs comprise a tiny fraction of the total number of blood cells, there are several different types of them, each with specific functions that protect the body in a variety of ways. Like RBCs, WBCs are produced in the bone marrow. WBCs are relatively large and have a variety of different features when viewed under a microscope. WBCs are signaled by chemical messengers to travel to areas where they are needed, and can migrate out of the blood vessels and into the tissue to perform their functions. The types of WBCs are neutrophils, eosinophils, basophils, monocytes, and lymphocytes.

Different types of WBCs respond preferentially to different kinds of antigens (pathogens and other foreign proteins). Examining which types of WBCs are increased in number can help physicians differentiate between different kinds of infections, such as viral, bacterial, and parasitic, or determine whether signs and symptoms are more likely due to allergies. Some WBCs act as nonspecific defenses for the body by responding to inflammation and injury. Monocytes, neutrophils, and eosinophils can ingest material by engulfing it in a process called *phagocytosis*. These cells have many complex functions to destroy and remove pathogens and debris. Lymphocytes (B lymphocytes and T lymphocytes) are involved in specific immunity by producing antibodies. Very few specific antibodies are present are birth. Most antibodies are acquired through a complex immune process after initial exposure to a pathogen, resulting in immunity to that pathogen.

Mast cells are basophils that migrate into the tissues, where they release histamine and heparin. Those substances play a critical role in body defense, but when released in

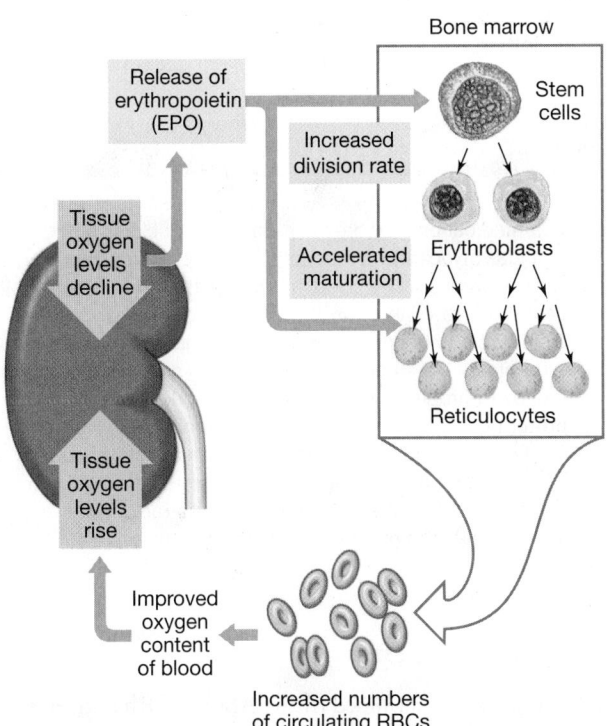

Bone marrow

Release of erythropoietin (EPO)

Increased division rate

Stem cells

Tissue oxygen levels decline

Accelerated maturation

Erythroblasts

Tissue oxygen levels rise

Reticulocytes

Improved oxygen content of blood

Increased numbers of circulating RBCs

FIGURE 26-1

Hypoxia triggers increased release of erythropoietin, a hormone that stimulates the bone marrow to produce red blood cells (RBCs). (Bledsoe, Bryan E.; Martini, Frederic H.; Bartholomew, Edwin F.; Ober, William C.; Garrison, Claire W.; Anatomy & Physiology for Emergency Care, 2nd Edition, © 2008. Reprinted with permission of Pearson Education, Inc., Upper Saddle River, NJ) excess, histamine produces many of the signs and symptoms of allergic and anaphylactic reactions. (See Chapter 27.) Macrophages are monocytes that have migrated into the tissues, where they play a role in engulfing pathogens and cellular debris. Some microphages are fixed, located in specific tissues such as the lung, liver, and spleen, where they perform specific defense functions. For example, the cells in the liver that engulf aged and damaged RBCs are one type of fixed macrophage.

Platelets

Platelets are fragments of thrombocytes (which exist only in the bone marrow), rather than complete cells. Platelets are activated by exposed tissue collagen in injured blood vessels. They are attracted to the injured area, where they become sticky and adhere to the injured tissue and to each other (platelet aggregation), creating a platelet plug. However, this plug is not stable and the hemostasis process must be completed by activation of the **clotting cascade**.

Hemostasis

Hemostasis is the process of stopping bleeding. The process occurs in three phases following vascular injury. First, the injured vessel constricts to slow the flow of blood through it. Next, platelets are attracted to the area, forming a platelet plug. The final stage is coagulation, or formation of a stable blood clot. The clotting (coagulation) cascade is a complex series of chemical reactions that occurs in response to injury (Figure 26-2). It requires a number of proteins, called *clotting factors*, plus calcium and vitamin K. The final outcome of coagulation is that a circulating substance called *fibrinogen* is converted to **fibrin**, which creates a meshwork to reinforce the blood clot and stabilize it.

Normally, the clotting process occurs locally, just at the area of injury. However, massive injury can result in systemic formation of blood clots, called *disseminated intravascular coagulation (DIC)*. This, in turn, can result in consumption of available clotting factors so that additional bleeding cannot be stopped. Deficiency in vitamin K or any of the clotting factors impairs blood clotting. Inherited deficiencies of specific clotting factors are the cause of various types of hemophilia. A number of medications can interfere with platelet aggregation or various parts of the clotting cascade, causing coagulopathies (Table 26-1).

IN THE FIELD

Aspirin inhibits a substance in platelets called *thromboxane A_2*, which plays a role in platelet aggregation. In patients who are prone to abnormal platelet aggregation, such as those with a history of cardiovascular disease or stroke, aspirin is given to reduce platelet aggregation and thus the formation of a clot that can obstruct blood flow.

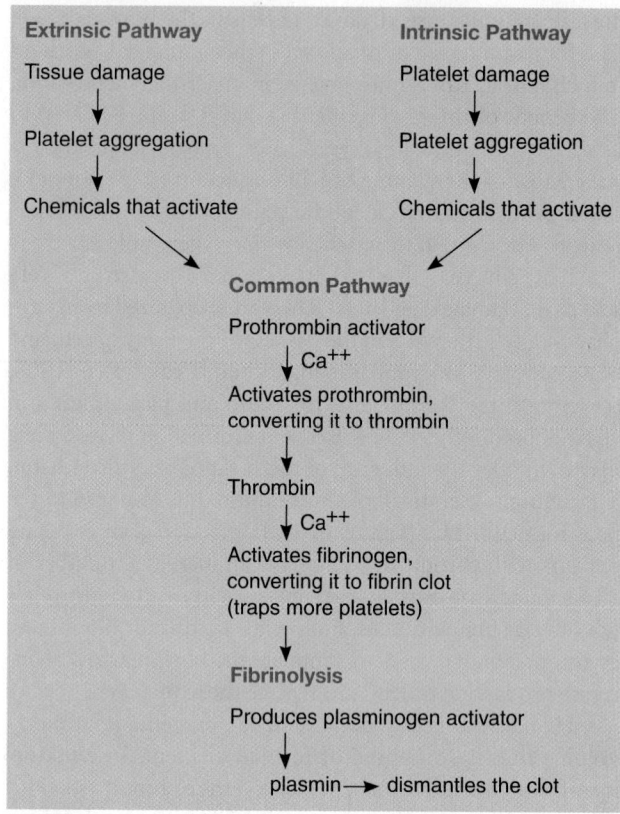

FIGURE 26-2

The clotting (coagulation) cascade.

IN THE FIELD

Some medications for breaking down blood clots in stroke and acute myocardial infarction (AMI) are called *fibrinolytics*. They work by taking advantage of the body's normal process of breaking down blood clots, or through the actions of a group of bacteria that cause clots to break down. Tissue plasminogen activator (tPA) is normally secreted by the body to break down blood clots. It works by converting a protein called *plasminogen* into plasmin, which breaks down fibrin (fibrinolysis). Streptokinase is a substance produced by a strain of streptococcal bacteria. Streptokinase also acts to break down fibrin clots, but is rarely given any more because of a high risk of allergic reactions.

Blood Groups

Blood types are determined by the ABO and Rh antigen systems, although there are more than 100 antigens on the surface of RBCs. The ABO and Rh antigens are on the surface of RBCs from birth (Figure 26-3). An individual may have either A, B, both A and B, or no (O) antigens on the surface of his RBCs. People with type A blood have only A antigens on the surface of their RBCs, and have anti-B antibodies in their blood. People with type B blood have only B antigens on their RBCs and have anti-A antibodies in the blood.

TABLE 26-1　Medications That May Indicate a Hematologic Disorder

Medication or Supplement	Use	Complications
alfalfa	Used as a tea for arthritis and multiple other conditions	Contains coumarin and vitamin K; excessive use can interfere with anticoagulant drug therapy
aspirin	Anti-inflammatory, analgesic, platelet aggregation inhibitor	Increased bleeding from impaired platelet function
borage oil	Used as an anti-inflammatory	Can prolong bleeding times
clopidogrel (Plavix)	Platelet aggregation inhibitor	Increased bleeding from impaired platelet function
dong quai	Taken for several reasons, including to treat premenstrual symptoms and menstrual cramps	Contains coumarins and can interact with warfarin, increasing bleeding risk
feverfew	Taken to prevent migraine headaches	Has antiplatelet and anticoagulant effects
garlic	Used in concentrated, capsule form as an anti-inflammatory, anti-infective, and to decrease risk of heart disease	Can cause increased bleeding when taken in conjunction with warfarin; decreases platelet aggregation
ginger	Used as an anti-inflammatory, antinausea, and analgesic supplement	Decreases platelet aggregation
gingko biloba	Taken to improve mental clarity and memory	Decreases platelet aggregation
guarana	Used as a stimulant, found in energy drinks	Inhibits platelet aggregation
horse chestnut	varicose veins	Contains coumarin and increases risk of bleeding
nonsteroidal anti-inflammatories (ibuprofen, naproxen, others)	Anti-inflammatory, analgesic	Irritates gastrointestinal tract, inhibits platelets
turmeric	Used to treat arthritis and inflammatory conditions	Antiplatelet effects
vitamin E	Antioxidant	Inhibits platelet aggregation
vitamin K	Dietary intake from green leafy vegetables	Can block effects of heparin and warfarin
warfarin (Coumadin)	Anticoagulant	Inhibits portions of clotting cascade
white willow bark	Taken as an anti-inflammatory and analgesic, has properties similar to aspirin	Can inhibit platelet aggregation and cause gastrointestinal irritation

People with both A and B antigens on their RBCs are type AB and have neither A nor B antibodies in the blood. Type O patients have neither A nor B antigens on the surface of RBCs and have both anti-A and anti-B antibodies.

A person with type A blood can receive type A blood, because he has no anti-A antibodies, and type O blood, because it has no antigens. However, if the patient receives type B or type AB blood, the anti-B antibodies in his blood will attack the foreign antigens, causing the RBCs to clump together, producing a transfusion reaction. In a similar manner, type B individuals can receive types B or O blood, but not type A or AB. The type AB individual can receive A, B, or O. He has no anti-A or anti-B antibodies, and type O has no antigens. Because type O has no antigens, it is considered

the universal donor type, and because type AB has no antibodies, it is considered the universal recipient type. Type O individuals, who have anti-A and anti-B antibodies, can only receive type O blood.

The presence or absence of the Rh factor must be considered in blood typing. Rh-positive individuals have an Rh antigen on their RBCs, and no anti-Rh antibodies in the blood. Rh-negative individuals do not have the Rh antigen on their RBCs, and do not initially have anti-Rh antibodies. However, if they are exposed to Rh-positive blood, they will develop anti-Rh antibodies. Type O negative blood is the universal donor type because it contains neither O nor Rh antigens. Type AB-positive blood is the universal recipient type because the individual does not have anti-A, anti-B, or

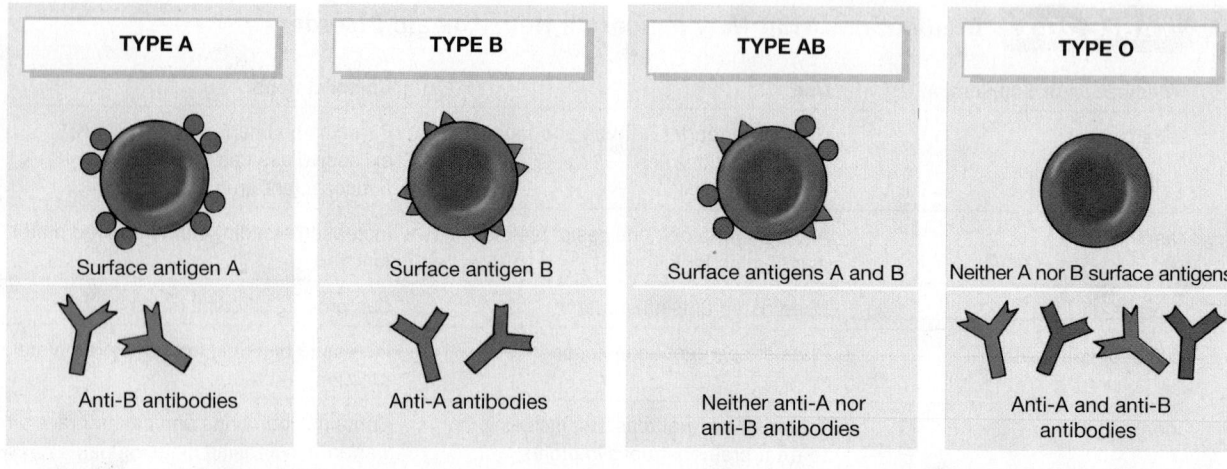

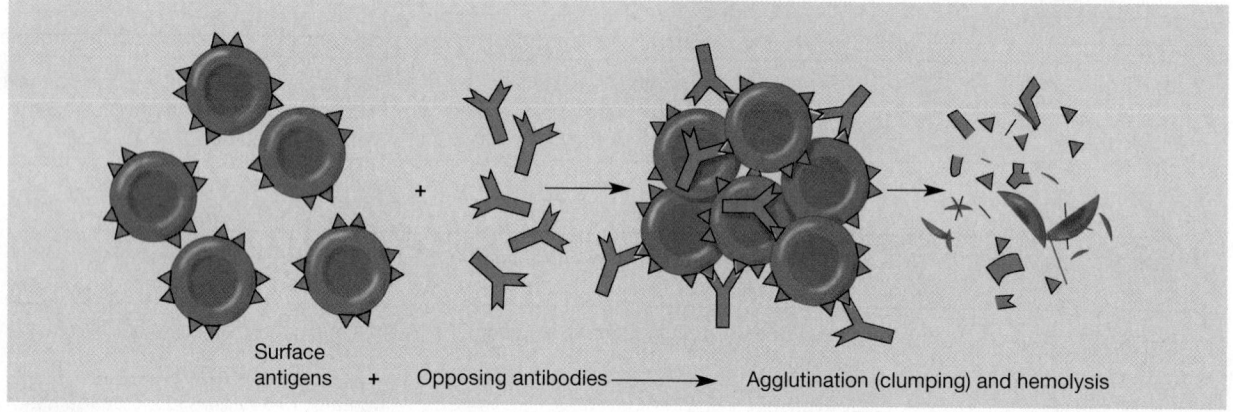

FIGURE 26-3

(A) Surface antigens on red blood cell membranes provide the basis of blood typing. (B) Antibodies in the recipient's blood recognize antigens of donor blood cells that do not match their own antigens and attack them. The foreign cells clump together (agglutinate) and are hemolyzed. (Bledsoe, Bryan E.; Martini, Frederic H.; Bartholomew, Edwin F.; Ober, William C.; Garrison, Claire W.; Anatomy & Physiology for Emergency Care, 2nd Edition, © 2008. Reprinted with permission of Pearson Education, Inc., Upper Saddle River, NJ)

anti-Rh antibodies. That phenomenon also explains hemolytic disease of the newborn.

In a first pregnancy in which an Rh-negative mother carries an Rh-positive fetus, fetal RBCs may come in contact with maternal blood during delivery. Because there are initially no anti-Rh antibodies in the mother's blood, the fetus is not affected. But, exposure to Rh-positive blood results in the mother's production of anti-Rh antibodies. In a subsequent pregnancy with an Rh-positive fetus, the maternal antibodies cross the placenta and attack the fetal RBCs.

Rh-negative women are given an injection of Rh immune globulin (Rhogam), an antibody that destroys any fetal Rh-positive blood cells that enter her blood before she can produce antibodies against them. However, the passively administered antibodies do not remain in the woman's blood indefinitely, meaning readministration with each pregnancy. The anti-A and anti-B antibodies do not cross the placenta, like the anti-Rh antibody, so that there is no problem, for example, with a blood type A mother carrying a type B baby. In transfusions, although the presence of antibodies in the donor's blood (for example, the anti-A and anti-B antibodies in type O blood) could result in

agglutination of an A, B, or AB recipient's RBCs, this typically does not occur to a significant extent.

In practice, blood transfusions are not quite as simple as selecting only on the basis of ABO and Rh antigens. As mentioned, there are many surface antigens on RBCs. Unless it is a dire emergency, blood is cross-matched for possible reactions before administration.

General Assessment and Management of Hematologic Emergencies

A variety of circumstances could lead to a hematologic emergency, and patient complaints will depend on the exact nature of the hematologic problem (Table 26-2). Patients with sickle cell disease suffer from painful vaso-occlusive crises that may prompt a call for EMS. A patient who is taking warfarin (Coumadin) may suffer an injury that bleeds profusely because warfarin interferes with the clotting

TABLE 26-2	**Signs and Symptoms of Hematologic Disorders**

- Tachycardia
- Tachypnea
- Dyspnea
- Fatigue, malaise, weakness
- Pallor
- Lymphadenopathy (swollen, tender lymph nodes)
- Fever
- Hematuria
- Petechiae (pinpoint hemorrhages that may appear like a rash)
- Purpura (hemorrhagic area in the skin > 3 mm in diameter)
- Unusual bruising or bleeding
- Pruritus (itching)
- Abdominal pain
- Joint pain and swelling
- Syncope
- Jaundice
- Severe night sweats

cascade. A patient with leukemia may bleed excessively from an injury because the abnormal cells in the bone marrow that are producing excessive WBCs can crowd out the cells that produce platelets. A patient with excessive platelets (thrombocytosis) may suffer a pulmonary embolism.

Many patients, such as those with sickle cell disease and hemophilia, will be aware of their disorder and provide you with this information. However, the patient with risk factors for abnormal bleeding or blood clotting may not be aware of the underlying problem. Your knowledge of anatomy, physiology, and pathophysiology will help you suspect a hematologic disorder.

Scene Size-Up

Approach the scene size-up as always, checking for possible hazards, multiple patients, and the need for additional resources. Note the patient's general appearance. Excessive bleeding from a minor mechanism of injury may be a clue that the patient is taking a medication that interferes with hemostasis.

Primary Assessment

Immediately check for a pulse in an apparently unresponsive patient who does not appear to be breathing. Otherwise, determine if the patient's airway is in jeopardy. **Epistaxis** (nose bleed), excessive bleeding from an injury, or **hematoma** formation can all interfere with the airway. Control bleeding and use suction as necessary to clear the airway. Assess the patient's ventilations and check for and control significant hemorrhage.

Secondary Assessment

For conscious patients, perform a focused history and exam as dictated by the patient's presentation and chief complaint. In unresponsive patients, perform a rapid medical or rapid trauma exam as indicated by the mechanism of injury or nature of the illness. In unresponsive patients in whom you cannot determine the problem, a head-to-toe examination may reveal additional information, such as the presence of **purpura** (Figure 26-4), **petechiae** (Figure 26-5), or **lymphadenopathy**. Obtain a set of baseline vital signs and use monitoring devices according to the situation. The patient's list of medications can be particularly helpful in determining whether the patient has, or is at risk for, a hematologic problem. If a hematologic problem is suspected, ask the patient about abnormal bleeding with tooth brushing or for small cuts, and ask about a family history of abnormal bleeding.

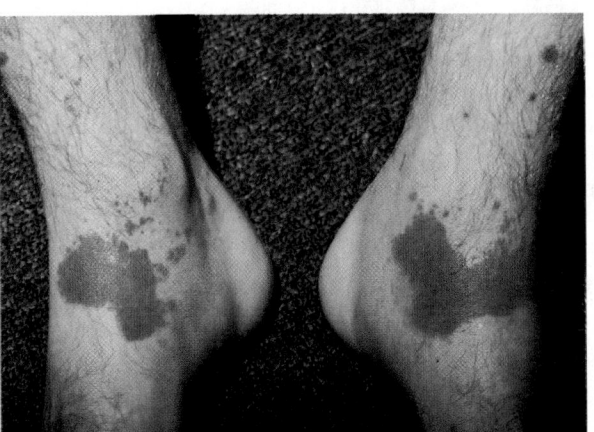

FIGURE 26-4

Purpura. (Courtesy of Jason L. Smith, MD)

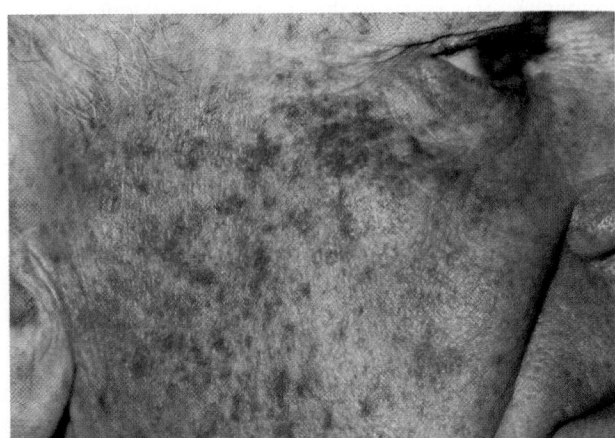

FIGURE 26-5

Petechiae. (© Dr. P. Marazzi/Science Photo Library/Custom Medical Stock Photo)

Clinical-Reasoning Process

The signs and symptoms of hematologic emergencies are unique to hematologic problems. Apply your knowledge of potential causes of various complaints, anatomy, physiology, and pathophysiology to guide your assessment and clinical-reasoning process. Together, the signs, symptoms, and history may increase your suspicion of a hematologic problem. Even when the presenting problem is not directly related to a hematologic problem, keep in mind the consequences of various hematologic problems in the patient's ability to maintain homeostasis.

Treatment

Select treatment based on the patient's presentation, complaints, history, and assessment findings. Consider the need for oxygen, fluid replacement, and analgesia.

Reassessment

Reassess critical patients every 5 minutes, or more frequently, if indicated. Reassess noncritical patients every 15 minutes, obtaining at least two sets of assessment findings. Determine the effects of interventions and evaluate the need for changes in treatment.

Blood Transfusion Reactions

If you perform interfacility transports as part of your Advanced EMT duties, or work in the emergency department, you might take part in the care of patients who are receiving blood or blood products, or who have received them shortly before transportation. Despite the care taken in typing and cross-matching blood and ensuring that patients receive the blood or blood products matched to them, the process is not perfect and mistakes can happen. In such cases, the patient's immune system reacts to the antigens in the donor blood, sometimes with severe signs and symptoms. You should be aware of indications of a transfusion reaction (Table 26-3).

TABLE 26-3 Signs and Symptoms of a Transfusion Reaction

- Flushing
- Pain at infusion site
- Chest pain
- Back or flank pain
- Restlessness or anxiety
- Nausea
- Fever
- Chills
- Renal failure

If the patient is still receiving the donor blood when exhibiting those symptoms, discontinue infusion of the blood product immediately.

Red Blood Cell Disorders

RBC disorders include polycythemia (too many RBCs), anemia (too few blood cells), and conditions in which RBCs are abnormally shaped. Polycythemia is indicated by an elevated hematocrit. In dehydration, the increase in RBCs is relative, because as water is lost from plasma, the other blood components become more concentrated. Polycythemia also results from chronic hypoxia or living at a high altitude, in which case it is a compensatory mechanism. Rarely, polycythemia is caused by an underlying disease process that increases the production of RBCs.

Anemia

Patients with anemia have an abnormally low hematocrit from one of three general causes, and generally become symptomatic when the hematocrit drops below 30 percent. The three causes are decreased production of RBCs, increased destruction of RBCs, or a loss of RBCs (hemorrhage), each of which decreases the oxygen-carrying capacity of the blood. As a result, the cells do not receive enough oxygen for energy production. Signs and symptoms include fatigue, pallor, tachycardia, and shortness of breath, particularly on exertion. In severe cases, the patient may have chest pain and signs of heart failure.

Causes of decreased RBC production include aplastic anemia, iron deficiency anemia, and pernicious anemia. Aplastic anemia occurs when the bone marrow does not produce an adequate number of RBCs, WBCs, or platelets. RBC production can be decreased by renal failure (the kidneys do not produce sufficient erythropoietin to stimulate the bone marrow), radiation or chemotherapy that suppresses or destroys bone marrow (reducing WBC and platelet production, as well), viruses, and autoimmune diseases. Pregnant women are frequently anemic. Bone marrow production of RBCs is sometimes decreased, but the large blood volume increase in pregnancy can also expand volume beyond the capacity of bone marrow to produce RBCs.

Pernicious anemia is due to a genetic deficiency in the ability of the stomach lining to produce intrinsic factor, which is needed to absorb vitamin B_{12} from the gastrointestinal tract. Vitamin B_{12} is needed in the Kreb's cycle. When it is deficient, energy production is reduced. This particularly affects rapidly dividing cells, such as those in the bone marrow that produce RBCs.

Anemia from increased destruction of RBCs is called *hemolytic anemia*. Sickle cell disease (discussed in the next section) is one cause of premature RBC destruction. Other causes include genetic and autoimmune problems and exposure to toxic chemicals or drugs.

Sickle Cell Disease

Sickle cell disease is a genetic disorder more common in people of African, Mediterranean, Middle Eastern, Caribbean, and South and Central American origin or descent. Patients who have inherited an abnormal gene from both parents have an abnormal form of hemoglobin that causes RBCs to take on an abnormal curved (sickle-shaped) appearance when oxygen dissociates from them in the tissues (Figure 26-6). It can regain its normal shape when reoxygenated, but the changes in the shape of the cell damage it, decreasing its life span. The abnormal RBCs live only 10 to 20 days, instead of the normal 120 days. Even though bone marrow production of RBCs is increased, it cannot keep pace with the rate of destruction, resulting in a low hematocrit.

The abnormal shape of sickle cells makes it difficult for them to move through capillaries, and they are more prone to clumping together. When clumps of sickle cells obstruct capillary beds, this is called a *vaso-occlusive crisis*. The tissues supplied by the obstructed capillaries become ischemic, resulting in pain and microinfarction of tissues. Vaso-occlusive crises can result in priapism in males. The intensity of crises varies, but can be excruciatingly painful, requiring narcotic analgesia. In the prehospital setting, administration of oxygen and hydration are critical elements of treatment. Consult with medical direction concerning analgesia, because it is an important part of sickle cell crisis management.

In splenic sequestration crisis, blood pools in the spleen, resulting in painful enlargement of the spleen and a decrease in circulating blood volume. Patients are at risk for stroke, blindness, leg ulcers, and renal failure, and the excessive amount of bilirubin from hemolysis can lead to gallstones and cholecystitis. Damage of the spleen makes the patient essentially asplenic, and more prone to certain kinds of infections. Ultimately, the life expectancy is shortened.

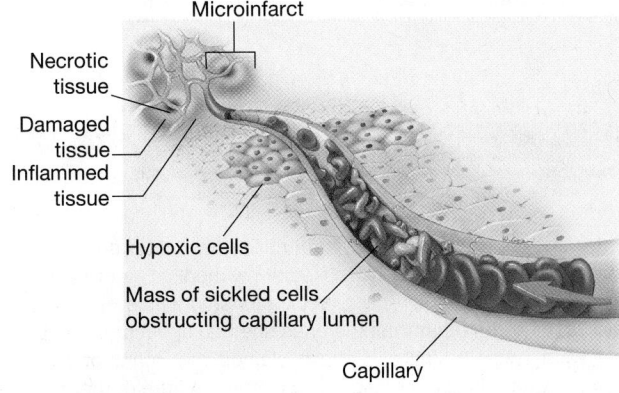

FIGURE 26-6

In sickle cell disease, abnormal hemoglobin proteins change shape after releasing oxygen, causing the red blood cells to become sickle shaped. The abnormally shaped red blood cells can cause vaso-occlusive crisis and have a short life span.

White Blood Cell Disorders

An increased WBC count (leukocytosis) is an indication of infection, inflammation, or blood cancers (leukemia). An examination of the types of WBCs responsible for the increase and their stage of maturity (differential) helps determine the type of infection (or inflammatory process) and its duration. Leukopenia is a decrease in WBCs, which can occur due to bone marrow suppression or destruction from chemotherapy or radiation therapy. Other causes include viral infections that suppress bone marrow function, cancers, and autoimmune diseases.

Leukemia

Leukemia is a cancer that causes the bone marrow to rapidly produce large numbers of abnormal WBCs. The abnormal cells can crowd out normal cells, resulting in anemia, bleeding, and infection. There are several types of leukemia, some of which are acute and others that are chronic. Leukemias are further named for the type of cell affected. Cells may be from the lymphocytic or myelocytic cell lines. Some types of leukemia, such as acute lymphoblastic leukemia (ALL) and acute myelogenous leukemia (AML) occur in children and adults, while others, such as chronic lymphocytic leukemia (CLL) and chronic myelogenous leukemia (CML) occur primarily in adults. Common signs and symptoms include easy bruising, bone pain, enlarged spleen, swollen lymph nodes, repeated infections, and fatigue. Life span after diagnosis and survival rates depends on the type of leukemia.

Lymphoma

Lymphomas are cancers of lymphocytes, either B lymphocytes or T lymphocytes, that are localized to the lymph notes. Lymphomas may either be Hodgkin's lymphoma or non-Hodgkin's lymphoma. Hodgkin's lymphoma involves specific types of B lymphocytes and non-Hodgkin's lymphoma can involve abnormal B lymphocytes or T lymphocytes. With treatment, the survival rate for Hodgkin's lymphoma is very high, and is relatively high for non-Hodgkin's lymphomas. Patients may give a history of profuse, abnormal night sweats (truly drenching the bed while sleeping) that is only seen in some lymphomas and in tuberculosis (TB) infections.

Multiple Myeloma

Multiple myeloma is a cancer of cells in the bone marrow in which abnormal cells multiply and crowd out normal cells. This results in decreased production of blood cells, and can result in **pathologic fracture** of the affected bone. Patients with multiple myeloma may present with a complaint of severe low back pain.

Clotting Disorders

Clotting disorders, also called *bleeding disorders,* are collectively known as *coagulopathies.* The underlying problem can involve platelets or the clotting cascade.

Platelet Disorders

Impaired hemostasis can occur from a low number of platelets (thrombocytopenia) or altered platelet function. Platelets can be reduced in number or impaired by leukemia or other bone marrow disorders. A number of drugs, either by themselves or because of interactions with other drugs, can reduce platelet function. In some cases, decreased platelet aggregation is desired, because it reduces the risk of stroke and acute myocardial infarction (AMI) in patients at risk. However, complications can occur, such as bruising, gastrointestinal bleeding, hemorrhagic stroke, and epistaxis. Increased platelet count can occur in some bone marrow disorders, resulting in risks for both bleeding and clotting (thrombocytosis).

Hemophilia

The complex clotting cascade requires approximately 20 different plasma proteins known as *clotting factors,* as well as other substances. Hemophilia is an inherited disease that leads to deficiencies in certain clotting factors. Hemophilia A is an X chromosome defect that results in deficiency of clotting factor VIII. Because females have two X chromosomes, they may carry one normal and one defective gene for factor VII, and can be carriers for the disease, but their blood clotting is normal. However, if a male inherits the defective X chromosome, he will have hemophilia A. Hemophilia B is also an X-linked inherited disorder. In this case, the deficient clotting factor is factor IX. There also are deficiencies of other clotting factors, which can result from liver disease, anticoagulant use, autoimmune disease, complications following childbirth, and vitamin K deficiency. Von Willebrand disease is an inherited deficiency of von Willebrand factor, which is important in both platelet aggregation and preventing breakdown of some clotting factors.

Patients with hemophilia and deficiencies of other clotting factors can have mild to severe impairment in blood clotting. In some cases, the disease can be treated with replacement of the specific clotting factor, especially after trauma or in conjunction with surgery. Signs and symptoms include painful, swollen joints (from bleeding into the joint space), abnormal menstrual bleeding, bleeding gums, bruising, epistaxis, rash, purpura, petechiae, prolonged bleeding from injuries and medical procedures, gastrointestinal bleeding, and urinary tract bleeding. Often, patients are aware of their disease and may have clotting factors at home that they self-administer in the event of traumatic injuries.

Blood Clots and Deep Vein Thrombosis

Deep vein thrombosis (DVT) occurs when blood clots form in the deep, large veins of legs, pelvis, or more rarely, the arms. Predisposing factors include fractures, abdominal surgery, immobilization (including sitting for long periods, especially with the legs crossed), pregnancy, hormones used for birth control or hormone replacement therapy after menopause, cancer, and heart and lung disease. DVT can present with a warm, painful, swollen lower extremity. In particular, if the DVT is in the lower leg, pain may increase in the calf with dorsiflexion of the foot. If a DVT breaks loose, it can travel to the right side of the heart and into the pulmonary circulation, causing a pulmonary embolism. Upper extremity DVTs are very rare, usually seen only in IV drug users, but their ability to cause pulmonary emboli is similar to that of lower extremity DVT. Patients diagnosed with, or at high risk for, DVT are usually prescribed anticoagulant medications.

PERSONAL PERSPECTIVE

Mr. Russell Parker: I hear now and then about different drugs and supplements that are good for reducing the risk of heart disease and stroke, improving memory, reducing cancer risk—all kinds of things. Little by little I added a medication here and a supplement there. Fish oil, garlic capsules, an aspirin a day, some gingko for my memory, and St. John's wort for my mood. I slipped and fell on my floor a few weeks ago. It's a hard stone tile floor and it hurt like you wouldn't believe, but I didn't break anything and I didn't think too much of it. A few hours later I had the beginnings of a really nasty bruise on my thigh. By the next morning the entire side of my leg was black and blue. I knew I fell hard, but I didn't expect that kind of bruise. I called my doctor and she saw me that afternoon. She looked at my medical record and asked me if I was taking any medications, vitamins, supplements, or herbs other than the ones she had on record. I told her what I was taking and she explained that many of the things I was taking decrease blood clotting. A little of that effect is good, she said, but too much means your blood can't clot normally when it needs to. She helped me find the right combinations and dosages of medications and supplements to meet my needs. Now, when I hear about a home treatment I am interested in, I research it a little harder before deciding whether or not to take it.

Disseminated Intravascular Coagulation

DIC results from systemic overactivation of clotting mechanisms. Systemic activation of clotting mechanisms can result from blood transfusion reactions, sepsis, surgery, and severe trauma. Small blood clots form that cause infarcts of affected organs, including the brain, liver, and kidneys. Because of the excess clotting, clotting factors are consumed and subsequent bleeding cannot be stopped. At this point, the patient has bleeding from multiple sites. Treatment is difficult because the patient is experiencing increased clotting and decreased clotting simultaneously.

CASE STUDY WRAP-UP

Clinical-Reasoning Process

Advanced EMTs Cecil and Eliza have just learned that their patient, nine-year-old Clancy, has sickle cell disease and a chief complaint of pain in the left upper quadrant of his abdomen for 45 minutes. In response to Cecil's questions, Clancy reveals that the pain is a 7 on a scale of 1 to 10, and that it is constant. He had just come home from school when the pain began. He has been unable to find anything that makes it better, and he says the pain is constant and has been getting worse. Clancy appears pale and his skin is moist and cool. He is alert, but restless. Clancy denies any other complaints, aside from the abdominal pain.

Cecil recognizes sickle cell disease as a hematologic disorder that can have painful and potentially life-threatening complications. His first thought is that, no matter what the cause of the pain, patients with sickle cell disease are made worse in conditions when there is increased need for oxygen in the tissues. He prepares a simple face mask to administer oxygen to Clancy at 8 L/min, while Eliza takes a set of vital signs. Cecil's examination of Clancy's abdomen reveals tenderness in the left upper quadrant with voluntary guarding.

Cecil suspects that Clancy's spleen is engorged with blood and that his lowered circulatory volume and pain are both contributing to his restlessness and pale, cool, moist skin. Eliza reports a blood pressure of 90/66, heart rate of 116, respirations of 24, and SpO$_2$ of 96 percent after oxygen administration.

"I'm really sorry you aren't feeling well, Clancy," says Cecil. "Eliza and I are going to get you ready to go to the hospital and your mom will be with you in the ambulance. I'm going to start some treatment before we get to the hospital and I will call the doctor on my radio to see what else we can do to make you feel better."

En route, Clancy says, "You said you've had an IV before and that it wasn't too bad. I'm going to start an IV on you now so we can give you some fluids. Are you warm enough? Do you need another blanket?"

After covering Clancy with another blanket and starting the IV, Cecil rechecks vital signs and checks to determine Clancy's pain level. A few minutes later, Cecil and Eliza wheel Clancy to the triage desk and give the nurse an update.

CHAPTER REVIEW

Chapter Summary

Knowledge of hematology, the study of blood and blood forming organs, helps you identify and understand a variety of blood disorders and their complications. This knowledge helps you anticipate patients' problems and plan appropriate treatment.

Blood is comprised of plasma, which serves as a transport medium, and formed elements. Plasma contains a variety of proteins, including albumin, antibodies, and clotting factors, as well as electrolytes, nutrients, and other substances. RBCs carry oxygen and carbon dioxide bound to hemoglobin for gas exchange. A decrease in RBCs from blood loss, decreased production, or increased destruction can lead to tissue hypoxia. The abnormal shape of RBCs in sickle cell disease leads to both increased hemolysis and microvascular occlusion by clumps of abnormal cells, resulting in sickle cell crisis. Antigens on the RBC surface provide the basis of blood typing. Exposure to antigens from donor blood can result in transfusion reactions.

An increase in WBCs can be a result of response to infection or inflammation, or a pathologic process, such as leukemia. Each type of WBC has specific functions, so that examination of the types of blood cells responsible for the increase provides valuable clues in the diagnosis of disease. A decrease in white blood cells, as may occur from chemotherapy or radiation, places a patient at increased risk of infection.

The hemostatic process involves vasospasm, platelet aggregation, and the clotting cascade. Platelet function and coagulation can be decreased by a number of medications. A patient's list of medications can provide information about the risk of impaired blood clotting, which can complicate trauma and planned medical procedures, such as IV access. Increased coagulation can occur in response to serious illness, such as cancer, or trauma. Abnormal localized blood clotting can cause DVT, which can lead to pulmonary embolism. Systemic over-activation of clotting mechanisms is called *DIC*.

In the general management of patients with hematologic disorders, consider the need for oxygen, intravenous fluids, and analgesia.

Review Questions

Multiple-Choice Questions

1. Which one of the following is a characteristic of RBCs?
   a. Large nucleus
   b. Spherical shape
   c. Hundreds of mitochondria
   d. Use anaerobic metabolism

2. The percentage of volume of blood comprised of formed elements is the:
   a. hemoglobin.
   b. saturation.
   c. differential.
   d. hematocrit.

3. Which one of the following best describes the function of platelets?
   a. They form stable blood clots.
   b. They clump together to form a temporary plug in an injured blood vessel.
   c. They engulf bacteria and debris as part of the immune response.
   d. They stimulate substances that break down fibrin clots.

4. A patient has type O negative blood. What blood types could he safely receive in a transfusion?
   a. AB negative and O negative
   b. A negative, B negative, and O negative
   c. O negative
   d. O negative and O positive

5. A patient has fine, pinpoint hemorrhages in the skin that look like a rash. This best fits the description of:
   a. petechiae.
   b. purpura.
   c. pruritus.
   d. priapism.

6. Which one of the following is the primary feature of anemia?
   a. Increase in abnormal WBCs
   b. Decrease in RBCs
   c. Decrease in platelets
   d. Increase in plasma albumin

7. Which one of the following occurs in sickle cell disease?
   a. Decreased RBC production
   b. Abnormally shaped WBCs
   c. Abnormal proteins that comprise part of the hemoglobin
   d. Platelets fragment into smaller portions

8. A 52-year-old male patient is recovering from surgery to remove part of his colon due to colon cancer. He presents with pain and swelling in his left lower leg. When you examine the leg, it is red, warm, and tender. He has no other complaints. He states the pain and swelling have become progressively worse since yesterday. Which one of the following is most consistent with the information provided?
   a. Lymphoma
   b. Hemophilia
   c. Deep vein thrombosis
   d. Vaso-occlusive crisis

Critical-Thinking Questions

9. Your patient has cirrhosis of the liver. What hematologic problems should you anticipate?

10. How can oxygen benefit a patient with vaso-occlusive crisis?

11. Your patient is a 23-year-old involved in a motor vehicle collision in which he was the driver of a small car struck in the driver's side by a large pick-up truck. He is complaining of left shoulder pain and gives a history of hemophilia. Describe your concerns about the patient's condition. What treatment will you provide?

12. Your patient is an 80-year-old woman with varicose veins. She says she bumped her leg on a coffee table an hour ago but she has not been able to stop the bleeding. You note smears of blood on carpet and sofa, as well as some saturated bandages. What are some theories about the cause of excessive bleeding in this patient? Describe your assessment and treatment.

Additional Reading

Centers for Disease Control and Prevention. (2010). *Blood disorders.* http://www.cdc.gov/ncbddd/blooddisorders/

Martini, F. H., Bartholomew, E. F, & Bledsoe, B. E. (2008). *Anatomy and physiology for emergency care* (2nd ed.). Upper Saddle River, NJ: Pearson.

27

Immunologic Disorders

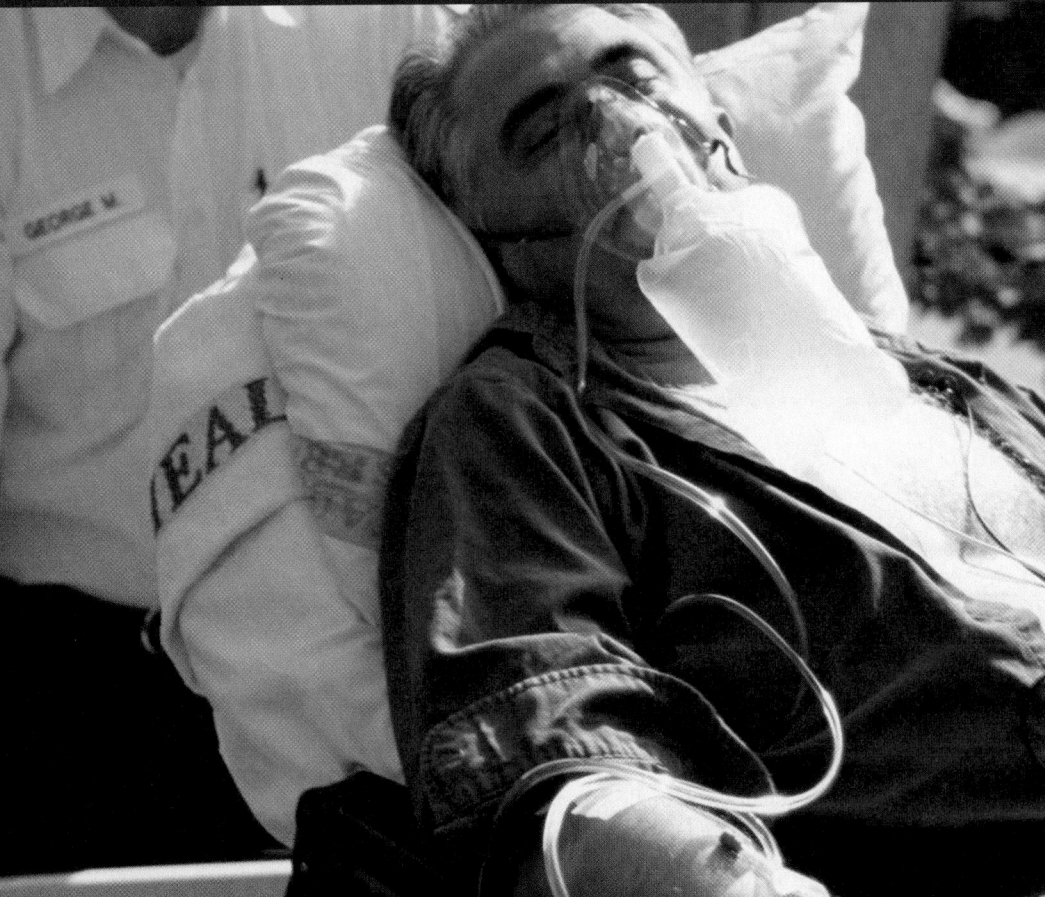

Content Area: Medicine

Advanced EMT Education Standard: Applies fundamental knowledge to provide basic and selected advanced emergency care and transportation based on assessment findings for an acutely ill patient.

Objectives

After reading this chapter, you should be able to:

27.1 Define key terms introduced in this chapter.

27.2 Explain the importance of being able to recognize and treat anaphylactic reactions.

27.3 Describe the pathophysiologic process by which exposure to an antigen results in anaphylaxis.

27.4 Recognize the signs, symptoms, and history associated with anaphylaxis.

27.5 Explain the life-threatening mechanisms of anaphylaxis, including airway compromise, impaired ventilation and oxygenation, and impaired perfusion.

27.6 Describe the effects of excessive histamine release on the body.

27.7 Describe the difference between an anaphylactic and an anaphylactoid reaction.

(continued)

Resource Central

To access Resource Central, follow the directions on the Student Access Card provided with this text. If there is no card, go to www.bradybooks.com and follow the Resource Central link to Buy Access. Under Media Resources, you will find:

• *What Is Allergic Rhinitis?* Watch and learn about allergic rhinitis and why it afflicts so many people.

• *Anaphylaxis.* Learn about the causes of anaphylaxis, signs and symptoms, and emergency treatment.

• *Autoimmune Diseases.* Discover the different types of autoimmune diseases and how they disrupt the normal functioning of the immune system.

CASE STUDY

"Ambulance 21, Engine 24, respond to the soccer field at Ehrlich Park, 3800 West 10th Street, for a child with an allergic reaction."

Firefighter/Advanced EMTs Erin Boomershine and Dale Arlen acknowledge the dispatch and leave their post, heading west on 10th Street. They arrive at the park in just under 2 minutes. They are met by an anxious soccer coach who explains that a boy on the team brought a treat for everyone after practice and one of the players with a peanut allergy ate a cookie, not realizing there was peanut butter in it. The patient is eight-year-old Jackson Lyles. He is sitting on the ground, looking anxious.

Problem-Solving Questions

1. What should Erin and Dale consider in the scene size-up for this situation?
2. What findings would confirm an allergic reaction?
3. What findings would differentiate a mild allergic reaction from an anaphylactic reaction?
4. How would the treatment for a mild allergic reaction differ from that of an anaphylactic reaction?

(continued from previous page)

27.8	Apply knowledge of substances that commonly cause anaphylactic and anaphylactoid reactions to develop an appropriate index of suspicion for these conditions.	
27.9	Discuss each of the ways that an antigen can be introduced into the body.	
27.10	Differentiate between patients who require prehospital treatment with epinephrine and those who do not.	
27.11	Explain the importance of limiting exposure to the antigen as a step in the treatment of the patient with an allergic or anaphylactic reaction.	
27.12	Describe the roles of airway management, fluid administration, and medications in the treatment of allergic and anaphylactic reactions.	
27.13	Given a variety of scenarios of patients with allergic and anaphylactic reactions, implement an appropriate treatment plan for each.	
27.14	Explain the necessity of ongoing evaluation of the patient having, or at risk for, an anaphylactic reaction.	
27.15	Recognize conditions that compromise immunity.	
27.16	Describe the basic pathophysiology of common autoimmune/collagen vascular diseases.	
27.17	Describe considerations for patients living with transplanted organs or tissues.	

Introduction

The body has both nonspecific and specific defenses against disease. They are remarkable mechanisms that protect us from the multitude of pathogens encountered every day. When any of the ways in which our bodies protect us against disease fails, illnesses that normally would not pose a serious risk can be life threatening. Patients whose immune systems are suppressed by chemotherapy, radiation, age, or illness, including human immunodeficiency virus (HIV), are more susceptible to infections and

cancer. Patients who have received organ transplants take medications that suppress the immune response to prevent rejection of the donor organ. Unfortunately, immune suppression is not highly selective and the patient is placed at increase risk of infection. Medications taken for other reasons, such as corticosteroids, also suppress the immune system.

What may seem less obvious is that life-threatening illnesses also can be caused by hypersensitivity of the immune system. Anaphylaxis and autoimmune diseases are both caused by reaction of the immune system to substances that do not normally cause an immune reaction. In an allergic reaction, the immune system recognizes an otherwise harmless foreign substance, such as a protein in shellfish, as harmful and launches an attack against it. In anaphylaxis, that attack is exaggerated, resulting in life-threatening events such as hypotension and airway swelling. Advanced EMTs are able to administer epinephrine, a simple but life-saving treatment. In patients with autoimmune diseases, the immune system recognizes the body's own tissues as foreign materials.

This chapter gives an overview of the anatomy and physiology of the immune system, and of the pathophysiology of selected immunologic disorders. You learn the importance of recognizing and protecting patients with immunosuppression, as well as how to recognize and manage patients with allergic and anaphylactic reactions.

Anatomy and Physiology Review

Nonspecific body defenses may recognize a substance as harmful, but do not have to recognize exactly what the substance is to protect the body against it. Nonspecific defenses include the following:

- Mechanical and chemical protection provided by the skin and mucous membranes

- Antimicrobial substances in the blood and interstitial fluid (such as interferons and the complement system)

- Natural killer cells (a type of lymphocyte)

- Phagocytosis (cellular ingestion of foreign material and debris)

- Inflammation

- Fever

Specific resistance to disease is called *immunity.* Substances that are recognized by the immune system as foreign and provoke an immune response are called **antigens,** which, in most cases, are proteins. The immune system has memory for most previously encountered antigens so that a second encounter stimulates a more rapid and robust response.

The functions of the immune system are carried out by white blood cells called *lymphocytes.* Both B lymphocytes and T lymphocytes develop from stem cells in the bone marrow. B cells mature in the bone marrow, but immature T cells migrate to the thymus for maturation. Both types of lymphocytes have surface proteins that act as antigen receptors. During an initial response to an antigen, very few cells have correct specificity for the antigen. The immune response results in the development of thousands of memory cells that can proliferate and differentiate rapidly upon subsequent exposure to the antigen. This is the basis for immunization by vaccination, as well as active natural immunity.

One way in which immunologic memory works is through the creation of specific **antibodies** that recognize specific antigens. There are five main classes of antibodies (also called *immunoglobulins*), each of which plays different roles. Immunoglobulin E (IgE), the antibody involved in allergic and anaphylactic reactions, comprises less than 0.1 percent of all antibodies. It has an affinity for binding to mast cells (in the tissue) and basophils (circulating). When there is recognition of a specific antigen by IgE, it causes the mast cells and basophils to release histamine, heparin, and other chemical mediators of inflammation from granules within the cells. The inflammatory response produced by histamine and heparin are usually localized and beneficial in ridding the body of the antigen. In anaphylaxis, the responses are systemic and exaggerated.

General Assessment and Management of Immunologic Emergencies

You may be called to care for patients who have a variety of immunologic problems, but the one that is most likely to present an immediate threat to life is an anaphylactic reaction. **Anaphylaxis** is a type of shock. Quick recognition of, and intervention for, problems with the airway, breathing, and circulation are the highest priorities for all patients, and can truly make the difference between life and death for patients with anaphylaxis.

Scene Size-Up

Occasionally, an allergic or anaphylactic reaction can be caused by a substance that provides a risk to others, as well as to the allergic patient. Bee and wasp stings are most often due to a single insect. But, sometimes, the stings are caused by a swarm of insects. When multiple stings occur, even patients who are not allergic can become quite ill. Do not enter an area with a swarm of bees or wasps. Instead, determine the number of patients and request resources needed to manage the situation. In other cases, if the substance does not pose a hazard to you, ensure that the patient is no longer in contact with the substance to which he is allergic. Continued exposure to the antigen will worsen the patient's condition.

Your first look at the patient may give you clues that an anaphylactic reaction is occurring. Swelling of the face and tongue, hives, stridor, and wheezing are signs of anaphylaxis. Determine from the patient or bystanders the nature of the illness and chief complaint. The onset of anaphylaxis usually begins within 30 to 60 seconds after exposure to the antigen, but it may take as long as an hour. As a general rule, the more rapid the onset is, the more severe the reaction.

Primary Assessment

If a patient is apparently unresponsive and not breathing, immediately check a pulse. If the pulse is absent, begin chest compressions and apply an AED. Otherwise, carefully assess the patient's airway status. Anaphylaxis can produce airway swelling, which can produce stridor (Figure 27-1). If the patient's face and lips are swollen, suspect that the tongue and airway tissues also may be swollen. Anaphylaxis can produce enough swelling to obstruct the airway. This is likely to render your usual approaches to airway management ineffective, and perhaps even dangerous. Insertion of an oropharyngeal airway can traumatize the already swollen mucous membranes, resulting in bleeding and increased edema. The size of devices such as Combitubes, LMAs, and King airways may prevent you from inserting them without causing trauma and additional swelling.

Unless you are able to perform an endotracheal intubation, it may be best to use manual airway maneuvers and a bag-valve-mask device. In patients with impending airway obstruction from edema, the person with the best intubation skills should perform the intubation. The intubation will be difficult and inexpert technique can increase airway edema. If available and indicated by severe airway obstruction, endotracheal intubation and cricothyrotomy (surgical airway) can be lifesaving. If ALS is available, request their assistance immediately. If ALS is not available, prepare to transport the patient to the nearest emergency department.

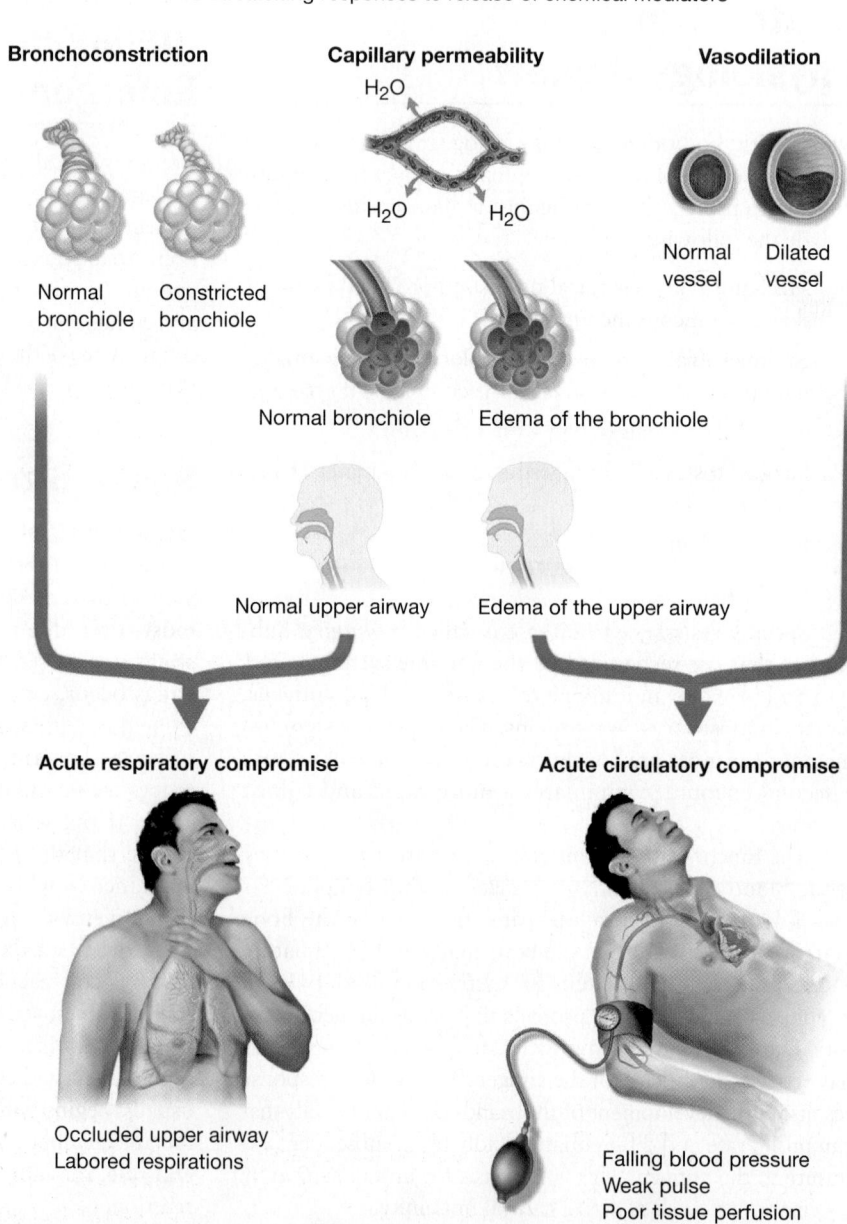

ANAPHYLAXIS
Life-threatening responses to release of chemical mediators

Bronchoconstriction

Normal bronchiole   Constricted bronchiole

Capillary permeability

H_2O

H_2O H_2O

Normal bronchiole   Edema of the bronchiole

Normal upper airway   Edema of the upper airway

Vasodilation

Normal vessel   Dilated vessel

Acute respiratory compromise

Occluded upper airway
Labored respirations

Acute circulatory compromise

Falling blood pressure
Weak pulse
Poor tissue perfusion

FIGURE 27-1

Life-threatening responses in anaphylactic reaction: bronchoconstriction, capillary permeability, vasodilation, and an increase in mucus production.

Observe the patient for signs of respiratory distress, including wheezing, grunting, drowsiness, use of accessory muscles, tachypnea, and cyanosis. Depending on the degree of distress, provide oxygen by nonrebreather mask or use a bag-valve mask with supplemental oxygen to assist ventilations.

Observe the patient for signs of shock. Check the pulse for presence, rate, and strength. Observe the patient for diaphoresis, pale skin or mucous membranes, and altered mental status. During this assessment, the finding of **urticaria**, or hives (Figure 27-2), will reinforce a hypothesis of anaphylaxis.

Although giving medications is not usually one of the priorities in the primary assessment, epinephrine is a way of managing airway, breathing, and circulation in a patient with anaphylaxis. The actions of epinephrine can help reduce airway edema, dilate bronchiolar smooth muscle, and constrict the peripheral vasculature. Once you determine that the patient's presentation is consistent with anaphylaxis, be prepared to administer epinephrine.

Secondary Assessment

For noncritical patients, perform a focused history and assessment. Check for edema and urticaria, and assess vital signs, breath sounds, and SpO₂. Obtain a SAMPLE history and use relevant parts of OPQRST to obtain details about the chief complaint. For critical patients, defer additional history and assessment until you have performed interventions for airway, breathing, and circulation. You should then perform a rapid medical assessment, including listening to breath sounds, and if indicated, a head-to-toe examination. Obtain a baseline set of vital signs, including SpO₂, and a SAMPLE history. If the patient has an altered mental status, perform blood glucose analysis.

Clinical-Reasoning Process

The signs and symptoms of anaphylaxis are usually obvious, if not always unique to anaphylaxis. By definition, anaphylaxis is life threatening. The patient will have a problem with airway, breathing, and circulation. As a result, the patient's mental status may be altered, and hypotension and tachycardia are likely. A specific sign of anaphylaxis is urticaria. Most often, there is a history of anaphylaxis and a known history of exposure. Sudden onset of abdominal cramps and diarrhea are also possible with anaphylaxis, particularly with ingested antigens. In most cases, it is not difficult to arrive at a clinical impression of anaphylaxis.

Treatment

Treatment decisions are different for patients with allergic reactions than they are for anaphylaxis. A patient with a mild allergic reaction, such as some hives without difficulty breathing or hypotension, may not require immediate prehospital treatment. A patient with an allergic reaction that produces mild to moderate wheezing without airway swelling or hypotension may be best served by giving an albuterol treatment. The patient with anaphylaxis needs airway management, possibly assisted ventilation, administration of epinephrine, and intravenous fluids.

In most other cases, patients with immunologic problems require whatever treatment is indicated by their specific complaints and presentations. A patient with HIV may present with sepsis, requiring oxygen and intravenous fluids. A patient taking immunosuppressant drugs may present with a mild fever and body aches, but with adequate SpO₂ and vital signs.

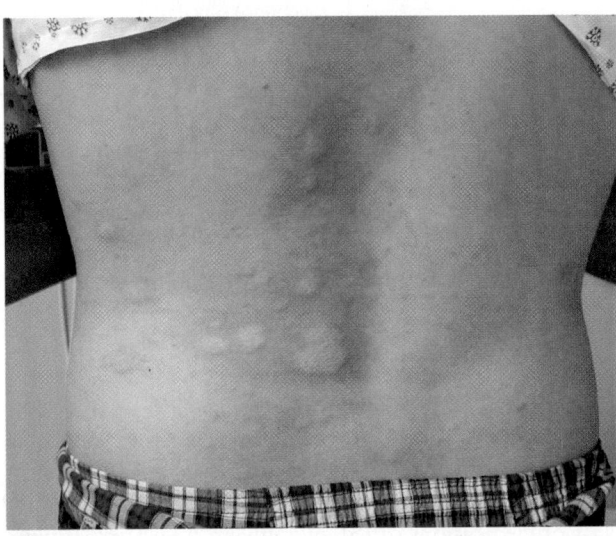

(A)

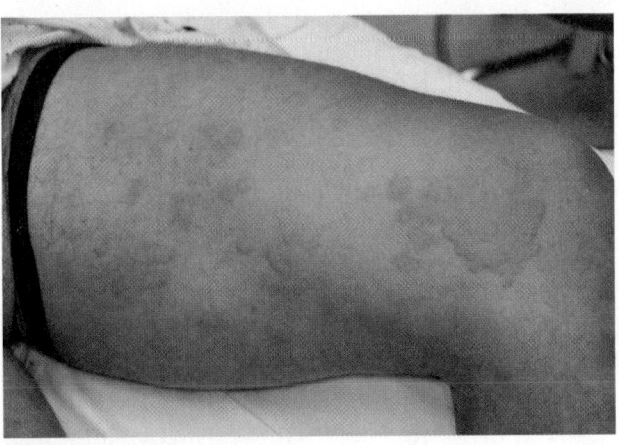

(B)

FIGURE 27-2

(A) Hives (urticaria) from an allergic reaction to a penicillin-derivative drug. (© Charles Stewart, MD, and Associates) (B) Hives on the lower extremity. (© Edward T. Dickinson, MD)

Reassessment

For patients in anaphylaxis, continually monitor the airway, breathing, and circulation, because they can deteriorate rapidly. Look for changes in mental status, edema, breath sounds, vital signs, and SpO_2. Anxiety and tachycardia may be a result of epinephrine administration, but are also signs of shock. Check with the patient about changes in complaints or additional complaints. Be aware that epinephrine can be very effective, but its duration of action is short; about 10 to 20 minutes when given intramuscularly. Patients may require an additional dose of epinephrine. Keep in mind, as well, that epinephrine has powerful effects on the cardiovascular system. Patients may experience tachycardia, tremors, and chest pain.

Allergies and Anaphylaxis

Both allergic reactions and anaphylactic reactions are known as *hypersensitivity reactions*. A mild allergic reaction is at one end of the spectrum and severe, life-threatening anaphylaxis is at the other. In both cases, the body is exposed to an antigen (also called an *allergen*) that normally does not provoke an immune response, and develops immunologic memory (Table 27-1). This is called *sensitization*, or a *primary response*. On subsequent exposure, there is a rapid response to the antigen, called a *secondary response*. On the milder end, some reactions are called *delayed cell-mediated hypersensitivity reactions*. The reaction is caused by T cell response. One example of this is poison ivy. The rash does not occur until several hours after exposure to the plant.

In other cases, antibodies produced by B cells during sensitization are carried by mast cells and basophils. The antigen is recognized by the antibodies, producing an antigen–antibody reaction. This is called an *immediate hypersensitivity response*. Some of the most common causes of immediate hypersensitivity responses include drugs (such as antibiotics and narcotics), foods (peanuts, sesame seeds, shellfish), and insects (bees, wasps). Like toxins, antigens can enter the body in a variety of ways, including ingestion (foods, medications), inhalation (pollen), injection (insect venom, medications), and skin contact (poison ivy, latex).

A similar type of reaction called an **anaphylactoid reaction** occurs in response to substances such as dyes used in radiology procedures. The signs and symptoms

TABLE 27-1	Common Allergens
Type of Allergen	**Examples**
Insect venom	▪ Bees, wasps, hornets, fire ants
Medications	▪ Antibiotics (penicillin, sulfa antibiotics, cephalosporin antibiotics) ▪ Aspirin ▪ Opiates (codeine) ▪ Local anesthetics (lidocaine, novocaine, procaine)
Foods	▪ Peanuts ▪ Tree nuts ▪ Shellfish ▪ Eggs ▪ Milk ▪ Sesame seeds ▪ Fruits (strawberries, kiwi, avocado) ▪ Chocolate
Pollen	▪ Trees ▪ Weeds ▪ Grasses
Latex	▪ Medical devices ▪ Medical gloves ▪ Elastic ▪ Rubber bands ▪ Carpet and rug backing

are the same as those of anaphylaxis, but the reaction is not a result of IgE reaction with an antigen. Another situation that can present as anaphylaxis is a reaction to a class of medications called *angiotensin converting enzyme (ACE) inhibitors*, used to treat hypertension. Examples include benazepril (Lotensin), captopril (Capoten), and enalapril (Vasotec), though there are many ACE inhibitors on the market. Patients can experience an acute onset

IN THE FIELD

The signs and symptoms of allergic reactions result from the body's attempts to rid the antigen from the body or prevent further exposure to the antigen. Coughing, sneezing, and watery eyes all work to remove the antigen from the body. When antigens are ingested, increased peristalsis, vomiting, and diarrhea work to rid the body of the antigen. With respiratory exposure, slight bronchoconstriction is aimed at limiting exposure. Angioedema allows antigens to be moved out of the circulation and into the tissues where the immune system can destroy them. In an anaphylactic reaction, these mechanisms go awry, resulting in life-threatening airway obstruction and fluid loss.

Pediatric Care

Children with food allergies may inadvertently be exposed to foods they are allergic to at birthday parties, school, and other situations where they are away from their parents.

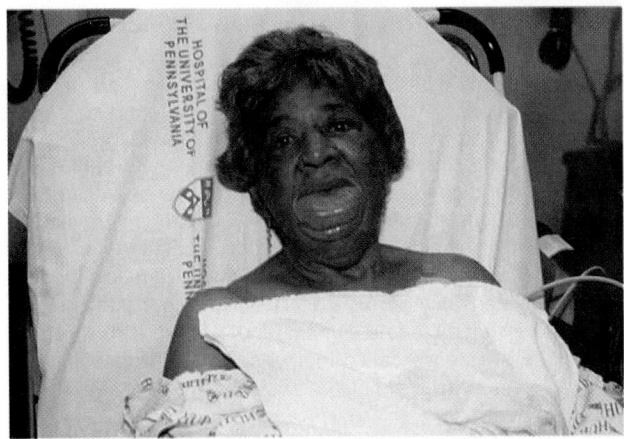

FIGURE 27-3

Angioedema of the tongue. (© Edward T. Dickinson, MD)

of **angioedema** (edema due to vasodilation and increased vascular permeability, also called *angioneurotic edema*) of the tongue and mouth (Figure 27-3).

An IgE-mediated allergic reaction causes a number of chemical mediators of the allergic reaction to be released from the cell. Among those substances is histamine, which is responsible for a number of the manifestations of allergic and anaphylactic reactions. In milder cases, such as seasonal allergies, the signs and symptoms are uncomfortable, but not life threatening. In more severe cases, the effects of histamine are more pronounced and widespread, and can be life threatening (Table 27-2).

Signs and Symptoms of Anaphylaxis

The effects of histamine include peripheral vasodilation, increased vascular permeability, and constriction of bronchiolar and gastrointestinal smooth muscle. The vasodilation and increased vascular permeability results in itching, hives, edema, distributive shock, and hypovolemic shock. Edema in the airway can cause varying degrees of airway obstruction, resulting in hoarseness, stridor, or complete obstruction. The smooth muscle constriction results in bronchospasm with restriction to airflow and wheezing, and sometimes results in abdominal cramping and diarrhea.

IN THE FIELD

Patients are often puzzled by hives because they arise in one area, causing concern, but by the time they are examined the hives in that area have disappeared, only to appear somewhere else on the body. That is the nature of hives. They are caused by transient vasodilation and increased vascular permeability. Hives are raised areas that can be widespread or localized, vary in size, and itch intensely. They often are paler in the center with a red flare around the border.

TABLE 27-2	Signs and Symptoms of Allergic Reactions	
	Mild Allergic Reaction	**Anaphylaxis**
Onset	Usually slower and more gradual than anaphylaxis	Usually rapid, often within 30 to 60 seconds of exposure, but up to 1 hour
Skin	Itching, hives	Itching and hives, may be widespread; diaphoresis, may be flushed; cyanosis with severe respiratory involvement
Angioedema	Mild	May be severe enough to cause airway obstruction; stridor indicates significant partial airway obstruction
Mental status	Normal, may be anxious	Anxiety, confusion, decreased responsiveness
Lungs	May have mild or scattered wheezing	May have significant wheezing in all lung fields
Vital signs	Normal	Hypotension, tachycardia, weak peripheral pulses, tachypnea, respiratory distress
Gastrointestinal system	Nausea, increased peristalsis	Nausea, vomiting, diarrhea

The severity of anaphylactic reactions tends to be related to their speed of onset, with more severe reactions developing more quickly after exposure to the antigen. However, you should anticipate that any patient with signs and symptoms of an allergic reaction has the potential to worsen. In general, the severity of signs and symptoms tends to increase with each subsequent exposure.

Most often, the patient knows what he is allergic to. Patients may wear medical identification jewelry that identifies their allergy and they might carry an epinephrine autoinjector for self-administration of epinephrine (Figure 27-4). Some autoinjectors come with one dose of epinephrine and some come with two doses. Autoinjectors are available in both pediatric and adult dosages.

PERSONAL PERSPECTIVE

dvanced EMT Gail Paul: I had a call a few weeks ago for a patient who experienced a sudden onset of hives and wheezing. I asked about allergies and the patient told me he was allergic to aspirin, but he hadn't taken any aspirin and didn't even keep any in the house. I asked him about any medications he used. He said he took some Tylenol for arthritis in his back about an hour before the hives and wheezing started. I knew that acetaminophen is not a common cause of allergies, so I kept asking about other substances the patient might have been exposed to. I asked about foods and if he used anything else for his arthritis. He said he used an extra-strength arthritis cream on his back. As he said it, I noticed the slight aroma of wintergreen. I made a note of it, but didn't know what it meant at the time. Later, I talked with one of the nurses at the hospital emergency department. She said she was glad I documented the arthritis rub, because the patient didn't consider it a medication and didn't mention it in his history. It turns out that a lot of topical arthritis creams contain oil of wintergreen, which contains a substance called methyl salicylate. It is closely related to aspirin and should be avoided by people with aspirin allergies.

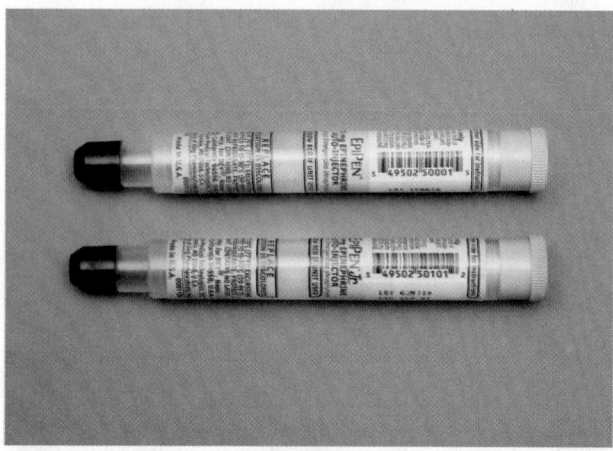

(A)

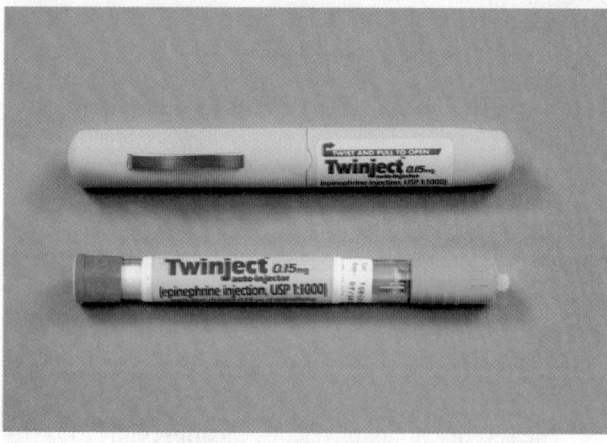

(B)

FIGURE 27-4

Epinephrine autoinjectors. (A) EpiPen autoinjectors for infant/child and adult. (B) Twinject autoinjectors for infant/child and adult.

Assessment and Management of Anaphylaxis

After ensuring scene safety, assess the patient's airway and determine the degree of airway compromise. Intervene as necessary, keeping in mind that airway edema can progress rapidly, but also that insertion of airway devices can exacerbate edema and result in bleeding into the airway. Anticipate vomiting and have suction available.

The patient may have audible wheezing and other signs of respiratory distress, including use of accessory muscles, tachypnea, and cyanosis. Administer high-flow oxygen by nonrebreather mask if ventilations are adequate and use a bag-valve-mask device if ventilations are inadequate.

For patients with significant airway edema, respiratory distress, or hypotension, administer epinephrine subcutaneously or intramuscularly (preferred) as directed by protocol. The usual dosage is 0.3 to 0.5 mg of 1:1,000 epinephrine for adults. For pediatric patients, the usual dosage is 0.01 mg/kg of body weight. For example, a child weighing 60 lb weighs 27.27 kg. Round this to 27 kg and multiply by 0.01. The dose would be 0.27 mg, which you would round to 0.3 mg.

Start an IV. If the patient is hypotensive, administer intravenous fluids (normal saline or lactated Ringer's solution) to increase the blood pressure. Use the patient's blood pressure as a guide for the rate and amount of fluid administration. Also consider any underlying medical conditions, such as heart failure. However, the need for fluid, overall, can be substantial. Up to 50 percent of the circulating volume can be lost in the first several minutes of anaphylaxis. Your protocols may call for two large-bore IVs and administration of fluid boluses while monitoring vital signs and lung sounds.

For patients without hypotension or significant airway edema, a nebulized albuterol (or levalbuterol) treatment can be administered to treat bronchospasm. The adult dosage of albuterol is 2.5 to 5 mg in 3 mL of normal saline. The usual dosage for children aged 1 to 12 years is 1.25 to 2.5 mg. Check with medical direction concerning the use of beta$_2$ agonists in conjunction with epinephrine.

If your protocols allow, the antihistamine diphenhydramine (Benadryl) can be used to prevent additional histamine from binding with histamine receptors.

(See Appendix 4.) The usual adult dose is 25 to 50 mg, and may be given intramuscularly or intravenously. The pediatric dose is 1 to 2 mg/kg of body weight.

Immunocompromise

Patients can be immunocompromised for a variety of reasons. Cancers that affect the bone marrow can prevent production of normal white blood cells. The chemotherapy that suppresses cancer cell reproduction also can suppress the rapidly dividing cells of the bone marrow. Medications given for one reason can have a side effect of suppressing immune function. For example, corticosteroids, which are given to reduce inflammatory reactions, impair the body's ability to respond to disease. Patients who have received organ transplants take medications to suppress the immune system. Otherwise, the immune system would attack the foreign donor tissue, destroying it. A number of diseases can temporarily or permanently impair immune function. The human immunodeficiency virus (HIV), which causes acquired immune deficiency syndrome (AIDS) is perhaps most well known to the general public.

Patients with immunocompromise are at risk for infectious diseases and cancers that are normally rare. In any patient with risk factors for immune compromise, assess for signs of infection, such as fever, cough, unexplained weight loss, and night sweats. Also remember that immunocompromised patients are at risk for infection from exposure to medical procedures, health care workers, the health care environment (including the ambulance), and other patients.

Autoimmune Diseases

Normally, the immune system effectively distinguishes molecules as being either "self" or "nonself." Nonself molecules are attacked by the immune system and self molecules are not. In **autoimmune diseases** the immune system fails to recognize certain molecules in the body as "self" and destroys them, affecting the function of the tissues involved. Often, the treatment for autoimmune diseases involves suppressing the immune system. The unfortunate side effect is that the person is also left less able to fight infectious diseases and cancers.

Autoimmune diseases include rheumatoid arthritis, psoriasis, systemic lupus erythematosus (SLE), Grave's disease (hyperthyroidism), Crohn's disease, multiple sclerosis (MS), and many others (Table 27-3) (Figure 27-5). SLE and rheumatoid arthritis are autoimmune diseases classified as collagen vascular diseases. Collagen vascular diseases affect tendons, bones, and other connective tissues. In addition, many other diseases, such as type 1

TABLE 27-3	Selected Autoimmune Diseases
Disorder	**Description**
Rheumatoid arthritis	A collagen vascular disease that affects the joints. Smaller joints, such as those in the hands, usually are affected first, but other joints are affected with time. There is joint pain, swelling, and stiffness with eventual deformity and loss of use. The patient also may experience fatigue, weight loss, and fever. Other organs can be affected. The disease is progressive, but patients can have long periods of remission with flare-ups from time to time.
Psoriasis	Rapid cell reproduction results in patches of scaly, thick skin with periods of worsening and improvement. Common areas affected include the elbows, knees, and scalp, but the lesions can be widespread in severe disease.
Scleroderma	Involves inflammation of the skin and blood vessels with formation of scar tissue. The skin and other organs become fibrotic from scar tissue. Patients have flare-ups and periods of remission.
Systemic lupus erythematosus (SLE)	More common in women (90 percent of patients). Signs and symptoms include fatigue, fever, joint pain, and rash. The disease can also affect the kidneys, heart, and lungs.

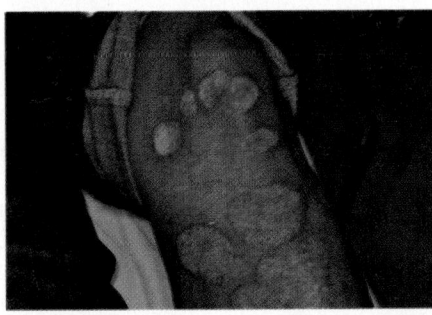

FIGURE 27-5

Psoriasis. (© Edward T. Dickinson, MD)

diabetes, have autoimmune components. Some drugs used to suppress immune functions in particular autoimmune diseases include methotrexate, etanercept (Enbrel), prednisone, adalimumab (Humira), and ustekinumab (Stelara).

CASE STUDY WRAP-UP

Clinical-Reasoning Process

Firefighter/Advanced EMTs Erin Boomershine and Dale Arlen are at a soccer field with eight-year-old Jackson Lyles, whose coach reported he has a peanut allergy and accidentally ate a cookie with peanut butter in it. Jackson is awake, sitting on the ground, looking anxious.

Erin scans the area to make sure the cookies are no longer near the patient. She kneels down next to Jackson, looking at his general appearance and level of distress. He has some hives on his face and neck, along with an occasional dry cough, but he is not pale or diaphoretic. "Hi, Jackson. I'm Erin and this is Dale. How are you feeling?"

"I'm scared," replies Jackson. "I'm allergic to peanuts and I ate a cookie with peanut butter."

"We're here to help you. Don't be scared, okay? Do you feel sick at all?"

"My throat feels itchy."

Erin knows this could be an early indication of airway swelling. "Is it hard to breathe at all?"

"No."

"Is it hard to swallow?"

"No."

"Can you open your mouth so I can look at your tongue?" Jackson complies and there is no edema of his tongue or mouth. Erin is satisfied that his airway is not in immediate jeopardy. "I'm going to use my stethoscope to listen to you breathe," says Erin. She places the diaphragm of the stethoscope on Jackson's upper left back and asks him to breathe in. Erin listens in four places on his back, noticing some slight, scattered wheezing on expiration. Meanwhile, Dale has obtained an SpO_2 of 99 percent on room air and reports that Jackson's radial pulse is 100, strong, and regular.

"Well, Jackson," says Erin, "I think you are having a mild allergic reaction, but it's not too bad. Has anyone called your parents?"

Jackson nods. "Yeah. My mom is on her way." The soccer coach confirms that Mrs. Lyles is just a few minutes away.

"Okay," replies Erin. "Do you know if you have any other medical problems besides a peanut allergy?" Meanwhile, Dale begins to set up an albuterol treatment with 2.5 mg of albuterol in 3 mL of normal saline.

Mrs. Lyles arrives and agrees to treatment, just as the ambulance pulls in and parks. Erin gives the ambulance crew a report as Dale begins the albuterol treatment and reassures Mrs. Lyles that it appears to be a mild allergic reaction.

Jackson is treated in the hospital emergency department and prescribed an epinephrine autoinjector. Before he is discharged, he and his mother receive specific instructions about the signs and symptoms of a severe allergic reaction requiring the use of the autoinjector.

CHAPTER REVIEW

Chapter Summary

Anaphylaxis is a severe type of hypersensitivity reaction in which the immune system initiates an extreme response against a foreign substance usually not recognized as harmful. In anaphylaxis, antibodies on mast cells and basophils bind with the antigen, resulting in release of several chemical mediators of anaphylaxis. One of these mediators, histamine, is responsible for many of the manifestations of anaphylaxis. The effects of histamine include vasodilation, increased capillary permeability, bronchoconstriction, and increased gastrointestinal motility. The results of these effects include urticaria, airway edema, wheezing, and hypovolemia.

Patients with anaphylaxis may require advanced airway management. If the patient has an airway obstruction or pending airway obstruction, request ALS, if available, or prepare to transport without delay to the nearest emergency department. Airway and ventilation can deteriorate quickly; monitor the patient closely for the need to intervene. The primary treatment for anaphylaxis is epinephrine, which you should administer intramuscularly. Patients may also require fluid resuscitation. Nebulized beta$_2$ agonists and diphenhydramine are adjunct treatments.

Patients with immunosupression, such as those on certain medications, cancer patients, and those with HIV, are at increased risk for infectious disease and cancer. Assess for signs of infection and be aware that contact with the health care system can increase the risk of infection in immunocompromised patients. Patients with autoimmune diseases have a condition in which their immune systems fail to distinguish between self and nonself molecules, resulting in destruction of affected tissues. Autoimmune diseases include rheumatoid arthritis and psoriasis. Medications taken by patients with autoimmune diseases can suppress the immune system, placing them at increased risk for infection and cancers.

Review Questions

Multiple-Choice Questions

1. Which one of the following is the mechanism by which anaphylaxis causes shock?

   a. Mechanical obstruction to blood flow from edema
   b. Vasodilation and increased capillary permeability
   c. Autoimmune destruction of the myocardium
   d. Blood loss

2. You respond to a hotel where a group is having a luncheon. A 25-year-old woman is lying on the floor with some coworkers kneeling next to her, fanning her. "She can't breathe," one of the coworkers tells you. You see that the patient is awake, has swelling of the face, and is in respiratory distress with stridor and wheezing. A coworker says the patient joked about not eating the shrimp gumbo because she has a seafood allergy, but the sandwich she ordered was supposed to be made with imitation crab. Your partner prepares to manage the airway and administer oxygen. Of the following, which one should have the highest priority in managing this patient?

   a. Performing chest compressions to relieve the airway obstruction
   b. Administering epinephrine intramuscularly
   c. Preparing for transport without delay
   d. Starting an IV

3. A 45-year-old has just left her dentist's office after having a routine cleaning and exam. She complains of itching in her throat and wheezing. You confirm wheezing but there is no evidence of upper airway edema. The patient is alert and oriented and has warm, dry, flushed skin. Her radial pulse is strong at 88, respirations are 20, blood pressure is 126/84, and SpO_2 is 96 percent on room air. She says she has a latex allergy, but thought the hygienist used a latex-free protocol during the procedure. Which one of the following should have the highest priority in the management of this patient?

   a. Nebulized albuterol
   b. Intravenous bolus of normal saline
   c. Glucagon
   d. Epinephrine

4. Which one of the following is an expected side effect of epinephrine administration?

   a. Decreased level of responsiveness
   b. Decreased blood pressure
   c. Increased anxiety
   d. Bronchoconstriction

5. For a 70-kg adult in severe anaphylaxis, the most appropriate IM dose of 1:1,000 epinephrine is:

   a. 0.4 mg.   c. 1.25 mg.
   b. 0.7 mg.   d. 2.5 mg.

6. Your patient is a four-year-old child who weighs 48 lb. An appropriate dosage of IM epinephrine for anaphylaxis in this patient is:

   a. 0.01 mg.   c. 0.2 mg.
   b. 0.02 mg.   d. 2 mg.

7. A class of medication with a known side effect of angioedema, particularly of the tongue, is:

   a. antihistamines.
   b. corticosteroids.
   c. $beta_2$ agonists.
   d. ACE inhibitors.

8. You have established an airway, begun bag-valve-mask ventilations, and administered IM epinephrine to an adult patient with severe anaphylaxis. Approximately 2 minutes after giving epinephrine, the patient's blood pressure is 70/48. Which one of the following is the best way to address this?

   a. Give an additional dose of epinephrine, 1:1,000 IM.
   b. Start an IV and give 0.5 mg epinephrine 1:1,000 IV.
   c. Start two large-bore IVs and give a 500-mL fluid bolus.
   d. Request an order for intravenous corticosteroids.

Critical-Thinking Questions

9. What is the benefit of giving epinephrine 1:1,000 intramuscularly, rather than subcutaneously, in patients with severe anaphylaxis?

10. What puts organ transplant patients at increased risk for infection? How can you reduce the chances that an organ transplant patient will acquire an infection from contact with the health care system?

11. What is the basic mechanism common to autoimmune diseases?

Additional Reading

Bledsoe, B. E., Porter, R. S., & Cherry, R. A. (2009). *Paramedic care: Principles and practice* (3rd ed., Vol. 3). Upper Saddle River, NJ: Pearson.

Martini, F. H, Bartholomew, E. F, & Bledsoe, B. E. (2008). *Anatomy and physiology for emergency care* (2nd ed.). Upper Saddle River, NJ: Pearson.

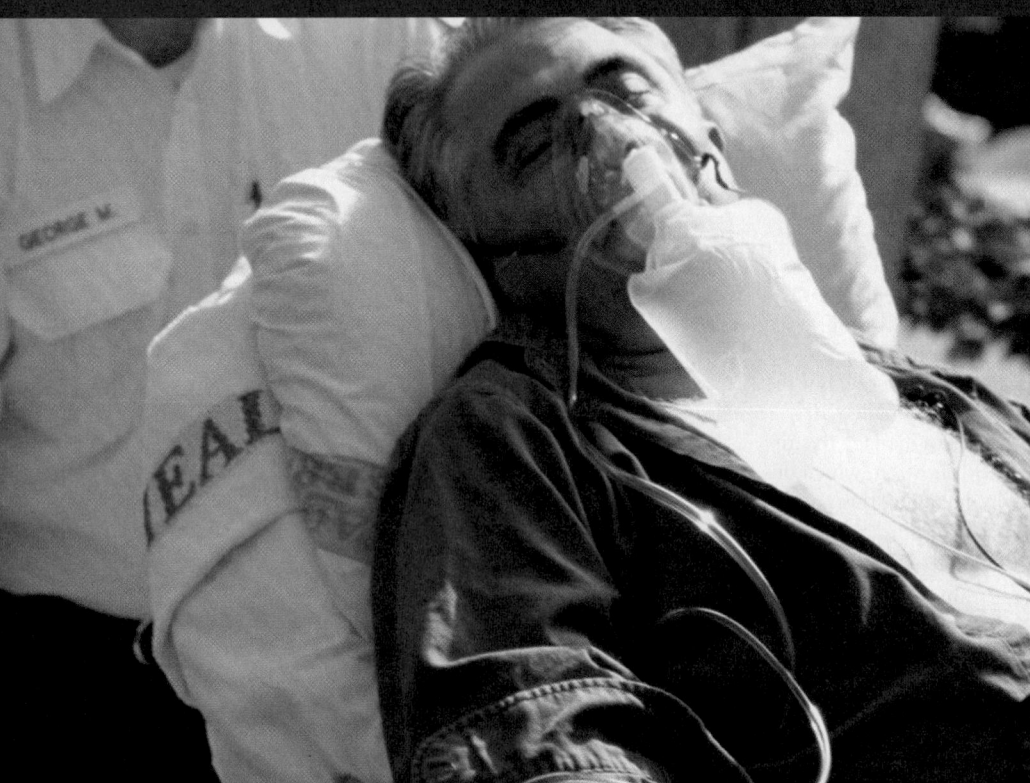

28

Infectious Illnesses

Content Area: Medicine

Advanced EMT Education Standard: Applies fundamental knowledge to provide basic and selected advanced emergency care and transportation based on assessment findings for an acutely ill patient.

Objectives

After reading this chapter, you should be able to:

28.1 Define key terms introduced in this chapter.

28.2 Describe the body's defenses against infectious illnesses.

28.3 Explain the actions health care providers must take to prevent the spread of communicable illnesses to themselves and others.

28.4 Describe the routes of transmission of infectious illnesses.

28.5 Discuss what constitutes a significant exposure to a communicable illness.

28.6 Describe the stages of infectious illnesses.

28.7 Identify the general signs and symptoms of infectious illnesses.

28.8 Describe the nature of agents of infectious illnesses, including bacteria, viruses, fungi, helminths, protozoa, and external parasites.

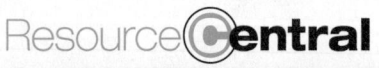

To access Resource Central, follow the directions on the Student Access Card provided with this text. If there is no card, go to www.bradybooks.com and follow the Resource Central link to Buy Access. Under Media Resources, you will find:

• *HIV and AIDS.* Why the disease is such a public health concern.

• *Tuberculosis.* Causes, signs and symptoms, and how to protect yourself as a health care professional.

• *Tickborne Illnesses.* Different types, signs and symptoms, prevention, and safe removal techniques.

CASE STUDY

Advanced EMTs James Sheridan and Marti Mathis have just arrived at an apartment building where they have received a request to assist law enforcement and child services with several siblings who are being placed in the care of the county. The four children range in age from 18 months to 7 years. The children are all awake and alert with no acute complaints and no signs of injury. All of the children have a pimple-like rash on their arms and torsos, with signs that they have been scratching at the rash.

Problem-Solving Questions

1. What are possible causes of a rash that fits this description?
2. What significance is there in all four children having the same rash?
3. What Standard Precautions would be appropriate in this situation?
4. What other signs and symptoms should James and Marti look for?

28.9   Discuss the causative agents, pathophysiology, routes of transmission, methods of prevention, and management of the following:
– Bacterial and viral meningitis
– Gastroenteritis and foodborne illnesses
– Hantavirus pulmonary syndrome (*sin nombre*)
– Hepatitis types A, B, C, D, E, and G
– HIV/AIDS
– Influenza
– Measles and rubella
– Mononucleosis
– Mumps
– Parasites and vector-borne illnesses, including scabies, lice, Lyme disease, viral encephalitis
– Pneumonia
– Rabies
– Sexually transmitted infections, including chlamydia, gonorrhea, and syphilis
– Staphylococcal infections, including MRSA; streptococcal infections, and VRE
– Tetanus
– Tuberculosis
– Upper respiratory infections
– Varicella and herpes infections

28.10   Discuss the significance and prevention of nosocomial infections and antibiotic-resistant infections.

28.11   Given various scenarios involving known or suspected infectious disease, obtain relevant history and assessment information, formulate and implement an appropriate treatment plan, and take precautions to prevent disease transmission.

Introduction

Prior to the mid-twentieth century, infectious illness was the leading cause of death in the United States. A number of public health developments, including vaccinations, and the creation of antibiotics caused a significant decrease in infectious illness morbidity and mortality. Though heart disease, stroke, cancer, and trauma deaths surpass infectious illness deaths, infectious diseases remain a public health concern in terms of morbidity, mortality, and cost. Infectious illnesses are caused by living organisms that invade the body. Those organisms include bacteria, viruses, fungi, and parasites.

Of the multitudes of organisms that reside in the environment and in and on the body, only a minority are pathogens (disease-producing organisms). Most pathogens result in relatively mild illnesses because it is not in a pathogen's best interest to kill its hosts. However, what is a mild illness in most people can be life-threatening in patients who are immunocompromised. In addition to community-acquired diseases, health care providers must be concerned with infections that are more prevalent among patients with exposure to the health care system. Many hospital-acquired infections are antibiotic resistant and extremely difficult to treat.

Of the many ways to reduce your risk of infectious illnesses, knowledge is among the most important. You must recognize general signs and symptoms of infection as well as signs and symptoms associated with some specific diseases. You must know what level of concern to have when caring for patients with particular infectious illnesses so that you can take appropriate steps to protect yourself and other health care providers and provide the patient with the best care.

Anatomy and Physiology Review

The body has many mechanisms to protect against infectious illness. The skin and mucous membranes provide a barrier between the external environment and the internal environment of the body. Body fluids contain antimicrobial substances and some white blood cells recognize foreign material, even without prior exposure, and defend the body against it. Inflammation and fever are also responses that fight infectious disease. The body even uses micro-organisms to prevent disease in the body. Numerous strains of bacteria are normally present in the mouth, nose, on the skin, and in the digestive tract. These **normal flora** prevent the growth of pathogens. Antibiotics can kill normal flora in the course of fighting an infection, resulting in an overgrowth of bacteria not susceptible to the antibiotic or an overgrowth of fungi, such as *Candida albicans*. Infections that occur from reduction of normal flora or in patients with compromised immune systems are called **opportunistic infections.**

Immunity is a response to specific pathogens. Passive immunity occurs without the activation of the immune system. Natural passive immunity, which lasts for the first few months of life, is conferred by the maternal antibodies passed on to the fetus through the placenta and to the infant through breastfeeding. Acquired passive immunity is provided by an injection of immunoglobulin (antibodies) for specific diseases. For example, a patient who has not been immunized against tetanus may receive an injection of tetanus immune globulin if he has an injury at high risk for tetanus.

Stimulating the immune system to produce immunologic memory develops active immunity. Natural active immunity occurs when a first exposure to a pathogen results in the body producing memory B cells and memory T cells. The first exposure may or may not produce signs and symptoms, but the body is protected against subsequent infection. Induced active immunity is developed through vaccination. Vaccines contain either live weakened pathogens or killed pathogens. When introduced to the body, the weakened or killed pathogens cannot produce disease, but the body develops immunologic memory for them. In many cases, active immunity is lifelong, but that is not the case with all pathogens.

Infection and Disease Transmission

Pathogens can be introduced to the body in many ways, such as through injured skin, through the mucous membranes, or through the respiratory, digestive, urinary, or reproductive tracts. Not every contact with disease constitutes an exposure, and not every exposure leads to illness. For example, contact between blood and intact skin is not an exposure, but contact between blood and non-intact skin or mucous membranes is an exposure. (See Chapter 3.) If the number of pathogens is large, if they are highly **virulent** (very strong and able to overcome body defenses), or if the patient's ability to resist disease has been compromised, infection may occur. Creating an environment that is inhospitable to pathogens and engaging in behaviors such as hand washing and using Standard Precautions can reduce the risk of infectious disease.

The body can be exposed to pathogens from a variety of sources, including food, water, soil, surfaces, insects, animals, and other people. When an infectious illness can be transmitted from one person to another, either directly or indirectly, it is classified as a **communicable disease.** Direct transmission occurs when the infected person is in contact with, or in close proximity to, another person. This includes being near a person who sneezes or coughs, kissing, or sexual contact. Indirect transmission occurs when the infected person contaminates a **fomite** (surface or object) that another person then comes in contact with, or when there is a **vector** (animal or insect intermediary).

Infectious illnesses are classified by their routes of entry and exit from the body. This includes direct contact, airborne diseases, sexually transmitted infections, bloodborne diseases, and diseases introduced through the gastrointestinal system. Illnesses transmitted through infected blood and body fluids inzclude HIV/AIDS and hepatitis types B, C, D, and G. Illnesses that enter through the respiratory tract include tuberculosis, influenza, and pneumonia. Illnesses spread through the gastrointestinal tract include hepatitis A and hepatitis E. Sexually transmitted infections include chlamydia, syphilis, herpes simplex type 2, and gonorrhea.

Once a pathogen gains access to the body, it must multiply, or colonize, in the body. From there, the course of infection can take different routes. With some types of infections, people can be infected, but never have signs and symptoms, yet a test for disease-specific antibodies reveals that the person was infected in the past. The patient may progress through several phases of a disease, or the disease can be **fulminant** (sudden and severe). An infection is asymptomatic, unapparent, or subclinical when colonization has occurred but there are no signs or symptoms. The infection may never become apparent, or may proceed to symptomatic illness.

The **incubation period** occurs between exposure and the onset of signs and symptoms. An illness is **latent** either between exposure and the onset of signs and symptoms, or between periods of active disease. For example, the herpes virus can be latent for varying periods between symptomatic episodes. Depending on the illness, transmission may or may not be possible during the latent period. The **window phase** is the period between exposure and the production of enough antibodies to be detected in the blood (seroconversion). The **disease period** is the period of time in which the patient has signs and symptoms. The disease period ends when the signs and symptoms resolve, or if the patient dies from the disease. Some infections, such as HIV/AIDS and hepatitis C, become chronic and patients may live many years with the infection. In some cases, for example in patients with hepatitis B, the patient is a **carrier** who remains capable of transmitting the disease, though signs and symptoms have resolved, or perhaps were never present.

Pathogens

The primary pathogens that cause disease in humans are bacteria, viruses, fungi, and parasites. Bacteria are single-celled organisms that are capable of reproduction. Examples of bacterial diseases include streptococcal diseases, staphylococcal diseases, gonorrhea, and *E. coli.* Bacteria can cause damage to the tissues directly, or can produce toxins that cause detrimental effects. For example, the bacterium that causes botulism produces a toxin that causes paralysis. *Staphylococcus aureus,* a common bacterium, can produce a toxin that leads to toxic shock syndrome.

Antibiotics are effective against many bacteria, but there are antibiotic-resistant strains of bacteria, such as methicillin-resistant *Staphylococcus aureus* (MRSA) and vancomycin-resistant enterococcus (VRE). There also are resistant forms of tuberculosis. The development of antibiotic-resistant strains of bacteria is largely due to the overuse of antibiotics. In addition, the administration of antibiotics is not without consequences, including allergic reactions and death of normal flora. Only use antibiotics when clearly indicated.

Viruses contain either DNA or RNA, but not both. They must gain access to a host's cell, where they use the cell's genetic material to replicate themselves, essentially turning the infected cell into a virus factory. Viral diseases include the rhinoviruses that cause the common cold, influenza, herpes viruses, HIV, and hepatitis viruses. Viral illnesses often result in immunologic memory, conferring lifelong immunity. Some viral infections, such as hepatitis B and hepatitis C, can become chronic, and others, such as herpes viruses, can lie dormant in the body but re-emerge under times of stress. There are drugs available that can inhibit viral replication, but antibiotics are not effective against viruses.

Fungi are simple plants, such as yeasts, that can live and reproduce in the body, and exist in the normal flora. When the immune system is compromised or body conditions otherwise provide a favorable environment, such as a decrease in normal bacterial flora, fungi can reproduce at a greater rate, causing opportunistic infection. Fungal infections include Candida strains that cause oral thrush, thrush infections of the skin, and vaginal yeast infections, ringworm, and various respiratory infections.

Protozoa are single-celled animals with the ability to move. The protozoa cryptosporidium and giardia lamblia are found in contaminated water, and can cause gastrointestinal illness. Malaria is caused by a parasite transmitted by mosquitoes. Parasites can either be internal or external. Internal parasites include helminths (worms), such as pinworms, hookworms, trichinella (the cause of trichinosis from eating undercooked pork or bear meat), and tapeworms. External parasites include scabies and lice.

Infection Control

You are responsible for your own safety, including protecting yourself from infectious disease through the use of Standard Precautions, hand washing, cleaning and disinfecting equipment and the work environment, immunizations, and maintaining general good health. If you are exposed to an infectious illness, follow your employer's policy for medical evaluation and reporting. Keep in mind that you have an obligation to protect patients from exposure to infectious diseases. Do not come to work when you have an infectious disease. Influenza, for example, can be fatal for the patient with immune compromise. Good hand washing, cleaning, disinfection, and disposal of used equipment are also measures to protect your patients.

IN THE FIELD

If you suspect a patient has a communicable disease that requires isolation from other patients, notify the receiving hospital.

General Assessment and Management of Infectious Illnesses

You may suspect infectious disease from a variety of clues from dispatch, the scene size-up, your assessment, and the patient's history. Fever is very often an indication of infectious disease, but there are other causes of increased body temperature, such as environmental emergencies; and not all infections result in fever. Cough, vomiting, diarrhea, and altered mental status can all be a result of infection, but have many other causes, too. Consider all findings in context. Compare your findings to the patterns associated with infectious and other causes of disease. Hone your skills by getting feedback from peers, physicians, and nurses, and by seeking follow-up on patients.

Scene Size-Up

Certain environments are associated with an increased risk for infectious disease. This includes residential facilities such as group homes, nursing homes, homeless shelters, and jails and prisons. When you are involved in the interfacility transportation of patients to and from hospitals, be aware of the increased risk of exposure to infectious disease. Patients with chronic illnesses, such as COPD, and patients with urinary catheters or central venous lines are at increased risk of infection. The presence of home oxygen, nebulizers, or other medical equipment should alert you to the patient's increased risk.

Several chief complaints are associated with infectious disease, including fever, cough, nausea, vomiting, diarrhea, muscle aches, fatigue, general malaise, runny nose, rash, headache, pain, swelling, and stiff neck (Table 28-1). Presentations that could indicate infectious disease include seizure and altered mental status, including confusion, delirium, jaundice, and decreased responsiveness.

Use findings from the scene size-up to determine if your use of Standard Precautions is appropriate to the situation. In addition to gloves, consider the need for respiratory protection.

Primary Assessment

Immediately assess the patient's pulse if he appears to be unresponsive and not breathing, and begin CPR and apply the AED if the patient is pulseless. If infectious illness is suspected, use appropriate respiratory protection for airway and ventilation procedures.

Some infectious diseases, such as epiglottitis and croup, can cause upper airway obstruction. Listen for stridor, observe for tripod positioning, and note any drooling. If you suspect airway edema from epiglottitis or croup, do not examine the airway or put anything in the mouth, because

TABLE 28-1   Signs and Symptoms of Infectious Illness

General signs and symptoms include:
- Fatigue
- Malaise
- Headache
- Muscle or joint pain
- Fever
- Chills
- Swollen lymph nodes
- Nausea
- Vomiting
- Rash

Signs and symptoms of respiratory illness:
- Nasal congestion
- Burning eyes, eye irritation
- Nasal discharge (rhinorrhea)
- Earache
- Sore throat
- Cough, productive or nonproductive
- Wheezing, rhonchi, crackles (rales)
- Respiratory distress
- Stridor
- Drooling
- Difficult or painful swallowing
- Hoarseness
- Signs of hypoxia, decreased SpO_2
- Tachypnea
- Altered mental status

Signs and symptoms of hepatitis:
- Upper right quadrant tenderness
- Jaundice
- Dark urine
- Clay-colored stools
- Anorexia

Signs and symptoms of meningitis:
- Stiff neck
- Photophobia
- Possible altered mental status
- Possible purpura

a complete airway obstruction can occur. Otherwise, use manual maneuvers and basic adjuncts, if necessary, to establish and maintain an airway. If the patient is unresponsive, consider the need for an advanced airway.

Respiratory distress can occur in childhood respiratory illnesses, pneumonia, and bronchitis. Observe for signs of fatigue, tachypnea, accessory muscle use, wheezing, coughing, diaphoresis, and cyanosis. Apply oxygen and assist ventilations as needed. Tachycardia can be an indication of fever, dehydration, or shock. If signs of shock, such as pallor, altered mental status, and diaphoresis are present, consider the need for fluid replacement.

Secondary Assessment

Perform a rapid medical assessment for critical patients, including listening to breath sounds. Perform a focused secondary assessment for noncritical patients, based on the chief complaint and presentation. Obtain a SAMPLE history, using OPQRST as relevant to explore the chief complaint. Obtain an SpO_2 and baseline vital signs. Check the blood glucose level in diabetics and patients with altered mental status.

Use your knowledge of pathophysiology and the patient's responses to develop your line of questioning and adapt your assessment as information emerges. If a patient denies having a cough, ask about other signs and symptoms. If your patient states he has had a cough, follow up with questions about the nature of the cough, and if you have not already done so, listen to his breath sounds.

Clinical-Reasoning Process

Adapt your assessment and history to the patient's complaint, presentation, and emerging information from the assessment and history. Test your hypotheses and determine whether infectious disease will be among your differential diagnoses. What mechanisms could explain the patient's presenting problems? Do the patient's signs and symptoms fit a particular pattern? Does he have risk factors that make infectious disease more likely? Are there signs and symptoms that do not fit? Does the patient have characteristics, such as age or **immunocompromise**, that might make infectious disease present atypically?

It is not possible to definitively diagnose a specific infectious disease in the prehospital setting, but you should be able to recognize if infectious disease is a possibility and what body systems are being affected. You may obtain information that makes you highly suspect pneumonia, urinary tract infection, meningitis, or other problems. In some cases, this information will cause you to reconsider your selection of Standard Precautions, or will prompt you to notify the receiving facility of your suspicions. Your suspicion may make you more aware of the possibility of dehydration, guiding your decisions about intravenous fluids.

Treatment

Treatment depends on the patient's complaints and problems, rather than a specific diagnosis. In addition to the interventions implemented in the primary assessment, consider the need for bronchodilators, intravenous fluids, and temperature regulation. Patients with some respiratory illnesses, with or without underlying chronic respiratory problems such as chronic obstructive pulmonary disease (COPD) or asthma, may have wheezing due to bronchoconstriction. If beta$_2$ agonists are permitted for this reason in your protocols, consider administering them, or check with

Pediatric Care

Never give aspirin to treat fever in pediatric patients. Though rare, there is an association between aspirin given for viral illness such as colds, influenza, and chicken pox, and Reye's syndrome. The American Academy of Pediatrics, Centers for Disease Control, and the U.S. Surgeon General recommend that aspirin and other salicylate products not be used in patients under 19 years old in illnesses that cause fever. Reye's syndrome is a potentially fatal disease with severe effects on the central nervous system and liver. The mortality rate is from 20 to 50 percent.

Geriatric Care

Elderly patients may present without a significant fever, even with serious infection. Always consider infection as a cause when an elderly patient has a new onset of confusion or other changes in behavior or mental status.

medical direction for an order. Patients with fever, infection, and tachypnea are prone to dehydration and may benefit from intravenous fluids, according to protocol. If you suspect sepsis, start an IV and administer fluids.

Low to moderate fever is usually not treated in the prehospital setting using acetaminophen or ibuprofen, but it may be included in protocols for services with long transport times. For high fever, follow protocols for medication administration and cover the patient only lightly to avoid further increasing the temperature. Patients with sepsis may be hypothermic. Prevent further heat loss by covering the patient with blankets and heating the patient compartment.

Reassessment

Reassess critical patients every 5 minutes or sooner. Reassess noncritical patients every 15 minutes or more often as needed. Reassess the patient's vital signs, SpO_2, complaints, relevant aspects of the assessment, and the effects of interventions.

Bloodborne Infections

Bloodborne infections are spread through contact between blood or body fluids and nonintact skin or mucous membranes. Always take Standard Precautions, such as using gloves when you may have contact with a patient's blood or body fluids and wearing eye protection when blood or body fluids are likely to splash. Carefully handling sharps, hand washing, and disinfecting contaminated surfaces also are important ways to minimize your risk of bloodborne infections at work.

HIV/AIDS

The human immunodeficiency virus (HIV) infects T lymphocytes by combining with a molecule on the cell surface so that it can gain entry. The virus uses the cell to replicate itself, producing thousands of copies of itself. In the process, the affected lymphocytes are damaged and their number decreases, resulting in immune suppression called *acquired immunodeficiency syndrome (AIDS),* which is referred to as *HIV/AIDS.* HIV is capable of mutating frequently so that the immune system cannot recognize and destroy it. The mutations make strains of HIV less susceptible to the effects of drugs intended to limit their replication (antiretroviral drugs). As a result, patients with HIV/AIDS are prone to numerous infections and cancers, including opportunistic infections and rare cancers, and the central nervous system is eventually affected as well (AIDS dementia complex). Signs and symptoms of HIV/AIDS include fever, night sweats, lymphadenopathy, and unexplained weight loss.

When caring for HIV/AIDS patients, the presenting problem is often due to another infectious illness or other complications. Any infection in a patient with HIV/AIDS is more serious because of immune compromise. Pneumonias and tuberculosis are common in patients with HIV/AIDS, as are oral thrush infections. A particular kind of cancer normally suppressed by the immune system, Kaposi's sarcoma, is frequently seen in patients with HIV/AIDS (Figure 28-1).

Treat the patient's signs and symptoms, assessing the need for airway management, ventilation, oxygenation, and intravenous fluids. HIV/AIDS is not spread through casual contact. Wear gloves if the patient's skin is not intact, you are going to start an IV, or you are to perform other procedures with a risk of exposure to body fluids. HIV/AIDS patients are at risk for illnesses transmitted by others, including health care providers and patients in the emergency department, and they are susceptible to infections from contaminated medical care areas.

Hepatitis

Hepatitis types A and E are spread through the fecal–oral route and may be contracted through contaminated food. Hepatitis types B, C, D, and G are spread through blood and body fluids. Hepatitis B can be contracted through contact with the blood and body fluids of infected individuals, including through sexual contact, medical procedures, and shared intravenous, tattoo, and acupuncture needles. Hepatitis B is a virulent virus that can survive for long periods of time outside the body. Hepatitis C is transmitted primarily through sexual contact and IV drug abuse. Both hepatitis B and C can become chronic and can lead to cirrhosis and liver failure. Vaccination against hepatitis B is available and is recommended for health care providers. There also is a vaccine for hepatitis A that is available to health care providers and is recommended for those who travel or who are in regular contact with children. There is not a vaccine for hepatitis C.

Hepatitis D occurs only in the presence of hepatitis B and has similar routes of transmission. Hepatitis G can occur either alone or in conjunction with other types of hepatitis. It was initially discovered in patients who developed post–blood transfusion hepatitis, and there is no vaccine.

Some patients with hepatitis are asymptomatic, and illness can range from mild to severe. Signs and symptoms include flu-like symptoms such as headache, fever, joint pain, general malaise, nausea, vomiting, and loss of appetite. Patients may have upper right quadrant pain. Urine may be dark because hemoglobin pigments from destroyed red blood cells cannot be broken down and eliminated by the liver. The stools may be clay colored because they lack the bile pigments that normally give them the characteristic color.

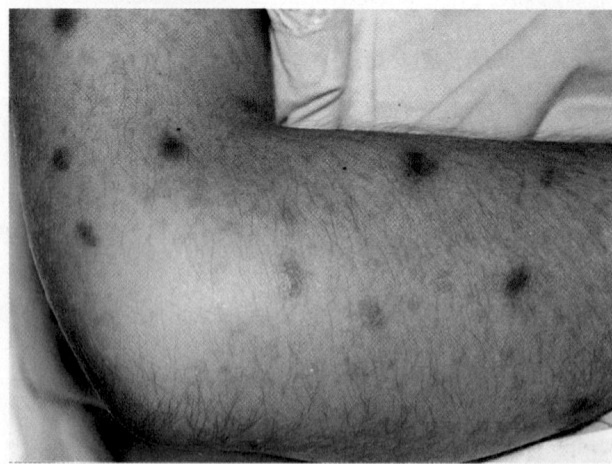

FIGURE 28-1

Kaposi's sarcoma. (Courtesy of Jason L. Smith, MD)

Respiratory Infections

Respiratory infections range from mild to lethal, depending on the infectious agent and the patient's underlying health. Respiratory infections include pneumonia, influenza, respiratory syncytial virus (RSV), bronchitis, croup, tuberculosis, sudden acute respiratory syndrome (SARS), and upper respiratory infections such as colds, pharyngitis, and epiglottitis. (Some of the illnesses, such as RSV and epiglottitis, are more prevalent in pediatric populations, and are discussed in Chapter 44.) The goal of management of patients with respiratory infections is to ensure an open airway and adequate breathing and oxygenation.

Tuberculosis

Tuberculosis (TB) was once a leading cause of death, and its prevalence in the United States is once again of concern. Tuberculosis is most often spread through the respiratory route and manifests as respiratory disease, but can affect many different parts of the body. Tuberculosis occurs at a higher rate among patients with HIV/AIDS and in recent immigrants from countries where the disease is more common. Tuberculosis often requires repeated, close contact, making it more prevalent in situations where people are in prolonged, close proximity to each other, such as jails, nursing homes, and homeless shelters.

Tuberculosis is treated with antibiotics, but there are multiple drug-resistant strains. A single occupational exposure is very unlikely to result in disease, but you should use Standard Precautions, including an N-95 respirator in cases of known or suspected active pulmonary tuberculosis and you should be routinely tested according to your employer's policy. Active pulmonary tuberculosis has a presentation similar to other infectious respiratory diseases, including fever, chills, night sweats, fatigue, and a chronic cough. Hemoptysis should increase your suspicion of tuberculosis.

Pneumonia

Many different infectious agents can cause pneumonia, including viruses, fungi, and many strains of bacteria. Different strains of bacteria are implicated in community-acquired and hospital-acquired pneumonias. Pneumonia may affect anyone, but the risk is increased in smokers, the elderly, those with chronic illnesses, and in immunocompromised patients. Typical signs and symptoms include a sudden onset of high fever with chills, difficulty breathing, pleuritic chest pain (sharp pain worse with inspiration), and a cough. The cough may be nonproductive or may produce sputum of varying character. Remember that elderly patients may not have a fever. The presenting problem can be a sudden onset of altered mental status.

Pneumonia infection and the body's response to it produce purulent material in the lungs. Pneumonia is often localized to one lobe of the lung, resulting in localized crackles and wheezes from the fluid produced and inflammation of the lung tissue. Accumulated fluid in the alveoli can result in collapse of the affected alveoli and oxygen saturation can be significantly reduced (Figure 28-2).

Carefully assess the patient's airway, work and quality of breathing, and oxygenation. Provide oxygen and assist ventilation as needed. Some protocols may allow administration of beta$_2$ agonists for suspected pneumonia patients who are wheezing. Consider the need for intravenous fluids, because fever, increased respiration, and decreased oral intake can all lead to dehydration.

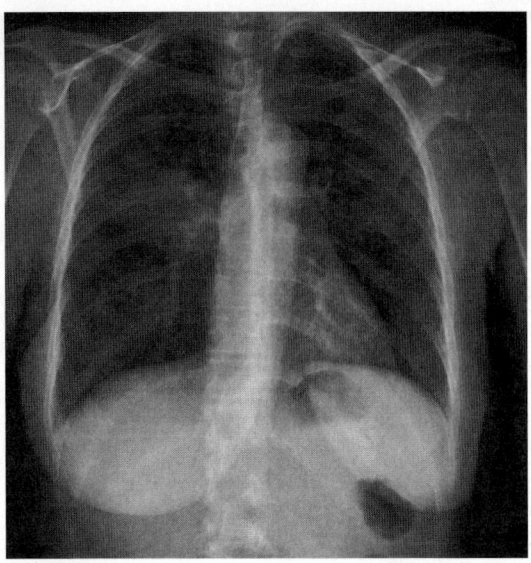

FIGURE 28-2

Pneumonia in the right lung. (© Edward T. Dickinson, MD)

Influenza, Colds, Pharyngitis, and Bronchitis

The common cold is caused by a multitude of rhinoviruses and coronaviruses that affect the upper airway, causing nasal congestion, runny nose, and sneezing. Complications include sinusitis and ear infection. Acute bronchitis is an inflammation of the bronchi, usually from viral infection with rhinoviruses, coronaviruses, influenza viruses, and RSV. In the pediatric population, RSV causes bronchiolitis. Less often, bronchitis is bacterial. Acute bronchitis also can be caused by inhalation or aspiration of irritants. Bronchitis usually begins with a dry cough that becomes productive. Often, the onset is within a few days of the onset of cold symptoms. Patients may be fatigued and have a low-grade fever. Bronchitis usually resolves spontaneously in two or three weeks, but can be complicated in patients with asthma, COPD, cystic fibrosis, or immunocompromise.

Pharyngitis is inflammation of the pharynx, commonly known as a sore throat, often caused by viruses, such as rhinoviruses, but also can be caused by streptococcal bacteria (strep throat). However, it may be caused by allergies and irritants. Most sore throats resolve on their own, but some causes are more serious. Strep throat can result in glomerulonephritis and untreated strep infection can lead to rheumatic fever and rheumatic heart disease. Strep throat is often accompanied by fever, swollen cervical lymph nodes, and **exudate** on the tonsils. Peritonsillar abscess is caused by bacterial infection in the capsule around the tonsil, producing swelling and pain. Occasionally, significant pharyngeal edema can lead to airway compromise.

Influenza, or the flu, occurs from infection with one of several influenza viruses through the airborne route. Flu viruses are highly contagious and some have a significant mortality rate from complications. There usually is a sudden onset of fever (often with chills), sore throat, muscle aches, headaches, cough, weakness, and fatigue. Complications include dehydration, pneumonia, and encephalitis. Influenza vaccines for the strains expected to infect patients in the United States are available each year at the start of the influenza season and they are suggested for health care workers and high-risk populations such as children and the elderly, and chronically ill, immunocompromised, and pregnant patients. Antiviral drugs are available and can be effective in some types of flu early in the illness, but some flu strains have become resistant to antiviral medications (Derlet, Sandrock, Nguyen, & Lawrence, 2011).

SARS

SARS, a coronavirus infection that causes acute pneumonia-like illness, has not been reported since an outbreak in 2004, but the high morbidity and mortality rate make continued surveillance and preparedness prudent. Respiratory protection is required when a SARS outbreak is suspected.

Pertussis

Pertussis, or whooping cough, which had decreased over previous decades, is increasing, with over 17,000 cases reported in 2009 (CDC, 2010a). Pertussis is a serious, sometimes fatal disease that causes coughing fits, which may last 10 or more weeks. Patients gasp for air following coughing fits with a characteristic "whooping" sound. Immunization with the DTaP vaccine is not recommended until two months of age, and requires a series of five vaccinations to confer immunity. Pertussis is increasing particularly among infants and school-age children. Both they and their family members should be vaccinated against pertussis (older children and adults receive the Tdap vaccine). It is suggested that adult health care workers be revaccinated for pertussis.

Infections of Regional Concern

Some regionally prevalent diseases include various arboviruses, hantavirus pulmonary syndrome (HPS), and bubonic plague. Bubonic plague and hantavirus, both carried by rodents, occasionally occur in the U.S. Southwest. The diseases are rare, but if you live in areas where cases occur you should be familiar with signs and symptoms. Hantavirus, also called *sin nombre* ("without name") because the cause of the illness was originally unknown, is carried by deer mice in the U.S. Southwest, and by rice and cotton rats in the U.S. Southeast. However, nearly all documented cases (193 between 2001 and 2008, according to the CDC [2011]) have occurred in the Four-Corners region (the area common to Utah, Colorado, New Mexico, and Arizona). Hantavirus is transmitted through the airborne route from the dried excrement of infected mice. It begins with flu-like signs and symptoms but progresses to a cardiopulmonary stage with hypotension, ARDS, and multiple organ failure.

Bubonic plague is generally transmitted from rodents to humans by fleas. It presents with fever, chills, and enlarged lymph nodes that may be hemorrhagic and necrotic. The largest concentration of infected animals in world is west of the 100th parallel, in New Mexico, Colorado, Utah, Arizona, and California. However, there are only about 13 human cases per year (Dufel & Cronin, 2009). Mortality is low with treatment, but high when the disease is untreated.

Domestic arboviruses, which are transmitted to humans by insects, are a cause of infectious encephalitis. The particular causative agent depends on the season and geographic location. Viruses in this group include West Nile Virus, Eastern Equine Encephalitis, and St. Louis Encephalitis.

PERSONAL PERSPECTIVE

Advanced EMT Ken Jones: Vaccines are a hotly debated topic right now. A lot of people are arguing that they cause more harm than good and that they get sicker from the vaccine than they would if they got the illness. I kind of bought into that and didn't get a flu shot for a couple of years. Last winter I got the flu and, with my history of asthma, I ended up getting pneumonia. I'm pretty healthy overall, but I was sick. I got so short of breath, I finally went to the hospital emergency department. My oxygen saturation was 86 percent. I was admitted to the hospital for five days, but it took me a couple of weeks to really feel good again and I missed a lot of work. On my follow-up visit, my doctor talked to me about the low risk of vaccines compared to the experience I just had. This year, I'm getting a flu shot!

Childhood Illnesses

A number of infectious illnesses are more prevalent in the younger pediatric population, but older children and adults occasionally contract them.

Croup

Croup is a viral illness that causes inflammation of the airways, including the vocal cords and subglottic area, and is also called *laryngotracheobronchitis*. The illness begins with upper respiratory symptoms, such as a sore throat, runny nose, and low-grade fever. After a day or two, the patient develops characteristic inspiratory stridor, hoarseness, and a "seal bark" cough, which generally are worse at night. The disease is mild in most cases, but can lead to respiratory distress and airway obstruction in severe cases. In milder cases the inspiratory stridor occurs during activity, while in moderate to severe cases it occurs at rest. Expiratory stridor occurs in more serious cases. Assess for airway obstruction, increased respiratory effort, suprasternal retractions, tripoding, accessory muscle use, fatigue, altered mental status, and cyanosis.

For mild to moderate cases, do not agitate the patient with unnecessary procedures because crying increases oxygen demand and may worsen edema. For patients with severe cases, treat hypoxia and hypoventilation. Humidified oxygen is preferred to prevent drying, irritation, and further swelling of the airway. Although rarely available in the prehospital setting, nebulized racemic epinephrine is used to treat severe cases. Intubation can be required in severe cases. If intubation is indicated and within your scope of practice, the provider who has the best intubation skills should perform it, because unnecessary manipulation of the airway can worsen edema. An endotracheal tube 0.5 to 1 mm smaller than normal should be used.

Although cool mist or steam were previously recommended as treatments for croup, there is no evidence that either treatment is effective (Muñiz, Molodow, & Defendi, 2010).

Epiglottitis

Epiglottitis is a bacterial infection that causes swelling of the epiglottis. The primary causative agent was the *Haemophilus influenzae* type B (Hib) bacterium, for which a vaccine has been available for several years. However, some cases of Hib epiglottitis do occur, and other bacteria also can cause it. Nonetheless, epiglottitis is rare. When epiglottitis does occur, the patient appears ill with fever, difficulty swallowing and breathing, and drooling. He is usually sitting in a tripod position. Stridor can occur, but decreases as airway obstruction increases. As with croup, keep the patient calm. If signs of hypoxia are present, administer oxygen, preferably

humidified, by the blow-by method. (See Chapter 44.) Ventilate patients with respiratory failure or arrest. Because of the risk of complete airway obstruction and the need for a cricothyrotomy (surgical airway), request ALS for patients with suspected epiglottitis or transport without delay to the nearest appropriate emergency department.

Mumps, Measles, Rubella, and Chickenpox

Mumps, measles (rubeola), rubella (German measles or three-day measles), and chickenpox have become unusual since vaccines became available. However, cases occasionally occur. They are usually mild in nature, but can have complications such as pneumonia and encephalitis. Mumps is a viral infection that affects glandular tissue, particularly the parotid salivary glands, causing painful swelling. Measles and rubella are viral illnesses that cause fever and rash. Both are usually mild, but rubella can cause severe birth defects when contracted by pregnant women in the first 20 weeks of pregnancy.

Chickenpox, or varicella, is a viral disease in the herpes family that causes general malaise and itchy, fluid-filled blisters on the skin that later crust and scab (Figure 28-3). It is highly contagious and easily spread between infected and nonimmune individuals. After recovery, the virus remains dormant in the body, usually in a dorsal spinal nerve, where it can be reactivated, causing a painful, unilateral rash called *shingles*. A person with shingles can transmit the virus to someone who has never had chickenpox or been immunized against varicella.

All health care providers should be vaccinated against the illnesses mentioned here. The illnesses themselves require no particular prehospital treatment. Notify the receiving facility that you are transporting patients suspected of having any of these illnesses.

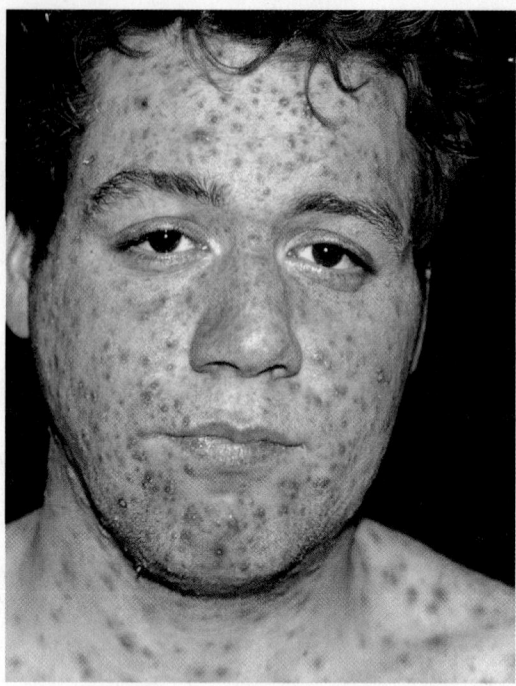

FIGURE 28-3

Chickenpox lesions (© SPL/Photo Researchers, Inc.)

Meningitis and Encephalitis

Meningitis can be viral or bacterial and is an inflammation and swelling of the meninges that surround the central nervous system. Viral meningitis tends to be less severe, while bacterial meningitis can be fatal. The incidence of childhood meningitis has decreased significantly since the Hib vaccine became available. There also is a vaccine for meningococcal meningitis, which is recommended for some high-risk populations.

The meningococcal bacterium commonly resides in the nasal passages, but rarely causes disease. Under certain circumstances, usually in the winter months, the bacteria gains access to the cerebrospinal fluid, causing meningitis. Viral meningitis occurs more often during the summer and fall. The early signs of viral and bacterial meningitis are similar, but bacterial meningitis can become much more severe. Signs and symptoms include fever, headache, photophobia, and stiff neck. In bacterial meningitis, seizures and altered mental status can occur.

Meningococcal bacteria can enter the blood (meningococcemia), causing damage to blood vessels with bleeding into the organs and skin (purpura). Other signs or symptoms include fever and chills, vomiting, diarrhea, joint, muscle, abdominal or chest pain, tachypnea, and cold hands and feet (CDC, 2010b). Meningococcemia can be fatal, or result in amputations and the need for skin grafts.

Bacterial meningitis is transmitted through contact with nasal and oral secretions and generally requires close contact with the infected person. It is not highly likely that it would be spread from patient to EMS provider, but the possibility exists and you should wear a mask, in addition to gloves, for Standard Precautions. In proven cases of meningococcal meningitis, all health care workers who were in significant contact with the patient must take prophylactic antibiotics.

Treat the patient symptomatically, recognizing the potential for hypoxia, sepsis, and hypotension in severe cases. Consider dehydration, even in mild cases. Report the findings suggestive of meningitis—fever, headache, photophobia, stiff neck, and purpural rash—to the emergency department so they can prepare for the patient's arrival.

Encephalitis is an inflammation of brain tissue. Common causes are domestic arboviruses, such as West Nile virus, St. Louis encephalitis, and Eastern Equine encephalitis, which are tickborne or mosquitoborne illnesses. Herpesvirus and toxoplasmosis (especially in immune compromised patients) are other causes. Signs and symptoms are similar to those of meningitis.

Other Vectorborne Illnesses

Lyme disease, tularemia, and Rocky Mountain spotted fever are tickborne illnesses. Of those illnesses, Rocky Mountain spotted fever, a bacterial infection, is the most severe. Within 5 to 10 days after being bitten by an infected tick (American dog tick or Rocky Mountain wood tick), patients may develop general signs of infectious illness, such as fever, nausea and vomiting, muscle aches, anorexia, and headache. Those signs and symptoms are followed by rash, abdominal pain, joint pain, and diarrhea.

Lyme disease is a bacterial infection transmitted by black-legged ticks. A characteristic sign is a red, circular, "bull's eye" rash that begins at location of the bite. Other signs and symptoms include general signs of infectious illness: fatigue, fever, chills, headache, muscle and joint pain, and swollen lymph nodes. The infection can lead to Bell's palsy, headaches, meningitis, and cardiac dysrhythmias. A majority of patients develop severe arthritis in the months following infection and a few patients develop chronic neurologic problems.

Tularemia is a bacterial disease of animals, such as rabbits and rodents, that can be transmitted to humans by deerflies and ticks, by handling infected dead animals, or through contaminated food and water. Only about 200 cases of tularemia occur in humans each year, but tularemia has been identified as a potential weapon of bioterrorism because it is highly infectious and has significant morbidity. The infection can be fatal if not treated. In addition to general signs and symptoms of infectious illness, patients may develop skin ulcers, sore throat, mouth sores, eye inflammation, a dry cough, weakness, and pneumonia with bloody sputum and respiratory failure.

Rabies is very rare, but fatal in humans, and is contracted through contact with the saliva of infected animals.

In the case of bats, aerosolization of urine in caves where large numbers of bats are present can result in transmission through mucous membranes. Animals in which rabies is common include bats, raccoons, skunks, coyotes, and foxes. It is a viral disease that attacks the central nervous system. Following the onset of general signs and symptoms of infectious illness, a number of neurologic signs and symptoms begin. Those include insomnia and anxiety, confusion, hallucinations, agitation, hypersalivation, and fear of water (hydrophobia). The rabies virus travels along nerves from the bite to the brain, where the virus multiplies and enters the salivary glands. The time of onset from infection to signs and symptoms varies. Immediate treatment with a combination of vaccination and immune globulin injection is highly effective in preventing illness. In the prehospital setting, thoroughly clean the wound, because this has been shown to significantly decrease the chances of rabies infection.

Gastrointestinal Infections and Botulism

Many gastrointestinal illnesses are caused by foodborne or waterborne pathogens or through the oral–fecal route of transmission. Although many people refer to gastrointestinal infections as "stomach flu," influenza is not the causative agent. Causes include salmonella, *E. coli,* norovirus, and staphylococcal bacteria, among others. Signs and symptoms include abdominal cramping, nausea, vomiting, diarrhea, and sometimes fever. Occasionally, outbreaks can be traced to a specific source, which may local, regional, or national. Most cases are self-limiting, but severe cases and cases in small children and the elderly can result in dehydration. Hemolytic uremic syndrome occurs in a minority of cases of *E. coli* infection. Red blood cells are destroyed, resulting in kidney failure. Cholera is a severe form of gastroenteritis that can occur following disasters that impact water sanitation, but is rare in the United States.

Check patients with gastroenteritis for signs of dehydration and shock, including checking skin turgor and vital signs. Start an IV for patients who can benefit from fluid replacement. If your protocols allow, consider administering an antiemetic, such as ondansetron (Zofran) for severe vomiting. Treat patients in shock by managing the airway and ensuring adequate ventilation and oxygenation.

Botulism is a bacterium that produces a neurotoxin. It can be found in low-acidity canned foods that are improperly processed, including home-canned foods. It causes paralysis by blocking the release of acetylcholine in motor neurons. Botulism is not common, but concern exists over the use of botulinum toxin as an agent of bioterrorism. Botulism can also infect the skin of intravenous drug abusers, especially among those who use black tar heroin. The cutaneous infection can become systemic.

Pediatric Care

Infants are at highest risk for infant botulism from about six weeks to six months of age, but it can occur anytime in the first year. Less than 100 cases per year occur, but the disease is serious. It is mostly contracted through honey, corn syrup, and dirt that contain botulism spores. As the gastrointestinal and immune systems mature, the small amounts of botulism that may be ingested from those sources is eliminated by the body without causing harm.

Mononucleosis and Herpes

Mononucleosis is a viral infection (Epstein-Barr virus) that causes fever and fatigue and affects the upper respiratory system, resulting in sore throat, swollen tonsils, and enlarged painful lymph nodes. The phagocytes in the spleen are affected, resulting in an enlarged spleen in many patients. It is transmitted through direct contact with saliva. By adulthood, about 95 percent of the population has been infected and developed antibodies.

Herpes simplex viruses primarily affect the mucous membranes and skin. Infection results in blisters that ulcerate (Figure 28-4). Herpes simplex type 1 usually affects the oral mucosa, resulting in cold sores. Herpes simplex type 2 usually affects the genitals. General signs and symptoms of infectious disease, including fever and malaise, often accompany primary infection. In both cases, the virus remains dormant between outbreaks, but does not go away. The viruses are spread through direct contact, and lesions may not be visible during the contagious period.

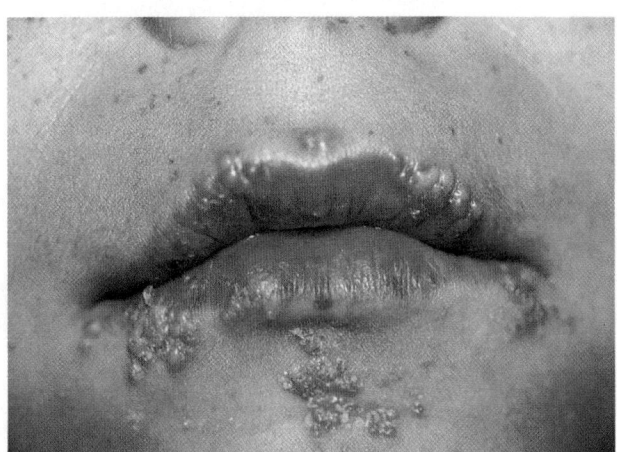

FIGURE 28-4

Typical appearance of herpes simplex type 1. (Courtesy of Jason L. Smith, MD)

External Parasites and Skin Infections

Scabies, lice, and ringworm can all present with intense itching and skin lesions. Both scabies and lice are external parasites. Scabies is caused by a mite that burrows under the skin and lays eggs, which causes a rash with intense itching (Figure 28-5). Scabies is transmitted through direct skin-to-skin contact with an infected person and is more common under crowded conditions, such as institutional settings. A particularly severe form of scabies, Norwegian scabies (crusted scabies), can affect the elderly and immunocompromised. In addition to direct contact, this type of scabies can be transmitted by contact with contaminated linens, clothing, and other items. Scabies is treated by application of a topical scabicidal lotion or cream that is available by prescription.

Lice are tiny insects that infest the body, using the hair shafts to deposit their eggs (nits). Infestation with lice is called *pediculosis* (Figure 28-6). Different types of lice prefer different areas of the body, and include head lice (*Pediculosis humanis capitis*), pubic lice ("crab" lice; pityriasis), and body lice (pediculosis corporis). Lice are spread by close contact with infected persons or, less commonly, through contact with their personal items, such as combs, bed linens, and hats. Head lice are not an indication of poor hygiene, and can affect anyone. Body lice typically live and lay their eggs in clothing, but feed from the skin, and are most common in conditions of crowding and poor hygiene. Pubic lice are usually spread through sexual contact, and can sometimes be found in other areas with coarse hair, such as the chest, axillae, or beard. Over-the-counter preparations are available to treat lice, but some infestations are resistant. Prescription preparations (such as lindane [Kwell]) can be toxic, particularly in smaller individuals and pregnant women. Other preparations can be prescribed, but have not been approved for this use by the FDA.

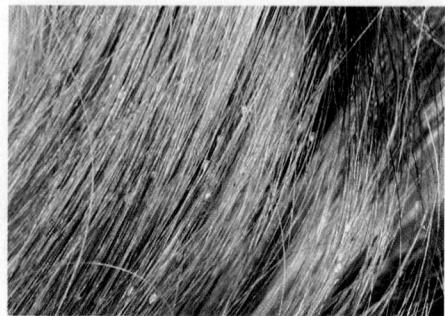

FIGURE 28-6

Infestation with head lice. (Courtesy of Jason L. Smith, MD)

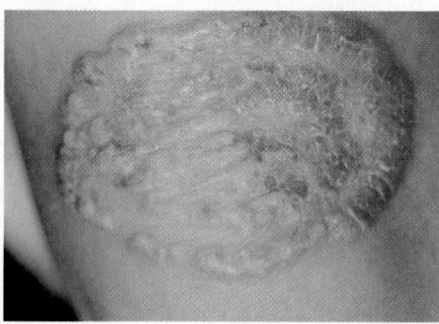

FIGURE 28-7

Ringworm. (Courtesy of Jason L. Smith, MD)

Ringworm (tinea corporis) is not a worm at all, but a fungus that results in itching, circular lesions on the skin (Figure 28-7). It is more common in warm, humid environments and in patients with immunocompromise. Ringworm is spread through direct contact with an infected person, but can be contracted through contact with contaminated soil or an infected pet. Over-the-counter antifungal medications such as miconazole and clotrimazole can be used to treat ringworm. Tinea capitis is a different fungal organism that causes ringworm of the scalp, which is more common in children than adults. Over-the-counter shampoos with selenium sulfide can be used to limit the spread of tinea capitis, but oral medications are required for treatment.

Impetigo is caused by streptococcal or staphylococcal bacteria. It is more common in children than in adults. Impetigo presents as a rash with fluid-filled vesicles that crust (Figure 28-8). The rash can be painful and itchy, and is contagious, particularly when there are breaks in the skin. Antibiotics are used to treat the infection.

Boils are painful abscesses that result from infection of hair follicles or oil glands (Figure 28-9). A cluster of boils is called a *carbuncle*. The most common cause of boils is staphylococcus. Very small boils can be treated at home in healthy individuals using warm compresses to promote drainage. Larger boils may require treatment with antibiotics and incision and drainage.

MRSA (methicillin-resistant *Staphylococcus aureus*) is resistant to antibiotics usually used to treat staphylococcal infections, and usually affects the skin. In the community

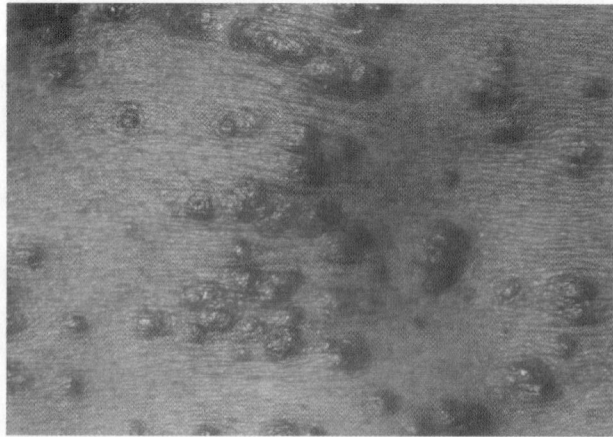

FIGURE 28-5

Scabies on the abdomen. (©Dr. P. Marazzi/Photo Researchers, Inc.)

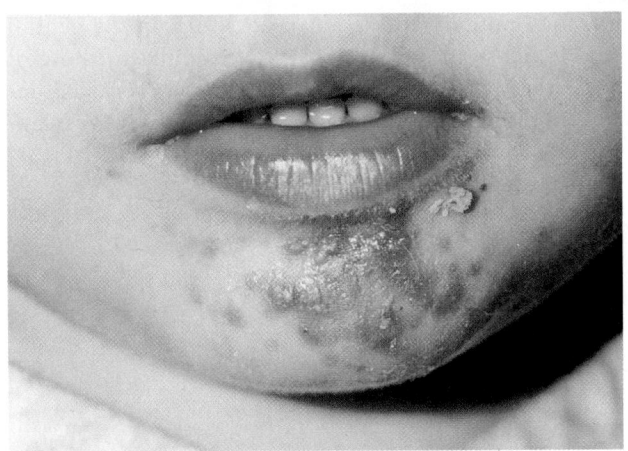

FIGURE 28-8

Impetigo. (Courtesy of Jason L. Smith, MD)

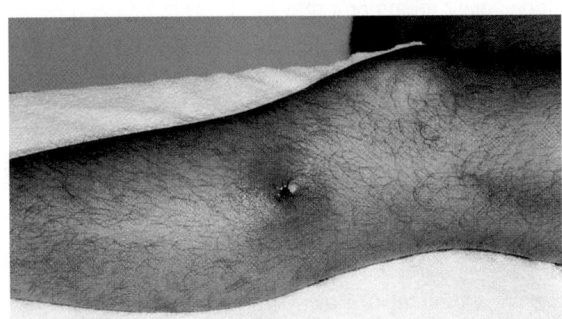

(A)

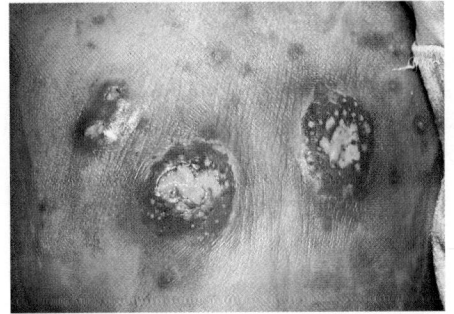

(B)

FIGURE 28-9

(A) A boil. (B) A carbuncle. (Both photos: Courtesy of Jason L. Smith, MD)

setting, MRSA presents as pustules or boils just like other staph infections, often at the site of an injury or other break in the skin. MRSA in health care settings is a **nosocomial infection** and can result in serious infections, including septicemia, surgical incision infection, and pneumonia. Some nursing homes may have a high prevalence of MRSA. Use Standard Precautions, including frequent hand washing, to prevent spread of MRSA between patients. Clean equipment, including the stretcher, between patients. Vancomycin-resistant enterococci (VRE) is another nosocomial infection of concern. Again, use Standard Precautions, hand washing, and cleaning and disinfection to prevent transmission.

Sexually Transmitted Infections

Primary signs and symptoms of most sexually transmitted infections (STIs) affect the genitals, but can infect other structures and have systemic effects. Always avoid contact with skin lesions and discharge and wash your hands after contact with an infected patient. Gonorrhea is a bacterial infection that causes painful urination and purulent urethral discharge in men, but which is often asymptomatic in women. Untreated gonorrhea can lead to infection of other genital structures and is a cause of pelvic inflammatory disease in women. Untreated gonorrhea can also lead to septic arthritis.

Syphilis is a bacterial infection that is transmitted sexually, but that can also be transmitted through other contact with its lesions. Contact with the blood of an infected person, such as through a needle stick, can result in disease transmission, but the risk is low. Untreated infected women can pass the infection to the fetus, resulting in congenital syphilis. Syphilis infection evolves through four stages if it remains untreated (Table 28-2).

Genital warts are fleshy growths caused by a number of human papillomaviruses (HPV). Certain strains of HPV are associated with cervical cancer in women. A vaccine against the most commonly implicated HPV viruses is available for cervical cancer prevention.

TABLE 28-2	**Stages of Syphilis**
Stage	**Description**
Primary syphilis	Approximately three to six weeks after exposure, a painless lesion called a *chancre* occurs at the site of exposure. The regional lymph nodes may be enlarged.
Secondary syphilis	Five to six weeks after the chancre heals, the patient may develop a rash on the palms of the hands or soles of the feet; a rash in warm, moist areas; and loss of hair in affected areas. The eyes, kidneys, or CNS can be affected.
Latent syphilis	Signs and symptoms disappear for a period of time that can last for months to years. During this time, secondary-stage symptoms can reappear. One third of cases develop tertiary syphilis.
Tertiary syphilis	Patient can develop painful lesions of the skin and bones. Cardiovascular infection can lead to aortic aneurysm. Appearance of neurologic signs and symptoms indicates neurosyphilis, which can include progressive dementia.

Chlamydia is caused by an organism that has characteristics of bacteria but lives within cells. It is a very common STI that can affect the eyes and respiratory system and is spread through transfer of infected secretions as well as through sexual contact. Chlamydia can cause blindness and pneumonia in babies born to infected mothers and is a cause of PID. In the genital system, its signs and symptoms are similar to those of gonorrhea. Trichomoniasis is a parasitic protozoan infection that is symptomatic in women but often asymptomatic in men. It causes a greenish-yellow, irritating vaginal discharge.

CASE STUDY WRAP-UP

Clinical-Reasoning Process

Advanced EMTs James and Marti are caring for four children who have a pimple-like rash on their arms and torsos, with signs that they have been scratching at the rash. They learn from children's services and law enforcement that the children were left alone by their parents who were later arrested. James and Marti will be transporting the children to the emergency department for evaluation. The children are hungry and live in generally poor conditions. There is no information available about whether the children have received routine vaccinations or if they have any health problems.

James and Marti realize that a rash is a sign of many infectious illnesses. The history of neglect makes them realize that the children may not be immunized, and may live in conditions that increase their risk for infectious illness.

The fact that all four children have the same rash increases their suspicion of infectious illness. The children have no other immediate indications of systemic illness. They are awake and alert with no cough or nasal discharge and their skin color is normal. James and Marti decide that gloves are sufficient PPE unless additional information becomes available.

James and Marti check the children's vital signs and take particular care to look for and ask about other signs and symptoms of infectious illness. The children do not have fevers or swollen cervical lymph nodes. They do not complain of sore throats, muscle or joint pain, nausea, vomiting, or diarrhea.

A more careful examination of the rash indicates that there are lines that radiate away from some of the lesions. James has seen this before in scabies. The lesions are not crusted, so he does not suspect Norwegian scabies, which can be transmitted from contaminated articles, as well as by direct contact.

James reassures the children and notifies the hospital emergency department that they are en route with four minors in the care of the county. He gives a description of the rash, along with the other history and assessment findings. After releasing the children to the emergency department staff, James and Marti place the used linens in the hamper, wash their hands, and put on new gloves to do routine cleaning and disinfection. They replace supplies and disposable equipment and go back inside to see if there is any additional information about the possibility of infectious illness. The pediatric nurse practitioner confirms that the children have scabies and will be treated before being released.

CHAPTER REVIEW

Chapter Summary

Advanced EMTs, like all health care providers, encounter patients with infectious illnesses. Recognizing general signs and symptoms of infectious illnesses guides your history taking, assessment, and decisions about protecting yourself and others from exposure to infectious disease. General signs and symptoms of infection include malaise, fever, chills, muscle or joint pain, and swollen lymph nodes.

Recognizing signs and symptoms of specific infectious illnesses allows you to anticipate particular complications and risks of those diseases. Cough, stridor, drooling, sore throat, nasal congestion, and adventitious lung sounds are indications of respiratory infection. In patients with those signs and symptoms, assess for hypoxia and ensure an adequate airway, breathing, and ventilation. Rashes are common in many illnesses, and some illnesses have characteristic rashes that can assist in differential diagnosis. Nausea, vomiting, and diarrhea are common with gastrointestinal illnesses. Those patients are prone to dehydration. Consider IV fluids for them.

Vaccination and good general health significantly reduce your risks of contracting an infectious illness through your work. Using Standard Precautions and communication with other health care providers reduce your risk of contracting infectious illness, the risk to other health care providers, and the risk to patients of nosocomial infection.

Review Questions

Multiple-Choice Questions

1. Organisms present in the body that do NOT cause disease and help protect against infections are called:

   a. opportunistic agents.
   b. immunoglobulins.
   c. pathogens.
   d. normal flora.

2. Which one of the following would confer natural active immunity against a specific illness?

   a. Having the illness
   b. Getting a vaccine against the illness
   c. Receiving maternal antibodies
   d. Getting an injection of immunoglobulin

3. Which one of the following is an example of a vector-borne illness?

   a. MRSA
   b. Hepatitis A
   c. Lyme disease
   d. Herpes simplex type 2

4. The time between exposure to a disease and the onset of signs and symptoms is the:

   a. incubation period.
   b. window phase.
   c. colonization time.
   d. carrier state.

5. Which one of the following is a bacterial disease?

   a. Oral thrush
   b. Influenza
   c. Tuberculosis
   d. Mononucleosis

6. What type of hepatitis is contracted through the fecal–oral route?

   a. A   c. C
   b. B   d. D

7. Which one of the following is a complication of untreated strep throat?

   a. Cirrhosis of the liver
   b. Rheumatic heart disease
   c. Kaposi's sarcoma
   d. VRE

8. The disease that causes severe coughing fits that leave patients gasping for air with a characteristic "whooping" sound is:

   a. rubella.
   b. croup.
   c. hantavirus pulmonary syndrome.
   d. pertussis.

9. Which one of the following diseases lies dormant in nerve roots after the initial infection and can re-emerge years later to cause shingles?

   a. Chickenpox
   b. Measles
   c. Botulism
   d. *Staphylococcus aureus*

10. A 17-year-old female patient at a boarding school presents with a fever, headache, sensitivity to light, and a stiff neck. You should highly suspect:

    a. mumps.
    b. Rocky mountain spotted fever.
    c. meningitis.
    d. rabies encephalitis.

11. Which one of the following has been identified as a likely weapon of bioterrorism?

    a. *Haemophilis influenza* type B
    b. Eastern Equine encephalitis
    c. Tularemia
    d. Herpes simplex type 1

12. Which one of the following has been identified as a causative agent of cervical cancer?

    a. Chlamydia
    b. Human papillomavirus
    c. Trichomonas
    d. Syphilis

Critical-Thinking Questions

13. You have arrived at a nursing home to transport a patient to the hospital emergency department. The nurse tells you the patient has MRSA. How should you proceed?

14. What are some patient populations who are at increased risk of infectious illness? What makes each of those groups more susceptible?

15. A four-year-old patient presents in a tripod position with stridor, drooling, and a poor overall appearance. What are possible causes of his presentation? What special concerns do you have in assessment and management of this patient?

16. What history, signs, and symptoms would make you suspect active pulmonary tuberculosis? What special concerns are there in assessing and managing a patient with active pulmonary tuberculosis?

17. A three-year-old presents with a "seal bark" cough, a hoarse cry, and stridor when agitated. The father gives a history of "cold" symptoms for two days and says the patient woke up with a terrible cough about 3 hours after going to bed. What are potential causes of the presentation? What considerations are there in treating this patient?

References

Centers for Disease Control and Prevention. (2010a). *Pertussis.* Retrieved July 18, 2011, from http://www.cdc.gov/pertussis/fast-facts.html

Centers for Disease Control and Prevention. (2010b). *Meningitis.* Retrieved January 11, 2011, from http://www.cdc.gov/meningitis/about/index.html

Centers for Disease Control. (2011). *Hantavirus.* Retrieved July 18, 2011, from http://www.cdc.gov/hantavirus/

Derlet, R. W., Sandrock, C. E., Nguyen, H. H., & Lawrence, R. (2011). *Influenza: Treatment & medication.* eMedicine.com.

Retrieved January 12, 2011, from http://emedicine.medscape.com/article/219557

Dufel, S. E, & Cronin, D. (2009). *CBRNE-Plague.* Retrieved January 12, 2011, from http://emedicine.medscape.com/article/829233-overview

Muñiz, A. M., Molodow, R. E., & Defendi, G. L. (2010). *Croup: Treatment & medication.* eMedicine. Retrieved January 12, 2011, from http://emedicine.medscape.com/article/962972-treatment

Additional Reading

Bledsoe, B. E., Porter, R. S., & Cherry, R. A. (2009). *Paramedic care: Principles and practice* (3rd ed., Vol. 3). Upper Saddle River, NJ: Pearson.

29

Nontraumatic Musculoskeletal and Soft-Tissue Disorders

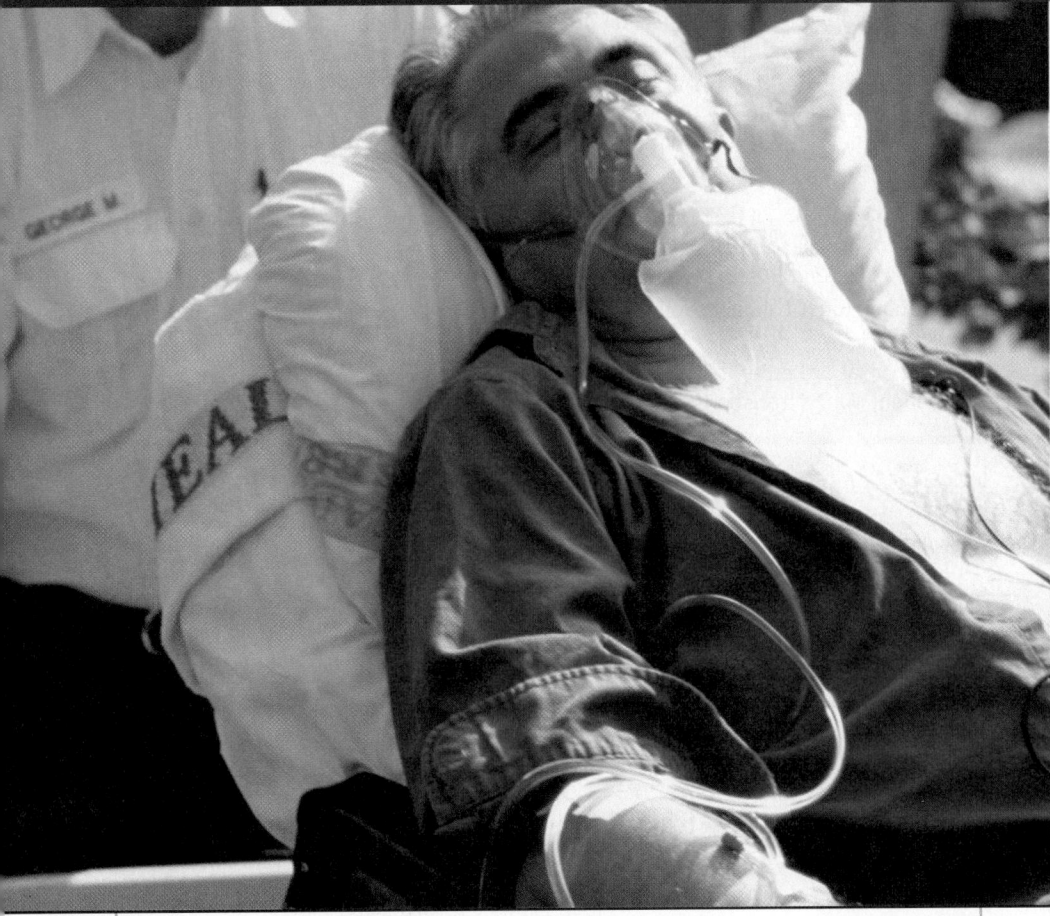

Content Area: Medicine

Advanced EMT Education Standard: Applies fundamental knowledge to provide basic and selected advanced emergency care and transportation based on assessment findings for an acutely ill patient.

Objectives

After reading this chapter, you should be able to:

29.1   Define key terms introduced in this chapter.

29.2   Obtain a relevant history from patients presenting with nontraumatic musculoskeletal disorders.

29.3   Describe the pathophysiology of, and concerns for, patients with osteoporosis.

29.4   List etiologies of nontraumatic back, neck, muscle, and joint pain.

29.5   Explain considerations in assessing and managing patients with nontraumatic musculoskeletal complaints.

29.6   Describe the pathophysiology of arthritis, including osteoarthritis, septic arthritis, rheumatoid arthritis, and gout.

(continued)

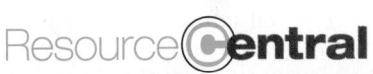
Resource **Central**

To access Resource Central, follow the directions on the Student Access Card provided with this text. If there is no card, go to www.bradybooks.com and follow the Resource Central link to Buy Access. Under Media Resources, you will find:

• *Bone Disorders.* Common types and how they develop.

• *Spinal Curvature Disorders.* Causes and how to prevent them.

• *Rhabdomyolysis.* How to treat this unusual condition in the prehospital setting.

CASE STUDY

Advanced EMTs Luis Garcia and Colin McDowell are en route to Hampton Hospital. They have been dispatched to transfer 70-year-old Mrs. Joelle Roudebush to University Hospital, nearly 2 hours away. Mrs. Roudebush, who has a history of osteoporosis, fell off a stepstool onto her kitchen floor, broke her right hip, and suffered a fracture and dislocation of her right shoulder. She was unable to get up and could not get to the phone. She lay on the floor for 20 hours before being discovered by a package delivery driver. She was transported to Hampton Hospital for initial stabilization, but must be transferred for definitive treatment. Luis and Colin have been informed that Mrs. Roudebush also has a history of type II diabetes.

Problem-Solving Questions

1. What complications could Luis and Colin predict from the patient's history?
2. What special considerations must Luis and Colin take into account when packaging and transporting this patient?
3. In addition to vital signs, what are other things Luis and Colin must consider in the continuing assessment of this patient during transport?

(continued from previous page)

29.7   List various etiologies of myalgia.

29.8   Describe the pathophysiology, progression, and needs of patients with muscular dystrophy.

29.9   Describe the pathophysiology and management of rhabdomyolysis.

29.10   Discuss various types of soft-tissue infection and inflammation, such as cellulitis, gangrene, and necrotizing fasciitis.

Introduction

Because musculoskeletal and soft-tissue signs and symptoms can originate in other body systems, there is overlap between some of the disorders in this chapter and those you were introduced to in other chapters. Muscle aches, weakness, rashes, changes in skin color, and other musculoskeletal and soft-tissue complaints can be signs and symptoms of other health problems, making them parts of a patient's overall medical history and your assessment of the patient's condition. There are also specific musculoskeletal and soft-tissue disorders that can result in a request for prehospital treatment and transport. Some of the conditions may be localized, while others can have systemic consequences. As a health care provider, you must have a basic understanding of how those disorders affect patients' health. In some cases, that understanding helps you make decisions about transport and special considerations in patient handling to avoid increasing the patient's discomfort.

Most nontraumatic musculoskeletal and soft-tissue disorders do not pose immediately life-threatening problems, but they can cause significant pain and disability. A few conditions are associated with potentially life-threatening problems. For example, rhabdomyolysis (breakdown of muscle with release of muscle cell contents) can cause renal failure and electrolyte disturbances. Some soft-tissue disorders, such as necrotizing fasciitis, can lead to death. Although it may seem that there is little you can do in the prehospital setting for those patients, there are important ways you can help them: Obtain a thorough history, including a complete list of medications; pay attention to patient comfort, and recognize that musculoskeletal and soft-tissue problems can be quite serious.

Anatomy and Physiology Review

The following text offers a brief review of the anatomy and physiology of the skin, skeletal muscle, and skeleton. For a more complete review, see Chapter 8.

The Skin

The skin is the protective outer covering of the body. Although we often think of the skin in cosmetic ways, the skin provides several essential functions. The functions of the skin include the following:

- Protecting the body from the environment, from fluid loss, and from infection
- Regulating temperature by increasing and decreasing blood flow to the body's surface
- Synthesizing and storing nutrients, such as vitamin D
- Providing sensory input from the environment
- Excreting wastes and secreting body substances

The skin consists of three layers: the outermost epidermis, the dermis, and the innermost subcutaneous (hypodermic) layer. The subcutaneous layer consists primarily of adipose tissue, which provides the body with a protective cushion, acts as insulation, and gives it shape. The dermis contains collagen and elastin fibers, blood vessels, glands, and hair follicles.

The epidermis is a bloodless layer, meaning that cells in its deeper layers must receive nutrients that diffuse from the dermis. As cells migrate toward the surface and become further removed from their nutrient supply, they die and act as a protective layer over the live cells until new cells replace them and they are shed. Epidermal cells arise in the deepest layer of the epidermis, which also contains the melanocytes that produce the pigment that gives skin its color. As skin cells migrate toward the surface, they produce and become filled with keratin, a protein that provides protection.

When skin is exposed to ultraviolet (UV) radiation from the sun, it synthesizes vitamin D_3. Vitamin D_3 is a precursor to the hormone calcitriol, which is vital to the absorption of calcium and phosphorus. Too little UV exposure results in vitamin D deficiency, but too much UV exposure leads to skin damage. Melanin production increases as sun exposure increases, providing a protective layer around the nucleus of dividing skin cells to protect DNA from damage. However, this protection is limited and excessive UV exposure results in cellular damage. The damage can manifest as decreased integrity of the connective tissues, with premature skin wrinkling and sagging, or as skin cancers.

In light-skinned individuals who have less melanin and less skin pigmentation, color changes are readily noticed. Normally, light-skinned individuals have a pinkish cast because of the oxygenated blood flowing through the skin. If blood vessels dilate, the skin becomes red, or flushed. With significant vasoconstriction or blood loss, the skin becomes pale. When the amount of deoxygenated hemoglobin in the blood increases, the skin takes on a bluish cast, called *cyanosis*, which is an indication of hypoxia. When the liver fails and excess bilirubin is deposited in the skin, the yellowish discoloration is easily seen in light-skinned individuals. As the amount of melanin in the skin increases, color changes become more difficult to detect. In darker-skinned individuals, color changes are more easily seen in areas with little or no

Geriatric Care

With age, a number of skin changes occur that make the elderly more prone to a variety of health problems. There are decreases in the number of skin macrophages (increasing risk of infection), vitamin D production (decreased bone and muscle strength), decreased oil production (dry, scaly skin), size of elastin fibers and collagen production (weak, thin, easily injured skin), circulation (decreased heat dissipation and slow healing), and decreased perspiration (decreased heat dissipation).

pigmentation, such as the nail beds, palms of the hands and soles of the feet, and mucous membranes (inside of lips or eyelids).

Skeletal Muscle

The more than 600 skeletal muscles in the body are each composed of individual muscle cells, or muscle fibers. Each muscle fiber receives its nerve supply from somatic nervous system axons that enter the muscle fiber to stimulate movement. Although skeletal muscles are under voluntary control, they also are influenced by autonomic control. For example, the diaphragm is under involuntary control, freeing us from having to think about the timing and depth of each breath, though we can over-ride the involuntary control for brief periods of time. Also under involuntary control are muscles that allow us to maintain posture and position without having to think about it, and muscles that respond to spinal reflexes, allowing withdrawal from painful stimuli without conscious processing.

Skeletal muscles provide several functions, including the following:

- Ability to move
- Maintaining position and posture
- Supporting soft tissues
- Regulating temperature through heat production
- Providing shape and protection

Skeletal muscle movement is controlled at the neuromuscular junction by the neurotransmitter acetylcholine (ACh). When a nervous impulse results in the release of ACh at the neuromuscular junction, ACh sets in motion changes in the muscle cell membrane (sarcolemma) that culminate in shortening the muscle fiber. Because a group of muscle fibers are stimulated at the same time, the overall effect is contraction of the muscle. If ACh was allowed to remain bound to the muscle receptors, it would result in continued muscle contraction. Acetylcholinesterase breaks down the ACh molecule so that it can be recycled within the neuron.

Muscle cells contain **myoglobin**, a protein similar to hemoglobin. Myoglobin binds to iron, which in turn binds with oxygen. Myoglobin allows muscles to perform work beyond the amount they would be able to perform if they could rely only on the amount of oxygen carried in the blood by hemoglobin. Myoglobin is normally found only within muscle cells. When myoglobin is released into the blood from injured muscle cells it can be toxic to the kidney tubules, resulting in renal failure. Muscle cells also contain potassium and other substances that are released when the cells are injured. Some of those substances, such as creatine phosphokinase (CK or CPK) can be measured in the blood as indicators of muscle damage.

Skeletal System

The skeletal system consists of bone, cartilage, tendons, and ligaments. Bone tissue consists of a matrix of collagen fibers embedded with minerals, such as calcium and phosphorus, which provide it with tremendous strength. Within the calcified matrix, there is living tissue: bone cells, blood vessels, and nerves. Bone cells are constantly remodeling bone by breaking it down and rebuilding it. A typical bone has a central cavity that contains marrow. Yellow marrow consists largely of fat, while red marrow consists of the stem cells that produce blood cells.

The skeletal system performs the following functions:

- Leverage, to allow movement in response to muscle contraction
- Support
- Protection
- Calcium and phosphorus storage
- Blood cell production

Joints are points at which two bones come together, or articulate. Joints have varying amounts of movement, depending on their structure, ranging from immovable to freely moveable. Joints can be classified as cartilaginous, such as the joints between the sacrum and ilia of the pelvis, or synovial, such as the shoulder, elbow, knee, and hip. The bone ends at a synovial joint are covered with articular cartilage. The joint itself is contained within a fibrous capsule that contains synovial fluid (Figure 29-1). Articular cartilage and synovial fluid function to decrease friction during movement and provide cushion. Ligaments connect bones at joints to provide stability. Tendons attach muscles to bones to allow movement. Bursae (singular, *bursa*) are small sacs of fluid that cushion surrounding soft tissues from ligaments and tendons. Some joints have additional structures to protect the bone ends. For example, the knee joint contains cartilaginous pads called *menisci* (singular, *meniscus*) to provide cushion.

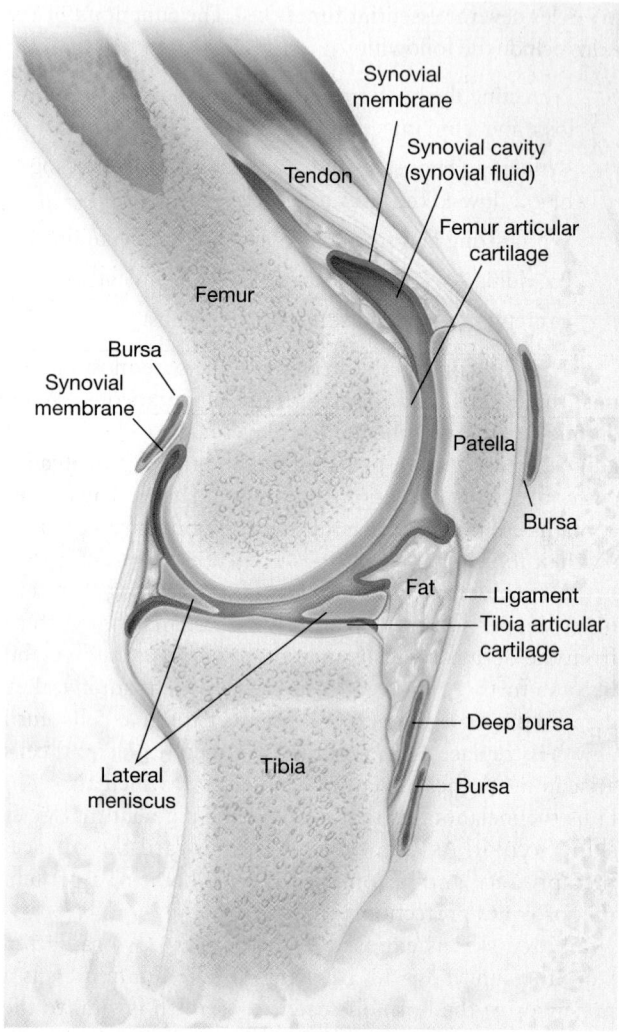

FIGURE 29-1

The knee joint.

General Assessment and Management of Nontraumatic Musculoskeletal and Soft-Tissue Disorders

Patients with nontraumatic musculoskeletal and soft-tissue problems can present with a variety of complaints, such as pain, weakness, swelling, redness, rash, or loss of use. Keep in mind that the problem may be localized or systemic. Use your knowledge of body systems, assessment findings, and pathophysiology to guide your history and examination. Perform a scene size-up to determine scene safety and the nature of the illness. Ensure the patient has an open airway and that his ventilation, oxygenation, and circulation are adequate.

Obtain vital signs and a SAMPLE history, using OPQRST to explore the chief complaint. In particular, a list of the patient's medication can be important in determining the cause of a musculoskeletal or soft-tissue complaint. In most cases, patients will be noncritical and a focused history and secondary assessment will be most appropriate. Check for **decubitus ulcers** (pressure sores or bedsores) in the secondary assessment of patients who are immobile or who have limited mobility. Use clinical reasoning to determine if a musculoskeletal or soft-tissue complaint is localized or due to a problem with another body system. Consider the impact of musculoskeletal and soft-tissue problems on patients presenting with other problems. Establish a baseline for the patient's condition, including level of responsiveness, vital signs, complaints, and pain level. Reassess critical patients at least every 5 minutes and noncritical patients every 15 minutes, obtaining at least two sets of observations.

Skin and Soft-Tissue Disorders

Skin and soft-tissue disorders may either be infectious or noninfectious. Disorders you should be aware of include **gangrene, necrotizing fasciitis, cellulitis,** and decubitus ulcers. Dry gangrene is the death of tissue due to ischemia, often in patients with poor circulation due to peripheral vascular disease. Patients with crushing injuries, frostbite, and severe burns can develop gangrene. The areas affected the most often are the fingers, hands, toes, and feet. The affected area becomes cold and discolored, and eventually blackens and sloughs away. This process may take days to weeks and the tissue may take on a mummified appearance.

Wet gangrene occurs as a result of an untreated infection, and is so called because the infected area oozes foul-smelling liquid. In patients with decreased peripheral circulation or peripheral neuropathy, such as diabetics, wound healing is prolonged and infection may occur. The infection causes swelling, which decreases capillary perfusion and increases ischemia. The bacteria involved (usually the clostridia species) are anaerobic and thrive in the ischemic tissue. Clostridia produce a putrid gas, resulting in the condition called **gas gangrene.** Severe pain and sepsis can occur, and the accumulation of gas in the tissues can cause a crackling sensation on palpation. Death occurs in hours to days without treatment. Even with treatment, mortality is significant. Treatment includes surgical excision of gangrenous tissue and aggressively treating infection.

Necrotizing fasciitis is a rapidly spreading infection, usually caused by group A hemolytic streptococci. In the popular media, this is referred to as the "flesh-eating bacteria," although other organisms are sometimes involved. The infection often begins at the site of an injury, which may be minor, or surgical procedure, or even at the site of an IM or IV injection. In some cases, a history of injury cannot be found. Diabetes and alcoholism are risk factors. A particularly significant complaint is pain that seems out of proportion with the appearance of the affected area. The **fascia** that surrounds muscle compartments is affected and as the infection progresses the skin and subcutaneous tissue become separated from the fascia. The infection can spread significantly within hours, and gangrene can develop. (Fournier's gangrene, discussed in Chapter 25, is an example.)

Cellulitis is an infection of the skin and subcutaneous tissues, resulting in the classic signs of inflammation: redness, swelling, warmth, and pain (Figure 29-2). It is a localized infection that can be caused by several different types of bacteria, but can progress to necrotizing fasciitis and sepsis. Cellulitis may begin at the site of a known skin injury, but sometimes a history of injury cannot be found. Immunocompromised patients, those with peripheral vascular disease, the elderly, and diabetics are at increased risk. Cellulitis can occur with or without an **abscess.**

Decubitus ulcers are commonly called *bedsores* or *pressure sores* (Figure 29-3). They can occur when an individual remains in one position for long periods of time, during which the tissue is compressed between bone and a surface. Usually, this kind of tissue compression becomes uncomfortable, causing the person to move. Patients with decreased sensation, such as diabetics and the elderly, may not feel the discomfort that prompts people to change positions. Patients who are weak or paralyzed are dependent on others to move them, and if they are not moved frequently

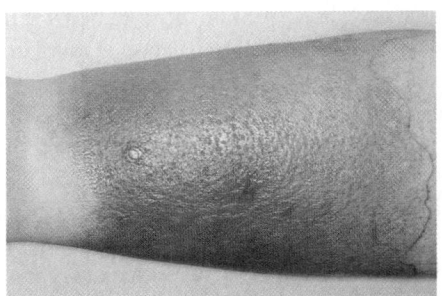

FIGURE 29-2

Cellulitis. (Courtesy of Jason L. Smith, MD)

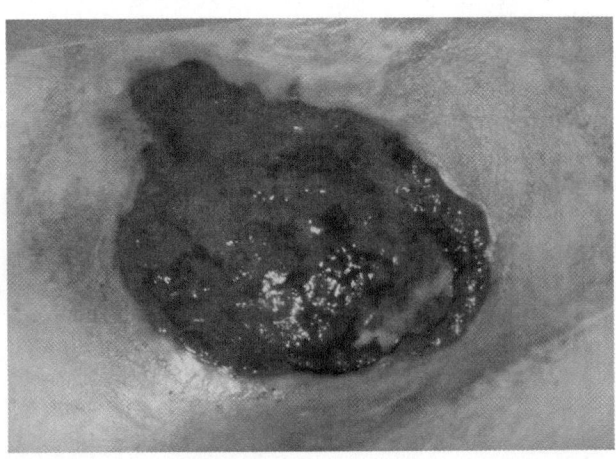

FIGURE 29-3

A decubitus ulcer. (© SPL/Photo Researchers, Inc.)

Keep in mind that the pressure caused by transportation on a long backboard, or even by a thin stretcher mattress, can lead to the irreversible changes that cause pressure sore formation in just 2 hours. Particularly if you work in an area where prolonged transports are common, do not place a patient on a long backboard unless it is indicated for spinal immobilization. If you must use a long backboard, provide adequate padding. The most common areas where decubitus ulcers develop include the sacral area, and tissues compressed by the ischial tuberosities, greater trochanter of the femur, and the heels. However, even with padding, pressure sores can occur. Remember that the duration of transport only accounts for part of the time that the patient remains in the same position. You also must consider any anticipated delays in removing patients from a long backboard once you reach your destination.

enough, decubitus ulcers can occur. The uninterrupted pressure on the skin and underlying tissues results in ischemia and tissue necrosis, which leads to ulcer formation. In susceptible individuals, the changes that eventually lead to decubitus ulcers can occur in as little as 2 hours.

Early decubitus ulcers may present as a localized area of redness over a bony prominence. At first the area may blanch when fingertip pressure is applied, but later it does not blanch, and may progress to a white, ischemic area before ulceration occurs. When you are assessing a decubitis ulcer, what is visible is often only the tip of the iceberg. Tissue destruction can include subcutaneous tissue, muscle, joint capsules, and bone. Reconstructive surgery is required for the management of severe decubitus ulcers. Always report any identified or suspected decubitus ulcer in your hand-off report to ensure nursing and medical staff are aware of it.

Decubitus ulcers are one type of nonhealing wound. Chronic, nonhealing wounds can occur in diabetics, immunocompromised patients, patients taking corticosteroids, and those who are hypoxic, malnourished, or have poor peripheral circulation. In the elderly, the normal time for a wound to heal can be six to eight weeks, instead of the normal three to four weeks. The longer a wound remains unhealed, the greater opportunity there is for infection. Diabetics are particularly prone to foot ulcers, and the homeless population may also have chronic foot ulcers.

Toxic epidermal necrolysis (TEN) and Stevens-Johnson syndrome (SJS) are two variants of a rare skin condition. In TEN and SJS, toxins lead to detachment of the epidermis and mucous membranes. SJS is the more limited form, with 10 percent or less of the total body surface area (TBSA) affected by epidermal detachment. In TEN, 30 percent or more of the epidermis may be detached. In those conditions, blisters form and progress until large sheets of epidermis detach. TEN and SJS are often drug induced, occurring within one to three weeks of starting drug therapy.

Drugs that have been associated with TEN and SJS include anticonvulsants, nonsteroidal anti-inflammatory drugs, sulfonamide antibiotics, antiretroviral medications, and allopurinol, a drug used to treat gout. SJS is also associated with products of certain viruses and bacteria. Because of the loss of epidermis, this condition is often is treated in a burn unit. In the prehospital setting, treat the patient as you would for burns, using dry sterile dressings and administering intravenous fluids and analgesics as needed.

Erythema multiforme (EM) has similar signs and symptoms, but is a separate disorder from TEN and SJS and is less severe. EM has two forms: EM minor and EM major. EM minor has raised, red lesions that primarily affect the trunk. EM major affects at least one mucous membrane in addition to the skin, but still affects less than 10 percent of the TBSA. A primary risk factor for EM is recent or recurrent infection with the herpes virus, but it also may be caused by the effects of drugs.

Joint Disorders

A common cause of nontraumatic joint pain is *arthritis*, which is a general term for inflammation of a joint. There are different types of arthritis, including rheumatoid arthritis, an autoimmune disorder discussed in Chapter 27. The most common type of arthritis, osteoarthritis, occurs from wear and tear on joints over time and is thus more common in middle-aged and older adults. In osteoarthritis, or degenerative joint disease (DJD), the articular cartilage is damaged and breaks down. Signs and symptoms include pain, warmth, tenderness, stiffness, swelling, and in severe cases, malalignment and deformity of the joint with accompanying muscle spasms.

Arthritis is common in the hands, spine, and weight-bearing joints, such as the knee and hip, but can occur in any joint (Figure 29-4). Infection (septic arthritis) and trauma can lead to arthritis. In severe cases that significantly impair quality of life and functioning, joint replacement can be performed.

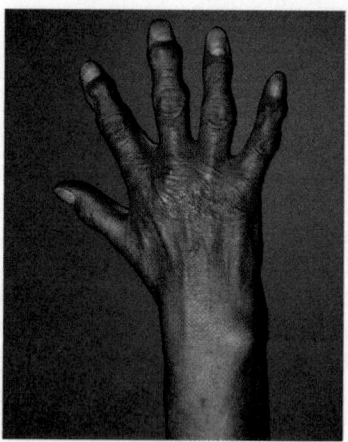

FIGURE 29-4

Osteoarthritis of the hands. (© Biophoto Associates/Photo Researchers, Inc.)

PERSONAL PERSPECTIVE

Advanced EMT Cindy Thompson: Like a lot of people I work with, I get low back pain from time to time. During one episode, my doctor ordered an X-ray of my lumbosacral spine. She was a little surprised when she got the radiology report. I'm in my early 40s, but I have facet syndrome, which is a kind of arthritis that affects the spine. Vertebrae each have a pair of facet joints that allow movement of the spine. These are synovial joints with articular cartilage, and the articular cartilage can be damaged, just like it can in other joints.

Apparently, the radiologic findings and clinical experience aren't always consistent with each other and the amount of pain experienced in facet syndrome varies. In my case, it may be due to occupational factors, but my sitting posture is poor, and that may contribute, too. I saw a physical therapist to learn some exercises to strengthen my spine and improve my posture and I am paying more attention to using proper body mechanics at work. I take ibuprofen when the pain flares up, but fortunately that is not too often.

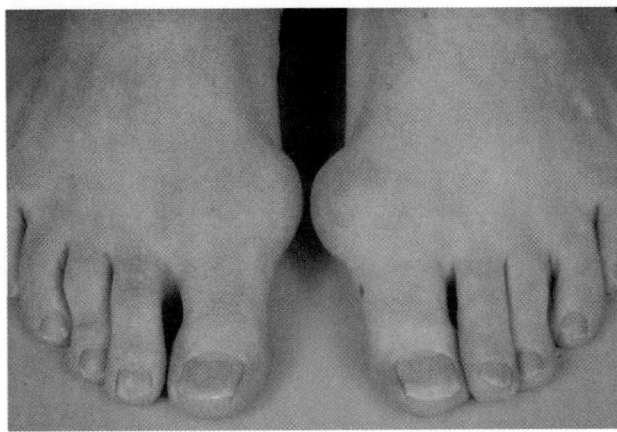

FIGURE 29-5

Gout. (© Biophoto Associates/Photo Researchers, Inc.)

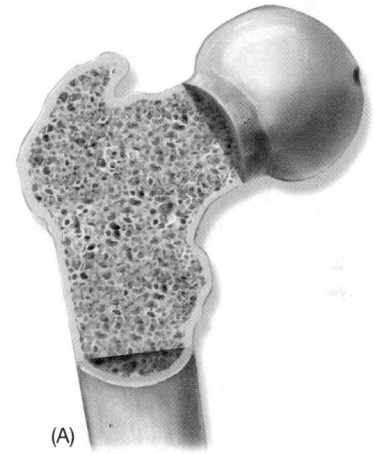

(A)

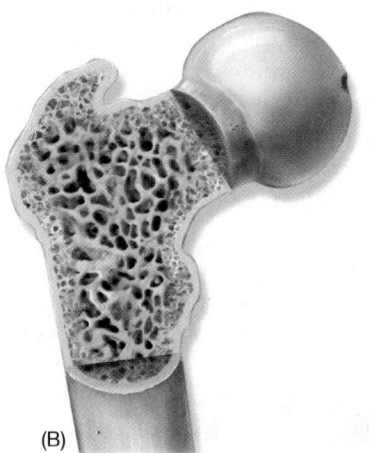

(B)

FIGURE 29-6

(A) Normal spongy bone. (B) Spongy bone in osteoporosis.

In some forms of arthritis, such as **ankylosing spondylosis**, the bones that form the joints (in this case, in the spine) can become fused, changing posture and limiting mobility. Gout is a form of arthritis that occurs from uric acid crystals being deposited in a joint, often in the foot (Figure 29-5). The disorder is a result of abnormal uric acid metabolism and is associated with a sudden onset of a hot, painful, swollen joint. Bursitis is an inflammation of the synovial fluid–filled sacs that protect the soft tissues adjacent to joints. Inflammation can be a result of infection within the synovial sac or irritation from excessive movement of the joint. Commonly affected joints are the shoulder, elbow, ankle, knee, and hip.

Bone Disorders

Nontraumatic bone disorders include **osteoporosis**, bone cancer, Paget's disease, and nonmalignant bone tumors. Increase in bone mass is supported by adequate amounts of vitamins A, C, and D. Deficiencies in those nutrients can result in scurvy (vitamin C deficiency) and rickets (vitamin D deficiency in childhood). Physical stress increases bone strength, because osteogenesis (bone production) adapts to the amount of stress placed on bones. The opposite is also true. In patients in whom bone stress is decreased—such as astronauts in weightless conditions, patients in casts, and immobilized patients—bone mass decreases. Exercise is an important factor in preventing osteoporosis.

Osteopenia, a decrease in bone mass, occurs with aging. When the decrease has pathologic consequences, it is called *osteoporosis* (Figure 29-6). Osteoporosis preferentially affects the jaws, vertebrae, and epiphyses of bones. It is more common in women, particularly Caucasian and Asian women of smaller stature. As the bones weaken, **pathologic fractures** (fractures that occur with minimal force) become common. Compression fractures of the vertebrae results in loss of height of the vertebrae. That, along with decreased thickness of intervertebral discs, can result in several inches in reduction of height in the elderly.

Kyphosis is an abnormal curvature of the spine that gives a "hunchback" appearance (Figure 29-7). Although some forms of kyphosis begin in adolescence, common causes include osteoporosis, degenerative arthritis of the spine, ankylosing spondylosis, and conditions in which the muscles are weakened or paralyzed. Kyphosis can pose difficulties in spinal immobilization. Always pad under the head and shoulders rather than trying to force the head, neck, and shoulders into alignment.

The most common primary bone cancers (osteosarcoma and Ewing's sarcoma) are more common in children and young adults, particularly in areas of rapid bone growth, such as around the knees and shoulders. Lymphomas and multiple myeloma are lymphatic cancers, but can affect the bones. Cancers from other sites, such as lung cancer, can metastasize to the bone. Bone cancers cause weakness of the bones and bone pain, and can result in pathologic fractures. Consider the possibility of

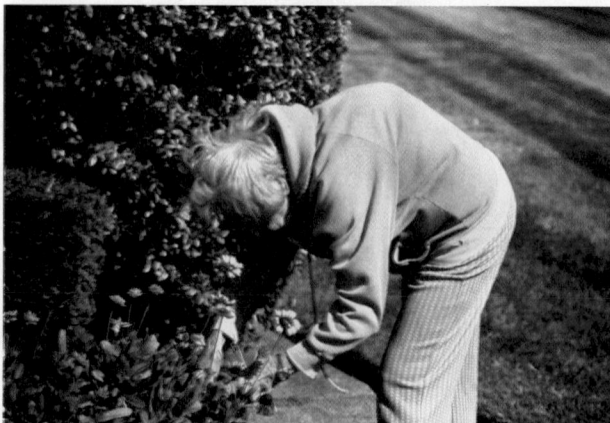

FIGURE 29-7

Kyphosis. (© Larry Mulvehill/Photo Researchers, Inc.)

pathologic fracture in patients with a history of cancer. A number of benign tumors, such as osteochondroma, can occur and result in pain and impaired growth. Paget's disease of the bone is an imbalance in the rate of normal bone destruction and rebuilding that results in enlarged, but weakened bones. It is more common with aging and most commonly affects the skull, spine, pelvis, and legs. Hereditary and viral mechanisms of disease have been suggested, but the underlying cause is not known. Fractures and arthritis are complications.

Muscular Disorders

Muscular dystrophies are genetic diseases that result in abnormalities of structural and functional muscle proteins, causing progressive muscle degeneration and weakness. The most common type of muscular dystrophy is Duchenne's muscular dystrophy, which affects males and has its onset between three and seven years of age. Most boys with Duchenne's muscular dystrophy must rely on a wheelchair by 12 years of age, and death often occurs by the early 20s due to respiratory failure. Other types of muscular dystrophies can affect females and elderly patients. In all cases, keep in mind that weakness of the respiratory muscles can lead to increased risk of pneumonia, and that immobile patients are at risk for decubitus ulcers.

Rhabdomyolysis is a breakdown of skeletal muscle that results in release of myoglobin and other muscle cell contents, which can enter the blood. There are both traumatic and nontraumatic causes of rhabdomyolysis. Traumatic causes include crushing injuries, electrocution, and severe burns. Nontraumatic cases can occur in patients who are immobile for long periods of time with resulting muscle ischemia. Scenarios include elderly patients who fall and are unable to get up, and alcoholics or those with a history of drug abuse who remain unconscious in the same position for prolonged periods. Rhabdomyolysis also can be caused by sepsis, seizures (particularly status epilepticus), prolonged exertion (running a marathon), and side effects of some drugs and toxins.

Some drugs associated with rhabdomyolysis include statins (used to lower cholesterol), neuroleptics (antipsychotics), antihistamines, and salicylates. Drugs of abuse and toxins associated with rhabdomyolysis include alcohol (ethanol), toxic alcohols (methanol, ethylene glycol, isopropanol), heroin, methadone, and cocaine. Significant toxic envenomations also can result in rhabdomyolysis.

Released myoglobin travels through the blood to the kidneys, where its color results in dark tea- or cola-colored urine. Myoglobin is toxic to the epithelium of the renal tubules and can result in acute renal failure. Hyperkalemia may occur, and can result in cardiac dysrhythmia. There can be massive fluid shifts into the injured muscle resulting in a significant decrease in circulating volume that compounds renal failure. One of the primary treatments for rhabdomyolysis is administration of isotonic crystalloid intravenous fluids to promote fluid excretion through the kidneys (Craig, 2010). Muscle edema can result in compartment syndrome, in which the pressure within the fascial compartment of the muscle increases above the capillary perfusion pressure, resulting in ischemia of the muscle within the compartment.

Fibromyalgia is a chronic inflammatory disease of the musculoskeletal system. Signs and symptoms include multiple tender points (11 out of 18 points identified by the American College of Rheumatology must be tender for a diagnosis of fibromyalgia), poor sleep, muscle stiffness, and muscle pain that have no other explanation. Fibromyalgia is commonly associated with chronic fatigue syndrome. It has been theorized that abnormal nerve transmission or neurotransmitter disorders may play a role in fibromyalgia. Some antidepressants that act on neurotransmitters and medications that affect the GABA receptors in the brain are used for treatment of symptoms.

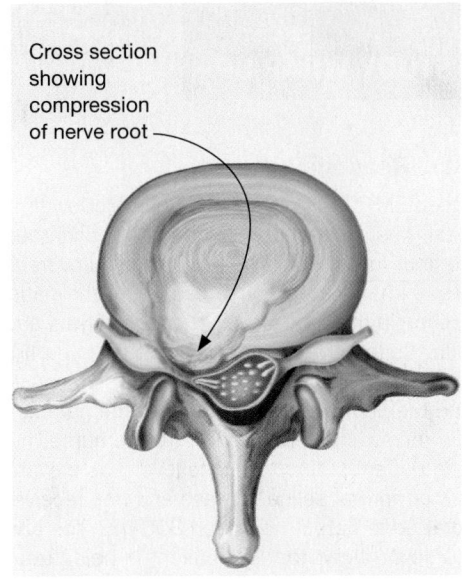

Cross section showing compression of nerve root

FIGURE 29-8

A herniated disc placing pressure on a spinal nerve.

Neck and Back Disorders

Several of the disorders discussed in this chapter, as well as a number of other problems, can lead to back pain. Back pain is one of the most common causes of time lost from work, but is sometimes difficult to diagnose and treat. In addition to the disorders already described, such as arthritis and pathologic fractures, lumbar strain and disc problems are common causes of low back pain. Nontraumatic back and neck pain can be a result of past injuries and poor posture. Neck stiffness and pain also can result from sleeping with the head turned or bent to the side. Lumbar strain, stretching or tearing the muscles in the lumbar area, occurs during activity, such as over-reaching or lifting, and is common in EMS providers. As a result, the injured muscles can spasm. Although it is painful, it can be treated with ice, rest, and anti-inflammatory medications. Other causes of low back pain include a herniated disc that impinges on a nerve. The intervertebral discs provide cushion between the vertebrae, but when they are subject to certain stresses, the disc material can be forced out of the disc space, which is called a *slipped disc* or *herniated disc* (Figure 29-8). The displaced disc material can place pressure on the nerves, resulting in pain. When the sciatic nerve is compressed, the pain can radiate through the buttocks and down the leg, resulting in **sciatica**.

Nontraumatic back and neck pain can be worsened by spinal immobilization and generally is not needed. In some cases, you should consider analgesia prior to moving patients with nontraumatic back pain.

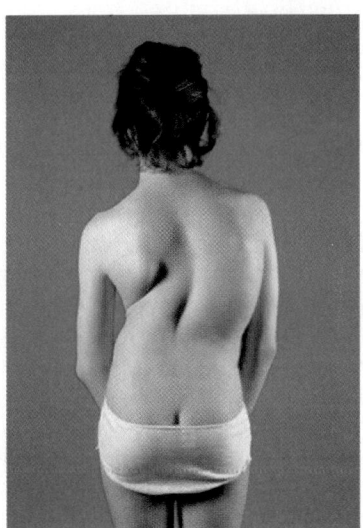

FIGURE 29-9

Scoliosis. (© SPL/Photo Researchers, Inc.)

Scoliosis is an abnormal lateral curvature of the spine, which can lead to an increased incidence of back pain later in life. Scoliosis can be slight and difficult to detect, or can be severe enough to result in unequal height of the shoulders or hips (Figure 29-9). Mild cases are usually monitored for changes, but are not actively treated. More severe cases may require braces or surgery. In severe, untreated cases, the shifting spine can alter the shape of the thoracic cavity, resulting in heart and lung impairment.

CASE STUDY WRAP-UP

Clinical-Reasoning Process

Advanced EMTs Luis Garcia and Colin McDowell are preparing Mrs. Roudebush for a nearly 2-hour transfer to University Hospital. Mrs. Roudebush broke her hip and shoulder when she fell at home. She was unable to call for help and was on the floor for 20 hours before being discovered.

Luis is immediately concerned about the patient's history of lying on the floor for 20 hours. He recognizes that tissue ischemia may have led to rhabdomyolysis and changes that could lead to decubitus ulcers. When he mentions this to Colin, Colin agrees and adds that the type II diabetes could be a complicating factor, both in the extent of tissue damage and the ability to heal. Luis is also concerned about dehydration and hypothermia from the patient's extended time on the floor. He anticipates that the patient will have IVs and a Foley catheter in place to monitor urine output.

Luis receives a verbal report from a nurse, along with a copy of the patient's chart and nursing notes. He notices that the patient's blood glucose level was elevated and that she has received insulin subcutaneously. The patient has two IVs of normal saline in place and has received a total of 2 L of fluid. The patient has a Foley catheter in place and her total urine output has been 800 mL. The urine looks dark and Luis asks about the possibility of rhabdomyolysis. The nurse confirms that the patient is being treated for rhabdomyolysis and has received diuretics to further promote urine output. Luis asks for some egg-crate foam to pad the stretcher and an extra blanket.

Louis introduces himself and he and Colin perform an assessment, including vital signs and a blood glucose level. Mrs. Roudebush is drowsy and the nurse confirms that she has administered a narcotic for pain. Their plan is to continuously monitor the patient's SpO_2 and pulse, and to program the automatic blood pressure cuff to take the blood pressure at 15-minute intervals. Luis also will monitor the patient's respirations, pain level, IV sites and rates, urine output, and blood glucose.

CHAPTER REVIEW

Chapter Summary

Nontraumatic musculoskeletal and soft-tissue complaints can have many underlying causes. Always consider systemic causes, as well as localized problems, in your history and assessment of the patient. Obtain a list of the patient's medications with those complaints, because several problems have been traced to the side effects of specific medications. Although most musculoskeletal and soft-tissue complaints are not life threatening, you can play a significant role in patient comfort. By understanding the mechanisms behind decubitus ulcers and rhabdomyolysis, you can anticipate the complications and avoid actions that can lead to their development. Understanding the consequences of specific disorders, such as gangrene and necrotizing fasciitis, helps you make appropriate transport decisions so that patients can rapidly receive the care they need. The rapid progression of those diseases means that an appropriate transport decision can truly be lifesaving.

Review Questions

Multiple-Choice Questions

1. A 62-year-old diabetic who does not receive regular medical care states that she stopped having feeling in the toes of her right foot a week ago and they have become progressively discolored. Her toes are blackened with a mummified appearance. The history and appearance are most consistent with:

   a. necrotizing fasciitis.
   b. decubitus ulcer.
   c. gangrene.
   d. cellulitis.

2. A 25-year-old patient who recently began taking an anticonvulsant for a new onset of seizures states that he developed large blisters on his skin followed by "peeling away" of large sheets of skin tissue. This description is most consistent with:

   a. gout.
   b. toxic epidermal necrolysis.
   c. wet gangrene.
   d. necrotizing fasciitis.

3. Arthritis that occurs in middle and older age from accumulated wear and tear on joints, resulting in loss of articular cartilage is called:

   a. osteoarthritis.
   b. ankylosing spondylosis.
   c. septic arthritis.
   d. rheumatoid arthritis.

4. The spinal deformity that results in exaggeration of the normal thoracic curve of the spine, eventually causing a "hunchback" appearance is:

   a. scoliosis.
   b. spondylosis.
   c. lordosis.
   d. kyphosis.

5. Breakdown of skeletal muscle with release of myoglobin and other cellular contents is called:

   a. Stevens-Johnson syndrome.
   b. fibromyalgia.
   c. rhabdomyolysis.
   d. toxic epidermal necrolysis.

6. A patient complains of low back pain with "shooting" pains through his buttocks and thigh. His complaint is most consistent with:

   a. sciatica.
   b. lumbar strain.
   c. compartment syndrome.
   d. scoliosis.

Critical-Thinking Questions

7. Why is fluid administration beneficial in patients with rhabdomyolysis?

8. Why are patients with poor circulation at risk for gas gangrene?

Reference

Craig, S. (2010). *Rhabdomyolysis: Treatment and medication.* eMedicine. Retrieved January 17, 2011, from http://medscape .com/article/827738-treatment

Additional Reading

Curtis, D. L. (2010). *Cellulitis.* eMedicine. Retrieved January 18, 2011, from http://emedicine.medscape.com/article/ 781412-overview

de la Torre, J. I., & Chambers, J. A. (2008). Wound healing, chronic wounds. eMedicine. Retrieved January 18, 2011, from http://emedicine.medscape.com/article/1298452-overview

Maynor, M. (2009). *Necrotizing fasciitis: Differential diagnoses & workup.* eMedicine. Retrieved January 17, 2011, from http:// emedicine.medscape.com/article/784690-diagnosis

Revis, D. R. (2010). *Decubitus ulcers.* eMedicine. Retrieved January 17, 2011, from http://emedicine.medscape.com/ article/190115-print

30 Disorders of the Eye, Ear, Nose, Throat, and Oral Cavity

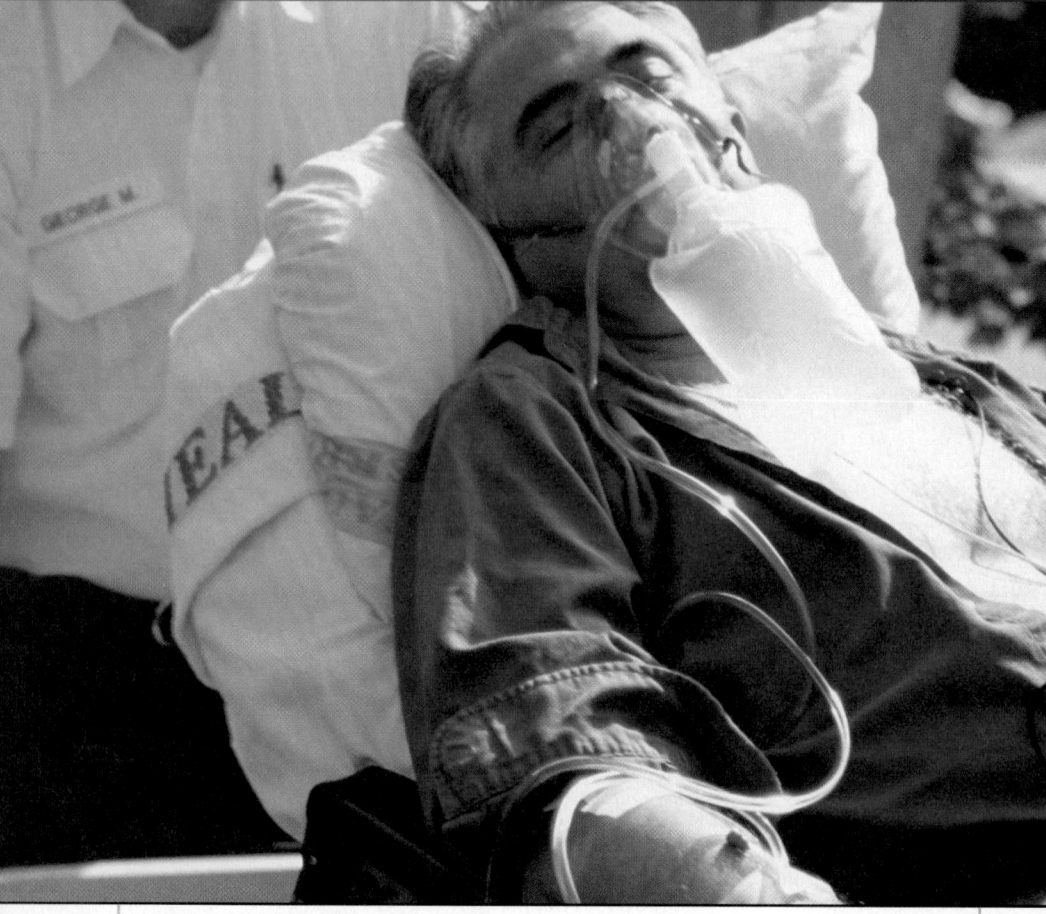

Content Area: Medicine

Advanced EMT Education Standard: Applies fundamental knowledge to provide basic and selected advanced emergency care and transportation based on assessment findings for an acutely ill patient.

Objectives

After reading this chapter, you should be able to:

30.1   Define key terms introduced in this chapter.

30.2   Describe the etiology and pathophysiology of the following:

– Chalazion

– Conjunctivitis

– Glaucoma

– Hordeolum

– Orbital cellulitis

– Periorbital cellulitis

30.3   Develop a list of differential diagnoses for patients presenting with eye complaints.

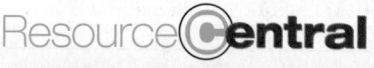

To access Resource Central, follow the directions on the Student Access Card provided with this text. If there is no card, go to www.bradybooks.com and follow the Resource Central link to Buy Access. Under Media Resources, you will find:

• *Epistaxis.* Learn about the common causes of epistaxis and how to manage it.

• *Vertigo.* Learn about the causes of and serious conditions manifested by vertigo.

• *Periorbital Cellulitis.* Determine when this strange condition may be an emergency.

Advanced EMTs Charlie Moore and Ben Paulson have just arrived on the scene at 6415 Broadmoor Road for a report of an elderly man with severe eye pain. The patient, 76-year-old Mr. Thaddeus Colson, is lying in bed with a damp washcloth over his forehead. Mr. Colson's neighbor called after finding him in severe pain. Mr. Colson's left eye is red and cloudy looking. He complains of severe eye pain and a headache with the pain rated a 9/10 with a sudden worsening in his vision, which he says is blurry. He is nauseated and has vomited three times. Although he is alert, he prefers not to speak or move because of the pain. He has a past medical history of high blood pressure, for which he takes captopril, an ACE inhibitor. His blood pressure is 148/90, heart rate 88, respirations 18, and SpO$_2$ is 97 percent on room air.

Problem-Solving Questions

1. What are some potential causes of the patient's presentation?
2. Under what circumstances could eye pain present a time-critical emergency?
3. What questions and assessments will help Charlie and Ben determine the nature of the underlying problem?

30.4 Develop a treatment plan for patients presenting with an eye problem in the prehospital setting.

30.5 Describe the etiology and pathophysiology of the following:
– Foreign body in the ear
– Otitis externa
– Otitis media
– Vertigo

30.6 Develop a list of differential diagnoses for patients presenting with ear complaints.

30.7 Develop a treatment plan for patients presenting with ear complaints in the prehospital setting.

30.8 Describe the etiology and pathophysiology of the following:
– Epistaxis
– Nasal foreign bodies
– Sinusitis

30.9 Develop a list of differential diagnoses for patients with nasal complaints.

30.10 Describe the etiology and pathophysiology of the following:
– Dentalgia and dental abscess
– Epiglottitis
– Peritonsillar abscess

30.11 Develop a list of differential diagnoses for patients with indications of problems of the throat and oropharynx.

30.12 Develop a treatment plan for patients presenting with problems of the nose, throat, or oropharynx in the prehospital setting.

Introduction

Areas of medical specialization are devoted to the specialized structures, functions, and unique problems of the eyes, ears, nose, oral cavity, and throat. However, in an emergency, patients may not have immediate access to those medical specialties and may require prompt care to prevent permanent damage, disability, or even death. Advanced

EMTs must have a basic understanding of disorders that affect the eyes, ears, nose, oral cavity, and throat. Human beings rely on the special senses of sight, hearing, and smell for critical information about the environment. The threat of loss of one of those senses is frightening for patients. Some of the disorders of those structures can be very painful. A few can be life threatening. But your actions and decisions can make a difference in the patient's outcome.

Anatomy and Physiology Review

A basic overview of the anatomy and physiology of the eye, ear, nose, oral cavity, and throat are necessary to understanding the problems associated with them.

The Eyes

The sense of vision is provided by special receptor cells in the eye that send nerve impulses to the visual cortex in the occipital lobes of the brain. Other parts of the eye function to focus the light that enters the eye so that light is detected in precisely the right way by those sensors (Figure 30-1). The bony orbits of the skull and accessory structures, such as the eyelids, eyelashes, and lacrimal (tear) ducts protect the fragile structures of the eye. Six extrinsic muscles control movement of the eyes.

Each eyeball is about 1 inch in diameter and weighs about one third of an ounce. The eye is a hollow globe with two fluid-filled chambers. The larger posterior

chamber is filled with a thick, viscous, gel called *vitreous humor*. Vitreous humor gives the eye shape and maintains the position of the retina. The smaller anterior chamber is filled with a watery fluid called *aqueous humor*. Aqueous humor is produced by cells of the ciliary body and drained by a structure called the *canal of Schlemm* to prevent excess buildup.

The structure of the eye is comprised of three layers, a tough outer fibrous layer, a middle vascular layer, and an inner neural layer. The fibrous layer is comprised of the white sclera and the clear cornea. The fibrous layer of the eye is continuous with the conjunctiva that lines the eyelids. The cornea has no direct blood supply, so it relies on the tears that flow onto its surface for oxygen. The lack of direct blood supply gives the cornea a limited ability to heal. Therefore, corneal injuries are serious and require prompt attention.

The vascular layer of the eye includes the circular, pigmented iris, which is composed of special smooth muscle. The pupil is not a physical structure, but an opening in the center of the iris that allows light to reach the lens of the eye. The two sets of muscles in the iris change the size of the pupil, either contracting or dilating it. Parasympathetic

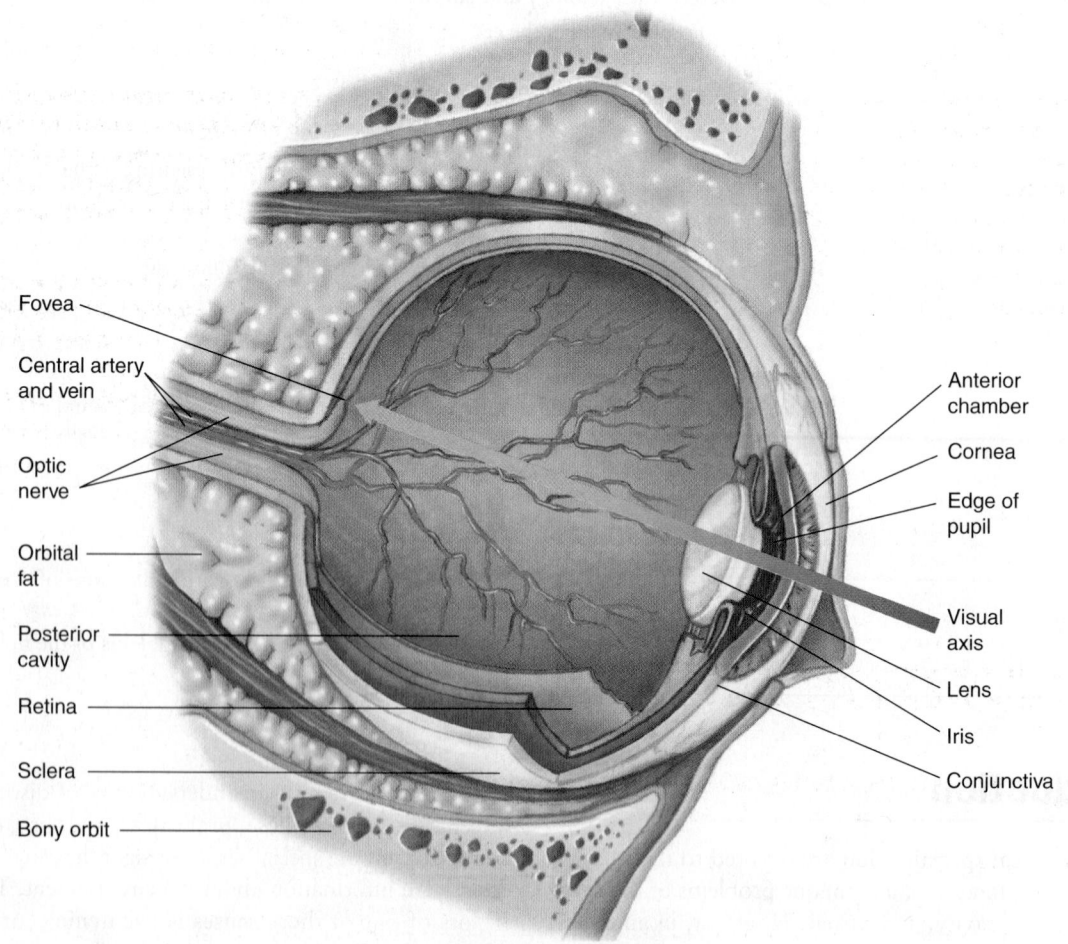

FIGURE 30-1

Anatomy of the eye.

innervation from CN III, the oculomotor nerve, allows pupils to constrict while sympathetic nerves allow the pupil to constrict. The ciliary body suspends the lens of the eye behind the pupil and acts to change the shape of the lens to allow the eye to focus at different distances.

The retina is the neural layer of the eye and is a direct outgrowth of the brain that is connected to the brain's visual centers. The retina has neural cells and pigmented cells. Two types of photoreceptor (light receptor) cells lay adjacent to the pigmented cells: rods and cones. Rods are very light sensitive, but not color sensitive, while cones are color sensitive. Vision is clearest when the light that passes through the lens is focused on an area of the retina with a high concentration of cones, called the *fovea*. The rods and cones, which are stimulated by the wavelengths of visible light, stimulate neural cells in the eye, resulting in the chain of events that results in transmission of information to the visual cortex.

The Ears

The complex structure of the inner ear allows for the senses of equilibrium and hearing (Figure 30-2). The pinna, or outer ear, directs sound waves into the external auditory canal, which is lined with cells that secrete cerumen (ear wax). Cerumen protects the ear canal from small foreign objects and pathogens. The tympanic membrane, or eardrum, separates the external auditory canal from the middle

Geriatric Care

With age, the lens of the eye is less able to change shape to focus on near objects. This condition, called presbyopia, often first becomes apparent in the 40s, gradually worsens from ages 50 to 70, and progresses more rapidly after the age of 70. Presbyopia often causes individuals who do not wear glasses to use magnifying reading glasses and individuals who once wore single-vision corrective lenses may need bifocal lenses. If a patient does not have his glasses, it may be difficult for him to read the print on any forms you want him to read and sign. Holding the forms slightly further away may help, but offer to retrieve the patient's glasses if you can.

ear. The middle ear is filled with air and communicates with the nasopharynx by way of the eustachian, or auditory, tube. The eustachian tubes allow equalization of pressure between the middle ears and the atmosphere. However, that pathway between the nasopharynx and middle ear can allow pathogens to enter the middle ear, resulting in an ear infection called **otitis media**. The middle ear also communicates with air cells within a portion of the temporal bone of the skull called the *mastoid process*. When an infection progresses to the air cells, the condition is called **mastoiditis**.

The auditory ossicles are three small bones of the middle ear. The malleus is connected to the tympanic

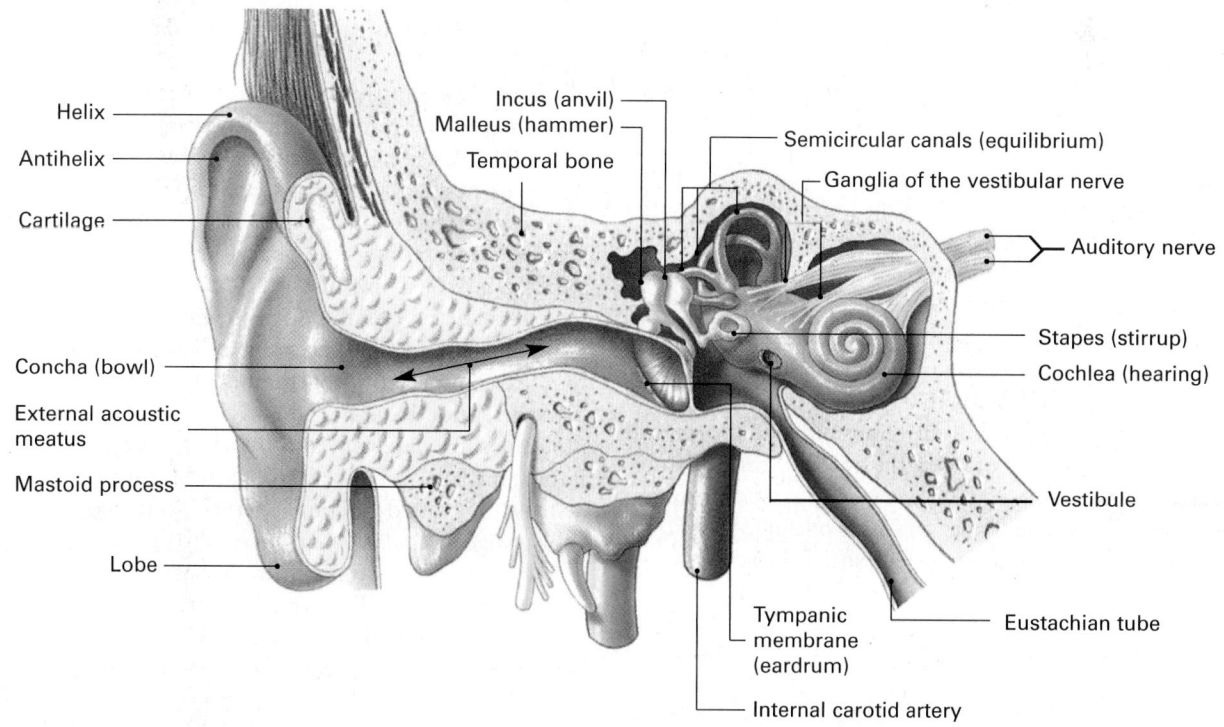

FIGURE 30-2

Anatomy of the ear.

membrane, and forms a chain with the incus and the stapes. The stapes connects to the oval window that separates the middle ear from the inner ear. When sound waves cause movement of the tympanic membrane, the movement is transmitted to the ossicles, thereby converting sound into a mechanical signal. The movement is then transmitted to the membrane of the oval window. Movement of the oval window is transmitted to the fluid that fills the bony *labyrinth* (the mazelike structure of the inner ear) of the cochlea.

The inner ear consists of a bony labyrinth that surrounds a membranous labyrinth within the temporal bone. The inner labyrinth is filled with fluid. Its membranous lining consists of special mechanoreceptors called *hair cells*. The first two sections of the labyrinth, the vestibule and semicircular canals, contain receptors that respond to changes in movement. Those sections are responsible for interpreting head position. When the head is moved too quickly, dizziness can occur. The last portion, the cochlea, contains receptors that respond to movements in the fluid within the inner ear. When sounds vibrate the tympanic membrane, the ossicles move and generate movement of the fluid in the cochlea. When hair cells in the inner ear are stimulated by the movement, they secrete neurotransmitters that stimulate nerve endings. Nerve impulses are transmitted to the central nervous system by way of CN VIII (also called the *vestibulocochlear, auditory,* or *acoustic nerve*). Prior to reaching consciousness, the impulses are conducted to the thalamus, explaining why we reflexively jump or turn our heads toward a loud noise. The auditory cortex in the temporal lobe of the brain permits recognition and interpretation of sounds. Damage to the auditory cortex impairs the ability to understand or make sense of sounds.

The Nose

In addition to the respiratory functions of warming, humidifying, and filtering air, the nose is the organ of olfaction, or smell. The olfactory organs are located deep in the nasal cavity (Figure 30-3). When molecules of odorants from the air come into contact with the mucus on the epithelium of the olfactory organ, they diffuse into the liquid medium where they can bind to receptors on olfactory receptor cells. When the odorant molecule binds to a receptor cell, it generates an action potential, which is then transmitted to the central nervous system by way of CN I, the olfactory nerve. Before reaching consciousness, the nerve transmissions stimulate the hypothalamus and limbic systems, explaining the strong emotional responses and memories associated with smells.

The Oral Cavity

The oral (buccal) cavity serves as part of the airway and digestive system. The digestive functions include the

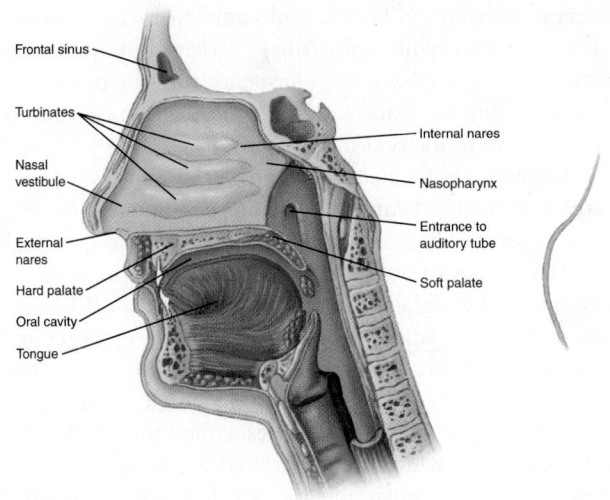

FIGURE 30-3

Anatomy of the nose.

gustatory sense, or taste, as well as mechanical breakdown of food through mastication (chewing) and the breakdown of complex carbohydrates into simple sugars by salivary amylase. The boundaries of the oral cavity are the lips anteriorly, cheeks laterally, hard and soft palates superiorly, oropharynx posteriorly, and the tongue (primarily) inferiorly. The gums are soft tissues that cover the surfaces of the upper and lower jaw, from which the teeth project. Both the upper and lower lips are partially attached to the gum behind them by a narrow band of tissue called a *frenulum*. The frenulum attaching the upper lip, especially, is easily torn with blunt trauma to the upper lip.

The surface of the tongue is covered with projections called *papillae*. Taste buds lie along the sides of the papillae, acting as receptors for the basic taste sensations: sweet, salty, sour, bitter, and umami (savory). There are fewer taste receptors in the pharynx and larynx, but there are water receptors in the pharynx. The water receptors explain how a drink of water can quench your thirst long before it is possible for the water to have reached the stomach and small intestine for absorption into the bloodstream (Martini, Bartholomew, & Bledsoe, 2008). Taste reception is similar to the sense of smell in the way molecules are detected, and olfactory receptors play an important role in the sense of taste. Information about taste is transmitted by cranial nerves VII (facial), IX (glossopharyngeal), and X (vagus).

Twenty primary teeth are eventually replaced by 32 secondary teeth. The arrangement of teeth is mirrored from left to right and top to bottom (Figure 30-4). Enamel covers the crown and neck of each tooth. The crown extends above the gum line, while the neck is normally surrounded by gum. The root section of the tooth extends

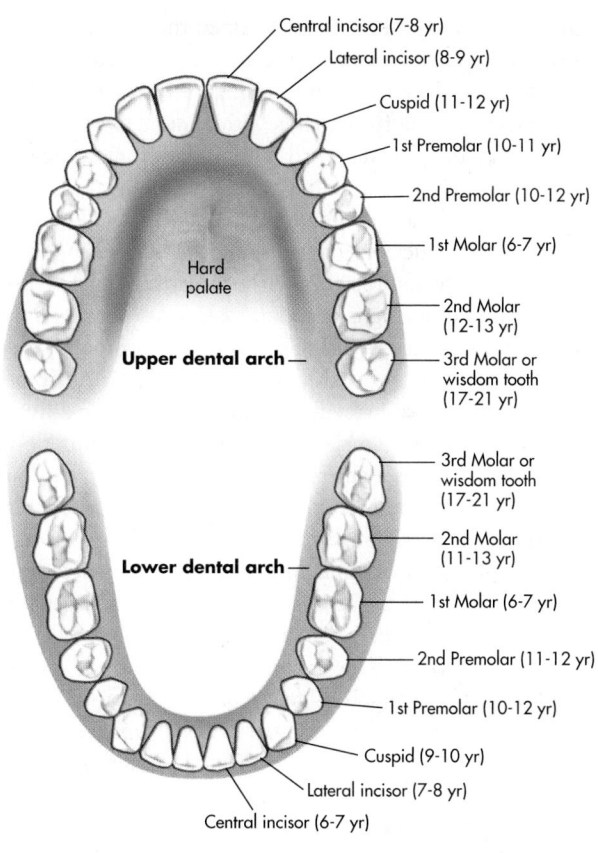

Central incisor (7-8 yr)
Lateral incisor (8-9 yr)
Cuspid (11-12 yr)
1st Premolar (10-11 yr)
2nd Premolar (10-12 yr)
1st Molar (6-7 yr)
2nd Molar (12-13 yr)
3rd Molar or wisdom tooth (17-21 yr)

Hard palate

Upper dental arch

3rd Molar or wisdom tooth (17-21 yr)
2nd Molar (11-13 yr)
1st Molar (6-7 yr)
2nd Premolar (11-12 yr)
1st Premolar (10-12 yr)
Cuspid (9-10 yr)
Lateral incisor (7-8 yr)
Central incisor (6-7 yr)

Lower dental arch

FIGURE 30-4

Dentition.

into the bone of the jaw. Beneath the enamel is a layer called *dentin*, which has microtubules that communicate with the pulp cavity, which contains the nerve and blood supply of the tooth. The root of the tooth is surrounded by a layer called *cementum*, which allows the tooth to be anchored in place by periodontal ligaments.

The Throat

The throat, or pharynx, is divided into three regions. From superior to inferior they are the nasopharynx, oropharynx, and hypopharynx (laryngopharynx) (Figure 30-5). The larynx and trachea are continuous with the hypopharynx anteriorly, by way of the glottic opening, which is guarded from the entry of solids and liquids by the epiglottis. Posteriorly, the hypopharynx is continuous with the esophagus, which leads to the stomach. All sections of the pharynx are covered by a mucous membrane. The oropharynx and hypopharynx have underlying muscles that are involved in the process of swallowing.

There are three sets of tonsils in the pharynx, the pharyngeal, palatine, and lingual tonsils, which are part of the lymphatic system. The pharyngeal tonsil is also known as the *adenoids* and is located in the superior nasopharynx. The palatine tonsils are the easily visualized pair of tonsils at either side of the entrance to the oropharynx. The lingual tonsils are located laterally at the base of the tongue.

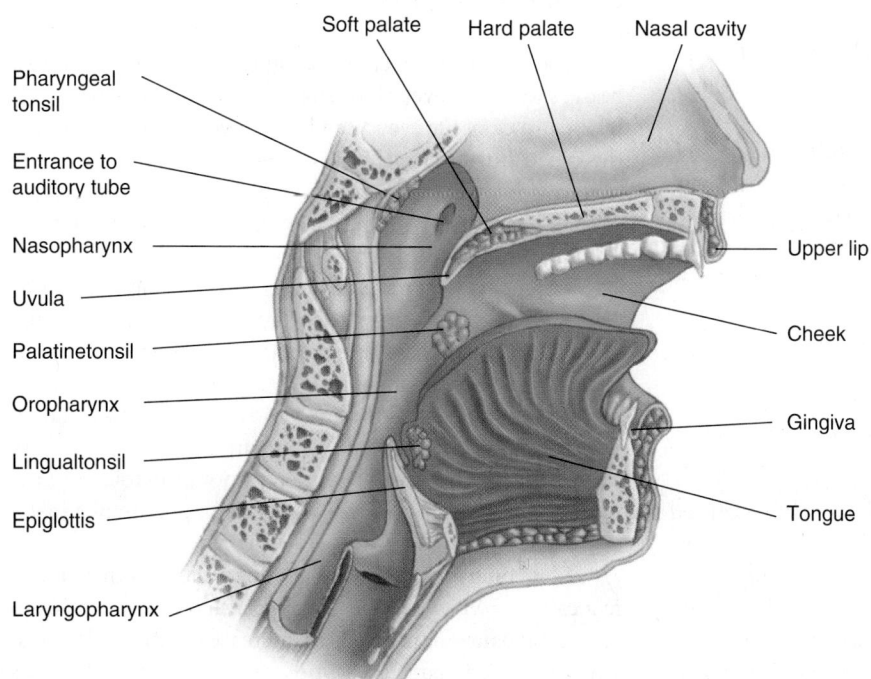

Soft palate   Hard palate   Nasal cavity

Pharyngeal tonsil
Entrance to auditory tube
Nasopharynx
Uvula
Palatinetonsil
Oropharynx
Lingualtonsil
Epiglottis
Laryngopharynx

Upper lip
Cheek
Gingiva
Tongue

FIGURE 30-5

The pharynx and tonsils.

General Assessment and Management of Eye, Ear, Nose, and Throat Disorders

Patients can present with a variety of complaints that may indicate a problem with the eye, ear, nose, throat, or oral cavity. Complaints are as diverse as pain and swelling of the affected area, loss function of the affected area, dizziness, headache, nausea, vomiting, and general signs of infection such as fever and malaise. It is particularly distressing when patients experience a sudden loss of hearing or seeing function. Reassure the patient that you are doing everything possible for him. Keep in mind that the problem may be localized or systemic. Use your knowledge of body systems, assessment findings, and pathophysiology to guide your history and examination.

Perform a scene size-up to determine scene safety and the nature of the illness. Ensure the patient has an open airway and that his ventilation, oxygenation, and circulation are adequate. Be particularly concerned with the airway in patients with complaints that involve the oral cavity and throat, because swelling of the structures can lead to complete airway obstruction. In severe cases, endotracheal intubation or cricothyrotomy (surgical airway) are necessary. Consider the need for ALS transport for patients with potential or actual airway compromise. If ALS is not immediately available, consider the possibility of intercepting with an ALS service or transport to the closest facility that can provide emergency airway access.

Obtain vital signs and a SAMPLE history, using OPQRST to explore the chief complaint. Establish a baseline for the patient's condition, including mental status, vital signs, complaints, and pain level. Assess for signs of shock and dehydration. Patients with infection or hemorrhage may require fluid replacement. Some emergencies of the eye, ear, nose, throat, and oral cavity are painful. Consider the need for analgesia according to your protocols or in consultation with medical direction. Reassess critical patients at least every 5 minutes and noncritical patients every 15 minutes, obtaining at least two sets of observations.

Disorders of the Eye

Conjunctivitis is an inflammation of the conjunctiva of the eye, resulting in a pink or red bloodshot appearance. It is a common nontraumatic eye problem, which may be caused by allergies, viruses, bacteria, or fungi. When patients have "pinkeye," they generally are referring to viral conjunctivitis. Conjunctivitis can lead to complaints of mild burning, a gritty feeling in the eye, and itching. Bacterial conjunctivitis may produce yellow exudate from the eye. Often, the exudate will form a crust along the eyelids and eyelashes while the patient is asleep, preventing him from opening the eye. Placing a wet compress over the eye will help relieve the crusting, allowing the patient to open the eye. The patient should be evaluated by a physician for diagnosis, and topical antibiotic drops or ointment may be prescribed. Wear gloves when caring for patients with conjunctivitis. Remove gloves immediately afterward without contaminating other surfaces and wash your hands with soap and water.

A hordeolum is, in lay terms, a sty. A hordeolum occurs when the ducts of glands along the margin of the eyelid become infected (usually with staphylococcus), causing swelling and other signs of inflammation. Generally, hordeolum can be treated by using a warm, wet compress several times a day to promote drainage of the gland. Antibiotics are sometimes prescribed, but most hordeola resolve on their own. When a hordeolulm results in accumulation of granular tissue, it is a chronic condition called a chalazion.

Orbital and periorbital cellulitis are serious bacterial infections of the tissues around the eye, which can occur as a complication of sinus infection, or other infection of the facial and eye tissues (including injuries, insect bites, and hordeolum). The periorbital area will be swollen and slightly discolored. The patient also might have systemic signs of infection such as fever, headache, and malaise. Patients may require hospitalization for aggressive management, and vision loss can occur. Orbital cellulitis is a deeper and far more serious infection, resulting in eye pain with any motion of the eye muscles.

Foreign bodies can affect the eye by irritating the cornea and conjunctiva, becoming imbedded in the cornea, or by penetrating the globe. Small foreign bodies in the eye are common and are often removed by tearing. Afterward, the eye may be red and irritated. A persistent feeling of a foreign body in the eye despite its removal can be an indication of corneal abrasion. Superficial foreign bodies are best treated by gentle irrigation with sterile saline or water, as for chemical exposure to the eye. (See Chapter 35.) A small foreign body, such as an eyelash or small insect, that adheres to the inner surface of the eyelid can be removed by gently everting the eyelid (turn the eyelid inside out) and wiping away the object with a wet cotton-tipped applicator, if your protocols permit. The patient should be evaluated by a physician for potential corneal abrasion.

Do not attempt to remove embedded foreign objects or objects impaled in the eye globe in the prehospital setting. Cover both eyes, stabilizing protruding objects as necessary (Chapter 37) and transport. Use metal eye covers that do not put any pressure on the eyelid or globe, if available. A small paper or plastic drinking cup can be used to help protect the eye if a metal eye cover is not available, or if the size of an impaled object does not permit the use of a metal eye cover.

Glaucoma is a vision-threatening condition that results in a call for EMS when there is an exacerbation that leads to severe eye pain. Glaucoma is an increase in intraocular pressure that can damage the optic nerve, leading to blindness if it is not treated. Intraocular pressure increases when the aqueous humor in the anterior chamber cannot drain normally. The increased pressure is transmitted to the posterior chamber. Glaucoma normally progresses over time, often beginning with loss of peripheral vision. However, the pressure can rise rapidly in some cases, resulting in eye pain and redness, headache, nausea, vomiting, seeing halos around lights, and a hazy-looking eye. In this case, the condition is an emergency and the patient requires prompt treatment.

Sudden partial or total loss of vision, in one or both eyes, can indicate very serious conditions, including stroke, retinal artery occlusion, and detached retina. Occasionally, sudden vision loss is a side effect of drugs used for erectile dysfunction. Occasionally migraine headaches can result in vision loss. Evaluate patients with sudden vision loss for other neurologic signs and symptoms and transport for further evaluation and treatment.

Disorders of the Ear

Otitis externa is an inflammation or infection of the external auditory canal. Factors that can precipitate bacterial infection of the external ear canal include trauma from placing an object in the ear, removing too much cerumen, and regular exposure of the ear canal to water, such as from swimming (swimmer's ear). Signs and symptoms of otitis externa include pain, a sensation of fullness or pressure in the ear, hearing loss, itching within the ear canal, and discharge from the ear canal. With otitis externa, the pain is usually increased by gently pulling on the external ear.

Otitis media is an inflammation or infection of the middle ear (behind the tympanic membrane), which may or may not be accompanied by a collection of fluid (effusion) in the middle ear. It is most common in pediatric patients and is often associated with viral upper respiratory infection. The upper respiratory infection can cause swelling and obstruction of the Eustachian tubes. This results in negative pressure within the middle ear, causing interstitial fluid to enter it. The fluid provides a medium for infection. Infants cannot provide specific complaints, but may be irritable or pull at the affected ear. In older patients, complaints include ear pain, fullness or pressure in the ear, decreased hearing, fever, and drainage from the ear. When examined with an **otoscope**, the tympanic membrane may be bulging in patients with an effusion of the middle ear. Rupture of the tympanic membrane is common, but usually heals without

complications. Although progression of the infection into the temporal bone is rare, it can occur. Whether antibiotics are indicated or not depends on the patient's age and severity of the infection.

Labyrinthitis is an inflammation of the inner ear that can occur from viral infections, bacterial infections, or other inflammatory processes. Some infections of the inner ear, particularly in the prenatal period, can lead to deafness. Signs and symptoms of inner ear involvement include vertigo, nausea, vomiting, and with some causes, hearing loss. **Ménière disease** and Ménière syndrome result from increased pressure that disrupts the mechanoreceptors of the inner ear, resulting in problems with balance and vertigo. In some cases, hearing is affected as well, and the patient may experience tinnitus (ringing or roaring in the ears). Not all vertigo is caused by labyrinthitis or Ménière disease. Benign paroxysmal positional vertigo (BPPV) is caused by head movements, and has several predisposing factors. Keep in mind that sudden vertigo can also be an indication of stroke.

Foreign bodies in the ear are most common in the pediatric population, although an insect, such as a cockroach, in the ear can occur at any age and can be quite distressing. Do not attempt to remove foreign objects from the ear in the prehospital setting. Doing so can cause pain and abrade the sensitive skin of the ear canal, or can result in forcing the object deeper into the ear. Flushing the ear can cause objects such as beans or seeds to swell and become more difficult to remove. If the object in the ear is an insect, there often will be a history of an insect flying into the ear or the patient will have the sensation of the insect moving or buzzing in the ear. If the patient is extremely distressed, check with medical direction about placing several drops of oil (such as olive oil) into the ear before transport, if feasible. The oil can sometimes kill the insect, reducing the patient's discomfort and anxiety.

A new onset of hearing loss can have several causes. Consider ear infection, inner ear disturbance, exposure to loud noise, ruptured tympanic membrane, cerumen impaction (accumulation of ear wax), and foreign body in the ear. A blow to the head can disrupt the ossicular chain, or fracture the temporal bone, interfering with sound conduction. Obtain a complete list of medications, because some drugs, including certain antibiotics and the common diuretic furosemide, are **ototoxic** and can cause hearing loss.

Advanced EMT Student Graham Blackstone: I was sitting in class one afternoon and had just turned to look out the window behind me. When I turned back to the front, I got dizzy. It lasted a minute or so, but every time I moved my head, the dizziness came back. I thought it would go away, but at break I was still feeling dizzy, and a little nauseated, so I laid my head down on the desk. Dr. Miller was guest lecturing that day and she asked if I was feeling alright. I was a little embarrassed, but I told her what happened. She explained that it sounded like benign paroxysmal positional vertigo. She had me lay down on a table with my head hanging over the edge slightly and gently moved my head around. She explained that there was a certain way to do it, and she called it the Epley maneuver. She said there are small calcium deposits in the inner ear, and sometimes they move to another area of the inner ear and cause dizziness. The maneuver she performed repositioned the deposits. It definitely worked in my case.

Disorders of the Nose

Epistaxis, or nosebleed, can occur spontaneously or as a result of trauma. Usually, the source of bleeding is the mucosa along the nasal septum, which is classified as an anterior nosebleed. The nasal mucosa is fragile and bleeds easily. One of the most common causes is trauma to the nasal mucosa, such as from picking the nose. Bleeding also might occur if the nasal mucosa is particularly dry, in patients with sinus infection, and in patients taking anticoagulant medications.

The bleeding can be significant, because the most common site of anterior bleeding receives blood supply from both the internal and external carotid arteries. Bleeding can be exacerbated in patients taking medications that interfere with platelet function or coagulation, those with hypertension, and those who have underlying medical problems, such as hepatic disease or hemophilia. Fortunately, you can compress the site of anterior bleeding by pinching the nostrils together. Posterior epistaxis is difficult to access, and you may suspect it if the patient has bleeding from both nares or has difficulty avoiding swallowing blood, even when leaning forward.

Assess the patient's airway and position him to keep blood from being aspirated or swallowed. The best position is sitting with the patient leaning forward over a basin. It is rare that the patient would be unable to protect his own airway, but if the bleeding is severe and the patient is at risk for aspiration, consider the need for advanced airway management. Pinch the nostrils together firmly to control bleeding. Instruct the patient not to swallow blood, which can cause nausea and vomiting. Once bleeding is controlled, caution the patient not to blow his nose, which will dislodge clots and cause re-bleeding.

Occasionally, epistaxis can be severe enough to cause shock. If bleeding is severe, start two large-bore IVs of isotonic crystalloid and administer fluids according to protocol.

Foreign bodies in the nose are more common in the pediatric population. Foreign bodies can be irritating to the nasal mucosa, resulting in swelling. The moist environment of the nasal cavity can lead to swelling of objects that absorb water. Button batteries may become corroded, leading to injury of the mucosa. There is also a risk that nasal foreign bodies can be swallowed or aspirated. As with foreign bodies in the ear, do not attempt removal in the prehospital setting.

Sinusitis often occurs after an upper respiratory system infection or in conjunction with seasonal allergies. It can result from several pathogens, leading to pain and pressure in the affected sinuses and often, a copious, purulent nasal discharge. Patients may have a headache that increases when lying down or bending over, pain in the eyes, postnasal drip (which can lead to sore throat and cough), fever, and halitosis (bad breath). Occasionally, sinusitis can spread to the orbit (orbital cellulitis), bone (osteomyelitis), and central nervous system (meningitis). There is no specific prehospital treatment for sinusitis. However, patients can feel very sick and experience significant pain, and complications are possible.

Disorders of the Oral Cavity and Throat

Patients with limited or no access to dental care often develop toothaches and dental abscesses, and may have nowhere to turn but to EMS when the pain becomes unbearable. Toothache can arise from several different tooth problems, but pain experienced in the tooth and jaw also can arise from other causes, including myocardial infarction, ear infection, and sinus infection. Painful dental problems include caries (cavities), abscess, cracked or broken teeth, and gum disease. Cavities are a result of erosion of tooth enamel, which is exacerbated by sweet, sticky foods that encourage the growth of bacteria that create an acidic environment. A deep cavity can lead to infection in the pulp cavity of the tooth, resulting in an abscess. The abscess can cause swelling and infection of the adjacent gum, and can extend into the bone. The patient may have fever, headache, and drainage from the tooth.

As with sinus infections, there is no specific prehospital treatment for dental pain. However, patients can feel very sick and experience significant pain, and complications are possible. Ludwig's angina is a cellulitis of the tissues of the floor of the oral cavity, which can be caused by an extension of dental abscess or an infection of an injury in the oral cavity. The swelling can involve the oral cavity, face, and neck, and airway obstruction is a possibility. Sepsis can occur as well, making this a life-threatening emergency.

There are several different possibilities to consider when a patient complains of throat pain. Although few causes are immediately life threatening, you must be aware of the causes that are serious and potentially life threatening. Sore throat can be caused by allergies, viral or bacterial infection, and gastroesophageal reflux.

Epiglottitis is a bacterial infection, commonly caused by *Haemophilis influena* type B (Hib). Although once more common in children, epiglottitis is now largely prevented by childhood vaccination. However, cases can occur in unvaccinated children and adults. Epiglottitis is a painful condition that results in drooling and difficulty swallowing. As the infection progresses, the patient may experience increasing airway obstruction with difficulty breathing and stridor. The patient is generally very ill with signs and symptoms of infection. If epiglottitis is among the differential diagnoses, do not attempt to inspect the throat or place anything in the mouth. Keep the patient calm and consider the need for ALS intervention for airway management.

Peritonsillar abscess, an infection in the capsule surrounding the palatine tonsils, is commonly caused by streptococcal and staphylococcal bacteria. The patient presents with general signs and symptoms of infection, sore throat, difficulty swallowing, and drooling. The pain may be referred to the ear on the affected side. Patients can present with a "hot potato" voice, speaking as though they are holding hot food in the mouth. Swelling and distortion of the soft tissues make airway obstruction a concern.

Diphtheria, a bacterial infection that was once largely controlled by vaccination, has begun to re-emerge in some populations. Patients with inadequate immunization, immunosuppression, and those living in poor and overcrowded conditions are at increased risk. The causative bacteria adhere to the nasopharyngeal mucosa where they excrete a toxin that destroys tissue, leading to necrosis and severe throat pain. The patient also may have other common signs and symptoms of upper respiratory infection.

The combination of tissue debris, inflammatory cells, and bacterial cells can form a pseudomembrane (a structure that looks like a membrane but is not) in any part of the respiratory tract. The infection can result in substantial swelling of the neck and asphyxiation can occur from airway obstruction or aspiration of the pseudomembrane. The patient may exhibit respiratory distress, drooling, and stridor with an obstructing pseudomembrane. The infection may spread to other locations in the body, including the heart and nervous system. There also is a cutaneous form of diphtheria that results in skin ulcers with a gray membranous covering.

Diphtheria is a contagious disease, and contact with the pseudomembrane or respiratory droplets is particularly infectious. Contact with cutaneous lesions also can result in either respiratory or skin infection. Add respiratory protection to your Standard Precautions, if diphtheria is suspected, and seek medical follow-up for exposure. Pay particular attention to the patient's airway status. Consider IV fluids for dehydration and suspected sepsis.

CASE STUDY WRAP-UP

Clinical-Reasoning Process

Advanced EMTs Charlie Moore and Ben Paulson are caring for Mr. Thaddeus Colson, a 76-year-old man who is complaining of severe eye pain, blurred vision, headache, nausea, and vomiting.

Charlie analyzes the information, determining that Mr. Colson is not critical, but that he has an urgent condition that requires prompt medical evaluation. The patient is slightly hypertensive, but otherwise his vital signs are within normal limits. Charlie is not sure whether the eye pain and vision change are part of the primary problem, leading to a headache, or whether something else, such as a stroke, is causing all of the signs and symptoms. The redness of the eye makes him think it may be an eye problem, but he performs a neurologic exam to look for indications of stroke. Mr. Colson has no neurologic deficits, and no past medical history of migraines or other severe headaches. Taking into account the patient's overall history and presentation, Charlie wonders if the problem is glaucoma.

Charlie and Ben reassure Mr. Colson and transport him to a large community hospital. Later in the day, they learn that Mr. Colson has glaucoma, and was admitted for treatment by an ophthalmologist. It is too soon to tell how much permanent vision loss Mr. Colson has, but prompt transport, hospital treatment, and follow-up all increase the chances of a good outcome from this episode.

CHAPTER REVIEW

Chapter Summary

Disorders of the eye, ear, nose, throat, and oral cavity, while usually not immediately life threatening, can be painful and distressing for patients. You must be aware of problems that are potentially life threatening, or threaten the loss of one of the special senses. Of particular concern are conditions that cause airway obstruction or lead to sepsis. Always keep in mind that a complaint about one of these structures, such as loss of sight or hearing, or vertigo, can have other causes, such as stroke.

Use a focused approach to history and assessment in most cases. Your knowledge of potential underlying causes of the complaints and pathophysiology will help you direct your questioning and assessment. Provide reassurance to the patient, pay particular attention to the need for airway management, and consider the need for intravenous fluids and analgesia.

Review Questions

Multiple-Choice Questions

1. The pigmented muscle that controls the amount of light that enters the eye is called the:
   a. ciliary body.
   b. photoreceptor.
   c. iris.
   d. pupil.

2. A patient tells you she was diagnosed a few days ago with labyrinthitis. Which symptom is most highly associated with this condition?
   a. Difficulty swallowing
   b. Headache
   c. Dizziness
   d. Sudden vision loss

3. Which one of the following should be your most immediate concern for a patient with suspected Ludwig's angina?
   a. Cardiac dysrhythmia
   b. Airway obstruction
   c. Blindness
   d. Uncontrollable hemorrhage

4. Another name for a hordeolum is:
   a. sty.
   b. orbital cellulitis.
   c. pink eye.
   d. glaucoma.

5. A patient complains she has a cockroach in her ear. She is very agitated and says she can feel and hear it crawling around in her ear. With permission from medical direction, which one of the following measures would be appropriate in decreasing the patient's discomfort?
   a. Pouring a few drops of olive oil in her ear
   b. Flushing the ear with copious amounts of warm water
   c. Using forceps or hemostats to grasp the insect and pull it out
   d. Pressing your hand over the ear and quickly releasing to create suction in the ear canal

Critical-Thinking Questions

6. A 42-year-old complains of a severe sore throat, mostly on the right side, right ear pain, and inability to swallow because of excruciating pain. Since yesterday he has had a fever and warm, flushed, moist skin and states that he thinks he has had "the flu or something." When he speaks, it sounds as if he is burning his tongue on a mouthful of hot food. What differential diagnoses should you consider? What assessments, history, and interventions would be appropriate?

7. A 30-year-old states she is homeless and has no access to medical or dental care. She complains of a severe toothache on the lower right side. Her lower right jaw is slightly swollen, and you can see swelling at the base of the tooth along her gum line. Why should this patient be transported to the emergency department?

8. A 50-year-old man complains of sudden loss of hearing in his left ear. What are some potential causes of this problem?

Reference

Martini, F. H., Bartholomew, E. F., & Bledsoe, B. E. (2008). *Anatomy and physiology for emergency care.* Upper Saddle River, NJ: Pearson Prentice Hall.

Additional Reading

Baminore, O., & Silverberg, M. A. (2010). *Epistaxis.* eMedicine. Retrieved January 21, 2011, from http://emedicine.medscape.com/article/764719-overview

Silverman, M. A., & Bessman, E. (2010). *Conjunctivitis: Treatment & medication.* eMedicine. Retrieved January 21, 2011, from http://emedicine.medscape.com/article/797874-treatment

31

Mental Illness and Behavioral Emergencies

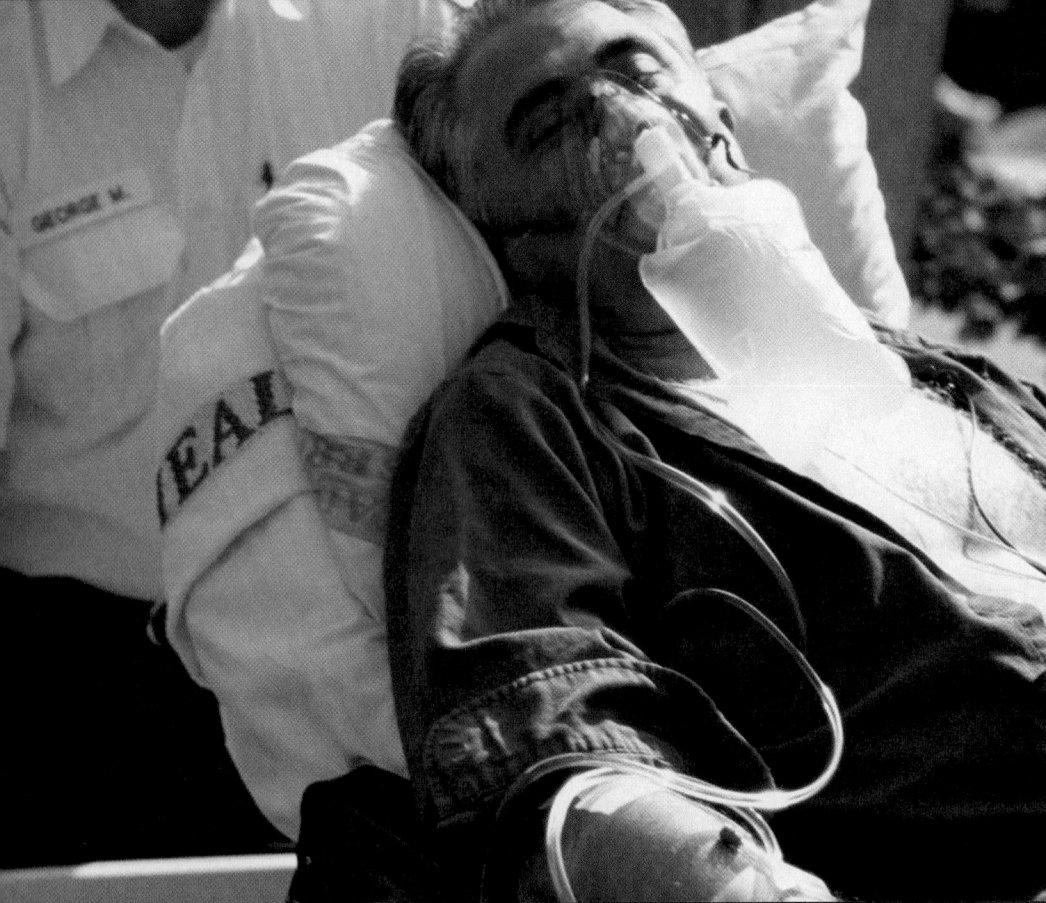

Content Area: Medicine

Advanced EMT Education Standard: Applies fundamental knowledge to provide basic and selected advanced emergency care and transportation based on assessment findings for an acutely ill patient.

Objectives

After reading this chapter, you should be able to:

31.1 Define key terms introduced in this chapter.

31.2 Explain the importance of being able to recognize and respond to patients suffering from behavioral emergencies.

31.3 Describe indications of danger associated with response to behavioral emergencies.

31.4 Discuss the underlying physical and psychological causes of behavioral emergencies.

31.5 Describe the focus of assessment and history taking for patients experiencing behavioral emergencies.

Resource Central

To access Resource Central, follow the directions on the Student Access Card provided with this text. If there is no card, go to www.bradybooks.com and follow the Resource Central link to Buy Access. Under Media Resources, you will find:

• *Suicide Intervention.* Learn about the warning signs of suicidal behavior, who is at risk and how to assist them.

• *Restraints.* Watch and learn about the different types of restraint devices and when to use them.

• *Schizophrenia.* Explore schizophrenia and what steps to take before caring for the schizophrenic patient.

CASE STUDY

Courtney Abbott and Albert Pearson, Advanced EMTs with McLean County Fire and Rescue, are providing special event coverage at the county fair. They are dispatched to the midway for a "possible heart attack." They respond on their specially equipped golf cart to find a woman in her mid 20s sitting on a bench, clutching her chest. She appears distressed, pale, and diaphoretic. Her sister is sitting next to her, looking very worried. "My sister said she thinks she's having a heart attack. She can't breathe! She needs help!" Courtney feels that the patient's age makes it less likely to be a cardiac problem than something else, but she can see that the patient is in a lot of discomfort and looks terrified.

Problem-Solving Questions

1. What are some hypotheses that immediately come to mind?
2. What line of questioning could Courtney use to determine the nature of the problem?
3. What assessments could prove useful in determining the nature of the problem?

31.6	Recognize behavioral characteristics of the following conditions:

    – Anxiety

    – Bipolar disorder

    – Depression

    – Panic attack

    – Paranoia

    – Phobias

    – Psychosis

    – Schizophrenia

31.7   Describe risk factors associated with violence toward others and suicide.

31.8   Incorporate the basic principles presented in the text into the assessment, communication, and management of patients with behavioral emergencies.

31.9   Prioritize patient care needs in terms of managing physical and behavioral problems.

31.10   Explain the importance of ongoing assessment of patients with behavioral emergencies.

31.11   Evaluate the need for law enforcement and medical direction involvement in a behavioral emergency situation.

31.12   Recognize indications for physical restraint of a patient.

31.13   Follow principles of safe physical restraint of patients.

31.14   Comply with legal and ethical principles when responding to patients with behavioral emergencies.

31.15   Document all information pertinent to calls involving behavioral emergencies and patient restraint.

31.16   Given a number of patient scenarios, assess and manage patients presenting with indications of a psychiatric disorder or behavioral emergency.

31.17   Consider physiologic differential diagnoses for patients presenting with indications of a psychiatric disorder.

31.18   Discuss substance abuse as a psychiatric disorder.

31.19   Describe the acute and long-term behavioral and physiologic effects of alcohol abuse and alcohol withdrawal.

Introduction

Mental illness remains a topic many patients are uncomfortable discussing, despite the significant changes in our understanding of it over the years. EMS providers are often uncomfortable managing patients with mental illnesses and behavioral emergencies because the skills and tools they commonly use for physical illnesses and trauma are not what the patient needs. In many cases, though, the most important way of interacting with patients with mental illnesses and behavioral emergencies is to use interpersonal skills and therapeutic communication.

Emergency calls involving mental illness and behavioral emergencies can have many elements. There can be scene safety issues; critical patients in need of immediate management of airway, breathing, and circulation; distraught patients who may feel hopeless; medical–legal considerations about consent and restraint; and ethical considerations. One of the most critical aspects is determining whether a patient's behavior or mental state is due to mental or emotional causes, or if there is an underlying physiologic cause. Some life-threatening problems, such as hypoglycemia, hypoxia, and others, can mimic behavioral emergencies.

This chapter presents basic information on behavioral emergencies, general assessment and management considerations for patients with mental illnesses and behavioral emergencies, and descriptions of specific common mental illnesses.

Overview of Mental Illness and Behavioral Emergencies

Mental illness is a broad term that refers to an emotional or mental state of dysfunction that may or may not be apparent in the patient's **behavior**. Behavior, unlike thoughts and feelings, is observable. Behaviors include facial expressions, posture, actions, and words. Social norms tell group members what behavior is acceptable and expected in certain situations and what behavior is considered abnormal. Because group members share, to great extent, the meanings associated with behaviors, behaviors are used to infer what we cannot directly see: the patient's mental state.

A behavioral emergency has been defined as behavior that is intolerable to the patient or those around him. Unfortunately, this definition leaves much to be desired. You may find someone talking loudly on his cell phone in the airport terminal intolerable, but it is not alarming and, unless the content of the conversation indicates otherwise, it rarely constitutes a behavioral emergency. In addition to being intolerable, there are usually elements of concern for the patient's safety and well-being and that of others, unusual behavior, and evidence of unusual thoughts in situations that comprise behavioral emergencies. Nonetheless, there is a subjective component to behavioral emergencies that can make them difficult to sort out. For instance, the individual on the street corner talking to himself was, in the past, psychiatrically ill; today, the person merely may be using a hands-free device to talk on the cell phone in his pocket.

All of us have had periods of time when our mental state has not been perfect and times when we do not understand or feel comfortable with the way we behaved in a situation. To diagnose mental illness, though, there are general criteria concerning how severely the disturbance interferes with the quality of life and ability to take care of oneself, and how long it persists. Your own experiences of emotional discomfort can open a window of understanding and compassion regarding mental illness and behavioral emergencies. Given the right circumstances, anyone can experience a behavioral emergency.

Patients with mental illness cannot be grouped together any more than patients with other medical problems. Mental illnesses are diverse, ranging from anxiety to depression, stress reactions, personality disorders, **psychotic** disorders, and addictive behaviors. Some mental illnesses are short term and successfully treated with therapy or medication, while others are more severe, long lasting, and difficult to treat.

Assessment and Management of Mental Illness and Behavioral Emergencies

A patient with a mental illness or behavioral emergency may call EMS, or EMS might be called by the patient's family, friends, coworkers, bystanders, or law enforcement, depending on the situation. Not every patient with a psychiatric or behavioral emergency presents an immediate danger to himself or others, but the fact that the situation has escalated to the point where EMS is requested often means that there is an element of violence or impending violence. For any report of a behavioral emergency, suicide attempt, domestic disturbance, altercation, or other situation in which the risk of violence is suspected, law enforcement should respond and secure the scene before you enter it. In other cases, if there is any indication that your safety could be at risk, take actions to protect yourself, including leaving the scene, if necessary, and request law enforcement (Figure 31-1).

You may determine from your first observations of the patient that he may need to be restrained. Patients who are more likely to be violent are psychotic (including schizophrenics, although the majority of schizophrenics are not violent), have a substance abuse history involving more than one substance, are delusional, or are in a state of delirium (including excited delirium). This is never a decision to make lightly. The only justifiable reasons for restraining a patient are to keep him from hurting himself or to keep him from hurting others. Methods and considerations in physically restraining a patient are discussed later in the chapter.

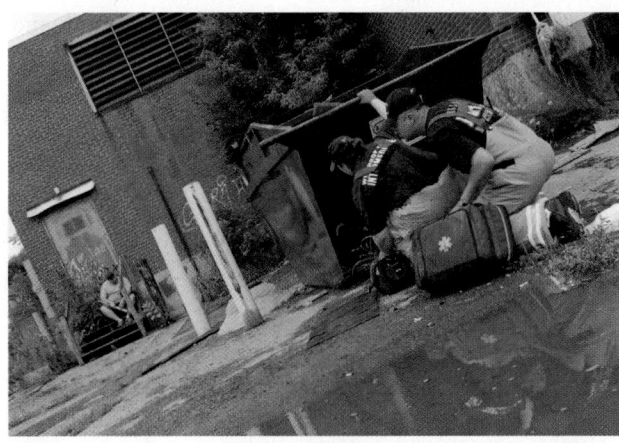

(A)

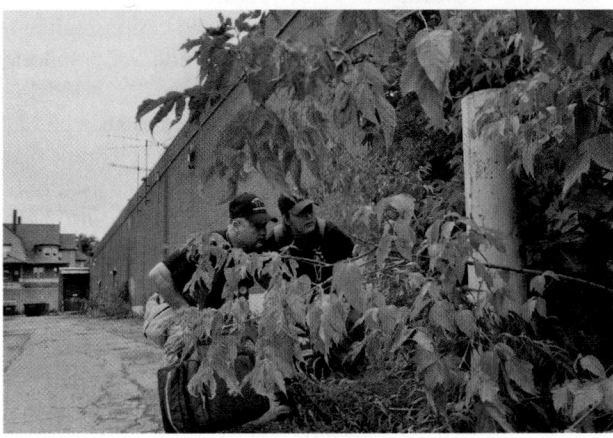

(B)

FIGURE 31-1

Be prepared to leave the scene, seeking cover (A) or concealment (B), if a patient becomes violent.

TABLE 31-1	Indications of Impending Violence

- Increased fidgeting or restlessness
- Pacing
- Profanity
- Loudness, yelling
- Destructive behavior
- Clenched fists, increased muscle tension
- Threats
- Intoxication
- Signs of past violence (scars)

Remember that scene safety is dynamic. A patient who is initially calm can become agitated. But, hostile patients usually do not randomly harm medical personnel. In most cases, violence against medical personnel is provoked by the way the provider treats the patient (Carney-Doebbeling, 2009). Behavior that can provoke the patient to violence includes arguing with him, invalidating his point of view, minimizing his concerns, threatening him (with restraint, calling law enforcement), being condescending, and being dishonest with the patient. Be empathetic to the patient and his situation and remove any aggravating factors, such as a specific person, too many bystanders, or too many EMS personnel. Be alert to changes in the patient's demeanor (Table 31-1), proactively remove items that could be used as weapons, and identify potential escape routes.

Scene Size-Up and Primary Assessment

Perform a scene size-up to ensure safety. Determine the nature of the illness and obtain the patient's chief complaint. Maintain a confident but relaxed approach. In developing your general impression, consider the patient's affect, posture, movements, and behaviors. Take note of the general living conditions. There may be clues to mental illness in the living environment, such as hoarding or disorganization. Look beyond the obvious to determine whether a patient may have attempted to harm himself. A call for an injured person or an unresponsive person, or what the patient claims to be accidental carbon monoxide exposure may, in fact, be suicide attempts. An injury that is inconsistent with the described mechanism can be a clue. For example, a patient with a very deliberate-looking laceration across his wrist may say that he cut himself in a kitchen accident, which would not be likely to produce that particular injury.

Vehicle collisions, particularly single-vehicle collisions, may be unrecognized suicide attempts. Absence of medication bottles or suicide note does not rule out a suicide attempt. However, if medication bottles are found, whether they belong to the patient or someone else, determine if the amount of medication present is consistent with the amount that should be present. Again, this can be deceiving, because suicidal patients can stockpile medications prior to the attempt.

If the patient appears to be unresponsive and not breathing, immediately confirm unresponsiveness and check the carotid pulse. If the pulse is absent, begin CPR according to protocol. If the patient has a decreased level of responsiveness, but appears to be breathing, check the airway, breathing, and circulation. Use manual airway maneuvers and basic adjuncts, if necessary. Assist ventilations and administer oxygen if needed. Look for and control any significant hemorrhage.

For responsive patients, balance patient privacy with your need for safety and respect the patient's personal space. When obtaining the chief complaint, it is often more effective to ask, "What happened?" rather than, "What is wrong?" Often, behavioral emergencies occur because many things are wrong about the patient's situation. When faced with the question of what is wrong, the patient may have difficulty knowing where to begin. However, there often is an event that immediately precedes the emergency, which the patient can identify. The event may be loss of a job, a threat to a relationship, or other stressor. An alternative way to begin conversation with the patient is to acknowledge his situation by saying something like, "You seem upset. How can I help?" Listen to the patient, but do not respond judgmentally. Do not lie to the patient or go along with **hallucinations** or **delusions**.

History and Secondary Assessment

An empathetic, nonjudgmental approach is essential in establishing rapport and gaining the patient's trust. You must have the patient's trust to obtain the information that is necessary for his medical care. If the patient's physical condition allows, be prepared to spend time with him. Use the techniques of therapeutic communication introduced in Chapter 6 to deal with silences, crying, excessive talking, and agitation. In fact, in the absence of injury or medical problems, therapeutic communication is the most effective tool you have for both assessing and treating patients with mental illness or behavioral emergency.

After establishing rapport, obtain a SAMPLE history. Determine the blood glucose level in all patients with altered mental status. Depending on how well the patient can relate his history, your exam may include looking for signs of trauma, stroke, renal failure, substance abuse, and infection. While assessing the history, notice the patient's emotional and cognitive states as part of a mental status exam (MSE). Following are things to pay particular attention to in the MSE:

- Level of responsiveness
- Orientation to person, place, and time
- Ability to sustain attention and concentrate (distractibility)

- Disorders of perception, including hallucinations and **illusions**
- Disordered thinking (assess speech content, speech patterns, suicidal or homicidal thoughts)
- **Affect** (visible emotional state) and mood (subjective emotional experience)
- Behavior, including appearance, increased or decreased psychomotor activity, and cooperation with EMS and law enforcement personnel

The list of medications is extremely important in the assessment of a patient with an apparent behavioral emergency (Table 31-2). The emergency may be due to medication toxicity, and many drugs used to treat mental illness can have significant side effects. Determine whether the patient has been compliant with his medication regimen. Suddenly discontinuing antidepressants and antipsychotic medications can have significant impact.

Never assume that a patient who denies that he has tried to hurt himself is being truthful, and never assume that patients who have tried to hurt themselves have used only one method. The patient who has cut himself may also have taken a drug overdose. Likewise, never assume that a patient who has taken an overdose only took one substance. Frequently, multiple substances are involved in intentional overdoses. When obtaining a list of medications, pay attention to those that may indicate a mental illness. Do not be afraid to ask the patient directly if he has attempted, or thought about, hurting or killing himself. If a patient has thought of harming himself, you will not give him an idea he has not already had; and if he has no intention of harming himself, your question will not suggest it to him.

It may be necessary to interview family or friends separately. However, if the patient is **paranoid** or hostile, this must be done discreetly.

TABLE 31-2 Selected Medications Used to Treat Mental Illness

Antidepressants	Antipsychotics	Other Medications Used for Mental Disorders
fluoxetine (Prozac)	chlorpromazine (Thorazine)	lithium
citalopram (Celexa)	haloperidol (Haldol)	clonazepam (Klonopin)
sertraline (Zoloft)	clozapine (Clozaril)	lorazepam (Ativan)
paroxetine (Paxil)	risperdone (Risperdal)	alprazolam (Xanax)
escitalopram (Lexapro)	olanzapine (Zyprexa)	buspirone (Buspar)
venlafaxine (Effexor)	quetiapine (Seroquel)	propranolol (Inderal)
duloxetine (Cymbalta)	ziprasidone (Geodon)	valproic acid (Depakote)
bupropion (Wellbutrin)	aripiprazole (Abilify)	carbamazepine (Tegretol)
trazodone (Desyrel)		gabapentin (Neurontin)
desvenlafaxine (Pristiq)		
St. John's wort (herbal remedy)		

Clinical Reasoning

You should make a clinical impression of mental illness as a cause of behavioral emergency or change in mental status only after assessing for medical and traumatic causes of the behavior change. Do not overlook the significance of unexplained vital signs or other exam findings as potential indications of medical emergencies or trauma. A drug overdose also can explain altered mental status, tachycardia, bradycardia, irregular pulse, depressed respirations, and hypotension. Several conditions, including some that are life threatening, can cause bizarre behavior (Table 31-3). Failure to recognize those conditions can prove fatal for the patient.

Also keep in mind that the patient's chief complaint may not be related, or at least not directly related, to a history of mental illness. Many patients with mental illness function very well with treatment and the history of mental illness is simply part of the patient's overall history. In fact, a common diagnostic error is to assume that, because a patient has a history of mental illness, his current problem is due to mental illness. This results in missed diagnosis of medical and traumatic disorders.

Treatment and Reassessment

Therapeutic communication is often the most effective prehospital treatment for behavioral emergencies uncomplicated by trauma or medical problems. Treat any injuries and medical conditions, as well. Establish a baseline for the patient's condition, including level of responsiveness, vital signs, and complaints. Reassess critical patients at least every 5 minutes and noncritical patients every 15 minutes, obtaining at least two sets of observations. If the patient has been physically restrained, assess him for injuries as soon as restraint is accomplished, monitor the patient continuously, and assess pulse, motor, and sensory function in the restrained extremities every 15 minutes, in addition to other reassessments.

TABLE 31-3	**Problems That May Present as Behavioral Emergencies**

- Infection
- Tumor
- Neurologic damage from substance abuse
- Recent or past traumatic brain injury
- Stroke
- Seizure
- Endocrine emergencies (hypoglycemia, hyperglycemia, thyroid conditions, adrenal conditions)
- Hypoxia
- Metabolic disturbances (uremia)
- Drugs, toxins

Anxiety Disorders

Anxiety is a state of fear and worry that everyone feels sometime. It is an important state to the extent that it helps people adapt to stressors. You are most likely familiar with the symptoms of anxiety, to at least a certain degree, and have specific stressors that trigger them. Excessive anxiety can interfere with social and occupational functioning and can be harmful. Anxiety disorders are common and are not always recognized or diagnosed. Anxiety disorders include panic disorders, **phobias**, obsessive–compulsive disorder, acute stress reactions, and post-traumatic stress disorder (PTSD). (See Chapter 3 for a review of stress and PTSD.)

No matter the trigger for anxiety, signs and symptoms can range from mild to severe, and can include tachycardia, chest pain or tightness, tachypnea, a feeling of fear, diaphoresis, a feeling of impending doom, and a sensation of choking or being suffocated. Shock, myocardial infarction, hyperthyroidism, adrenal disorders, asthma, cocaine, caffeine, amphetamines, and withdrawal syndromes cause those same symptoms. This underscores the importance of taking all such complaints seriously and taking a history and performing an assessment designed to narrow down the most likely causes of the patient's presentation. Medications that suggest a history of an anxiety disorder include benzodiazepines, antidepressants, and beta blockers. Whether the patient's anxiety is from a situational or psychosocial cause or a result of an underlying medical disorder, provide reassurance and display a composed, confident demeanor to calm the patient.

A panic attack is a brief period of intense fear, anxiety, and discomfort. The patient might fear that he is going to die, having a heart attack, going crazy or losing control, or he may have a sensation of unreality (depersonalization). In addition to those signs and symptoms of anxiety, patients may experience numbness and tingling, nausea, palpitations, and tremors. Panic attacks can occur in any patient with an anxiety disorder. Patients who have repeated panic attacks have panic disorder. The fear of having a panic attack may prevent the patient from participating in normal activities. Panic attacks pass quickly, usually within 10 minutes. Help the patient having a panic attack focus on slow, controlled breathing, reassure him that you are there to take care of him, and let him know the sensations will pass.

Cognitive Disorders

Cognitive disorders, or disorders of thinking, include delirium and dementia. (See Chapter 22 for a review.) Delirium is an acute onset of a confusional state with an underlying correctable cause, such as infection, drug toxicity, and other medical problems. Delirium tends to be less noticeable earlier in the day, worsening toward evening. Dementia is a progressive deterioration of mental function, including memory impairment. Causes include Alzheimer's disease and multi-infarct dementia. Delirium and dementia can involve confusion leading to fear and combative behavior. The patient's age should not be a factor in determining whether his behavior can be a risk to your safety. In a study by Shah et al. (2011), a higher proportion of elderly patients with cognitive impairment arrive at the emergency department by ambulance than by other means. The Mini Mental State Exam (MMSE) presented in Chapter 22 can be a helpful tool in recognizing cognitive impairment.

Eating Disorders

Anorexia nervosa, bulimia nervosa, and binge eating are eating disorders more prevalent in young women but are increasingly affecting men as well. Patients with anorexia nervosa are extremely thin (emaciated), yet obsessed with losing weight and controlling food intake. They use dietary restriction and may use excessive exercise, laxatives, diuretics, and induced vomiting to prevent weight gain. The risk of death is increased approximately 10 times over that of the general population due to physical complications of starvation.

Patients with bulimia nervosa are often of normal weight, but are obsessed with losing weight. Over the course of a week, they repeat a cycle of binge eating and then taking measures to counteract it, such as excessive exercise, vomiting, and use of laxatives and diuretics. Physical complications include fluid and electrolyte disorders, gastrointestinal problems, and problems in the oral cavity, such as persistent sore throat and erosion of dental enamel. Often, they can be identified by the teeth scrapes on their knuckles from the ongoing process of gagging themselves in order to vomit.

Patients with binge eating disorder are generally obese. Binge eating is not followed by attempts to lose weight. Instead, the feelings of loss of control and disgust generated by binge eating often leads to further binges.

Factitious Disorders and Somatoform Disorders

A factitious disorder is characterized by intentional infliction of either physical or psychological signs and symptoms, either in one's self (Munchausen syndrome) or others (Munchausen syndrome by proxy). The behavior is motivated by the desire to assume the sick role, or caretaker of a sick person, and receive the associated attention. There is no external gain from the behavior, such as time off work or financial compensation. If an external gain exists, the behavior is considered malingering and does not fit in this category. Patients may inject themselves with or ingest toxins or contaminants, produce false signs and symptoms by contaminating urine samples with blood, and report false events such as syncope or seizures. Patients are deceptive

and evasive; may have an extensive history of medical procedures, medications, or surgeries performed in response to the fictitious disorder; and may be aware of textbook presentations of disorders. They readily accept the risks of surgeries and procedures, and can become controlling, hostile, and attention seeking, particularly when diagnostic tests are negative and treatment is not initiated.

Somatoform disorders result in physical symptoms without apparent physiologic cause. The most familiar to most people is hypochondriasis, which may result from an unusual awareness of normal bodily sensations. Patients often have multiple, unexplained chronic problems and sources of pain. They are preoccupied with, and fearful of, serious illnesses and their symptoms are consistent with their perceptions of how a particular illness presents. Their concern continues despite negative diagnostic tests and reassurance.

Conversion disorder is a sudden loss of specific neurologic function following a severe stressor. Patients may have a pseudoseizure, sudden onset of paralysis, or sudden blindness.

In body dysmorphic disorder, patients are preoccupied with a physical defect that is not apparent to others, often seeking multiple plastic surgeries to correct the perceived defect.

Impulse Control Disorders

Consistent with the name, patients with impulse control disorders cannot control their impulses to engage in certain behaviors. Disorders include kleptomania (stealing), pyromania (fire setting), pathologic gambling, and intermittent explosive disorder (angry outbursts).

Mood Disorders

Mood disorders are common, affecting at least 10 to 15 percent of the population, and include depression and bipolar disorder. A major depressive episode manifests with depressed mood, decreased interest in things once found pleasurable, weight loss or gain, insomnia or excessive sleeping, and increased or decreased psychomotor activity. The patient often experiences feelings of worthlessness and guilt, may complain of an inability to think and concentrate, inability to make decisions, and recurrent thoughts of death or suicide. Physical symptoms without identifiable physical cause, such as pain, are common. The patient who is having a depressive episode often looks sad or dejected, presents with a slumped posture, and may make poor eye contact. Depression is a serious health concern, both because of the impact the disease has on the quality of life, and because depression is associated with an increased risk for cardiovascular disease and stroke. Some antidepressant therapy is based on the theory that depression is caused by changes in neurotransmitter activity. A variety of antidepressants works to increase the levels or effects of one or more neurotransmitters, including serotonin, norepinephrine, and dopamine.

Bipolar disorder is uncommon, affecting less than 1 percent of the population. It is characterized by periods of persistent, abnormally elevated mood interspersed with periods of depression. During the manic phase of bipolar disorder, patients often exhibit a sense of inflated self-esteem, decreased need for sleep, pressured speech, flight of ideas, distractibility, and increased goal-directed activity. Patients often engage in risky behavior with high potential for negative consequences, such as extravagant spending, gambling, and promiscuous sexual activity. The patient may have delusional thoughts and grandiose ideas and plans. Medications used to treat bipolar disorder include antipsychotics, antidepressants, anticonvulsants, and lithium, which acts as a mood stabilizer.

Personality Disorders

Patients with personality disorders have persistent maladaptive ways of perceiving, thinking, and relating to others. They are ill equipped to function adequately in society, and often have difficulty maintaining jobs and relationships. They typically lack insight into their behavior and tend not to perceive themselves as having a problem, but often cause difficulty for others.

Personality disorders are clustered into three types. The cluster A disorders include being emotionally distant and isolated, often with odd or eccentric behavior, such as the paranoid personality disorder. The cluster B disorders are characterized by emotional instability, impulsiveness, and intensity in behavior or relationships. This group includes some of the more commonly known personality disorders, such as antisocial personality disorder, borderline personality disorder, histrionic personality disorder, and narcissistic personality disorder. Cluster C is comprised of the anxious or fearful personality disorders, including obsessive–compulsive personality disorder.

Schizophrenia

Schizophrenia and related disorders are psychotic disorders, in which the patient is said to have lost contact with reality. Patients often have delusions, disorganized

thoughts and behavior, hallucinations (visual or auditory), flat affect, and impaired reasoning. Some patients exhibit **catatonic** behavior (rigidity or slackness of the extremities). Contrary to popular belief, most schizophrenics are not violent. This risk increases, however, in patients who have hallucinations in which they are being persecuted or commanded to do things, in patients who are not compliant with their medications, and in patients with substance abuse problems.

Schizophrenia usually has an onset in early adulthood, but may improve with age. There is a strong hereditary and biologic component, with specific brain changes that are noticeable in brain imaging studies. Patients with schizophrenia have approximately a 10 percent incidence of suicide. Treatment includes the use of various antipsychotic medications.

Substance Abuse, Addiction, and Withdrawal

Addiction, substance abuse, and dependence can involve legal or illegal substances, prescription substances, and easily obtained substances such as alcohol and tobacco. Substance abuse is defined in terms of what is considered socially unacceptable. Many of society's norms are defined by law. However, some substance abuse is not illegal, but still is socially unacceptable. For example, alcohol is not illegal but its use can interfere with family obligations or work, which constitutes abuse. Substance abuse also can be thought of as use of a substance in a way not intended. The **Diagnostic and Statistical Manual (DSM-IV TR)** of the American Psychological Association lists substance abuse as a mental illness.

Addiction is characterized by preoccupation with obtaining and using a substance, which can occur with or without physical dependence. Physical dependence results in physical signs and symptoms when a drug is discontinued, called *withdrawal*. Psychological dependence is said to exist when the patient needs the drug to feel satisfied and when his use of the substance continues even though he is aware of the negative actual or potential consequences of doing so. Drugs that have an increased likelihood of resulting in psychological dependence are those that have pleasurable effects such as decreasing anxiety, euphoric mood, increased ability to concentrate or perform physical activity, or those that alter perception or behavior. Examples include alcohol, marijuana, amphetamines, cocaine, benzodiazepines, and narcotics.

Intoxication is a state of mental and behavioral changes induced by a substance usually including euphoric mood, changes in perception, impaired judgment, and sometimes, confrontational behavior. Significant intoxication with CNS depressants, such as alcohol and narcotics, can lead to respiratory depression and the loss of ability to protect the airway. Intoxication with CNS stimulants, such as cocaine and methamphetamine, can lead to tachycardia, hypertension, seizures, and hyperthermia. (Assessment and treatment of overdose and toxicity are discussed in Chapter 32.)

Alcohol

Beverage alcohol, or ethanol, is absorbed quickly from the stomach and small intestine. Once in the bloodstream, alcohol binds with GABA receptors in the brain, resulting in sedation and CNS depression. Alcohol is metabolized mostly in the liver, but at a slower rate than it is absorbed from the gastrointestinal system. Alcohol is converted by a liver enzyme called *alcohol dehydrogenase* into acetaldehyde, which is then broken down into substances that can be eliminated by the body. A certain amount of alcohol is excreted by the body unchanged. It is the excretion of alcohol through the respiratory membrane that gives the breath the odor of alcohol after it is ingested.

The blood alcohol concentration (BAC) is used to legally define intoxication. Medically, the BAC is expressed as mg/dL. A BAC of 50 mg/dL is equivalent to a BAC of 0.05 percent. In inexperienced drinkers, a BAC of 300 to 400 mg/dL (0.3 to 0.4 percent) results in unconsciousness; and a BAC greater than 400 mg/dL can result in death from respiratory depression and dysrhythmia. Hypotension and hypoglycemia also can occur. The effect of BAC is less predictable in experienced drinkers who have developed tolerance for the effects of alcohol. Intoxicated patients are at risk for decreased responsiveness, vomiting, and aspiration.

Binge drinking has become a serious health concern among teenagers and young adults in recent years. When alcohol is consumed quickly, it is not all absorbed from the gastrointestinal tract by the time the person becomes so intoxicated that they can no longer drink. However, the alcohol in the stomach continues to be absorbed, increasing the BAC further, to potentially lethal levels. The effects of chronic alcohol abuse include cirrhosis of the liver, pancreatitis, gastrointestinal bleeding, Wernicke-Korsakoff syndrome, alcoholic dementia, and malnutrition. (See Chapter 22.)

Alcohol withdrawal, in a physically dependent patient, can begin in as little as 6 hours with tremors, headache,

weakness, sweating, and, sometimes, seizures. In 12 to 24 hours the patient may begin to experience frightening hallucinations and vivid nightmares. **Delirium tremens (DTs)** begin in 48 to 72 hours after abstaining from alcohol. Delirium tremens include anxiety, confusion, sleep disturbances, hallucinations and nightmares, hyperthermia, tachycardia, and diaphoresis. Dysfunction of the autonomic nervous system can lead to death.

Treat the acutely intoxicated patient by managing the airway, breathing, and circulation. Be particularly alert to the possibility of vomiting and aspiration. Obtain IV access in patients with a decreased level of responsiveness, and administer 50 percent dextrose for hypoglycemia. Alcoholics may require the administration of 100 mg thiamine in conjunction with 50 percent dextrose, if allowed in your protocols. Alcohol withdrawal can be fatal. Those patients should have IV access, if possible, in anticipation of complications.

Suicide

Suicide is the eighth leading cause of death in the United States, taking more than 32,000 lives annually (Andrew, 2010). In adolescents, suicide is the third leading cause of death (Russinoff & Clark, 2004). Under-reporting of suicide is likely substantial. Therefore, the actual incidence of suicide is probably significantly higher. It is estimated that there are between 8 and 25 suicide attempts for every suicide completed. Approximately 90 percent of all patients who commit suicide have a mental illness, such as depression, schizophrenia, or a personality disorder. Drug and alcohol abuse figure substantially in suicide, as well. Alcoholics have up to 120 times greater risk of suicide, and 40 to 60 percent of patients who commit suicide are intoxicated with drugs or alcohol. Access to a lethal method, feelings of hopelessness, and lack of social support also are risk factors.

Method of suicide and the lethality of suicide attempt methods vary by gender. White males account for 78 percent of all successful suicides, with 56 percent of them involving a firearm. Females are more likely to use poisoning/overdose. Suicide is prevalent in the elderly, and you should not overlook this in the differential diagnosis process with elderly individuals. The rate of suicide in those over the age of 85 years is 1.8 times that of the general population (Russinoff & Clark, 2004).

The nature of the dispatch may or may not alert you to the possibility of a suicide attempt. A call for an unresponsive person, sick person, or injured person may turn out to be a suicide attempt. Keep in mind that apparent accidents, such as carbon monoxide exposure and motor vehicle collisions, may not be accidents at all, but suicide attempts.

After ensuring scene safety, your first priority is managing life threats. In the absence of immediate life threats, or after you have managed them, you must care for the behavioral aspect of the situation, as well as the medical or traumatic problems resulting from the suicide attempt. In doing so, it is critical that you realize that most suicide attempts are not simply, "cries for attention." A suicide attempt is an indication that the person can no longer cope with his situation and sees no other alternatives.

Violent Patients

Signs that a patient may become violent include increasing fidgeting or restlessness, pacing, profanity, increasing voice volume, and destructive behavior, such as throwing things or punching a wall. In the prehospital setting, restraint is best used in conjunction with law enforcement, and is only done if the person is a threat to himself or others. You must clearly document the behavior and statements (such as threats of violence) that played a role in the decision to restrain. Key considerations include preserving the patient's dignity, monitoring patient safety, and not using restraints punitively. Four-point restraints (both arms and both legs) are used to restrain the patient in a supine position. *Never restrain a patient in a prone position.*

At least five people are needed to safely restrain a patient. One person is assigned to each extremity and one applies the restraints. Explain to the patient that he is being restrained to protect himself and others, but do not negotiate. Once the decision is made, follow through with it, and do not remove the restraints until the situation is secure, which generally involves the use of medications to sedate the patient. The approach is coordinated so that the extremities are controlled simultaneously. Use only the amount of force needed to restrain the patient, and no more. The restraints are attached to each of the four limbs and to the stretcher or bed frame. Leather restraints are best to prevent inadvertent tightening, stretching, or injury. However, sheets or roller gauze can be used if leather restraints are not available.

Immediately after securing the patient, assess him for injury. Monitor airway, breathing, and circulation and check vital signs. Check the circulation, sensation, and motor function in each of the four extremities distal to the restraints every 15 minutes, and document your findings. Never apply restraints over the head, neck, or chest. Do not place anything in the mouth to prevent spitting (wear a mask and eye protection to avoid exposure). Do not place patients prone or use "hobbling" or "hog-tying" approaches, which have been associated with deaths due to excited delirium. (See Chapter 22 for a review of excited delirium.)

CASE STUDY WRAP-UP

Clinical-Reasoning Process

Advanced EMTs Courtney and Albert were dispatched to the midway of the county fairgrounds for a possible heart attack. Their patient is a woman in her mid-twenties named Donna Axelrod. She is sitting on a bench, clutching her chest and appears distressed, pale, and diaphoretic. Although Donna's sister is concerned that the patient is having a heart attack, Courtney decides she needs more information.

The patient's age and gender do not put her in a high-risk category for a myocardial infarction, yet her signs and symptoms appear consistent with myocardial infarction. "Hi, my name is Courtney. What happened?"

"We were standing in line to ride the Scrambler. I don't like rides, but I didn't want to chicken out. The closer we got, the more I felt like I was having heart attack."

"What makes you say it feels like a heart attack?"

"My chest is tight. It feels like I can't breathe. I was afraid if I got on the ride I was going to die."

Courtney feels that the situation of anticipating the sensation of the ride might have caused the patient to panic, but she doesn't want to overlook possible medical conditions. "Has anything like this ever happened before?"

(continued)

"A few months ago. My fiancé and I went to a national park where there are some caves. We got about a quarter mile into the cave and all of the sudden it narrowed. It was so dark, I didn't know what was ahead, but there were people behind me, so I couldn't turn back."

"Do you have any medical problems, like asthma or heart problems?"

"No. I'm hardly ever sick."

"Okay. My partner, Albert, is going to check your pulse, blood pressure, and oxygen level while I listen to your breath sounds. I don't think you are having a heart attack, but we are going to check some things out and go from there, alright? In the meantime, try as best you can to relax and slow your breathing. We are right here to help you."

Courtney determined that Donna is alert and oriented, though anxious. She is sweating and a little pale, but there is no cyanosis, no evidence of injuries, and no edema. The patient's heart rate is 100 and regular, her respirations are 24, blood pressure 122/78, and SpO_2 is 100 percent. Her breath sounds are clear and equal. There are no immediately life-threatening conditions.

Courtney reassures Donna and tells her she thinks her discomfort will begin to pass in a few minutes. "I know it is a scary feeling, but I think the problem may be related to your anxiety about the ride. With your permission, we'd like to take you over to the medical tent where a physician can take a look at you and check things out." Donna agrees, and they take Donna and her sister to the medical tent. By the time they get there, Donna is feeling much better. Her color is better, she has stopped sweating, and her repeat vital signs are a pulse of 94, respirations of 16, blood pressure of 118/76, and SpO_2 of 100 percent. The physician monitors her for a period of time and dismisses her with a referral for follow-up.

CHAPTER REVIEW

Chapter Summary

Behavioral emergencies can have situational, mental, or physical causes. Regardless of the underlying cause, your safety, the patient's safety, and bystanders' safety can be at risk. Perform a scene size-up, including assessing the patient for indications of impending violence. Be alert to items that can be used as weapons, identify and maintain escape routes, and be prepared to leave the scene, if necessary, and request law enforcement. Restrain patients only if necessary to protect him from harming himself and others. Follow your protocols for restraint, including indications, methods, assessment, and documentation of restraint.

One of the key responsibilities of EMS personnel in the assessment of patients with behavioral emergencies is identifying medical or traumatic causes of the behavior and managing them accordingly. Hypoglycemia, hypoxia, shock, infection, endocrine emergencies, and toxic exposures can all cause behavioral changes. Once you are addressing medical and traumatic problems, use therapeutic communication as an essential element of both assessment and management of patients with behavioral emergencies and mental illness. Be nonjudgmental and empathetic in your approach to patients with behavioral emergencies and mental illness.

Review Questions

Multiple-Choice Questions

1. A 45-year-old male patient says he sees spiders and snakes crawling all over his bed. You do not see anything that would explain this, but he seems truly terrified. This is most consistent with:

   a. delusion.
   b. paranoia.
   c. hallucination.
   d. illusion.

2. Your patient tells you she wants to be transported to a certain emergency department because the physician who is working is secretly in love with her, but cannot admit it or he will lose his job. You are sure this is not the case. The patient's behavior is consistent with:

   a. delusion.
   b. paranoia.
   c. hallucination.
   d. illusion.

3. Post-traumatic stress disorder is a type of _____ disorder.
   a. mood
   b. personality
   c. psychotic
   d. anxiety

4. A patient has injected herself with insulin obtained from a medication cart at the nursing home where she works in order to produce a sudden onset of severe hypoglycemia and seizure. This type of behavior is consistent with_____ disorder.
   a. somatoform
   b. factitious
   c. impulse control
   d. cognitive

5. A patient has episodes of despair and hopelessness that alternate with periods of increased energy, overconfidence, excessive talkativeness, and perceived great creativity. This behavior is most consistent with:
   a. schizophrenia.
   b. bipolar disorder.
   c. antisocial personality disorder.
   d. delirium tremens.

6. Which one of the following medications is often indicated, in conjunction with 50 percent dextrose, for treatment of hypoglycemia in alcoholics?
   a. Thiamine
   b. Naloxone
   c. Glucagon
   d. Cyanocobalamin

7. Four-point restraint means that the patient is restrained:
   a. at the head, chest, hips, and legs.
   b. at the shoulders, torso, thighs, and ankles.
   c. by each arm at the wrist and each leg at the ankle.
   d. with the right arm behind the back, tied to the right leg, and the left arm behind the back, tied to the left leg.

Critical-Thinking Questions

8. A woman has called for EMS because she says her son is "out of control." The adult son is upset and there obviously has been some kind of conflict between him and the mother. What criteria will help you determine if there is a behavioral emergency or not?

9. Your patient seems agitated. What actions can you take to prevent her from escalating to violence?

References

Andrew, L. B. (2010). *Depression and suicide.* eMedicine. Retrieved January 24, 2011, from http://emedicine.medscape.com/article/805459

Carney-Doebbeling, C. (2009). *Behavioral emergencies. The Merck manual for healthcare professionals.* Retrieved January 24, 2011, from http://www.merckmanuals.com/professional/sec16/ch206/ch206d.html?qt=behavioral%20emergencies&alt=sh

Russinoff, I., & Clark, M. (2004). Suicidal patients: Assessing and managing patients presenting with suicidal attempts or ideation. *Emergency Medicine Practice: An Evidence-Based Approach to Emergency Medicine, 6*(8)

Shah, M. N., Jones, C. M., Richardson, T. M., Conwell, Y., Katz, P., & Schneider, S. M. (2011). Prevalence of depression and cognitive impairment in older adult emergency medical services patients. *Prehospital Emergency Care, 15*(1), 4–11.

Additional Reading

Soreff, S. (2011). *Suicide.* eMedicine. Retrieved January 24, 2011, from http://emedicine.medscape.com/article/288598-overview

32 Toxicologic Emergencies

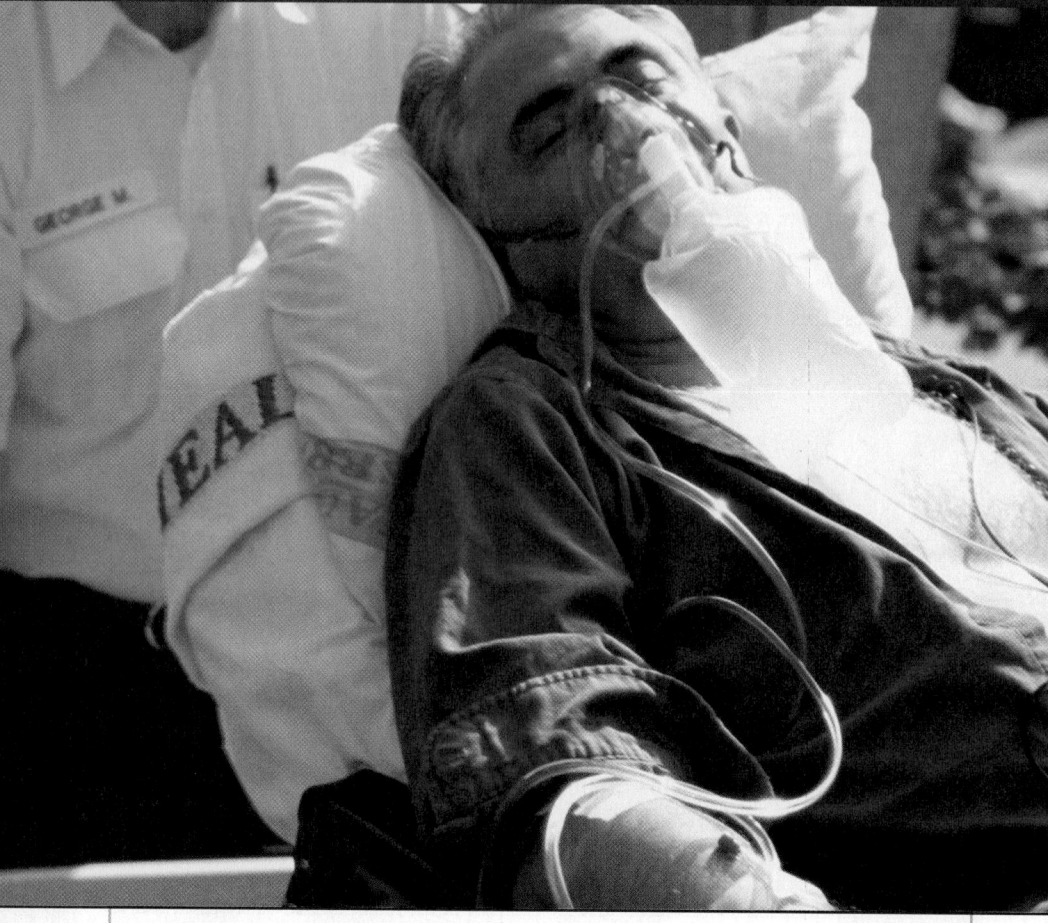

KEY TERMS

ataxic *(p. 737)*

cardiac glycosides *(p. 739)*

confabulate *(p. 737)*

myoclonus *(p. 744)*

nystagmus *(p. 737)*

scombroid fish poisoning *(p. 738)*

toxidromes *(p. 728)*

toxins *(p. 728)*

Content Area: Medical

Advanced EMT Education Standard: The Advanced EMT applies fundamental knowledge to provide basic and selected advanced emergency care and transportation based on assessment findings for an acutely ill patient.

Objectives

After reading this chapter, you should be able to:

32.1 Define key terms introduced in this chapter.

32.2 Describe the importance of understanding the pathophysiology and assessment-based management of patients with toxicologic emergencies.

32.3 Give examples of common substances involved in intentional and unintentional toxicologic emergencies in adults and children.

32.4 Describe each of the four routes by which a poison can enter the body:
– Absorption
– Ingestion
– Inhalation
– Injection

(continued)

Resource Central

To access Resource Central, follow the directions on the Student Access Card provided with this text. If there is no card, go to www.bradybooks.com and follow the Resource Central link to Buy Access. Under Media Resources, you will find:

• *Poison Control Centers.* Learn about prevention and how to treat poisoning in the prehospital setting.

• *Cocaine.* Watch and learn how cocaine affects the brain and causes dependence.

• *Alcohol.* Discover how alcohol affects the body and common conditions that can mimic alcohol abuse.

Ambulance 47 has just arrived at a residence for a report of an attempted suicide by overdose. Law enforcement officers have secured the scene and tell the Advanced EMTs, Alice Blackledge and Cosette Mayfield, that the patient is a 32-year-old man who is unresponsive but breathing. An officer hands Alice two medication bottles, one for hydrocodone and one for alprazolam, and states that it also appears the patient has ingested a large amount of alcohol. Entering the house, the Advanced EMTs find the patient supine on a sofa and immediately hear snoring respirations. A nearly empty liter bottle of 100-proof vodka sits on the coffee table next to a cocktail glass.

Problem-Solving Questions

1. What immediate patient care actions must Alice and Cosette take?
2. What information do Alice and Cosette need about the medications the police officer handed to them?
3. What information do they need about the patient's history?
4. What type of physical examination should they perform?

(continued from previous page)

32.5 Perform a scene size-up to identify indications that a patient may be suffering from a toxicologic emergency.

32.6 Given a scenario involving a patient with a toxicologic emergency, anticipate special considerations in protecting your safety and that of other personnel, the patient, and bystanders.

32.7 Given a series of scenarios, demonstrate the assessment-based management of patients suffering a variety of toxicologic emergencies.

32.8 Anticipate the effects of various classifications of toxins and commonly abused substances on the respiratory, nervous, cardiovascular, and gastrointestinal systems.

32.9 Explain the limited role of specific antidotes in toxicologic emergencies.

32.10 Explain the importance of identifying the following historical information for patients who have been exposed to a toxin:
   – Substance or substances involved, including ingestion of alcohol with other substances
   – Amount of substance(s) involved
   – Length of time since exposure, and time period over which exposure occurred
   – Any attempted treatment of the poisoning
   – Underlying psychiatric or medical conditions
   – Patient's weight
   – Types of substances available to the patient
   – Medications

32.11 Anticipate pitfalls in obtaining an accurate and complete history from patients with toxicologic emergencies.

32.12 Describe the indications, contraindications, mechanism of action, side effects, dosage, and administration of activated charcoal.

32.13 Describe special considerations in assessing and managing patients with each of the following:
   – Carbon monoxide poisoning
   – CNS stimulants (cocaine, amphetamines, methamphetamine)
   – Cyanide poisoning
   – Delirium tremens

(continued)

(continued from previous page)

- Ethanol ingestion
- Ethylene glycol ingestion
- Exposure to acid or alkali substances
- Exposure to hydrocarbons
- Exposure to poisonous plants
- Food poisoning
- Hallucinogens
- Huffing
- Isopropanol ingestion
- Methanol ingestion
- Prescription and over-the-counter medication overdose
- Withdrawal syndromes

32.14 Explain the importance of contacting the poison control center with as complete a patient history as possible.

32.15 Explain the importance of careful assessment and conscientious management of patients who have ingested a toxin.

32.16 Explain the purpose and process of reassessing patients with a toxicologic related emergency.

Introduction

Exposure to toxins, accidental and intentional, is a common reason for emergency medical care. There were nearly 2.5 million poisoning emergencies reported to poison control centers in 2009, with 65 percent of them occurring in patients under 20 years old (Bronstein et al., 2010). However, the greatest proportion of fatal exposures occurs in the 40- to 49-year old age group. The vast majority of toxin exposures (82 percent) are unintentional, but intentional poisoning accounts for the majority of suicide attempts, and accounts for the majority of poisoning deaths. Intentional exposure also occurs in the abuse or misuse of substances, and as a mechanism of intentionally harming another person. Unintentional exposures include accidental exposures and therapeutic errors, as well as occupational and environmental exposures.

Ingestion of toxins is the most common route for both fatal and nonfatal exposures (84 percent of cases). The most common substances involved in toxic exposures include analgesics, personal and household substances, sedative–hypnotics, pesticides, and antidepressants. The substances most frequently involved in fatal exposures include sedative–hypnotics, opioids, cardiovascular drugs, acetaminophen, antidepressants, anticonvulsants, alcohol, stimulants, and street drugs. In the pediatric population, analgesics, batteries, hydrocarbons, plants, cough and cold preparations, and other medications comprise the majority of fatalities.

The study of toxicology provides important information for EMS providers about the effects of toxins, allowing you to anticipate the consequences of specific poison exposures on the body, and develop treatment strategies. In most cases, your interventions will be general, including ensuring your own safety from exposure to the toxin and making sure the patient has an open airway, and adequate ventilations, oxygenation, and circulation. The general approach to management of poisoned patients includes decreasing exposure to the toxin, decreasing absorption of the toxin once exposure occurs, and promoting its elimination from the body. A few toxins have specific antidotes or antagonists. In particular, the narcotic antagonist naloxone (Narcan) is used to treat patients with respiratory depression due to narcotic overdose.

Toxicology and Poison Control Centers

Toxicology is a broad field that includes the study of prescription and illegal drugs, and plant, animal, and many other types of **toxins**. Some substances are toxic in minute quantities, while others are considered safe or even therapeutic in smaller doses, but toxic in larger doses. The vast number of toxic substances and the amount of information related to each substance make the topic seem daunting. Yet, knowledge gained from the study of those many substances allows them to be grouped into categories by their effects, making understanding the field simpler. The categories are called **toxidromes**. While there are still specific considerations for each substance, knowledge of toxidromes helps in identifying the cause of poisoning based on signs and symptoms, and in determining treatment (Table 32-1).

Toxins can gain access to the body by four routes: ingestion, inhalation, surface absorption, and injection. Ingested substances enter the body by being swallowed.

TABLE 32-1	Selected Toxidromes		
Toxidrome	**Example Toxins**	**Signs and Symptoms**	**Treatment**
Cholinergic: Stimulates parasympathetic nervous system action.	Betel nut (from palm trees [*Areca catechu*] native to parts of Asia, Malaysia, and Indonesia; the nut contains a stimulant that stains the teeth red; can be grown in other tropical areas). Used in Ayurvedic medicine and other forms of traditional medicine. Bethanechol (medication used for difficulty in urination). Carbachol (used in treatment of glaucoma). Muscarine (found in poisonous mushrooms). Pilocarpine (medication used to treat dry mouth). Jaborandi (Pilocarpus species plant used in homeopathic medicine). Organophosphate pesticides such as Diazinon and Trithion (acetylcholinesterase inhibition).	Feeling of warmth, tachycardia or bradycardia, sweating, constricted pupils, increased salivation, blurred vision, confusion, urinary incontinence, diarrhea. Can cause bronchoconstriction and increased bronchial secretions. (SLUDGE: salivation, lacrimation, urinary incontinence, diarrhea, gastric distress, emesis.)	Airway management with suctioning to control secretions; atropine and pralidoxime for organophosphate poisoning. Treat bronchospasm with bronchodilators, in consultation with medical direction.
Anticholinergic: Inhibits parasympathetic nervous system action, allowing increased sympathetic nervous system effects.	Bella donna alkaloids, atropine, scopolamine (used for motion sickness), Datura (jimson weed), Amanita muscaria (mushrooms), a component of Donatal, used for treatment of intestinal cramping, hyoscyamus niger (black nightshade or black henbane, used in homeopathic medicine). Tricyclic antidepressants, phenothiazines, and antihistamines also have anticholinergic effects.	Dry skin and mucous membranes, flushed skin, hyperthermia, blurred vision, dilated pupils, urinary retention, delirium, ataxia, seizures. (Mad as a hatter, dry as a bone, red as a beet, blind as a bat, hot as hell.)	Supportive: manage airway, breathing, and circulation.
Sympathomimetic: Stimulates sympathetic nervous system action.	Caffeine, cocaine, amphetamine, ephedra.	CNS stimulation, excitement, seizures, tachycardia, hypertension, chest pain, cardiac dysrhythmia, stroke.	Treat supportively: manage the airway, breathing, and circulation.
Narcotic: Binds with CNS opiate receptors, causing CNS depression.	Heroin, morphine, codeine, hydromorphone, hydrocodone, oxycodone, propoxyphene, opium fentanyl, meperidine.	CNS depression, pinpoint pupils, respiratory depression, hypotension.	Manage airway, breathing, and circulation; administer naloxone for respiratory depression.
Extrapyramidal: The extrapyramidal tracts of the nervous system are involved in motor control; antipsychotic and chemically similar drugs can cause extrapyramidal side effects.	Haldol, droperidol, chlorpromazine, other antipsychotics and antiemetics.	Muscle spasm, rigidity, tremor, oculogyric crisis, torticollis, neuroleptic malignant syndrome.	Manage airway, breathing, and circulation; provide reassurance that acute dystonic reactions can be reversed with medication (diphenhydramine); treat hyperpyrexia.

Plants, medications, alcohols, and household substances are all commonly ingested poisons. Caustic substances, such as strong acids and alkalis, can cause immediate damage to the soft tissues of the oral cavity, pharynx, esophagus, and stomach. Most substances are absorbed from the gastrointestinal tract once they reach the stomach and small intestine. Inhaled toxins, such as fumes and gases, can cause tissue damage on contact with the respiratory mucosa (such as anhydrous ammonia) or can cross the respiratory membrane to exert their effects (such as cyanide

Pediatric Care

Factors contributing to pediatric poisonings include curiosity, an underdeveloped sense of taste, inability to recognize the consequences of behavior, poor supervision, and poor childproofing.

Geriatric Care

Factors contributing to geriatric poisonings include taking multiple medications, depression, poor cognitive function, poor judgment, and poor eyesight.

and carbon monoxide gases). Many toxins can either cause damage directly to the skin and mucous membranes, or can be absorbed through them to enter the bloodstream and cause systemic effects. For example, organophosphates are toxins that can readily enter the body through surface absorption, and cocaine can be readily absorbed through mucous membranes. Toxins can be injected into the subcutaneous or muscular tissues, or directly into the venous system. Envenomated bites and stings and intravenous drugs are examples of toxins that can enter the body through injection.

Toxins can have a number of effects, depending on their nature. Some have primarily local effects, causing irritation of the exposed tissues. Other toxins have profound effects on a particular system, such as the cardiovascular or nervous systems. Others, such as cyanide, affect the function of all systems by causing cellular asphyxia.

There are 60 poison control centers distributed throughout the United States and its territories. Poison control centers are staffed 24 hours a day by pharmacists, physicians, nurses, and other health care professionals who are specialists in medical toxicology. The American Association of Poison Control Centers (AAPCC) operates the centers, which provide timely and accurate identification of the toxins involved in exposures. Poison control centers serve as important resources for medical providers, both in hospital and out of hospital. The poison control hotline is available through the national toll-free phone number 1-800-222-1222.

Poison control staff can help the Advanced EMT determine the severity of an exposure and suggest how best to manage exposures to specific toxins. In cases of low-level exposures where the substance is known, and the patient is asymptomatic, you may contact poison control to determine whether a patient needs to be transported. An example may include an unintentional pediatric exposure to a small amount of a known household chemical. If the substance is

unknown, or the amount of substance to which the patient has been exposed is in question, the safest approach is to transport any patient who has been poisoned. Begin treatment as appropriate.

The National Poison Data System (NPDS) is a large computerized database that can help track exposures. Uses of the database, which is operated by the AAPCC, include linking multiple exposures to a specific substance, following recalls and banned products, and identifying acts of chemical and biologic terrorism. The database can also work as a powerful research tool for those involved in researching and analyzing exposures.

General Assessment and Management of Toxicologic Emergencies

As with many calls, sometimes the nature of a toxicologic emergency is clear from dispatch and initial scene information. In those cases, it makes sense to discuss how to assess a toxicologic emergency. In other cases, though, the cause of the problem is initially unknown, and requires a process of clinical reasoning to identify poisoning as a differential diagnosis. For them, you must identify the problem before it makes sense to assess it as a toxicologic emergency. To do this, you must recognize patterns of behavior and signs and symptoms, and must know how to explore various hypotheses for the patient's presentation. Particular instances in which you should suspect toxic exposure, either as the primary problem or in conjunction with another situation, include fires, motor vehicle collisions, industrial settings, environments with high incidences of drug abuse, behavioral emergencies, and patients with altered mental status. Given any type of toxicologic exposure, you should be able to begin stabilizing the patient's condition, providing supportive care, and anticipating whether an ALS intercept or physician consult is necessary.

Scene Size-Up

Scene safety involves early identification of the hazard, activation of appropriate resources, and utilization of personal protective equipment (PPE). Some resources available at the request of the Advanced EMT include law enforcement, fire department, hazmat, search and rescue, and additional transport units (Figure 32-1). Intentional poisoning, overdoses, and substance abuse often go hand in hand, with an increased potential for violent behavior. Involvement of more than one patient, unusual odors, the presence of vapors or spills of unknown substances, unresponsive patients, behavioral emergencies, and patients presenting with altered mental status should all increase your suspicion of a toxicologic emergency.

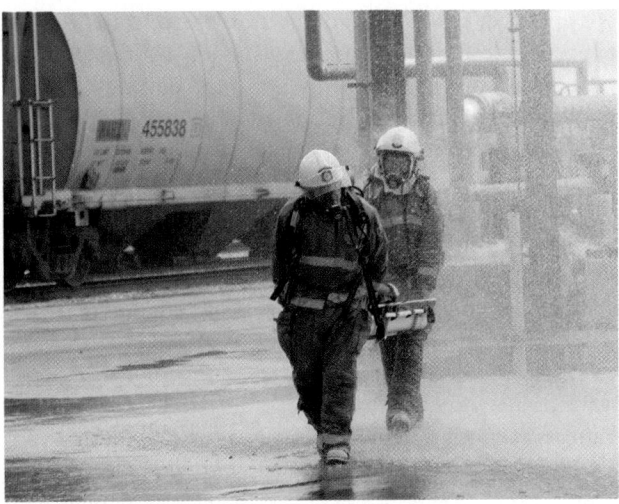

FIGURE 32-1

Only trained rescuers with appropriate PPE should rescue patients from toxic environments. (© Kevin Link)

Once you identify a toxicologic emergency, you must obtain the following information:

- The name of the substance or substances. If the name is not known, collect as much information about it as you can. If it is safe to do so (not a hazardous material), bring the substance or a sample of it to the hospital. If a plant is involved, bring a large enough sample to identify it. Taking a picture of the whole plant may be helpful.

- The quantity involved.

- The time of exposure.

- The patient's weight.

- What, if anything, has been attempted in the treatment of the patient prior to your arrival.

- If relevant (such as a skin exposure or inhalation), the duration of exposure.

- Label information. Bring the container to the hospital, if possible.

- If applicable, use the Department of Transportation *Emergency Response Guide* or Material Safety Data Sheet to obtain more information.

- Identify the potential for polysubstance overdoses. Do not overlook the ingestion of alcohol or over-the-counter drugs in combination with prescription drugs or street drugs.

Primary Assessment

Toxins can affect level of responsiveness, airway, breathing, and circulation in many ways. CNS depressants can impair the gag reflex, result in unresponsiveness deep enough to cause airway obstruction, and depress respiratory rate and depth. Vomiting is anticipated with exposure to many types of toxins, further jeopardizing the airway. Some toxins cause soft-tissue damage of the upper airway, inflammation of the lower airways and lungs, or pulmonary edema. Check breath sounds early, and again during reassessments. Toxins with cardiovascular effects can cause vasodilation or impair cardiac output, reducing perfusion. Constant evaluation of the airway, breathing, and circulation are cornerstones of managing toxicologic emergencies.

IN THE FIELD

Poisoning and overdose patients can deteriorate quickly. The patient who is initially awake and oriented can progress quickly to unresponsiveness and respiratory depression or respiratory arrest. Maintain constant awareness of the patient's mental status, airway, and breathing.

PERSONAL PERSPECTIVE

Advanced EMT Timothy Lloyd: The scene size-up is definitely critical, but it doesn't always tell you everything you need to know. I went on a call a couple of years ago for an unresponsive patient. His house was a mess, but nothing I hadn't seen before. There was no alcohol, no medication containers, or evidence of street drugs. The patient was snoring and was responsive only to painful stimuli. His pulse was fast, but normal in strength and regular. His respirations were adequate once his airway was positioned, and all we could find on the exam was a laceration on his head. It was superficial and the blood had dried some time ago. His pupils were slightly dilated, but equal and reacted to light. It was puzzling. The head wound didn't explain the unresponsiveness, especially with his pupils, respirations, and heart rate. I was running through all the possible causes of altered mental status in my mind. I checked his blood glucose level, and it was normal.

There was no odor of alcohol or anything else suspicious for ingestion on his breath. There was no evidence that he had a seizure, but I couldn't rule it out. There were no medications to give us a clue to his medical history, and the friend who had found him didn't know much about his medical history either. The only things I could find for sure were that he was responsive only to pain, he had minor trauma to his scalp but no other indications of traumatic brain injury, and a heart rate of 120. His other vital signs were within normal limits. I followed up with the emergency department physician later that day. It turns out the patient had taken a significant overdose of tricyclic antidepressants. There wasn't anything we would have done differently in his treatment, but it really hit home that day—that when you learn something from the scene size-up, it's great, but not finding anything doesn't mean you can rule anything out either!

For apparently unresponsive patients who do not appear to be breathing, immediately check the carotid pulse and, if necessary, begin CPR and prepare to apply the automated external defibrillator (AED). If the patient has a pulse, use manual airway maneuvers, suction, and basic airway adjuncts as needed to open and maintain the airway. Begin thinking about the need for advanced airway devices, such as a Combitube or supraglottic device. You can use Fowler's position in conscious patients who are vomiting. You can use a left lateral recumbent position to help protect the airway in patients who have a gag reflex but a decreased level of responsiveness. Administer oxygen for patients with increased metabolic rate; for example, in cocaine or methamphetamine overdoses, inhaled toxin exposure, and those who are hypoxic or at risk for hypoxia.

Assess the patient for shock. Check for cool, pale skin, diaphoresis, pulse rate, strength, and regularity. Some toxins place patients at particular risk of cardiac dysrhythmia and cardiac arrest. Once the primary assessment is completed, applying a cardiac monitor, if permitted in your EMS system, and gaining IV access are important considerations.

Syrup of ipecac is an emetic agent that formerly was commonly used to induce vomiting in instances of ingested poisoning. It is no longer recommended in most cases and its availability has become more limited because the substance has been abused by persons with bulimia nervosa to induce vomiting. However, it is still possible to obtain syrup of ipecac in small amounts without a prescription. It is important to know if the patient has taken or been given syrup of ipecac. It produces repeated episodes of forceful vomiting.

In the patient whose level of responsiveness is declining, the risk of aspiration is high. It is important to quickly obtain this information, in addition to as much other pertinent history as possible, because of the potential for poisoning and overdose patients to deteriorate quickly.

History and Secondary Assessment

Obtain a SAMPLE history from the patient, keeping in mind that you may need to verify or supplement the information with other sources, such as the patient's friends and family. Find out as much about the exposure as possible, as previously discussed. Find out what substance or substances are involved, the route and duration of exposure, time of exposure, dose of the substance, and any actions taken to try to treat the exposure. Determine the patient's medications, last oral intake, and events leading up to the problem. Determine if the exposure was intentional or unintentional. Obtain vital signs and the results of monitoring devices, such as pulse oximetry. Determine the blood glucose level in any patient with a history of diabetes or who has an altered mental status. Perform a focused or head-to-toe exam, depending on the situation and the patient's condition.

Clinical Reasoning

Patients with toxicologic emergencies can present in a variety of ways. A patient may present without a clear history of exposure. It may not occur to the elderly patient with nausea, abdominal pain, and other signs and symptoms that he has unintentionally developed toxic medication levels. A person found alone and unresponsive may have taken an overdose at another location, leaving no telltale empty bottles or drug paraphernalia as clues. A child with abdominal pain may have ingested part of a plant without his parents' knowledge. A patient may present with a behavioral emergency, yet deny that there is anything wrong. Without careful questioning and a high index of suspicion for a toxicologic emergency, poisoning can go undetected until the patient suddenly deteriorates. In fact, many patients who attempt suicide do so with mixed methods. A patient from a single-vehicle crash or with superficial lacerations to his wrists may have poisoned himself or taken an overdose, in addition to the more obvious, but less serious problem. In some types of poisoning, the presence of more than one affected patient provides a strong clue.

Treatment

The prehospital care for most poisoned patients is supportive: managing the airway, breathing, ventilation, oxygenation, and circulation, which you will have begun in the primary assessment. Intravenous access is recommended for patients with significant exposures. Patients with hypotension may require fluid infusion. In addition, you must minimize the amount of toxin to which the patient is being exposed. The way in which this is done depends on the toxin and route of exposure. For example, removing a patient from an area with fumes to fresh air limits exposure (Figure 32-2). To slow absorption, an extremity with an envenomated snake bite is *not* elevated as most injured extremities are. Activated charcoal is sometimes given to adsorb some ingested toxins.

Most toxins do not have specific antidotes, but in one particular case, in narcotic overdoses with respiratory depression, Advanced EMTs can give naloxone to compete with the drug for opiate receptor sites, thereby reducing the drug's effects. Advanced EMTs also may use an organophosphate antidote kit containing atropine and pralidoxime. (See Chapters 13 and 49.)

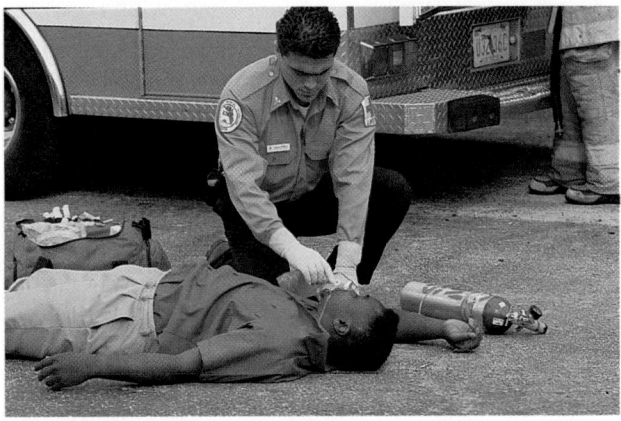

FIGURE 32-2

Remove toxic inhalation patients to fresh air and administer oxygen.

Activated charcoal is an adsorbent, which means it binds to most types of toxins in the gastrointestinal tract. Activated charcoal is not recommended for substances that do not form strong bonds to it, such as lithium, methanol, ethanol, and ethylene glycol; or for caustics or hydrocarbons. To be effective, you must administer activated charcoal within 1 to 2 hours after ingestion of the substances. Do not give anything by mouth, including activated charcoal, to a patient who cannot control his airway or whose level of responsiveness is likely to decrease before reaching the hospital, because activated charcoal can cause vomiting as a side effect. Activated charcoal usually comes premixed in a slurry containing sorbitol, a sugar alcohol that adds flavor and acts as a cathartic (Scan 32-1). The typical dosage of activated charcoal is 1 gram/kg, with a minimum of 30 grams. In some cases, multiple doses of activated charcoal are given over time.

Whether or not the poison control center is contacted or not depends on your protocols, the substance, and the patient's condition and history. Many busy emergency

Pediatric Care

Do not give pediatric patients more than one dose of products containing sorbitol. The large sugar molecule causes water to osmotically enter the bowel, resulting in diarrhea. Dehydration and electrolyte imbalance can occur.

IN THE FIELD

The most important actions in the management of a poisoned patient are recognition; scene safety; managing the airway, breathing, and circulation; and minimizing additional exposure, absorption, and distribution of the toxin.

departments routinely handle common types of overdoses, such as narcotics, acetaminophen, alcohol, and common antidepressants.

Reassessment

Remember, the level of toxin in the patient's system may be increasing, even as you speak with him. Anticipate deterioration and monitor the patient closely. Pay close attention to the patient's mental status, airway, breathing, and circulation and be alert to any changes. Monitor the vital signs and SpO₂, as well as the patient's complaints and the effects of any treatment. Be prepared to upgrade the patient's priority for treatment and transport, if needed, and to take any additional measures based on changes in the patient's condition.

Carbon Monoxide

Carbon monoxide is a colorless and odorless gas created during incomplete combustion of fuels such as petroleum products, wood, and other carbon-containing fuels. Carbon monoxide is particularly dangerous in enclosed spaces, such as vehicles with faulty exhaust, homes with a faulty gas furnace or in which alternative heat sources such as kerosene heaters are used, or in garages in which a vehicle is left running. Campers using fires or gas-fueled stoves or heaters are at increased risk, as are persons in stationary running vehicles.

Having a garage door open while a vehicle is running is not sufficient to prevent carbon monoxide poisoning. Carbon monoxide is also one of the toxins involved in smoke inhalations in fires. Carbon monoxide poisoning kills over 400 people each year, not including those who die in fires, and each incident has the potential for multiple patients (Centers for Disease Control, 2005). But, poisoning can be prevented through safety measures, such as maintaining furnaces and avoiding situations that can lead to the accumulation of carbon monoxide. Carbon monoxide detectors are available, as well.

Once inhaled, carbon monoxide is quickly absorbed across the respiratory membrane, where it binds readily with hemoglobin. Carbon monoxide has about 250 times the affinity for hemoglobin as oxygen does, meaning that hemoglobin preferentially binds with carbon monoxide, rather than oxygen. Rather than forming oxyhemoglobin, carboxyhemoglobin is formed. This leads to poor oxygen-carrying capacity and cellular hypoxia. Organs initially affected are those that have the highest demand for oxygen, such as the brain, accounting for the headache, dizziness, confusion, and sleepiness associated with carbon monoxide poisoning. Other signs and symptoms include vomiting, shortness of breath, and general malaise.

The symptoms of carbon monoxide poisoning, the insidious nature of the gas, and the fact that the increase in

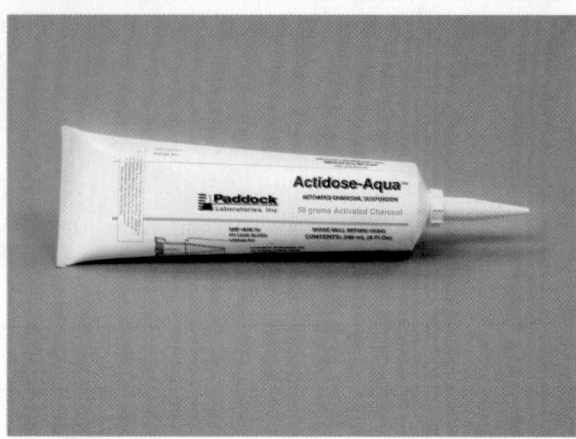

Medication Name

Activated charcoal is the generic name. Some of the better-known trade names of activated charcoal are:

- SuperChar
- InstaChar
- Actidose
- Actidose-Aqua
- Liqui-Char
- Charcoaid

Indications

Activated charcoal may be used for a patient who has ingested poison by mouth, upon specific orders from medical direction. It is most effective when administered within 1 hour after the ingestion of the poison and only in very specific cases of poisoning.

Contraindications

Do not administer activated charcoal to a patient who:

- Has an altered mental status (is not fully alert) because it may cause aspiration
- Has swallowed acids or alkalis (such as hydrochloric acid, bleach, ammonia, or ethyl alcohol)
- Is unable to swallow
- Has overdosed on cyanide

Medication Form

- Premixed in water, frequently available in a plastic bottle containing 12.5 grams of activated charcoal
- Powder, which should be avoided in the field

Dosage

Unless directed otherwise by medical direction, give both adults and children 1 gram of activated charcoal per kilogram (1 gram/kg) of body weight. The usual adult dose is 30 to 100 grams. The usual dose for infants and children is 12.5 to 25 grams.

Administration

Directions that follow are general. Consult medical direction or the poison control center, according to local protocol, before administering activated charcoal to any patient.

1. The activated charcoal settles to the bottom of its container and needs to be evenly distributed. So shake the activated charcoal in the bottle thoroughly. If it is too thick to shake well, remove the cap and stir it until it is well mixed.
2. Activated charcoal looks like mud. The patient may be more willing to drink it if he cannot see it, such as through a straw from a covered opaque container.
3. If the activated charcoal settles, shake or stir it again before letting the patient finish the dose.
4. Record the time and the patient's response.
5. If the patient vomits, notify medical direction to authorize one repeat of the dose.

Once you have given a patient activated charcoal, do not let him have milk, ice cream, or sherbet. They all decrease the effectiveness of activated charcoal.

Actions

Activated charcoal adsorbs poisons in the stomach (it prevents their absorption by the body and enhances their elimination from the body). The ability of activated charcoal to adsorb poisons is due to the preparation process that makes it extremely porous. Activated charcoal does not bind to (is not effective for) alcohol, kerosene, gasoline, caustics, or metals such as iron. It is not routinely used for ingested poisoning. Only administer activated charcoal based on medical direction.

Side Effects

The most common side effect is blackening of the stools. Some patients, especially those who are already nauseated, may vomit. If the patient vomits, repeat the dose of activated charcoal once. Be alert for further vomiting, and transport as soon as possible. Other side effects are rare.

Reassessment

During administration, ensure that the patient's airway and mental status are adequate so that he or she does not aspirate the medication. Check for abdominal pain or distress upon administration. Watch for possible vomiting after administration and prevent aspiration by placing the patient in a sitting or lateral recumbent position and being prepared to suction.

use of gas heat sources coincides with flu season lead to patients frequently mistaking carbon monoxide poisoning for influenza. Other signs and symptoms include tachycardia, tachypnea, hyperthermia, memory problems, agitation, and impaired judgment. Signs and symptoms of severe poisoning include chest pain, confusion, ataxia, seizures, and unconsciousness. Rhabdomyolysis and renal failure can occur with prolonged exposure.

Scene safety involves early identification of the hazard, activation of appropriate resources, and removing patients from the source, if it is safe for you to do so. Always keep in mind the potential for multiple patients and perform a thorough search of the structure. For unresponsive patients, open and maintain the airway and assist with ventilation as needed. Anticipate vomiting in all patients with carbon monoxide poisoning. All patients exposed to carbon monoxide require administration of oxygen by nonrebreather mask. Keep in mind that the use of pulse oximetry (without CO-oximetry) and skin color are unreliable indicators of oxygenation in patients exposed to carbon monoxide.

The half-life of carbon monoxide in an ambient air environment is 3 to 4 hours. High-flow oxygen can reduce the half-life to 30 to 90 minutes, and hyperbaric oxygen therapy can reduce the half-life even more dramatically. Start an IV and consider fluid administration for hypotension.

Cyanide

Cyanide is found in several products and items, including silver polish, fruit pits and seeds, and as gas formed when common household products, such as acrylics, nylon, wool, cotton, some plastics, paper, and wood, among other items, are burned. The most prevalent route of cyanide poisoning is from home fires, and often occurs in conjunction with carbon monoxide poisoning in such cases. Cyanide is a cellular asphyxiant that stops energy production at the cellular level and keeps the mitochondria from processing oxygen, resulting in anaerobic metabolism. Death occurs in seconds to minutes after inhalation or ingestion, and in minutes to hours after absorption through the skin.

Scene safety involves using the same principles as carbon monoxide poisoning. Suspect additional patients were involved in home fires until proven otherwise. In situations in which the exposure is smaller or more chronic, or in which the onset is delayed, patients generally have weakness, malaise, headache, dizziness, confusion, seizures, shortness of breath, pulmonary edema, and coma. The odor of bitter almonds may be detected on the patient's breath, but this is not a reliable finding because many people cannot detect it. Pulse oximetry may be high, because oxygen is present, but cannot be used at the cellular level. Signs and symptoms reflect hypoxia and acidosis despite the presence of oxygen.

Treatment focuses on managing airway, breathing, and circulation. Provide high-flow oxygen and be prepared to encounter severe dyspnea and pulmonary edema. Activated charcoal may be indicated for ingested cyanide. Consult with medical direction. As with all critical patients, constantly monitor vital functions and obtain venous access. Two types of antidotes are available for cyanide: hydroxocobalamin (vitamin B12), and a three-part cyanide antidote kit containing amyl nitrite, sodium nitrite, and sodium thiosulfate.

Caustic Substances

Acids and alkalis are caustic substances that can cause chemical burns when they come into contact with the body. Caustic household substances include toilet bowl cleaners, rust removers, drain cleaners, batteries, bleach, laundry detergents, dishwashing detergents, oven cleaners, swimming pool chemicals, ammonia, and hair relaxer solutions. Additionally, concentrated acids and alkalis are used in many industrial settings. Exposure to the substances may result in dermal, ocular, inhalation, or ingestion injuries.

Often, household chemicals containing acids or alkalis are ingested in an attempted suicide. When strong acids contact the skin, they generally result in coagulation necrosis, in which a thick layer of damaged tissue helps to limit deeper exposure. Significant ingestions of acids can result in metabolic acidosis. One particular acid, hydrogen fluoride, leeches calcium from the body, causing life-threatening hypocalcemia. Strong alkalis result in liquefaction necrosis, in which the exposed tissues are liquefied, allowing the alkali to penetrate into deeper tissue layers. If ingested, acids and, particularly, alkalis, can result in erosion of the esophagus and stomach. This can cause hemorrhage and severe pain. Never induce vomiting in patients with caustic ingestion because it results in a second exposure of the esophagus and oral mucosa to the substance.

Patients may complain of skin irritation, and exhibit burns of the mouth and tongue, with drooling and difficulty swallowing, hematemesis, stridor, hoarseness, and difficulty breathing. Follow scene safety guidelines, being careful not to expose other providers, and remove all contaminated clothing and jewelry before beginning treatment. Flush dermal and ocular exposures with copious amounts of water to reduce injury. Use water only; do not attempt to use a chemical antidote to neutralize the substance, because this can result in significant heat release, increasing the damage. Activated charcoal is not indicated in the treatment of caustic ingestion. The use of water to dilute or wash away particles of solid alkali adherent to the esophagus is sometimes recommended. Consult with poison control and medical direction.

During management of the patient, focus on supportive care and the treatment of immediate life threats. Airway management may be complicated in the case of extensive tissue damage. Nonvisualized airways, such as

Combitube, are contraindicated. Consider the need for ALS response or intercept, if available. If available, choose a hospital with a burn center for patients with significant tissue damage.

Hydrocarbons

Hydrocarbons include gasoline, butane, kerosene, lamp oils, mineral oil, and toluene. They are found in lighter fluids, laundry stain removers, spray lubricants (such as WD-40) glues, paints, and aerosol propellants (fluorocarbons), and exposure can occur through any route. The intentional inhalation of hydrocarbons is informally known as "huffing" (Figure 32-3). The toxicity of hydrocarbons varies. Many do not result in significant problems with a single exposure, but a few, including halogenated or aromatic hydrocarbons (such as chlorofluorocarbons, or CFCs), can be

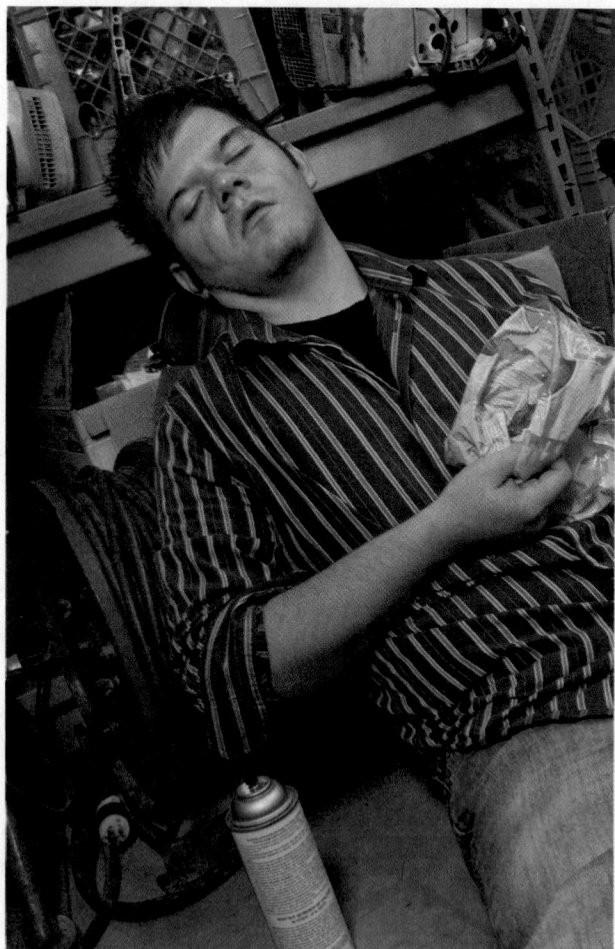

FIGURE 32-3

Huffing is the deliberate concentration and inhalation of vapors or fumes to achieve intoxication. Users may saturate a cloth with volatile liquid substances and place it over the mouth and nose or concentrate aerosols in a bag for inhalation.

very serious. Symptoms vary depending on the toxicity of the substance, route and amount of exposure, and history of repeated exposure.

Hydrocarbon exposure has a toxic effect on multiple body systems. Nervous system damage may include dizziness, confusion, ataxia, altered mental status (AMS), unresponsiveness, and apnea. Cardiovascular findings may include hypotension and sudden cardiac arrest. Gastrointestinal problems generally arise from the caustic nature of hydrocarbons on the stomach and intestines. Signs and symptoms following an ingestion may include nausea, vomiting, diarrhea, and burning of the oropharynx. When an exposure has occurred to the skin, erythema, dermatitis, and burns may occur. Cases of renal and hepatic system failure have been documented. Ingestion of liquid forms of hydrocarbons carries a high risk of aspiration, leading to pneumonitis, dyspnea, and hypoxia.

Huffing is the deliberate inhalation of hydrocarbons for the purpose of intoxication. Some commonly abused substances include gasoline, kerosene, spray paint, paint thinner, gun cleaner, typewriter correction fluid, and glue. The substance is soaked in a rag, held around the mouth and nose, and inhaled. When spray paint or another gaseous hydrocarbon is sprayed into a paper sack and inhaled, it is called "bagging." Huffing hydrocarbons affects the same body systems as other routes of hydrocarbon exposure; however, symptoms are more acutely focused in the respiratory system. The patient may be wheezing, tachypneic, complain of shortness of breath, and develop hypotension. Erythema and dried paint may be present around the mouth and nose area from huffing or bagging spray paint. When severe wheezing is heard upon auscultation, aspiration pneumonitis (inflammation of the lungs) may have developed.

Some hydrocarbons commonly used in intentional inhalation can sensitize the myocardium, making it susceptible to the effects of catecholamines and leading to a phenomenon known as *sudden sniffing death syndrome*. For this reason, even if inhalation of hydrocarbons results in wheezing, check with poison control and medical direction before administering sympathetic agonists, such as albuterol. Monitor the cardiac rhythm, if permitted in your scope of practice, and anticipate cardiac dysrhythmia.

Organophosphates

Organophosphates are primarily found in pesticides, but have gained attention as a possible weapon of terrorism. Exposure may occur through inhalation, absorption, or ingestion. Although organophosphates may be found around the home, also consider organophosphate exposure when responding to agricultural settings and greenhouses. Organophosphates are potent cholinergics that produce prolonged, unopposed stimulation of the parasympathetic nervous system by inhibiting acetylcholinesterase, the enzyme that breaks down acetylcholine in synapses and the neuroeffector junctions.

The effects are remembered by the acronym SLUDGE:

S – Salivation

L – Lacrimation (tearing)

U – Urination

D – Defecation

G – Gastric distress

E – Emesis

Other effects include muscle twitching, paralysis, seizures, altered mental status, bradycardia, hypotension, bronchospasm, and pulmonary edema.

Treatment considerations include scene safety, avoiding exposure of EMS personnel or bystanders, and decontaminating the patient. Irrigate with copious amounts of water, using soap if available. Airway management can be complicated by copious bronchial and oral secretions. Use suction as needed and request ALS, if available. In most cases, the organophosphate antidote kits carried by Advanced EMTs are intended for self-use or administration to your partner in the event of a terrorism event. However, the treatment for organophosphate poisoning is the same for exposures in other settings: atropine and praladoxime (2-pam). Consult with medical direction about administering these medications.

Ethanol and Toxic Alcohols

Ethanol, or beverage alcohol, is a widely used and culturally accepted intoxicating substance in the United States and many other countries. Ethanol is a CNS depressant, and patients may have slurred speech, **ataxic** gait, poor coordination, **nystagmus**, altered mental status, and behavioral changes. Severe alcohol intoxication may present with respiratory depression, emesis potentially with aspiration, and unconsciousness. There is generally an odor of alcohol to the breath, but this can sometimes be difficult to distinguish from the odor of ketones produced in diabetic ketoacidosis. In some cases, your suspicion of ethanol ingestion is increased by the presence of alcoholic beverages at the scene. However, do not assume that the patient's only problem is acute alcohol intoxication. Intoxicated patients are at increased risk of injury, but may have a decreased sensation of pain or lack of appropriate concern for the injury. Medical emergencies can occur in the context of acute intoxication as well. As always, check a blood glucose level in any patient who has changes in cognition or behavior.

There are numerous detrimental effects to the body after years of alcohol abuse, including neurologic, cardiovascular, and gastrointestinal diseases. Wernicke-Korsakoff's syndrome is an alcohol-related psychosis resulting from a combination of thiamine deficiency and permanent neurologic damage. The patient may have amnesia and may **confabulate**. Cardiovascular diseases include alcoholic cardiomyopathy, hypertension, and high cholesterol. Gastrointestinal problems may include pancreatitis, cirrhosis, stomach cancer, and decreased blood-clotting factors, among others. With chronic alcohol abuse, males may suffer testicular atrophy and feminizing characteristics.

Try to verbally calm down intoxicated patients who are uncooperative, but do not place providers at risk by not restraining those who are physically combative. Due to the chances of aspiration among unconscious patients, treatment emphasizes management of the patient's airway.

Delirium tremens (DTs) usually occur two to three days following the sudden cessation, or significant decrease, of alcohol among those with a long history of dependence. DTs have a mortality rate ranging from 5 to 15 percent, even with current treatment therapies (Catlett, 2004). Patients may present with tachycardia, hypertension, sweating, delusions, and visual, auditory, or tactile hallucinations. Sudden alcohol withdrawal may precipitate generalized seizures from 6 to 48 hours from the time of the last drink. Treat the patient in DTs cautiously because behavior can be erratic and violent. The patient is in a state of metabolic hyperactivity and is desperately in need of medical treatment.

Like other patients with addictions, alcoholics are preoccupied with obtaining and using their drug. When ethanol is not available, particularly in the homeless population and among underage alcohol consumers, alternatives may be sought. However, those substitutes are toxic alcohols, which can cause severe illness and may be fatal in small doses.

Methanol was originally produced from the cooking of wood in an oxygen-free environment; thus, it is sometimes called *wood alcohol*. Methanol is used in many commercial products including windshield de-icing solution, fuels, and some illegally produced alcoholic drinks. The solvent is also used in the illegal manufacturing of methamphetamine. It is extremely flammable, leading to safety hazards associated with locations where illegal methamphetamine is manufactured ("meth houses" or "meth labs").

In addition to the signs associated with ethanol ingestion, patients exposed to methanol may develop acute blindness or blurred or cloudy vision, which is a characteristic finding of methanol poisoning; abdominal pain; and altered mental status, including coma. A rapid respiratory rate, or tachypnea, may be present as the body attempts to correct metabolic acidosis, a byproduct of the breakdown of methanol. Activated charcoal is ineffective in the treatment of toxic alcohol ingestion. Manage the airway, breathing, and circulation of the poisoned patient. Provide oxygen at a flow rate to maintain normal oxygen saturation. Start an IV and consult with medical direction about a fluid bolus to maintain renal perfusion and prevent renal failure.

Isopropanol, also known as *isopropyl alcohol* or *rubbing alcohol*, is used as a disinfectant in the household and a solvent in industrial settings. It also is used in easily available products such as cough and cold medications, hand sanitizer, mouthwash, and ointments. Because of the wide distribution of isopropanol, the potential for exposure is high. Anticipate altered mental status, ataxia, slurred speech, and abnormal behavior. Isopropanol is a powerful intoxicant that produces similar signs and symptoms to ethanol ingestion, but as is often said the effects are, "twice as drunk, twice as sick, twice as long." Patients who have consumed isopropanol may complain of abdominal pain and may have upper gastrointestinal bleeding due to its effects on the gastric mucosa.

Obvious or hidden (under the bed, for example) containers of isopropanol-containing products should increase your suspicion of intoxication, but check for other causes of altered mental status, such as stroke, trauma, and hypoglycemia. Manage the patient's airway, with anticipation of vomiting. Monitor for respiratory depression, and anticipate hypotension and dysrhythmia. Obtain IV access and consider the need for fluids to maintain perfusion.

Ethylene glycol is used as an ingredient in vehicle radiator antifreeze. It is very sweet tasting when unaltered by bittering agents, and often has an iridescent green color in antifreeze solutions. Ethylene glycol is lethal in small amounts. Even an amount as small as 30 mL can be lethal to an adult (DynaMed, 2010). The sweet taste makes ethylene glycol attractive to pediatric patients (and pets), and figures in suicide attempts, as well as accidental ingestions, in adults. Signs and symptoms include neurologic changes, such as unconsciousness, ataxia, slurred speech, and seizures; tachypnea, tachycardia, nausea, and vomiting. Patients are also at risk of renal failure.

Manage the patient's airway, with anticipation of vomiting. Monitor for respiratory depression, and anticipate hypotension and dysrhythmia. Obtain IV access and consider the need for fluids to maintain perfusion.

Food and Plant Toxins

Food Toxins

Food poisoning was presented in Chapter 28, but remember that in addition to the direct effects of infectious agents, some types of food poisoning, such as botulism, are caused by the toxins produced by infectious agents. Therefore, patients with food poisoning can present with systemic signs and symptoms of toxicity, as well as gastrointestinal signs and symptoms.

Some seafoods, such as grouper, snapper, eel, sea bass, barracuda, and Spanish mackerel, also can contain dangerous toxins (Arnold, 2010). The toxin, ciguatera (ciguatoxin), accumulates in older fish from ingestion of certain types of organisms called *dinoflagellates*. Unfortunately, the toxin does not affect the smell, appearance, or flavor of affected fish, and it is not destroyed by heat or gastric acid. The availability of foods once restricted to other parts of the globe means that the once-exotic foods are readily found in most locations. Nonetheless, ciguatera poisoning is unusual in the United States, with most cases noted in Hawaii and Florida. It is seldom fatal, but can induce gastrointestinal symptoms within one to two days,

including abdominal pain, nausea, vomiting, and diarrhea. Neurologic symptoms can begin in as little as 3 hours, but sometimes last for months. Paresthesias, reversal of the sensations of hot and cold, itching, joint and muscle pain, tooth pain, weakness, lack of coordination, and dizziness may occur. Rarely, respiratory arrest and coma occur. Bradycardia and hypotension are less common, but can occur.

Histamine fish poisoning, formerly called **scombroid fish poisoning**, accounts for 37 percent of seafood-related foodborne illnesses (Noltkamper, 2009). The signs and symptoms can mimic an allergic reaction but the underlying cause of the problem is ingestion of toxins in the fish. Scombroid fish include tuna, mackerel, swordfish, and marlin. However, the toxin implicated in reactions is present in other common fish as well, including mahi-mahi, sardine, and herring. When susceptible fish is inadequately processed or refrigerated, a substance present in certain types of bacteria converts a naturally occurring compound in fish tissue to histamine. As the bacteria in improperly stored fish multiply, the amount of histamine present in the tissues can increase to levels that well exceed the amount needed to cause toxicity. There likely is a second substance in contaminated fish that plays a role in the development of histamine fish poisoning, because histamine on its own is not well absorbed from the gastrointestinal tract.

Signs and symptoms of histamine fish poisoning include flushing of the skin, usually on the upper half of the body; a severe, throbbing headache; nausea, vomiting, and diarrhea; abdominal cramping; palpitations; itching and hives; dizziness; and dry mouth. Hypotension, bronchospasm, and angioedema can occur. Respiratory distress and chest tightness can also occur, but are rare (Noltkamper, 2009). There will be a history of recent ingestion of fish. Ask the patient if the fish tasted or appeared unusual. Affected fish can have an "off" flavor, such as a metallic taste, and perhaps an unusual, honeycomb appearance.

Because angioedema and bronchospasm can occur, pay careful attention to assessing and managing the airway, breathing, and circulation. Administer IV fluids for hypotension and consider administering a nebulized beta$_2$ agonist for wheezing. The preferred treatment is antihistamines. If diphenhydramine (Benadryl) administration is in your scope of practice, consult with medical direction. If in doubt and the patient has severe signs and symptoms, such as airway obstruction, respiratory distress, or hypotension, treat the patient for anaphylaxis according to your protocol.

Plant Toxins

Many types of poisonous plants are found in the home and garden, at the roadside, in fields, and in the wild (Table 32-2). Household and garden plants pose a threat to children because they are readily available. Some people intentionally abuse plants for their hallucinogenic and intoxicating properties, such as jimsonweed (*Datura*), which grows abundantly in many parts of the country. Jimsonweed, which is smoked or drunk as a tea, has potent anticholinergic effects,

TABLE 32-2	Poisonous Plants	
Toxin	**Plant**	**Signs and Symptoms**
Cyanide	Stone fruit pits (peaches, apricots, plums) and fruit seeds (pears, apples)	Weakness, nausea, vomiting, seizures, coma
Colchicine	Autumn crocus, meadow saffron	Cramps, nausea, hematuria, shock, coma
Calcium oxylate/ oxalic acid	Diffenbachia (Dumb cane), philodendron, rhubarb leaves	Severe gastroenteritis, burning and swelling of oral mucosa, anuria
Amygdalin	Parts of wild and cultivated cherry trees, including seeds	Stupor, vocal cord paralysis, seizures, coma
Bella donna alkaloids	Jimson weed (Datura), nightshade	Anticholinergic effects; fever; tachycardia; dilated pupils; red, hot, dry skin
Glycosides	Purple foxglove, lily of the valley	Cardiac dysrhythmia, nausea, shock, gastroenteritis
Solanine	Potato plant leaves; green parts of potato, horse nettle	Severe gastroenteritis, headache, apnea, shock

Other poisonous plants: hyacinth, narcissus, and daffodil (cholinergics); mistletoe; oleander; poinsettia; iris; azaleas and rhododendrons; wisteria; castorbean (source of ricin); buttercups; hemlock

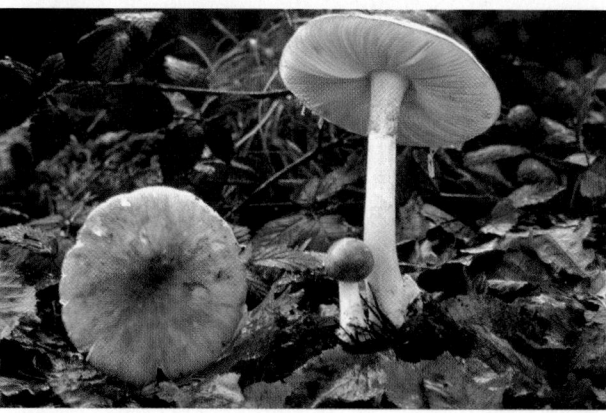

medication, digitalis. An overdose of cardiac glycosides may lead to cardiac arrhythmias, such as bradycardia, and changes in visual perception, including color changes and loss of visual acuity. Most poison mushroom deaths are from one group, *Amanita*, which causes liver failure (Figure 32-4). Other toxic mushrooms are less deadly; however, *Galerina* is particularly toxic. Poison ivy usually causes a delayed hypersensitivity reaction, but in patients who are especially sensitive, exposure to smoke from burning plants can produce anaphylaxis.

Initiate supportive care for victims of a poisonous plant overdose by ensuring adequate airway, ventilation, and oxygenation. Anticipate vomiting and establish an IV in anticipation of hypotension. Provide fluids corresponding to the patient's hemodynamic status. Identification of the plant is critical, as is determining what part of the plant was ingested or otherwise caused exposure (leaves, bark, fruit, roots, bulbs). Bring a sample of the plant large enough to allow identification. Taking a digital picture of the plant may help speed identification if it can be transmitted to poison control or medical direction. Consider contacting an ALS intercept in symptomatic patients because there may be cardiac changes that are treatable within the paramedic scope of practice.

Venom

Many venomous insects and animal bites cause local discomfort and swelling without producing systemic effects. However, in cases of allergy, exposure to the bite or sting of multiple insects or animals, or exposure to particular potent toxins, life-threatening problems can occur. Among the types of venomous bites and stings that EMS providers may encounter are bees and wasps (discussed in Chapter 27), spiders, marine animals, and snakes. Hymenoptera (bees and wasps) cause the most deaths related to envenomation, but mostly due to anaphylaxis, rather than the direct effects of the toxins. Fire ants are also in the hymenoptera family, but their venom is somewhat different. It contains toxins

with signs and symptoms including altered mental status, flushed and dry skin, dilated pupils, and hyperventilation on physical exam. The effects are said to be unpleasant enough that there are few repeat exposures. Consistent with the anticholinergic toxidrome, the presentation is summarized as the following:

- Mad as a hatter (chemicals used to make hats in past centuries led to changes in mentation and behavior)
- Dry as a bone (dry skin and mucous membranes, decreased urine output and difficult urination)
- Red as a beet (flushed skin)
- Blind as a bat (pupil dilation causes blurred vision)
- Hot as hell (hyperthermia)

Several widely cultivated plant species, including purple foxglove, oleander, wallflower, and dogbane contain **cardiac glycosides**, the active ingredient of the antidysrhythmic

that cause pustule formation, as well as proteins similar to the proteins that cause bee-sting anaphylaxis. Fire ants can cause several burning, itching stings in a very short period of time.

In most cases, the patient will be able to relate a clear history of the bite, or will have easily identified localized effects to aid in recognition. However, in some cases, such as the brown recluse spider and, sometimes, coral snakes, the patient may not be aware of the bite until several hours later. In addition to the effects of venom, also be aware that infection is a risk with insect and animal bites.

Spiders and Scorpions

The two types of spiders of greatest concern are the black widow and brown recluse. The brown recluse tends to be found in the Midwest and South, and as its name implies, prefers seclusion in woodpiles, sheds, and other outbuildings, plus closets, mailboxes, and dark, hidden areas (Figure 32-5).

The spider is small, with a violin-shaped band on its back. Although the bite may initially be painless, the venom results in massive localized tissue destruction. Within 8 hours of the bite, there is increasing pain, swelling, and redness (Figure 32-6). Tissue destruction can continue for days to weeks. Patients also may develop nausea and vomiting, chills and fever, and joint pain. There is no specific prehospital treatment, but Advanced EMTs must recognize that this spider's bite can lead to substantial necrosis.

The black widow spider is found in most parts of the country and is readily recognized as a shiny black spider with a red or orange hourglass-shaped mark on her (only

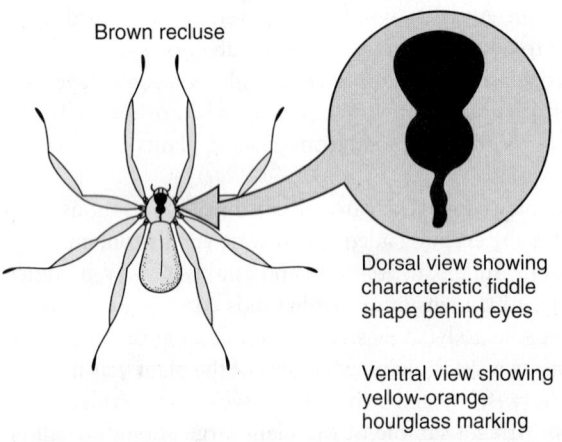

Brown recluse

Dorsal view showing characteristic fiddle shape behind eyes

Ventral view showing yellow-orange hourglass marking

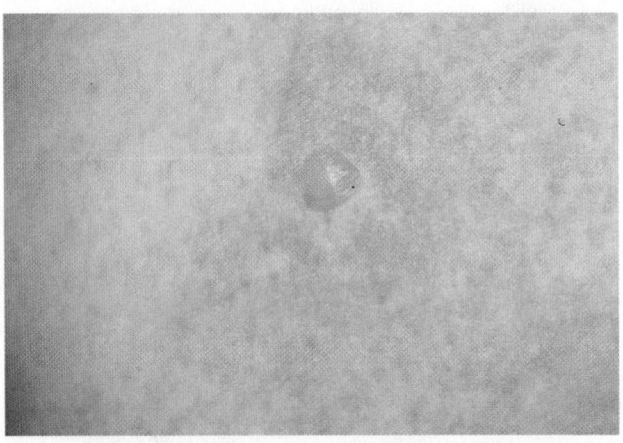

(A)

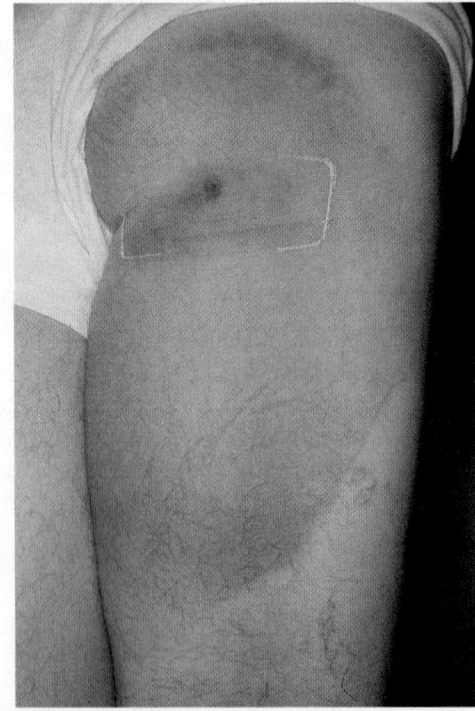

(B)

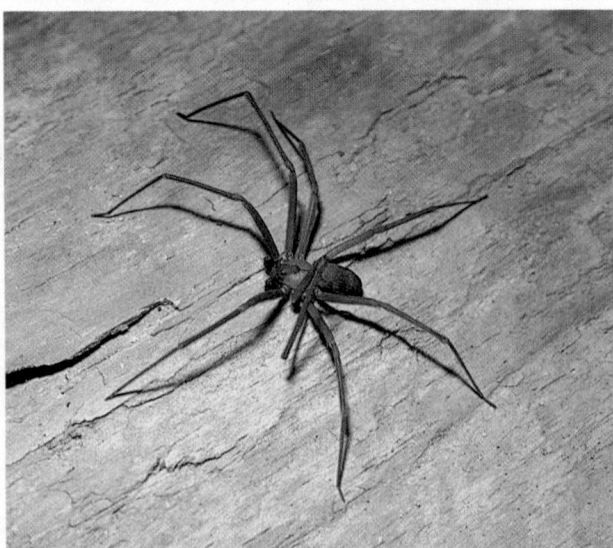

FIGURE 32-5

A brown recluse spider. (Bottom photo: © Breck P. Kent)

FIGURE 32-6

(A) A brown recluse bite 24 hours after envenomation.
(B) A brown recluse bite four days after envenomation.
(Both photos: Courtesy of Scott and White Health Care)

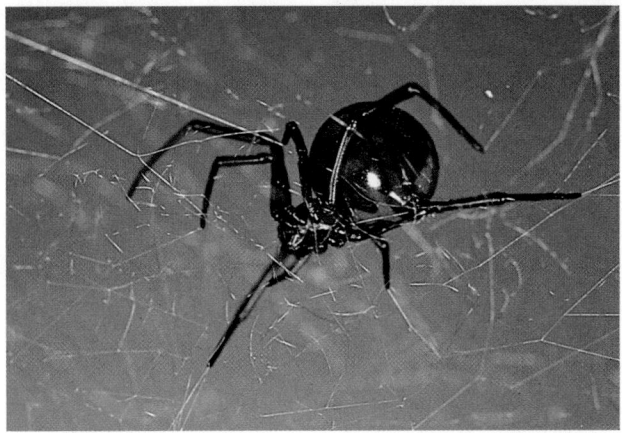

FIGURE 32-7

A black widow spider. (© Joseph T. Collins/Photo Researchers, Inc.)

the female bites are dangerous) abdomen (Figure 32-7). Black widow spider venom is a potent neurotoxin that causes painful spasms in the large muscles, nausea, vomiting, diaphoresis, seizures, paralysis, and altered mental status. Provide support treatment, including management of the airway, breathing, and circulation. Obtain IV access and monitor the patient closely for changes.

Scorpions are common in the Southwestern states, but of the several types of scorpions, the bark scorpion is the only one known to have caused fatalities, though this is rare. Scorpions are mostly seen at night, but can be found beneath objects during the day. The venom is a neurotoxin that can cause altered mental status, muscle twitching, cramping, and seizures. If approved in your protocols, you can apply a loose constricting band above the site to slow distribution of the toxin.

Snakes

The most common classification of venomous snake, pit vipers, is found throughout the United States (Figure 32-8). Pit vipers include rattlesnakes, water moccasins, and copperheads. Those snakes have an elliptical pupil, like a cat's, and a pit (a heat-sensitive organ) between the eye and nostril, as well as a distinctive triangular head. Pit

vipers have noticeable fangs through which they inject venom into their prey. Their venom is potent because it is designed to kill sizeable animals by breaking down their body tissues. The most common scenario of a human bite is that of a person stepping on or near the snake, or of attempting to pick up the snake.

The envenomated bite exhibits both localized and systemic effects. Not all bites are envenomated (25 percent do not result in envenomation), or envenomated to the same degree. A minimal envenomation has only localized effects. A moderate envenomation will result in some systemic effects, while a severe envenomation results in shock. An envenomated bite results in pain, discoloration, and swelling at the site. Tissue necrosis may occur. Bleeding from the wound, although minor, generally does not clot. Systemic effects include weakness, chills, diaphoresis, nausea, vomiting, diarrhea, shock, and respiratory failure.

If the patient is still in the area where the bite occurred, ensure the snake is not nearby. Get as accurate a description of the snake as possible. Prehospital care is supportive, depending on the severity of the patient's presentation. Neither ice nor constricting bands are applied, because both will increase tissue destruction. However, splinting the extremity and keeping it immobilized may help reduce the distribution of venom. Do not elevate the extremity; keep it in a neutral position. Manage the airway and breathing, and apply oxygen for patients with moderate to severe signs and symptoms. Establish IV access, and if possible, transport the patient to a facility that has or can rapidly obtain antivenin, particularly for severe envenomations.

Coral snakes are found mostly in the Southwest, but are not pit vipers. Instead of large fangs, they have smaller, backwards oriented fangs that require the snake to hang on and use a chewing motion to inject venom. As a result of this inefficient mechanism, only about 40 percent of bites are envenomated. Coral snakes resemble many harmless snakes in their appearance. In North America, coral snakes have red and black bands separated by thinner yellow stripes, so that the red and black bands do not directly contact each other. You can use the mnemonic, "Red on yellow harms a fellow; red on black, pat his back," to remember this, but in other geographic locations this pattern does not necessarily hold true.

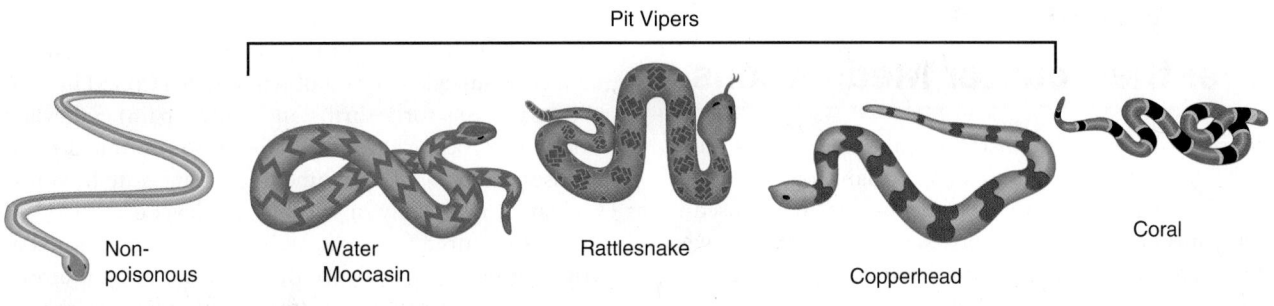

FIGURE 32-8

Typical features of nonpoisonous snakes, pit vipers, and coral snakes.

Overall, coral snake bites are rare, and generally occur in those who are deliberately handling them. Nonetheless, their venom is a very potent neurotoxin. Yet, no deaths have been reported since antivenin became available (Norris, 2008). Signs and symptoms can be delayed by many hours, but include paresthesias, altered mental status, impairment of cranial nerve function, weakness, muscle twitching, respiratory failure, hypotension, and tachycardia. In addition to supportive treatment, a compression bandage (elastic bandage or crepe bandage) is applied starting distal to the bite and working proximally to include the entire extremity to limit absorption and distribution of the toxin. After wrapping the extremity, splint it and keep it level with the body. As with pit viper bites, do not apply ice.

Marine Animals

Both freshwater and saltwater marine animals can be venomous. In most cases, they are painful, but do not cause serious illness. In warmer salt water, beachgoers may encounter jellyfish, Portuguese man-of-war, stingrays, corals, or sea urchins. The stings or punctures are very painful. There also may be localized itching and a raised wheal, or welt. In severe cases, there may be nausea, vomiting, diarrhea, abdominal pain, paresthesias, lymphadenopathy, difficulty breathing or swallowing, chest pain, and muscle cramps. Some jellyfish species in Indonesian and Australian areas are deadly. Catfish, which can be found in freshwater and saltwater, also can produce painful stings.

For saltwater bites and stings, flush the area with saline, 70 percent isopropyl alcohol, or vinegar (fresh water may cause remaining nematocysts to discharge venom). Remove stingers or nematocysts from the skin by scraping. The edge of a plastic card works well, or you can shave the area with a razor. Scrubbing the area or tweezing the stingers may result in release of more venom. Follow by flushing again with vinegar, alcohol, or saline. The application of heat inactivates the venom and relieves pain in local reactions. In more severe cases, with weakness, nausea, vomiting, respiratory distress, or shock, a loose constricting band can help slow the distribution of venom. If you work in an area where marine animal envenomation is common, you will likely have protocols to direct the specific care of patients.

Prescription and Over-the-Counter Medications

Pharmacology is a mainstay of modern medical treatment. Many pharmaceuticals are available over the counter, allowing patients to treat themselves. When used in recommended therapeutic doses, prescription and over-the-counter medications are relatively safe and have many benefits. However, drug side effects, interactions, overdoses, misuse, and cumulative effects can lead to the need for emergency medical care.

Over-the-Counter Medications

Because they are readily available, over-the-counter (OTC) medications figure prominently in suicide attempts, because one of the determinants of the method of suicide or suicide attempt is availability. People also underestimate the potency of OTC medications, reasoning that they must have a wide margin of safety because they are available without a prescription. OTC medications that figure prominently in toxicity are the analgesics acetaminophen, aspirin, and other nonsteroidal anti-inflammatory drugs (NSAIDs), sleep aids, cough and cold preparations, and vitamins and dietary supplements.

Analgesics

Acetaminophen (Tylenol) is a widely used pain reliever found in many OTC preparations. Preparations of acetaminophen are within the top five of medications with the largest number of associated fatalities. Acetaminophen does not have a wide margin of safety. This is complicated by the availability of mixed preparations, such as those for coughs, colds, allergies, and premenstrual symptoms that patients do not realize contain acetaminophen. Patients may take acetaminophen in addition to the mixed medication, without realizing they are ingesting a relatively large amount of it. Poisonings may occur unintentionally, or in an intentional overdose. Acetaminophen is sometimes used in suicidal gestures because the patient believes it is relatively safe, allowing the patient a way to express his distress through a method he believes has a lower possibility of death. Unfortunately, acetaminophen is hepatotoxic at relatively low levels of about 7.5 to 15 grams in an adult and 150 milligrams per kilogram in a pediatric patient (Chun, Tong, Busuttil, & Hiatt, 2009). Keep in mind that the normal adult dosage of two extra-strength acetaminophen tablets or capsules is 1 gram.

In the short term, acetaminophen overdose is relatively asymptomatic, although nausea is common. However, within 24 hours, signs of liver failure can begin. Fortunately, if administered in time, there is an effective antidote available. N-acetylcysteine, a drug used for cystic fibrosis, also serves as an antidote for acetaminophen toxicity.

Aspirin, used as an analgesic as well as a platelet aggregation inhibitor, is a salicylate. Other drugs that fall into the salicylate family and have similar presentations in toxicity include bismuth subsalicylate (PeptoBismol) and methyl salicylate, or oil of wintergreen (found in topical preparations for arthritis and muscle pain). Salicylate toxicity may occur chronically, because continued regular doses accumulate over time at a greater rate than it is eliminated, or acutely in overdose. A level of about 300 mg/kg is required for toxicity. As with acetaminophen, patients often are not aware that they are using multiple products that contain salicylates. In the elderly, who may take aspirin as part of their daily medication regimen, a combination of rote routine and forgetfulness may lead to taking multiple doses on a single day, perhaps more days than not.

Salicylates are acidic (acetylsalicylic acid) and toxicity can lead to metabolic acidosis and impair cellular energy production. As a compensatory mechanism, respirations may be increased. Other signs and symptoms include gastrointestinal distress, dizziness, ringing in the ears (tinnitus), hyperpyrexia, confusion, abdominal pain, and vomiting. In severe cases, heart failure, dysrhythmia, and pulmonary edema may occur. Also anticipate the effect for which aspirin is often taken: decreased platelet aggregation.

Signs and symptoms of toxicity from other OTC (and prescription) NSAIDs (ibuprofen [Advil, Motrin], naproxen [Aleve], and others) vary. Be alert to complaints of abdominal pain, nausea, vomiting, tinnitus, headache, dyspnea, wheezing, and pulmonary edema.

Antihistamines and Sleep Aids

Many OTC sleep aids are, in fact, antihistamines. One of the most common OTC sleep aid ingredients is diphenhydramine, the same substance marketed as Benadryl. Antihistamines have anticholinergic properties, accounting for the side effects you may be familiar with, including dry mouth and thirst. There also may be blurred vision, tachycardia, hyperthermia and flushed skin, confusion or excitement, and hypertension. Both antihistamines and sleep aids may be combination products with NSAIDs, aspirin, or acetaminophen.

Vitamins and Dietary Supplements

Many vitamins have a fairly wide safety margin, but the addition of iron to vitamin preparations gives them a much narrower safety margin. Iron is notoriously toxic, and is a leading cause of unintentional poisoning and poisoning death in small children. Iron toxicity can cause severe gastrointestinal disturbance, including nausea, vomiting, pain, hematemesis, and hypovolemia. Systemically, iron interferes with cellular energy production. The end result is metabolic acidosis, and the liver, heart, kidneys, and lungs can be severely damaged. Gastrointestinal symptoms may occur with an ingestion of 20 mg/kg, and death may occur at levels of 60 mg/kg and higher. Patients with iron overdose can become critically ill and require treatment with supportive measures, including IV access for anticipated hypotension. Hospital treatment is aimed at binding the iron with a chelating agent called *deferoxamine*. Any substance can be toxic with a large enough dosage. In patients who take vitamins or dietary supplements in overdose, check with poison control.

Prescription Medications

Some prescription medications commonly involved in toxicity and overdose include benzodiazepines and other sedative–hypnotics, narcotics, antidepressant and psychotropic medications, and cardiac medications.

Benzodiazepines

Benzodiazepines are widely available to treat anxiety and promote sleep. Examples include diazepam (Valium), alprazolam (Xanax), and lorazepam (Ativan). Rohypnol, or "Ruffies," is also a benzodiazepine. Drugs that act similarly to benzodiazepines, but which are classified as sedatives, include zolpidem (Ambien) and eszopiclone (Lunesta). Benzodiazepines bind to GABA receptors in the central nervous system and inhibit the reticular activating system. Because GABA receptors are complex, different benzodiazepines preferentially act in certain ways. Some, such as alprazolam, mostly reduce anxiety, while others, such as midazolam (Versed) and Rohypnol prevent formation of short-term memories (and long-term memory, because information must first be processed in short-term memory), resulting in an amnestic effect.

On their own, benzodiazepines rarely result in death in overdose. They can result in altered mental status, slurred speech, sedation, respiratory depression, and hypotension. In the hospital there is a benzodiazepine antagonist, flumazenil, that is used when benzodiazepines (used in procedural sedation) are given in excess. However, it is not recommended that flumazenil be used in intentional overdoses, because the sudden withdrawal of benzodiazepine action in dependent individuals may cause seizures. In addition, many intentional benzodiazepine overdoses include other substances, such as antidepressants or alcohol, which may cause seizures when the benzodiazepine is reversed.

Narcotics

Narcotics include opiates, such as morphine, codeine, and heroin, and synthetic and semi-synthetic narcotics, such as fentanyl (Sublimaze, Duragesic), meperidine (Demerol), oxycodone (Oxycontin, Percocet, Tylox), hydrocodone (Vicodin, Lortab), propoxyphene (Darvon), and hydromorphone (Dilaudid). Narcotics are controlled substances used to relieve pain, treat coughs, and slow gastrointestinal activity (Lomotil). Several narcotic preparations are compounded with aspirin or acetaminophen. Check the name of the medication and use a reference guide or contact poison control to determine if the drug taken is a narcotic-only, or if it contains other substances.

Overdosage causes CNS depression, respiratory depression, constricted pupils (in most cases), bradycardia, and hypotension. In some cases, pulmonary edema may occur. Untreated, significant narcotic overdoses are fatal. In addition to managing the patient's airway, breathing, and circulation, the use of naloxone, a narcotic antagonist, is recommended for patients with a narcotic overdose who have respiratory depression. The adult dosage is 0.4 to 2 mg, with 1 to 2 mg typically given. Larger doses, up to 5 mg, may be required for propoxyphene overdose. Titrate the dose to improved respiratory status, but continue to monitor respirations. The intravenous route is usually used in the prehospital setting, but a special preparation for intranasal administration is available.

Other Sedative–Hypnotics

Other drugs that depress CNS function include alcohol and barbiturates (phenobarbital, butalbital [Fiorinal], secobarbital [Seconal]). Slurred speech, altered mental status, respiratory depression, hypotension, and death can occur from both substances. Treatment is supportive, aimed at managing the airway, breathing, and circulation. For deeply unresponsive patients without a gag reflex, consider the use of an advanced airway device. Obtain IV access and treat hypotension with fluids.

Antidepressants

Antidepressants are available to a population at increased risk for suicide, and there is some evidence that initial treatment with antidepressants, particularly in children, adolescents, and young adults, can increase the risk of suicide. Therefore, those drugs figure prominently in overdoses.

Antidepressants fall into three main categories: cyclic antidepressants (most often called *tricyclic antidepressants (TCAs)*, monoamine oxidase inhibitors (MAOIs), and newer antidepressants, which include drugs such as trazodone (Desyrel), bupropion (Wellbutrin), and selective serotonin reuptake inhibitors (SSRIs), serotonin and norepinephrine reuptake inhibitors (SNRIs) and norepinephrine reuptake inhibitors (NRIs). Recently, drugs used as antipsychotics, such as aripiprazole (Abilify), have begun to be added to treatment regimens for depression in some cases.

TCAs are older drugs, and there are concerns about their safety in overdose, but they are cheap and have other uses, such as treating chronic pain, headaches, and insomnia. Examples include amitriptyline (Elavil), nortriptyline (Pamelor), and desipramine (Norpramin), just to name a few. TCAs work by inhibiting reuptake of serotonin and norepinephrine. Flexeril (cyclobenazaprine) is prescribed as a muscle relaxant, but is closely related to TCAs and has the same effects in overdosage. TCAs have a narrow therapeutic index, meaning that the therapeutic and toxic levels are not separated by a wide margin. In overdosage, TCAs can cause anticholinergic signs and symptoms, confusion, hallucinations, hyperthermia, respiratory depression, seizures, tachycardia, and specific types of cardiac dysrhythmias and

heart blocks. If you suspect TCA overdose, apply the cardiac monitor if permitted in your scope of practice, or request ALS, if available.

MAOIs consist of an older generation of drugs (Marplan, Nardil, Parnate) and a newer generation of drugs (selegiline, which is also used in treatment of Parkinson's disease). MAOIs have significant potential for side effects and interactions with foods containing tyramine, such as beer, red wine, chocolates, aged cheeses, and processed meats. Ingestion of those substances in a patient on MAOIs, or the use of many OTC cold and allergy preparations can result in hypertensive crisis. MAOIs work by inhibiting the enzyme (monoamine oxidase, or MAO) that breaks down norepinephrine in brain synapses, thereby increasing the action of norepinephrine. MAOIs are generally not used unless treatment with other types of antidepressants has been unsuccessful.

SSRIs include citalopram (Celexa), fluoxetine (Prozac), sertraline (Zoloft), paroxetine (Paxil), and escitalopram (Lexapro). SNRIs include venlafaxine (Effexor), duloxetine (Cymbalta), and desvenlafaxine (Pristiq). NRIs are less common, and include atomoxetine (Strattera). Overdoses of those categories of medication are much less likely to result in death, but serotonin syndrome can occur. When death occurs, it is often due to a mixed overdose.

Signs and symptoms of serotonin syndrome include agitation, anxiety, insomnia, headache, sleepiness, nausea, diarrhea, excess salivation, goose bumps, flushed skin, hyperthermia, tachycardia, and muscle rigidity, shivering, ataxia, and **myoclonus**. Prehospital management is symptomatic and supportive.

Neuroleptics

Neuroleptics are used as antipsychotics, sedatives, and antiemetics, and include medications such as haloperidol (Haldol) and droperidol (Inapsine), and phenothiazines, such as chlorpromazine (Thorazine) and prochlorperazine (Compazine). Newer agents, such as ziprasidone (Geodon), olanzepine (Zyprexa), and aripiprazole (Abilify) are considered safer, but can result in the same problems as the older medications. Effects include anticholinergic effects, extrapyramidal symptoms such as dystonia, tardive dyskinesia, and other movement disorders; neuroleptic malignant syndrome; seizures; cardiac dysrhythmia; and hypotension. Neuroleptic malignant syndrome consists of altered mental status, muscular rigidity, fluctuating blood pressure, tachycardia, hyperpyrexia, and diaphoresis. Rhabdomyolysis can occur. A black box warning was issued for droperidol by the Food and Drug Administration because it can cause a potentially lethal cardiac dysrhythmia called *torsades de pointes* in some patients.

Lithium is used in bipolar disorder as a mood stabilizer, but it has a narrow therapeutic index and toxicity can occur easily. Signs and symptoms include gastrointestinal complaints, dry mouth, tremors, lethargy, confusion, seizures, coma, muscle tremors, and bradycardia. In many cases, toxicity is chronic, rather than acute. Even in acute cases, activated charcoal is of very limited value and is generally not recommended. Prehospital treatment is supportive.

Cardiac Medications

Cardiac medication toxicity can occur in several different scenarios. The toxicity may be insidious, due to therapeutic error, issues with patient compliance, failure to use child-resistant caps (elderly patients often request caps that are not child resistant, because it is difficult for the patient to open them). Patients may be forgetful about their medication regimen, accidentally taking more than intended, may not understand that they need to discontinue one medication when they are prescribed another, or may believe that "more is better" when it comes to a particular medication. Finally, the elderly and chronically ill are at increased risk for depression and suicide, for which the medications provide a readily accessible means.

Even with intentional overdose, the call may be for a sick person or unknown problem. Without a high index of suspicion for a toxicologic emergency, you may miss the actual problem. Suspect poisoning and overdose of cardiac medications in patients who have altered mental status, bradycardia, or tachycardia. The particular risks and signs and symptoms depend on the class of medications involved.

Beta blockers—such as atenolol, metoprolol, and propranolol—may cause bradycardia, hypotension, and even asystole in cases of overdose. Depending on the exact nature of the beta blocker, patients may also have hypoglycemia, seizures, bronchospasm, or pulmonary edema. Treatment can be difficult, because the beta blocker prevents the action of many of the drugs (catecholamines) that would ordinarily be given to treat bradycardia, hypotension, and bronchospasm. Glucagon has direct cardiostimulatory effects and can be used to treat beta blocker overdose, but the amount needed is generally not available in the prehospital setting. If available, request ALS, because other drugs and transcutaneous pacing may be helpful in increasing cardiac output.

Calcium channel blockers are used to treat hypertension, tachycardias, and angina through smooth muscle relaxation. Medications in this class include verapamil, diltiazem, and nifedipine. Signs and symptoms include bradycardia, hypotension, and hyperglycemia. In some cases, hypotension can result in a reflex tachycardia. Specific dysrhythmias can occur, and you should request ALS, if available. As with beta blockers, glucagon can be used in the hospital setting, along with calcium.

Digitalis (digoxin, Lanoxin) is a medication that has long been used to treat patients with atrial fibrillation and heart failure. In therapeutic doses, it both controls the heart rate and strengthens cardiac contraction. However, digoxin has a very narrow therapeutic index and toxicity can occur easily. Signs and symptoms of toxicity include loss of appetite, nausea, vomiting, headache, diarrhea, weakness, blurred vision, yellow-green vision, mood changes, confusion, bradycardia, and cardiac dysrhythmia. Prehospital treatment is supportive, and ALS may be needed to treat dysrhythmia.

Street Drugs

Commonly abused drugs are classified as stimulants, such as amphetamines and cocaine; narcotics–opiates, such as heroin and prescription narcotics; sedative–hypnotics, such as benzodiazepines and barbiturates; hallucinogens, such as LSD and PCP; marijuana; and inhalants.

Stimulants

Cocaine is derived from the leaves of the coca plant, which grows in South America. Cocaine is produced by chemically processing the leaves into cocaine hydrochloride powder. It is a controlled substance, which is used by physicians as a topical anesthetic, particularly in some nose and throat surgeries. Recreationally, cocaine can be inhaled in the powder form, or injected as a liquid. Crack cocaine, in particular, is smoked.

The effects of cocaine are immediate, but relatively short acting. In the central nervous system, cocaine leads to an increase in dopamine at synapses, causing users to feel euphoric, energetic, and alert. Users often feel that cocaine enhances performance of physical and mental tasks. Generally, both appetite and the need for sleep are decreased.

Cocaine is a vasoconstrictor and can increase the heart rate, body temperature, and blood pressure. In higher doses, cocaine can lead to agitation, irritability, paranoia, psychosis, and violent behavior. Stroke (especially hemorrhagic), myocardial infarction, cardiac dysrhythmia, and seizures can occur. Cocaine can result in tolerance and psychological dependence, as well as physical addiction withdrawal. Chronic use can result in erosion of the nasal mucosa from inhalation and complications of IV drug abuse when injected. If cocaine is ingested, including in the case of "body packing," the result can be massive sympathetic nervous system stimulation with seizures, cardiac arrest, and death. In cases that are not immediately fatal, the vasoconstrictive properties can lead to gangrene of the bowel.

Amphetamines are stimulants that have been used by prescription as diet pills, to increase mental alertness, and to treat attention deficit disorder (ADD)/attention deficit hyperactivity disorder (ADHD). Amphetamines increase the levels of both dopamine and norepinephrine in the brain, and have effects similar to those of cocaine. Forms of amphetamine include methamphetamine, Dexedrine, Ritalin, and Adderall. Street names include *speed, crystal, crystal meth, meth, crank,* and *ice.* Ecstacy (MDMA) or X, is a form of amphetamine used as a club drug. Amphetamines can be ingested, injected, inhaled as a powder (absorbed across the nasal mucosa), and smoked. As with cocaine, amphetamines can cause tolerance and psychological and physiologic dependence.

Anticipate behavioral changes and the potential for violence in patients who have used cocaine or amphetamines, as well as seizures, hypertension, hyperthermia, dysrhythmia, and cardiac arrest. Both cocaine and amphetamines have been implicated in deaths due to excited delirium.

Hallucinogens

Phencyclidine (PCP) is a dissociative anesthetic that was developed in the 1950s for use during surgery. It is a close relative of ketamine, which is still commonly used for dissociative anesthesia. Dissociative anesthetics provide analgesia and amnesia during medical procedures without causing respiratory arrest, as some other anesthetics. The medication was discontinued from production due to the side effects patients developed when they regained consciousness. PCP is only available today as an illegal street drug. It can be smoked (often with marijuana), injected, ingested in tablet or liquid form, or snorted. The hallucinogenic effects of PCP may cause patients to become belligerent, agitated, violent, psychotic, and have a diminished response to pain. Signs of a PCP overdose include nystagmus, ataxia, slurred speech, hypertension, tachycardia, and behavioral changes.

Patients who have taken PCP are at risk of excited delirium, rhabdomyolysis, hypertensive crisis, respiratory depression, unresponsiveness, and seizures. Activate law enforcement early, or have the scene secured prior to arrival, when it becomes apparent PCP use is involved. Physical and/or chemical restraints may become necessary to prevent harm to providers or patients themselves. Cool the hyperthermic patient with washcloths soaked in water, and in severe cases, cold packs may be placed at the armpits and groin.

LSD is derived from ergot, a fungus that grows on rye, and was discovered by Albert Hoffman in 1938. It was developed as a drug used in psychiatric treatment, and the U.S. government researched its uses for various purposes. It became popular as a recreational drug in the 1960s. Recreationally, LSD is called *acid*, after its chemical name. The psychological effects of LSD are highly variable, depending on the user, external stimuli, and dose. Usually, LSD is ingested. Fatal overdose is extremely rare, but the psychological effects can be frightening, and the patient may experience anxiety, panic, or paranoia.

Mescaline is obtained from the peyote cactus, as well as a few other cactus species. It has been used for thousands of years in Native American rituals and religious ceremonies. Mescaline can cause illusions (sensory misperceptions) and hallucinations and a sensation of expanded consciousness. Psilocybin is a hallucinogen derived from mushrooms that grow in some regions of the United States, Mexico, and Central and South America. The mushrooms are ingested and metabolized to a substance called *psilocybin*. In addition to its psychedelic effects, psilocybin can cause nausea, vomiting, muscle weakness, and ataxia.

Narcotics

Opiates are derived from the opium poppy plant, and have been used by humans for thousands of years. The pharmacology works on opiate receptors in the CNS to control pain, and has a direct effect on the gastrointestinal tract. Opiates are used both legally as prescription pain relievers and often illegally as drugs of abuse. Opiates and other narcotics can be ingested or injected.

Based on the processing of the chemical compound, opiates are considered either natural, such as morphine, codeine, and heroin; or synthetic, such as oxycodone and fentanyl. The opiate toxidrome includes constricted pupils, respiratory depression, and sedation. Constricted pupils, however, are not a universal sign in an opiate overdose. A patient who has been severely hypoxic may present with dilated pupils, and some synthetic opiates do not cause pupillary constriction. Other signs that can help you recognize the possibility of an opiate overdose include "track marks," or evidence of IV drug use, and prescription bottles (Figure 32-9).

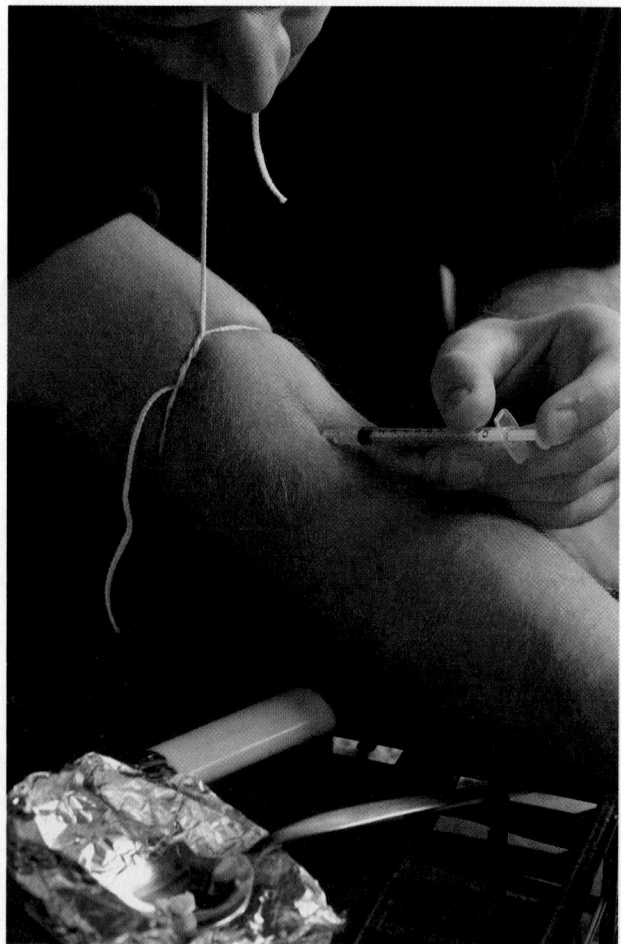

FIGURE 32-9

Intravenous drug abuse.

Treatment is identical to that described for prescription narcotic overdose, but scene safety deserves special consideration due to the possibility of hypodermic syringes or other illegal activity at the scene.

Other Drugs of Abuse

GHB (gamma hydroxybutyric acid), originally used as an anesthetic agent, is a drug often used at raves and as a club drug, and has been implicated as a date rape drug. It is classified as a sedative–hypnotic and known for creating disinhibition of behavior and enhanced sensuality. It is known in street terms as *Georgia Home Boy*, *liquid ecstasy*, *liquid X*, and *liquid G*. Ketamine, whose slang names include *Special K*, *Vitamin K*, and *K*, is a dissociative anesthetic used in medicine and veterinary medicine, but is used recreationally for effects such as hallucinations and a sense of dissociation or depersonalization/unreality. GHB can cause a dramatic respiratory depression requiring immediate airway management, with an equally dramatic improvement minutes to hours later.

Dextromethorphan is an agent available in OTC cough and cold medications, such as NyQuil and Robitussin, which is also used as a dissociative. Its use is sometime referred to as "Robo-tripping." Sedative–hypnotic overdose is treated as described previously under prescription drug overdoses.

Marijuana overdose is rare, but occasionally paranoia, anxiety, and panic can occur. In addition, the patient may complain of dry mouth, have altered sensation (illusions), and dilated pupils. In most cases, reassurance is all that is needed.

CASE STUDY WRAP-UP

Clinical-Reasoning Process

Advanced EMTs Alice and Cosette have a 32-year-old male patient suspected of taking a mixed medication overdose with a large amount of alcohol. The patient is apparently unresponsive and snoring. Alice recognizes hydrocodone as a narcotic, and notices the label also includes acetaminophen. She knows that alprazolam is a benzodiazepine. Both medications and the alcohol are CNS depressants, immediately raising concern about the patient's respiratory status. Cosette has determined that the patient is unresponsive to painful stimulus, and performs a head-tilt/chin-lift maneuver to open the airway, which relieves the snoring. The patient's respirations are shallow at 8 breaths per minute. Alice assembles the bag-valve-mask device and attaches to oxygen. She passes it to Cosette, who begins ventilating the patient at a rate of 10 per minute and a tidal volume of about 500 mL. The patient's radial pulse is weak at a rate of 60. As Alice obtains the pulse, she hears the squad arrive. A quick check shows constricted pupils.

She decides that the patient is at high risk for vomiting because of his depressed respirations and the medications ingested, along with the alcohol. She is not sure how much of the respiratory depression is due to the narcotic and how much is due to the benzodiazepine and alcohol. She starts an IV and administers 1 mg of naloxone. Within a few minutes the patient's respirations increase to 12 with better volume, and he is responsive to painful stimuli. Cosette places a nonrebreather mask on the patient with 12 L/min of oxygen, and continues to closely monitor his respirations.

With the squad's help, they obtain vital signs, apply the pulse oximeter, and obtain a blood glucose level. The patient has respirations of 12, a pulse of 60, blood pressure of 94/58, SpO$_2$ of 97 percent on 12 L/min of oxygen, and a blood glucose level of 90 mg/dL. Alice increases the IV rate to give a 500-mL fluid bolus. While one of the Advanced EMTs from the squad gets information from the patient's girlfriend, Alice performs a head-to-toe assessment. The patient's skin is cool, pale, and dry. His breath sounds are clear and equal, and there are no signs of injury or intravenous drug use.

Working as a team, they place the patient on the stretcher and transfer him to the ambulance. Meanwhile, Alice has determined that the prescription for hydrocodone and acetaminophen was filled the previous day with 20 tablets. The alprazolam belongs to the patient's girlfriend, and she states that there were four or five 0.5-mg tablets in the bottle the last time she checked. The girlfriend also provided information that the patient was fine about 90 minutes earlier when she left for the store, although he had been drinking steadily through the afternoon. She said that the patient has been depressed about his bills and the loss of his job. When she came back from the store the medication bottles were on the coffee table and she could not wake up the patient. The patient was prescribed hydrocodone and acetaminophen for back pain, but has no other medical problems, medications, or allergies.

The patient is initially managed in the emergency department, with careful attention to monitoring his respirations. He receives two additional doses of naloxone to manage his respirations. The patient has ingested an amount of acetaminophen just below the level considered hepatotoxic. However, the concomitant ingestion of alcohol and benzodiazepine place him at greater risk of liver damage. He is monitored in the intensive care unit for three days before being admitted for inpatient psychiatric evaluation and care.

CHAPTER REVIEW

Chapter Summary

Poisoning and overdose are common reasons for seeking emergency care. There is a wide variety of toxic substances of which you must be aware. These substances can be classified into toxidromes to make remembering their effects and treatments easier. Toxins can enter the body through four routes: ingestion, injection, inhalation, and absorption.

A thorough scene size-up is essential in both establishing the safety of the scene and gaining information about the possibility of a toxicologic emergency. Once the scene is safe, the goals of treating toxicologic emergencies are decontamination, establishing and maintaining an airway, and ensuring adequate ventilation and oxygenation. IV access is important in toxicologic emergencies; fluids often benefit patients with hypotension. Consider the need for ALS in patients in whom airway

management is complicated and in which cardiac dysrhythmia are anticipated.

Decontamination includes reducing the amount of toxin by limiting exposure, reducing absorption and distribution, and enhancing elimination. Two medications that Advanced EMTs can give in toxicologic emergencies are activated charcoal, which can adsorb many ingested toxins, and naloxone, a narcotic antagonist.

Always consider the possibility of polysubstance overdoses, and the presence of trauma and medical conditions that may occur in the context of toxicologic emergencies. The poison control center and medical direction are valuable resources in determining the level of concern and recommended treatment in specific toxicologic emergencies.

Review Questions

Multiple-Choice Questions

1. A medication used specifically to antagonize the effects of narcotics is:

   a. flumazenil.
   b. activated charcoal.
   c. atropine.
   d. naloxone.

2. The typical dosage of activated charcoal is _____/kg of body weight.

   a. 1 mg
   b. 30 mg
   c. 1 gram
   d. 30 grams

3. The mechanism of action by which activated charcoal works to reduce the effects of toxins is by:

   a. having a laxative effect.
   b. causing vomiting.
   c. binding substances to prevent absorption.
   d. breaking down substances to harmless components.

4. Carbon monoxide causes death by:

   a. preferentially binding to hemoglobin, displacing oxygen.
   b. acting as a direct pulmonary irritant.
   c. promoting the release of insulin, resulting in hypoglycemia.
   d. poisoning the cytochrome oxidase system in the cell.

5. The specific prehospital treatment for carbon monoxide exposure is:

   a. high-flow oxygen.
   b. nitrous oxide.
   c. hydroxocobalamin.
   d. sodium thiosulfate.

6. The most prevalent cause of cyanide poisoning is:

   a. ingestion of fruit pits.
   b. house fires.
   c. industrial exposure.
   d. product tampering.

7. The acronym SLUDGE describes the effects of exposure to:

   a. opiates.
   b. cholinergics.
   c. anticholinergics.
   d. sympathomimetics.

8. A characteristic finding in methanol toxicity is:

   a. blindness.
   b. tinnitus.
   c. sweet breath odor.
   d. sudden sniffing death.

9. A 14-year-old male admits that, on a dare, his friend smoked some jimson weed. Which one of the following signs or symptoms is most consistent with this history?

   a. Paresthesia of the extremities
   b. Pupil constriction
   c. Cool, pale, sweaty skin
   d. Delirium

10. The primary consideration in most brown recluse spider envenomations is:

   a. neurotoxicity.
   b. muscle spasms.
   c. cardiotoxicity.
   d. tissue necrosis.

11. Which one of the following actions is recommended in the treatment of a pit viper envenomation of an extremity?

   a. Application of ice
   b. Application of a tourniquet
   c. Application of a splint in a neutral position
   d. Elevation

12. As part of the treatment for a jellyfish sting, you should:

   a. flush the area with cool, fresh water.
   b. flush the area with sea water.
   c. scrub the area with soap and water.
   d. apply ice.

13. The primary concern in acetaminophen overdose is:

   a. liver failure.
   b. acute renal failure.
   c. cardiac dysrhythmia.
   d. respiratory depression.

14. A 55-year-old patient with arthritis presents with tinnitus, fever, tachypnea, and gastric distress. Of the four medications you find in the home, which one would best explain the patient's presentation?

   a. Aspirin (Excedrin)
   b. Acetaminophen (Tylenol)
   c. Antihistamine (Benadryl)
   d. Antidepressant (Effexor)

15. The date rape drug Rohypnol is classified as a(n):

   a. amphetamine.
   b. sedative–hypnotic.
   c. hallucinogen.
   d. narcotic.

16. A patient presents with a history of taking three times his normal dose of escitalopram (Lexapro) every day for 10 days. He presents with agitation, shivering, teeth chattering, goose bumps, muscle jerking, insomnia, and diarrhea. The history and presentation are most consistent with:

   a. extrapyramidal reaction.
   b. sympathomimetic toxidrome.
   c. beta blocker overdose.
   d. serotonin syndrome.

17. Ecstasy, or "X," is a type of:

   a. amphetamine.
   b. dissociative anesthetic.
   c. sedative–hypnotic.
   d. hallucinogen.

Critical-Thinking Questions

18. A patient has overdosed on a combination of three medications. What information do you need to determine the nature of the overdose, anticipate problems, and develop a treatment plan?

19. Explain the rationale for transporting patients with toxin exposure, even if they are asymptomatic when you arrive.

20. Why do OTC medications, antidepressants, and cardiac medications figure prominently in suicide attempts?

References

Arnold, T. C. (2010). *Toxicity, ciguatera.* eMedicine. Retrieved January 29, 2011, from http://emedicine.medscape.com/article/813869-overview

Bronstein, A. C., Spyker, D. A., Cantilena, Jr., L. R., Green, J. L., Rumack, B. H., & Giffin, S. L. (2010). 2009 annual report of the American Association of Poison Control Centers' national poison data system (NPDS): 27th annual report. *Clinical Toxicology, 48*(10), 979–1178.

Catlett, C. L. (2004). Seizures and status epilepticus in adults. In J. E. Tintinalli, G. D. Kelen, & J. S. Stapczynski (Eds.). *Emergency medicine: A comprehensive study guide* (p. 1416). New York, NY: McGraw-Hill.

Centers for Disease Control. (2005). Unintentional non—fire-related carbon monoxide exposures United States 2001–2003. *Morbidity and Mortality Weekly Report, 54*(2), 36–39.

Chun L. J., Tong M. J., Busuttil R. W., & Hiatt J. R. (2009). Acetaminophen hepatotoxicity and acute liver failure. *Journal of Clinical Gastroenterology, 43*(4), 342–349.

DynaMed. (2010). *Ethylene glycol poisoning.* Ipswich, MA: EBSCO Publishing.

Noltkamper, D. (2009). *Toxicity, marine – histamine in fish: Treatment & medication.* eMedicine. Retrieved March 31, 2011, from http://emedicine.medscape.com/article/1009464-overview

Norris, R. L. (2008). *Snake envenomation, coral.* eMedicine. Retrieved January 28, 2011, from http://emedicine.medscape.com/article/771701

Additional Reading

Centers for Disease Control. (2007). Carbon monoxide--related deaths—United States, 1999—2004. *Morbidity and Mortality Weekly Report, 56*(50), 1309–1312.

SECTION

6

Trauma

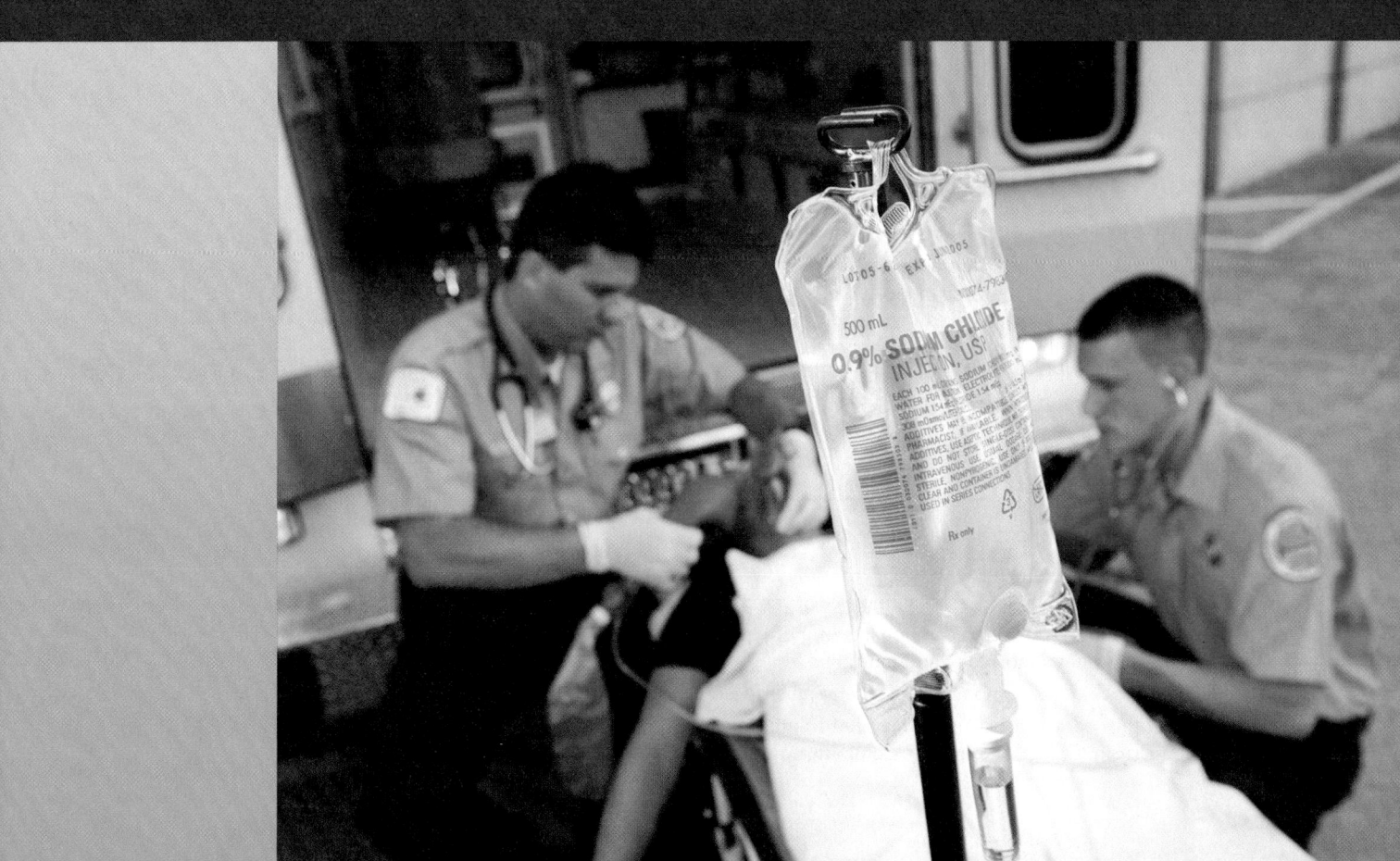

33

Trauma Systems and Incident Command

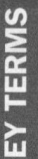

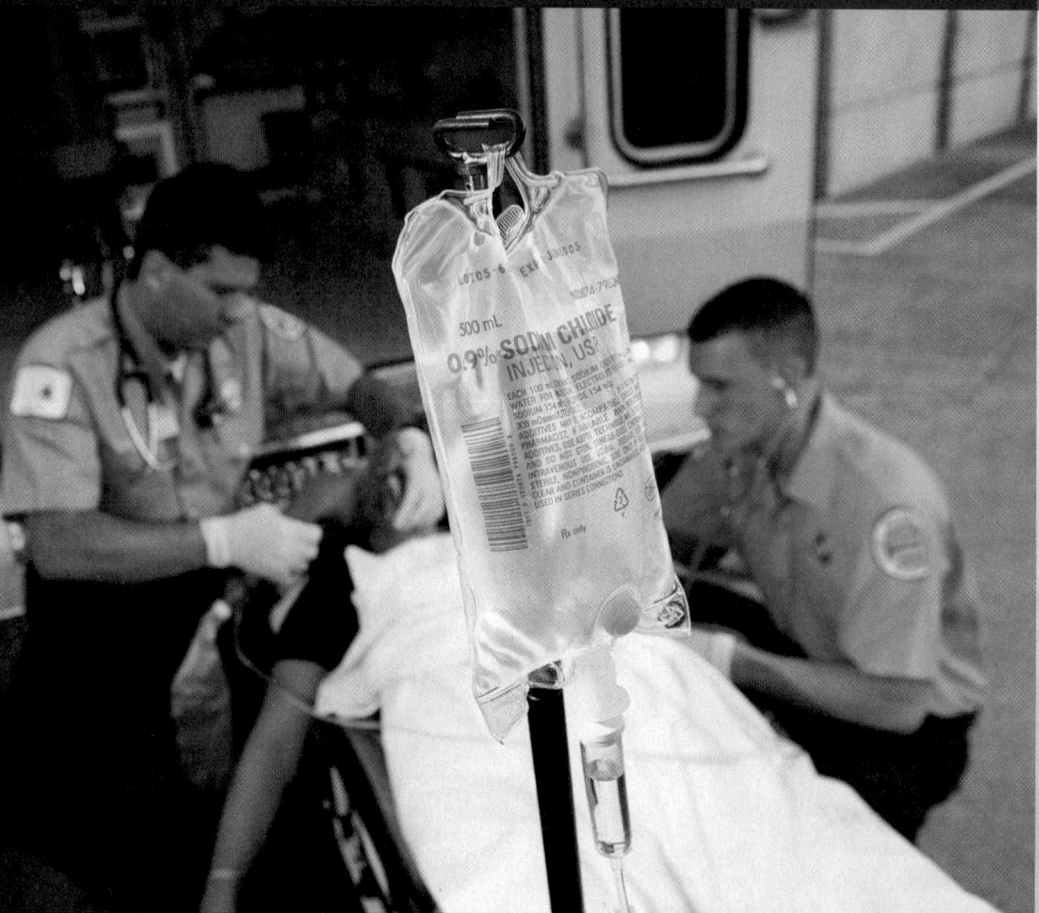

Content Area: Trauma; EMS Operations

Advanced EMT Education Standard:

- Applies fundamental knowledge to provide basic and selected advanced emergency care and transportation based on assessment findings for an acutely injured patient.
- Applies knowledge of operational roles and responsibilities to ensure patient, public, and personnel safety.

Objectives

After reading this chapter, you should be able to:

33.1 Define key terms introduced in this chapter.

33.2 Describe the epidemiology and significance of trauma.

33.3 Explain the importance and components of injury prevention programs in reducing trauma morbidity and mortality.

33.4 Describe each of the components of a comprehensive trauma care system.

33.5 Identify the characteristics of each level of trauma center as designated by the American College of Surgeons Committee on Trauma.

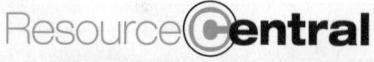

To access Resource Central, follow the directions on the Student Access Card provided with this text. If there is no card, go to www.bradybooks.com and follow the Resource Central link to Buy Access. Under Media Resources, you will find:

- *Multiple System Injuries.* Learn about common mechanisms of injury and the types of injuries they produce.

- *Gunshot Wound.* Watch and learn about how gunshot wounds can cause different injuries.

- *FEMA.* Discover FEMA's role in disaster planning and implementation.

CASE STUDY

On a windy and rainy afternoon, Advanced EMTs Steve Abercrombie and Jason Bailey have just entered back into service after transporting a patient to the local ED when they are dispatched to another emergency. "Unit 34, be en route to I-10 at mile marker 122 for a bus collision. You are the closest unit, so please advise on resources needed upon arrival."

As they make their way past the stopped traffic on the interstate, they see a large tour bus on its side in the median. Fire and law enforcement units are arriving as well.

Problem-Solving Questions

1. What does the information provided tell you about the potential for a multiple-casualty incident?
2. What are Steve and Jason's primary responsibilities once on scene?
3. What is the importance of knowing the number and capabilities of hospitals in the immediate area?

33.6	Explain the importance of having an understanding of how to manage situations in which there are multiple patients.
33.7	Explain the importance of immediately identifying the number of patients at a scene.
33.8	Compare the needs of an event to the resources available to identify multiple-casualty incidents in a given EMS system.
33.9	Differentiate between the management goals of single-patient and multiple-patient incidents.
33.10	Discuss some common issues with communications in multiple-casualty incidents and disaster situations.
33.11	Prioritize your actions as the first provider on the scene of a multiple-casualty incident.
33.12	Describe the principles of an incident command system.
33.13	Identify the roles and responsibilities that may be assigned to EMS units at a multiple-casualty incident.
33.14	Describe the principles of a triage system.
33.15	Given a scenario with multiple patients, categorize patients according to a color-coded triage system.
33.16	Explain the principles used in the START triage system.
33.17	Describe adaptations of START triage to JumpSTART for pediatric patients.
33.18	Perform primary and secondary triage in a multiple-casualty incident.
33.19	Use triage tags to document assessment and care of patients in a multiple-casualty incident.
33.20	Describe considerations in determining the transport destination for patients in a multiple-casualty incident.

Introduction

Unintentional injury is the fifth leading cause of the nearly 2.5 million deaths reported annually in the United States. In 2007, unintentional injury claimed the lives of 182,479 people (Jiaquan Xu, Kochanek, Murphy, & Tejada-Vera, 2010). Death from injury in the United States is substantial but pales in comparison with the 2.8 million hospitalizations and more than 40 million emergency department visits annually. Cost estimates of injury can run as high as $325 million annually (McSwain, Salomone & Pons, 2007).

As an Advanced EMT you will often respond to emergency calls involving injured patients. You can take many actions to reduce the impact of injury on those patients, but that is only the beginning of trauma care. Organized trauma systems are key in reducing trauma morbidity and mortality by providing readily accessible surgical care for trauma patients.

Unfortunately, even the best trauma systems cannot save the most severely injured patients. The only way to prevent deaths in such cases is to prevent the incident that caused the injuries, or to reduce the severity of injuries caused by the incident. For example, it is better to educate children and their parents about the use of helmets to prevent head injuries in recreational activities than it is to try to reverse the damage caused by traumatic brain injury. Trauma systems play a critical role in injury prevention through community education programs.

EMS providers must understand the trauma system to know which patients can benefit from transport to a trauma center, and which facilities can provide the best trauma care for patients. EMS providers can also participate in the trauma system's injury prevention programs, since they often have a unique opportunity to interact with patients and the public.

Medical calls usually involve only one patient. Trauma scenes can sometimes involve multiple patients and the need for multiple types of resources. Such scenes can be chaotic if not properly managed, leading to delays in patient care and improper prioritization of injured patients for transport. The various responding agencies must work together in a coordinated manner to facilitate patient care while maintaining responders' safety. To effectively manage multiple-casualty incidents (MCIs) Advanced EMTs must understand and be able to operate within an organized structure called the *incident command system (ICS)*.

Injury Prevention

The most dramatic impact that can be made to reduce the morbidity and mortality associated with injury is through prevention. It is easier to educate people on how to prevent becoming injured than it is to treat the following injury. The goal of injury prevention is to change the knowledge, attitude, and behaviors of individuals and society.

The *Three Es of Injury Prevention* provide strategies for reducing injuries. The Three Es of Injury Prevention are as follows:

- *Education.* This is an active strategy that requires the cooperation of the target audience. The target audience must be receptive to information being delivered and willing to make changes in behavior based on the information. An example of this strategy is EMS professionals teaching the general public about proper child safety seat use.

- *Enforcement.* This strategy uses the law to persuade individuals to behave in ways that reduce the likelihood of injury. An example of an enforcement strategy is seatbelt laws. Individuals who do not believe that seatbelts prevent injuries may be motivated to wear a seatbelt to avoid receiving a traffic citation.

- *Engineering.* Engineering controls do not require the active cooperation of the target group to have an impact. Instead, engineering controls rely on the design of equipment, vehicles, roadways, and other structures to reduce injuries. The use of safety glass, rather than regular glass, in automobile windows is an example of engineering as a method of reducing injuries.

The public health approach to injury prevention is an effective way to address problems within the community. It simply asks "who, what, when, where, and why" a specific injury is occurring so a prevention plan can be developed and implemented.

The public health approach to injury prevention includes four steps, as follows:

- *Define the problem.* Before a problem can be effectively addressed, the scope of the problem must be identified. This is done by collecting data related to the problem from within the community. For example, the number of intoxicated pedestrians struck by vehicles, along with the days and times when most of the incidents occur, helps in understanding the problem.

- *Identify risk and protective factors.* This step involves identifying why a certain type of injury is occurring, what factors place people at risk for injury, and what factors could protect people from injury. For example, long stretches of streets without crosswalks may prompt pedestrians to cross the street under unsafe conditions.

- *Develop prevention strategies.* The knowledge gained from the two previous steps is used to identify prevention strategies. For example, if long stretches of streets do not have crosswalks, building elevated pedestrian bridges may reduce the number of pedestrians struck by vehicles.

- *Implement, evaluate, and share.* The prevention plan is put into action, the effects of the plan are evaluated for effectiveness, and results of the plan are shared through public presentations or publication.

The "Children Can't Fly" campaign that was implemented in the early 1970s is an excellent example of how the public health approach is utilized. The New York City Department of Health implemented the program in an effort to address an alarmingly high incidence of death and serious injury in children as a result of a fall from a window. The program involved passing a law requiring window guards to be installed in high-rise apartments where young children lived. A reporting system was set in place that required all fall-related injuries be reported. Once reported, a consultant would visit the home to provide education and assistance with creating a safe environment for children. The campaign resulted in a significant decrease in the incidence of falls. Some areas of the city had a decline in fall-related injuries of more than 50 percent. Other cities around the world have since implemented similar campaigns with positive results.

In addition to the lives of children saved, the campaign showed to be cost effective compared to the cost of hospitalizations, rehabilitation, and care for injured or permanently disabled children (World Health Organization, n.d.).

Trauma Systems

A **trauma system** is a set of components and services specifically designed to provide definitive care for patients with serious injuries. The National Highway Traffic Safety Administration (NHTSA) has identified the components of a comprehensive trauma care system in its Trauma Care Agenda for the Future. They are as follows:

- *Leadership.* It is necessary for an identified council to advise the federal government on the need to support existing trauma systems and to fund the development of much-needed systems. After systems are established, they must be supported and run by an identified lead agency.

- *Professional resources.* For a trauma system to work, there must be adequately trained individuals to work within it. This includes physicians, nurses, and prehospital providers who have been adequately trained in trauma care. Funding for the recruitment and retention of these providers is scarce; thus, trauma system leadership must lobby to address this issue.

- *Education and advocacy.* The general public is poorly informed and educated in injury prevention. One of the responsibilities of a trauma system is to educate the general public in injury prevention and trauma care.

- *Information management.* For trauma systems to move forward and improve care, they must have the ability to gather data. The data should be collected to enable research, improve the management of trauma care, and enhance performance.

- *Finances.* Trauma systems rely on federal and state funding, reimbursement from insurance companies, and private-pay patients. Unfortunately, government funding does not cover the operating costs of a trauma system; thus, the cost is shifted to the private insurance industry, leading to a rise in insurance rates for companies and individuals.

- *Research.* Trauma systems should research existing trauma care and make recommendations to improve care.

- *Technology.* There have been many technologic advances that play a role in the care provided to patients within a trauma system. Examples include global positioning systems (GPS), automatic collision notification (ACN), and wireless E-911 systems. Those technologies allow for faster responses by EMS to the patient; thus, patients enter into the trauma system more quickly.

Hospitals that are part of a trauma system have a specific trauma center designation based on criteria set forth by the American College of Surgeons Committee on Trauma (Figure 33-1). That designation is based on the services available at each facility. Trauma center designations are defined in Table 33-1.

Trauma systems include more than just a specialized emergency department. Many specialty services, such as

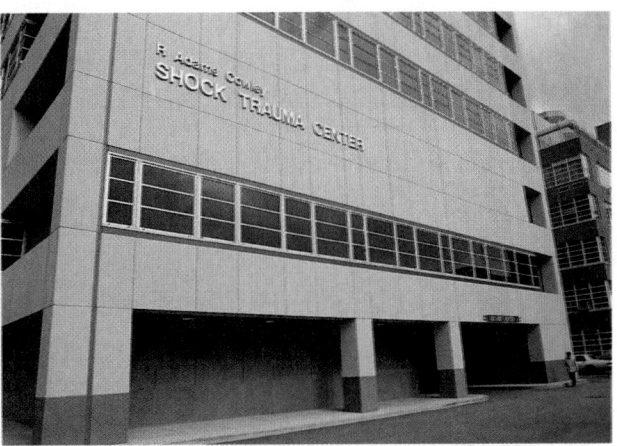

FIGURE 33-1

The R. Adams Crowley Shock Trauma Center in Baltimore is a Level I trauma center.

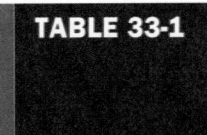

TABLE 33-1 | American College of Surgeons Committee on Trauma, Trauma Center Designations

Level Designation	Capabilities
Level I regional trauma center	Capable of managing any type of traumatic injury 24 hours a day, 365 days a year.
Level II area trauma center	Capable of managing most traumatic injuries 24 hours a day, 365 days a year. Capable of stabilizing trauma patients that cannot be managed and transferring them to a Level I trauma center.
Level III community trauma center	Provides some surgical capability and specially trained ED staff to manage trauma. The focus is on stabilization of the trauma patient and transferring to a higher-level center.
Level IV trauma facility	Smaller hospitals located in remote areas that are capable of stabilizing trauma patients for transfer to a higher-level center.

surgical specialties (including neurosurgery, vascular surgery, orthopedic surgery, and others), rehabilitation facilities, pediatric trauma specialists, critical and intensive care units are required to provide comprehensive trauma care. EMS plays a vital role in the trauma system because EMS professionals make initial contact with the patient and provide **triage**, emergency treatment, and transport to the most appropriate medical facility where definitive care can be provided.

Managing Multiple-Casualty Incidents

A **multiple-casualty incident (MCI)** is any event in which the number of patients exceeds the capabilities of the resources on scene. An event that constitutes an MCI in a relatively small community, where limited resources are available, may not necessarily be an MCI in a larger city, where more resources are available. For example, a rural area with four ambulances will not be able to provide enough resources for a tour bus collision with 20 patients, whereas a larger EMS agency with 20 ambulances in service and the capability to put five more in service at any given time would be able to manage the 20 patients.

Examples of potential MCIs include the following:

- School bus crash
- Plane crash
- Passenger train derailment
- Explosion in a populated space
- Mass shootings
- Building collapse
- Industrial accidents
- Toxic chemical release

As an Advanced EMT, you are likely to be the first medically trained person on the scene of an MCI. The key to successful management is to request additional resources early. Once on scene, you should overestimate the amount of resources that you believe you will need. It is easy to cancel resources that are not needed. So, be sure that you have resources en route to the scene in the event that you identify later that they are needed.

Successful mitigation of an MCI also depends on decisions that are made early on about the proper staging of vehicles, placement of triage and treatment areas, providing care, and transporting patients from the scene in an efficient manner. Failure to properly identify staging and treatment areas could result in inefficient transport of patients from the scene.

The emergency care you provide to patients during an MCI will differ from the care that you ordinarily provide. The goal at the scene of an MCI is to provide the most good for the greatest number of patients. So, provide treatment only to those patients who have a chance of survival. As callous as that sounds, you simply cannot allow one patient to occupy resources at the expense of other patients. You will learn how to prioritize patients (triage) and provide treatment during an MCI later in this chapter.

Communications

One of the most vital aspects of successfully managing an MCI is the ability of responders to communicate with each other effectively. On arrival, the scene will most likely be very chaotic, making communication between responders even more important. Many EMS agencies have MCI kits in sprint vehicles that contain multiple portable radios with which responders can communicate.

In closed or contained incidents, such as a bus crash or explosion, radio or cell phone communication will more than likely be unaffected, allowing for various modes of communication. However, during a large event, such as a natural disaster, radio and cell phone towers may be inoperable; therefore, normal communication may be nonexistent. In the first few days following Hurricane Katrina, for example, there was little communication in and around the city of New Orleans. The radio and cellular towers were down or were inoperable because there was no electrical power. Portable radios could be used, but the absence of repeaters made them ineffective over long distances. The only reliable mode of communication was through the use of satellite phones. The lack of communication between responding agencies and individual responders made coordinated efforts very difficult.

Many lessons have been learned from incidents such as Hurricane Katrina, including how to quickly establish radio communication by using self-contained mobile command centers and portable repeaters. Until those communications are established, you must rely on whatever means are at your disposal. It will be important for multiple agencies to communicate with one another. To accomplish this, some areas have a dedicated radio frequency to be used during an MCI response.

National Incident Management System

President George W. Bush signed Homeland Security Presidential Directive 5 in February, 2003, which led to the development of the **National Incident Management System (NIMS)**. NIMS was designed for use by all agencies during a disaster so different agencies—including fire, EMS, and law enforcement—could work together effectively under the same organizational structure using the same terminology.

In 2006, the federal government required all agencies that may be called to respond to a disaster to become NIMS compliant. NIMS compliance requires all responders to obtain certification in basic incident command systems. That means as an Advanced EMT, you will be required to obtain certification so the organization you are affiliated with remains compliant.

Obtaining certification is only the beginning of being prepared to effectively manage a disaster response. As with

IMS EMS BRANCH

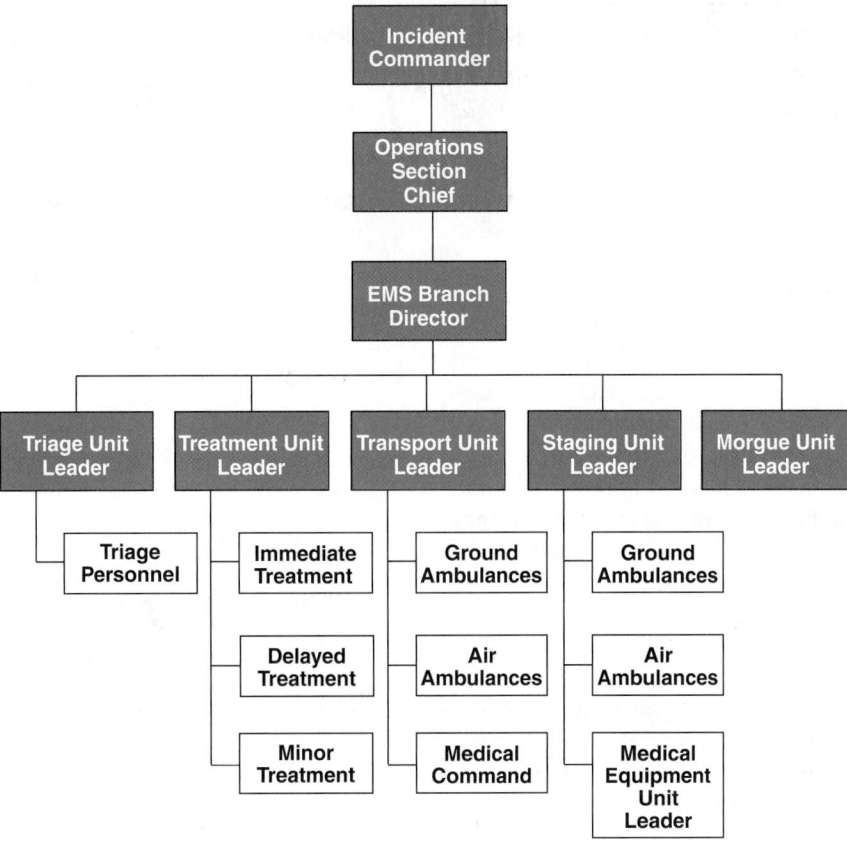

FIGURE 33-2

EMS branch organization used for larger-scale responses.

any other skill, you must practice the application of knowledge, or you will not be prepared to use it when necessary. For this reason, organizations must participate in disaster drills to practice application of the incident command system. Disaster drills allow responders and agencies to identify strengths and weaknesses of their response plans so they can be addressed prior to an actual event.

Incident Command System

The **incident command system (ICS)** is a standardized command system used by all agencies involved in an incident response. There are five sections of the ICS, which are referred to by the acronym CFLOP:

C – Command

F – Finance/administration

L – Logistics

O – Operations

P – Planning

The five sections work together to successfully manage MCIs or disasters while ensuring the safety of all responders involved, achievement of objectives, and efficient use of

available resources. The complexity of the command structure used during an incident response depends on the size and scope of the incident. For large responses, the IMS EMS Branch may be used (Figure 33-2). For smaller responses, the Basic ICS Organization for EMS Operations may be used (Figure 33-3).

BASIC ICS ORGANIZATION EMS OPERATIONS

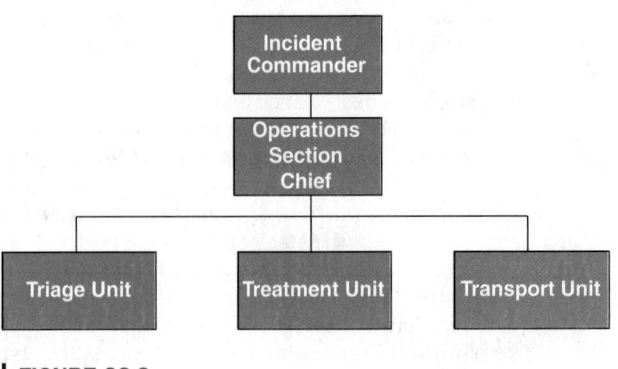

FIGURE 33-3

Basic ICS organization used for smaller-scale responses.

Command

Command is the most important section of the ICS. The **incident commander (IC)** is the individual responsible for the coordination of the entire response. You may be the first individual on scene; in such a case, you will establish command and begin to coordinate the response. As other more qualified individuals arrive on scene, incident command will be relinquished to them after you provide a complete report, including what you have done thus far and all information that you have obtained.

There are two types of command structures that may be used depending on the size and scope of the incident: singular command and unified command. **Singular command** is used for smaller incidents, when one agency assumes command of the response. **Unified command** is used for large-scale incidents or disasters that are complex and require the concerted response of multiple agencies. In a unified command system, managers representing each agency work as a team and make decisions regarding the response together. If required, the IC may name officers to assist in managing the incident. Officers that may be named include the following:

- *Safety officer.* Responsible for the safety of responders and patients alike, the **safety officer (SO)** ensures that all response activities are being carried out using the proper safety equipment.

- *Liaison officer.* The liaison officer (LO) coordinates all activities with outside agencies, such as government agencies and private industry.

- *Information officer.* The **information officer (IO)** is responsible for communicating information regarding the response to the public and press.

Finance/Administration

The **finance/administration** section is generally used in large-scale responses and is responsible for accounting and administrative activities.

Logistics

The **logistics section** is responsible for acquiring and distributing essential supplies and equipment needed during the response.

Operations

The operations section consists of triage, treatment, and transportation of patients from an MCI.

Planning

The **planning section** analyzes data collected from responses and makes recommendations to change the response plans in order to improve future responses.

PERSONAL PERSPECTIVE

Advanced EMT David Finley: At 0530, just before our 0600 crew change, my partner and I were startled by a loud explosion. We looked in the direction of the explosion and could see a large cloud rising into the air. Dispatch called our station and advised us to respond to a nearby industrial plant for an explosion.

On arrival at the main gate to enter onto the plant property, we were advised by law enforcement to proceed to the next gate but to not enter the plant. When we reached the next gate, a company representative ran toward us, stating that there was one patient out of the explosion area and he was being decontaminated in a building next to where we were parked. He advised that there should be about 35 employees who were in the area of the explosion. The one employee who was dragged out was badly burned with a liquid caustic chemical. The other workers would probably be burned as well.

I immediately advised dispatch that we would have 35 patients with chemical burns and requested additional ambulances and aeromedical support. I established command and identified treatment and staging areas and a landing zone for the helicopters that would arrive. The plant rescue team, with the assistance of the local fire department, began initial triage of the workers and set up a decontamination area.

One of my supervisors arrived on the scene as the first patient was being carried toward us following decontamination.

I gave him a report of what had happened and advised him of where the staging, treatment, and landing zone areas would be.

Because additional units were beginning to arrive and command had been turned over to my supervisor, I began treatment, waiting for the first helicopter to arrive. As the workers were brought out of the plant, they were decontaminated by the fire department and brought to the appropriate treatment area based on their triage category, where care was initiated. Staged ambulances pulled up to the treatment areas where patients were loaded and transported to designated hospitals.

The operation ran very efficiently because everyone knew their role and resources were properly positioned and utilized. Because of the teamwork between plant employees, law enforcement, fire departments, and EMS agencies, we were able to rapidly triage, decontaminate, treat, and transport all 35 patients in a timely manner. Five of the workers had critical burns and were flown to a burn unit, 15 were transported by ground and air to a trauma center, and the remaining workers were transported to two smaller hospitals in the area. We felt as though we were prepared to mitigate an incident such as this because we had participated in disaster drills with the industrial plants on an annual basis in this particular community. Preparation is the key to being able to respond to MCIs.

CASE STUDY (continued)

Steve and Jason park their ambulance in a position on the shoulder next to the median of the interstate to protect themselves from passing traffic. They notice approximately 15 patients who have exited the bus. Some are lying and sitting in the grass, and others are walking around.

They approach the bus after determining that it is safe to do so. The bus driver is located and advises them that there were 40 passengers on the bus. The driver states that the bus must have hydroplaned, which caused him to lose control and enter the median, where the bus rolled onto its side.

Problem-Solving Questions

1. What should be Steve and Jason's next immediate action?
2. Who will assume the role of incident commander?
3. What additional resources are needed?

On the Scene

When you have established that it is safe to enter the scene, notify dispatch and exit your ambulance. Continue to size up the area and obtain an estimate of the number of patients and resources needed at the scene. Remember that overestimating is better than underestimating when requesting resources. After you have sized up the scene and obtained your estimates, notify dispatch so resources can be directed.

As an Advanced EMT on the scene of an MCI, it is likely that you will be assigned to emergency medical care. Once command has been established and the organization of the scene response is set, be prepared to see patients. However, much like your other actions on the scene of an MCI, your interactions with patients will not be the same as it would be on a typical emergency call. Instead, you will be assigned to a particular aspect of patient care: triage, treatment, or transport.

During your time on scene, you will be assigned to one of the three groups. Although you may end up performing each of the jobs during the duration of the event, you will never perform them simultaneously. This is the essence of an MCI response and the incident command system: specialization of resources to prevent duplication of effort while maximizing resource capabilities.

Triage

The word *triage* comes from the French word *trier*, which means "to sift, sort, or select." It is the process by which you prioritize the treatment of patients at an MCI. By definition, an MCI involves more than one patient. However, it also assumes, at least at the outset, that there are more patients than responders, and therefore requires responders to prioritize treatment and transport based on severity of injury or illness. Triage provides the tools to sort patients into categories in the most efficient manner possible.

Triaging is a quick sorting process. Your goal is to triage many patients in the shortest amount of time. It is critical for you to realize that triaging patients is not the same as treatment. You should not consider the treatment of patients, and the intervention associated with it, during your triaging assessment. Triage is simply a process of categorizing a patient's priority for later treatment.

There are two phases of triage that occur: primary and secondary triage. **Primary triage** is performed immediately by the first EMS responders on scene. **Secondary triage** is a second assessment of the patient; at this time, the triage category may remain the same or be increased or decreased. Secondary triage usually occurs when the patient arrives at a treatment area.

In primary triage, patients will be placed into one of four different categories: immediate, expectant, delayed, or minor. "Immediate" patients have life-threatening injuries that require immediate attention and rapid transport. Deceased or "expectant" patients are either dead or have injuries that make it unlikely they will survive. "Delayed" patients have care needs that do not require immediate attention, but should be seen as soon as possible. Finally, "minor" patients are those who require little or no care. They also are known as the "walking wounded," and typically can simply walk away from a scene without any further medical care.

As you assign patients into the four categories, you must communicate to other responders on scene how you have categorized them. Your ambulance, as part of its MCI kit,

IN THE FIELD

In preparation for triage, make sure you and your partner equip yourselves with enough gloves. A good method of doing so is to wear multiple pairs of gloves simultaneously. This will allow you to remove your gloves quickly as you move from patient to patient. Mark the bottom pair with an "X" so that you have a visual signal when you are on your last pair. This is when you and your partner will switch positions.

should have **triage tags** placed for easy deployment during an MCI. Triage tags are essentially colored tags that correspond to the various categories: red (immediate), yellow (delayed), green (minor), and black (expectant). Be aware that not all the triage tags on the market have assigned those same colors, and there may be some variance in the word assigned to each group. But generally, the ones mentioned here are what you will probably see while on an MCI (Figure 33-4).

The triage tag itself consists of the marked portions and a small lanyard, usually made of string or rubber. The lanyard is the part of the tag that is attached to the patient. You should hang it on an extremity, usually the arm or foot, where it can be found easily. You should never tie the lanyard around the neck, because this can potentially restrict the patient's airway.

Triage is usually not performed alone. Ideally, responders should work in isolated teams of two as they work through the group of patients on the scene. If you find yourself assigned to the triaging area, you and your partner will take turns triaging the patients while the other one handles the documentation.

As with all other aspects of EMS response, documentation is critical. First, you will be carrying all the triage tags to prevent cross contamination. On many triage tags, there are two bar codes very similar to the ones on the boxes of commercial products you might buy at a store. The bar codes will act as a tracking mechanism when patients are treated and transported. Each bar code also should include a number, in case the bar code is somehow damaged or inoperable. The first bar code is usually located at the top of the tag, and will stay with the patient throughout his journey through treatment and transport. You will retain the other tag, and you will use this tag as the comparison for the authorities on scene who will be keeping track of patients. It is usually located at the bottom of the tag, and can be easily torn off. As you collect the tags, you should place them in a separate plastic bag so they may be easily retrieved later. Try your best to keep the tags organized, although the pace of the scene may not allow you to do much beyond a cursory movement of the tags.

Ensure that you are standing behind your partner, facing the patient. Determine the side at which your partner wishes to receive the tags by simply asking before patient triage begins. Do not assume a right-hand orientation or predisposition. Listen to your partner. Once you have determined a priority, tear the tag along the appropriate line and hand the

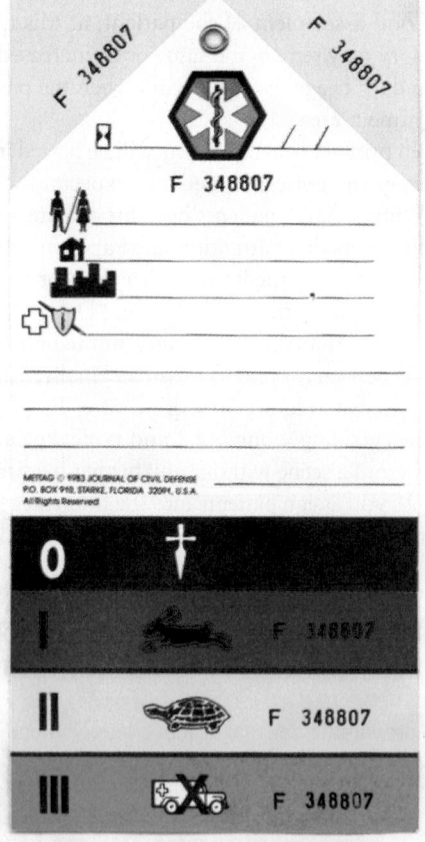

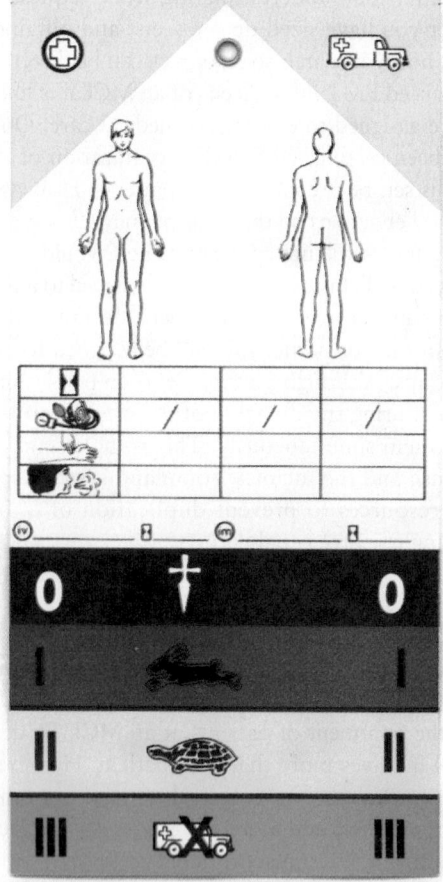

FIGURE 33-4

Triage tag, front and back.

tag to your partner. Depending on the number of patients, if you have not done so already, you and your partner will eventually switch positions, and you will be in charge of the primary triage while your partner handles the documentation.

START Triage

Simple Triage and Rapid Treatment (START) is the most commonly accepted form of triage in the United States. Through a systematic series of steps, you will be able to prioritize the treatment and transport of patients according to specific signs and symptoms. It is this process that maximizes the ability of EMS responders on an MCI to make the best treatment decisions, given limited resources (Figure 33-5).

The first step simply involves providing a command to all patients who can walk on their own to move themselves to the treatment area of the MCI response. Any individual who can follow your command is automatically placed on the lowest treatment priority, and would be marked "Minor." The reason is those patients are breathing, are not experiencing an altered mental state, do not have a debilitating injury that would prevent them from walking, and most likely do not have any life-threatening injuries. Therefore, they are categorized simply as the "walking wounded."

The second step of START triage affects all patients who do not respond to the initial command. It begins when you approach your first patient. Immediately check for breathing, as you would with any other patient. If you do not detect a breath, quickly reposition the patient's airway. It may be that the patient's fallen position has closed the airway. If, after you reposition the airway, you still

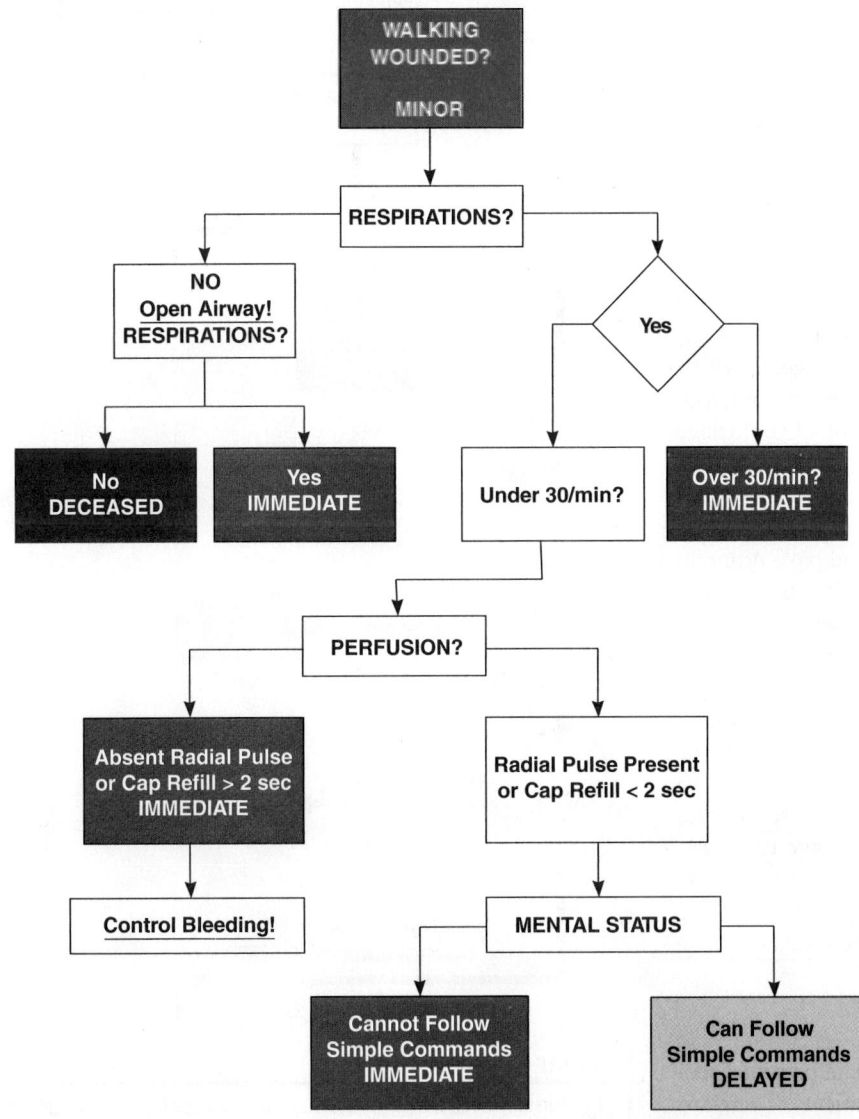

START TRIAGE SYSTEM

FIGURE 33-5

The START triage system.

do not detect a breath, you should tag the patient as "Deceased," denoted with a black tag. If, however, you are able to identify a breath after repositioning the airway, this patient should receive an "Immediate" category tag, which is typically red. However, the situation is much different if, when you first approach the patient, you are able to detect a breath without repositioning the airway. In that case, the only important element is to determine if the patient is breathing more or less than 30 breaths per minute. If the patient is breathing at a rate higher than 30, then he is automatically considered "Immediate," and you move on to the next patient. If the patient is breathing at a rate less than 30, you should move on to Step 3.

The third step of START triage begins after determining the patient's ventilation rate. Next, determine the level of perfusion in that patient's body. If the patient is bleeding, you can take steps to control it. If the patient continues to bleed excessively, you should label the patient "Deceased." However, if the bleeding is controlled, examine the patient's perfusion. The two-part test is a simple one that you will be introduced to in Chapter 35: radial pulse and capillary refill. First, check for a radial pulse. If there is no radial pulse, that patient receives a red tag. You will also consider the patient "Immediate" for a capillary refill longer than 2 seconds. If the refill rate is less than 2 seconds, however, then you must move on to Step 4, the final step in the process.

The final step of the START triage process is the assessment of the patient's mental status. If the patient is unconscious, or is unable to follow simple commands, that patient receives a red tag. By contrast, if the patient is conscious and is able to follow your commands, then you will categorize the patient as "Delayed."

After all the patients have gone through a complete triage, there will most likely be a secondary triage, in which all the patients will be re-examined for change in condition. However, this does not necessarily relieve you of your triage responsibility. As new patients are discovered, you and your partner will perform a primary triage and tag them accordingly. Keep in mind during the triage steps that once you have determined the tag for the patient and have properly documented the fact, you should move on to the next patient. The initial triage is not the time for interventions; it is simply to gather information about the patients' conditions to categorize them for later responders.

When you have completed the initial triage, you may be asked to stay in triage to wait for additional patients or to complete secondary triage, or you may be reassigned to the treatment staff. Expect patient conditions to change, which will result in you changing their triage category. For instance, if a patient who was initially categorized as "green" suddenly begins to complain of difficulty breathing and chest pain, the patient's category would escalate.

JumpSTART Triage

The START triage system described in the previous section is not designed to triage pediatric patients. There are physiologic differences between the adult and pediatric patient that make the START system inappropriate for pediatric triage. To account for this, the **JumpSTART triage system** was created for use on any patient who appears to be a child. The START triage system is for use on adolescents and adults.

The JumpSTART triage system is based on the same three categories as START triage: respiratory status, perfusion status, and mental status. The JumpSTART triage system is illustrated in Figure 33-6.

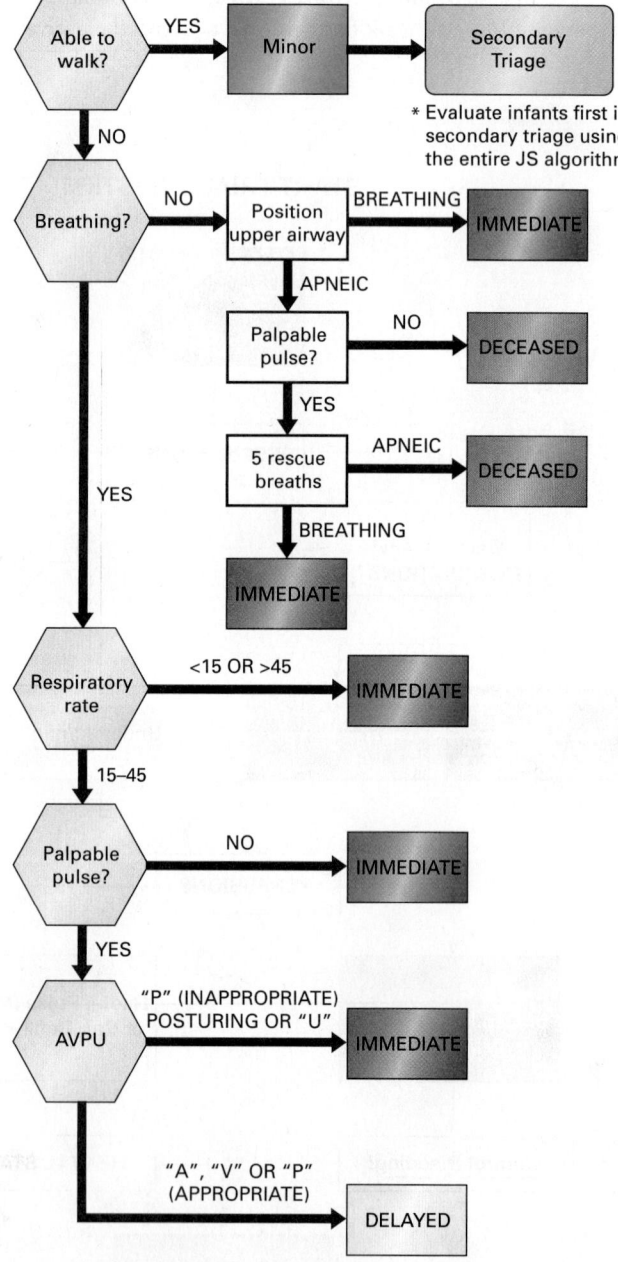

JumpSTART Pediatric MCI Triage

FIGURE 33-6

The JumpSTART triage system. (© Lou Romig, MD, FAAP, FACEP)

Treatment

One of the most important rules of an EMS MCI response is that you should not start treatment until the patient has gone through triage. This is a critical component of the overall response, because the sheer number of patients demands an efficient utilization of resources.

Treatment on scene should be as minimal as possible. The overwhelming number of patients demands that the priority is to transport patients off scene to area hospitals that have access to vastly more resources and personnel than is available on a typical MCI. Injury and illness patterns will follow the mechanisms involved. For instance, following a terrorist bombing, you should expect trauma injuries associated with a blast. However, you also should be aware of injuries that may not be as obvious, which will be revealed in your patient assessment. The critical element to remember is that you should base the time of treatment on scene on the patient's initial triage and condition, which may have changed since the first triage. Some patients may require additional assistance; others may have slightly recovered. In most cases you will remain in the treatment area but you may be reassigned to transport patients from the scene (Figure 33-7).

Transport

The transport of patients will vary widely, depending on the kind of MCI you encounter. However, most well-organized scenes will have a clear ingress and egress point, where you will be positioned with your stretcher. Take advantage of this opportunity and make sure that you place yourself in a position to easily take a patient out of the treatment area and back to your ambulance.

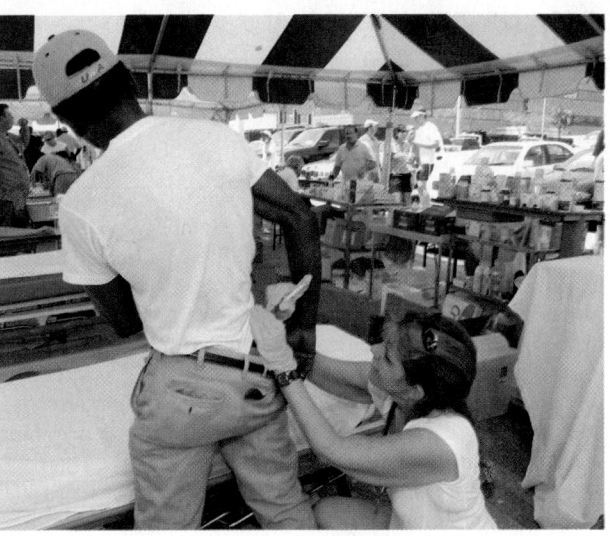

FIGURE 33-7

Field treatment area. (© Barry Williams/Getty Images)

During this time, it is critical that you follow medical direction and determine where your patient will be received. Hospitals receiving patients from an MCI can become overwhelmed quickly. Therefore, ensure that you stay in constant communication with your dispatch and with medical direction so you do not inadvertently take a patient to a hospital that is already at capacity or one that cannot handle the type of patient you are transporting. Remember, some illnesses or injuries require specialized care, such as a hyperbaric chamber, that is not readily available at all receiving facilities.

CASE STUDY WRAP-UP

Clinical-Reasoning Process

Jason tells Steve to notify dispatch that there are 40 patients on scene. Firefighters inform Jason that the state police have established traffic control and asks how he would like to proceed. Jason quickly scans the area and decides that the staging area should be established on the other side of the Interstate, where units can enter and exit the scene without traffic concerns.

Steve notifies dispatch of the staging area: "Dispatch, have responding units stage on the westbound lanes of the interstate." State police block the inside lane of traffic on the westbound side of the interstate to prepare for the arriving units.

Jason asks the firefighters to establish and mark treatment areas in the median near the staging lane. Steve gathers other firefighters to begin triage. All patients who are able to walk are directed to walk to the marked green treatment area, where they will be assessed and triaged. Dispatch advises that aeromedical units cannot respond because of the weather.

As additional units arrive, Jason designates one medic as the treatment officer and another as the transportation officer. Once all the patients have been triaged, the firefighters begin carrying patients to the appropriate marked treatment areas where emergency care is provided. After initial triage is complete, a firefighter advises Jason that there are 31 green patients, 6 yellow patients, and 4 red patients. Hospitals in the area are contacted and notified of the situation. The patients are transported, according to the severity of their condition, to the most appropriate facility until all patients have been transported from the scene.

CHAPTER REVIEW

Chapter Summary

As an Advanced EMT, you may or may not work within an established trauma system. This will depend on the area in which you work. In the future, more trauma systems will be formed as funding is acquired in different communities across the country. Even if a trauma system is not established in the area in which you work, you will participate in aspects of a trauma system, such as providing injury prevention education and advocacy. Recall that this is a key element in a trauma system that can be established in any community.

Chances are that at some point in your career you will participate in an MCI. It is imperative that you understand what must be done in order to successfully mitigate an MCI.

Establishing command is the first step; therefore, if you are the first responder to arrive on scene, you must establish command and begin setting the foundation that the response will build on. After command is established at an MCI, START and JumpSTART triage of the patients on scene must begin in order to determine number and acuity.

Response to MCIs can be very stressful; therefore, you must remain focused and task oriented to provide the greatest chance of survival to the greatest number of patients. Whatever role you play during an MCI, that role is vital to successful mitigation of the incident and you must perform your task to the best of your ability.

Review Questions

Multiple-Choice Questions

1. Unintentional injury is the _____ leading cause of death in the United States.

   a. second
   b. third
   c. fourth
   d. fifth

2. Which one of the trauma system components listed below deals with the gathering of data to enable research, improve the management of trauma care, and enhance performance?

   a. Professional resources
   b. Leadership
   c. Information management
   d. Research

3. Upon arrival at an MCI, which one of the following should occur first?

   a. Establish communication.
   b. Request additional resources.
   c. Perform triage.
   d. Establish treatment and staging areas.

Categorize the following patients in questions 4 through 7 using the START and JumpSTART triage systems:

4. A 34-year-old male patient, confused with respirations at 32 breaths per minute, has an angulated fracture to his lower right leg.

   a. Green
   b. Yellow
   c. Red
   d. Black

5. A 22-year-old female is not breathing. You manually open her airway and she is still not breathing. She has no obvious signs of trauma.

   a. Green   c. Red
   b. Yellow   d. Black

6. An approximately six-year-old girl has respirations of 30 breaths per minute and no palpable pulses. She has a large contusion on the right lateral abdominal wall.

   a. Green   c. Red
   b. Yellow   d. Black

7. A 45-year-old female has respirations of 24 breaths per minute, a capillary refill time of less than 2 seconds, and is able to follow simple commands. She cannot walk because of a fractured left lower leg.

   a. Green   c. Red
   b. Yellow   d. Black

8. Which individual in the ICS is responsible for communicating information regarding an MCI to the press?

   a. Incident commander
   b. Safety officer
   c. Liaison officer
   d. Information officer

9. JumpSTART triage is for use in patients ages:

   a. newborn to nine years.
   b. one to eight years.
   c. two to nine years.
   d. one to ten years.

Critical-Thinking Questions

10. Give examples of each of the "three Es of injury prevention."

11. Explain the responsibilities of the officers that an incident commander may name to assist him in managing an MCI.

12. Explain each of the four steps of the public health approach to address issues within a community.

References

Jiaquan Xu, M., Kochanek, K. D., Murphy, S. L., & Tejada-Vera, B. (2010). *Deaths: Vital data for 2007*. Hyattsville, MD: U.S. Department of Health and Human Services, National Center for Health Statistics.

McSwain, N. E., Salomone, J. P., Pons, P. T. (Eds). (2007). *Prehospital trauma life support* (6th ed.). St. Louis, MO: Elsevier.

World Health Organization. (n.d.). *Programmes and projects: World Health Organization*. Retrieved March 15, 2011, from http://www.who.int/violence_injury_prevention/child/injury/world_report/USA_falls/en/

34

Mechanisms of Injury, Trauma Assessment, and Trauma Triage Criteria

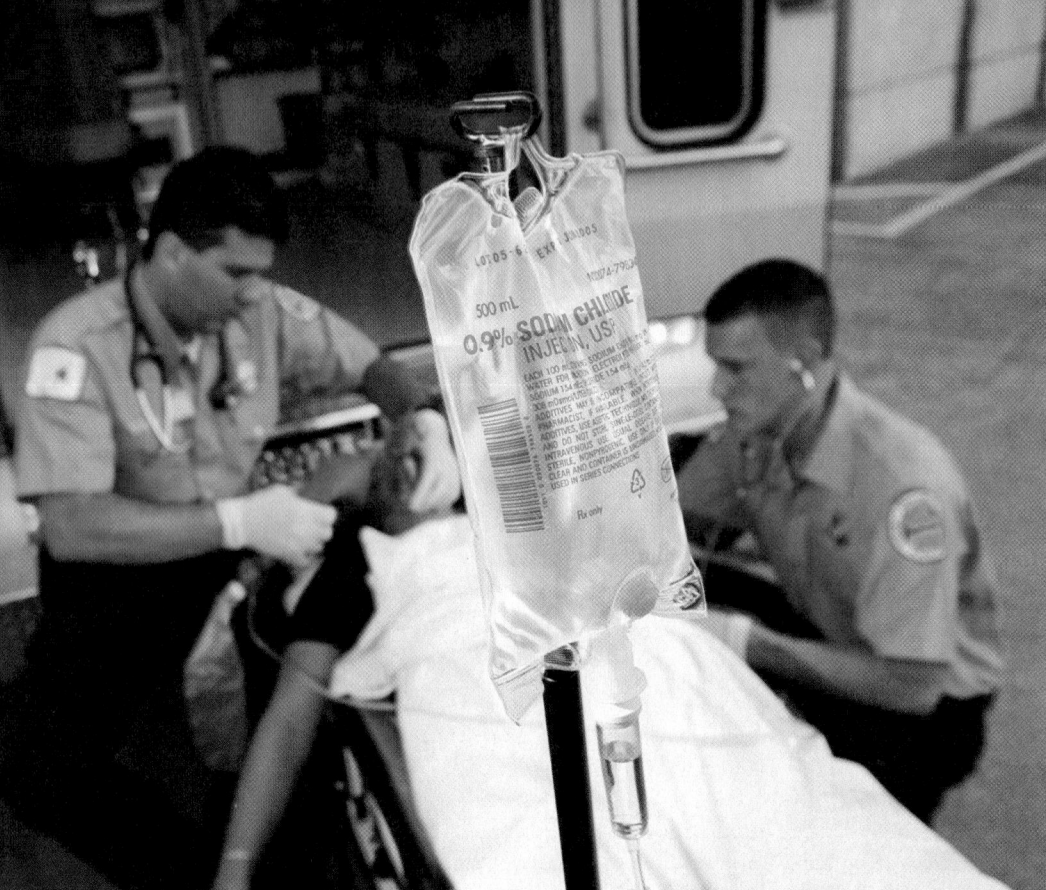

Content Area: Trauma

Advanced EMT Education Standard:
- Applies fundamental knowledge to provide basic and selected advanced emergency care and transportation based on assessment findings for an acutely injured patient.
- Pathophysiology, assessment, and management of the trauma patient.
  - Trauma scoring
  - Rapid transport and destination issues
  - Transport mode

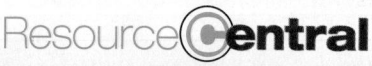

Objectives

After reading this chapter, you should be able to:

34.1 Define key terms introduced in this chapter.

34.2 Describe the purpose and goals of trauma patient assessment.

34.3 Describe the components of the trauma patient assessment process.

CASE STUDY

It is a warm Sunday afternoon when Advanced EMTs John "Mac" MacPherson and Courtney Anders are dispatched to a single-vehicle motor vehicle crash in a rural area just outside of town. While en route, they are advised by dispatch that first responders are on scene and report one unrestrained patient who is unconscious. Emergency medical responders are requesting air transport by the local air service, AirMed, for the patient.

Problem-Solving Questions

1. What can the information provided so far tell Mac and Courtney about the potential severity of the patient's injuries?
2. What should Mac and Courtney include in their initial plans for approaching the scene and assessing the patient?

34.4 Discuss the decisions that must be made during the trauma patient assessment process.

34.5 Explain the importance of various decision-making and problem-solving approaches in the trauma patient assessment and patient care processes.

Introduction

Trauma is an injury to the body resulting from external forces. The injury can be minor such as a puncture wound to the foot, or life threatening, such as being crushed beneath an automobile. Traumatic injury affects people of all age groups and can occur in any environment at any time (Figure 34-1). You must be prepared to respond to and properly assess and manage trauma patients. In this chapter, you will learn how to analyze specific mechanisms of injury and integrate the analysis into assessment of trauma patients (Figure 34-2). You also will learn to use the mechanism of injury and assessment findings to categorize trauma patients and make appropriate destination decisions.

Kinematics of Trauma

One of the most common ways in which the body sustains injury is the application of **kinetic energy**, the energy of motion, to the body. **Kinetics** is a branch of physics that studies how objects in motion are affected by outside forces and how energy is distributed when objects collide. In reference to mechanisms of injury, the term kinematics is often used, as well. Understanding basic principles of kinetic energy and its effects when applied to the body is important to being able to anticipate the injuries patients sustain when they are subjected to kinetic injury. For example, understanding how the speed and mass of an object striking various types of tissues in the body, such as in an assault or motor vehicle

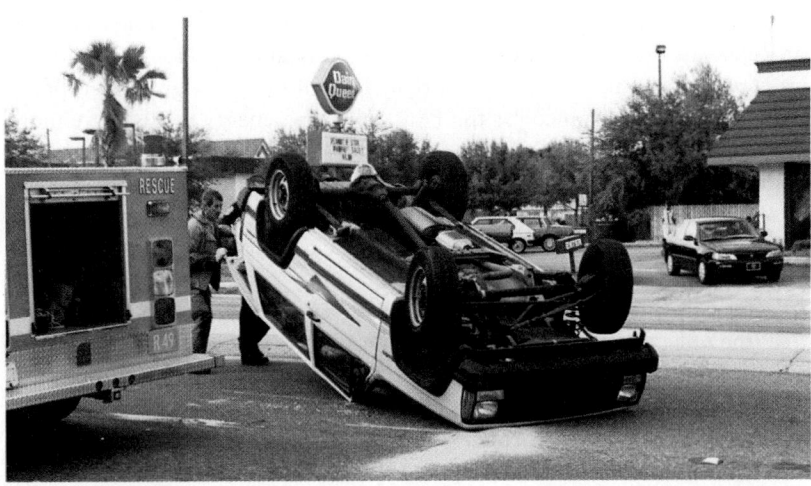

FIGURE 34-1

Because injury can occur to anyone at any time, you must be prepared to respond and properly manage trauma patients. (© Eddie Sperling Photography)

Trauma Assessment Flowchart

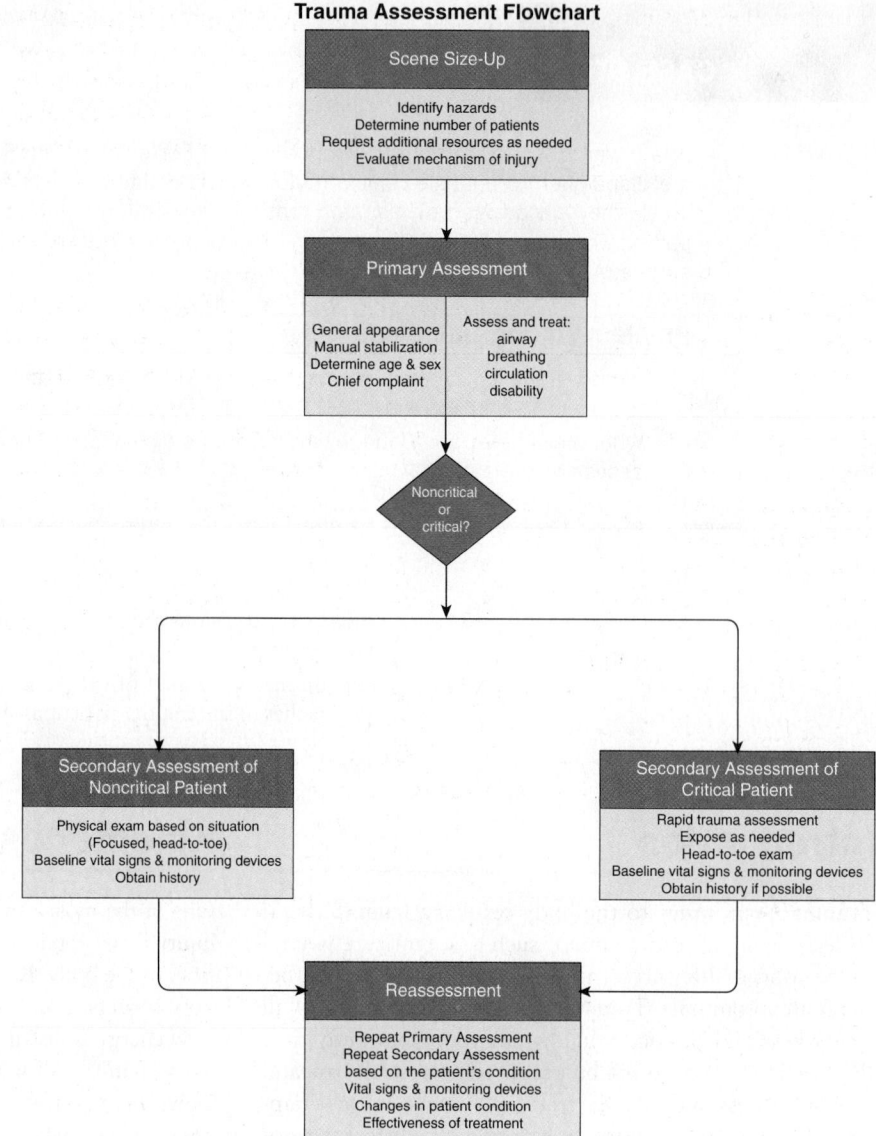

FIGURE 34-2

Trauma assessment flowchart.

collision (MVC), helps you predict the severity and types of injuries a patient has.

Kinetics

In order to understand how kinetics apply to particular situations, you must understand some general laws of physics and energy. The first is Newton's first law of motion, or the **law of inertia**. It states that a body in motion will remain in motion and a body at rest will remain at rest unless acted upon by an outside force.

Consider the following scenario: An unrestrained driver of a car is traveling 65 mph when the car leaves the road and strikes a large tree head-on. The car's forward movement stops due to the impact with the tree (the outside force in this case). The tree stops the car through direct impact, but the body has not yet been acted upon by an outside force. The driver will continue moving forward until it is acted upon by an outside force, which may be an

airbag, seatbelt and shoulder harness, or steering wheel, windshield, and dashboard.

The less dense of the objects involved in the collision will absorb the most energy and sustain the greatest damage. An airbag has very low density and is able to absorb the kinetic energy of the body and decrease the injury to the body. (The airbag also allows for a greater stopping distance for the body, allowing energy to dissipate more gradually before the body comes to a stop.) Compared to the windshield, though, the body has lower density and will absorb a greater amount of energy and sustain greater damage. Of course, the windshield will also be damaged in the collision (Figure 34-3).

The **law of conservation of energy** states that energy can neither be created nor destroyed. Energy can, however, be changed from one form to another. For example, as a driver applies the brakes in a moving vehicle kinetic energy is transformed to heat (another form of energy) through friction. An impact between the driver of the car and the

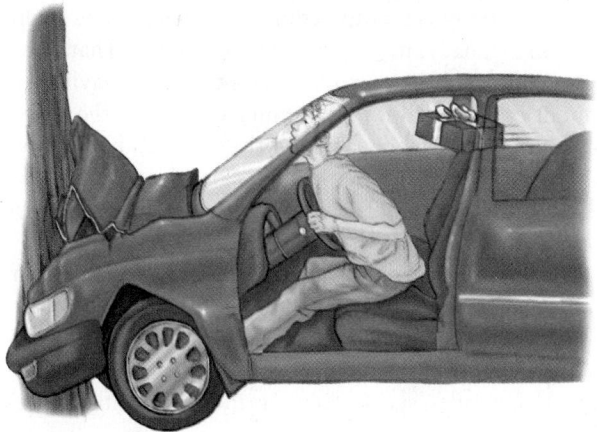

FIGURE 34-3

The law of inertia: A body in motion will remain in motion and a body at rest will remain at rest unless acted upon by an outside force.

steering wheel, windshield, and dashboard results in energy being transferred to the driver. Kinetic energy is transformed to tissue deformity.

Kinetic energy is a function of mass (weight) and velocity (speed). Units of kinetic energy are calculated by the following formula:

$$\text{Kinetic energy} = \text{mass} \times \text{velocity}^2/2$$

This formula illustrates that velocity is the factor that influences the production of energy most. If a 1-pound ball is traveling at 80 mph when it strikes an individual in the head, 3,200 units of kinetic energy are produced, calculated as follows:

$$3{,}200 = 1 \times 80^2/2$$

If the velocity of the ball is changed to 90 mph, the number of units produced significantly increases to 4,050 units, calculated as follows:

$$4{,}050 = 1 \times 90^2/2$$

Just as an increase in velocity results in an increase in energy produced, so does an increase in mass. If you double the weight of the ball and calculate the energy produced with a velocity of 80 mph, you will see the units of energy increase from 3,200 to 6,400 units. Note in the following calculation that increasing mass causes an increase in energy but not nearly as much as an increase in velocity:

$$6{,}400 = 2 \times 80^2/2$$

Newton's second law of motion illustrates how forces are distributed during a collision. The formula for this law is as follows:

$$\text{Force} = \text{mass} \times \text{acceleration or deceleration}$$

This law emphasizes the importance of the rate of change of the speed of an object involved in a collision. When changes in speed occur slowly, less force is generated than when changes in speed occur abruptly. When you are

driving and gradually slow your vehicle as you approach a stop sign, there is not much force exerted on your body. When a driver loses control of his vehicle and strikes a large tree, he experiences a very rapid deceleration and a tremendous amount of force applied to his body. The greater the force applied, the greater the potential for injury.

Classifying Trauma

Trauma is classified as either blunt trauma or penetrating trauma. Blunt trauma occurs when the surface area and velocity of an object striking the body are not sufficient to penetrate the tissues. Penetrating trauma occurs when the velocity and surface area of an object, such as a knife or bullet, allows the object to penetrate the tissues.

Blunt Trauma

Blunt trauma results when an object contacting the body causes energy to be transferred either directly or indirectly. Blunt trauma caused by contact between the body and an object is called a **direct injury**. For instance, if you dropped a can of soup on the top of your bare foot, the impact would cause a crushing of the skin and underlying tissues. That may lead to capillary injury within and beneath the skin, resulting in bleeding. The damage caused by the can was a result of direct contact with the injured tissues.

If enough energy is involved in the contact with the body, energy is transmitted through the tissues and injury occurs deeper within the body as well as at the point of impact. This is called an **indirect injury**. Consider this example: A man fell from a height of 10 feet and landed on his feet. Because of the rapid deceleration upon contact with the ground, you would expect to see direct injury where his feet struck the ground. Because the fall was from a significant height, substantial force was applied to the body. You also would consider the possibility of injuries to the knees, hips, and spine. Energy is transferred from one point to another until it has been completely absorbed. In the previous example in which the man fell 10 feet, the energy will travel up his legs toward the hips and spine until all of it is absorbed. The direct injury would be to his feet, and the indirect injuries would be to his legs, hips, and spine.

Penetrating Trauma

When an object is driven into the body creating a break in the skin, the injury is called **penetrating trauma**. Blunt trauma can cause lacerations to the tissues as the force of the object striking the body splits the tissues. The difference with penetrating trauma is that the object enters the tissues.

IN THE FIELD

You should be suspicious of underlying internal injury when a significant MOI and external injury are present.

Penetrating trauma results from sources of energy such as a stab or bullet wound. When an object penetrates the skin and travels into the underlying tissues, a permanent cavity is created. As the object passes through the tissues, energy is dispersed to the surrounding tissues creating a temporary cavity and additional internal injury (Figure 34-4).

Penetrating trauma is caused by low-, medium-, or high-velocity mechanisms. Low-velocity penetrating injuries include those created by a hand-driven object such as sticks, ice picks, or knives. Because there is not a significant amount of energy involved with these injuries, the potential for immediate injury other than the direct injury is low as compared to medium- or high-energy penetrating trauma. However, all penetrating trauma is associated with a high risk of infection, which can affect the patient's overall condition following injury.

It is also important to determine the length and width of an object that penetrates the patient's body. That information allows you to estimate the permanent cavity and amount of potential internal injury present. If the object was manipulated while inside of the patient's body, more injury will occur. The cone of injury provides you with an idea of how much internal damage the object could have caused (Figure 34-5).

Handguns and some smaller caliber rifles are considered medium-velocity weapons because they produce enough energy to cause injury beyond the immediate pathway of the projectile. High-velocity injuries are caused by high velocity rifles, such as hunting and assault rifles, which often use large caliber ammunition.

The combination of the increased mass of large caliber ammunition and the high velocity provided by a powerful

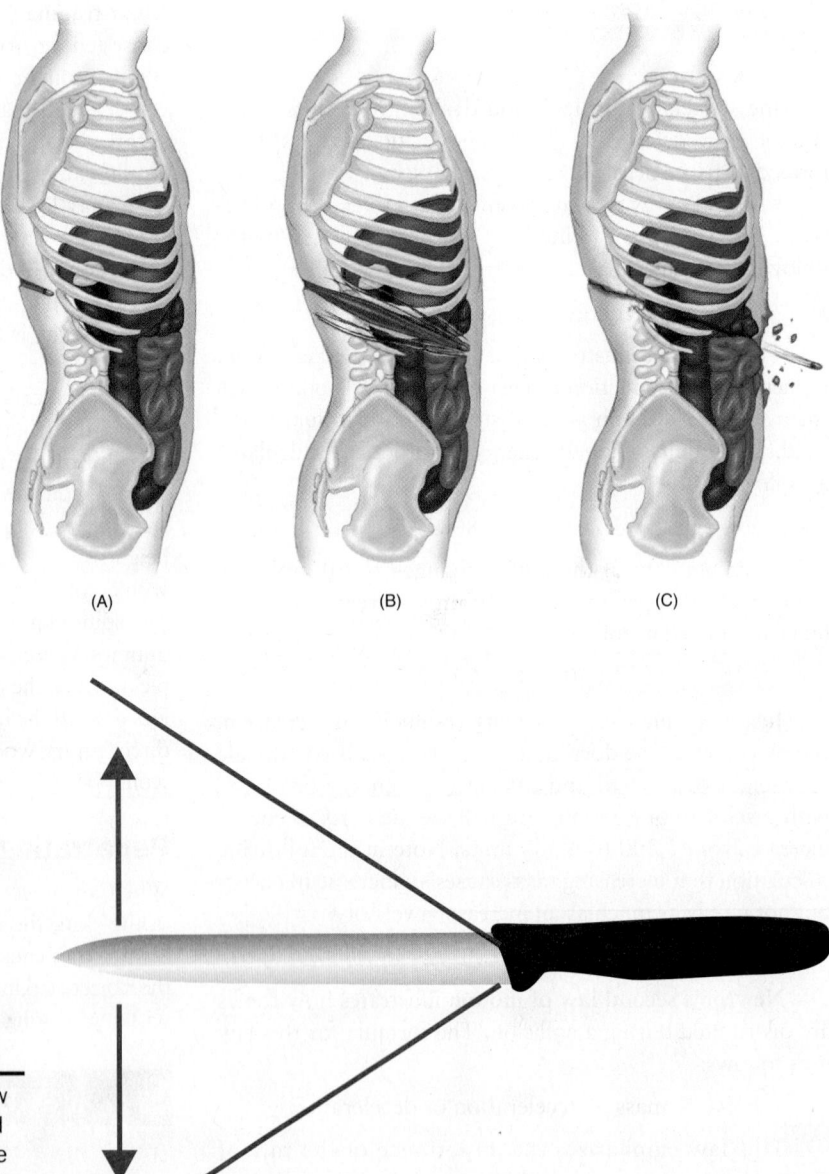

FIGURE 34-4

As an object passes through the tissues, a permanent cavity is created (A and C). As the object continues, energy is dispersed to the surrounding tissues, creating a temporary cavity (cavitation) and additional internal injury (B).

(A)   (B)   (C)

FIGURE 34-5

The cone of injury provides an idea of how much internal damage may have occurred through movement of the object within the tissues. It is for this reason that you must identify the object that has caused the patient's injury.

rifle increase the kinetic energy delivered by these weapons. Those weapons can cause massive direct and indirect injuries.

During patient assessment, you should attempt to determine the caliber of the weapon that created the injury and the distance between the weapon when fired and the patient. High-velocity weapons fired in close proximity to the patient will result in higher energy injuries because the projectile is at maximum velocity as it exits the weapon and velocity decreases as it travels over distances.

When penetrating trauma is present, it is vital that you identify both entrance and exit wounds on the patient. Identifying these wounds will provide you with an idea of what underlying body structures are injured. While it is not necessary to differentiate between entry and exit wounds, they do have different characteristics that will be discussed further in Chapter 35.

Assessment of the Trauma Patient

The assessment of a trauma patient involves the same basic steps as the assessment of a medical patient—scene size-up, primary assessment, secondary assessment, and reassessment. Analyzing the mechanism of injury (MOI) in the scene size-up is a critical step in determining the potential for injury.

Scene Size-Up

As you approach the scene of a traumatic injury, you must take Standard Precautions. Due to the likelihood of blood and other bodily fluids being present, you should be prepared to don gloves, eye protection, face protection, disposable gown, and a reflective vest as necessary. Once on the scene, perform a scene size-up. The scene size-up consists of

ensuring that the scene is safe to enter, identifying the number and location of the injured, assessment of the MOI, and considering the need for additional resources. If hazards exist at the scene, you should not approach. Instead, call and wait for the arrival of additional resources necessary to eliminate the hazards present. Hazards may include uncontrolled traffic, fire, downed power lines, risk of explosion, hazardous materials, or the presence of individuals with weapons. If additional resources are required but it is safe to approach patients, call for the additional resources and begin assessing the injured patients (Figure 34-6).

Mechanism of Injury

The forces and energy that cause injury to the patient are called the **mechanism of injury (MOI)**. It is important to identify the forces that the patient sustained. Because you

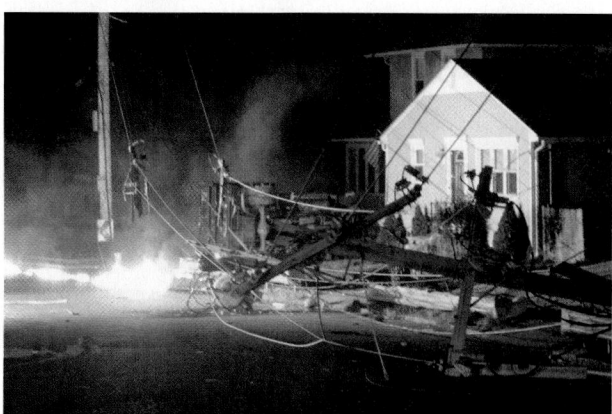

FIGURE 34-6

You must not approach a scene unless it is safe to do so. If a scene is not safe upon arrival, you must call for appropriate additional resources to mitigate the hazards prior to approaching the scene. (© Mark C. Ide)

PERSONAL PERSPECTIVE

Janice Jones, Advanced EMT: My partner and I were dispatched to a head-on collision on a two-lane highway just outside of town. En route to the scene, we heard fire rescue calling for extrication.

Upon arrival, we approached the vehicles where firefighters advised us that the driver of one car was dead on arrival (DOA) and the other is ambulatory and refusing transport. Both cars had massive damage to their front end. My partner confirmed that the other driver was in fact DOA, as I approached the other driver who was now sitting on the side of the highway wiping blood from his face. The driver stated that he did not want to go to the hospital by way of an ambulance and would go later if he felt that he needed to.

While performing my primary assessment, I explained to the patient that he was in a very serious collision and he should be evaluated by a physician. His only complaint was a stiff neck and upper left chest pain and tenderness from the seatbelt. His respiratory rate was slightly elevated

and his pulse rate was 110 strong and regular. His blood pressure was 110/90, which I thought was a little low for a man his size. After much convincing, he agreed to treatment and transport. His condition remained the same throughout transport. When we arrived at the hospital emergency department, we rolled the patient into the trauma bay and provided a patient report.

Later in the shift, we returned to that same ED with another patient when the ED physician approached me and stated that it was a good thing that we did not allow the patient from the MVC earlier to refuse. He went on to explain that the patient had a dissected aorta and would have surely died if it hadn't been identified and repaired.

It was the MOI that led my partner and me to convince the patient that he should be transported directly to the ED via ambulance. The patient survived due to recognition of a significant MOI and potential for life-threatening injury, and transport to the most appropriate facility.

are at the scene, you have a unique opportunity to assess the MOI that is not available to hospital personnel. Each mechanism of injury has a predictable pattern of potential injuries associated with it. The predictability allows you to formulate a list of potential injuries based solely on the MOI. You will deliberately assess the patient for the predicted injuries during the patient assessment process.

Motor Vehicle Crashes

Motor vehicle crashes (MVCs) are the leading cause of death among 5- to 44-year-old people in the United States. The Centers for Disease Control and Prevention reported that more than 2.3 million patients were treated in emergency departments following an MVC (Centers for Disease Control and Prevention, 2011). An MVC occurs when vehicles collide with objects or other vehicles. MVCs can result in both blunt and penetrating trauma.

There are three impacts associated with a rapid-deceleration MVC (Figure 34-7), as follows:

- When the patient's vehicle collides with an object or another vehicle

- When the patient inside the vehicle is forced to decelerate by restraint systems, such as seatbelts and airbags, or collides with the interior of the vehicle

- When the internal organs of the patient collide with one another and the inside wall of the body

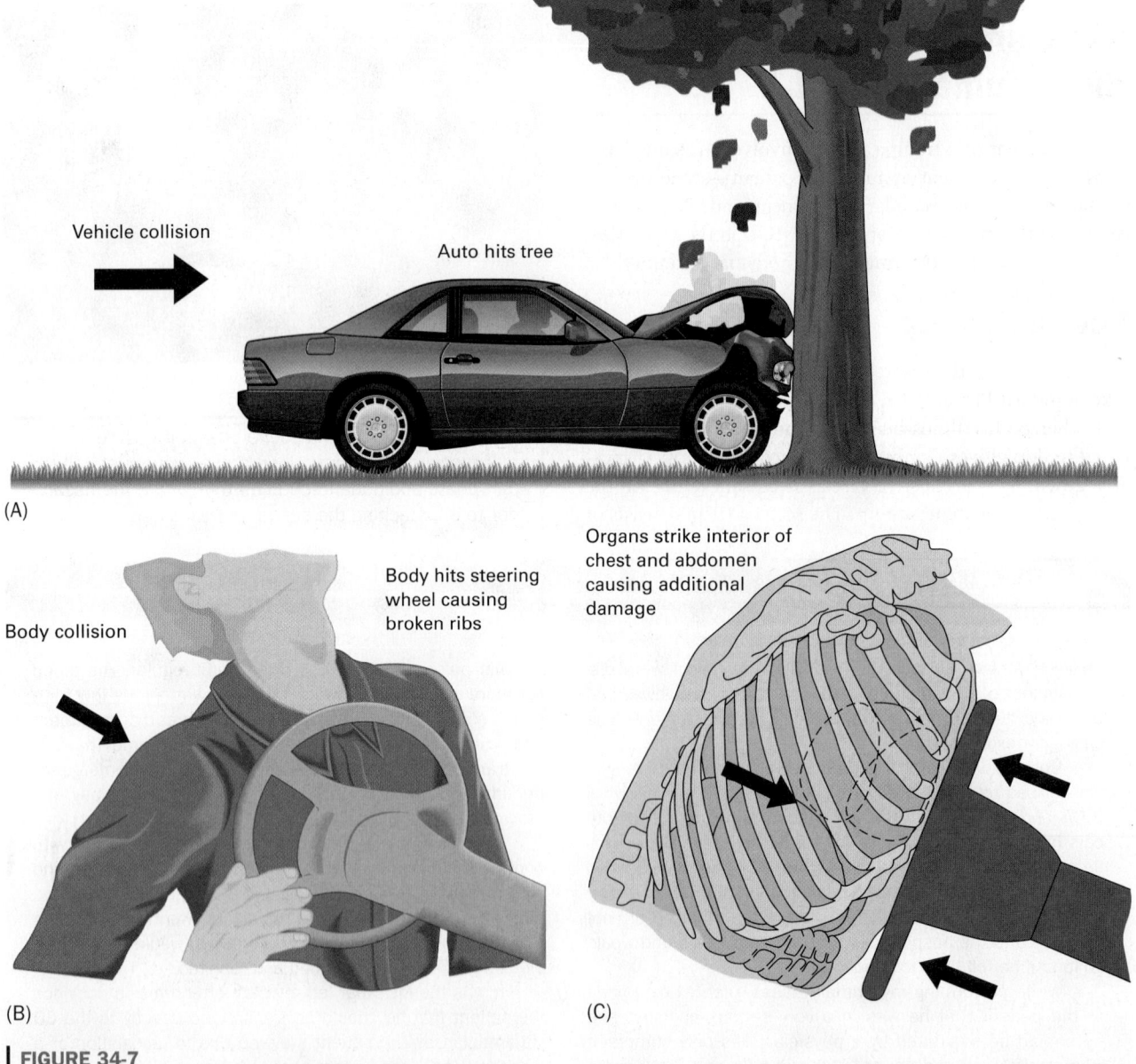

FIGURE 34-7

There are three collisions that occur with a rapid-deceleration MOI: (A) The vehicle collides with an object, (B) the driver collides with steering wheel, and (C) the organs collide with the inside of the body.

If an unrestrained driver of a car strikes a large concrete post, the car will rapidly decelerate (Newton's first law of motion). As the car decelerates, the unrestrained driver continues forward movement until he strikes the airbag, seatbelt, steering wheel, dashboard, and/or windshield. Once the driver decelerates from contact with the interior of the car, internal organs continue the forward movement until they collide with one another or the inside wall of the body. As the organs continue forward, they may tear at the points where they are restrained within the body. For example, as the aorta continues forward, it is stopped by ligaments at its arch that are inelastic. This results in stretching and tearing of the aortic tissues. The liver is an inelastic organ that is restrained from forward motion at the ligamentum teres. As the liver continues forward motion it can be torn at the point where it is restrained by the ligament.

The collisions of internal organs can cause bruising, lacerations, and tearing, which can lead to massive internal bleeding that is not visible on external examination. In these situations, you must rely on the assessment of the MOI and indirect indications of injury and bleeding, such as pale, diaphoretic skin and abnormal vital signs, to identify potential internal life-threatening injuries.

MVCs can be divided into the following five categories of impact: frontal, rear, lateral, rotational, and rollover. The best method to identify the potential injuries a patient may have is to look at the damage to the patient's vehicle and determine which of the five types of crashes occurred.

Frontal Impact

In a **frontal impact** MVC, or head-on collision, the vehicle collides with an object causing damage to the front of the vehicle (Figure 34-8). The extent of damage to the vehicle provides insight to the forces that were exerted on the patient. Damage to the vehicle is directly related to the potential for patient injury. The greater the vehicle damage, the greater the likelihood of patient injury. With a frontal impact collision, the unrestrained patient will follow one of two possible paths: up and over, or down and under. Although supplemental restraint systems (SRS) known as airbags can greatly reduce impact with the interior of the vehicle, they are only deployed once. If there is more than one impact to a vehicle from the same direction, the airbags have already been deployed in the initial impact.

With an up-and-over pathway, the patient collides with the steering wheel and his head moves upward toward the windshield (Figure 34-9). This can result in chest, head, neck, abdominal trauma, and partial ejection of the patient through the windshield.

With a down-and-under pathway, the patient collides with the bottom of the steering wheel and in some cases, his legs collide with the dashboard (Figure 34-10). This can result in chest, abdominal, and lower extremity injuries.

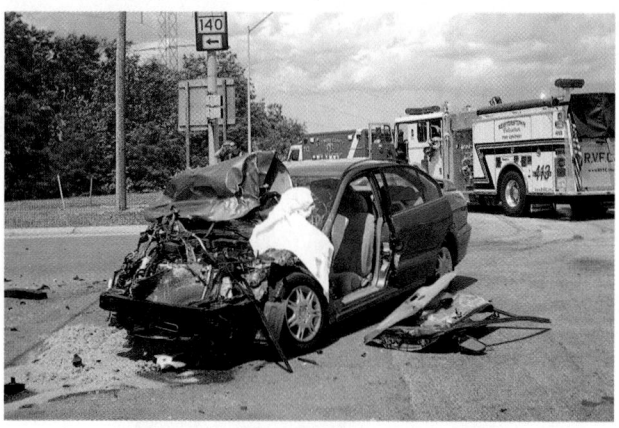

(A)

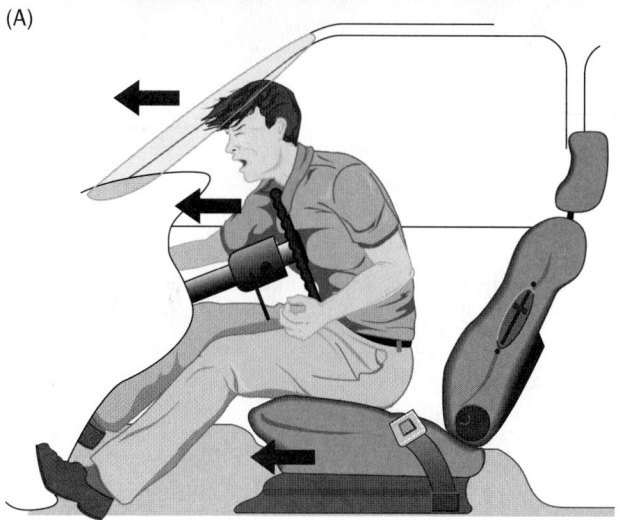

(B)

FIGURE 34-8

(A) In a frontal impact collision, the vehicle collides with another object, causing damage to the front of the vehicle. (© Mark C. Ide) (B) In a frontal impact collision, the occupant continues traveling at the same speed after the initial impact.

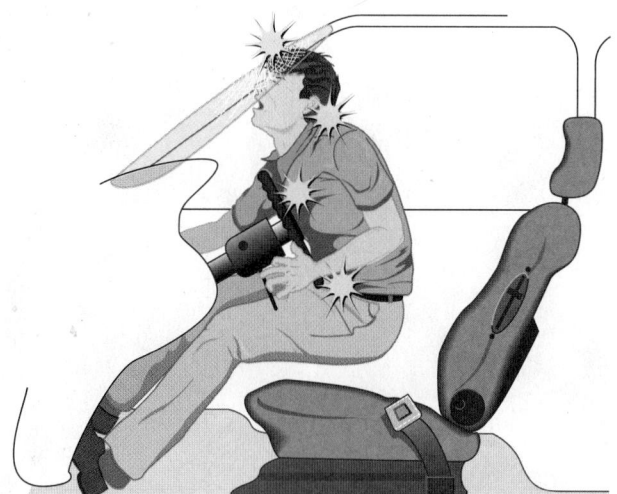

FIGURE 34-9

It is important to consider the predictable injuries of the head, neck, chest, and abdomen associated with a patient's up-and-over pathway.

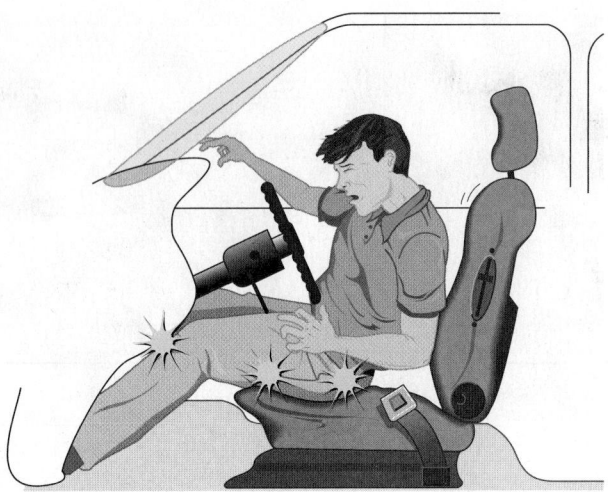

FIGURE 34-10

It is important to consider the predictable injuries of the abdomen, hips, spine, and lower extremities associated with a patient's down-and-under pathway.

Often, the lower legs, ankles, and feet are forced into the floorboard and pedals, creating injury.

In frontal impact MVCs, you should look for the following damage to the vehicle, which will assist in predicting potential significant injury to the patient (Figure 34-11):

- The amount of damage to the front of the vehicle. More than 18 inches of damage is considered significant.
- Starring or shattering of the windshield
- Bending of the steering wheel or collapsing of the steering column
- Damage to the dashboard

The presence of any of those signs indicates that significant forces were involved in the collision and the potential

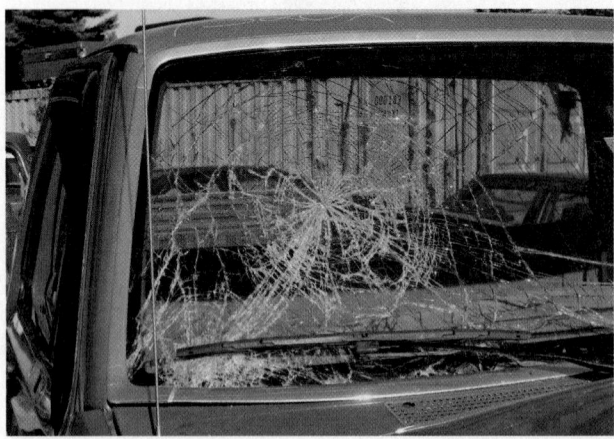

FIGURE 34-11

You should look for damage to the vehicle to predict potential injury to the patient. Starring of the windshield indicates possible head injury to the patient.

IN THE FIELD

The presence of a deployed airbag indicates that the forces involved in the impact were significant. Also consider the potential for injury caused by an airbag with the unrestrained patient. If the patient was unrestrained and traveled forward with the airbag in the process of deploying, the result can be blunt injury to the face. You also should be aware of an undeployed airbag with a frontal impact. Never position yourself in front of an undeployed airbag because this may result in significant injury to you if it suddenly deploys.

for injury is high. Also be alert to the presence of objects inside the patient's vehicle, which could have been thrown from the rear of the vehicle to the front upon impact. Those objects can cause serious injury or death to anyone inside the vehicle.

Look for the following injuries to the chest, abdomen, head, and neck with patients who have been involved in a frontal impact collision regardless of whether they took an up-and-over or a down-and-under pathway.

- *Chest.* On impact, the chest will strike the steering wheel or dashboard affecting the bones and soft tissues. The sternum and ribs may break, which can lead to significant internal bleeding. Because the heart and lungs are within the chest cavity, they are susceptible to injury from an impact to the chest. When the chest is compressed from the impact, the heart and lungs are compressed between the sternum and ribs and the spine. In addition, those organs also are susceptible to shearing forces from a rapid deceleration, which can lead to massive internal bleeding and death. The lungs also can be injured by air that is trapped within them upon impact. If the epiglottis suddenly closes as the lungs are being compressed due to the impact, the air pressure within the lungs rises tremendously and this can lead to rupture of lung tissue. This type of injury is known as a "paper-bag injury," because it is similar to blowing up a paper bag and popping it by compressing it between your hands.
- *Abdomen.* Damage to the steering wheel and/or dashboard should cause a high index of suspicion for internal abdominal injury. Vital organs within the abdominal cavity can be subject to compression and shearing injury with frontal impacts. The liver and spleen are solid, highly vascular organs that, when injured, can lead to massive internal bleeding and death.
- *Head.* When the patient strikes the windshield, the head is often injured. Those injuries can range from mild lacerations to massive skull fractures. If you note "starring," which is a broken area in a starlike

> **IN THE FIELD**
>
> You should expect to see injury to the patient's face when an airbag has been deployed, whether the patient was restrained or not. Airbags inflate at a very rapid rate and can cause burning, bruising, and lacerations.

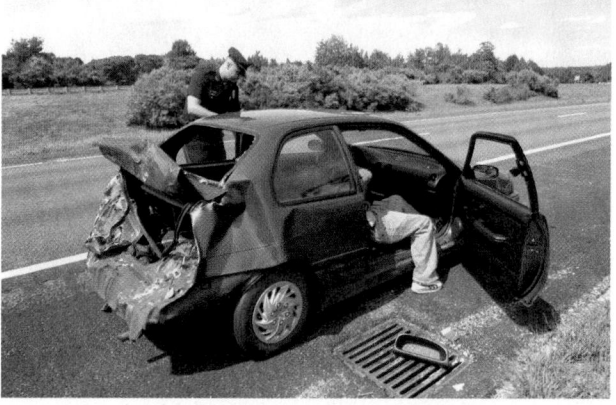

(A)

pattern of the windshield, assume that the patient's head caused it. In some cases, the forces applied to the skull upon impact lead to massive fractures and direct injury to the brain (bone fragments can be pushed into the brain). The position of the patient's head upon impact will determine if the patient's face will sustain injury, as well. When the head strikes the windshield, the patient also is susceptible to indirect injury to the neck, which can include fractures and damage to the spinal cord.

Rear Impact

With a **rear impact** MVC, the patient's vehicle is struck from behind, driving the vehicle forward (Figure 34-12). This acceleration of the vehicle causes acceleration injuries. If the patient's seat does not have a headrest or the headrest is not properly positioned, the head lags behind as the body accelerates, causing severe hyperextension of the neck. This hyperextension can lead to serious injury of the soft tissues, spine, and even the spinal cord, and is commonly referred to as "whiplash." Remember, the amount of damage to the vehicle is directly related to the forces that were applied to the patient.

Lateral Impact

In **lateral impact** MVCs, the patient's vehicle is struck on the side (Figure 34-13). This type of impact is commonly called a "T-bone" collision. Determine if intrusion into the passenger compartment of the vehicle occurred and in what location. If intrusion is present at the same location the patient was seated in the vehicle, the patient may have sustained significant injury. These injuries could include fractured extremities on the side of impact, lateral chest trauma, hip fractures, and head and neck injury.

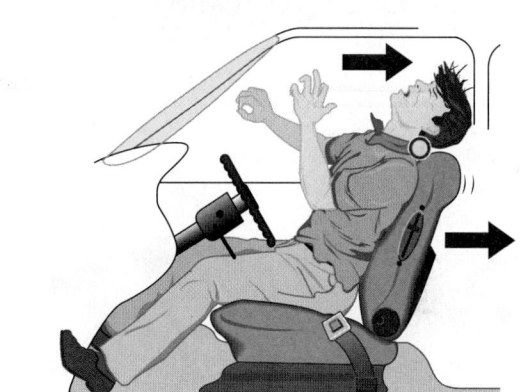

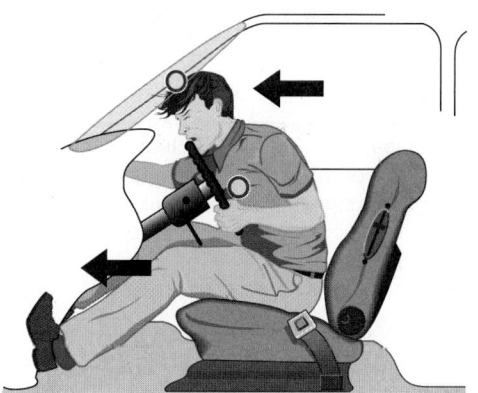

(B)

FIGURE 34-12

(A) Rear impact. A rear impact MOI results in rapid-acceleration injuries such as "whiplash," or hyperextension injuries. (© Mark C. Ide) (B) Following the acceleration the occupant decelerates, moving forward and causing injury to the head and chest.

> **IN THE FIELD**
>
> Headrests are designed to limit the amount of hyperextension of the neck with rear impact collisions. If headrests are not present in a vehicle that sustained a rear impact, you should suspect hyperextension injury to the patient's neck.

Rotational Impact

A **rotational impact** MVC occurs when a lateral impact causes the patient's vehicle to rotate or spin (Figure 34-14). The lateral impact causing rotation usually occurs at either the front or rear fender locations. In a rotational impact MVC, the patient is subjected to twisting forces that can lead to significant injury, particularly the neck and internal organs.

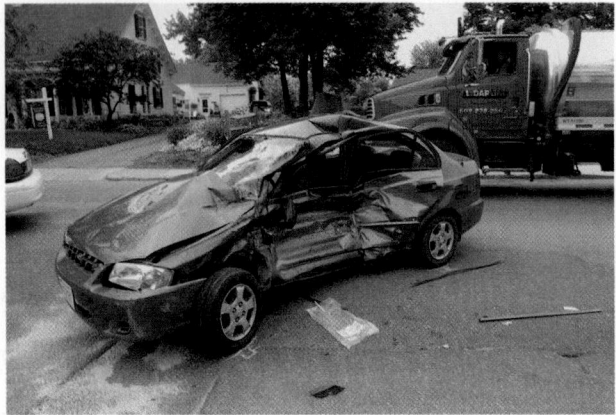

(A)

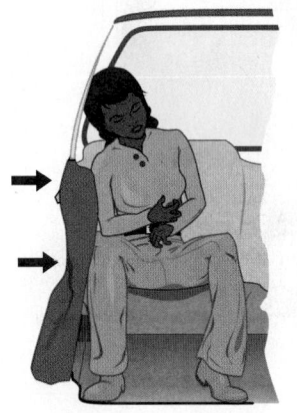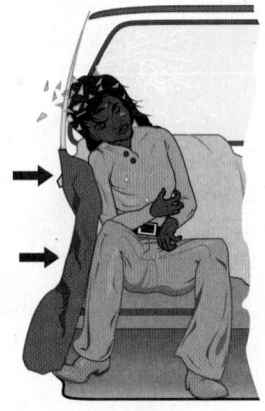

(B)

FIGURE 34-13

(A) Lateral impact. (© Mark C. Ide) (B) In a lateral impact MOI, you must consider the potential for injury to the side of the patient that sustained the energy from impact.

Rollover

Rollover MVCs subject the patient to forces of every kind and can lead to significant injury (Figure 34-15). During a rollover MVC, unrestrained individuals inside the vehicle may be ejected from the vehicle. **Ejection** refers to a patient being thrown from the vehicle, usually through a window. Patients who have been ejected usually sustain serious injury or death.

Pedestrian–Vehicle Collisions

When a pedestrian is struck by a vehicle, the extent of injury sustained by the patient depends upon the following (Figure 34-16):

- Speed of the vehicle impact
- Part or parts of the patient's body struck
- Distance the patient was thrown following impact
- Body parts that struck the ground following impact
- Type of surface on which the patient landed

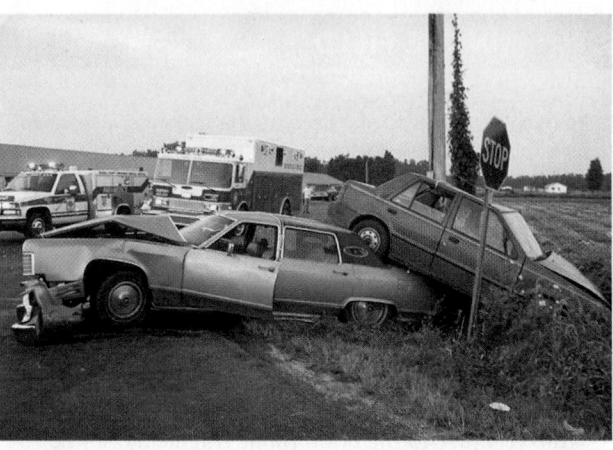

FIGURE 34-14

A rotational impact occurs when a lateral impact causes the patient's vehicle to rotate or spin. This rotation results in twisting forces to the patient. (© RGB photo)

When a person realizes that he is about to be struck by a vehicle, he will tend to turn his back to the coming impact, absorbing it either on the lateral or posterior side of his body. As the vehicle impacts the person, he is lifted off his feet and the forward movement of the vehicle causes him to impact the windshield of the vehicle. If the speed of the vehicle is substantial, the person will travel completely over the vehicle. If the driver of the vehicle decelerates by applying the brakes, the person will roll off of the hood of the car and strike the ground, causing additional injury. The further the person is thrown from the vehicle, the more forces were applied to his body. It is important to identify each of these collisions and the potential for injury as a result.

Motorcycle Crashes

Advanced EMTs respond to many MVCs involving motorcycles (Figure 34-17). Because the driver of a motorcycle is exposed, he is at much more risk for injury than the driver of an automobile. Motorcyclists who are involved in an

Pediatric Care

When a child is struck by a vehicle, he tends to sustain injury from the vehicle impact on the anterior surface of his body. This results from the child's tendency to look directly toward the vehicle before impact. Children are more likely to sustain life-threatening injury because their bodies are smaller, which means more of their body surface area sustains a direct impact as compared to the adult. Because of a child's height, he or she may be thrown to the ground upon impact and dragged beneath the vehicle instead of traveling onto the hood and into the windshield.

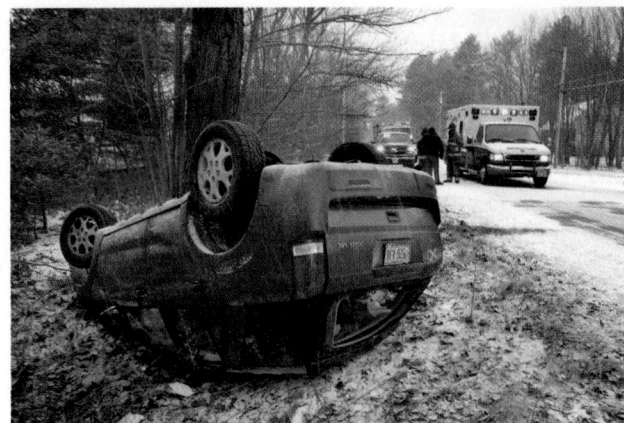

(A)

FIGURE 34-15

(A) Rollover impact. (© Daniel Limmer) (B) A rollover MVC subjects the patient to forces of every kind and can lead to significant patient injury.

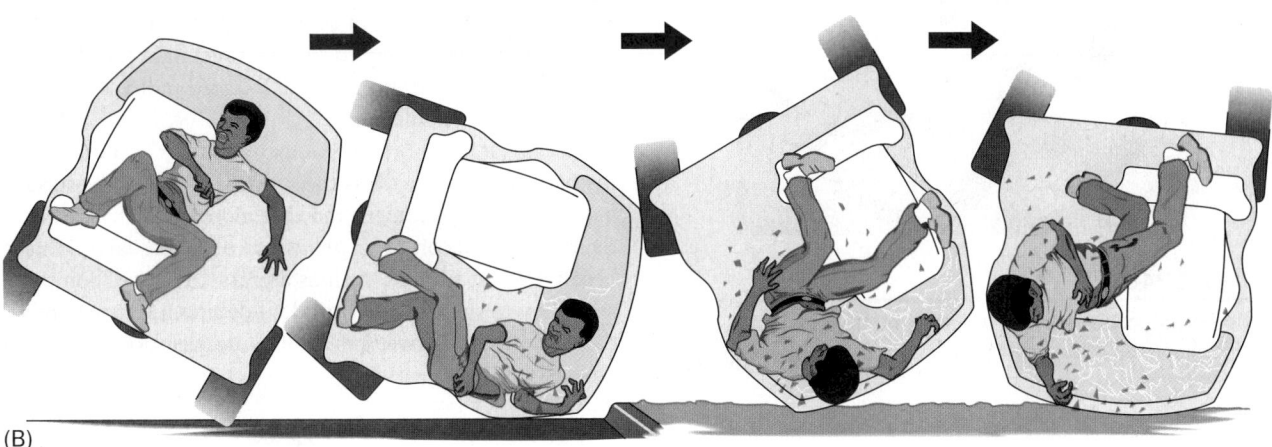

(B)

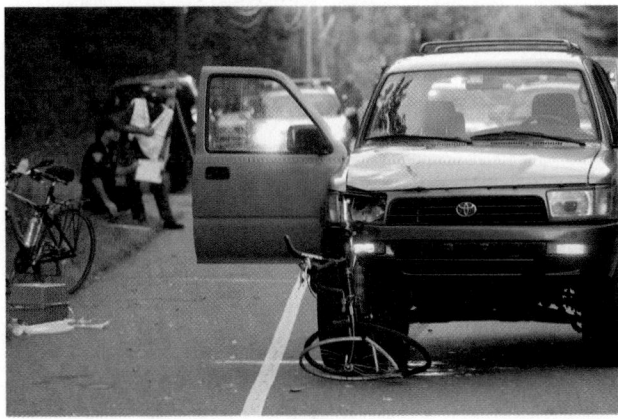

FIGURE 34-16

Adults tend to turn away from an approaching vehicle, whereas children tend to turn and face directly toward it. (© Mark C. Ide)

MVC and are not wearing a helmet are at a much greater risk of sustaining head injury, increasing morbidity and mortality. There are three types of motorcycle collisions: head-on, lateral, and "lying the motorcycle down."

In a head-on motorcycle collision, the rider is thrown into and over the handlebars and continues until he comes to rest after striking the ground. When the rider impacts the handlebars, it is common for fractures of the lower extremities to occur. After impacting the handlebars, the rider continues over them and impacts other objects such as another vehicle or the ground where even more injury occurs.

With a lateral impact motorcycle collision, the rider is struck by another vehicle, sustaining injury to the leg on the side of impact. After impact, the rider then will lose control of the motorcycle and crash, causing more injury as he impacts other objects and the ground.

IN THE FIELD

If a motorcyclist is involved in a collision and was wearing a helmet, you should inspect the helmet and note any damage to it. Significant damage to the helmet suggests significant energy absorption by the helmet and potentially the patient's head.

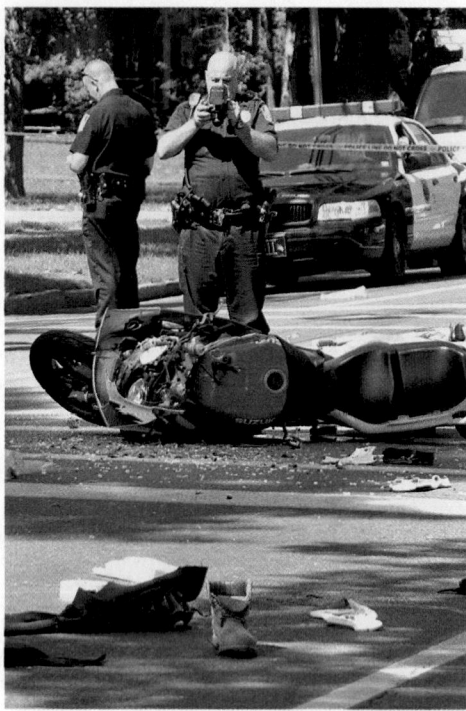

FIGURE 34-17

Motorcycle collisions can result in multiple impacts that injure the rider. (© CW McKean/Syracruse Newspapers/ The Image Works)

Ejection of a motorcyclist occurs when the rider is separated from the motorcycle. If the motorcyclist is wearing the proper personal protective equipment (PPE) such as a helmet, gloves, boots, and leather jacket the severity of injury will be less than if he is not. This is particularly true about helmets. When a helmet is not worn, the likelihood of significant head trauma occurring is much higher. In some cases, a rider who has been ejected from a motorcycle will only sustain "road rash," or severe abrasions, and musculoskeletal injury.

Falls

In 2009, emergency departments treated 2.2 million nonfatal fall injuries among older adults; more than 582,000 of those patients had to be hospitalized (Centers for Disease Control and Prevention, 2010).

When faced with a patient who has fallen, there are three things that you should take into consideration:

- Height of the fall
- Body part that impacted the landing surface first
- Surface fallen onto

To understand the amount of force applied to the patient, determine the height of the fall. A trip and fall from a standing position can cause injury, but will not cause as serious of an injury as if the patient had fallen from a height of 10 feet.

When a patient falls, determine what part of the patient's body impacted the landing surface first. Recall that

direct injury occurs where the patient's body contacts the ground but energy continues to be absorbed by the body until it has been absorbed totally. This energy can lead to additional indirect injury to the patient (Figure 34-18). For instance, when a patient trips and falls forward, he usually extends his hands in front of him to break the fall. In some cases, this will cause him to sustain direct injury to the hand or wrist. But it also can cause associated indirect injury to the forearm or shoulders.

Lastly, it is important to identify the surface onto which the patient has fallen. Was the surface soft? Was the surface hard? It is easy to understand that more injury will occur if the patient lands on concrete instead of a grass lawn. This is because a soft surface, such as a grass lawn, will compress and allow a slightly more gradual deceleration (remember the relationship between the rate of deceleration and force)

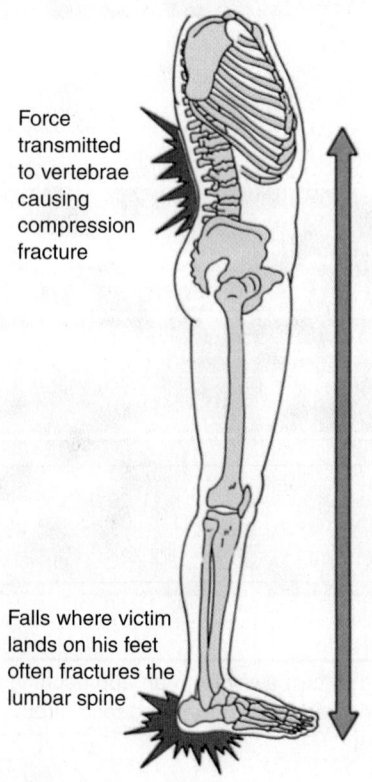

Force transmitted to vertebrae causing compression fracture

Falls where victim lands on his feet often fractures the lumbar spine

FIGURE 34-18

Direct injury occurs with contact with the ground, and indirect injury occurs as energy is transferred to other parts of the body.

Pediatric Care

Children are more likely to strike their head during a fall. This is because a child's head is larger than an adult's in proportion to the rest of the body.

Geriatric Care

As people get older, their reflexes begin to slow and their skeletal system weakens. (You will learn more about this process later.) When geriatric patients fall, their reflexes are often too slow for them to try to either prevent or break the fall by extending their hands in front of them. When this occurs, they can strike the ground without slowing before impact. Because their bones are weaker, they are at high risk for fractures and internal bleeding.

than an unyielding surface such as concrete or asphalt. The density of the concrete as compared to the density of human tissues also means that the body will absorb more energy than the concrete. As that occurs the kinetic energy is converted to the potential energy of tissue deformity.

Blast Injuries

Blast injuries occur as a result of explosions from natural gas, fireworks, improvised explosive device (IED), and others. When responding to an explosion, first ensure that the scene is safe prior to entering. Regardless of the cause of explosions, each produces three phases of injury. The four phases are the **primary blast injury**, the **secondary blast injury**, **tertiary blast injury**, and the **quaternary blast injury**, described as follows:

- *Primary blast injury.* This phase is caused by the pressure wave from the explosion. The extent of the pressure wave is directly related to the force of the explosion. When a patient is exposed to the pressure wave from an explosion, the hollow organs of his body—such as the lungs, stomach, intestines, bladder, and ears—may rupture due to extreme changes in pressure. Severe injury or even death can occur from this rapid increase in pressure caused by the pressure wave.

- *Secondary blast injury.* This phase results from debris that is thrown from the explosion as a result of the pressure wave. This debris can include the material of the casing of the explosive device or container, objects from the environment around the explosion, and even other victims. The most common types of secondary injuries include lacerations, impaled objects, burns, and musculoskeletal injuries.

- *Tertiary blast injury.* This phase occurs when the pressure wave and debris impact the patient and he is thrown away from the explosion. Tertiary injuries can produce injuries identical to those sustained by a patient who has been ejected from a vehicle during an MVC.

- *Quaternary blast injury.* In this phase, injuries are caused by environmental conditions following an explosion. Examples of quaternary blast injuries include crush injuries following structural collapse, toxic fume inhalation injuries resulting from breathing fumes in the air following the explosion, or burns as a result of fire following the explosion.

Significant Mechanisms of Injury (MOIs)

Significant MOIs are those which have been associated through research with life-threatening injuries. Consider the MOI of your patient in order to determine if the potential for life-threatening injury exists. MOIs that are considered significant are as follows (Table 34-1):

- Ejection from a vehicle
- Death of someone in the same vehicle
- Rollover MVC
- High-speed collisions, defined as greater than 40 mph
- Pedestrian struck by a vehicle
- Falls from greater than 20 feet (10 feet for pediatric patients)
- Motorcycle and rider separation
- Penetrating trauma to the head, neck, torso, or proximal extremity
- Significant blunt trauma to the head, neck, or torso

TABLE 34-1	Mechanisms That Indicate High Potential for Significant Injury

	Significant Mechanisms of Injury
Maintain a High Index of Suspicion	Ejection from a vehicle
	Death of someone in the same vehicle
	Rollover MVC
	High-speed collisions (>40 mph)
	Pedestrian struck by a vehicle
	Falls of >20 feet (>10 feet for pediatrics)
	Motorcycle and rider separation
	Penetrating trauma to the head, neck, torso, or proximal extremity
	Significant blunt trauma to the head, neck, or torso

Advance EMTs Mac and Courtney were dispatched to a single-vehicle MVC for which first responders are requesting air transport for the patient. Upon arrival at the scene, Mac and Courtney grab their gear and approach the vehicle, which has impacted a tree with a frontal impact. The car has significant damage to the front and the Advanced EMTs see that the windshield is shattered in a star pattern on the driver side. Emergency Medical Responders have placed the patient on high-flow oxygen via nonrebreather mask and applied a cervical collar.

Problem-Solving Questions

1. What pattern of injuries should Mac and Courtney anticipate?
2. How should they begin their assessment and management?

When you identify any of these significant MOIs, you must have a high index of suspicion that life-threatening injury exists. These patients often require surgical intervention to correct life-threatening injuries and therefore must be transported to a facility with surgical services available.

Nonsignificant Mechanisms of Injury

Not all calls for injured patients involve significant MOIs. But, patients with less-severe injuries can require EMS care, too. Those patients may be in severe pain and require evaluation and treatment in the hospital setting. Your role is to assess the patient, treat and package him, and provide transport to an appropriate facility.

Primary Assessment

The goal of the primary assessment is to identify immediate life threats and treat them as they are identified so that the patient's condition does not deteriorate. Use a systematic approach when performing the primary assessment and complete the primary assessment before performing a head-to-toe exam and treating non–life-threatening injuries. In some cases, trauma patients have gruesome injuries that can be distracting. Do not allow the injuries to distract you from performing a systematic primary assessment.

The primary assessment of a trauma patient consists of the following six steps:

1. Manually stabilizing the head and neck if the MOI is consistent with the potential for cervical spine injury
2. Determining airway status
3. Determining breathing status
4. Determining circulation status
5. Determining disability or level of consciousness

If you encounter a patient who appears to be unresponsive, immediately check the patient's pulse at the carotid artery. Depending on your trauma protocols, the patient may or may not be a candidate for attempted resuscitation. In some systems, patients with blunt trauma who are in cardiac arrest, or patients with unsurvivable injuries, such as mid-section transection, are not resuscitated. If the patient is a candidate for resuscitation according to your protocols and you do not feel a pulse, place the patient in the supine position as quickly as possible while maintaining manual inline stabilization of the head and neck, and begin CPR. For patients who are responsive, even with decreased responsiveness, follow the steps as outlined earlier.

Manual Stabilization of the Head and Neck

Prior to beginning the assessment of a trauma patient, you must consider the possibility of injury to the spine. It is not possible to determine in the field if injury to the spine exists; thus, you must consider the possibility. As a general rule, perform and maintain manual stabilization of the head and neck when any one of the following exists:

- Forces have been applied to the head, neck, or back.
- Neurologic deficits of the extremities are present.
- The patient has altered mental status.

Manual stabilization of the head and neck is accomplished by placing your hands on both sides of the head and holding it in a neutral inline position (Figure 34-19). Inline manual stabilization is an important consideration, but you must never let it interfere with airway management.

Airway

After considering manual stabilization of the head and neck, assess the patient's airway. When a patient is conscious, it is easy to determine if the airway is patent. If the patient is able to speak without difficulty and in full sentences, consider the airway to be patent.

If blood, vomit, or other fluids are in the airway, clear it by suctioning the airway prior to manually opening it.

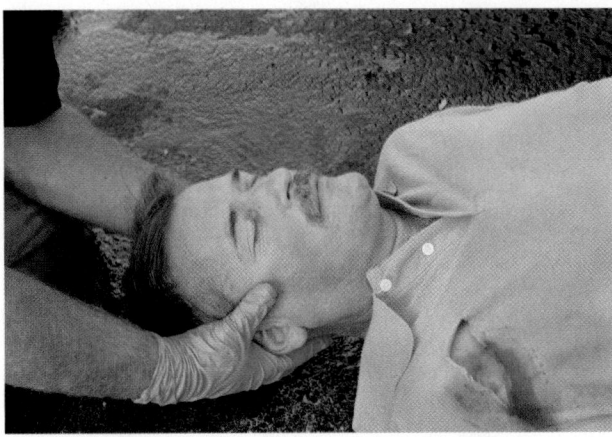

FIGURE 34-19

When a trauma patient has the potential for spine injury, manually stabilize his head and neck to restrict motion as soon as you make contact with him.

IN THE FIELD

Patients who have sustained significant traumatic brain injury are prone to projectile vomiting, so you must have suction readily available and be prepared to clear the airway.

Remember, abnormal respiratory sounds such as gurgling, snoring, or stridor are indicative of a partially obstructed airway and you must manage them.

If the patient is unconscious or has a decreased level of consciousness, assessment of the airway is more difficult. In order to determine if the airway is patent, look, listen, and feel for breathing. This is accomplished by positioning yourself at the patient's head and manually opening the airway using a modified jaw-thrust maneuver while maintaining manual stabilization of the head and neck. Place your ear about 6 inches from the patient's mouth and nose. While in this position, look for rise and fall of the patient's chest, listen for air entering and exiting the airway, and feel for air exiting the patient's airway. If you cannot open and maintain the airway using a modified jaw-thrust maneuver, use a head-tilt/chin-lift maneuver. Once the airway is open, insert a nasal or oral airway adjunct to help maintain an open airway.

Breathing

Once the patient's airway is open, ensure adequate breathing. If breathing is adequate, apply oxygen, if needed, to maintain an SpO_2 of 95% or higher. If breathing is not adequate, ventilate the patient using a bag-valve mask attached to high-flow oxygen. Consider both the rate and depth of breathing when determining adequacy. Rates of less than 8 to 10 breaths per minute or shallow breaths mean that breathing is inadequate and requires intervention.

If the patient complains of difficulty breathing or if there is inadequate rise and fall of the chest, auscultate for lung sounds. If lung sounds are diminished or absent on one side of the chest, pneumothorax or hemothorax may be present. Tension pneumothorax is an immediately life-threatening situation involving breathing that must be treated without delay. (This is discussed further in Chapter 38.)

Circulation

When assessing circulation in the trauma patient, follow these three steps:

- Pulse check
- Skin condition (and capillary refill in pediatric patients)
- Blood sweep

Quickly feel for a radial pulse. If you cannot feel a radial pulse, immediately feel for a carotid pulse. Assess the pulse for rate, rhythm, and quality.

While assessing the patient's pulse, simultaneously assess skin condition. Is the patient's skin cool, clammy, and diaphoretic? If so, the patient is exhibiting signs of shock.

Performing a blood sweep consists of visually inspecting the patient for visible bleeding. To assess the entire posterior of the patient to identify serious bleeding, quickly slide your gloved hands beneath the patient and then slide them out to see if blood is present on your gloves. If life-threatening bleeding is present, control it immediately before you perform any other treatment. Once bleeding is controlled, continue the primary assessment.

Disability

Disability is the patient's level of responsiveness. By the time you have assessed the patient's airway, breathing, and circulation, you will have also assessed the patient's level of responsiveness. Initially, use the AVPU mnemonic to describe the level of responsiveness. You also will have gained information needed to determine the patient's Glasgow Coma Scale score (GCS). The GCS is a quick and simple method to determine level of consciousness (Table 34-2).

A patient can have a maximum score of 15 and a minimum score of 3. There can be many combinations of scores, which you should always document by category. For example, if a patient has spontaneous eye opening, provides inappropriate responses, and follows commands, document his score as follows: E-4, V-3, M-6. A GCS of less than 14 is considered significant and you should consider the patient a priority patient.

Expose

Once the primary assessment is completed, expose critical trauma patients, or those with significant MOIs, to prepare for a rapid trauma exam in the secondary assessment. Remove, move, or cut clothing so that you can see the head, neck, chest, abdomen, back, and extremities to look for signs

TABLE 34-2   Glasgow Coma Scale

EYE OPENING	Points	VERBAL RESPONSE	Points	MOTOR RESPONSE	Points
Spontaneous	4	Oriented	5	Obeys commands	6
To voice	3	Confused	4	Localizes pain	5
To pain	2	Inappropriate words	3	Withdraws	4
None	1	Incomprehensible sounds	2	Abnormal flexion	3
		None	1	Abnormal extension	2
				None	1

of significant injury. If it is necessary to expose the patient, keep in mind that hypothermia occurs easily in the patient in shock, even in warm temperatures, and hypothermia worsens the outcome of severely injured patients. For that reason, and to protect the patient's modesty, consider performing this step in the back of the ambulance if you are able to load the patient into the ambulance without delay. If you must expose the patient in the open where people have gathered, you should take steps to shield the patient from bystanders. For example, you could direct firefighters or law enforcement officers to hold up sheets around the patient. You cannot treat what you cannot see, so it is important to visually inspect the patient. Once you have completed the rapid trauma exam, keep the patient warm by covering him with blankets.

Secondary Assessment

The secondary assessment is performed to identify life-threatening injuries that were not identified in the primary assessment. This assessment consists of the following:

- A rapid trauma assessment for critical patients and those with a significant MOI
- Baseline vital signs
- Medical history
- Either a focused or head-to-toe exam, depending on the patient's MOI, complaints, and overall condition

Rapid Trauma Exam

The rapid trauma exam is a quick visualization and palpation of vital areas of the body to identify life-threatening injuries that may not have been evident in the primary assessment. During the rapid trauma assessment, you will visualize and palpate the head, neck, chest, abdomen, pelvis, extremities, and the posterior of the patient. The following **DCAP-BTLS** mnemonic serves as a reminder of the signs of injury you will assess for:

D – *Deformity.* A deformity is the abnormal shape or size of a body part typically caused by broken bones, dislocated joints, and swelling.

C – *Contusions or crepitus.* Contusions result from bleeding beneath intact skin and are characterized by a discoloration of the skin. **Crepitus** is a grating sound, such as that made by bone fragments or subcutaneous air.

A – *Abrasions.* Abrasions result from skin tissue being removed from the body as a result of friction.

P – *Penetrating trauma.* Penetrating trauma results from an object puncturing the skin. It is important to attempt to identify how deep the puncture wound is in order to determine if underlying structures may have been affected.

B – *Burns.* Burns are tissue destruction that results from thermal, electrical, or chemical contact. You should assess the amount of body surface area affected. This will be discussed in detail in Chapter 35.

T – *Tenderness.* Tenderness is pain that is felt with palpation.

L – *Lacerations.* Lacerations are cuts in the skin that may be jagged or very precise, depending on the object that created the wound.

S – *Swelling.* Swelling is the enlargement of a body part caused by the accumulation of blood and other body fluids within the tissues surrounding an injury.

You will only treat life-threatening injuries during this assessment. You will note any non–life-threatening injuries so that you can address them while en route to the hospital.

To perform the rapid trauma assessment, do the following (Figure 34-20):

- *Head.* Palpate and inspect the head for signs of injury, including the posterior skull and facial structures.
- *Neck.* Palpate and inspect the neck for signs of injury. Assess for jugular venous distension and tracheal deviation. Once your assessment of the neck is

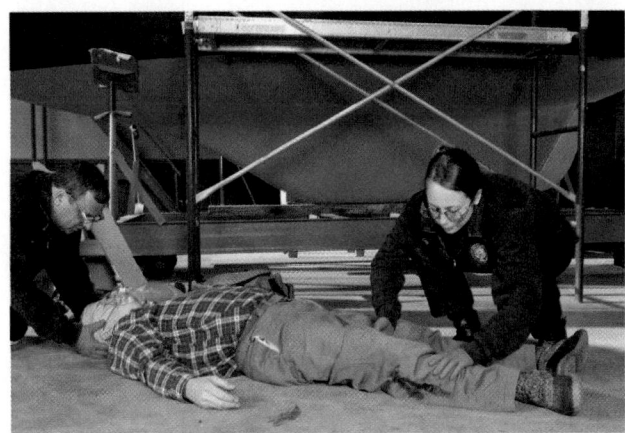

FIGURE 34-20

The rapid trauma assessment is performed to identify life-threatening injuries that were not identified during the primary assessment.

TABLE 34-3	SAMPLE History
S	Signs and symptoms
A	Allergies
M	Medications
P	Past medical history
L	Last oral intake
E	Events leading up to the injury

complete, properly size and apply a cervical collar to the patient, if indicated.

- *Chest.* Palpate and inspect the chest for signs of injury, paradoxical movement of the chest wall, and subcutaneous emphysema. Reassess breath sounds at this time, as well.

- *Abdomen.* Palpate and inspect the abdomen for signs of injury.

- *Pelvis.* Palpate and inspect for signs of injury and loss of bladder or bowel control. Assess the pelvis by placing one hand on each of the hips and applying gentle pressure in a downward and inward direction. Do not "rock" the hips back and forth or apply a significant amount of pressure to the hips.

- *Posterior.* Palpate and inspect the posterior for signs of injury. In order to access the posterior of the patient, perform a log roll while maintaining manual stabilization of the head and neck.

- *Extremities.* Palpate and inspect all extremities for signs of injury. Assess the hands and feet for circulation, movement, and sensation.

Baseline Vital Signs

Obtain a set of baseline vital signs to use as a comparison for subsequent vital signs. The baseline vital signs consist of the following:

- Respiratory rate
- Pulse rate
- Blood pressure

A single set of vital signs only indicates the patient's condition at that point in time. It is the subsequent vital signs compared to the baseline vital signs that will allow you to identify trends. Those trends may indicate that the patient's condition is improving, remaining unchanged, or deteriorating. Retake vital signs as part of the reassessment process.

Patient History

Part of the secondary assessment is obtaining the patient's history. Follow the SAMPLE mnemonic as described in Chapter 19 (Table 34-3).

Critical Trauma Patients

At this point in the assessment process, you will have gathered enough information to determine whether the patient is critical or non-critical. The following findings indicate that the patient is critical:

- Glasgow Coma Scale less than 14
- Systolic blood pressure less than 90 mmHg
- Respiratory rate less than 12 or greater than 29 (less than 20 in an infant under one year of age)

If the patient is critical your goal is to efficiently treat and package the patient and begin transport as soon as possible. Proper scene management when caring for a patient who is unstable includes minimizing scene time. Ideally, the scene time for a critical trauma patient is less than 10 minutes. However, the need to transport without delay is not an excuse for not carrying out needed assessments and interventions. Entrapment, scene characteristics, and other situations can extend the scene time, as well. Do your best to initiate transport without delay, but without jeopardizing your safety or the patient's care.

Focused Trauma Exam

When caring for patients who have an isolated injury without significant MOI, such as a twisted ankle from stepping in a hole, it is only necessary to examine the area of the patient's chief complaint. While performing a focused trauma exam, you should use the applicable components of the head-to-toe exam discussed in the next section.

Head-to-Toe Exam

For critical patients, after you have identified and addressed all life threats, package the patient for transport. Once en route to the most appropriate hospital, perform a

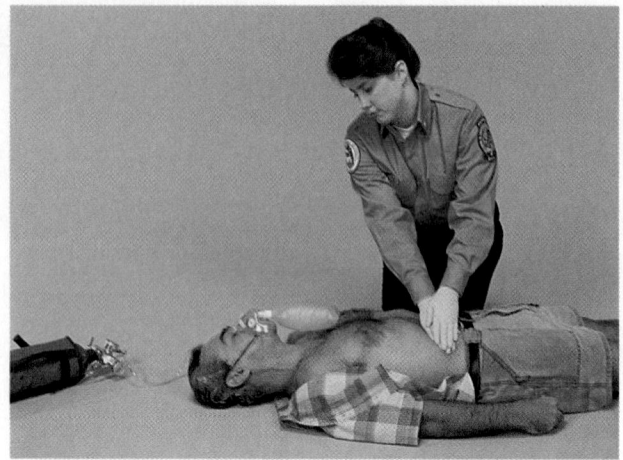

FIGURE 34-21

The head-to-toe exam is a complete head-to-toe assessment in which all injuries are identified. This assessment should not delay transport; rather, you should perform it en route to the hospital emergency department.

head-to-toe exam. (Figure 34-21). The head-to-toe exam is performed to identify all injuries. Begin at the patient's head and look for injuries by systematically inspecting and palpating the entire body. Use the DCAP-BTLS mnemonic to remember what signs of injury you are looking for. Proceed as follows (Scan 34-1):

- *Head.* Gently palpate the entire head and look inside the ears for blood and/or cerebrospinal fluid.

- *Face.* Gently palpate the bones of the face and inspect the nose and mouth for the presence of fluids. Inspect the eyes for equality and reactivity using a penlight.

- *Neck.* Palpate the anterior and posterior neck. Assess the trachea to identify if it is midline or not. Assess for jugular venous distention (JVD).

- *Chest.* Gently palpate and inspect the chest wall.

- *Abdomen.* Gently inspect and palpate the four quadrants of the abdomen.

- *Pelvis.* Palpate both sides of the pelvis and gently press downward and inward.

- *Posterior.* Log roll the patient and gently palpate and inspect the posterior surfaces of the body.

- *Extremities.* Assess for circulation, motor function, and sensation in all four extremities. Gently palpate and inspect each extremity.

Maintain awareness of the patient's airway, breathing, and circulation while you are performing the head-to-toe exam. If the patient requires immediate attention regarding the ABCs, immediately discontinue the head-to-toe exam and address them. In some cases, you do not have time to perform a head-to-toe exam on your patient. If the patient

is critical, you may spend all of your time with them addressing life-threatening injuries and not have time to complete the head-to-toe exam.

Once the head-to-toe exam is complete, you will address any non–life-threatening injuries as time permits.

Reassessment

Once you have addressed all injuries, it is important to continually reassess the patient en route to the hospital. For critical patients, reassess vital signs and interventions every 5 minutes, or more frequently. For non-critical patients, reassess every 15 minutes.

Mode of Transport and Destination Decision

When faced with a critical trauma patient, you must make decisions regarding mode of transport and transport destination. In years past, EMS professionals would quickly package patients and provide rapid transport to the closest emergency department. In today's EMS systems, transporting the patient to the *most appropriate facility* is part of the care that you provide to the patient. You must weigh both the distance of the facility and the capabilities it can provide when you are making transport mode and destination decisions. Ensuring transport to an appropriate hospital may decrease morbidity and provide the patient the best chance at survival.

Mode of Transport

Mode of transport refers to the method used to transport a patient to the closest, most appropriate facility. The most appropriate facility is the destination where the services meeting the needs of the patient are present. The most appropriate facility for critical trauma patients is one with surgery readily available. When working in an urban EMS system, the decision for mode of transport usually does not apply because transport by ground via ambulance is the fastest mode, unless there are extenuating circumstances. Advanced EMTs who work in rural communities must determine whether transport by ground or air would be most appropriate for the patient (Figure 34-22).

Your EMS system's policies and protocols give guidance regarding requesting air medical transport. In general, consider the following when determining if air transport is indicated:

- The patient's condition
- Estimated time of arrival (ETA) of the aircraft
- Weather conditions
- Ground transport time
- Location of potential landing zones

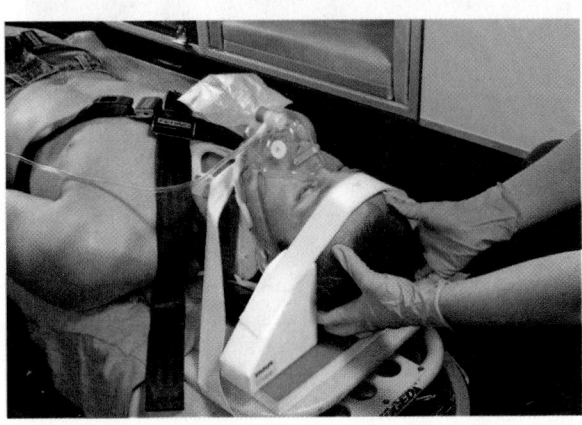

1. Run your gloved hands over the scalp and through the hair. Note any blood on your gloves.

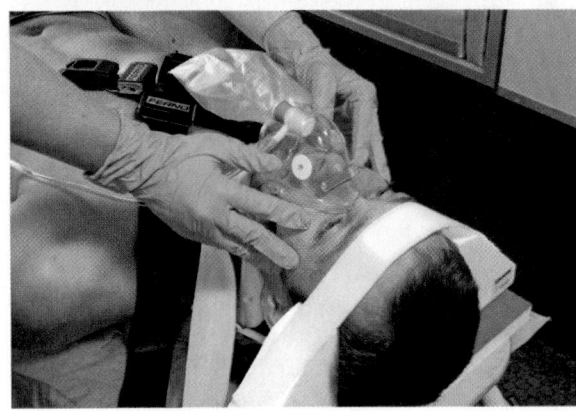

2. Palpate the face, forehead, and jaw.

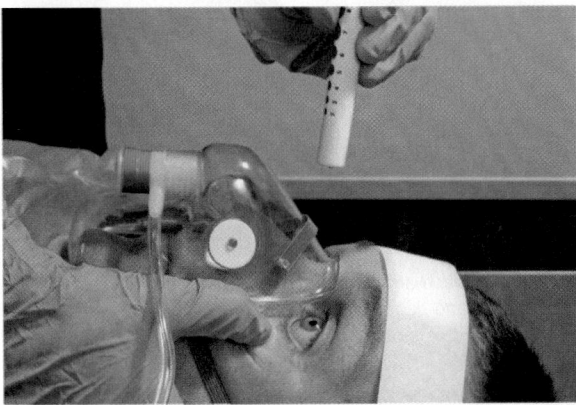

3. Observe the pupils using an appropriate light source.

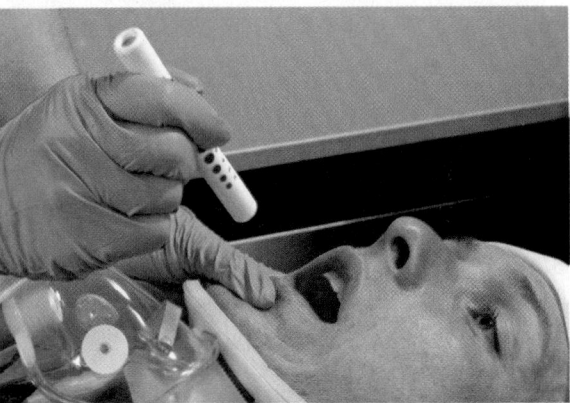

4. Observe for drainage of blood or cerebrospinal fluid, flaring of nostrils, and damage to teeth. Look behind the ears for bruising (Battle's sign).

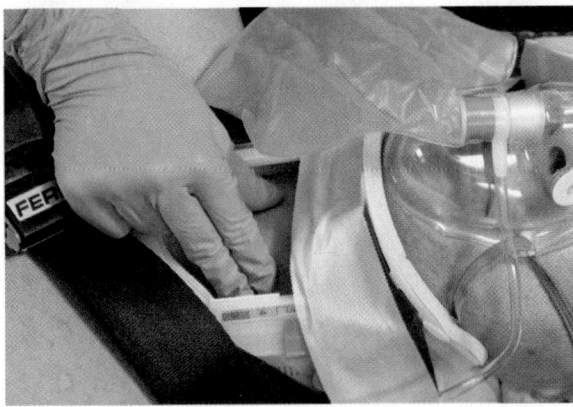

5. Observe for JVD and run your thumb and forefinger along both sides of the trachea to confirm proper alignment. Note any retractions above the clavicles.

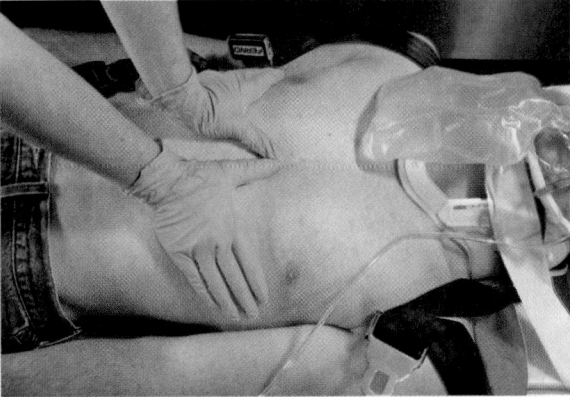

6. Palpate the chest with both hands, feeling for crepitus or subcutaneous emphysema, then listen for equal breath sounds and observe for paradoxical movement of the chest.

(continued)

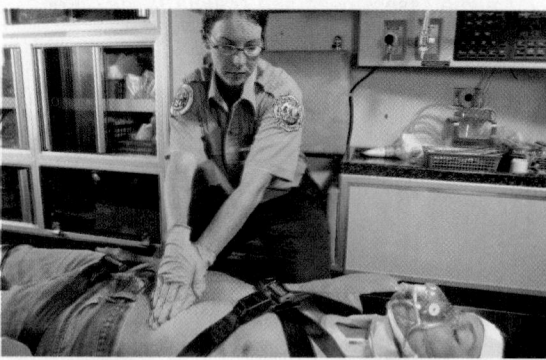

7. Palpate each quadrant of the abdomen with both hands. Observe the patient's face for signs of grimacing, and note body language for evidence of guarding.

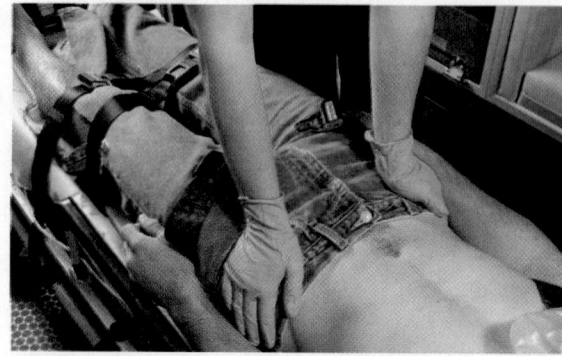

8. Palpate both sides of the pelvis gently with both hands. Press downward and outward gently. Observe for signs of wetness that may be blood or urine.

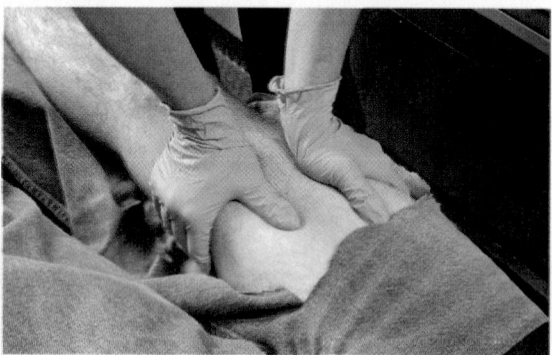

9. Palpate each leg with both hands and assess distal pulses, and sensation. Have the patient push and pull against the resistance of your hands to test for motor function.

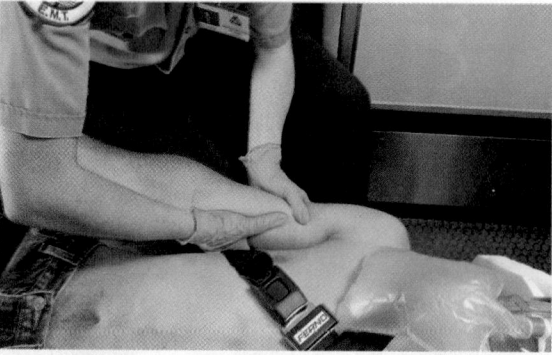

10. Palpate each arm with both hands, and assess distal pulses, and sensation. Have the patient squeeze both hands with his simultaneously to test for motor function.

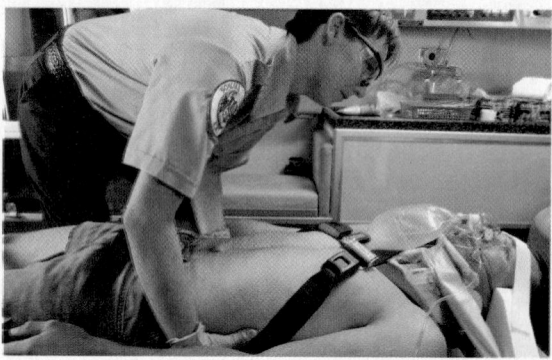

11. Palpate as much of the back as you can with both hands, feeling for soft spots (paradoxical movement) and crepitus (subcutaneous emphysema or rib fractures).

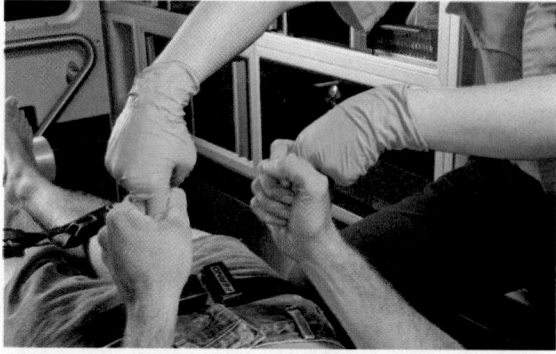

12. Use both hands to perform the grip test.

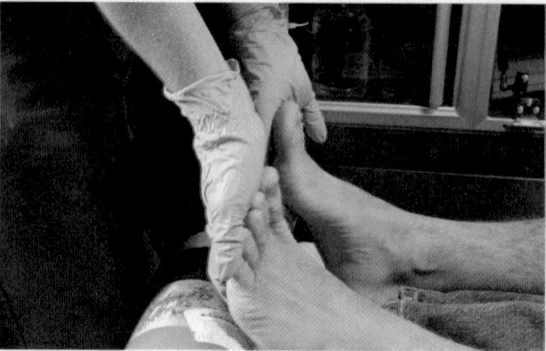

13. Perform the foot-flex test against both feet.

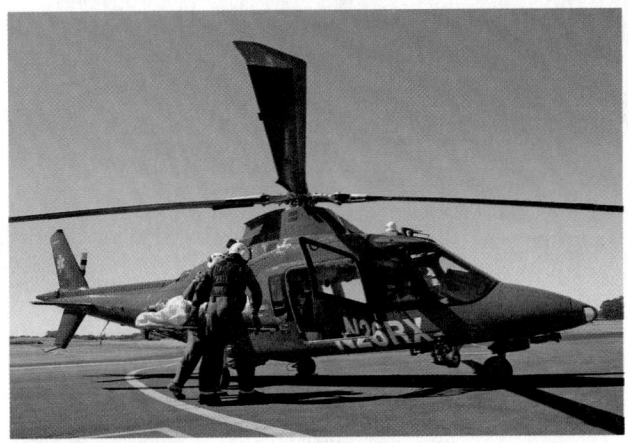

FIGURE 34-22

You must determine the most appropriate mode of transport of the patient.

It may not be the best decision to remain on scene with a critical trauma patient waiting for the arrival of the aircraft. In some cases, it will be faster to transport by ground.

Destination Decision

Today there are many specialty care hospitals that provide specific services. These include trauma centers, pediatric centers, and burn centers. When making a **destination decision,** you must identify the needs of the patient and provide transport to the nearest, most appropriate facility that meets those needs. For instance, if the patient has internal bleeding, the patient will not benefit from transport to a facility that does not have surgical services available. If the patient is transported to this nonsurgical facility, he will have to be transferred to a facility that does have surgical services, causing a significant delay in definitive care that could lead to an increase in morbidity and possibly even death.

IN THE FIELD

Each year, the approximately one million EMS providers have a substantial impact on the care of injured persons and on public health in this country. The profound importance of daily on-scene triage decisions made by EMS providers is reinforced by CDC-supported research showing that the overall risk of death was 25 percent lower when care was provided at a Level I trauma center than when it was provided at a nontrauma center.

The "Field Triage Decision Scheme: The National Trauma Triage Protocol" (Decision Scheme) (Figure 34-23) educational initiative was developed to help EMS providers, EMS medical directors, trauma system leadership, and EMS management learn about and implement the revised Decision Scheme. This Decision Scheme was developed in 2006 in partnership with the American College of Surgeons–Committee on Trauma and the National Highway Traffic Safety Administration (NHTSA) and is grounded in current best practices in trauma triage. It has been endorsed by 17 organizations, along with concurrence from NHTSA, and is intended to be the foundation for the development, implementation, and evaluation of local and regional field triage protocols.

As part of this initiative, CDC has developed easy-to-use materials for EMS professionals. Each of these materials provides information that EMS professionals can use to take an active role in improving the health outcomes for persons injured in their communities.

Additional information on the Field Triage Decision Scheme: The National Trauma Triage Protocol can be found on the Centers for Disease Control website at the following web address: http://www.cdc.gov/fieldtriage/

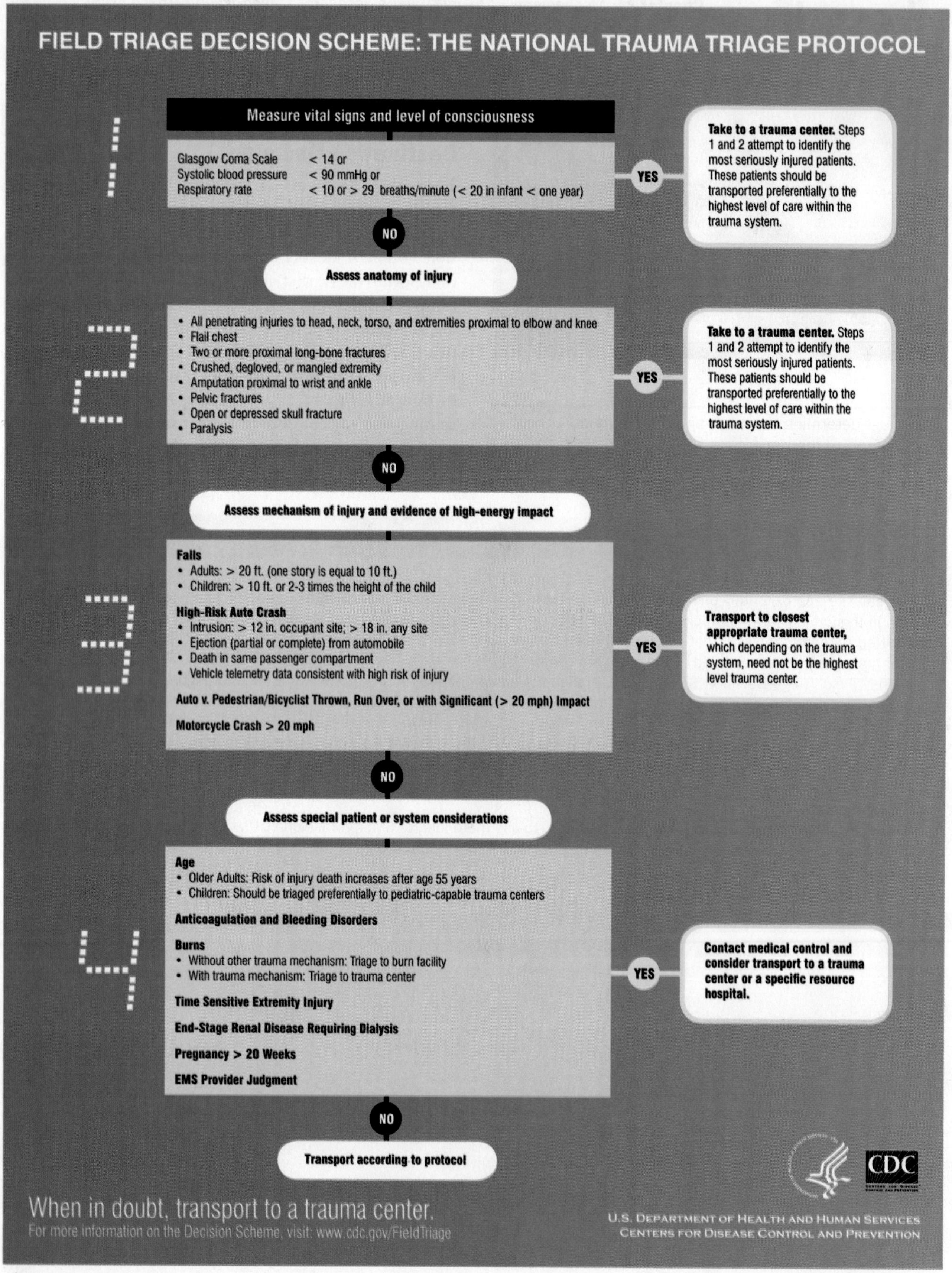

FIELD TRIAGE DECISION SCHEME: THE NATIONAL TRAUMA TRIAGE PROTOCOL

1

Measure vital signs and level of consciousness

Glasgow Coma Scale	< 14 or
Systolic blood pressure	< 90 mmHg or
Respiratory rate	< 10 or > 29 breaths/minute (< 20 in infant < one year)

YES → **Take to a trauma center.** Steps 1 and 2 attempt to identify the most seriously injured patients. These patients should be transported preferentially to the highest level of care within the trauma system.

NO ↓

2

Assess anatomy of injury

- All penetrating injuries to head, neck, torso, and extremities proximal to elbow and knee
- Flail chest
- Two or more proximal long-bone fractures
- Crushed, degloved, or mangled extremity
- Amputation proximal to wrist and ankle
- Pelvic fractures
- Open or depressed skull fracture
- Paralysis

YES → **Take to a trauma center.** Steps 1 and 2 attempt to identify the most seriously injured patients. These patients should be transported preferentially to the highest level of care within the trauma system.

NO ↓

3

Assess mechanism of injury and evidence of high-energy impact

Falls
- Adults: > 20 ft. (one story is equal to 10 ft.)
- Children: > 10 ft. or 2-3 times the height of the child

High-Risk Auto Crash
- Intrusion: > 12 in. occupant site; > 18 in. any site
- Ejection (partial or complete) from automobile
- Death in same passenger compartment
- Vehicle telemetry data consistent with high risk of injury

Auto v. Pedestrian/Bicyclist Thrown, Run Over, or with Significant (> 20 mph) Impact

Motorcycle Crash > 20 mph

YES → **Transport to closest appropriate trauma center,** which depending on the trauma system, need not be the highest level trauma center.

NO ↓

4

Assess special patient or system considerations

Age
- Older Adults: Risk of injury death increases after age 55 years
- Children: Should be triaged preferentially to pediatric-capable trauma centers

Anticoagulation and Bleeding Disorders

Burns
- Without other trauma mechanism: Triage to burn facility
- With trauma mechanism: Triage to trauma center

Time Sensitive Extremity Injury

End-Stage Renal Disease Requiring Dialysis

Pregnancy > 20 Weeks

EMS Provider Judgment

YES → **Contact medical control and consider transport to a trauma center or a specific resource hospital.**

NO ↓

Transport according to protocol

When in doubt, transport to a trauma center.
For more information on the Decision Scheme, visit: www.cdc.gov/FieldTriage

CDC

U.S. DEPARTMENT OF HEALTH AND HUMAN SERVICES
CENTERS FOR DISEASE CONTROL AND PREVENTION

FIGURE 34-23

The Field Triage Decision Scheme: Use the National Trauma Triage Protocol to identify and categorize trauma patients. (Courtesy of the Centers for Disease Control)

CASE STUDY WRAP-UP

Clinical-Reasoning Process

Upon arrival at the patient's side, Mac introduces himself, but the patient does not respond. The patient is breathing 14 times per minute with good chest expansion. His skin is pale, cool to the touch, and diaphoretic. While the patient has multiple lacerations to his face, scalp, and arms there is no life-threatening bleeding present. To assess level of responsiveness, Mac elicits a painful response and though the patient pulls away and groans, his eyes do not open.

The crew works together to perform a rapid trauma exam. Courtney points out to Mac that there is a large hematoma on the patient's forehead and bruising to his right chest wall. Mac says, "He also has fractures with deformity to both of his legs."

Meanwhile, dispatch advises that AirMed has a 17-minute ETA but will have to land about a quarter mile from the scene. "With cool-down, loading, and a roof-helipad landing at the hospital, we can get the patient to the trauma center before AirMed can," says Mac. "Go ahead and cancel them."

"Agreed," says Courtney. After cancelling AirMed, she says, "It looks like he took an up-and-over pathway. That's consistent with his head injury and could be why he has decreased responsiveness."

"A steering wheel impact to the chest and abdomen could explain why he's shocky, too," says Mac. "I suspect he has some internal bleeding." With the help of the EMRs, the crew rapidly extricates the patient and immobilizes him on a long backboard while monitoring his airway, breathing, and circulation. One of the EMRs volunteers to drive so that Courtney and Mac can focus their full attention on the patient.

En route the crew continues to monitor the patient's airway, breathing, and circulation. Courtney obtains a set of baseline vital signs and applies the pulse oximeter while Mac performs a head-to-toe exam. As Mac begins a preliminary radio report to the trauma center, Courtney prepares to start two IV lines.

During the 20-minute transport, Courtney and Mac keep the patient warm and reassess him every 5 minutes. A 1,000 mL of normal saline keeps the patient's heart rate in the range of 112 and his blood pressure stays around 104/72.

The patient was diagnosed with a cerebral contusion and a liver laceration, as well as bilateral tibia and fibula fractures, and a right femur fracture. Courtney and Mac's decision to transport by ground was an important factor in minimizing the time to get the patient to surgery and stop the bleeding from his liver and insert a monitor to measure his intracranial pressure. The patient was released from the hospital two weeks after the collision, and is undergoing rehabilitation.

CHAPTER REVIEW

Chapter Summary

While the assessment process for all patients follows the same principles, there are some differences when assessing patients with traumatic injury. The scene of a critical trauma patient will be hectic. You must remain focused on organized, systematic assessment, treatment, packaging, and making decisions about transport. Failure to manage the emergency in an efficient manner can lead to an increase in morbidity and possible death. The goal is to minimize scene times and begin transporting the patient to the nearest appropriate medical facility. You will learn to be efficient and minimize scene times through practice and proper utilization of resources available to you on scene.

Review Questions

Multiple-Choice Questions

1. Injury that occurs to a part of the body as a result of energy being transmitted through the body is called:
   - a. indirect injury.
   - b. direct injury.
   - c. significant MOI.
   - d. blunt trauma.

2. An "up-and-over" path is one that could have occurred during which type of MVC impact?
   - a. Lateral impact
   - b. Rotational impact
   - c. Rear impact
   - d. Frontal impact

3. In which type of MVC is the potential for ejection of the patient most likely?

   a. Rollover
   b. Lateral impact
   c. Rotational impact
   d. Rear impact

4. High-energy penetrating trauma can cause significant internal injury resulting from:

   a. direct injury.
   b. indirect injury.
   c. small-caliber guns.
   d. blunt trauma.

5. You should perform the head-to-toe exam:

   a. after you have managed all life threats.
   b. immediately after the scene size-up.
   c. in conjunction with the primary assessment.
   d. upon arrival at the emergency department.

6. The goal of the _____ is to identify immediate life threats and treat them as they are identified so that the patient's condition does not deteriorate.

   a. scene size-up
   b. primary assessment
   c. secondary assessment
   d. mechanism of injury

Critical-Thinking Questions

7. You arrive on the scene of an MVC and note that there is approximately 18 inches of intrusion to the driver side door of a car that was struck with a lateral impact. What types of injuries would you suspect the driver to have sustained?

8. Explain the potential injuries a patient who was ejected from a vehicle that was involved in a rollover collision could have sustained.

9. List and describe the four phases of blast injuries.

10. Calculate the GCS for this patient: You arrive to find a patient who was ejected from a vehicle involved in a rollover MVC. Once at the patient's side, you note that his eyes are closed and open only to painful stimulus. When you elicit the painful stimulus, the patient groans and reaches out to grab the hand used to elicit the stimulus. When questioned, the patient does not respond verbally. What is this patient's GCS?

References

Centers for Disease Control and Prevention. (2010). *Injury prevention and control: Home and recreational safety.* Retrieved March 15, 2011, from http://www.cdc.gov/HomeandRecreationalSafety/Falls/fallcost.html

Centers for Disease Control and Prevention. (2011. *Injury prevention and control: Motor vehicle safety.* Retrieved March 15, 2011, from http://www.cdc.gov/Motorvehiclesafety/seatbelts/facts.html

35
Soft-Tissue Injuries and Burns

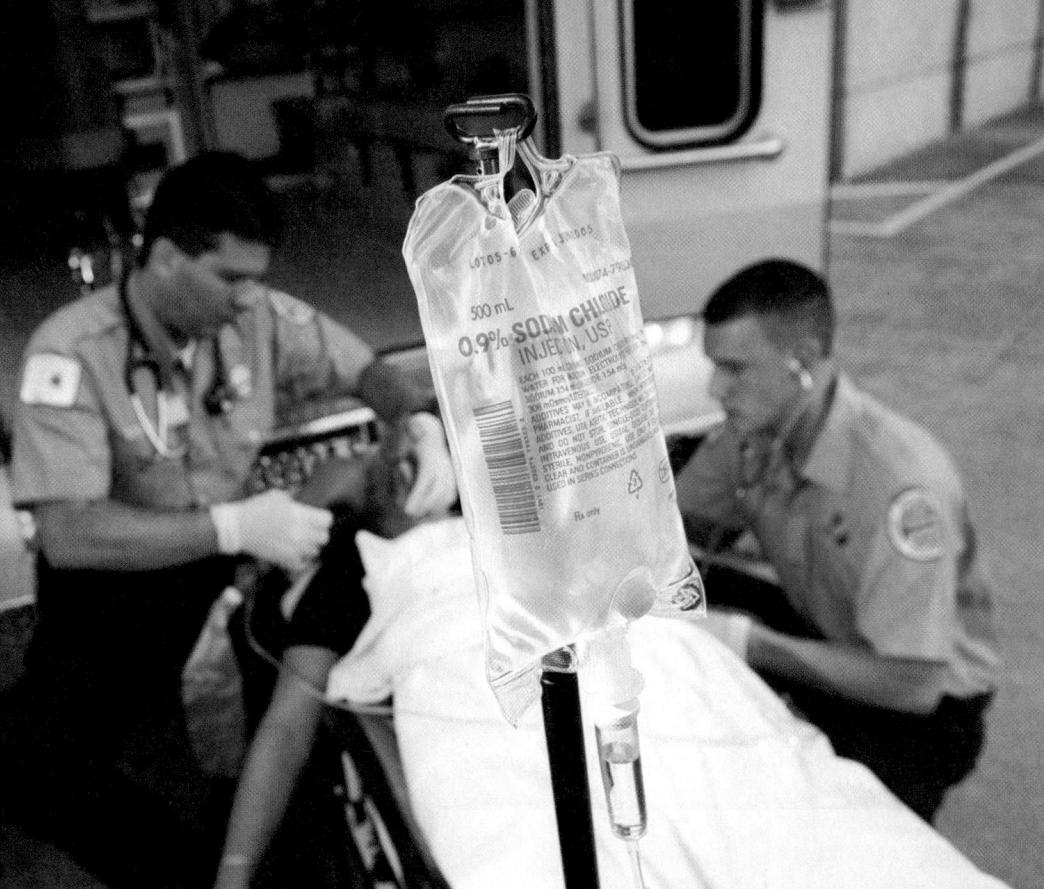

Content Area: Trauma

Advanced EMT Education Standard: The Advanced EMT applies fundamental knowledge to provide basic and selected advanced emergency care and transportation based on assessment findings for an acutely injured patient.

Objectives

After reading this chapter, you should be able to:

35.1 Define key terms introduced in this chapter.

35.2 Discuss the epidemiology and significance of burns and soft-tissue injuries.

35.3 Describe the structure and function of the skin.

35.4 Describe the consequences of damage to the skin.

35.5 Describe special considerations in the scene size-up when responding to calls involving burned patients.

35.6 Describe the effects of burns on the circulatory, respiratory, renal, nervous, and musculoskeletal systems.

35.7 Identify indications of inhalation injury in the burned patient.

(continued)

Resource Central

To access Resource Central, follow the directions on the Student Access Card provided with this text. If there is no card, go to www.bradybooks.com and follow the Resource Central link to Buy Access. Under Media Resources, you will find:

• *Electrical Injury.* The causes and management of electrical injuries.

• *Burns.* Learn about common causes and management of burns in children.

• *Fluid Resuscitation.* Learn how to calculate percent of burned body surface area and how much fluid to administer to these patients.

KEY TERMS (continued)

rule of palm *(p. 808)*	stellate laceration *(p. 799)*	venous bleeding *(p. 801)*	zone of hyperemia *(p. 804)*
scalds *(p. 805)*	subcutaneous layer *(p. 794)*	zone of coagulation *(p. 804)*	zone of stasis *(p. 804)*
steam burns *(p. 805)*	superficial burns *(p. 806)*		

CASE STUDY

At 0200 hours Advanced EMTs Wilson Connery and Paige White are dispatched to a single-vehicle MVC on an interstate that runs directly through the center of the city. "Fire is requesting an EMS ETA," dispatch advises. Paige gives dispatch an 8-minute estimated time of arrival (ETA) as they respond to the scene.

As Wilson and Paige approach the scene, they see the patient's car on fire. A firefighter waves them toward a small group of people gathered around a man lying on the ground approximately 20 yards from the burning car. As they head toward the group, they note that it was a head-on collision with a concrete pole and the car has about 24 inches of intrusion to the front end. The posted speed limit is 55 mph.

A firefighter tells Wilson and Paige that the patient was pinned beneath the steering wheel and dashboard when they arrived. During extrication the car caught fire and the patient sustained burns to his face and arms before he could be freed.

Problem-Solving Questions

1. What does this mechanism of injury suggest?
2. How should Wilson and Paige determine whether the injuries from the MVC or the burns are more critical?
3. What additional information should they obtain from the firefighters?

(continued from previous page)

35.8   Describe procedures for stopping the burning process when responding to a burned patient.

35.9   Given a description or picture of a burn, classify the burn by depth and body surface area involved, for both adult and pediatric patients.

35.10   Consider burn depth, location, body surface area involved, the patient's age, and any pre-existing medical conditions in determining the severity of burn injuries.

35.11   Discuss each of the following types of burns:
- Chemical
- Electrical
- Inhalation
- Radiation
- Thermal

35.12   Discuss each of the following mechanisms of burn injuries:
- Contact
- Electrical
- Flame
- Flash
- Gas
- Scald
- Steam

35.13 Describe special considerations in responding to, assessing, and managing patients with chemical and electrical burns.

35.14 Demonstrate the ability to calculate proper volumes of fluid to be infused into the burn patient using the Parkland burn formula.

35.15 Describe each of the following types of soft-tissue injury:
  – Abrasions
  – Amputations
  – Avulsions
  – Closed injury
  – Contusion
  – Crush injury
  – Hematoma
  – Impaled objects
  – Incisions and lacerations
  – Open injury
  – Punctures

35.16 Describe the pathophysiology and management of complications of soft-tissue injuries and burns, including the following:
  – Bleeding
  – Blood and fluid loss
  – Compartment syndrome
  – Toxic inhalation
  – Traumatic rhabdomyolysis

35.17 Engage in a process of clinical reasoning to effectively prioritize the steps in management of patients with burns and soft-tissue injuries.

35.18 Demonstrate effective methods of controlling bleeding and dressing and bandaging wounds and burns, using a variety of dressing and bandaging materials.

35.19 Describe considerations in retrieving, caring for, and transporting amputated parts.

Introduction

Soft-tissue injuries and burns affect the integumentary system and have some similarities. Open soft-tissue injuries and burns compromise the integrity of the body's largest organ: the skin. Compromised skin leaves patients vulnerable to infection. When large areas of the skin are affected, patients can lose large amounts of fluid and their thermoregulatory mechanisms are impaired. Burns are more than just an injury to the skin. Serious burns affect the function of many vital body systems, such as the respiratory, renal, and cardiovascular systems.

Though most soft-tissue injuries and burns are not life threatening, some are. Soft-tissue injuries and burns are often isolated injuries, but they also can be just one type of injury suffered by a patient with multisystem trauma. The most frequent life-threatening complication of soft-tissue injuries is hemorrhage. Knowing how to properly treat critically injured patients can reduce morbidity and can mean the difference between life and death. Controlling life-threatening bleeding is a basic skill that can save a patient's life.

Beyond the potential for life-threatening injury, patients with soft-tissue injuries often worry about the potential for scarring and disfigurement that can accompany such injuries. Your skills are important here, too, in reassuring patients that many injuries can be repaired with a good cosmetic result and that complete healing takes several months, during which the appearance of the wound will improve.

According to the American Burn Association, an estimated 500,000 burn injuries are treated in the hospital or clinic setting annually, with 40,000 of them requiring admission to a hospital. An estimated 4,000 people die each year as a result of burn injuries (Campbell, 2008).

Major burn injuries are one of the most catastrophic and painful types of soft-tissue injury a person can endure, and can be very stressful for the Advanced EMT to manage. Even though you will not encounter critically burn-injured patients very often, it is important to correctly identify and categorize them to ensure that the patient receives proper care and transport to an appropriate medical facility.

Anatomy and Physiology Review

The skin is the largest organ of the body. It contributes to regulation of fluid balance, protects the body from the environment, provides sensory information about the

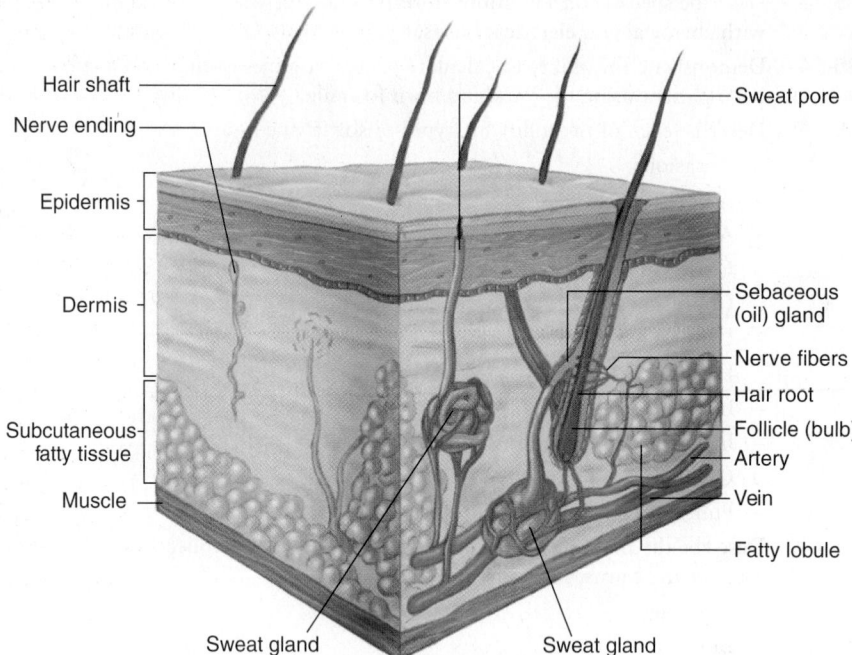

FIGURE 35-1

Cross section of the skin, showing its detailed anatomy.

Labels: Hair shaft, Nerve ending, Epidermis, Dermis, Subcutaneous fatty tissue, Muscle, Sweat gland, Sweat pore, Sebaceous (oil) gland, Nerve fibers, Hair root, Follicle (bulb), Artery, Vein, Fatty lobule, Sweat gland

environment, and assists with the regulation of body temperature. The skin has three layers (Figure 35-1). The **epidermis** is the outermost layer of skin and serves as a barrier between the body and the environment. Just beneath the epidermis is a thick layer of tissue called the *dermis*. The dermis contains blood vessels, oil and sweat glands, hair follicles, and sensory nerves. The innermost layer of skin is the **subcutaneous layer** and is predominantly fatty tissue that assists with body temperature regulation.

Soft-Tissue Injuries

During traumatic injury, the skin becomes damaged; in some cases, the underlying structures of the body may be injured, as well. Injuries to soft tissues are classified as either open or closed injuries. Many mechanisms of injury result in a patient who has both open and closed soft-tissue injuries. Mechanisms of injury that cause soft-tissue injury can also lead to other, more serious injuries. Always look beyond the obvious to assess for other injuries that may be indicated by the presence of soft-tissue

injuries. For example, a contusion, abrasion, or laceration on the head can indicate a skull fracture or traumatic brain injury.

General Assessment and Management of Soft-Tissue Injuries

Begin with a scene size-up to assess the safety of the scene and the mechanism of injury (MOI). Determine the number of patients and request any resources you may need. Violence very frequently results in soft-tissue injuries. When responding to a report of an injured person, perform a careful scene size-up for indications of violence. Obtain additional details about the MOI from the patient or bystanders, if possible. Use the MOI to guide your index of suspicion for the potential for serious injuries. Do not let a dramatic-appearing, yet non-life-threatening injury distract you from fully analyzing the MOI and assessing the patient. Becoming distracted can cause you to lose sight of priorities and cause harm to the patient.

IN THE FIELD

When contusions or hematomas are located on the skin over vital organs, maintain a high index of suspicion that internal injury has occurred and closely monitor the patient for signs and symptoms of shock.

IN THE FIELD

Soft-tissue injuries can be very dramatic looking. Do not be distracted from addressing life threats. Keep your composure and focus when caring for patients with distracting injuries.

Take Standard Precautions to protect yourself from contact with blood and body fluids. Complete a primary assessment, determining the patient's level of responsiveness and evaluating the airway, breathing, and circulation. Again, do not let a dramatic injury distract you from recognizing the need for airway management and ventilation. With open soft-tissue injuries, bleeding can be substantial, meaning that controlling bleeding in the primary assessment is a critical step in patient care.

Patients with minor mechanisms of injury and isolated soft-tissue injuries require only a focused exam, vital signs, and medical history. Patients who have an altered mental status, a problem with airway or breathing, a significant mechanism of injury, or significant bleeding require a rapid trauma exam. Once en route to the hospital, obtain vital signs and a medical history and perform a head-to-toe exam.

Suspect closed soft-tissue injury if you see the following signs during your assessment:

- Pain and tenderness at the injury site
- Edema at the injury site
- Discoloration of the skin at the injury site
- Evidence of internal bleeding, such as signs of hypoperfusion

Suspect open soft-tissue injuries if you see the following during your assessment:

- Break in the integrity of the skin
- Bleeding
- Edema
- Signs and symptoms of hypoperfusion

Reassess the patient for changes in condition and adjust your care accordingly. Reassess critical patients every 5 minutes and reassess noncritical patients every 15 minutes.

General care of soft-tissue injuries starts in the primary assessment if there is life-threatening bleeding. Opening and maintaining an airway, ensuring adequate ventilation and oxygenation, and controlling significant bleeding are the first steps in caring for soft-tissue injuries.

Remove gross contamination and debris from open wounds and control minor bleeding with direct pressure. Irrigation with sterile saline or water can help remove gross contamination (such as small bits of gravel or grass) from

IN THE FIELD

Do not delay transport to initiate intravenous access on scene. Obtain intravenous access en route to an appropriate facility.

Your goal is to treat immediate life threats on scene and minimize on-scene time by initiating transport to an appropriate facility as soon as possible.

minor wounds. Cover open wounds with a dressing and bandage. The pain and swelling from both open and closed wounds can be reduced by immobilizing the injured part, elevating it, and applying a cold pack.

Closed Soft-Tissue Injuries

In **closed soft-tissue injury** the skin remains intact. This type of injury can be caused by blunt trauma or crushing of the tissues. Closed soft-tissue injuries are classified as either contusions or hematomas.

A **contusion** is the black-and-blue discoloration, or bruising, of the skin as a result of bleeding within the dermis. Although contusions turn black and blue with time, eventually changing to green and brown as the blood beneath the skin breaks down, they initially are reddish in color. Some contusions are initially tender to the touch, but the tell-tale mark may not appear for a few hours.

Contusions are rarely life threatening, but may be an indication of injury to underlying tissues and organs. Because of this, it is important to consider the underlying organs beneath the location of a contusion. For instance, you arrive on a scene to find a 28-year-old man who fell 18 feet out of a tree. There is a large contusion to the right upper quadrant of his abdomen. When you attempt to palpate the area, the patient grimaces and pushes your hand away. This is cause for concern, because the liver is located in this region and a contusion indicates blunt trauma resulting from the patient striking a limb as he fell.

This patient has a mechanism of injury and physical findings indicating the potential for injury to his liver and ribs. Although it may take several hours for the actual contusion to form within the skin, you can identify blunt trauma by a patient's complaints of pain and tenderness and by reddening of the skin at the injury site (Figure 35-2).

When bleeding within the tissues is significant enough to accumulate in an area resulting in edema, it is called a

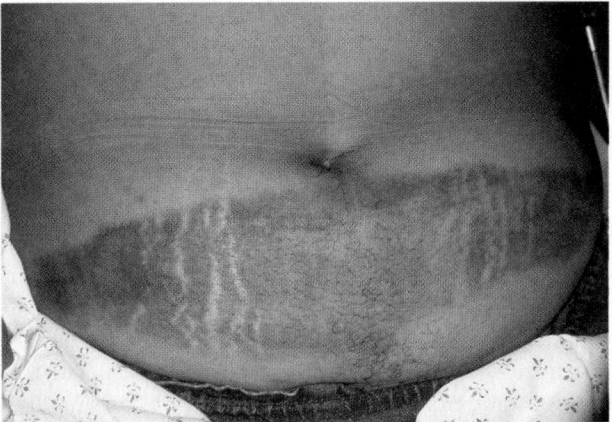

FIGURE 35-2

Contusion of the lower abdomen. (© Charles Stewart, MD, and Associates)

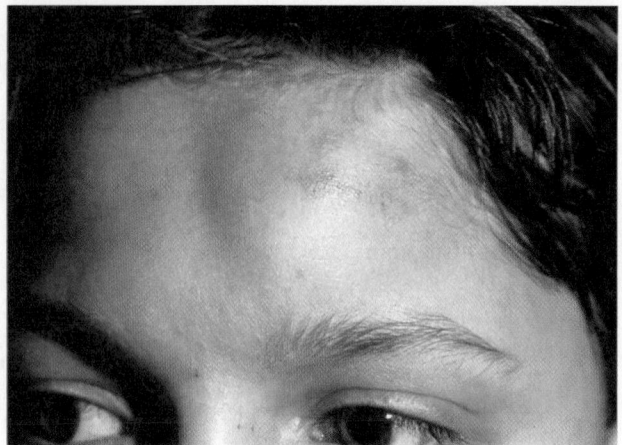

FIGURE 35-3

Hematoma superior to the left eye. (© Dr. P. Marazzi/Photo Researchers, Inc.)

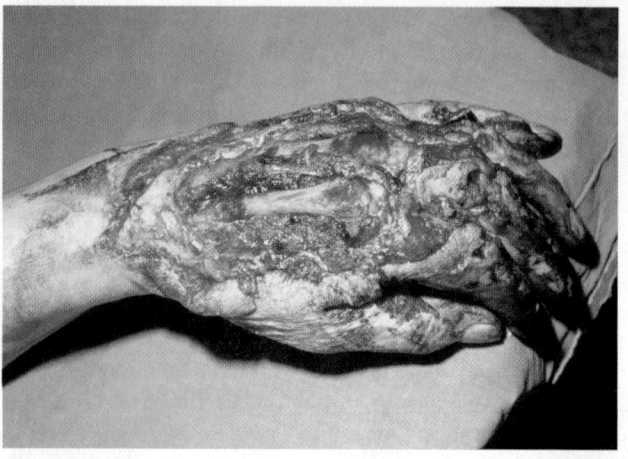

FIGURE 35-4

Crush injury to the hand. (© John Callan/Shout Pictures)

hematoma. The size of the hematoma is directly related to the amount of bleeding that has occurred and presents as a lump with discoloration to the skin at the site of injury (Figure 35-3). Remember to consider the possibility of underlying injury to organs and bone.

Crush injuries are a result of considerable blunt forces that compress the tissues, (Figure 35-4). Patients who are inside buildings that collapse are susceptible to crush injuries by being pinned beneath falling rubble.

Because of the forces that are involved with such injuries, you must consider the potential for injury to underlying structures, including blood vessels, bones, nerves, and organs. Injury to internal structures often leads to internal bleeding and sometimes death. Depending on the forces that cause a crush injury, you may find the injury to be either open or closed. Extensive crush injuries can lead to traumatic rhabdomyolysis, the breakdown of skeletal muscle. Myoglobin and potassium from the damaged skeletal muscle cells are released into the tissues and blood. The excess potassium can cause hyperkalema with associated cardiac dysrhythmias. The myoglobin is toxic to the renal tubules and can lead to acute renal failure. Patients with extensive crush injury can require large amounts of normal saline to prevent renal failure. Make sure you adequately describe any crushing mechanisms when consulting with medical direction about an IV infusion rate.

Compartment syndrome occurs when edema of the extremity reaches a point at which nervous function and circulation to the remainder of the extremity are compromised as a result of being compressed. Muscles and muscle groups are surrounded by fascia forming a compartment of muscle, nerves, and blood vessels. The fascia does not expand; thus, when injury occurs leading to edema within a compartment the muscle, nerves and blood vessels within the compartment become compressed by the increase in pressure. This can lead to permanent damage to the nerves and vessels. Apply cold packs and

TABLE 35-1	The "Five Ps" of Compartment Syndrome

- Pain
- Pallor
- Paralysis
- Paresthesia
- Pulselessness

elevate injured extremites to reduce the edema. Signs and symptoms, the "Five Ps" of compartment syndrome, are listed in Table 35-1.

Open Soft-Tissue Injuries

When an injury breaks the integrity of the skin, it is called an **open injury.** Open injuries can be caused by either penetrating or blunt trauma. When the force of blunt trauma exceeds the strength of the skin, the skin can tear under the blunt force, resulting in a laceration. Open injuries put the patient at risk for bleeding and infection. As with closed injuries, you must consider the possibility of underlying injuries with open injuries. They could include fractured bone, injury to blood vessels, injury to nerves, and injury to organs.

Types of Open Soft-Tissue Injuries

There are five different types of open soft-tissue injuries, as follows:

- Abrasions
- Avulsions
- Amputations
- Punctures/penetrations
- Lacerations

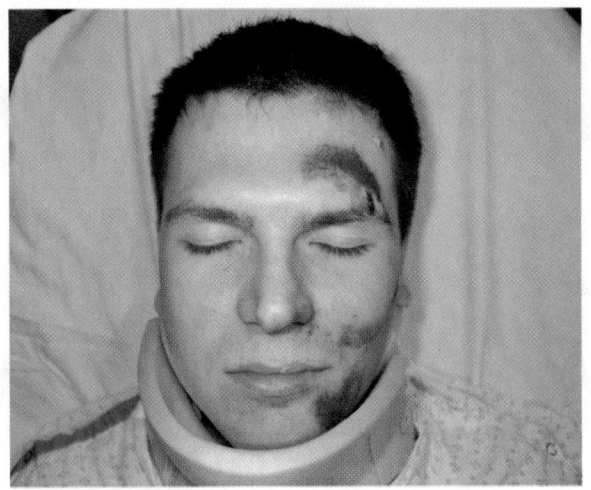

FIGURE 35-5

Abrasions to the face. (© Edward T. Dickinson, MD)

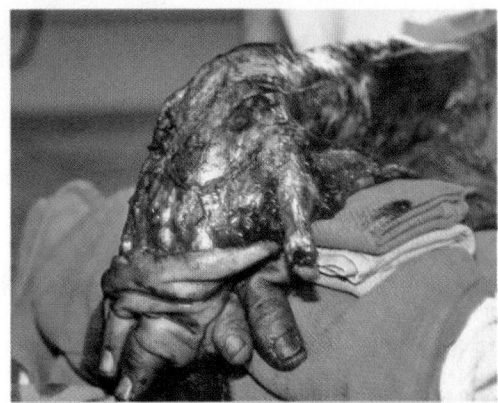

FIGURE 35-6

An avulsion injury that caused a degloving. (© Edward T. Dickinson, MD)

Each of these injuries has its own characteristics that differentiate it from the others.

Abrasions

An **abrasion** is an open injury that results from the skin being removed from the body as a result of friction (Figure 35-5). In most cases, abrasions will affect only the epidermis. In more significant mechanisms of injury, deeper layers of the skin, and even muscle, could be affected.

An example of a more significant mechanism of injury resulting in abrasions of the deeper tissues is a motorcyclist who is not wearing protective clothing and who crashes and skids across an asphalt surface on his back. You would expect to see deep abrasions to the patient's back.

Abrasions are not generally considered to be life threatening, because bleeding from such wounds tends to be a slow oozing of blood from capillaries and will usually stop without treatment. In severe cases, however, abrasions can cover a large body surface area, leading to a greater amount of blood loss and a reason for the Advanced EMT's concern.

Even though bleeding from abrasions is generally not life threatening, do not underestimate the amount of pain the patient may be experiencing. Nerve endings are located in the dermis, which lies just beneath the epidermis. If the epidermis is removed in an abrasion, the nerve endings are exposed, causing pain.

Abrasions carry a risk of infection, because dirt or other foreign substances are often ground into the tissues as the abrasion occurs.

Avulsions

An **avulsion** occurs when a flap of skin, and possibly underlying tissue such as muscle, has been partially removed (partial avulsion) or completely torn away (complete avulsion) (Figure 35-6). Bleeding as a result of an avulsion depends on

the depth of injury. If the avulsion is deep enough to cause injury to larger vessels, bleeding will be more significant. In some cases arteries also can be damaged, leading to life-threatening blood loss. Avulsions that are the result of accidents involving machinery often affect the fingers, hands, and arms.

Amputations

An **amputation** occurs when a body part, usually a digit or extremity, is severed from the body (Figure 35-7). A **partial amputation** refers to a body part that has not been completely detached from the body. Amputations can result from ripping, crushing, or cutting of the tissues and can cause life-threatening hemorrhage. With amputations you will treat the patient, but the amputated part will require proper handling to preserve it for possible surgical reattachment. Amputations are very dramatic events, especially when an entire extremity is involved. You must not let yourself become distracted by the gruesome injury. Doing

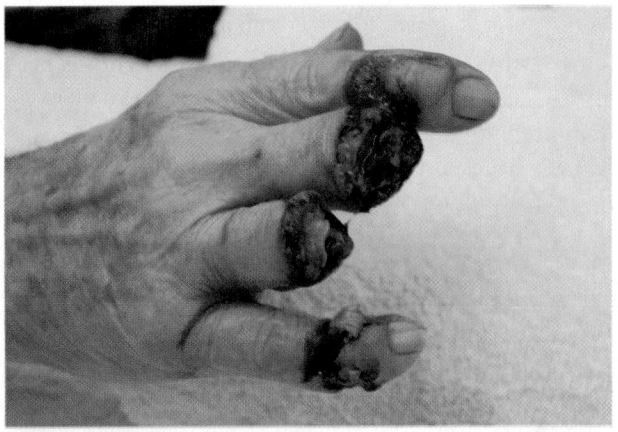

FIGURE 35-7

A hand with three amputated fingers. (© Edward T. Dickinson, MD)

IN THE FIELD

Sometimes an amputation caused by a clean cut with a sharp object does not result in massive hemorrhage, because the elasticity of the vessels causes them to contract and stop or slow the bleeding. In contrast, amputations resulting from a crushing or ripping injury are more likely to produce massive hemorrhage.

In partial amputations the part remains attached by a small amount of tissue Do not cut or tear the remaining tissue to complete the amputation. You will treat the part as described here and immobilize it as best you can.

If the partially amputated part is trapped in machinery or wreckage, contact medical direction. In some cases, a surgeon may respond to the scene for surgical removal of the part in order to free the patient.

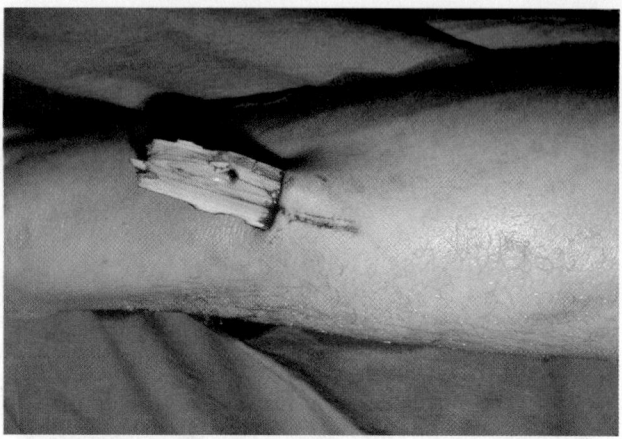

FIGURE 35-8

Penetrating injury to the forearm. (© Charles Stewart, MD, and Associates)

so may lead to your failure to identify a life-threatening problem, which will result in deterioration of the patient's condition.

The steps for proper handling of an amputated part include the following:

1. After taking Standard Precautions, ensure that you have managed all life threats to the patient.

2. Perform gross decontamination of the part by flushing with sterile water and brushing debris away using gauze. Do not immerse the part in any type of fluid, because it may cause damage to the tissues.

3. Wrap the amputated part with sterile dressings. Some systems direct the use of wet dressings, whereas others direct the use of dry dressings. It is important to follow your protocol. If the part is too large to be wrapped, such as an entire arm or leg, decontaminate the open injury end of the part and cover according to protocol.

4. Place the amputated part in a plastic bag or wrap it with plastic to preserve moisture.

5. Keep the part cool by using cold packs or ice, but do not place the part directly on ice, because it may result in tissue damage.

6. Transport the amputated part with the patient to an appropriate facility.

IN THE FIELD

Do not be misled by a puncture/penetrating wound that has minor or no external bleeding. The injury could have caused damage to underlying structures, causing life-threatening internal bleeding that you cannot see.

Punctures/Penetrations

Puncture/penetration injury results from an object being forced into the tissues of the body (Figure 35-8). This can include injuries resulting from stepping on a nail, stab wounds, animal bites, or even gunshot wounds.

Attempt to identify the object that caused the puncture wound and determine its length and diameter. This provides you with an idea of whether there is underlying injury. If the wound is a gunshot wound, attempt to identify the caliber of the bullet and the distance from which the shot occurred. If the object is still in the patient, ask about the length of the object. If the object has been removed, attempt to see it to determine its length and width. This is particularly important in cases in which a puncture wound has occurred to the head, neck, torso, or proximal extremities, because the potential for life-threatening underlying injury exists.

Bleeding can be minor or major, depending on the extent of injury and structures involved. Because dirt and bacteria could be introduced into the tissues during the injury, puncture/penetration injury patients are at high risk for infection.

Bites are puncture/penetrating injuries, the result of teeth being forced into the tissues. Animal bites present additional potential complications to those listed previously, such as infection from bacteria and exposure to diseases such as rabies. Human bites also can result in exposure to diseases such as hepatitis.

An **impaled object** is an object that has penetrated the skin and remains embedded in the tissues (Figure 35-9). Examples of this include, but are not limited to, the following objects that remain embedded in the tissues:

- Knives
- Sticks
- Glass
- Other debris, such as shrapnel from an explosion

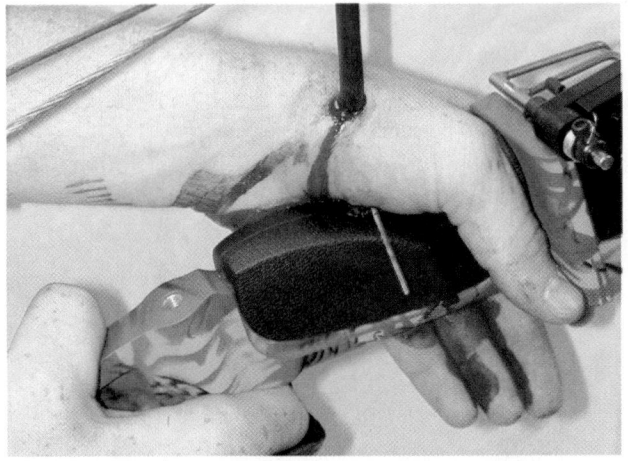

FIGURE 35-9

An impaled object in the hand. (© Charles Stewart, MD, and Associates)

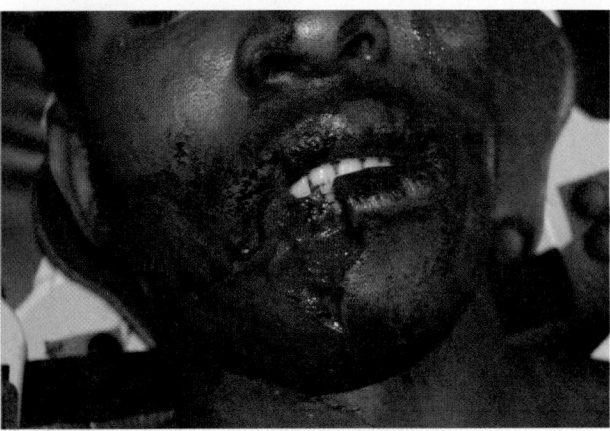

FIGURE 35-10

Lacerations to the face. (© Edward T. Dickinson, MD)

When presented with an impaled object, you will not remove it unless it prevents you from managing the patient's airway and breathing. The impaled object may restrict bleeding while in place. If the object is removed, the injury may begin to bleed. This bleeding may be minor or life threatening, so it is best to leave the object in place and stabilize it for transport.

Stabilizing an impaled object means dressing the wound by applying dressings such as roller gauze or bulky dressings completely around the wound to prevent movement of the object and additional injury. The dressings will then be secured in place using gauze, triangular bandages, or tape.

In some cases, you may be presented with an impaled object that is too large to remain intact or in place for transport. In those cases, you should attempt to cut the object while stabilizing it manually. If it is not possible to shorten the object, you may have to remove it to facilitate transport. You should contact medical direction in those rare situations.

An impaled object through a patient's cheek is the only impaled object that is acceptable to be removed in the field without compromising the patient's condition. Access to both sides of the wound allows direct pressure to be applied from both sides to control bleeding. You should remove an impaled object through the cheek if it poses a threat to airway patency. When removing an impaled object from a patient's cheek, be sure to have dressings and suction available to protect the patient's airway.

Lacerations

Lacerations are open injuries to skin—and, in some cases, underlying tissues—that result from a cutting of the tissues (Figure 35-10). They are categorized as either linear or stellate. A **linear laceration**, also called an *incision*, is an injury in which the cut in the tissues is in a straight line, such as a cut from a knife. The term **stellate laceration**

refers to a starlike laceration, and is a jagged cut in the tissues. Stellate lacerations are commonly the result of blunt trauma that compresses the skin against underlying bony prominences, which cause a jagged or nonlinear laceration to occur from the inside out. An example of this is a boxer who is punched in the nose, resulting in a laceration. In this example, the skin was compressed against the bony prominence of the nasal bone, increasing the tissue pressure to a point beyond its tensile strength, tearing it.

Lacerations or punctures to the neck carry some special considerations. Recall that the jugular veins and carotid arteries are located on either side of the neck. Open neck injuries (Figure 35-11) can involve those large vessels. The bleeding can be immediately life threatening. The bleeding can also result in hematomas in the soft tissue of the neck that jeopardize the airway and circulation. Air can also enter the cut ends of the large vessels. When air enters into the vessels, a bubble in the bloodstream called an *air embolism* will result. This is a potentially life-threatening condition. To properly treat an open neck

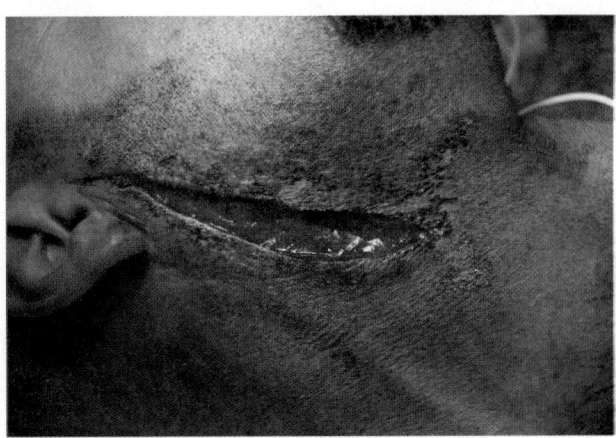

FIGURE 35-11

Open injury to the neck. (© Edward T. Dickinson, MD)

TABLE 35-2 Classes of Hemorrhage

	Class 1	Class 2	Class 3	Class 4
Blood Loss	<15 percent	15–30 percent	30–40 percent	>40 percent
Heart Rrate	↑	↑↑	↑↑↑	↑↑↑↑ or ↓
Vasoconstriction	↑	↑↑	↑↑↑	↑↑↑↑ or ↓↓
Ventilatory Rate	Normal	↑	↑↑	↑↑↑↑
Systolic BP	Normal	Normal		↓↓↓
Skin	Normal to slightly cool	Pale, cool, and clammy	Severely pale and cool	Severely pale, cool, and mottled

Note: In this table, the ↓ and ↑ symbols indicate an increase or decrease; the number of symbols indicates a greater degree of increase or decrease.

injury and reduce the possibility of air embolism, you should use the following steps:

1. Immediately cover the open injury with a gloved hand until you can apply an occlusive dressing completely covering the wound.
2. Cover the occlusive dressing with gauze or bulky dressings.
3. Control the bleeding by providing gentle direct pressure, taking care not to occlude the patient's airway. Never apply a circumferential bandage around a patient's neck.
4. Monitor the patient for problems with airway, breathing, or the reoccurrence of bleeding.

Bleeding

Bleeding is a complication of soft-tissue injuries. Although most of the bleeding injuries you will encounter as an Advanced EMT are not life threatening, some are. Uncontrolled bleeding can cause rapid deterioration of the patient and death. Significant bleeding is a threat to life and you must control it in the primary assessment (Table 35-2).

Bleeding can occur with all types of open soft-tissue injury and can vary in severity and difficulty to control. The amount of bleeding is directly related to the following two things:

- *Size of the vessel.* Larger vessels contain more blood and will bleed more than smaller ones.
- *Pressure within the vessel.* Arteries are under high pressure as the ventricle contracts and forces blood through them. Arterial bleeding is more profuse and more difficult to control because of the pressure behind it. Lower-pressure venous bleeding can be life threatening but is generally easier to control in the healthy patient.

There are three types of **external bleeding** (Figure 35-12):

- *Capillary bleeding.* Slowly oozing blood that can be either bright or dark red is characteristic of **capillary bleeding** from a wound. In most cases, it stops by itself and seldom requires treatment. But remember that cases in which capillary bleeding is occurring from a large body surface area, the patient can have a significant amount of blood loss.
- *Venous bleeding.* Dark red in color because it is depleted of oxygen, **venous bleeding** flows steadily

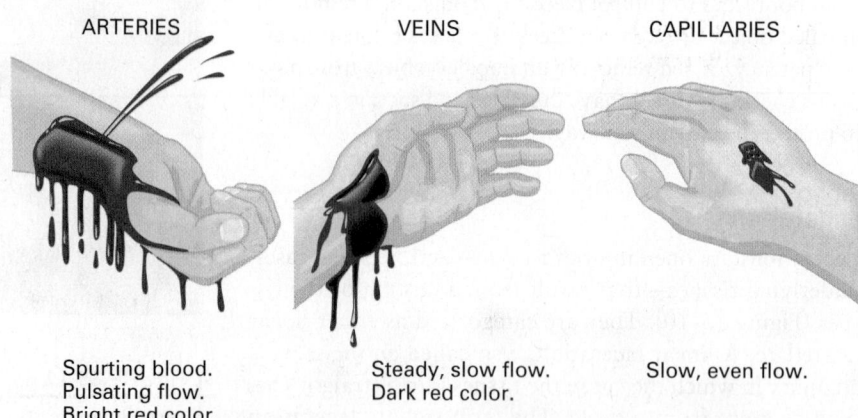

FIGURE 35-12
Types of bleeding.

ARTERIES — Spurting blood. Pulsating flow. Bright red color.

VEINS — Steady, slow flow. Dark red color.

CAPILLARIES — Slow, even flow.

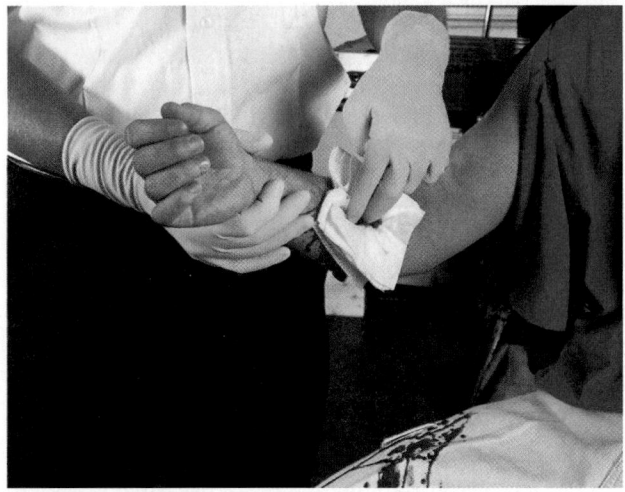

FIGURE 35-13

Applying direct pressure to a bleeding wound.

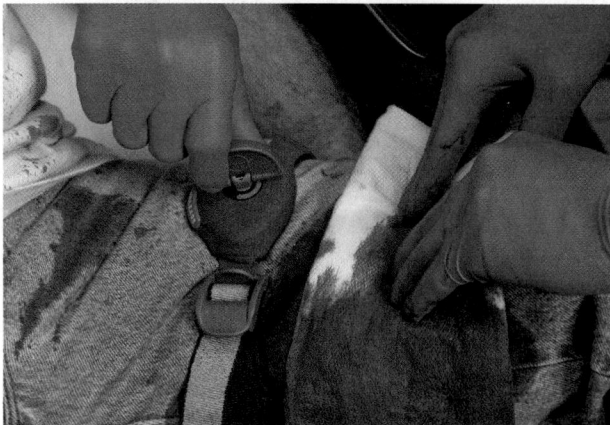

FIGURE 35-14

A commercial tourniquet being applied.

from injured vessels. It can be life threatening but is much easier to control than arterial bleeding.

- *Arterial bleeding.* Under pressure by the contractions of the heart, **arterial bleeding** is recognized by spurting blood that corresponds to the patient's pulse. It also is bright red, because it is saturated with oxygen. Arterial bleeding can be more difficult to control than any other kind.

To control bleeding, you should first apply firm direct pressure. If you cannot control bleeding with direct pressure, then you should apply a tourniquet. Elevation of the injured extremity while applying direct pressure was thought to be effective but no research has shown that to be true. However, because no research has shown that it is *not* effective, elevate the extremity when it is possible to do so.

Direct pressure is compression that is applied directly to an injury in an effort to control bleeding (Figure 35-13). After you have employed appropriate Standard Precautions, cover your fingertips or palm of your hand with dressings and apply steady pressure directly to the origin of the bleeding. If dressings are not immediately available, use your gloved hand. For larger, gaping wounds, it may be of benefit to pack the wounds with dressings before applying direct pressure.

If the dressings become soaked with blood, do not remove them because doing so can disrupt blood clots that

may have begun to form. Add clean dressings on top of them and continue applying direct pressure. However, this can only be done to a point. Piles of saturated dressings will eventually make the application of direct pressure over them ineffective. After bleeding is controlled, apply a pressure dressing to maintain pressure on the injury. Bandage the injury and transport the patient to an appropriate facility.

If life-threatening bleeding from an extremity is not successfully controlled with direct pressure, you must apply a tourniquet to stop the bleeding. There are many commercial tourniquets available (Figure 35-14), but a folded triangular bandage may be used instead. The process for applying a tourniquet is as follows:

1. Ensure that the tourniquet is at least 4 inches wide to prevent it from cutting into the skin while tightening.
2. Wrap the tourniquet around the extremity proximal to the injury but as close to it as possible without covering it. When the wound is near a joint, do not apply a tourniquet at the joint such as an elbow or knee. Instead, apply the tourniquet just above the joint.
3. Tighten the tourniquet until bleeding ceases.
4. Secure the device so that it does not loosen.
5. Document the time of application on a piece of tape and attach it to the tourniquet. You should document the time of application with the following method: TK (to indicate tourniquet) 1432 (to indicate that it was applied at 1432 hours).
6. Advise the receiving facility of the application of a tourniquet.

Hemostatic agents are substances that promote the clotting process of blood when applied to a bleeding injury. Hemostatic dressings have chemicals within the dressing that promote clotting when exposed to a bleeding wound, which assists in bleeding control (Figure 35-15).

IN THE FIELD

Never cover a tourniquet; it must be visible so that it is easily identified. Continuously reassess the injury for bleeding during patient transport. If it begins to bleed again, you must tighten the tourniquet until bleeding stops once again.

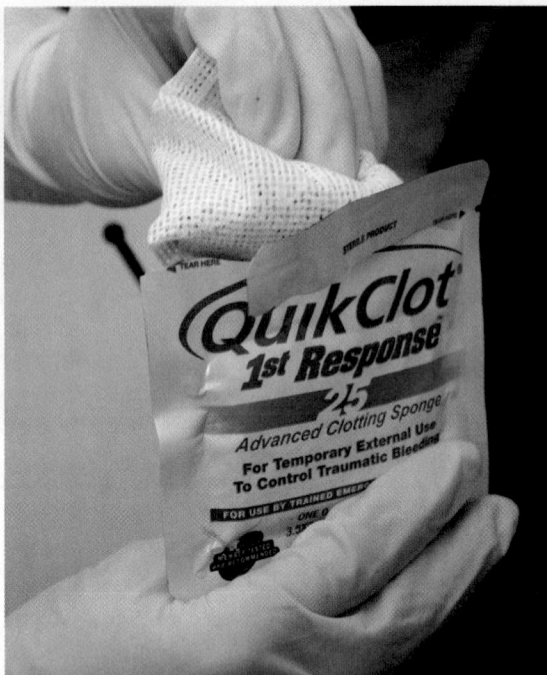

FIGURE 35-15

A hemostatic agent used to control bleeding.

In addition to hemostatic dressings, there are hemostatic agents that are poured directly into a wound to control bleeding. These agents all contain agents that promote clotting.

After applying the hemostatic dressing or substance and you have controlled the bleeding, you should apply a pressure dressing and bandage as usual.

Nosebleeds

Bleeding from the nose, called *epistaxis*, can be caused by trauma, hypertension, sinusitis, or blood clotting disorders. Nosebleeds also can compromise the patient's airway, because blood from inside the nose may begin to flow through the nasopharynx into the patient's oropharynx. The patient can aspirate the blood, resulting in airway compromise.

Whenever a patient sustains a nosebleed secondary to trauma, you must consider the mechanism of injury because other injuries, such as spine injury, may be present.

Emergency care for nosebleeds is as follows:

1. If it is not contraindicated by other injuries, have the patient sit in an upright position, leaning slightly forward. Remember to maintain manual stabilization of the head and neck for suspected spine injury.
2. The patient's head should be in a neutral position. Do not have the patient lean his head back, because it will facilitate blood flow down the throat and toward the airway. Swallowing large amounts of blood can result in vomiting.

3. Provide direct pressure by pinching the nostrils together and holding with steady pressure.
4. You can apply cold packs to the nose during direct pressure. The cold packs may assist in controlling the bleeding by causing vasoconstriction of the vessels within the nose.

Dressings and Bandages

Dressing and bandaging injuries are an important skill that you must master in order to manage soft-tissue injuries and bleeding.

A **dressing** is made of absorbent gauze and is applied directly to an open injury. Dressings placed on open wounds should be sterile. Dressings come in a multitude of sizes and types, to assist in controlling bleeding and preventing infection. The following are some types of dressings and their uses:

- *Adhesive dressings.* Self-adhering dressings such as the popular Band-Aid brand are used for dressing smaller open injuries, such as lacerations and abrasions.
- *Gauze pads.* Layered fabric pads that come in a variety of sizes such as 2"×2", 4"×4", and larger sizes are available for use on small- to medium-size open injuries (Figure 35-16).
- *Universal or trauma dressings.* Similar to the smaller gauze pads but thicker and larger, universal or trauma

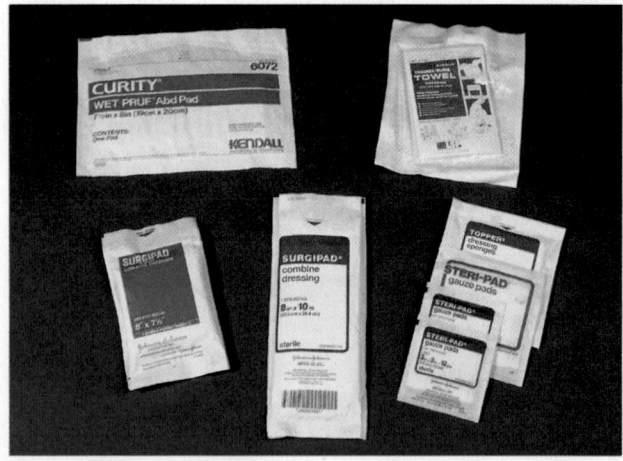

FIGURE 35-16

Sterile gauze pads.

dressings are usually 10"×30" and are for use on large open injuries (Figure 35-17). They are ideal for injuries of the chest and abdomen.

After a dressing is applied directly to an injury, a **bandage** is applied to hold a dressing in place. As with dressings, bandages are available in various sizes in sterile and nonsterile packaging. The following are examples of some bandages that you may use as an Advanced EMT:

- *Gauze rolls.* Rolls of thin gauze are available in various widths, ranging from 1 to 6 inches (Figure 35-18).

- *Triangular bandages.* Commonly used as slings but also used as bandages, these triangular bandages are folded, and then tied around a dressing to secure it (Figure 35-19).

- *Self-adhering bandages.* These are bandage rolls that adhere to themselves when they are overlapped.

- *Air splints.* These are used to secure a dressing in place on an injured extremity (Figure 35-20).

There are guidelines for applying dressings and bandages, but no hard-and-fast rules exist. The goal is to control bleeding and cover the injury to prevent contamination.

The following are general steps for dressing and bandaging open injuries:

1. Remove any clothing or jewelry that may constrict the area as a result of edema or prevent the injury from being covered.

2. Cover the entire injury with the dressing.

3. After you have controlled active bleeding with direct pressure, apply a **pressure dressing**. A pressure dressing is secured snugly directly above the dressings used to control the bleeding to prevent a recurrence of bleeding.

4. Select the most appropriate available method to bandage the injury. For injuries to the

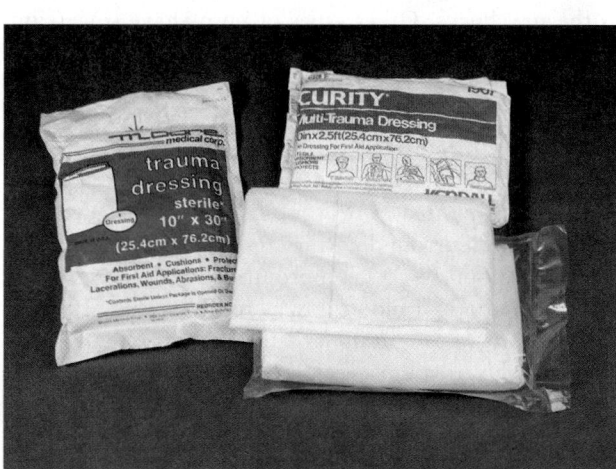

FIGURE 35-17

Universal or trauma dressings.

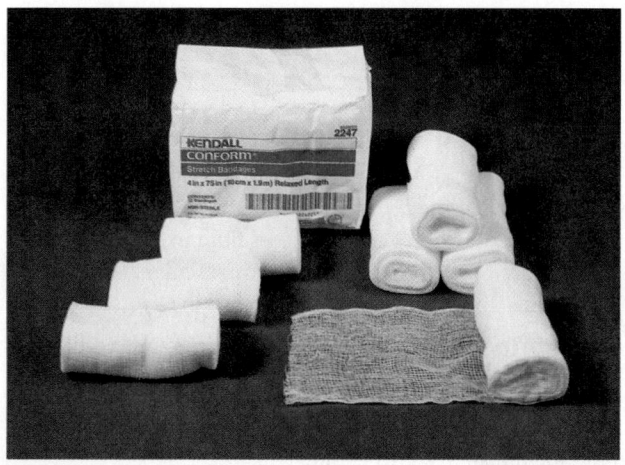

FIGURE 35-18

Gauze rolls.

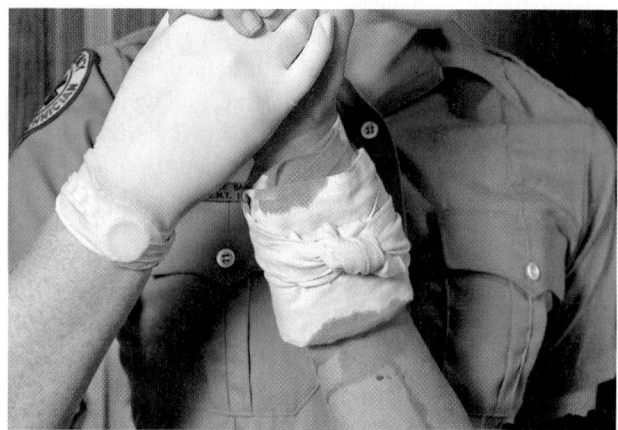

FIGURE 35-19

Triangular bandage used as a pressure bandage.

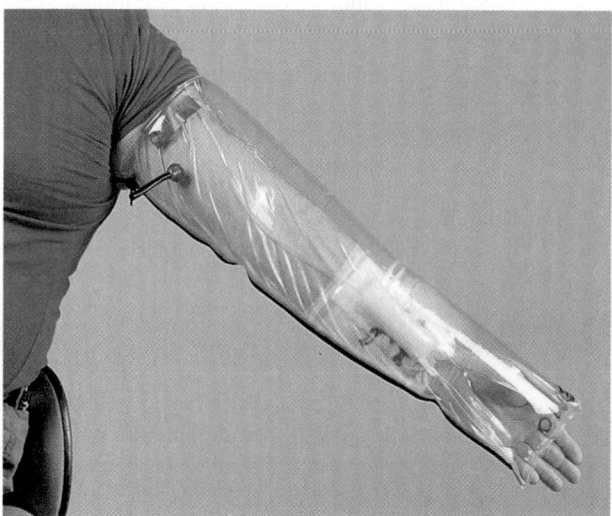

FIGURE 35-20

Inflatable air splint used as a bandage.

Advanced EMTs Wilson and Paige have responded to a patient whose vehicle caught fire after a collision. They place their gear on the ground and form a general impression of the patient. He is lying supine on a long backboard with all his clothes removed except his underwear. An EMT is manually stabilizing his head and neck and he is receiving high-flow oxygen by nonrebreather mask.

The patient, 55-year-old Todd Griffin, has second-degree burns to both arms, neck, and face. He also has bilateral angulated femur fractures. There is no external bleeding. There also is a large contusion to his abdomen. The patient is in obvious pain and is screaming.

Problem-Solving Questions

1. What should be Wilson and Paige's priorities, given the available information?
2. Are the patient's burn injuries critical? Why or why not?
3. Does the information available suggest critical traumatic injury? Why or why not?

extremities, use roller gauze by wrapping the extremity from distal to proximal beginning at least 1 inch from the dressing and wrap until the bandage covers at least 1 inch beyond the dressing. The dressing should be at least three wraps thick. Secure the roller gauze bandage with tape or by tying it. Tape works well for dressings on smaller injuries or on flatter parts of the body such as the chest and abdomen.

5. Ensure that distal circulation, motor function, and sensation are present after application of the bandage. Remove the bandage if distal circulation, motor function, or sensation have been compromised by the bandage and reapply, taking care not to apply the bandage too tightly.

6. Immobilize the extremity in the position of function or as indicated for suspected joint injuries or fractures. (See Chapter 36.)

7. Monitor for recurrence of bleeding during transport. Check distal neurovascular function of bandaged extremities during your reassessment of the patient.

Dressing and bandaging eye injuries require special consideration and will be discussed in Chapter 37.

Burns

Some of the most devastating calls that you will encounter as an Advanced EMT will include patients with burn injuries. Not all burn injuries are significant, but you must properly care for those that are in order to reduce morbidity and mortality of the patient.

Burn injury occurs when the skin is damaged by thermal energy, radiation, or caustic chemical contact. The most common type of burn that EMS providers care for is thermal burns. Other types of burns have some similarities to thermal burns, but have special considerations, as well.

The body responds to a burn by initiating an inflammatory response to the affected tissue that can lead to further injury. When a thermal burn is severe enough, it results in an area of necrotic tissue called the **zone of coagulation**. Surrounding this area is the **zone of stasis**, in which blood flow is compromised but tissue may not become necrotic if blood flow is restored to it. The outermost zone of a burn injury is called the **zone of hyperemia**. In this area, an increase of circulation to the skin results in redness and edema.

In addition to the physical pain and scarring, many burned patients experience psychological effects that last a lifetime.

Effects of Burns on the Body

Burns cause injury not only to the skin, but to other body systems as well.

Effects on the Circulatory System

Burn injuries cause destruction of the tissues, resulting in fluid loss. This fluid loss occurs as a result of increases in capillary permeability, which allows fluid to escape from the vasculature of the body into the extravascular tissues, causing edema. In turn, edema can increase the pressure within the tissues and reduce circulation. In the first 24 hours following a large burn, fluid can continue to leak into tissues, resulting in massive edema. The result of the fluid leaving the intravascular space is a decrease of circulating blood volume, which can lead to shock.

In some cases, patients who sustain burn injuries also sustain traumatic injury in the process. Do not let the burns distract you to the point that you fail to recognize the potential for traumatic injury. For example, a patient who has jumped from a third-story window because he was being burned in a structure fire is likely to have sustained traumatic injury. Yes, you must care for his burn injuries. But recall that a fall from more than 20 feet is a significant mechanism of injury and has the potential to produce life-threatening injury.

As an Advanced EMT, you must consider the mechanisms of injury and be prepared to provide the best possible care, including the fluid therapy required for the patient's burn injuries. (Fluid therapy is discussed later in this chapter.)

Effects on the Respiratory System

Burns can produce life-threatening effects on the respiratory system. This occurs when a patient inhales either hot air or chemicals that cause burns. When the tissues of the airway are burned, edema results, which causes the airway to narrow and fluid to accumulate in the lungs. The narrowing of the airway often occurs in the larynx, which is called *laryngeal edema.*

If the patient was in an enclosed burning structure, he may also inhale poisonous gases produced by the materials that are burning, causing a multitude of complications.

Another risk to the respiratory system occurs when there are circumferential burns of the torso. If the torso is circumferentially burned, **eschar** may prevent adequate expansion of the chest and lead to respiratory compromise. Eschar is burned tissue that has no elasticity and takes on the appearance of dry leather.

You must be aware of the possibility of burn injury to the respiratory system and be prepared to protect the airway in order to prevent the patient from deteriorating. Signs and symptoms of an airway burn include singed nasal hair, carbonaceous sputum, hoarse voice, sore throat, and difficulty breathing.

Effects on the Renal System

If the patient experiences a significant amount of fluid loss from the intravascular space, shock may ensue. If shock progresses, the first vital organ system that is affected by hypoperfusion is the renal system. Recall that the renal system is responsible for the elimination of waste from the body. Damage to the renal system can cause renal failure, which can cause edema, anemia, metabolic acidosis, hyperkalemia, and difficulty breathing as a result of congestive heart failure.

Effects on the Nervous System

Burn injuries can cause damage to the nerves in the affected area and ultimately cause motor, sensation, and joint dysfunction. Patients will require extensive physical

and occupational therapy to regain or preserve normal function.

Sources of Burns

Burn injuries can occur as a result of various sources, including:

- Exposure to a heat source
- Inhalation of heated gases or noxious fumes
- Exposure to chemical agents
- Exposure to electrical sources
- Exposure to radiation sources

Burn injury may occur as a result of a number of mechanisms, as follows:

- *Flame burns.* Burns that occur when skin is exposed to an open flame are called **flame burns**. In some cases, the open flame causes the patient's clothing to ignite, resulting in further exposure and injury.
- *Contact burns.* Burns that occur when the skin comes into contact with a hot surface are called **contact burns**. They are usually isolated to the area of contact, but edema may be extensive.
- *Scalds.* **Scalds** are burns that occur when skin comes into contact with hot liquids.
- *Steam burns.* **Steam burns** tend to be more severe than flame burns, because steam has the capacity to achieve higher temperatures than open flames.
- *Gas burns.* Burns that occur when tissues are exposed to hot gases—**gas burns**—tend to be the cause of airway burns.
- *Electrical burns.* Burns may occur as a result of the heat generated by electrical current as it passes through tissues that offer resistance. **Electrical burns** are often more extensive than they appear to be because injury occurs wherever electrical current passes, externally and internally.
- *Flash burns.* Burns that occur as a result of exposure to a flammable gas or liquid that ignites and burns very rapidly are called **flash burns**. Areas of the body that are covered with clothing are often uninjured, whereas areas that are not, sustain injury. If the flash occurs in an enclosed space, the air may be heated enough to produce airway burns.
- *Chemical burns.* **Chemical burns** occur as a result of exposure of the skin to chemicals that are either acidic or alkaline.

Classification of Burn Severity

The severity of burns is determined by the depth of tissue affected and the amount of body surface area (BSA) affected. The severity of burn is affected by the initial exposure and injury and the body's inflammatory response to

them. The inflammatory response can result in progressive tissue injury for up to two days following the injury, increasing burn depth.

When a decrease in circulation to the injured tissue occurs, it leads to progression of injury and increasing burn depth. For this reason, it is important for you to determine the depth and extent of burn injury. That information will indicate whether the patient should be treated at a burn center or a hospital emergency department.

Burns are classified as superficial (first degree), partial thickness (second degree), or full thickness (third degree) (Table 35-3). Burns develop over time. That is, burns that appear superficial or partial thickness in the prehospital setting may later be determined to be deeper than they originally appeared to be.

Superficial burns, also called *first-degree burns*, involve only the epidermis (Figure 35-21). They are identified by reddening of the skin and minor to no edema at the burn site. Those burns cause minor to moderate pain to touch and generally heal on their own without treatment. Sunburn is an example of a superficial burn.

Partial-thickness burns, also called *second-degree burns*, involve the epidermis and dermis (Figure 35-22).

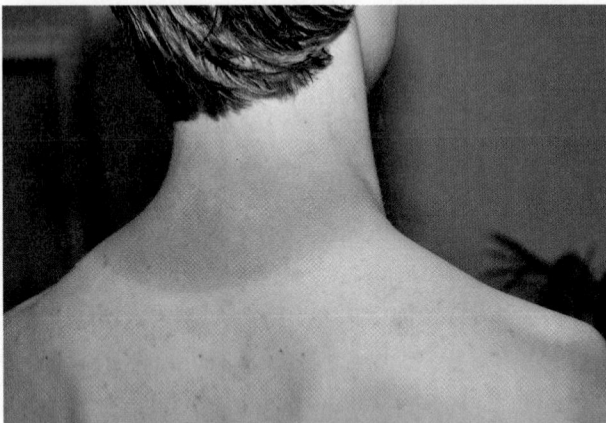

FIGURE 35-21

A superficial (first-degree) burn. (© Edward T. Dickinson, MD)

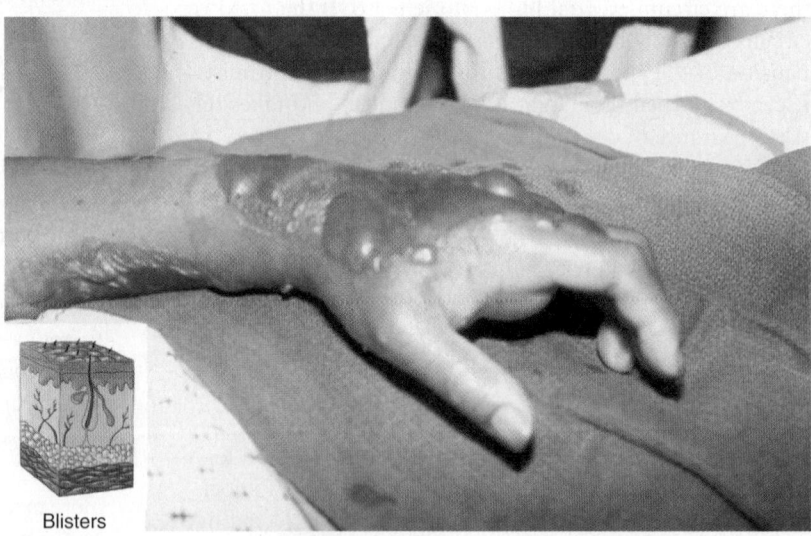

FIGURE 35-22

A partial-thickness (second-degree) burn.
(© Roy Alson, MD, courtesy of ITLS)

Blisters

TABLE 35-3	**Characteristics of Burn Injuries**		
	Superficial (First Degree)	**Partial Thickness (Second Degree)**	**Full Thickness (Third Degree)**
Mechanism	Sun or minor flash	Hot liquids, flash, or thermal	Chemicals, thermal, electricity
Skin Color	Red	Mottled red	White and waxy or dark and charred
Skin Surface	Dry without blisters	Moist/weeping with blisters	Dry and leather-like

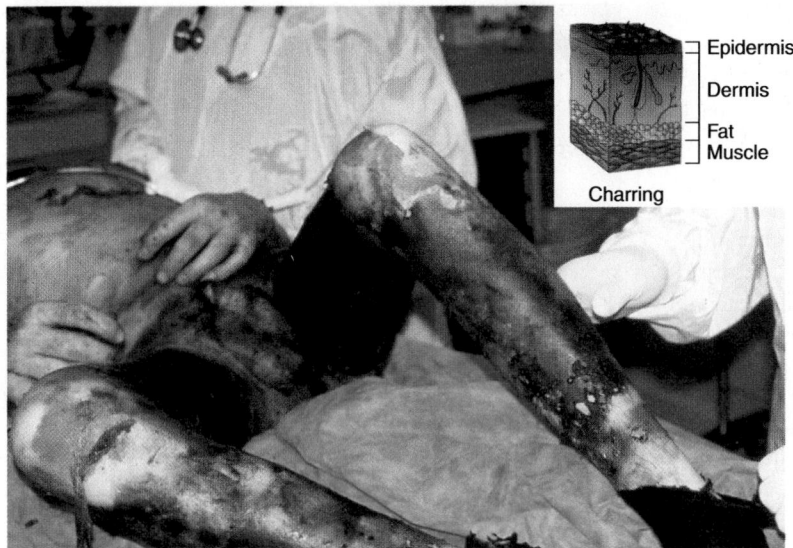

FIGURE 35-23

A full-thickness (third-degree) burn. (© Roy Alson, MD, courtesy of ITLS)

They are identified by reddening of the skin, the presence of blisters, edema, and a mottled appearance. They cause severe pain. Although edema and blisters usually appear rapidly, they may worsen over hours to days after the injury. Partial-thickness burns will generally heal by themselves when treated appropriately, leaving little scarring.

Full-thickness burns, also called *third-degree burns*, involve all layers of the skin and in some cases muscle tissue (Figure 35-23). They are identified by tissue that is dry and hard, with a leather-like appearance, which is either white and waxy or dark and charred in color. The affected tissue from the burn is called *eschar*.

The burned tissue does not cause pain to the patient because the nerves in the affected tissue have been destroyed. However, in nearly all cases of full-thickness burns, there will be areas of partial-thickness and superficial burns,

IN THE FIELD

You may hear other health care providers refer to a fourth-degree burn. Fourth-degree burns affect all layers of the skin, muscle, and bone. Those burns are typically the result of electrical injuries and are devastating to the patient.

which will cause the patient severe pain. Full-thickness burns may require extensive treatment, such as skin grafting, to reduce disfiguration of the patient. Scarring may be severe even with skin grafting.

The **rule of nines** (Figure 35-24) is used to determine the amount of BSA affected by partial- or full-thickness burns. The rule of nines divides the body into areas of either

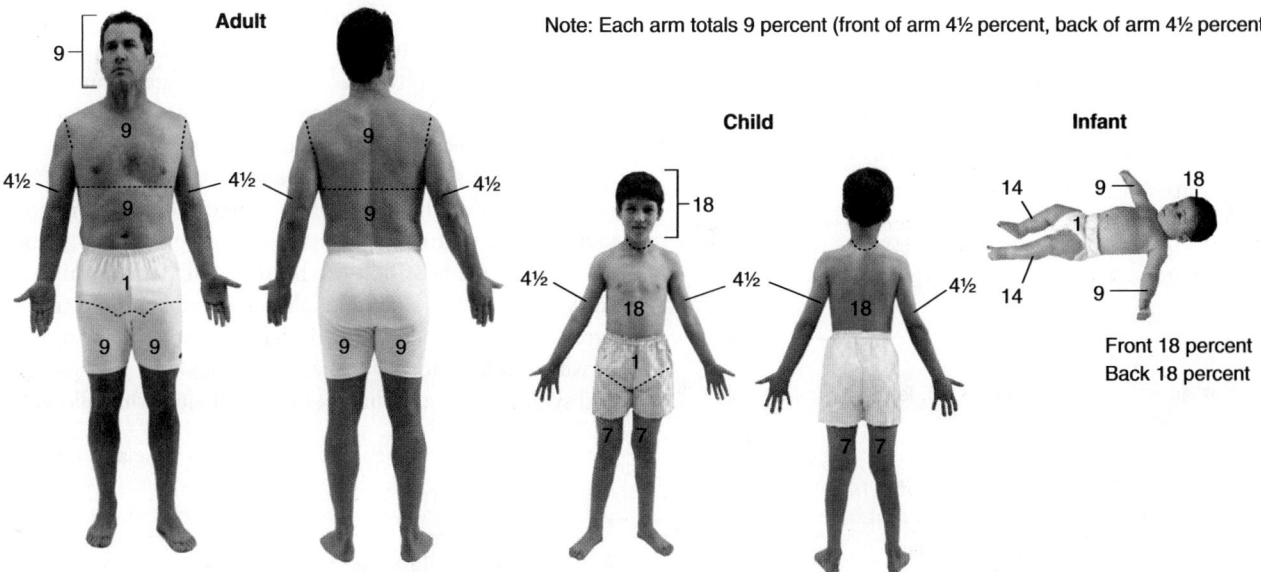

FIGURE 35-24

The rule of nines.

9 percent or 18 percent of total BSA, which is used to calculate an approximate total BSA affected.

In an adult patient, the head and neck (combined), each upper extremity, chest, abdomen, upper back, lower back, anterior of each lower extremity, and the posterior of each lower extremity each represents 9 percent BSA. The genitalia represent 1 percent BSA.

In infants and children, the BSA percentages are different because the head is larger in proportion to the rest of the body. In patients under the age of one year, the head and neck, chest and abdomen, and entire back each represent 18 percent BSA. Each upper extremity represents 9 percent and each lower extremity represents 14 percent.

An alternative method of determining total BSA affected is to use the **rule of palm**. The rule of palm uses the size of the patient's palm as an approximate representation of 1 percent BSA. This method works well when estimating the BSA of smaller burns.

Factors other than BSA and depth of burns contribute to the severity of burn injuries. Patient age and pre-existing medical conditions also play a role in determining burn severity.

Pediatric and geriatric patients may have difficulty recovering from burn injuries. Pediatric patients do not have mature body systems and cannot recover as well compared to healthy adults. Geriatric patients do not recover as well because the functionality of their body systems has begun to deteriorate.

Severity of burn injury is classified as minor, moderate, or critical. Tables 35-4 and Table 35-5 outline the classification of burns by severity for adults and children.

TABLE 35-5	Classification of Burns by Severity: Children < 5 Years
MINOR BURNS	
Partial-thickness burns < 10 percent	
MODERATE BURNS	
Partial-thickness burns 10–20 percent	
CRITICAL BURNS	
Full-thickness burns of any extent or partial-thickness burns > 20 percent	

Source: American Burn Association SCALD INJURY PREVENTION Educator's Guide A Community Fire and Burn Prevention Program Supported by the United States Fire Administration Federal Emergency Management Agency.

Pediatric Care

Pediatric patients cannot compensate for fluid and heat loss as well as adults, making them more susceptible to shock and hypothermia. You must continuously monitor these patients for deterioration in condition.

Geriatric Care

All burns that are classified as moderate are considered critical in patients 55 years old or older.

TABLE 35-4	Classification of Burns by Severity: Adult
MINOR BURNS	

- Full-thickness burns of < 2 percent, excluding face, hands, feet, genitalia, or respiratory tract
- Partial-thickness burns < 15 percent
- Superficial burns > 50 percent

MODERATE BURNS

- Full-thickness burns of 2–10 percent, excluding face, hands, feet, genitalia, or respiratory tract
- Partial-thickness burns of 15–30 percent
- Superficial burns > 50 percent

CRITICAL BURNS

- All burns complicated by injuries to the respiratory tract and traumatic injury
- Partial- or full-thickness burns involving the face, hands, feet, genitalia, or respiratory tract
- Full-thickness burns > 10 percent
- Partial-thickness burns > 30 percent
- Circumferential burns

All burns that are classified as moderate are considered critical in patients 55 years old or older.

Burn Injury Assessment

Ensure that the scene is safe prior to approaching the patient. Never enter a space where fire, chemicals, or electricity are the cause of burn injury unless you have the proper training and equipment to handle the situation. Identify the mechanism of injury and pay attention to the possibility of associated trauma. For example, a patient burned in an explosion or vehicle collision has additional mechanisms of injury that you must consider.

After the scene size-up is complete, immediately remove the patient from the burn source if he is still in contact with it. Perform a primary assessment, paying close attention to the possibility of burns to the patient's airway. Airway burns and smoke inhalation greatly complicate the care of a burn patient. Ensure that the patient has an open airway and look for evidence of an inhalation injury. Signs and symptoms of an inhalation injury include the following:

- Presence of soot beneath the patient's nose and inside the mouth and nose
- Sore throat
- Hoarseness while speaking
- Shortness of breath

If any one of those findings is present, you must carefully monitor the patient's status and be prepared to secure the airway. Consider requesting ALS assistance because airway management can be extremely difficult in patients with inhalation burns. Ensure adequacy of breathing and provide supplemental oxygen and positive pressure ventilations as indicated. Check for and control significant bleeding.

If the patient is critical, perform a rapid trauma exam. Follow the rapid trauma exam with vital signs, a patient history, and head-to-toe exam. For patients with isolated injuries, perform a focused exam and obtain baseline vital signs and a medical history. You should ask the following questions to obtain necessary details of injury:

How did the burn occur?

Did the burn occur indoors or outdoors?

Did the patient's clothes catch fire?

How long did it take to extinguish the flames on the patient?

How were the flames on the patient extinguished?

Was an accelerant involved?

Was there an explosion?

Was the patient in a smoke-filled room?

How did the patient escape?

Has the patient sustained a traumatic injury?

Were others killed at the scene?

Was the patient unconscious at the scene?

Determine the severity of the patient's injuries and make a transport decision. You should directly transport patients who have sustained critical burn injuries to a burn center, if possible. If the patient has a traumatic injury with burns, you should transport him to a facility where his traumatic injuries can be managed prior to transport to a burn center.

Emergency Management for Burn Injuries

Assessing and maintaining an airway and adequate ventilation in burned patients is a frequent consideration because thermal burns can also result in inhalation injuries. Inhalation injuries account for more than half of burn-related deaths in the United States (Campbell, 2008). Inhalation injuries are classified as the following:

- Carbon monoxide poisoning
- Heat-inhalation injury
- Smoke-inhalation injury

Those injuries typically occur when a patient was in an enclosed space where fire was present.

Carbon monoxide poisoning occurs when the air that a person breathes contains high amounts of carbon monoxide. This is by far the most common cause of death with burn injury (American Burn Association, 2007). Carbon monoxide is one of the chemicals found in smoke, so when a person breathes smoke-filled air, he is being exposed to

IN THE FIELD

Pulse oximetry can lead you to believe that a patient has adequate oxygenation, when in fact he does not. This is because pulse oximetry measures the percent of hemoglobin that is saturated but it cannot determine what it is saturated with. Therefore, a patient may have carbon monoxide poisoning and have a pulse oximetry reading of 99 percent.

Special devices are now available for use in the prehospital environment that measure carboxyhemoglobin levels in the bloodstream, allowing the Advanced EMT to identify carbon monoxide poisoning in patients and themselves.

IN THE FIELD

Lactated Ringer's solution is recommended by the American Burn Association for fluid therapy in burn patients (American Burn Association, 2007). Normal saline may also be used in some EMS systems. Always follow your protocol.

this chemical. It is colorless, tasteless, and odorless, and therefore cannot be detected without special equipment.

Carbon monoxide binds with hemoglobin, and its affinity is 257 times stronger than that of oxygen. When the hemoglobin has carbon monoxide bound to it, oxygen cannot bind to it; therefore, hypoxia ensues (Table 35-6).

Immediately remove patients with carbon monoxide exposure from the poisonous environment and treat with high-flow oxygen by nonrebreather mask or positive pressure ventilations as indicated. Your goal is to provide

TABLE 35-6	**Signs and Symptoms of Elevated Carboxyhemoglobin Levels**
Carboxyhemoglobin Level (percent)	**Signs and Symptoms**
20	Throbbing headache, exertional shortness of breath
30	Headache, altered judgment, irritability, dizziness, altered vision
40–50	Major central nervous system dysfunction, including confusion, collapse, exertional syncope
60–70	Convulsions, unconsciousness, apnea with prolonged exposure
80	Death with prolonged exposure

Source: From The Merck Manual of Diagnosis and Therapy, Online Medical Library, edited by Robert Porter. Copyright 2004–2011 by Merck Sharp & Dohme Corp., a subsidiary of Merck & Co., Inc., Whitehouse Station, NJ. Available at: www.MerckManuals.com/professional.

oxygenation and supportive care as necessary. Transport the patient to an appropriate facility. With significant carbon monoxide exposure, the patient may benefit from hyperbaric oxygen treatment. Medical direction may request transport to a facility where hyperbaric treatment is available.

Heat-inhalation injury occurs when a person inhales heated gases. This usually occurs when a person is trapped in an enclosed space that is on fire. When the person inhales, the heated gases travel through the airway and cause injury. Laryngeal edema results from burns to the tissues within the larynx, leading to rapid narrowing of the airway. Burns to the airway also can result in fluid accumulation in the lungs. Signs of possible heat-inhalation injury include the following:

- Singed facial and nasal hair
- Soot under and inside the nose and mouth
- Burns to the face
- Stridor
- Sore throat
- Hoarseness

If any of these signs and symptoms are present, apply high-concentration oxygen by nonrebreather mask and be prepared to secure the airway in the event of deterioration. Provide rapid transport to an appropriate facility.

Smoke-inhalation injuries are the result of inhaling noxious chemicals that cause injury to the alveoli. Remember that there is no way for you to know what types of products are burning in a structure fire. Smoke from burning plastics produce cyanide gas, which can cause death in a short period of time with significant exposure. Household chemicals can produce toxic fumes when burned and pose a serious threat to the patient and responders. The chemicals are irritating to the airway and may lead to bronchospasm, which should be treated with beta agonists and high-flow oxygen.

In addition to chemical exposure that produces immediate effects to the patient, there are several chemicals, such as those found in furniture, wallpaper, vinyl flooring, and even cotton, that can produce signs and symptoms of injury up to two days following exposure (delayed toxin-induced lung injury).

After you have managed all immediate life threats, you will care for burn injuries. Follow these steps when managing thermal burn injuries:

1. *Treat for shock as indicated.* Do not delay transport of a critical patient to initiate intravenous access on the scene. Obtain intravenous access while en route to an appropriate facility.

2. *Stop the burning process.* After the patient is removed from the source of the burn, his clothes may be on fire or smoldering. Remove all clothing from the area of the burn. If clothing adheres to the patient, do not pull it from the patient; cut around the adherent part, leaving it in place. Cool the burn to stop the progression of the burn by applying sterile water for no longer than a minute or two. Avoid cooling for long periods of time, because this puts the patient at risk for hypothermia.

3. *Remove clothing and jewelry from the burn area.* As edema progresses, jewelry and constrictive clothing can reduce circulation by acting as a tourniquet. If jewelry is not removed early, it may not be possible to remove it later without cutting it off.

4. *Cover the burn with dry sterile dressings or burn sheets to help prevent infection and reduce the pain associated with airflow over the burned area.* Avoid covering the patient directly with materials, such as wool blankets, that will leave particles stuck to the wound when removed. Remember that burn-injured patients are at risk for hypothermia, so they must be covered to preserve body heat. Some agencies have protocols that allow the use of moist sterile dressings for smaller burns (usually 10 percent BSA or less) as a pain relief measure. If in doubt, use a dry dressing. Always follow your protocol.

   Avoid breaking blisters. When burns to the hands and feet also involve the fingers and toes, first remove any jewelry and then separate the digits with dry sterile dressings to prevent them from adhering to one another. Finally, wrap the entire area with dry sterile dressings (Figure 35-25).

5. *Do not force the eyes open to assess them.* When burns to the eyes occur, eyelids can swell closed. Determine whether the burns are from a thermal or chemical source. If from a thermal source, apply dry sterile dressings to both eyes to prevent movement. Flush chemical burns with water. If adequate flushing has been done prior to your arrival, dress the eyes and prepare for transport. If flushing has not occurred or may have been inadequate, flush the eyes en route to the hospital.

6. *Transport to an appropriate facility.* Consider the use of air transport when ground transport time to definitive care is long. See Table 35-7 for burn center referral criteria.

7. *Initiate fluid therapy en route* using the Parkland burn formula, or another formula approved in your EMS system.

The **Parkland formula** is used to identify the amount of fluid a patient with extensive burns should receive within

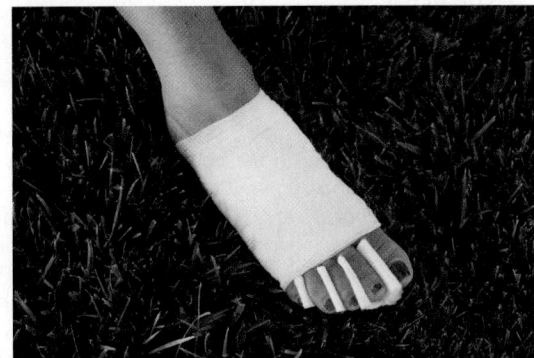

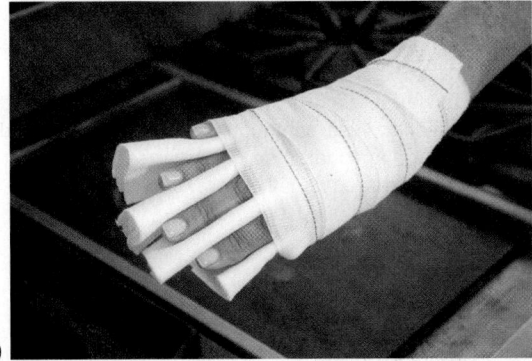

FIGURE 35-25

(A) Place dry sterile dressings between the toes. (B) Place dry sterile dressings between the fingers.

IN THE FIELD

When responding to a chemical burn at an industrial facility, such as an oil refinery or chemical plant, you will likely be greeted by a responder who will have a material safety data sheet (MSDS) for you that provides all the information regarding the chemical that the patient was exposed to. This information is used as a guide to decontaminate and treat the patient.

You may arrive to find that the patient has already been decontaminated and treatment has been started. It is generally not the responsibility of an Advanced EMT to decontaminate patients. Care is administered after the patient has been decontaminated by those trained to do so.

TABLE 35-7	Burn Center Referral Criteria

- Inhalation injury
- Partial-thickness burn >10 percent BSA
- Full-thickness burn
- Burns of the hands, feet, face, genitalia, perineum, or major joints
- Electrical burns (including lightning strikes)
- Chemical burns
- Burns in patients with pre-existing medical conditions

Source: American Burn Association SCALD INJURY PREVENTION Educator's Guide A Community Fire and Burn Prevention Program Supported by the United States Fire Administration Federal Emergency Management Agency.

the first 24 hours postinjury. Use it to identify the correct amount of fluids to be administered, as follows:

- *Adults:* Lactated Ringer's solution 2–4 mL × kg body weight × percent BSA burned (partial- and full-thickness burns)

- *Children:* Lactated Ringer's solution 3–4 mL × kg body weight × percent BSA burned (partial- and full-thickness burns)

Once the total amount of volume to be infused in the first 24 hours post–burn injury is determined, divide it by 2 to identify the volume to be infused in the first 8 hours

postburn. The remaining half will be delivered over the next 16 hours after the burn.

Proper fluid resuscitation is vital to the survival of patients with extensive burn injuries. The body loses a significant amount of circulating blood volume in the first 24 hours of the burn injury. It is important to anticipate this and provide fluid resuscitation to the patient to prevent hypovolemia from occurring. If hypovolemia occurs, organ dysfunction and damage will soon follow. In some cases, a burn center may order more or less fluid than calculated using the Parkland burn formula based on the type of burn, past medical history, and patient age.

Specific Burn Injuries

Some burn injuries—such as chemical, electrical, and radiation burns—require special consideration when treating them.

Chemical Burns

With chemical burns, the burning process will continue as long as the chemical is in contact with the skin (Figure 35-26). The two mechanisms by which chemical

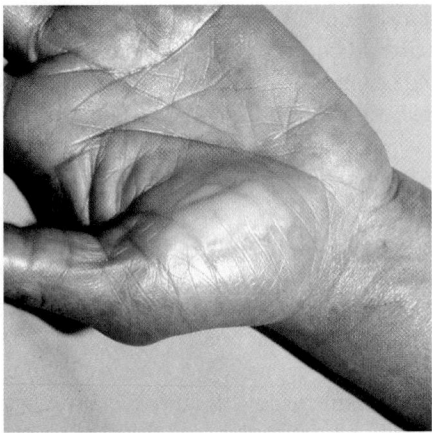

FIGURE 35-26

Chemical burn to the hand. (© David Effron, MD, FACEP)

PERSONAL PERSPECTIVE

Advanced EMT Sandra Sherman: Every now and then, you will run an emergency and afterward think to yourself, "Wow . . . now that was a good call." One of those calls occurred to me early one morning.

My partner and I were dispatched to an MVC just outside of town. We arrived on scene to find firefighters working to free the driver of the car, whose legs were pinned beneath the steering wheel and dashboard. He was driving his car down the highway when he drifted across the center line, striking a garbage truck head-on.

When I arrived at the patient's car, I noticed a firefighter holding direct pressure to the patient's left shoulder. The dressings were soaked in blood. The patient was disoriented, on high-flow oxygen, and breathing normally. He was pale and cool, tachycardic, and hypotensive.

Knowing that the closest hospital was 15 minutes away but did not have surgical services, I chose to call for air transport to the nearest surgical facility, a little farther away. The firefighter explained to me that the patient's left arm was amputated at the shoulder in the collision and he believed that the bleeding was now controlled. The arm was properly wrapped and being cooled with ice packs prior to our arrival.

By the time we got the patient freed from the car and packaged for transport, Air Med had landed at the scene. The flight medic was given a report and the patient, along with his amputated arm, was transported by air to the surgical facility.

This patient survived his injuries because of the quick thinking and appropriate actions of the firefighters, who were first on scene. Had the patient's bleeding not been controlled immediately, he would have surely died. The amputated part was properly packaged and everyone on scene worked as a team to get the patient packaged and transported to the appropriate facility. Also contributing to the survival of the patient was the appropriate use of air transport to the closest facility that was equipped to provide definitive care to the patient.

---

burns occur are **coagulation necrosis** and **liquefaction necrosis**. Coagulation necrosis is death of the tissue caused by protein coagulation as a result of exposure to an acid. This coagulation process forms eschar, which limits the depth of injury. Liquefaction necrosis is the denaturing of proteins, which leads to a "melting" of tissues as a result of alkali exposure. Liquefaction necrosis has the ability to create very deep burns into tissue.

You will find that in many cases, the injury will have been decontaminated prior to your arrival. If it has not, you must stop the burning process by removing the chemical from the patient. The processes for removing liquid chemicals and dry chemicals are different.

As a general rule, when removing liquid chemicals, remove any contaminated clothing from the patient, taking care not to spread the chemical. Then flush him with copious amounts of water. Prior to doing so, consult a Material Safety Data Sheet or a Department of Transportation *Emergency Response Guidebook* for hazardous materials because some liquid chemicals react to water. If a guidebook is readily available, follow the instructions for the specific chemical.

When removing dry chemicals, first brush the chemical from the skin and then flush the skin with copious amounts of water (Figure 35-27). Once again, if a hazardous materials guidebook is readily available, follow the instructions for the specific chemical.

When flushing chemicals from the eyes, place the patient in a supine position and have him turn his head in the direction of the injured eye to prevent chemicals from entering the unaffected eye (Figure 35-28). Once the patient is positioned, gently pour sterile water or saline into the corner of the affected eye while holding it open with your other hand. Continue to flush the eye until the burning process has stopped or you have arrived at a hospital.

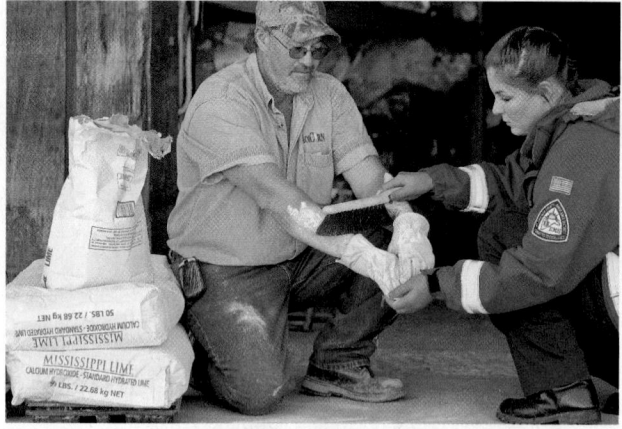

FIGURE 35-27

Brush dry chemicals from the skin.

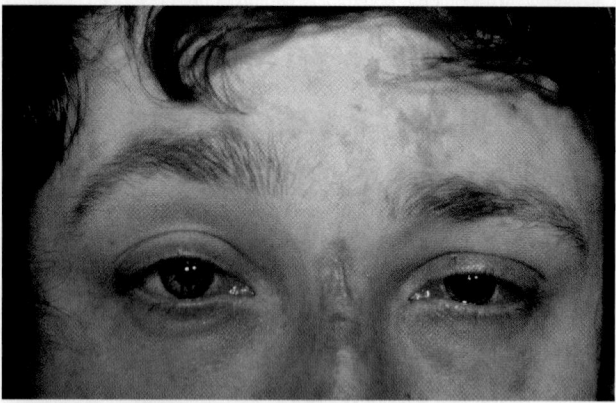

FIGURE 35-28

Chemical burn to the eyes. (© Western Ophthalmic Hospital/Photo Researchers, Inc.)

Some EMS systems use a device called a Morgan lens, which is designed to fit onto the surface of the eye like a large contact lens, to irrigate eyes.

When managing chemical burns, identify the chemical involved and, if possible and safe to do so, bring the container with you to the hospital.

Electrical Burns

Electrical burns can occur in situations that pose a risk to rescuers, such as lightning storms and situations with downed power lines. *Never attempt to access a patient who is in contact with electrical lines or within a vehicle with power lines contacting it.* Call for the power company to disconnect the electricity traveling through the lines and allow them to remove the electrical contacts from the patient or the vehicle.

With electrical burns, injury occurs as the electricity enters the body and travels through the tissues until it exits. This injury occurs as a result of the electrical damage to organs of the body and heat generated as the current of electricity travels through the tissues. When a patient is exposed to electrical shock, whether from household electricity or a lightning strike, you should locate the contact burn and exit burn. However, keep in mind that the burns may not be the most severe of the patient's injuries. Electrical current can cause severe damage to the internal organs and cause respiratory arrest and cardiac dysrhythmias.

Entry burns tend to be smaller in relation to exit burns. After entry, the current will continue to travel through the body until it exits at a point where the person is grounded. There is no way to determine the extent of internal injuries, so you should assume the worst and transport the patient to a burn center. When the electrical current exits the body, it does so violently and may produce massive tissue damage (Figures 35-29 and 35-30).

Burns from entrance and exit points are caused by the electrical arc, which can reach temperatures of 2,500 degrees Celsius. In some cases, you will see large areas of tissue completely destroyed or detached.

In the history, ask the following questions to obtain specific details of the injury:

What was the source of the current involved?

What was the duration of contact?

Did the patient fall?

What was the estimated voltage?

Was there loss of consciousness?

In addition to managing the airway, ensuring adequate ventilation, oxygenation, and circulation, and consider requesting ALS response. Cardiac dysrhythmia is a common complication of electrical injury. Assess for an entrance and exit wound and treat as you would a thermal injury.

Pediatric Care

When children reach the age at which they are crawling, they are very curious and explore the world around them using their senses, such as taste. Many homes are not adequately childproofed and power cords are in places accessible to children. If a child is able to pull a power cord out of an appliance and put it in his mouth while it is still plugged into the wall, it will result in electrical shock. The shock could be very minor if the current is small, but it could be serious with higher currents. With these serious electrical shocks, you may see a burn to the child's mouth. Remember always to look for an exit burn when assessing an electrical injury patient.

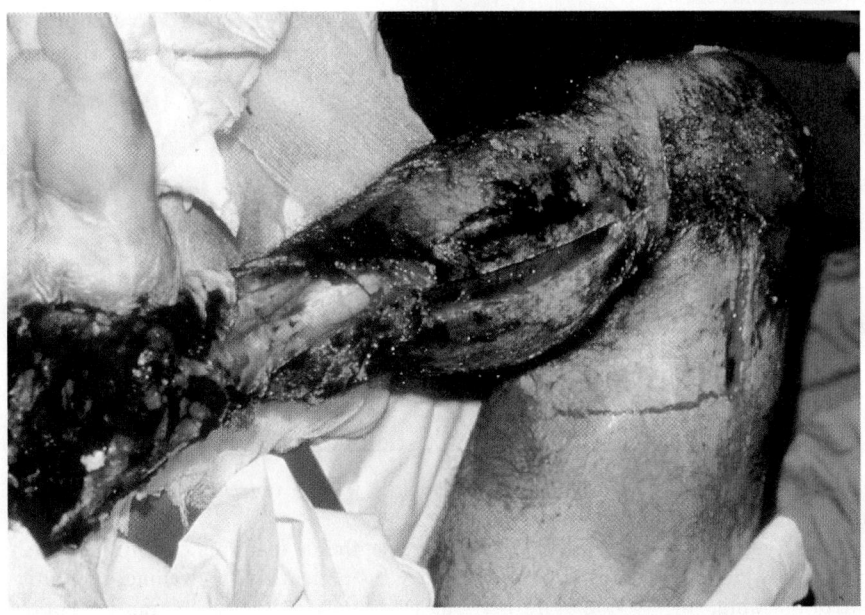

FIGURE 35-29

Electrical burn to a lower extremity.
(© Roy Alson, MD, courtesy of ITLS)

Clinical-Reasoning Process

Wilson's primary assessment of the patient reveals no life-threatening external bleeding. The patient's airway and breathing are adequate. Wilson and Paige are unable to obtain a patient history because the patient's pain makes it impossible for him to cooperate. Vital signs are stable at this point. The secondary assessment reveals only non–life-threatening injuries in addition to the life threats already identified. Wilson realizes they need to spend as little time on the scene as possible.

Paige and the firefighters rapidly immobilize the patient using a long backboard and load him into the ambulance, immediately beginning treatment for shock. Wilson estimates the patient's burns to be approximately 27 percent of BSA with no evidence of airway involvement.

Because of the traumatic injuries and possible internal bleeding, Wilson instructs the EMT who has been designated to drive to begin the 15-minute transport to a Level 1 trauma center. En route, Paige initiates two large-bore IVs and begins fluid administration. Upon arrival at the trauma center, the patient's care is transferred to emergency department staff without incident.

A few days later, Paige and Wilson learn that the patient had a lacerated liver in addition to the bilateral femur fractures. The injuries were surgically repaired and the patient was transferred to a burn center for treatment.

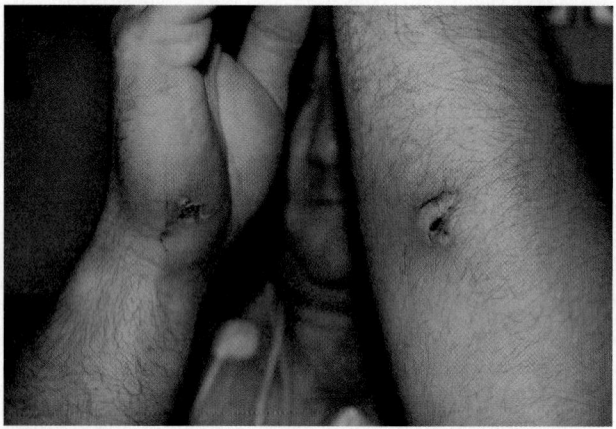

FIGURE 35-30

Entrance and exit electrical burns. (© Edward T. Dickinson, MD)

Radiation Burns

Ionizing radiation causes burn injuries by breaking the molecular bonds in the cells of the body. Those burns look identical to thermal burns and are cared for in the same way. The major difference between thermal burns and radiation burns is the onset. Radiation burns develop very slowly over days, as opposed to the rapid onset of thermal burns.

Think scene safety and personal protection with suspected radiation burns. A person cannot be radioactive and contaminate you unless he has been contaminated with radioactive material, as opposed to exposed to a radiation source without contamination. Because of the slow onset of radiation burn injuries, it is not likely for those burns to be called in as an emergency. (The response to and proper management of radiation contaminated patients is discussed in Chapter 48.)

CHAPTER REVIEW

Chapter Summary

In this chapter, you learned to identify the different types of soft-tissue injuries and bleeding and how to properly manage them. The control of life-threatening bleeding is one of the single most important skills that you possess as an Advanced EMT. If you cannot control bleeding, the patient will surely deteriorate, increasing morbidity and mortality rates.

A key point to remember is that even though fluid therapy is often necessary for patients with bleeding, the initiation of intravenous access should never delay transport of the patient. You should obtain IV access en route to an appropriate facility.

You also learned to categorize burns by severity and manage specific burn injuries. It is important to not allow yourself to become distracted by gruesome injuries and the patient's emotional distress when managing a burn-injured patient. You must complete a systematic approach to assessment and management in order to reduce morbidity and mortality associated with burn injury.

The three most important aspects of managing burn patients are:

- Maintain a patent airway.
- Identify traumatic injury in conjunction with the burn and treat the traumatic injury first.
- Initiate fluid resuscitation using the Parkland burn formula.

Review Questions

Multiple-Choice Questions

1. The condition of an extremity that results from edema reaching a point that nervous function and circulation are compromised is called:
   a. compartment syndrome.
   b. crush injury.
   c. clamping injury.
   d. compression syndrome.

2. Which one of the following types of open injury is most prone to infection?
   a. Laceration   c. Avulsion
   b. Abrasion   d. Amputation

3. Identifying the blade length and width of a knife that was used in a stabbing will:
   a. provide you an idea of what internal organs may have been injured by the knife.
   b. provide you with an idea of how much force was involved with the injury.
   c. assist you in determining how critical the patient is.
   d. determine the medical facility that you will transport the patient to.

4. Complications of traumatic rhabdomyolysis occur following:
   a. significant superficial burn injuries.
   b. initiation of intravenous access.
   c. renal failure and hyperkalemia.
   d. the reperfusion of the affected tissues.

5. Impaled objects are immobilized as found in order to:
   a. reduce the patient's pain while moving them to and from your stretcher.
   b. allow the receiving physician to assess the mechanism of injury.
   c. prevent increases in bleeding from the puncture wound.
   d. reduce the possibility of infection.

6. Which one of the statements about amputations is correct?
   a. Immerse the amputated part in sterile water to remove debris, if possible.
   b. Do not place the amputated part directly on ice.
   c. All amputated parts can be surgically reattached.
   d. Wrap a tourniquet just distal to the open injury to control bleeding.

7. Which one of the following steps should you take first when caring for a patient with an open neck injury?
   a. Cover the injury with your gloved hand.
   b. Provide high-flow oxygen to the patient.
   c. Locate an occlusive bandage in your gear to cover the injury.
   d. Identify the most appropriate facility to transport the patient.

8. Which one of the following is applied directly on an open injury?
   a. Dressing
   b. Pressure dressing
   c. Bandage
   d. Air splint

9. Which one of the following statements about external bleeding is true?
   a. It is the most common chief complaint that you will experience as an Advanced EMT.
   b. It will not pose a risk to you.
   c. The severity of bleeding has nothing to do with the size of the injured vessel.
   d. The size of a vessel determines how much bleeding will occur.

10. The best way to determine whether bleeding was significant to the patient is:
    a. by relying on the patient's clinical signs and symptoms.
    b. to estimate the volume of blood on the scene.
    c. to ask the patient how much blood he has lost.
    d. to assess the patient's blood pressure.

11. You should suspect internal bleeding:
    a. if the mechanism of injury suggests a possibility of it.
    b. whenever your patient loses consciousness following head trauma.
    c. if the patient complains of lower back pain.
    d. whenever the patient complains of difficulty breathing.

12. Which one of the following mechanisms of injury should cause you to have a high index of suspicion for internal injury?
    a. MVC while traveling 30 mph
    b. Falls of greater than 20 feet
    c. Penetrating trauma distal to the knee
    d. Rear-end collision from a vehicle traveling 35 mph

13. Your goal while on the scene with a patient exhibiting signs and symptoms of internal bleeding is to:
    a. address life threats and transport as soon as possible.
    b. address life threats and obtain intravenous access.
    c. obtain intravenous access and provide fluid therapy.
    d. obtain a SAMPLE history as soon as possible in case the patient becomes disoriented or cannot speak.

14. The area of a burn injury where blood flow is compromised but may not become necrotic if blood flow is restored is called the zone of:
    a. coagulation.
    b. hyperemia.
    c. stasis.
    d. hypertrophy.

15. Which classification of burns is most painful?
    a. Partial-thickness burns
    b. Full-thickness burns
    c. Superficial burns
    d. Airway burns

16. A hand-to-hand electrical burn constitutes approximately what percent of BSA?
    a. 30 percent
    b. 25 percent
    c. 35 percent
    d. 20 percent

17. A patient with partial-thickness and full-thickness burns to his anterior right arm and chest represents what percent of BSA burned?
    a. 12.5 percent
    b. 27 percent
    c. 18 percent
    d. 14.5 percent

18. Which one of the following is considered to be a critical burn injury?
    a. Circumferential burn
    b. Superficial burn greater than 50 percent
    c. Full-thickness burn greater than 5 percent
    d. Partial-thickness burn greater than 20 percent

19. Significant burn-injury patients are prone to:
    a. hypothermia.
    b. hypoglycemia.
    c. hypokalemia.
    d. hypercalcemia.

Critical-Thinking Questions

20. List the seven burn center referral criteria.

21. You arrive on the scene of a structure fire where a firefighter is complaining of difficulty breathing. He states that he had been inside the structure while not wearing respiratory protection. You determine that his vital signs are blood pressure 128/90, heart rate 92, respiratory rate 18 unlabored, SpO_2 98 percent. What do you believe has caused the patient's current complaint and how would you treat it?

22. Describe the process of controlling life-threatening external bleeding.

23. You and your partner arrive on the scene of a rollover collision with one patient who was ejected from the vehicle and is now exhibiting signs and symptoms of shock. Explain why it is important to minimize scene times and provide rapid transport for this critically injured patient to the most appropriate facility.

References

American Burn Association. (2007). *Advanced burn life support course provider manual.* Chicago, IL: American Burn Association.

Campbell, J. E. (2008). *International trauma life support* (6th ed.). Upper Saddle River, NJ: Pearson Prentice Hall.

Additional Reading

Williams, B., & Boyle, M. (2007). Estimation of external blood loss by paramedics: Is there any point? *Prehospital and Disaster Medicine, 22*(6), 502–506.

36

Musculoskeletal Injuries

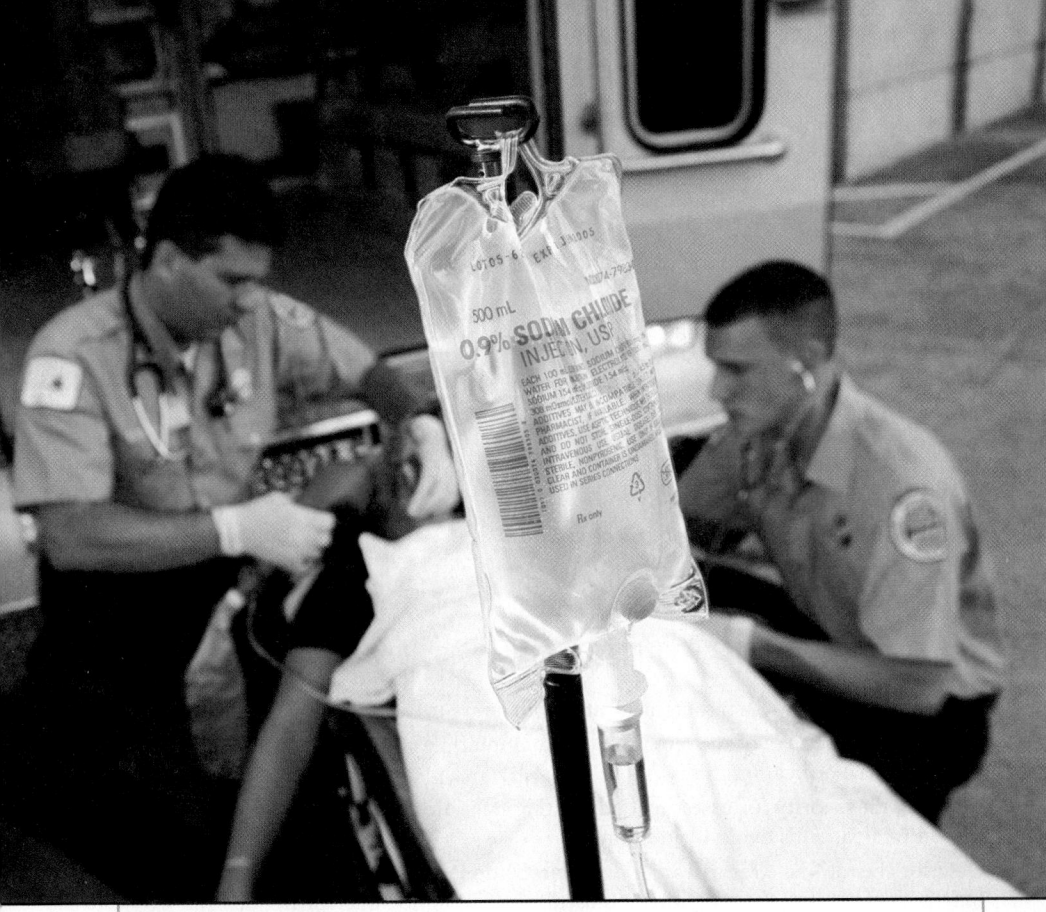

Content Area: Trauma

Advanced EMT Education Standard: The Advanced EMT applies fundamental knowledge to provide basic and selected advanced emergency care and transportation based on assessment findings for an acutely injured patient.

Resource **Central**

Objectives

After reading this chapter, you should be able to:

36.1   Define key terms introduced in this chapter.

36.2   Describe the structures and functions of the musculoskeletal system, including:

- Bones
- Cartilage
- Joints
- Ligaments
- Skeletal muscle
- Tendons

36.3   Give examples of direct, indirect, and twisting forces that can produce musculoskeletal injuries.

(continued)

CASE STUDY

Advanced EMTs Mark Ducote and Joey Galliano are dispatched to a fall in a local shopping mall parking lot. As they approach the scene in their vehicle, they see a woman lying on her side near the curb. They park their unit and advise dispatch that they have arrived on the scene. A man runs toward them.

"My wife fell and her leg looks like it is broken," says the man. As they grab their gear and head toward the woman, Mark and Joey can hear the woman crying.

Joey introduces himself to the patient, who is holding her lower right leg. "My name is Joey and this is my partner, Mark. What is your name?"

"My name is Janice," she whispers. Then exclaims, "My leg is killing me!"

Problem-Solving Questions

1. What should Joey and Mark's next immediate steps entail?
2. What questions should Joey and Mark ask at this point?
3. What are some potential injuries that could have occurred?

(continued from previous page)

36.4 Describe each of the following types of injuries:
- Dislocations and subluxations
- Fractures
- Sprains
- Strains

36.5 Describe the signs and symptoms associated with injury to the musculoskeletal system.

36.6 Explain why fractures of the femur, pelvis, and multiple concomitant long bones are considered critical fractures.

36.7 Establish the priority for assessing and treating musculoskeletal injuries with respect to a patient's overall condition.

36.8 Describe the rationale for assessing distal circulation, sensation, and motor function before and after splinting a musculoskeletal injury, and for frequently reassessing for changes in distal neurovascular function.

36.9 Recognize signs and symptoms of compartment syndrome.

36.10 Describe the pathophysiology of compartment syndrome.

36.11 Consider the need for fluid replacement and pain management in patients with musculoskeletal injuries.

36.12 Explain the rationale for splinting musculoskeletal injuries.

36.13 Describe special considerations for splinting pelvic fractures.

36.14 Discuss pitfalls associated with improper splinting.

36.15 Compare and contrast the characteristics and uses of various types of splints, including the following:
- Formable splints
- Improvised splints
- Pressure (air or pneumatic) splints
- Rigid splints
- Sling and swathe
- Long backboard
- Traction splints
- Vacuum splints

36.16 Given a variety of scenarios involving patients with musculoskeletal injuries, manage the injury using general rules of proper splinting.

Introduction

Isolated musculoskeletal injuries generally are not life threatening. However, in some cases, severe internal or external hemorrhage may occur, resulting in a life-threatening condition. Also remember that musculoskeletal injuries can be sustained as part of multisystem trauma. The musculoskeletal injury may be the first thing to catch the patient's attention, and yours. Do not be distracted from the priorities of patient assessment and care by a dramatic-appearing musculoskeletal injury. As an Advanced EMT, your priorities when caring for a patient with musculoskeletal injuries include identifying immediate problems with the airway, breathing, and circulation, recognizing potentially life-threatening musculoskeletal injuries but not letting lesser ones distract you, and recognizing mechanisms of injury that can produce additional injury to the patient.

In the absence of a life-threatening condition, you will focus on immobilizing the injured extremity, or splinting. When life-threatening injury is present, you will focus on managing immediate life threats, packaging the patient, and transporting to an appropriate facility where definitive treatment can be provided.

In addition to extremity injuries, a common musculoskeletal complaint is back pain, particularly low back pain. Back pain is is a common type of musculoskeletal injury that can lead to temporary or permanent disability. Among individuals under 45 years old, back pain results in approximately 95 million workdays lost annually with a cost of up to $50 million (Dailey, 2010).

In this chapter, you will learn to recognize and manage various types of musculoskeletal injuries.

Anatomy and Physiology Review

The musculoskeletal system consists of 206 bones and more than 700 skeletal muscles (Figure 36-1). Following are the functions of the musculoskeletal system:

- Provide shape to the body
- Protect internal organs
- Provide for movement of the body
- Produce red blood cells

Skeletal Muscles

Skeletal muscles are the muscles of the body that provide for voluntary movement. These muscles allow for movement because of their attachment to bones. When a skeletal muscle contracts, it pulls the attached bones together. Opposing skeletal muscles contract and move the bones apart. When muscles are overexerted, they can become injured, or strained, resulting in pain and loss of function.

Ligaments and Tendons

Ligaments and tendons are specialized connective tissues within the body. Ligaments are connective tissues that connect bone to bone (Figure 36-2). Tendons are connective tissue that connects muscle to bone (Figure 36-3). Just as any other tissue in the body, ligaments and tendons can become injured, or sprained, resulting in pain and loss of function.

Cartilage

Cartilage is connective tissue found between two bones, such as the cartilage that covers the ends of the bones that comprise the knee joint. Cartilage provides shock absorption and allows the bones to move against one another without friction. Cartilage also serves other functions, such as providing structure without the rigidity of bone, such as the cartilage of the external ear and nose. Varying amounts of cartilage connect the ribs to the sternum, with larger areas of cartilage connecting the lower ribs to the sternum. The flexibility of this cartilage allows for expansion of the rib cage during ventilation. Cartilage can be injured, resulting in pain and loss of function. It is avascular (having little direct blood supply) and heals poorly when injured.

Bones

The 206 bones that comprise the skeletal system are divided into the axial and appendicular skeletons. The axial skeleton consists of the head, bones of the thorax, and the spine. The appendicular skeleton consists of the pelvis, shoulder girdles, and bones of the extremities.

Bones of the skeletal system are categorized by shape, as follows:

- *Long bones.* The **long bones** include the femur, humerus, radius, ulna, tibia, and fibula.
- *Short bones.* The **short bones** include metacarpals, metatarsals, and phalanges.
- *Flat bones.* **Flat bones** include the sternum, scapula, and ribs.
- *Sesamoid bones.* **Sesamoid bones,** so called for their resemblance in shape to sesame seeds, are located within a tendon and include the patella and the pisiform of the wrist.

Being familiar with the bones of the skeletal system assists you in assessing and caring for patients with musculoskeletal injuries (Figures 36-4 and 36-5) and in communicating these injuries in precise terms to the emergency department (ED) physician.

Bone is living, metabolically active tissue with blood supply and nerves. The structure of bone is continually remodeled as calcium and other minerals are deposited in the bone and released to the blood as needed. The bone marrow in the cavity of certain bones produces blood cells.

FIGURE 36-1

The skeletal system.

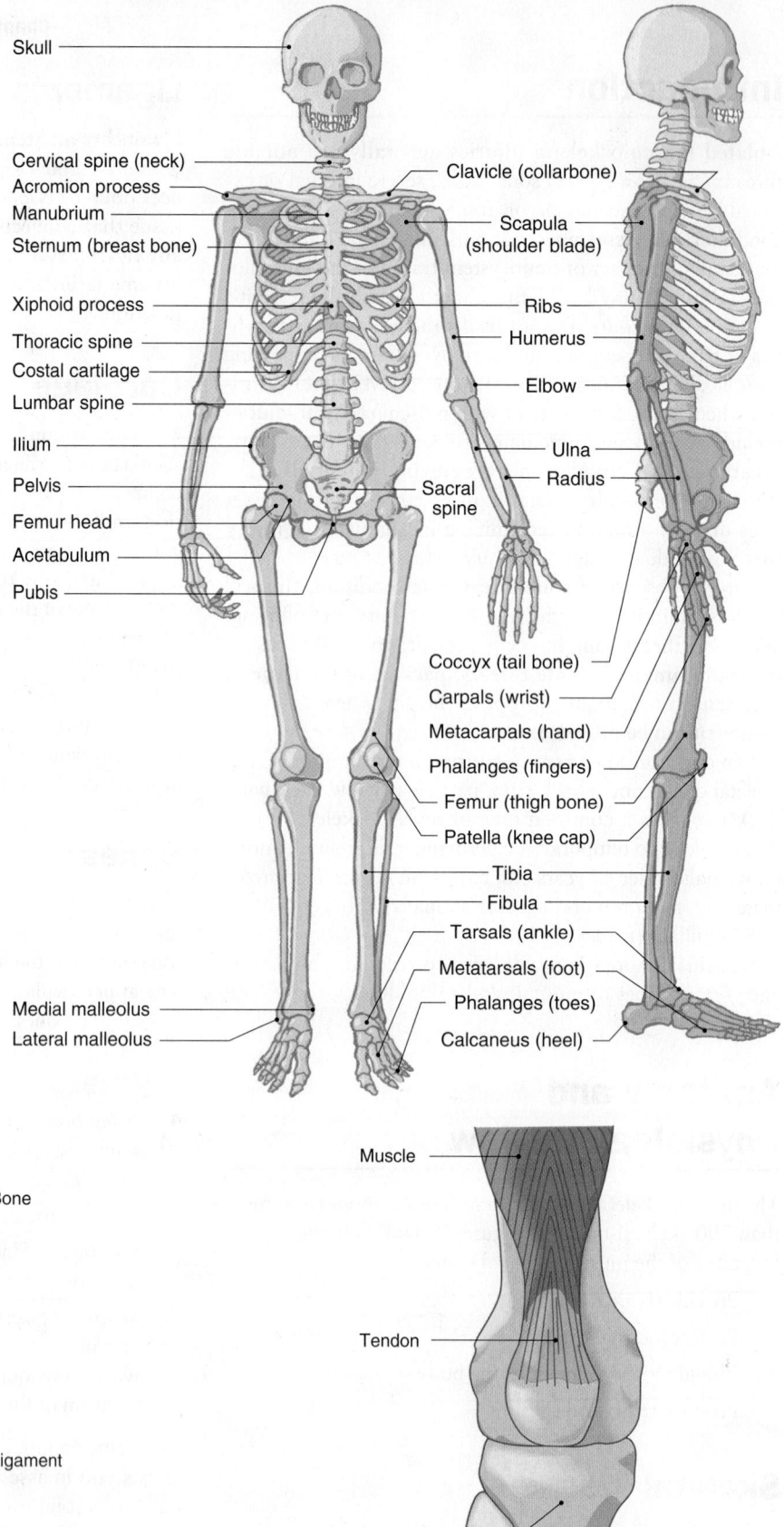

Skull

Cervical spine (neck)
Acromion process
Manubrium
Sternum (breast bone)

Xiphoid process
Thoracic spine
Costal cartilage
Lumbar spine
Ilium
Pelvis
Femur head
Acetabulum
Pubis

Clavicle (collarbone)

Scapula
(shoulder blade)

Ribs
Humerus
Elbow

Ulna
Radius

Sacral
spine

Coccyx (tail bone)
Carpals (wrist)
Metacarpals (hand)
Phalanges (fingers)
Femur (thigh bone)
Patella (knee cap)

Tibia
Fibula
Tarsals (ankle)
Metatarsals (foot)
Phalanges (toes)
Calcaneus (heel)

Medial malleolus
Lateral malleolus

Bone

Ligament

Bone

Muscle

Tendon

Bone

FIGURE 36-2

Ligaments attach bone to bone.

FIGURE 36-3

Tendons connect muscle to bone.

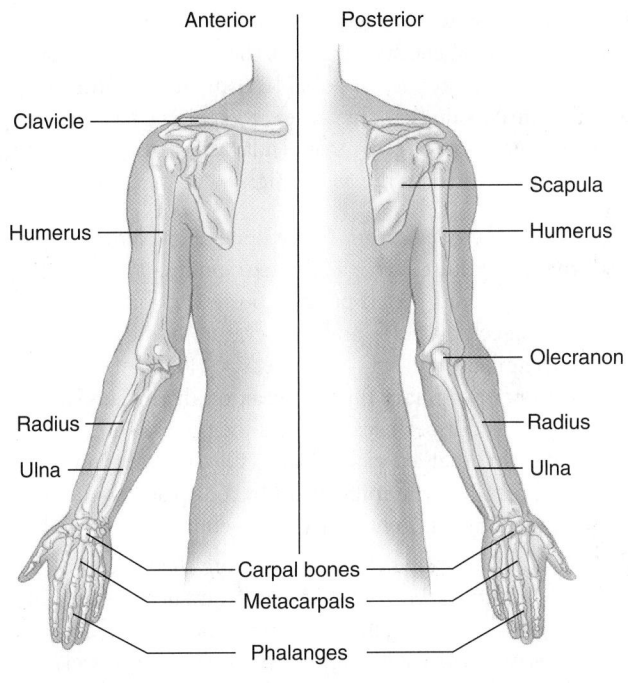

Anterior | Posterior

Clavicle

Humerus

Radius

Ulna

Scapula

Humerus

Olecranon

Radius

Ulna

Carpal bones
Metacarpals
Phalanges

FIGURE 36-4

Bones of the upper extremities.

Joints

Joints are the points at which the bones meet and articulate to allow motion. Joints allow for various types of movement, including flexion, extension, adduction, abduction, circumduction, and rotation. They are complex structures of bone, cartilage, and ligaments. Nerves and blood vessels pass in close proximity to joints. Any of these tissues may be injured when there is a joint injury.

General Assessment and Management of Musculoskeletal Injuries

As with most calls, you will not know the exact type of injuries a patient has until you arrive on the scene. In the scene size-up, determine the mechanism of injury, look for indications of dangers at the scene, determine if there are additional patients, request any additional resources needed, and gain a general impression of your patient's condition.

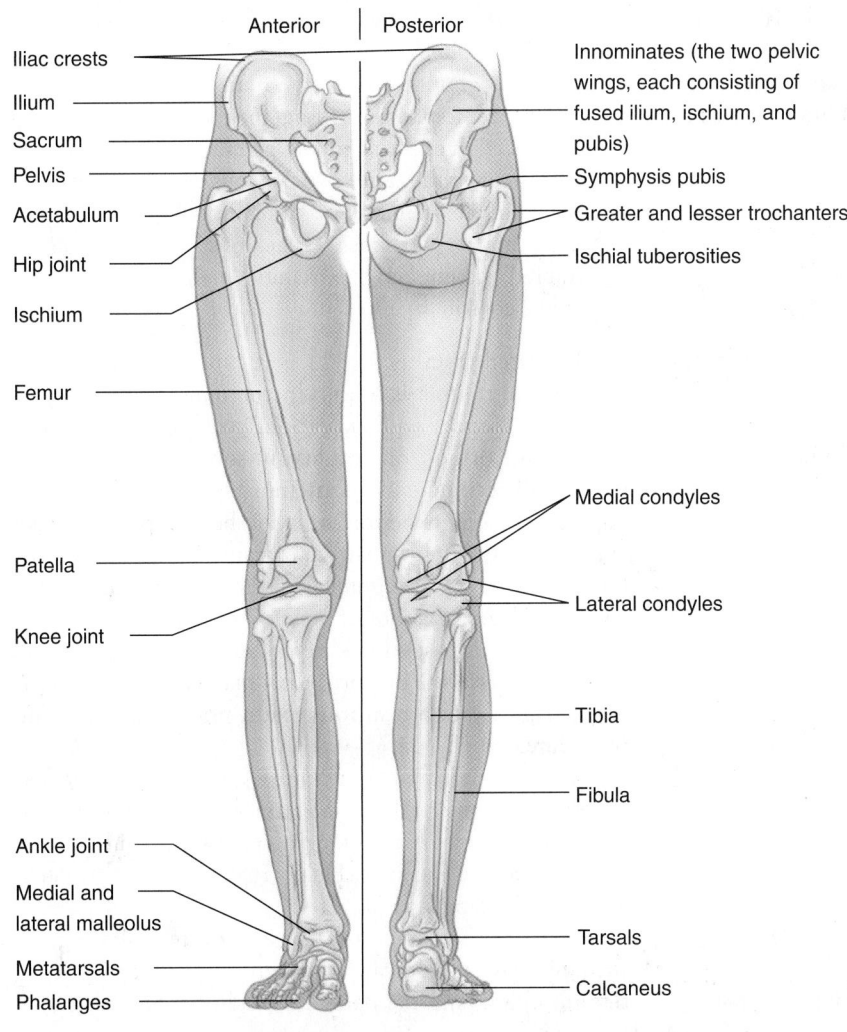

Anterior | Posterior

Iliac crests
Ilium
Sacrum
Pelvis
Acetabulum
Hip joint
Ischium

Femur

Patella
Knee joint

Ankle joint
Medial and
lateral malleolus
Metatarsals
Phalanges

Innominates (the two pelvic wings, each consisting of fused ilium, ischium, and pubis)
Symphysis pubis
Greater and lesser trochanters
Ischial tuberosities

Medial condyles

Lateral condyles

Tibia

Fibula

Tarsals

Calcaneus

FIGURE 36-5

Bones of the lower extremities.

Musculoskeletal injuries can be very dramatic. Never let the appearance of those injuries distract you from performing a systematic assessment and identifying life threats.

In most cases, patients with musculoskeletal injuries have experienced isolated injury of a bone, joint, or muscle from a minor mechanism of injury, such as tripping and falling onto an outstretched hand. The pain associated with these injuries can be severe and your proper assessment and management will help reduce the patient's pain and anxiety, but such patients do not require expedited transport. Take your time before packaging and transport to properly perform a focused exam and manage the patient's injury. Also obtain baseline vital signs and a medical history, which you can do en route.

You must, however, always consider the mechanism of injury. A patient who has fallen from a height or who has been involved in a significant motor vehicle collision (MVC) must receive a rapid trauma exam and detailed head-to-toe exam. If the patient is critical, prepare to transport while managing the airway, breathing, and circulation. Use a long backboard as a single means of providing immobilization for all musculoskeletal injuries the patient may have. If the patient's condition and time allow, you can manage individual injuries en route to the hospital.

Focused Assessment of Musculoskeletal Injuries

When assessing a specific musculoskeletal injury, use the DCAP-BTLS mnemonic as a guide to looking for signs and symptoms of injury. Expose the injured area and use the techniques of examination and palpation and look specifically for the following signs and symptoms of musculoskeletal injuries:

- Pain
- Deformity or abnormal positioning
- Swelling
- Loss of function
- Discoloration
- Bleeding
- Crepitus
- Exposed bone
- Bruising, hematoma, abrasions, or lacerations over the bone
- Decreased circulation distal to the injury
- Decreased motor function distal to the injury

In addition to assessing the patient's general cardiovascular and neurologic status, assess the neurovascular status of the injured extremity. If possible, compare the findings to the uninjured side (in some cases, the patient has bilateral injuries). Assessment of neurovascular function distal to the side of injury includes the following:

- *Assess the circulation.* In the upper extremities, check the radial pulse. In the lower extremities, check the dorsalis pedis (pedal) pulse or posterior tibial pulse. Also check the color and temperature of the skin and the capillary refill of the nailbeds. Cold, pale skin with poor capillary fill or a weak or absent pulse are signs of poor perfusion beyond the point of injury, indicating that arterial blood supply is compromised by direct injury, impingement by a displaced bone or bone fragment, joint injury, or swelling.

- *Assess tactile sensation by touching the hand or foot distal to the site of injury.* Numbness, decreased sensation, and tingling sensations (paresthesia) are signs of sensory nerve injury. As with blood vessels, the nerves can be damaged directly, compressed by bone, trapped within an injured joint, or compressed by general edema of the extremity.

- *Assess motor function in the upper extremities by having the patient grasp your fingers and squeeze with both hands simultaneously, to identify weakness.* For the lower extremities, have the patient use his feet to dorsiflex (bring the toes upward in the direction of the shin) and plantar flex (push the toes downward) against your hands. Weakness of the injured extremity indicates injury to the nerves of the extremity. Weakness or lack of sensation in both injured and uninjured extremities indicates a possible spinal cord injury.

Impaired distal neurovascular function due to musculoskeletal trauma is a limb-threatening injury and you must transport the patient without delay to a facility that can manage orthopedic trauma. In some cases, your protocols will recommend an attempt to grossly realign the injured extremity to restore function before splinting. This is particularly important if your transport times are prolonged. However, realignment of deformed extremities is painful (although pain relief may follow once the deformity is reduced) and poses a risk of further injury to the nerves and blood vessels. Your protocols may allow you to provide analgesia, such as nitrous oxide, prior to the splinting procedure.

You should splint some injuries, such as a dislocated knee joint, in the position they are found. Posterior knee dislocations carry a high risk of injury of the popliteal artery that runs behind the knee. Hemorrhage from the popliteal artery can be rapidly fatal.

Reassess the neurovascular status after splinting the extremity and periodically throughout transport to identify any changes in the patient's condition. Splinting may inadvertently cause additional injury to a blood vessel or nerve, although the primary reason for obtaining a baseline before splinting and reassessing is to document that there was no deterioration in neurovascular function as a result of splinting. As the injury progresses, additional swelling can cause impairment of neurovascular function. You must quickly detect and treat that condition, which is compartment syndrome. Frequent reassessment is the best way to detect developing compartment syndrome. Reassessment also allows you to identify an improperly placed splint. Often, a splint was properly applied, but additional swelling afterward makes the splint too tight.

Splinting and Care of Musculoskeletal Injuries

Care of musculoskeletal injuries includes immobilization and reducing pain, bleeding, and swelling. Immobilization decreases additional injury and pain. Adjuncts to immobilization to decrease pain, bleeding, and swelling include elevating injured extremities and applying a cold pack to the injured area.

Splinting uses an external device to stabilize an injured extremity and prevent it from moving. Splinting reduces additional injury from movement of the injured part and reduces pain. **Splints** come in many varieties and also can be improvised, if necessary. Commercial devices include rigid splints, pressure splints, traction splints, formable splints, vacuum splints, sling and swathe, and long backboards.

General Principles of Splinting and Types of Splints

No matter which type of splint is best in a given situation, there are several general principles of splinting to consider, as follows:

- Treat life-threatening conditions first; splint individual injuries only if the patient's condition allows.

- Assess the distal neurovascular status before and after splinting.

- Pad splints or otherwise make them so that they do not cause injury to the skin and soft tissues.

- Immobilize an injury to a bone to include the joint proximal to the injury and the joint distal to the injury.

- Immobilize an injury to a joint to include the bone proximal to the injury and the bone distal to the injury.

Rigid Splints

Rigid splints are made of wood, plastic, cardboard, or metal. They may be straight, unformed boards or formed aluminum or plastic designed to fit the contours of a specific part of an extremity. They are very effective in immobilizing injured body parts, but require padding to provide comfort and prevent soft-tissue injury. If the splint does not have integrated padding, use roller gauze as padding by wrapping the splint until padding is adequate. Rigid splints come in various lengths and widths. Select the splint that allows you to immobilize adequately. Rigid splints are secured in place with roller gauze. As you wrap the extremity to secure the splint,

PERSONAL PERSPECTIVE

Advanced EMT Greg Niles: While standing by at the last local high school football game of the season, my partner and I were watching as the running back for the home team broke a few tackles before being hit in the legs and brought down. When he was hit, we saw that his right leg buckled half way between his knee and ankle. We knew that we would be heading onto the field to treat the player.

Immediately after the tackle, the player began screaming, while players and coaches near him along the sideline called for us to come to his side. We grabbed our stretcher, with our gear on it, and headed for the player.

The player had a severely angulated and open right tib-fib fracture. We carefully splinted the fracture in the position found as best we could and began transport to the closest hospital with orthopedic services.

En route to the hospital I spoke to the player and to his mother, who was accompanying him. The player was in obvious pain, despite the nitrous oxide we gave him, and was crying. His mother was also crying. I attempted to reassure them, but was not being effective.

His mother then explained to me that this was his last high school game and he had committed to play football at a major university with a full scholarship. His mother went on to explain that no one in their family had ever gone to college, and the only way that he would be able to attend was with a scholarship, because she could not afford to pay his tuition.

We arrived at the hospital and transferred care to the emergency department staff.

About two weeks following that night, I was contacted by my supervisor and advised that she had a letter that was addressed to me. I picked the letter up later that day.

The letter was from the football player's mother. In the letter she expressed her thanks for our caring for her son. She went on to explain that the orthopedic surgeon told her that it was a good thing that the medics who cared for her son did not attempt to straighten his leg and instead splinted it in the position found, because manipulation of the fracture could have produced additional injury.

The player made a full recovery and went on to play college football the next year.

Although this patient's injury was not life threatening, it could have been life changing. Because we properly managed the injury, this young man was able to make a full recovery and carry on with his life.

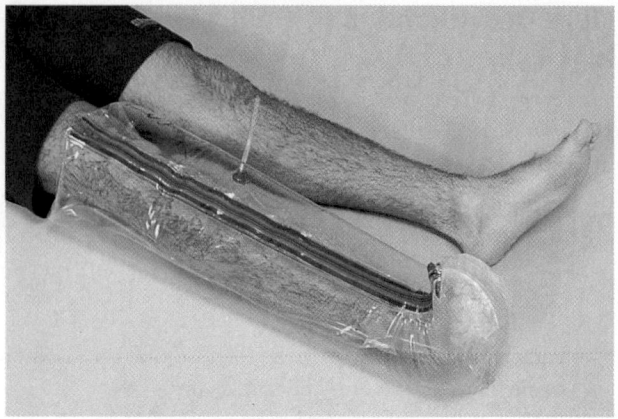

FIGURE 36-6

Air splint applied to the lower leg.

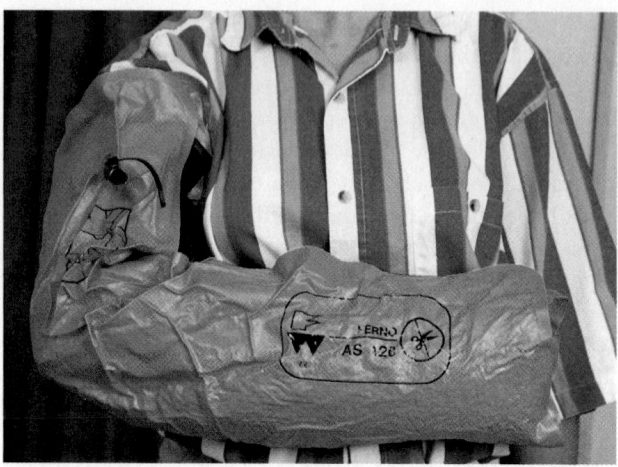

FIGURE 36-7

A vacuum splint immobilizing an injured arm.

make sure you allow access to check the distal neurovascular status. Secure the splint to immobilize the extremity, but do not secure it so tightly that circulation is compromised.

Moldable Splints

Moldable splints are similar to board splints, but they are pliable in order to be molded to fit the extremity. They are sturdy, yet can be fitted to a specific patient's needs.

Pressure Splints

Pressure splints are also called *air splints* or *pneumatic splints* (Figure 36-6). Air splints are made of pliable material, such as vinyl. They are made like a sleeve to be slipped onto the extremity, or have a zipper that allows them to be placed around the extremity and then zipped. Pressure splints are double walled to create air chambers that are inflated after the splint is applied. When the splint is inflated, it provides stabilization and support to the injured area. A disadvantage to the use of air splints is that once applied, they may not allow access to reassess the pulse.

Vacuum Splints

Vacuum splints are constructed of pliable material that, when applied, conforms to the shape of an injured extremity (Figure 36-7). The splint is applied and a pump is used to suck the air out of it. As the air is sucked out, the splint collapses upon itself, conforms to the shape of the extremity, and becomes rigid.

Sling and Swathe

A sling and swathe can be used as a standalone splint for a shoulder or clavicle injury, or as an adjunct to supporting a splinted arm, elbow, forearm, or hand. It is a splinting method used to assist with the immobilization of an injured arm or shoulder (Figure 36-8). Slings are available

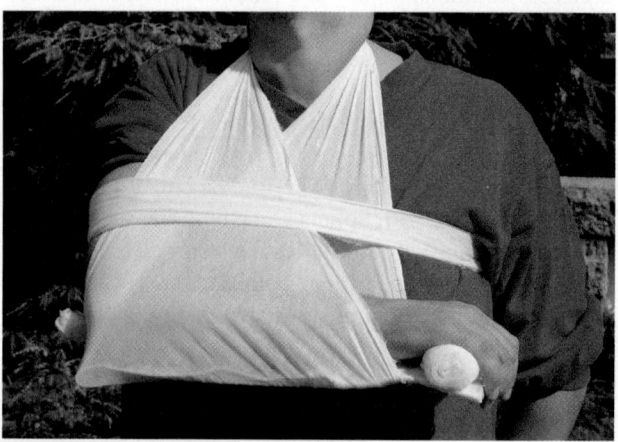

FIGURE 36-8

A sling and swathe applied to immobilize the shoulder and arm.

commercially or can be made from a triangular bandage or improvised from a similarly shaped piece of cloth. The sling supports the arm by suspending it from the shoulder. A swathe is a bandage or strap that is wrapped or tied around the patient's torso holding the arm firmly against the body. The sling and swathe reduce the potential for movement of the arm and shoulder. The proper procedure for applying a sling and swathe is illustrated in Scan 36-1.

Long Backboard

In addition to immobilizing the spine, you can use a long backboard as a patient handling device and as a device to grossly immobilize the extremities of a patient who is critical and must be transported without delay. In such cases, improper handling can worsen the patient's condition, but so will delaying critical interventions and transport

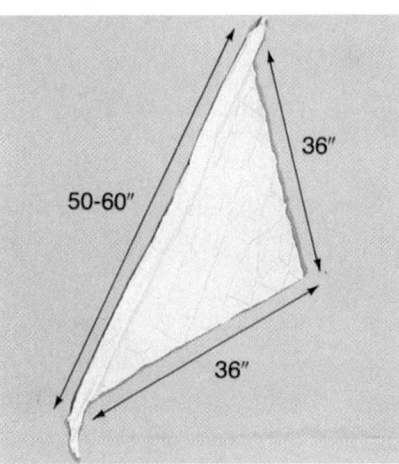

1. Prepare the sling by folding cloth into a triangle. A triangle bandage makes an ideal arm sling.

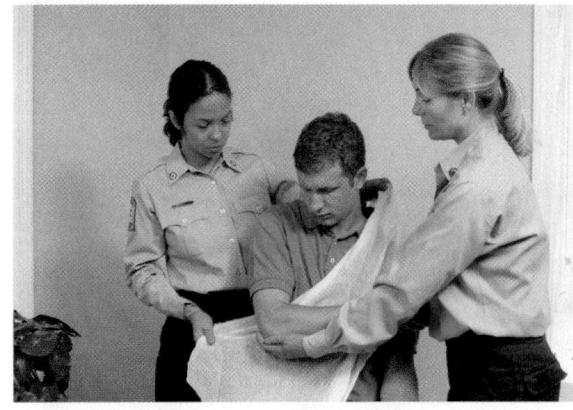

2. Position the sling over the top of the patient's chest as shown. Fold the patient's injured arm across his chest.

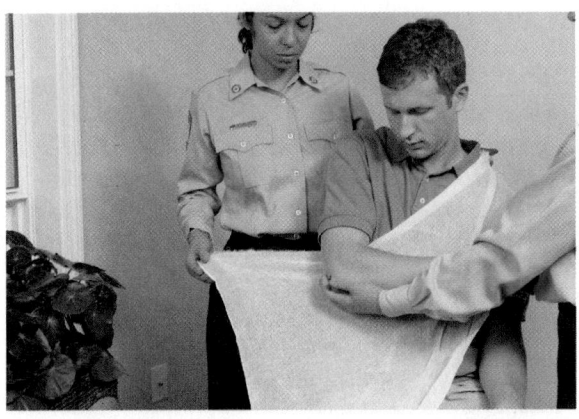

3. If the patient cannot hold his arm, have someone assist until you tie the sling.

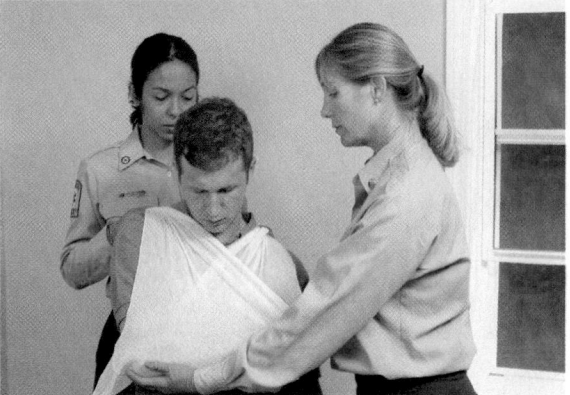

4. Extend one point of the triangle beyond the elbow on the injured side. Take the bottom point and bring it up over the patient's arm. Then take it over the top of the injured shoulder.

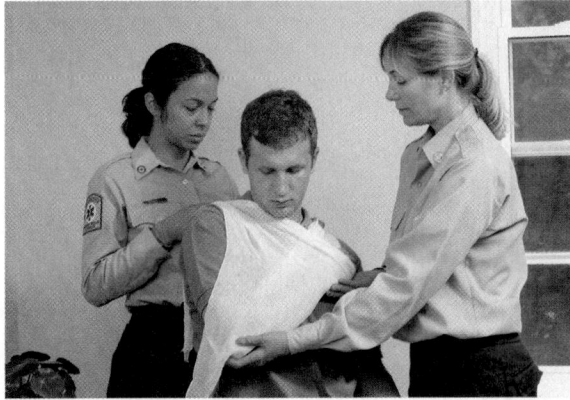

5. If appropriate, draw up the ends of the sling so the patient's hand is about 4 inches above the elbow.

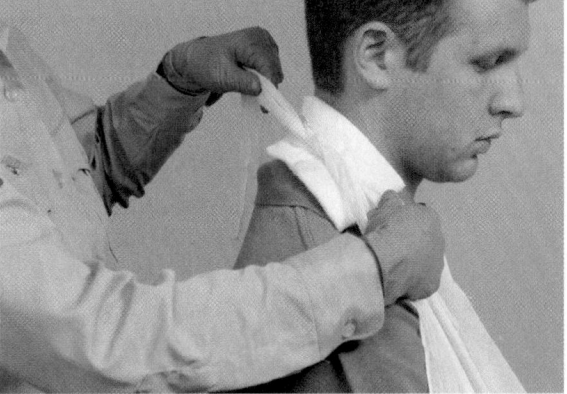

6. Tie the two ends of the sling together, making sure that the knot does not press against the back of the patient's neck. Pad with bulky dressings. (If spine injury is possible, pin ends to clothing. Do not tie around the neck.)

(continued)

Properly Applied Sling and Swathe (continued)

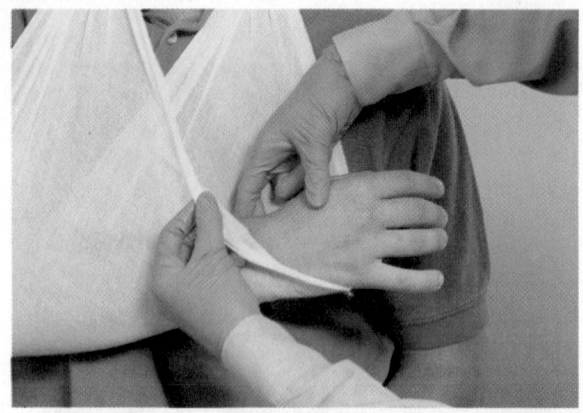

7. Check to be sure you have left the patient's fingertips exposed. Then assess distal neurovascular function. If the pulse is absent, take off the sling and repeat the procedure. Then check again.

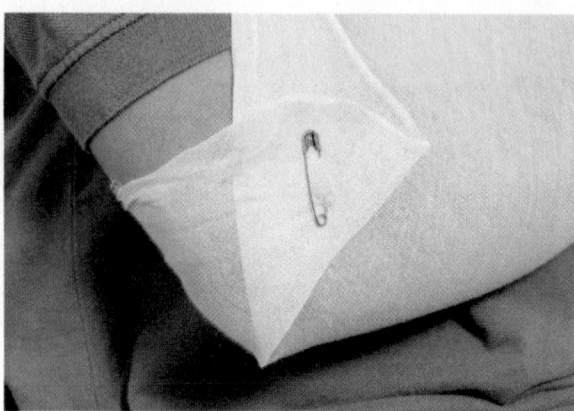

8. To form a pocket for the patient's elbow, take hold of the point of material at the elbow and fold it forward, pinning it to the front of the sling.

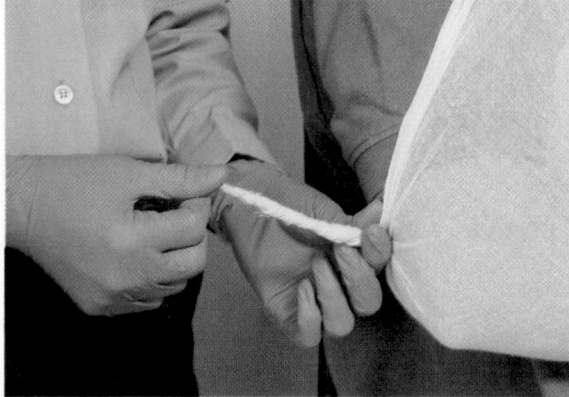

9. If you do not have a pin, twist the excess material and tie a knot in the point.

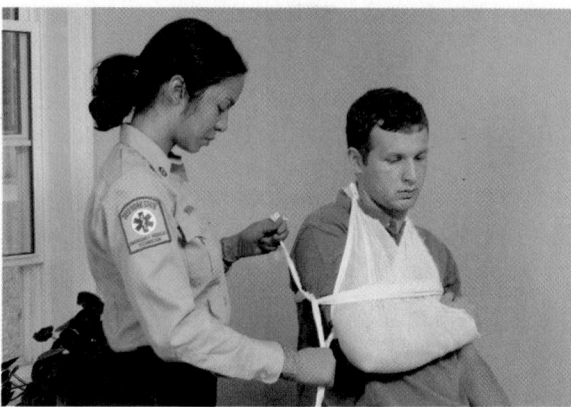

10. Form a swathe from a second piece of material. Tie it around the chest and the injured arm, over the sling. Do not place it over the patient's arm on the uninjured side.

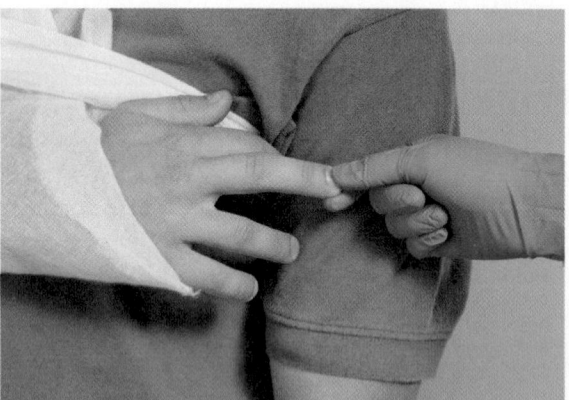

11. Reassess distal neurovascular function. Treat for shock and provide high-concentration oxygen. Take vital signs. Perform detailed assessments and reassessments as appropriate.

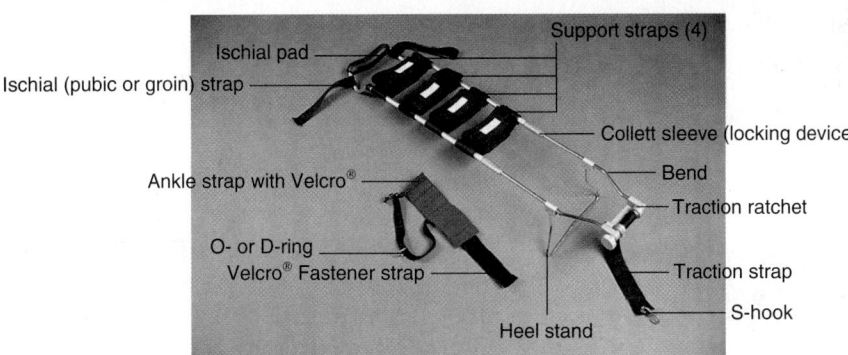

FIGURE 36-9

Traction splint.

to care for individual injuries. The long backboard allows you to move the patient without complicating any extremity injuries he may have.

Traction Splints

Traction splints are used only to immobilize fractures of the femur in certain patients. In addition to immobilization, they apply traction to the extremity to overcome the spasms of the powerful thigh muscles that can accompany femur fractures. Restoring the thigh muscles to their normal length accomplishes several goals. It decreases the volume of space available to collect blood from the large blood vessels of the femur and thigh that can be injured, reducing the overall amount of hemorrhage. It grossly aligns the ends of the femur, reducing pain, and it uses the thigh muscles to help provide stability to the fractured bone to prevent movement.

Traction splints consist of a frame that fits against a fixed point of the skeleton, such as the ischical tuberosity of the pelvis. The frame is attached at a second point that is used to apply traction against the fixed point, such as the ankle. Once the frame is secured against a fixed point, a ratchet device is used to lengthen the extremity (Figure 36-9).

There are two types of traction splints: bipolar frame and unipolar frame. A bipolar frame traction splint has two rails that comprise its frame. A unipolar traction splint frame consists of only one rail. The application of each is discussed later in this chapter.

Formable splints are constructed of a malleable material that allows the splint to be formed to the shape of an injured extremity. Once the splint is formed to the shape of the extremity, it is secured using tape, Velcro, or cravats.

Improvised Splints

When a commercial splint is not available or does not meet the unique demands of a situation, you may need to improvise a splint from materials available at the scene. An improvised splint is any object or material that is used to immobilize an injured extremity. You can be creative as long as you adhere to the general principles of splinting. Examples include sticks, a towel, cardboard boxes, a pillow, or a rolled-up magazine (Figure 36-10).

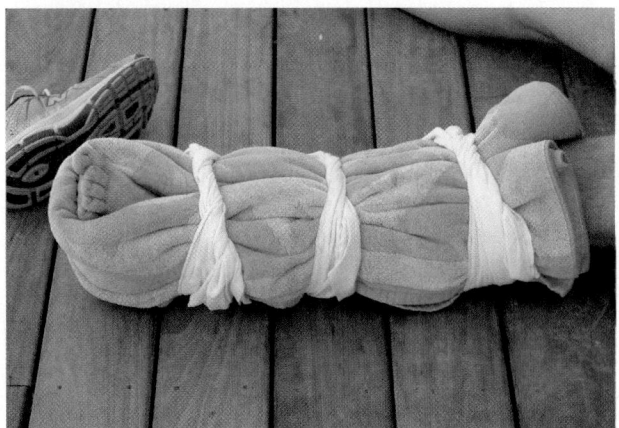

FIGURE 36-10

A towel used as an improvised splint.

Fractures

A **fracture** is a break in a bone and includes everything from a small, hairline crack in the bone's surface to a severely fragmented bone. Fractures result from a variety of forces, including direct, indirect, and twisting forces (Table 36-1). Mechanisms include assaults, falls,

TABLE 36-1	Types of Forces That Can Cause Fractures
Type of Force	**Examples**
Direct force	Being struck by a baseball bat in the upper arm, resulting in a fracture to the humerus
Indirect force	Falling on outstretched hands, resulting in a fracture to the radius and ulna
Twisting force	Stepping into a hole while running, causing a twisting of the lower leg, and resulting in a fracture to the tibia and fibula

gunshot wounds, MVCs, and other substantial forces. A weakened bone requires minimal force to break. When a bone breaks because it is weakened by disease, such as severe osteoporosis or cancer, it is called a *pathologic fracture.*

Geriatric Care

Elderly patients are more susceptible to fractures because their bones are not as rigid and dense as those of a healthy younger adult. Additionally, they may develop osteoporosis, a degenerative disease of the bones that results in bone weakness.

Pediatric Care

Pediatric patients are not as susceptible to fractures as adults are. This is because of the flexibility of their bones, which are not fully developed and rigid. If fracture is present, you must assume that the mechanism of injury was significant.

Types of Fractures

The various types of fractures include the following (Figure 36-11):

- *Comminuted fracture.* A **comminuted fracture** is one in which the bone is broken into multiple pieces.
- *Impacted fracture.* An **impacted fracture** results from bone being compressed along its axis.
- *Greenstick fracture.* A partial fracture of the bone, the **greenstick fracture**, is typically seen in pediatric patients.
- *Oblique fracture.* The **oblique fracture** runs at an angle other than 90 degrees to the axis of the bone.
- *Spiral fracture.* A fracture that runs spirally around the bone, the **spiral fracture**, is usually caused by twisting forces.
- *Transverse fracture.* A **transverse fracture** is at a 90-degree angle to the axis of the bone.

Fractures are classified as either open or closed. An **open fracture** is a fracture in which a broken bone end causes a break in the integrity of the skin. As with any open wound, open fractures carry a risk of infection. A **closed fracture** is a fracture in which a broken bone end does not break the integrity of the skin (Figure 36-12).

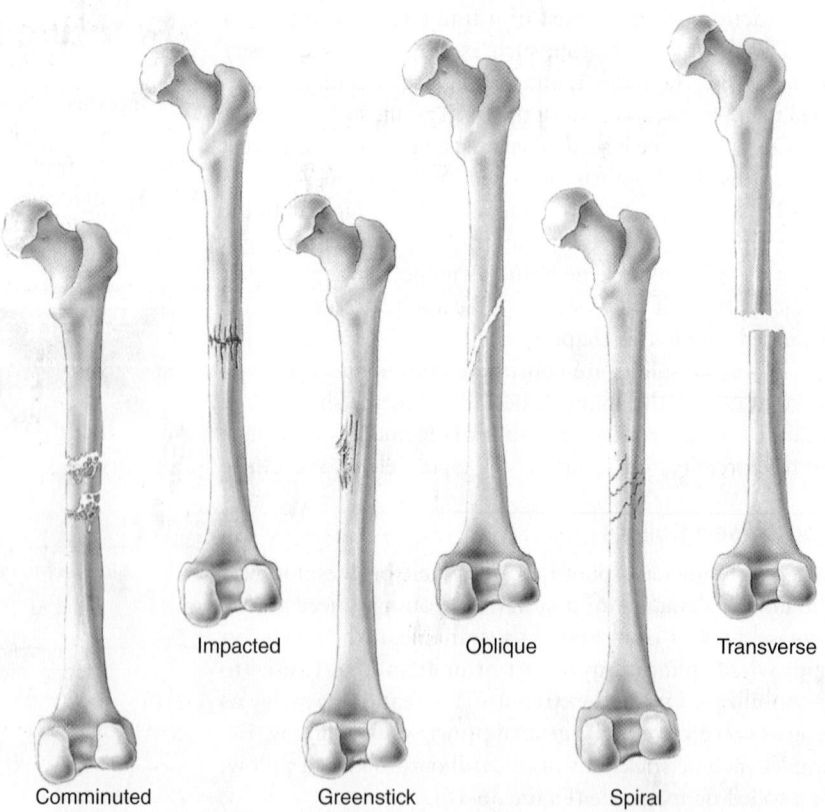

FIGURE 36-11

Types of fractures.

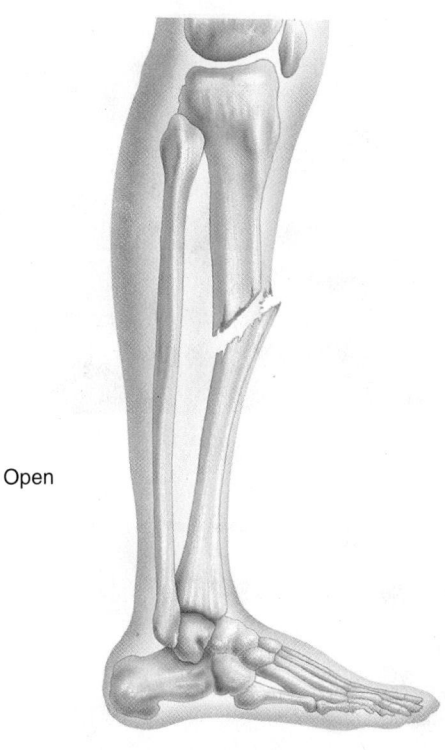
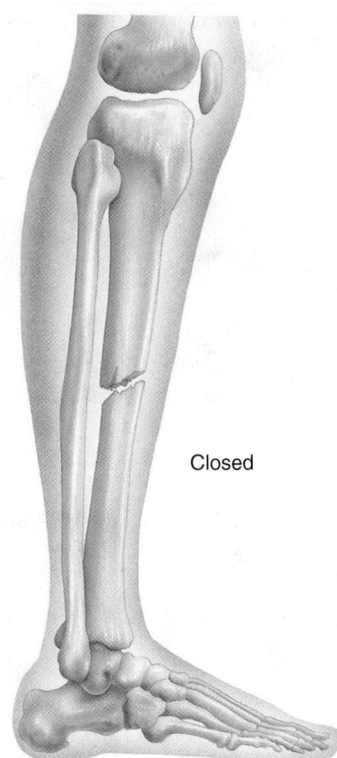

Open

Closed

FIGURE 36-12

Open and closed fractures.

Complications of Fractures

When fractured bone ends are displaced and move around inside the tissues, they can lacerate blood vessels and nerves. Bleeding can be substantial, even life threatening. Specific injuries with increased potential for hemorrhagic shock include fractures of femur and pelvis, and multiple long-bone fractures. Injury to nerves by broken bone ends may result in permanent loss of sensation, weakness, or paralysis.

Although compartment syndrome can be caused by other means, long bone fractures, particularly of the lower leg, are one cause of compartment syndrome. One study concluded that 69 percent of compartment syndrome diagnosis involves a fracture, most frequently the tibia (Paula, 2009).

As swelling increases within the muscle compartment, pressure in the compartment increases because the fascia surrounding the muscle compartment is tough and inelastic. As the pressure in the muscle compartment increases, it begins to exceed the pressure in the capillaries so that the cells cannot receive capillary blood flow. At this early stage, a pulse is still present distal to the site of injury because the pressure in the compartment has not yet exceeded arterial pressure. Despite the presence of a pulse, the tissue is not being perfused. However, as the pressure increases, venous pressure and then arterial pressure can also be exceeded.

As tissue ischemia and hypoxia progress, the injured cells result in additional tissue edema, further increasing the pressure in the compartment. Although compartment syndrome develops over time, it is possible that you will treat a patient whose injury occurred hours before and he is seeking treatment only as pain increases; or the patient may have received treatment, such as a splint or cast, but swelling continued after discharge, resulting in compartment syndrome.

The increasing pressure in the compartment results in what are called the *5 Ps* of compartment syndrome:

- Pain (increasing pain out of proportion with the severity of the original injury)
- Paresthesia (tingling sensations)
- Pallor (pale skin of the affected area due to decreased perfusion)
- Paralysis (weakness or loss of use)
- Pulselessness (loss of a pulse distal to the affected site is a later sign; perfusion is affected before pulselessness occurs)

Managing Long-Bone Fractures

You can splint most long-bone injuries with a rigid, moldable, pneumatic, or vacuum splint. Femur fractures, discussed in the following section, often require a traction splint.

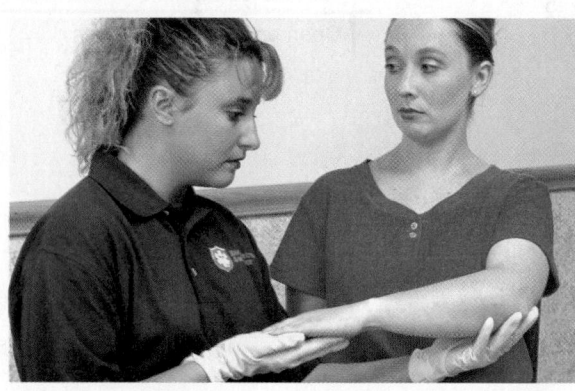

1. Apply manual stabilization to the injured extremity. Cover open wounds before applying the splint.

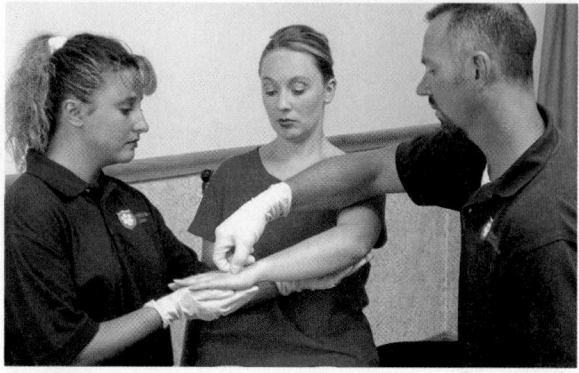

2. Assess the distal neurovascular function.

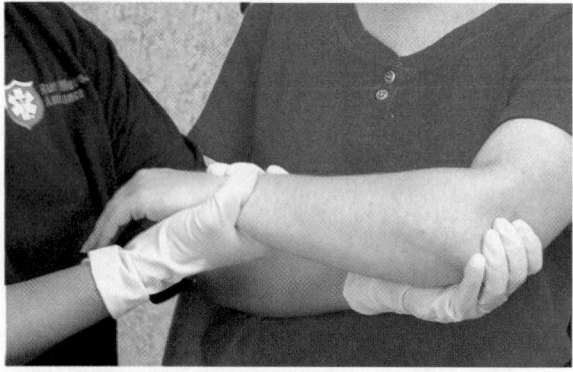

3. If the deformity is severe, distal pulses are absent, or the distal extremity is cyanotic, align with gentle manual traction.

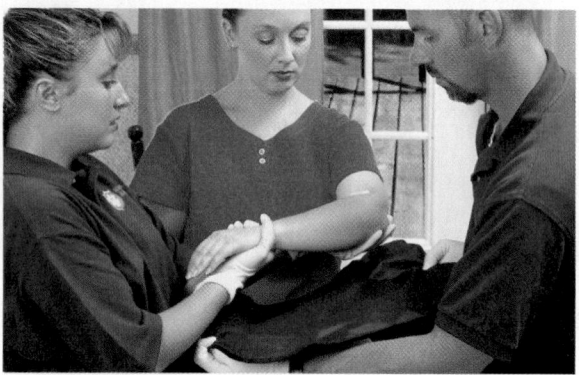

4. Measure the splint for proper length.

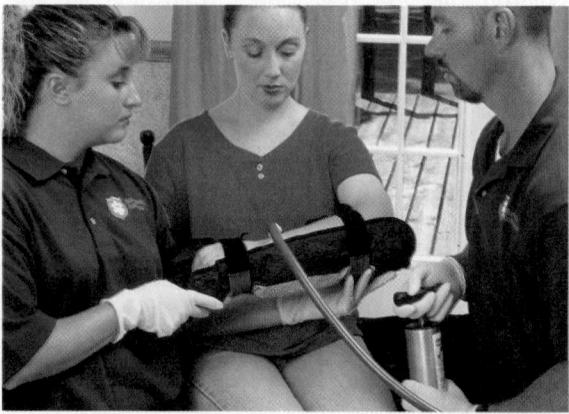

5. Secure the entire injured extremity. Immobilize the hand (or foot) in the position of function.

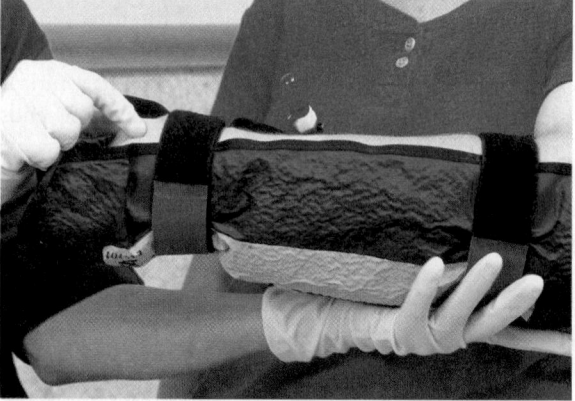

6. Reassess the distal neurovascular function.

To splint a long-bone injury, first control bleeding from, and place dressings on, any open wounds. Do not attempt to replace broken bone ends or fragments back into the wound. Follow the steps in Scan 36-2 for long-bone splinting. If the procedure increases pain or you meet resistance to gross alignment of the extremity, stop and splint the extremity in the position it is in.

After immobilizing the extremity with a splint and reassessing distal neurovascular function, elevate the extremity and apply a cold pack. Reassess the patient en route to the hospital.

Some ways of splinting specific injuries are as follows:

- *Humerus and forearm.* Splint with a rigid, moldable, pneumatic, or vacuum splint and use a sling and swathe to support and further immobilize the arm, elbow, and shoulder. When splinting the humerus, do not allow the edge of a rigid splint to rest in the axilla because doing so may cause damage to nerves and blood vessels. Make sure to support the wrist and hand with the hand placed in the position of function. The position of function of the hand is with the fingers slightly flexed as if holding a baseball in the hand. Placing a bulky roll of gauze in the hand helps achieve this position.

- *Femur, if a traction splint is contraindicated.* Use a rigid splint and be generous with padding. If the patient is critical, a long backboard will adequately splint the femur to prevent delay on the scene.

- *Lower leg.* Use a rigid, moldable, pneumatic, or vacuum splint. Ensure the foot is in a neutral position, neither plantar flexed or dorsiflexed. Ensure adequate padding behind the knee to prevent compression of nerves and blood vessels.

Critical Fractures

Some fractures are associated with higher mortality, either because of hemorrhage, the amount of force needed to cause a particular type of fracture, injury of underlying structures, or a combination of these. Critical fractures include fractures of the femur, pelvis, scapula, and first rib.

Fractures of the scapula and first rib are associated with higher mortality because these bones are well protected and require significant force to break. The force required usually results in injury to the intrathoracic organs.

Another fracture that can cause complications is a fractured clavicle. Although the clavicle can be fractured with indirect force or minimal direct force, displacement of the ends of the clavicle can result in pneumothorax or laceration of large blood vessels.

The iliac arteries extend through the pelvis where they continue to become the femoral arteries that run alongside the femurs. These are large arteries that have the potential to produce life-threatening hemorrhage when damaged. The pelvis has a large volume and can hold a tremendous amount of blood, whereas the pressure created by bleeding into a small, closed space helps reduce bleeding. A pelvic fracture resulting from anterior–posterior compression of the pelvis can result in what is called an *open-book fracture*, which increases the volume of the pelvis even further. A fractured pelvis can result in up to 2,000 mL of blood loss.

Stabilizing the pelvis is essential to minimizing further injury to the blood vessels and decreasing the volume

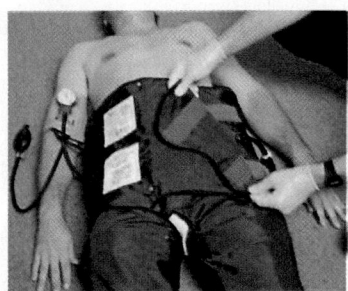
(A)

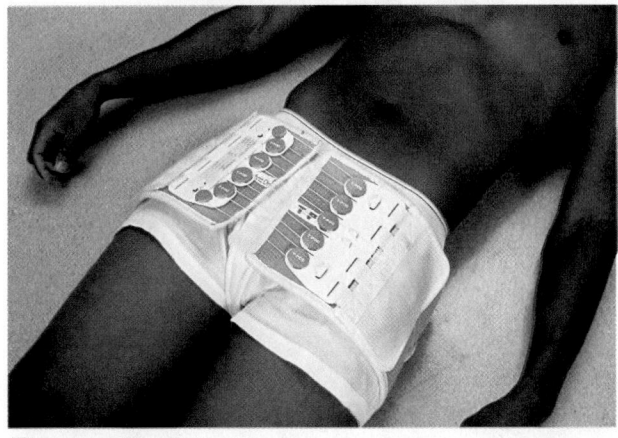
(B)

FIGURE 36-13

Pelvic fractures can be splinted by (A) a PASG, or (B) a commercial pelvic splint.

of the pelvis. You can use commercial pelvic binders, an improvised pelvic binder (such as a Kendrick Extrication Device [KED] or a bed sheet), or PASG to help stabilize the pelvis, in addition to placing the patient on a long backboard (Figure 36-13).

A single fractured femur can result in up to 1,500 mL of blood loss, while bilateral femur fractures could result in loss of up to 50 percent of the blood volume (Campbell, 2008). When there is a complete fracture of the femur, the tension of the leg muscles pulls the broken bone ends toward each other, allowing them to override and shorten the length of the leg. A fractured femur will often present as a shortened, deformed leg that is internally or externally rotated and with increased thigh diameter.

IN THE FIELD

An isolated femur fracture can cause up to 1,500 mL of blood loss. The average adult has 4,000 to 5,000 mL of blood volume. When treating a patient with bilateral femur fractures, you must consider the need to treat shock, because the patient may experience up to 3,000 mL of blood loss from the fractures alone.

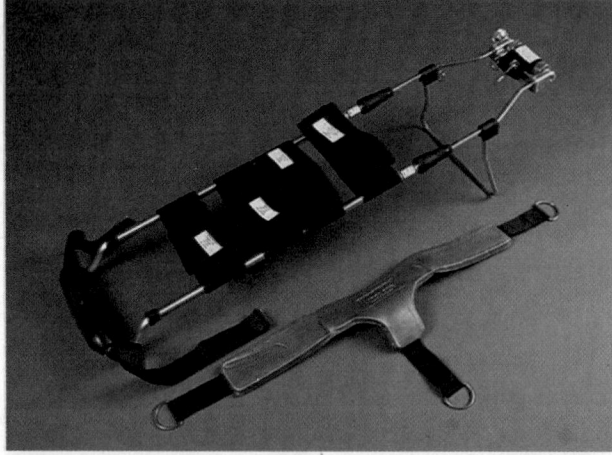

(A)

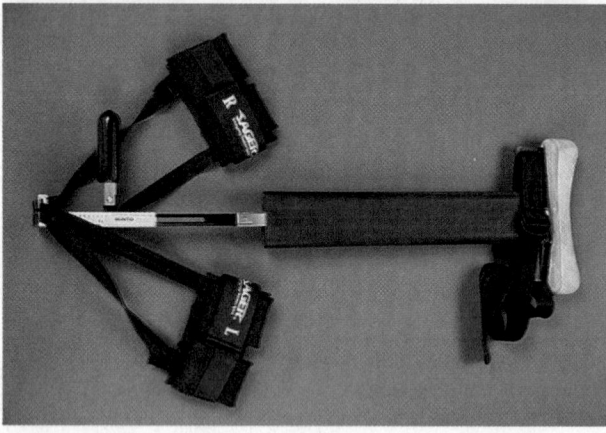

(B)

FIGURE 36-14

Types of traction splints: (A) a bipolar traction splint; (B) a unipolar traction splint.

Although traction splints are generally indicated for suspected femur fracture, there are some cases in which their use is contraindicated. Do not apply a traction splint in the following situations:

- The injury is within 2 inches from the knee or hip.
- A hip or pelvic injury is suspected.
- There are injuries to the knee, ankle or lower leg.

Bipolar and unipolar traction splints have different application procedures (Figure 36-14). Scan 36-3 shows the procedure for a unipolar splint and Scan 36-4 shows the procedure for a bipolar splint.

Joint Injuries

Joint injuries include sprains and dislocations. A **sprain** occurs when the joint is forced beyond its normal range of motion, stretching or tearing the ligaments around the joint. Joints that are most susceptible to sprains include the ankle and knee. Although many sprains heal with a period of resting the joint and treating it with cold

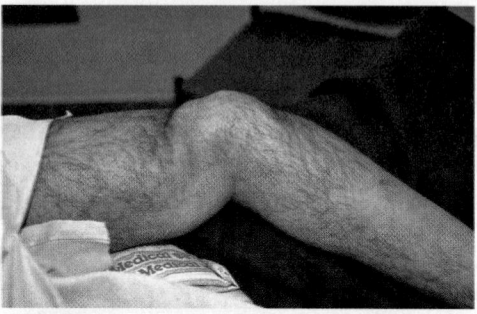

(A)

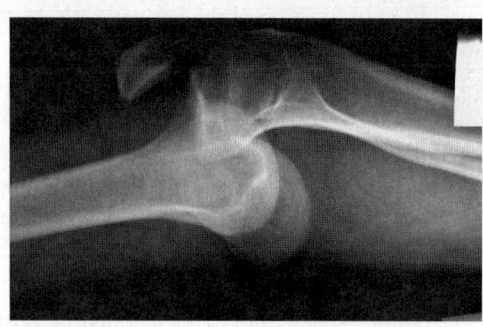

(B)

FIGURE 36-15

(A) Dislocation of the knee. (B) X-ray of the dislocation.
(Both photos: © Edward T. Dickinson, MD)

packs and elevation, a severe sprain can take longer to heal and be more complicated than a fracture. In some cases, the torn ligament tears away a piece of bone as it is stretched and torn. That is known as an *avulsion fracture*, so keep in mind that sprains and fractures can occur in the same injury.

A **dislocation** is a complete displacement of a joint (Figure 36-15). Dislocations are caused by overstretching of the ligaments through stress that allows a bone to slip out of place. Dislocations produce obvious deformity to the affected joint. This type of injury poses serious risk to vessels and nerves, because they may become compressed by the bones of the dislocated joint. Fractures and sprains can accompany dislocations.

A **subluxation** is a partial displacement of a joint. Unlike dislocation, subluxation may not be obvious because the joint is only partially displaced. Subluxation is caused by the overstretching of ligaments under stress, allowing bones to partially slip out of place. Subluxations are commonly caused by hyperflexion, hyperextension, extreme lateral rotation, and extreme axial forces to the joint.

In general, joint injuries are treated by immobilizing them in the position in which they are found, following the

IN THE FIELD

Never attempt to reduce, or replace, a dislocation. This is an injury that requires treatment in the hospital setting. Immobilize the extremity as best you can and transport.

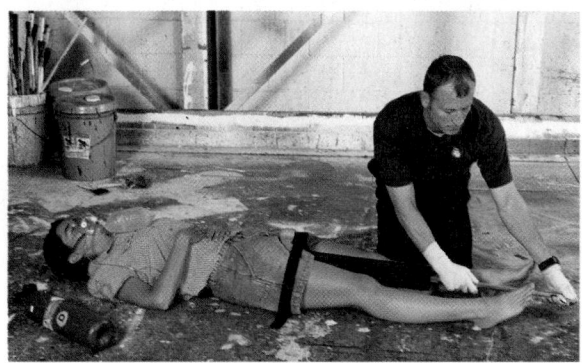

1. Assess distal neurovascular function. Place the splint along the medial aspect of the injured leg. Adjust it so that it extends about 4 inches beyond the heel.

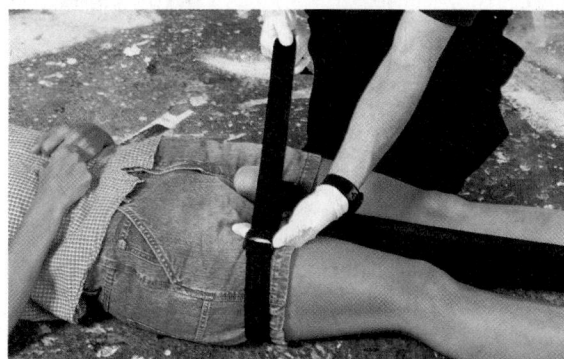

2. Secure the strap to the thigh.

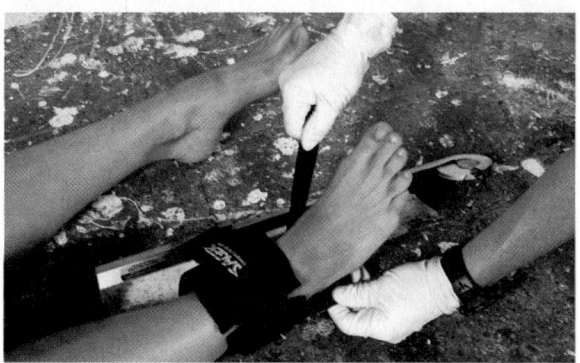

3. Apply the ankle hitch and attach it to the splint.

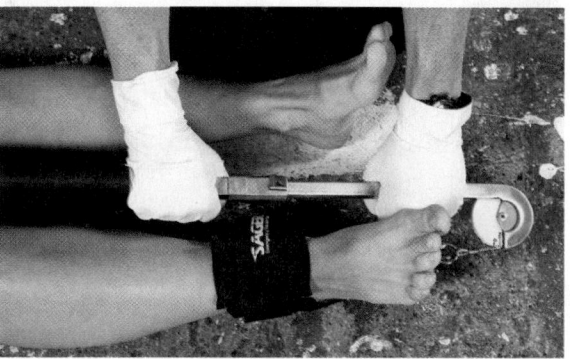

4. Apply traction by extending the splint. Adjust the splint to 10 percent of the patient's body weight.

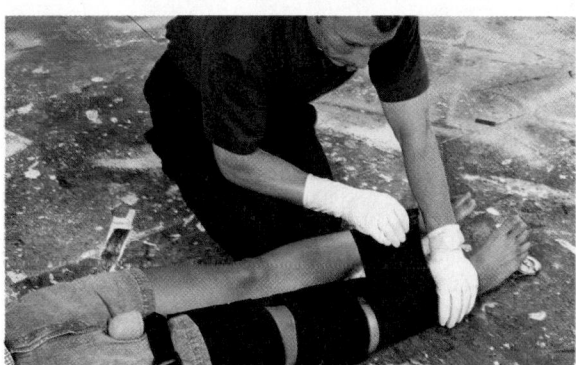

5. Apply the straps to secure the leg to the splint. Reassess distal neurovascular function.

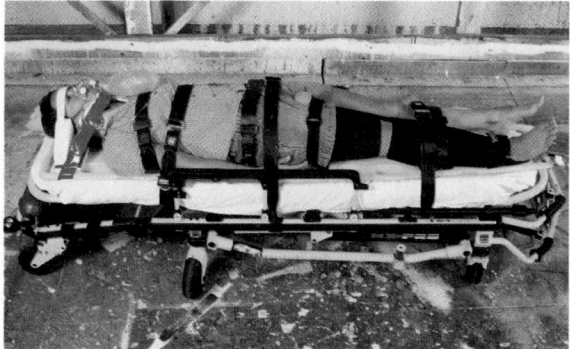

6. Place the patient onto a long backboard. Strap the ankles together and secure to the board.

general principles of splinting (Scan 36-5). A clavicle fracture is treated as a shoulder injury, which is best immobilized using a sling and swathe.

Hip Fractures and Dislocations

Hip fractures typically involve the proximal femur. Hip dislocations can either be anterior, in which the head of the femur is displaced to the front of the pelvis, or posterior, in which the head of the femur is displaced behind the pelvis. A common scenario of a hip fracture involves an elderly patient who falls at home. In a younger person, it would take significant force to fracture the proximal femur. It can take just minimal force in an elderly patient.

Hip dislocations can occur from falls or forcing the joint beyond its normal range of motion. In both hip fractures and dislocations, the injured extremity is shortened, compared to the uninjured extremity. In a fracture,

Applying a Bipolar Traction Splint

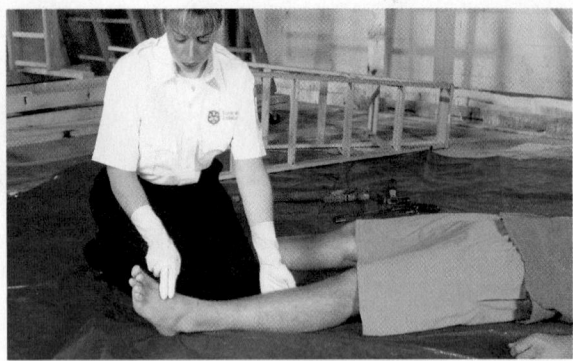

1. Assess distal neurovascular function.

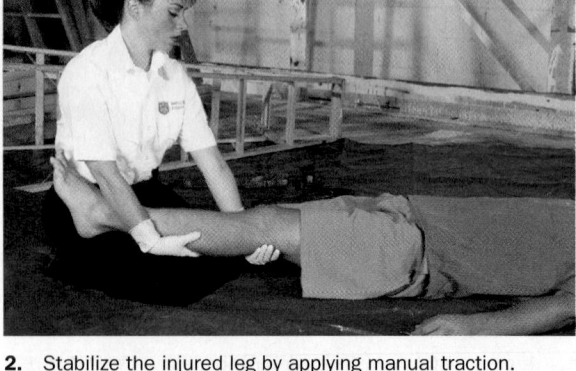

2. Stabilize the injured leg by applying manual traction.

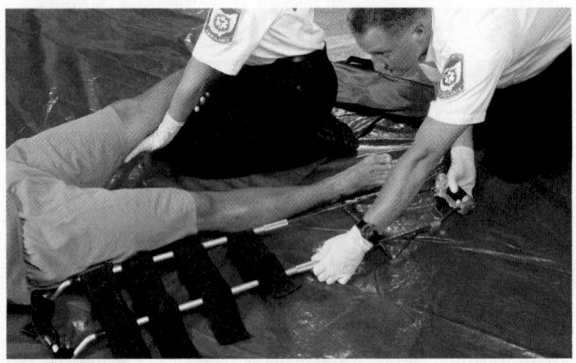

3. Adjust the splint for proper length, using the uninjured leg as a guide.

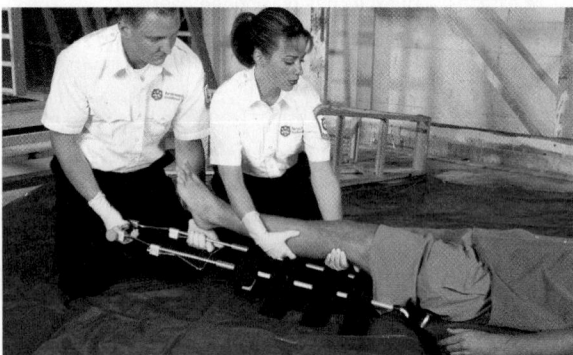

4. Position the splint under the injured leg until the ischial pad rests against the bony prominence of the buttocks. When the splint is in position, raise the heel stand.

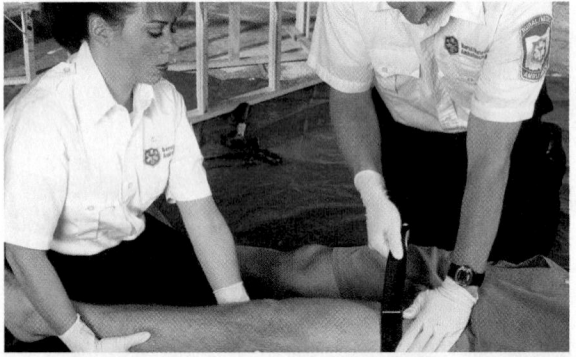

5. Attach the ischial strap over the groin and thigh.

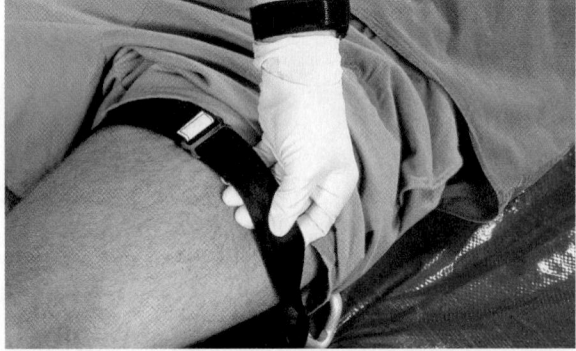

6. Make sure the ischial strap is snug but not tight enough to reduce distal circulation.

Geriatric Care

Elderly patients are at a much higher risk than other patients for hip fractures and dislocations. Geriatric patients have a higher pain tolerance than other adults, because pain perception decreases with age. Some elderly patients will walk around on a newly fractured hip and not even know it.

the foot is often rotated externally. In a posterior dislocation, the hip is flexed, adducted, and internally rotated. In an anterior dislocation, which is more uncommon, there is minimal hip flexion with abduction and external rotation.

Hip injuries are extremely painful, and you must take care when moving the patient. To splint the hip, log roll the patient onto his uninjured side. Slide a

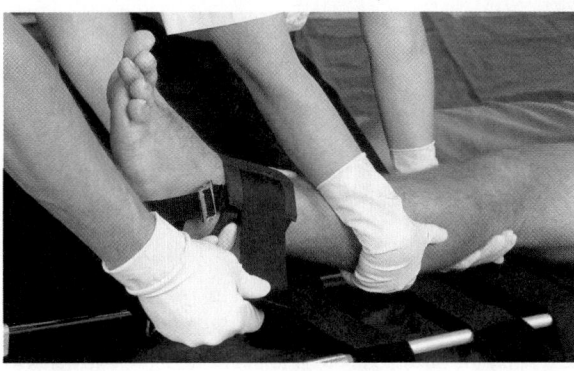

7. With the patient's foot in an upright position, secure the ankle hitch.

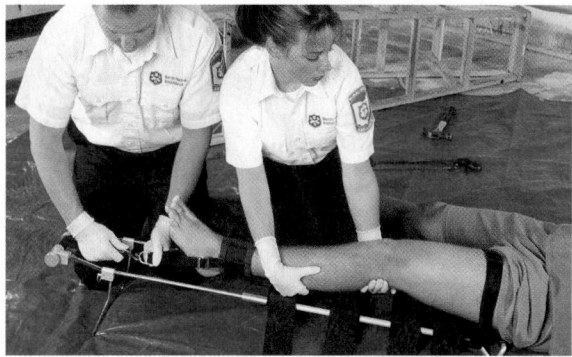

8. Attach the "S" hook to the "D" ring and apply mechanical traction. Full traction is achieved when the mechanical traction is equal to the manual traction and the pain and muscle spasms are reduced. In an unresponsive patient, adjust the traction until the injured leg is the same length as the uninjured leg.

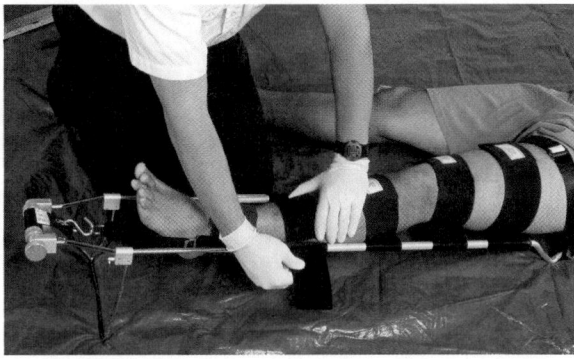

9. Fasten the leg support straps.

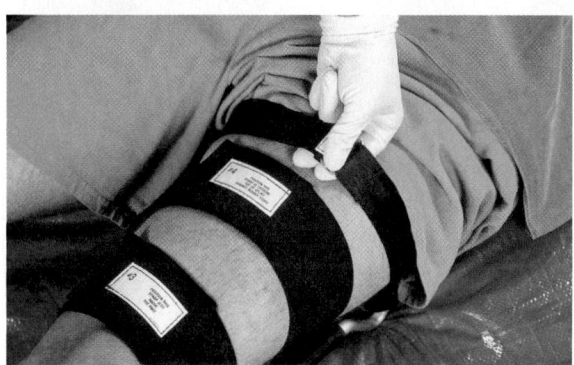

10. Re-evaluate the ischial strap and ankle hitch to ensure that both are securely fastened.

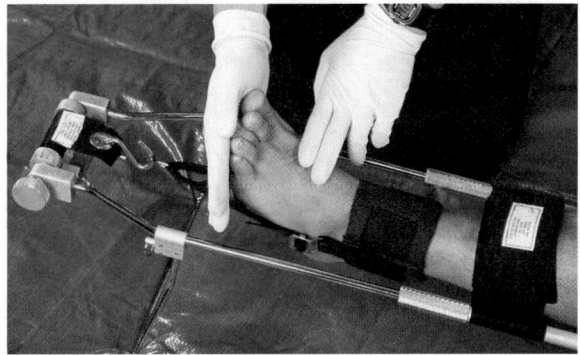

11. Reassess distal neurovascular function.

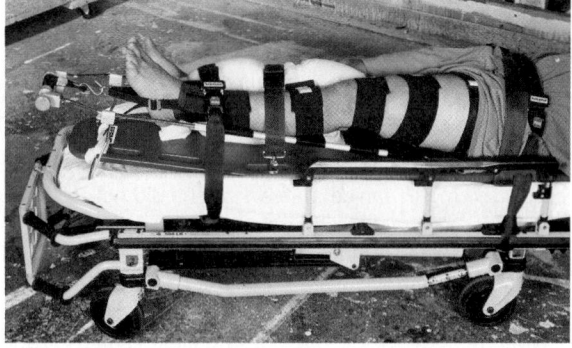

12. Place the patient on a long backboard and secure with straps. Pad between the splint and the uninjured leg. Secure the splint to the backboard.

scoop stretcher beneath the patient. Once the scoop stretcher is in place, secure the hip by wrapping a pillow across the hip and securing it snugly in place using straps. Pad beneath the knee if it is flexed. Secure the straps across one another to form an "X" across the pillow.

Muscle Injuries

A **strain** occurs when muscle fibers are stretched beyond their limitations, resulting in tearing of the fibers. Generally, a person is susceptible to a strain when muscles are under extreme stress, such as when lifting a heavy weight.

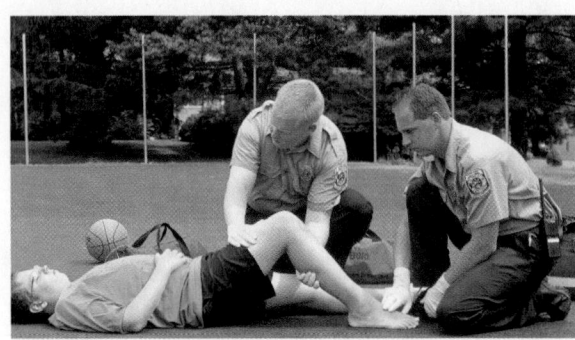

1. Manually stabilize the joint in the position found. Then assess the distal neurovascular function.

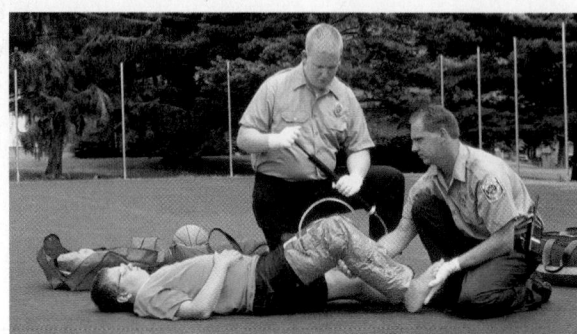

2. Apply the splint to immobilize the bone above and below the joint.

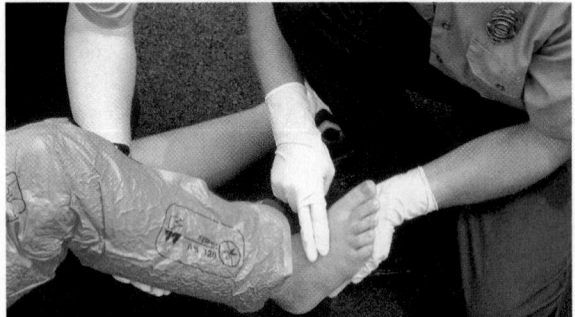

3. Reassess distal neurovascular function.

CASE STUDY WRAP-UP

Clinical-Reasoning Process

Joey completes a primary assessment and determines that the patient, Janice, does not have any life-threatening injuries. Furthermore, Janice states that she did not fall to the ground and denies striking her head. She was not expecting the curb to be there as she stepped off it, and her leg twisted as she stepped down. Her husband grabbed her before she hit the ground and assisted her down.

As Joey is cutting Janice's pants leg to expose the injury, she tells him that she felt and heard a "pop" just above her ankle when her leg twisted.

When her leg is exposed, Joey notices significant edema and ecchymosis to her lower leg and ankle. There is tenderness to palpation, but no deformity noted to the injured area or ankle. Janice states that she is unable to move her ankle and it hurts.

Mark reports that Janice's vital signs are: blood pressure 128/88 mmHg, pulse rate 100, and respirations 20. Mark advises Joey that he is going to fetch splinting material from their ambulance. Joey assesses pulse, motor function, and sensation while completing a secondary assessment and finds them to be normal. Janice rates her pain as a 9 on a scale of 1 to 10 and continues to cry.

Based on Janice's description of the incident, Mark and Joey rule out the need for spinal immobilization and prepare to splint the injury. Joey contacts medical direction and receives orders to administer Nitrox prior to splinting Janice's injury. Once splinting is completed, Janice is moved to the stretcher and Mark and Joey initiate transport to the nearest hospital with orthopedic services. En route to the ED, Joey reassesses Janice's vital signs and pulse, motor function, and sensation in the injured extremity.

CHAPTER REVIEW

Chapter Summary

Musculoskeletal injuries consist of a group of injuries involving bones and joints. Some injuries may be obvious and very gruesome. You must not allow these injuries to distract you from managing life-threatening injuries, because this may lead to deterioration of the patient and possibly even death.

When life-threatening injuries are not present, assess and manage musculoskeletal injuries by splinting. Recall that there is a multitude of splints available. Choose the most appropriate one for a particular injury.

The purpose of splinting is to reduce pain and prevent additional injury from occurring. When splinting injuries to bone, you will immobilize the joints above and below the injury site. When splinting injuries to joints, you will immobilize the bones above and below the injury.

Take care to splint the injury appropriately, because failure to do so may lead to further injury to the patient. Remember to assess distal neurovascular status before and after splinting and document your findings.

Review Questions

Multiple-Choice Questions

1. Which one of the following is *not* a function of the musculoskeletal system?

   a. Provides shape to the body
   b. Protects internal organs
   c. Provides for movement
   d. Provides for insulin reabsorption

2. Which one of the following statements is true?

   a. Ligaments attach muscle to bone.
   b. Cartilage reduces friction between bones as they move against one another.
   c. Tendons attach bone to bone.
   d. Skeletal muscle is found in the vessels of the body.

3. A patient falls from a 15-foot ladder and lands on his feet. Upon impact, the patient's left calcaneus was fractured. This fracture is the result of which type of force?

   a. Direct
   b. Indirect
   c. Twisting
   d. Compression

4. A patient's leg is crushed between a utility pole and the rear bumper of a large truck when the truck backs into the patient. Which type of fracture would you suspect the patient has sustained?

   a. Greenstick
   b. Spiral
   c. Impacted
   d. Comminuted

5. Which one of the following bones is likely to produce significant hemorrhage when fractured?

   a. Hip
   b. Fibula
   c. Pelvis
   d. Radius

6. You arrive at the scene of an emergency to find a patient with an angulated fracture of the right tibia and fibula. Which one of the following splints would be best to use on this particular injury?

   a. Vacuum splint
   b. Rigid splint
   c. Traction splint
   d. Improvised splint

7. Which one of the following is *not* a contraindication for the use of a traction splint?

   a. An injury that is less than 2 inches from the ankle
   b. An associated injury to the knee of the same leg
   c. A suspected pelvic injury
   d. An injury that is more than 2 inches from the knee

Critical-Thinking Questions

8. Joe and Lisa arrive at the scene of a critically injured multisystem trauma patient. The patient has suspected internal bleeding and is exhibiting signs and symptoms of shock. Following immobilization of the patient onto a long backboard, Lisa applies a traction splint to the patient's right leg, because the thigh is severely swollen and crepitus is felt upon palpation. What critical error have Joe and Lisa made regarding the appropriate treatment of this patient?

9. Joe and Lisa respond to a state park in a rural area outside of town for a traumatic injury call. Upon arrival, they find a hiker with a severely swollen right lower leg. The patient states that he fell off of a large rock and thinks that he broke his leg upon landing. He goes on to explain that the injury was about 2 hours ago. He was stranded until other hikers heard his screams and found him. He was carried to his current location and 911 was called once their cell phones were able to pick up a signal. Upon assessment, the patient's leg is very firm to the touch and extremely painful. The skin distal to the injury site is pale and cool. What injuries and/or complications do you suspect the patient to have sustained?

10. Explain how the application of a traction splint assists in the control of internal bleeding associated with femur fractures.

References

Campbell, J. E. (2008). *International trauma life support* (6th ed.). Upper Saddle River, NJ: Pearson Prentice Hall.

Dailey, B. (2010). *Health and safety: JEMS.* Retrieved March 15, 2011, from http://www.jems.com/article/health-and-safety/musculoskeletal-injury-prevent

Paula, R. (2009). *Compartment syndrome in emergency medicine: eMedicine.* Retrieved March 16, 2011, from http://emedicine.medscape.com/article/828456-overview

37

Head, Brain, Face, and Neck Trauma

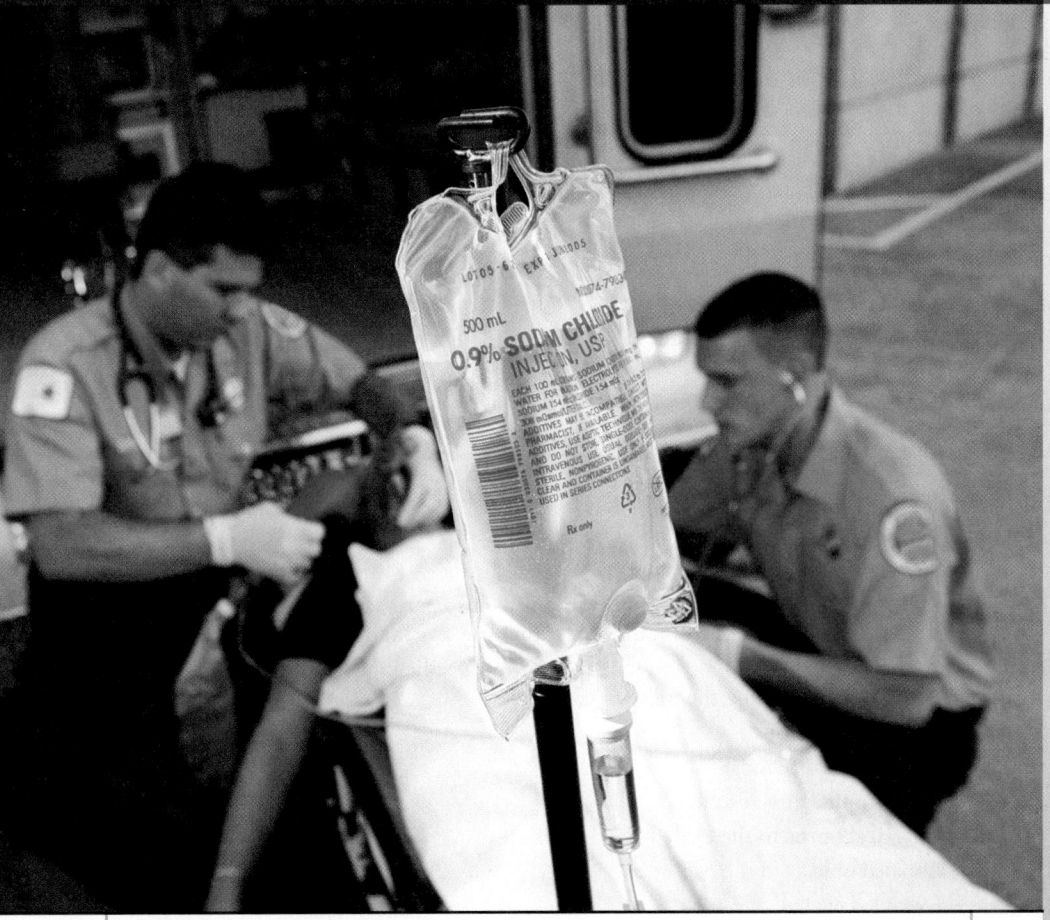

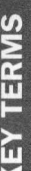
Content Area: Trauma

Advanced EMT Education Standard: Applies fundamental knowledge to provide basic and selected advanced emergency care and transportation based on assessment findings for an acutely injured patient.

Objectives

After reading this chapter, you should be able to:

37.1   Define key terms introduced in the chapter.

37.2   Describe the anatomy and function of the brain, skull, meninges, intracranial blood vessels, eye, facial structures, and structures of the neck.

37.3   Discuss special considerations in the assessment and management of patients with injuries to the head, face, and neck, including the following:

 – Airway compromise

 – Profuse bleeding

 – Potential that injuries may be self-inflicted or the result of violence

 – Patient fears associated with the injuries

(continued)

Resource(C)entral

CASE STUDY

On a sunny Saturday afternoon, Advanced EMTs Chuck Benedict and Matt Meyers are standing by at a local parade. They are staged at a corner of the parade route, standing at the rear of their ambulance watching the people, when they hear dispatch call them on the radio. "Unit 72, respond to the corner of Victor Boulevard and Sandra Street for an MVC."

"10-4, Unit 72 en route," Matt says.

The intersection is only three blocks away, so they arrive on the scene quickly. As they pull up, they notice a police officer waving them toward a woman lying supine on the street and a bystander holding manual stabilization of her head and neck. Chuck and Matt also notice a motorcycle lying in the street approximately 30 feet from the woman. The woman is not wearing a helmet.

Problem-Solving Questions

1. What does this information tell Chuck and Matt about the mechanism of injury?
2. How would the mechanism of injury assist them in determining the potential for injury to this patient?
3. What additional information should they obtain?

(continued from previous page)

37.4   Given a variety of scenarios, demonstrate the assessment-based management of patients with injuries to the brain, skull, scalp, face, eye, and neck.

37.5   Demonstrate the assessment and management of specific injuries of the eye, scalp, face, and neck, including the following:
  - Injury to the orbit
  - Injury to the eyelid
  - Injury to the globe of the eye
  - Chemical burns to the eye
  - Impaled objects in the eye
  - Extruded eyeball
  - Facial fractures
  - Avulsed tooth
  - Impaled object in the cheek
  - Injury to the nose
  - Injury to the ear
  - Penetrating injury to the neck
  - Blunt injury to the neck

37.6   Explain the indications and procedure for removing contact lenses from an injured eye.

37.7   Explain the pathophysiology and significance of the following with respect to traumatic brain injury:
  - Scalp lacerations and avulsions
  - Open and closed skull fractures
  - Cerebral concussion and diffuse axonal injury
  - Cerebral contusion
  - Coup–contrecoup injury
  - Cerebral and intracranial hematomas
  - Cerebral hemorrhage

37.8   Explain the compensatory mechanisms, and the resulting symptoms, for increased intracranial pressure.

37.9 Explain the limitations of the compensatory mechanisms for increased intracranial pressure.

37.10 Describe the pathophysiology and key signs of increased intracranial pressure and brain herniation.

37.11 Identify and, where possible, manage factors that can worsen traumatic brain injuries, including the following:
- Hyperglycemia
- Hyperthermia
- Hypoglycemia
- Hypotension
- Hypoxia
- Hypercarbia
- Hypocarbia

37.12 Document information relevant to the assessment and management of patients with injuries to the head.

Introduction

As an Advanced EMT, you will be called on to care for many patients who have sustained injuries to the head, brain, face, or neck. The injuries may be minor and require simple care, or they may be life threatening.

Head injuries account for approximately 1.6 million emergency department visits annually. Of those patients, around 500,000 sustain traumatic brain injury (TBI). Although 80 percent of them are diagnosed as having mild injuries, about 50,000 are pronounced dead on arrival at the emergency department. Patients with moderate and severe TBI could face months to years of rehabilitation and long-term or permanent disability. TBI in patients who have sustained multisystem trauma contributes to nearly half of all trauma-related deaths (McSwain, Salomone & Pons, 2007).

As an Advanced EMT, you must be able to identify the potential for TBI by evaluating the mechanism of injury and assessing the patient for signs and symptoms of injury. Failure to recognize and appropriately treat brain injury significantly increases the chances of severe disability or even death of the patient.

Injuries to the face and neck also can range from minor to life threatening. Significant trauma to the face can occlude the airway or cause profuse bleeding into the patient's airway, compromising its patency. Although eye injuries are not life threatening, the care you provide helps to prevent further injury and permanent loss of sight. Be sensitive to patients. They will experience fear and panic at the idea of living the rest of their lives without the ability to see or being disfigured by scarring. Do what you can to calm and reassure them, even if the loss of vision or disfigurement seems certain. Do not lie to your patient if asked about the potential for scarring or disfigurement but be tactful and supportive. Tell them it is not possible to determine the extent of injury in the prehospital setting and that many injuries can be repaired with good cosmetic results, though healing may take several months.

Injury to the neck, especially to the trachea or larynx, can be life threatening because of airway obstruction. Trauma to the neck may involve the major blood vessels, causing serious bleeding and decrease in perfusion.

In this chapter, you will learn to identify mechanisms of injury that indicate the potential for the injuries described here, as well as the appropriate management for each.

Anatomy and Physiology Review

The brain is surrounded by the protective structure of the skull, which consists of two parts, the cranium and the face. The skull is covered by soft-tissue structures. The face contains some of the structures of the special senses, as well as structures of the airway, and provides identity. Within the skull, the brain is covered by the meninges and surrounded by cerebrospinal fluid.

The Skull

The skull is part of the skeletal system and provides protection for the brain. It consists of large plates of bone that are fused together to form the cranium, the "helmet-like" covering of the brain. The plates of bone include the frontal bone, temporal bones, parietal bone, sphenoid bones, and the occipital bone. The base of the skull is formed by portions of those bones as well as additional bones. The facial bones include the bones of orbits and nose as well as the maxillae, zygomatic bones, and mandible.

The **basilar skull** is the floor of the skull that is composed of several thinner bones and is weaker than the heavy bones that make up the upper part of the skull. As a result, it can be fractured with less force than some of the other cranial bones. The spinal cord passes through an opening in the posterior basilar skull called the *foramen magnum.*

The brain occupies approximately 85 percent of the total space within the skull. Under normal circumstances, the remainder of the space is occupied by cerebrospinal fluid and the volume of blood perfusing the brain. This leaves little room for swelling or accumulation of blood with the brain or skull.

The Brain

Cerebrospinal fluid (CSF) serves as a cushion for the brain but also plays additional roles in protecting the brain from infection and serving metabolic functions. CSF is continuously produced in the ventricles of the brain and is reabsorbed at a steady rate that prevents accumulation of excess CSF. As a temporary measure, if the volume of blood increases in the brain or skull, or if the brain swells, CSF is shunted into the spinal canal to keep pressure within the cranium at normal levels. However, that, like all compensatory mechanisms, has limits.

The brain is surrounded by three layers of meninges, which are layers of tissue that encapsulate the brain and the spinal cord. The tough, fibrous outermost layer is the *dura mater*; the middle layer is the *arachnoid layer*, which is laced with blood vessels; and the innermost layer is the *pia mater*, which is a thin and fragile layer of tissue. Between the dura mater and arachnoid mater is a potential space called the *subdural space*. The *subarachnoid space* between the arachnoid and pia mater contains cerebrospinal fluid.

The brain consists of three parts: the cerebrum, cerebellum, and the brainstem. The *cerebrum* is the largest part of the brain and is divided into right and left hemispheres, which together are responsible for cognitive function and most sensory functions, motor functions, and emotion. The *cerebellum* is a smaller part of the brain, located in the posterior skull beneath the posterior lobes of the right and left cerebrum, and is primarily responsible for coordination and equilibrium. The *brainstem* consists of the pons, midbrain, and the medulla oblongata and is continuous with the spinal cord. It is located beneath the cerebrum, extending through the foramen magnum, and is responsible for autonomic body functions, including blood pressure, heart rate, and respiratory rate. Injury to the brainstem can lead to circulatory and respiratory failure and death of the patient (Figure 37-1).

The Neck

The neck contains structures that are vital to sustaining life. They include the trachea and larynx, which are vital to air exchange, and major blood vessels, which are responsible for transporting blood to and from the brain. The vessels include the external and internal jugular veins and the carotid arteries. Injury that results in significant bleeding from the large vessels may lead to rapid deterioration and death of the patient. The cervical spine and esophagus are also located within the neck.

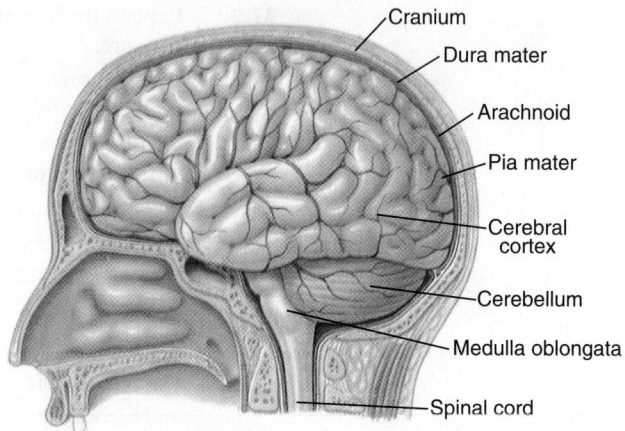

FIGURE 37-1

The brain.

The Face

The face consists of 14 facial bones (Figure 37-2): the orbits that surround the eyes, nasal bones, zygomatic bones, and maxilla. Most of the facial bones are immovable; the only movable facial bone is the mandible. The facial bones provide protection for the eyes and form the framework of the airway and face. The facial bones also serve as attachment points for the facial muscles that are responsible for chewing food, speaking, and facial expressions. Trauma that is significant enough to cause fractures of the face may also cause brain injury.

The Eye

The globe of the eye (Figure 37-3) is a spherical shape approximately 1 inch in diameter. Its tough outer layer is the *sclera*. The clear covering over the front of the eye is the *cornea*, which covers the *pupil*. The colored portion of the eye is a pigmented muscle called the *iris*, which gives people their eye color. The pupil is an opening in the center of the iris that allows light into the eye. The iris dilates and constricts to change the size of the pupil to let in more or less light.

The lens is located just behind the pupil and focuses the light entering the eye onto the retina. The retina is the light-sensitive posterior portion of the eye where the optic nerve receives impulses and sends them to the brain. Within the brain the impulses are interpreted as an image. The eye is protected and lubricated by a clear mucous membrane called the *conjunctiva*, which lines the inner eyelids and covers the sclera.

The interior of the eye consists of two fluid-filled cavities that give the eye its shape. The anterior cavity is located between the cornea and lens and is divided into anterior and posterior chambers, both filled with aqueous humor. The vitreous cavity is located between the lens and retina, filling most of the globe of the eye. The vitreous cavity is filled with viscous vitreous humor.

The eye is surrounded by the cup-shaped orbits formed by several of the facial bones. Muscles attach the eye to the orbit and allow movement of the eye.

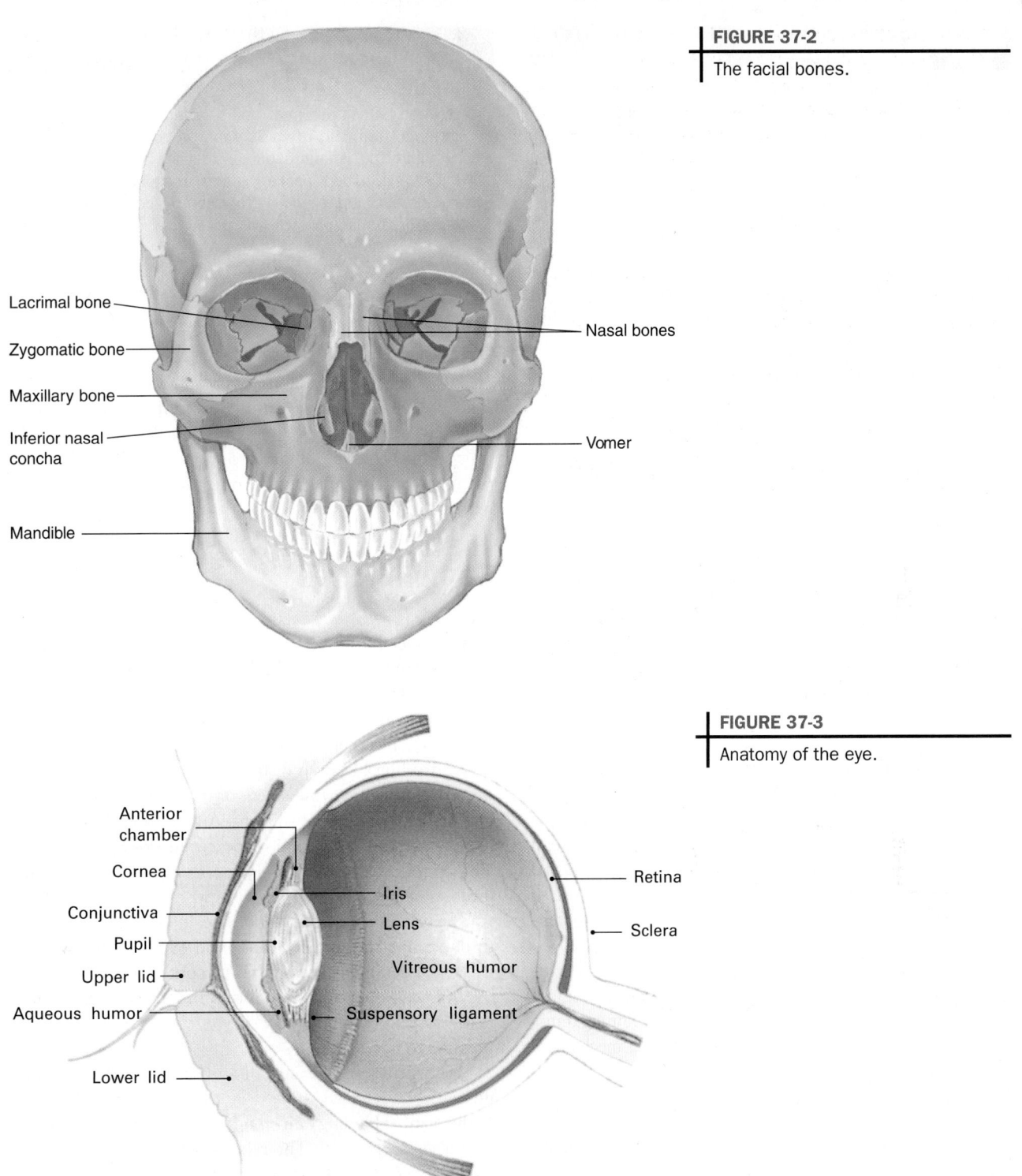

FIGURE 37-2

The facial bones.

Lacrimal bone

Zygomatic bone

Maxillary bone

Inferior nasal concha

Mandible

Nasal bones

Vomer

FIGURE 37-3

Anatomy of the eye.

Anterior chamber

Cornea

Conjunctiva

Pupil

Upper lid

Aqueous humor

Lower lid

Iris

Lens

Vitreous humor

Suspensory ligament

Retina

Sclera

General Assessment and Management of Injuries to the Head, Brain, Face, and Neck

Patients can present with a variety of mechanisms of injury and complaints that may indicate an injury of head, brain, face, or neck. Falls, assaults, motor vehicle collisions (MVCs),

and being struck by a projectile are all mechanisms that can potentially injure those structures. Some signs, such as altered mental status, bleeding, or substantial edema or discoloration, may be seen as you approach the patient in the scene size-up. Complaints that accompany the mechanisms include pain and swelling of the affected area, loss of function of the affected area, dizziness, headache, nausea, and vomiting.

Perform a scene size-up to determine scene safety and the mechanism of injury. If the mechanism of injury is consistent with the possibility of cervical-spine injury, provide or direct an assistant to provide in-line manual stabilization of the head and neck to restrict spinal motion.

Do not let the sometimes dramatic appearance of head and facial injuries distract you from the priorities of patient assessment and care. Ensure the patient has an open airway and that ventilation, oxygenation, and circulation are adequate. Be particularly concerned with the airway in patients with significant facial bleeding, vomiting, altered mental status, and complaints that involve the oral cavity and throat, because swelling of the structures and bleeding can lead to complete airway obstruction or aspiration. In severe cases, endotracheal intubation or cricothyrotomy (surgical airway) are necessary. Consider the need for ALS transport for patients with potential or actual airway compromise. If ALS is not immediately available, consider the possibility of intercepting with an ALS service or transport to the closest emergency department where an emergency airway can be secured.

The face and scalp have a rich blood supply. Both open and closed injuries can result in substantial bleeding. For open wounds, use direct pressure to control bleeding and keep blood from entering the airway. Hematomas of the head, face, and neck can be large. Cold packs can help decrease bleeding into the hematoma. Both open and closed injuries of the neck require special considerations because of the large amount of bleeding that can occur and the potential for airway damage or obstruction.

Make a determination of whether the patient is critical or noncritical and begin planning how you will integrate needed interventions without undue delay in beginning transport. If the patient is critical or has a substantial mechanism of injury, expose him and perform a rapid trauma exam, followed at an appropriate time by a head-to-toe exam. Perform a focused exam for patients with isolated injuries.

Obtain vital signs and a SAMPLE history, using OPQRST to explore the chief complaint. Establish a baseline for the patient's condition, including mental status, vital signs, complaints, and pain level. Reassess critical patients at least every 5 minutes and noncritical patients every 15 minutes, obtaining at least two sets of observations. Remain alert for signs and symptoms of shock during reassessment throughout transport to the hospital emergency department.

With injuries to the head, face, and neck, the best position in which to transport the patient is the one that allows him to maintain his own airway, if possible. Consider placing the patient in a sitting position unless it is contraindicated by altered mental status, neurologic deficit, or other conditions.

Injuries to the Head

Head injury is a general term that can be confusing because it is not exact. There are differences in the nature of an injury to the scalp or skull and a traumatic brain injury (TBI). This section describes injuries to the scalp and skull, which often accompany TBI, but are much more complex in their management.

Scalp Injuries

The scalp is highly vascular. Even a relatively minor laceration can bleed profusely. The scalp vessels do not vasoconstrict as other vessels in the body do, so profuse bleeding can result. In some patients, this bleeding can be substantial enough to cause or contribute to hypovolemia. You must control the bleeding in the primary assessment, but do not let controlling bleeding distract you from either other aspects of the primary assessment or the secondary assessment and need for other interventions. Always consider an injury to the scalp an indication of potential skull fracture and TBI, so follow through with your assessment to determine if those injuries exist.

Significant bleeding from the scalp can make it difficult to determine the size, location, and extent of the wound. Careful assessment is essential to control the bleeding. It may be necessary to rinse clotted blood from the hair to help you find the injury so that you can better apply direct pressure to it.

The structure of the skull and scalp can lead to some unique injuries called *scalping injuries*, in which a large flap of the scalp, including hair, skin, and underlying soft tissues, is avulsed from skull. The relatively thin layer of soft tissue over the skull also results in full-thickness lacerations in which the skull can be seen through the laceration. With scalping injuries in which the scalp remains attached as a flap, grossly align the flap into its anatomical position and apply direct pressure. If a portion of the flap is folded over on itself, it can restrict blood supply to the remainder of the flap, making successful reattachment less likely. If the avulsed portion of scalp is no longer attached, treat it as an amputated part.

Closed scalp injuries occur from blunt trauma and may result in the formation of a hematoma that is visible and easily palpated. If a hematoma is present, you must consider the possibility of underlying injury to the skull and brain. The application of a cold pack may reduce bleeding into the hematoma, which can reduce swelling and pain. Occasionally, hematomas give the tissues a "mushy" feeling that is mistaken for a massive skull fracture with instability of the skull bones.

Skull Injuries

The skull consists of thick plates of fused bone that provide protection to the brain. The bones of the skull can be fractured as a result of forceful impact, such as may occur from a fall, gunshot wound, being kicked by a horse's hoof or by a heavy boot, in an MVC, or in recreational activities—particularly when the patient is not wearing a helmet. Impact forceful enough to fracture the bones of the skull also can injure the brain. The most important considerations in managing a patient with a skull fracture are to maintain the airway, breathing, and circulation and assess carefully for indications of TBI. A forceful impact to the skull can cause movement of the neck beyond its normal range of motion, resulting in cervical-spine injury.

Skull fractures can be classified as either linear or depressed and as open or closed (Figure 37-4). In a **linear skull fracture** the fracture appears as a thin line across the bone on X-ray. Linear fractures do not result in displaced segments of bone, meaning there is no obvious deformity of the skull.

A **depressed skull fracture** occurs when an impact to the skull results in multiple cracks that are pushed, or depressed, into the skull. Depressed skull fractures may be identified through palpation during assessment and perhaps by direct visualization. Palpate the skull gently to avoid pushing broken bone into the brain tissue. In some cases, a hematoma masks an underlying depressed skull fracture; therefore, you must consider the mechanism of injury and the potential for underlying injury to the skull.

In a **closed skull fracture** the scalp remains intact. Conversely, in an **open skull fracture** an open injury to the scalp is present. If an object is impaled in the skull, do not remove it because doing so can cause injury to the brain and blood vessels. Immobilize an impaled object in the skull as you would any other impaled object.

A fracture to the base, or floor, of the skull is called a *basilar skull fracture.* Depending on the location of the basilar skull fracture, the fracture may allow cerebrospinal fluid (CSF) to flow through the fracture site and into the nares or ear canal. When you see clear or bloody fluid draining from the ears, nose, or mouth in a patient with trauma to the head, suspect it is cerebrospinal fluid (CSF) and a basilar skull fracture is present. Do not obstruct the drainage of CSF. Instead, cover a draining ear lightly with a sterile dressing to prevent contamination, because there is now a passageway between the environment and the normally sterile cranial vault. Do not cover the nose or mouth because doing so can result in airway obstruction. Use gentle suction to clear secretions that interfere with the patient's airway.

Basilar skull fractures also result in "raccoon eyes" (ecchymosis around the eyes) and "Battle's sign" (ecchymosis behind the ears). It generally takes hours for this ecchymosis to develop, so if it is seen in the prehospital environment, assume the injury occurred hours prior to your arrival at the patient's side.

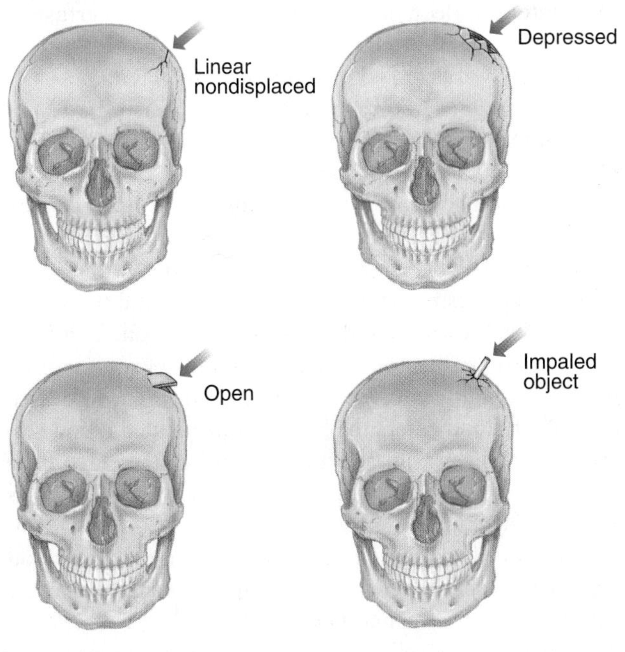

Traumatic Brain Injuries

The rigidity of the skull is an important anatomic feature in protecting delicate brain tissue from injury. However, if the brain is injured within the skull, the inability of the skull to expand means that swelling of the injured brain or accumulation of blood within the skull will increase the intracranial pressure (ICP), the pressure within the skull. The body can compensate for small increases in intracranial pressure through vasoconstriction of cerebral blood vessels and by shunting some of the CSF into the spinal canal. However, these compensatory mechanisms are limited and are often insufficient in the presence of significant intracranial bleeding or cerebral edema.

FIGURE 37-4

Types of skull fractures.

IN THE FIELD

It is vital that you anticipate the need for suction when managing patients with suspected brain injury, because vomiting is common. Ensure that suction is readily available at all times.

TBIs occur in two phases. Primary brain injury occurs at the time of impact with the skull. **Secondary brain injury** results from cerebral edema, ischemia, and hypoxia. EMS providers cannot change the severity of the primary injury, but can do much to limit the severity of secondary brain injury. To understand how you can help limit secondary brain injury, you must understand what happens when the brain is injured and the intracranial pressure begins to increase.

Cerebral Edema and Increased Intracranial Pressure

Because brain tissue is compressed by increasing ICP, there is progressive brain dysfunction. The vomiting center of the brain may be stimulated, resulting in projectile vomiting. Pressure on the blood vessels in the cranium causes headache. Altered mental status occurs and often patients become combative, which makes treatment very challenging. Pressure on the cranial nerves results in their dysfunction. A common indication of increased ICP and impending **brain herniation** is unequal pupils. As cerebral edema shifts the brain unevenly within the skull, pressure increases on cranial nerve III (the oculomotor nerve) on the affected side. The pupil controlled by the oculomotor nerve on that side becomes widely dilated and unresponsive to light. Both oculomotor nerves can be affected, which results in bilateral dilated, unresponsive pupils.

The increase in pressure on the brain means that the blood pressure must increase to overcome it to deliver oxygen and nutrients to, and remove wastes from, the cellular level. As a reflex response to hypertension, the heart rate slows. This phenomenon, increasing blood pressure—particularly systolic blood pressure—and decreasing heart rate, is called **Cushing's reflex. Cushing's triad** includes the two findings of Cushing's reflex and altered mental status, and is an indication of increasing ICP.

Unfortunately, the increase in blood pressure worsens intracranial bleeding and cerebral edema. The result is a cycle of increasing blood pressure and increasing cerebral edema. As the brain is compressed, the tissue becomes ischemic and additional cerebral edema occurs. The patient enters a downward spiral that can only be corrected by decreasing the intracranial pressure with surgical interventions and medications.

As ICP increases unchecked, the brain tissue is forced through areas of lowest resistance in the cranium. The tissue may be forced through structures within the cranium called the *tentorium cerebelli* of the *falx cerebri*, or through the foramen magnum and into the spinal column. When this occurs, it is called *herniation*, which is a terminal event. Signs of impending herniation include Cushing's triad, pupillary changes, altered respirations, trismus (clenched jaw, which can make airway management difficult), and *posturing* in response to painful stimuli. Rigid extension of the extremities in response to painful stimuli is called *decerebrate*

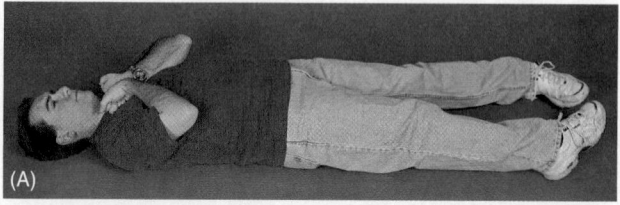
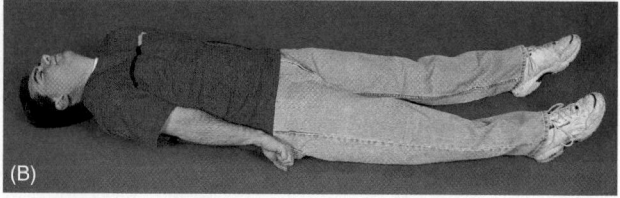

FIGURE 37-5

(A) Flexion (decorticate) posturing and (B) extension (decerebrate) posturing. (Both photos: © Carl Leet)

posturing. Rigid flexion of the upper extremities in response to pain is called *decorticate posturing* (Figure 37-5).

Factors that worsen cerebral edema and ischemia—thus increasing brain dysfunction and the risk of herniation—are hypoperfusion, hypoxia, hyperoxia, hypocapnia, hypercapnia, hypoglycemia, and hyperglycemia. Your actions can influence each of those factors.

There must be a substantial enough difference between the blood pressure (as determined by mean arterial pressure [MAP]) and the intracranial pressure to allow adequate perfusion of the brain tissue. Maintaining an adequate MAP in patients with cerebral edema is critical. Whereas most trauma patients are resuscitated to a level of permissive hypotension (systolic blood pressure of 80 mmHg) to minimize internal bleeding while improving tissue perfusion, patients with TBI should receive IV fluids, if necessary, to maintain a systolic blood pressure of 90 mmHg.

Both oxygen and carbon dioxide are vasoactive substances, meaning that they influence the degree of constriction of blood vessels, particularly the arterioles. The CSF and the blood circulating to the brain must contain enough oxygen to prevent hypoxia of the tissues. However, higher-than-normal PaO_2 causes vasoconstriction in the brain, which decreases tissue perfusion. The ischemic tissue will further swell, worsening the patient's condition. You must ventilate the patient adequately to remove excess carbon dioxide. A high $PaCO_2$ causes vasodilation. The increased volume of blood enters the brain via the dilated blood vessels increases the volume within the fixed structure of the skull, increasing intracranial pressure. Low $PaCO_2$ causes vasoconstriction.

Brain cells are extremely sensitive to a drop in blood glucose levels because they cannot rapidly switch to another fuel source. As ischemia increases and delivery of glucose and oxygen to the cells decrease, the level of responsiveness decreases rapidly. Increased perfusion of the brain must be accompanied by an adequate blood glucose level. However, an increased blood glucose level is detrimental to the outcomes of patients with TBI. Glucose readily enters brain cells. In excess, the osmotic property of glucose pulls water into the brain cells, causing the brain to swell even further, increasing cerebral edema.

Assessment and Management of Traumatic Brain Injury

In addition to the standard components of trauma assessment, you must perform a neurologic exam. Key components of the neurologic exam include the following:

- Determine if there is a history of altered mental status or loss of consciousness after the injury.

- Assess the level of responsiveness and mental status. In particular, obtain a Glasgow Coma Scale (GCS) score.

- Check the pupils for size, equality, and reactivity to light.

- Look for neurologic deficits such as slurred or difficult speech and weakness or paralysis of the face or body on one or both sides.

Management of TBI includes the following:

1. Consider the need for restricting motion of the cervical spine.

2. Open and maintain the airway using positioning, suctioning, manual maneuvers, basic airway adjuncts, and advanced airways as indicated by the patient's condition.

3. Ensure normal ventilation. If ventilations are less than 8 or more than 30 per minute, assist with a bag-valve-mask device at a rate 10 per minute, using a normal tidal volume (5 to 7 mL/kg) based on the patient's size. If available, monitor $ETCO_2$, and adjust ventilations to maintain an $ETCO_2$ of 30 to 35 mmHg.

4. Administer oxygen, if needed, to maintain an SpO_2 of 95 percent or higher.

5. Control bleeding to preserve the oxygen-carrying capacity of the blood and maintain adequate perfusion.

6. Start IVs, if needed, en route to the hospital (or on the scene if the patient is entrapped and transport is unavoidably delayed) to maintain a systolic blood pressure of 90 mmHg.

7. Maintain the patient's normal body temperature. (Patients with severe TBI can have impaired thermoregulation.)

8. Check the blood glucose level and treat hypoglycemia.

9. Transport the patient without delay by the most appropriate mode to the most appropriate facility based on the patient's needs and the transport time.

Patients with signs of impending brain herniation require more aggressive ventilation. Although hyperventilation causes vasoconstriction that may ultimately decrease brain perfusion and increase swelling, it also may decrease the cerebral volume, slowing the rate of increase of ICP long enough to get the patient to a facility where burr holes (drilling holes in the cranium to relieve pressure) or a craniotomy (removing a portion of skull to allow the brain to expand without being compressed) can be performed.

If signs of impending herniation are present, aim for a brief period (a few minutes) of moderate hyperventilation, which means ventilating at a rate of 12 to 20 times per minute with a normal tidal volume.

Specific Brain Injuries

Brain tissue can be injured in several specific ways. The brain tissue itself can be directly injured, or injuries to cranial blood vessels can cause an accumulation of blood within the cranium that compresses the brain tissue.

Concussion

Concussion is a brain injury caused by blunt force trauma in which no structural damage to the brain can be identified through imaging technology. That is, the function of neurons is disrupted by the blow, but there is no gross physical injury that shows up on a CT scan or MRI.

Often there is a brief loss of consciousness followed by a period of anterograde amnesia. *Antero-* is a prefix that means *forward*. In anterograde amnesia, the patient cannot remember what happens *forward* in time from the point of injury. He cannot form memories of events after the injury. He will not remember what you have said to him or the questions he has asked you. The result, frequently, is a patient who asks repetitive questions or makes repetitive statements. Because memory formation requires a period of cognitive processing, the patient also may not remember the event that caused the injury or things that happened just before it.

The prefix *retro-* means backward or past. **Retrograde amnesia** is the inability to remember past events and facts. That is, events backward in time from the point injury, such as one's address, date of birth, what happened the day before, or similar items. It usually is not associated with a concussion. Rather, it is associated with damage to particular areas of the brain responsible for those memories.

A cerebral concussion is relatively mild, compared to other types of TBI. However, thinking of a concussion as a minor injury is misleading. Concussions can be severe and can lead to a prolonged period of postconcussive syndrome in which the patient experiences headaches, memory problems, depression, and other signs and symptoms. There has been much in the media in recent years about the effects of repeated concussions on behavior, personality, memory, and cognitive function. This has led to calls for changes in policies and practices in high school, college, and professional sports, because athletes in some sports, such as boxing and football, are prone to repeated incidents of head trauma.

Concussion can occur in conjunction with other TBIs, such as an epidural hematoma or **subdural hematoma**. Do not let a field impression of concussion give you a false sense of security that the patient does not have a more severe injury that is developing even as you are assessing him and preparing him for transport.

Cerebral Contusion

Cerebral contusion is bruising of the brain, usually with prolonged loss of consciousness or confusion. Edema to the brain is a concern, because it can lead to secondary brain injury.

One scenario in which cerebral contusions occur is **coup–contrecoup injuries**. This injury occurs when the brain "bounces" back and forth in the skull. There is an injury to brain tissue in the area of initial impact with the head as well as an injury to tissue on the opposite side of the brain when it rebounds off the inside of the skull. For example, if someone is struck in the forehead with a baseball bat, the brain will sustain injury at the point of impact. This is the coup injury (*coup* is a French word for *blow* or *impact*). The force of impact will then drive the brain toward the back of the skull, resulting in an additional injury. This is called the *contrecoup* (counter-impact) *injury* (Figure 37-6).

It is not possible, in the prehospital setting, to differentiate between cerebral contusion and several other types of significant TBIs because the mechanisms of injury and signs and symptoms are similar. Typical signs and symptoms of TBI are as follows:

- Altered mental status, ranging from confusion to unresponsiveness
- Weakness
- Altered respiratory rate or pattern
- Bradycardia
- Hypertension (especially the systolic blood pressure)

- Impaired speech
- Unusual behavior
- Unequal pupils
- Nausea
- Vomiting
- Seizures
- Posturing
- Trismus

Diffuse Axonal Injury

Diffuse axonal injury is an injury to the brain caused by shearing or tearing forces associated with acceleration/deceleration injuries. The axons of the nerves are stretched, causing them to dysfunction. The prognosis for such injuries is generally poor. The brain tolerates forward–backward acceleration and deceleration better than side-to-side acceleration and deceleration. A common scenario for diffuse axonal injury is a lateral-impact MVC. Shaken baby syndrome is a form of diffuse axonal injury. In most cases, patients with diffuse axonal injuries have decreased responsiveness or are unresponsive without focal (localized) neurologic dysfunction.

Intracranial Hemorrhage

Intracranial hemorrhage is bleeding within the cranial vault resulting in formation of a hematoma. It may occur between the skull and dura mater (epidural hematoma), between the dura mater and arachnoid mater (subdural hematoma), between the arachnoid and pia mater (subarachnoid bleeding is more common from stroke than from trauma), or within the brain tissue itself (intracerebral hematoma).

A blow to the temporal area of the skull, even a blow of relatively low velocity, can fracture that thin area of bone. The middle meningeal artery runs through a channel in a portion of the temporal bone. A fracture through the channel can tear the artery, resulting in brisk bleeding into the epidural space (Figure 37-7). Because the blow needed

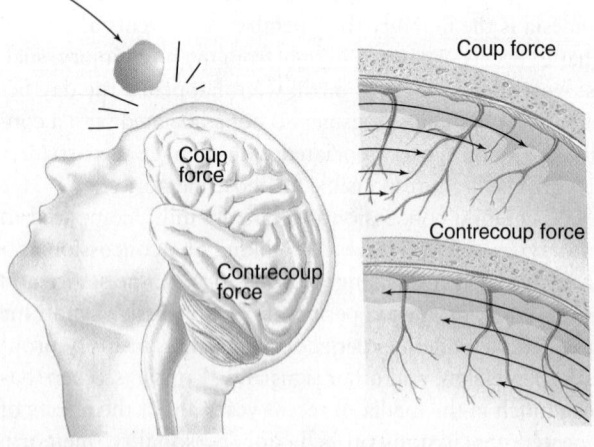

FIGURE 37-6

Coup and contrecoup injury to the brain.

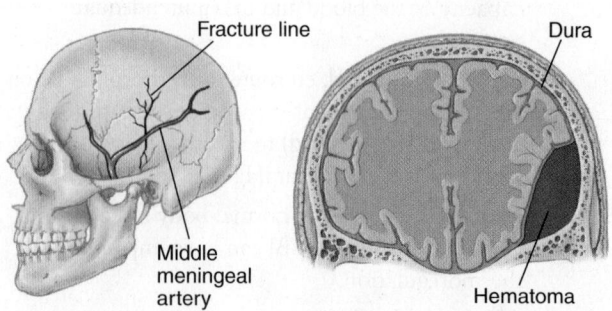

FIGURE 37-7

Epidural hematoma. Linear fractures can cause laceration of the middle meningeal artery, which leads to the accumulation of blood between the skull and dura mater.

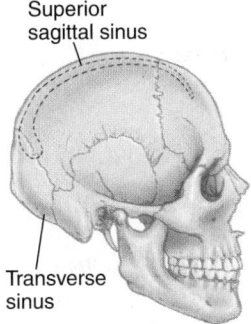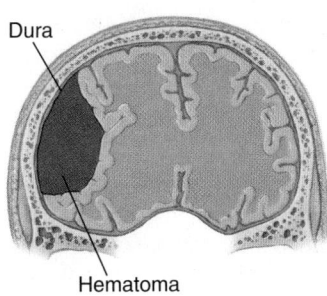

Superior sagittal sinus

Dura

Transverse sinus

Hematoma

FIGURE 37-8

Subdural hematoma. Venous bleeding between the dura mater and arachnoid mater usually leads to the formation of a hematoma.

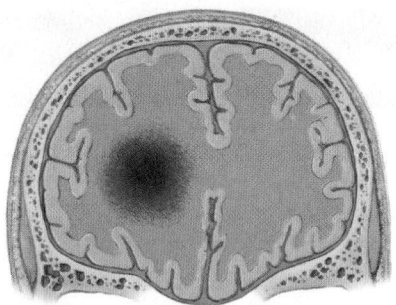

FIGURE 37-9

Intracerebral hemorrhage.

> **IN THE FIELD**
>
> It is vital that all patients who experience a loss of consciousness following an injury be evaluated by a physician in the emergency department as soon as possible.

> **IN THE FIELD**
>
> Always suspect subdural hematoma in patients who present with altered mental status following a head injury, even if the injury occurred days earlier.

> **IN THE FIELD**
>
> The earlier signs and symptoms of increased intracranial pressure include altered mental status, unequal pupils, increased systolic blood pressure, and vomiting. As ICP worsens and the brainstem is forced down into the foramen magnum, bradycardia, abnormal breathing patterns, and posturing will present.

to cause fracture of the temporal is not necessarily a severe impact, the patient sometimes suffers a brief loss of responsiveness due to concussion, and then regains consciousness. Meanwhile, blood from the torn artery is rapidly accumulating in the epidural space. Following a brief period of responsiveness, called a *lucid interval*, the patient's level of responsiveness rapidly deteriorates. That sequence of events is suspicious for an epidural hematoma. However, keep in mind that a patient need not suffer a brief loss of responsiveness and lucid interval to have an epidural hematoma. Consider the possibility of epidural hematoma with injury to the temporal or adjacent parietal region of the skull.

The source of subdural bleeding is usually venous (Figure 37-8). ICP can rise more gradually than with epidural bleeding, which is arterial, so the onset of signs and symptoms can be gradual. In some cases, an accumulation of blood significant enough to cause signs and symptoms can take hours, days, or even weeks or months to occur. That most commonly happens in alcoholics or the elderly with a relatively minor blow to the head. However, the bleeding can be severe.

Subdural hematomas are often accompanied by other traumatic injuries to the brain, giving them a high mortality rate of 60 to 90 percent if the patient is found unconscious (Campbell, 2008). Signs and symptoms may occur days, weeks, or even months after the initial injury.

Intracerebral hemorrhage is bleeding within the brain tissue (Figure 37-9). Intracerebral hemorrhage may result from either blunt or penetrating trauma or from stroke. With intracerebral hemorrhage, patients will present with focal neurologic deficits similar to those of stroke. The focal deficit can be clouded by signs and symptoms of other TBIs, such as concussion or cerebral contusion, or generalized cerebral edema and ischemia from increased intracranial pressure. The bleeding is localized in a specific region of the brain; therefore, deficits will depend on the area of injury.

Injuries to the Face

Injuries to the face can be very frightening for the patient. Patients may be concerned about temporary or permanent loss of vision when eye injuries are present, or permanent disfigurement as a result of fractures or facial scarring. As an Advanced EMT, you will do your best to calm and comfort them, but your primary concern will be maintaining a patent airway.

Bleeding, fractures, and edema can be an immediate threat to airway patency. Oral trauma can cause airway compromise because of associated bleeding. Broken teeth may become airway obstructions.

Matt and Chuck pull up to the scene where a woman is lying in the street. They notify dispatch that they have arrived, grab their gear, and proceed to the patient's side.

The man holding manual stabilization of the head and neck tells them that he witnessed the injury. He says that the woman had an initial loss of consciousness that lasted about a minute or so. He also reports that the woman had convinced the owner of the motorcycle to let her ride it despite the fact that she had been drinking. She was not wearing a helmet when she attempted to take off on the motorcycle. She apparently gave it too much gas because the motorcycle rose up on its rear wheel, causing the woman to fall backward and strike her head on the pavement. She has moderate bleeding to the posterior head with no signs of deformity.

Chuck begins to immobilize her C-spine as Matt obtains the following vital signs: blood pressure, 142/92; respirations, 12 nonlabored; pulse, 110; Glasgow Coma Scale score, 4, 4, 6.

The patient states that she has pain in the back of her head and that she feels like she is going to throw up.

Problem-Solving Questions

1. What are the pertinent pieces of information gathered from the mechanism of injury?
2. How does the mechanism of injury and the clinical presentation of the patient assist in making a transport decision?
3. What are Matt and Chuck's major concerns at this point?

Facial Fractures

Trauma to the face resulting in facial fractures may produce both open and closed injuries. Profuse bleeding may affect airway patency, but deformity as a result of facial fractures may compromise the airway as well. Because the facial bones provide protection to the airway and give it its shape, the airway can be compromised when these bones are fractured, especially when there is deformity.

Fractures of the mandible are painful and may result in airway compromise because teeth can be dislodged and become foreign airway obstructions. If the mandible is fractured and dislocated, rendering it unable to support the tongue, the tongue can obstruct the airway. This is of particular concern when the patient is placed in the supine position.

Fractures to the midface are classified according to **Le Fort criteria** (Figure 37-10). **Le Fort I fractures** involve the maxilla only and may result in slight instability and deformity. **Le Fort II fractures** include fractures of the maxilla and nasal bones. **Le Fort III fractures** involve the entire midfacial region. Le Fort II and III fractures usually result in the leakage of cerebrospinal fluid from the skull, produce significant instability of the region, and put the patient at high risk for airway compromise because of bleeding.

Fractures to the nasal bone alone are generally not life threatening unless bleeding is profuse enough to pose a risk to the airway. They do, however result in significant deformity because of edema. In such cases, ensure that the airway remains patent through suctioning or directing the patient to spit the blood from his mouth into a basin or biohazard bag.

Orbital fractures generally involve the zygoma and maxilla. The fractures may also affect the muscles of the eye, resulting in limited movement. Patients with orbital fractures commonly complain of blurred or double vision, or diplopia.

Eye Injuries

Injuries to the eyes can occur as a result of blunt trauma, penetrating trauma, or chemical exposure. When treating a patient with an eye injury, be sensitive to the fact that the injury may be very frightening to the patient. The thought of becoming blind, even in one eye, will be of major concern to the patient.

Even though the eyes are fairly well protected by facial bones, they are susceptible to blunt trauma if something applies direct pressure to the eye. Recall that the anterior surface and chamber of the eye consist of specialized tissues; injury to them can lead to blindness. In some cases, enough force can be applied to the eye to cause separation of the retina from the posterior wall of the eye. This type of injury is called a *detached retina* and is a true emergency. Patients with a detached retina will usually complain of dark areas within their vision.

Penetrating trauma to the eyes can be caused by larger objects, such as sticks, or smaller objects, such as small shards of metal (Figure 37-11). In either case, the eye can sustain injury that places the patient at risk of blindness.

The extent of injury is directly related to the mechanism of injury. For example, if a small shard of metal gets

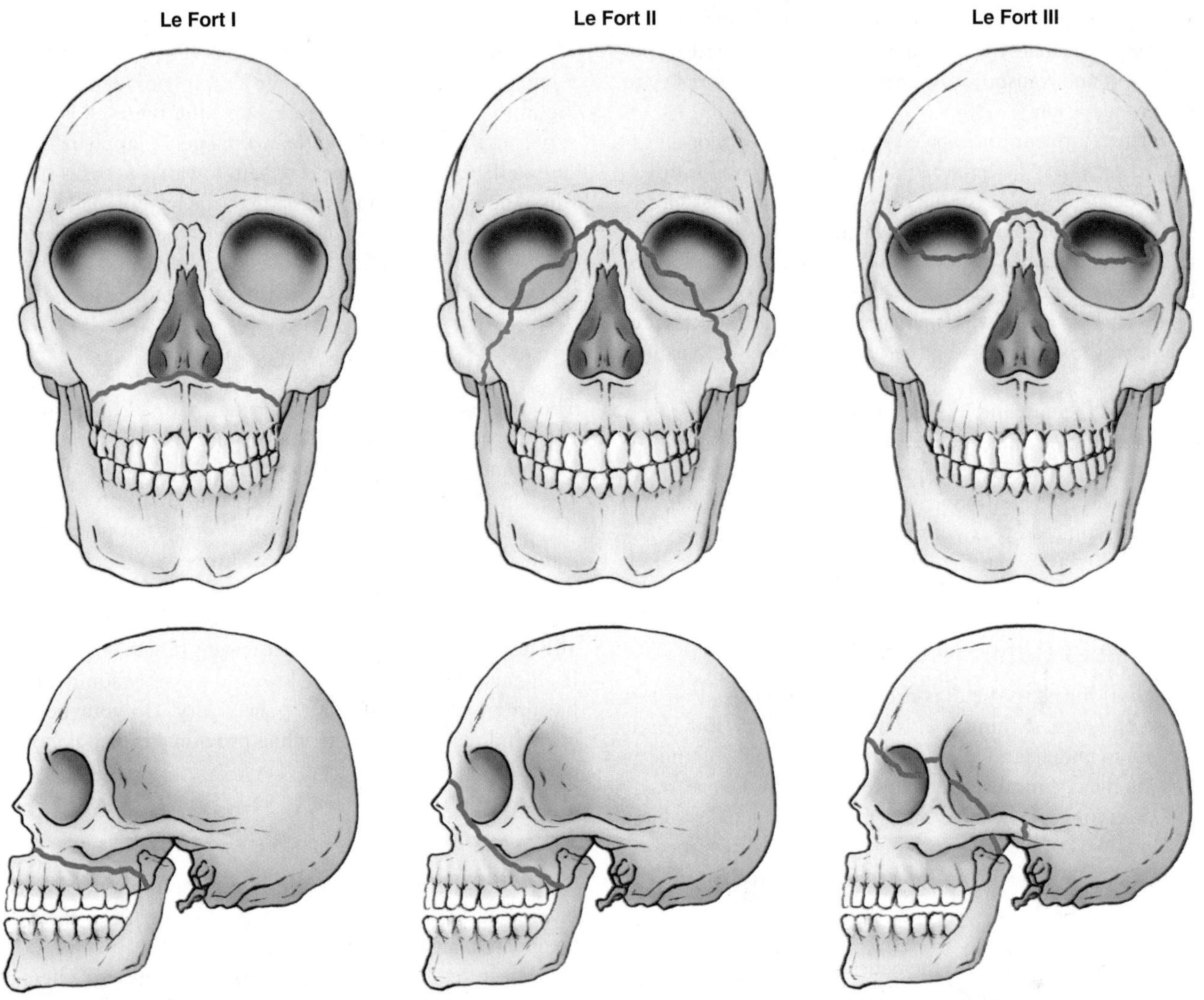

Le Fort I **Le Fort II** **Le Fort III**

FIGURE 37-10

Le Fort facial fracture classification.

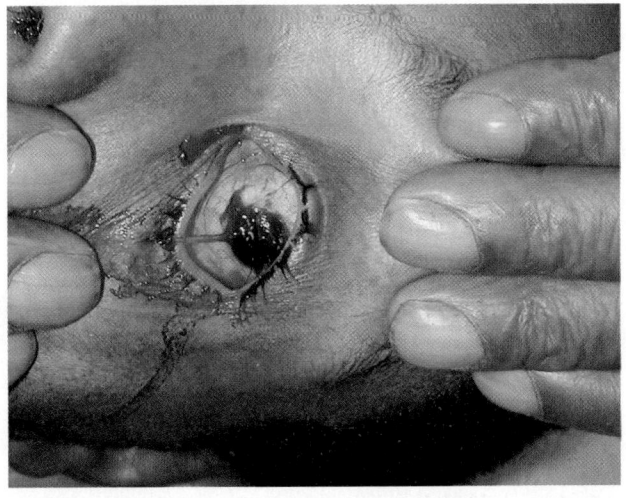

FIGURE 37-11

Penetrating trauma to the globe of the eye, resulting in blindness. (© Charles Stewart, MD, and Associates)

into the eye, it can cause a laceration or abrasion to the conjunctiva or cornea. If someone is shot in the eye with a pellet rifle, the extent of injury will be much more significant. There may be damage to the anterior tissues of the eye and possibly a leak of intraocular fluid. Additionally, if the pellet goes deep enough in the eye, the posterior structures such as the retina also may be affected.

In some cases, the eyelid is injured but the eye itself is not. An example of this type of injury is an avulsed eyelid. Recall that the inside of the eyelid protects the eye and provides lubrication. If it is not intact, the eye may sustain injury if not treated appropriately.

Impaled Objects in the Eye/Extruded Eyeball

Stabilize impaled objects in the eye in place, because removal can cause additional injury. In some cases, trauma to the eye leads to extrusion of the eyeball from its socket.

Never attempt to replace the eyeball in its socket. For an impaled object to the eye or an extruded eyeball, rapid treatment and transport to an appropriate facility are key to preserving vision.

The treatment for impaled objects in the eyes or an extruded eyeball is the same. First, stabilize the object or extruded eyeball with a sterile dressing such as roller gauze. For extruded eyeballs, moisten the dressing with saline so the eyeball does not dry out, which would result in further injury. Once the object or eyeball is stable, cover it with an object such as a crushed paper cup. For impaled objects, cut a hole in the cup, allowing the object to protrude through the bottom.

Hold the cup and dressing in place while you apply a bandage that encircles the head and covers both eyes. It is important to cover the uninjured eye as well. Because both eyes move together, movement of the uninjured eye can cause the injured eye to move as well, possibly causing additional injury. When the injury is dressed and bandaged, transport the patient immediately to an appropriate facility.

Chemical Burns to the Eyes

Chemical burns to the eyes are true emergencies that can cause blindness within seconds of exposure. It is important for you to understand that injury to the eyes will continue as long as the chemical remains in contact with the eye. Signs and symptoms of chemical burns to the eyes include redness or cloudiness of the eyes, swelling, blurred or diminished vision, pain, and, in some cases, redness or burns around the eyes (Figure 37-12).

When a chemical is in the eyes, immediately begin to provide emergency care to the patient by flushing the chemical from the affected eye with water. Place the patient in a supine position and hold the eye open wide with your fingers. Continuously irrigate the eye with water or normal saline for at least 20 minutes. This is done by pouring the water or normal saline into the eye at the inside corner and allowing it to flow across the eye and out the other side.

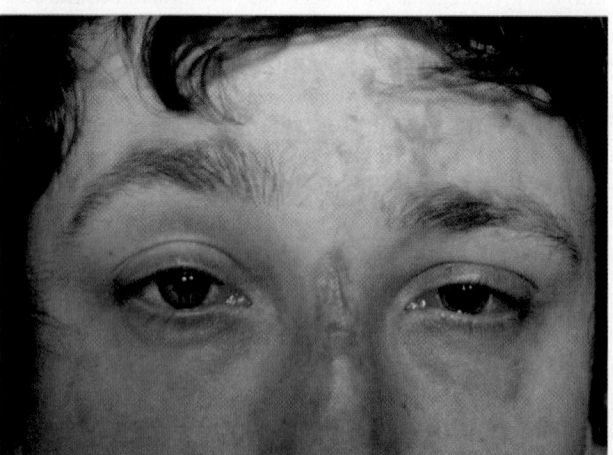

FIGURE 37-12

Chemical burn to the eyes. (© Western Ophthalmic Hospital/Photo Researchers, Inc.)

If soft contact lenses are in the eye, remove them by opening the eye and gently pinching the lens with your thumb and forefinger, and then removing the lens. If hard contact lenses are in the eye, remove them by opening the eyelids wide, exposing the entire contact lens, then gently applying pressure to the eyelids as you close them toward the edges of the lens. Apply slightly more pressure to the lower eyelid as you close them, which will cause the lower lid to slide under the lens. After the lens is lifted by the lower lid, continue to close the eyes until you can grasp the lens and remove it.

Ear Injuries

The external ear is composed primarily of cartilage and is not very vascular. Therefore, bleeding as a result of injury is minor and does not pose a life threat.

The internal structures of the ear are well protected by the skull. Therefore, injury results only from penetrating trauma or through rapid changes in pressure, such as with diving accidents or explosions. Ruptures to the tympanic membrane (eardrum) are not life threatening and will usually heal without treatment. However, the patient may be frightened, because hearing loss and possibly some minor bleeding will be present after the injury. Do your best to calm and reassure patients while providing transport to an emergency department.

Avulsed Teeth

Trauma to the face may result in teeth becoming dislodged or avulsed. It is important that you consider these teeth to be potential airway obstructions.

When teeth are avulsed, transport them with the patient to the emergency department, because the doctors may be able to reimplant them. Hold an avulsed tooth by the crown, never by the roots, and rinse it with saline to gently remove any debris. After rinsing the tooth or teeth, place them in a container of balanced electrolyte solution. In the prehospital setting, sterile normal saline is usually the most feasible solution.

Injuries to the Neck

The neck contains many vital structures. Therefore, injury to the neck demands careful assessment to identify potential life-threatening injuries. Neck trauma, whether caused by blunt or penetrating trauma, can result in injury to the cervical spine, blood vessels, and the airway.

Injuries to the Cervical Spine

The vertebrae of the cervical spine provide protection to the spinal cord. If blunt or penetrating trauma occurs to this region of the spine, the patient is at risk for paralysis, shock, respiratory compromise, and even death. (You will learn more about cervical spine injuries in Chapter 40.)

Injuries to Blood Vessels

Penetrating trauma to the neck usually is obvious and can cause life-threatening hemorrhage if the large vessels of the neck are injured (Figure 37-13).

Recall that the external jugular veins, internal jugular veins, and carotid arteries are located on the lateral sides of the neck; therefore, open and closed soft-tissue injuries to those regions are of concern. Although injury to

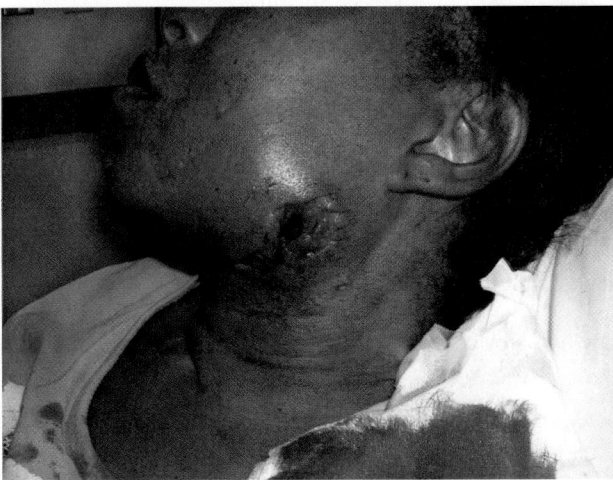

FIGURE 37-13

Laceration to the lateral neck. (© Edward T. Dickinson, MD)

the large veins of the neck may produce significant hemorrhage, injury to the carotid arteries may result in life-threatening bleeding in a matter of minutes. Hematomas from closed injuries can obstruct the airway or impair blood flow.

With a vascular injury, you must consider the possibility of air entering the vessels of the neck, producing an air embolism. To prevent this from occurring, immediately cover open neck wounds with your gloved hand, then apply an occlusive dressing.

Blunt trauma to the neck also can result in life-threatening injury to blood vessels within the neck. If blunt trauma is significant enough to cause internal bleeding, a hematoma may begin to form. Hematomas can continue to increase in size and lead to compression of the structures within the neck, such as the trachea and blood vessels.

Injuries to the Airway

Blunt or penetrating trauma can result in injury to the trachea or larynx, which can affect airway patency. In some cases, edema of the neck, resulting from soft-tissue injury, can create enough pressure to compress the airway. In penetrating trauma, blood can enter the trachea through an opening caused by the injury. Regardless of whether blunt or penetrating trauma to the neck has occurred, frequently assess the patient's adequacy of airway and breathing status.

PERSONAL PERSPECTIVE

Advanced EMT Hannah West: While working one day, my partner and I were called to the scene to find a man in his early 30s who had been assaulted in a graveyard while placing flowers on his mother's grave. He was repeatedly struck in the head with an object and his wallet was taken.

Bystanders witnessed the attack and advised law enforcement and us that the patient was struck in the head three times with what appeared to be a large stick. When bystanders arrived at the patient's side, he was unconscious, so they called 911.

Upon our arrival, the patient was still unconscious and bleeding profusely from the head. During my assessment, I quickly decided that we had to rapidly transport the patient to the nearest neurosurgical facility, which was about 15 minutes

away. Firefighters on the scene assisted us in packaging the patient while my partner provided positive pressure ventilations, because the patient was not breathing adequately.

En route to the hospital emergency department, the patient began to exhibit decorticate posturing, which continued throughout the transport. Upon arrival, the patient was quickly evaluated and taken to radiology so a CT scan could be obtained. My partner and I got our equipment ready for the next call and left the hospital.

Later, I was told by another crew that the patient we had transported was placed on a ventilator. His injuries were very severe and his family eventually decided to take him off life support and donated his organs. His injuries were apparently too severe despite the treatment provided by us and the hospital staff.

CASE STUDY WRAP-UP

Clinical-Reasoning Process

Advanced EMTs Matt and Chuck arrived on scene and immediately determined that the patient had a significant mechanism of injury (MOI) and experienced a loss of consciousness. The MOI suggests a high potential for brain injury. The loss of consciousness and nausea further support the possibility for such an injury. Matt and Chuck recognize the need for rapid transport to a neurosurgical facility. Because the nearest neurosurgical facility is over an hour away, they initiate transport to the closest facility where the patient can be assessed by a physician and transferred to an appropriate facility.

Matt and Chuck get the patient fully immobilized and begin the short 5-minute transport to the hospital emergency department. Matt initiates IV access and reassesses the patient. Matt knows that the patient may vomit and prepares his suction equipment so that he is ready to act if necessary. Patients with closed head injury and an increased ICP often are at risk for airway compromise. This is due to altered mental status and the potential for vomiting.

En route, the patient vomits into the nonrebreather mask. Matt quickly removes the mask and suctions her airway. By the time her airway is cleared, they have arrived at the hospital. The patient is taken inside and Matt gives his report to the receiving physician just as the patient vomits again.

Within an hour, the emergency department physician diagnoses the patient with an epidural hematoma and sends her to a neurosurgical facility.

Matt and Chuck managed this particular patient appropriately and provided her with the best chance for a positive outcome.

CHAPTER REVIEW

Chapter Summary

Managing patients with injuries to the head, brain, face, and neck involves your identifying life threats related to these specific injuries. Additionally, you must also consider the potential for associated trauma to other parts of the body. Keep in mind that internal injuries may produce internal bleeding, which causes hypotension.

Caring for a patient with a head injury may be very challenging, because these patients will frequently have an altered level of responsiveness and may be combative. If this occurs, it is vital that you have additional help on scene and en route to the emergency department in order to properly care for them.

TBI patients are also very susceptible to deterioration in condition as a result of hypotension, hypoxia, hypercapnia, and hypocapnia, so you must ensure adequate ventilation. If necessary, you must provide positive pressure ventilations with high-flow oxygen. Always be prepared to use suction when bleeding into the airway and/or vomiting are present. Failure to do so can lead to the loss of airway patency.

Your ability to manage those patients relies on strong assessment and management skills, which will only get better through experience.

Review Questions

Multiple-Choice Questions

1. Which region of the skull is the thinnest and more easily fractured than the others?

   a. Parietal   c. Basilar
   b. Occipital   d. Frontal

2. What percent of the space within the skull does the brain occupy?

   a. 70 percent   c. 90 percent
   b. 85 percent   d. 75 percent

3. Which one of the following is the most fragile layer of the brain?

   a. Pia mater   c. Arachnoid mater
   b. Dura mater   d. Meninges

4. What region of the brain is responsible for coordination and equilibrium?

   a. Cerebrum   c. Pons
   b. Brainstem   d. Cerebellum

5. Injury to what part of the brain can lead to immediate life-threatening inability to maintain adequate blood pressure, heart rate, and respiratory rate?

    a. Cerebrum　　　　c. Meninges
    b. Brainstem　　　　d. Cerebellum

6. Which chamber of the eye is located between the iris and lens?

    a. Anterior chamber　　c. Vitreous chamber
    b. Posterior chamber　　d. Optical chamber

7. Which one of the following is true about bleeding from the scalp?

    a. It is generally minor and will not produce significant blood loss.
    b. It is more persistent than bleeding in other regions of the body due to the vessels' lack of ability to retract and constrict.
    c. It should be controlled by persistent direct pressure in every situation.
    d. It is generally controlled by clotting that takes place in the patient's hair.

8. Which one of the following is true about a depressed skull fracture?

    a. It generally does not produce underlying injury to the brain.
    b. It may be hidden by the formation of a hematoma over the area of the fracture.
    c. It is usually linear in nature.
    d. It is generally a closed fracture.

9. Which type of skull fracture would you suspect if cerebrospinal fluid is found to be leaking from the ears and nose?

    a. Open skull fracture
    b. Depressed skull fracture
    c. Basilar skull fracture
    d. Linear skull fracture

10. As an Advanced EMT, you can most effectively minimize the amount of secondary brain injury to the patient by:

    a. controlling external bleeding.
    b. placing the patient in the Trendelenburg position.
    c. transporting the patient to a neurosurgical facility.
    d. ensuring adequacy of the airway and ventilations.

11. Coup–contrecoup injuries usually result in what type of injury to the brain?

    a. Cerebral contusion
    b. Subdural hematoma
    c. Epidural hematoma
    d. Intracranial hemorrhage

Critical-Thinking Questions

12. Explain why hypertension associated with TBI is not treated in the prehospital environment.

13. Explain the importance of properly ventilating a patient who is exhibiting signs and symptoms of brain herniation.

14. With which type of head injury could direct pressure to the bleeding site cause injury to the underlying brain tissue?

References

Campbell, J. E. (2008). *International trauma life support* (6th ed.). Upper Saddle River, NJ: Pearson Prentice Hall.

McSwain, N. E., Salomone, J. P., Pons, P. T. (Eds). (2007). *Prehospital trauma life support* (6th ed.). St. Louis, MO: Elsevier.

Additional Reading

Brain Trauma Foundation. (n.d.). *Prehospital severe TBI guidelines/ treatment: Cerebral herniation: Brain Trauma Foundation.* Retrieved March 16, 2011, from http://tbiguidelines.org/ glHome.aspx?gl=2

38

Thoracic Trauma

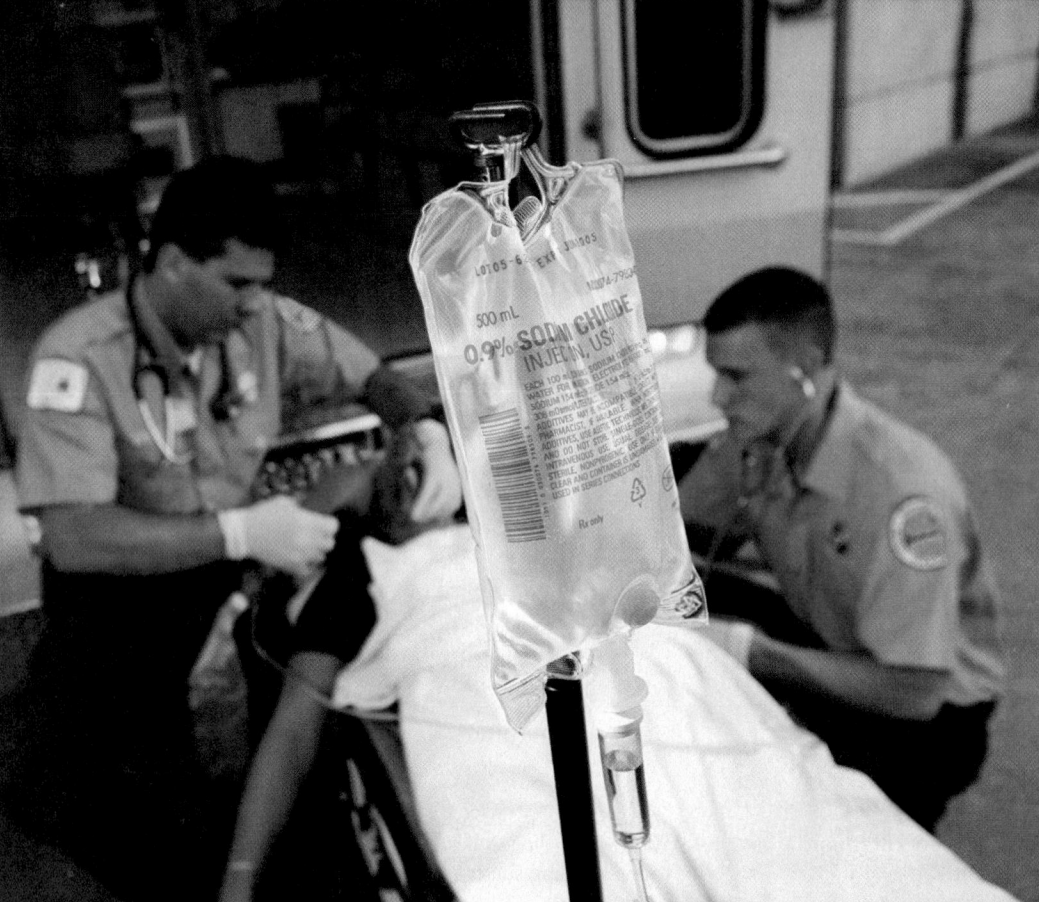

Content Area: Trauma

Advanced EMT Education Standard: The Advanced EMT applies fundamental knowledge to provide basic and selected advanced emergency care and transportation based on assessment findings for an acutely injured patient.

Objectives

After reading this chapter, you should be able to:

38.1 Define key terms introduced in this chapter.

38.2 Explain the relationship between an intact thoracic cavity and lungs, and ventilation, oxygenation, and respiration.

38.3 Relate mechanism of injury to the potential for specific types of chest trauma.

38.4 Relate assessment findings to suspicion for specific types of chest injuries.

Resource Central

To access Resource Central, follow the directions on the Student Access Card provided with this text. If there is no card, go to www.bradybooks.com and follow the Resource Central link to Buy Access. Under Media Resources, you will find:

• *Commotio Cordis.* How to identify this strange condition.

• *Chest Decompression Procedure.* How to perform a needle chest decompression.

• *Traumatic Asphyxia.* How to manage this traumatic injury.

CASE STUDY

On a warm, sunny afternoon, Advanced EMTs Byron Johnson and Angela Soriano are dispatched to a single-victim shooting. Dispatch advises that law enforcement is en route. They know the area where the shooting took place well, because they have responded there many times for emergencies ranging from drug overdoses to shootings.

About two blocks from the scene, dispatch advises that law enforcement is on scene and it is secure. When Byron and Angela arrive, a police officer tells them that there is one patient with a gunshot wound to the upper chest.

Problem-Solving Questions

1. What injuries might the patient have sustained as a result of the gunshot wound?
2. What additional information do Byron and Angela need at this point?
3. How does the mechanism of injury play a part in Bryon and Angela's transport destination decision?

38.5 Explain the pathophysiology and management of the following types of chest injuries:
  - Blunt cardiac injury
  - Commotio cordis
  - Flail chest
  - Hemothorax
  - Myocardial contusion
  - Open pneumothorax
  - Penetrating cardiac injury
  - Pericardial tamponade
  - Pulmonary contusion
  - Rib fractures
  - Simple pneumothorax
  - Tension pneumothorax
  - Traumatic asphyxia

Introduction

Thoracic injuries range from uncomplicated contusions of the chest wall and minor rib fractures to severe injuries of the chest wall and underlying vital organs. Because the organs of the thoracic cavity are responsible for ventilation, respiration, and circulation, injury to them can quickly lead to death from hypoxia, hypercarbia, or blood loss.

Thoracic injury can occur on any surface of the thorax: anterior, lateral, or posterior. Impact or penetration of any of those surfaces can result in injury to the vital organs contained in the thoracic cavity. Failure to assess all surfaces of the thorax can result in missing clues to potential vital organ injuries and adversely affect the patient's outcome.

Blunt thoracic trauma can result from mechanisms of injury such as motor vehicle collisions, falls, assaults, or crush injuries and accounts for 20 to 25 percent of all trauma deaths (Mancini, 2008). Penetrating trauma includes mechanisms such as shootings, stabbings, and flying debris from explosions.

Regardless of the mechanism of injury, you must recognize and treat thoracic injuries promptly and properly to address problems with breathing and circulation.

This chapter offers a review of the anatomy and physiology of the thoracic cavity. It also will help you learn to differentiate between specific thoracic injuries and how to properly care for each.

Anatomy and Physiology Review

The thoracic cavity, also called the *chest cavity*, is the cavity within the upper torso. It is separated from the abdominal cavity by the diaphragm (Figure 38-1). The mediastinum is the section of the thorax immediately behind the sternum. It contains portions of the esophagus, trachea, and great vessels, and the heart. The lungs lie on either side of the mediastinum. Despite the protection provided by bones and muscle of the thoracic cage, injury can occur when force is transmitted through those protective structures.

The organs within the thoracic cavity are protected on the anterior surface by the sternum, clavicles, ribs, and pectoral muscles of the chest. The lateral walls of the thorax are protected by the ribs, which extend from the spine toward the anterior surface of the chest. The ribs of the lateral walls of the thorax provide protection for intrathoracic organs but are susceptible to injury because they are not protected by muscle. The posterior wall of the thorax is protected by the spine, scapula, and posterior ribs.

The Lungs and Ventilation

Providing oxygen for cellular metabolism and eliminating carbon dioxide produced by cellular metabolism requires ventilation, the movement of air into and out of the lungs, and respiration, the exchange of gases. Respiration consists of two phases. During external respiration, oxygen and carbon dioxide are exchanged across the respiratory membrane composed of the alveolar–capillary interface in the lungs. In internal respiration, gases are exchanged between the systemic capillaries and the cells of the body.

Ventilation requires an intact brainstem, nerve pathways, and an intact chest wall, pleura, and lungs. External respiration requires adequate perfusion and ventilation and a small distance across which gases must diffuse. That is, the alveoli and pulmonary capillaries must be in close contact with each other. Internal respiration requires adequate on-loading of oxygen to hemoglobin, adequate circulation to the tissues, and adequate off-loading of oxygen at the cellular level.

The thoracic cavity is lined with the pleura, which consists of two layers—the visceral pleura and the parietal pleura. The parietal pleura is the outermost layer that is in direct contact with the inside of the thoracic wall while the visceral pleura is the innermost layer that is in contact with the lungs. A potential space, the pleural space, lies between the two pleural layers. The pleural space contains a few milliliters of serous fluid that seal the layers to each other to allow expansion of the lungs on inspiration and act as a lubricant, reducing friction between the two pleura during ventilation.

During inspiration, the diaphragm and intercostal muscles between the ribs contract, increasing the volume of the thoracic cavity. The negative pressure created by an increase in the size of the thoracic cavity creates negative pressure in the pleural space, which allows the lungs to expand, creating negative intrapulmonary pressure. As intrapulmonary pressure decreases, air moves from the higher pressure of the atmosphere, through the nose or mouth into the upper and lower airways, filling the lungs, where external respiration takes place. During external respiration, oxygen diffuses across the respiratory membrane and enters the blood, and carbon dioxide diffuses out of the blood and enters the alveoli for expiration.

During expiration, the diaphragm and rib cage return to their original positions, decreasing the volume of the thoracic cavity. The decreased volume creates positive pressure within the pleural and intrapulmonary spaces. Under higher pressure, air flows out of the lungs and is exhaled into the atmosphere.

Anything that impairs the motion of the chest wall, contact between the pleural layers, the integrity of the lung, alveolar surface area available for gas exchange, or pulmonary perfusion interferes with tissue oxygenation and elimination of carbon dioxide.

The Heart

The heart is located at the center of the chest just below the sternum where it is fairly well protected. The heart is responsible for perfusing the entire body with nutrients, chemical messengers, and oxygen-rich blood and with bringing carbon dioxide back to the lungs for elimination. In order to sustain life, the heart must be able to pump an adequate amount of blood throughout the body. Any injury

CHEST CAVITY

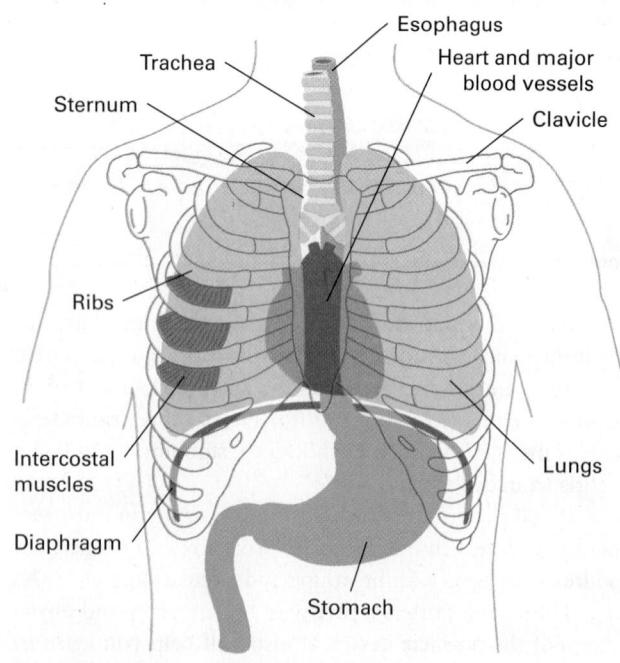

Esophagus
Trachea
Sternum
Heart and major blood vessels
Clavicle
Ribs
Intercostal muscles
Diaphragm
Lungs
Stomach

FIGURE 38-1

The thoracic cavity.

to the heart that reduces its ability to adequately circulate blood creates a life-threatening condition.

The heart is surrounded by a tough membrane called the *pericardium.* The pericardium consists of two layers, visceral pericardium and parietal pericardium. Approximately 30 mL of pericardial fluid between those layers provides lubrication as the heart contracts and moves within the pericardial sac.

The superior and inferior vena cava carry deoxygenated venous blood from the systemic circulation back to the right side of the heart. Blood from the right ventricle is circulated to the lungs by way of the pulmonary arteries. Once the blood is circulated through the lungs for gas exchange, it returns to the left side of the heart via the pulmonary veins. Blood leaves the left side of the heart to be circulated through the systemic circulation through the aorta.

The myocardium receives its blood supply during diastole, the relaxation phase of the cardiac cycle, through the coronary arteries that arise from the aorta just as it leaves the left ventricle. Blood flow through the heart is controlled by valves between the atria and ventricles and between the ventricles and the large arteries they supply.

General Assessment and Management of Thoracic Trauma

Patients can sustain injury to the thorax through a number of mechanisms of injury, blunt and penetrating alike. For example, an unrestrained driver who is involved in a frontal impact is likely to strike his chest on the steering wheel. The impact may be significant enough to cause injury to internal organs of the thorax. Penetrating trauma may cause injury to the internal thoracic organs as well. When a patient sustains a stab or gunshot wound to the thorax, injury to the internal organs is likely to occur. Regardless of the specific mechanism, injuries to the thorax can be classified as either open or closed. During your assessment, inspect and palpate the thorax on all sides—anterior, posterior, and lateral walls. When penetrating trauma is present, carefully assess the entire thorax so that you do not overlook additional wounds. This is particularly important when the patient has sustained a gunshot wound. The bullet may have entered the anterior surface of the thorax and travelled completely through the patient, leaving an even larger exit wound on the posterior surface.

General guidelines for the management of thoracic trauma patients include the following:

1. Ensure an open airway.
2. Assist ventilations as needed.
3. Provide supplemental oxygen to maintain an SpO_2 of at least 95 percent.
4. Monitor ECG, SpO_2, and $EtCO_2$.
5. Treat for shock when indicated.
6. Consider the need for immediate surgical intervention and transport the patient to an appropriate facility utilizing the most appropriate mode of transport available.

Scene Size-Up

Always ensure that the scene is safe prior to entering it. This is particularly true when responding to any call that may involve violence. Identify the number of patients and call for additional resources as needed. Take a moment to ensure that the Standard Precautions you have selected are adequate to the situation.

Consider the mechanism of injury (MOI). MOIs such as falls, penetrating trauma, significant impact to the chest, and MVCs all have the potential to cause thoracic injury. Consider the need for manual stabilization of the spine.

Form a general impression of the patient. How does the patient look? Does he appear to have a decreased level of responsiveness? Does he appear to have dyspnea? Your general impression of the patient provides your first indication of how quickly you must prepare for transport.

> **IN THE FIELD**
>
> The primary assessment and rapid trauma assessment should flow together. Complete both within the first minute of caring for a critical trauma patient. If possible, you should package and prepare the patient for transport as soon as the primary and rapid trauma assessments are complete. Aim for a total scene time of less than 10 minutes, but do not neglect components of the primary assessment, or interventions to establish and maintain airway and ventilation, and control bleeding.

Primary Assessment

A decreased level of responsiveness in a trauma patient can indicate traumatic brain injury, shock, or hypoxia. If the patient is unresponsive and does not appear to be breathing adequately, immediately check for a pulse. If a pulse is not present, begin CPR. If a pulse is present, continue on with your primary assessment.

Ensure that the patient has a patent airway. Open the airway using manual maneuvers and suction as necessary. If those techniques are ineffective, insert a simple airway adjunct. Assess breathing and assist with a bag-valve-mask device and supplemental oxygen if needed. Impaired breathing should increase your suspicion of chest trauma.

Check the pulse and control significant bleeding with direct pressure. Administer oxygen to patients with an SpO_2 less than 95 percent, poor initial impression, decreased responsiveness, inadequate breathing, or indications of significant blood loss. Maintain the patient's SpO_2 at 95 percent or above. These patients are critical and a high priority for transport.

Rapidly extricate critical trauma patients in vehicles. Make decisions about the need and feasibility for ALS response and air medical transportation early in order to get the resources en route to your location.

Secondary Assessment: Rapid Trauma Assessment

Immediately after addressing issues with the airway, breathing, and circulation, perform a rapid trauma assessment. Expose the patient and check the head, neck, chest, abdomen, pelvis, and extremities for potentially life-threatening injuries. The rapid trauma assessment includes quickly palpating and auscultating the chest to check for injury and equality of breath sounds.

Expose areas of the body as much as possible, given the circumstances. For example, it may be difficult to completely expose a patient who is entrapped in a badly damaged vehicle. In dim or dark conditions, use a flashlight, but plan for reassessment in adequate light.

Signs of chest trauma include the following:

- Cyanosis
- Tachypnea
- Dyspnea
- Soft-tissue injury to the thorax (including the anterior, lateral, and posterior aspects)
- Penetrating trauma to the thorax with or without the presence of a sucking chest wound
- Decreased or absent breath sounds in a lung field
- Paradoxical movement of the chest
- Hemoptysis, or bloody sputum
- Subcutaneous emphysema
- Jugular venous distention (JVD)
- Tracheal deviation (late sign)
- Shock

Immediately cover any open injury of the neck or chest. Do not forget that the back is also part of the chest.

Secondary Assessment: Vital Signs, Monitoring Devices, History, and Physical Exam

For critical patients, the remainder of the secondary assessment is completed en route to the hospital, if possible. If transport is delayed due to extrication or other factors, complete the secondary assessment on scene, as soon as it is feasible.

Obtain a set of baseline vital signs, including pulse, respiratory rate, and blood pressure. Pulse oximetry is very valuable in assessing patients with chest injuries. Initiate continuous pulse oximetry as soon as possible. An ECG and $EtCO_2$, if available, provide additional useful information.

Keep in mind that patients with thoracic trauma may have multisystem trauma. Perform a thorough head-to-toe assessment, searching for signs of injury.

Treat additional life-threatening injuries as soon as they are identified. Manage less serious injuries after the secondary assessment, according to the resources available. For example, if you are by yourself with a critical patient and have a transport time of 4 or 5 minutes, you may not be able to apply dressings to minor wounds.

Perform a head-to-toe assessment or focused assessment depending on the patient's injuries. Assess the neck, looking for jugular venous distention (JVD), tracheal deviation, or subcutaneous emphysema. Palpate and inspect the chest (anterior, lateral, and posterior) and assess lung sounds for equality and adequate depth of ventilation.

If the patient is alert and oriented, obtain a medical history en route to the hospital. If the patient's mental status is altered, search for any indications of a medical history, such as medical identification jewelry or medications in the patient's personal belongings.

Communication and Documentation

Serious thoracic injuries require immediate physician evaluation and intervention, possibly including surgical

IN THE FIELD

When signs and symptoms of life-threatening injury are present or if significant mechanism of injury is present, transport the patient without delay. Only treat life-threatening injuries on the scene.

intervention. For patients to receive that care, you must notify the receiving hospital as quickly as possible about patients with serious injuries or mechanisms of injury. Report the patient's age and gender, mechanism of injury, level of responsiveness, significant injuries and physical findings, vital signs, treatment implemented, response to treatment, and estimated time of arrival. Remember to request any specific orders from medical direction at this time, as well.

The hospital does not require a complete listing of injuries and findings in the radio report. Include what is pertinent to convey the urgency of the patient's situation so that preparations can be made, if necessary. Fill in additional details on arrival, including any changes in the patient's condition since your radio report. Record the details in the patient care report (PCR).

Reassessment

Anticipate the potential for developing problems with the patient's ventilation and perfusion. Perform your reassessment every 5 minutes for critical patients and every 15 minutes for noncritical patients. Pay close attention to trends in vital signs and appearance for signs of patient deterioration. Check any interventions performed as part of the reassessment.

Types of Thoracic Injuries

The two general categories of thoracic trauma are open and closed chest injuries.

CASE STUDY (continued)

When Byron and Angela arrive at the patient's side, they notice that he appears to be having difficulty breathing. The patient, 22-year-old Nick Mina, has a gunshot wound to the left anterior chest, just inferior to the clavicle at the midclavicular line. The wound is sucking air into it upon inspiration. Byron immediately covers the wound with his gloved hand and then secures an occlusive dressing over the wound. As he places his hand on the patient's chest, he notices that the patient's skin is diaphoretic, but his skin color and temperature are good.

Angela administers high-flow oxygen to the patient by nonrebreather mask. The patient has a strong, regular, though slightly rapid radial pulse. Byron and Angela perform a rapid trauma exam, including the patient's back, and do not find any other injuries. The mechanism of injury and difficulty breathing make the patient a high priority for transport.

"He doesn't have any neurologic deficits and has isolated penetrating trauma, so our protocols don't require spinal immobilization," says Byron. "Let's get him on the stretcher and load him into the ambulance. We can finish our assessment and treatment en route." Because the patient is not hypotensive but is having difficulty breathing, they place him in semi-Fowler's position on the stretcher.

Problem-Solving Questions

1. What further assessments and/or treatments should Byron and Angela perform en route?
2. What additional information is important for Byron and Angela to know?

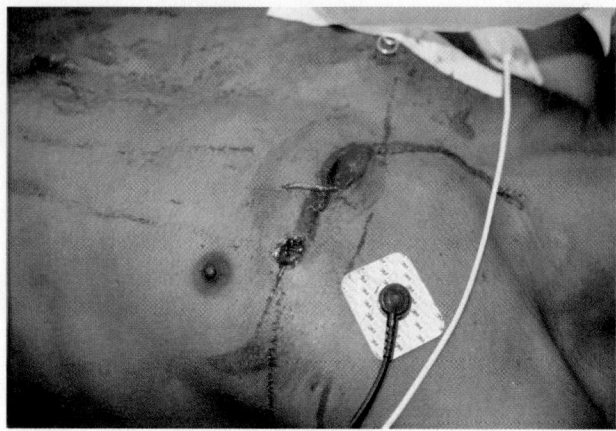

FIGURE 38-2

Penetrating trauma to the anterior chest.

(© Edward T. Dickinson, MD)

Open Chest Injury

An **open chest injury**—is the result of penetrating or blunt trauma to the thorax in which the integrity of the thoracic wall is broken (Figure 38-2). Penetrating trauma may be the result of forces applied to the outside of the body, such as a bullet wound. An open wound also can result from blunt trauma if a fractured rib lacerates the chest wall.

When an open chest injury is present, identify the mechanism of injury that caused the injury. If the patient has been stabbed, try to identify the weapon's length and width. Doing so gives you an idea of the extent of internal injury. Bullet wounds can produce a small entrance wound but can be accompanied by massive internal damage. Look not only for entrance wounds, but exit wounds as well. Failure to perform a thorough assessment may result in overlooking a life-threatening injury.

Injuries that can accompany open chest wounds include injury to the trachea, esophagus, diaphragm, heart, and great vessels. Damage to these structures can result in a very rapid deterioration of the patient, and result in death from hypoxia and massive blood loss.

The active process of ventilation occurs as a result of decreases and increases of pressure within the pleural space and lungs, causing air to enter through the nose and mouth. If an opening in the chest wall is approximately two-thirds the diameter of the trachea or larger, the pressure changes in the pleural cavity allowing air to enter the pleural cavity during inspiration. When air accumulates in the pleural space in the presence of an open chest wound, it is called an **open pneumothorax**. These wounds also are called **sucking chest wounds**, because as the patient breathes in, outside air is drawn into the thoracic cavity, making a sucking sound. During expiration, you may see bubbling of blood as air escapes through the wound. The patient's ventilation is

impaired by disruption in the integrity of the chest wall and the accumulation of air or blood within the pleural space. In such cases, you will immediately cover the open injury with a gloved hand followed by the application of an occlusive dressing.

Closed Chest Injury

Closed chest injury is caused by blunt trauma. You must evaluate the mechanism of injury to appreciate the potential for injury to the heart, lungs, great vessels, trachea, esophagus, and diaphragm. Patients with a significant mechanism of injury to the thorax have the potential to deteriorate rapidly because of the inability to breathe adequately, adequately circulate blood, or because of massive blood loss.

Broken bones from blunt trauma may lacerate or penetrate internal organs, which can cause massive internal hemorrhage. Consider the following: A patient is struck on the ribs with a baseball bat. The impact does not result in penetration of the chest wall; however, a rib was fractured and driven into the liver. Evidence of a closed chest injury includes contusions and/or fractures to the anterior, lateral, and posterior chest wall.

Specific Thoracic Injuries

This section covers specific thoracic injuries, their clinical significance, and the appropriate management of each.

Rib Fracture

Rib fractures can result from blunt or penetrating trauma. The ribs of the lateral chest wall are more vulnerable to fracture than the rest of the ribs, because they are not as well protected by muscle. The ribs that are attached directly to the sternum are vulnerable to fracture, because a rigid connection reduces their ability to flex, resulting in an increase in fractures. Rib fractures can cause internal bleeding, severe pain, hypoxia, and lung injury.

Pediatric Care

When thoracic trauma occurs in pediatric patients, consider the possibility of abdominal injury, because the pediatric torso is smaller and more flexible than that of the adult. This increase in flexibility makes internal organs susceptible to injury, sometimes without the presence of rib fractures. Because of the smaller thorax, the abdominal and thoracic organs are closer together.

If a force applied to the chest wall was significant enough to break one or more ribs, suspect underlying injury. The force that was applied can be great enough to fracture the bone and force jagged broken bone into internal structures, such as vessels and organs. Even without rib fracture, blunt trauma to the chest can transmit forces to the underlying structures, causing injuries such as pulmonary contusion. This is particularly true in children, whose ribs are pliable and less prone to fracture, yet provide less protection, overall, to the underlying organs.

The presence of rib fracture increases the mortality rate of the thoracic trauma patient. In particular, fractures of the first rib and scapula are associated with higher mortality because the amount of force needed to cause those fractures increases the likelihood of underlying organ injury. Rib fractures can be complete or partial, depending on whether the break extends through the bone. Rib fractures produce substantial pain, especially while breathing, which can result in hypoventilation and hypoxia. During the primary assessment, assess for and ensure adequate ventilation and oxygenation of the patient.

Signs and Symptoms of Rib Fractures

The following are signs and symptoms of rib fractures:

- Pain or tenderness at the injury site
- Contusions
- Open wounds
- Crepitus (if a complete fracture is present)
- Guarding
- Pain on inspiration
- Hypoventilation
- Hypoxia
- Hypercarbia

Emergency Management of Rib Fractures

There is no definitive treatment in the prehospital environment for rib fractures. Your role when treating a patient with rib fractures is to maintain adequate airway, breathing, and circulation. Allow the patient to sit in a position of comfort (if spine injury is not suspected). The patient may "splint" the rib fracture by holding a hand over the site. Monitor the patient's ECG, SpO_2, and $EtCO_2$. If necessary, you may apply a sling and swathe to the arm on the injured side, which will reduce pain by limiting movement. Even though patients are often in significant pain, remember that pain management with nitrous oxide is contraindicated because of the potential for pneumothorax.

If pain severely limits ventilation, you may need to assist the patient with a bag-valve-mask device to maintain adequate ventilation.

Arteries and veins run along the inferior edge of the ribs. Laceration of one of the vessels can allow blood to accumulate in the pleural space, causing a hemothorax. If the patient has signs and symptoms of shock, expedite transport and obtain intravenous access en route to an appropriate facility.

Flail Chest

A **flail chest** occurs when two or more ribs are broken in two or more places, resulting in a segment being detached from the rib cage. The flail segment floats freely during inspiration and expiration, causing **paradoxical movement** of the chest (Figure 38-3). Initial muscle spasm following injury may prevent paradoxical chest wall movement. While the precise frequency of flail chest is not currently known, the American College of Surgeons estimate that level 1 and level 2 trauma centers treat one to two flail chest injuries each month. The number of flail chest injuries treated outside of trauma centers is not known (Bjerke, 2009).

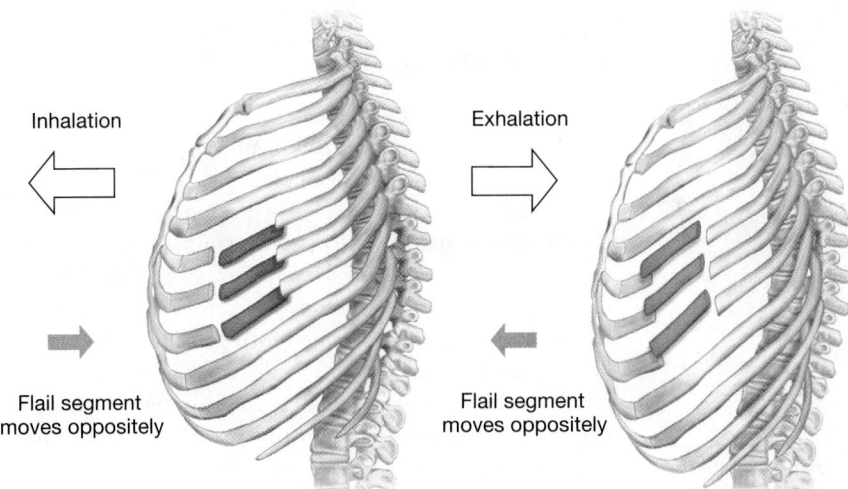

Inhalation

Exhalation

Flail segment moves oppositely

Flail segment moves oppositely

FIGURE 38-3

Paradoxical movement of a flail segment.

Paradoxical movement of the chest occurs when the flail segment appears to sink as the chest wall expands during inspiration. During exhalation, the segment protrudes out as the chest wall returns to its resting position.

Flail chest is a life-threatening injury, because it interferes with ventilation and often coexists with underlying injury. The amount of force necessary to result in a flail chest is usually significant enough to drive the flail segments into the lungs, resulting in **pulmonary contusion** or laceration (Figure 38-4).

Pulmonary contusion is injury to the lung tissue that decreases the ability of gas exchange to take place, leading to hypoxemia. For external respiration to take place, the alveoli must be inflated and there must be close contact between the pulmonary capillaries and alveoli. When lung tissue is contused, swelling and bleeding in the lung tissues occur. The swelling and accumulation of blood increase the distance between the alveolar walls and pulmonary capillaries, reducing gas exchange. The larger the injury, the more lung tissue is involved, and the greater the decrease in gas exchange.

Additionally, the flail segment will reduce the amount of negative pressure generated by inspiration, resulting in smaller inspiratory volumes. If the flail segment is large enough, it can lead to hypoventilation and hypoxia.

Signs and Symptoms of Flail Chest

The following are signs and symptoms of flail chest:

- Pain or tenderness at the injury site
- Dyspnea
- Contusions
- Crepitus
- Paradoxical movement of the chest (may not always be obvious)
- Guarding
- Pain on inspiration
- Hypoxia
- Hypercarbia

Emergency Management of Flail Chest

When treating a patient with flail chest, your care will include immediately ensuring adequacy of airway, breathing, and circulation. Consider the use of CPAP or assisted ventilations for patients who exhibit signs and symptoms of hypoxia and hypoventilation.

Pneumothorax

Pneumothorax occurs when air enters the pleural space between the visceral and parietal pleura. Pneumothorax is divided into three categories: simple, open, and tension.

Simple pneumothorax is the presence of air within a closed pleural space. Patients with simple pneumothorax may not experience any dyspnea or shortness of breath initially, but as the pneumothorax develops further, signs and symptoms become more profound. Symptoms become increasingly evident as the volume of air accumulation in the pleural space increases. Simple pneumothorax may occupy a significant portion of the hemithorax, but is self-limiting and there is no increase in air pressure within the chest.

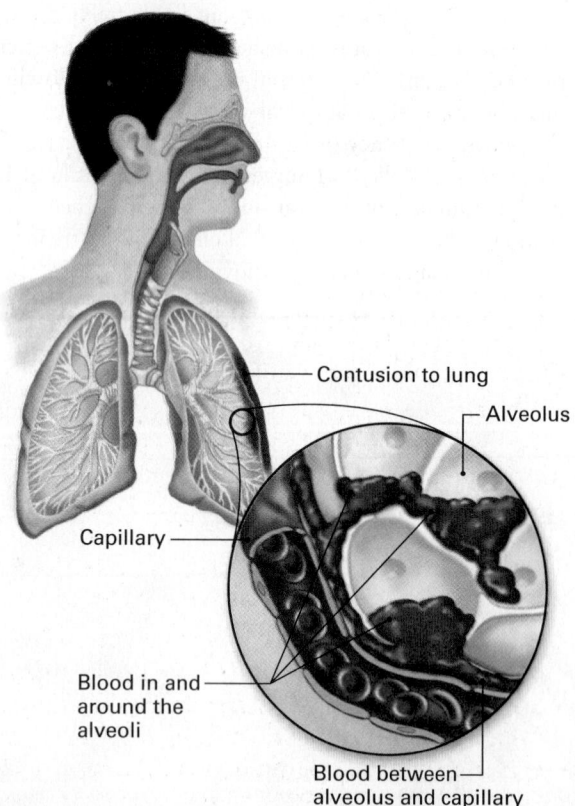

Contusion to lung
Alveolus
Capillary
Blood in and around the alveoli
Blood between alveolus and capillary

FIGURE 38-4

Pulmonary contusion results in bleeding into and around the alveoli, reducing the ability of gas exchange to take place.

Open pneumothorax occurs when an open chest injury allows air from the outside to be sucked into the pleural space during ventilation. If this air is not allowed to escape during exhalation, pressure in the pleural space will increase. If not identified and treated immediately, the pressure will intensify, leading to a life-threatening condition called *tension pneumothorax*.

Tension pneumothorax is relatively uncommon, but is an immediate threat to life. It occurs when air accumulates within the pleural space and cannot escape. Unlike in simple pneumothorax where the defect in the lung is self-sealing, limiting the escape of air, tension pneumothorax involves a large defect, such as a laceration of a bronchus, that is not self-sealing. This leads to significant pressure increases in the affected side of the thoracic cavity. As pressure rises, the structures of the mediastinum shift toward the unaffected side and the lung on the opposite side begins to collapse.

As the mediastinal structures shift, the vena cava may become partially obstructed by kinking, resulting in a reduction in venous return to the heart. As pressure within the chest rises, it can exceed the pressure in the vena cava, further reducing blood return to the heart. As blood backs up behind the right side of the heart, the jugular veins may become distended. However, jugular venous distention (JVD) may not be pronounced if the patient also has significant hypovolemia.

As the mediastinal shift continues, it may be identified by **tracheal deviation**. Tracheal deviation results from significant mediastinal shift associated with tension pneumothorax. It is a late sign and not always evident. *You must not rely on presence of tracheal deviation to suspect tension pneumothorax.* In some cases, you may see **subcutaneous emphysema,** or air that has been trapped in the skin, resulting in tiny bubbles that have a crackling feeling when palpated. Patients will experience increasing hypoxia and hypoperfusion despite oxygen therapy and positive pressure ventilation.

Resistance to positive pressure ventilation will increase as tension pneumothorax progresses. Tension pneumothorax can occur with both open and closed thoracic injuries. Recall, for instance, that blunt trauma to the chest resulting from an unrestrained driver's chest striking the steering wheel during a frontal impact may result in a "blow out" or "paper bag" injury of the lungs because the lungs are compressed against a closed glottis on impact. You must

---

IN THE FIELD

Tracheal deviation is a late sign of tension pneumothorax, and may not be noticeable in all cases. Absence of tracheal deviation does not rule out tension pneumothorax. The presence of dyspnea, increasing respiratory distress despite oxygen therapy, and decreased or absent breath sounds on the affected side indicates the presence of a developing tension pneumothorax.

---

identify mechanisms of injury that suggest the potential for pneumothorax and monitor the patient closely for development of signs and symptoms (Figure 38-5).

Signs and Symptoms of Pneumothorax

The following are signs and symptoms of pneumothorax:

- Tachypnea
- Diminished or absent breath sounds on the affected side
- Tachycardia
- Hypoxia
- Juguluar venous distention (JVD)
- Cyanosis
- Subcutaneous emphysema
- Unequal chest expansion
- Extreme anxiety
- Increasing resistance to positive pressure ventilation
- Tracheal deviation (late sign)
- Shock
- Worsening condition despite appropriate treatment

Emergency Management of Pneumothorax

Your goal when treating a patient with a suspected pneumothorax is to prevent the condition from progressing to a tension pneumothorax. Whenever possible, request ALS response for patients with open pneumothorax or tension pneumothorax. Tension pneumothorax is a condition with which just a few minutes' delay in ALS care can make the difference between life and death.

If a sucking chest wound is present, immediately cover it with a gloved hand to prevent air from entering into the wound. Then cover it with an occlusive dressing and secure it on three sides (Figure 38-6). During inspiration, negative pressure will pull the dressing down over the injury, preventing air from entering the thorax. During exhalation, air will be allowed to escape through the unsecured side. This will assist in preventing the development of tension pneumothorax.

If the patient's condition is deteriorating after the application of an occlusive dressing and he begins to show signs and symptoms of tension pneumothorax, lift one side of the occlusive dressing to ensure that accumulated pressure can escape. This is sometimes called *burping the dressing*. After pressure is relieved, secure the dressing on three sides once again.

Hemothorax

Hemothorax is the accumulation of blood in the pleural space. Hemothorax can be the result of blunt or penetrating

HEMOTHORAX

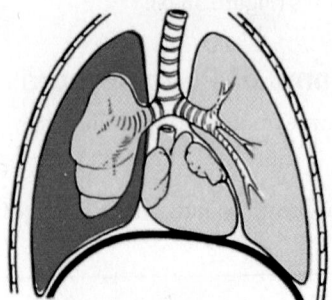

Blood leaks into the chest cavity from lacerated vessels or the lung itself and the lung compresses.

PNEUMOTHORAX

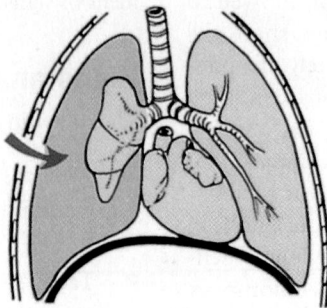

Air enters the chest cavity through a sucking wound or leaks from a lacerated lung. The lung cannot expand.

SPONTANEOUS PNEUMOTHORAX

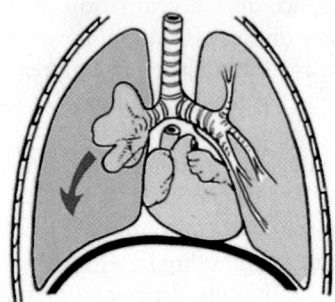

Air leaks into the chest from a weak area in the (nontrauma) lung surface and the lung collapses.

HEMOPNEUMOTHORAX

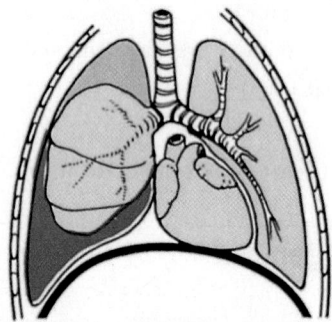

Air and blood leak into the chest cavity from an injured lung putting pressure on the heart and uninjured lung.

TENSION PNEUMOTHORAX

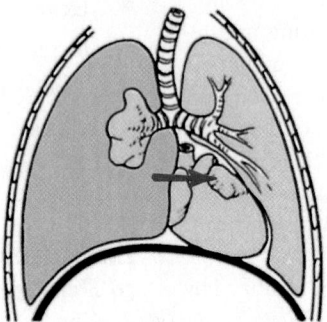

Air continuously leaks out the lung. It collapses, pressure rises, and the collapsed lung is forced against the heart and other lung.

MEDIASTINAL SHIFT

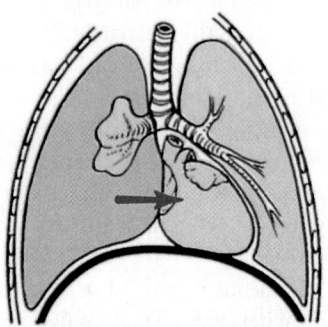

Shifting of the internal chest structures away from the tension pneumothorax.

FIGURE 38-5

The progression of pneumothorax.

trauma and has the same emergency management as pneumothorax. Because each side of the chest can hold a significant amount of blood, signs and symptoms of hypovolemic shock may be present before significant impairment of ventilation.

If enough blood accumulates within the pleural space, a tension hemothorax may develop. Treatment for tension hemothorax is the same as for tension pneumothorax.

Traumatic Asphyxia

Traumatic asphyxia occurs as a result of sudden massive compression forces being applied to the chest. That pressure

IN THE FIELD

Patients with massive hemothorax may present with signs and symptoms of shock more prominent than signs of respiratory distress because of the amount of blood that can be contained within the chest.

IN THE FIELD

The presence of traumatic asphyxia suggests a high potential for intrathoracic injury and bleeding. Be prepared to treat the patient for shock while providing rapid transport to an appropriate facility.

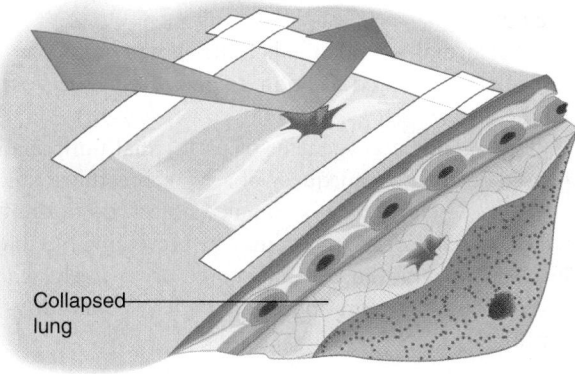

On inspiration, dressing seals wound, preventing air entry

Collapsed lung

Expiration allows trapped air to escape through untaped section of dressing

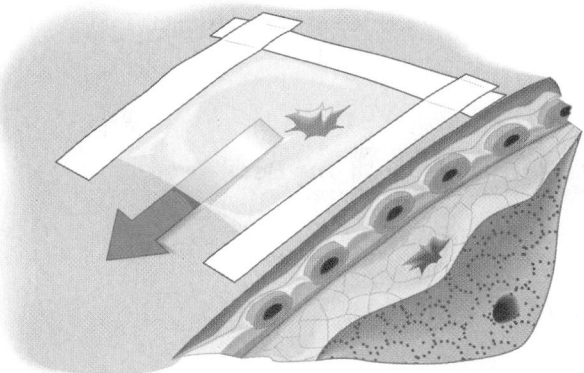

FIGURE 38-6

Securing the occlusive dressing on three sides assists with preventing the development of tension pneumothorax.

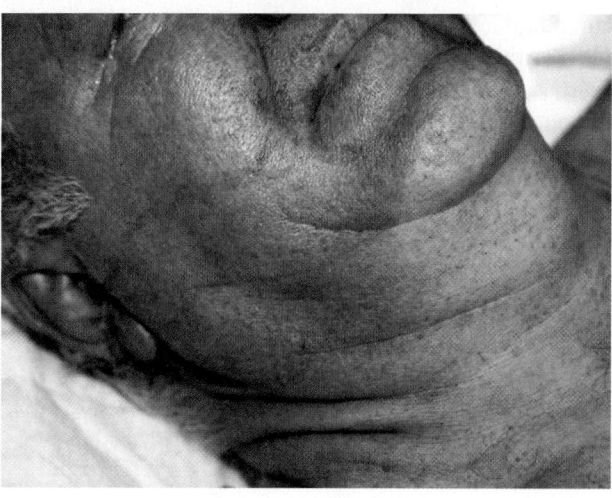

FIGURE 38-7

Signs of traumatic asphyxia. (© Edward T. Dickinson, MD)

causes the patient to appear to be asphyxiated, but asphyxiation does not actually occur. The compression of the mediastinum causes forceful retrograde (backward) blood flow that results in capillary engorgement in the upper chest, neck, and head, resulting in discoloration and edema. Emergency management is focused on supporting airway, breathing, and circulation.

Signs and Symptoms of Traumatic Asphyxia

Signs and symptoms of traumatic asphyxia include the following (Figure 38-7):

- Bluish-purple discoloration of the upper chest, neck, and head
- Jugular venous distention (JVD)
- Conjunctival hemorrhage
- Edema of the tongue and lips

Blunt Cardiac Injury

When blunt trauma to the chest occurs with enough force, the heart can be injured by impact with the sternum or from being compressed between the sternum and spine. The heart can sustain contusion, and with forceful compression, blood in the chambers can be forced backward, damaging the heart valves, which can lead to decreased cardiac output and shock. In severe cases, the myocardium can rupture. In addition to compression injury to the heart, electrical conduction may be disturbed resulting in dysrhythmia.

Myocardial Contusion

A **myocardial contusion** is bruising of the heart muscle that can occur with significant chest trauma. As with contusions that occur in other parts of the body, myocardial contusions occur as a result of a force causing vessels within the myocardium to rupture. The resultant ischemia in areas of disrupted circulation make myocardial contusion similar to acute coronary syndrome (ACS) in some ways. Emergency management of myocardial contusion is focused on ensuring adequacy of airway, breathing, and circulation.

Along with a significant mechanism of injury to the chest and general indications of chest trauma, you may see the following specific signs and symptoms of myocardial contusion:

- Chest pain
- Signs of heart failure or cardiogenic shock
- Cardiac arrhythmias

Commotio Cordis

Commotio cordis is sudden cardiac arrest resulting from a sudden blow to the center of the chest. A specific combination of circumstances seems to be required for a blow to the chest to result in commotio cordis. The condition seems to be associated with impacts of certain velocity during a particularly vulnerable phase in the cardiac electrical cycle.

Commotio cordis has occurred in martial arts, baseball, and other sports—for instance, when a baseball player is struck in the chest by a line drive. If the baseball strikes the chest with enough force, the impact can cause ventricular fibrillation and death.

The cardiac arrest is managed as any other cardiac arrest, but even with immediate defibrillation, mortality is very high. Nonetheless, you must provide full resuscitative efforts.

Pericardial Tamponade

Pericardial tamponade is the condition in which pressure increases inside the pericardial sac as a result of the accumulation of blood, leading to a decrease in cardiac output. The typical cause of pericardial tamponade is low-velocity penetrating trauma to the chest that causes an injury to the heart that bleeds within the fibrous pericardial sac that surrounds the heart. A small opening is created in the pericardium, and an injury to the heart causes bleeding into the pericardial sac. If the rate of bleeding exceeds the rate at which blood can escape from the opening in the pericardial sac, blood begins to accumulate.

The pericardial sac is not pliable, especially with rapid accumulation of blood. It will not stretch as blood accumulates within it. This causes a rise in the pressure within the pericardial sac that offers resistance when the heart expands during diastole, resulting in a decrease in cardiac output.

Pericardial tamponade is a life-threatening condition that must be treated as soon as possible in the hospital setting.

Emergency management of pericardial tamponade is focused on ensuring adequacy of airway, breathing, and circulation. When there is an impaled object, do not remove it. The presence of the object may be preventing bleeding. If the object is removed, bleeding could occur freely, leading to very rapid deterioration in the patient's condition, and death.

Signs and Symptoms of Pericardial Tamponade

The classic signs and symptoms of pericardial tamponade (Figure 38-8) are referred to as **Beck's triad** (Table 38-1).

TABLE 38-1 **The Beck Triad**
■ Hypotension
■ Distended neck veins
■ Muffled heart sounds

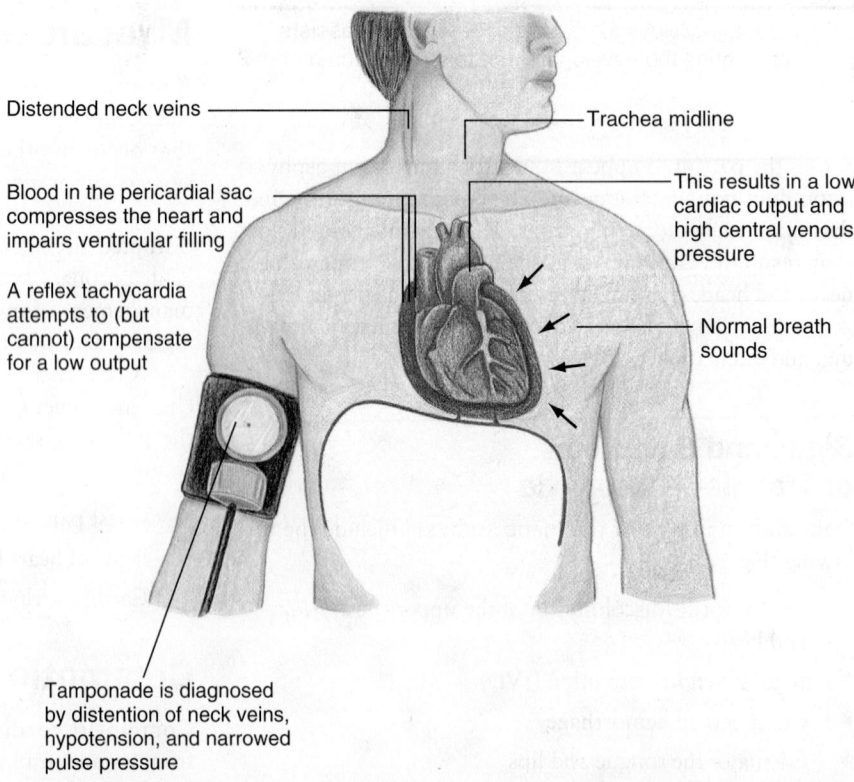

Distended neck veins

Blood in the pericardial sac compresses the heart and impairs ventricular filling

A reflex tachycardia attempts to (but cannot) compensate for a low output

Trachea midline

This results in a low cardiac output and high central venous pressure

Normal breath sounds

Tamponade is diagnosed by distention of neck veins, hypotension, and narrowed pulse pressure

FIGURE 38-8

Signs and symptoms of pericardial tamponade.

CASE STUDY WRAP-UP

Clinical-Reasoning Process

Advanced EMTs Angela and Byron are en route to a nearby trauma center with 22-year-old Nick Mina, who has a gunshot wound to the anterior left chest. As they load the patient into the ambulance, the police officer who agreed to drive the ambulance tells them that other officers caught the shooter a few blocks away, and the weapon used was a .38-caliber handgun.

As Byron applies an occlusive dressing sealed on three sides over the wound, Angela listens to breath sounds and obtains baseline vital signs. "He has a slight decrease in breath sounds in the right upper lung fields," says Angela.

The patient's vital signs are blood pressure 112/88; heart rate 108; respiratory rate 24; and SpO$_2$ 95 percent on high-flow oxygen. Byron performs a head-to-toe assessment, and is especially alert to potential signs of tension pneumothorax, cardiac injury, and shock. Byron does not find any additional injuries. Meanwhile, Angela has started two IVs of normal saline, both at keep-open rates. Byron calls in a report to the trauma center.

When they arrive at the trauma center, Angela and Byron are directed to the trauma bay in the emergency department. The patient is transferred to the hospital bed and Angela and Byron give their report to the attending physician. As Byron finishes up his documentation in the trauma bay, the physician inserts a chest tube for a developing tension pneumothorax.

CHAPTER REVIEW

Chapter Summary

When thoracic trauma is present, pay close attention to the mechanism of injury and the patient's clinical signs and symptoms. Because the organs and vessels contained within the thoracic cavity are vital to sustaining life, maintain a high index of suspicion that underlying injury is present.

When life-threatening injury to the thorax exists, act immediately to prevent the deterioration of the patient's condition. Your assessment skills and knowledge of appropriate treatment will reduce morbidity and mortality associated with thoracic injuries.

Review Questions

Multiple-Choice Questions

1. A patient who has been stabbed in the chest with an ice pick presents with hypotension, jugular venous distention (JVD), and muffled heart sounds. Based on the MOI and the patient's signs and symptoms, you suspect:

a. tension pneumothorax.
b. open pneumothorax.
c. pericardial tamponade.
d. pulmonary contusion.

2. A patient with a single gunshot wound to the left anterior chest presents with increasing dyspnea despite treatment, decreased breath sounds on the left, and severe anxiety. Based on the MOI and signs and symptoms described, you suspect:

a. pulmonary contusion.
b. pulmonary laceration.
c. pneumothorax.
d. tension pneumothorax.

3. The injury that you would suspect if a patient is crushed beneath a car for 20 minutes and has discoloration of the chest, neck, and head is:

a. pulmonary contusion.
b. pneumothorax.
c. traumatic asphyxia.
d. pericardial tamponade.

4. Tension pneumothorax has occurred when:

a. air is allowed to enter the pleural space.
b. air accumulates in the pleural space, causing lung collapse and a decrease in cardiac output.
c. blood accumulates around the heart, resulting in a decrease in cardiac output.
d. penetrating trauma causes internal bleeding within the pleural space.

5. Flail chest occurs when:

   a. two or more ribs are broken in two or more places.
   b. one or more ribs are broken in two or more places.
   c. one or more ribs become detached from the sternum as a result of blunt trauma.
   d. cardiac arrest results from blunt trauma to the chest.

6. You respond to the scene of an assault in which a patient was kicked in the center of his chest and is now in cardiac arrest. The patient sustained no additional trauma. Based on this information, you conclude that the patient's condition is a result of:

   a. commotio cordis.
   b. tension pneumothorax.
   c. pericardial tamponade.
   d. tension hemothorax.

7. Immediate action that will reduce the mortality risk of a patient with a sucking chest wound includes:

   a. placing the patient on high-flow oxygen.
   b. treating the patient for shock.
   c. covering the wound with a gloved hand.
   d. immediate transport to the closest emergency department.

Critical-Thinking Questions

8. Describe the progression from simple pneumothorax to tension pneumothorax.

9. List the signs and symptoms for which you should be alert when assessing the neck of a thoracic trauma patient.

10. Explain how the progression of blood accumulation in the pericardial sac leads to hypotension.

References

Bjerke, M. F. (2009). *Flail chest.* eMedicine. Retrieved March 25, 2011, from http://emedicine.medscape.com/article/433779-overview

Mancini, M. C. (2008, October 23). *Blunt chest trauma.* eMedicine. Retrieved March 25, 2011, from http://emedicine.medscape.com/article/428723-overview

39

Abdominal Trauma

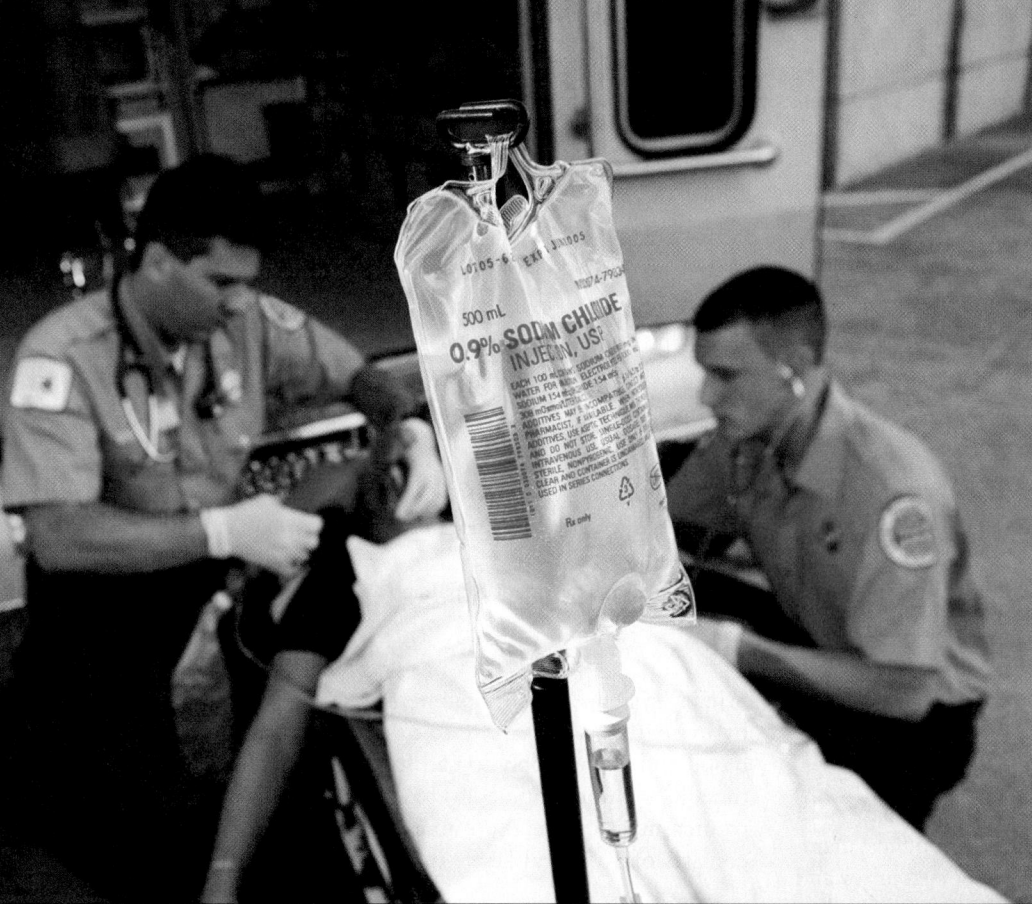

KEY TERMS

abdominal evisceration
(p. 876)

Cullen's sign (p. 875)

diaphragmatic rupture
(p. 877)

Grey Turner's sign (p. 875)

involuntary guarding (p. 875)

Kehr's sign (p. 875)

parietal peritoneum (p. 873)

peritoneal cavity (p. 873)

peritoneum (p. 872)

retroperitoneal space (p. 873)

visceral peritoneum (p. 872)

voluntary guarding (p. 875)

Content Area: Trauma

Advanced EMT Education Standard: Applies fundamental knowledge to provide basic and selected advanced emergency care and transportation based on assessment findings for an acutely injured patient.

Objectives

After reading this chapter, you should be able to:

39.1   Define key terms introduced in this chapter.

39.2   Describe the gross anatomy of the abdominal cavity and its contents.

39.3   Differentiate between the characteristics of solid and hollow organs in the abdomen.

39.4   Give examples of both blunt and penetrating mechanisms of abdominal trauma.

39.5   Recognize signs and symptoms associated with injuries to the abdomen.

39.6   Describe the association between abdominal injury and the potential for life-threatening hemorrhage.

39.7   Demonstrate an assessment-based approach to management of the patient with open and closed abdominal injury, including evisceration and impaled objects.

(continued)

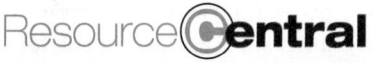

To access Resource Central, follow the directions on the Student Access Card provided with this text. If there is no card, go to www.bradybooks.com and follow the Resource Central link to Buy Access. Under Media Resources, you will find:

• *Penetrating Abdominal Trauma.* Using field technology to identify abdominal injuries.

• *Cullen's Sign.* How it can help identify abdominal trauma in the field.

• *Blunt Abdominal Trauma.* How blunt trauma is different from penetrating trauma.

It is a cool and rainy afternoon when Advanced EMTs Jack Sullivan and Jamal Weathers are dispatched for an injured person at a horse stable outside town. On their arrival, a teenage girl runs to meet the ambulance. She is yelling, "Come quick! My dad got kicked in the stomach by a horse and he's badly hurt!"

Jack and Jamal don't identify any hazards at the scene so they quickly grab their gear and follow the girl into the stables. Upon entering, they see a man in his early 40s lying on the ground with his knees drawn toward his chest and holding his abdomen. As they approach him, they notice that he appears pale and sweaty. He makes eye contact with Jamal when he says, "One of the horses kicked me. My stomach is killing me."

Problem-Solving Questions

1. What types of injuries could the patient have sustained from this mechanism?
2. What potential injury would concern Jack and Jamal the most if present? Why?
3. What additional information would assist Jack and Jamal in their decision making at this point?

(continued from previous page)

39.8   Explain the special considerations for airway management in the care of patients with abdominal injuries.

39.9   Explain the process and elements of reassessment of patients with abdominal injuries.

Introduction

Unrecognized abdominal trauma is one of the leading causes of death in trauma patients. In patients with a mechanism of injury (MOI) that suggests abdominal injury you must maintain a high index of suspicion for intra-abdominal injury and remain alert for the signs and symptoms of internal bleeding and shock. In some cases, there will be no visible external injuries to the abdomen, but the patient may be bleeding internally as a result of blunt trauma or deceleration injury.

Abdominal injury can be the result of both penetrating and blunt trauma. With penetrating trauma, the certainty of injury is more readily identified than in blunt trauma. Both penetrating and blunt trauma can produce life-threatening internal bleeding and a risk for serious infection.

Your role as an Advanced EMT is to identify the potential for abdominal injuries, treat life threats, assess the patient for signs and symptoms of abdominal injury, and provide both injury-specific and supportive care while en route to a hospital with immediate surgical capabilities.

Anatomy and Physiology Review

The abdominopelvic cavity is inferior to the diaphragm and contains the abdominal organs, including organs of the circulatory, digestive, endocrine, reproductive, and urinary systems. The abdominal organs are held in place by mesenteries, which are folds of tissue that carry the blood and nerve supply to and from the organs. The **peritoneum** is a thin, double-layered epithelial lining that surrounds most of the abdominal organs (Figure 39-1). It consists of a visceral layer, the **visceral peritoneum**, that

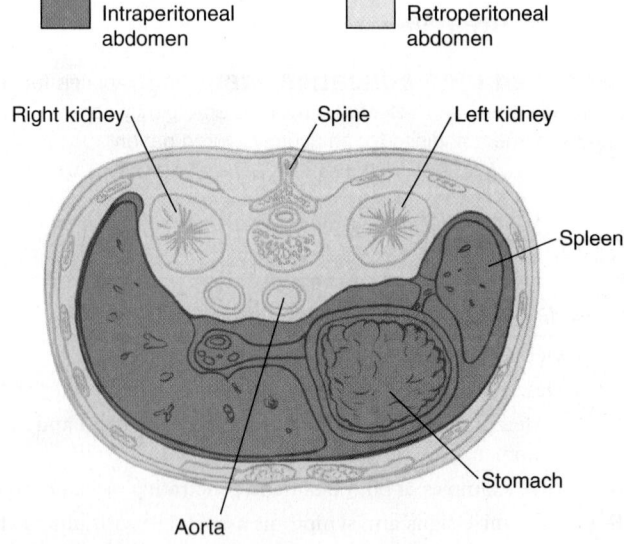

Intraperitoneal abdomen

Retroperitoneal abdomen

Right kidney   Spine   Left kidney

Spleen

Aorta

Stomach

FIGURE 39-1

The abdomen is lined by the parietal and visceral peritoneum and consists of the peritoneal and retroperitoneal cavities.

Geriatric Care

Geriatric patients may have less musculature and weaker bones than younger adults have to protect the abdominal organs. So, they are at higher risk for internal abdominal injury.

Pediatric Care

Pediatric patients do not have musculature mature enough to provide protection for abdominal organs. The organs, particularly the liver, are large for the size of the abdominal cavity, making them more prominent. This puts them at higher risk for intra-abdominal injury.

adheres to the organs. The visceral layer folds over itself, forming a second layer called the **parietal peritoneum**. A small amount of serous fluid between the layers allows for movement of the abdominal organs without friction. Some organs, such as the kidneys, ureters, and portions of the duodenum, colon, and pancreas are behind the posterior-most layer of peritoneum and are considered to be in the **retroperitoneal space.**

The abdominal organs are afforded some protection by the musculature of the torso as well as the bones of the inferior thorax and the pelvis, but the organs are relatively vulnerable to injury.

For assessment and documentation purposes, the abdomen is divided into four quadrants: two lower and two upper quadrants. The right and left quadrants are divided by the midline, which extends from the xiphoid process to the symphysis pubis. The upper and lower quadrants are divided by a transverse line that intersects the midline at the umbilicus. The location of organs within the abdomen is shown in Figure 39-2. The abdominal aorta and inferior vena cava are located along the midline of the retroperitoneal space. These vessels, along with other arteries and veins, pose a serious risk for massive internal bleeding and rapid deterioration if they are injured.

The organs of the abdominal cavity are classified as either hollow or solid organs (Table 39-1). Hollow and solid organs are prone to different types of injuries that have different consequences for patients.

Hollow organs are not as vascular as solid organs. Therefore, they do not produce as much risk of internal bleeding when injured. However, they contain digestive enzymes and waste that can cause inflammation and infection of the peritoneum called *peritonitis*. When acidic digestive enzymes are released into the **peritoneal cavity**, it typically results in immediate pain. Infection takes time to develop and can complicate the patient's recovery.

The solid organs are inelastic and highly vascular. When injured, severe internal bleeding is possible and, ultimately, death may occur if the injury cannot be surgically repaired in time. So, recognize abdominal injury in

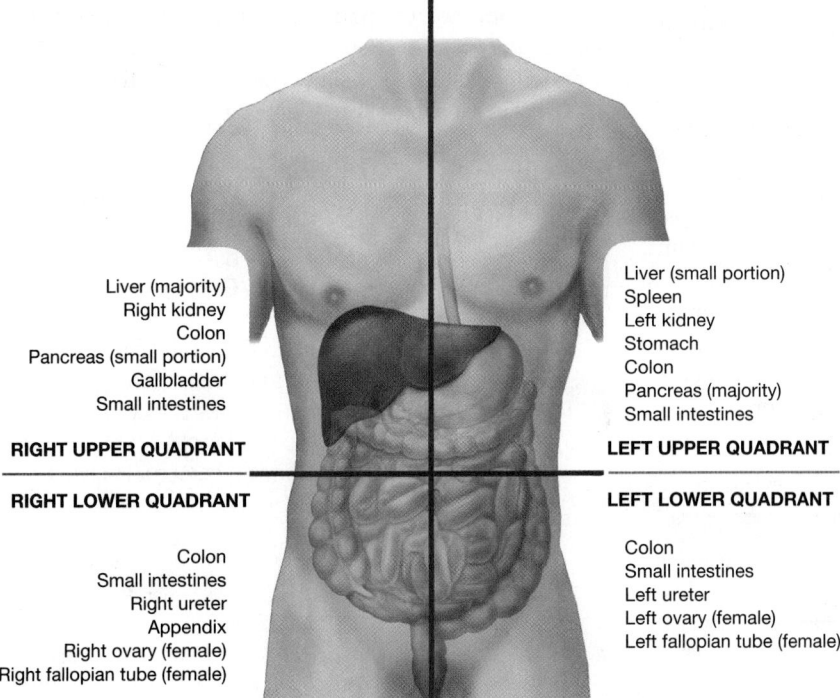

FIGURE 39-2

The four quadrants of the abdomen and their contents.

TABLE 39-1	Hollow and Solid Abdominal Organs

Hollow Abdominal Organs	Solid Abdominal Organs
Stomach	Liver
Small intestines	Spleen
Large intestines	Kidneys
Ureters	Pancreas
Gallbladder and bile ducts	
Urinary bladder	

your patient quickly, and be alert for signs and symptoms of shock. Rapidly transport the patient to a facility with immediate surgical capabilities.

General Assessment and Management of Abdominal Trauma

Assessment of the patient with abdominal injury will always consist of ensuring the adequacy of airway, breathing, and circulation, but you also should identify the MOI or potential for underlying injury.

Note that it is relatively easy to overlook abdominal injury in patients with distracting injuries or an altered level of responsiveness. For example, imagine a patient falling from a tree and striking his abdomen on a limb during the fall. Upon landing, his femur is fractured. The pain associated with the femur fracture may distract the patient's attention from less severe pain to his abdomen.

If the patient is intoxicated or suffers head injury, causing a decrease in responsiveness, it may be difficult to obtain information regarding pain or tenderness to the abdomen. Those patients may not feel pain associated with abdominal injury or may be unresponsive. You must maintain a high index of suspicion for intra-abdominal injury in patients with an MOI that suggests it, regardless of the presence or absence of pain.

IN THE FIELD

When a patient presents with signs and symptoms of shock in the absence of obvious external injury, assume intra-abdominal hemorrhage as the cause until proven otherwise.

IN THE FIELD

On the scene of shootings and stabbings, remember that the scene is a crime scene and take precautions to preserve it as best you can. In some cases, you will obtain information about objects used in stabbings or caliber of guns used in shootings from law enforcement on scene.

You should never delay transport to obtain this information. In most cases, law enforcement will go to the receiving facility to continue their investigation, and information can be obtained at that time.

Scene Size-Up

The scene size-up can provide you with valuable information related to the potential for injury to the patient. Once the scene is safe to approach, look around the scene for objects that created the injury. Was the patient stabbed? If so, identify the object used. Was the patient shot? If so, identify the caliber of the gun used. Was the patient struck with an object? If so, identify the object and determine how hard the patient was struck.

If the injury was a result of an MVC, inspect the vehicle and gather additional information (Table 39-2). Other MOIs that could lead to abdominal trauma include crush injuries, falls, explosions, and assault with objects such as sticks, pipes, and bats.

Primary Assessment

As you approach the patient, form a general impression, including level of responsiveness. In many cases, patients with abdominal injury will be lying on their side with knees drawn toward their chest. This is a position of comfort,

TABLE 39-2	Pertinent Information Regarding the MOI of an MVC

How fast was the patient's vehicle traveling on impact?

What types of vehicles were involved in the MVC?

If more than one vehicle was involved, how fast were the other vehicles traveling on impact?

What type of collision occurred? (head-on, lateral, rotational, rear, rollover)

Was the patient ejected?

Was the patient restrained?

What path did the patient follow on impact? (up and over vs. down and under)

Are there deformities to the steering wheel and/or dashboard?

because it reduces the tension of the abdominal muscles, which helps to reduce the patient's pain.

If spine injury is suspected, you must manually stabilize the head and neck. Ensure adequacy of airway and breathing. Provide positive pressure ventilations with high-flow oxygen as indicated. Assess for and control any life-threatening external bleeding. Place the patient on oxygen, if needed, to maintain an SpO$_2$ of 95 percent or higher.

Assess the skin for color and temperature. Pale, cool, and diaphoretic skin indicates the onset of shock and warrants rapid transport to a surgical facility. Assess pulse rate and quality.

Secondary Assessment

Determine the patient's chief complaint and expose the patient to perform a focused exam or rapid trauma assessment as indicated. Inspect the abdomen using the DCAP-BTLS mnemonic. (Signs and symptoms of abdominal injury are given in Table 39-3.) Palpate the abdomen in all four quadrants to assess for abnormalities such as masses, tenderness, or rebound tenderness. If the patient complains of pain in a particular area, palpate that area last to prevent him from becoming anxious. Palpate with enough pressure to feel abnormalities, but not so deep as to unnecessarily increase the patient's pain.

Because penetrating trauma can result in evisceration, you may see organs, usually a loop of intestine, protruding from an open wound. **Cullen's sign** (ecchymosis around the umbilicus) and **Grey Turner's sign** (ecchymosis around the

flanks) indicate retroperitoneal bleeding. They are not usually seen in the prehospital environment because they take hours to develop. In some cases though, such as an assault, you may not be called to care for the patient until several hours have elapsed.

The abdominal cavity allows for the accumulation of a significant amount of blood, approximately 1.5 liters, before distention occurs (McSwain, Salomone & Pons, 2007). If abdominal distention is present, assume that the patient has lost a massive amount of blood and expedite transport to an appropriate facility as soon as possible.

Kehr's sign is referred pain to the left shoulder caused by diaphragmatic irritation, which is caused by the presence of blood and may indicate splenic injury.

Observe the patient for abdominal guarding. When palpating a tender area of the abdomen, the abdomen may tense up in anticipation of palpation. This is called **voluntary guarding** and is a natural response to reduce pain associated with palpation. **Involuntary guarding** is uncontrolled spasm of the abdominal muscles as a response to peritonitis.

After assessing the anterior abdomen, assess the posterior surface of the patient using the DCAP-BTLS mnemonic. Obtain a SAMPLE history and baseline vital signs, and then make a transport decision.

The emergency management for abdominal trauma begins with management of the patient's airway, breathing, and circulation. In many cases, the best care that you will provide to a patient with abdominal trauma is prompt recognition of life-threatening internal bleeding and rapid transport to an appropriate facility.

Management of Abdominal Trauma

After managing immediate life threats, the goal of treatment of the patient with abdominal trauma is to treat for shock, if present, make the patient as comfortable as possible, and manage specific injuries, such as impaled objects or evisceration.

Keep the patient warm. If it is not contraindicated by other injuries, the patient may be most comfortable with the hips and knees flexed to reduce tension on the abdominal muscles. Start IVs en route, according to your protocols. Although general prohibition of pain management for patients with abdominal pain has relaxed, do not administer nitrous oxide to a patient with suspected abdominal trauma.

TABLE 39-3 General Signs and Symptoms of Abdominal Injury

- Contusions, lacerations, and/or penetration of the abdomen
- Pain and/or tenderness to palpation
- Distended abdomen (indicates significant blood loss)
- Lying in a position of comfort; knees drawn toward the chest
- Ecchymosis to the umbilicus or flank (late finding)
- Signs of shock
- Presence of MOI for abdominal injury

Reassessment

Reassessment of the abdominal trauma patient is key to identifying shock. If you overlook the subtle signs and symptoms of shock, the patient's condition will continue to deteriorate. The failure to identify and treat a life-threatening condition will lead to increases in morbidity and mortality risks for the patient. Reassess critical patients at intervals of no more than 5 minutes, and reassess noncritical patients every 15 minutes.

Specific Abdominal Injuries

Penetrating and blunt trauma produce different types of injury. Blunt trauma is the most common type of abdominal injury and has mortality rates of 10 to 30 percent. The mortality rates are likely the result of accompanying trauma to the head and chest in as many as 70 percent of MVC patients who die (Campbell, 2008).

Regardless of the mechanism or type of organ involved, abdominal trauma is classified as either open or closed injury. Open injuries are easier to identify, because bleeding and/or pain will be present at the site of injury. For instance, a patient who is shot in the abdomen with a .38-caliber handgun will have an obvious open injury and pain at the injury site.

When there is a potential closed abdominal injury, you must rely on your assessment skills to identify the potential for underlying internal injury. For example, imagine that you have arrived on the scene of a front-impact MVC to find a restrained driver complaining of pain and tenderness to the lower abdomen. While exposing the abdomen, you notice a large contusion across the lower quadrants, which is the result of a compression injury from the lap belt. In this case, you must suspect internal compression injury to the organs of the lower abdomen (Figure 39-3).

Penetrating Trauma

Penetrating trauma to the abdomen can produce minor to severe injuries. Overall, about 15 percent of patients with

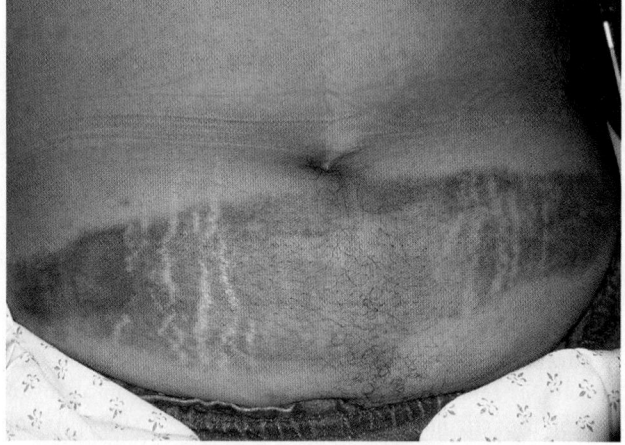

FIGURE 39-3

Contusion of the abdomen from a lap belt. (© Charles Steward, MD, and Associates)

abdominal stab wounds require surgical intervention, as compared with about 85 percent of abdominal gunshot wound patients (McSwain, Salomone & Pons, 2007). This difference is directly related to the energy that is transferred to the body by the mechanism.

Determine the size of the object used in a stab wound and the caliber of the bullet with a gunshot wound. Look for multiple wounds, including entrance and exit wounds. The extent of internal injury cannot always be determined, even when it appears that a bullet made a "through and through" (through one aspect of the body and then through the opposite side) injury. The energy transmitted from a high-velocity projectile creates both a permanent and temporary cavity. The temporary cavity can extend well beyond the immediate track of the bullet, causing injury to nerves, blood vessels, and other structures.

Open wounds to the abdomen can be very dramatic. In some cases, abdominal organs (usually the small intestines) protrude through the opening. This is called an **abdominal** evisceration (Figure 39-4). Although they are gruesome, evisceration injuries are seldom life threatening.

Emergency care for abdominal evisceration is as follows (Scan 39-1):

1. Expose the entire abdomen.

2. Place the patient in a supine position with knees flexed toward the chest if lower extremity or spinal trauma is not suspected. Transport with legs flat in the presence of those injuries.

3. Apply a sterile dressing soaked with sterile water or normal saline directly over the eviscerated organs. Do not attempt to push eviscerated organs back into the abdominal cavity, because it can result in additional complications to the patient.

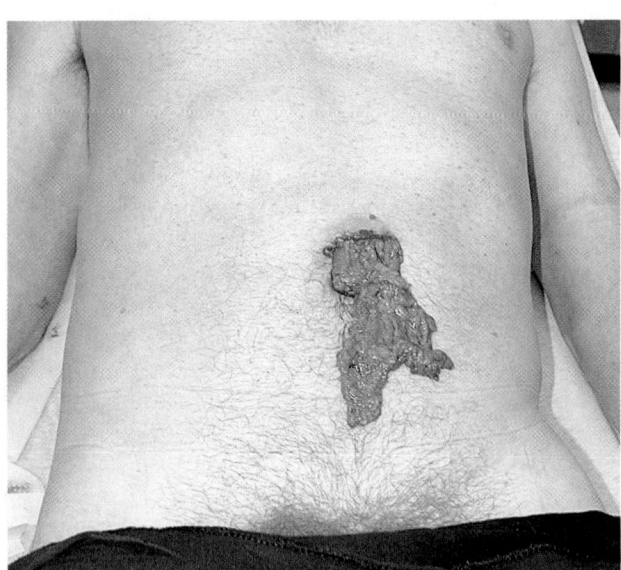

FIGURE 39-4

An abdominal evisceration resulting from penetrating trauma. (© Charles Stewart, MD, and Associates)

4. Cover the dressing with an occlusive dressing to preserve moisture and heat.

5. Monitor and treat for shock as indicated. Do not delay transport to initiate IV access on the scene. Obtain IV access en route to an appropriate facility.

Impaled Objects

Do not remove an object impaled in the abdomen, because doing so can result in uncontrollable hemorrhage. Your goal is to prevent further injury by stabilizing the object in place by stacking roller gauze or bulky dressings around the object and taping them securely in place. You may need to shorten long objects in order to transport the patient and decrease the amount of motion transferred to the patient.

Blunt Trauma

Internal bleeding is the primary concern for patients with blunt abdominal trauma. Blunt trauma can result from direct injury, such as being struck in the abdomen with a bat or through deceleration injury. Although the presence of blood inside the peritoneal cavity does not cause immediate irritation, it sometimes results in referred pain. Recall the impact and shearing and tearing forces that are applied to internal organs with deceleration injury secondary to an MVC. The best emergency care for patients with internal hemorrhage from blunt abdominal trauma is to focus on the airway, breathing, and circulation, treat for shock, and transport without delay to a facility with immediate surgical capabilities.

Diaphragmatic Rupture

The diaphragm is the primary muscle of ventilation that separates the thoracic and abdominal cavities. **Diaphragmatic rupture** occurs when a hole or tear in the diaphragm results in an opening between the thoracic and abdominal cavities, through which abdominal contents can become herniated. This creates two problems with ventilation. First, the muscle itself is impaired. Second, the volume of the lungs is decreased by the presence of abdominal organs in the chest cavity. The abdominal organs can become strangulated, suffering ischemic damage.

Pediatric Care

The thorax of the pediatric patient is smaller or more compact in comparison with that of the adult. The abdominal and thoracic cavities consist of a much smaller surface area of the body. So, always consider the potential for thoracic injury in the presence of abdominal injury.

Take standard precautions first!

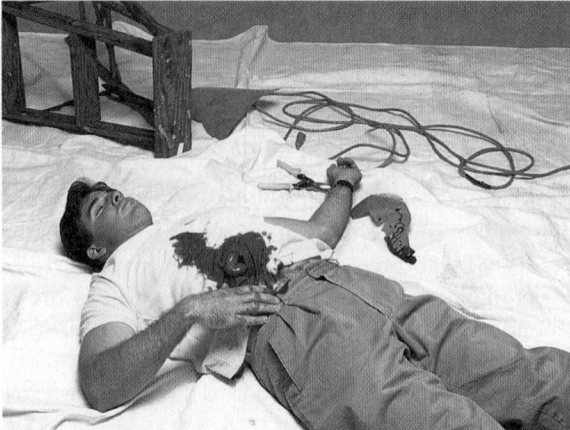

1. An open abdominal wound with evisceration.

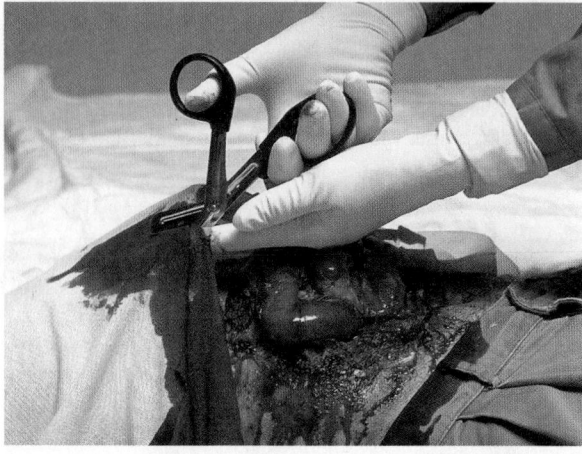

2. Cut away clothing from the wound.

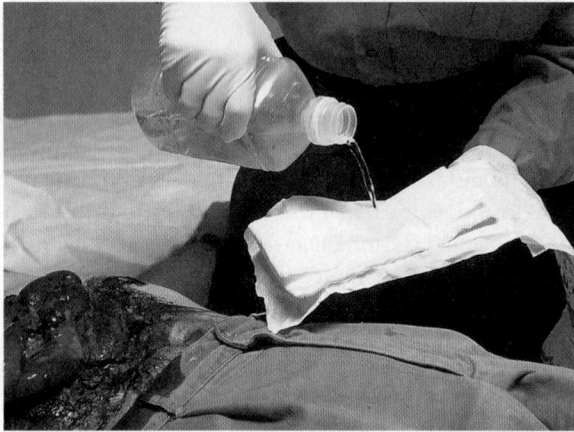

3. Soak a dressing with sterile saline.

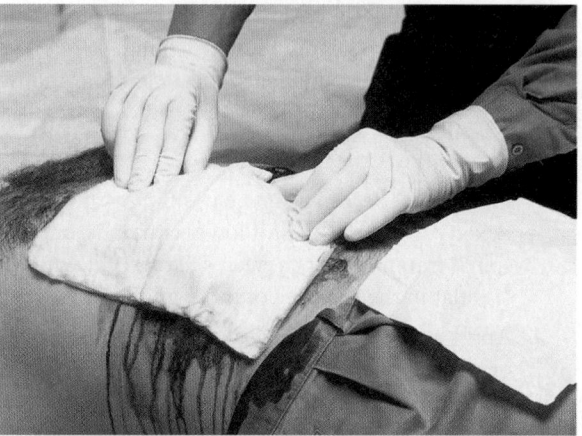

4. Place the moist dressing over the wound.

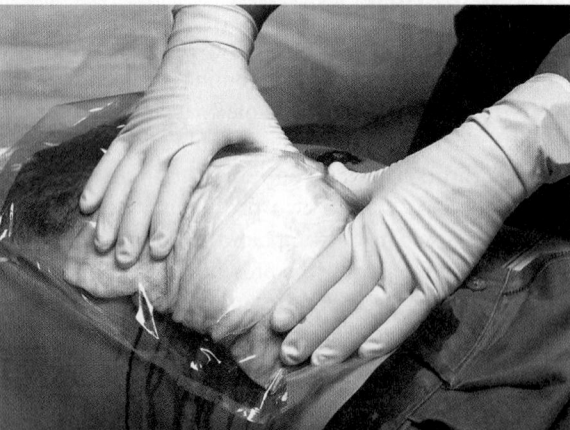

5. Apply an occlusive dressing over the moist dressing if your protocols recommend that you do so. Cover the dressed wound to maintain warmth. Secure the covering with tape or cravats tied above and below the position of the exposed organ.

Smaller diaphragmatic defects may not be found until weeks, or even months, after the injury. The patient may present as a medical patient with abdominal pain. This underscores the importance of obtaining a thorough history in all patients.

Deceleration Injuries

Another MOI that can result in internal abdominal injury is a deceleration injury. Recall Newton's first law of motion, which states that an object in motion will remain in motion until acted on by an outside force. Consider the following scenario: A car leaves the highway and strikes a concrete bridge support travelling at 50 mph. The car decelerates rapidly. Simultaneously, the restrained driver, including his internal organs, rapidly decelerates as he pushes against the seatbelt. The internal

organs continue in a forward motion until they are stopped by impacting the interior surfaces of the body. The impact of organs can result in laceration and rupturing of the organs and massive hemorrhage. Additionally, the forward motion of the organs puts tension on the vessels, which can result in vessel laceration and massive internal hemorrhage.

Explosion Injury

Blasts from explosions can injure the hollow organs of the body, including the hollow organs of the abdomen. If an explosion is powerful enough, a pressure wave is generated and causes a very rapid increase in hollow organ pressure. This can result in tearing or rupture of the hollow organs. In some cases, the patient may not have sustained any visible external trauma.

CASE STUDY WRAP-UP

Clinical-Reasoning Process

When Jack and Jamal expose the patient's abdomen, they see a softball-sized area of ecchymosis to the RUQ that is tender to palpation. The patient denies any other areas of pain and says he did not strike his head. The patient's skin is slightly pale, moist, and cool to the touch.

Jack and Jamal recognize that the MOI has potential for causing internal bleeding and the patient's vital signs indicate the patient has signs of shock, so they immediately place the patient on the stretcher. Because Jack and Jamal know that the patient will require surgery to repair any internal bleeding, they initiate rapid transport to a trauma center 15 minutes away. En route, Jamal obtains vital signs. The patient's vital signs are: blood pressure 105/88, heart rate 108, respiratory rate 18 nonlabored. As Jamal gathers additional information from the patient, Jack obtains an SpO$_2$ of 97 percent on room air. However, because the patient has some early indications of shock, Jack places a nasal cannula on the patient at a flow rate of 4 L/min.

Jack initiates two large-bore IVs, while Jamal calls in a report to the trauma center. Medical direction orders a 500-mL bolus of normal saline if the patient's systolic blood pressure falls below 100 mmHg. The patient's blood pressure holds at greater than 100 mmHg throughout transport. Shortly following arrival at the trauma center, the patient is taken to surgery, where internal bleeding is repaired, resulting in the patient's complete recovery.

CHAPTER REVIEW

Chapter Summary

The threat of life-threatening injury is high with abdominal trauma. Your ability to identify obvious and potential abdominal trauma will allow you to adequately care for and provide appropriate transport for the patient.

Although abdominal evisceration and impalement have unique care considerations, all other abdominal trauma patient care includes supportive care and transport without delay to an appropriate facility. In cases of intra-abdominal hemorrhage,

the patient may deteriorate quickly. Therefore, your goal is to treat life threats while minimizing on-scene time.

Once life threats are addressed, rapidly transport the patient to a surgical facility where definitive care is available. Take time to identify the most appropriate mode of transport. Use aeromedical transport when indicated to reduce the time between injury and definitive care. Your ability to do this will make the biggest difference in the patient's chances of survival.

Review Questions

Multiple-Choice Questions

1. In many cases, the best treatment that you will provide for an internal abdominal injury is:

   a. initiating fluid therapy en route to the emergency department.
   b. identifying the injured abdominal organ.
   c. estimating the amount of blood loss and relaying this information to the receiving physician.
   d. providing rapid transport to a surgical facility.

2. When you palpate your patient's abdomen, he grimaces in pain as you release pressure in the RLQ. This is best described as:

   a. RLQ pain.
   b. RLQ tenderness.
   c. RLQ rebound tenderness.
   d. diffuse abdominal tenderness.

Critical-Thinking Questions

3. Why would a single stab wound made with a 3-inch pocketknife blade to the RUQ of the abdomen be of concern?

4. Explain how hollow and solid organ injuries differ regarding life threats.

5. Explain the steps of emergency care for evisceration.

References

Campbell, J. E. (2008). *International trauma life support* (6th ed.). Upper Saddle River, NJ: Pearson Prentice Hall.

McSwain, N. E., Salomone, J. P., Pons, P. T. (Eds). (2007). *Prehospital trauma life support* (6th ed.). St. Louis, MO: Elsevier.

40 Spine Injuries

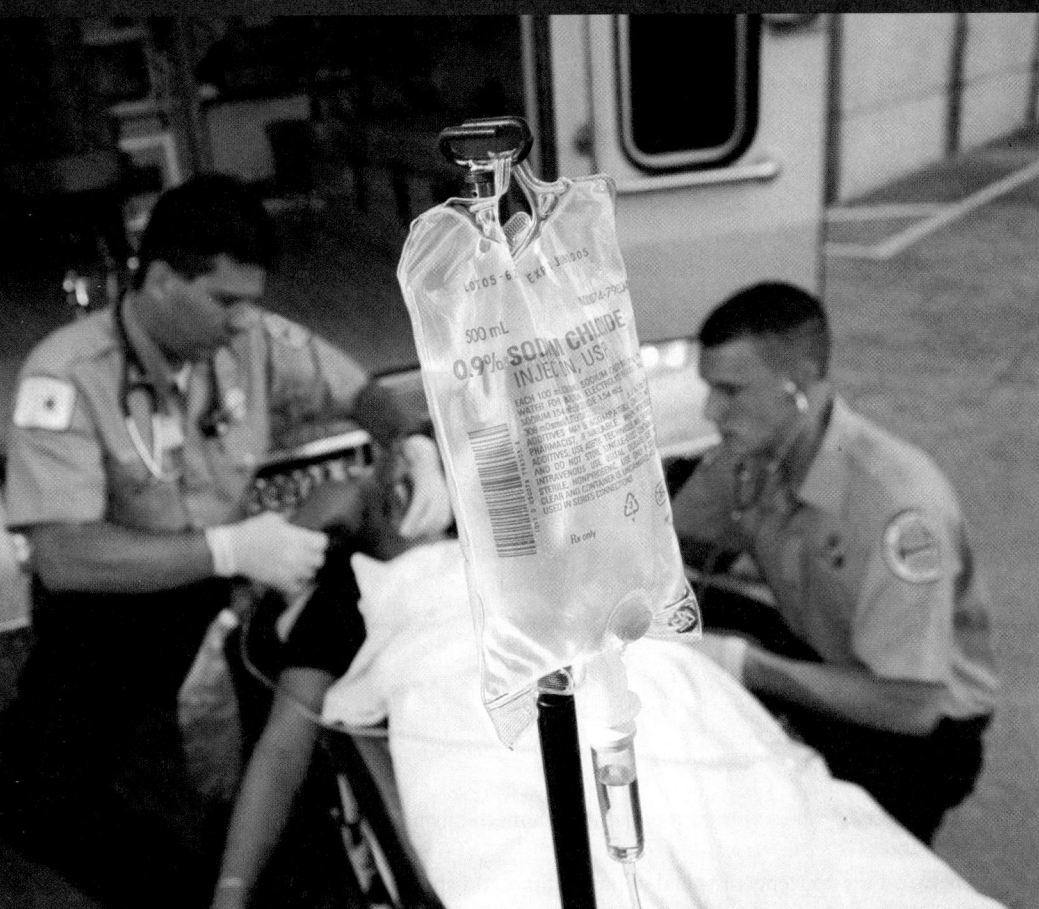

Content Area: Trauma

Advanced EMT Education Standard: Applies fundamental knowledge to provide basic and selected advanced emergency care and transportation based on assessment findings for an acutely injured patient.

Resource Central

Objectives

After reading this chapter, you should be able to:

40.1   Define key terms introduced in this chapter.

40.2   Describe the structure and function of the spinal column, spinal cord, and spinal nerves.

40.3   Use scene size-up, understanding of mechanisms of injury, patient assessment, and patient history to develop an index of suspicion for spine injuries.

40.4   Describe the incidence of neurologic deficit in patients with injury to the spinal column.

40.5   Explain the threat to ventilation associated with injuries to the spinal cord at the cervical level.

(continued)

CASE STUDY

While waiting to order lunch at a favorite restaurant, Advanced EMTs Ashley Davis and Sarah Smith are dispatched to a helicopter crash at a heliport. "Looks like we're going hungry today, huh?" says Sarah.

As they enter their ambulance, dispatch reports over the radio, "Unit 72, the caller advises that there is one patient on scene. The patient is ambulatory."

"That's strange," says Ashley.

After the 13-minute response to the heliport, they are waved through the gate and directed toward the downed helicopter, located in the grass approximately 50 yards from a helipad. Fire service personnel are on scene, though the helicopter does not appear to have been on fire.

As they approach, they notice a man in a flight suit standing next to the rescue truck, speaking to firefighters. Because the scene is safe to approach, they drive closer to the location of the patient.

As Ashley and Sarah walk toward the patient, a firefighter approaches them and begins providing information. The patient is 57-year-old Bruce Hadley, a helicopter pilot for one of the city news channels. Just after takeoff, the aircraft lost oil pressure and rapidly began to lose altitude and air speed. Mr. Hadley circled back toward the heliport hoping to make it out of the wooded area below him. He had just cleared the trees at an altitude of 60 feet, when the aircraft dropped and crashed.

Problem-Solving Questions

1. Given this mechanism of injury, what types of injuries might the pilot have sustained?

2. The patient was ambulatory on the scene. What does that tell Ashley and Sarah about the potential for significant injury?

(continued from previous page)

40.6   Anticipate the presence of other injuries in patients with mechanisms of injury that can produce spine injury.

40.7   Differentiate between the concepts of spinal-column injury and spinal-cord injury.

40.8   Give examples of forces that would produce each of the following mechanisms of spine injury:
- Compression
- Distraction
- Extension
- Flexion
- Lateral bending
- Penetration
- Rotation

40.9   Describe the concepts of complete and incomplete spinal-cord injury.

40.10   Differentiate between the concepts of spinal shock and neurogenic hypotension.

40.11   Recognize signs and symptoms of spinal-cord and spinal-column injury.

40.12   Given a series of scenarios, demonstrate the assessment and management of patients suspected of having an injury to the spine.

40.13   Describe the importance of padding and filling voids between the patient and spinal immobilization devices.

40.14   Demonstrate the following skills associated with management of the patient with a suspected spine injury:
- Inline manual stabilization of the cervical spine in seated and supine patients
- Modified jaw-thrust maneuver
- Repositioning the patient
- Application of a cervical collar

(continued)

(continued from previous page)

       – Immobilization to a long backboard or other full-body spinal immobilization device

       – Application of a short spinal-immobilization device

       – Rapid extrication

       – Spinal immobilization of patients found in seated, standing, supine, and prone positions

       – Managing patients wearing helmets or football equipment

       – Immobilizing infants and children

40.15   Describe the purpose and process of reassessing patients with suspected injury to the spine.

40.16   Discuss current trends and controversies in the assessment and management of patients with suspected spine injuries.

Introduction

Approximately 11,000 people sustain spine injury in the United States annually. Individuals between 16 and 35 years of age sustain spine injury more frequently than others, a result of high-risk activities. Common causes of spine injury include motor vehicle crashes (48 percent), falls (20 percent), penetrating injury (15 percent), sports injuries (14 percent), and others (2 percent) (McSwain, Salomone & Pons, 2007).

Spinal-cord injuries can lead to permanent disability, sometimes leaving the patient paralyzed for life. Although the potential is low, it is possible for improper handling of a patient with a spinal-column injury to result in injury to the spinal cord. When the potential for spinal-column injury exists, you must restrict the motion of the spine, first manually, and then by securing the patient to a long backboard with a cervical collar in place. As an Advanced EMT, identify the potential for spine injury by considering the mechanism of injury and assessing signs and symptoms.

The cervical spine is delicate, compared to the rest of the spinal column, and is more prone to injury. A risk factor for injury of the cervical spine is injury to the head or face. But not all patients who sustain trauma to the head, face, and neck will have a spinal-column or spinal-cord injury. It is actually quite the contrary. According to a nationwide review of patients with head and facial trauma, 6.7 percent of patients with facial fractures and 7.8 percent of patients with combined facial fracture and head injury had associated cervical-spine injury (Mulligan, Friedman, & Mahabir, 2010). Another study found that 3.69 percent of patients with craniomaxillofacial fractures had associated cervical-spine injury (Elahi, Brar, Ahmed, Howley, Nishtar, & Mahoney, 2008). In a study of trauma above the clavicles as predictor of spine injuries, 4.2 percent of patients with facial injuries had associated cervical-spine injury, but only 0.75 percent had cervical spinal-cord injuries (Williams, Jehle, Cottington, & Sufflebarger, 1992). The same study suggests that a Glasgow Coma Scale score of less than 14 might be a better predictor of cervical-spine injury than the presence of head or facial trauma alone.

Anatomy and Physiology Review

The nervous system consists of two anatomical divisions: the central nervous system and the peripheral nervous system, which communicate with each other. Motor neurons exit the spinal cord from its anterior (ventral) surface, and sensory neurons enter it from its posterior (dorsal) surface. Tracts of gray matter, consisting of nerve cell bodies, and white matter, consisting of nerve fibers (axons), allow nervous signals to be transmitted up and down the spinal cord, between the brain and peripheral nervous system. Those tracts, or columns, are arranged so that certain types of impulses travel up the anterior portion of the spinal cord, and other types travel up the lateral and posterior aspects of the cord. When the spinal cord is completely severed, all communication from that point in the cord downward ceases. When the cord has an incomplete injury, the signs and symptoms will reflect which of the columns is injured. In some cases, nerve fibers cross over from one side of the spinal cord to the other, so that some functions will be impaired on one side of the body, and others will be impaired on the opposite side (Figure 40-1).

The central nervous system consists of the brain and spinal cord. The peripheral nervous system consists of all nervous tissue outside the central nervous system. Efferent, or motor, neurons originate in the brain or spinal cord and travel to effector cells, such as those of skeletal muscle. Afferent, or sensory, neurons sense stimuli throughout the body, initiating signals that travel toward the brain or spinal cord.

The efferent portion of the peripheral nervous system is divided into the autonomic and voluntary divisions. The autonomic nervous system is further divided into sympathetic and parasympathetic divisions.

The ability of the sensory and motor signals to be transmitted to and from the brain requires the system to be intact. When there is a disruption in the ability of these signals to travel to and from the brain, normal bodily function is affected. Nerves do not have the ability to regenerate

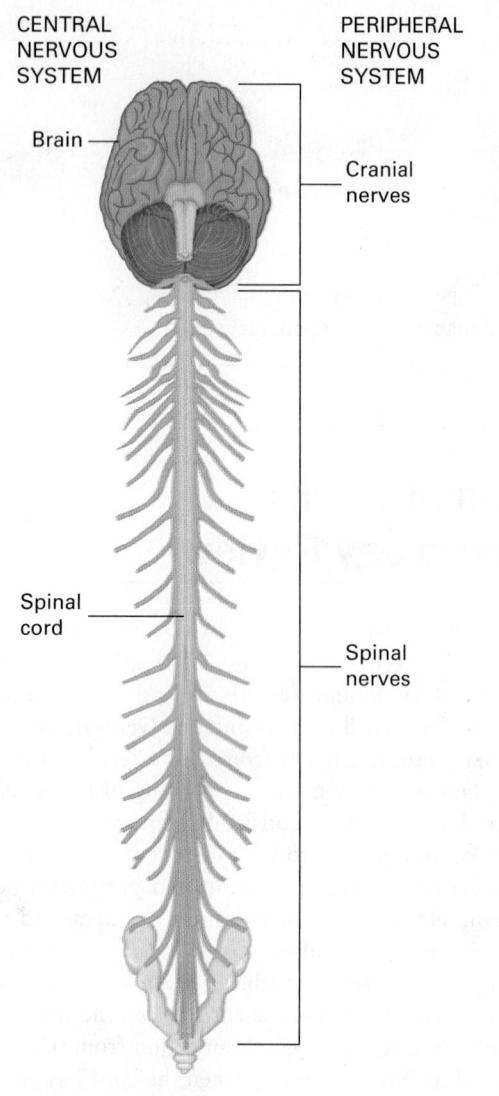

CENTRAL NERVOUS SYSTEM

PERIPHERAL NERVOUS SYSTEM

Brain

Cranial nerves

Spinal cord

Spinal nerves

FIGURE 40-1

The central and peripheral nervous systems.

themselves; therefore, when injury occurs, the results are permanent.

The brain and spinal cord are protected by the skull and spinal column, respectively. When significant forces are applied to these protective structures, the brain and spinal cord are susceptible to injury.

The Spinal Column

The spinal column extends from the base of the skull to the pelvis. It consists of 33 vertebrae, which are stacked on top of one another or (in the case of the sacral and coccygeal vertebrae) fused together. Each vertebra is separated from the others by a fibrous **intervertebral disk**. This intervertebral disk acts as a shock absorber, preventing the vertebrae from contacting one another and causing damage. Each vertebra has a hole through its center called a *vertebral foramen,* which houses and protects the spinal cord.

The spinal column is divided into five regions (Figure 40-2): the cervical spine, thoracic spine, lumbar spine, sacral spine, and coccyx, which are described as follows:

- *Cervical spine.* This part of the spine is within the neck and consists of seven vertebrae (C-1 through C-7). The skull rests atop the first cervical vertebra (C-1), called the **atlas.** The atlas sits on the second cervical vertebra (C-2); it is called the **axis.** The atlas allows free forward and backward nodding movement of the head and the axis allows the head to rotate in an approximately 180-degree range of motion.

- *Thoracic spine.* This part of the spine is below the cervical spine and consists of 12 vertebrae (T-1 through T-12) that attach to the ribs.

- *Lumbar spine.* The lumbar spine consists of five vertebrae and is distal to the thoracic spine (L-1 through L-5).

- *Sacral vertebrae and coccyx.* These two parts of the spine form the inferior region of the spine. The sacrum is the fused sacral vertebrae supporting the majority of the body's weight.

The spine is more susceptible to injury in some areas than in others. The susceptibility of injury to those regions is due to the size of the vertebrae, the extent of supporting musculature and ligaments, and the curvature of the spine. Approximately 55 percent of spine injuries occur in the cervical spine, 15 percent in the thoracic spine, 15 percent in the thoracic spine, and 15 percent in the lumbar spine (McSwain, Salomone & Pons, 2007).

Muscles and ligaments together support and hold the spine in its normal position and allow for movement. If the ligaments and muscles are torn, the spine becomes susceptible to excessive movement. The excessive movement may result in dislocation of a vertebra, which can result in pressure being exerted on the spinal cord and injury to the spinal cord or nerves that extend from between the vertebrae.

Cervical-spine injuries are more prevalent because the weight of the head has the potential to cause hyperflexion, hyperextension, and rotation when forces are applied to the body. The muscles of the neck are simply not strong enough to support the head and prevent this movement when significant forces are applied.

The Spinal Cord

The spinal cord begins at the base of the brainstem and continues through the vertebral foramen of each vertebra to the second lumbar vertebra (L-2), where it separates into nerves. At the level of each vertebral disk are nerve roots that extend from the spinal cord, through small tunnels called **neural foramina,** which are located on each side of the spinal column. These nerve roots form nerves that continue to the body and carry impulses from the body to the brain and vice versa.

FIGURE 40-2

The spinal column.

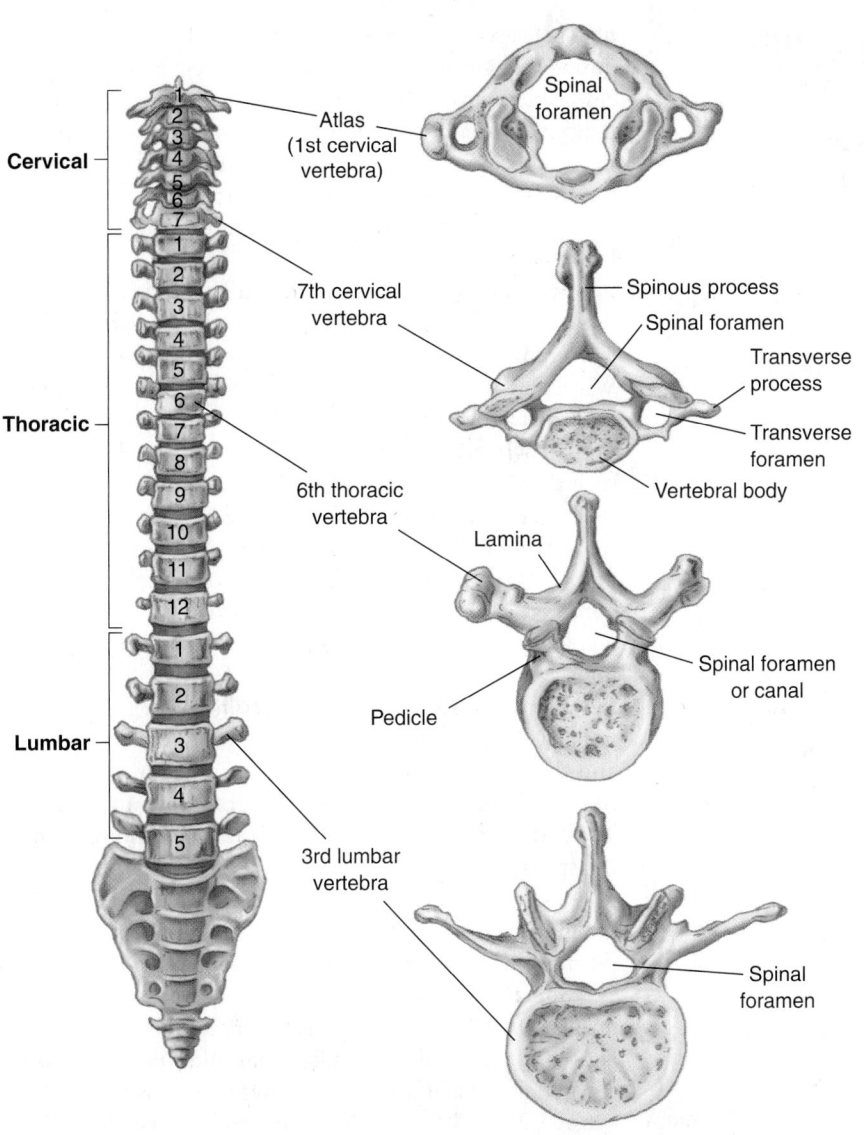

Spinal foramen

Atlas (1st cervical vertebra)

Cervical

7th cervical vertebra

Spinous process

Spinal foramen

Transverse process

Transverse foramen

Vertebral body

Thoracic

6th thoracic vertebra

Lamina

Spinal foramen or canal

Pedicle

Lumbar

3rd lumbar vertebra

Spinal foramen

Front view of vertebral column

Vertebrae from above

All muscle functions, voluntary and involuntary alike, result from nerve impulses. Recall that the primary muscle of ventilation is the diaphragm. The contraction of the diaphragm results from nervous impulses that are generated in the brainstem. The nervous impulses then travel to the diaphragm by way of the phrenic nerves, which exit the spinal column at the C3-C5 region. Therefore, injury to the spinal cord in the high cervical-spine region may result in injury to the phrenic nerves and cause failure of the diaphragm to contract, resulting in life-threatening ventilatory insufficiency. With this in mind, it is important to pay particular attention to the patient's breathing status when high cervical-spine injury is suspected.

Reflexes are defense mechanisms that assist us in preventing injury to ourselves. The nerve roots of the spinal cord provide for reflex actions to take place. A reflex is an action that results from nervous stimulation within the spinal cord, not the brain. For example, if you touch a hot surface, the heat results in a sensory impulse that is sent to the spinal cord through the nerve roots. When this very strong impulse reaches the spinal cord, a motor impulse is immediately generated and sent to your arm, resulting in the removal of your hand from the heat source. This action does not require the involvement of the brain.

The spinal cord contains two types of spinal tracts—ascending and descending. **Ascending spinal tracts** carry impulses from the body to the brain. Ascending nerve tracts can be further divided into tracts that carry various types of sensations, such as light touch, pressure, pain, temperature, and vibration. **Descending spinal tracts** carry motor impulses from the brain to the body and control muscle activity and tone.

Mechanisms of Spine Injury

Even though the spinal cord is well protected from injury by the spinal column, injury may result when enough force is applied. In situations in which the mechanism of injury suggests the potential for spine injury, such as a "starred" windshield after an MVC, you should assume that injury exists.

Although not all injury to the spinal column results in injury to the spinal cord, you must take the necessary steps to immobilize the spine so that movement does not worsen any injury that does exist.

Spine injury can result from any of the following mechanisms (Figure 40-3):

■ *Compression.* With this mechanism, pressure is applied to the top of the head or pelvis, leading to axial loading to the spinal column. If enough force is applied to the vertebrae, **compression** fractures may occur.

■ *Hyperflexion.* With **hyperflexion**, the spine is forced anteriorly, beyond its normal range of motion.

■ *Hyperextension.* The spine is forced posteriorly with **hyperextension**, beyond its normal range of motion.

■ *Rotation.* Excessive rotation of the spine will cause injury.

■ *Lateral bending.* Excessive bending of the spine to one side or another also causes injury.

■ *Distraction.* With **distraction**, excessive stretching of the spine occurs.

■ *Penetration.* For penetration to occur, an object must be forced into the spine.

When any of these mechanisms is present, assume that spine injury exists and treat the patient accordingly.

Spinal-Column Injury Versus Spinal-Cord Injury

Spinal-column injury refers to damage to musculoskeletal structures—the vertebrae or ligaments of the spine. This can result from a multitude of mechanisms and can be a complete fracture, incomplete fracture, or compression fracture of the vertebrae. Typically, a patient will complain of pain and tenderness to the location of the spine that is injured.

IN THE FIELD

Observing the mechanisms of injury to the patient, such as those involved in a particular type of MVC impact or a fall, will allow you to determine which specific mechanism of spine injury was applied to the patient.

In some cases, deformity can be palpated or may be visible during assessment.

As a rule, you should treat the patient for spinal-column injury when pain or tenderness is present to any portion of the spinal column. Spinal-column injury does not mean that a spinal-cord injury exists—only that the potential exists. Proper management of spinal-column injury is discussed later in this chapter.

Spinal-cord injury refers to damage to the spinal cord itself. As you learned earlier, the spinal cord is responsible for impulse transmission to and from the body or brain. When spinal-cord injury is present, the patient will present with **neurologic dysfunction** (abnormal neurologic function). There are various degrees of neurologic dysfunction, such as tingling sensations, numbness, weakness, or paralysis. Injury to the spinal cord is classified as either primary or secondary injury.

Primary injury to the spinal cord is the result of compression or shearing of the cord. This is the direct result of the mechanism of injury. Consider the following scenario: A patient is in a vehicle that is struck from the rear and a headrest is not present. As a result of the impact, the body moves forward rapidly with the vehicle and the head does not. This results in hyperextension of the neck. If the hyperextension is dramatic, it may result in fractures to the cervical vertebrae and compression of the spinal cord.

Secondary injury to the spinal cord occurs after the initial injury and is usually the result of swelling, ischemia, or the movement of bone into or against the spinal cord.

Spinal-cord concussion is the temporary disruption of normal spinal-cord function distal to the site of injury. This is usually the result of swelling that takes place following the initial incident and subsides over time. As the swelling subsides, so will neurologic dysfunction—or at least some of the dysfunction. There is no way to determine the extent of permanent injury, if any, until swelling subsides.

Complete and Incomplete Spinal-Cord Injury

Complete spinal-cord injury refers to the total disruption of the spinal cord and results in a total loss of neurologic function distal to the injury site.

When complete disruption occurs, swelling also will occur. Recall that this swelling can result in neurologic dysfunction but, as swelling subsides, some neurologic function will return. Neurologic dysfunction from the initial injury will remain, whereas temporary dysfunction resulting from swelling will subside. For this reason, the full extent of injury cannot be determined until at least 24 hours following injury.

Incomplete spine injury refers to an injury involving a portion of the spinal cord. Because only a portion of the cord is involved, the tracts that are not affected continue to function. Types of incomplete spinal-cord injuries

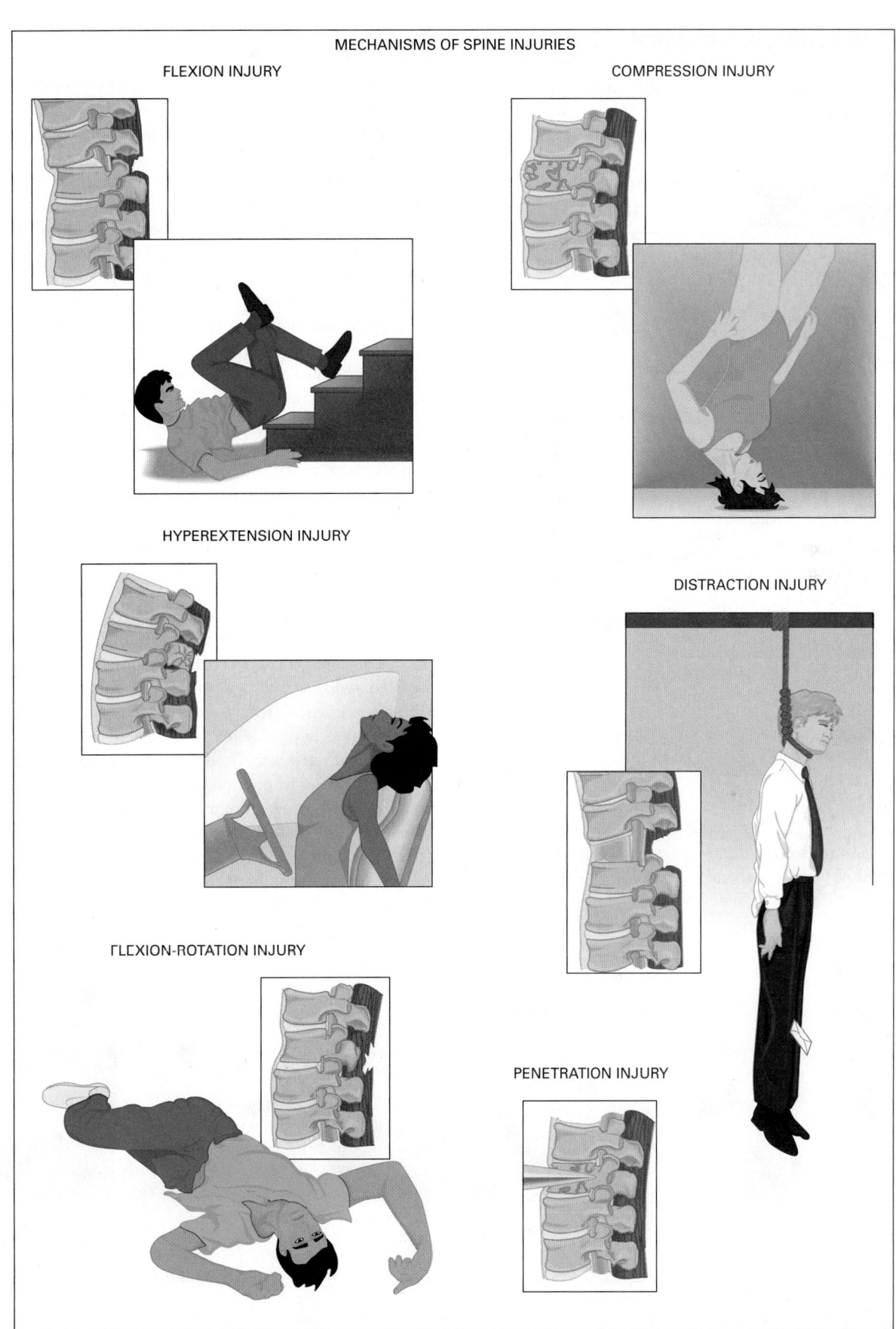

FIGURE 40-3

Mechanisms of spine injury.

include **anterior-cord syndrome, central-cord syndrome,** and **Brown-Séquard syndrome.** Those specific incomplete spine injuries, common mechanisms of injury for each, and their signs and symptoms are listed in Table 40-1 and Figure 40-4.

TABLE 40-1	Types of Incomplete Spine Injuries	
Type of Injury	**Mechanism of Injury**	**Signs and Symptoms**
Anterior-cord syndrome	Bone fragment introduction or pressure to blood vessels of the anterior cord	Loss of motor function and pain, temperature, and light touch sensation at and below the level of injury. Normal vibration and position senses.
Central-cord syndrome	Usually occurs with hyperextension of the cervical spine	Weakness to upper extremities, while lower extremities maintain strength. Variable sensory changes.
Brown-Séquard syndrome	Penetrating injury causing hemitransection of one side of the cord	Loss of motor function and vibration and position sense on the affected side of the body with loss of pain and temperature sensation on the other side.

Source: This article was published in Publication, Prehospital Trauma Life Support, 6ed, Salomone, J.P., Pons, P.T.; Copyright Elsevier.

Spinal Shock

Spinal shock results from a concussion-like injury to the spinal cord that causes neurologic deficits below the level of injury. When spinal-cord injury occurs, there is a loss of muscle tone or paralysis below the level of the injury.

Recall that the vasculature and sphincters of the body consists of smooth muscle. Just as skeletal muscle tone is lost, so is smooth muscle tone. The relaxation of smooth muscle, which commonly causes patients to lose bowel and bladder sphincter control, should be evident during your assessment of the patient. Additionally, the smooth muscle walls of the vasculature relax, resulting in the dilation of vessels and the loss of temperature regulation, making the patient susceptible to hypothermia.

If enough vasculature is affected, as with a high cervical-spine injury, hypotension occurs. This hypotension as a result of spinal shock is called **neurogenic hypotension**. In most cases, spinal shock resolves within 24 hours post-injury, but it can sometimes last for several days.

Neurogenic hypotension resulting from spinal shock is referred to as **neurogenic shock**. As described in the previous section, the dilation of vasculature results from injury to the spinal cord in the high cervical-spine region. The dilation results in a state of hypovolemia, not from blood loss but from the significant increase in volume of the vasculature. This particular type of hypovolemic state is called *relative hypovolemia,* as opposed to *absolute hypovolemia,* which results from the loss of blood volume. With relative hypovolemia, the patient becomes hypotensive. Ordinarily, the body is able to respond to this condition through its compensatory mechanisms. With spinal shock, however, the most effective of those mechanisms to cause smooth muscle contraction and vasoconstriction—namely, the sympathetic response that leads to the release of norepinephrine and epinephrine into the bloodstream—is lost.

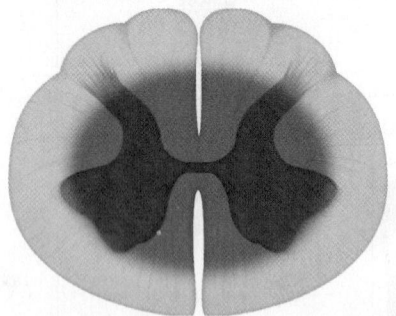 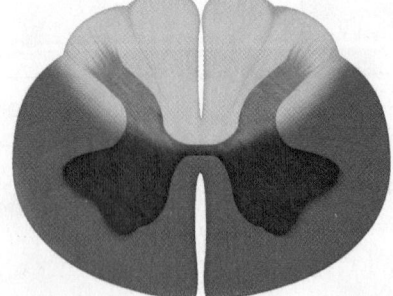 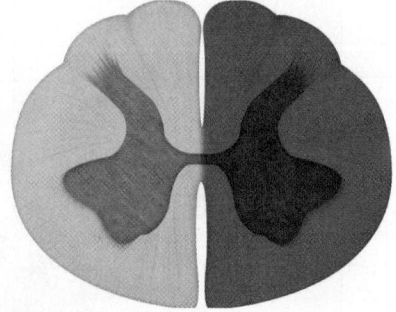

(A) Central-cord syndrome   (B) Anterior-cord syndrome   (C) Brown-Séquard syndrome

FIGURE 40-4

Incomplete spine injuries: (A) Central-cord syndrome results from injury to the central region of the cord. (B) Anterior-cord syndrome results from injury to the anterior cord. (C) Brown-Séquard syndrome results from injury to one side of the cord, either right or left.

TABLE 40-2	Comparison of Neurogenic and Hypovolemic Shock*		
	Neurogenic Shock	**Hypovolemic Shock**
Skin condition	Pale and cool above the level of injury, flushed and warm below the level of injury	Skin of the entire body is pale and cool
Heart rate	Remains within normal range	Tachycardia

*The difference in signs and symptoms of the neurogenic shock patient is due to the loss of sympathetic stimulation, which is a compensatory mechanism for hypovolemic states.

TABLE 40-3 Mechanisms of Injury Indicating the Potential for Spine injury

- Motor vehicle collisions
- Motorcycle or bicycle crashes
- Falls
- Blunt trauma to the head, neck, or back
- Penetrating trauma to the head, neck, or torso
- Pedestrians struck by a vehicle
- Sports-related injuries of the neck and back
- Hangings
- Diving accidents
- Any unresponsive trauma patient

Typically, a patient who is exhibiting signs and symptoms of shock will be pale, with cool skin and tachycardia. This is because of the sympathetic response, which causes peripheral vasoconstriction and an increase in heart rate. Because the sympathetic response is lost with spinal shock, the patient will present differently. Those differences are illustrated in Table 40-2.

General Assessment and Management of Spine Injuries

You will be called to care for an injured patient with the potential for spine injury frequently as an Advanced EMT. Injury to the spinal column and spinal cord may occur as a result of a fall, MVC, assault, and penetrating trauma. Your ability to identify potential injuries to the spine is directly related to the thoroughness of your assessment.

Scene Size-Up

As with every patient, begin your assessment by ensuring that the scene is safe prior to entering. Once on scene, assess the mechanism of injury. Maintain a high index of suspicion when the mechanism of injury indicates the potential for spine injury. Those mechanisms are listed in Table 40-3.

With motor vehicle collisions, remember to assess the vehicle for indications that spine injury might have occurred, such as starring of the windshield or broken door windows.

Primary Assessment

If the mechanism of injury suggests a potential for spine injury, immediately take—or direct someone else to perform—manual stabilization of the head and neck by grasping either side of the head with gloved hands

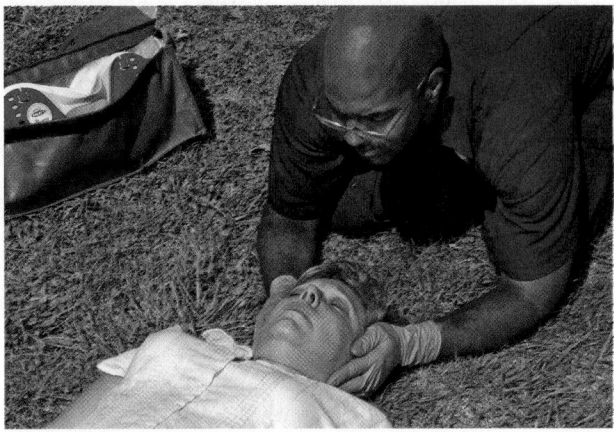

FIGURE 40-5

Manual stabilization of the head and neck.

IN THE FIELD

Do not rule out spine injury in patients who are ambulatory at the scene. The ability to ambulate does not rule out spine injury.

(Figure 40-5). Instruct the patient to remain still and do not allow him to move. If possible, position yourself in the patient's line of sight so he will not attempt to turn his head toward you as you speak.

Maintain manual stabilization of the head and neck until the patient's spine is fully immobilized or until it is determined that spinal immobilization is not indicated (discussed later in this chapter).

If the patient is ambulatory, have him stand still while manual stabilization of the head and neck is held. Once the head and neck are stabilized, complete your primary assessment, ensuring adequacy of airway, breathing, and circulation. If you must manually open the patient's airway, use the modified jaw-thrust maneuver, because this allows the opening of the airway without compromising the spine.

In rare situations, you may find it difficult to maintain a patent airway using a modified jaw-thrust maneuver. In such cases, allow for only as much movement of the spine as necessary to maintain a patent airway. Remember, the patient must have a patent airway or he will die within minutes. If you must choose between moving the spine to establish an airway and not establishing an airway, you always must choose to establish an airway.

Pay particular attention to the patient's level of responsiveness, because alterations may indicate head injury, intoxication, shock, or hypoxia. Patients with decreased level of responsiveness are considered unreliable in terms of giving information that can help you make decisions about spinal immobilization.

Patients with associated injuries, such as extremity fractures, may not readily notice neurologic problems resulting from spine injury, such as tingling, numbness, or weakness, because they are distracted by the painful extremity injuries. As an Advanced EMT, treat your patient based on the mechanism of injury and clinical signs and symptoms. It is important that you do not become distracted by dramatic-appearing injuries and overlook the potential of an associated spine injury.

Determine if the patient is critically injured or noncritically injured and make a transport destination decision accordingly.

Secondary Assessment

Perform the secondary assessment while maintaining manual stabilization of the head and neck. Begin by performing a rapid trauma exam. During this assessment, quickly assess for life-threatening injuries not identified during the primary assessment. During the head-to-toe exam, assess neurologic, motor, and sensory function in all four extremities (Scan 40-1). In male patients, the presence of a persistent erection of the penis, called *priapism*, is indicative of spine injury.

Obtain baseline vital signs and a patient history.

CASE STUDY (continued)

Ashley knows that the patient's airway, breathing, and circulation are not grossly impaired at the moment because she has noted his skin color (good) and that he has been speaking with the firefighters. "Hi, Mr. Hadley. I'm Ashley, an Advanced EMT with the ambulance service. How are you feeling?"

"My lower back is killing me," replies Mr. Hadley.

Ashley can hear the discomfort in his voice and asks, "On a scale from 1 to 10, with 10 being the worst pain you've ever had, how do you rate this pain?"

"I was shot down in Vietnam," he says, "and had some fractures. This isn't quite that bad. I'd call it a 6."

"Do you have any weakness, numbness, or tingling in your arms or legs?" asks Ashley.

"No. Nothing like that."

Problem-Solving Questions

1. Would Ashley and Sarah determine this patient as critical or noncritical? What factors would support their decision?

2. Combining the information from the scene size-up with the patient's initial information, what injuries would Ashley and Sarah suspect?

3. How will Ashley and Sarah integrate assessment, management, and preparation for transport in this situation?

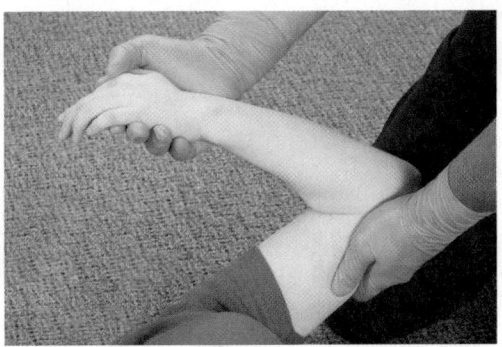

1. Assess flexion.

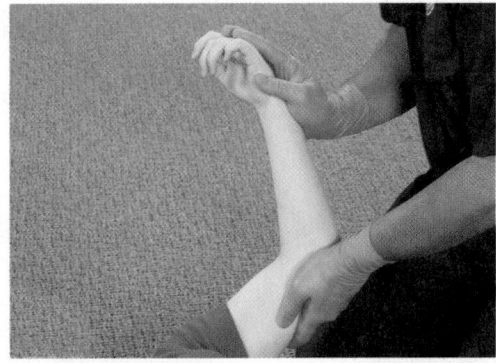

2. Assess extension.

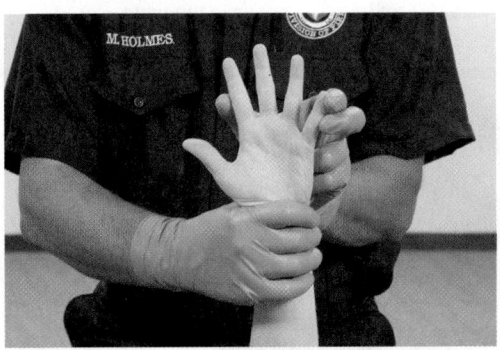

3. Assess finger abduction.

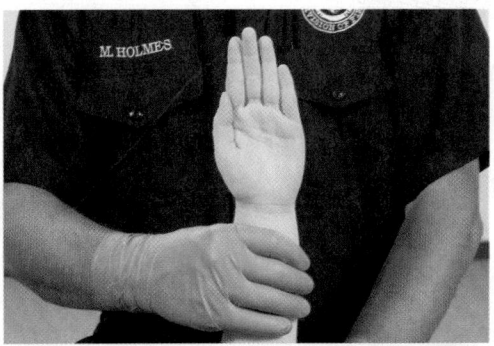

4. Assess finger adduction.

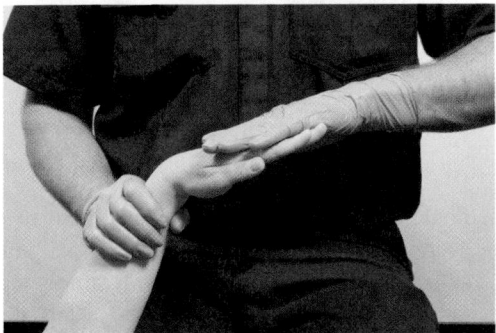

5. Assess the wrist and hand.

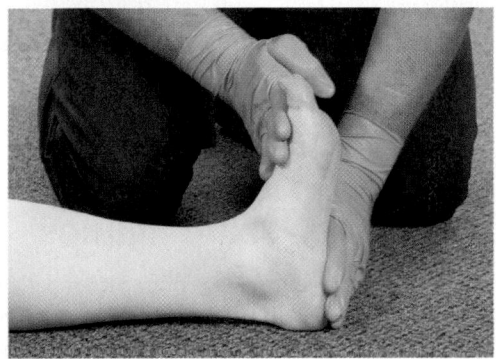

6. Assess plantar flexion.

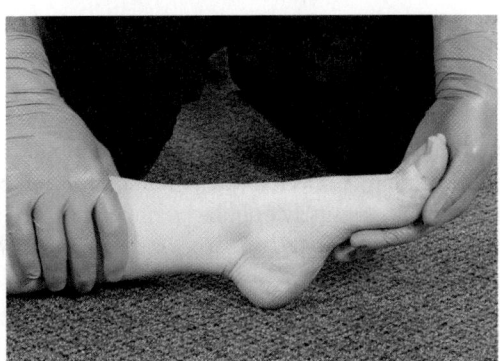

7. Assess dorsiflexion.

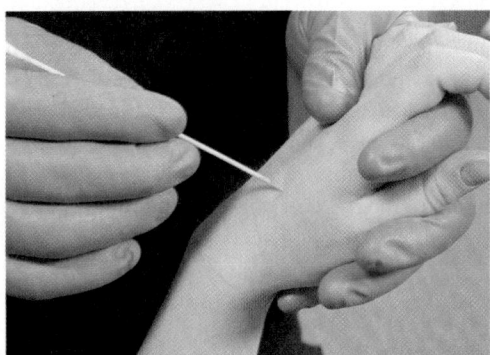

8. Assess pain response in the hand.

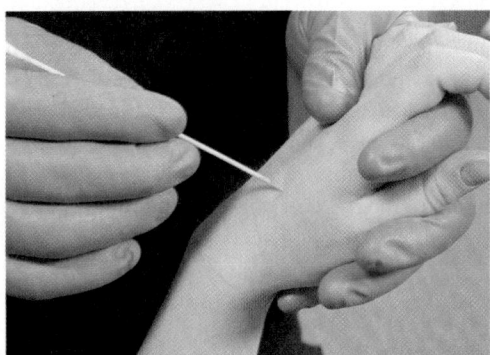

(continued)

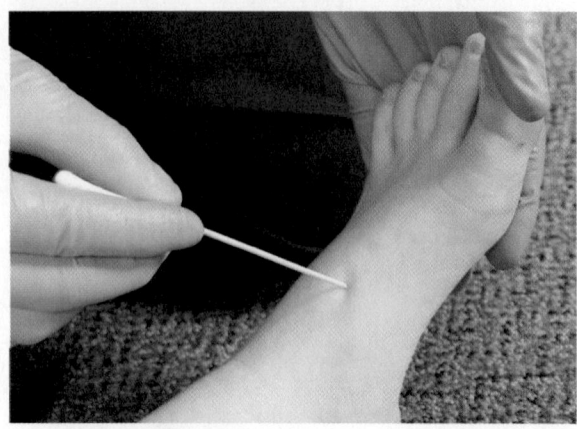

9. Assess pain response in the foot.

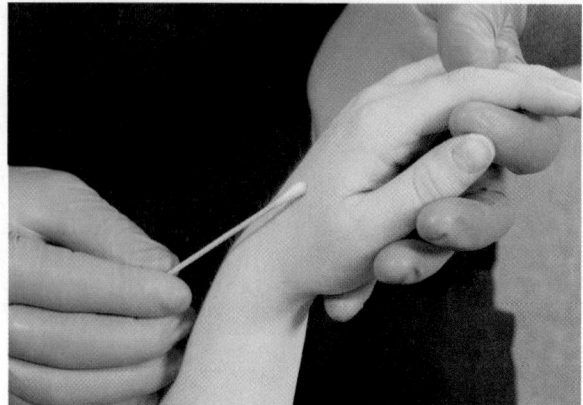

10. Assess light touch response in the hand.

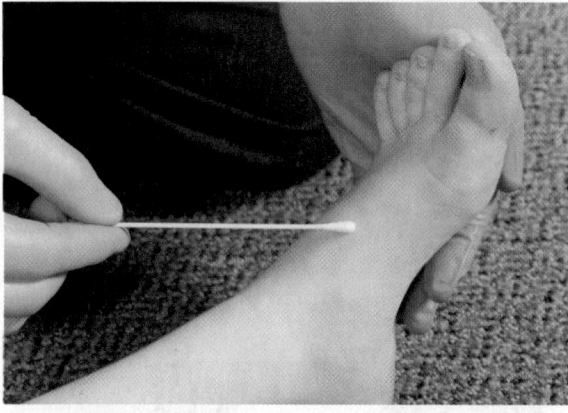

11. Assess light touch response in the foot.

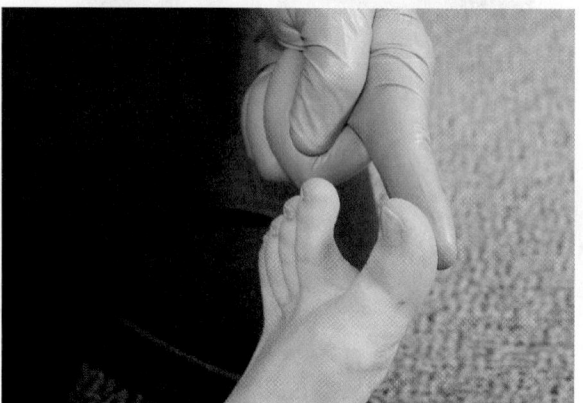

12. Assess flexion of the great toe on the same foot.

Management of Spine Injuries

The process of spinal immobilization is different for patients who are standing, seated, or lying down. The process for immobilizing patients found seated inside vehicles depends on whether their condition is stable or unstable. In this section, the various methods of immobilizing the spine are covered.

Size and apply a rigid cervical collar to restrict the motion of the head and neck (Scans 40-2 and Scans 40-3). The application of a rigid cervical collar does not immobilize the head and neck, but it does assist. Therefore, you must maintain manual stabilization of the head and neck even after the application of the rigid cervical collar, until the patient is completely secured to a long backboard.

Reassessment

Reassess motor function and sensation in all four extremities. In some cases swelling will occur, exerting pressure on the spinal cord. Swelling can be extensive enough to produce neurologic deficits. The presence of new neurologic deficits during subsequent assessments when none were noted initially does not necessarily mean that you managed the patient incorrectly. It simply means that deficits are now present and may be the result of swelling. This can be a frightening experience for the patient, so make an effort to reassure and comfort him. Document any changes in your patient care report upon arrival at the hospital emergency department.

Selective Spinal Immobilization

Not all injured patients require spinal immobilization. The implementation of selective spinal immobilization protocols has become increasingly popular in the prehospital environment. It is vital that you incorporate specific criteria into these protocols and strictly adhere to them in order to use the technique properly. Review the spinal immobilization decision protocol (Figure 40-6).

In order to determine whether to perform spinal immobilization on a patient, you must consider the mechanism of injury, the patient's signs and symptoms, patient age, and the patient's level of responsiveness.

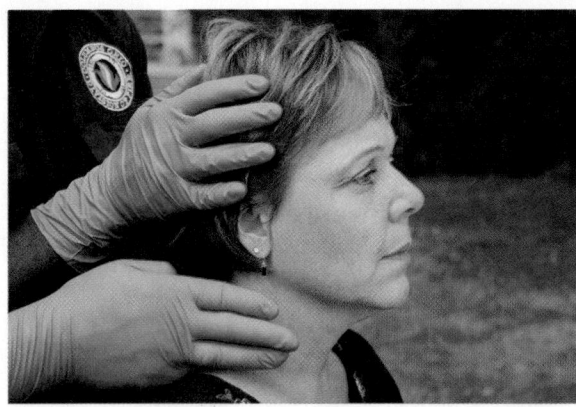

1. To size a cervical spine immobilization collar, first draw an imaginary line across the top of the shoulders and the bottom of the chin. Use your fingers to measure the distance from the shoulder to the chin.

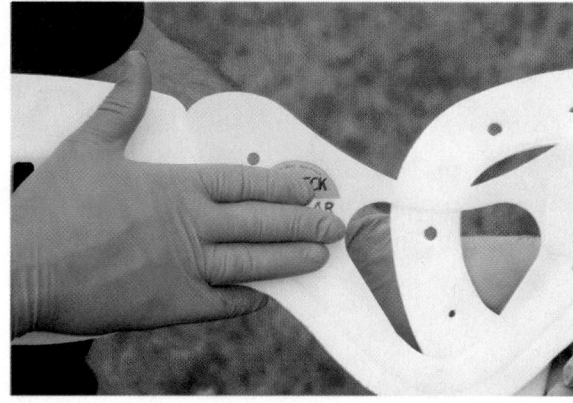

2. Check the collar you select. The distance between the sizing post (black fastener) and lower edge of the rigid plastic should match that of the number of stacked fingers previously measured against the patient's neck.

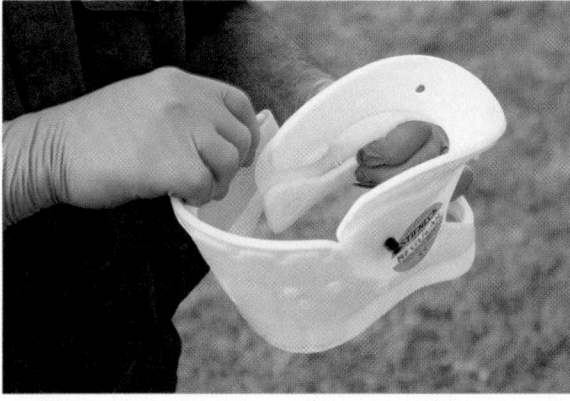

3. Assemble and preform the collar.

Mechanisms of injury that are positive indications for spinal immobilization include the following:

- Motor vehicle collision
  - Ejection of the patient
  - Death of another occupant in the same vehicle
  - Rollover
  - High-speed collision (greater than 40 miles per hour)
  - Extrication time of greater than 20 minutes
  - Bumper displacement of greater than 18 inches
  - Intrusion into the passenger compartment of greater than 20 inches
- Auto versus pedestrian collision greater than 5 miles per hour
- Motorcycle collisions
  - Collision speed of greater than 20 miles per hour
  - Motorcycle and rider separation
- Obvious or depressed skull fracture

- Any blast or explosion injury
- Gunshot wound to the neck or torso
- Fall from greater than 10 feet or less than 10 feet if the patient struck an object during the fall
- Blunt trauma above the level of the clavicles
- Unresponsiveness due to trauma

As an Advanced EMT, you must understand that spinal immobilization is indicated with the presence of a mechanism of injury not considered a positive indication for immobilization and signs and symptoms of spine injury. Such mechanisms of injury are considered questionable and warrant further assessment to determine whether the patient requires spinal immobilization. You must assess the patient and make a determination based on not only the mechanism of injury but also the patient's signs and symptoms. The proper assessment of the patient in order to determine whether spinal immobilization is indicated will always follow the application

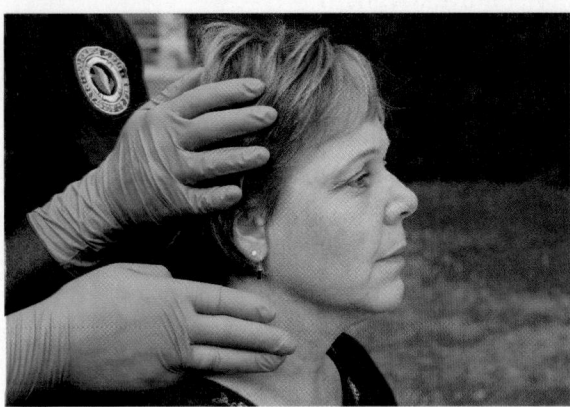

1. After selecting the proper size, slide the cervical spine immobilization collar up the chest wall. The chin must cover the central fastener in the chin piece.

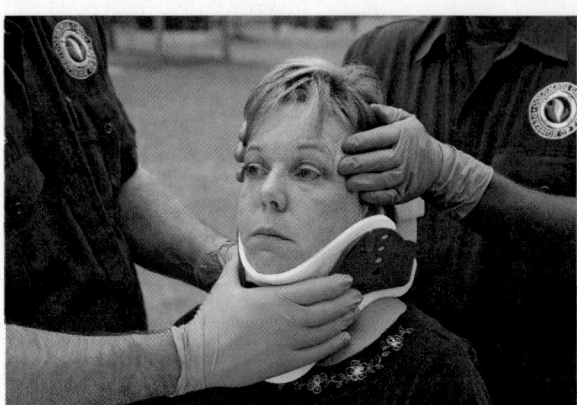

2. Bring the collar around the neck and secure the Velcro. Recheck the position of the patient's head and collar for proper alignment. Make sure the patient's chin covers the central fastener of the chin piece.

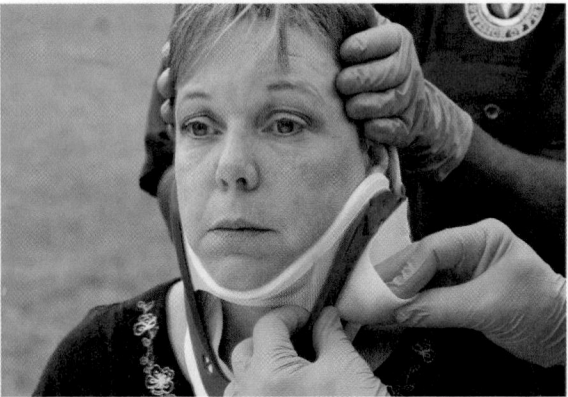

3. If the chin is not covering the fastener of the chin piece, readjust the collar by tightening the Velcro until a proper sizing is obtained. If further tightening will cause hyperextension of the patient's head, select the next smaller size.

of manual stabilization of the head and neck and the primary assessment.

Assessment to determine the indication for spinal immobilization with questionable mechanisms of injury will include the following:

1. Assess the patient's level of responsiveness. If any alteration is present or if there is a communication barrier such as with a deaf patient or a patient who does not speak English, you must immobilize the patient.

2. Ask the patient if his neck or back hurts. If pain is present, you must immobilize the patient.

3. Palpate the entire spine and ask if tenderness is present. If tenderness is present, you must immobilize the patient.

4. Assess for motor and sensory deficits. If deficits are present, you must immobilize the patient.

In some cases, the patient has a **distracting injury** such as an extremity fracture. A distracting injury is an injury that may make the patient less sensitive to the presence of other symptoms such as tingling or numbness as a result of the pain from the injury. For example, if a patient falls from a 4-foot ladder and has an obvious arm fracture, the pain from this injury may reduce the patient's ability to notice tingling to his arms as a result of an associated spine injury. The presence of those injuries, along with the potential for spine injury, indicates the need for spinal immobilization.

Negative mechanisms of injury indicating that spinal immobilization is not required include but are not limited to isolated extremity trauma, gunshot wounds to the extremities, industrial trauma to the hand, and so on.

Protocol, policy, and procedure among EMS agencies vary, so as always, follow your protocol regarding indications for spinal immobilization.

Spinal Immobilization Decision

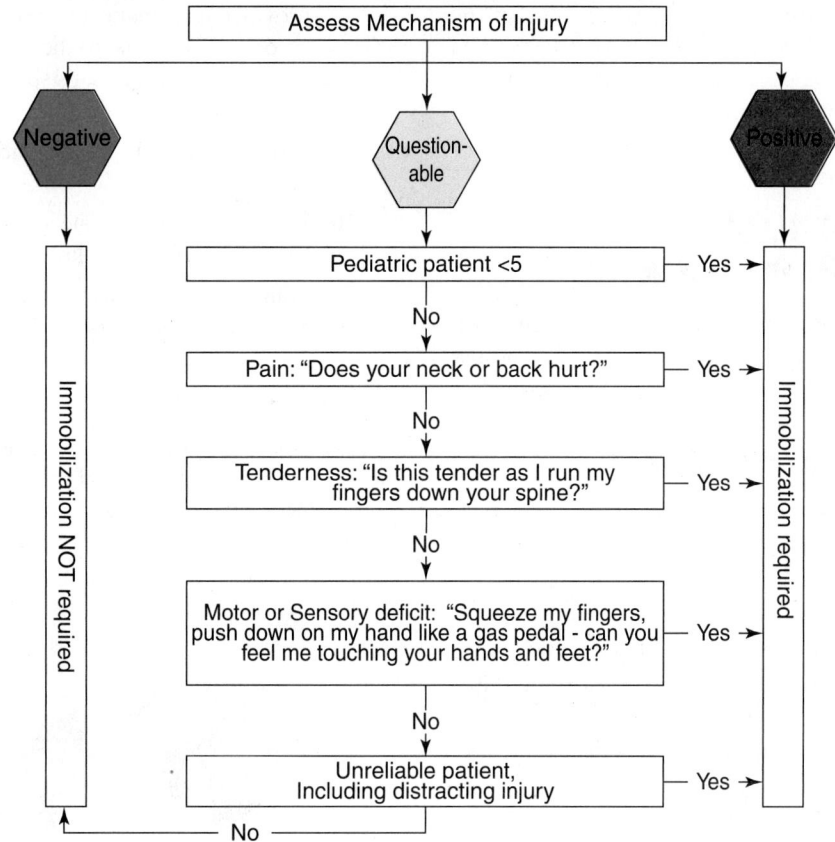

Guidelines:

o **Positive** Indications:

   1. MVC: Ejection, death of another occupant in same vehicle, rollover, high speed (>40 mph), extended extrication time (>20 minutes), bumper displacement >18 inches, Intrusion of >12 inches into passenger compartment
   2. Pedestrian: Auto vs. pedestrian / bicycle (>5 mph) & pedestrian struck and thrown or rolled over
   3. Motorcycle collision with speed >20 mph or bike rider separation
   4. Skull fracture or depression
   5. Blast or explosion injury
   6. GSW to neck or torso
   7. Fall from >10 feet or falls <10 feet if patient contacting objects during the fall (i.e., tree branches, scaffolding, etc.)
   8. Injury to clavicle or above
   9. Unresponsiveness due to trauma

o **Negative** Indications: GSW to foot, tibial fracture from stepping in pothole, industrial trauma to hand, etc.

o **Questionable** Indications: Minor MVC, falls <10 feet, elderly person falls, helmet to spine tackle, etc.

o Unreliable patients include altered mental status (brain injury, intoxication, etc.), acute stress reaction, distracting injury, or communication barrier. These patients cannot accurately report signs/symptoms.

o Distracting injury produces a level of pain that would "mask" the pain from a spine injury. Because pain severity is subjective, the medic must use clinical judgment to determine if a minor injury is distracting.

o Support your decision to forego spinal immobilization by documenting pertinent information.

FIGURE 40-6

Spinal immobilization decision protocol.

Once you suspect spine injury in your patient, manually stabilize the patient's head and neck. Maintain stabilization until the patient is fully immobilized. Note that the process of spinal immobilization is different for patients who are standing, seated, or lying. The process also may be different, depending on whether the patient's condition is critical or noncritical.

Spinal Immobilization: Supine and Prone Patients

You must log roll the patient who is found in a supine position in order to place him on a long backboard. The proper procedure for immobilizing such a patient is described as follows (Scan 40-4):

1. Perform manual stabilization of the head and neck.

2. Size and apply a rigid cervical collar.

3. Position the long backboard alongside the patient and be prepared to pad the voids between him and the board.

4. Position yourselves alongside the patient, opposite the long backboard, and grasp the patient at the shoulder, hip, and leg.

5. The EMT holding the head should direct the others to gently roll the patient toward him at the count of three.

6. Once the patient is rolled onto his side, position the long backboard so that the foot end of the board is located at the level of the patient's knees or slightly lower. Place a blanket on the backboard; it provides padding, as well as a way to move the patient up into position on the backboard.

7. Roll the patient onto the long backboard.

8. Grasp the patient or the blanket beneath him at the shoulders and hips. On the count of the provider at the patient's head, slide the patient up on a slight angle so the patient is centered on the board. (The patient's spine should be at the midline of the board.)

9. Pad the voids between the patient and the long backboard.

10. Secure the patient to the long backboard at the chest, hips, above the knees, and below the knees.

11. Immobilize the patient's head to the board using a head immobilization device.

12. Transfer the patient onto a stretcher and secure him to the stretcher.

Note that the patient's body is immobilized to the long backboard first, not the head. If the head were to be secured first, the neck would become a pivot point for any motion of the body as it is secured.

If the patient is found in a prone position, perform manual stabilization of the head and neck (Figure 40-7).

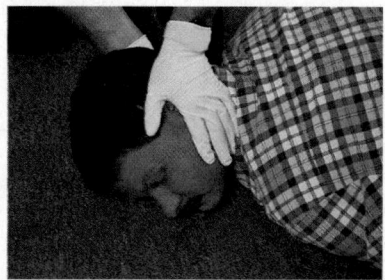

FIGURE 40-7

Stabilize the head and neck of a prone patient and allow the head to rotate into a neutral position as the body is log rolled. (© Carl Leet)

PERSONAL PERSPECTIVE

Advanced EMT Victor D'Angelo: In EMS, you will respond to emergencies that will challenge you in ways you won't expect. I once responded to an injured-person call at a shipyard to find a worker who had been pinned beneath a large sheet of iron. It was being raised into place to be welded when the rigging slipped, allowing the sheet to fall. It struck the patient across his shoulders and pinned him beneath it.

Prior to our arrival, the sheet had been removed from the patient. My partner and I arrived to find several coworkers gathered around him. The patient was positioned as if he was seated on the ground, but his chest was resting on his right upper leg. He was alert and oriented and was complaining of pain to his upper back. While cutting his shirt away, I noticed that his spine appeared to be folded in half in the lumbar spine region. Two vertebrae were protruding outward,

appearing as if they were about to puncture the skin. The patient had no sensation or movement from the waist down.

In order to position him on a long backboard, my partner and I had to straighten him out as best we could. Because there was no pain or resistance felt when moving the patient, we were able to position him in the left lateral recumbent position on a long backboard and immobilize him.

The patient was transported to the hospital emergency department, where it was determined that he suffered a complete transection of the spinal cord in the lumbar region. He was paralyzed from the waist down as a result of the injury but he was lucky that the sheet of iron did not strike him in the head, because that could've been fatal.

In EMS, you will be faced with situations where you'll have to improvise. Always treat the patient appropriately to the best of your ability, given the circumstances.

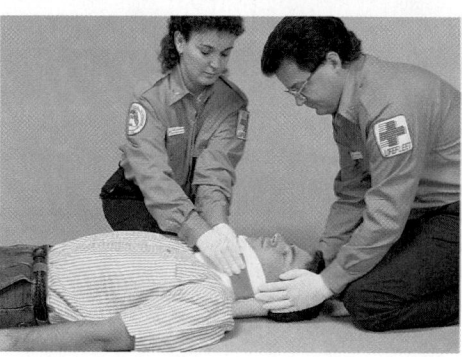

1. Establish and maintain inline stabilization. Apply a rigid cervical spine immobilization collar.

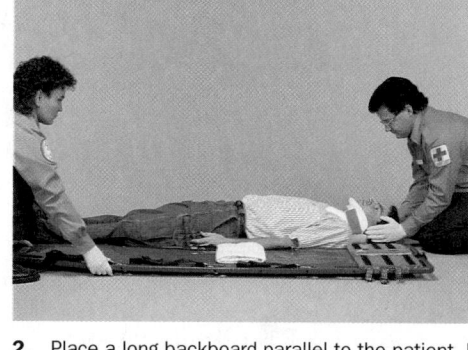

2. Place a long backboard parallel to the patient. If possible, pad the voids under the head and torso.

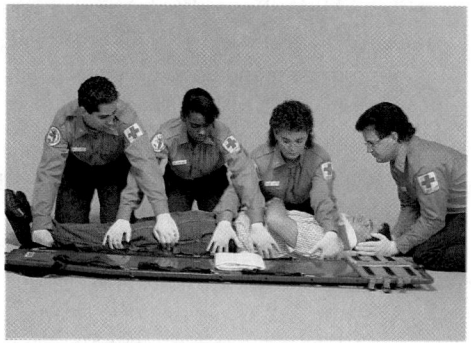

3. Three EMTs kneel at the patient's side opposite the board, leaving space to roll the patient toward them.

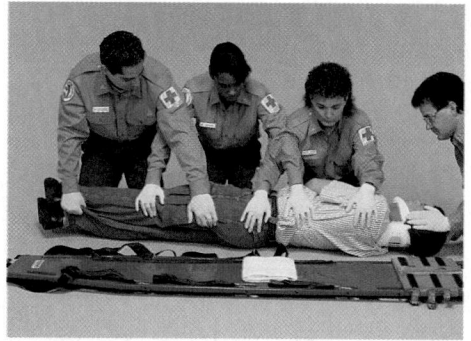

4. The EMT at the head directs the others to roll the patient, as a unit, onto his side. Assess the patient's posterior side.

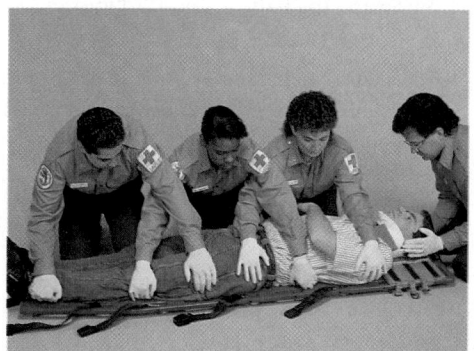

5. The EMT at the waist reaches over, grasps the backboard, and pulls it into position against the patient. (This can also be done by a fifth rescuer.) The EMT at the head instructs the rescuers to roll the patient onto the backboard.

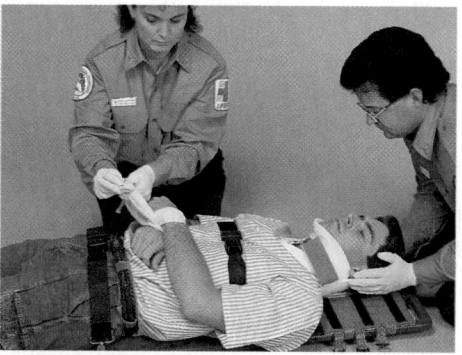

6. Secure the patient to the board with straps. Tie the wrists together loosely.

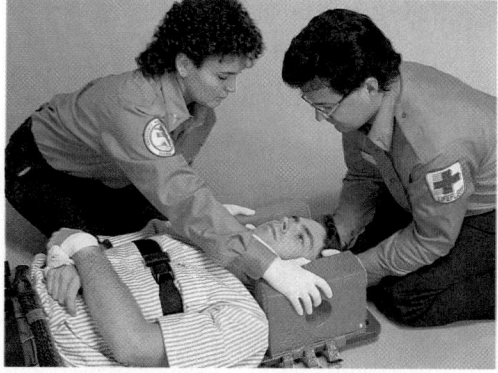

7. Using a head/cervical immobilizer, secure the patient's head to the backboard.

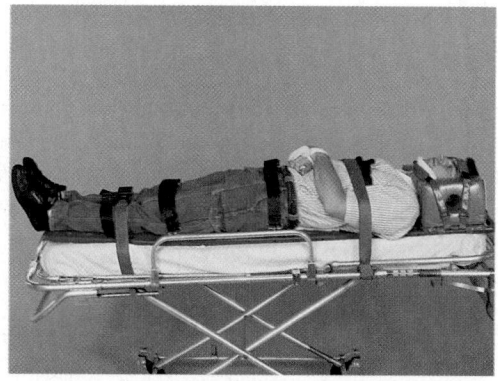

8. Transfer the patient and the backboard as a unit. Secure the patient and the backboard to the cot.

Pediatric Care

Because of the larger size of the pediatric patient's head in relation to the rest of his body, padding is required beneath the shoulders to maintain the head in a neutral position.

Geriatric Care

Geriatric patients sometimes develop kyphosis, or "hunchback," which results in a large void in the lumbar spine region and causes the neck to be hyperextended when the patient is placed in the supine position. You should be prepared to apply additional padding beneath the lumbar spine and head in these cases.

The head should gently rotate into a neutral position as the body is log rolled. Once the patient is in the supine position, immobilize him to the long backboard as if he were found supine.

In most cases, once the patient is log rolled onto the long backboard, he will not be centered on it. In order to address this, place the long backboard beside the patient with the foot end of the board positioned approximately at the patient's knees. Doing so will allow you to slide the patient up the long backboard, toward the head end as a single unit, and at a slight angle, which will center him on the board.

Once the patient is properly positioned on the long backboard, pad the voids between the patient and the board to support the spine and to provide comfort and support. Common voids requiring padding include the lower back (lumbar spine region) and behind the knees. After you have completely immobilized the patient to the long backboard, reassess and document pulses, motor function, and sensation in all four extremities.

Spinal Immobilization: Seated Patient

In many cases, you will find a patient who has the potential for spine injury in the seated position. Such patients are usually found seated inside a motor vehicle following an MVC. To immobilize the patient's spine, you will need the following equipment:

- Rigid cervical collar
- Short spinal immobilization device, such as a short board or vest-type immobilization device
- Long backboard
- Straps

On rare occasions, you will encounter a patient who will not tolerate lying flat. This may be due to pre-existing medical conditions that cause shortness of breath when lying flat. In such cases, it is appropriate to immobilize the patient using a short board or vest-type immobilization device and transport him seated on the stretcher with his head elevated.

To immobilize a seated patient, follow the steps listed below (Scan 40-5):

1. After manual stabilization of the head and neck is performed and a rigid cervical collar is applied, position the Kendrick extrication device (KED) carefully behind the patient.
2. Align the KED by centering it and wrapping the sides around the patient's torso.
3. Ensure that the sides of the device are placed in the armpits when wrapped around the patient. Once placed, secure the torso straps.
4. Secure the leg straps, ensuring that the straps are located beneath the patient's buttocks and through the crotch.
5. Secure the patient's head to the device using straps or roller gauze.
6. Secure the patient's hands to prevent him from grabbing interior parts of the vehicles while he is being removed.
7. Pivot the patient onto a long backboard and recline him onto it.

Spinal Immobilization: Standing Patient

From time to time, you will encounter a patient with suspected spine injury who is ambulatory at the scene. When a patient is found in a standing position, you will need the following equipment in order to immobilize the spine:

- Rigid cervical collar
- Head immobilizer
- Long backboard
- Straps

The procedure for immobilizing a standing patient with three rescuers is as follows (Scan 40-6):

1. One EMT performs manual stabilization of the head and neck from behind the patient while another sizes and applies a rigid cervical collar.
2. Position the long backboard behind the patient while manual stabilization of the head and neck are being maintained.

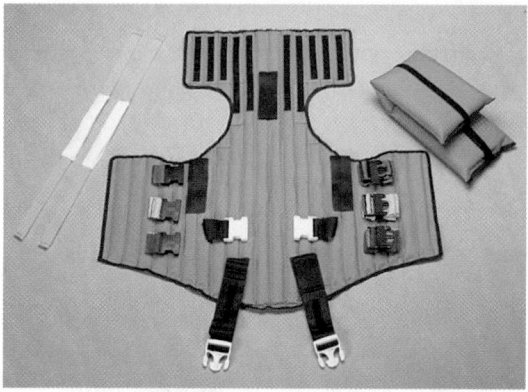

1. The Ferno Kendrick Extrication Device (KED).

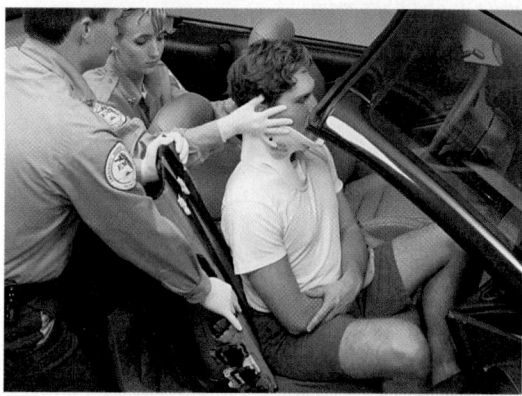

2. After a cervical spine immobilization collar has been applied, slip the KED behind the patient and center it.

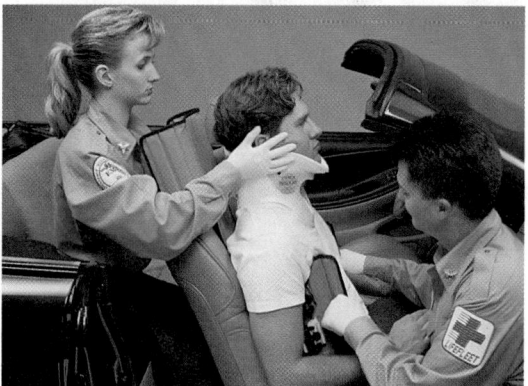

3. Align the device properly, then wrap the vest around the patient's torso.

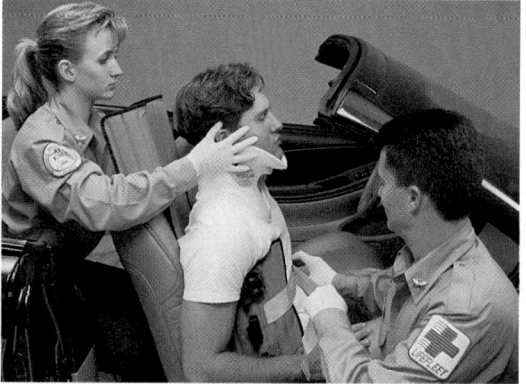

4. When the device is tucked well up into the armpits, secure the chest straps.

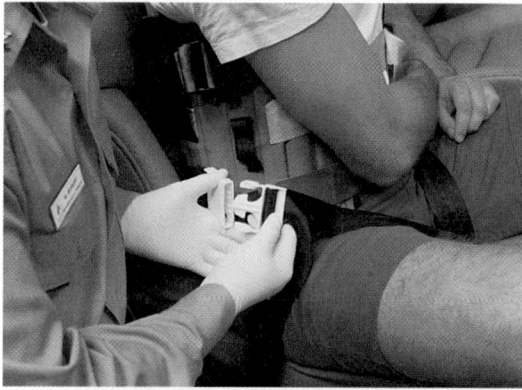

5. Secure the leg straps.

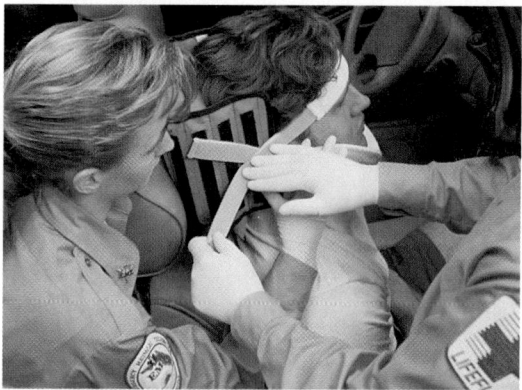

6. Secure the patient's head with the Velcro head straps.

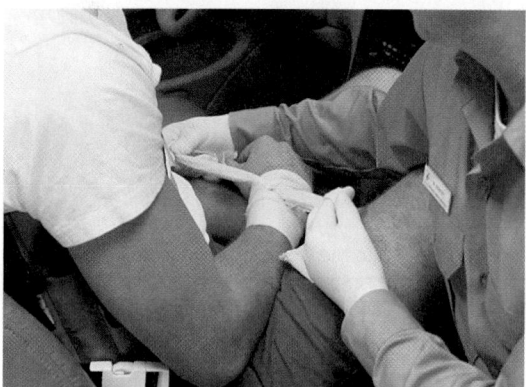

7. Tie the hands together.

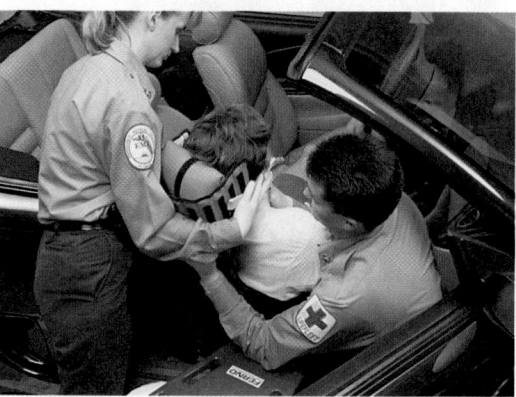

8. Pivot the patient onto the backboard while maintaining inline stabilization.

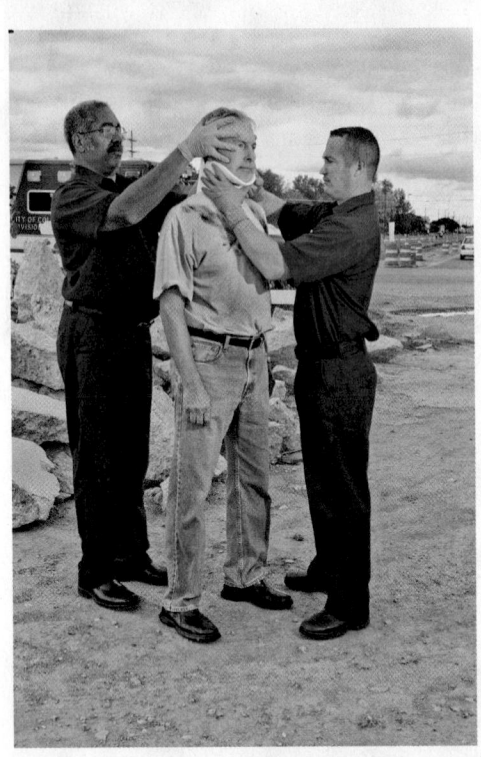

1. Apply a cervical spine immobilization collar while holding inline stabilization.

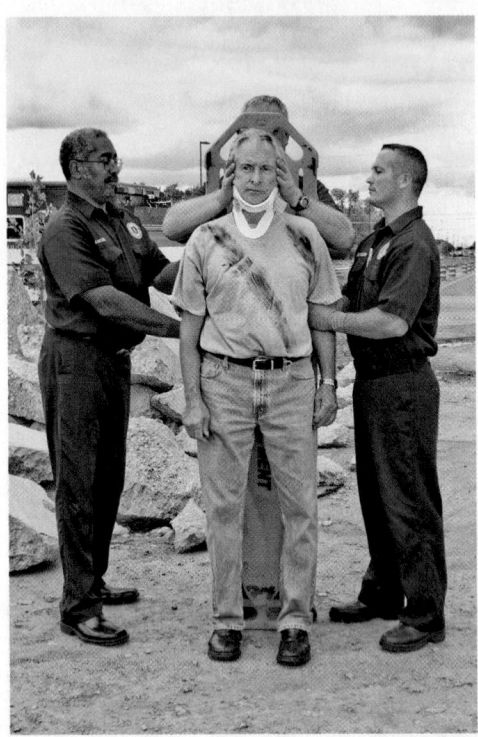

2. Position the backboard behind the patient and align it properly. Check the position of the board from the front of the patient.

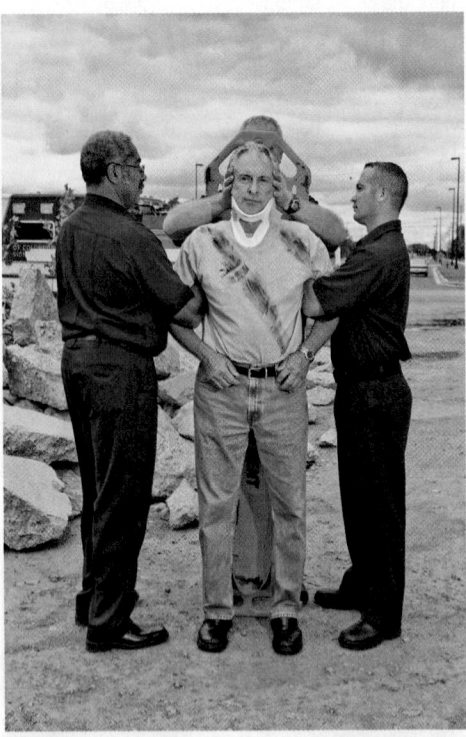

3. The EMTs at the sides of the patient place their hands under each arm and grasp the next highest handhold. Their other hands grasp the elbows of the patient to provide additional stabilization on the board.

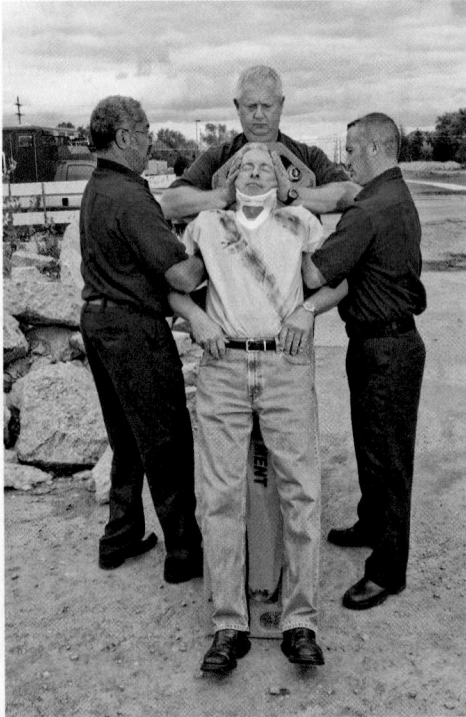

4. Lower the patient to the ground. Continue holding inline stabilization until the patient is completely immobilized to the backboard with a head/cervical immobilization device and straps.

3. Two EMTs position themselves at opposite sides of the patient and grasp the highest handhold by reaching beneath the patient's armpits. Their free hands then grasp the patient's elbows to provide additional stabilization.

4. At a count given by the EMT holding the patient's head, the others gently lower the board to the ground.

5. Once on the ground, the patient is immobilized to the long backboard.

Spinal Immobilization: Rapid Extrication

Rapid extrication is the procedure used for removing a patient from a vehicle rapidly while maintaining manual stabilization of the spine. There are three situations that indicate the use of rapid extrication:

- Patient is critically injured and must be moved immediately.
- Patient is blocking access to a critically injured patient.
- Patient is in immediate danger.

Rapid extrication does not simply mean to grab the patient and pull him from the vehicle without regard to maintaining spinal alignment. There is a procedure that you must follow for rapid extrication that includes maintaining spinal alignment.

When preparing to perform the rapid extrication of a patient, you will need the following equipment:

- Rigid cervical collar
- Head immobilizer
- Long backboard
- Straps

Rapid extrication proceeds as follows (Scan 40-7):

1. Perform manual stabilization of the head and neck from behind the patient while a second EMT sizes and applies a rigid cervical collar.

2. On the count of the EMT holding the patient's head, rotate the patient in small increments until his back is facing where the long backboard will be placed.

3. Position the long backboard behind the patient with one end against the patient's buttocks.

4. Gently recline the patient onto the long backboard while maintaining manual stabilization of the head and neck.

5. Gently slide the patient onto the long backboard.

6. Move the long backboard onto the stretcher and secure the patient's torso, then secure his head.

The rapid extrication procedure will allow you to rapidly move a patient from a vehicle while simultaneously maintaining spinal alignment. Use it only in the three cases listed earlier. Remove any other patient with the potential for spine injury from the vehicle using a short backboard or a vest-type extrication device.

Special Considerations

Helmet Removal

There are many activities for which people wear protective helmets that may cause difficulty in proper management of the patient. Those activities include bicycle riding, roller skating, and motorcycle riding.

As always, complete a primary assessment while maintaining manual stabilization of the head and neck. In addition to the primary assessment, determine whether the helmet fits the patient well enough to prevent movement of the head within it, whether the helmet allows for access to the patient's airway should airway management be required, and whether the patient can be properly immobilized with the helmet in place.

If the helmet fits well, allows for access to the airway, and you can properly immobilize the patient using padding beneath the torso, you may leave the helmet in place. If the helmet does not fit well enough to prevent movement of the head within it, access to the patient's airway is not possible, or you cannot properly immobilize the patient with the helmet in place, you must remove the helmet.

If you must remove the helmet, follow these procedures for proper helmet removal:

Removal of full-face motorcycle helmets:
1. EMT #1 grasps the face mask portion of the helmet and maintains manual stabilization of the head and neck.
2. EMT #2 removes or cuts the chin strap.
3. EMT #2 gently grasps the mandible of the patient with one hand and supports the posterior neck with the other.
4. EMT #1 removes the helmet slowly and gently.
5. EMT #2 hands over manual stabilization of the head and neck to EMT #1.

Removal of open-face helmets:
1. EMT #1 performs manual stabilization of the head and neck.
2. EMT #2 removes or cuts the chin strap.
3. EMT #2 removes the helmet while EMT #1 maintains manual stabilization of the head and neck.
4. EMT #2 sizes and applies a rigid cervical collar while EMT #1 maintains manual stabilization of the head and neck.

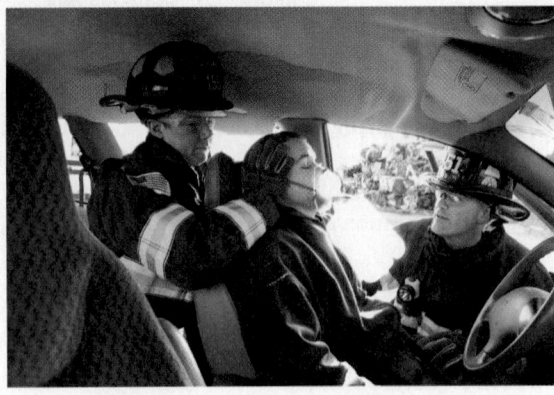

1. In some cases, the vehicle may be damaged to the point at which access to perform extrication is limited. In such cases, the use of extrication resources to remove the roof of the vehicle will make extrication of the patient much easier.

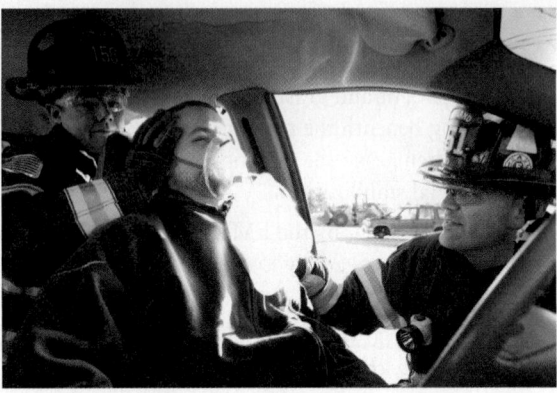

2. The patient's head is held in a neutral position; this is best done from the rear. While stabilizing the head, obtain the primary assessment.

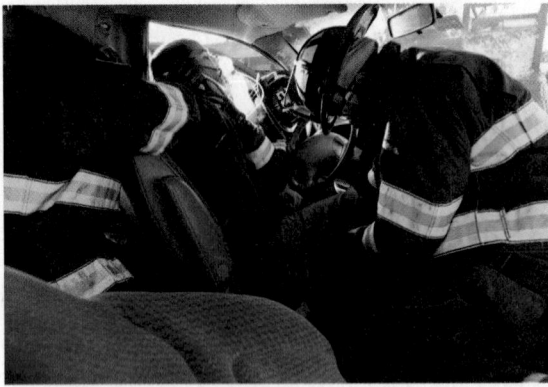

3. While one EMT maintains manual stabilization of the head, other EMTs rotate the patient in small increments by communicating with one another.

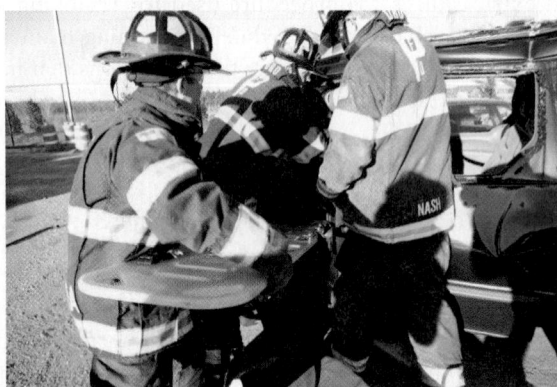

4. When the patient is in position to be reclined onto the long backboard, it is placed on the seat of the vehicle, against the patient's buttocks. The head end of the board can either be held by additional EMTs or placed on the stretcher for support. Communicate the slow and steady reclining of the patient onto the board while maintaining manual stabilization of the head and supporting the torso.

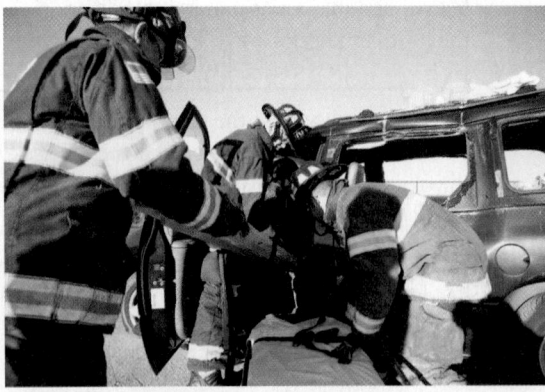

5. Ensure that the head is maintained in a neutral position and the torso remains supported as the patient is reclined onto the LSB.

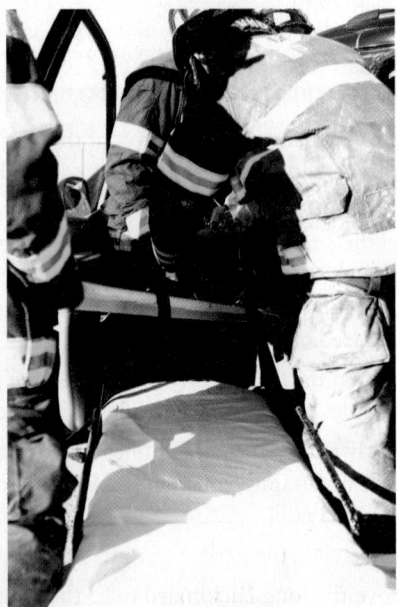

6. Slide the patient into correct position with short calculated movements.

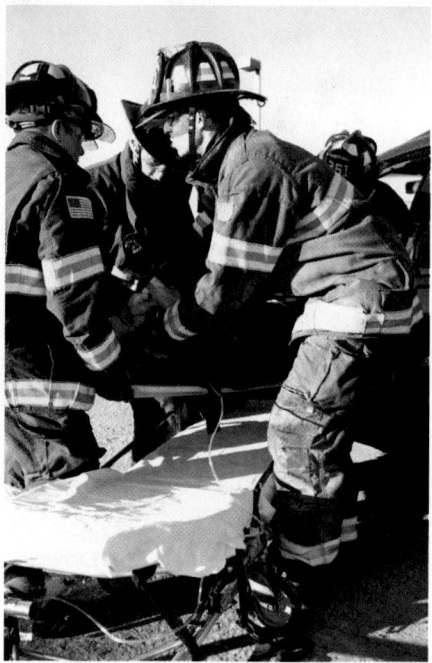

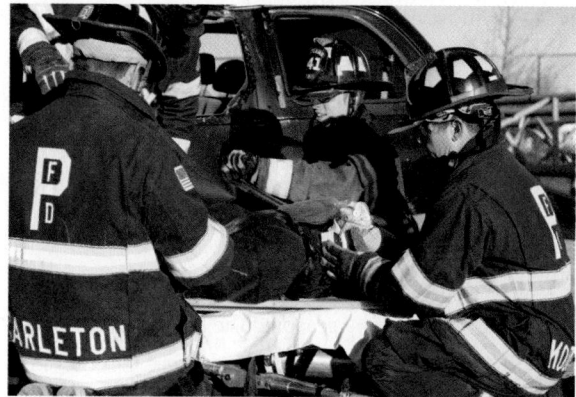

8. Maintain manual stabilization of the head as the torso is secured. Once the torso is secured, the head is then secured to the LSB.

7. The LSB should then be slid into proper position on the stretcher.

Football-Related Injuries

As an Advanced EMT, you will likely stand by at football games as a public service or be called to manage an injury at a game in your area. In many cases, there will be athletic trainers present to assist the players with injuries during the game. They will have the tools necessary to remove helmet facemasks in their kits and will be there to assist you in the event of an injury that requires you to treat a player. Those professionals are, in most cases, trained at the EMT level and can be a valuable resource to you. Many of the injuries

sustained in football involve the potential for spine injury, and the equipment worn in football presents unique problems regarding patient care.

For example, when a player is wearing shoulder pads and helmet, he will be in a neutral position when lying supine. If the helmet is removed and the player is placed in the supine position, the head will be hyperextended due to the thickness of the shoulder pads (Figure 40-8). It is important that you remember this if you remove the patient's helmet and intend to immobilize him. As discussed in the previous section, you must determine whether the

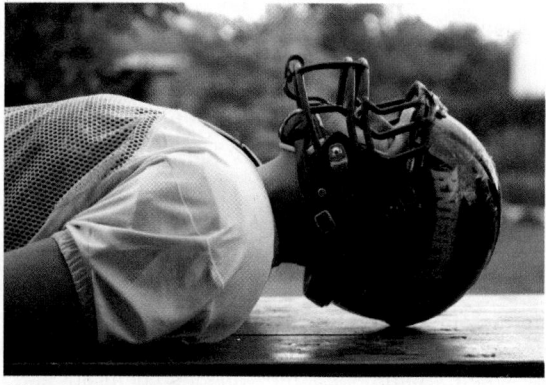

(A)   (B)

FIGURE 40-8

(A) When the patient's helmet and shoulder pads are on, the patient will be in a neutral position. (B) When the helmet is removed, the patient's neck will be hyperflexed due to the thickness of the shoulder pads.

helmet fits well enough to prevent movement of the head within it. In most cases, football helmets are fitted to the player and will not allow for movement.

Another point to consider is whether the helmet will allow for easy access to the airway. Football helmets all have face masks that will not allow adequate access to the airway. You must remove these face masks. The proper procedure for removing a face mask from a football helmet is as follows:

1. EMT #1 performs manual stabilization of the head and neck by grasping the helmet at the sides.

2. EMT #2 removes the face mask clips. Cut the side clips first, because it will allow the face mask to be tilted up for immediate access to the airway. You can then cut the top clips. It is sometimes recommended that a power screwdriver be used, but in many cases the screws will not easily be removed in a timely manner without manipulating the head and neck. In such cases, you should cut the clips using a pair of anvil shears or a face mask extractor (Figure 40-9).

3. Once the clips are cut, remove the face mask. You can then immobilize the patient onto a long backboard.

In some cases, you may need to immediately manage the patient's airway. It is appropriate then to remove the helmet, taking care as much as possible not to manipulate the spine. When faced with this situation, you should follow

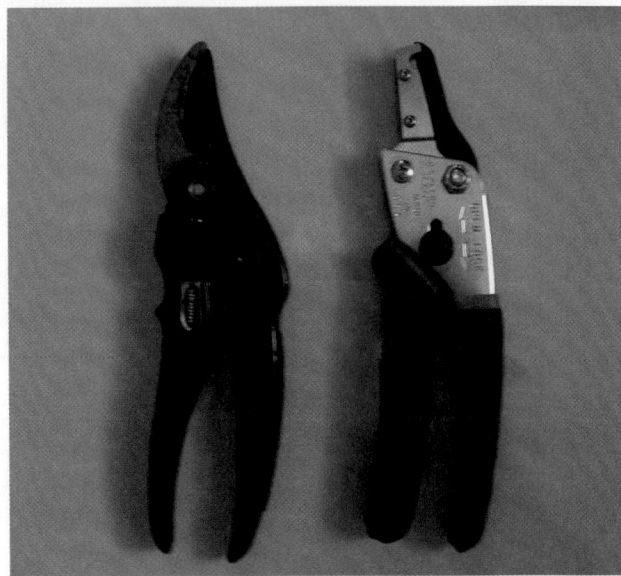

(A) Anvil Shears   (B) Extractor

FIGURE 40-9

(A) Anvil shears or (B) a face mask extractor can be used to cut the clips securing a face mask. (© Jeff Hinshaw, MS, PA-C, NREMT-P)

the same steps for removing a full-face helmet described earlier in this chapter. Remember that if the helmet is removed and the shoulder pads are not, you must pad beneath the patient's head during the immobilization process so that the spine will be in a neutral position.

CASE STUDY WRAP-UP

Clinical-Reasoning Process

Sarah and Ashley are on the scene of a patient involved in a helicopter crash, in which the helicopter made a sudden 60-foot vertical drop. The patient, Mr. Hadley, is ambulatory and complaining of low back pain. A firefighter is providing manual cervical-spine stabilization.

Sarah and Ashley recognize that the mechanism of injury was sudden vertical deceleration. Not only is the mechanism consistent with a compression injury to the lumbar spine, but it is also consistent with shearing injury to internal structures. Although the patient's vital signs are not an immediate concern and there is no known anatomical injury that meets trauma triage criteria, the mechanism of injury is consistent with a high-energy impact. In addition, the patient is older than 55 years, which statistically increases his risk of injury. Although the patient is alert and does not have immediate life threats, the potential for injury is significant.

"Mr. Hadley," Ashley begins, "I'm going to check your ability to move your hands and feet. When I'm finished we are going to place a stiff collar around your neck and lower you to the ground on the long backboard the firefighters are setting up behind you. Okay?"

"I'm ready when you are," replies Mr. Hadley.

Once the patient is completely immobilized and loaded into the ambulance, Sarah obtains a set of vital signs while Ashley completes a head-to-toe secondary assessment. There are no abnormal physical findings, but the patient reports that his back pain is increasing. Climbing into the driver's seat, Sarah notes the patient's complaint and recognizes the need for a smooth ride. "It's going to take us about 20 minutes to get the hospital," Ashley tells Mr. Hadley. "I'll recheck your vital signs on the way in, but in the meantime, if your pain increases or anything else doesn't seem right, let me know, okay? I'm going to let the hospital know we're on our way and see if I can get you some medication for pain."

If the patient's condition requires access to the chest such as with cardiac arrest or chest injury, you must cut the front strings that secure the shoulder pads, spread the pads apart, and gently slide them from beneath the patient. Remember that removing the shoulder pads will cause the head to be hyperflexed if the helmet is not removed. Either remove the helmet or pad beneath the torso of the patient so that the neck is in a neutral position.

Immobilizing Infants and Children

Use the same procedure for immobilizing infants and children as with adults. However, you must be aware of some specific differences in order to immobilize them properly. For example, you must use an appropriately sized board

or commercial pediatric immobilization device and appropriately sized rigid cervical collars.

Note also that infants and children have larger heads than adult patients. Therefore, when they are in a supine position, their necks will be slightly flexed. To adjust for this, you will apply padding beneath the patient's torso so the neck is in a neutral position.

Often, you will find an infant or child restrained in a car safety seat following an MVC. In such cases, you should take or direct another EMT to perform manual stabilization of the head and neck. Size and apply a rigid cervical collar. Then remove the patient from the seat onto a long backboard or commercial pediatric immobilization device.

CHAPTER REVIEW

Chapter Summary

The decisions that you must make about the appropriate management of suspected spine injuries are relatively straightforward. If a significant mechanism of injury is present, or if the patient exhibits signs and symptoms of spine injury, you will immobilize him. If immobilization is not indicated, you will not immobilize him, because doing so will cause undue stress and discomfort.

When immobilizing a patient, it is vital that you do so appropriately. Always follow your protocol. Inappropriate immobilization techniques can lead to additional injury to the patient and leave the patient permanently disabled. The care that you provide to spine-injured patients will reduce the likelihood of worsening the patient's condition and reduce the possibility of devastating, lifelong disability.

Review Questions

Multiple-Choice Questions

1. Which one of the following is the most common mechanism of spine injury?
   a. Penetrating trauma
   b. Motor vehicle collisions
   c. Falls
   d. Sports injuries

2. What region of the spine consists of seven vertebrae?
   a. Lumbar
   b. Sacral
   c. Cervical
   d. Thoracic

3. In which region of the spine do most spine injuries occur?
   a. Cervical
   b. Thoracic
   c. Lumbar
   d. Sacral

4. Which one of the following conditions would be considered the primary concern for patients who have a high cervical-spine injury?
   a. Neurogenic shock
   b. Quadriplegia
   c. Neurogenic hypotension
   d. Paralysis of the diaphragm leading to respiratory insufficiency

5. Descending spinal tracts of the spinal cord are responsible for:
   a. sensation of light touch.
   b. sensation of pain.
   c. muscle activity and tone.
   d. sensation of temperature.

6. Secondary injury to the spinal cord is a result of:
   a. hyperflexion.
   b. lateral bending.
   c. swelling.
   d. distraction.

Critical-Thinking Questions

7. Use your knowledge of anatomy, physiology, and pathophysiology to explain how neurologic shock occurs and what its signs are.

8. What factors could make a patient's information about the possibility of spine injury unreliable?

9. Explain how it is possible for a spine-injured patient to initially present without neurologic deficits but develop signs and symptoms over the next few hours.

10. What should you consider in determining whether rapid extrication is appropriate for a patient involved in an MVC?

11. How is it possible for a patient with a spine injury to present with loss of movement only on one side and loss of sensation only on the other?

References

Elahi, M. M., Brar, M. S., Ahmed, N., Howley, D. B., Nishtar, S., & Mahoney, J. L. (2008). Cervical-spine injury in association with craniomaxillofacial fractures. *Plastic and Reconstructive Surgery, 121*(1), 201–208.

McSwain, N. E., Salomone, J. P., Pons, P. T. (Eds). (2007). *Prehospital trauma life support* (6th ed.). St. Louis, MO: Elsevier.

Mulligan, R. F., Friedman, J. A., & Mahabir, R. C. (2010). A nationwide review of the associations among cervical spine injuries, head injuries, and facial fractures. *Journal of Trauma, 68*(3), 587–592.

Williams, J., Jehle, D., Cottington, E., & Sufflebarger, C. (1992). Head, facial, and clavicular trauma as a predictor of cervical-spine injury. *Annals of Emergency Medicine, 21*(6), 719–722.

41

Environmental Emergencies

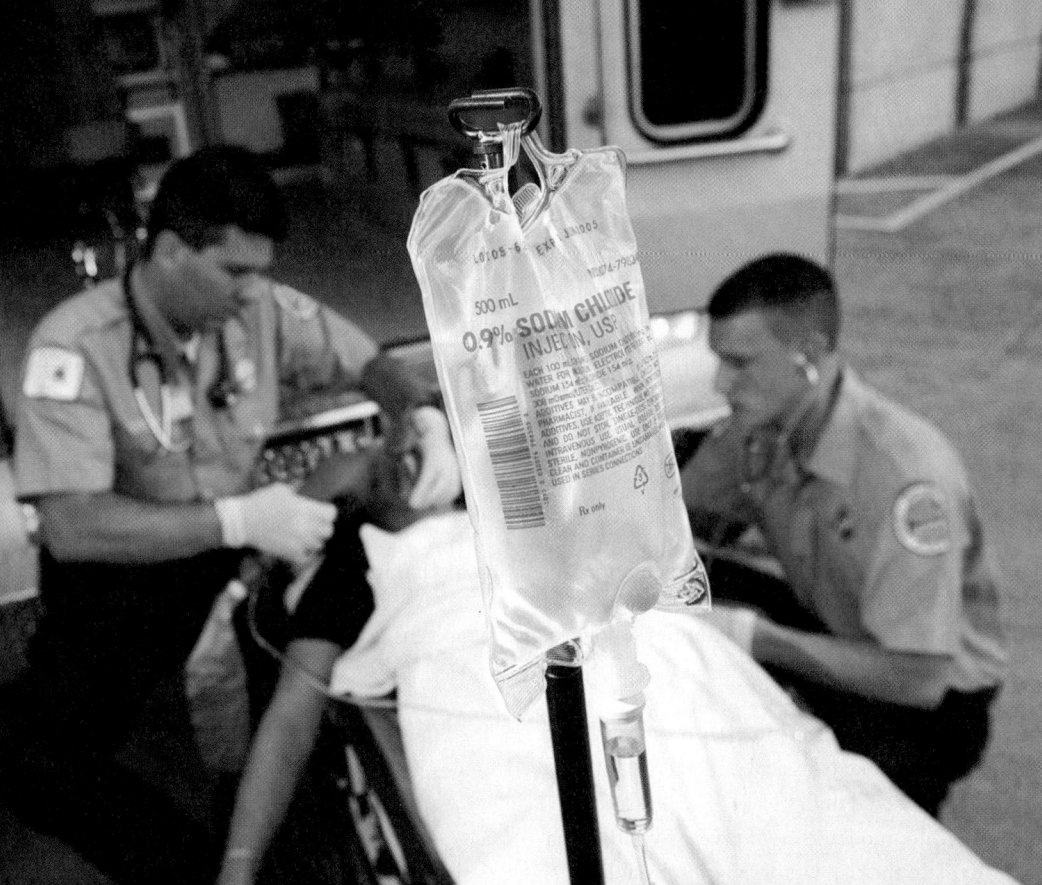

Content Area: Trauma

Advanced EMT Education Standard: The Advanced EMT applies fundamental knowledge to provide basic and selected advanced emergency care and transportation based on assessment findings for an acutely injured patient.

Objectives

After reading this chapter, you should be able to:

41.1   Define key terms introduced in this chapter.

41.2   Explain actions you should take to protect your own safety when responding to environmental emergencies.

41.3   Describe the scene size-up, primary and secondary assessment, and management of environmental emergencies, to include the following:

– Deep-water diving injuries

– High-altitude sickness

– Lightning strike

– Local cold injuries

– Drowning

– Systemic heat and cold injuries

(continued)

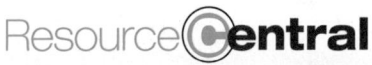

To access Resource Central, follow the directions on the Student Access Card provided with this text. If there is no card, go to www.bradybooks.com and follow the Resource Central link to Buy Access. Under Media Resources, you will find:

• *Effects of Venomous Snake Bites.* Effects and management.

• *Information about Hypothermia.* Types, effects, and high-risk people.

• *Hyperthermia.* Types and prevention.

• *Emergency: Near Drowning.* Reasons it occurs and its effects.

• *How to Remove a Tick.* Removing a tick, plus more on Lyme disease.

CASE STUDY

It is 1500 hours when Advanced EMTs Jennifer Mitchell and Harry Cole are at their station relaxing for a few minutes between calls. The air conditioned station is a welcome relief from the 96°F temperature and 80 percent humidity outside. After just a few minutes inside the station, dispatch calls, "Unit 36, respond to a heat-related emergency at 500 Tunnel Boulevard."

The address that the two Advanced EMTs respond to is a construction site where concrete is being poured for a parking lot adjacent to a new department store. As they approach the scene, they notice a man lying on the concrete while others are pouring water on him and fanning his body. The man does not appear to be conscious or moving.

Problem-Solving Questions

1. What problems do you think Jennifer and Harry have identified so far?
2. What hypotheses should Jennifer and Harry be developing?
3. What information supports each hypothesis they may be developing?
4. What will they need to find out to test each hypothesis?
5. What should be their immediate actions?

(continued from previous page)

41.4   Explain the process of thermoregulation, including mechanisms by which the body gains and loses heat.

41.5   Explain the risk factors, pathophysiology, signs, symptoms, assessment, and management of the following:
   – Heat cramps
   – Heat exhaustion
   – Heatstroke (classical and exertional)
   – Local cold injury
   – Mild, moderate, and severe hypothermia

41.6   Explain the risk factors, pathophysiology, signs, symptoms, assessment, and management of lightning strike injuries.

41.7   Explain the following gas laws as they relate to high altitude and deep-water diving emergencies:
   – Boyle's law
   – Charles' law
   – Dalton's law
   – Henry's law

41.8   Explain the risk factors, pathophysiology, signs, symptoms, assessment, and management of high-altitude sickness and dysbarism to include the following:
   – Acute mountain sickness
   – Arterial gas embolism
   – Barotrauma
   – Decompression sickness
   – High-altitude cerebral edema
   – High-altitude pulmonary edema
   – Nitrogen narcosis

41.9   Explain the risk factors, pathophysiology, signs, symptoms, assessment, and management of drowning.

41.10 Recognize additional mechanisms of injury and illness that are associated with drowning, such as trauma and hypothermia.

41.11 Explain factors that affect the likelihood of survival from drowning.

Introduction

Environmental emergencies occur when normal body processes are affected by external conditions such as temperature, submersion in water, lightning, and changes in atmospheric pressure. When cold, the body conserves heat, and when hot, the body eliminates heat. The mechanisms by which the body regulates temperature have limitations; therefore, when the environmental conditions are such that the mechanisms are no longer effective, an emergency situation occurs. Calls for environmental emergencies can involve risks to emergency personnel, who can be subject to the same environmental conditions that led to the patient's emergency. Be aware of the risks and take measures to protect yourself. Then protect your patient from further exposure to the environment.

Heat- and Cold-Related Emergencies

Despite wide variations in environmental temperature, the body maintains a normal core temperature through thermoregulation as a result of its ability to recognize how hot or cold it is. In extreme environmental temperatures, particularly with prolonged exposure, the body's thermoregulatory mechanisms are overwhelmed and the body temperature can increase or decrease, leading to illness. In hot conditions, sweating and vasodilation can lead to hypovolemia and loss of electrolytes. In cold conditions, the tissues can be affected locally, as well, resulting in frostbite and related conditions. A number of risk factors can increase a patient's susceptibility to changes in environmental temperature.

Anatomy and Physiology Review

Thermoregulation is the process by which the body regulates its core body temperature. Core temperature is not the same as skin, or shell temperature. Core temperature is the temperature of the blood and internal organs. The body detects core temperature through **thermoreceptors**, which are sensory nerve endings that monitor temperature within the body. Thermoreceptors have two classifications: central thermoreceptors and peripheral thermoreceptors. Central thermoreceptors are located on or near the hypothalamus within the brain. Peripheral thermoreceptors are located in the mucous membranes of the body and skin. When the thermoreceptors send signals to the brain about core temperature, the hypothalamus reacts by activating temperature regulatory mechanisms.

A **thermal gradient** is the difference between body and environmental temperatures. Very seldom is the ambient temperature (room temperature or the actual temperature of an environment) the same as normal body temperature, 98.6°F (37°C), which means that the body must regulate the amount of heat lost and gained to maintain a normal core temperature. This regulation is accomplished through two processes: thermogenesis and thermolysis.

Thermogenesis is the process of generating heat. Heat is a product of energy production within the cells. Heat is generated by contraction of muscles, such as shivering or moving about, increasing heart rate and force of contraction, and increasing the metabolic rate of the body (through the release of nonepinephrine and epinephrine into the bloodstream).

Thermolysis is the process of transferring heat from the body to the environment. This transfer of heat is accomplished by five mechanisms (Figure 41-1), described as follows:

- *Conduction.* Heat transfer from the body to a cooler object by direct contact is called **conduction**. For example, during a hot summer day, you may sit on the shaded ground under a tree. The ground is cooler than your body temperature; therefore, heat will be transferred from your body to the cooler ground.

- *Convection.* Heat transfer to air molecules that are passed across the skin due to a moving air current is called **convection**. For example, fanning yourself when you feel warm assists in cooling your body. As heat is transferred from your body to the immediately surrounding air, fanning removes the warmer air, replacing it with cooler air, increasing the thermal gradient and facilitating further heat loss. In the winter, the wind chill factor is figured into the weather forecast. The *wind chill factor* is the effect that wind has on how we perceive how cold it is. As wind speed increases, so does the rate at which we lose body heat. High wind speeds can cause a moderately cold winter day feel much colder, and the body to lose heat faster than in the same temperature with no wind.

- *Radiation.* Heat transfer from the body without physical contact is called **radiation**. It is the primary means of heat loss from the body that, under normal conditions, accounts for approximately 60 percent of total heat loss. When core body temperature increases, vasodilation occurs in the skin allowing for more blood to flow closer to the skin where heat can be eliminated through radiation. When vasodilation occurs, the skin becomes "flushed," or red in color. In colder temperatures, vasoconstriction occurs to prevent the blood from losing heat near the surface of the skin. The areas of the body that radiate the most heat are the head, hands, and feet. Removing layers of clothing that trap heat against your skin—especially at the head, hands, and feet—will allow you to cool off.

- *Evaporation.* Sweat vaporizing and dissipating from the skin carrying the heat with it is called **evaporation**. The amount of evaporation depends on the relative humidity of the environment. In conditions where the relative humidity is 75 percent or higher, evaporation is significantly reduced. Undoubtedly, you have noticed that on humid days it feels hotter

MECHANISMS OF HEAT LOSS

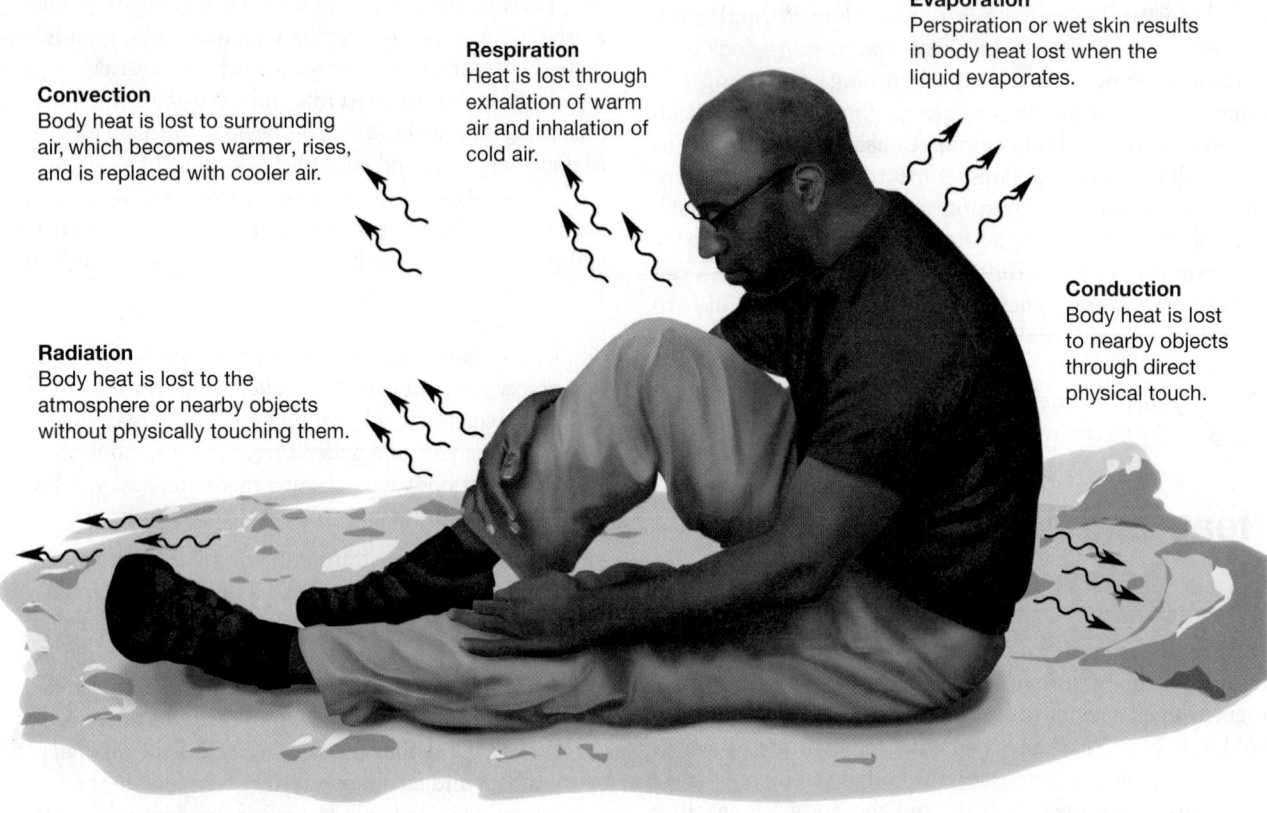

Convection
Body heat is lost to surrounding air, which becomes warmer, rises, and is replaced with cooler air.

Respiration
Heat is lost through exhalation of warm air and inhalation of cold air.

Evaporation
Perspiration or wet skin results in body heat lost when the liquid evaporates.

Conduction
Body heat is lost to nearby objects through direct physical touch.

Radiation
Body heat is lost to the atmosphere or nearby objects without physically touching them.

FIGURE 41-1

Mechanisms of heat loss.

than the actual temperature. Sweat does not evaporate to cool you, and your skin and clothes remain wet. Heat index is a calculation of how hot it feels at specific temperatures and relative humidity levels. As evaporation is reduced as a result of increasing relative humidity, the temperature feels hotter to us. For example, at a temperature of 90°F with a relative humidity of 40 percent, the heat index is 95°F. When the relative humidity increases to 70 percent, the heat index increases to 106°F, which places individuals at increased risk for heat-related emergencies.

■ *Respiration.* When air enters the body through the nose and mouth and travels through the airway into the lungs, it is warmed and humidified. When the air is

Geriatric Care

Geriatric patients often suffer a decrease in their ability to regulate core body temperature through thermoregulation. This makes them susceptible to extremes in temperature and at a higher risk for heat- and cold-related emergencies.

exhaled, it includes the heat and water transferred to it by the body. The body loses heat and water with every breath. Normally, the heat is replaced quickly with metabolically generated heat and the water is replaced through normal fluid intake.

Risk Factors for Heat- and Cold-Related Emergencies

Some factors contribute to a person's ability to regulate core body temperature. The following factors increase a person's likelihood of heat- and cold-related emergencies:

■ *Patient age.* Pediatric and geriatric patients cannot tolerate extremes of temperature as a healthy adult patient can. Pediatric patients do not have mature

Pediatric Care

Cover a child or infant's head as well as the body in a cold environment because large amounts of heat can be lost from the head through radiation. This is due to the relatively large size of a child's or infant's head in relation to the rest of the body.

thermoregulatory mechanisms to assist them in temperature regulation. Conversely, geriatric patients' thermoregulatory mechanisms have declined with age.

- *Patient health.* Patients with pre-existing medical conditions, such as diabetes, lose the efficiency of their autonomic nervous system, which can interfere with normal thermoregulatory mechanisms. Patients who are immobile cannot remove themselves from an unsuitable environment, increasing the duration of exposure. Kidney disease, cardiovascular disease, extensive diseases of the skin, and other chronic illnesses can impact thermoregulation.

- *Medications.* Some medications can inhibit thermoregulatory mechanisms. They include diuretics, antihistamines, antipsychotics, and beta blockers. Medications or other substances that impair judgment, such as alcohol and drugs of abuse, also increase the risk of heat- and cold-related emergencies.

- *Length of exposure.* The longer a patient is exposed to extremes in temperature, the more likely it is that they will suffer a heat- or cold-related emergency.

- *Intensity of exposure.* The hotter or colder the environment, the more likely it is that the patient will suffer an environmental emergency.

- *Socioeconomic factors.* People with limited incomes may not have adequate heat or cooling in their homes and may not have transportation to places with adequate heat or cooling. Malnutrition also decreases the ability to compensate for extremes in environmental temperature.

General Assessment and Management of Heat- and Cold-Related Emergencies

While an unusually hot or cold environment is a clue to a possible heat- or cold-related emergency, the environment does not necessarily have to be extreme for those problems to occur. Patients with impaired thermoregulation are at increased risk for environmental emergencies even in more moderate environments. For example, an elderly patient who has fallen onto a tile floor and cannot get up is losing heat by conduction to the coolness of the floor, as well as by radiation to the environment. In addition, the immobility prevents generation of heat through muscle movement and prevents the patient from getting a sweater or blanket that could help conserve body heat. Maintain an increased index of suspicion for heat- and cold-related emergencies in patients with risk factors, particularly when you cannot find another explanation for the patient's presentation.

Scene Size-Up

The presence of an environmental emergency may not be known from the dispatch information. Keep an open mind

during all scene size-ups for clues to the nature of the emergency, no matter what dispatch information was provided. Remember: the dispatcher relies on information from the caller, who may not be able to give exact information about the nature of the emergency. A call for a sick person or intoxicated person at a bus stop may very well involve a heat- or cold-related emergency. Also keep in mind that an environmental emergency can accompany another emergency. Patients involved in motor vehicle collisions (MVCs) may become hypothermic in a very short period of time while awaiting response. Every minute spent in the environment increases their risk of environmental emergencies in addition to their injuries.

During the scene size-up, look for potential hazards. The same environment that has been detrimental to the patient's condition can affect you and your partners. As a general rule, consider temperatures of 90°F or greater and relative humidity of greater than 75 percent an environment that is ideal for heat emergencies to occur (Figure 41-2). Identify the number of patients, determine the need for additional resources, and form a general impression of the patient. Does he seem to be responsive or unresponsive? Is he flushed, pale, mottled, sweating, or shivering? Is he dressed appropriately for the environment?

You may be very busy responding to heat-related emergencies during extended heat waves. To prevent yourself from becoming ill do the following:

- Maintain adequate fluid intake

- Allow time for gradual acclimatization to the heat prior to physical exertion

- Limit time of exposure

In cold weather, dress appropriately, which should include your footwear, a hat, and warm gloves in addition to your coat and layered clothing.

Primary Assessment

Heat- and cold-related emergencies can be accompanied by a decreased level of responsiveness, which in turn jeopardizes the patient's ability to maintain his airway. Central nervous system depression also can impair breathing effort. Extremes in temperature can affect circulation by affecting heart function and through fluid loss. Ensure the adequacy of the patient's airway, breathing, and circulation. Once all immediate life threats have been addressed, remove the patient from the extreme environment and take measures to stabilize the patient's body temperature. Determine

---

IN THE FIELD

As an Advanced EMT, you will be called to work in hot environments, sometimes for extended periods of time. You are not immune to becoming a patient yourself, so you must take the necessary steps to prevent hyperthermia.

Temperature (°F) versus Relative Humidity (%)						
°F	90%	80%	70%	60%	50%	40%
80	85	84	82	81	80	79
85	101	96	92	90	86	84
90	121	113	105	99	94	90
95		133	122	113	105	98
100			142	129	118	109
105				148	133	121
110						135

HI	Possible Heat Disorder:
80°F - 90°F	Fatigue possible with prolonged exposure and physical activity.
90°F - 105°F	Sunstroke, heat cramps, and heat exhaustion possible.
105°F - 130°F	Sunstroke, heat cramps, and heat exhaustion likely, and heatstroke possible.
130°F or greater	Heat stroke highly likely with continued exposure.

FIGURE 41-2

The risk of heat-related emergencies increases with increased heat and humidity.

if the patient is critical or non-critical and make decisions about your next steps in assessment, management, and transport according to the patient's condition.

Secondary Assessment

If the nature of the problem is not known, perform a rapid secondary exam to identify potentially life-threatening conditions that may not have been evident in the primary assessment. Obtain baseline vital signs, obtain a medical history, and perform either a head-to-toe or focused examination, depending on the patient's condition. Although a body temperature is not usually obtained in prehosptial care, it can be helpful to assess the patient's body temperature if you suspect a heat- or cold-related emergency. The use of monitoring devices can give valuable information. Use pulse oximetry, blood glucose monitoring, end tidal CO_2 monitoring, and cardiac monitoring as directed by your protocols. If a heat- or cold-related emergency is possible, obtain information related to the events leading up to the emergency including the temperature, humidity, wind, and length of exposure to the environment

Reassessment

En route to the emergency department, reassess critical patients at least every 5 minutes and every 15 minutes for non-critical patients to detect trends in condition, including level of responsiveness; airway, breathing, and circulation; vital signs, including body temperature; and the effects of interventions.

Specific Heat-Related Emergencies

Heat-related emergencies are categorized as heat cramps, heat exhaustion, and heatstroke. Although heat cramps are usually not accompanied by hyperthermia, heat exhaustion can be, and heatstroke is always accompanied by hyperthermia. If an individual is working in a hot environment and becomes ill he can progress from heat cramps to heat exhaustion or from heat exhaustion to heatstroke if he does not take steps to cool down and replace fluids and electrolytes. However, some individuals present initially with heatstroke. As the body attempts to cool itself, you will see signs of thermolysis including sweating and hot, flushed skin. Paradoxically, the patient with heat exhaustion, which is a mild form of shock, may have cool, clammy skin. Patients with classic heatstroke may have hot, dry skin because the body's thermoregulatory mechanism of sweating has ceased to function.

Heat Cramps

Heat cramps are the least severe of all heat-related emergencies. Muscle groups, often those of the lower extremities, cramp in response to overexertion and dehydration in a hot environment. The primary problem is loss of electrolytes, such as sodium and chloride. Profuse sweating leads to an electrolyte imbalance, which causes the cramping of

As an Advanced EMT, you will likely be required to stand by at festivals, parades, or other public events all day long. In such cases, you and your partner should be prepared by ensuring that you have access to shade and adequate amounts of water to drink.

muscles. The signs and symptoms of heat cramps include the following:

- Cramping of the larger muscles of the body (generally the abdominal muscles and muscles of the arms and legs)
- Weakness
- Possible complaints of lightheadedness or dizziness

If the patient is alert and is not nauseated the preferred management is to remove the patient from the hot environment and administer an oral electrolyte replacement fluid, such as a non-caffeinated sports drink. Some services have their response units carry coolers of oral fluids during extremely hot, humid weather. In some cases, your protocols may specify the use of a half-strength sports drink. Gentle massage and stretching may help with the muscle cramps. If the patient is nauseated or so uncomfortable that he cannot drink, or has a decreased level of responsiveness, start an IV of isotonic fluid, such as normal saline, and infuse according to your protocols.

Heat Exhaustion

Heat exhaustion is a moderate heat-related illness characterized by inadequate perfusion that results in a mild state of shock. This state of mild shock is the result of increased vasodilation in the peripheral circulation, which leads to pooling of blood in the vessels of the skin. Prolonged and profuse sweating leads to loss of circulating blood volume and results in inadequate circulation.

Signs and symptoms of heat exhaustion include the following:

- Body temperature greater than 100°F (37.8°C)
- Cool and diaphoretic skin
- Tachypnea
- Weak pulses
- Possible muscle cramping
- Weakness
- Headache
- Dizziness
- Anxiety
- Altered mental status (possible loss of consciousness)

Remove the patient from the hot environment and remove heavy clothing that prevents heat loss to the environment. Do not allow the patient to become chilled. Shivering will increase heat production by the muscles. Management of heat exhaustion includes the administration of fluids orally, as described for heat cramps, if the patient is alert and is not nauseated.

Heatstroke

Heatstroke is a life-threatening condition that occurs when the body's thermoregulatory mechanisms cease to work. Heatstroke is characterized by a core body temperature of greater than 104°F (greater than 40°C) and has a mortality rate that ranges from 20 to 80 percent. Because the thermoregulatory mechanisms no longer work, the core body temperature rises uncontrollably resulting in the destruction of brain cells, which leads to permanent disability or death.

Heatstroke occurs in two circumstances, referred to as classic heatstroke and exertional heatstroke. The history of classic heatstroke is often that of an elderly or ill person who is unable to escape a hot environment, such as a poorly ventilated apartment without air conditioning during a heat wave. **Exertional heatstroke** occurs in those who are working in a hot environment, which may be outdoors during a heat wave, or indoors in a factory or other hot setting. This type of heatstroke is a concern for firefighters, who wear heavy clothing to work near intense sources of heat; and in athletes.

Signs and symptoms of heatstroke include the following:

- Altered mental status
- Cessation of sweating, although the skin can still be moist or wet in exertional heatstroke
- Hot, flushed skin
- High core body temperature
- Deep, rapid respiration that can become slow and shallow
- Tachycardia that can proceed to bradycardia
- Hypotension
- Possible seizures

Rapid identification and rapid, effective treatment of heatstroke can decrease morbidity and mortality rates. After the primary assessment and removing the patient from the hot environment, begin rapidly cooling him by removing his clothing and either covering him with a wet sheet or misting the skin with water and fanning him. Your goal is to decrease the core temperature to 102°F (39°C). Place cold packs in the groin (on either side of the genitalia), under the arms, and on either side of the neck, because these are areas where large blood vessels are located just beneath the skin. Do not cool the patient to the point at which shivering occurs. (Shivering generates heat.) If shivering begins, cover the patient lightly until the shivering stops. Initiate two

CASE STUDY (continued)

Jennifer and Harry advise dispatch that they are on scene, grab their gear, and approach the patient who is lying supine in the direct sunlight. When they get to the patient's side, the patient's coworker tells Harry that the patient had been complaining of dizziness and weakness for the past hour or so but continued to work. They saw the patient stagger a little bit and then sit down on the ground. When they ran to him, he was speaking with slurred speech and breathing very fast.

Jennifer begins to assess the patient and notes that his skin is very flushed, hot, and dry. His heart rate is 110, strong and regular, at the radial pulse and his respiratory rate is 24 with adequate depth. He is not responding to verbal stimuli and only moans to painful stimulus.

Problem-Solving Questions

1. What hypotheses might have moved higher on Jennifer and Harry's list, and which might have moved lower?
2. How might the information obtained have changed Jennifer and Harry's priorities for patient care and transport?
3. What should be their next actions?

large-bore IVs of isotonic crystalloid solution, such as normal saline. Fluid losses may exceed 1 to 1.5 liters. Follow your protocols in determining the total amount of fluids to be administered and the rate of administration. Be prepared to manage seizures.

Specific Cold-Related Emergencies

Cold temperature exposure can produce two types of emergencies. Generalized hypothermia affects the body as a whole. Local cold injuries affect isolated areas of the body that are exposed to freezing or near-freezing conditions.

Generalized Hypothermia

Generalized hypothermia is a condition where the core body temperature drops below 95°F (35°C). Severe hypothermia is a life-threatening condition that can have a mortality rate of more than 80 percent under given circumstances.

When core body temperature drops to 95°F (35°C), the body's thermoregulation mechanisms fail and core body temperature falls quickly. As the core body temperature falls, cardiac output decreases and ultimately leads to cardiac arrest. Death can occur quickly. Prehospital care is a critical phase of resuscitaiton of hypothermic patients.

PERSONAL PERSPECTIVE

Advanced EMT Brian Bishop: On a pleasant spring day we were called to respond to an injured person at the river. It was sunny with a slight breeze and the temperature was in the low 70s. We found the patient seated on a bench wrapped in a blanket. He was confused, shivering, and his skin was pale. He told us that he was driving his boat in the river when he hit something under the water causing him to be thrown from the boat. He was wearing a flotation device and managed to swim to the bank where he remained for a few hours before flagging down a passing boat. The people in the other boat called 911 and brought him to the boat launch.

The patient was still wearing his wet clothing. I assisted the patient in removing them, and completed a primary assessment, which revealed slow respirations, bradycardia, and mild hypotension. We began rewarming the patient by wrapping him in blankets and placing warm packs in the blankets. We transported him to the closest hopsital, a level II trauma center. By the time we arrived, the patient's vital signs were beginning to improve and he had stopped shivering.

This patient was hypothermic because he was thrown into cold water and remained wet in a cool breeze for a substantial amount of time. Luckily, another boat passed and he was able to flag them down. Had he remained in the cool environment longer he would have certainly become more unstable and, if he had been stranded overnight, would have probably died.

Management of this emergency is very simple but you must understand how contributing factors affect patient condition. In this case, it was cold water temperature, cool ambient temperature, presence of a breeze, the length of exposure, and the fact that he remained wet.

Hypothermia can be classified as mild or severe, as follows:

- *Mild hypothermia* occurs when the core body temperature is between 90°F (32°C) and 95°F (35°C).

- *Severe hypothermia* occurs when core body temperature is less than 90°F (32°C)

As a person progresses from mild to severe hypothermia, the signs and symptoms are grouped into five stages, shown in Figures 41-3 and 41-4.

Treatment of hypothermic patients depends on the degree of hypothermia. After completing a primary assessment, managing the airway, breathing, and circulation, and removing the patient from the cold environment, you must stabilize his temperature. The way this is done depends on how cold the patient is. There are other differences in the assessment and management of severely hypothermic patients, as well.

For all hypothermic patients, do the following:

- Handle gently. Rough handling can induce cardiac dysrhythmias in hypothermia.

- Remove wet clothing to prevent further evaporative heat loss.

- Prevent further heat loss and exposure to wind or water by covering with blankets and moisture barriers.

- Monitor the core temperature, if equipped to do so.

- Monitor the cardiac rhythm, if equipped to do so.

For mild hypothermia, you also should do the following:

- Apply heat packs. Insulate the heat packs so they do not burn the skin.

- Start IVs with warmed fluids (95°F to 100°F or 35°C to 38°C).

- If available, particularly if warmed IV fluids are not available and transport is delayed, you can give warm, sweetened fluids orally to patients who are alert and not nauseated. Do not give beverages that contain alcohol or caffeine. Alcohol causes vasodilation, which can increase heat loss. Caffeine causes vasoconstriction, which can increase local cold injury.

IN THE FIELD

You should never attempt to rescue a patient from cold water unless you have the proper equipment and have been trained to do so. Your first priority regarding safety is always your own safety.

STAGES OF HYPOTHERMIA

Stage 1: Shivering is a response by the body to generate heat. It does not typically occur below a body temperature of 90°F.

Stage 2: Apathy and decreased muscle function. First fine motor function is affected, then gross motor functions.

Stage 3: Decreased level of responsiveness is accompanied by a glassy stare and possible freezing of extremities.

Stage 4: Decreased vital signs, including slow pulse and slow respiration rate.

Stage 5: Death.

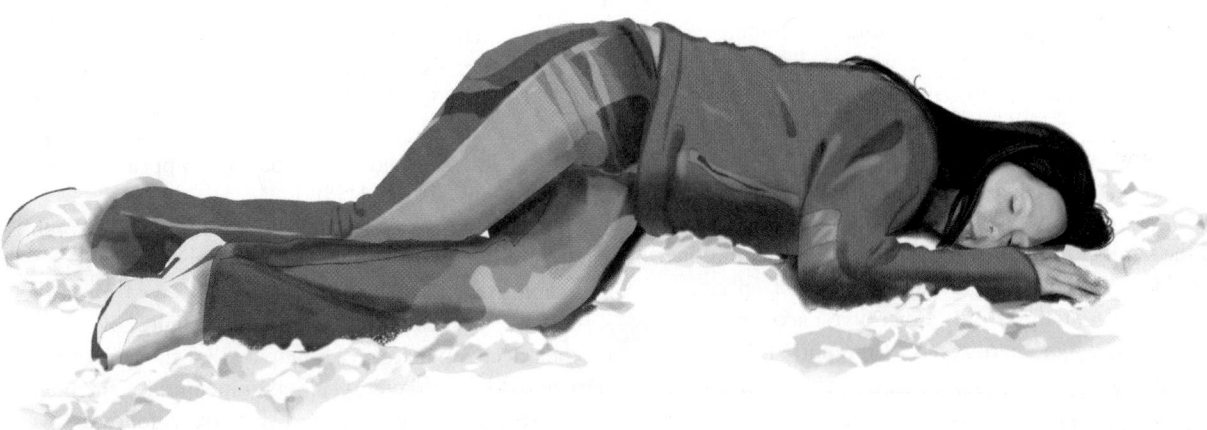

FIGURE 41-3

Five stages of hypothermia.

SIGNS AND SYMPTOMS OF HYPOTHERMIA

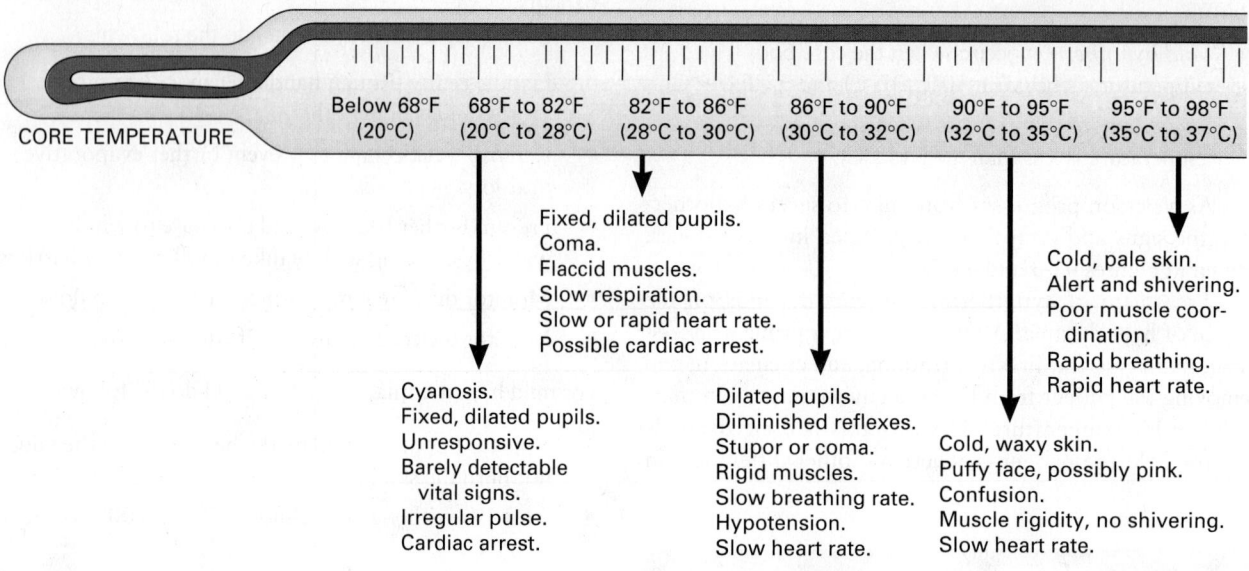

| CORE TEMPERATURE | Below 68°F (20°C) | 68°F to 82°F (20°C to 28°C) | 82°F to 86°F (28°C to 30°C) | 86°F to 90°F (30°C to 32°C) | 90°F to 95°F (32°C to 35°C) | 95°F to 98°F (35°C to 37°C) |

Fixed, dilated pupils.
Coma.
Flaccid muscles.
Slow respiration.
Slow or rapid heart rate.
Possible cardiac arrest.

Cold, pale skin.
Alert and shivering.
Poor muscle coor-
dination.
Rapid breathing.
Rapid heart rate.

Cyanosis.
Fixed, dilated pupils.
Unresponsive.
Barely detectable
vital signs.
Irregular pulse.
Cardiac arrest.

Dilated pupils.
Diminished reflexes.
Stupor or coma.
Rigid muscles.
Slow breathing rate.
Hypotension.
Slow heart rate.

Cold, waxy skin.
Puffy face, possibly pink.
Confusion.
Muscle rigidity, no shivering.
Slow heart rate.

FIGURE 41-4

Signs and symptoms of hypothermia as related to core body temperature.

For severe hypothermia, consider the following, according to the patient's condition:

- Do not attempt active rewarming with hot packs or IV fluids unless transport is delayed. If transport is delayed, follow your protocols regarding active rewarming. Application of external heat and warm peripheral IVs can cause rewarming shock, which leads to a further drop in core temperature. As cold, low-pH blood from the extremities returns to the central circulation, the core temperature drops.

- If the patient is pulseless and has no signs of life, start CPR and apply the AED. Your protocols may recommend checking the pulse of a hypothermic patient for longer than the 10 second maximum usually used because profound bradycardia can exist and the pulse may be difficult to detect due to the poor compliance of cold tissues and low cardiac output. The ideal number of defibrillation attempts in hypothermic patients has not been established (American Heart Association, 2010a). Follow your protocols with regard to the number of defibrillation attempts. Resuscitation should be started even if the downtime is not certain, because resuscitation from cardiac arrest accompanied by prolonged hypothermia has been reported.

- Use an advanced airway to provide an adequate airway and ventilation.

- Consider transportation to a facility with cardiac bypass capabilities, because cardiac bypass is an important step in core rewarming.

Local Cold Injury

Local cold injury can range from mild to severe, with the more severe form referred to as *frostbite*. Localized cold injuries can occur by themselves or in conjunction with hypothermia. Frostbite usually occurs in the distal extremities, the nose, and ears.

Frostbite occurs when the intracellular fluid freezes. The frozen fluid crystallizes and expands, causing tissue damage. Cells rupture and blood flow is interrupted. Early in frostbite, the superficial layers of tissue are affected. This is called *superficial frostbite* or *frostnip*. Tissues feel firm superficially, but soft beneath. The skin color first becomes red, then blanches. Initially, there is a loss of sensation, but as the part rewarms, burning and tingling can occur. With increased intensity of cold and increased duration of exposure the deeper tissues are affected, resulting in deep frostbite. The tissues feel hard and frozen and the area appears white. There is a loss of sensation, but pain can be excruciating as thawing begins. The part can appear mottled as thawing begins (Figure 41-5).

In general, frostbitten areas are not thawed in prehospital management. An exception would be having a patient in a remote area in which transport is delayed. Even then, if there is a possibility that the patient might have to walk on the affected part to reach help or that the part might be refrozen, do not thaw it. General guidelines for the prehospital care of the patient with frostbite are as follows:

- Do not massage the area or rub it. This will cause the ice crystals in the cells to do more damage to the tissues.

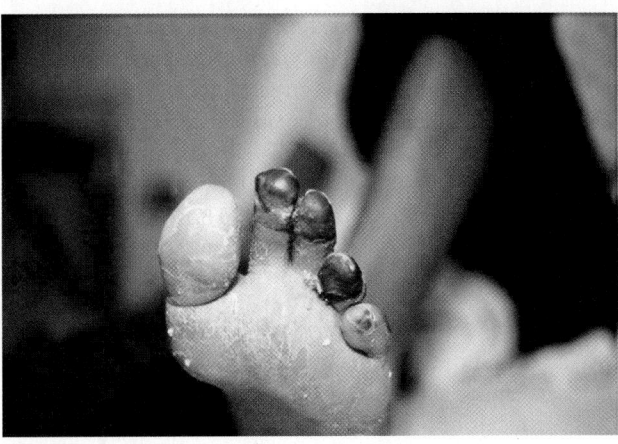

FIGURE 41-5

Deep local cold injury. (© Edward T. Dickinson, MD)

To protect yourself from frostbite, be aware of the following:

- Tight shoes or boots reduce circulation to the feet, increasing the risk of frostbite.

- Windy conditions increase the rate of heat loss. Be aware of the wind chill factor and cover exposed parts (Figure 41-6).

- Caffeine and nicotine cause vasoconstriction and increase the risk of frostbite.

Trench foot, also called *immersion foot*, is a localized cold injury that occurs when the feet are immersed in cold water, just above freezing temperatures, for prolonged periods. Although it is primary a problem in the military, it also can occur in hunters and others engaged in outdoor activities that involve having the feet wet in cold conditions for prolonged periods.

- If you must allow the area to thaw, first administer analgesia.

- Transport the patient to the hospital for rewarming. If you must rewarm the frostbitten body part in the field, immerse it in water that is 102°F to 104°F (39°C to 40°C). Add warm water as needed to maintain this temperature throughout thawing.

- Cover the frozen or thawed part with dry, sterile dressings, placing dressings between the fingers and toes and bandage loosely. Take care to avoid breaking any blisters that form.

- Keep the part elevated.

Drowning

According to the Utstein criteria for uniform reporting of data from drowning, "Unintentional **drowning** [emphasis added] is a process resulting in primary respiratory impairment from submersion/immersion in a liquid medium. Implicit in this definition is that a liquid/air interface is present at the entrance of the victim's airway, preventing the victim from breathing air. The victim may live or die after this process, but whatever the outcome, he or she has been involved in a drowning incident" (Idris, Berg, Bierens, Bossaert, Branche, et al., 2002). The use of older terms such as *submersion incident, near-drowning, wet drowning,* and *dry drowning* is no longer recommended.

WIND-CHILL INDEX

WIND SPEED (MPH)	WHAT THE THERMOMETER READS (degrees °F)											
	50	40	30	20	10	0	−10	−20	−30	−40	−50	−60
	WHAT IT EQUALS IN ITS EFFECT ON EXPOSED FLESH											
CALM	50	40	30	20	10	0	−10	−20	−30	−40	−50	−60
5	48	37	27	16	6	−5	−15	−26	−36	−47	−57	−68
10	40	28	16	4	−9	−21	−33	−46	−58	−70	−83	−95
15	36	22	9	−5	−18	−36	−45	−58	−72	−85	−99	−112
20	32	18	4	−10	−25	−39	−53	−67	−82	−96	−110	−121
25	30	16	0	−15	−29	−44	−59	−74	−88	−104	−118	−133
30	28	13	−2	−18	−33	−48	−63	−79	−94	−109	−125	−140
35	27	11	−4	−20	−35	−49	−67	−82	−98	−113	−129	−145
40	26	10	−6	−21	−37	−53	−69	−85	−100	−116	−132	−148

Little danger if properly clothed	Danger of freezing exposed flesh	Great danger of freezing exposed flesh

FIGURE 41-6

Wind chill index. (Courtesy of U.S. Army)

Demographics

Unintentional drowning is the seventh leading cause of death for all age groups, the second leading cause of death for ages 1 to 14 years, and the fifth leading cause of death for those under one year of age. Drowning accounts for approximately 3,500 deaths annually in the United States (American Heart Association, 2010b). The most common place that drowning occurs in children under one year of age is in the bathtub. In those cases, the parent or caregiver reported leaving the child alone for less than 5 minutes. In children 1 to 5 years of age, the most common place that drowning occurs is in swimming pools (McSwain, Salomone, & Pons, 2007).

Adolescents and adults drown most often in ponds, lakes, rivers, and oceans. In some of those cases, trauma such as cervical-spine injuries resulting from diving accidents, alcohol, or medical problems contribute to the drowning. However, spine injury is rare in drowning. If the patient has obvious signs of trauma, a known mechanism such as diving into shallow water head-first, or intoxication, spinal immobilization may be considered but must not delay removal of the patient from the water to begin CPR. Chest compressions are ineffective until the patient has been removed from the water and placed on a firm surface (American Heart Association, 2010a).

When called for a drowning consider underlying medical conditions that may have led to being submerged, including the following:

- Hypoglycemia
- Seizures
- Syncope
- Myocardial infarction
- Stroke
- Anxiety disorders
- Exhaustion
- Hypothermia
- Alcohol or drug use

Deliberate hyperventilation and breath holding prior to attempting to swim is also associated with drowning.

Pathophysiology of Drowning

Following submersion in a liquid medium, the patient first voluntarily holds his breath. Often, reflex swallowing of water occurs at this point. If the patient aspirates a small amount of water, laryngospasm occurs, which constricts the airway. If the patient is not removed from the water and breathing is restored, the carbon dioxide level in the blood increases and the oxygen level decreases. As the patient deteriorates, laryngospasm relaxes and there may be active respiratory movements, but gas exchange cannot

occur. The amount of liquid that enters the airway varies from patient to patient. Hypoxia, hypercapnea, and acidosis lead to cardiac arrest and organ injury. The factor that has the most dramatic impact on the patient's prognosis is the duration of submersion. The longer a patient is submerged, the poorer the prognosis. However, other factors can influence the outcome, as well. Those factors include the following:

- *Water cleanliness.* When water is aspirated, it accumulates in the smaller airways of the lungs and alveoli. If the aspirated water contains pathogens, it can cause pneumonia. Contamination of water with chemicals or debris can also lead to pneumonitis and pneumonia.
- *Water temperature.* When core body temperature drops, the heart rate and metabolism also drop. Because the body as a whole slows, it does not have the same oxygen demand as when core body temperature is normal. Patients can be apneic for longer periods of time while hypothermic than when normothermic without brain damage occurring. There have been some cases where patients, usually pediatric patients, have been successfully resuscitated after being submerged in cold water for long periods of time.
- *Patient health.* Patients with pre-existing medical conditions cannot tolerate hypoxia due to submersion as well as a healthy patient can.

General Assessment and Management of a Drown Patient

Drown patients may or may not be out of the water when you arrive at the scene. If the patient is out of the water, your approach will begin differently than if the patient is still in the water. If you are not trained in water rescue and do not have the proper equipment, you must not enter the water to attempt a rescue. If water rescue resources have not already been dispatched, request them immediately.

During rescue efforts, patients must be removed from the water as quickly as possible. Remember, injury to the spine is uncommon in drowning. However, delaying resuscitation to perform spinal immobilization in the water will result in further hypoxia. Although it is possible to perform mouth-to-mouth or mouth-to-mask breathing in the water, chest compressions are not effective until the patient is out of the water.

The primary considerations in assessment and management of drowning patients is detecting and correcting any threats to the airway, breathing, and circulation; correcting hypoxia, and assessing for underlying medical problems, hypothermia, and injuries.

Scene Size-Up

Assess the scene for hazards as you would at any other scene and take measures to ensure your safety and the safety of your crew, patient, and bystanders. Occasionally, drownings involve more than one patient. Question bystanders to determine the number of patients and request additional EMS units, if needed. Also determine from bystanders what circumstances led the patient to be submerged and decide if there is a mechanism of injury that requires cervical-spine stabilization.

If the patient is out of the water when you arrive, or once he is removed from the water, develop a general impression. Is the patient awake and alert? Is he unconscious? Does he appear to be breathing? Is he cyanotic?

Primary Assessment

If your general impression from the scene size-up is that the patient is unresponsive and not breathing normally, immediately check the patient's carotid pulse. If you do not feel a pulse within 10 seconds, begin chest compressions as your partner applies the AED. Be sure to dry the patient quickly before applying the AED pads. Keep in mind that the cause of cardiac arrest is likely to be hypoxia.

If the patient is unresponsive with a pulse, assess the airway, breathing, and circulation, correcting life-threats any life-threatening problems as soon as you identify them. Even if water was aspirated into the lungs, it does not act as a foreign body. However, suction water and emesis from the mouth, if necessary. Use manual position and basic airway adjuncts as needed. Assist ventilations, if necessary, using a bag-valve-mask device with supplemental oxygen. As resuscitation proceeds, consider using an advanced airway device. Check for and control external bleeding.

If the patient is responsive, you must assess for any problems with his airway, breathing, and circulation and treat them accordingly. Assess the patient's oxygen saturation early in your assessment and apply oxygen as needed to maintain an SpO_2 of 95 percent or greater.

Secondary Assessment

Perform a rapid trauma exam for patients who are unresponsive or have a decreased level of responsiveness. Obtain baseline vital signs and a patient history, if possible. Perform a focused exam for patients who are conscious and oriented. Perform a head-to-toe exam for patients with a decreased level of responsiveness.

Management and Reassessment

Even patients who are alert and in no distress after being submerged can later develop respiratory distress and must be transported to an emergency department for evaluation. Management is aimed at improving oxygenation and perfusion. Also be alert to the possibility of hypothermia. Heat loss occurs 30 times faster in water than in dry air. Patients can quickly become hypothermic, even in water temperatures of 70 degrees Fahrenheit.

En route to the emergency department reassess the patient's vital signs at least every 5 minutes for critical patients and at least every 15 minutes for noncritical patients. Check the effectiveness of any interventions performed and record your findings in the patient care report.

Diving Emergencies

Diving emergencies occur due to the effects of pressure exerted on the body in deep water, particularly when the diver breathes compressed air from a self-contained underwater breathing apparatus (SCUBA). A diving emergency can occur anywhere there is water that is deep enough, not just in the ocean. Inland stone quarries and lakes are often deep enough to allow recreational scuba diving or commercial diving operations. Occasionally, a patient who has dived and then flown to a location far away from water can still suffer a complication of the dive, underscoring the need for a thorough history.

Understanding the physics of gases, including the effects of pressure as stated in Boyle's, Dalton's, and Henry's laws helps you understand the pathophysiology and management of diving emergencies.

Effects of Pressure

Water is an incompressible liquid that exerts weight on anything that is in it. Under water, depth and pressure are directly related, meaning the deeper you go, the more pressure, or weight, is exerted on you and on the gases you breathe. **Dysbarism** refers to medical conditions resulting from changes in pressure.

At sea level, air has a pressure (atmospheric pressure) of 760 mmHg at sea level. The pressure decreases at high altitudes. You are likely more familiar with the barometric pressure expressed in inches of mercury, as given in the weather report. 760 mmHg is equal to approximately 30 inches of mercury. That amount of pressure is known as one atmosphere. It is the pressure of the entire atmosphere of the earth exerting force. Water exerts more pressure than air. Every 33 feet of water exerts one atmosphere of pressure.

Boyle's Law

Boyle's law states that the volume of a gas is inversely proportional to its pressure. At a constant temperature, as the pressure of a gas increases, its volume decreases. If the pressure on a gas is doubled, its volume will decrease by half. Another way of expressing the pressure of the atmosphere is in terms of pounds per square inch (psi). At sea level, air has a pressure of 14.7 psi. That pressure is equal to 1 "atmosphere absolute," or 1 ata. The pressure at a depth of 33 feet beneath water is 2 ata, the pressure at 66 feet is 3 ata, and so on.

Following this principle, 1 liter of air at the surface of water will be compressed to 500 mL of air at 33 feet. At 66 feet, it will be compressed to 333 mL.

Dalton's Law

Dalton's Law states that the total pressure of a gaseous mixture is equal to the sum of the partial pressures of each of the individual gases in the mixture. The air we breathe is a mixture of 78 percent nitrogen, 21 percent oxygen; and trace amounts of carbon dioxide and other gases. Because atmospheric pressure at sea level is 760 mmHg, the pressure of nitrogen is 593 mmHg (78 percent of 760 mmHg is 593 mmHg), the pressure of oxygen is 160 mmHg, and the pressure of carbon dioxide is about 4 mmHg. Each gas exerts its own pressure toward the total pressure of the mixture. Increases in altitude or diving to depths beneath the water change atmospheric pressure; but the component gases of the mixture will still account for the same proportion of whatever the total pressure is.

Henry's Law

Henry's Law states that the solubility of a gas in a liquid at a particular temperature is proportional to the pressure of that gas above the liquid. As you descend underwater, the pressure that water exerts on you will increase with depth. This pressure also compresses the gases that are breathed in, forcing it to be dissolved in liquids, mainly the blood, and tissues of the body. Air is composed of only 21 percent oxygen. This oxygen is used as fuel for the cells of the body, leaving only small amounts to be dissolved into the blood. Nitrogen, however, comprises 78 percent of the air that we breathe and is not used in the metabolism of the body. Therefore, a greater amount of nitrogen is dissolved into the blood and tissue with increasing depth. As a person ascends toward the surface of the water, gases that have been dissolved into the blood and tissues enter back into the bloodstream. If ascent occurs too rapidly, bubbles are formed.

When a diver descends underwater, the gases within his body are compressed and dissolved into the blood and tissues. During ascent, those same gases (mostly nitrogen, because the majority of oxygen has been used for metabolism) exit the tissues. During a rapid ascent, nitrogen bubbles can form in the blood, brain, spinal cord, inner ear, skin, muscles, and joints. Think of opening a soda can. The can is pressurized and the gases are dissolved in the soda. When the can is opened, the pressure rapidly decreases, causing bubbles to form.

Charles' Law

Charles' law states that all gases will expand equally when heated. Water temperature decreases as a diver descends; therefore, inhaled and exhaled gases will contract with the change in temperature. As a diver ascends, the opposite occurs: Gases will expand as water temperature increases.

General Assessment and Management of Diving Emergencies

Assessment and management of diving emergencies follows the same sequence of scene size-up, primary assessment, secondary assessment, management, and reassessment. There also is some specific, very important information you must obtain about the dive history, which includes the following:

- Time of onset of signs and symptoms (as accurate as possible)
- Type of breathing equipment used
- Depth of the dive
- Number of dives
- Duration of each dive
- Whether aircraft travel followed the dive and whether the cabin was pressurized or unpressurized
- Rate of ascent
- Experience of the diver
- Previous decompression illnesses
- Medications
- Alcohol or drug use

Specific Diving Injuries

Types of diving injuries that result from diving include barotrauma, decompression sickness, arterial gas embolism, and nitrogen narcosis.

Barotrauma

Barotrauma occurs when air pressure in the hollow spaces of the body (such as the middle ear and sinuses) rises too high or drops too low. During descent diving, barotraumas is commonly called *the squeeze*. As a diver descends, pressure increases and the volume of gas in airspaces decreases, creating a vacuum. If pressure between the nasopharynx and eustachian tube cannot be equalized during descent, injury to the middle ear can occur. A common cause of this is a diver who has an upper respiratory infection with congestion that prevents the equalization of pressure. Sinus infections can prevent the equalization of pressure within the sinus cavities, as well. When pressure within the sinuses cannot be equalized, injury can occur.

Signs and symptoms of descent barotraumas include the following:

- Mild to severe pain in the ears or sinus regions
- Discharge of clear fluid or blood from the nose or ears (due to ruptured sinuses or eardrums)
- Dizziness
- Tinnitus
- Hearing loss

Decompression Sickness

Decompression sickness, also called *the bends*, occurs as nitrogen gas bubbles are produced and accumulate in the blood and tissues as a result of rapid ascent during a dive. This occurs according to Henry's law, if a diver ascends too rapidly. Any time a diver descends below 40 feet, a controlled ascent must occur to prevent bubbles from forming. A controlled ascent is sometimes called a *staged ascent,* meaning that the diver will ascend a certain amount and then pause to allow equilibrium of pressure to occur. Those bubbles can affect the body in two ways: First, they can act as an air embolism in the bloodstream and, second, they stretch blood vessels and nerves of the body. The bends result in severe pain usually in the joints and abdomen.

Decompression sickness has two classifications, as follows:

- *Type I decompression sickness.* A mild form of decompression sickness, **Type I decompression sickness,** is also called the bends. As the diver ascends too rapidly, nitrogen bubbles form in the blood within the capillaries of the skin, resulting in itching or a burning sensation of the skin and a rash. Type I decompression sickness also may present with pain in the joints and limbs (most commonly the knees, elbows, and shoulders) as a result of nitrogen bubble formation.

- *Type II decompression sickness.* A condition caused by nitrogen bubble formation within the nervous, respiratory, and circulatory systems, **Type II decompression sickness** presents with signs and symptoms that include the following:
  - Low back pain
  - Weakness
  - Paralysis
  - Incontinence of the bladder or bowel
  - Headache
  - Visual disturbances
  - Dizziness
  - Nausea and vomiting
  - Tinnitus
  - Substernal burning upon inhalation
  - Nonproductive cough
  - Respiratory distress
  - Signs of shock
  - Pulmonary edema
  - Seizure
  - Edema

Decompression illness is generally treated through recompression of the patient. Recompression is accomplished by placing the patient in a hyperbaric chamber, where the patient is subjected to pressurized oxygen therapy to force the nitrogen to redissolve, then gradually decompressing to allow the nitrogen to escape again without the formation of bubbles (Figure 41-7). Obviously, hyperbaric treatment is provided in the hospital setting. However, initial

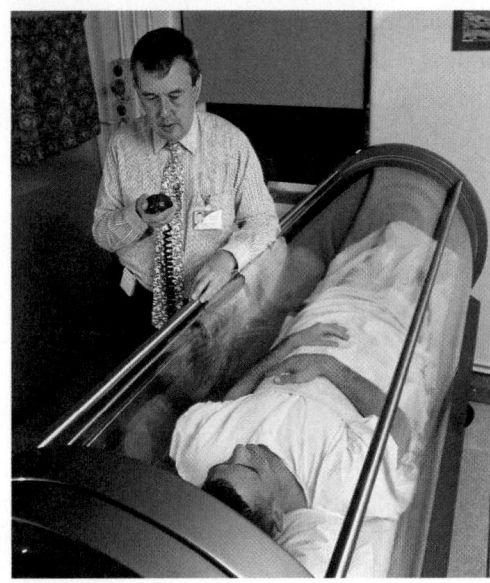

FIGURE 41-7

Hyperbaric chamber. (© James King-Holmes/Photo Researchers, Inc.)

management of the patient in the prehospital setting includes management of airway, breathing, and circulation. Provide high-flow oxygen to the patient and transport him in the supine position. IV access should be initiated and provide fluid therapy as indicated by the patient's condition.

If air transport is used, the patient must not be exposed to decreased barometric pressure (high altitude flight without a pressurized cabin) because it will precipitate the condition. In fact, sport divers are recommended by the Diver's Alert Network (DAN) to the follow these guidelines:

- A minimum of 12 hours should be spent at surface level before flying in a commercial aircraft.

- An extended period of time (beyond 12 hours) should be spent at surface level following daily, multiple dives for several days or dives that require decompression stops.

Arterial Gas Embolism

Arterial gas embolism. If ascent occurs too rapidly or if the diver holds his breath during ascent, nitrogen bubbles will form in the arterial bloodstream and become an **arterial gas embolism (AGE).** The condition can be rapidly fatal. Signs and symptoms include the following:

- Respiratory distress
- Altered mental status
- Dizziness
- Chest pain
- Severe pain in the muscles and joints
- Visual disturbances
- Hearing loss

- Nausea and vomiting
- Paralysis
- Numbness
- Lack of coordination
- Frothy and bloody sputum
- Edema of the neck
- Memory loss
- Stroke
- Coma
- Respiratory arrest
- Cardiac arrest

Treatment for AGE is supportive, consisting of treating problems with the airway, breathing, and circulation, and treating any other injuries the patient has. In the past it was recommended that patients with suspected AGE be placed in Trendelenburg position. This is no longer recommended because it increases cerebral edema and injury to the blood-brain barrier.

Nitrogen Narcosis

Nitrogen narcosis, commonly called *rapture of the deep,* is a state of stupor resulting from nitrogen's effect on cerebral function. With nitrogen narcosis, the diver may act as if he is intoxicated and take risks that he ordinarily would not take. In some cases, the affected diver will remain underwater until his oxygen runs out, resulting in asphyxiation or drowning. Divers refer to the *martini effect,* because, they say, it feels like you have had one martini for every 33 feet of depth descended.

High-Altitude Illness

High-altitude illness is caused by a decrease in atmospheric pressure. According to Dalton's law, the air we breathe consists of 21 percent oxygen. This proportion remains constant despite the changes in atmospheric pressure. As altitude increases and barometric pressure decreases, air still contains 21 percent oxygen, but the partial pressure of oxygen is lower. If PaO_2 is 160 mmHg at sea level (21 percent of 760 mmHg), it is only about 133 mmHg at 5,000 feet, where the atmospheric pressure is 632 mmHg. Keeping in mind that oxygen onloading is favored in conditions of high PaO_2, hemoglobin saturation levels are lower at higher atmospheres where the PaO_2 is lower. That is not a problem for those who are acclimated to higher altitudes. But significant increases in altitude over short periods of time can cause illness, even in healthy adults, and exacerbate pre-existing illnesses such as CHF, angina, and COPD.

When ascending to high altitudes (4,500 to 11,500 feet) you must do so gradually to allow the body to acclimate along the way. Failure to allow acclimation to the hypoxic environment of higher altitude may result in illness. In addition to gradually ascending to high altitudes, you can decrease the likelihood of high-altitude illness by minimizing physical exertion until acclimated. Complete acclimation to an altitude generally takes up to one week but after a few days most individuals are able to function normally unless they exert themselves too much.

As a general rule, the rate of ascent, altitude ascended to, amount of physical activity at high altitude, and individual susceptibility are contributing factors to the incidence and severity of high-altitude illness.

A key part of the treatment of patients with any type of altitude illness is quickly bringing the patient to a lower altitude.

Acute Mountain Sickness

Acute mountain sickness occurs when a person ascends to an altitude of 2,000 meters (6,600 feet) too rapidly. Signs and symptoms produced by acute mountain sickness can be classified as mild or severe as follows:

Mild

- Lightheadedness
- Mild shortness of breath
- Weakness
- Headache
- Nausea and vomiting

Severe

- Profound weakness
- Severe vomiting
- Significant shortness of breath
- Altered mental status

Patients who experience mild signs and symptoms but continue to ascend run the risk of developing severe signs and symptoms as altitude increases. If ascent is discontinued after mild signs and symptoms present, the patient generally will improve within two days. Treatment priorities include ensuring adequacy of airway, breathing, and circulation. Make arrangements to bring the patient to a lower altitude. If your protocols permit, administer antiemetic medication for nausea and vomiting.

High-Altitude Pulmonary Edema

High-altitude pulmonary edema (HAPE) is noncardiogenic pulmonary edema that occurs at altitudes of 2,500 meters (8,200 feet) or greater. Its actual cause is still not well understood but is believed to be the result of increased permeability of the alveolar capillary membrane. Signs and symptoms of HAPE are as follows:

- Tachycardia
- Shortness of breath
- Rales

- Coughing (sometimes frothy sputum)
- Weakness
- Coma
- Death

High-Altitude Cerebral Edema

High-altitude cerebral edema (HACE) is an increase of fluid in the brain leading to an increase in intracranial pressure. HACE usually occurs in conjunction with AMS or HAPE and its cause is unknown. Signs and symptoms of HACE include the following:

- Lack of coordination
- Decreased level of responsiveness
- Seizure
- Headache
- Vomiting
- Coma

Treatment consists of maintaining an open airway, assisting ventilations, administering oxygen to maintain an SpO₂ of 95 percent or higher, ensuring adequate circulation, and arranging for transport to a lower altitude. Consult with medical direction about the administration of IV fluids and medications.

Lightning Injuries

According to a review of medical examiner death certificates listing lightning as the cause of death, there were 1,318 lightning deaths between 1980 and 1995 in the United States. Analysis of lightning injuries revealed that 30 percent of victims die and 74 percent of survivors suffer permanent disability (McSwain, Salomone, & Pons, 2007).

Before continuing on, you should know some terms used to describe electricity. The first is *voltage*; it is a representation of the electric potential energy per unit charge. In other words, it is a measurement of energy within an electric circuit at a given point. *Current* is the flow of an electric charge through a conductive material, such as an electrical wire. Current is referenced by a unit of measure called *amperes*. To put those terms into perspective, an average household electrical circuit is 120 volts with a current of 20 amperes.

The voltage and current of lightning is extraordinarily high—in excess of 1,000,000 volts with 200,000 amperes of current. Think of this in comparison to standard household electricity, which is 110 volts and 100 amperes of current. The temperatures generated by lightning can be up to 60,000°F at the point of contact.

Injury from lightning can be the result of the following four types of strike:

- Direct strike occurs when lightning hits the victim first, before making contact with any other object.
- Contact strike refers to lightning hitting an object with which the patient is in contact.
- Side flash strike refers to lightning hitting an object and then jumping to the victim who is located nearby.
- Ground current strike occurs when lightning energizes the ground, affecting people standing in the area of the strike.

The same concepts that apply to electrical burn injuries also apply to lightning strike. In some cases, the lightning strike patient will have associated traumatic injury if the strike caused them to fall or be thrown as a result of the strike. Be alert for associated traumatic injuries during your assessment of the patient.

General Assessment and Management of Lightning Injuries

Prior to approaching the patient, ensure that the scene is safe. When it is safe to do so, begin a primary assessment followed by a secondary assessment and transport of the patient. Lightning strike affects many body systems because electricity travels through the body, causing injury to muscle, nerves, organs, and bones before exiting. Injuries include injury to the respiratory drive center in the brain, resulting in respiratory arrest. Patients may be apneic following lightning strike long enough to produce cardiac arrest if rescue breathing is not provided to the patient. Cardiac arrest following lightning strike is often secondary to apnea. The energy produced by lightning strike causes injury along its path through the body.

Signs and symptoms of lightning strike include the following (Figure 41-8):

- Altered mental status
- Amnesia
- Weakness
- Pain
- Tingling and numbness
- Paralysis
- Dizziness
- Fixed pupils

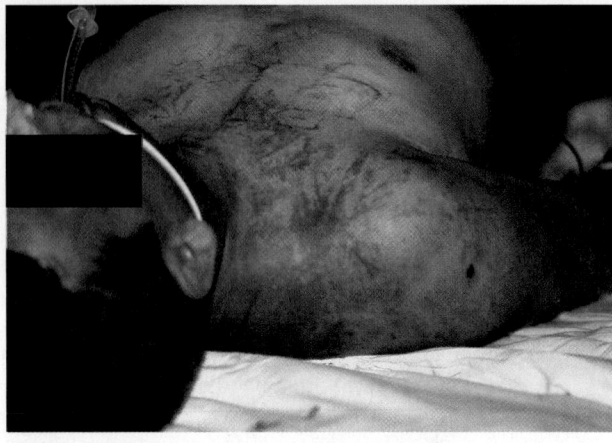

FIGURE 41-8

Lightning strike injury. (Courtesy of David Effron, MD)

- Seizures
- Burns to the skin that tend to be superficial but in areas where conductive materials such as metal jewelry are located, you may see partial- and full-thickness burns as a result of the metal heating during the strike.
- Joint dislocations
- Fractures
- Tinnitus
- Ruptured ear drums
- Respiratory failure
- Respiratory and cardiac arrest

Management of lightning strike patients is mainly supportive but also may include treatment of burn injuries, musculoskeletal injuries, spine injuries, and cardiac arrest.

CASE STUDY WRAP-UP

Clinical-Reasoning Process

Based on the history of the present illness, Jennifer and Harry quickly recognize that the patient is experiencing heat stroke. Despite the patient's decreased level of responsiveness, he is maintaining a patent airway and breathing adequately. With the assistance of bystanders, Harry removes the patient's clothing. Jennifer obtains a core body temperature of 106°F. Knowing that the patient needs supplemental oxygen and cooling, they immediately apply high-flow oxygen by nonrebreather mask and soak the patient with sterile water from their unit.

The patient is placed on the stretcher and loaded into the air-conditioned module of the ambulance. Harry asks one of the patient's coworkers to accompany the patient to the hospital emergency department. Jennifer sets up an IV line as Harry exits the ambulance module. They begin rapid transport to the nearest emergency department, which is approximately 10 minutes away. En route, Jennifer applies cold packs to the patient's armpits, sides of his neck, and in his groin. She knows that it is important to monitor the patient for shivering and discontinue active cooling if present, so she watches him closely. IV access is obtained and fluid therapy is initiated.

The patient's level of responsiveness improves significantly en route. Upon arrival at the hospital, Jennifer notes that the patient's temperature has decreased to 99.7°F and his level of responsiveness has improved significantly. They roll the patient inside and provide a patient report to the receiving physician.

CHAPTER REVIEW

Chapter Summary

People spend time outdoors everyday and can become victims of the environment in many different ways. In some cases, injury is minor but it also can be life threatening. This is especially true for the pediatric and geriatric populations.

Respect the environment and ensure that you are prepared for the conditions to which you will be exposed. As an Advanced EMT, you are not immune to injury or illness. Always take precautionary measures. Your goal is to identify the environmental cause of illness or injury. After doing so, you will manage the patient's condition appropriately, preventing deterioration and providing transport to a medical facility where the patient can receive definitive care.

Review Questions

Multiple-Choice Questions

1. The process by which the body produces heat is called:

   a. thermolysis.
   c. thermocreation.
   b. thermoregulation.
   d. thermogenesis.

2. Which one of the mechanisms listed below is the primary means of heat loss under normal body conditions?

   a. Convection
   c. Radiation
   b. Conduction
   d. Evaporation

3. Which one of the heat-related conditions listed below occurs when core body temperature is between 100°F and 104°F?

   a. Heat cramps
   b. Classic heatstroke
   c. Heat exhaustion
   d. Exertional heatstroke

4. Following the primary assessment of a heat-related emergency patient, which one of the following is your first priority related to patient care?

   a. Removal of the patient from the cold environment
   b. Providing fluid therapy
   c. Initiating active cooling
   d. Immediately transporting to an appropriate facility

5. Which one of the following signs differentiates deep local cold injury from superficial local cold injury?

   a. Cold skin
   b. Redness to the affected tissues
   c. Numbness to the affected tissues
   d. Presence of blisters to the affected tissues

6. Which type of injury results in an influx of fluids into the alveoli as a result of diffusion?

   a. Dry drowning
   b. Saltwater drowning
   c. Submersion injury
   d. Freshwater drowning

7. Which one of the laws related to diving injuries states that there is an inversely proportional relationship between pressure and volume, assuming that temperature remains constant?

   a. Boyle's
   c. Dalton's
   b. Henry's
   d. Charles'

8. Which type of bite or sting results in ulceration of the injury site that gets progressively worse with time?

   a. Black widow bite
   c. Stingray sting
   b. Brown recluse bite
   d. Any bite

Critical-Thinking Questions

9. You arrive on scene to find a 28-year-old patient who has been pulled from a pond. The temperature is 65°F with a 10 miles per hour breeze. The patient is standing in the sun to try to warm himself. He is wearing wet clothes, including a jacket. What should your initial actions include?

10. Explain the pathologic difference between heat exhaustion and heatstroke.

11. Describe the relationship between rate of ascent and risk for illness during a dive.

References

American Heart Association. (2010a). Part 12: Cardiac Arrest in Special Situations: 2010 Guidelines for Cardiopulmonary Resuscitation and Emergency Cardiac Care. *Circulation*, 122 S829–861 DOI: 10.1161/CIRCULATIONAHA.110.971069

American Heart Association. (2010b). Part 5: Adult Basic Life Support: 2010 Guidelines for Cardiopulmonary Resuscitation and Emergency Cardiac Care. *Circulation*, 122 S685–705 DOI: 10.1161/CIRCULATIONAHA.110.970939

Idris, A. H., Berg, R. A., Bierens, J., Bossaert, L., Branche, A., et al. (2003). *Circulation*, 108: 2565–2575 DOI 10.1161/01. CIR.0000099581.70012.68

McSwain, N. E., Salomone, J. P., Pons, P. T. (Eds). (2007). *Prehospital trauma life support* (6th ed.). St. Louis, MO: Elsevier.

Additional Reading

American Burn Association. (2007). *Advanced burn life support course provider manual.* Chicago, IL: American Burn Association.

Campbell, J. E. (2008). *International trauma life support* (6th ed.). Upper Saddle River, NJ: Pearson Prentice Hall.

42

Multisystem Trauma and Trauma Resuscitation

KEY TERMS

coagulopathy *(p. 933)*

multisystem trauma *(p. 927)*

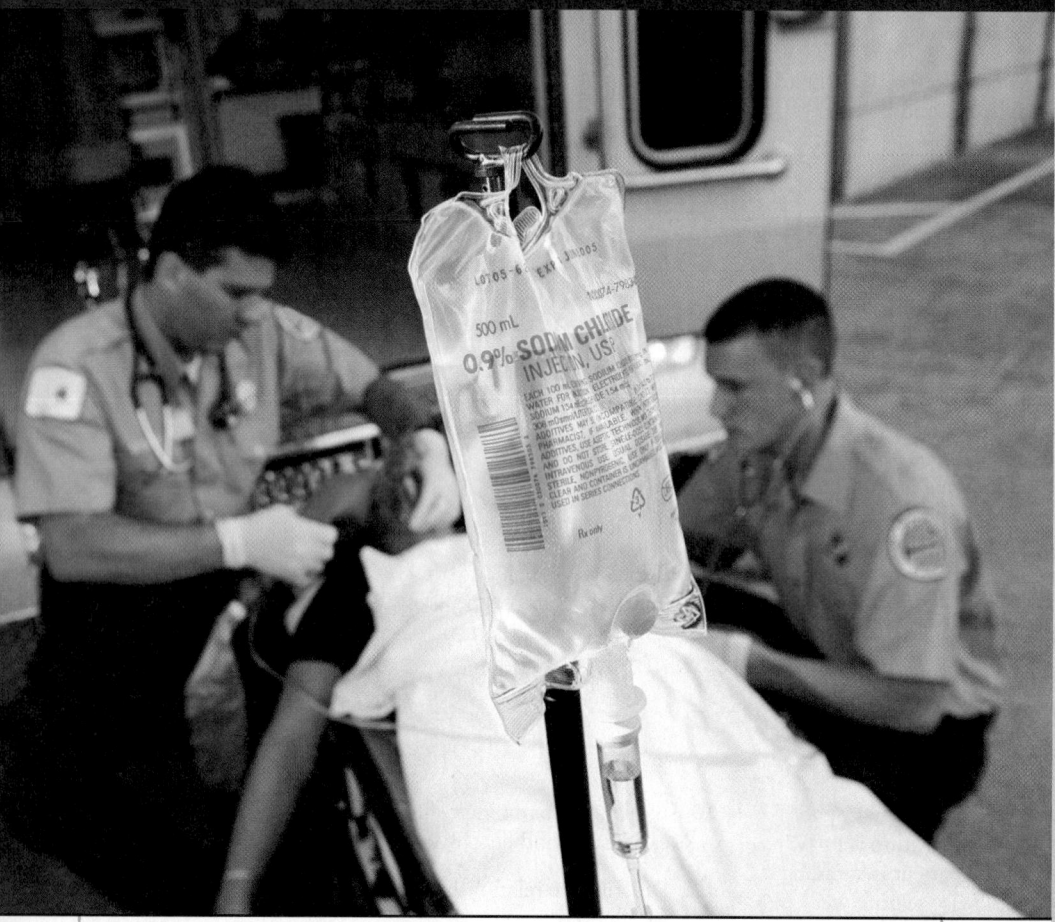

Content Area: Trauma

Advanced EMT Education Standard: The Advanced EMT applies fundamental knowledge to provide basic and selected advanced emergency care and transportation based on assessment findings for an acutely injured patient.

Objectives

After reading this chapter, you should be able to:

42.1 Define key terms introduced in this chapter.

42.2 Discuss the increased morbidity and mortality associated with multisystem trauma.

42.3 Describe the importance of each of the following principles of out-of-hospital multisystem trauma care:

- Ensure safety of rescue personnel and the patient.
- Determine the need for additional resources.
- Understand mechanism of injury.
- Identify and manage life threats.
- Manage the airway while maintaining cervical-spine immobilization.

(continued)

Resource Central

To access Resource Central, follow the directions on the Student Access Card provided with this text. If there is no card, go to www.bradybooks.com and follow the Resource Central link to Buy Access. Under Media Resources, you will find:

- *Trauma Resuscitation.* The most recent trauma resuscitation guidelines.
- *Pediatric Trauma.* The complexities of pediatric trauma.
- *Geriatric Trauma.* Managing the special considerations related to geriatric trauma.

Advanced EMT William Turnley and his EMT partner Terri Pierce have just left the emergency department after transporting a patient there, when dispatch calls. "Unit 77, respond to an MVC involving a motorcycle at the intersection of Riverside Drive and Renwick Boulevard."

When William and Terri arrive at the scene, police officers are directing traffic away from the area where a motorcycle rider lost control and struck a large tree. The posted speed limit on this roadway is 45 miles per hour. Two police officers are near the motorcycle waving William and Terri toward them. The crew notices as they approach that the motorcycle has significant damage to it and the patient is lying prone approximately 30 feet from the motorcycle and is not wearing a helmet. Terri advises dispatch that they are on scene. William and Terri exit the ambulance and move toward the patient with their gear in hand.

Problem-Solving Questions

1. What does the mechanism of injury tell William and Terri about potential injuries to the patient?
2. How will they prioritize actions at this scene?
3. What additional information do William and Terri need to collect to make decisions and determine the appropriate interventions?
4. How should they balance the patient's need for intervention with the need for transport?

(continued from previous page)

- Support ventilation and oxygenation.
- Control external hemorrhage and treat for shock.
- Perform a secondary assessment.
- Splint musculoskeletal injuries and maintain spinal immobilization.
- Make transport decisions.

Introduction

Many trauma patients have isolated injuries. However, particularly with significant mechanisms of injury such as high-speed motor vehicle collisions (MVCs), falls from heights, and gunshot wounds, the patient sustains injuries to more than one body system. When **multisystem trauma** occurs, morbidity and mortality are increased. Instead of focusing only on a specific injury, you must consider the overall impact of multisystem trauma, manage immediate life threats, and begin transport to the closest appropriate facility. For instance, imagine that a patient was ejected from a vehicle during a high-speed MVC. He sustained a closed head injury and is presenting with signs and symptoms of brain herniation. He also is hypotensive as a result of having sustained internal hemorrhage from a vessel or organ injury. On their own, each injury is life threatening. The hypotension further impairs cerebral perfusion, which increases cerebral hypoxia and edema

and increases intracranial pressure (ICP). The impaired neurologic function impairs the ability to compensate for hypovolemia. If the patient also has a lung injury or impaired airway, leading to hypoxia, his condition is even more critical. The combination of two or more life-threatening conditions in the same patient increases his risk of death substantially.

The principles of assessing and managing multisystem trauma patients are those that you have already learned: Perform a scene size-up, perform a primary

IN THE FIELD

If at any time you feel that you are becoming overwhelmed or are uncertain about how to proceed with a multisystem trauma patient, take a deep breath and systematically reassess the patient, beginning with the patient's airway followed by breathing and circulation.

assessment with interventions for problems with airway, breathing, and circulation while considering the need for manually restricting cervical-spine motion. Perform a rapid trauma exam, package as indicated by the mechanism of injury; and transport without delay with additional assessment and intervention en route to the closest appropriate facility.

Potential pitfalls are failing to recognize multisystem trauma and the increased risk to the patient, letting one type of injury distract you from managing the patient's overall condition, and failing to deal with individual injuries that are contributing to the patient's condition. Managing patients with multisystem trauma requires the ability to rapidly recognize the situation and incorporate an understanding of both specific and multiple injuries into the process of establishing priorities for assessment, management, and transport.

General Assessment and Management of Multisystem Trauma Patients

As an Advanced EMT, your early identification of life-threatening injuries, proper management of airway, breathing, and circulation, and rapid transport to the closest appropriate facility can reduce morbidity and mortality associated with multisystem trauma. Your goal is to minimize your time on scene, and initiate transport as soon as possible. This does not mean that you will omit completing a primary assessment or managing immediately life-threatening conditions of the airway, breathing, and circulation for the sake of transporting quickly. You, your partner, and other rescuers who may be available on scene must work efficiently as a team to properly assess, treat immediate life threats, and package the patient for transport. Working well as a team reduces scene time and allows for expeditious transport to an appropriate facility.

In some cases, such as when prolonged extrication of the patient is required, you will not be able to transport until the patient is disentangled. In such cases, manage the airway, breathing, and circulation and make preparations for further care and transport while you wait for the patient to be extricated. While waiting, advise the receiving facility so they can begin preparations for receiving the patient.

Scene Size-Up

As with all emergency responses, your first priority is your own safety and the safety of your partner. Never attempt to access the patient until all hazards have been controlled by individuals trained to do so. Request additional resources, such as extrication teams, rescue teams for confined spaces

or high angles, hazmat teams, law enforcement, the utility company, and additional EMS providers.

You and your partner can care for only one critical patient at a time. With just one patient you need, at a minimum, either another EMS provider to assist you while your partner drives, or someone to drive so you and your partner can care for the patient. Always follow your EMS service's policies with regard to who is approved to accompany you during transport or drive the ambulance. If you arrive on scene to find more than one critical patient, call for as many additional EMS resources as necessary to care for them all.

If ALS is available, consider requesting them, according to your protocols, for critical trauma patients. ALS can help with airway management, particularly in patients who need to be sedated or paralyzed to achieve control of the airway and those with suspected tension pneumothorax.

Determining the most appropriate facility and the best way of transporting the patient requires excellent clinical judgment, knowledge of the capabilities of emergency care facilities in your area, and knowledge of your EMS service's protocols and policies. You always must balance the need for immediate stabilization of life-threatening conditions with the need for specialized diagnostic tests and surgical interventions. Although the closest hospital may not have sophisticated surgical capabilities, it does no good to transport the patient to a Level I trauma center 45 minutes away if he dies en route because he needs immediate decompression of a tension pneumothorax, which could be performed at the closest facility. In some cases, it is best to go to the closest facility for immediate stabilization and then transfer the patient by ground or by air to a facility with more sophisticated capabilities. In other cases, it makes more sense to extend transport time by 10 minutes to reach a facility with higher-level capabilities.

Consider the distance to the most appropriate facility for the patient and whether there will be any delays in transport in determining whether air medical transport could be beneficial. In addition to being able to transport the patient to a more distant facility for appropriate care, air medical personnel can perform many interventions, such as administering blood products and inserting chest tubes, to help stabilize the patient's condition. If air medical transport is needed and feasible, make the request as soon as possible.

The forces applied to the patient during injury provide clues to the likelihood of life-threatening injury and multisystem trauma. Mechanisms of injury that can lead to multisystem trauma include the following:

- Ejection from a vehicle
- Pedestrian struck by a vehicle
- Fall from a height greater than 10 feet in an adult or greater than twice the height of a child
- Motorcycle and rider separation in an MVC
- MVC impact greater than 40 mph

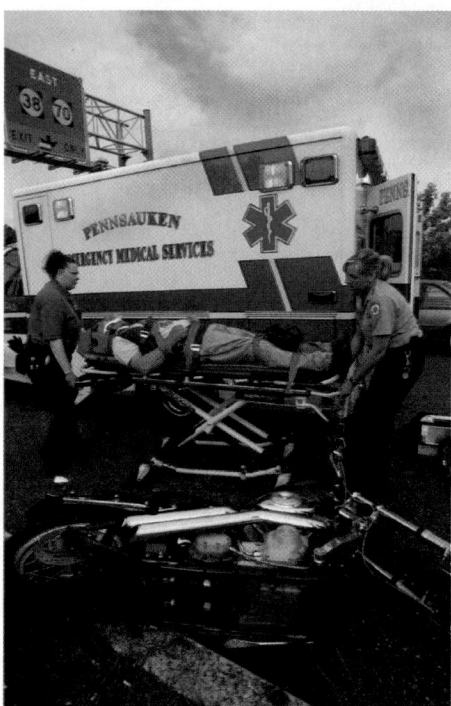

FIGURE 42-1

Motorcycle collisions can result in multisystem trauma.
(© Mark C. Ide)

- Explosion
- Multiple penetrating trauma injuries (especially to the head, neck, and torso)

When you identify any of these mechanisms of injury, suspect the presence of multisystem trauma. As you perform your patient assessment, be alert for signs and symptoms of potential injuries to the patient (Figure 42-1).

Use the mechanism of injury to help you determine the need for manual stabilization of the head and neck as you approach the patient.

Primary Assessment

A systematic primary assessment allows you to identify immediate life threats related to airway, breathing, and circulation. During the primary assessment, manage life threats as soon as they are identified, before moving on to other components of the assessment.

Teamwork is essential to giving the patient the care he needs. Rather than approaching assessment and management linearly, teamwork allows you to accomplish many tasks simultaneously for the patient's benefit. Aspects of assessment are performed simultaneously with aspects of treatment, patient packaging, and transport.

Many multisystem trauma patients who you encounter have a decreased level of responsiveness that places them at risk for an inadequate airway. Patients with trauma to the face or neck also may have an inadequate airway. Be prepared to clear the airway manually and with suction, because blood, loose teeth, vomit, or other airway obstructions may be present.

Use manual airway maneuvers, basic adjuncts, and advanced airways as needed to establish and maintain an open airway. If the patient is unresponsive, you may use a Combitube, supraglottic airway, or endotracheal tube, according to your protocols. If you cannot establish and maintain the patient's airway, request ALS or air medical transport or transport the patient without delay to the closest facility at which an airway can be established. Some particularly challenging situations in which you must consider this are when a patient requires an airway adjunct but has trismus (clenched jaw muscles), a gag reflex, or when there is massive facial trauma that obstructs the upper airway, requiring a surgical intervention (cricothyrotomy) to establish an emergency airway.

The level of responsiveness and airway status of a patient with multisystem trauma can deteriorate, sometimes rapidly. Anticipate changes and be vigilant to detect them.

Assess the adequacy of breathing. If the patient is breathing adequately, apply supplemental oxygen according to his level of respiratory distress and SpO_2. If breathing is inadequate, perform positive pressure ventilations using a bag-valve-mask device with supplemental oxygen. If ventilations are inadequate, consider causes including decreased responsiveness, traumatic brain injury, spinal cord injury, and injuries of the chest wall or lungs. Cover open wounds of the chest immediately with an occlusive dressing sealed on three sides (use your gloved hand first, then quickly apply the dressing). If you suspect tension pneumothorax, request ALS or transport without delay to the closest facility where the chest can be decompressed.

Assess the patient's pulse to determine whether perfusion is adequate and immediately control external hemorrhage. Even a source of bleeding that is not immediately life threatening contributes to the overall amount of blood loss. Direct pressure controls most external bleeding. If you cannot control external bleeding from an extremity by direct pressure, apply a tourniquet. Part of treating a patient in shock is keeping him warm. Keep that in mind as you prepare to expose the patient for a rapid trauma exam and make decisions about packaging and transporting the patient.

IN THE FIELD

When signs and symptoms of impending brain herniation are present (such as posturing and unequal pupils), the patient should be slightly hyperventilated at a rate of 20 breaths per minute. When end-tidal CO_2 monitoring is being utilized, the patient will be ventilated to maintain an end-tidal CO_2 reading of 35 mmHg.

Transport Decision

Whether as a result of an isolated injury or multisystem trauma, critical trauma patients are best cared for by transporting without delay to a Level I trauma center. However, not all areas have a Level I trauma center available within a reasonable transport distance. If ground transport to a Level I trauma center is not feasible given the patient's condition, consider transporting the patient to a closer facility for immediate intervention and stabilization before transport to a Level I trauma center, or consider requesting air medical transportation (Figure 42-2). Use the Centers for Disease Control and Prevention (CDC) Field Triage Decision Scheme: The National Trauma Triage Protocol (Figure 42-3) to determine if the patient is a candidate for direct transport to a trauma center. As stated on the CDC protocol, when in doubt, transport to a trauma center (CDC, 2010). Follow your EMS system's protocols and policies when making transport decisions. Patients with any of the following life-threatening conditions are considered critical:

- Inadequate airway
- Inadequate ventilations, which may be indicated by any of the following:
  - Abnormally fast (>30 per minute) or slow (<8 per minute) ventilatory rate
  - Signs of hypoxia (altered mental status, cyanosis, tachycardia, bradycardia)
  - Dyspnea

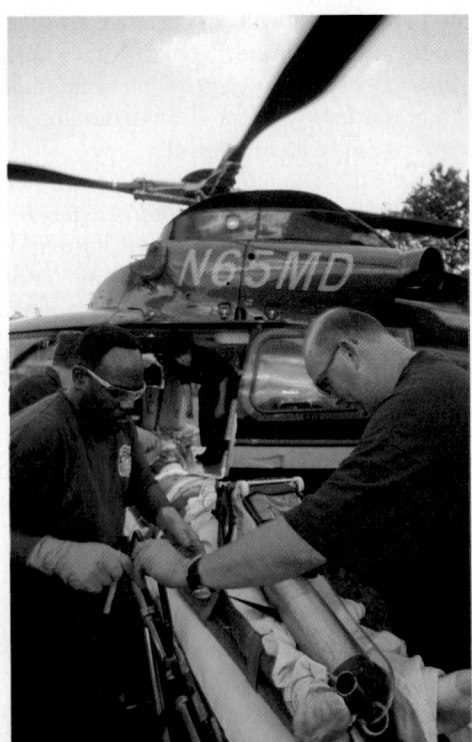

FIGURE 42-2

Use aeromedical transport when necessary to transport multisystem trauma patients directly to a trauma center.
(© Mark C. Ide)

- Suspected pneumothorax
- Flail chest
- Significant external hemorrhage
- Suspected internal hemorrhage
- Decreased level of responsiveness (GCS less than 14)
- Penetrating trauma to the head, neck, torso, or proximal extremities
- Amputation proximal to the wrist of ankle
- Combination of trauma with significant burns
- Two or more long-bone fractures. (Even a single femur fracture can result in enough blood loss to cause shock.)
- Suspected pelvic fracture
- Signs and symptoms of shock

Secondary Assessment

Immediately after the primary assessment, perform a rapid trauma exam for critical trauma patients. Ideally, adequate personnel are available to simultaneously prepare to package the patient and load him into the ambulance for transport. During transport (if adequate resources were not available to complete these steps sooner) obtain baseline vital signs and pulse oximetry, complete a head-to-toe exam, obtain a medical history, perform other monitoring (such as end-tidal CO_2 and blood glucose determination as indicated), and contact the receiving facility to provide a patient report.

Reassessment

Once en route to the hospital, assess the patient at least every 5 minutes for a critically injured patient and every 15 minutes for a noncritically injured patient. Look for trends in patient condition and adjust your interventions accordingly. Advise the receiving facility of significant improvement or deterioration in the patient's condition.

Multisystem Trauma Patient Packaging

Whether a patient has suspected spine injuries, using a long backboard is an efficient way to package a patient for transport. If you suspect spine injuries, secure the patient to the board, with a cervical collar in place, in a manner that restricts spinal motion as much as possible. Do not splint extremity fractures separately on the scene as you would with a noncritical patient. This delays transport and is inappropriate for a critical patient. Instead, carefully stabilize extremities by securing them to the body using the backboard straps to prevent them from moving. It also is improper to allow fractured extremities to move freely during packaging

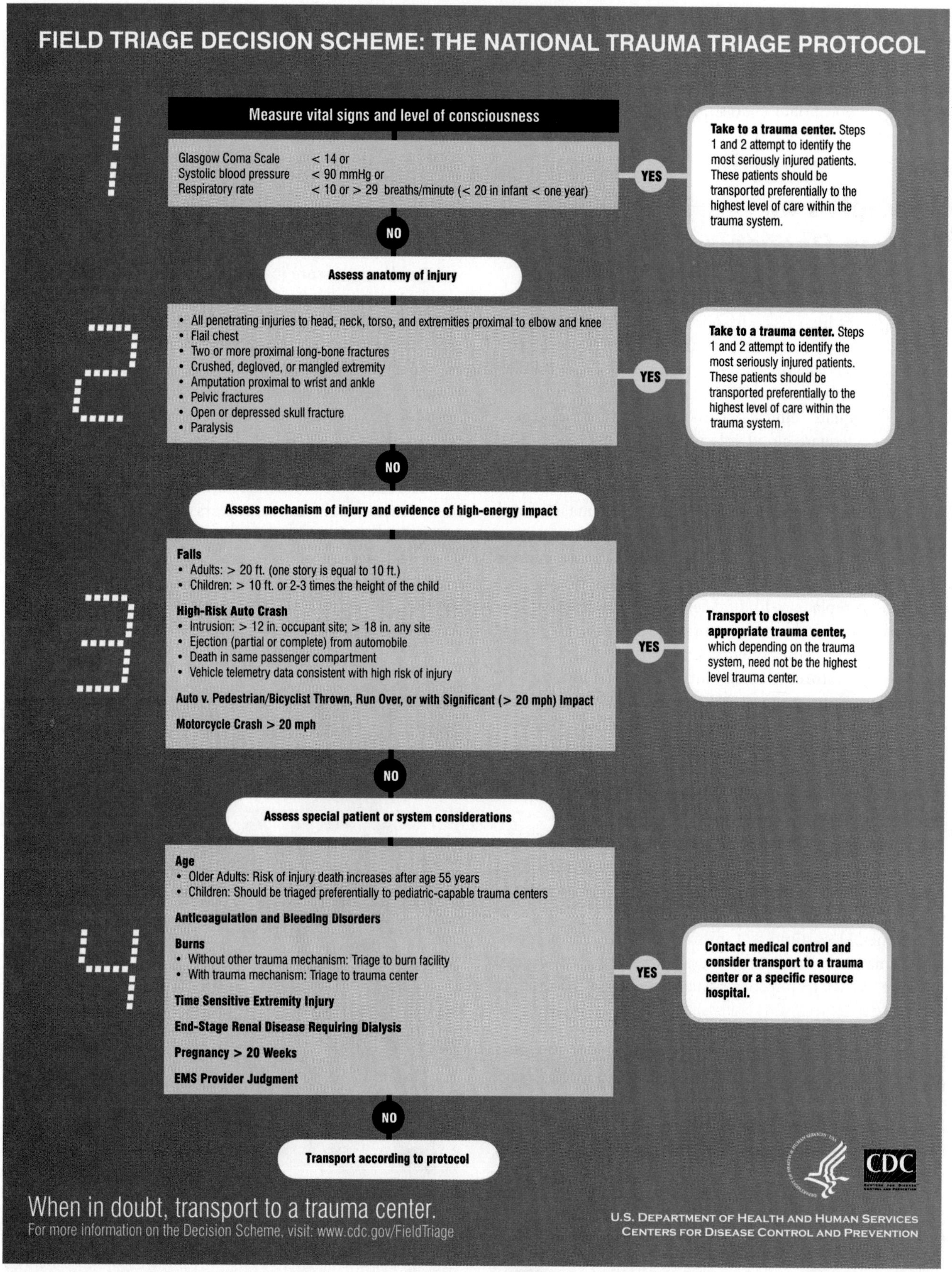

FIELD TRIAGE DECISION SCHEME: THE NATIONAL TRAUMA TRIAGE PROTOCOL

1

Measure vital signs and level of consciousness

Glasgow Coma Scale	< 14 or
Systolic blood pressure	< 90 mmHg or
Respiratory rate	< 10 or > 29 breaths/minute (< 20 in infant < one year)

YES → **Take to a trauma center.** Steps 1 and 2 attempt to identify the most seriously injured patients. These patients should be transported preferentially to the highest level of care within the trauma system.

↓ NO

2

Assess anatomy of injury

- All penetrating injuries to head, neck, torso, and extremities proximal to elbow and knee
- Flail chest
- Two or more proximal long-bone fractures
- Crushed, degloved, or mangled extremity
- Amputation proximal to wrist and ankle
- Pelvic fractures
- Open or depressed skull fracture
- Paralysis

YES → **Take to a trauma center.** Steps 1 and 2 attempt to identify the most seriously injured patients. These patients should be transported preferentially to the highest level of care within the trauma system.

↓ NO

3

Assess mechanism of injury and evidence of high-energy impact

Falls
- Adults: > 20 ft. (one story is equal to 10 ft.)
- Children: > 10 ft. or 2-3 times the height of the child

High-Risk Auto Crash
- Intrusion: > 12 in. occupant site; > 18 in. any site
- Ejection (partial or complete) from automobile
- Death in same passenger compartment
- Vehicle telemetry data consistent with high risk of injury

Auto v. Pedestrian/Bicyclist Thrown, Run Over, or with Significant (> 20 mph) Impact

Motorcycle Crash > 20 mph

YES → **Transport to closest appropriate trauma center,** which depending on the trauma system, need not be the highest level trauma center.

↓ NO

4

Assess special patient or system considerations

Age
- Older Adults: Risk of injury death increases after age 55 years
- Children: Should be triaged preferentially to pediatric-capable trauma centers

Anticoagulation and Bleeding Disorders

Burns
- Without other trauma mechanism: Triage to burn facility
- With trauma mechanism: Triage to trauma center

Time Sensitive Extremity Injury

End-Stage Renal Disease Requiring Dialysis

Pregnancy > 20 Weeks

EMS Provider Judgment

YES → **Contact medical control and consider transport to a trauma center or a specific resource hospital.**

↓ NO

Transport according to protocol

When in doubt, transport to a trauma center.
For more information on the Decision Scheme, visit: www.cdc.gov/FieldTriage

U.S. DEPARTMENT OF HEALTH AND HUMAN SERVICES
CENTERS FOR DISEASE CONTROL AND PREVENTION

CDC

FIGURE 42-3

The Centers for Disease Control and Prevention (CDC) Field Triage Decision Scheme: The National Trauma Triage Protocol.
(Courtesy of the Centers for Disease Control)

931

and transport of the patient because this can cause additional tissue injury and bleeding, leading to the progression of shock. If time and resources allow for more appropriate splinting en route to the emergency department or trauma center, it is appropriate to do so.

Principles of Trauma Resuscitation

Critical trauma patients, including those with multisystem trauma, are at high risk for shock. Shock leads to cellular hypoxia and death, which can ultimately lead to the patient's death. Your goal is to maintain an adequate cellular perfusion to prevent irreversible organ damage from occurring. Adequate cellular perfusion means that the patient must have adequate blood volume, mass of red blood cells, cardiac output and blood pressure, ventilation, and internal and external respiration.

The best way to maintain the patient's mass of red blood cells and intravascular fluid volume is to control hemorrhage. Once hemorrhage is controlled, intravenous fluids can play a role in restoring vascular volume, but they cannot replace red blood cells, platelets, clotting factors, proteins needed for oncotic pressure, electrolytes, and other blood components. Oxygen-carrying capacity can only be restored through infusion of red blood cells. The addition of even modest volumes of IV fluid also reduces the patient's core temperature, which increases his cellular energy needs when cellular energy production is already impaired and impairs blood clotting. Only one third of the volume of isotonic fluids infused remain in the vascular space after 1 hour.

In patients with internal hemorrhage, the bleeding is inaccessible except through surgery. Increasing the blood pressure increases the rate of blood loss, in addition to the other complications of fluid administration.

Nonetheless, fluid administration still can play a role in trauma resuscitation by increasing the mean arterial pressure (MAP) to improve tissue perfusion, if you follow certain guidelines. Ideally, the MAP should be 60 mmHg. Because information about MAP is not always immediately available in the prehospital setting, it is recommended that fluid administration is titrated to maintain a systolic blood pressure of 80 to 90 mmHg. In patients with traumatic brain injury, your protocols may call for a systolic blood pressure of 100 mmHg to improve brain perfusion.

Remember: Despite the fact that intravenous fluids raise the blood pressure, the increase in blood pressure may come at the cost of increasing bleeding, hemodilution, and hypothermia. You must achieve a balance between increasing the blood pressure in severely hypotensive patients and avoiding worsening their condition.

A reasonable approach to fluid resuscitation in the prehospital setting is to use large-bore (16- or 14-gauge), 1.25-inch needles to start two IVs of either normal saline or lactated Ringer's solution using macrodrip tubing. Infuse a bolus of 500 mL and recheck the blood pressure. If blood pressure is still inadequate, infuse an additional 500 mL. Follow your protocols for the volume of fluid to infuse.

The use of the pneumatic antishock garment (PASG) has been controversial for several years and many EMS agencies have removed them from their ambulance inventory. Other agencies have protocols that allow inflation of PASGs to immobilize pelvic fractures (Figure 42-4) (McSwain, Salomone & Pons, 2007). Always follow your protocol.

IN THE FIELD

Rapid identification and management of life threats and rapid transport of the patient to an appropriate facility provide the patient with the best chance of survival. Minimize time on the scene and begin transport in less than 10 minutes when at all possible. You should only address immediate life threats on the scene. It is never acceptable to delay transport of the patient in order to obtain IV access on the scene. Obtain IV access en route to the emergency department except for situations where transport will be delayed such as with prolonged extrication times.

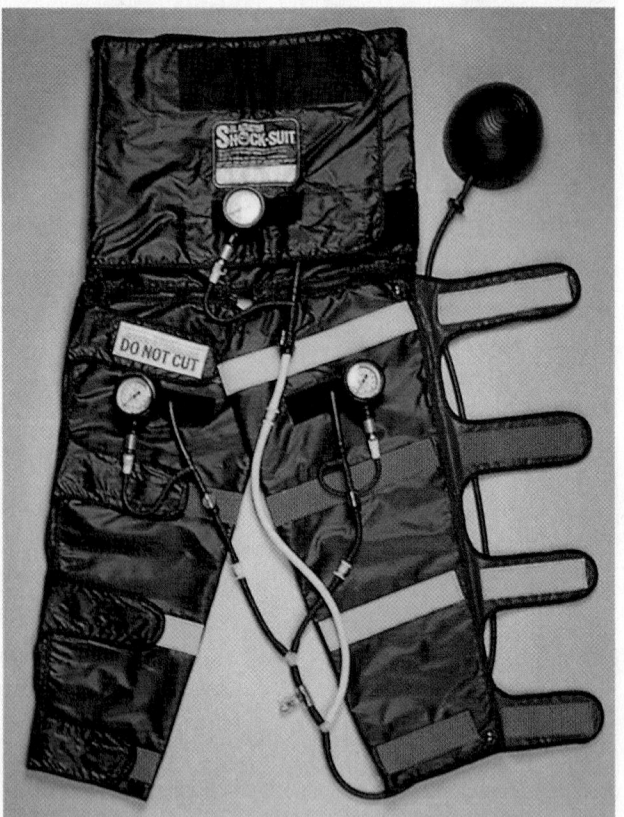

FIGURE 42-4

Pneumatic antishock garment (PASG).

The concept behind PASGs is to force blood from the abdominal cavity and lower extremities into the central circulation in order to maintain perfusion to the vital organs. However, keep in mind that the patient in shock is already maximally vasoconstricted through the body's compensatory mechanisms, leaving very little blood in the lower extremities to potentially return to the central circulation. The abdominal section of the PASG applies pressure to the abdominal organs when it is inflated. Although it is thought that the pressure could reduce internal bleeding below the level of the PASG, it also could increase internal bleeding above the level of the PASG, such as bleeding into the thoracic cavity. In addition, pressure on the abdominal organs reduces the volume of the thoracic cavity, which can impair ventilation. This is particularly concerning in patients who may have a ruptured diaphragm.

If your protocols allow the use of PASGs, you must be aware of the complications that can be associated with them, as well as the indications and contraindications for using them. The indications for using the PASG are as follows:

- Decompensated shock (systolic blood pressure less than 90 mmHg)
- Suspected pelvic fracture with hypotension
- Suspected intra-abdominal hemorrhage with hypotension

Contraindications for PASG use include the following:

- Cardiogenic shock
- Abdominal evisceration
- Penetrating thoracic trauma
- Pregnancy
- Cardiac arrest

Once a PASG is inflated, do not deflate it unless you are advised to by medical direction because of complications, such as impaired ventilation. Usually, PASGs are deflated in the hospital under physician supervision, either in surgery or when adequate volume replacement has been achieved.

Keep the trauma patient warm by minimizing exposure time, removing any wet clothing (including clothing that is wet with blood), moving him to a warm environment, and covering him with blankets following exposure for assessment. If the temperature in the back of the ambulance is comfortable to you, it is probably not warm enough for the patient in shock. Patients who are in shock are susceptible to hypothermia due to the significant blood loss because blood carries body heat with it when it leaves the body. Impaired cellular energy production prevents the patient from increasing the body temperature through metabolism. If the environment is cool, the rate of heat loss is accelerated. Allowing a critical trauma patient to become hypothermic can be fatal. Hypothermia reduces the effectiveness of the body's blood-clotting mechanisms, resulting in **coagulopathy**. Coagulopathy reduces the body's ability to stop active bleeding, which leads to more blood loss.

Successful trauma resuscitation takes place in the context of a well-functioning trauma care system. Part of the care that you provide to the trauma patient includes

PERSONAL PERSPECTIVE

Advanced EMT Carlos Sanchez: One evening, I was working in a suburb of a large city when my partner and I were called to an MVC where a motorcycle struck a pickup truck in a T-bone collision. When we got to the scene, I noticed that the motorcycle was embedded into the truck between the cab and truck bed. The rear corner of the truck's cab was dented where the patient struck it as he was thrown over the truck. The patient was about 45 feet from truck.

We were about 40 minutes from the nearest trauma center, so I requested aeromedical assistance. Dispatch advised me that they were already en route.

When I got to the patient, he was on his back with large blood clots and vomit in his airway. All of his extremities were grossly deformed due to fractures and his torso was twisted 180 degrees at the waist. He had a closed head injury, internal bleeding, and extensive musculoskeletal trauma.

After suctioning and inserting an oropharyngeal airway, my partner began ventilating the patient because he had agonal breathing at a rate of about 8 breaths per minute. My partner continued to manage airway and breathing as firefighters assisted me in immobilizing and packaging the patient. We established two large-bore IVs and initiated fluid therapy. The

fire department advised the responding aeromedical crew of the landing zone location, which was about 100 yards from the scene.

We loaded the patient into our ambulance and arrived at the landing zone just as the helicopter landed. I flew in with the patient to assist en route to the trauma center. Near the end of our flight, the patient's heart rate was steadily falling. The trauma center staff met us on the helipad and we rushed the patient into the trauma center where physicians and nurses were awaiting our arrival. The patient was prepared and taken into surgery in a very short time.

I don't know if the patient survived but I do know that through our actions, we provided him with the best chance of survival. From the time of the collision to the time the patient was taken into surgery, it was approximately 50 minutes. This was accomplished through teamwork, which involved me and my partner, the firefighters, law enforcement, the aeromedical crew, and the staff at the trauma center.

Those types of calls are always hectic. It is your responsibility to remain focused on the goal, which is managing life threats and providing rapid transport to an appropriate facility.

selecting the best hospital destination for the patient's circumstances, selecting the best method of transporting the patient to that facility, and communicating with the receiving facility as early as possible so that they can prepare for the patient's arrival by notifying the necessary personnel. Paint a concise and accurate picture of the

patient's condition so that the appropriate services within the hospital can be alerted.

Finally, improving trauma care requires feedback on your performance through a continuous quality improvement process and making every effort to remain abreast of changes in trauma care recommendations.

CASE STUDY WRAP-UP

Clinical-Reasoning Process

Advanced EMT William and his EMT partner Terri have just arrived at the scene of a motorcycle collision into a tree. They have a single patient who was found 30 feet beyond the point of impact. He is lying prone and not wearing a helmet.

William and Terri immediately recognize that the mechanism of injury is consistent with a high risk of multisystem trauma involving the head, spine, and chest, as well as abdominal and long-bone injuries. They immediately associate those injury patterns with a high probability of life-threatening problems with the patient's airway, breathing, and circulation.

"Take the head and airway," Terri tells William. "Let's get him supine and take care of the ABCs." William confirms that the patient is unresponsive to painful stimuli, giving him a GCS of 3. With the help of the engine crew who pulled up right behind them, Terri and William log roll the patient onto a long backboard while maintaining manual cervical-spine stabilization. Before William could even ask, an EMT from the engine turns on the suction and begins suctioning blood out of the airway.

"He's got some minimal respiratory effort," says William, "But he's not moving any air." The first EMT inserts an oropharyngeal airway while another connects the bag-valve-mask device to oxygen and prepares to hand it to him. As the first EMT delivers a breath, the second quickly checks breath sounds, noting a decrease on the right side, as well as some paradoxical movement of the right anterior chest wall.

Meanwhile, Terri has palpated a weak, rapid radial pulse and prepared an absorbent dressing to stop bleeding from a large scalp laceration. The EMTs place a cervical collar, prepare backboard straps, and lower the stretcher next to the patient. Terri performs a rapid trauma exam, noting massive facial swelling, instability of the right anterior chest wall, and bilateral open femur fractures.

"He's still got blood in the airway," says William. Let's suction before we lift him, and as soon as we get him loaded let's put in a Combitube. In the back of the ambulance, William inserts the Combitube and confirms correct placement in the esophagus by listening to breath sounds and auscultating over the epigastrium. The EMTs obtain vital signs, a pulse oximetry reading, and set up for capnometry.

As they depart for the hospital emergency department with a driver and tech borrowed from the engine, Terri completes a head-to-toe assessment, noting several additional, but less serious, injuries. Meanwhile, the EMTs have set up two IVs of normal saline. One of the EMTs takes over ventilations so William can start the IVs as Terri contacts the trauma center.

CHAPTER REVIEW

Chapter Summary

Successful management of a multisystem trauma patient begins with the scene size-up, including the identifying mechanisms of injury that are likely to produce life-threatening injury. Perform a systematic primary assessment and manage all immediate life threats. Through a rapid trauma exam and head-to-toe exam, identify injuries and manage each appropriately, in the context of the patient's overall condition.

During resuscitation of the trauma patient, your first priorities are always to maintain a patent airway, ensure adequate ventilations and oxygenation, and control life-threatening external bleeding. Maintain the patient's body temperature, and ensure that the patient's systolic blood pressure is adequate to allow tissue perfusion without worsening bleeding and other complications of fluid resuscitation. In general, it is desirable to maintain a systolic blood pressure of 80 to 90 mmHg, although a systolic blood pressure of 100 mmHg may be required in patients with traumatic brain injury.

Because the definitive treatment for multisystem trauma patients is surgery, minimize your on-scene time while managing the airway, breathing, and circulation. Transport the patient by the most appropriate means available to the most appropriate facility available, given the circumstances. Do not delay transport of the critical trauma patient to splint extremity fractures or initiate IV access on the scene. In cases of extended transport times, consider the use of aeromedical transport to definitive care. Simply stated, you should do the following:

- Identify and manage life threats.

- Initiate transport as soon as possible.

- Provide rapid transport to a facility where the patient can receive definitive care.

Following these guidelines will provide the patient with the best chance of survival and recovery from injuries.

Review Questions

Multiple-Choice Questions

1. When administering an initial fluid bolus, how much fluid should be infused?
   a. 100 mL
   b. 250 mL
   c. 500 mL
   d. 1,000 mL

2. A rapid trauma assessment of a critical multisystem trauma patient should take place:
   a. immediately after obtaining a SAMPLE history.
   b. simultaneously with the primary assessment.
   c. simultaneously with treatment of life threats and packaging of the patient.
   d. en route to the hospital emergency department.

3. A multisystem trauma patient with internal hemorrhage must maintain a MAP of at least _____ mmHg in order to maintain perfusion to his vital organs.
   a. 40
   b. 50
   c. 60
   d. 80

4. You arrive on the scene of a construction site to find a patient who was pinned against a concrete wall by a very large forklift. The patient is complaining of shortness of breath and severe pain to the right side of his chest. His vital signs are as follows: blood pressure 78/P, heart rate 110 (absent at the radial artery, palpated at the carotid artery), respirations 30 and shallow. In your initial treatment of this patient, your next action is to:
   a. initiate IV access.
   b. assist ventilations with a bag-valve-mask device attached to high-flow oxygen.
   c. immobilize the patient's spine using a long backboard and transport immediately.
   d. apply a PASG and inflate it.

Critical-Thinking Questions

5. Explain how Advanced EMTs can apply knowledge of pathophysiology to reduce morbidity and mortality in patients with multisystem trauma.

6. How does injury to more than one body system increase morbidity and mortality?

7. What is the importance of maintaining the patient's MAP?

8. Discuss the pros and cons of fluid administration in the multisystem trauma patient.

9. What is the relationship between trauma, heat loss, and patient outcome?

References

Centers for Disease Control and Prevention. (2010). *Injury prevention and control: Field triage.* Retrieved April 25, 2011, from http://www.cdc.gov/fieldtriage/

McSwain, N. E., Salomone, J. P., Pons, P. T. (Eds). (2007). *Prehospital trauma life support* (6th ed.). St. Louis, MO: Elsevier.

43 Obstetrics and Care of the Newborn

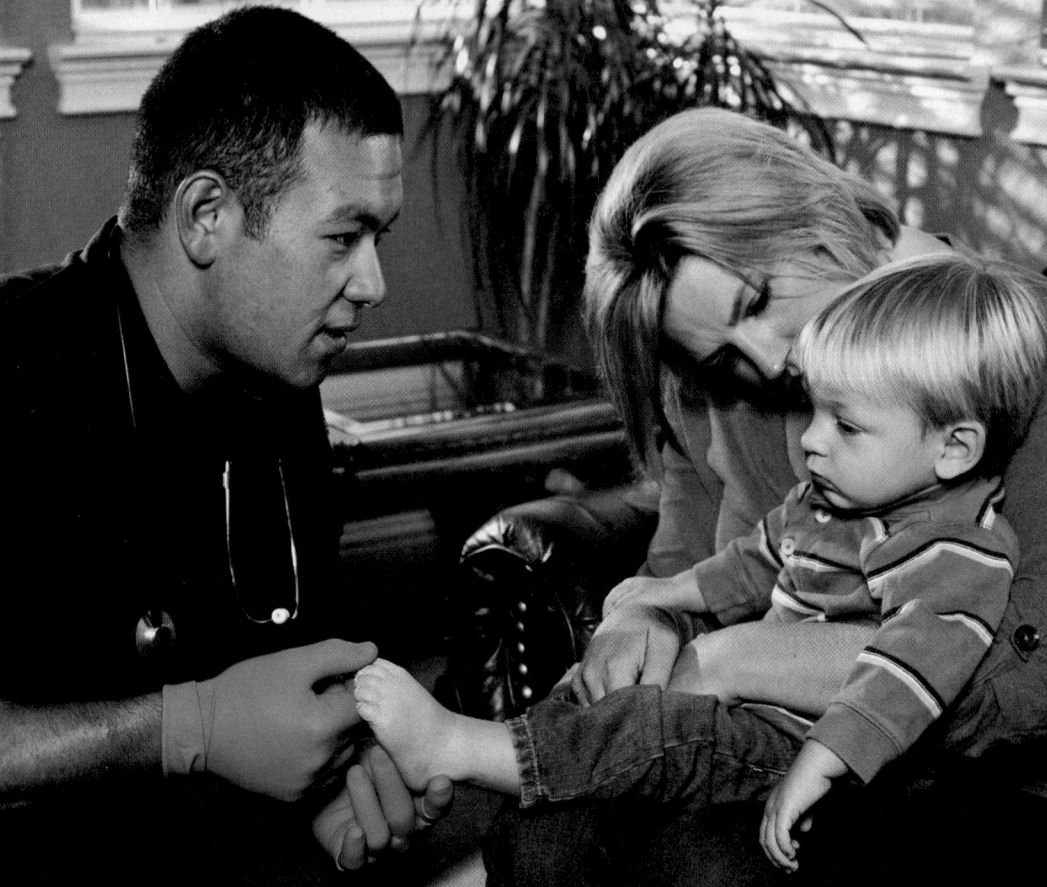

Content Area: Special Patient Populations

Advanced EMT Education Standard: Applies a fundamental knowledge of growth, development, and aging and assessment findings to provide basic and selected advanced emergency care and transportation for a patient with special needs.

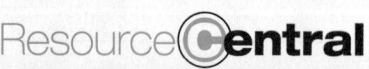

To access Resource Central, follow the directions on the Student Access Card provided with this text. If there is no card, go to www.bradybooks.com and follow the Resource Central link to Buy Access. Under Media Resources, you will find:

- *APGAR.* Scoring and assessment.
- *Childbirth.* Stages of labor and delivery and post-delivery responsibilities.
- *Preeclampsia.* Signs and symptoms, complications, and high-risk factors.
- *Ectopic Pregnancy.* Risk factors and relevant history-taking questions.
- *Trauma in Pregnancy.* Common causes and how to assess the pregnant patient.

Objectives

After reading this chapter, you should be able to:

43.1 Define key terms introduced in this chapter.

43.2 Describe the anatomy and physiology of the female reproductive system.

43.3 Describe the anatomy and physiology of pregnancy, including the following:

- Fertilization of an ovum
- Gestational age
- Placenta
- Umbilical cord
- Amniotic sac

(continued)

CASE STUDY

Just as Advanced EMT Steve Gore tells his partner, Scott Guidry, that the ice storm they are experiencing seems to be keeping people off the roads, they are dispatched to an apartment for a 27-year-old female patient in labor. When they arrive at the address, the patient's husband greets them at the door.

"My wife is in labor," he tells them, "but she is only 35 weeks. The baby isn't supposed to be here for another month! I can't take a chance of driving her to the hospital myself in this weather. What if we end up in a ditch, you know?"

Scott and Steve find the patient, Claire Velez, lying on a sofa. Mrs. Velez appears to be uncomfortable and is experiencing a contraction as the crew approaches.

Problem-Solving Questions

1. At 35 weeks gestation, what is the risk of distress if the baby is born now?
2. How should Scott and Steve prioritize the order of the information they need?
3. What factors determine how they should conduct the physical exam?
4. What treatment should they anticipate for the mother and, if a field delivery is performed, the newborn?

(continued from previous page)

- Changes in the reproductive system
- Changes in the respiratory and cardiovascular systems
- Changes in the gastrointestinal and urinary systems
- Changes in the musculoskeletal system
- Normal labor and delivery

43.4 Elicit a pertinent history from the patient with an obstetric emergency.

43.5 Describe the assessment and emergency management of patients with antepartum emergencies, including the following:
- Abruptio placentae
- Ectopic pregnancy
- Placenta previa
  Pre-eclampsia/eclampsia
- Pregnancy-induced hypertension
- Ruptured uterus
- Spontaneous abortion
- Supine hypotensive syndrome
- Trauma in pregnancy

43.6 Describe the assessment and management of a patient in active labor.

43.7 Describe the steps of assisting with an out-of-hospital obstetric delivery.

43.8 Take steps to manage abnormal out-of-hospital obstetric deliveries, including the following:
- Breech and limb presentations
- Meconium staining
- Multiple births
- Preterm labor/premature rupture of membranes
- Precipitous delivery
- Prolapsed umbilical cord
- Shoulder dystocia

(continued)

(continued from previous page)

43.9   Take steps to manage postpartum complications, including the following:
- Postpartum hemorrhage
- Pulmonary embolism

43.10   Demonstrate the steps of assessing and managing a neonate, including the following:
- APGAR scoring
- Assessing breathing and circulation
- Positioning
- Preventing heat loss
- Suctioning

43.11   Recognize signs that indicate the need for neonatal resuscitation.

43.12   Apply the concepts of the neonatal resuscitation pyramid to the care of neonates in need of resuscitative measures.

43.13   Effectively communicate to other health care providers a pertinent patient history, assessment findings, and interventions for pregnant patients and neonates.

Introduction

Caring for an obstetric patient and assisting with the delivery of her child can be one of the most rewarding experiences you can have as an Advanced EMT. Although the majority of obstetric calls are uncomplicated, you must be aware of signs, symptoms, and history that indicate potential problems with the pregnancy or delivery. Occasionally, a baby is born with medical problems that must be immediately corrected. You must be able to recognize indications of emergencies related to pregnancy and childbirth and emergencies in the newborn, or neonate. This chapter provides information you need to properly assess and care for an obstetric patient and a **neonate** following birth.

Anatomy and Physiology Review

The anatomy and physiology of pregnant women is different from that of typical adult patients. The anatomy and physiology of the neonate is different from that of older infants and children. Understanding those differences forms a foundation for understanding assessment findings, obtaining a pertinent history, and anticipating and managing problems.

Female Reproductive System

The female external genitalia consist of the mons pubis, labia majora, labia minora, and clitoris (Figure 43-1). The urethral meatus lies between the clitoris and the introitus, the entrance to the vagina. The vagina is a hollow tubular passageway that connects the external genitalia with the internal genitalia. In childbirth, the vagina serves as part of the birth canal.

The uterus is a small muscular organ lined with endometrium tissue that thickens each month during the reproductive years in preparation for the possible implantation of a fertilized ovum (Figure 43-2). Anatomically, the uterus is divided into three sections, from superior to inferior. The uppermost portion is the fundus and the lowest portion is the cervix, with the body of the uterus lying between. The cervix projects into the upper vagina, where it provides a passageway (os cervix and cervical canal) for sperm to enter the uterus and travel to the fallopian tubes.

The outer portion of each fallopian tube drapes around an ovary, providing a passageway for ova to travel toward the uterus. If sperm are present, fertilization normally takes place in the outer third of the fallopian tube. The fertilized ovum continues to travel toward the uterus, where it may be implanted in the endometrium (uterine lining).

The ovaries and endometrium undergo cyclical monthly changes under the influence of the endocrine system, called the *menstrual cycle*. Day 1 of the menstrual cycle is the day that bleeding begins as the endometrium is shed from the uterus in nonpregnant women. The bleeding lasts about five days, but ranges from three to seven days. The total amount of blood lost over this time is about 30 mL.

After the uterine lining is shed, hormonal changes influence it to be rebuilt. Meanwhile, several follicles containing immature ova have already begun developing in the ovaries. In a typical cycle, the development of one of the follicles outpaces that of the others. About 14 days after the first day of

FIGURE 43-1

(A) Female external genitalia.
(B) Cross-section of female internal and external reproductive organs.

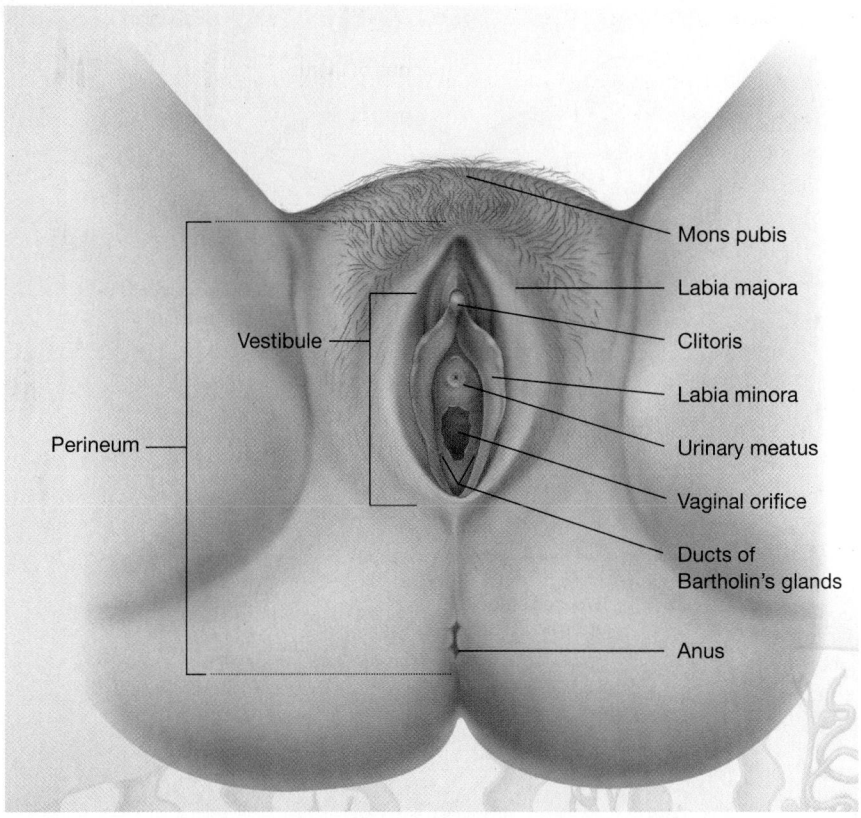

Mons pubis

Labia majora

Clitoris

Labia minora

Urinary meatus

Vaginal orifice

Ducts of
Bartholin's glands

Anus

Vestibule

Perineum

(A)

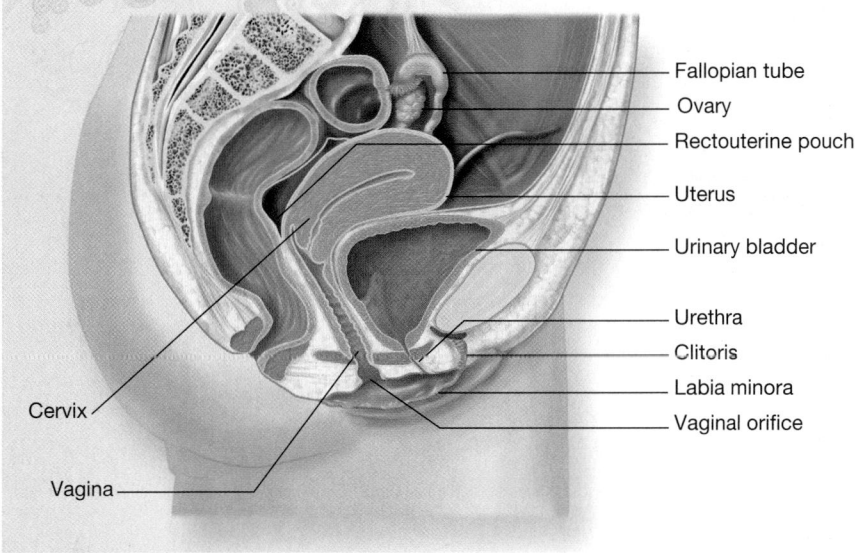

Fallopian tube

Ovary

Rectouterine pouch

Uterus

Urinary bladder

Urethra

Clitoris

Labia minora

Vaginal orifice

Cervix

Vagina

(B)

menstrual bleeding, the mature follicle ruptures, discharging the ovum into the pelvic cavity near the entrance of the adjacent fallopian tube. This is called *ovulation*.

Pregnancy

If sperm arrive in the fallopian tube during a short window of time surrounding ovulation, fertilization may occur, resulting in pregnancy (Figure 43-3). If pregnancy occurs,

the rapidly dividing fertilized egg must travel to the uterus, where it will be implanted in the thickened endometrium. Hormones released by the developing **embryo** induce changes that preserve the endometrium and prevent new follicles from beginning to develop. If pregnancy occurs, the follicle that discharged the ovum, the corpus luteum, is maintained, rather than degenerating. The corpus luteum secretes hormones that support the pregnancy until the placenta develops.

FIGURE 43-2

Frontal view of the uterus, fallopian tubes, and ovaries.

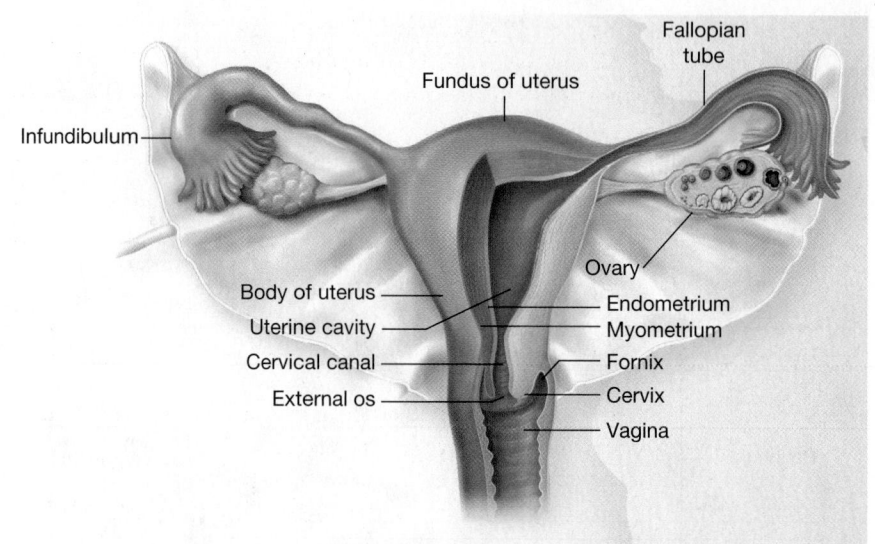

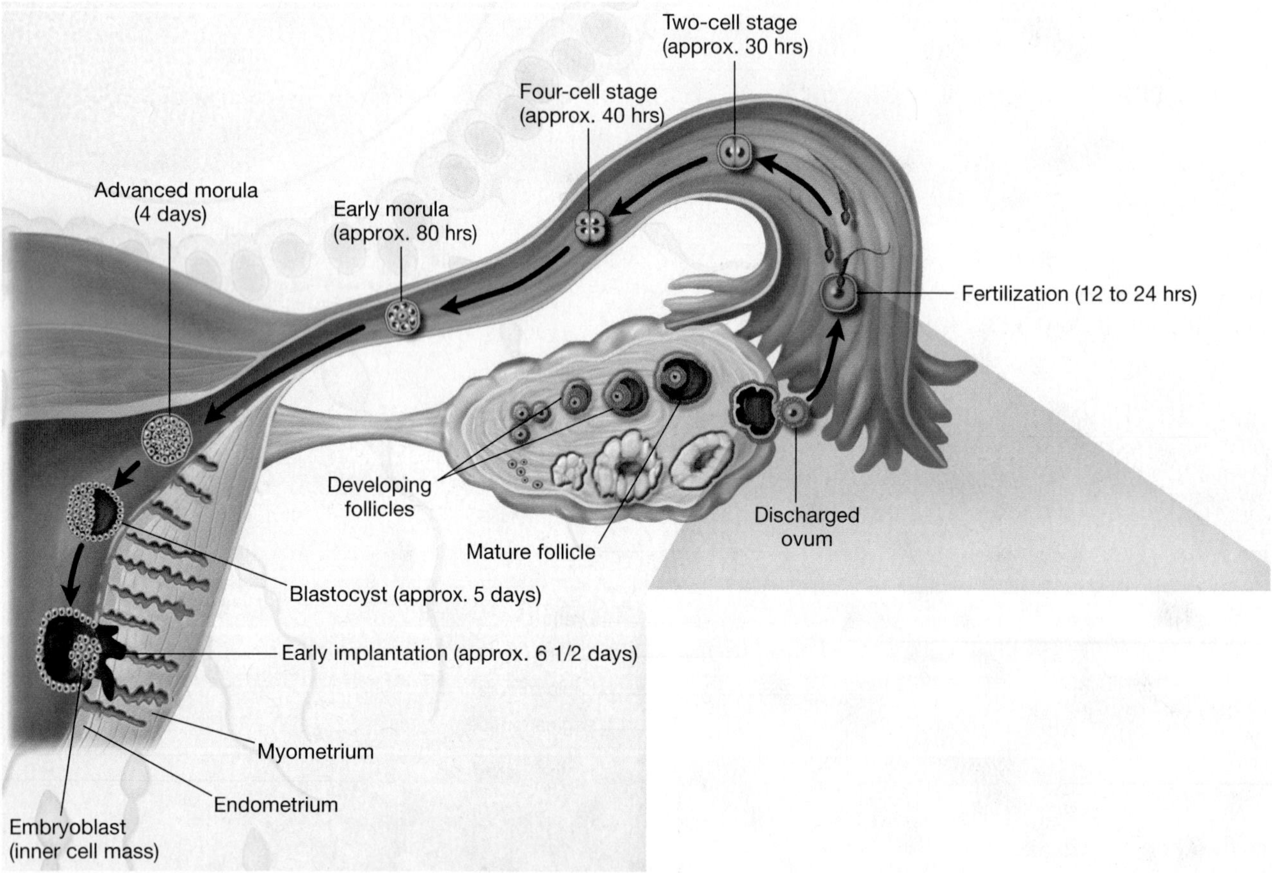

FIGURE 43-3

Fertilization, early development of the zygote, and implantation.

Fertilization and Embryonic Development

Fertilization, or conception, is the union of a spermatozoon and an ovum, which produces a **zygote**. The entry of a single spermatozoon into the ovum triggers changes in the ovum that prevent entry of additional spermatozoa. Each spermatozoon and ovum contain only 23 chromosomes, half the normal number in human cells. The zygote contains 46 chromosomes, 23 from the ovum and 23 from the spermatozoon.

The fertilized ovum begins to divide about 30 hours after fertilization. By six days after fertilization, the zygote enters the uterine cavity and the dividing cells have formed a hollow ball of cells called a *blastocyst*. The outer layer of the blastocyst cells allow for implantation into the endometrium, while the inner layer of cells will become an embryo. The inner cell mass separates from the outer cell mass, creating a cavity that becomes the amniotic cavity as it enlarges. As cells divide and migrate, the extraembryonic membranes, including the amnion (amniotic sac) are formed.

The chorion, a layer of the extraembryonic membranes, develops blood vessels within finger-like projections called *villi*. The villi extend into the endometrium, allowing maternal blood to pass in close proximity to the villi, which allows for fetal gas exchange. The thickened area of chorion that is attached to the endometrium is called the **placenta**. The placenta is a temporary organ of pregnancy, to which the fetus is attached by the umbilical cord. The umbilical cord contains two umbilical arteries that carry deoxygenated blood to the placenta, and one umbilical vein that carries oxygenated blood from the placenta to the embryo.

Fetal Development

During the first 60 days of pregnancy, the developing organism is called an *embryo* (Figure 43-4). From 60 days **gestation** to birth, the organism is called a **fetus** (Figure 43-5). The normal duration of pregnancy is from 37 to 41 weeks and is divided into 13-week trimesters. The due date, or estimated date of confinement (EDC), is calculated as 280 days, or approximately 40 weeks, from the date of the mother's last menstrual period (LMP). A full-term infant weighs 3.0 to 3.5 kg (6.6 to 7.7 pounds) and is, on the average, 50 cm (20 inches) in length.

Rudimentary organs form by the end of the second month of gestation, but must continue to develop throughout pregnancy. In particular, the lungs do not produce surfactant until the 28th week of gestation (Table 43-1). A fetus has the greatest chances for survival when the pregnancy

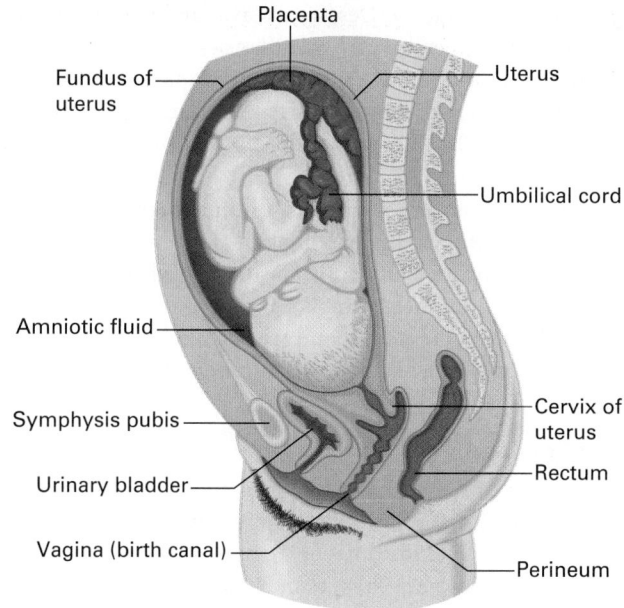

FIGURE 43-5

A fetus near term.

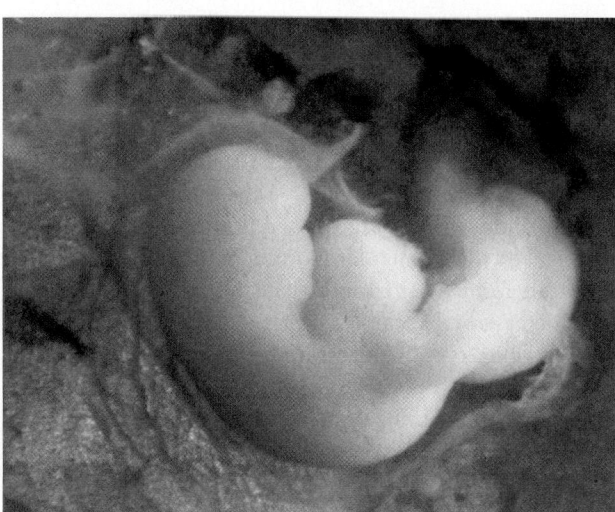

FIGURE 43-4

A 28-day embryo. (© Petit Format/Photo Researchers, Inc.)

TABLE 43-1	Milestones in Fetal Development	
Gestational Age in Months	**Approximate Size**	**Development**
1	0.25 in.; less than 1 oz	Rudimentary formation of vital organ systems. Heartbeat begins.
2	1.5 in.; less than 1 oz	Skin, muscle, and skeletal tissue begin to develop.
3	3 in.; about 1 oz	Basic central nervous system structure is complete.
4	5 in.; 5 oz	Mother can feel movements. Hair is beginning to develop.
5	10 in.; 1 lb	Continued development of systems; nares open.
6	13 in.; 1.5 lb	Continued nervous system development; reflexes are developing, alveoli are forming. Fat deposits are being stored.
7	16 in.; 3.3 lb	Eyelids open and in males, the testes begin to descend.
8	18 in.; 5 lb	Alveoli are formed. Fat deposits increase as birth approaches.
9	20 in.; 7 lb	Systems formed and functioning at newborn level.

continues to full term. Despite the availability of sophisticated neonatal medical care, most fetuses born before 25 to 27 weeks gestation have a birth weight under 600 g (just over 1 pound) and do not survive (Martini, Bartholomew, & Bledsoe, 2008). Those that do survive often have developmental abnormalities.

Preterm delivery is birth that occurs between 28 and 36 weeks gestation, at which time the fetus weighs at least 1 kg. However, an infant has a low birth weight if he weighs less than 2.5 kg (5.5 pounds). Chances of survival and normal development are good with specialized advanced medical care in a neonatal intensive care unit (NICU).

Maternal Changes

The body of a pregnant woman must undergo many changes to support the developing fetus and prepare for childbirth. Beyond the obvious changes in the reproductive system, there also are changes in blood volume, cardiovascular and respiratory function, nutritional needs, demands on the urinary system, and in the gastrointestinal and musculoskeletal systems.

Reproductive System

By the end of pregnancy, the uterus has increased from a small, 2-ounce organ that does not rise above the level of the pubic bone to a 2-pound organ that extends nearly to the lower costal margin of the thoracic cavity. Later in pregnancy, the uterus receives about 16 percent of the maternal blood volume. A mucus plug forms in the cervix, where it protects the uterine cavity and developing fetus.

The breasts begin to change early in pregnancy in preparation for lactation (milk production). Enlarged, tender breasts are a common early indication of pregnancy.

Later in pregnancy, as the uterine fundus rises above the level of the pubis and changes the profile of the abdomen, the abdomen becomes more prone to injury. Balance, posture, and gait are affected and, in combination with musculoskeletal changes, make low back pain a common complaint. The distended uterus and abdomen are more prone to trauma.

Cardiovascular System

The pregnant woman's blood volume increases by 45 percent to almost 50 percent by the time she reaches term. There is a greater increase in plasma volume than in red blood cells, which results in a lower hematocrit. Although stroke volume declines in late pregnancy, the heart rate increases by 10 to 15 beats per minute, increasing cardiac output to 6 to 7 L/min. The blood pressure may be lower during the first two trimesters, but returns to normal in the third trimester. Hypertension in a pregnant woman should make you suspicious of the presence of a hypertensive disorder of pregnancy, such as pre-eclampsia.

The increased maternal blood volume delays the findings associated with shock. As much as 30 to 35 percent of the blood volume may be lost before there are changes in vital signs. Maintain a high index of suspicion for shock in pregnant patients with trauma or who present with nontraumatic bleeding.

Respiratory System

The maternal respiratory system must provide a mechanism of gas exchange for the developing fetus in addition to meeting the needs of the mother. The effect of pregnancy hormones reduces airway resistance, allowing the increased needs to be met. The combined needs of the fetus and mother result in a 20 percent increase in oxygen consumption by term. The tidal volume increases substantially, but there is only a small increase in respiratory rate. The expanding uterus displaces the abdominal organs and elevates the diaphragm. As a result of anatomical and physiological changes, slight shortness of breath is a common complaint in late pregnancy.

Gastrointestinal System

The gastrointestinal system is associated with one of the most unpleasant side effects of pregnancy: the nausea and vomiting of early pregnancy known as *morning sickness*. Severe nausea and vomiting leading to dehydration and weight loss occurs in a minority of pregnancies and may persist throughout the entire pregnancy. That condition is known as **hyperemesis gravidarum**, which must be treated with antiemetics, sometimes with limited success. Patients with hyperemesis gravidarum may receive IV fluids and intravenous or subcutaneous administration of antiemetics at home.

The gastrointestinal system slows during pregnancy, which may contribute to bloating and constipation. Always anticipate that the pregnant patient's stomach is full and be prepared to protect the airway if vomiting occurs. The size and position of the uterus make assessment of the abdominal organs difficult as pregnancy advances.

Urinary System

The increasing size and changed position of the uterus in the first trimester make urinary frequency a common sign of pregnancy. Although urinary frequency may decrease in the second trimester, it returns in the third trimester as the uterus continues to enlarge. Blood flow to the kidneys is increased and the glomerular filtration rate (GFR, the amount of filtrate formed per minute) increases by up to 50 percent. The increased GFR can result in poor reabsorption of glucose and excretion of glucose in the urine. However, glucose in the urine also may be an indication of gestational diabetes. Protein in the urine is an indication of pre-eclampsia.

Musculoskeletal System

One of the hormones of pregnancy, *relaxin*, causes the joints to loosen. Although the goal of this process is to allow flexibility of the pelvic girdle, all joints are affected. Sprains and joint injuries occur more readily and should be anticipated according to the mechanism of injury. Relaxation of the joints contributes to the low back pain often experienced in pregnancy.

Labor and Delivery

The mechanism that results in the onset of labor involves a complex interaction between increased levels of hormones and mechanical stress on the uterine muscle (myometrium) and cervix. Throughout pregnancy, the increase in estrogen levels makes uterine smooth muscle more sensitive to the effects of **oxytocin**. Mild, irregular uterine contractions occur throughout pregnancy. However, later in pregnancy the contractions stimulate the release of more oxytocin and the release of prostaglandins, both of which, in turn, increase uterine contractions.

Late in pregnancy, the mother experiences intense, but painless, tightening of the uterus, known as **Braxton-Hicks contractions**. At the same time, prostaglandin plays a role in softening and thinning the cervix so that uterine contractions can cause it to dilate. At some point, the level of oxytocin increases to the point where contractions are regular and sustained. Often, much of the work of labor is done before the mother experiences the onset of regular, intensifying contractions, particularly in women who have previously given birth.

Labor is divided into four stages, each characterized by certain events.

- *Stage one.* Stage one is known as the **dilation** stage (Figure 43-6). It begins with the onset of regular contractions and ends when the cervix is completely dilated. During this stage, the fetus descends further into the pelvis. This is called *station,* which is determined (by a physician or obstetric nurse) by the position of the fetal head with reference to the mother's pelvic outlet. Early in stage one, contractions may be 10 or more minutes apart, but increase in frequency and intensity. The amniotic sac may rupture late in this stage, although sometimes the amniotic membranes can rupture spontaneously prior to the onset of contractions. In the hospital, the obstetrician may use a small hook, called an

THE THREE STAGES OF LABOR

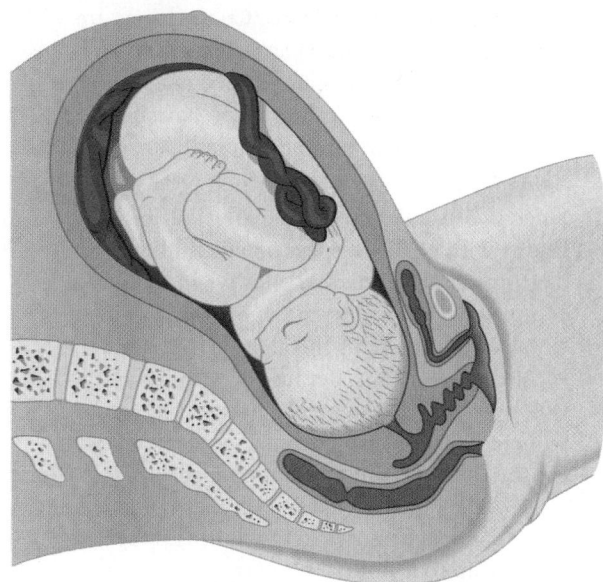

(A)　**FIRST STAGE:**
First uterine contraction to dilation of cervix

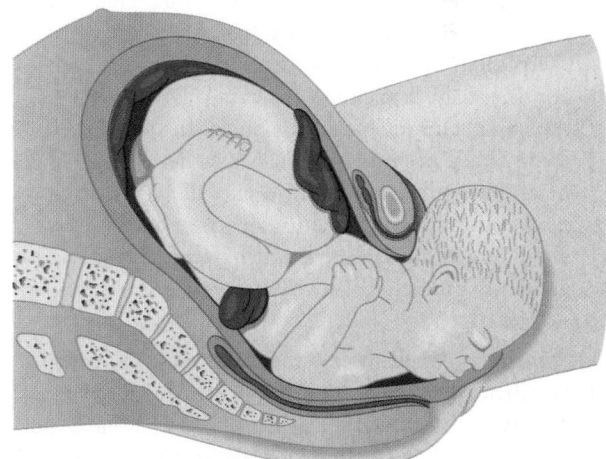

(B)　**SECOND STAGE:**
Birth of baby or expulsion

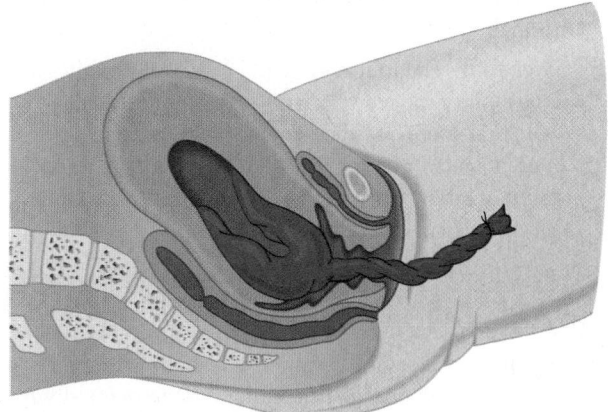

(C)　**THIRD STAGE:**
Delivery of placenta

FIGURE 43-6

(A) The first stage of labor begins with regular uterine contractions and ends with complete dilation and effacement of the cervix. (B) The second stage of labor begins with complete cervical dilation and effacement and ends with expulsion of the fetus. (C) The third stage of labor begins with expulsion of the fetus and ends with expulsion of the placenta.

amniotome, to rupture the membranes after the cervix has dilated sufficiently. Contractions are intensified after the membranes are ruptured. Stage one lasts about 8 hours, but can be much shorter in **multiparous** women (those who have delivered previously) and can be longer in nulliparous women (those who have not given birth before).

- *Stage two.* Stage two is the expulsion stage. It begins with complete **effacement** (thinning) and dilation of the cervix and ends when the fetus has completely emerged from the birth canal. The expulsion of the fetus through the birth canal is called **parturition**. Because cervical dilation is not checked in the prehospital setting, you will recognize this stage by its intense, frequent contractions. Often, as the mother progresses from stage one to stage two, she becomes irritable and may experience nausea and vomiting. Stage two can last up to 2 hours, but may be much shorter in multiparous women. As the fetus descends from the upper part of the birth canal to the vaginal opening, the perineum will bulge with each contraction. When the fetus' scalp is visible at the vaginal opening, first with contractions, then continuously, it is called **crowning**. Delivery of the head is imminent at this point. In some cases, it may take several more pushes to deliver the head, but in others, the head may deliver with the next contraction as the mother pushes. The fetus' shoulders and body are smaller than the head and generally are delivered with the next contraction or two.

- *Stage three.* Stage three is the placental stage, which lasts from delivery of the fetus (now called a *neonate,* or newborn) through the delivery of the placenta. The placenta may be delivered within a few more contractions, but can take up to an hour. Detachment and expulsion of the placenta are accompanied by blood loss. Up to 500 mL blood loss during delivery is normal.

- *Stage four.* The fourth stage of labor begins with expulsion of the placenta and ends 1 hour later. Note that some classifications of labor, particularly in prehospital literature, may list only the first three stages of labor, because they are the most relevant to out-of-hospital delivery.

The Role of Prenatal Care

Regular **prenatal** visits to an obstetrician or obstetric nurse practitioner during pregnancy are associated with better maternal and fetal outcomes. Routine examinations and testing can detect many problems early so that they can be managed in order to decrease risks to the mother and fetus (Figure 43-7). Conditions such as

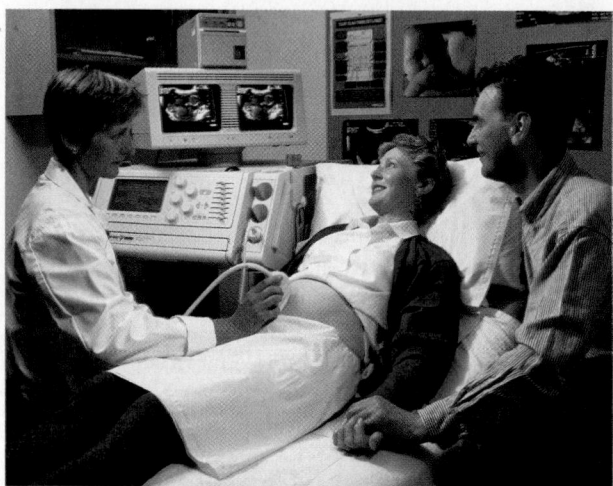

FIGURE 43-7

At least one ultrasound is part of routine prenatal care.
(© SPL/Photo Researchers, Inc.)

gestational diabetes, hypertensive disorders of pregnancy, risks for **preterm labor**, abnormal placement of the placenta, poor fetal growth, and certain fetal abnormalities can be identified through good prenatal care, and the mother can receive advice about nutrition, medications, rest, activities, and health behaviors in order to support a healthy pregnancy.

Neonatal Anatomy and Physiology

A developing fetus has several anatomic and physiological differences that allow him to develop in a watery environment without ingesting food or breathing air. At birth, the fetus becomes a neonate whose body systems must immediately adjust to doing work that his mother's body did for him before he was born.

Ventilation and Circulation

Because the fetus does not breathe air into his lungs, they are filled with fluid. Much of that fluid is expelled as the fetus squeezes through the birth canal. The neonate will continue to rid the airway of additional fluids in the first several hours after birth. Upon birth, he must work to take the first breath into his airless lungs. Taking air into the lungs for the first time results in changes in pulmonary pressure. These changes redirect the blood flow that bypassed the fetal lungs.

During prenatal life, fetal blood cannot be oxygenated by passing through the pulmonary circulation. Instead, blood receives oxygen from the mother's circulation (Figure 43-8). The umbilical arteries, which branch from the internal iliac arteries, carry deoxygenated blood containing higher carbon dioxide and waste levels from the fetal circulation, through the umbilical

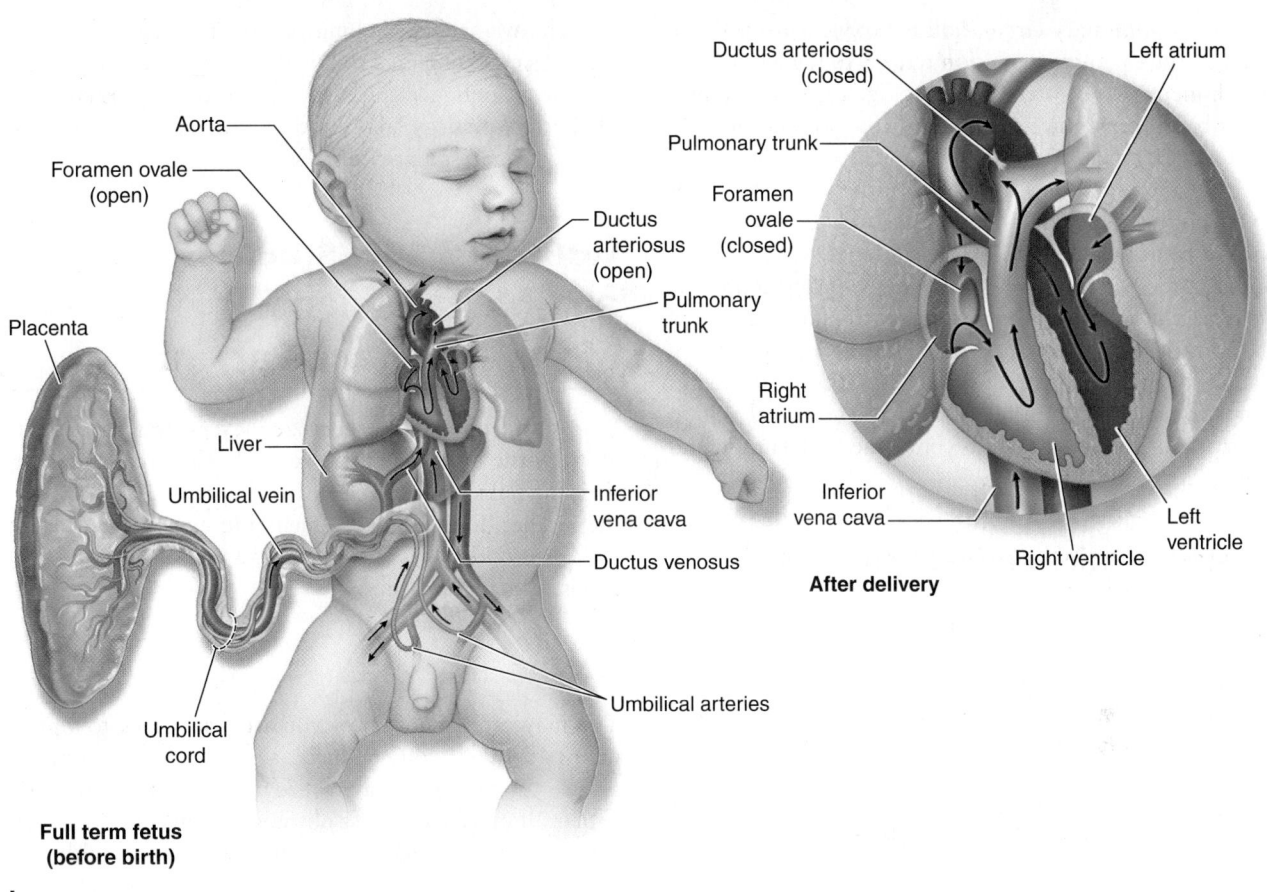

Aorta

Foramen ovale (open)

Placenta

Liver

Umbilical vein

Umbilical cord

Full term fetus (before birth)

Ductus arteriosus (open)

Pulmonary trunk

Inferior vena cava

Ductus venosus

Umbilical arteries

Ductus arteriosus (closed)

Pulmonary trunk

Foramen ovale (closed)

Right atrium

Inferior vena cava

Left atrium

Left ventricle

Right ventricle

After delivery

FIGURE 43-8

Fetal circulation bypasses the pulmonary circulation. Gas exchange occurs in the placenta. Blood is delivered to the placenta by the umbilical arteries and returns to the fetal circulation through the umbilical vein.

cord, and into the circulation of the chorionic villi of the placenta. The villi are surrounded by maternal blood that is higher in oxygen and lower in carbon dioxide than fetal blood, allowing gas exchange. Blood that is higher in oxygen and nutrients and lower in carbon dioxide and wastes returns to fetal circulation through the umbilical vein. The umbilical vein passes through the liver, where some of the blood enters the hepatic circulation to deliver nutrients. The rest of the blood in the umbilical vein returns to the inferior vena cava by way of the *ductus venosus.*

The oxygenated blood continues through the inferior vena cava to the right atrium of the heart. About 25 percent of the blood entering the right atrium is diverted directly to the left atrium through an opening in the intra-atrial septum called the *foramen ovale.* A flap over the foramen ovale acts as a one-way valve that allows blood to flow from right to left, but prevents it from flowing from left to right during atrial systole.

The remainder of the blood entering the right atrium enters the right ventricle. When the right ventricle contracts, blood enters the pulmonary artery as usual, but is diverted into the aorta by a vessel called the *ductus*

arteriosus. Only a small amount of blood passes through the pulmonary arterial system. Some of the blood leaving the aorta circulates to the tissues, but some is once again diverted through the umbilical arteries to travel back to the placenta.

To allow a sufficient gradient for gas exchange between the maternal circulation and fetal circulation, the fetal PaO_2 must be lower than maternal PaO_2 and fetal $PaCO_2$ must be higher than maternal $PaCO_2$. Recall from Chapter 8 that onloading of oxygen onto hemoglobin is enhanced by a high PaO_2 and offloading of oxygen at the tissue level is enhanced by a low PaO_2. To compensate for differences in oxygenation, the fetus has a form of hemoglobin, fetal hemoglobin, that is adapted to the lower-oxygen environment. Fetal hemoglobin is more saturated with oxygen at a lower PaO_2 than adult hemoglobin.

Ventilatory movements prior to birth fill the fetal lungs with amniotic fluid. After passing through the birth canal and expelling fluid from the lungs, the neonate's ventilatory movements allow air to enter the lungs. When air fills the alveoli the resistance to pulmonary circulation is greatly reduced, allowing blood that bypassed the pulmonary circulation by way of the ductus arteriosus to enter the pulmonary circulation for oxygenation. Blood from the pulmonary circulation returns to the left atrium, which increases the pressure in the right atrium and prevents blood from the right atrium from passing through the foramen ovale.

When circulation through the umbilical cord ceases as the cord is clamped, blood bypasses the umbilical arteries and continues through the iliac arteries. With time the ductus arteriosus closes and becomes the ligamentum arteriosum, which attaches the pulmonary trunk to the arch of the aorta. The foramen ovale closes, leaving a depression on the intra-atrial septum called the *fossa ovalis*. The ductus venosus, which allowed blood from the umbilical vein to enter the inferior vena cava, becomes the ligamentum teres (round ligament) of the liver.

Characteristics of the Neonate

Normal newborns have several characteristics that impact assessment and management. (See Chapter 9.) At birth the infant is wet and slippery, and some of the waxy substance that protected his skin from the amniotic fluid, called *vernix caseosa*, remains on the skin. The head, which was molded as it passed through the birth canal, is elongated and is large in proportion to the body. The bones of the skull are thin and are separated by membranes called *fontanels*. Some peripheral cyanosis (acrocyanosis) may linger for a short time after birth as respiratory and cardiovascular systems adjust.

The neonate cries for a short time immediately after birth, but then remains quietly alert, although stimulation such as suctioning and drying may cause him to cry. The normal heart rate of the newborn is between 100 and 180 beats per minute. The normal respiratory rate is between 30 and 60 breaths per minute. Some amniotic fluid may continue to be expelled from the airway after birth and should be suctioned using a bulb syringe. Blood pressure is not normally assessed in neonates in the prehospital setting, but the normal systolic pressure is between 70 and 90 mmHg. The body temperature should be between 98°F and 100°F.

Developmental priority is given to the organs that must be most functional at birth. The immature kidneys cannot concentrate urine, increasing the neonate's fluid loss and risk of dehydration. Immature temperature regulation, higher respiratory rate, less subcutaneous fat, and large body surface area put the neonate at risk for hypothermia. Decreased glycogen stores can result in hypoglycemia, particularly in the distressed neonate whose energy requirements are increased.

Several anatomical differences contribute to the need for special techniques of airway management and ventilation. The head is proportionally large with a prominent occiput, the neck is short, the tongue is proportionally large, and the diameter of the airway is small and funnel shaped. The nose is small, flat, and soft, and neonates are primarily nose breathers. The tiny nares can be easily obstructed, leading to respiratory distress.

The average tidal volume of a full-term newborn is just 18 to 28 mL, compared to the 500 mL of an average adult. The lungs are fragile and easily damaged by aggressive ventilation. Respiratory failure and respiratory arrest can ensue quickly from respiratory distress.

General Assessment and Management of the Pregnant Patient

Illness and injury during pregnancy place two patients at risk—the mother and the fetus. In the prehospital setting, the fetus can only be treated indirectly, by managing the mother. Excellent assessment and management of the mother is critical because the most common cause of fetal demise is maternal demise.

Scene Size-Up

You may or may not know you are responding to a pregnant patient. As you conduct a scene size-up for a motor vehicle collision, you may realize that you have a pregnant patient. If pregnancy is less obvious, you may not be aware of it until you obtain a history from the patient, although most pregnant women will offer this information early out of concern for the fetus. When responding to a call for a pregnant patient, keep in mind that domestic violence is not uncommon during pregnancy. Look for indications of hazards and violence as you would when approaching any scene. If there are indications of domestic violence, be alert to indications of continuing danger at the scene and to the potential for injuries that the mother may not disclose, especially in the presence of the abuser.

Do not assume that an obviously pregnant patient has a chief complaint that is directly related to the pregnancy. She may have a medical emergency, such as asthma, appendicitis, or cholecystitis, or she may have suffered an injury. Complete the scene size-up by forming a general impression, including determining whether the patient is responsive or apparently unresponsive and whether the patient appears to be breathing normally.

Primary Assessment

The primary assessment of a pregnant woman has the same components and takes the same approach as in other patients. If the patient is apparently unresponsive and not breathing normally, check the carotid pulse for no more than 10 seconds. Begin CPR if a pulse is not detected. If the patient is unresponsive but breathing, or is not breathing normally but has a pulse, ensure an open airway, adequate ventilation and oxygenation, and adequate circulation.

A common cause of hypotension in the third trimester of pregnancy is **supine hypotensive syndrome**

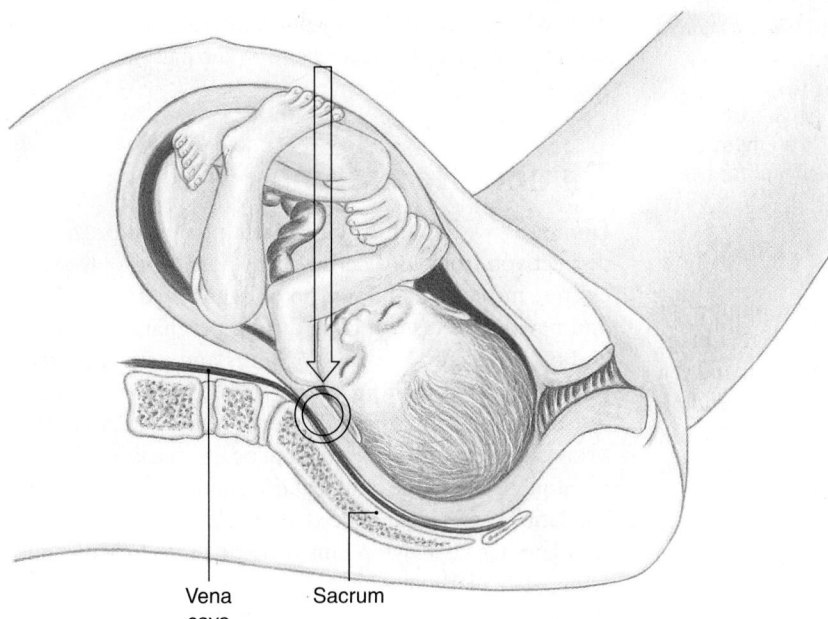

Vena
cava

Sacrum

FIGURE 43-9

Supine hypotensive syndrome
occurs in the third trimester of
pregnancy when the inferior vena
cava is compressed by the gravid
uterus, reducing blood return to
the heart and compromising
cardiac output.

(Figure 43-9). The gravid (pregnant) uterus compresses the inferior vena cava when the patient is supine, reducing the return of blood to the heart and decreasing cardiac output. Supine hypotensive syndrome is easily relieved by allowing the mother to sit up, if her condition allows, or placing her on her side. If spinal immobilization is required or there is another reason the mother must be supine, you must position her so that she is tilted slightly onto her left side. If she is on a long backboard, place a folded blanket under the right side of the backboard. Otherwise, place a pillow or folded blanket under the mother's right side.

Secondary Assessment

The secondary assessment proceeds according to the mechanism of injury or nature of the illness, chief complaint, and whether the patient is critical. Perform a rapid medical exam or rapid trauma exam if the patient is critical. If the patient is not critical, perform a focused exam according to the chief complaint. Perform a detailed head-to-toe exam for critical trauma patients and for critical medical patients in whom the problem has not been identified.

An internal examination of the genitalia is never performed in the prehospital setting. The only indications for

inspecting the external genitalia are (1) when you suspect that trauma to the external genitalia may be causing significant hemorrhage that can be controlled by direct pressure, and (2) to check for perineal bulging or crowning in the patient in active labor with indications of imminent delivery.

Obtain a complete set of vital signs. Analyze the vital signs in the context of the patient's overall presentation to identify any concerning findings and use the first set of vital signs as a baseline against which you can compare subsequent vital signs.

Fetal heart sounds can be heard in the hospital or physician's office with the aid of a Doppler device to amplify the sounds at about 10 to 12 weeks gestation. The use of a fetoscope (a specialized listening device that is similar to a stethoscope but has largely been replaced by the availability of Doppler devices) usually cannot detect fetal heart sounds before 20 weeks gestation. A traditional stethoscope is not as useful in auscultating fetal heart sounds. The ability to hear fetal heart sounds can be affected by background noise, examiner experience in auscultating fetal heart sounds, maternal obesity, and an increased amount of amniotic fluid. Keep in mind that the mother will be understandably alarmed when an attempt to auscultate fetal sounds is unsuccessful. Auscultation of fetal heart sounds in the prehospital setting has not been studied. The potential usefulness and limitations are not known. The practice is not currently listed as an expected skill of the Advanced EMT.

Regardless of whether the chief complaint seems to be directly related to the pregnancy, you must collect information in addition to that which you would collect in a patient who is not pregnant. If the patient's chief complaint indicates that she is in labor, additional questions are required. The answers to those additional questions may require that you follow up with additional physical examination.

IN THE FIELD

Keep in mind that in some cultures it is not permissible for a female patient to be attended to by a male health care provider, particularly for gynecologic and obstetric problems. If necessary, enlist the help of a female relative to assist you.

A basic obstetric history includes the total number of pregnancies the mother has had, including the current pregnancy, and the number of times she has given birth and the number of pregnancies that did not result in birth, including **spontaneous abortion** (miscarriage) or induced abortion. The total number of pregnancies, regardless of outcome and including the current pregnancy is referred to as **gravida**, abbreviated by the letter G. A woman pregnant for the first time is known as a *primagravida*, and one who has been pregnant more than once is known as a *multigravida*.

The number of times the mother has given birth is called **para**, abbreviated by the letter P. A mother who has given birth once is called a *primapara*, while the mother who has given birth more than once is called a *multipara*. The total number of abortions is abbreviated *Ab*. A woman who is pregnant for the third time with one previous live birth and one previous miscarriage is *G3, P1, Ab1*.

Ask whether the patient is receiving prenatal care and when her last prenatal visit was. Ask about problems with the current pregnancy and with previous pregnancies, including a history of preterm labor.

Determine the date of the last menstrual period (LMP). Women receiving regular prenatal care will most likely be able to tell you how many weeks pregnant they are, but if necessary, use the LMP to estimate the length of gestation. The due date is estimated by counting backward three months from the LMP and then counting forward two weeks. *This method does not account for a change in the year. It is only used to determine the month and day.* If the LMP is March 8, 2011, first count backward three months, which would be December 8 and then add two weeks, which gives an estimated due date of December 22, 2011. If you respond to a call for that patient on October 30, 2011, you would estimate that she is about 32 to 33 weeks pregnant.

Asking about fetal movement can be helpful in cases where the pregnancy may be jeopardized, such as in significant trauma or placental abruption. The first fetal movements, known as *quickening*, are usually felt by the mother at about 16 weeks gestation, but may not be noticed until later, especially in a first pregnancy. The presence of fetal movement is a reassuring sign, but does not rule out problems. The absence of fetal movement may or may not be significant, because the fetus normally has periods of inactivity and sleep.

In addition to a SAMPLE history and an exploration of the chief complaint using OPQRST, the history is guided by the nature of the patient's chief complaint. The questions will be determined by your knowledge of the anatomy and physiology of pregnancy and of the pathophysiology of pregnancy-related problems.

Clinical-Reasoning Process

Do not allow the knowledge that a patient is pregnant to distract you from considering other possible problems. Pre-existing medical conditions can be aggravated by pregnancy and new problems can arise during pregnancy. However, you must recognize chief complaints and patient presentations associated with pregnancy-related problems and active labor with imminent delivery. Altered mental status, seizures, hypertension, abdominal or low back pain, vaginal bleeding or discharge, and leaking amniotic fluid can all be indications of pregnancy-related problems.

The signs and symptoms of some pregnancy complications, particularly those in early pregnancy, overlap with gynecologic emergencies and other causes of abdominal pain. Consider those possibilities when obtaining a history.

Patients with pregnancy complications and neonates in need of resuscitation require specialized care. Consider your transport destination carefully with regard to your patients' needs. Call for additional personnel if a field delivery is anticipated, because you will have two patients to care for and transport. Consider the need for ALS transport. If transport times are long, consider requesting air medical transport according to your protocols.

Treatment

Medical problems in pregnancy are treated much as they are in nonpregnant patients. If medications are required, remember that the benefits of treating the mother must outweigh the risks of administering medication. In a true medical emergency, such as severe asthma or anaphylaxis, the biggest risk to the fetus is in *not* treating the mother. However, if time permits, consult with medical direction, even if your standing orders otherwise allow you to treat the condition without consultation.

The rich vascular supply to the reproductive organs means that many complications of pregnancy and childbirth are accompanied by hemorrhage and may result in hypovolemic shock. Anticipate shock and be prepared to treat it. Unlike external bleeding, the hemorrhage associated with most obstetrical emergencies cannot be accessed and controlled by direct pressure (the exception is perineal tearing associated with delivery). Heavy bleeding requires intervention in the hospital, which may include medication administration and surgical procedures. Transport the patient without delay.

Use a lower threshold for deciding to administer oxygen and intravenous fluids, keeping in mind that the mother's homeostatic mechanisms are aimed at saving her life at the potential cost of the life of the fetus. The pregnant woman in hypovolemic shock may have few signs and symptoms despite significant blood loss, yet placental blood flow can be severely compromised, jeopardizing the fetus.

To treat for shock, manage the patient's airway, ventilation, and oxygenation as indicated by her overall condition. For patients in the third trimester, avoid supine hypotensive syndrome by positioning the patient tilted slightly onto her left side. Establish intravenous access, preferably in two sites with large-bore catheters. Infuse fluids according to your protocol for treating hemorrhagic shock. As with all patients in shock, keep the patient warm.

Specific considerations for managing out-of-hospital delivery and complications of pregnancy are discussed in the next sections.

Reassessment

The patient's condition may change quickly. Maintain an ongoing assessment of your general impression of the patient's condition. Reassess the chief complaint and associated complaints. Repeat vital signs according to the patient's condition and monitor the effects of interventions.

Obstetrical Complications and Emergencies

Complications may occur during pregnancy, some of which can be life threatening. Complications of pregnancy include trauma (including trauma associated with domestic violence), spontaneous abortion, complications of induced abortion, ectopic pregnancy, preterm labor, gestational diabetes, hypertensive emergencies of pregnancy, placental abruption, and placenta previa. The presentation of many obstetric emergencies overlaps with that of gynecologic problems and other causes of abdominal pain, particularly in early pregnancy (Table 43-2).

Ectopic Pregnancy

An **ectopic pregnancy** occurs when a fertilized ovum is implanted and begins to develop somewhere other than in the endometrium within the uterine cavity. Most often, an ectopic pregnancy occurs in a fallopian tube. One risk factor for ectopic pregnancy is scarring of the fallopian tubes from prior pelvic inflammatory disease (PID), but there are other risk factors as well, including endometriosis and some forms of contraception. Fertilization normally takes place in the outer third of the fallopian tube. As the fertilized ovum begins to develop, it may not be able to pass through the narrowed lumen of a scarred fallopian tube, and may implant in the fallopian tube. The developing embryonic tissues erode and stretch the fallopian tube, resulting in lower abdominal pain. Unless the condition is recognized and

TABLE 43-2	Differential Diagnoses to Consider with Obstetric Emergencies

- Spontaneous abortion
- Complications of abortion
- Dysmenorrhea
- Pregnancy
- Pregnancy complications
- Ectopic pregnancy
- Appendicitis
- Cholecystitis
- Trauma
- Dysfunctional uterine bleeding
- Urinary tract infection
- Pelvic inflammatory disease
- Endometriosis
- Ovarian cyst
- Ovarian torsion

managed surgically, the fallopian tube ruptures with accompanying hemorrhage, which can be fatal.

The chief complaint in ectopic pregnancy may be lower abdominal pain or syncope, with or without a history of a missed menstrual period. The most common complaint is abdominal pain, which occurs in 98.6 percent of cases (Chi, 2009). Abdominal pain is frequently, but not always, accompanied by a history of a missed period and irregular vaginal bleeding. Those symptoms are similar to those of spontaneous abortion, and not diagnostic of ectopic pregnancy. The patient also may complain of referred shoulder pain from peritoneal irritation. With severe blood loss, the patient may present in shock or in cardiac arrest. Patients in hemorrhagic shock from ruptured ectopic pregnancy may not exhibit tachycardia (Chi, 2009). Abdominal examination findings are nonspecific.

Maintain a high index of suspicion for ectopic pregnancy in any female of childbearing age who presents with lower abdominal pain, syncope, otherwise unexplained shock, or cardiac arrest. Anticipate and be prepared to treat for shock. Transport to a hospital with surgical capabilities.

Abortion

The term **abortion** often has negative connotations to the lay public, although it refers to the termination of pregnancy from any cause prior to the 20th week of gestation. A spontaneous abortion is what most laypersons refer to as a *miscarriage,* and occurs in 5 to 15 percent of pregnancies (Gaufberg, 2010). If the pregnancy terminates spontaneously after 20 weeks without survival of the fetus, it is considered a **stillbirth.** Spontaneous abortions have several potential causes but many of them are thought to occur due to genetic abnormalities.

Spontaneous abortion may occur without the patient having suspected that she was pregnant or after one or more missed periods and a positive pregnancy test. Signs and symptoms include lower abdominal cramping and vaginal bleeding. The bleeding is often heavier than that of a normal menstrual period and may contain tissue or clots. In some cases, hemorrhage can be severe enough to result in hypovolemia. When a patient gives a history of vaginal bleeding heavier than that associated with her normal menstrual period, it is helpful to ask how many pads or tampons have been used. When cramping and bleeding occur in early pregnancy but the pregnancy is maintained, it is called a *threatened abortion.*

An induced abortion is what most people think of when they hear the term *abortion.* Induced abortions may be carried out legally or illegally. In particular, induced abortions carried out illegally may occur in unsanitary conditions and be performed by untrained personnel. An induced abortion is called a *therapeutic abortion* when it is medically necessary. Complications can arise from spontaneous and induced abortion and from medical treatment for spontaneous abortion. Complications include immediate or delayed hemorrhage and infection (endometritis). Endometritis may present with fever, lower abdominal pain, and a foul-smelling vaginal discharge within 48 to 72 hours of a gynecologic procedure or spontaneous abortion. Without treatment, the condition can progress to sepsis and cause death.

A patient may be reluctant to give a history of induced abortion because of the social stigma associated with it. Regardless of your beliefs about the issue, your role as a health care provider is to remain nonjudgmental and to provide excellent medical care and emotional support.

Assess the patient with suspected spontaneous abortion or abortion complications for hypovolemic shock. Ensure adequate airway, ventilation, and oxygenation. Administer IV fluids according to your protocol for hypovolemic shock. Provide emotional support because spontaneous abortion can be emotionally devastating. Even when pregnancy was not suspected, spontaneous abortion can represent the loss of a child. When reassuring the patient, do not make statements about being able to have another child, because it trivializes the loss of the current pregnancy.

Gestational Diabetes

Pre-existing diabetes may be more difficult to manage during pregnancy and increases the risks of complications to both the mother and fetus. In some cases, patients without a prior history of diabetes develop gestational diabetes during pregnancy, which also increases the risk of complications to the mother and fetus. Patients at higher risk for gestational diabetes are those who are over 35 years of age, obese, with a family history of diabetes, and a history of stillbirth.

In the absence of regular prenatal care, gestational diabetes may be present but undiagnosed. Include diabetic emergencies among your hypotheses when a pregnant patient, particularly after the 20th week of pregnancy, presents with altered mental status, and check the blood glucose level.

Hyperglycemia also may be associated with signs of untreated diabetes, including nausea, vomiting, abdominal pain, thirst, and increased urination. Hypoglycemia may result in seizure. There is no difference in the prehospital management of diabetic emergencies in pregnant patients. Manage the airway, breathing, and circulation. Start an IV of normal saline and give fluids for hyperglycemia. Administer oral glucose to the conscious patient who can protect her airway and administer intravenous 50 percent dextrose to a patient with a decreased level of responsiveness.

Hypertensive Emergencies

There are several classifications of hypertensive disorders of pregnancy (HDP). **Pre-eclampsia** is a progressive disorder that can progress to **eclampsia.** The disorder usually begins in the last trimester of pregnancy but can develop up to 48 hours after delivery. Pre-eclampsia is diagnosed when there is an increase of 30 mmHg in the systolic blood pressure or an increase in diastolic blood pressure of 15 mmHg that is sustained across two readings at least 6 hours apart. Without a baseline blood pressure from early in the pregnancy, it is more difficult to diagnose pre-eclampsia. In those cases, pre-eclampsia is suspected when the blood pressure is 140/90 mmHg or greater.

A likely factor in pre-eclampsia is maternal vasospasm, which raises the blood pressure and decreases placental circulation. There is protein in the mother's urine in pre-eclampsia and edema. In severe pre-eclampsia, hypertension, protein levels in the urine, and edema are all increased. As pre-eclampsia progresses, the mother may complain of headache, visual disturbances, and decreased urine output. The physical exam may reveal exaggerated deep tendon reflexes (such as the patellar reflex) and pulmonary edema can occur.

A number of complications can result from pre-eclampsia, including hemorrhagic stroke, placental abruption, and renal failure. The onset of seizures or coma marks the transition from pre-eclampsia to eclampsia, which has high maternal and fetal mortality.

Other hypertensive disorders of pregnancy include chronic hypertension, in which the blood pressure is elevated before pregnancy or early in pregnancy, or persists after pregnancy. Patients with chronic hypertension may develop pre-eclampsia, which may occur earlier in pregnancy and progress more rapidly than in patients without chronic hypertension. Transient hypertension can occur during labor or immediately after delivery, but resolves within 10 days.

Be suspicious of pre-eclampsia when the patient has edema, sudden weight gain (which indicates fluid retention), visual disturbances, pain in the epigastric area or right upper quadrant of the abdomen, or headache. Seizure, particularly in the presence of a history consistent with pre-eclampsia or in a patient without a prior history of seizures is consistent with eclampsia.

Prehospital treatment of hypertensive emergencies of pregnancy include management of airway and breathing, administering supplemental oxygen, placing the mother in the left lateral recumbent position to facilitate circulation, obtaining IV access, and monitoring blood pressure. During transport, keep the patient calm and reduce sensory stimulation, which may precipitate a seizure, by dimming the lights and avoiding use of the siren. If pre-eclampsia or eclampsia is suspected, request ALS ground transport or air medical transport, if available, according to protocols. Keep in mind the risk for seizures, placental abruption, and pulmonary edema and reassess the patient frequently. The patient requires specialized care in a facility with advanced obstetrical capabilities and neonatal intensive care.

Placenta Previa

Placenta previa refers to implantation of the placenta in the proximity of or directly over the cervix (Figure 43-10). As part of prenatal care, pregnant women receive at least one ultrasound, during which, among many other things, the position of the placenta is determined. Placenta previa may be partial or complete, but in either case, will cause bleeding during labor as the cervix dilates and will interfere with delivery. When placenta previa is detected, a cesarean section (c-section) is scheduled.

If a woman with placenta previa goes into labor outside of the hospital, the neonate cannot be delivered in the field. Bleeding may begin as the patient approaches term. The patient presents with bright red vaginal bleeding that is usually painless. Place the patient in left lateral recumbent position, provide oxygen, establish IV access, and transport without delay to a facility where an emergency cesarean section can be performed.

Placental Abruption

Placental abruption, also called **abruptio placentae**, occurs when the placenta prematurely detaches, partially or completely, from the uterine wall, compromising fetal perfusion (Figure 43-11). The condition is life threatening for both the mother and fetus. Fetal mortality ranges from 20 percent with lesser degrees of placental separation, to 100 percent with complete separation. Increased maternal age, multiparity, hypertension, trauma, and cocaine use all increase the risk of placental abruption.

Signs and symptoms of placental abruption depend on the degree of placental separation and whether the separation begins around the edges of the placenta (marginal) or in the center (central). In marginal separation there is vaginal bleeding, but often no pain. In central separation, the bleeding is trapped by the attachment of the placenta at the edges, but the condition is accompanied by sudden sharp, tearing pain with abdominal rigidity. A complete separation is accompanied by massive vaginal bleeding and hypotension.

Place the patient in left lateral recumbent position, provide oxygen, establish IV access, treat for hypovolemic shock, and transport without delay to a facility where an emergency cesarean section can be performed.

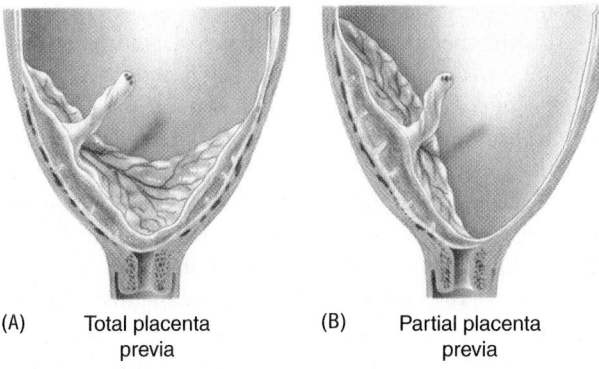

(A) Total placenta previa (B) Partial placenta previa

FIGURE 43-10

Placenta previa. (A) Total placenta previa. (B) Partial placenta previa.

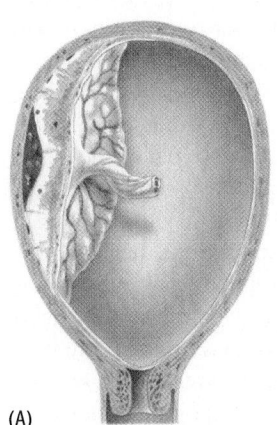 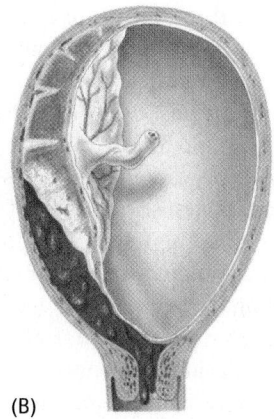 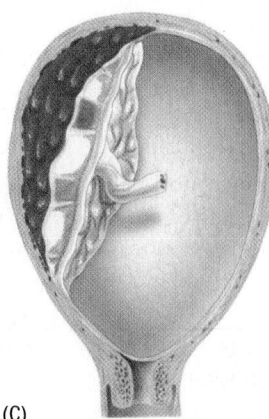

(A) Partial separation (concealed hemorrhage) (B) Partial separation (apparent hemorrhage) (C) Complete separation (concealed hemorrhage)

FIGURE 43-11

Abruptio placentae. (A) Partial abruption with concealed hemorrhage. (B) Partial abruption with hemorrhage. (C) Complete abruption with concealed hemorrhage.

Trauma in Pregnancy

Trauma in pregnancy is commonly due to motor vehicle collisions and falls, but may also occur due to domestic violence. The position and increased vascularity of the uterus, particularly beyond 20 weeks gestation, increases the risk of serious maternal injury and hemorrhage. Although the fetus is somewhat protected from blunt trauma, it is jeopardized by maternal hemorrhage, placental abruption, premature labor, and uterine rupture. Encourage pregnant trauma patients, especially those who are beyond the first trimester, to be transported for evaluation in the emergency department.

Remember that shock can be well concealed in the pregnant woman, presenting with few signs and symptoms. You must anticipate shock based on the mechanism of injury and initiate treatment at a lower threshold than for nonpregnant patients. To prevent supine hypotensive syndrome and further impairment in maternal and fetal perfusion, never transport a patient in the third trimester of pregnancy in a supine position.

Normal Labor and Delivery

Although it is not a common call, EMS providers are sometimes called to care for a patient in labor. In contrast to dealing with illness, injury, and death, assisting a patient with a normal labor and delivery can be an exciting, positive experience, provided you are prepared with the knowledge and resources to do so. Keep in mind that delivery should preferably take place in a labor and delivery unit. If there is no time to transport the patient for delivery, delivering at the patient's home or other fixed location is preferable to delivering in the ambulance. Take a few minutes to obtain the information that helps you make a decision about whether you should transport the patient or prepare for delivery on the scene.

Signs and Symptoms of Labor

Several events occur in the days and hours prior to the onset of active labor, in preparation for delivery. Braxton-Hicks contractions and increasing levels of pregnancy hormones and prostaglandins allow the cervix to begin to soften, efface (thin), and dilate. Those events are accompanied by an increase in vaginal secretions and, sometimes, noticeable loss of the mucus plug that protected the opening of the cervix during pregnancy. A discharge of blood-tinged mucus is known as *bloody show*. Labor generally begins within 24 to 48 hours of losing the mucus plug.

Prior to active labor, but occasionally not until after contractions begin, the fetus will noticeably drop lower into the pelvic cavity as his head engages in the pelvis. This process is called **lightening**. A pregnant woman may be able to give you information from her last prenatal visit, including the degree of effacement and dilation and the fetal station.

In its normal state, the cervix is thick and long and the cervical os is closed. However, it must thin and dilate to allow for birth. The degree of effacement is given in percentages. Effacement at 100 percent means the cervix is paper thin. Dilation is measured in centimeters, with full dilation being 10 cm. Station is measured from -3 to 5. Negative 3 station means the fetal head has not yet descended into the pelvic cavity and is 3 cm above the ischial spines at the pelvic floor. By zero station, the head is even with the ischial spines. Positive numbers indicate the number of centimeters the head is past the ischial spines, with $+5$ indicating crowning. Keep in mind that this information can only be obtained by a physician or obstetric nurse by manual examination of the cervix, which is not performed by prehospital personnel.

During pregnancy the mother experiences irregular contractions that may be intense, but are not painful, and which subside after a short time. Those contractions are Braxton-Hicks contractions and not active labor. The contractions of active labor are regular and increase in intensity. In the beginning, the contractions may be 10 or more minutes apart, each lasting about 20 seconds. Most obstetricians advise patients to go to the hospital when contractions are 5 minutes apart.

Toward the end of the first stage of labor, contractions are 2 to 3 minutes apart and last a minute or more. In the second stage of labor, contractions are very intense, occur approximately every 2 minutes, and each may last more than 1 minute. The bag of water usually breaks late in the first stage of labor, or during the second stage, prior to delivery. Occasionally, the amniotic membranes rupture prematurely, increasing the risk of maternal and fetal infection, if labor does not begin spontaneously within 24 hours.

If the water breaks, determine whether it was clear, or if it was yellowish or greenish in color, indicating the presence of **meconium**. Meconium is the contents of the fetal bowel, consisting of a small amount of digested cells and products and from ingested amniotic fluid. Normally, the first bowel movement does not occur until after delivery. However, it can occur if the fetus is distressed prior to or during labor, or if he is post-term. If meconium, particularly thick meconium, is aspirated into the neonate's airway, it can cause respiratory distress. If possible, the delivery should take place in the hospital. If delivery must take place out of the hospital, request additional resources in anticipation of the need for neonatal resuscitation.

To time the frequency of contractions, begin timing at the beginning of one contraction and stop timing at the beginning of the next contraction. The mother will be able to tell you when each contraction starts. If you place your hand on the abdomen over the uterine fundus, you will feel the uterus tighten and contract, and as contractions increase in intensity, you will be able to see the abdomen take on a rounder shape during contractions.

Deciding to Transport or Prepare for Delivery

To determine whether you should transport or prepare for delivery on scene, you must assess whether delivery is imminent. Keep in mind that some labors will progress much more quickly than others, particularly in multiparous women. If the mother has had a previous vaginal delivery, ask how long she was in labor, because subsequent labors are likely to proceed more quickly. Signs of imminent delivery include the following:

- Indications that the mother is in the second stage of labor, particularly with multiparous women, in whom this stage may take only 20 to 30 minutes. If contractions are frequent and intense, determine if the mother feels an urge to push and check for crowning.

- The mother feels an urge to bear down or push, or feels pressure similar to that felt when needing to have a bowel movement. If the mother complains of those symptoms, check for crowning.

- Perineal bulging or crowning.

If you do not think it is possible to transport the mother and turn her care over to emergency department personnel before delivery, prepare to deliver on the scene. If you make the decision to deliver at the scene, request additional personnel, if necessary, so that there will be at least one provider to care for the mother and one to care for the neonate.

If you decide to transport the mother, continue to monitor her for indications of imminent delivery. If you must deliver in the back of the ambulance, have the driver select a safe place and stop the ambulance. Keep the doors to the ambulance closed and keep the patient compartment warm. If the delivery is complicated (prolapsed umbilical cord, abnormal presentation, or suspected uterine rupture, placenta previa, or placental abruption) or does not occur within 20 minutes of contractions that are 2 to 3 minutes apart, begin transport.

Preparing for Delivery

Ideally, you will have a few minutes to prepare the patient and the needed equipment before delivery. However, if the presenting part, which is the head in a normal delivery, is crowning, be prepared to gently place your gloved hand over the head to prevent explosive delivery. Uncontrolled expulsion of the head can increase the severity of trauma to the mother's perineum and result in fetal injury.

Prepare a suitable place for delivery, out of the sight of bystanders. Allow the mother to have one or two support persons of her choice at her side, if room permits. A bed is ideal, but you can use the ambulance stretcher. The mother should be supine, with someone to help her elevate her head

CASE STUDY (continued)

Advanced EMTs Steve and Scott have just arrived at the home of 27-year-old Claire Velez, who is 35 weeks pregnant and appears to be in labor. The situation is complicated by an ice storm that has made the roads hazardous. "Hi, Mrs. Velez, my name is Steve and this is my partner, Scott. Are you having contractions?"

"Yes," she replies.

"When did the contractions start?"

"About an hour ago. At first I thought it was just false labor, but the contractions didn't stop and they are getting worse."

"How far apart are the contractions?"

"About 5 minutes, I think."

"Okay," says Steve. "I need to ask you a few more questions. Let me know if you start to have a contraction, alright? We will time them to see exactly how far apart they are. Is this your first pregnancy?"

"No. I had a miscarriage a few months before I found out I was pregnant with this baby."

"So, just one other pregnancy, but it ended in a miscarriage? You haven't given birth before?"

"Yes. Just the one pregnancy before. This will be our first baby."

"Do you feel any pressure, like you would if you had to move your bowels, or feel like you need to push?"

"No."

Problem-Solving Questions

1. What other information do Steve and Scott need to determine if delivery is imminent?
2. How does the weather affect their decision making?
3. If delivery is not yet imminent, what can Steve and Scott do about the preterm labor?

FIGURE 43-12

Contents of an OB kit.

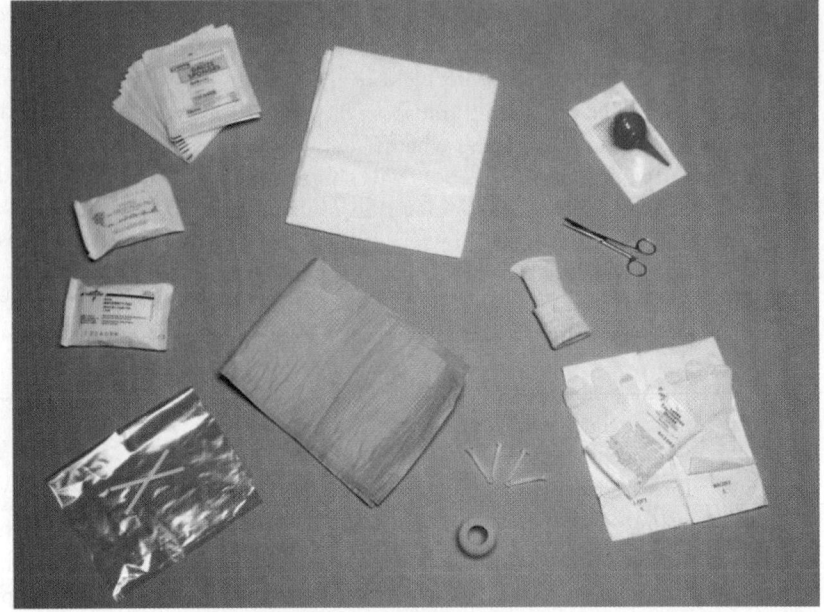

and shoulders to push. If the mother is sitting up, as opposed to elevating the shoulders, it is difficult for the fetus to make the turn from vertical to horizontal to get past the pubic bone.

The mother should have the hips and knees flexed. When she pushes, she may wish to grasp her knees, or a support person or assistant on each side may support and lift under the knees as she pushes.

If possible, place a folded towel beneath the buttocks to elevate the vaginal opening a few inches, allowing space for you to grasp the baby as he emerges.

Make sure the equipment you need is ready. It should be prepackaged in an obstetrical (OB) kit. You will need the following (Figure 43-12):

- Drapes or towels
- Bulb syringe
- Umbilical cord clamps (2)
- Scissors
- Infant receiving blankets (2 to 3)
- 4″ × 4″ gauze squares
- Perineal pad (sanitary pad)

If time and the number of personnel on the scene allow, start an IV at a keep-open rate. If there are any complications or anticipated complications, administer oxygen to the mother.

Assisting with the Delivery

The provider directly assisting with the delivery should, in addition to gloves, wear a fluid-impervious gown and a face shield or mask and goggles. Once you have prepared for the delivery, if crowning is present, you can instruct the mother to push during contractions (Scan 43-1). To assist with the delivery, do the following:

1. As the head emerges from the birth canal, gently place your gloved hand over it to prevent explosive delivery. Once the head emerges, usually face down, the fetus rotates to the side. When the head is fully delivered, tell the mother to stop pushing.

2. Check to see if the umbilical cord is wrapped around the neck (nuchal cord). If it is, try to gently slip it over the head and shoulder. If it is wrapped tightly, instruct the mother not to push. Clamp the cord in two places, about 2 inches apart, and cut the cord between the clamps.

3. Use a bulb syringe to clear the mouth and then the nose (Table 43-3). Current recommendations (American Heart Association [AHA], 2010)

TABLE 43-3	**Using a Bulb Syringe**

1. Squeeze the bulb.
2. Place the tip in the newborn's mouth.
3. Release the bulb to suction.
4. Discharge the suctioned contents by squeezing the bulb over a towel or basin.
5. Squeeze the bulb.
6. Place the tip of the syringe in the nares.
7. Release the bulb to suction.
8. Discharge the contents by squeezing the bulb over a towel or basin.
9. Repeat for the other nare.
10. Repeat suctioning for excessive secretions.

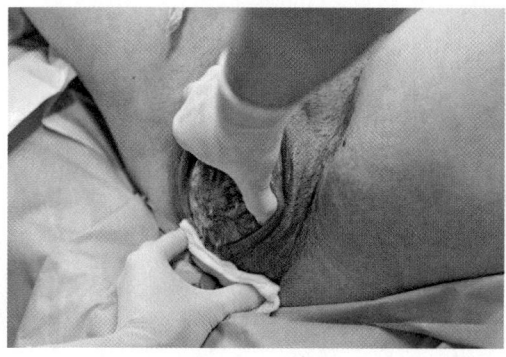

1. Crowning.

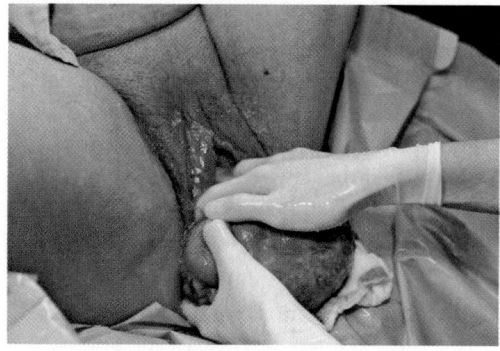

2. Head delivers and turns.

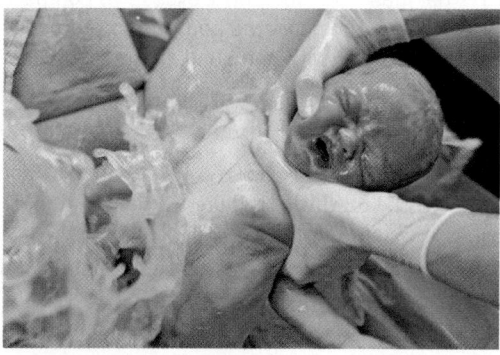

3. Body delivers.

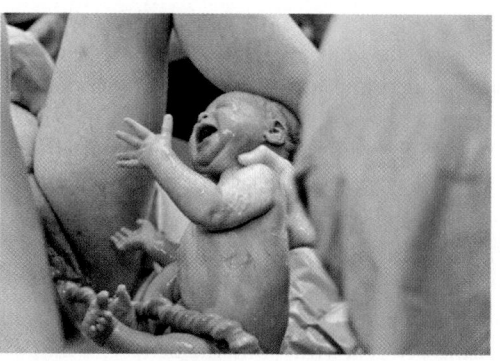

4. Grasp the newborn firmly as he is delivered.

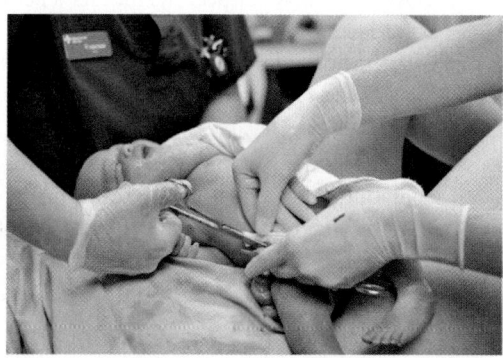

5. Clamp and cut the umbilical cord.

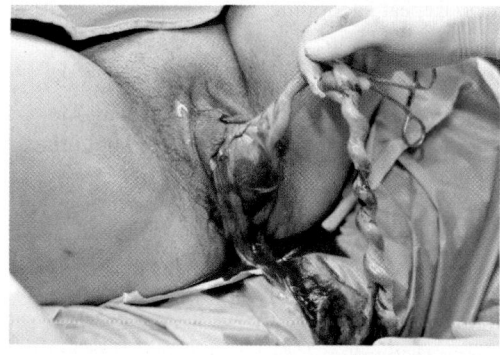

6. Placenta delivers.

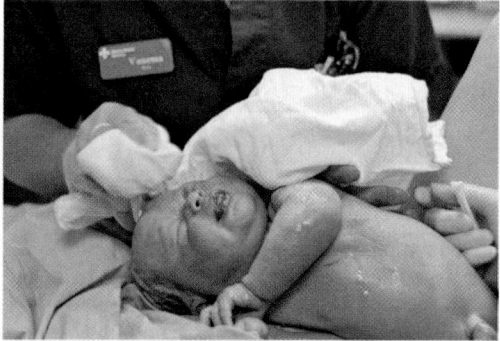

7. Clean and dry the newborn.

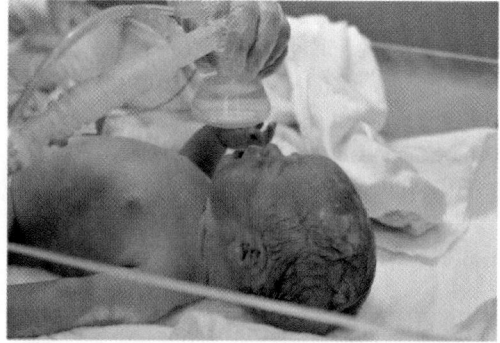

8. Administer blow-by oxygen if needed.

are to avoid additional suctioning of the airway unless there is an obvious obstruction or a need for positive pressure ventilation. Meconium staining is not treated by additional oropharyngeal suctioning prior to delivery of the shoulders, and suctioning is not performed after delivery, if the newborn is vigorous. Meconium aspiration in nonvigorous newborns must be treated by endotracheal intubation and suctioning (AHA, 2010).

4. With the next contraction, gently guide the head downward to facilitate delivery of the upper shoulder. Do not use force! Gently guide the head upward to facilitate delivery of the lower shoulder.

5. The rest of the body is narrower than the head and shoulders and will emerge rapidly. Support the head and body, keeping in mind that the baby is slippery. Once the baby has completely emerged, keep him at the level of the vagina until the umbilical cord is clamped.

6. Within 30 to 45 seconds of delivery, place an umbilical clamp about 10 cm (4 inches) from the baby and then place a second clamp about 5 cm (2 inches) further away from the baby. Cut the cord between the two clamps.

7. Wipe the baby's face to clean away any blood and mucus. Repeat suctioning with a bulb syringe, if necessary.

8. Dry the baby gently and wrap him in warm, dry blankets. If there are no complications with the mother or neonate, allow the mother to hold the baby.

9. Record the time of birth.

10. Assign an EMS provider to assess and care for the baby, including obtaining APGAR scores at 1 minute and 5 minutes after delivery (discussed in a later section).

11. Contractions will begin again after delivery, although with less intensity, to expel the placenta. Separation of the placenta will cause the exposed portion of the umbilical cord to lengthen. *Do not pull on the umbilical cord to speed expulsion of the placenta!*

12. You may begin to prepare the mother for transport while awaiting delivery of the placenta.

13. Place the placenta in a biohazard bag and transport it with the mother for inspection and disposal.

14. If excess bleeding, more than 500 mL, occurs either before or after the placenta is delivered, perform fundal massage as follows: Support the body of the uterus by placing the side of one hand firmly against the abdomen, just above the pubic

Control Bleeding

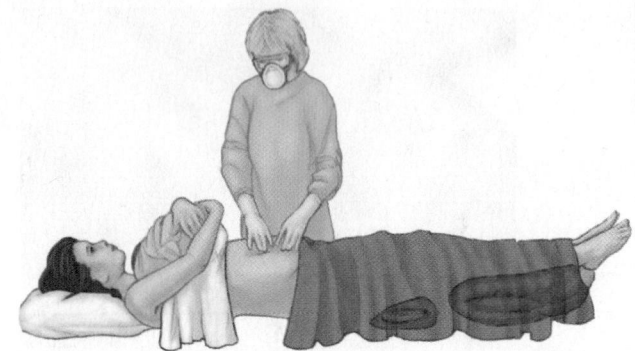

FIGURE 43-13

Fundal massage. To control excessive postpartum hemorrhage, support the body of the uterus just above the pubic bone with one hand and massage the fundus with the other hand.

bone (Figure 43-13). Use the other hand to locate the fundus of the uterus, which should be at about the level of the umbilicus. Massage the uterus until it contracts and becomes hard. The muscular contraction constricts the blood vessels in the uterus, slowing bleeding. If the mother is able and agrees, allowing the newborn to feed at the breast also stimulates uterine contraction.

15. After delivery, inspect the mother's perineum for lacerations. Apply direct pressure to external lacerations with ongoing bleeding. Place a sanitary pad over the perineum and help the mother lower her legs.

16. Reassess the patient's vital signs and monitor the amount of bleeding during transport, applying additional fundal massage if excessive bleeding occurs. If bleeding continues and an IV was not started previously, start an IV and infuse fluids.

Notify the receiving hospital as soon as feasible. It is preferable to admit the patients directly to the labor and delivery unit, rather than the emergency department, if possible.

IN THE FIELD

Newborns easily become hypothermic without the signs and symptoms that usually indicate hypothermia. Newborns do not shiver. Possible indications of hypothermia include irritability (early), with lethargy in later stages, pale or cyanotic skin, respiratory distress or respiratory arrest, and bradycardia. Prevent heat loss in all newborns by drying them promptly and wrapping them in blankets. Do not unnecessarily open ambulance doors and keep the temperature at a minimum of 75°F. Keep hypothermia in mind as a possible cause of respiratory depression and bradycardia.

Advanced EMT Patricia McDonough: My first field delivery was a term neonate to a mother who had five children. Clearly, she was more of a pro at the process than I was, and probably not nearly as nervous! My partner was a little more experienced than I was; he had delivered one baby in the field before. When we arrived, the patient said she felt like she needed to push, and a quick check showed that the perineum was bulging with contractions. We quickly prepared and my partner did the delivery. I clamped and cut the cord and my partner handed the newborn to me, a baby girl.

I remember briefly thinking, "What am I supposed to do with this?" But I had good training. We practiced newborn assessment and care frequently in labs in my Advanced EMT class. I quickly dried the baby and did a 1-minute APGAR score, which was a nine. I wrapped her up and handed her to her mom for a few minutes while we finished taking care of her and prepared to transport them. I think I was almost as excited as the mom and dad! My partner tried to act like he wasn't all that excited about it, but I know him; he was definitely excited about it, too!

Be sure that your documentation includes the time of birth and gender of the infant.

Complications of Labor and Delivery

Complications of labor and delivery include preterm labor, uterine rupture, uterine inversion, abnormal fetal presentation, precipitous delivery, shoulder dystocia, prolapsed umbilical cord, multiple births, and maternal pulmonary embolism. Notify the receiving hospital as soon as possible for complications of labor and delivery. Consult with medical direction as needed for assistance with the situation.

Preterm Labor

Preterm labor is the onset of labor prior to 37 weeks gestation. Newborn complications are related to immaturity of the organ systems and low birth weight (Figure 43-14). The greater the gestational age, the greater the newborn's chance of survival and the less likely he is to have significant problems, which include inadequate respirations, poor thermoregulation, and cerebral hemorrhage. The goal is to stop preterm labor to allow the fetus to develop as much as possible before delivery.

Although Advanced EMTs do not administer tocolytics (medications that stop labor), there is one treatment available to Advanced EMTs that can be successful in stopping preterm labor. The hormone oxytocin, which is the hormone responsible for inducing uterine smooth contraction, is secreted from the posterior pituitary gland from cells adjacent to those that secrete antidiuretic hormone (ADH), also called *vasopressin*. ADH is secreted when the circulating blood volume is low, to prevent diuresis (the loss of water). When circulating volume is increased, ADH is inhibited. It appears that inhibiting the cells that secrete ADH also may inhibit the release of oxytocin. Therefore, administration of IV fluids, in consultation with medical direction, may stop premature contractions.

Abnormal Presentations

Normally, the fetal head is the presenting part. Occasionally, the fetus will not have turned and assumed a head-down presentation prior to birth. On those occasions, the fetus most often is in a **breech position**, with either the buttocks or both feet presenting first in the birth canal (Figure 43-15). Preterm birth and small fetal size, such as in multiple births, increase the chances of breech presentation. Breech presentation increases the risk for maternal and fetal trauma, fetal hypoxia, and compressed or prolapsed umbilical cord.

Breech deliveries are best managed in the hospital, where cesarean section is often necessary. However, if delivery is imminent, you must intervene. Request ALS response, if available. The body is usually delivered easily, but the shoulders or head may be difficult to deliver.

If the shoulders or head are not easily delivered, position the mother so that her buttocks are on the edge of the bed, if possible. Have the patient lie back and use her hands to grasp her legs behind the knees and hold them up

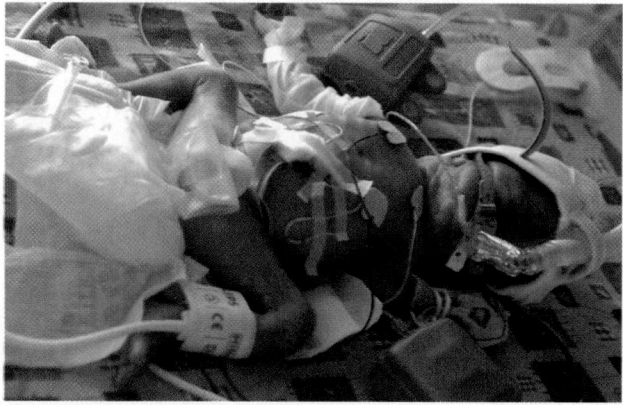

FIGURE 43-14

A premature newborn. (© BSIP/Photo Researchers, Inc.)

FIGURE 43-15

Breech presentation. Support the body as it delivers. If the head does not deliver spontaneously and the fetus begins breathing, insert the index and middle fingers of your gloved hand around the fetal nose and mouth to allow him to breathe.

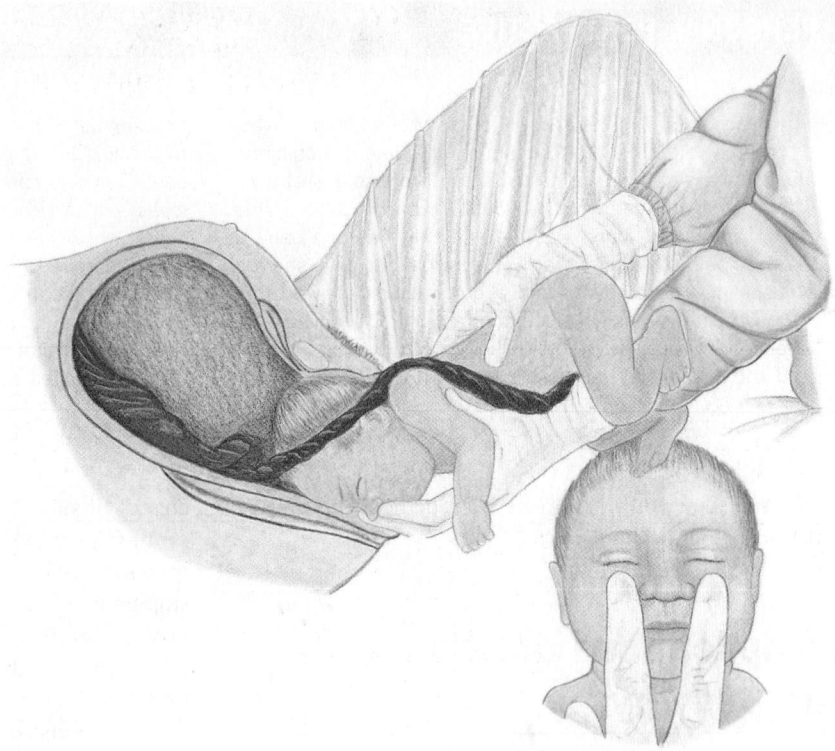

and apart in a flexed position, with the knees as close to the shoulders as possible.

In a breech presentation, support the legs and body as they emerge, but do not pull on them. Either the shoulders or the head may present an obstacle to delivery. If the body has delivered but the head does not deliver, apply gentle upward traction to assist the head in clearing the pubic bone. If the head does not deliver but the baby begins to breathe spontaneously, slide your index and middle fingers into the vaginal opening to create a "V" around the baby's nose and mouth and push the vaginal tissue away from the nose to allow him to breathe.

If the shoulders present an obstacle to delivery, the body will emerge to the level of baby's umbilicus, but not further. Ensuring that there is adequate slack in the umbilical cord, gently rotate the body so that the shoulders are in an anterior–posterior orientation with respect to the mother's pelvis. If necessary, use a towel to better grasp the body. Very gently apply traction until the axillae are visible. Then guide the body upward to deliver the posterior shoulder, then downward to deliver the anterior shoulder. Then deliver the head.

Rarely, an arm or leg is the presenting part (limb presentation). Those situations cannot be managed in the prehospital setting. Place the mother in left lateral recumbent position, administer oxygen, and transport without delay to a facility capable of emergency cesarean section. If transport time is prolonged, request air medical transport, if available.

Prolapsed Umbilical Cord

A **prolapsed umbilical cord** occurs when the umbilical cord emerges before the presenting part of the fetus (Figure 43-16). The condition is more common with preterm and breech deliveries and with premature rupture of the amniotic membranes. As the presenting part descends into the birth canal, it compresses the cord, compromising fetal circulation. The prehospital goal is to prevent the cord from being compressed before the patient can be transported to the hospital.

Place the mother in knee–chest position (Figure 43-17). Insert two fingers of your gloved hand into the vagina and lift the presenting part off of the cord. Apply oxygen by nonrebreather mask. Cover the exposed cord with sterile, moist dressings. Transport without delay.

Shoulder Dystocia

Shoulder dystocia occurs when the baby's shoulders are larger than its head and become lodged between the mother's pubic bone and sacrum. The problem is associated with very large fetuses, such as those born to diabetic mothers and those who are post-term. Shoulder dystocia can be recognized when the head delivers normally, but then retracts back into the birth canal. While preparing for immediate transport, have the mother lay with her buttocks at the very edge of the bed and use her hands to pull her knees back as close to her shoulders as possible.

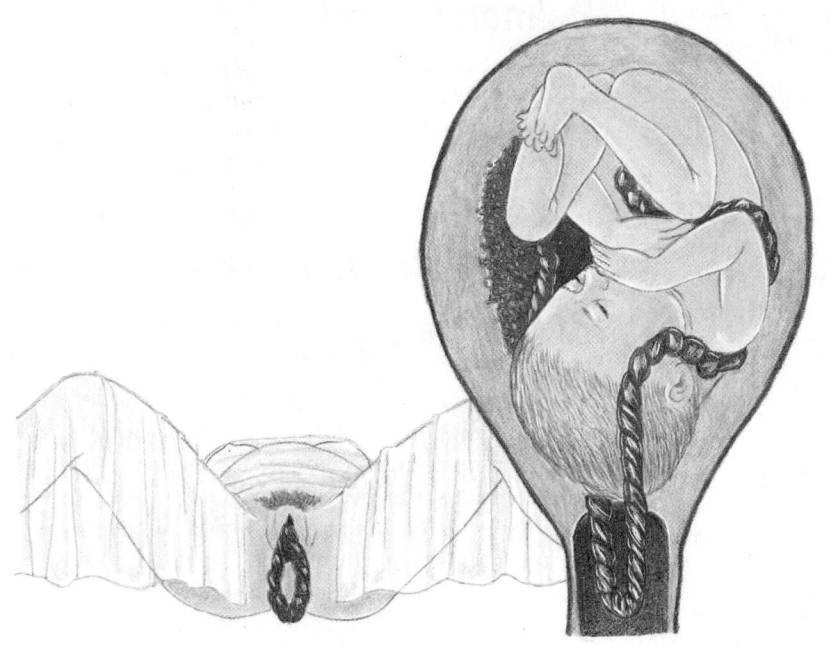

FIGURE 43-16
A prolapsed umbilical cord.

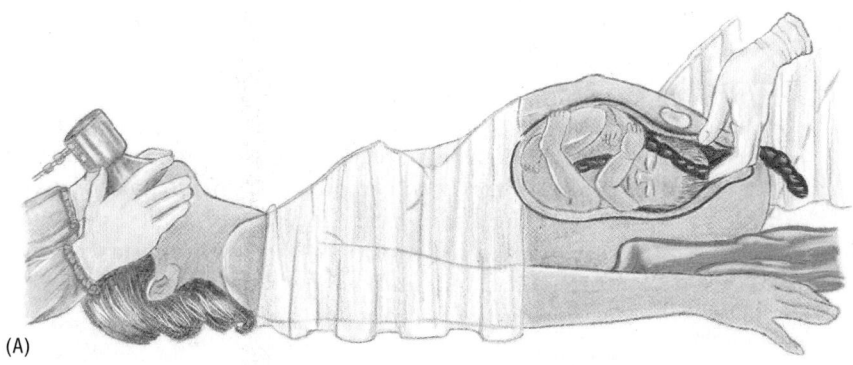

(A)

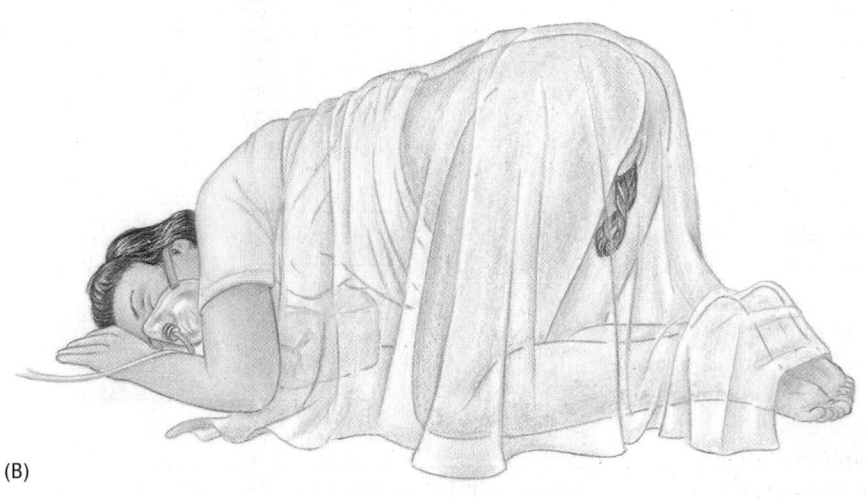

(B)

Use your open hand to apply firm pressure just above the pubic bone. If delivery does not occur, initiate transport without delay.

Precipitous Delivery

Precipitous delivery is delivery that occurs within 3 hours of the onset of labor. It is more common in grand multiparas (women who have had several children) and in preterm labor with small newborns. Risks include increased possibility of maternal and fetal trauma. There is no specific prehospital treatment for precipitous delivery, but be aware of the increased risk for complications.

Multiple Births

Although modern fertility treatments have increased the incidence of multiple births, they still are uncommon. Twins occur in about 1 in 90 pregnancies, and other multiples occur much less frequently. In most cases, the mother will be aware of a multiple pregnancy. Multiples are frequently premature and smaller than single-birth infants. With twins, one usually presents in normal, head-down (vertex) position, and the other is in breech position. Deliver the first infant normally and clamp and cut the cord. Then deliver the second infant. There may be one placenta (identical twins), or two placentas. Smaller size and prematurity of the infants requires special attention to maintaining body temperature.

Uterine Rupture

Uterine rupture is a tearing of the uterus that may occur during labor or as a result of trauma. A previous cesarean section with a vertical incision into the uterine wall and prolonged labor are risk factors. Maternal and fetal mortality are high. The patient experiences extreme abdominal pain and uterine contractions stop. Hypovolemic shock is common. The pain may decrease if the rupture is complete. Transport without delay to a facility with immediate surgical capabilities. Manage the patient for hypovolemic shock.

Uterine Inversion

Uterine inversion occurs rarely, but its risk is substantially increased by pulling on the umbilical cord in an attempt to speed delivery of the placenta and by aggressive fundal massage without supporting the body of the uterus above the pubic bone. When uterine inversion occurs, the uterus is turned inside out and pulled through the cervix. Bleeding associated with the trauma to the supporting tissues can be substantial and hypovolemic shock is likely. Transport without delay and manage the patient for hypovolemic shock. Cover the exposed tissue with moist sterile dressings and consult with medical direction about making an attempt to replace the uterus in position by applying pressure to the fundus.

Pulmonary Embolism

Pulmonary embolism can occur anytime during pregnancy or after delivery, and is more common in patients who have had a cesarean section. Treat the patient as you would any other patient with pulmonary embolism. (See Chapter 20.)

Assessment and Management of the Neonate

At birth, the neonate is wet and slippery and can easily become hypothermic. In the first few moments, cyanosis is common but his color should improve quickly. Key considerations in neonatal management are assessing the need for resuscitation and employing simple methods to maintain body temperature and improve respiration and heart rate if needed. In most cases, neonates do not require more than routine care: suctioning excess secretions, drying, and keeping them warm. Additional steps include tactile stimulation to improve respiration. Supplemental oxygen, assisted ventilation, and chest compressions are indicated less frequently. The relative frequency with which those interventions are needed is represented by an inverted pyramid called the *neonatal resuscitation pyramid* (Figure 43-18).

In some cases, you should anticipate the need for neonatal resuscitation. If possible, those deliveries should take place in the hospital. If field delivery is anticipated, request additional assistance. Neonates born to mothers with high-risk pregnancies (those with pre-existing medical problems, complications of pregnancy, or of very young age or over 35 years old), who are premature, or who are born to mothers with substance abuse during pregnancy and those without prenatal care are at increased risk of problems.

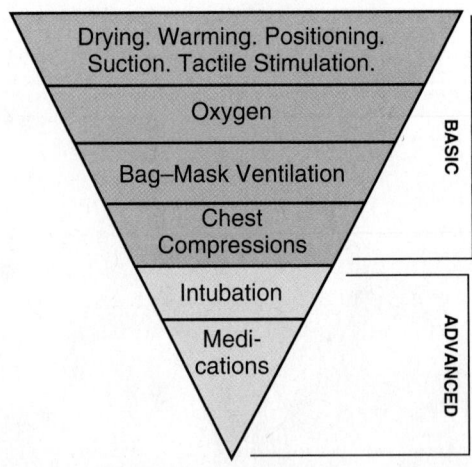

FIGURE 43-18

An inverted pyramid represents the relative frequencies of interventions required in neonatal resuscitation.

Determining the Need for Resuscitation

The American Heart Association (2010) guidelines for neonatal resuscitation recommend a rapid assessment of every newborn to differentiate between newborns who require resuscitation and those who do not require resuscitation. The three characteristics of those who *do not* require resuscitation include being full-term gestation, crying or breathing, and with good muscle tone. The newborn is placed with the mother and covered to maintain body temperature, and observation of the breathing, muscle tone, and color continues.

If any of the characteristics is not present, then one or more of the following four steps are taken in the order shown here:

1. *Initial steps for stabilization.* Provide warmth, clear the airway if necessary, dry, and stimulate. This should take 60 seconds, including time for re-evaluating the newborn's condition and beginning the next step, if needed.

2. *Ventilation.* If respirations are absent, gasping, or labored and the heart rate is less than 100 per minute (determined by auscultation), then you should provide oxygen and initiate ventilations. Use a neonatal oropharyngeal airway if prolonged ventilation is anticipated. Place a small folded towel or blanket under the shoulders to position the patient's head properly.

3. *Chest compressions.* If the heart rate is less than 60, begin chest compressions.

4. *IV or IO access.* If chest compressions do not improve the patient's condition, medications and fluids are indicated (for ALS providers and in the hospital). Intravenous access is difficult in neonates and you must not delay on the scene to establish IV access. If time and personnel permit it during transport, establish IV or IO access, according to your protocol. (See Chapter 12.) Suitable IV sites for neonates include the dorsum of the hand or foot. Although scalp veins or the umbilical vein are cannulated in the hospital setting, do not attempt those procedures unless you have been specifically trained and authorized by your medical director to do so. Generally, a 24-gauge catheter is required for neonatal IV access.

APGAR Score

Newborns are assessed using the APGAR score (Table 43-4). APGAR is a mnemonic based on the name of the physician who developed the system, Dr. Virginia Apgar. The APGAR score assesses the newborn's appearance (A), pulse (P), grimace (G), activity (A), and respiratory effort (R). Each

TABLE 43-4	APGAR Scoring		
A — Appearance			
	0	**1**	**2**
	Cyanotic head, body, and extremities	Head and body pink, extremities cyanotic	Completely pink
P — Pulse			
	0	**1**	**2**
	Absent	Less than 100	Over 100
G — Grimace			
	0	**1**	**2**
	No reaction to stimuli	Grimaces in response to stimuli	Cries
A — Activity			
	0	**1**	**2**
	Limp	Some flexion of extremities	Active movement
R — Respirations			
	0	**1**	**2**
	Absent	Weak or irregular	Strong cry

dimension on the scale is assigned a score of zero, one, or two, with a maximum of 10 points possible. The APGAR score is assessed at 1 minute and at 5 minutes after delivery. Include the APGAR scores in your report to the receiving hospital and in your documentation.

Appearance refers specifically to the newborn's skin color. A newborn that is completely pink receives a score of 2. If the extremities are dusky or cyanotic, but the face and body are pink, the score is 1. A newborn who has cyanosis of both centrally (central cyanosis) and in the extremities (acrocyanosis) receives a score of 0.

A pulse rate above 100 beats per minute is assigned a score of 2, a pulse below 100 is assigned a score of 1, and a 0 is given if the pulse is absent.

Grimace, also known as *reflex irritability*, is an evaluation of the neonate's response to stimuli. If the newborn cries, sneezes, or coughs, he receives a score of 2. A facial grimace without a cry, sneeze, or cough is assigned a score of 1. A lack of response receives a score of 0.

Activity is a measure of the newborn's muscle tone. A newborn with active movement receives a score of 2. If there is some flexion of the extremities, the score is 1. If the newborn is limp, the score is 0.

Respirations are evaluated in terms of respiratory effort. A strong cry is assigned a score of 2. Slow (less than 30 breaths per minute), irregular respirations receive a score of 1. A 0 is assigned if respiratory effort is absent.

Most newborns score between 7 and 10 and need only to be dried and kept warm, and if excess secretions are present, suctioned with a bulb syringe. A score between 4 and 6 indicates moderate distress. Newborns scoring in that range require supplemental oxygen and tactile stimulation, such as rubbing the back or flicking the soles of the feet. In most cases, the repeat APGAR score will be between 7 and 10. Newborns who score a 3 or less are in severe distress and require bag-valve-mask ventilations with supplemental oxygen. If the heart rate is below 60 and does not respond to ventilations, start chest compressions. (See Chapter 17.) Hypoxia is the most common cause of bradycardia in newborns and can often be corrected with oxygen and bag-valve-mask ventilations.

Assessing Vital Signs

Although the newborn's pulse may be assessed at the brachial artery, it is preferable to assess the heart rate by auscultating the chest over the apex of the heart. The ideal range for the heart rate is 140 to 160, but should be between 100 and 180 beats per minute. Skin color and capillary refill are also useful in assessing the neonate's perfusion.

Respirations

A strong cry indicates adequate respirations. Signs of respiratory distress include grunting, subcostal, intercostal or supracostal retractions, and seesaw respirations (alternating movement of the chest and abdominal wall). Lung sounds are assessed as normal using an infant stethoscope. Avoid using an adult stethoscope to ensure you do not pick up extra chest and abdominal sounds.

Oxygen Saturation

Pulse oximetry can be reliably used in the neonate if an oximeter with a disposable adhesive infant or neonatal sensor is available. Pulse oximetry is recommended when the need for resuscitation is anticipated, for example, if there is persistent cyanosis, more than a few breaths with positive pressure ventilation are required, or when supplemental oxygen is administered. The neonate's SpO_2 will not reach expected infant values for approximately 10 minutes after birth. It is typical for the SpO_2 to remain between 70 and 80 percent for several minutes, consistent with the cyanotic appearance typical in the first few minutes of life. It has been suggested that skin color may not be a good indicator of oxygenation status in a newborn who is breathing well and has good muscle tone.

Temperature

If possible, take an axillary temperature. The neonate's temperature should be between 98°F and 100°F. To prevent heat loss, the room temperature or temperature in the back of the ambulance should be at least 75°F. Dry the newborn and wrap him in blankets, including covering his head (Figure 43-19).

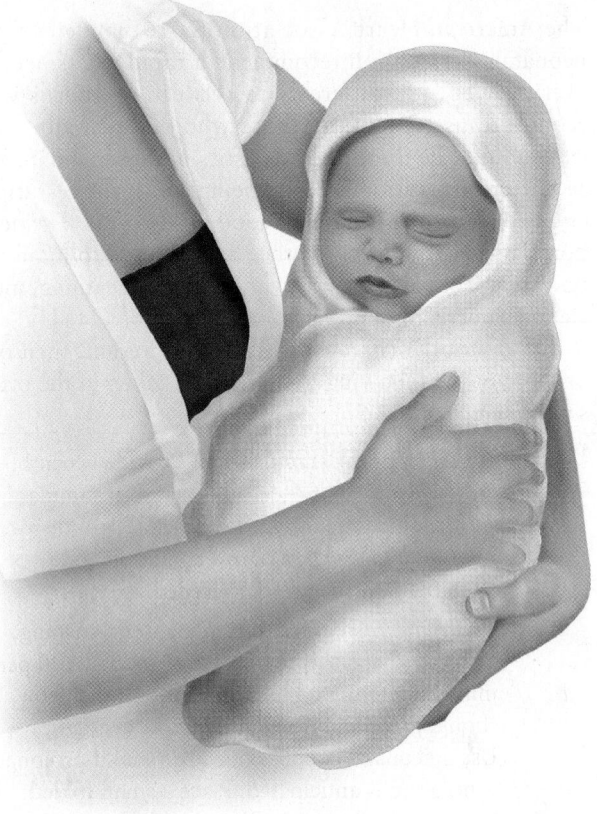

FIGURE 43-19

Wrap the newborn in receiving blankets to prevent heat loss. Make sure to cover the head, as well as the body.

Blood Glucose Level

It is not necessary to routinely assess the newborn's blood glucose level in the prehospital setting. If the newborn is severely distressed and does not respond to simple resuscitative efforts, obtain a blood glucose level from the outer surface of the heel (if permitted by your protocols). If the blood glucose level is below 60 mg/dL, consult with medical direction about starting an intravenous or intraosseous line and administering 10 percent dextrose solution.

Considerations in Neonatal Resuscitation

As indicated previously, simple techniques, beginning with tactile stimulation, are frequently sufficient in neonatal resuscitation. However, occasionally, oxygen administration, assisted ventilations, and chest compressions are required.

Oxygen Administration

Both an inadequate amount of oxygen and excess oxygen can be harmful in newborns. If you must administer supplemental oxygen, the goal is to maintain an SpO_2 of 96 percent because long-term administration of high concentrations of oxygen can cause complications in newborns. Keep in mind, however, that hypoxia is the primary reason for neonatal bradycardia. If you must administer oxygen, do not give it directly by mask or nasal cannula. Instead, use oxygen tubing to enrich the newborn's immediate atmosphere with oxygen. This is sometimes called administering oxygen by *blow-by*.

Airway Management and Ventilation

Although the mouth and nose are suctioned with a bulb syringe immediately after the head is delivered, additional suctioning may not be beneficial, and may be harmful (AHA, 2010). In the past, the recommendation was to perform oropharyngeal suctioning in the presence of thick meconium. However, this has not been found to be beneficial. If meconium is aspirated, the neonate requires endotracheal intubation and suction. If thick meconium is noted when the water breaks or at delivery, request ALS assistance. If ALS is not available, be prepared to transport as quickly as possible after delivery.

Meconium aspiration syndrome (MAS) may occur in the presence of thick meconium. The thick secretions act like a one-way valve in the lower airways, allowing air in, but not allowing it out. Hyperinflation of the chest, hypoxia, and pneumothorax can result.

Do not use battery-powered or fixed electric suction in the neonate. Further suctioning with a bulb syringe is indicated only if secretions are excessive.

Keeping in mind the anatomical differences of the neonate, position the airway by placing a small folded towel or receiving blanket under the shoulders to compensate for the large occiput. Consider a neonatal oropharyngeal airway for prolonged ventilation. Neonatal laryngeal mask airways (LMA) may be useful in neonates delivered at 34 weeks gestation or greater, or weighing over 2,000 g (4.5 pounds). The use of an LMA may be considered if ventilation by facemask is not effective.

To assist or provide ventilations, use a neonatal bag-valve-mask device. The neonate's flat face may make achieving a seal difficult, particularly if there is too much air in the cuff of the mask. Avoid excessive pressure to achieve a seal.

The neonate's tidal volume is small, just 18 to 28 mL. Ventilate at a rate of 40 to 60 breaths per minute. If more than a few ventilations are required, use supplemental oxygen until the neonate's condition improves.

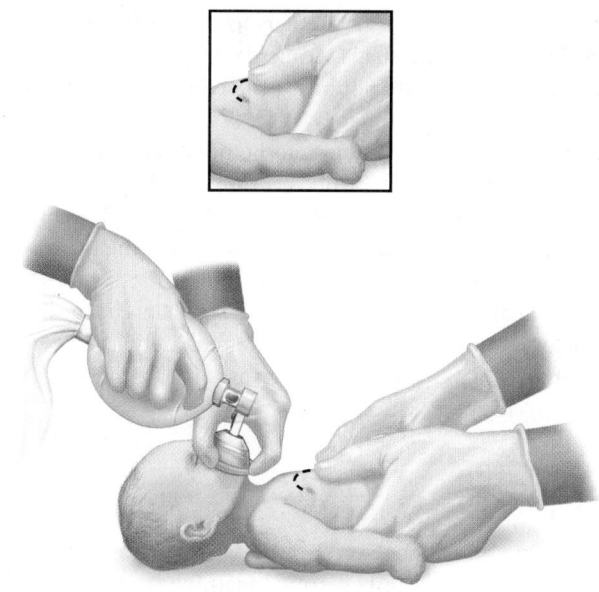

FIGURE 43-20

Proper position for CPR in the neonate.

Chest Compressions

Initiate chest compressions if the heart rate is less than 60 beats per minute and has not improved after assisted ventilation with supplemental oxygen for 30 seconds (Figure 43-20). Encircling the chest with the hands and using both thumbs over the lower third of the sternum is the preferred technique, but if space or other circumstances do not allow that, the use of two fingers of one hand over the lower third of the sternum is acceptable.

Use a compression-to-ventilation ratio of 3:1 at a rate of 90 compressions and 30 breaths per minute, with a compression depth of one third the anterior–posterior dimension of the chest. Reassess periodically, because hypoxia is the primary cause of bradycardia in neonates.

Fluids and Medications

Medications are rarely used in newborn resuscitation, although 2 mL/kg of 10 percent dextrose, IV or IO, may be indicated during postresuscitation care, based on blood glucose levels. Only consider IV or IO fluid infusion if blood loss is known or suspected and other measures have not been effective in improving the neonate's status. The dosage is 10 mL/kg, but do not infuse the fluids rapidly, particularly in premature newborns because brain hemorrhage may result.

Neonatal Complications and Defects

Prematurity is a serious problem. The course and outcome is largely dependent on the gestational age and weight at birth. Birth defects ranging from mild to severe occur in about 1 in every 33 births (Centers for Disease Control and Prevention [CDC], 2011). Some defects are not immediately apparent and do not pose problems in the immediate postnatal period. Fortunately, more severe birth defects are uncommon. However, they can be potentially lethal, accounting for more than 20 percent of infant deaths. There are a few defects that prehospital providers should be aware of, because of their dramatic appearance and the increased risks they pose to the neonate.

Premature newborns and those with significant birth defects require specialized care immediately after birth. Carefully weigh the options for transport to ensure the patient gets the care he needs.

Prematurity

A neonate that is born prior to 37 weeks gestation is premature. Neonates can be born prematurely for a variety of reasons, many of which are not well understood. Some of the reasons can include the following:

- Placental anomalies
- Maternal infections
- Medically induced due to maternal health problems

The longer the duration of pregnancy, the lower the risk of complications to the newborn and the better the newborn's chances for survival. Generally, a neonate is not considered viable until 24 weeks gestation and 450 grams in weight. Neonates born at this age and weight still have a high chance of mortality and complications. However, you should resuscitate any newborn delivered after 20 weeks gestation, unless death is obvious (such as softening and decomposition of the fetus). Do not withhold resuscitative measures from any fetus delivered with signs of life, regardless of suspected gestational age.

Premature newborns require specialized care in a NICU. If a facility with a NICU is not within reasonable transport distance, transport to the closest facility capable of initially stabilizing the newborn. A neonatal transport team, with specialized training and equipment, can be dispatched to transfer the neonate from the receiving facility to a NICU.

The immaturity of premature newborns is related to several potential immediate complications. The lungs are underdeveloped and may lack surfactant (resulting in atelectasis), fat deposits are inadequate to maintain body temperature, the thermoregulatory mechanism is immature, glycogen stores may be inadequate (increasing the risk for hypoglycemia), and the brain is less protected and more fragile, putting the premature newborn at risk for intracranial hemorrhage.

Simply preventing heat loss may not be sufficient for the premature newborn, who cannot generate sufficient heat on his own. It may be necessary to wrap the newborn in blankets and place warm packs around the blankets. Specialized thermal infant wraps are available. If you do not have access to one, place aluminum foil or plastic wrap around the receiving blankets the baby is wrapped in to better prevent heat loss.

If resuscitation is needed, keep in mind that the smaller lungs have an accordingly smaller tidal volume and will be damaged by excessive ventilation pressures.

Airway Abnormalities

Neonates can be born with defects to the airway that may make airway management difficult. *Choanal atresia* is a rare defect characterized by a complete blockage of both nares that occurs in about 0.82 out of every 10,000 births (Tewfik, Alrajhi, & Hagr, 2009). Choanal atresia prevents the neonate, a nasal-obligate breather, from being able to breathe effectively. Without treatment, asphyxia can occur. Cleft lip or cleft palate can also make airway management difficult (Figure 43-21). *Pierre Robin Syndrome* occurs in about one in 8,500 births (Tewfik, Trinh, & Teebi, 2010) and is characterized by a shorter-than-normal chin and large tongue. The large tongue easily obstructs the airway. Good airway positioning and an OPA, if necessary, will help resolve the airway obstruction.

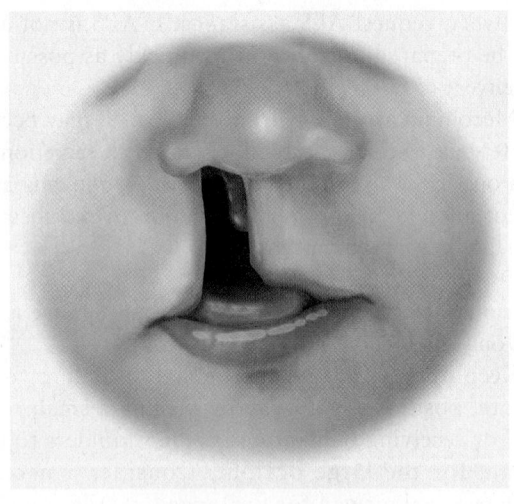

(A)

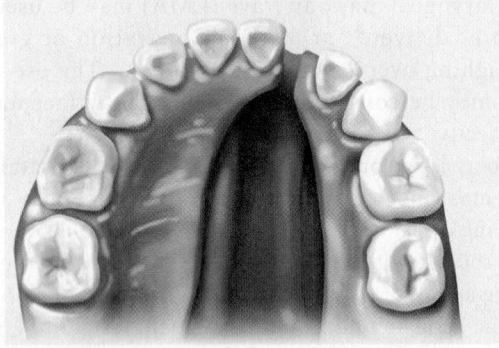

(B)

FIGURE 43-21

(A) Cleft lip. (B) Cleft palate.

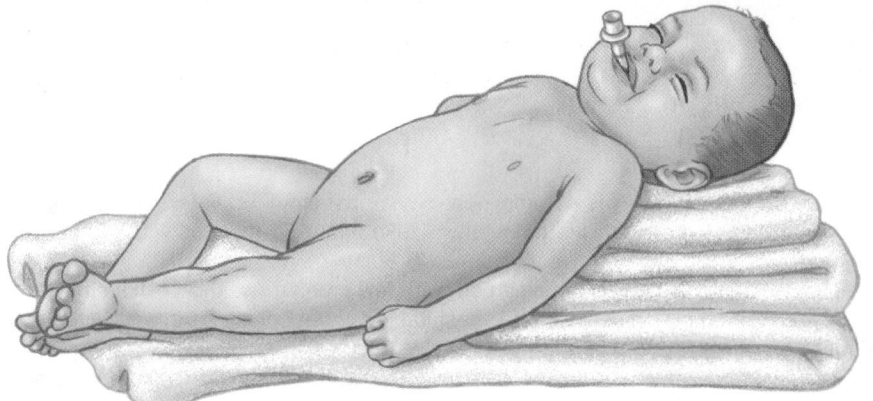

FIGURE 43-22

Elevate the head and shoulders of a newborn with congenital diaphragmatic hernia to decrease compression of the lungs by the abdominal organs.

Defects of the Abdomen

Congenital diaphragmatic hernia (CDH) is an abnormal opening in the diaphragm that allows the abdominal contents to migrate into the chest. Impairment of the diaphragm and the space occupied in the thoracic cavity by the abdominal organs impair respiration (Figure 43-22). Suspect CDH in newborns with respiratory distress and an unusually flat abdomen. *Gastroschisis* is an abdominal wall defect in which the abdominal contents extrude through an abdominal wall defect. An *omphalocele* is a similar condition, but the organs are contained within a translucent sac outside the abdominal wall. Cover the exposed organs with a moist, sterile dressing and avoid placing pressure on the exposed organs.

Defects of the Nervous System

A myelomeningocele is a form of spina bifida in which the meninges are exposed over the lumbar spine and may or may not contain portions of the spinal cord (Figure 43-23). Transport a neonate with a suspected myelomeningocele prone and take extreme care to not disrupt the defect. A defect that does not remain intact can damage the spinal cord and can lead to meningitis.

Defects of the Skin

Ichthyosis is a skin defect characterized by flaking and sloughing skin, and which may resemble a burn. Impairment of the skin increases heat and fluid loss.

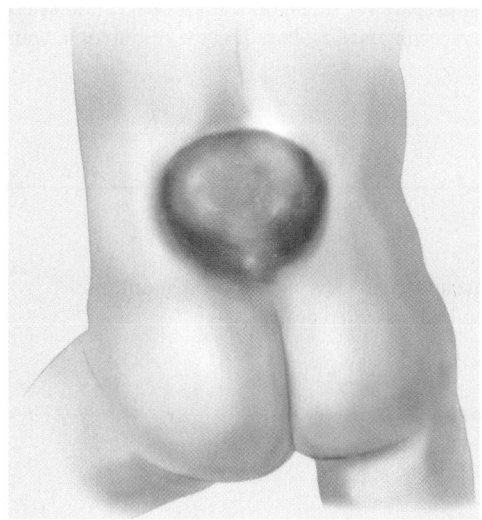

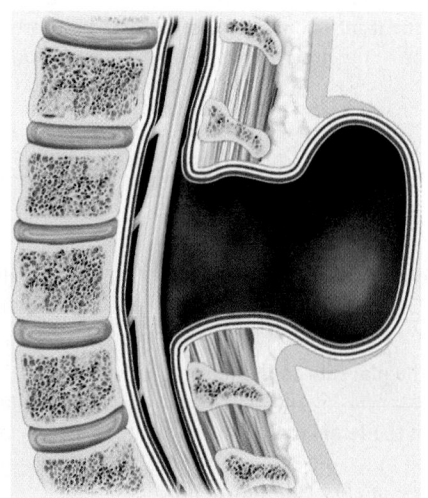

(A)   (B)

FIGURE 43-23

Myelomeningocele.

Clinical-Reasoning Process

Advanced EMTs Steve and Scott have determined that delivery is not imminent in their patient, Mrs. Velez, but they are concerned that she is just 35 weeks pregnant and their trip to the hospital will take about 50 minutes with the poor weather conditions.

Steve knows that, at 35 weeks, the baby has a good chance of being born with few problems, although his smaller size will make him more prone to hypothermia. Nonetheless, he knows the hospital is the best place for this baby to be born, preferably a couple of weeks from now.

Steve starts an IV as Scott obtains a complete set of vital signs. Steve explains to Mrs. Velez, "Sometimes getting some IV fluid can slow down premature labor, so let's give it a shot, ok? We will get you ready to go to the hospital and I will get some more information from you on the way. I will keep a close watch on your contractions and take good care of you. Your husband can ride with us, okay?"

Mrs. Velez' contractions continue at 5 minutes apart throughout transport and there are no other changes in her condition, although she remains anxious that her baby isn't supposed to born for a few weeks yet. Steve notifies the hospital of the patient's condition and they are able to admit her directly to the labor and delivery unit. Mrs. Velez is administered medications to stop labor. A week later, she gives birth to a healthy 6-pound baby girl with no complications.

CHAPTER REVIEW

Chapter Summary

Obstetric calls can be fast paced and exciting, resulting in the field delivery of a newborn. However, complications can occur during pregnancy or labor and delivery, requiring the Advanced EMT to have excellent knowledge about assessing and managing emergencies involving pregnancy, childbirth, and care of the newborn.

Pregnancy complications include trauma, spontaneous abortion, placental abruption, gestational diabetes, and hypertensive emergencies. You must not only expertly assess and manage those conditions, but you also must be prepared to provide reassurance and emotional support to the mother.

When you are called for a patient in labor, you must determine if delivery is imminent and make a decision whether to transport or prepare for a field delivery. If a field delivery is anticipated, ensure you have enough personnel to dedicate to the assessment and care of both the mother and the neonate.

In most cases, the delivery is uncomplicated and the neonate is not distressed. However, preterm labor, abnormal fetal presentations, prolapsed umbilical cord, uterine rupture, or distress in the newborn can turn a routine call into a critical situation that calls for quick thinking and action. In addition to managing the airway, breathing, and circulation of both patients, you must prepare for transport without delay and select an appropriate receiving facility, based on the resources in your community.

Review Questions

Multiple-Choice Questions

1. The role of the umbilical arteries in the fetus is to carry:
   a. deoxygenated blood from the placenta to the fetal inferior vena cava.
   b. oxygenated blood from the placenta to the fetal inferior vena cava.
   c. deoxygenated blood from the fetal circulation to the placenta.
   d. oxygenated blood from the fetal circulation to the placenta.

2. By the time a woman is two months pregnant, the developing baby is called a(n):
   a. embryo.
   b. fetus.
   c. neonate.
   d. zygote.

3. A typical full-term newborn weighs about _____ pounds.
   a. 5
   b. 7
   c. 9
   d. 10

4. By the end of pregnancy, the maternal blood volume increases by up to nearly:
   a. 10 percent
   b. 30 percent.
   c. 50 percent.
   d. 70 percent.

5. A woman in late pregnancy may lose _____ percent of her blood volume before exhibiting signs and symptoms of shock.
   a. 15
   b. 35
   c. 45
   d. 50

6. Which one of the following events occurs in the first stage of labor?
   a. The cervix thins and dilates.
   b. Crowning occurs.
   c. Irregular, painless contractions occur.
   d. The placenta is delivered.

7. In normal fetal circulation, blood flows from the:
   a. right atrium to the left atrium.
   b. umbilical arteries to the right atrium.
   c. right ventricle to the left ventricle.
   d. umbilical vein to the ductus arteriosis.

8. The minimum acceptable heart rate in a newborn is _____ beats per minute.
   a. 60
   b. 80
   c. 100
   d. 150

9. The neonatal respiratory rate should be at least _____ breaths per minute.
   a. 12
   b. 20
   c. 30
   d. 45

10. During a delivery, the water breaks and you notice it is heavily stained with meconium. When the head delivers, you notice a small amount of meconium in the mouth. You should:
    a. use mechanical suction with a flexible suction catheter to suction the mouth and oropharynx.
    b. insert an oropharyngeal airway in preparation for bag-valve-mask ventilations.
    c. use mechanical suction with a rigid suction catheter to suction the mouth and oropharynx.
    d. use a bulb syringe to suction the mouth and then the nose.

11. The normal tidal volume for a newborn is no more than _____ mL.
    a. 10
    b. 30
    c. 50
    d. 100

12. A woman who is 25 weeks into her first pregnancy is documented as:
    a. G0, P0.
    b. G0, P1.
    c. G1, P1.
    d. G1, P0.

13. A patient who is 32 weeks pregnant complains of a headache; increased swelling of her hands, feet, and face; and difficulty with her vision. She is alert and oriented, but anxious. Her vital signs are: blood pressure 142/88, heart rate 92, respiratory rate 18, SpO_2 98 percent on room air. Her blood glucose level is 118 mg/dL. The patient's presentation is most consistent with:
    a. gestational diabetes.
    b. pre-eclampsia.
    c. eclampsia.
    d. hyperemesis gravidarum.

14. When clamping the umbilical cord, a clamp should not be placed closer than _____ inches from the newborn.
    a. 2
    b. 4
    c. 6
    d. 8

15. At 1 minute after birth, a newborn is pink except for his feet and hands, he is crying vigorously, and is kicking his feet and flexing his arms. His heart rate is 162. His APGAR score is:
    a. 7.
    b. 8.
    c. 9.
    d. 10.

16. During active labor, your patient, a 35-year-old G3 P2 whose last delivery was by cesarean section, complains of sudden, excruciating abdominal pain. Contractions stop and the abdomen is tender and rigid. The patient's presentation is most consistent with:
    a. uterine inversion.
    b. placental abruption.
    c. placenta previa.
    d. uterine rupture.

17. The most commonly needed intervention in newborn resuscitation is:
    a. tactile stimulation.
    b. oxygen.
    c. bag-valve-mask ventilations.
    d. intravenous dextrose.

18. Chest compressions should be started in a newborn whose heart rate is less than:

a. 150.
b. 100.
c. 80.
d. 60.

19. The most common cause of bradycardia in newborns is:

a. maternal narcotic use.
b. hypoxia.
c. congenital heart defects.
d. hypoglycemia.

20. A newborn has an unusually flat abdomen and is in respiratory distress. You should suspect:

a. gastroschisis.
b. omphalocele.
c. myelomeningocele.
d. diaphragmatic hernia.

Critical-Thinking Questions

21. Explain how you would determine whether to transport a pregnant patient or prepare for field delivery.

22. You respond to a call for a woman in labor. She is 32 weeks pregnant and states she feels like she is about to deliver. Your exam shows that both fetal feet are presenting at the vaginal opening. Explain the concerns in this situation and how you should handle them.

23. A newborn has both central and peripheral cyanosis, respiratory effort at 30 per minute, a weak cry, and weak flexion of the extremities. Outline a treatment plan for this patient.

References

American Heart Association. (2010). Part 15: Neonatal resuscitation: 2010 American Heart Association guidelines for cardiopulmonary resuscitation and emergency cardiovascular care. *Circulation, 122,* S909–S919.

Centers for Disease Control and Prevention. (2011). Birth defects: Leading cause of infant death. Retrieved March 10, 2011, from http://www.cdc.gov/Features/dsInfantDeaths/

Chi, T. J. (2009). *Pregnancy, ectopic.* eMedicine. Retrieved March 9, 2011, from http://emedicine.medscape.com/article/796451-overview

Gaufberg, S. V. (2010). *Early pregnancy loss: Differential diagnoses & workup.* eMedicine. Retrieved March 9, 2011, from http://emedicine.medscape.com/article/795085-diagnosis

Martini, F. H., Bartholomew, E. F., & Bledsoe, B. E. (2008). *Anatomy and physiology for emergency care* (2nd ed.). Upper Saddle River, NJ: Pearson.

Tewfik, T. L., Alrajhi, Y. A., & Hagr, A. A. (2009). *Choanal atresia.* eMedicine. Retrieved March 11, 2011, from http://emedicine.medscape.com/article/872409-overview

Tewfik, T. L., Trinh, N., & Teebi, A. S. (2010). *Pierre Robin syndrome.* eMedicine. Retrieved March 11, 2011, from http://emedicine.medscape.com/article/844143-overview

Additional Reading

Bledsoe, B. E., Porter, R. S., & Cherry, R. A. (2009). *Paramedic care: Principles and practice* (3rd ed., Vol. 3.). Upper Saddle River, NJ: Pearson.

Ma, O. J., Cline, D. M., Tintinalli, J. E., Kelen, G. D., & Stapczynski, J. S. (Eds.) (2004). *Emergency medicine manual* (6th ed., Updated). New York, NY: McGraw Hill.

44

Pediatric Emergencies

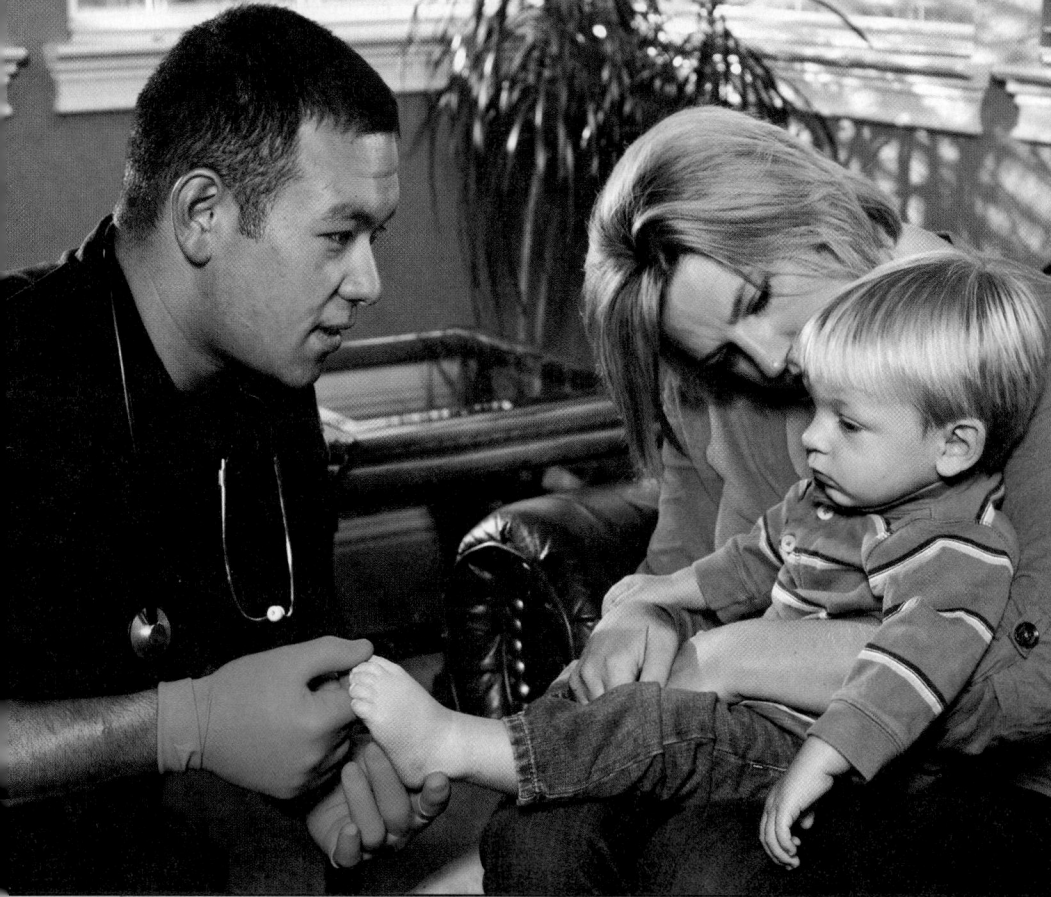

Content Area: Special Patient Populations

Advanced EMT Education Standard: Applies a fundamental knowledge of growth, development, aging, and assessment findings to provide basic emergency care and transportation for a patient with special needs.

Objectives

After reading this chapter, you should be able to:

44.1   Define key terms introduced in this chapter.

44.2   Discuss the leading reasons that pediatric patients require medical attention.

44.3   Explain the special considerations in dealing with the caregiver of a sick or injured child.

44.4   Describe the major anatomic, physiological, and developmental characteristics of pediatric patients in each of the following age groups:
- Infant
- Toddler
- Preschooler
- School age
- Adolescent

(continued)

Resource Central

To access Resource Central, follow the directions on the Student Access Card provided with this text. If there is no card, go to www.bradybooks.com and follow the Resource Central link to Buy Access. Under Media Resources, you will find:

- *Pediatric Trauma Considerations.*
- *Communicating with Toddlers.*
- *SIDS.* What it is and its causes.
- *Caring and Empathy.* How to express genuine care.
- *The Pediatric Assessment Triangle (PAT).* How to use it.

CASE STUDY

Advanced EMTs Vic Gagne and Marcel Sager are attending a continuing education class at their station when they receive a call for an infant not breathing. "Oh, man," says Vic. "I hate the feeling I get in my stomach when I hear calls like that. Let's talk about our approach on the way." En route, the crew talks about possible scenarios, ranging from an over-reaction to the baby coughing or gagging, to a foreign body airway obstruction, respiratory illness or trauma, to an apparent life-threatening event or sudden infant death syndrome. When they arrive at the home, they find two very anxious and upset parents, with the mother holding a crying infant.

Problem-Solving Questions

1. What criteria should Vic and Marcel use to develop a general impression of the patient's condition?
2. What questions should they ask of the parents?
3. How should they proceed with the assessment of an infant?

(continued from previous page)

44.5   Give examples of modifications of patient assessment and management techniques that increase the likelihood of cooperation by patients in each of the following age groups:
- Infant
- Toddler
- Preschooler
- School age
- Adolescent

44.6   Given a description of vital signs for pediatric patients of various ages, classify the values as normal or abnormal.

44.7   Use the pediatric assessment triangle to determine a pediatric patient's status.

44.8   Recognize signs of respiratory distress, respiratory failure, and respiratory arrest in pediatric patients.

44.9   Describe the presentation and assessment-based prehospital management of the following conditions:
- Altered mental status
- Anaphylaxis
- Apparent life-threatening emergencies (ALTE)
- Asthma
- Bronchiolitis
- Cardiac arrest
- Complications of cystic fibrosis
- Congenital heart disease
- Croup
- Drowning
- Epiglottitis
- Fever
- Gastrointestinal disorders
- Meningitis
- Pneumonia
- Poisoning
- Seizures, including status epilepticus
- Shock
- Sudden infant death syndrome (SIDS)

44.10 Demonstrate emergency medical care techniques for pediatric patients including the following:
- Airway management
- CPR
- Fluid resuscitation
- Management of partial and complete foreign body airway obstruction
- Medication administration
- Oxygen administration
- Ventilation

44.11 Describe special considerations in the scene size-up in suspected SIDS.

44.12 Describe special considerations in assisting family members in suspected SIDS.

44.13 Describe the importance of the presence of parents during pediatric resuscitation.

44.14 Integrate consideration of a pediatric patient's size and anatomy into the assessment of mechanism of injury.

44.15 Demonstrate removal of a pediatric patient from a child car seat.

44.16 Demonstrate proper spinal immobilization of a pediatric patient.

44.17 Explain the importance of injury prevention programs to reduce pediatric injuries and deaths.

44.18 Recognize indications of child abuse and neglect.

44.19 Explain special considerations in managing situations in which you suspect child abuse or neglect.

44.20 Discuss ways in which you can manage the stress that can be associated with pediatric calls, both during and after the call.

Introduction

Caring for a critically ill or injured child can be a stressful experience for EMS providers. However, you must never forget that, regardless of your feelings and stress level, the patient and his caregivers are depending on you to remain calm and in control and to perform your job well. Nonetheless, you must recognize the potential stress associated with calls for pediatric patients. Ways of recognizing and managing that stress were discussed in Chapter 3.

Although there is overlap between adults and children in the types of emergencies they may experience, there are differences, too. For example, fever is an unusual cause of seizures in adults, but a common cause in pediatric patients. When adults suffer cardiac arrest, the usual cause is sudden cardiac arrest (SCA) from underlying coronary heart disease. In contrast, the most frequent cause of cardiac arrest in children is respiratory failure and arrest. Children are a generally healthy group, making acute illnesses and injuries much more frequent than problems related to chronic illnesses.

Your assessment, clinical reasoning process, and treatment must take into account the differing epidemiology of illness and injury in children, and anatomic, physiological, and psychosocial differences as you evaluate the presenting problem. Keep in mind that, despite the differences, you are still able to call on a vast amount of your knowledge of emergencies in adult patients. Refer back to the chapters where the topics were introduced for review.

Pediatric Development Review

The rapid growth and development that takes place during childhood make pediatric patients differ vastly from each other according to age and size. Those differences, introduced in Chapter 9, are reviewed in this section.

Infants

From one month of age to one year of age, a child is referred to as an *infant*. Overall, the body systems are immature and do not function the way they will as the child continues to grow and develop (Figure 44-1). The liver is large for the size of the abdomen, meaning it is not as well protected by the ribs as in adults. The abdominal wall is thin, composed of less muscle and fat, also creating less protection. The ribs are pliable, which allows forces to be transmitted to the organs beneath, rather than absorbing the energy as well as in adults. The kidneys do not efficiently concentrate urine, which increases the risk of dehydration. The bones are softer and less well formed.

FIGURE 44-1

Anatomic and physiologic considerations in infants and children.

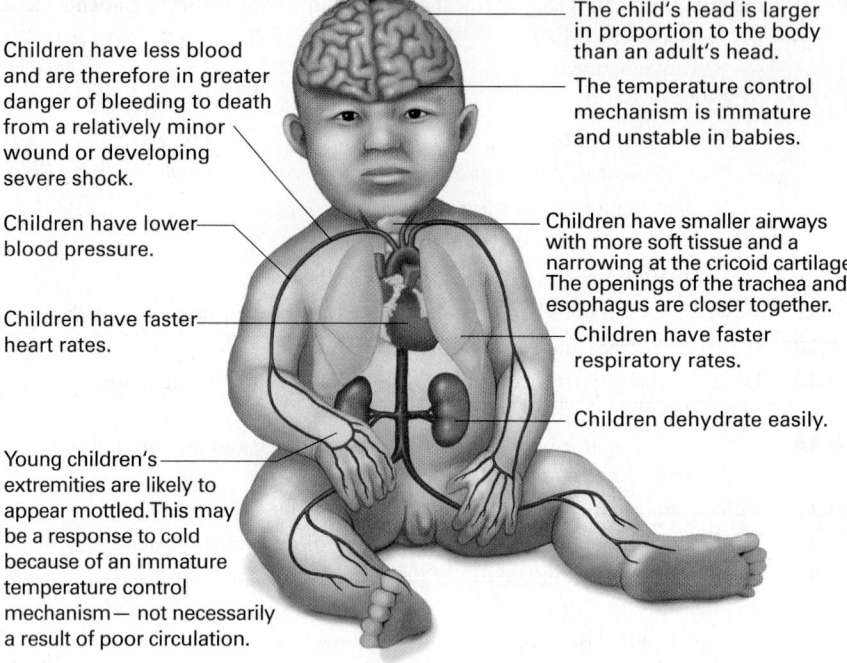

Children have less blood and are therefore in greater danger of bleeding to death from a relatively minor wound or developing severe shock.

Children have lower blood pressure.

Children have faster heart rates.

Young children's extremities are likely to appear mottled. This may be a response to cold because of an immature temperature control mechanism— not necessarily a result of poor circulation.

The child's head is larger in proportion to the body than an adult's head.

The temperature control mechanism is immature and unstable in babies.

Children have smaller airways with more soft tissue and a narrowing at the cricoid cartilage. The openings of the trachea and esophagus are closer together.

Children have faster respiratory rates.

Children dehydrate easily.

The skeletal muscle mass is small, providing less strength, protection, and heat production.

The infant's head is disproportionately large, making up about 25 percent of the body weight, and the neck is weak. The soft fontanels do not provide the protection to the brain that the harder bones of the skull will provide as the infant grows.

Infants have a greater surface area-to-volume ratio. That means neonates and infants have a large surface area compared to their body size, which allows for increased heat loss from the body. Heat loss and water loss also are increased with the increased respiratory rate of infants. The heat and water transferred to air as it passes through the airway is lost at an even greater rate during respiratory distress. Coupled with an immature thermoregulatory system, infants are prone to hypothermia and must be kept warm. Covering the head prevents heat loss from the large surface area of the scalp.

The differences in pediatric airway anatomy compared to that of adults means that airway obstruction can occur very easily. The tongue takes up a relatively larger portion of the oral cavity than in adults. The airway is slightly funnel shaped, with the narrowest point at the cricoid ring, and it is proportionately shorter and softer than in adults. The nose is small and soft. The occipital region of the skull is prominent compared to the torso. When an infant is supine, the large occiput causes flexion of the neck. Older infants learn to grasp objects and put them in their mouths.

There are fewer alveoli in the lungs and the lungs are fragile and easily damaged. The tidal volume is small, approximately 6 to 8 mL/kg. The chest wall is pliable and the ribs have a more horizontal orientation, increasing reliance on the diaphragm for breathing. The respiratory muscles are immature and glycogen stores are minimal. Respiratory failure and respiratory arrest can occur quickly in an infant with respiratory distress.

The water vapor lost with every breath leads to dehydration with increased respirations during respiratory distress. The blood volume of neonates and infants is small to begin with (approximately 80 mL/kg). Just a few milliliters of fluid loss can lead to shock. Poor feeding, vomiting, diarrhea, and fever can result in significant dehydration.

The infant's immune system is immature and less able to fight infection. Immaturity of the nervous system means that a young infant may not have a high fever, even with serious infection. Fever in infants is always concerning.

Crying is the young infant's only way of communicating. Parents and caregivers often recognize the difference in cries for different reasons. Parents may be concerned because of a change in the infant's cry or because the infant is inconsolable. The best way to prevent crying from

IN THE FIELD

Although you must expose the pediatric patient for examination, inspect one part of the body at a time, covering the patient again before moving to the next part.

separation is to allow the parent to hold the child while you examine him. If an infant does not cry when he is separated from his parents, consider the possibility of illness, injury, or developmental issues.

Toddlers and Preschool Children

A toddler is a child from one to three years of age. Preschoolers are three to six years of age. The head is still proportionally large, but not as disproportionate as an infant's. The airway is still relatively small and can be obstructed easily. Levels of maternal antibodies decrease in infancy, and toddlers and preschoolers are exposed to more people, making them vulnerable to communicable diseases. Most of the diseases are minor, and are an important part of developing immunity. Ear infections and upper and lower respiratory tract infections are common. Some diseases, such as croup, **bronchiolitis**, pneumonia, and epiglottitis can lead to respiratory distress in this age group.

Strangers, including health care providers, can provoke anxiety in children this age. Establish rapport and gain the child's trust and communicate with him in a way he can understand. Demonstrating the techniques of assessment you plan to use on a doll or stuffed animal can decrease anxiety, as can allowing the child to handle the equipment, if appropriate, before you use it.

School-Age Children

The school-age years are from 6 through 12 years of age. Physical proportions become more adult-like. Approval and acceptance are important. Problem-solving ability is developing, but reasoning skills remain relatively concrete. Children in this age group are beginning to develop an understanding of illness, loss, death, and dying, but still need adults' assistance in coping with the fears associated with those issues. Modesty and the need for privacy are developing and must be kept in mind when caring for school-age children. School-age children appreciate being kept informed, in terms they can understand, about what you are doing.

Adolescents

Between 12 and 18 years of age, children's vital signs approach adult values, and toward the later years physical growth is nearly complete. It is during this period of development that children complete puberty. They want to be regarded as adults, but are not legally capable of making medical decisions. The teenage brain has not yet developed adult judgment and handles emotions differently than the adult brain.

Adolescents become more challenging to parental authority and family conflict often increases with an adolescent in the home. Teens can have a sense of invulnerability. This, along with immature judgment and the experimentation that emerges during identity development, can lead to risky behaviors, including unsafe driving; use of tobacco, alcohol, and drugs; and unsafe sexual behavior. Rates of depression and suicide increase in this age group.

In most prehospital situations involving adolescents, assessment and management of the anatomic and physiological aspects of injury and illness are similar to that of young adults. But, you must keep in mind the psychosocial differences in the approach to patients, and the differing epidemiology of illness and injury in adolescents, as compared to older adults. Keep in mind the adolescent's possible reluctance to be forthcoming with relevant health information in the presence of family and peers.

General Assessment and Management of Pediatric Patients

Assessment and management of pediatric patients requires the appropriate equipment, in addition to knowledge of differences between adults and pediatric patients (Table 44-1). Otherwise, you will rely on many of the same principles of assessment and management you have already learned. In fact, in some situations, you may not know that you have a pediatric patient until you have already begun your scene size-up.

TABLE 44-1 **Equipment for Pediatric Prehospital Care**

- Length-based resuscitation tape, such as a Broselow tape
- Pediatric stethoscope
- Pediatric blood pressure cuffs
- Pediatric pulse oximeter sensor
- Pediatric oropharyngeal and nasopharyngeal airways
- Pediatric advanced (supraglottic) airways
- Pediatric oxygen masks
- Pediatric bag-valve-mask device
- Pediatric cervical collars in a variety of sizes
- Bulb syringe
- Blankets for warmth and padding
- 60-gtts/mL IV tubing
- Volumetric IV device, such as a Buretrol
- 24-, 22-, and 20-gauge IV catheters
- 25 percent dextrose
- 10 percent dextrose
- Pediatric long-bone splints
- Pediatric car seat and restraint devices for transport

Scene Size-Up

The principles of scene size-up remain the same. Do not allow knowledge that you are responding for a pediatric patient to distract you from looking for hazards, determining the total number of patients, evaluating the need for additional resources, and determining the nature of the problem.

When responding to pediatric trauma calls, keep in mind that anatomical differences of the pediatric body alter the patterns of trauma you should suspect. The head is large, and is often the point of impact in falls. The organs are less protected than in an adult. The bones have more flexibility, meaning that serious underlying organ injury can occur without evidence of a fracture.

A special consideration on pediatric calls is that you must take into account the reactions and needs of the parents or caregivers. Having a sick or injured child can be terrifying. Unless the parent is unable to cooperate and interferes with providing care (and if abuse is suspected), there is no reason to separate the child from the parents. It will increase their distress. Provide reassurance to the parents or caregivers, as well as to the patient. Allow the parents to participate in the child's care as much as possible.

Child abuse and neglect are sometimes the reason EMS is needed. There are particular indications of abuse and neglect that may begin to be evident in the scene size-up (Table 44-2). Scenes involving potential abuse or neglect require law enforcement presence. If law enforcement is not on the scene, request them. Keep in mind that it may be best for you or your partner to request law enforcement out of the hearing of the parents or caregiver to avoid a potential escalation of violence. When child abuse or neglect or **sudden infant death syndrome (SIDS)** is suspected, there are particular observations you must make and document. (Those observations are discussed in later sections of this chapter.)

During the scene size-up, formulate a general impression to guide your approach to the primary assessment. A general impression is facilitated by the use of the **pediatric assessment triangle (PAT)**. Using the principles of the pediatric assessment triangle, develop a general impression of the patient's overall appearance, work of breathing, and circulation to the skin, as follows (Figure 44-2):

- Appearance
  - *Muscle tone.* Does the child appear to have normal muscle tone or is he flaccid or limp?
  - *Interactiveness.* Does the child interact with you or want to know what is going on (if expected for the child's developmental age)?
  - *Consolabilty.* Can the child be consoled by you or his caregiver?
  - *Eye contact.* Is the child able to maintain eye contact?
  - *Speech or crying.* Is the child able to speak and tell you what is wrong or does the child cry and hold onto parent or caregiver?
- Work of breathing
  - *Abnormal airway noise.* Do you hear obvious sounds like wheezing, grunting, or stridor as you approach the patient? Those sounds indicate a respiratory problem that may require immediate intervention.
  - *Abnormal positioning.* Does the child appear to be sitting upright in a tripod position? This is often a sign of a significant respiratory problem.
  - *Retractions.* Do you notice that the suprasternal or intercostal tissues retract while breathing? Does it

TABLE 44-2	Indications of Child Abuse and Child Neglect

- Injuries inconsistent with history provided
- Bruises over soft areas (buttocks, abdomen, cheeks, thighs, upper arms), as opposed to bony areas such as the forehead or shins
- Multiple injuries in various stages of healing
- Unusually fearful child
- Specific wound patterns such as cigarette burns, hand marks, belt buckle impression, human bite marks
- Clearly delineated burn marks, burn marks in the shape of a specific object
- Lack of adequate supervision
- Injuries to the genitals
- Untreated illness
- Delay in reporting illness or injury
- Malnourishment, lack of food
- Sexual behavior or unusual knowledge of sexual activity
- Unsafe living environment

General appearance	Does the child appear to be flaccid or limp? Is the child interacting with people appropriately? Can the crying child be consoled? Does the child make appropriate eye contact?
Ventilatory effort	Are there abnormal sounds while breathing? Is the patient positioning themselves to make breathing easier? Are there signs of accessory muscle use?
Skin perfusion	Are there any abnormal findings suggesting hypoperfusion?

FIGURE 44-2

Rapid visual assessment of the pediatric patient.

appear that the child is using accessory muscles to breathe?

- *Nasal flaring.* Do you notice flaring of the child's nares during inspiration?

■ Circulation to the skin
- What is the child's skin color? Pallor, mottling, and cyanosis all are signs of poor perfusion in an infant or child.

End the preliminary scene size-up with an impression of how sick the child is and determine the patient's priority for transport. If you determine a poor overall appearance such as lethargy, limpness, or cyanosis, increased work of breathing (or diminished breathing), and poor circulation to the skin as indicated by poor skin color, make the patient a high priority for treatment and transport.

Primary Assessment

If the patient is apparently unresponsive and not breathing normally, confirm unresponsiveness and check for a pulse. The best place to check the infant's pulse is at the brachial artery over the medial aspect of the humerus. Check the carotid pulse of an older child. If a pulse is not detected within 10 seconds, begin chest compressions according to the American Heart Association (AHA) guidelines for the patient's age (Table 44-3). (See Chapter 17.)

Keep in mind that the most common cause of cardiac arrest in pediatric patients is hypoxia due to respiratory

failure and respiratory arrest. If a clear respiratory cause is suspected, such as drowning, the AHA allows for EMS provider judgment in making ventilation a higher priority during CPR. For example, if you arrive on the scene first, or if you are off duty and no other personnel are present, you may consider changing your approach. If hypoxia is the suspected underlying cause of cardiac arrest, it may be best to perform 1 to 2 minutes of CPR prior to attaching the AED. Follow your protocols with regard to any potential deviations from the standard CPR sequence of circulation, airway, and breathing. If you are alone, consider performing 1 to 2 minutes of CPR before calling for help.

If the patient is responsive, or is unresponsive but breathing, carefully assess the patient's airway, breathing, and circulation, keeping in mind that you must address any problem found in the primary assessment before moving on to the secondary assessment.

Carefully assess the patient for indications of partial or complete airway obstruction. Upper respiratory illness and foreign bodies can easily obstruct the pediatric airway. (See Chapter 16 for treatment of partial and complete airway obstruction.) Use padding under the shoulders of smaller patients to compensate for the large size of the occiput and maintain alignment of airway structures (Figure 44-3). Assess the need for assisted ventilations, keeping in mind that respiratory distress can progress quickly to respiratory failure and respiratory arrest in pediatric patients. Be prepared to intervene

TABLE 44-3

Age	Initiation	Positioning of hands	Depth of compression	Rate of compression	Compressions to ventilations ratio
1 to 8 years of age	If unresponsive, not breathing or inadequate breathing is present, no palpable pulse, or pulse rate of <60 with signs of inadequate perfusion begin 2 minutes of CPR	1 or 2 hands over the lower half of the sternum	At least 1/3 the thickness of the chest cavity; approximately 2 inches	At least 100 per minute	30 compressions to 2 ventilations with one rescuer; 15 compressions to 2 ventilations with 2 rescuers
Less than one year of age	If unresponsive, not breathing or inadequate breathing is present, no palpable pulse, or pulse rate of <60 with signs of inadequate perfusion begin 2 minutes of CPR	Two finger widths below the nipple line	At least 1/3 the thickness of the chest cavity; approximately 1 ½ inches	At least 100 per minute	30 compressions to 2 ventilations with one rescuer; 15 compressions to 2 ventilations with 2 rescuers

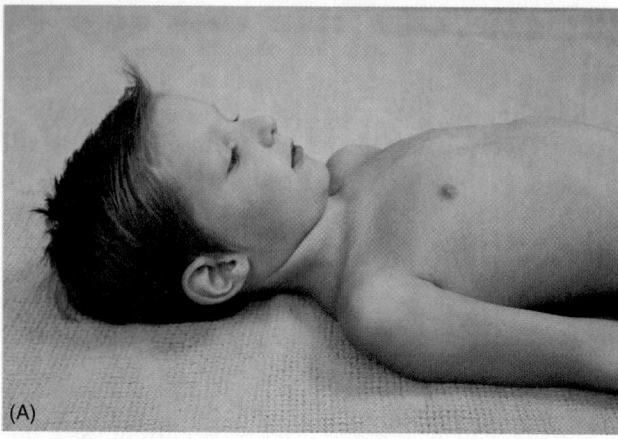 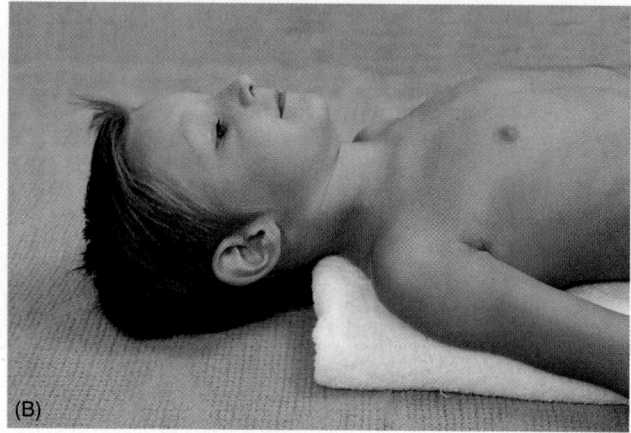

FIGURE 44-3

(A) When a child is supine without padding beneath the shoulders, the neck can flex, resulting in airway obstruction. (B) Pad beneath the shoulders to maintain proper alignment of airway structures with the neck in a neutral position.

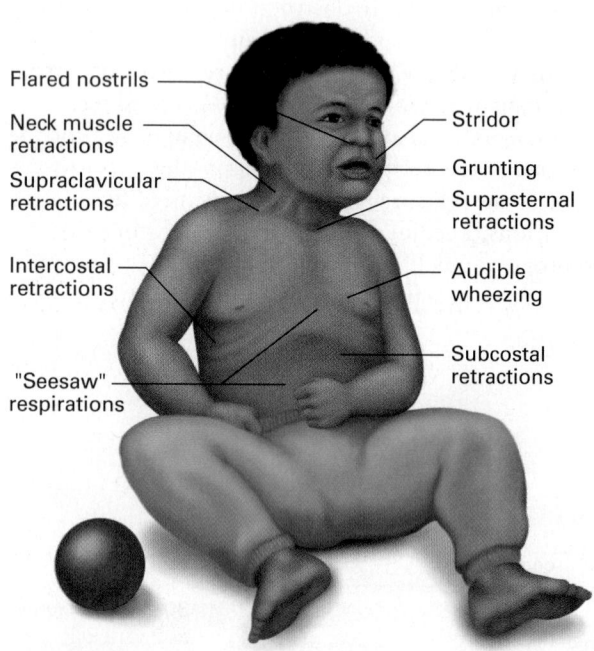

Flared nostrils

Neck muscle retractions

Supraclavicular retractions

Intercostal retractions

"Seesaw" respirations

Stridor

Grunting

Suprasternal retractions

Audible wheezing

Subcostal retractions

FIGURE 44-4

Signs of respiratory distress in a pediatric patient.

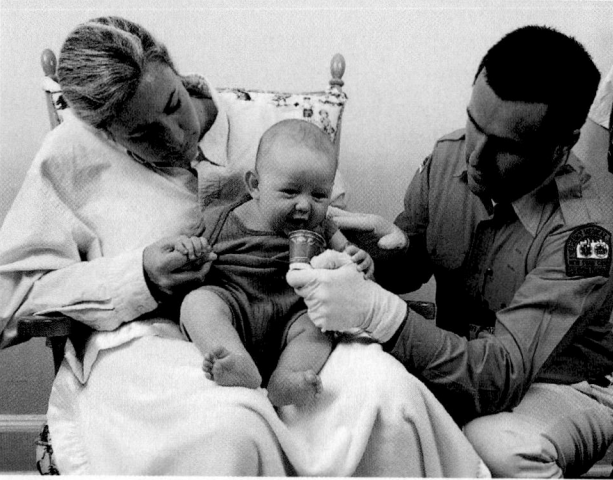

FIGURE 44-5

Administering oxygen to an infant using the blow-by method.

IN THE FIELD

With a blood volume of about 80 mL/kg, a one-year-old child weighing 10 kg (22 pounds) has a blood volume of just 800 mL, which is less than 1 L. A loss of just 125 mL (about half a cup, or 4 ounces) of blood amounts to 15 percent of the blood volume, enough to result in compensated shock.

quickly, should the need arise, with any child who has signs of respiratory distress (Figure 44-4).

If hypoxia is evident or likely, provide supplemental oxygen. While older children may tolerate a facemask, a facemask is not appropriate for infants and may not be tolerated by toddlers. In such cases, use blow-by oxygen (Figure 44-5). Some EMS services have a device shaped like an animal or other toy that attaches to the oxygen tubing to make receiving blow-by oxygen more acceptable to the patient. If your service does not have those devices, consider punching a hole into the bottom of a paper cup and feeding the oxygen tubing through the hole and allowing the child, or his parent, to hold the cup close to his face.

Children's blood volume is small and shock can occur with seemingly little volume loss (Figure 44-6). Yet, children compensate well early in the process, which can mask signs of shock. Control hemorrhage and maintain a high index of suspicion for internal bleeding based on mechanism of injury. Keeping a patient with blood loss warm is always important, but keep in mind that children are especially prone to hypothermia.

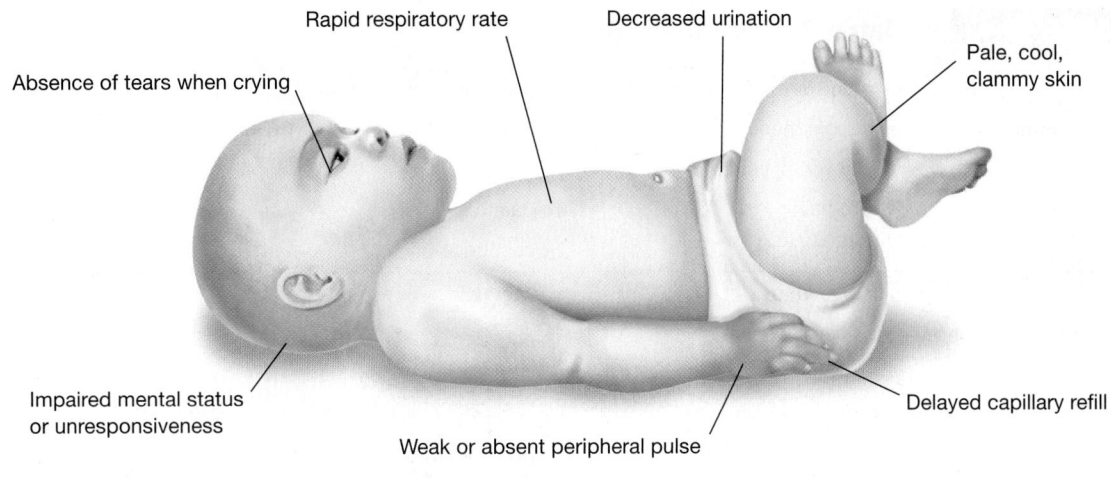

Rapid respiratory rate

Decreased urination

Absence of tears when crying

Pale, cool,
clammy skin

Impaired mental status
or unresponsiveness

Delayed capillary refill

Weak or absent peripheral pulse

FIGURE 44-6

Signs of shock (hypoperfusion) in an infant or child.

Secondary Assessment

There are some special considerations in obtaining a pediatric patient history and vital signs and in conducting a physical exam. One particular difficulty you may encounter is the younger pediatric patient's inability to give a chief complaint, or the limited language skills to elaborate on a chief complaint. In younger pediatric patients, the ability to localize pain may not be well developed, further contributing to vagueness of the chief complaint.

Medical History

Obtaining a medical history may be difficult if the child is in daycare or with a babysitter. If the parents are not able to arrive on the scene before you depart, attempt to contact them by phone to obtain a history.

In addition to the questions formulated to obtain a SAMPLE history and explore the chief complaint using OPQRST, there are some specific questions to ask, based on the child's presentation, as follows:

- Is the child's activity level normal for him, or does he seem unusually active or lethargic?

- Has the child had a fever or been sick recently? If there was a fever, how high was it and how long did it last? What were the signs and symptoms of any recent illness?

- Does the child have a rash?

- What has the amount of oral intake been? Have there been changes in urinary output (number of wet diapers or number of trips to the bathroom)? Has the child had diarrhea or vomiting?

- Are there any current or past medical problems? For infants and toddlers, ask about any problems with gestation or birth, such as prematurity or other complications. If birth was premature, to what degree (how many weeks or months)?

- Is the child up to date on recommended vaccinations? This question, in particular, is helpful in increasing or decreasing the index of suspicion for specific infectious diseases.

Level of Responsiveness

Initially, the level of responsiveness is determined using the AVPU method. Apply the Pediatric Glasgow Coma Scale to obtain a more precise assessment of the level of responsiveness (Table 44-4).

Vital Signs

You must know the normal values of pediatric vital signs in order to interpret the findings (Table 44-5). As with all patients, you must interpret the findings in context. Consider the following example:

You have just arrived at an urgent care center to transport a 22-month-old male who presented with fever, cough, and dyspnea. The urgent care physician made a provisional diagnosis of bronchiolitis with possible pneumonia. When the child first presented at urgent care, he had a respiratory rate of 60, heart rate of 134, SpO₂ of 95 percent, and tympanic temperature of 104.2°F. The patient just completed an

TABLE 44-4   Pediatric Glasgow Coma Scale

	> One Year	< One Year	
Eye opening	4 Spontaneous	Spontaneous	
	3 To verbal command	To shout	
	2 To pain	To pain	
	1 No response	No response	
	> One Year	**< One Year**	
Best motor response	6 Obeys		
	5 Localizes pain	Localizes pain	
	4 Flexion withdrawal	Flexion withdrawal	
	3 Flexion abnormal (decorticate rigidity)	Flexion abnormal (decorticate rigidity)	
	2 Extension (decerebrate rigidity)	Extension (decerebrate rigidity)	
	1 No response	No response	
	Five Years	**Two to Five Years**	**0–23 months**
Best verbal response	5 Oriented and converses	Appropriate words and phrases	Smiles, coos, cries appropriately
	4 Disoriented and converses	Inappropriate words	Cries
	3 Inappropriate words	Cries and/or screams	Inappropriate crying and/or screaming
	2 Incomprehensible sounds	Grunts	Grunts
	1 No response	No response	No response

TABLE 44-5   Normal Pediatric Vital Signs

Age Group	Respiratory Rate (per minute)	Heart Rate (per minute)	Systolic Blood Pressure in mmHg	Temperature in °F
Newborn	30 to 60	100 to 180	70 to 90	98 to 100
Infant	25 to 40	100 to 160	70 to 90	98 to 100
Toddler	24 to 30	80 to 130	72 to 100	98.6 to 99.6
Preschooler	22 to 34	80 to 120	78 to 104	98.6 to 99.6
School age	18 to 30	70 to 110	80 to 115	98.6
Adolescent	12 to 20	60 to 105	88 to 120	98.6

albuterol treatment as you arrived. As you attempt to get baseline vitals prior to transport, the nurse comes in with the intent of administering oral ibuprofen for the fever. The patient begins screaming and thrashing in response. You observe the pulse oximeter reading, which gives a heart rate of 200 beats per minute. While this rate would quickly lead to compromised cardiac output and heart failure in an adult, it is not immediate cause for alarm in the 22-month-old child, unless it does not return to the baseline at rest. Keep in mind that you must consider the fever, albuterol, and activity in interpreting the heart rate. Is the SpO$_2$ acceptable? Is his skin color good? Is there any sign of partial airway obstruction, such as stridor, when the child cries? Is he consolable once the noxious stimulus is removed?

Blood pressures are normally not obtained in the prehospital setting in patients under three years of age. Readings are difficult to obtain and interpret. Capillary refill time is a reliable indication of perfusion status in young children. The capillary refill time is normally less than 2 seconds. Consider compensated shock if the capillary refill time is between 2 and 4 seconds, and decompensated shock if the capillary refill time is greater than 4 seconds.

Physical Exam

Base the physical exam on the chief complaint, as well as the child's overall presentation and history. Use a lower threshold for performing a detailed head-to-toe exam in the patient who cannot give a specific chief complaint or in whom you cannot obtain an adequate history. Be alert to some specific indications of illness and injuries in pediatric patients, as follows:

- Unusual lethargy, flat affect, lack of interest in surroundings.

- Unusual patterns of bruising, injuries that are unusual in a child, or that have an unusual pattern or location. Once infants begin to pull themselves to a standing position and then walk, some bumps on the forehead, a split lip, and bruises to the shins are not unusual. However, significant bruising or cuts, burns, or welts; bruising to the torso, thighs, or buttocks; or injuries with the pattern of an object or handprint should raise your index of suspicion of child abuse or inadequate supervision.

- Rashes and petechiae, which could indicate an infection or allergic reaction.

- Does the child produce tears when he cries? Absence of tears can be a sign of dehydration.

- Drainage or bleeding from the ear, which can indicate an ear infection or trauma.

- Are there signs of a possible toxic ingestion, such as discoloration or burns around or in the mouth, or an odor indicative of toxic ingestion?

- If the patient is an infant, are the fontanels either bulging or depressed? Although the anterior fontanel may bulge slightly with crying in younger infants, it should otherwise be more or less flush with the surrounding skull. A bulging fontanel may indicate increased intracranial pressure, from either medical or traumatic causes. A depressed fontanel is an indication of dehydration.

- Check the abdomen for distention. Look for bruises, discoloration, and tenderness. Although it is normal for infants and toddlers to have a "pot belly," the abdomen should be soft and nontender.

- Note whether the child favors, protects, or refuses to use an extremity. Check the extremities for signs of injury, including swelling, deformity, bruises, tenderness, impaired motion, and crepitus.

Clinical-Reasoning Process

Throughout your assessment, be prepared to change your general impression and the patient's priority for transport. The epidemiology of illnesses and injuries is different in children than in adults, making some problems more probable and some less probable. Your hypotheses and process of differential diagnosis must reflect your knowledge of those differences. The pediatric population is a generally healthy population that can compensate well for many illnesses and injuries in the short term. But, their energy stores (liver and muscle glycogen) are limited and they can deteriorate with little warning. Maintain a high index of suspicion for shock and impending respiratory failure based on the mechanism of injury or nature of the illness, rather than waiting for obvious signs and symptoms of distress or shock. Whenever possible, transport pediatric patients to a facility with a pediatric emergency department and, if serious illness or injury is present, consider facilities with specialized pediatric trauma and critical care capabilities.

Treatment

Always use equipment and supplies appropriate for pediatric patients. Use basic life support measures for managing the patient's airway, breathing, and circulation. Remember that the large size of the pediatric occiput may require padding under the patient's shoulders to maintain correct alignment of airway structures. If basic measures, such as manual airway position and a basic airway adjunct with supplemental oxygen or bag-valve-mask ventilations are not effective, consider using a pediatric-size advanced airway, such as an LMA. Keep in mind the lower volume and higher rate of ventilations appropriate to pediatric patients (Table 44-6).

If spinal immobilization is required, place adequate padding under the patient's body to avoid hyperflexion of the cervical spine. Use cervical collars and splinting devices appropriate to the child's size.

If the patient is dehydrated, has lost blood volume, or requires intravenous medications, start an IV. Keep in mind that IVs are often best started en route to the hospital, rather than delaying on the scene. If IV access is

TABLE 44-6	Pediatric Bag-Valve-Mask Ventilation	
Age	**Ventilations per Minute**	**Approximate Volume per Breath**
Neonate	30	6 to 8 mL/kg (approximately 20 to 30 mL), use bag-valve-mask with no greater than 250 mL volume
Infant	20 to 25	6 to 8 mL/kg (approximately 20 to 80 mL), use a bag-valve-mask device with 250 to 500 mL volume
Child one to eight years	12 to 20	7 mL/kg (approximately 70 to 200 mL)

difficult, follow your protocols concerning intraosseous (IO) access. Administer medications as indicated according to the patient's condition and your protocols. Consult with medical direction as needed for orders. When administering any drug to a pediatric patient, obtain the most accurate information about his weight as possible to determine the correct dose.

Manage the patient's body temperature, keeping in mind that pediatric patients are particularly prone to hypothermia. Use blankets as necessary and adjust the temperature in the patient compartment of the ambulance. If the patient has a high fever and you have prolonged transport times, your protocols may allow you to administer ibuprofen or acetaminophen.

Reassessment

Keeping in mind that pediatric patients can deteriorate quickly, reassess them frequently. Compare subsequent findings to baseline findings to identify trends in the patient's condition. Monitor the effects of any treatments initiated.

Pediatric Medical Emergencies

You have been introduced to many of the medical emergencies that can affect children in previous chapters. However, some emergencies are more common in children, or have special considerations in their assessment and management when they occur in children.

Respiratory Emergencies

Common respiratory emergencies in children include asthma and infectious respiratory illnesses. Cystic fibrosis, which affects the lungs, first becomes apparent in childhood. Anaphylaxis can also be a cause of respiratory emergencies in the pediatric population. Some respiratory emergencies that are common in adults, such as COPD, are uncommon or rarely expected in the pediatric population. (See Chapter 20 for a review of respiratory emergencies.)

Assessment of Respiratory Emergencies

As with adults who have respiratory problems, pediatric patients can deteriorate rapidly from respiratory distress to respiratory failure to respiratory arrest unless you quickly identify the problem and take measures to restore ventilation and oxygenation. In addition to the signs and symptoms of respiratory distress noted in adults, pediatric patients may also display grunting with expiration in an attempt to create positive end expiratory pressure to keep the alveoli and bronchioles open (Table 44-7). You also may see nasal flaring, and retraction of the tissue above the clavicles and between the ribs may be prominent. Because pediatric patients

TABLE 44-7	Indications of Pediatric Respiratory Distress

- Abnormal sounds, such as stridor, crowing, wheezing, grunting, hoarseness, snoring, coughing, gagging, gasping
- Tachypnea
- Bradypnea
- Tachycardia
- Bradycardia
- Diminished air movement
- $SpO_2 < 95\%$
- Tripod position
- Suprasternal or intercostal retractions
- Use of neck muscles
- Nasal flaring
- Head bobbing
- Cyanosis or pallor
- Fatigue/lethargy
- Seesaw breathing
- Unresponsiveness or limp muscle tone

rely preferentially on the diaphragm, "belly breathing" may be prominent. The struggle to breathe can make the chest and abdomen appear to "seesaw" during breathing.

As hypoxia develops, pediatric patients can exhibit bradycardia, rather than tachycardia, as expected in adults. Be prepared for immediate intervention in the pediatric patient who appears lethargic, limp, or cyanotic.

When listening to pediatric breath sounds, be aware that sounds are transmitted easily throughout the chest and it can be difficult to localize sounds or recognize the absence of sounds. Often, it is difficult to distinguish between lower airway sounds and upper airway sounds in pediatric patients. What may seem to be crackles or rhonchi may actually be sounds produced by air moving past mucous in the upper airway.

Asthma

Pediatric asthma patients may exhibit a dry cough that indicates inflammation of the lower airways, either instead of or in addition to obvious wheezing.

For asthma patients who are awake and able to maintain their airways, begin oxygen administration as you complete assessment and obtain a history. Humidified oxygen, if available, is preferred. Base oxygen administration on the patient's level of distress, vital signs, and SpO_2. Follow your protocol in administering a beta$_2$ agonist or combined beta$_2$ agonist–anticholinergic by small-volume nebulizer. The typical dose for nebulized albuterol in pediatric patients is 0.15 to 0.3 mg/kg.

For patients in respiratory failure, immediately establish an airway, assist with ventilations, and provide supplemental oxygen. The patient must be transported without delay with an IV established en route. For status asthmaticus, contact the receiving facility for notification and consult with medical direction about the possibility of using subcutaneous (SC) or intramuscular (IM) epinephrine.

Intravenous fluids can be beneficial to patients with asthma to reverse or prevent dehydration. Follow protocols in the amount of fluids to administer, keeping in mind the overall smaller blood volume of pediatric patients. Use 60-gtt/mL tubing for small pediatric patients. If available, use a volumetric device, such as a Buretrol, for small children to prevent fluid overload. Frequently reassess the asthma patient, including mental status, airway, breathing, vital signs, breath sounds, level of distress, and SpO$_2$. Keep in mind the possibility of deterioration and be prepared to provide an airway and start ventilations by bag-valve-mask device.

Respiratory Infections

Both upper and lower respiratory tract infections are common in the pediatric population. (See Chapters 20 and 28.) A few that deserve special mention in this section include epiglottitis, croup, **pertussis**, bronchiolitis, and pneumonia.

Epiglottitis

Fortunately, widespread vaccination against *Haemophilis influenza B* (Hib) has all but eradicated epiglottitis in this age group. Keep in mind that a history of the patient's vaccinations is an important part of your differential diagnosis process. In particular, ask about the Hib vaccine. In the unvaccinated patient, suspect epiglottitis in the patient who is acutely ill with a febrile illness and dysphagia (difficulty swallowing) to the point of avoiding swallowing (which is why drooling occurs). The patient may have stridorous respirations, present in the tripod position, and may be drooling.

If epiglottitis is suspected, do not place anything in the mouth and do not agitate the patient. Transport him without delay in a position of comfort, which will usually be sitting up. Request advanced life support if available, if transport time is more than a few minutes.

Croup

Laryngotracheobronchitis, or croup, is a viral infection of the lower airway that often presents with mild signs and symptoms during the day, but worsens at night. Croup causes inflammation of the airways, including the vocal cords and subglottic area. The illness begins with upper respiratory symptoms, such as a sore throat, runny nose, and low-grade fever. After a day or two, the patient develops characteristic inspiratory stridor, hoarseness, and a "seal bark" cough, which generally are worse at night. The disease is mild in most cases, but can lead to respiratory distress and airway obstruction in severe cases. In milder cases, the inspiratory stridor occurs during activity, while in moderate to severe cases it also occurs at rest. Expiratory stridor occurs in more serious cases. Assess for airway obstruction, increased respiratory effort, suprasternal retractions,

tripoding, accessory muscle use, fatigue, altered mental status, and cyanosis.

For mild to moderate cases, do not agitate the patient with unnecessary procedures because crying increases oxygen demand and may worsen edema. For severe cases, treat hypoxia and hypoventilation. Humidified oxygen is preferred to prevent drying, irritation, and further swelling of the airway. Although rarely available in the prehospital setting, nebulized racemic epinephrine (a form of epinephrine in which its chemical structure is a mirror image of the normal epinephrine structure) is used to treat severe cases. However, there is debate over whether racemic epinephrine is superior to other beta$_2$ agonists, such as albuterol or levalbuterol. Intubation can be required in severe cases. If intubation is indicated and within your scope of practice, it should be performed by the provider who has the best intubation skills, because unnecessary manipulation of the airway can worsen edema. An endotracheal tube 0.5 to 1 mm smaller than normal should be used.

Although exposure to cool mist or steam was previously recommended for croup, there is no evidence that either treatment is effective (Muñiz, Molodow, & Defendi, 2010).

Pertussis

Pertussis is a serious, sometimes fatal disease that causes coughing fits that may last 10 or more weeks. Patients gasp for air following coughing fits with a characteristic "whooping" sound (thus, the term whooping cough). Immunization with the DTaP vaccine is not recommended until two months of age, and requires a series of five vaccinations to confer immunity. Pertussis is increasing particularly among infants and school-age children. Be sure to ask whether the patient has received the DTaP vaccine. Prehospital management is aimed at maintaining adequate ventilation and oxygenation.

Bronchiolitis

Bronchiolitis is an acute viral lower airway disease that occurs most commonly in children between two months and two years of age. The virus (usually respiratory syncytial virus, or RSV) causes cell death and increased mucus secretion in the lower airways, along with lower airway edema. The combination of edema, mucus, and sloughing of the dead cells creates lower airway obstruction. Airway constriction results in expiratory wheezing, tachypnea, and signs of respiratory distress. Respirations may be in the range of 50 to 60 breaths per minute, or higher. The early signs and symptoms present as an upper respiratory infection, which may progress within one to two days to include fever, cough, wheezing, and respiratory distress. Lung sounds include expiratory wheezing and inspiratory crackles. Most cases occur between November and April, and reinfection is possible (Louden, 2010). **Respiratory syncytial virus (RSV)** is the most common cause, but other viruses have been implicated as well. Differentiating between bronchiolitis and pneumonia can be difficult in the prehospital setting.

Prehospital treatment includes keeping the patient in an upright position, giving oxygen to maintain an SpO$_2$ greater than 95 percent, and, often, a nebulized beta$_2$ agonist. If available, humidified oxygen is preferred. Assess the patient for signs of significant dehydration and consider the need for fluid replacement if dehydration is severe and transport time is prolonged.

Pneumonia

Except in newborns, cough and fever are common early signs of pediatric pneumonia. Newborns may exhibit neither cough nor fever, despite being very ill with pneumonia. Other signs and symptoms include tachypnea, respiratory distress, lethargy, irritability, and vomiting. Lung sounds can include crackles, but they are not always heard. Often, what may seem to be crackles are actually sounds transmitted from the presence of secretions in the upper airway (Neuman, 2010). Localized wheezing and decreased breath sounds also may be present. The prehospital management of suspected pneumonia includes supplemental oxygen to maintain an SpO$_2$ of 95 percent or higher. Assist ventilations if respiratory failure or arrest is present. CPAP, if permitted in your pediatric protocols, may be beneficial for patients in severe respiratory distress.

Upper Respiratory Infections

Upper respiratory infections with rhinorrhea and cough are common in children. Those infections are often accompanied by low-grade fever and can result in otitis media. In infants, nasal secretions can significantly obstruct breathing. Use a bulb syringe, if necessary, to clear the nares.

Anaphylaxis

Anaphylaxis may present as a respiratory emergency with signs of upper or lower airway obstruction, including dyspnea, stridor, wheezing, and other signs of respiratory distress. Anaphylaxis also may be accompanied by vasodilation and loss of intravascular volume, leading to hypoperfusion. (See Chapter 27.) Be sure to include questions about allergies and possible exposure to allergens associated with anaphylaxis, such as antibiotics, nuts, and bee stings. Children with a history of anaphylaxis may have been prescribed an epinephrine autoinjector. Determine if the child has an epinephrine autoinjector and whether it has been used.

To treat hypoperfusion, stridor, or wheezing that has not responded to inhaled beta$_2$ agonists, administer subcutaneous or intramuscular epinephrine 1:1,000 at a dosage of 0.01 mg/kg, according to your protocol or online medical direction.

Cystic Fibrosis

In **cystic fibrosis (CF)** the presence of two defective genes, one inherited from each parent, results in the production of extremely viscous mucus. In the respiratory tract, the thick secretions can obstruct the airways and lead to life-threatening infection. Until recent years, patients with CF died as children or very early in adulthood.

Treat the patient for his signs and symptoms. Administering oxygen without humidification may aggravate the tenacious mucus in the lungs, making it harder to expectorate (clear from the lungs by coughing). However, do not withhold oxygen if the patient has an SpO$_2$ of less than 95 percent. IV fluids may assist in hydrating the mucus. Consult with medical direction for the type of fluid and rate of administration. CPAP may be useful for patients with impending respiratory failure. Administer a nebulized bronchodilator for wheezing, if allowed by medical direction.

Pediatric Cardiovascular Disorders

Because coronary artery disease progresses over many years, children are not at high risk for acute coronary syndrome (ACS). When cardiac arrest occurs, it is usually due to hypoxia. However, adolescents have been known to suffer cardiac arrest during strenuous activity. Many times, the patient is a well-conditioned athlete with no known medical problems. The underlying problem is sometimes traced to a cardiac conduction abnormality or left ventricular hypertrophy. Many high schools and colleges have public access defibrillation programs in place, particularly in areas where sports are played, increasing the potential for rapid defibrillation in those cases.

Cardiac arrest also may occur from commotio cordis in the school-age and adolescent age groups. Commotio cordis occurs when there is a direct blow to the chest at a vulnerable point in the cardiac cycle, leading to cardiac arrest. Commotio cordis may occur in baseball, martial arts, football, soccer, and other sports in which the patient is vulnerable to a blow to the chest.

In cases involving cardiac arrest in adolescent patients, manage the situation as you would for an adult patient. Focus on effective, early chest compressions with minimal interruption and rapid defibrillation. (See Chapter 17.)

Most pediatric cardiac problems are due to congenital abnormalities, which are often diagnosed and surgically corrected shortly after birth or in early childhood. A longitudinal scar over the sternum is an indication of prior heart surgery and should prompt specific questions about heart problems if the patient or parents have not already mentioned it. Uncorrected congenital heart defects can lead to poor perfusion and hypoxia. Treat the patient for shock, paying particular attention to correcting hypoxia and improving circulation.

Sudden Infant Death Syndrome

Sudden infant death syndrome (SIDS) is the sudden death of an infant under one year of age that cannot be explained despite a thorough case investigation and autopsy. Thus, SIDS is a diagnosis of exclusion. Some proposed mechanisms of SIDS include long QT syndrome, an abnormality of the cardiac cycle, apnea from a variety of possible causes, poor autonomic nervous system regulation, and other physiological and developmental hypotheses. There are approximately 2,000 SIDS deaths per year, but the rate has been decreasing. The majority of SIDS deaths occur in infants younger than five months of age, with most of those occurring between two and four months of age. The typical history of SIDS is that of a healthy infant who was put to bed or put down for a nap and is later found dead.

An **apparent life-threatening event (ALTE)** occurs when there is a combination of apnea, color change (cyanotic or pale), limpness, and choking or gagging. Infants with ALTE are at increased risk of SIDS, but it is not known whether ALTEs are witnessed, interrupted SIDS, or a different type of event (Burnett & Adler, 2011). Often, the infant with a described ALTE will have no signs and symptoms of distress once EMS arrives. However, *you must transport all infants with a reported ALTE to the emergency department for evaluation.*

In the absence of signs of presumptive death, such as livor mortis or rigor mortis, begin CPR in the suspected SIDS patient and transport the patient with continuing resuscitative efforts.

There is often concern about the exact nature of death when there is a sudden, unexpected death of an infant. All cases of sudden, unexpected death fall under the jurisdiction of the medical examiner (or coroner, depending on the state). If the child is not a candidate for resuscitation, treat the scene as a potential crime scene. However, keep in mind that it is only a *potential* crime scene. It is devastating for the parents of a SIDS infant to be treated as suspects in their child's death. Contact law enforcement if they are not already on the scene. Do not disturb the body or move anything, and document observations about the scene (Table 44-8).

Do not treat the parents as if they are at fault in the patient's death. Be careful how you form your questions to avoid implying blame. Do not misinterpret normal signs of death, such livor mortis or frothy, potentially pink-tinged discharge from the mouth or nose, as signs of abuse (Burnett & Adler, 2011).

In cases of pediatric resuscitation, allow parents to be in attendance if possible. The parents have a strong need to be with their child and to be kept informed about what is going on. In the event that the patient does not survive, the parents are helped to realize that everything that could be done for the child was done. In all cases, whether resuscitation is attempted or not, the parents require your emotional support.

TABLE 44-8	Documenting the Scene in Suspected Sudden Infant Death Syndrome

- How was the child found on your arrival?
- Where was the child when the parents found him? What kind of surface was the child on when found?
- Were there any pillows, loose bedding, stuffed animals, or other objects where the child was found that could have posed an asphyxiation hazard?
- What clothing was the child wearing? Could it have posed an asphyxiation hazard?
- If the child was in a crib, were there any signs of defect, such as an opening in which the child could have become wedged?
- What was the general condition of the residence?
- Who was present at the scene, and what were their demeanors?
- Was rigor mortis or livor mortis present?
- What was the skin temperature of the patient?
- Were there any apparent injuries or marks?

Responding to a patient with SIDS can be particularly traumatic for health care providers. Recognize signs of acute stress reaction in yourself and others who responded and be prepared to seek assistance, if necessary. Excessive acute stress can impair the ability to focus and perform your job. Take a deep breath and refocus your energies on addressing the patient's and parents' needs, recognizing that you can and should take time to examine your feelings about the situation when the call is over.

Remember: One of the most important things you can do to combat stress is to be prepared. Develop and maintain solid knowledge and skills in handling pediatric emergencies. Draw on the stress management techniques discussed in Chapter 3. If signs of cumulative stress or post-traumatic stress disorder develop, seek assistance from a mental health professional.

Infectious Diseases

Although vaccinations have significantly reduced the incidence of childhood infectious illnesses—such as measles, chickenpox, and mumps—they do still sometimes occur. Many of those illnesses present with general malaise, fever, and often, a rash. Remember to ask about vaccinations in the history.

Meningitis can be viral or bacterial and is an inflammation and swelling of the meninges that surround the central nervous system. Viral meningitis tends to be less severe, while bacterial meningitis can be fatal. The incidence of childhood meningitis has decreased significantly since the Hib vaccine became available.

The meningococcal bacterium commonly resides in the nasal passages, but rarely causes disease. Under certain circumstances, usually in the winter months, the bacteria gains access to the cerebral spinal fluid, causing meningitis. Viral meningitis occurs more often during the summer and fall. The early signs of viral and bacterial meningitis are similar, but bacterial meningitis can become much more severe. Signs and symptoms include fever, headache, photophobia, and stiff neck. In bacterial meningitis, seizures and altered mental status can occur.

Meningococcal bacteria can enter the blood (meningococcemia), causing damage to blood vessels with bleeding into the organs and skin (purpura). Other signs or symptoms include fever and chills, vomiting, diarrhea, joint, muscle, abdominal or chest pain, tachypnea, and cold hands and feet (Centers for Disease Control, 2010). Meningococcemia can be fatal, or result in amputations and the need for skin grafts.

Follow up on the diagnosis of patients with suspected bacterial meningitis so that you can receive appropriate prophylactic care if you were exposed to a patient with the disease.

Neurologic Disorders

Altered mental status (AMS) in children has many causes, as it does in adults. The mnemonic AEIOU-TIPS is useful in remembering the potential causes of AMS (Table 44-9). The first priority in any patient with AMS is ensuring adequate airway, ventilation, oxygenation, and circulation. However, you also must search for reversible causes, including possible hypoglycemia, hypoxia, and narcotic overdose.

Children may have seizures for a variety of reasons. Causes include epilepsy, toxins, drugs, metabolic disturbances (check for hypoglycemia), trauma, intracerebral hemorrhage, and tumors; but a common cause is fever. As in adults, seizures may be generalized, including tonic–clonic and absence or partial seizures. In general, the assessment and treatment are the same as in adult

TABLE 44-9	**AEIOU-TIPS Mnemonic for Altered Mental Status**

A – Alcohol, anoxia

E – Environment, epilepsy

I – Insulin (diabetes and other endocrine disorders)

O – Overdose

U – Uremia (renal failure)

T – Trauma (shock, traumatic brain injury)

I – Infection

P – Psychosis, poisoning

S – Stroke (for example, pediatric patients may have intracranial hemorrhage from a ruptured arteriovenous malformation)

patients. However, be particularly alert to the possibilities of hypoglycemia and fever.

Febrile seizures tend to be related to the rate at which the fever increases and are typically short in duration with a limited postictal state. Nonetheless, a febrile seizure (or any seizure) can be terrifying for the parents or caregiver. Do not bundle a febrile child in blankets, because that will prevent heat from dissipating and increase the body temperature. The child should be dressed lightly, but do not allow the child to become chilled, which would increase shivering. The increased muscle activity of shivering will increase the body temperature.

Follow your protocols or consult with medical direction concerning administration of acetaminophen or ibuprofen to febrile pediatric patients. Key information the physician will need includes a brief report on the patient's presentation and history, the child's age, temperature, weight, allergies, and when the last time was that acetaminophen or ibuprofen was administered and how much was given.

Hydrocephalus occurs when there is an imbalance between formation and outflow or absorption of cerebrospinal fluid (CSF), resulting in an accumulation of excess CSF within the ventricles of the brain. Hydrocephalus is often evident in the neonatal period, but presentation can be delayed until the child is older. In infants, the presentation includes a large head with bulging fontanels and separation of the cranial sutures. The eyes may appear to bulge with increased visibility of the superior part of the globe, resulting in "sunset eyes." Increased intracranial pressure (ICP) can lead to vomiting and apnea. Once the fontanels are closed, increased ICP can lead to headaches, changes in vision, cognitive difficulties, decreased responsiveness, and respiratory arrest.

Hydrocephalus is often treated with a ventriculostomy shunt that drains excess CSF. (See Chapter 46.) The child's caregiver is often very knowledgeable about the shunt. Sometimes, the shunt can become displaced, resulting in an increase in intracranial pressure. Signs and symptoms can include headache, neurologic complaints, decreased responsiveness, and seizures. Prehospital treatment is aimed at supporting the airway, ventilation, oxygenation, and circulation.

Children with ventriculostomy shunts may have other medical problems. Do not let the history of hydrocephalus and ventriculostomy divert you from a full assessment and history and consideration of other differential diagnoses, such as hypoglycemia, infection, and trauma.

Diabetes

Diabetes in children is usually insulin-dependent diabetes mellitus (IDDM), but non–insulin-dependent diabetes can occur also and its incidence in pediatrics is increasing due to high rates of childhood obesity in the United States. Increased risk of death from diabetes tends to occur in the toddler and preschool ages and in adolescence. Death may occur due to complications of undiagnosed diabetes resulting in diabetic ketoacidosis (DKA), cerebral edema from untreated or poorly treated diabetes, or hypoglycemia. Be particularly alert to signs of untreated diabetes, because diagnosis may not yet have been made and the history of diabetes may not be known by the patient or parents.

Maintain a high index of suspicion for diabetic emergencies in patients presenting with altered mental status, with or without a known history of diabetes, and obtain a blood glucose level in all patients with altered mental status. Other signs and symptoms include severe, persistent diaper rash from yeast organisms, lethargy or malaise, weight loss, thirst, and frequent urination.

Children with hyperglycemia may be irritable and complain of weakness, and may complain of abdominal pain. Look for severe dehydration, the presence of a ketone odor, Kussmaul's respirations, vomiting, and decreased level of responsiveness. The child also may have an infection, particularly a urinary tract or respiratory infection.

Hypoglycemia generally occurs in patients being treated for diabetes and usually occurs suddenly with irritability; behavioral changes; pale, cool skin; seizures; and decreased level of responsiveness. Hypoglycemia can occur in nondiabetic pediatric patients whose oral intake has been severely decreased or in whom the metabolic needs are significantly increased (respiratory distress, trauma, burns) when glycogen stores are not adequate to meet the increased needs. Other causes of pediatric hypoglycemia include poisoning and metabolic diseases. Prolonged hypoglycemia has a significant impact on subsequent cognitive and neurologic development and you must treat this without delay.

When hypoglycemia is confirmed in the pediatric patient, administer 25 percent dextrose 1 mL/kg (0.25 g/kg). Use 10 percent dextrose in neonates.

Gastrointestinal Disorders

Gastroenteritis, with accompanying vomiting and diarrhea are common in the pediatric age group, and can lead to dehydration. Signs of dehydration include the following:

- Poor skin turgor (tenting)
- No or few wet diapers or infrequent urination
- No tears when crying
- Sunken-appearing eyes
- Dry mucous membranes
- Sunken anterior fontanel
- Lethargy
- Tachycardia
- Tachypnea
- Pale, cool skin

Constipation is also common among pediatric patients. Vomiting and diarrhea are often due to viruses and foodborne illness, but can occur in other illnesses as well, such as

IN THE FIELD

If a pediatric patient is fearful and uncooperative with an abdominal exam, instruct the parent how to palpate the abdominal quadrants while you watch for the child's reaction.

with urinary tract infections and febrile illnesses. Abdominal pain can be related to gastroenteritis, or may be due to appendicitis. Other causes of abdominal pain to consider are urinary tract infection and DKA. Hernias may occur in the pediatric age group. Bowel obstruction is unusual, but intussusception, volvulus, and pyloric stenosis can occur in newborns and infants. (See Chapter 24.) Keep in mind that swallowed foreign bodies are common in the pediatric age group, and the history of ingestion may be known or unknown.

Eye, Ear, Nose, and Throat Disorders

Children are prone to a variety of eye, ear, nose, and throat disorders. Conjunctivitis is particularly common in that age group, as are styes and chalazia. Orbital and periorbital cellulitis may occur as a complication of sinus infection or other infection of the eye and facial tissues and constitute medical emergencies. Foreign bodies in the eye also are common in pediatric patients. Otitis externa and otitis media are common in pediatric patients, as are foreign bodies in the ear. Epistaxis is common in pediatric patients, as well, and is usually from an anterior site. Foreign bodies in the nose also may occur in pediatric patients. Pharyngitis, often due to viral or bacterial infection is common, too. In general, eye, ear, nose, and throat disorders in the pediatric population are treated in the prehospital setting in the same way they are in the adult population. (See Chapter 30).

Behavioral Emergencies

School-age children and adolescents can suffer from behavioral emergencies and psychological disorders including depression and other mood disorders, substance abuse and addiction, anxiety disorders, eating disorders, and impulse control disorders. The risk of suicide increases in the adolescent years, but can affect younger, school-age children, as well. (See Chapter 31.) Unfortunately, various forms of bullying and harassment, including cyber bullying, have been implicated in child and adolescent suicides.

Do not overlook the possibility of behavioral emergencies and psychological disorders in pediatric patients. Do not forget: Your safety can be jeopardized by a child or adolescent with a behavioral emergency, just as it can be by an adult patient.

Toxicologic Emergencies

Toxicologic emergencies in pediatric patients can arise from intentional and unintentional exposures. Factors in unintentional pediatric poisonings include curiosity, an underdeveloped sense of taste, inability to recognize the consequences of behavior, poor supervision, and poor childproofing. Toxicologic emergencies also may occur from drug and alcohol abuse and suicide attempts.

Particular signs and symptoms depend on the substance involved. (See Chapter 32.) Keep in mind that poisoning and overdose patients can deteriorate quickly. A patient who is initially awake and oriented can progress quickly to unresponsiveness and respiratory depression or respiratory arrest. Maintain constant awareness of the patient's mental status, airway, and breathing.

If activated charcoal is included in your protocol, do not give pediatric patients more than one dose of products that contain sorbitol. Sorbitol osmotically attracts water into the lumen of the bowel, causing diarrhea, which may result in dehydration and electrolyte imbalance. The pediatric dosage of activated charcoal is 1 gram/kg with a minimum of 30 grams. Follow your protocols or the advice of poison control or online medical direction for the administration of activated charcoal.

Shock and Trauma in Pediatric Patients

Traumatic injury is the leading cause of death in children over one year of age. Trauma is also a significant cause of morbidity and disability in that age group. The vast majority of those deaths are preventable through a combination of injury prevention and rapid, appropriate management when injury occurs.

Pediatric Mechanisms of Injury

The most common mechanisms of injury in pediatric patients are due to blunt, rather than penetrating forces. Blunt mechanisms of injury in pediatric patients include motor vehicle collisions, being struck by a vehicle, and falls. Blunt trauma is often associated with multisystem trauma. The anatomic and physiologic differences in children also should increase your index of suspicion for multisystem trauma. The anatomy and physiology of pediatric patients is such that life-threatening traumatic brain injury and internal organ injury can occur with few external signs of injury, reinforcing the importance of analyzing the mechanism of injury carefully (Table 44-10).

In motor vehicle collisions, maintain a high index of suspicion for multiple injuries, including head and neck injuries in unrestrained pediatric occupants. Restrained pediatric occupants can suffer serious injury from airbag deployment and seatbelts, particularly when seatbelts are improperly placed. With restrained pediatric vehicle occupants, suspect spinal fractures (thoracic, in particular) and abdominal and chest injuries. Airbag deployment can result in head, chest, and upper extremity injuries.

The injuries of a child struck by a vehicle depend on the speed of the vehicle and the patient's height in relation to the vehicle. With older, taller, children low-speed impact tends to produce lower extremity injuries. With smaller children, the head and torso receive the impact of

IN THE FIELD

The American Academy of Pediatrics recommends that children should be secured in rear-facing car seats until age two years or until they exceed the height and weight recommendations for the car seat being used (35 to 45 pounds for most car seats). Children should use a belt-positioning booster seat until they are 4 feet 9 inches tall, which is usually between 8 and 12 years of age. The center of the rear seat is the safest place in a vehicle for a child. Children under 13 years of age should not ride in the front seat. Never assume that a car seat offered maximum protection for a child, because studies have indicated that car seats are often installed incorrectly.

PERSONAL PERSPECTIVE

Advanced EMT Lance Ringer: I was working in the emergency department on a Friday evening when we received a call from an ambulance service transporting a two-year-old child who had fallen head first from a set of bleachers at a raceway onto the gravel parking lot 20 feet below. One of the nurses and I went to the ambulance bay to assist with unloading the patient. The patient was unresponsive and had abnormal breathing. I noticed that the EMS crew had not taken time to perform spinal immobilization or even to secure the patient to the stretcher, and the position of the patient's airway interfered with ventilation. The EMT ventilating the patient was ventilating at a depth appropriate to an adult, not a two-year-old child, and the patient's stomach was terribly distended, probably with air, further impairing ventilation. I felt bad that the EMTs were so rattled by the call. It was a call that no one wants to go on and that would be upsetting to anyone. It was tragic. But what was even more tragic was that the patient's condition was further compromised by errors in care because the EMTs panicked. It is always better to take 2 seconds to take a deep breath and focus your thoughts and actions than to provide inadequate care for, in this case, 35 minutes.

TABLE 44-10 National Trauma Triage Protocol

Vital Signs and Level of Responsiveness
- Glasgow Coma Scale < 14 or
- Systolic blood pressure < 90 mmHg or
- Respiratory rate < 10 or > 20 breaths per minute (< 20 in infant < one year old)

Anatomy of Injury
- All penetrating injuries to head, neck, torso, and extremities proximal to elbow and knee
- Flail chest
- Two or more proximal long-bone fractures
- Crushed, degloved, or mangled extremity
- Amputation proximal to wrist or ankle
- Pelvic fracture
- Open or depressed skull fracture
- Paralysis

Mechanism of Injury and Evidence of High-Energy Impact
- Falls
  - Adults > 20 ft (1 story = 10 ft)
  - Children >10 ft or two to three times patient's height
- High-risk auto crash
  - Intrusion > 12 in. occupant site; > 18 in. any site
  - Ejection (partial or complete) from automobile
  - Death in same passenger compartment
  - Vehicle telemetry data consistent with high risk of injury
- Auto v. pedestrian/bicyclist thrown, run over, or with > 20 mph impact
- Motorcycle crash > 20 mph

Special Patient or System Considerations
- Age
  - Risk of injury death increases after age 55 years
  - Children should be preferentially triaged to pediatric-capable trauma centers
- Anticoagulation and bleeding disorders
- Burns
  - Without other trauma: Triage to burn facility
  - With trauma mechanism: Triage to trauma center
- Time-sensitive extremity injury
- End-stage renal disease requiring dialysis
- Pregnancy > 20 weeks
- EMS provider judgment

Data from Centers for Disease Control. (2006). Field triage decision scheme. Retrieved August 5, 2011, from http://www.cdc.gov/fieldtriage/

the vehicle, resulting in head and internal injuries. With high-speed impact, both older and younger children are prone to head and neck injuries, as well as multiple internal organ injuries.

The active lifestyle of many pediatric patients makes sports and recreational injuries likely. The injury patterns vary according to the type of sport and impact and the appropriateness of protective equipment.

Assessment and Management of Pediatric Trauma

The three most common causes of pediatric trauma death in the immediate period following injury are hypoxia, massive hemorrhage, and traumatic brain injury (McSwain, Salomone, & Pons, 2011). Thus, the most immediate needs in pediatric trauma resuscitation are establishing and maintaining an airway, ensuring adequate ventilation and oxygenation, and controlling bleeding and treating shock. Although you cannot alter a primary brain injury, your attention to the patient's airway, ventilation, oxygenation, and circulation can limit secondary brain injury from hypoxia and hypoperfusion.

In the pediatric patient with suspected cervical-spine trauma, maintain the head in a neutral position, placing a small folded towel or blanket under the shoulders, if necessary, based on the patient's size. In the absence of suspected cervical-spine trauma, slightly elevate the chin and face to maintain a "sniffing position." If the child does not have a gag reflex, insert an oropharyngeal airway to help maintain the airway. If the oropharyngeal airway is inadequate to maintain the airway, use an appropriately sized supraglottic airway device. Endotracheal intubation is difficult in children and you should not attempt it in the prehospital setting unless it is otherwise not possible to establish and maintain an adequate means of ventilation. Prehospital endotracheal intubation in pediatric patients has been associated with worse outcomes.

Traumatic brain injury, shock, and chest trauma can result in the need for assisted ventilations. If bag-valve-mask ventilations are required, use supplemental oxygen and adjust the rate and depth according to the patient's size. Hyperventilation is a common mistake in all trauma patients and can worsen cerebral edema and impair cardiac output. In spontaneously breathing patients, administer oxygen if needed to maintain a SpO_2 of 95 percent or higher.

Control external hemorrhage and maintain a high index of suspicion for internal bleeding, according to the mechanism of injury. Treat the patient for shock with a lower threshold than for adult patients, because early signs are subtle and easily missed. Keep the patient warm. Pediatric patients are at increased risk of hypothermia and hypothermia significantly worsens patient outcomes by increasing metabolic needs in the context of tissue hypoxia and impairing blood clotting mechanisms.

Frequently monitor the pediatric trauma patient's mental status, vital signs, and other signs of perfusion to detect emerging shock. Bradycardia and tachycardia are both causes of concern. Be concerned if the heart is above or below the following guidelines for the patient's age:

- Newborns greater than 160 or less than 100 beats per minute
- Infants greater than 150 or less than 80 beats per minute
- Toddlers greater than 140 or less than 60 beats per minute
- Preschool age greater than 130 or less than 60 beats per minute
- School age greater than 120 or less than 60 beats per minute
- Adolescent greater than 100 or less than 60 beats per minute

Capillary refill is a reliable sign of perfusion in pediatric patients, as follows:

- Less than 2 seconds: normal
- 2 to 4 seconds: compensated shock
- Greater than 4 seconds: decompensated shock

If shock is suspected, infuse IV or IO fluids (normal saline or lactated Ringer's solution) in a bolus of 20 mL/kg. If the patient does not improve after a single bolus, give a second 20-mL/kg bolus. If the patient does not improve, or improves but then deteriorates, give a third 20-mL/kg bolus. A patient who requires two or three fluid boluses is unstable and you should consider this patient critical.

Considerations in Spinal Immobilization

There are a few special considerations in spinal immobilization in pediatric patients. In the past, it was recommended that trauma patients presenting in an infant car seat be immobilized in the seat. However, once a car seat has been involved in a vehicle collision, it is no longer considered safe for use. Instead, the car seat can be used to assist in manual stabilization of the spine during extrication because the seat and child are removed from the vehicle as a unit. Then tilt the seat as manual stabilization of the cervical spine is maintained and move the patient along the longitudinal axis of

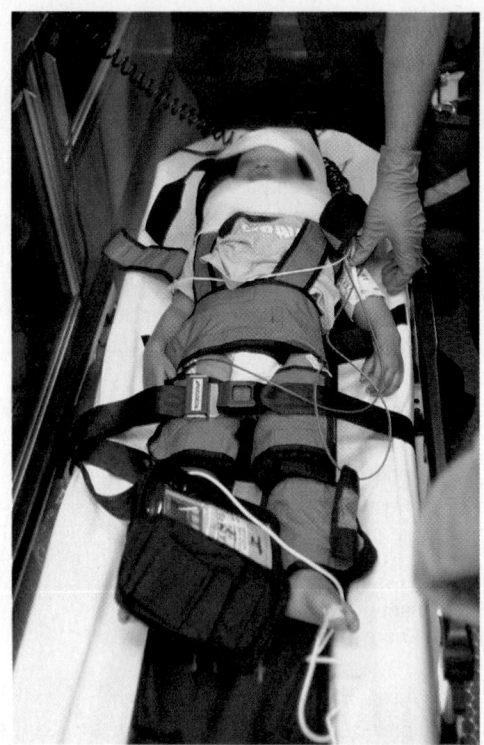

FIGURE 44-7

Spinal immobilization of a pediatric patient using a commercial restraint device. (© Mark C. Ide)

the body onto a spinal immobilization device. Padding may be required under the shoulders to properly align the cervical spine during immobilization. The child's smaller size increases the need for padding along the sides of the body to prevent him from sliding from side to side on the backboard. A special safety harness is ideal for immobilizing a pediatric patient to a long backboard (Figure 44-7). If such a device is not available, you must use additional backboard straps to secure the patient.

Burns

Children have thin skin that can be burned at a much lower temperature and shorter duration of exposure to heat than in an adult. Scald burns may occur accidentally, particularly if the hot water heater in the home is on a setting that is too high. Many accidental childhood burns can be prevented through safety measures such as making sure that electrical cords from hot appliances do not dangle within the child's reach, turning pot handles away from the edge of the stove to keep them out of reach, keeping children at a safe distance when cooking, and keeping matches, lighters, candles, and other sources of heat and flame out of children's reach.

There are two special considerations in caring for the pediatric burn patient. First, it is estimated that one in five burns in children is a result of child abuse or child neglect. Particular burn patterns should increase your suspicion, as should a history that is inconsistent with the nature of the

Note: Each arm totals 9 percent (front of arm 4½ percent, back of arm 4½ percent)

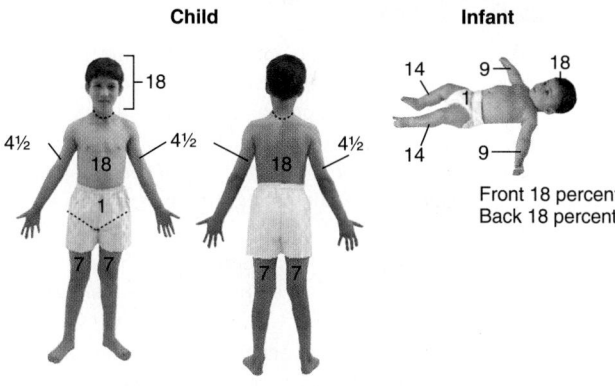

FIGURE 44-8

The Rule of Nines used to calculate the percent of body surface involved in burns is altered in infants and children to account for their proportionately larger heads.

injury (see "Child Abuse and Neglect"). For instance, "stocking foot" burns are burns of the feet and lower legs that have a socklike appearance with a clear line of demarcation (no splash burns) from a child having his feet dipped into or held in hot water. Second, the Rule of Nines is altered for pediatric patients to account for the greater proportion of body surface area comprised by the head (Figure 44-8).

Drowning

Drowning is primary respiratory impairment resulting from submersion in a liquid medium (Moore Shepherd & Shoff, 2010), and is largely preventable. About 1,500 children die from drowning each year in the United States. The incidence of drowning is higher in toddlers, who are mobile and curious, but often unable to swim; and in adolescent males. Most toddler drownings occur in bathtubs and swimming pools when the child is left unattended, even momentarily. Risk-taking behavior and alcohol are implicated in the adolescent male group.

Drowning is a form of asphyxia resulting in hypoxia and acidosis. Often, the asphyxia begins with an involuntary laryngospasm as water begins to enter the airway. As hypoxia progresses, laryngospasm may relax and water can enter the lungs if the patient attempts to breathe at that point. Continued hypoxia results in cardiac arrest. Ingestion of large amounts of freshwater from reflex swallowing can result in electrolyte imbalances.

In young children who are suddenly immersed in cold water, the mammalian diving reflex can result in reflex apnea, bradycardia, and shunting of peripheral circulation to the vital organs. The mammalian diving reflex decreases oxygen demand in the tissues and can confer a survival advantage. Otherwise, hypothermia is a complication of many drownings.

Most children who survive drowning are rescued within 2 minutes of submersion, while most who do not survive have been submerged 10 minutes or longer. Death may occur immediately due to asphyxia and cardiac arrest, or may occur in the hospital due to acute respiratory distress syndrome (ARDS) or multiple organ dysfunction syndrome (MODS). Factors affecting survival also include water temperature, water contamination, and associated injuries (for example, injuries involved in boating and personal watercraft collisions).

If the patient is still in the water, perform a rescue only if it is safe to do so. Otherwise, await trained water rescue personnel. Remove the patient from the water as quickly as possible. Consider rescue breaths with the patient in the water if removal from the water is delayed (for example, the patient is some distance from the shore of a water of body). Otherwise, remove the patient from the water immediately and, if he is unresponsive and does not have normal breathing, begin chest compressions according to the CPR guidelines for the patient's age. (See Chapter 17.) In the absence of a known history of diving head first into shallow water or trauma associated with watercraft collision, cervical-spine injury is unusual in drowning. In the absence of those mechanisms, do not delay removal from the water for spinal immobilization, because this delays CPR. Chest compressions will be ineffective as long as the patient is in the water. Even when cervical-spine injury is a possibility, you must weigh the need for spinal immobilization against the delay it will cause in beginning CPR.

Transport all patients who have been submerged in water with subsequent respiratory impairment to the hospital emergency department for evaluation, even if they are asymptomatic on EMS arrival.

For patients in cardiac arrest, begin chest compressions immediately, but consider airway management and ventilation early, because the primary problem is asphyxia and hypoxia. In patients with a pulse—but who have respiratory distress, respiratory, failure, or respiratory arrest—prehospital management is directed at establishing and maintaining an airway, assisting ventilation, and ensuring adequate oxygenation.

Traditionally, part of the management of drowning has been to prevent worsening of hypothermia. However, with ongoing research into potential neuroprotective benefits of therapeutic hypothermia following cardiac arrest, that practice may be re-evaluated. Keep up to date on best practices through continuing education and journal articles. Follow your protocols regarding measures to treat hypothermia in drowning patients.

Child Abuse and Neglect

Child abuse is an improper, intentional, or excessive action that causes injury or harm to a child. Child neglect is the inadequate provision of attention or respect to a person entitled to it. Unfortunately, both are common. Be aware that, in many states, you are considered a mandatory reporter of suspected child abuse or neglect. In any case, even if you are not legally obligated to report, you are ethically obligated to report your suspicions. The exact mechanism of reporting depends on your protocols and the laws in your jurisdiction. (See Chapter 4.) There are several indications of possible abuse or neglect (Figure 44-9).

If abuse or neglect is suspected, your first priorities are scene safety and providing medical treatment for the child. Notify law enforcement if you believe that you, the child, or anyone else at the scene is in danger. Do not confront the suspected abuser. Carefully document, without drawing conclusions, all pertinent information (Table 44-11).

TABLE 44-11	**Documenting Suspected Child Abuse or Neglect**

- Document objectively. Do not make assumptions or draw conclusions. For example, you could document that the patient stated he was struck with a belt buckle, or that the patient has a 3-in. by 2-in. "U-"shaped bruise on his back, but you cannot state that (in your opinion) the patient was beaten with a belt buckle.
- Objectively document and precisely describe all injuries by their appearance and locations. Make drawings if possible.
- Place in quotation marks any relevant statements made by the patient, witnesses, or caregivers.
- Document the conditions of the surroundings.
- Document relevant aspects of the child's appearance, such as what he was wearing, for example, if he was found outside in cold weather but not wearing a coat, or if the child is unkempt or appears thin or emaciated.
- Document the behavior of the child and caregivers.

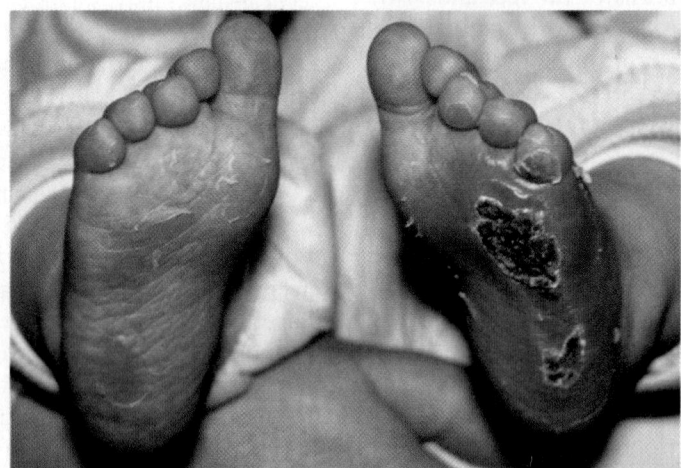
(A)

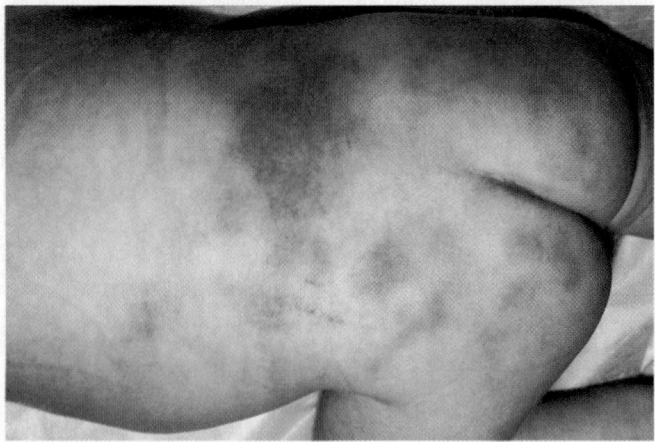
(B)

FIGURE 44-9

Indications of child abuse: (A) burns to the feet caused by dunking the child's feet in hot water (© SPL/Photo Researchers, Inc.), (B) bruising resulting from physical abuse. (© Biophoto Associates/Photo Researchers, Inc.)

Significant injury and illness in a child are very often distressing, but feelings of distress can be even more pronounced in instances of suspected child abuse or neglect. You may feel tremendous anger or sadness at the situation, but you must control your emotions at the scene and remain professional. Focus on the task at hand: providing medical care and transportation to the patient.

Acknowledge your feelings but temporarily put them aside in order to provide the best care possible to the patient, with the understanding that you will examine the feelings at an appropriate time. Recognize signs of acute stress reaction, cumulative stress, and post-traumatic stress disorder in yourself and others who responded to the scene, and seek professional mental health assistance, if needed.

CASE STUDY WRAP-UP

Clinical-Reasoning Process

Advanced EMTs Vic and Marcel have arrived at the home of an infant who was reported to be not breathing. When they arrived, the patient, three-month-old Paisley Johnson, was crying and being held by her mother.

Vic quickly forms a general impression using the pediatric assessment triangle. The patient's appearance, work of breathing, and circulation to the skin all are normal. "Hi, I'm Vic and this is my partner, Marcel. Sit down and hold Paisley. I'll take a look at her while Marcel gets some information from the two of you."

As Mrs. Johnson sits with Paisley in her lap, Vic assesses her airway, noting a little mucus in the nose, which he clears away using a bulb syringe. Vic confirms that there are no signs of respiratory distress: no nasal flaring, no retractions, no abnormal sounds after the nares were cleared, and no cyanosis or pallor. As Paisley calms down and stops crying, Vic listens to breath sounds, which are clear, and obtains a heart rate of 142 and a respiratory rate of 30. Paisley's skin is warm and dry with normal color and she has a capillary refill time of less than 1 second.

Looking from head to toe, Vic notices that the fontanels look normal and there are no rashes or signs of injury. As he completes his exam, talking softly to Paisley, she begins to smile at him.

Meanwhile, Marcel has reassured the parents that Paisley's breathing is normal and asks what happened that caused them to call 911. "She was feeding but her nose was a little stuffy and all of the sudden she started choking and coughing and couldn't catch her breath. Her lips turned blue and we were so scared! Barry, my husband, called 911 and I turned her over and started patting her back. She started breathing again. I'm sure it was just a few seconds, but it seemed like forever."

Marcel determines that Paisley was born four weeks prematurely but was dismissed from the hospital with no apparent problems after four days. She has been gaining weight normally and is seen regularly by her pediatrician and has received vaccinations as scheduled. Mrs. Johnson has just returned to work and she is afraid that Paisley caught a cold at day care, causing her congestion. Mrs. Johnson states that Paisley has not had a fever, but started having "a stuffy nose" the day before and seemed a little irritable.

Vic observes that the parents are appropriately concerned. Surveying the immediate environment, he sees only the signs of a "lived in" home of two working parents with an infant to care for. "Paisley looks fine right now," he tells the Johnsons. "But we never take a report of a baby not breathing lightly. We would like to transport her and you can ride with her, of course, to be evaluated by a physician. What hospital do you go to?"

The Johnsons readily agree to transport. En route, Paisley falls asleep. She is breathing easily, her appearance remains normal, including her skin color. Vic continues to reassess her breathing and perfusion en route. Paisley is released from the emergency department later in the evening. After evaluation and observation, the physician diagnoses her with an upper respiratory infection and advises the parents to make sure they use a bulb syringe to clear her nose before, and if necessary, during feeding and to follow up with their pediatrician the next day.

CHAPTER REVIEW

Chapter Summary

Pediatric patients are different in important ways from adult patients. They are not only smaller, but have anatomic, physiological, and psychosocial differences that you must consider in the assessment and management of emergencies involving pediatric patients. In addition, the epidemiology of injury and illness is different in the pediatric age group. Keys to successfully managing pediatric calls include knowledge of pediatric differences, using equipment designed for pediatric patients, and the ability to maintain composure.

Key differences in pediatric patients include differences in the airway and airway management techniques, increased susceptibility to hypothermia and dehydration, and subtle signs and symptoms of shock despite significant blood loss. Pediatric patients are more vulnerable to the effects of some infectious illness, several of which can lead to airway obstruction or respiratory distress, respiratory failure, or respiratory arrest. Hypoxia is the leading cause of cardiac arrest in pediatric patients, underscoring the need to vigilantly monitor the patient's airway, breathing, and oxygenation and intervene quickly.

SIDS and ALTE affect the infant age group and can pose particular difficulties for EMS providers. In addition to being stressful, signs related to those disorders can mimic indications of possible child abuse. You must document the scene carefully as a potential crime scene without implying that the parents are in any way at fault for the situation. You must also recognize, document, and report suspected child abuse and neglect.

Pediatric patients can receive different patterns of trauma than adults subjected to the same mechanisms because of their anatomical differences. Blunt mechanisms of injury are the most common in the pediatric population and are likely to produce multisystem trauma. Whenever possible, transport critically ill or injured pediatric patients to a facility capable of specialized pediatric care.

Review Questions

Multiple-Choice Questions

1. Which one of the following is the most common cause of cardiac arrest in the pediatric population?
   a. Congenital heart defects
   b. Sudden cardiac arrest
   c. Commotio cordis
   d. Hypoxia

2. Which one of the following positions best maintains alignment of the airway structures in a pediatric patient, allowing for an open airway?
   a. Hyperextension of the neck with a modified jaw-thrust maneuver
   b. Moderate flexion of the neck with a tongue-jaw lift maneuver
   c. Neutral position of the neck with the head in the sniffing position
   d. Hyperflexion of the neck by placing a folded towel beneath the head

3. You are ventilating a three-year-old patient who weighs approximately 35 pounds. Which one of the following is the best tidal volume for this patient?
   a. 250 mL   c. 80 mL
   b. 120 mL   d. 50 mL

4. Your patient is an 18-month-old child who was restrained in a rear-facing child car seat in the center of the rear seat of a vehicle that was struck at about 40 mph in the driver's side by another vehicle. You should be concerned if the patient's heart rate is higher than _____ per minute.
   a. 140   c. 120
   b. 130   d. 100

5. A two-year-old patient who has had a fever with vomiting and diarrhea for 36 hours has a capillary refill time of 3 seconds. You should suspect that he:
   a. has not lost a significant amount of fluid.
   b. is in compensated shock.
   c. is in decompensated shock.
   d. is in irreversible shock.

6. A 60-pound pediatric patient with suspected shock should receive an initial fluid bolus of _____ mL.
   a. 100   c. 500
   b. 250   d. 750

7. Which one of the following vaccines is given to prevent pertussis (whooping cough)?
   a. DTap   c. MMR
   b. Hib   d. HPV

8. You respond on a January afternoon for a 15-month-old child who presents with lethargy, dyspnea, breath sounds characterized by inspiratory crackles and expiratory wheezing, a temperature of 103.4°F, heart rate of 134 beats per minute, respiratory rate of 60 breaths per minute, and SpO_2 of 95 percent on room air. His mother states that he has had a minor cough and runny nose beginning the previous afternoon. The presentation is most consistent with:
   a. ALTE.   c. epiglottitis.
   b. croup.   d. bronchiolitis.

9. A 15-month-old patient presents awake but lethargic, with dyspnea, breath sounds characterized by inspiratory crackles and expiratory wheezing, a temperature of 103.4°F, heart rate of 134 beats per minute, respiratory rate of 60 breaths per minute, and SpO_2 of 95 percent on room air. In addition to preparing the patient for transport without delay to a pediatric-capable emergency facility, which of the following has the highest priority?
   a. Start an IV and give a fluid bolus.
   b. Start a nebulized albuterol treatment.
   c. Give ibuprofen elixir in the dosage permitted by your protocols.
   d. Assist ventilations by bag-valve-mask device.

10. The proper ratio of chest compressions to ventilations in one-rescuer infant CPR is:
    a. 15:1.   c. 30:1.
    b. 15:2.   d. 30:2.

11. A 16-year-old patient has fever, chills, joint and muscle pain, a headache, stiff neck, photophobia, and purpuric rash. Those signs and symptoms are most suspicious for:
   a. bacterial meningitis.
   b. pneumonia.
   c. cystic fibrosis.
   d. measles.

12. A seven-year-old patient with a history of peanut allergy presents with stridor and wheezing after eating some cookies at a friend's house. He weighs approximately 55 pounds. The dose of 1:1,000 epinephrine for this patient, to be administered subcutaneously or intramuscularly, is _____ mg.
   a. 2.5
   b. 5
   c. 0.25
   d. 0.5

13. A nine-month-old child has partial-thickness burns to both feet and both lower legs, circumferentially, to the level of the knees. The estimated total body surface area involved is:
   a. 7.
   b. 9.
   c. 14.
   d. 18.

14. A six-year-old patient with a history of hydrocephalus with a ventriculostomy shunt presents with decreased level of responsiveness, vomiting, and seizure. The skin temperature is normal, the breath sounds are clear and equal, and the vital signs are as follows: respirations 12 and irregular, pulse 80 and regular, blood pressure 126/84, and SpO_2 96 percent on room air. The patient's father says that the child complained of a headache and blurred vision early in the day, but otherwise has had no complaints or problems. There are no other findings in the physical exam. Those findings are most consistent with:
   a. bacterial meningitis.
   b. increased intracranial pressure.
   c. anaphylaxis.
   d. diabetic ketoacidosis.

15. An eight-year-old child with a history of type 1 diabetes presents with an altered mental status and a blood glucose level of 48 mg/dL. He weighs approximately 65 pounds. Proper treatment includes the administration of dextrose in which one of the following concentrations and dosages?
   a. 50 percent, 30 mL
   b. 25 percent, 30 mL
   c. 50 percent, 15 mL
   d. 25 percent, 120 mL

16. A three-year-old child fell into a swimming pool after leaving the house unsupervised. He may have been submerged for as long as 15 minutes before being pulled from the water by a relative. The patient is pulseless and apneic. Which one of the following is the highest priority in the management of this patient?
   a. Correcting hypothermia
   b. Cervical-spine immobilization
   c. Performing a detailed head-to-toe exam
   d. Beginning CPR

Critical-Thinking Questions

17. Explain how pediatric anatomic differences can increase the risk of abdominal injuries.

18. Explain why pediatric patients with respiratory distress are at increased risk of dehydration.

References

Burnett, L. B., & Adler, J. (2011). *Sudden infant death syndrome in emergency medicine: Treatment & medication.* eMedicine. Retrieved March 21, 2011, from http://emedicine.medscape.com/article/804412-overview

Centers for Disease Control. (2006). Field triage decision scheme. Retrieved August 5, 2011, from http://www.cdc.gov/fieldtriage/

Centers for Disease Control and Prevention. (2010). *Meningitis.* eMedicine.com. Retrieved January 11, 2011, from http://www.cdc.gov/meningitis/about/index.html

Louden, M. (2010). *Pediatric bronchiolitis: Treatment & medication.* eMedicine. Retrieved March 21, 2011, from http://emedicine.medscape.com/article/800428-overview

McSwain, N. Salomone, J., & Pons, P. T. (Eds.). (2011). *Prehospital trauma life support* (7th ed.). St. Louis, MO: Elsevier.

Moore Shepherd, S., & Shoff, W. H. (2010). *Drowning: Treatment and medication.* eMedicine. Retrieved March 21, 2011, from http://emedicine.medscape.com/article/772753-treatment

Muñiz, A., Molodow, R. E., & Defendi, G. L. (2010). *Croup: Treatment & medication.* eMedicine. Retrieved January 12, 2011, from http://emedicine.medscape.com/article/962972-treatment

Neuman, M. I. (2010). *Pediatrics, pneumonia: Treatment & medication.* eMedicine. Retrieved March 21, 2011, from http://emedicine.medscape.com/article/803364-overview

Additional Reading

Centers for Disease Control. (2011). *Diseases and conditions index.* Retrieved April 29, 2011, from http://www.cdc.gov/DiseasesConditions/

Cystic Fibrosis Foundation. (2009). *About cystic fibrosis.* Retrieved October 7, 2010, from http://www.cff.org/AboutCF/

45

Geriatrics

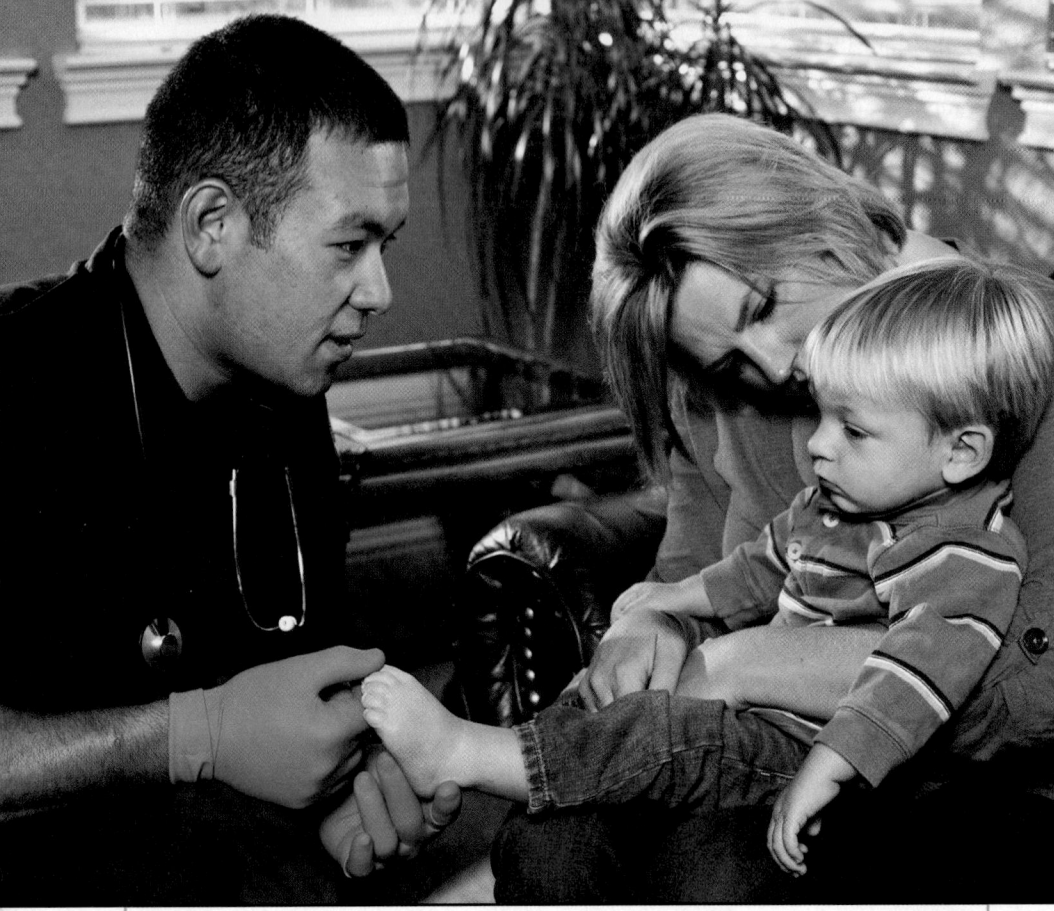

Content Area: Special Patient Populations

Advanced EMT Education Standard: Applies a fundamental knowledge of growth, development, and aging and assessment findings to provide basic and selected advanced emergency care and transportation for a patient with special needs.

Resource Central

To access Resource Central, follow the directions on the Student Access Card provided with this text. If there is no card, go to www.bradybooks.com and follow the Resource Central link to Buy Access. Under Media Resources, you will find:

- *Alzheimer's Disease.* The challenges of managing geriatric patients with this disease.

- *Elder Mistreatment and Abuse.* How to identify important signs of elder abuse.

- *Polypharmacy.* Why geriatric patients are susceptible to the effects of polypharmacy and how prehospital professionals can help.

Objectives

After reading this chapter, you should be able to:

45.1   Define key terms introduced in this chapter.

45.2   Summarize age-related anatomic and physiologic changes for each of the following systems:
  – Cardiovascular
  – Endocrine
  – Gastrointestinal
  – Integumentary
  – Musculoskeletal
  – Nervous and sensory
  – Renal
  – Respiratory

CASE STUDY

Advanced EMTs Eddie Veach and Harper Conlin are counting down the minutes until shift change when a call for a motor vehicle collision comes in. They acknowledge the call, climb into the cab of the ambulance, buckle their seat belts, and cautiously pull into traffic for the 6-minute response. En route, an EMT from the rescue squad updates Eddie and Harper that they have a single patient, an 86-year-old female who was driving a car that struck a tree in the buffer strip next to the street. The patient is confused and seems to be having trouble breathing.

As Eddie and Harper arrive at the scene, they confirm that the scene is safe and that they have only one patient. The rescue squad crew has accessed the patient through the driver's door. The vehicle has moderate damage to the front end and the front air bags deployed. An accident investigator with the sheriff's office tells Harper he estimates the speed at impact was 25 mph and that it does not appear that the patient tried to brake or avoid the tree.

One of the EMTs is setting up for oxygen administration and a second EMT is listening to the patient's breath sounds. Eddie notices some abrasions on the patient's face and sees that she has a nosebleed.

Problem-Solving Questions

1. How does knowledge of the patient's age and details of the collision contribute to the clinical reasoning process?
2. What age-related differences should Eddie and Harper consider in the assessment and management of this patient?
3. What are some initial thoughts about potential causes of the patient's reported confusion and difficulty breathing?

45.3 Relate the anatomic and physiologic changes associated with aging to anticipated differences in complaints and assessment findings for geriatric patients.

45.4 Discuss the presentation, assessment, and management of common medical emergencies in the elderly population, including the following:
   – Altered mental status
   – Congestive heart failure
   – COPD
   – Delirium and dementia, including Alzheimer's disease
   – Drug toxicity
   – Environmental emergencies
   – Gastrointestinal problems
   – HHNC
   – Myocardial infarction
   – Pneumonia
   – Pulmonary embolism
   – Seizures
   – Stroke and TIA
   – Syncope

45.5 Describe the elderly patient's altered response to trauma.

45.6 Recognize signs and risk factors of elder abuse.

45.7 Describe modifications that may be necessary to effectively assess and treat geriatric patients.

Introduction

The segment of the U.S. population age 65 years and older is increasing and is expected to continue to increase in the coming decades. As of 2008, there were nearly 37 million people in the United States aged 65 and older, comprising 12.3 percent of the population (U.S. Census Bureau, 2008a). The Census Bureau (2008b) projects that by 2015, there will be nearly 47 million people in that age group, and nearly 64 million by 2025. Two factors are primarily responsible for that change in demographics: the post–World War II "baby boom" and increasing life expectancy.

Although most older people live independent, active lives, the prevalence of many diseases and disabilities increases in the older population. That means older adults comprise a sizeable proportion of EMS patients. Common reasons that older adults require EMS include cardiac and respiratory problems, neurologic problems such as stroke and altered mental status, injuries from falls, and nonspecific complaints like dizziness, weakness, and fatigue.

The approaches to patient assessment and care that you learned in this textbook are generally applicable when caring for older patients, but you also must keep in mind some special considerations. The effectiveness of body systems gradually declines with age. The changed responses of the body to disease and injuries can increase the severity of illness and injury in older patients and can alter the expected presentation and course of illnesses and injuries. Beyond its physical aspects, aging also has psychosocial impacts that affect health and access to health care.

Geriatrics is the branch of medicine that specializes in treating elderly patients. Gerontology is a more general term that refers to the study of aging and the elderly. In this chapter, the terms elderly, geriatric, and older adult are used interchangeably. This chapter presents the common changes associated with aging, common illnesses and injuries in the elderly, and differences in complaints, assessment findings, and interventions.

Anatomy and Physiology Review

The maximum *life span* of human beings is about 120 years. But, our *life expectancy* is much lower, currently 77.9 years on the average in the United States (Centers for Disease Control and Prevention, National Center for Health Statistics, 2010). Factors that influence life expectancy include gender, genetics, environment, and lifestyle. Life expectancy is different for different cohorts of individuals, depending on their year of birth and is influenced by diet, sociocultural factors, and health behaviors.

Aging is a process that takes place gradually over time. The incidence of certain conditions statistically increases at a given age, but it does not mean that every person of that age has the same level of health. Simply categorizing those age 65 years or older as elderly does not account for the wide variation in lifestyles and health statuses of older patients. Every patient, regardless of age, is an individual who is likely very different from other patients of the same age. For example, the onset of age-related hearing loss depends on many factors, including exposure to occupational and other sources of noise.

Some age-related changes become noticeable in middle adulthood and become more pronounced in late adulthood. Age-related decline of body system function results in decreased ability to maintain homeostasis in the face of anatomical and physiologic changes (Figure 45-1). The same illnesses and injuries the body could easily overcome in young adulthood pose a greater risk of morbidity and mortality to older adults (Table 45-1). In middle adulthood, there commonly are changes in vision as the lens of the eye loses its ability to focus (presbyopia), creating problems in seeing objects that are close. Some age-related hearing loss (presbycusis) may occur, as well. The incidence of cardiovascular disease and risk factors increases, hypercholesterolemia and hypertension are more common, and cardiac output declines. Weight control becomes more difficult beginning in middle age and obesity is associated with the onset of type II diabetes. There also is an increase in the incidence of cancer.

Menopause occurs in women in their late 40s to early 50s, at an average age of 51 years of age. The decline in endogenous (from within the body) estrogen, which is protective against cardiovascular disease, results in an increased incidence of cardiovascular disease in postmenopausal women.

From the seventh decade onward, body systems continue to decline, including worsening of the vision and hearing changes that began in middle age. Signs of aging become more visible at this stage. The skin is thinner and the loss of elasticity of connective tissues leads to sagging and wrinkling of the skin. The skin becomes fragile and can easily be torn. Pruritus (persistent itching) can occur from eczema, medication side effects, or kidney or liver failure. Scratching the thin, dry skin can lead to excoriations (scratching or abrading the skin), which can become infected and heal poorly.

IN THE FIELD

The loss of connective tissue and skin elasticity can make starting an IV more difficult in elderly patients. Because they are no longer as well anchored by connective tissue, veins may roll away from the tip of the IV needle. The veins are fragile and IV attempts may result in venous injury with bruising, hematoma formation, and infiltration of IV fluids. Use as small an IV catheter as possible, given the situation.

CHANGES IN THE BODY SYSTEMS OF THE ELDERLY

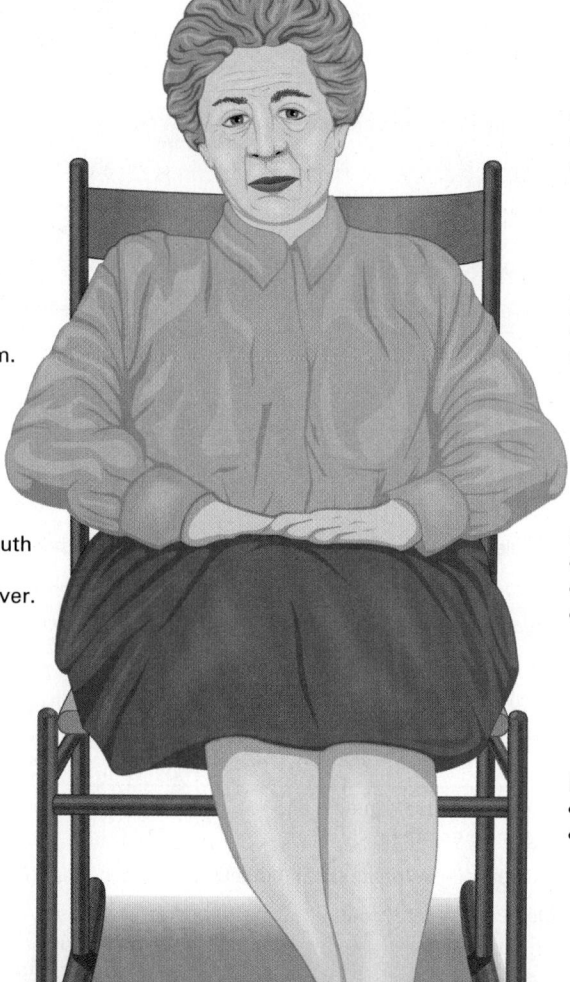

Neurologic System
• Brain changes with age.
• Clinical depression common.
• Altered mental status common.

Cardiovascular System
• Hypertension common.
• Changes in heart rate and rhythm.

Gastrointestinal System
• Constipation common.
• Deterioration of structures in mouth common.
• General decline in efficiency of liver.
• Impaired swallowing.
• Malnutrition as result of deterioration of small intestine.

Musculoskeletal System
• Osteoporosis common.
• Osteoarthritis common.

Respiratory System
• Cough power is diminished.
• Increased tendency for infection.
• Less air and less exchange of gases due to general decline.

Renal System
• Drug toxicity problems common.
• General decline in efficiency.

Skin
• Perspires less.
• Tears more easily.
• Heals slowly.

Immune System
• Fever often absent.
• Lessened ability to fight disease.

FIGURE 45-1

Age-related changes in the body systems.

Less pigment is produced by melanocytes and the skin is paler. The hair usually gradually becomes gray or white. Thinning of the hair and hair loss is common in both genders, but often more noticeable in males. Muscle mass decreases and skeletal muscles may weaken. Loss of body fat tends to occur as age progresses. The overall loss of soft tissue mass and decreased mobility can lead to **decubitus ulcers** (pressure sores or bedsores).

Osteoporosis can occur in both genders, but is especially common in women. The combination of muscle weakness,

vision changes, and changes in balance can lead to falls. Muscle weakness can prevent the elderly person who has fallen from getting up or from reaching the phone to call for help. Fractures can occur with minimal force. For example, compression fractures of the spine can occur from forceful coughing in patients with osteoporosis. A seemingly minor fall can result in rib or hip fractures. Hip fractures, in particular, in the elderly are associated with increased mortality.

The blood vessels thicken, which increases systemic vascular resistance, decreases organ perfusion, and

TABLE 45-1 Age-Related Changes and Their Significance

Body System	Change	Possible Consequences
Senses	Thickening of the lens of the eye	Decreased accommodation resulting in difficulty with near vision
	Cataracts	Clouding of vision, difficulty seeing
	Macular degeneration	Loss of central vision
	Glaucoma	Loss of peripheral vision
	Change in inner ear structures	Decreased hearing, especially for high tones; dizziness
	Decreased pain sensitivity	Decreased ability to detect illness and injury
	Decreased taste and smell	Decreased enjoyment of food
Neurologic	Structural and functional brain changes	Brain atrophy (shrinkage), dementia, memory impairment, slowed learning, depression, slowed reactions, and impaired proprioception
Cardiovascular	Atherosclerotic changes	Hypertension, acute coronary syndrome, stroke, mesenteric infarction, renal infarction, aortic dissection or aneurysm
	Cardiac conduction system changes	Dysrhythmia, decreased maximum heart rate
	Myocardial changes	Decreased cardiac output
Respiratory	Changes in chest wall compliance	Impaired ventilation
	Decreased cough and gag reflexes; decreased ciliary function	Increased risk aspiration and infection
	Decreased gas exchange	Decreased ability to compensate for increased oxygen demand
Gastrointestinal	Decreased stomach acid and digestive enzymes	Impaired digestion and nutrient absorption
	Decreased gastrointestinal motility	Constipation, bowel obstruction
	Decreased liver function	Decreased production of proteins and enzymes, decreased clearance of drugs metabolized by the liver; may contribute to drug toxicity
Genitourinary and renal	Decreased renal function	Decreased clearance of substances eliminated in the urine; may contribute to drug toxicity
	Impaired bladder function	Urinary retention, urinary tract infection
Immune system	General decline in function	Increased risk of infection, may lack fever with infection
Musculoskeletal system	Loss of muscle mass, weakness	Decreased mobility, increased risk of falls, may not be able to get up after falling
	Osteoporosis	Pathologic fractures
	Osteoarthritis	Pain, decreased mobility
Integumentary	Loss of elasticity; thinning of skin	Skin is easily injured; decubitus ulcers
Thermoregulation	Decreased sweating, decreased shivering	Heat- and cold-related emergencies

increases the workload of the heart. At the same time, the heart functions less efficiently, is less able to respond to increased physical activity, and becomes less tolerant of tachycardia. Anemia and decreased response to infection can occur. Some forms of leukemia are more prevalent in this age group.

Decline in the respiratory system puts older adults at risk for health problems, including decreased ability to increase oxygenation to meet increased demands during illness and injury. Lung capacity decreases, as does gas diffusion through the respiratory membrane. Respiratory muscle function declines and the chest wall becomes less compliant. Ribs and costal cartilage become weakened and brittle. The cough and gag reflexes are diminished, providing less protection to the lower airway.

Decreased senses of taste and smell, along with isolation and decreased mobility and financial means can lead to decreased food intake. Diminished salivation and gastric secretions decrease digestive function and nutrients are not as well absorbed, leading to vitamin and mineral deficiencies. A lifetime of dental issues may creep up on the elderly, leading to tooth loss and the need for dentures. Constipation is common and bowel impaction and obstruction may occur. Diminished activity of the endocrine system results in less insulin production and decreased glucose metabolism. Liver function decreases as well, and substances (including medications) may not be efficiently eliminated from the body. Loss of up to 50 percent of the nephrons and glomerular abnormalities result in decreased urine production. Substances that normally are excreted through the kidneys, including drugs and wastes, may accumulate.

Changes in the nervous system include decreased sensory function, reaction time, and **proprioception** (sensation of the orientation of the body or body parts without visual input). A common scenario involving elderly drivers related to the decrease in proprioception is the driver mistakenly pressing the accelerator instead of the brake, leading to a collision. Levels of neurotransmitter decrease, which may contribute to depression in the elderly. The cumulative effects of vascular disease and inflammatory processes can lead to **dementia**. Pain perception decreases and even serious injury and illness may not produce the expected degree of pain. Neurons function less efficiently and problem-solving ability and new knowledge assimilation can slow. Overall, cognitive decline, including Alzheimer's disease and other forms of dementia, is not a normal consequence of aging, but of pathologic processes. The sleep–wake cycle may become impaired as levels of melatonin (a hormone that helps regulate sleep) drop, and is common in patients with dementia.

Psychosocial Aspects of Aging

Although better health in older age has contributed to an increased number of people aged 65 and older in the workforce, there is another factor that has led to an increased number of elderly in the workforce. The economic recession of recent years and increased costs of living make it difficult for retired persons on fixed incomes to make ends meet. Nearly six million people age 65 years and older work part-time or full-time jobs, and 116,000 people aged 85 years or older work part-time or full-time jobs (U.S. Census Bureau, 2008a). For those unable to work beyond mandatory retirement age, economic hardship can mean being underinsured and making tough choices between paying for housing and food and paying for medicine and medical care. Currently,

9.7 percent of those 65 years and older and 13 percent of those 85 years and older live below the poverty line. Despite programs such as **Medicare, Medicaid,** and Social Security, it still can be a struggle to pay for medical care, prescription drugs, food, housing, utilities, transportation, and other expenses.

Lack of adequate income and social support can result in elderly patients living in potentially dangerous situations. An unsafe space heater may be used to supplement the inadequate heat of a faulty furnace that is too costly to repair or replace. Without the means to repair or replace the furnace, it may become a fire or carbon monoxide hazard, or leave the home without heat at all. An elderly patient may not have smoke detectors, or may not be able to change the batteries in them. Lack of air conditioning in hot climates, combined with lack of opportunity to seek relief from the heat, can lead to heat-related emergencies. Stairs, steps, and banisters in poor repair can lead to falls. Slippery floors, loose throw rugs, bathtubs, and showers can pose hazards, as well.

With maturity, individuals learn to face problems more as challenges than as threats. However, losses of function, independence, and companionship and financial burdens are common in this age group. Financial and physical dependence on others increases vulnerability of the elderly and the risk of abuse and neglect (Table 45-2). Abuse may include being restrained, physical abuse (hitting, kicking), sexual abuse, and financial abuse. Neglect may mean that

TABLE 45-2 Factors Associated with Increased Risk for Elder Abuse

Patient Factors	Abuser Factors
Age 80 or older	May have numerous stressors in addition to caring for the patient
Female	
Physically or financially dependent on others	May be a family member or other caregiver (nursing home, hospital personnel)
Immobile	
Incontinent	
Dementia	
Sleep disturbances	
Multiple medical problems	

the patient is not being helped to the bathroom, moved or turned to prevent decubitus ulcers, kept clean, or given adequate food, medications, or medical care. Depression is common among the elderly and suicide may occur. Nonetheless, the majority of elderly patients live independently, with minimal assistance, or with family members.

General Assessment and Management

Follow the same steps for assessing geriatric patients as you do other patients. However, there are some potential challenges and considerations you must be aware of.

Scene Size-Up

You may not know that your patient is an older adult until you have begun the scene size-up, so perform the scene size-up as you would on any other call. Look for potential hazards, including indications of violence. Determine the number of patients and the need for additional resources, and determine the nature of the illness or mechanism of injury. Obtain the chief complaint and develop a general impression of the seriousness of the patient's condition.

Once you determine that the patient is an older adult, pay particular attention to the patient's surroundings when you respond to a residence. Notice any indications of chronic illness, such as the presence of oxygen tanks or tubing, nebulizers, a hospital bed, or other medical equipment. Assess the patient's degree of mobility. Is there a walker, cane, wheelchair, or electric mobility device in the patient's environment? Does the environment appear as if the patient is able to take care of himself or, if he is dependent on others, that he is well cared for? Is there an odor that indicates urinary or bowel incontinence? Is the environment excessively hot or cold? Older people cannot regulate their body temperatures very well. They need an environment that may feel uncomfortably warm to younger people. Even in warmer temperatures, some older people still wear several layers of clothing to retain sufficient heat. This can result in a heat-related emergency if the temperature rises and the patient fails to realize it.

For responsive patients, obtain the chief complaint as you complete the scene size-up. Two factors can pose a challenge to that task. First, there may be communication issues, such as hearing impairment, altered mental status, poor dentition, or speech difficulties due to a prior stroke. Do not assume that the patient cannot communicate with you, or that he cannot give a reliable history. *Always attempt to communicate directly with the patient first, turning to others only if you cannot obtain a history from the patient, or to collect additional information.* Give the elderly patient a bit longer to process your questions and formulate answers. If the patient has a hearing aid but is not wearing

it, offer to retrieve it for him. If the patient has difficulty speaking or hearing, he may be better able to communicate through writing or reading. (See Chapter 6.)

The second challenge may be getting a single, specific chief complaint. Older patients can have vague or multiple complaints, or may give information about all current illnesses when you ask about the reason for needing medical care. It is helpful to ask what is bothering the patient most or what has changed that is causing him concern. It can be difficult for patients to differentiate between age-related changes and the onset of disease. A patient may attribute aches and pains or shortness of breath to "old age" when, in fact, those symptoms may indicate an acute problem that should be treated. Advanced EMTs also must avoid the pitfall of attributing signs and symptoms of disease to the aging process. Always determine what a patient's normal or baseline condition is. Ask the patient how things are different now than they were a week ago. For example, "Mrs. Schuster, is there anything different about the way you feel today than the way you felt last week?" That information can be very helpful in differentiating a chronic condition from a new problem.

Primary Assessment

By the end of the scene size-up you have a general impression of the patient's level of distress, including whether he appears to be responsive or unresponsive. If the patient is unresponsive and does not appear to be breathing normally, confirm unresponsiveness and check the carotid pulse. If you do not detect a pulse within 10 seconds, begin chest compressions, unless you are presented with a current, valid, signed do not resuscitate (DNR) order in a timely manner.

If the patient is responsive, or is unresponsive but has a pulse, assess the patient's airway, breathing, and circulation. Treat airway compromise, difficulty breathing, hypoxia, and bleeding before continuing to the secondary assessment.

Opening and maintaining an airway can be made difficult by the absence of teeth or the presence of poorly fitting dentures, or **kyphosis**, an exaggerated curvature of the thoracic spine. Never force the head, neck, or back into position. Instead, a jaw-thrust maneuver or modified jaw-thrust maneuver may be necessary. You also may need to place padding under the patient's head. Leave dentures in place unless they interfere with airway management. Use basic or advanced airway adjuncts as necessary.

Consider the possibility of aspiration and foreign body airway obstruction. Difficulty swallowing, diminished cough and gag reflexes, difficulty chewing, and muscle weakness all increase the risk of aspiration and foreign body airway obstruction. Use positioning, suction, manual maneuvers, and basic and advanced airway adjuncts as needed.

Look for signs of respiratory distress, such as tripod position, increased respiratory effort, abnormal noises with breathing, increased or decreased respiratory rate, pursed lips, anxiety, confusion, and cyanosis. Assist with or provide ventilations as needed. The absence of teeth or missing dentures can make achieving a good seal with a bag-valve-mask difficult. If you are unable to maintain an adequate seal between the mask and face, consider using an advanced airway device, such as a Combitube, LMA, or KingLTD airway.

An irregular pulse is a common finding in elderly patients. The incidence of atrial fibrillation increases with age. In the absence of chest pain, altered mental status, respiratory distress, and signs of hypoperfusion, a pulse that is irregular but at a rate of between 60 and 100 per minute, may not be cause for concern. However, there are other causes of an irregular pulse that are associated with increased risks for hypoperfusion and lethal dysrhythmia. The patient's history, perfusion status, and overall condition help you determine whether the irregular heart rate is causing or contributing to the current problem, or is a pre-existing condition.

Control bleeding using direct pressure, but keep in mind that some medications can interfere with platelet function and coagulation, necessitating applying pressure for a longer period of time.

Determine the patient's priority for treatment and transport. Any patient with a concerning chief complaint, such as chest pain or dyspnea (see Chapter 15), an overall poor general impression, or problem with the airway, breathing, or circulation is a high priority for treatment and transport (Table 45-3). The priority for transport may change. The elderly can present with vague complaints that, after a more thorough history and exam, turn out to be more concerning than initially thought.

Secondary Assessment

The approach to the secondary assessment is determined by whether the nature of the problem is medical or traumatic and whether the patient is critical or noncritical. Medical problems and trauma can overlap in the elderly patient. For example, syncope, a transient ischemic attack (TIA), stroke, dysrhythmia, or other medical problem can lead to a motor vehicle collision or fall. When examining an elderly trauma patient, always consider underlying medical emergencies. Even if a medical emergency did not lead to the incident that caused trauma, the presence of medical conditions and medications can alter the patient's response to injury and lead to additional complications.

Mental Status

Assessing mental status is an important part of the assessment of all patients. In the elderly, assessing mental status can be especially challenging because older people with dementia have an altered mental status as part of their baseline condition. If family members or caregivers are available, it is important for you to find out from them what normal status is for that patient. A recent or sudden onset

TABLE 45-3 Common Complaints in the Elderly and Their Significance

Complaint or Presentation	Conditions to Consider
Abdominal pain or discomfort	Acute coronary syndrome Aortic dissection or aneurysm Bowel infarction or obstruction Gastroenteritis Gastrointestinal bleeding Pneumonia
Altered mental status	Dementia Delirium Hepatic failure Hypoglycemia or hyperglycemia Hypoperfusion (shock, acute coronary syndrome, heart failure) Hypothermia or hyperthermia Hypoxia Infection Medications or toxins Renal failure Seizure Stroke Substance abuse (alcohol, prescription drugs, recreational drugs) Trauma (traumatic brain injury, hypoperfusion, hypoxia)
Dyspnea	Acute coronary syndrome Anemia Asthma COPD Heart failure Infection (pneumonia, influenza) Lung cancer Pneumothorax Pulmonary embolism
Chest pain or discomfort	Acute coronary syndrome Hiatal hernia Musculoskeletal pain Pneumonia Pulmonary embolism
Syncope	Acute coronary syndrome Cardiac dysrhythmia Hypovolemia Medications Vasovagal syncope
Weakness, fatigue	Acute coronary syndrome Anemia Dehydration Electrolyte imbalance Infection Medications Hypothyroidism Stroke

of confusion or other deterioration in mental status should make you consider a serious acute medical condition rather than Alzheimer's disease or other forms of dementia.

As part of the scene size-up and primary assessment, grossly determine the patient's level of responsiveness according to the AVPU mnemonic. As you explore the chief complaint and obtain a history, determine if it is likely that the patient is giving an accurate history. If there is any doubt as to the patient's mental status (for example, if he is not oriented or gives unusual responses), perform a Mini Mental State Exam (MMSE) as part of the secondary assessment. (See Chapter 22.)

History

Introduce yourself, speak slowly and clearly, and position yourself where the patient can easily see you. If the patient is answering your questions slowly and your primary assessment did not reveal any immediate threats to life, give him additional time. Make sure you are asking only one question at a time. If the patient's speech is slurred from a prior or current stroke, allow him time to communicate with you and try to understand him. If the patient's speech is difficult to understand because his dentures are not in place, ask him to put them in if appropriate. Depression also is a reason that a patient's answers can be delayed, and can interfere with memory and concentration.

Throughout your interaction with the patient, use his responses to monitor his mental status. But be cautious when assessing his orientation to time. Consider the geriatric patient oriented to time if he is able to tell you what year it is. Knowing the day or month can be a function of participating in the workforce, reading newspapers, or watching the news on television. A person who does not do those things may not have a good sense of day or month but can still be considered oriented to time.

Orientation to person, place, and time may not be a sensitive enough indication of mental status. The MMSE is a more sensitive indication of mental status. That tool can be particularly important when a patient does not want to consent to treatment and transport. You must make sure the patient is competent to make that decision.

In some cases, a family member may tell you that some of the information given by the patient is incorrect. That might be a result of a neurologic condition, but it can also be caused by medications the patient is taking, especially if there are many of them or the dose for some is too high. **Confabulation** occurs when a patient unknowingly fills in

gaps in memory with information that seems to fit. Sometimes confabulation is obvious because the information given is implausible. In other cases, the information is plausible and you may not realize that it is incorrect unless you verify with a family member. A spouse, other family members, or caretakers can be an excellent source of information about a patient's medications, past medical history, and history of the present illness.

Obtain a complete history, using the mnemonics SAMPLE and OPQRST as guides. Apply your knowledge of pathophysiology and age-related changes to help develop the line of questioning based on the patient's chief complaint. Pay particular attention to obtaining a complete medication history. Ask about all prescription and over-the-counter medications and herbal or homeopathic remedies the patient is using. **Polypharmacy** (taking multiple drugs) is common in the elderly.

Drugs can have unexpected effects in the elderly and can interact in unexpected ways. A decrease in kidney or liver function, decreased total body water, decreased plasma proteins, and decreased fat stores all can contribute to an unexpectedly high level of the medication despite normal dosage. Always consider medications as a potential cause of, or contributing factor to, the patient's problem.

Vital Signs

Vital signs of the elderly should be similar to those of other adults. When they are not, it is an indication of illness or injury. Even so, normal vital signs do not rule out the presence of significant illness or injury. For example, the maximum heart rate decreases with age and as a side effect of some medications. Beta blockers, taken to treat dysrhythmias and hypertension, can prevent the heart rate from increasing in response to fever, shock, or other conditions. A seemingly normal blood pressure may, in fact, be low for a patient who has chronic, poorly controlled hypertension.

Medications taken for hypertension, as well as those taken for other conditions, can lead to hypotension, orthostatic hypotension (inability to compensate for the effects of gravity when standing up), syncope or near syncope. Even a normal dosage of medications can result in side effects that affect the vital signs. But the problem may be more complicated. The patient may be forgetful about having taken his medication and may have taken more than the prescribed dosage, or the medication may be interacting with another medication.

Physical Exam

For a critical patient, perform a rapid medical exam or rapid trauma exam. The chief complaint and medical history guide a focused physical exam for noncritical medical complaints. For trauma patients, the mechanism of injury and chief complaint guide the focused physical exam. Perform a detailed head-to-toe exam for patients with significant trauma and for critical medical patients in whom the nature of the problem has not been determined.

When performing a physical exam on an older person, there are a few things to keep in mind. Some elderly patients have difficulty staying warm and may wear several layers of clothing, even in warm weather. The layers of clothing can make taking a blood pressure, watching chest wall movement to assess respirations, and other aspects of the physical exam challenging. Do not cut the patient's clothing unless absolutely necessary, such as you would need to for a patient in a significant motor vehicle collision. It may be hard for the elderly patient on a limited income to replace the clothing you cut. Instead, if appropriate for the patient's condition, work with him to remove his arm from a sleeve or take off an extra shirt.

Elderly patients may have limited range of motion and some movements can be painful, so be patient and gentle. Remember that the skin is easily injured. Also, keep in mind the patient's dignity and modesty. Explain what you are going to do before you do it and replace any clothing you remove as soon as possible.

The physical exam is approached in the same order as for other patients, but there are special considerations. Some elderly patients can have decreased sensitivity to pain and may not complain of the level of pain expected with certain conditions. An elderly patient can have a serious abdominal emergency or extremity fracture without complaining of severe pain or tenderness. On the other hand, pre-existing conditions can increase the patient's level of pain on exam. As always, you must consider all findings in context and be aware of the possibility of altered pain perception.

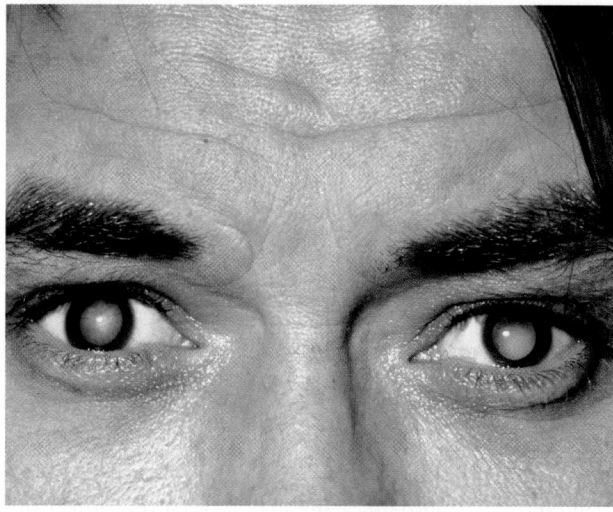

FIGURE 45-2

Cataracts appear as cloudiness of the lens of the eye.
(© SPL/Photo Researchers, Inc.)

When examining the head and neck, you might find that the pupils are not round or do not react normally to light. Pre-existing eye problems and eye surgery can result in pupil changes or cloudiness of the lens (Figure 45-2). Consider the finding in the context of the patient's overall presentation and ask the patient if he has a history of eye problems, such as **cataracts**, glaucoma, or eye surgery. The neck may be stiff, with limited range of motion and pain with movement. Kyphosis may require modifications to airway management and spinal immobilization. Do not force the neck beyond the patient's normal range of motion. Use towels beneath the head to maintain alignment if necessary (Figure 45-3).

Breath sounds can be diminished because of decreased lung capacity and decreased chest wall movement. Wheezes, rhonchi, and crackles (rales) are indications of respiratory

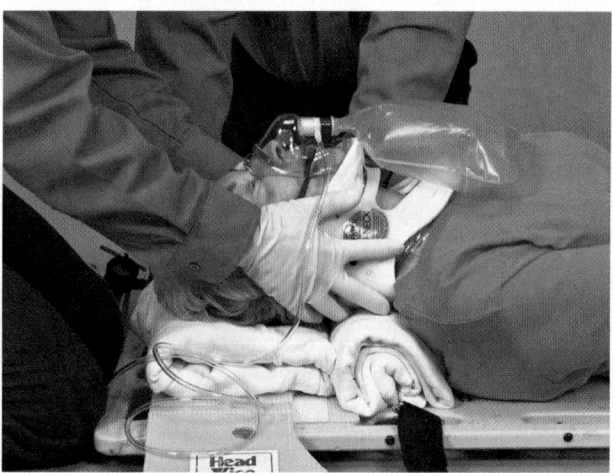

FIGURE 45-3

Place padding beneath the head of a patient with kyphosis when placing him supine or securing him to a backboard.

or cardiac problems. In some cases, an elderly patient can have crackles in the bases of the lungs that disappear after the patient has taken a few deep breaths. If faint crackles are heard in the bases, recheck the breath sounds after the patient has taken a few deep breaths. Check the lower extremities for edema, which can be an indication of cardiovascular, renal, or liver disease.

Clinical-Reasoning Process

The elderly are affected by many of the injuries and illnesses that affect middle-aged and younger adults. However, the signs and symptoms can present differently. You must be aware of variations in the presentations of illnesses and injuries in the elderly. The elderly can be very ill, yet complain of little pain. They may have severe infections without fever. Never take an elderly patient's complaints lightly because the complaint seems mild or vague. Many factors can interact to exacerbate or confound the patient's presentation. Consider the effects of aging on the body systems and the possibility of drug side effects and interactions. When deliberating the meaning of individual findings, remember that they are best interpreted in light of the patient's overall presentation.

Do not assume that an elderly patient is an unreliable source of information. Still, carefully assess the mental status. If it is not clear that the patient is oriented to person, place, and time, perform a MMSE. If needed, confirm information with the patient's family or caretakers.

Treatment

In general, treatment for illnesses and injuries are the same in elderly patients as in younger patients. Airway management and ventilation can be challenging due to loss of dentition or poorly fitting dentures, or changes in the alignment of the spine. If possible, keep dentures in place to achieve a good seal between a ventilation mask and the face. Use padding under the head for airway positioning. Controlling bleeding can be complicated by

coagulopathies (blood clotting disorders), but you can still control most external bleeding by direct pressure. The elderly patient can easily be overloaded with fluids. Use caution when administering IV fluids, even when the patient is hypovolemic. Spinal immobilization requires special attention to padding to avoid increasing tissue pressure, which leads to decubitus ulcers. Padding is also required to achieve proper immobilization and to increase patient comfort.

Reassessment

Base the frequency of reassessment on the patient's condition. Reassess critical patients every 5 minutes or sooner. Reassess noncritical patients at intervals of no longer than 15 minutes. Monitor the patient for changes in mental status, complaints, and vital signs, and assess the effects of treatment. Compare the trends of reassessments to the baseline findings. Adjust your clinical impression, the patient's priority, and treatment plan as needed.

Additional Considerations

Although it is difficult to imagine what life might be like at an older age, do your best to see things from the patient's perspective. Give the elderly patient the respect he deserves. Do not speak to family or caregivers instead of speaking to the patient. Use Mr., Ms., or Mrs. and the patient's last name, unless he or she asks you to use his or her first name. Make eye contact with the patient and listen patiently to his responses.

A serious injury or illness is a major stressor for most people. For the elderly, the ability to live independently can evaporate in an instant, leaving him dependent on others. Hospitals can trigger painful memories. Many friends and family may have been admitted to the hospital for serious illnesses, some of them never to return. You can help by being empathetic and not minimizing the patient's fears. Reassure the patient that you are there to take good care of him. If the patient's demeanor suggests

PERSONAL PERSPECTIVE

Mrs. Dianna Jennings: My husband, Herb, is 89 years old and has developed many health problems over the past few years. He has heart failure and kidney failure, and he gets urinary tract infections a lot. He normally is pretty with it, mentally, but when he gets an infection, he gets confused. He doesn't know who I am or where he is and he tries to walk out the door to "go home." He is a big guy, but he is weak and he has fallen a few times when he has gotten confused. He has gotten a few really bad bruises and he broke two ribs last fall, and then he got pneumonia because of that.

It has gotten so I can't handle him by myself when he gets confused. I have had to call the ambulance three times in the past year. The Advanced EMTs are always so nice. They are professional and respectful to both Herb and me. They always take good care of Herb, even though he can be difficult. They make sure I am doing okay and help me figure out whether I should ride with them and call somebody to pick me up later, or meet them there. It is such a relief to know that help is there when we need it.

that it would be welcome, a comforting hand on the forearm or shoulder can reassure the patient.

Patients who live alone may have many concerns about leaving their residence unattended. The patient could be the primary caregiver for an elderly spouse who cannot be left alone. There might be pets that need to be tended to or other worries. Ask the patient if he would like you to lock up before you leave the house, or if he needs you to check on anything before you leave the scene. If there is an elderly spouse or other family member who will be left alone or if there are pets, ask whether there is a neighbor who can take care of them for a while, or if there is someone you can call for them.

Keep the patient warm and protect him from the elements. Handle the patient gently and respectfully, telling him what you are going to do before you do it. Talking with the patient during transport about what he has done over the course of a lifetime can be beneficial for the patient and informative for you.

Respiratory Disorders

Ventilatory capacity and oxygen uptake decrease with aging. In the presence of a respiratory disorder, the elderly patient can easily become hypoxic. Always consider hypoxia as a cause of altered mental status in the elderly. The patient who is drowsy, confused, or combative may be suffering from an underlying respiratory problem, such as pneumonia or a pulmonary embolism. Causes of dyspnea and hypoxia in the elderly include the following:

- Anemia
- Asthma
- COPD
- Heart failure with pulmonary edema
- Lung cancer (and complications, such as pleural effusion)
- Myocardial infarction
- Pneumonia
- Pneumothorax
- Pulmonary embolism

Sometimes the signs and symptoms of those disorders are the same as in younger patients, but they also may present atypically.

Pneumonia is a common cause of death in the elderly, and may be community acquired or nosocomial (acquired in the health care setting). Immobility and respiratory system changes increase the risk of pneumonia. (See Chapter 28.) The patient may have fever, chills, pleuritic chest pain (pain that is worse with inspiration), tachypnea, dyspnea, a productive cough, and altered mental status. However, fever can be absent and pain can be referred to the abdomen. The treatment goals are to support the airway, ventilation, and oxygenation to maintain an SpO_2 of 95 percent or higher and to treat dehydration with careful administration of IV fluids, according to your protocol.

The elderly have many risk factors for pulmonary embolism, including deep vein thrombosis; immobility; cancer; fractures of the pelvis, femur (hip), or leg; recent major surgery; indwelling catheters; and atrial fibrillation. Suspect pulmonary embolism with a sudden onset of dyspnea. Massive pulmonary embolism can quickly lead to hypoxia and cardiac arrest. Other signs and symptoms include pain in the lower leg (possibly indicating deep vein thrombosis), often with a positive Homan's sign (increased calf pain with dorsiflexion of the foot), and pleuritic chest pain. Treat the patient for hypoxia and hypotension and transport without delay to the closest appropriate facility.

Pulmonary edema in the elderly is often a result of left-sided heart failure. The patient may have a history of heart failure, or may have suffered a myocardial infarction with subsequent failure of the left ventricle. Pulmonary edema can occur at any time, but patients often awake with severe dyspnea a few hours after lying down to sleep. The patient may have severe pulmonary congestion with the production of copious amounts of frothy, sometimes blood-tinged, sputum. The patient often has tachypnea and is anxious, with signs of severe respiratory distress. Respiratory failure, respiratory arrest, and cardiac arrest can ensue rapidly. The physical examination may reveal crackles in the lungs, sometimes accompanied by wheezing and rhonchi; hypertension; jugular vein distention; and edema in the lower extremities.

Patients with pulmonary edema can be challenging to treat. They can be in respiratory failure, requiring ventilatory assistance, yet their level of responsiveness does not permit the insertion of an advanced airway device. CPAP can be helpful in improving oxygenation through positive end-expiratory pressure. Use a bag-valve-mask device, if necessary, to assist ventilations. Unless the patient's level of responsiveness is substantially decreased, keep the patient in a sitting position. Administer supplemental oxygen with a goal of maintaining an SpO_2 of 95 percent or higher. Obtain IV access, but do not administer IV fluids. A saline lock is an excellent option for patients with pulmonary edema. If transport time is long, medical direction may order administration of nitroglycerin, if allowed in your scope of practice for treatment of pulmonary edema.

Cardiovascular Disorders

Cardiovascular diseases in the elderly include acute coronary syndrome (ACS), hypertension, heart failure, cardiogenic shock, dysrhythmia, and aortic aneurysm or dissection. A common presentation in the elderly patient with a cardiovascular problem is syncope. Even though there are other causes of syncope, you must always consider a cardiovascular emergency in the elderly patient with syncope or near syncope.

Although the elderly patient can present with the same signs and symptoms of cardiovascular disease as younger patients, the incidence of silent myocardial infarction and atypical presentations increases substantially with age. An elderly patient with acute myocardial infarction (AMI) can present with epigastric or abdominal pain or discomfort instead of chest pain or discomfort. The patient also may complain of pain in the neck, jaw, or teeth. The elderly patient may not experience pain at all when experiencing an AMI. He may suddenly become weak or short of breath with physical activity, complain of generalized weakness or fatigue, have a syncopal episode, or present with dyspnea, faintness, or altered mental status.

Treat chest pain of suspected cardiac origin in an elderly patient the same as you do in younger patients. Maintain an SpO_2 of 95 percent or higher. Administer nitroglycerin and aspirin according to your protocols. (See Chapter 21.) Start an IV and transport without delay to a hospital capable of managing cardiac emergencies. If the patient does not complain of chest pain, yet ACS is high on your list of differential diagnoses, administer oxygen, if the SpO_2 is less than 95 percent, and start an IV. Check with medical direction for further orders. In the absence of chest pain or discomfort, the presence of ACS is much less certain and the medical direction physician may prefer to obtain an ECG prior to initiating treatment.

Consider aortic aneurysm or dissection in patients who present with abdominal pain, back pain, unexplained shock, or loss of pulses, sensation, or function, particularly of one or both of the lower extremities. A palpable pulsating mass can sometimes be felt in the midline of the lower abdomen in patients with aortic aneurysm, but absence of that finding does not rule it out. Check and document the characteristics of the pulses in all four extremities.

Consider all causes of shock in the elderly patient presenting with signs of hypoperfusion. (See Chapter 17.) In addition to cardiogenic shock, septic shock is common in the elderly. Also consider hypovolemic shock, which may be caused by trauma, internal bleeding (gastrointestinal bleeding, aortic dissection, or aortic aneurysm), or dehydration. Obstructive shock can occur due to cardiac tamponade, tension pneumothorax, or pulmonary embolism.

Neurologic Disorders

There are many causes of altered mental status in the elderly. (Remember AEIOU TIPS from Chapter 22.) Consider hypoxia, infection, hypoperfusion, hyperthermia, hypothermia, endocrine disorders, poisoning, overdose, and trauma in addition to neurologic causes of altered mental status. Neurologic causes of altered mental status include stroke, transient ischemic attack (TIA), seizures, and dementia. Always search for immediately reversible causes of altered mental status, including hypoxia, hyperthermia, hypothermia, and hypoglycemia.

The elderly have several risk factors for stroke, including atherosclerotic disease, atrial fibrillation, hypertension, and coagulopathies. For suspected stroke, complete a stroke screening tool (Los Angeles Prehospital Stroke Screen or Cincinnati Prehospital Stroke Scale). Manage hypoxia and hypoglycemia, if they are present. Transport the patient without delay to the closest hospital capable of definitive stroke care.

Seizures may occur in the elderly for a variety of reasons, including epilepsy, stroke (especially hemorrhagic stroke), traumatic brain injury (current or past), medications, hypoglycemia, alcohol withdrawal, or tumor. Syncope and cardiac arrest also can be interpreted by witnesses as being seizures. When responding to a call for a seizure, keep those possibilities in mind.

Vertigo (dizziness) can occur for many reasons in the elderly, including stroke, sudden changes in position, and Ménière's disease. (See Chapter 22.) Vertigo can be accompanied by diaphoresis, nausea, and vomiting and can either be of short duration or ongoing. Patients often use the term *dizziness* to mean faintness or lightheadedness. Be sure to ask the patient to explain the nature of the sensation. Vertigo is a spinning or tumbling sensation of moving through space although stationary, while faintness usually involves a temporary narrowing or loss of vision, sounds becoming distant, and sensation of almost "passing out" or "blacking out"

Both **delirium** and dementia occur commonly in the elderly. Delirium is a sudden onset of altered mental status, often with changes in behavior, such as aggressiveness, due to an underlying medical cause such as infection, renal failure, hypoperfusion, hypoxia, hypoglycemia, or medications. Delirium tends to be less pronounced earlier in the day, becoming worse toward evening. Dementia is a progressive, irreversible, global impairment of cognitive function. A common cause of dementia is **Alzheimer's disease**. Many studies indicate that exercise, maintaining social relationships, a healthy diet, and engaging in challenging cognitive activities can protect against or delay the onset of the signs and symptoms of age-related cognitive decline.

Parkinson's disease is more common in patients over the age of 50, and is related to a degeneration of dopamine-producing cells in the brain. Signs and symptoms include postural rigidity, tremors, and loss of facial expression. Depression is common in patients with Parkinson's disease.

Renal and Genitourinary Disorders

Renal failure and urinary problems are common in the elderly. Urinary tract problems include urinary retention, urinary incontinence, and urinary tract infections. Urinary retention increases the risk of urinary tract infection and can be caused by medications, neurologic problems, and in males, an enlarged prostate gland. (See Chapter 25.)

Poor hygiene due to physical disability, cognitive decline, and other factors increases the risk of urinary tract infection, as does placement of a Foley catheter. There is a high prevalence of urinary tract infection in patients with a Foley catheter, and you should assume infection as part of your differential diagnosis process.

Urinary **incontinence** (loss of bladder control) may occur due to poor pelvic muscle tone, decreased sensation, cognitive impairment, or immobility. Treat the patient with urinary incontinence with respect and in a manner that preserves his dignity. If possible, remove and replace wet clothing before transporting the patient.

Gastrointestinal Disorders

Many gastrointestinal complaints in the elderly are indications of other disease processes or side effects of medications. Nausea, vomiting, diarrhea, and constipation are common side effects of many drugs. Nausea, vomiting, and diarrhea can lead to decreased fluid intake and increased fluid losses, leading to dehydration. Constipation can lead to bowel obstruction, if not treated. Abdominal bloating also can be a sign of bowel obstruction and other serious disorders. The elderly have several risk factors for mesenteric infarction, which can lead to bowel ischemia and necrosis, and the release of intestinal bacteria into the abdominal cavity with resultant sepsis and death.

A complaint of abdominal pain, regardless of severity and no matter how vague or specific, can be an indication of several serious, potentially life-threatening disorders in the elderly and you must never take it lightly. Also keep in mind that pain can be referred to the abdomen from pneumonia and AMI, so keep those problems in mind as you perform your assessment. Gastrointestinal bleeding is a common problem in the elderly, and can lead to hypovolemia and death. Upper gastrointestinal bleeding can also compromise the airway.

Bowel incontinence (loss of control of the bowels) is less frequent than urinary incontinence, but can occur. Contributing factors include diarrhea; neurologic problems, such as loss of sensation and loss of sphincter tone; immobility; and cognitive impairment. If bowel incontinence occurs, help the patient maintain his dignity. Clean up the patient because prolonged contact with fecal matter can lead to skin breakdown.

Endocrine Disorders

The incidence of type 2 diabetes increases with age, and the cumulative effects of both type 1 and type 2 diabetes can result in a number of complications in the elderly, including impaired vision, atherosclerotic disease, infection, and lower extremity amputations. Consider diabetic emergencies as a cause of altered mental status in the elderly and obtain a blood glucose level as you would in any patient with altered mental status. Major surgery, infection, or illness, such as myocardial infarction, can increase the risk of diabetic ketoacidosis (DKA) and hyperosmolar hyperglycemic nonketotic coma (HHNC). Treat diabetic emergencies as you would for younger patients. Administer 50 percent dextrose intravenously for hypoglycemia or, if you cannot obtain IV access, administer glucagon intramuscularly. Give IV fluids for DKA and HNKC, but carefully monitor breath sounds and vital signs for indications of fluid overload.

Also consider endocrine disorders such as hyperthyroidism (including Grave's disease), hypothyroidism (myxedema), and complications of corticosteroid treatment or withdrawal.

Infectious Disease

Decreased immune system function makes infectious disease a significant cause of death among the elderly. You should consider pneumonia, influenza, and sepsis (from a variety of sources) as causes of illness in the elderly. Herpes zoster (shingles) is a reactivation of the chickenpox virus, which often occurs in patients over the age of 50 years. The virus lies dormant along a dorsal nerve root and manifests as severe, unilateral pain, often with a vesicular (having fluid-filled blisters) rash, along the dermatome that corresponds to the affected nerve. Herpes zoster most often manifests on the trunk, but also can affect cranial nerves, affecting the head and face.

The cough reflex can be impaired, resulting in a diminished cough, and the elderly patient may not have a fever, despite severe infection. Altered mental status is a frequent presentation in the elderly patient with a serious infection. Consider infection among your hypotheses in elderly patients presenting with altered mental status, generalized weakness or fatigue, or signs of poor perfusion (which may indicate septic shock).

The medical history is important in your clinical reasoning process, too. Risk factors for infection include having a Foley catheter or indwelling catheter in place, residing in an extended care facility, immunosuppressant medications (such as corticosteroids and medications for autoimmune disease and to prevent transplanted organ rejection) and pre-existing illnesses such as COPD, diabetes, heart failure, and cancer.

Musculoskeletal Disorders

Musculoskeletal pain is common in the elderly. Disorders include osteoarthritis, osteoporosis, and pain and decreased range of motion due to immobility and injury. Fractures can occur with little force in weakened bones (pathologic fractures). A minor fall can result in fractures of the vertebrae, ribs, or long bones. In some cases, it can be unclear whether a fall resulted in a fracture, or whether a pathologic fracture of the hip (proximal femur, femoral trochanter, or femoral neck) sustained upon standing or walking resulted in a fall.

The extremity with a fractured hip often presents as being shortened, compared to the uninjured side, and externally rotated (hip dislocations usually result in an internally rotated extremity). The patient may complain of severe pain, or may complain of little pain, despite having a fracture. As part of the assessment, check the distal neurovascular status of the extremity. Often, the best way to splint a hip fracture in the elderly patient is to use pillows for padding and support. A scoop stretcher is an ideal way to lift and move the patient with minimal movement of the injured site. If your protocols allow and the patient has no contraindications, consider administering nitrous oxide before moving the patient. If you must use a long backboard because of suspected associated spine injury, pad the board well to protect against increasing tissue pressure and to minimize patient discomfort.

Fractures can result in many complications in the elderly. Pain that restricts deep breathing and coughing, and immobility increase the risk for pneumonia. Immobility also increases the risk for pulmonary embolism. The patient who was, just moments ago, independent and able to care for himself, may suddenly be faced with hospitalization, surgery, and dependence on others. Injury prevention is important in the elderly. A few minor repairs and changes in the home, such as good lighting, removing throw rugs, and repairing steps, thresholds, and banisters, can prevent many injuries. Maintaining muscle strength and flexibility are also keys to preventing injuries.

Arthritis is a major source of discomfort and can substantially interfere with activities of daily living. Osteoarthritis can affect any joint, but commonly affects the neck, back, hands, hips, and knees. **Spondylosis**, degeneration of the vertebrae and intervertebral discs, can affect the neck and back, limiting mobility and increasing the risk for spine injury. Some medications taken for arthritis can increase the risk of upper gastrointestinal bleeding. In severe cases, the diseased joint may be replaced with a prosthetic (artificial) joint.

Be gentle when assessing, treating, and moving elderly patients. Abrupt movements or moving joints beyond their range of motion can be painful and can cause injury. Allow patients extra time to move in compliance with your requests.

Hematologic Disorders

Hematologic disorders in the elderly include anemia, leukemia, and coagulopathies. Anemia can result from many underlying causes, including renal disease, decreased nutrient intake and absorption, occult (unnoticed) gastrointestinal bleeding, and other illnesses. The anemic patient may present with weakness, fatigue, and dyspnea on exertion. The

skin and mucous membranes may be pale. In anemia the SpO_2 may be normal, but the overall lack of hemoglobin results in tissue hypoxia. In severe cases, patients may have chest pain and heart failure.

Coagulopathies may result from immobility and circulatory stasis with increased risk for blood clotting, or from medication side effects or illnesses, such as liver disease, that decrease blood clotting. Keep in mind that many medications can impair blood clotting. Obtain a complete list of medications, including prescription and over-the-counter medications and supplements. The presence of bruising or purpura can be an indication of coagulopathy. Patients may present with epistaxis, or can be at increased risk for bleeding after injury.

Behavioral Emergencies

Behavioral emergencies in the elderly can result from underlying psychiatric illness, dementia, or delirium due to illness or medications. Always consider hypoxia, hypoglycemia, stroke, infection, toxicologic emergencies, trauma, and other medical causes of behavior change. Never assume that abnormal behavior in an elderly person is a result of dementia. Determine the patient's baseline behavior and mental status and find out what the progression of behavior change was. A sudden change in behavior is often the result of a medical emergency. The patient with a behavioral emergency is often confused, disoriented, and frightened. Stay calm and do your best to calm and reassure the patient using techniques of therapeutic communication. However, do not underestimate the ability of an elderly patient to harm himself or others, and be prepared to restrain the patient, if necessary. Use only the force necessary, maintaining awareness of the ease with which the elderly patient can be injured.

Depression and suicide are common in the elderly. Do not overlook the possibility of depression in the patient with flat or sad affect or who gives slow, halting responses to questions. Suicide attempts in the elderly come in many guises. Cardiac arrest, dysrhythmia, or altered mental status may be the result of an overdose. What appears to be an accidental collision may, in fact, be a suicide attempt. In other cases, such as with self-inflicted gunshot wounds, the suicide attempt may be more obvious.

Toxicologic Emergencies

There are several factors that contribute to toxicologic emergencies in the elderly. Diminished liver and kidney function, decreased plasma proteins, decreased total body water, and decreased adipose tissue all can result in increased plasma levels of drugs. Polypharmacy can result in unanticipated drug interactions. When more than one protein-bound drug competes for protein binding sites, or when more than one drug uses the same liver enzymes in its metabolism, the free levels of the drugs increase. Forgetfulness can lead to taking multiple doses of medications. Finally, you must not overlook intentional overdose as a cause of toxicologic emergency. Although specific signs and symptoms of toxicologic emergencies are related to the substances involved, suspect a toxicologic emergency in any patient with an altered mental status, behavioral change, or abnormal vital signs. Be sure to collect a thorough medication history. Checking the dates when prescriptions were filled and comparing the amount of medication present with the expected amount can give clues to possible inadvertent or intentional overdose.

Trauma in the Geriatric Population

Mechanisms of Injury

Motor vehicle collisions and falls are major causes of injury in the elderly. As age increases, falls become an even more significant cause of injury, with falls in the home accounting for many injuries in the elderly population. Crimes are committed against the elderly, as well, and injuries can be a result of abuse, being injured as a result of a mugging or robbery, or sexual assault. Burns can occur easily in the elderly.

Shock

Consider all causes of shock in the elderly patient presenting with signs of hypoperfusion. Sepsis and cardiogenic shock should be high on your list of hypotheses, as well as hypovolemic shock. Decreased protection afforded by the musculoskeletal system and amount of adipose tissue can increase the potential for organ injury in blunt trauma. Impaired blood clotting can exacerbate blood loss. An early sign of hypoperfusion is altered mental status. The homeostatic mechanisms of elderly patients may not respond to blood loss with the efficiency of younger patients. The heart rate may not be increased and the patient might not exhibit diaphoresis. What appears to be a normal blood pressure may actually be low for a patient with pre-existing unmanaged hypertension.

Rely heavily on mechanism of injury in determining the potential for shock. Ensure that the patient has an open airway and adequate ventilation and oxygenation. Administer

---

IN THE FIELD

Tissue pressures high enough to cause ischemia and set in motion the events that eventually lead to decubitus ulcer can occur in as little as 30 minutes. If the elderly patient does not have a mechanism of injury consistent with spinal trauma, do not use a long backboard. Pad all hard surfaces with which the patient may come in contact and avoid creating friction on the skin.

---

oxygen, if needed, to maintain an SpO_2 of 95 percent or higher. Obtain IV access, preferably in two sites, using large-bore catheters. Infuse isotonic crystalloids according to protocol, but carefully monitor breath sounds and vital signs for signs of fluid overload.

Fractures

As discussed previously under musculoskeletal disorders, fractures can occur easily in the elderly. Maintain a high index of suspicion for fracture in the elderly, based on mechanism of injury. Assess and treat fractures as you would in other patients. Pay particular attention to padding splints to prevent injury to the skin. Remember that a long backboard is a splint and you must also pad it to prevent the increase in tissue pressure that leads to ischemia and later development of decubitus ulcers.

For patients who require a cervical collar, ensure that placement of the device does not force the neck into a position that is unnatural for the patient and does not interfere with opening the mouth or airway management. If a suitable cervical collar cannot be found, make a collar using a folded towel or thin blanket rather than using an improperly fitting collar. Pad under the head, if necessary, to prevent spinal extension in the patient with kyphosis.

Burns

The elderly may be burned as a result of residential fires, cooking accidents, falling asleep smoking, or smoking while using oxygen. Hot tap water is also a cause of burns in the elderly. Like pediatric patients, the skin of the elderly is thin. Lower temperature and shorter exposure time are needed to cause significant burns in the elderly. In addition, decreased sensation may not allow the elderly person to realize he is being burned until substantial tissue damage has occurred. The elderly patient with impaired mobility may be unable to remove himself from a source of heat, such as a heating pad or wrap that has been overheated.

All patients with extensive burns are at risk for hypothermia. The elderly patient's decreased thermoregulatory ability increases the risk for hypothermia. Elderly patients may have pre-existing dehydration, contributing to the complication of fluid loss with burns. Administer fluids, as indicated by the extent of body surface area involved, but monitor the patient closely for signs of fluid overload. Also remember that large amounts of IV fluids lower the body temperature. Keep the patient compartment of the ambulance warm and keep the patient covered to prevent heat loss. If your service allows, use an IV fluid warmer to prevent hypothermia.

The threshold for transporting an elderly patient to a burn center is lower than that for younger patients. (See Chapter 35.) The presence of heart, lung, kidney, or liver disease also increases the severity of burns and complicates the patient's ability to recover from them.

Environmental Emergencies

The impaired thermoregulatory function of the elderly increases their risk for heat- and cold-related emergencies. Housing with inadequate heating and cooling increase the risk, as well. Elderly patients who are

CASE STUDY WRAP-UP

Clinical-Reasoning Process

Advanced EMTs Eddie and Harper are on the scene of a single-vehicle collision. The patient is an 86-year-old woman whom they determine is Mrs. Priscilla Ottinger. It appears that Mrs. Ottinger did not brake before striking the tree, a factor that makes Eddie consider that she might have experienced a medical problem that caused the collision. Although the damage to the vehicle is not extensive, the patient's age and the fact that she is presenting with confusion and difficulty breathing increase Eddie's suspicion that Mrs. Ottinger may have sustained significant injury in the collision.

Eddie categorizes the patient as critical and recognizes that she meets criteria for transport to a trauma center. The EMT assessing the patient tells Eddie that the patient has crackles in her lower lung fields bilaterally, that her skin is cool and moist, and that she has a weak, thready, rapid radial pulse. Eddie leads the team in coordinating rapid extrication from the vehicle. Eddie performs a rapid trauma assessment, during which he notices the neck veins are flat, there are abrasions to the chest and abdomen consistent with the seat belts, and no other signs of injury. The patient does not know what happened, what the day, month, or year is, or where she is.

After ensuring that the patient is properly immobilized, with attention to padding the backboard and supporting the patient's head in its slightly anterior normal position, the team places the patient in the ambulance. One of the EMTs from the rescue squad agrees to drive the ambulance. While taking a set of vital signs and performing a detailed head-to-toe exam, Eddie and Harper discuss potential causes of confusion with pale, cool skin, and a rapid, weak, thready pulse. They agree that the findings indicate poor perfusion, so they discuss causes of shock.

"If a medical problem came before the collision, I'm thinking cardiac is a likelihood," Harper says. "The abdomen is soft, I don't feel any masses and there doesn't seem to be any tenderness, so I don't think it's an aortic aneurysm, and there hasn't been any vomiting or stools that would tell us it is a GI bleed."

"Agreed," responds Eddie. "The weak, rapid pulse could be the cause of the problem, not the result. It could be a cardiac dysrhythmia that led to confusion or syncope and the collision. A dysrhythmia also could explain the crackles in the bases of her lungs."

"Let's get a blood glucose level to be sure she isn't hypoglycemic, which could explain the collision. In that case, I would be more inclined to think that shock is a result of injury, not a medical problem," says Harper.

The crew completes the vital signs and head-to-toe exam and obtains a blood glucose level and pulse oximetry reading. There are no indications of significant injury. There are no other injuries to the face and head aside from the abrasions and epistaxis. The pupils are equal and react to light, although a slight cloudiness hints at cataracts. The neck veins are flat and the trachea is in the midline. The patient's lung sounds are present and equal, with crackles in the bases. Chest wall movement is symmetrical and there is no instability, tenderness, or crepitus. The abdomen is soft, nontender, and nondistended. The pelvis is stable and compressing it does not result in pain. There are no obvious injuries to the lower extremities and the patient moves both legs. The lower extremities are cool and slightly mottled, consistent with overall poor perfusion. The upper extremities show no signs of injury and the patient is able to squeeze with both of her hands on command.

The pulse is regular at 168 beats per minute, respirations are 24 breaths per minute, the blood pressure is 100/58, pulse oximetry is 95 percent with oxygen by nonrebreather mask, and the blood glucose level is 124 mg/dL. Eddie comments that the heart rate is more consistent with a dysrhythmia than shock, and Hunter agrees.

Based on their radio report, the trauma team meets the crew and patient in one of the resuscitation rooms. One of the nurses attaches the patient to the cardiac monitor and states, "She's in ventricular tachycardia." Before continuing the trauma assessment, the emergency department physician treats the patient for the dysrhythmia, using synchronized cardioversion. Mrs. Ottinger's heart rhythm converts to normal, and her mental status improves. The continued trauma workup reveals only minor injuries, but Mrs. Ottinger is admitted for treatment of the dysrhythmia, which may have been the cause of the collision.

immobile may not be able to remove themselves from an environment that is too hot or too cold. Cognitive impairment can lead to an elderly patient wandering away and becoming lost. If temperatures are extreme, he may suffer from an environmental emergency in addition to suffering injuries, becoming dehydrated, and suffering from medical problems. In addition, a number of medical conditions and medications contribute to the risk of heat- and cold-related emergencies. Keep in mind the more limited ability of the elderly to maintain homeostasis in response to environmental changes and maintain a high index of suspicion for hyperthermia and hypothermia, even when the environment does not seem extreme to you.

CHAPTER REVIEW

Chapter Summary

The number of elderly people in the United States is at the highest level in history and is projected to rapidly increase over the coming years. Although many elderly patients enjoy good health, increasing age is associated with increasing risk for certain illnesses and injuries. As a result, Advanced EMTs frequently are called to care for elderly patients. Patience, respect, gentleness, and efforts to overcome potential challenges to communication all are important parts of providing high-quality, professional care to elderly patients. Communication difficulties can sometimes be minimized by retrieving the patient's hearing aid or dentures.

The combination of normal age-related changes, medications, and illnesses can create a diagnostic challenge. In some cases, illness and injuries can present differently in the elderly than in younger patients. The elderly patient might not complain of the level of pain expected and might not exhibit the expected homeostatic responses. The elderly also are at increased risk for complications from illnesses and injuries.

Common complaints among the elderly population include dyspnea, weakness, chest pain or discomfort, dizziness, and injuries from motor vehicle collisions and falls. Medication side effects, toxicity, and interactions are common in the elderly, making a thorough medication history an essential part of the assessment process.

For the most part, the principles of assessment and management that you learned throughout the text apply to the elderly, although there are some special considerations. For example, airway management and spinal immobilization can require padding to properly position the head and neck and you must administer intravenous fluids cautiously and monitor the patient closely to prevent fluid overload. Always consider the patient's perspective and what the illness or injury may mean to him. Understand that the elderly patient may be very reluctant to leave his home. Attempt to understand what his concerns are and do your best to address them.

Review Questions

Multiple-Choice Questions

1. You should consider an elderly person to be disoriented to time if he is unable to tell you what _____ it is.
   a. hour
   b. day of the week
   c. month
   d. year

2. On the average, people in the United States can expect to live to be about _____ years old.
   a. 65   c. 91
   b. 78   d. 120

3. Age-related changes of the lens of the eye can lead to difficulty seeing:
   a. up close.
   b. at night.
   c. far away.
   d. colors.

4. An 82-year-old woman says she started walking down some steps and when she put weight on her left leg she felt a "pop" in her left hip. She is complaining of pain in her left hip. The left leg appears shorter than the right and the foot is turned outward. The history and findings listed are most consistent with:
   a. deep vein thrombosis.
   b. osteoarthritis.
   c. pathologic fracture.
   d. spondylosis.

5. A patient has severe kyphosis. To compensate during airway management, you should:
   a. pad beneath the head.
   b. ask a family member to find the patient's dentures.
   c. use a long backboard to immobilize the spine in a position of extension.
   d. avoid the use of airway adjuncts and devices.

6. The federally funded and administered program to provide health care benefits to patients aged 65 years and older is called:

   a. supplemental insurance.
   b. Medicaid.
   c. Medicare.
   d. Social Security.

7. A pleasant but slightly confused elderly woman presents with a laceration over her right tibia. She tells you that she hurt her leg while picking strawberries. You find this doubtful, because the ground is covered with snow and outdoor temperatures are below freezing. You glance at the patient's daughter, who shakes her head and tells you that she isn't sure how her mother injured her leg, but that she has not been out of the house for a few days. The information provided to you by the patient is an example of:

   a. excited delirium.
   b. confabulation.
   c. dysphasia.
   d. perseveration.

8. Upon examining the pupils of a 75-year-old man, you notice that the right eye appears cloudy behind the pupil. That finding is most consistent with:

   a. hordeolum.
   b. cataract.
   c. presbyopia.
   d. retinal detachment.

9. An 85-year-old male complains of pain in his lower left jaw, weakness, and nausea for the past 12 hours. He tells you he thinks he has a "bad tooth." The jaw and surrounding soft tissues appear normal and are not tender to palpation. His skin is cool and dry, he has a heart rate of 88 beats per minute with a slight irregularity to the rhythm, his respirations are unlabored at 16 breaths per minute, his blood pressure is 142/96, and his SpO_2 is 97 percent on room air. He is alert and oriented to person, time, and place. He gives a past medical history of arthritis, for which he takes acetaminophen as needed. Which one of the following conditions should you most highly suspect?

   a. sepsis
   b. pneumonia
   c. acute coronary syndrome
   d. stroke

10. Until it is ruled out by a physician, you should always suspect that syncope in an elderly patient is caused by:

   a. a cardiac problem.
   b. vagal stimulation.
   c. medication side effects.
   d. hypoglycemia.

Critical-Thinking Questions

11. A 91-year-old woman presents with changes in mental status and behavior over the past 4 hours. Outline and explain your clinical reasoning process with respect to the patient's history and physical exam.

12. Explain how the same illness or injury that a younger person can easily recover from can be more complicated in an older patient.

References

Centers for Disease Control, National Center for Health Statistics. *FastStats*. (2010). Retrieved March 25, 2011, from http://www.cdc.gov/nchs/

U.S. Census Bureau. (2008a). Current population survey, annual social and economic supplement. Retrieved March 25, 2011, from http://www.census.gov/population/www/socdemo/age/older_2008.html

U.S. Census Bureau. (2008b). Table 2: Projections of the population by selected age groups and sex for the United States: 2010 to 2050. Retrieved March 25, 2011, from http://www.census.gov/population/www/projections/summarytables.html

46 Patients with Special Challenges

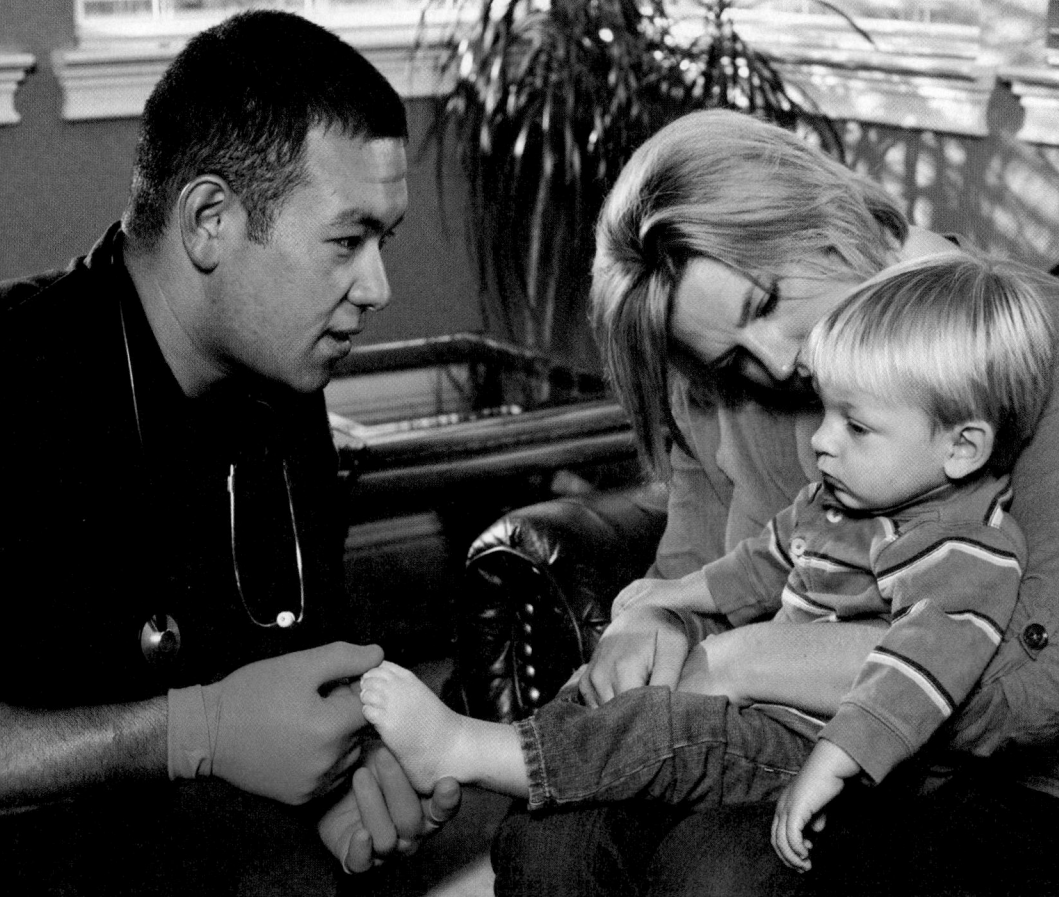

Content Area: Special Patient Populations

Advanced EMT Education Standard: The Advanced EMT applies a fundamental knowledge of growth, development, and aging and assessment findings to provide basic and selected advanced emergency care and transportation for a patient with special needs.

Objectives

After reading this chapter, you should be able to:

46.1 Define key terms introduced in this chapter.

46.2 Explain the importance of understanding the care of patients with special challenges.

46.3 Demonstrate empathy and respect when caring for patients with special challenges.

46.4 Advocate for the empathetic treatment of patients with a variety of special challenges.

46.5 Give examples of special challenges.

(continued)

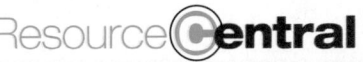

To access Resource Central, follow the directions on the Student Access Card provided with this text. If there is no card, go to www.bradybooks.com and follow the Resource Central link to Buy Access. Under Media Resources, you will find:

- *Autism.* The challenges of managing patients with autism.

- *Tracheostomy.* How to manage the tracheostomy patient's airway.

- *Intimate Partner Violence.* Why patients are victims of intimate partner violence and how prehospital professionals can help.

CASE STUDY

It is a Saturday afternoon and Advanced EMT Robert Mitchell and his partner Al Benson are dispatched to a residence for a "sick person."

"Unit 33 en route, sick person at 512 St. Mary Street," answers Al.

As they arrive at the residence, the Advanced EMTs notice that there is a wheelchair ramp leading up to the porch. Neither of them has responded to this residence before. They are met at the front door by a woman who introduces herself as the patient's mother. She states that her son Bobby is confined to a bed and is running a high fever with a pulse oximeter reading much lower than normal. "I'd like him to be brought to the hospital so a doctor can evaluate him," says the mother.

Problem-Solving Questions

1. What are the first actions that Robert and Al should take?
2. What are some potential causes of the patient's condition?
3. What additional information would assist Robert and Al in determining the cause of the patient's condition?

(continued from previous page)

46.6   Describe the special physiologic, medical, and psychosocial concerns, and accommodations and modifications to patient assessment and management that are required when caring for patients with each of the following types of challenges:
- Abused patients
- Bariatric patients
- Brain-injured patients
- Dialysis patients
- Homeless/impoverished patients
- Patients with mental, emotional, or developmental impairments
- Paralyzed patients
- Patients with gastrointestinal and genitourinary devices
- Patients with intraventricular shunts
- Patients with sensory impairments
- Technology-dependent patients
- Terminally ill patients

46.7   Describe common types of home medical equipment, including the following:
- Apnea monitors
- CPAP and BiPAP
- Feeding tubes
- Intraventricular shunts
- Mechanical ventilators
- Medical oxygen
- Ostomy bags
- Tracheostomy tubes
- Urinary catheters
- Vascular access devices

46.8   Describe the philosophy of hospice care.

Introduction

Special challenges that patients face can be the result of obesity, sensory impairments, paralysis, reliance on medical equipment such as a mechanical ventilator, or social conditions such as abuse, neglect, homelessness, or poverty. You can encounter patients with special challenges in a variety of settings, including homes, institutions, and public settings. In some cases, patients with disabilities are cared for by family members, and in others, by home health nurses. In other cases, patients with special challenges live in group homes, extended care facilities, or other institutions.

Not all special challenges that you encounter involve physical or intellectual challenges. Patients who are homeless, impoverished, or abused all face unique challenges. You must be empathetic to the patient's condition, not judgmental. Your job is to care for the patient regardless of his or her history, mental state, physical state, or living conditions.

When called upon to care for a patient with special challenges, he often is the most reliable source of information about his condition. In other cases, you may need to rely on his caregiver, either a family member or health care professional, for information. Family members who care for a relative with a disability or medical problem are usually very knowledgeable about the condition, the patient's history, and any medical equipment in the home.

Sensory and Speech Impairments

Sensory impairments involve one or more of the patient's senses. When a patient has a sensory or speech impairment, it can make communicating with him difficult. For instance, when caring for a deaf patient, it may be difficult or impossible for the patient to understand what you are trying to communicate verbally. In such cases, you can try writing down what you need to communicate, or using an interpreter or caregiver to assist with communication.

Hearing Impaired

Hearing impairment, also called *deafness*, is classified by either partial or total loss of hearing. Partial-loss deafness can involve one ear or both ears. Deafness, either partial or total, can be the result of a congenital condition, a brain injury, or an illness such as meningitis.

To assist them with hearing, many hearing impaired patients rely on hearing aids, which are sometimes worn behind the ear. Hearing aids may be obvious but in some cases they may be covered by the patient's hair and not visible. Patients also might rely on cochlear implants, which are electronic devices that are surgically implanted. An outside unit, worn behind the ear, attaches to the implanted unit by way of a magnetic connection through the skin. You may notice the small magnet attached to the patient's scalp

a couple of inches behind the ear. It is connected to the outside unit by a small wire.

When communicating with a patient who is partially deaf, it may be necessary for you to speak in a louder than normal voice so that you are understood, but shouting is not helpful because it distorts the sound of words. In order to improve the likelihood of a completely deaf patient understanding you, speak normally while looking directly at the patient, because many deaf patients rely on lip reading. This is true even for patients who use hearing aids and cochlear implants. Exaggerating pronunciation or speaking slowly will only make it more difficult for the patient to understand you.

Though some deaf patients cannot speak clearly, others are able to speak quite well and are easily understood. In situations where verbal communication is not possible, you should either utilize a family member or friend who can communicate with the patient through sign language. If that is not possible, use a pen and paper to communicate with the patient.

Vision Impaired

Vision impairment, also called *blindness*, is classified by either partial or total loss of vision. It is possible for a patient to have vision loss in only one eye, vision loss in specific visual fields, or total loss involving both eyes. Blindness can be congenital or the result of illness, infection, injury, or degenerative conditions involving the eye or optic nerve.

It is not uncommon to encounter a blind patient, or patient with another disability, who uses a service dog. If you encounter a patient with a service dog, do not attempt to pet the dog. Service animals are professionally trained to assist the patient in day-to-day living and are not meant to be pets. Unless the animal poses a threat to you, which would be extremely unusual, you must allow the animal to accompany the patient in the ambulance.

When caring for a patient who is blind, announce yourself to the patient as you approach, letting him know that you are an Advanced EMT and are there to assist. You should not touch the patient without first letting him know what you are going to do. Keep the patient abreast of what you are doing at all times, so that he is not startled by touch or noises associated with your actions.

Speech Impairment

In some cases, the patient you have been called to care for may not be able to effectively communicate with you. This lack of effective communication can be the result of one of the following four types of speech impairment: language disorders, articulation disorders, voice production disorders, and fluency disorders:

- *Language disorders.* A **language disorder** is the inability to understand spoken or written communication. It can be the result of impairments such as learning disorders, cerebral palsy, deafness, stroke, traumatic brain injury, or brain tumor.

- *Articulation disorders.* An **articulation disorder**, also known as *dysarthria*, is the inability to speak clearly. Articulation disorders can be the result of deafness or a disturbance of nerve impulses from the brain to the muscles used to articulate words. If you find that you are not able to understand the patient, enlist the assistance of family or friends, or ask the patient to use pen and paper to communicate with you.

- *Voice production disorders.* A voice production disorder is an impairment of normal voice in which hoarseness or unusual pitch results from damage to the larynx or vocal cords.

- *Fluency disorders.* A **fluency disorder** presents as stuttering speech. Patients repeat syllables or sounds while speaking or cannot appropriately put words together during speech. Do not interrupt these patients while they are attempting to speak to you. Instead, patiently allow them to complete what they are attempting to say.

Cognitive Impairment

Cognitive impairment can be the result developmental disorders, past traumatic brain injury or stroke, dementia, or mental illness.

When initially encountering these patients, it may not be obvious that they suffer from impairment. It is sometimes during your primary assessment when their impairment will become evident. For example, when you approach the patient, he may seem to be alert and oriented but once you begin to ask him questions, you may recognize that he is having difficulty communicating with you or his statements do not seem to make sense. When dealing with a patient who is severely cognitively impaired it may not be possible to effectively communicate with him. In such cases, you may have to rely on caregivers to provide you with information. In some types of cognitive impairment, judgment and inhibition are affected. So be alert to the potential for violent or otherwise inappropriate behavior.

Developmental Impairments

Patients with developmental impairments are those who have difficulty learning or a limited ability to learn. Those patients are encountered in a variety of settings such as private residences, nursing homes, or group homes. In some

IN THE FIELD

Treat developmentally impaired patient with respect and dignity. Enlist the assistance of caregivers and family members when needed and have them accompany the patient to the hospital with you. Doing so will reduce patient fear and anxiety as well as assist the hospital staff in obtaining information and care for the patient.

cases, it may not be evident that the patient has a developmental impairment until you begin your assessment. Many of them have mild impairment and can generally answer questions normally, but those with severe impairment cannot communicate effectively, which leads to difficulty in assessment, particularly when attempting to obtain a history of the present illness or injury and medical history. When called to care for a patient with severe developmental impairment, you may have to rely on primary caregivers or others on the scene to provide patient information to you.

If the patient is afraid of you, take extra time to gain trust prior to beginning your assessment. You are a stranger to the patient and the back of your ambulance is an unfamiliar environment. If possible, allow a caregiver to accompany the patient in the ambulance to provide a sense of familiarity and comfort. (Figure 46-1).

Brain-Injured Patients

Brain-injured patients can present with unique challenges because they sometimes have impairments in cognition, emotions, and behavior. Brain injury can be the result of a number of causes such as brain trauma, encephalitis, and meningitis. Those causes can result in minor to severe disability, ranging from subtle emotional changes to chronic unresponsiveness and the need for around-the-clock care.

Brain-injured patients often require the use of medical devices such as ventilators, catheters, and pumps for their

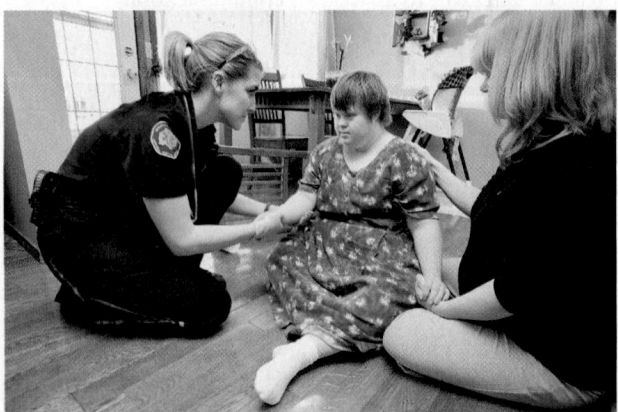

FIGURE 46-1

Developmentally impaired patients are often difficult to communicate with, so you should enlist the assistance of caregivers whenever possible.

day-to-day care. The individuals responsible for the care of the patient are well versed in proper use of the devices and their assistance to you can be invaluable. They also can provide you with the patient's medical history and the history of the present illness or injury.

Paralyzed Patients

Paralysis may be the result of trauma such as a spine injury or medical causes such as stroke or neuromuscular disease. The level of care required by patients for day-to-day living depends upon the extent of their paralysis. Some patients have paralysis of only one extremity. Others are paraplegic (paralysis from the waist down) or quadriplegic, also called tetraplegic (paralysis of all four extremities).

Patients who are paralyzed are susceptible to specific medical problems, including pressure sores, pneumonia, and urinary tract infections. You may see mechanical ventilators, urinary catheters, colostomy bags, and feeding tubes, all of which will be discussed later in this chapter. When caring for and transporting a patient who utilizes such equipment, you must take care not to allow device tubing to become caught on an object when transferring them to your stretcher and transporting them in the ambulance.

Bariatric Patients

Bariatrics is the branch of medical care that specializes in the care of obese patients. Over the past several years, there has been an alarming increase in the prevalence of obesity in the United States. According to the Centers for Disease Control and Prevention, in 2009 there were 33 states that had a prevalence of obesity of 25 percent or more (Mississippi being the highest with 34.4 percent). Only two states had a prevalence of obesity less than 20 percent: Colorado and the District of Columbia. Nearly all of the United States had an increase in prevalence of 10 percent or more since 1999 (Centers for Disease Control and Prevention, 2010).

Individuals who are obese not only suffer from limited mobility but are at higher risk for many serious medical conditions, such as coronary artery disease, diabetes, congestive heart failure, stroke, chronic obstructive pulmonary disease, and hypertension. As a result of an increasing prevalence of obesity and its medical implications, EMS is being called to care for and transport bariatric patients more frequently. Because of this increase, many EMS agencies have placed specialized bariatric ambulances into service. They are equipped with stretchers capable of holding very heavy

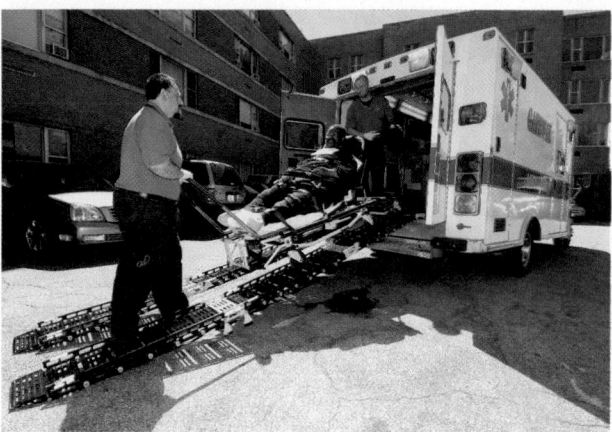

FIGURE 46-2

Many EMS agencies use specialized bariatric ambulances to transport obese patients. (© Ray Kemp/Triple Zilch Productions)

loads, ramps made for those stretchers, and motorized winches designed to pull a stretcher up the ramps and into the back of the ambulance (Figure 46-2).

Obesity occurs when the individual's caloric intake exceeds the amount of calories required to meet the body's needs. This is often the result of overeating or inadequate physical activity, but the underlying problem that causes the imbalance can be complex in some cases. An example of a medical condition resulting in low metabolic rates is hypothyroidism. Other causes of low metabolic rate may include medications such as anticonvulsants and certain antidepressants.

There are special considerations in caring for extremely obese patients. Placing an obese patient in supine position can lead to respiratory difficulty and a partially obstructed airway as a result of the weight of the patient's own tissues compressing the neck and thorax. The adipose tissue accumulation between the patient's shoulder blades can cause hyperextension of the neck that results in airway obstruction. In order to prevent this, allow the patient to assume a position of comfort or place rolled towels or sheets beneath the patient's shoulders and neck. Prior to attempting to lift an obese patient, ensure that you have adequate assistance to do it safely. This helps prevent you from being injured. It also will reduce the possibility of dropping the patient.

Homeless and Impoverished Patients

While it is difficult to get accurate data on the number of homeless individuals, there have been studies that provide a good estimate of the prevalence of homelessness in the United States. According to one study, there are 3.5 million people, 1.35 million of them children, who experience homelessness in any given year (National Coalition for the Homeless, 2009). Another study revealed that on one night there were approximately 672,000 homeless people on

---

IN THE FIELD

If you are unfamiliar with how to handle the patient's medical equipment, enlist the assistance of the caregiver because he or she will be very familiar with it.

one given night in January of 2007. Approximately 124,000 of them were chronically homeless. **Chronic homelessness** is defined as an unaccompanied individual with a disabling condition who has been continuously homeless for a year or more or has experienced four or more episodes of homelessness over the past three years (U.S. Department of Housing and Urban Development, 2009). Several factors contribute to an individual being homeless, including the following:

- Poverty
- Mental illness
- Lack of affordable housing
- Substance abuse
- Domestic violence
- Forced evictions (mortgage foreclosures)

Most of the time a homeless person may be focused on where their next meal will come from or locating shelter to escape from the weather, rather than making long-term plans to change their situation (Figure 46-3). Because of the environment they live in, the homeless are at risk for the following:

- Illness and disease (many have medical conditions and do not have the means to obtain proper medication)
- Violence
- Abuse
- Discrimination
- Unemployment (may be seen as not suitable for employment)

The homeless may sleep on the ground or on benches in public places. Because they do not have a residence, they must resort to finding shelter wherever they can. Such places include in parking garages, in abandoned buildings, beneath bridges, in vehicles, or in covered doorways to buildings.

Individuals who are impoverished, though they still have a home, often cannot afford to pay for necessities required to maintain a healthy lifestyle. According to the U.S. Census Bureau, in 2009 the poverty threshold was defined as an annual income of $21,954 for a family of four. In 2009,

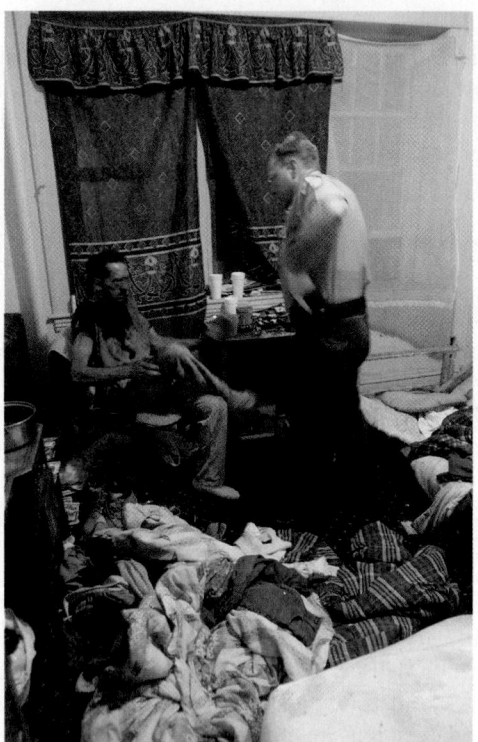

FIGURE 46-4

Impoverished individuals live in poor conditions and cannot afford basic necessities. (© Mark C. Ide)

the family poverty rate and the number of families in poverty were 11.1 percent and 8.8 million respectively, up from 10.3 percent and 8.1 million in 2008 (U.S. Census Bureau, 2009). Some of the necessities that those individuals cannot afford, placing them at risk for illness or injury, include the following:

- Prescription medications
- Medical care
- Utilities such as heat, air conditioning, and running water
- Proper clothing such as coats and shoes
- Nutritious food

In addition to these risks, homeless people often live in high-crime areas, which place them at greater risk to injury and abuse (Figure 46-4).

IN THE FIELD

When caring for individuals who are homeless or impoverished, care for him as you would anyone else. Do not be judgmental or prejudiced. You do not know the individual's circumstances. Be aware of special healthcare needs of the homeless and impoverished, such as lack of access to routine medical care or prescription medications.

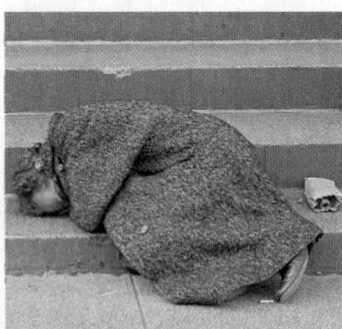

FIGURE 46-3

Homeless people are often seen in public with little to no personal belongings. (© Michal Heron)

Abused Patients

Individuals of every age are abused each day in the United States. The exact number of abuse instances cannot be determined because in many cases the abuse is not reported. Following are some statistics on abuse in the United States to give you an idea of the scope of the problem:

- One **child abuse** case is reported every 10 seconds and nearly five children die as a result of abuse each day in the United States (Childhelp, 2010).
- Approximately 4 to 6 percent of the elderly are abused annually in the United States (National Committee for the Prevention of Elder Abuse, 2010).
- Approximately 25 percent of women are victims of domestic violence once in their lifetime (Domestic Violence Resource Center, 2010).

Children and adults alike can be victims of abuse. Abuse can be categorized as the following:

- Physical force that results in bodily injury is called **physical abuse.**
- The willful infliction of mental or emotional anguish through threat, humiliation, or other verbal or nonverbal means is called **psychological abuse.**
- Sexual contact of any kind, nonconsensual for the competent adults and any kind for children, is called **sexual abuse.**
- The illegal or improper use of an individual's money, property, or resources is called **financial abuse.** It most often involves the elderly.
- Violence used to intimidate a partner to gain power or control is called **domestic abuse.**
- The failure of a caregiver to provide proper care to an individual for whom they are responsible is called **neglect.**

In many cases of abuse, the abuser is not reported. You must maintain a high index of suspicion to potential abuse or neglect. While it is not your role to confront the potential abuser, it is your role to report your suspicions to the proper authorities according to your state's guidelines.

Your goal is to remove the patient from the environment, care for him or her, and report your suspicions so that the authorities can intervene. Confronting the suspected abuser may lead to their refusal to allow you to transport the patient to the hospital. When documenting your patient

IN THE FIELD

You may find it difficult to maintain your composure when you suspect abuse of children or the elderly. Maintain emotional control so that you can remove the patient from the environment. After the patient is safe, report your suspicions to the proper authorities.

care report, include as much detail as possible, but be objective and factual and do not draw conclusions. Your report could be called into evidence if charges are pressed against the accused abuser.

Child Abuse

Child abuse affects children up to 18 years of age (Figure 46-5). The abuser of the child is most often someone the child knows and trusts, including the child's own parents. Other potential abusers include a family member (including step-relatives), babysitter, coaches, or anyone else who spends time with the child (Figure 46-6).

Characteristics of the Abuser

Child abuse occurs within all races and socioeconomic groups. Abusers tend to be male more often than female. Physical forms of discipline tend to become more severe over time and, in some cases can be severe enough to cause

Types of Child Abuse

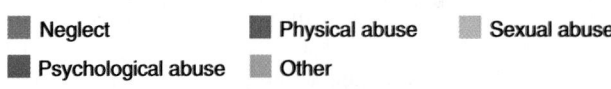
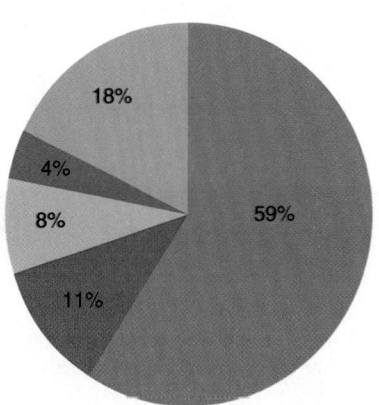

■ Neglect   ■ Physical abuse   ■ Sexual abuse
■ Psychological abuse   ■ Other

18%
4%
8%
11%
59%

FIGURE 46-5

Types of child abuse.

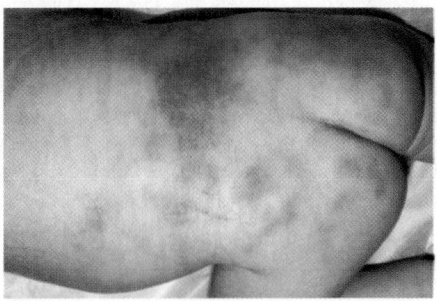

FIGURE 46-6

Bruising resulting from physical abuse. (© Biophoto Associates/ Photo Researchers, Inc.)

death. Some traits that are typical of an abuser include the following:

- Drug and/or alcohol abuse
- Obvious lack of concern for the child (no attempt to comfort the child)
- Lack of concern for the child's injuries or condition
- Blaming the child for the child's injuries or condition
- Open criticism of the child

If you observe any of these traits, suspect that the child is a victim of abuse and be alert for signs during your physical assessment.

Characteristics of Abuse

A child's behavior can be an important indicator of abuse. Behaviors that should alert you to the possibility of abuse include avoiding or pulling away from the parent or caregiver, wary or fearful of physical contact, and lack of normal crying or emotion consistent with the injury or situation.

You also may find that the parent or caregiver is evasive or provides contradictory information when answering questions about the child's injury or condition. In some cases the parent or caregiver may give information about how an injury occurred that is not consistent with the injury. For example, imagine a four-year-old patient has a fractured humerus and the parent is reporting that the patient fell off of a sofa onto the floor. This mechanism is not consistent with the child's injury. In other cases, the parent or caregiver may report that the patient injured himself intentionally. Children do not typically injure themselves

intentionally and such information should raise your suspicion to the possibility of abuse.

Elder Abuse

Elder abuse can occur in the patient's home, in nursing homes, and in other medical care facilities. Caring for an elderly person demands tremendous amounts of patience and time. Typically, elder abuse occurs when the caregiver is under additional stress such as financial burdens, job stress, and caring for other family members. Adult male children who are caring for an elderly parent are most likely to commit elder abuse.

The types of elder abuse are similar to those perpetrated on children (Figure 46-7). Financial abuse can occur with children but in most cases it occurs with the elderly. This type of abuse typically occurs when the caregiver and elderly person live in a private residence. Elderly people become incapacitated and dependent upon others but in many cases still have revenue from social security, pensions, or dividends from investments. When the caregiver takes advantage of the elderly person by misusing his money, financial abuse occurs.

As with child abuse, the characteristics of elder abuse may be evident in the patient's actions or in physical signs. The following is a general list of signs of elder abuse (Figure 46-8):

- Changes in personality or behavior
- Tension or frequent arguing between the patient and caregiver

PERSONAL PERSPECTIVE

Advanced EMT Bill Davis: My partner and I were called to a residence for an unknown emergency. Dispatch advised us that the caller was incoherent on the phone and no information could be obtained.

When we arrived on scene, law enforcement had already arrived. The residence was in a blighted neighborhood scattered with houses in poor condition. My partner and I advised dispatch that we had arrived at the scene and got out of the ambulance. As we were retrieving our gear, a female police officer approached us. "Oh my god, this is the worst thing I've seen in my life," she said.

Not knowing what could possibly be awaiting us inside the residence, my partner and I just looked at one another waiting for further information from the officer. As we walked toward the residence, the officer explained that there was a deceased male lying on the sofa and an elderly woman who looked very bad in a recliner. As we approached the front door of the residence, we could smell a horrible stench. In the front room of the house we found a dead man who appeared to be in his 30s on a sofa with obvious signs of death. Drug paraphernalia was visible on the table next to the sofa. In a corner of the room sat an elderly woman in a recliner who appeared to be very malnourished and weak. She could barely speak. She was

hypotensive and appeared to be very dehydrated. She must have been sitting in that chair for a very long period of time, because the chair was soaked in urine and feces.

We began assessment and treatment and attempted to move her to the stretcher, when we realized that the back of her legs and buttocks were actually stuck to the material of the chair. When we lifted her, it appeared to hurt the patient, so we decided to cut the material from the chair and transport her with it attached.

Later we were told by the police and hospital emergency department staff that the woman was living with her nephew who was her only surviving relative and a known drug user. The nephew apparently kept the woman in the chair for days to weeks on end, knowing that she could not walk, forcing her to sign her social security checks so he could cash them. It was determined that the nephew had been dead for approximately three days when neighbors, knowing the woman was in the home, called the police. The woman was admitted into the hospital and transferred to a nursing home when she was discharged.

This was a very difficult call for my partner and me. This woman had special challenges and relied on her nephew to properly care for her needs, but instead she was neglected and abused so that her nephew could support his drug habit.

Types of Elder Abuse

■ Neglect   ■ Physical abuse   ■ Financial abuse
■ Emotional abuse   ■ Sexual abuse   ■ Unknown
■ Other types

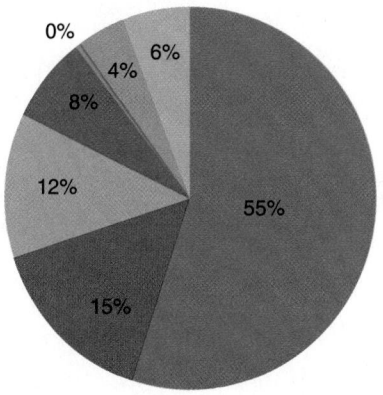

0%
6%
4%
8%
12%
55%
15%

FIGURE 46-7

Types of elder abuse. (Courtesy of the National Center on Elder Abuse)

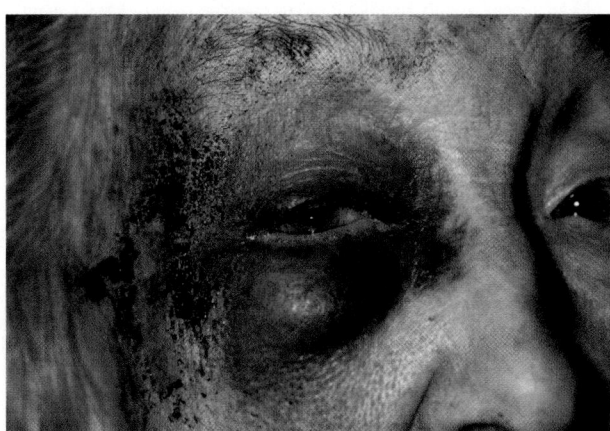

FIGURE 46-8

Signs of elder abuse should be reported to the appropriate authorities so that they may intervene as appropriate. (© Dr. P. Marazzi/Photo Researchers, Inc.)

- Unexplained injuries (especially if the patient is bed confined)
- Evidence of restraints, such as contusions or lacerations of the wrists and ankles
- Caregiver's refusal to let you be alone with the patient
- Unexplained vaginal or anal bleeding
- Malnourished appearance

As with suspected child abuse, do not confront the caregiver. Your main priority is to remove the patient from the environment, care for him, and report your suspicions to the proper authorities per your state's guidelines.

Technology-Dependent Patients

Advances in medical technology have made it possible for more and more patients to be cared for in the home than in past years. Because of this, EMS providers are being called to care for these patients more frequently. Some medical equipment allows the patient to maintain independence, such as with urinary catheters, while others are required to sustain life, such as mechanical ventilators. You must be familiar with the various types of medical equipment that you are likely to encounter.

Regardless of what types of medical equipment the patient uses in the home, first address the reason that you are called to the scene. Do not let the presence of this equipment distract you from performing an appropriate assessment of the patient.

Medical equipment commonly encountered in the field is categorized as airway and respiratory devices, vascular access devices, and gastrointestinal and genitourinary devices.

Medical Oxygen

The use of medical oxygen by patients increases their ability to live independent and normal lives, because they are able to transport the oxygen with them wherever they go. Most home oxygen devices that patients use are very similar to the oxygen devices that you use on the ambulance. They consist of a nasal cannula connected to a humidifier and oxygen cylinder. However, there are other types of oxygen delivery devices that patients use in their homes, including an oxygen concentrator and liquid oxygen, which are described as follows:

- An oxygen concentrator is a device that captures and concentrates oxygen from the ambient air and then delivers it to the patient. Because this device is limited by the amount of oxygen available to it, it is only capable of supplying low-flow oxygen (up to 6 L/min) to the patient.
- Liquid oxygen is oxygen that has been cooled and compressed into a cylinder about the same size as an ordinary thermos. In its liquid state, a large amount of oxygen can be stored in a very small cylinder.

Because those are very simple systems, few problems arise and when they do, they are usually rectified by the patient without assistance. However, if the system fails, the patient will be without oxygen and will require assistance. If the patient is not able to receive oxygen for a length of time, his condition can deteriorate and require intervention. Other times, you may be called to care for a patient on home oxygen whose condition has worsened, resulting in difficulty breathing; assess and treat the patient according to your protocol.

Apnea Monitors

An apnea monitor is a device that constantly monitors the patient's breathing and alarms when the patient ceases to breathe. The devices are often used for infants who are at risk for sudden infant death syndrome (SIDS) or have suffered an apparent life-threatening event (ALTE). When the device alarms, it produces a very loud, high-pitched tone. When called to a location where an apnea monitor alarm has been activated, assess the patient and intervene as indicated. Do not waste time trying to diagnose the monitor. Immediately assess the patient and act accordingly. Determine how long the alarm has been sounding prior to your arrival because this will tell you how long the patient has been apneic.

Tracheostomy Tubes

A tracheostomy is a procedure during which a hole is surgically created through the tissues of the neck and into the trachea in order to provide an alternative airway for the patient. Tracheostomies are performed as a temporary or permanent airway. If the tracheostomy is to provide a permanent airway for the patient, it is called a *stoma*.

Tracheostomies are performed on patients who have chronic upper airway problems or are going to be on a mechanical ventilator long term. This eliminates the need for an endotracheal tube to remain in place. Not all patients who have undergone a tracheostomy are confined to the home or in a medical facility. In some cases, tracheostomies are performed on patients who have had laryngeal or throat cancer. The patients maintain a normal life, breathing through the stoma. Some patients, however, do not have the ability to maintain a patent airway with just a stoma. Patients who are in a coma, paraplegic from spinal-cord injury, or suffering from neuromuscular disorders have a tracheostomy tube placed in their stoma to maintain a patent airway.

There are two basic types of tracheostomy tubes used. A single-lumen tracheostomy tube is used for infants because of its small diameter. For larger children and adults, a tube that has an inner cannula and an outer cannula is used (Figure 46-9). The outer cannula ensures that the stoma remains open. It is secured by a strap that is secured around the patient's neck. The inner cannula is smaller in diameter, which allows it to be inserted into the outer cannula. At the distal end of the inner cannula is a small inflatable cuff, which when inflated, assists with holding it in place and provides a seal between the cannula and the inner walls of the trachea. At the proximal tip of the cannula is an adapter that accommodates a mechanical ventilator circuit or bag-valve-mask device in the event positive pressure ventilations must be performed.

In some cases, the patient encounters complications associated with the tracheostomy tube. They include the following:

- Obstruction (usually from a mucus plug in the tube)
- Air leakage around the cuff

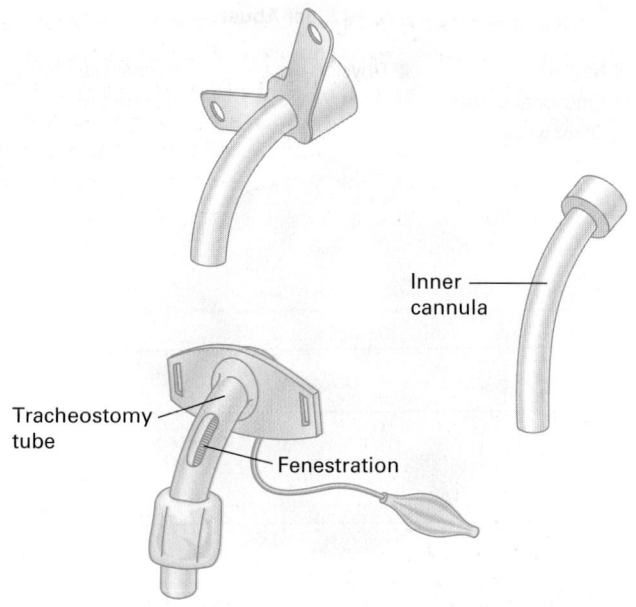

FIGURE 46-9

Tracheostomy tubes. Top: a single-lumen tube used for infants. Bottom: a tracheostomy tube and inner cannula used for larger children and adults.

- Tube dislodgement
- Infection

Of those complications, obstruction is the most common. This is because when a tracheostomy tube is in place, the normal filtering and humidifying functions of the upper airway are not used. That results in a need for regular suctioning of the tube. If a tracheostomy tube is obstructed, you must suction it in order for the patient to regain a patent airway. Instilling a few milliliters of sterile normal saline into the stoma can help hydrate mucus, making it easier to suction. Suction no longer than 10 to 15 seconds when attempting to clear the tube.

CPAP and BiPAP

Continuous positive airway pressure (CPAP) and **bilevel positive airway pressure (BiPAP)** devices provide positive airway pressure for spontaneously breathing patients through tubing attached to a mask that covers

IN THE FIELD

When a patient with a tracheostomy tube is coughing, you should ensure that you are not in front of the opening of the tube. To minimize the chances of exposure to airborne illnesses, stand to the side and use Standard Precautions.

the patient's mouth and/or nose. CPAP devices provide a continuous level of positive pressure during the inspiratory and expiratory phases of ventilation, while BiPAP devices provide higher positive pressure during inspiration and lower positive pressure during expiration. Both devices are designed to keep the lower airways open during expiration, which assists in ventilation and oxygenation. The amount of positive pressure applied by the device can be adjusted to meet the individual patient's needs.

The use of CPAP and BiPAP in the home is common for patients who have been diagnosed with chronic obstructive pulmonary disease (COPD) and sleep apnea. Many EMS agencies use CPAP devices to treat patients who are in respiratory distress from exacerbation of COPD or congestive heart failure (CHF). Patients can benefit greatly from CPAP, with or without the use of medications and in many cases endotracheal intubation can be avoided as a result.

Mechanical Ventilators

Mechanical ventilators are devices used both in the medical care facilities and at home by patients who require breathing assistance. Several different medical conditions can require mechanical ventilation, including COPD, lung cancer, stroke and traumatic brain injury.

Many different types of mechanical ventilators may be used in a patient's home. Newer models are very small and weigh just a couple of pounds, while others are larger and can weigh 20 to 30 pounds. Mechanical ventilators are set to provide positive pressure ventilation at a specific rate and to deliver a specific tidal volume with each ventilation. In addition to providing the ventilation itself, the device can be set to deliver a specific concentration of oxygen to the patient. In order to prevent injury to the patient's lungs and to ensure that the patient receives the specific rate and depth of ventilation required, the device has a built-in alarm that will sound when the preset parameters are exceeded. Ventilations are delivered to the patient by way of a large-diameter tubing called a *ventilator circuit*. The ventilator circuit attaches to the adapter of a tracheostomy tube.

Following are common mechanical ventilator alarms that alert the caregiver or Advanced EMT that a problem with the ventilator exists:

- *High-pressure alarm.* A high-pressure alarm is activated when the pressure required to ventilate a patient's lungs exceeds the preset parameter. Some causes include kinking of the ventilator circuit, obstruction of the tracheostomy tube, bronchospasm, the patient coughing during the inspiratory phase, or conditions that result in a decrease in lung compliance such as pulmonary edema, pneumothorax, or atelectasis.

- *Low-pressure alarm.* A low-pressure alarm is activated when the tidal volume falls 50 to 100 mL below the preset parameter. Some causes include a disconnected ventilator circuit or air leakage around the cuff of the tracheostomy tube.

- *Apnea alarm.* An apnea alarm is activated when the patient fails to initiate spontaneous ventilation. Causes may include decreased mental status or fatigue.

- *Low FiO$_2$ alarm.* A low FiO$_2$ alarm is activated when the preset FiO$_2$ falls below the preset parameter. Causes include a disconnected or depleted oxygen source.

When called to care for a patient who is on a mechanical ventilator, assess the patient as you would any other. Is the ventilator providing adequate ventilation and oxygenation for the patient? As with other medical devices, the

IN THE FIELD

If you are in doubt that the patient is being adequately ventilated and oxygenated on a ventilator, disconnect it and ventilate the patient using a bag-valve-mask device attached to high-flow oxygen.

CASE STUDY (continued)

Robert and Al follow the mother to the child's room where they find a 12-year-old boy lying in a hospital bed on a mechanical ventilator. Robert touches the boy's head and confirms that he is hot to the touch. "The urine in the catheter bag is clear," says Al. While Robert performs his primary assessment, he notices a feeding tube in the boy's abdomen. Al attaches a pulse oximeter, which gives a reading of 90 percent. There are multiple medication bottles on a nightstand next to the bed. The boy begins to cough and the mechanical ventilator alarms.

Problem-Solving Questions

1. What could be causing the ventilator to alarm?
2. How should Robert and Al proceed with the care of this patient?
3. Given this additional information, what do you think could be causing the patient's condition?

patient's caregiver will be very familiar with the equipment, so enlist his or her assistance when needed. Changes in patient condition can cause ventilator alarms to be activated, so thoroughly assess the patient and treat him accordingly.

Vascular Access Devices

A **vascular access device (VAD)** is a device that allows for readily available vascular access when patients require ongoing intravenous medication administration for a length of time. Frequently, patients with VADs are those who require hemodialysis, chemotherapy, total parenteral nutrition (TPN), or long-term intravenous antibiotic administration. In most EMS agencies, protocols do not allow for the Advanced EMT to access a VAD because some require special needles and others require special procedures prior to use. While you will not use the devices, you should be aware of them because you will encounter them from time to time (Figure 46-10).

Central Intravenous Catheters

Central intravenous catheters (sometimes called *central lines*) are usually placed into the large subclavian vein below the clavicle, or, less commonly, the internal jugular vein is used. Central intravenous catheters are very similar to peripheral intravenous lines that an Advanced EMT uses, but they are designed for long-term access (several weeks to months). The tubing is secured with sutures to the chest wall just beneath the clavicle. Suturing the line in place prevents

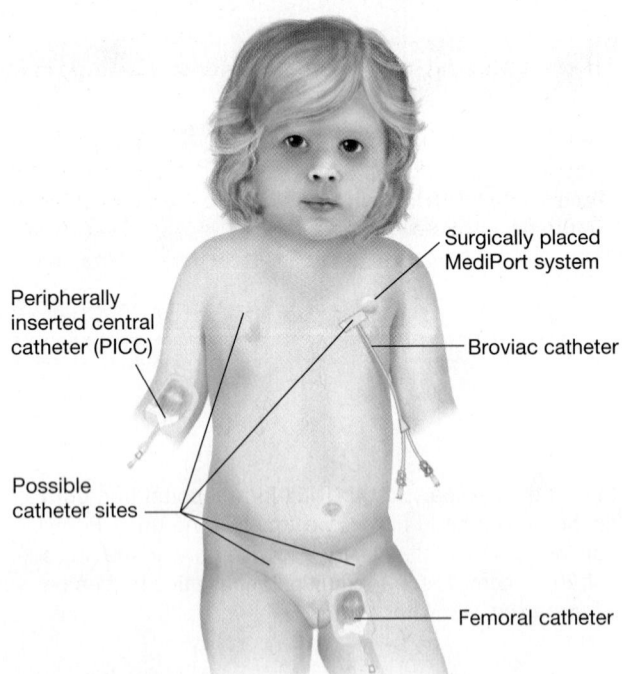

Peripherally inserted central catheter (PICC)

Possible catheter sites

Surgically placed MediPort system

Broviac catheter

Femoral catheter

FIGURE 46-10

Vascular access devices (VADs) include central IV catheters such as a PICC line, central venous lines such as a Broviac catheter, and implanted ports such as a MediPort.

it from becoming easily dislodged. The line will have one or more medication access ports for the administration of medications. Some common types of central venous lines include Broviac, Hickman, and Groshong lines.

A common type of central intravenous catheter you will encounter is a peripherally inserted central catheter (PICC) line. PICC lines are usually inserted into a vein in the forearm or antecubital fossa and fed into the central circulation.

Implanted Venous Access Ports

Implanted venous access ports are disk-shaped devices that are surgically implanted just beneath the skin of the upper chest. Some common types include Port-A-Cath, MediPort, and Infuse-a-Port.

Dialysis Shunts

Patients who require hemodialysis as a result of a loss of kidney function do so by way of a surgically implanted arteriovenous (AV) shunt, AV fistula, or AV graft. Though you will not use those devices, you must be aware of some issues when caring for such a patient. For example, never attempt to obtain a blood pressure in a patient's arm where an AV shunt, AV fistula, or AV graft is placed. Doing so can cause significant damage to the device because the pressure of the blood pressure cuff will cause an increase in pressure within the device.

Also, a patient who has a damaged AV shunt, AV fistula, or AV graft may present with significant bleeding. This bleeding may be external or internal and observed as a large hematoma beneath the skin. In either case, control the bleeding by applying constant direct pressure, providing high-flow oxygen, and treating for shock if indicated.

Gastrointestinal and Genitourinary Devices

When patients suffer a loss of gastrointestinal or genitourinary function, they may have to rely on medical devices to receive nutrition or eliminate waste. Those devices include feeding tubes, ostomy bags, and urinary tract devices. Even though malfunction or damage to those devices does not produce life threats, you may be called to care for a patient who uses them. Therefore, you must be familiar with their function.

Feeding Tubes

Feeding tubes are used to provide nutrition directly into stomach or small intestine in patients who cannot chew or swallow. Feeding tubes are thin, long, flexible tubes that are named according to how they are inserted. If a tube is inserted through the nose, it is called a *nasogastric (NG)* tube. If the tube is inserted through the patient's mouth, it is called an *orogastric (OG)* tube. Patients who are administered oral medications through a feeding tube do so after the medications have been crushed. Failure of the caregiver to adequately crush the medication can result in the tube becoming clogged.

NG and OG tubes may be used for the administration of nutrients as well as to suction stomach when it is desirable to keep the stomach empty to reduce vomiting, such as with a minor gastrointestinal bleed. When used for the administration of nutrients, they are considered to be short-term devices. If a patient will require long-term nutritional administration by way of a feeding tube, a tube will be surgically inserted through the abdominal wall directly into the GI system. That surgical procedure is called a **gastrostomy** (Figure 46-11). If the surgically implanted tube is inserted into the stomach, it is called a *gastric (G)* tube, while a feeding tube placed through the gastric wall and into the jejunum is called a *jejunal (J)* tube.

Ostomy Bags

Ostomy bags are devices that are connected to an opening in the abdominal wall. They collect feces directly from the patient's colon. Patients who require the use of an ostomy bag do so as a result of medical conditions such as diverticulitis, colon cancer, or Crohn's disease. Ostomy bags are a very simple system and generally have few complications, but you may be called to transport these patients for other reasons. When called to do so, take care not to compress or pull the ostomy bag because doing so can cause it to become disconnected.

Urinary Catheters

A urinary catheter is a device used to empty urine from the patient's urinary bladder through a tube and into a collecting bag. There are two basic types of urinary catheters that you may encounter. The least invasive of the two is called an *external catheter*, or *condom catheter*. Condom catheters are placed on the penis just as a prophylactic condom would be. A catheter at the tip of the condom allows urine to flow into a collecting bag (Figure 46-12).

The second type of urinary catheter is a Foley catheter. It is somewhat invasive because it must be threaded into the urinary bladder through the patient's urethra. Once inside the urinary bladder, a small balloon is inflated, which prevents the catheter from being pulled out (Figure 46-13). Foley catheters are generally for long-term use. In other cases, patients may catheterize themselves to empty the bladder several times a day, but the catheter is not kept in place.

The most common complication associated with urinary catheters is the development of a urinary tract infection (UTI) because the catheter provides a route of entry for bacteria. Some patients may develop a UTI severe enough to cause life-threatening sepsis. UTI causes lower abdominal pain and cloudy, "tea-colored" urine, which will be visible in the catheter collecting bag.

Ventriculostomy Shunts

Some patients, mainly pediatric patients, have a medical condition that causes either an overproduction of cerebrospinal fluid (CSF) in the brain, poor reabsorption of CSF, or inadequate flow of CSF within the meninges and ventricles of the brain. Those problems lead to an overaccumulation of CSF in the brain, called *hydrocephalus*, and leads to an increase in intracranial pressure (ICP).

A device called an **ventriculostomy shunt** is surgically placed in one of the ventricles in the brain, allowing pressure to be relieved. Ventriculostomy shunts drain into the abdomen, heart, pleural space, or a blood vessel in the neck.

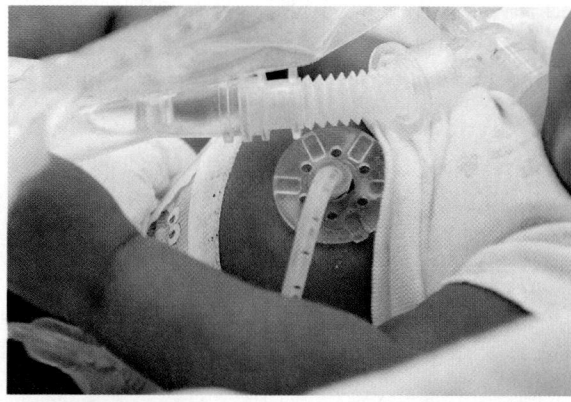

FIGURE 46-11

Surgically inserted feeding tubes are used for long-term nutritional support. (© Ray Kemp/Triple Zilch Productions)

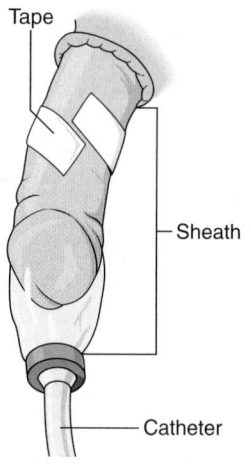

FIGURE 46-12

An external, or condom catheter.

FIGURE 46-13

An internal catheter system.

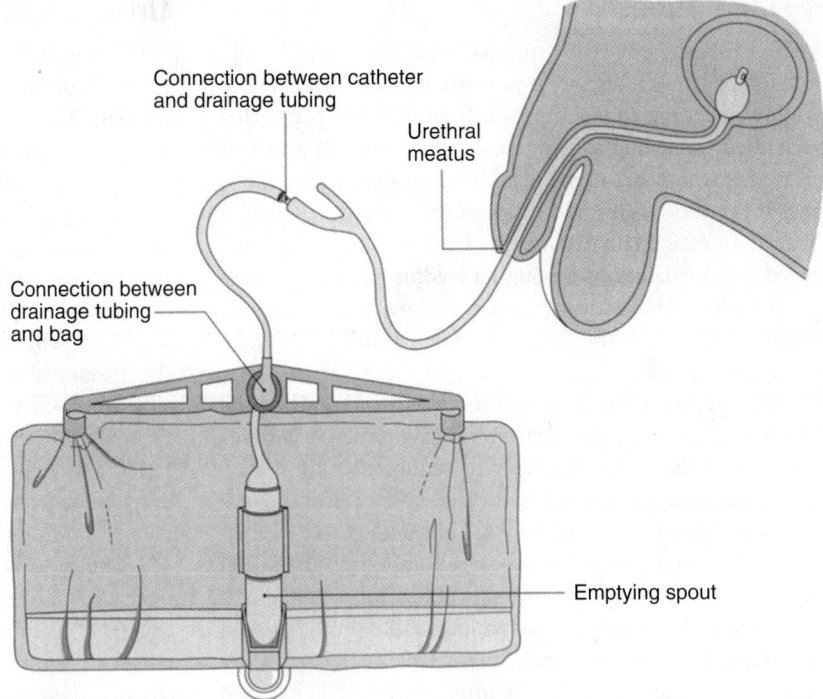

Connection between catheter and drainage tubing

Urethral meatus

Connection between drainage tubing and bag

Emptying spout

In some cases a small reservoir is surgically placed between the skull and scalp where fluid can be collected for laboratory examination (Figure 46-14).

While complications can occur, they do not produce life threats very often, although the potential is there. Common types of complications related to ventriculostomy shunts include infection, subdural bleeding, and occlusion. Infection can result in encephalitis or sepsis. Occlusion of the shunt can lead to the accumulation of CSF within the brain and an increase in ICP. When called to care for a patient with

IN THE FIELD

When called to care for and transport a patient with a ventriculostomy shunt, it may be necessary to transport the patient to a medical facility where neurosurgical services are available.

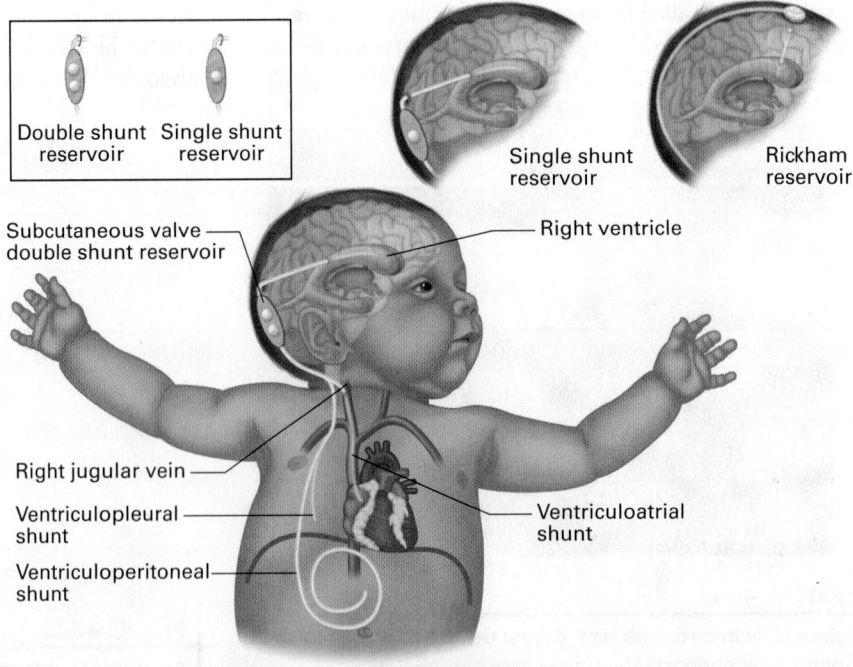

Double shunt reservoir   Single shunt reservoir

Single shunt reservoir

Rickham reservoir

Subcutaneous valve double shunt reservoir

Right ventricle

Right jugular vein

Ventriculopleural shunt

Ventriculoatrial shunt

Ventriculoperitoneal shunt

FIGURE 46-14

Intraventricular shunts originate within a ventricle in the brain and drain into the abdomen, heart, pleural space, or a blood vessel in the neck to relieve ICP.

CASE STUDY WRAP-UP

Clinical-Reasoning Process

As the boy continues to cough, the mother approaches the boy's side. "Excuse me," she says as she gently pushes Robert aside. She immediately takes a suction catheter and removes the ventilator circuit from the boy's tracheostomy tube and suctions thick greenish-brown mucus from it. She then reattaches the ventilator circuit, the ventilator ceases to alarm, and the boy calms down. "Happens all the time, but his mucus is definitely an odd color," says the mother.

"When you finish doing what you need to do, let me know and I'll help move Bobby over to your stretcher so we can be on our way," she says.

Robert suspects pneumonia, and en route to the hospital emergency department, Robert calls in his patient report and asks the ED physician if he should increase the patient's FiO_2 setting on the ventilator. The physician agrees and the patient's SpO_2 increases to 94 percent.

Robert continues to monitor the patient's SpO_2 and other vital signs en route.

As a precautionary measure, Robert retrieves a French suction catheter from the ambulance cabinet and sets it beside the suction unit just to be prepared in the event that the patient needs more suctioning before they arrive at the hospital.

---

complications of an intraventricular shunt, assess and treat the patient based on his clinical presentation.

Hospice Care

Hospice is care that focuses on comfort care of terminally ill patients. Pain management is a common goal, as is providing the patient and his family with support. Terminal illness is defined as an illness that leads to the deterioration of the patient and results in death. When a patient is diagnosed with a terminal illness, the physician may refer the patient for evaluation by hospice. Hospice will evaluate the patient on a regular basis and make recommendations to the physician regarding the patient's care.

It is common for hospice patients to receive pain management medications and, as their condition worsens, the dose of medications may be increased. The hospice staff contacts the physician to obtain orders to make such changes in the patient's treatment. In addition to medical treatment, hospice personnel also explain to the patient and his or her family what to expect as death approaches. Social workers or other mental health care providers also may

IN THE FIELD

In some cases, the family of a hospice patient will call EMS to transport the patient to the hospital, not for treatment but simply because they do not want the patient to die in the home, potentially causing other family members uneasiness about remaining in the home after the patient's death.

visit the patient and family to assist them with coping and acceptance.

Even though the family of a hospice patient has been directed to contact hospice as the patient nears death, they may call for EMS instead. If you respond in this situation, ensure that hospice is contacted. Provide emotional support to the family. If the family insists that the patient be transported, determine whether there is a do not resuscitate (DNR) order available and provide care to the patient accordingly. Communicate with the hospital and consult with medical direction for guidance, if needed.

CHAPTER REVIEW

Chapter Summary

During your career as an Advanced EMT, you will encounter patients with special challenges that range from hearing disability to homelessness to the utilization of life-sustaining medical technology. In order for you to provide them with the best care, you must understand their needs and how their challenges relate to the reason you were called.

Always remain a patient advocate and avoid the temptation to give into your feelings under the stress of a difficult situation such as with elder or child abuse.

When called to care for a patient who relies on medical technology to maintain an independent lifestyle or to sustain life, do not allow the presence of the equipment to distract you from performing a systematic assessment and appropriately treating your patient. When faced with medical equipment that you are not familiar with, enlist the assistance of the patient's caregiver because he or she will prove to be a

valuable resource. Caregivers can provide you with a wealth of knowledge about the patient's medical equipment, medical history, and needs. Ask questions and allow the caregiver to assist you when necessary.

Review Questions

Multiple-Choice Questions

1. A 26-year-old female patient answers you with incomprehensible, slurred speech. This patient has a(n) _____ disorder.
   a. language
   b. articulation
   c. voice production
   d. fluency

2. In order to avoid breathing difficulty, obese patients should be transported in which position?
   a. Supine
   b. Prone
   c. Position of comfort
   d. Lateral recumbent

3. According to studies, which type of child abuse occurs most frequently in the United States?
   a. Physical abuse
   b. Psychological abuse
   c. Sexual abuse
   d. Neglect

4. Which mechanical ventilator alarm is commonly associated with occlusion of the tracheostomy tube by an accumulation of mucus?
   a. Low-pressure alarm
   b. High-pressure alarm
   c. Low FiO$_2$ alarm
   d. Apnea alarm

5. Intraventricular shunts are placed in order to prevent:
   a. infection.
   b. hydrocephalus.
   c. increased intracranial pressure.
   d. stroke.

6. When communicating with a hearing-impaired patient, you should:
   a. speak slower than normal.
   b. speak in a loud, clear voice.
   c. shout.
   d. exaggerate how you articulate your words.

Critical-Thinking Questions

7. Explain the steps that can be taken in order to prevent breathing difficulty when transporting an obese patient.

8. Explain why it is important to avoid confronting the parents of a child who you suspect is the victim of child abuse.

9. Describe the difference in tracheostomy tubes that are used for infants and those used for larger children and adults.

10. Describe the difference between CPAP and BiPAP.

11. What is the intended purpose of CPAP and BiPAP?

12. What is the difference between a nasogastric tube and an orogastric tube?

References

Centers for Disease Control and Prevention. (2010). *U.S. obesity trends*. Retrieved January 3, 2011, from http://www.cdc.gov/obesity/data/trends.html#State

Childhelp. (2010). *National child abuse statistics*. Retrieved December 29, 2010, from http://www.childhelp.org/pages/statistics

Domestic Violence Resource Center. (2010). *Domestic violence statistics*. Retrieved December 29, 2010, from http://www.dvrc-or.org/domestic/violence/resources/C61/

National Coalition for the Homeless. (2009). *How many people experience homelessness?* Retrieved December 28, 2010, from http://www.nationalhomeless.org/factsheets/How_Many.html

National Committee for the Prevention of Elder Abuse. (2010). *What is elder abuse?* Retrieved December 29, 2010, from http://www.preventelderabuse.org/elderabuse/

U.S. Census Bureau. (2009). *Income, poverty and health insurance coverage in the United States: 2009*. Retrieved December 29, 2010, from http://www.census.gov/prod/2010pubs/p60-238.pdf

U.S. Department of Housing and Urban Development. (2009). *ResearchWorks—A clearer national perspective on homelessness*. Retrieved December 28, 2010, from http://www.huduser.org/periodicals/Researchworks/decjan_09/RW_vol6num1t3.html

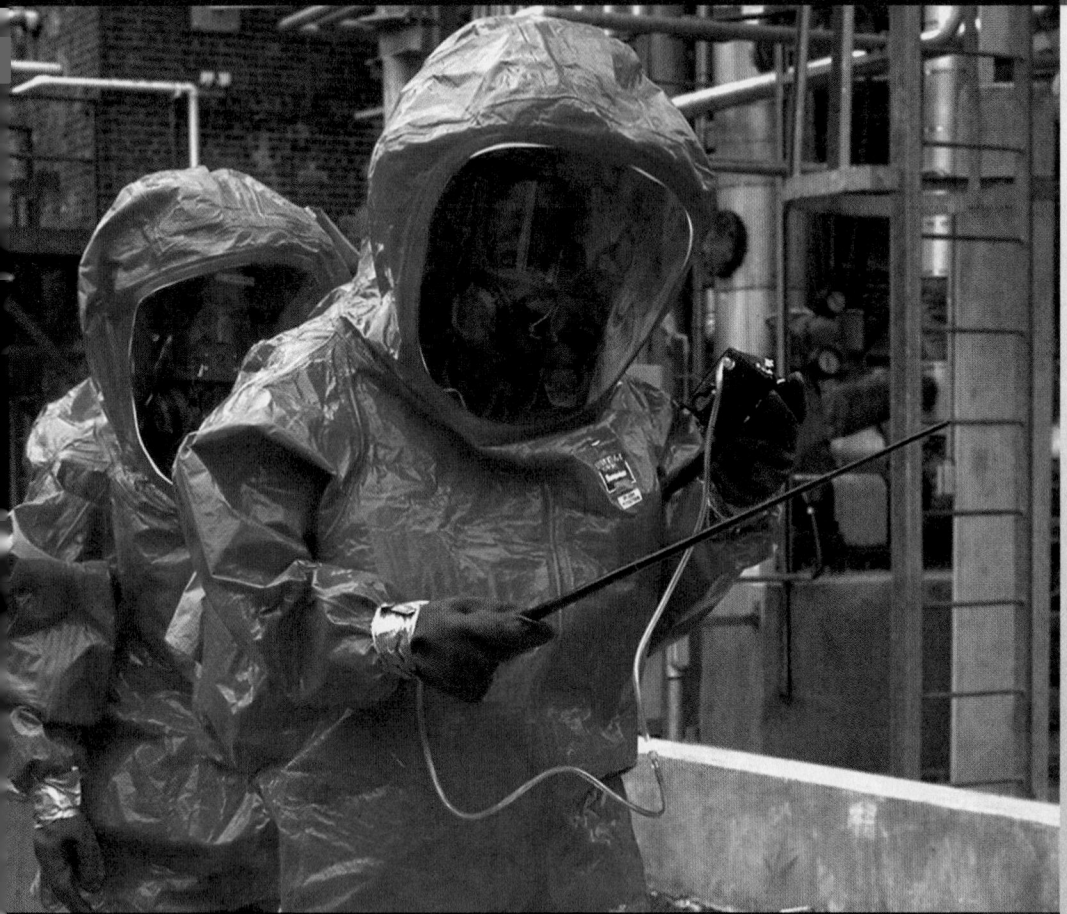

47 Rescue Operations and Vehicle Extrication

Content Area: Rescue Operations and Vehicle Extrication

Advanced EMT Education Standard: The Advanced EMT applies knowledge of operational roles and responsibilities to ensure patient, public, and personnel safety during rescue and vehicle extrication.

Objectives

After reading this chapter, you should be able to:

47.1 Define key terms introduced in this chapter.

47.2 Use scene size-up information to anticipate potential problems in accessing patients.

47.3 Determine what types of resources may be needed in rescue situations.

47.4 Explain the integration of medical care and rescue operations through teamwork.

47.5 Establish personnel, patient, and public safety as priorities in rescue situations.

47.6 Recognize equipment used for water, rough terrain, confined space, and vehicle rescue.

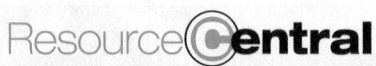

To access Resource Central, follow the directions on the Student Access Card provided with this text. If there is no card, go to www.bradybooks.com and follow the Resource Central link to Buy Access. Under Media Resources, you will find:

• *Body Substance Isolation and Equipment.* Anticipate the use of BSI equipment.

• *Air Medical Service.* How to prepare the landing zone.

• *Electric Vehicle Safety Training.* Electric and hybrid vehicles and how they differ from traditional combustion vehicles.

The weather is terrible. It snowed the day before and the melted snow is turning to ice as Advanced EMTs Jay Maxwell and Al Davis start their shift. The temperature outside is 19°F when Jay and Al are alerted to a one-car motor vehicle collision (MVC) about a mile from the station. After an extended response time due to the weather and road conditions, they arrive at the scene. Jay and Al find one automobile that drove off the road, hit a tree, and slid down a 10-foot embankment. The automobile's front and driver side have significant damage. With a flashlight aimed at the vehicle, Al informs Jay, "I can see at least one patient in the driver compartment and he doesn't appear to be moving."

Problem-Solving Questions

1. What additional resources should Jay and Al call for at this point?
2. Based upon the MVC description, what might be their thoughts about the stability of the vehicle where it rests?
3. How should they attempt to access the patient, if at all?

47.7	Select appropriate personal protective equipment for use during vehicle extrication.
47.8	Identify the safest, most effective ways of gaining access to patients in given motor vehicle collision scenarios.
47.9	Protect the patient from further harm during vehicle extrication.
47.10	Explain how to minimize risk of injury from extrication hazards, such as airbags that have not deployed, fuel leaks, traffic, weather, and other hazards.
47.11	Describe the processes used to stabilize a vehicle prior to beginning extrication.
47.12	Discuss the impact on extrication procedures of damage to specific parts of the vehicle.
47.13	Explain specific extrication safety considerations for hybrid vehicles.
47.14	Discuss the uses of particular types of hand and hydraulic extrication tools.

Introduction

As an Advanced EMT you will be called to emergency scenes where access to the patient is not readily available. Some of those scenes include MVCs, bodies of water, and hazardous atmospheres and terrain. While the majority of rescue operations are performed by personnel assigned to a dedicated rescue unit, sometimes, as an Advanced EMT, you may be required to assist in rescue operations such as the **extrication** or disentanglement of patients from wreckage. However, your primary responsibility during any rescue operation is your safety, the safety of your partner, followed by the welfare of the patient or patients.

Personal Protective Equipment

The use of personal safety equipment must be paramount at every scene. Proper application of personal protective equipment (PPE) is vital to your safety and to the continuation of your career in EMS. It is well known that noncompliance in using Standard Precautions such as gloves, mask, gown, and other precautions can lead to a transfer of disease. It is also true that compromising the use of PPE during rescue operations can lead to injury or even death of the rescuer. It is important to note that you must use Standard Precautions and PPE that are specific to the type of rescue operation. Personnel not wearing appropriate PPE should not be permitted to operate on the scene of the rescue operation. Your focus may be the medical care of the trauma patient; however, like other rescuers, you must protect your head, eyes, ears, hands, feet, and body from cutting forces, falling objects, and other hazards associated with rescue operations (Figure 47-1). That protection includes the following:

- *Head and face protection.* Helmets protect your head from flying debris and provide protection from protruding sharp objects that have the potential to cause skull fractures and soft-tissue injuries. Helmets should have a nonelastic, four-point suspension system that provide more protection than standard hard hats typically worn by construction workers. For vehicle and structural extrication, a compact firefighting

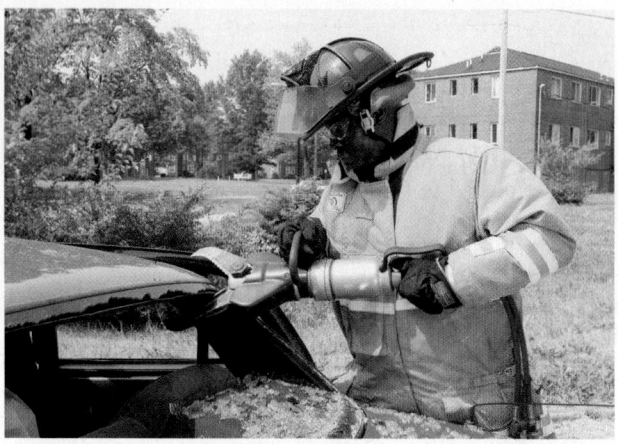

FIGURE 47-1

You must wear proper personal protective equipment during vehicle extrication to prevent injury.

helmet that meets National Fire Protection Association (NFPA) standards is adequate. Other types of helmets used in rescue operations include climbing helmets for high-angle and confined-space rescue and kayaking helmets for water rescue.

- *Eye protection.* Two types of eye protection are available during rescue operations: goggles and safety glasses. Ensure that goggles are vented to prevent fogging while performing operations such as vehicle extrication and confined-space rescue. Use safety glasses approved by the American National Standards Institute (ANSI) for operations in which a potential for debris or fluid may be directed toward your face.

- *Ear and hearing protection.* Use hearing protection, including ear plugs inserted directly into the ear canal, because some scenes, such as a vehicle extrication scene, can be extremely loud. Amplified sound of the extrication symphony includes engine noise from multiple rescue vehicles, generators, hydrolytic and pneumatic extrication tools, and the combined voices of all those involved in the rescue.

- *Hand protection.* Leather gloves provide the best protection against twisted metal and broken glass, which you will encounter during some rescue operations. In most situations, you should wear close-fitting leather gloves that provide the dexterity to provide unrestricted patient care but are sturdy enough to protect hands from soft-tissue injuries. In addition, you should wear medical exam gloves beneath the protective leather gloves to provide protection from blood and body fluids.

- *Foot protection.* When selecting footwear, consider the hazards and potential injuries that may be present at an emergency scene. Leather boots with steel toe and metatarsal protection are recommended and a proper fit is necessary to reduce fatigue and blister formation.

- *Body protection.* Firefighting turnout coat and pants will provide you protection against flying debris, sharp objects, and other hazards at the scene. However, not all Advanced EMTs are employed by a fire service, so an acceptable alternative for turnout coat and pants are extrication jump suits. The suits are manufactured by all of the structural firefighting turnout gear companies and are made from a cotton/Nomex blend for protection from flame. The jumpsuits are outfitted with reflective striping for high visibility. The greatest advantage of this type of protection is their lightweight construction and better fit, giving the Advanced EMT better mobility while providing care to the injured patient.

- *Personal flotation devices (PFDs).* If you work in an area where bodies of water are located, your service may provide you with PFDs to be worn while on or near water. PFDs used during rescue operations must meet the U.S. Coast Guard standards for flotation.

Patient Safety

After you and the rescue team are safe and protected, you must shield your patient from the same elements. Following are some items that will help to create a safe environment for your patient:

- Wool blankets for warmth and to protect from debris
- Tarp
- Helmet
- Hearing protection
- Goggles
- Dust mask, unless the patient is having difficulty breathing or is on oxygen
- Shielding, such as a backboard used to form a barrier between the patient and sharp objects or equipment

Rescue Operations

The importance of safety on the scene of a rescue operation cannot be stressed enough. You must understand that rescue operations should always be performed by trained individuals. Performing tasks such as the disentanglement of a patient from a vehicle requires the operation of potentially dangerous equipment. Do not attempt to perform tasks that you are not qualified to perform because doing so will place you and others at risk for injury.

A successful rescue operation involves cooperation and teamwork usually between multiple agencies including law enforcement, firefighters, and EMS. It is important that each individual knows and performs his or her specific tasks because doing so will allow the patient to be accessed, treated, disentangled, packaged, and transported with no unnecessary delay.

A general approach to rescue operations identifies seven phases of operation: arrival and size-up, hazard control, patient access, medical treatment, disentanglement, patient packaging, and removal/transport of the patient from the scene.

Phase One: Arrival and Size-Up

You may be the first rescuer to arrive on the scene. Remember to ensure that the scene is safe prior to approach. Once on the scene, identify the number of patients and any additional resources needed. Notify dispatch of your findings and make applicable requests for resources as soon as possible. In many cases, dispatch will send specific resources based upon information gathered by the caller. For example, if someone falls into a well, it will be necessary to have individuals trained in that type of rescue to access the patient. Additionally, if ground transport time will be prolonged, an aeromedical response may be utilized. Promptly recognizing the need for specific rescue teams will allow for treatment and transport of the patient in a shorter period of time. Have those resources dispatched to assist and avoid placing yourself, partner, and bystanders at risk to gain access to a patient.

Phase Two: Hazard Control

Remain alert when approaching a scene and identify hazards quickly by scanning the area to find clues to the presence of a hazard. When hazards are present, stay clear of danger and keep others away. Remember that the environment itself can pose a risk to your safety. For instance, the presence of dangerous wildlife, lightning, rock slides, and so on should be avoided. Immediately notify dispatch of the need for specific resources. Table 47-1 lists some of the potential hazards you may encounter while working as an Advanced EMT and the specific resources that you may request.

Phase Three: Patient Access

Once it is safe to access the patient, determine the safest possible way to do so while ensuring your own safety. Be alert for hazards that may present themselves during the

TABLE 47-1	Resources Necessary for Potential Hazards
Hazard	**Resources**
Fire	Fire services
Entrapped patient	Extrication team
Chemical release	Hazmat team
Dangerous individuals	Law enforcement
Dangerous animals	Animal control
Downed power lines	Utility company

process of gaining access to the patient. For example, if the patient is in a cave-in situation, it may be necessary to remove debris to access and move him. However, doing so could cause further cave-ins and pose a risk to you and others in the area. Immediately notify the appropriate rescue personnel on the scene and allow them to address the situation.

In many situations, you will likely be directed to stand by and prepare to treat patients as they are removed from the environment by specialized rescue professionals.

Phase Four: Medical Treatment

Once access to the patient is obtained, you will be responsible for the following:

- Assessing the patient
- Initiating treatment
- Continuing treatment until the patient can be transported
- Transporting the patient to an appropriate facility

When the potential for spine injury exists, which is likely in rescue operations, you will immediately take manual stabilization of the head and neck and maintain cervical-spine alignment. Perform a primary assessment and treat life threats as they are identified. Rescue from a confined space, water, or a severely damaged vehicle can be a very stressful and scary experience for the patient. Do your best to calm and reassure the patient during the rescue process. This is best accomplished through constant communication. Tell the patient exactly what is going on around him and keep him abreast of how the rescue operation is progressing. Learn the patient's name and use it when speaking to or referring to him. Remain calm and professional because the patient can detect nervousness on your part, which will increase his anxiety.

Phase Five: Disentanglement

Disentanglement is the act of freeing a patient from entrapment. For example, a hydraulic ram is used to lift a collapsed dashboard from a patient's legs, allowing him to be removed from the vehicle. Disentanglement is a

---

IN THE FIELD

You will be called to MVCs where disentanglement will take a prolonged period of time due to the complexity of the wreckage. In such cases, you will initiate treatment as soon as practical and prepare to transport the patient as soon as possible when freed. Consider the use of aeromedical transport when indicated and available.

technical skill that requires specific expertise to be performed effectively and safely. During this phase of the rescue operation, you may be directed to stand by and prepare to treat the freed patient. Other times you may enter the space with the patient and initiate treatment there. When doing so, it is imperative that you wear the appropriate PPE. Protect the patient as well.

Phase Six: Patient Packaging

Once the patient is freed, he must be properly packaged. In some situations, rapid extrication will be indicated by the presence of an immediate danger, a critically injured or ill patient, or to gain access to other critically injured or ill patients. Other patients may not require spinal immobilization. No matter the case, you must consider how the patient will be moved. If the patient must be removed from a confined or hazardous space, specially trained rescuers will package and bring the patient to you. When patients must be lifted from a small space, such as a man hole, they are packaged using a device that allows a vertical lift. Once the patient is secured to the device, ropes are used for rigging the patient for removal. In situations in which the patient is in a location away from a roadway or walkway, you will have to carry him to your stretcher. Most patients are placed in a Stokes basket to be carried by multiple rescuers to a stretcher.

Phase Seven: Removal/Transport

The actual removal of the patient from the scene often is difficult even after he is freed. Patients who have fallen into holes, from cliffs, or into crevices must be safely lifted by using specialized vertical lift devices called *rescue tripods* or a *ladder truck*. In some situations, the patient must be lowered from a height such as from a cliff face. High-angle rescue refers to the method in which rescuers are totally dependent on the use of ropes to access an individual. Rescuers access the patient, package him for removal, and prepare him to be lowered by using rope rigging. Other times, the patient who has been packaged in a Stokes basket will have to be carried over difficult terrain with unstable footing. Always choose a method to move the patient that offers the least risk to your own safety, as well as the safety of other rescuers and the patient.

The mode of transport is considered as part of the secondary assessment and preparations should have been made while the patient is being freed and packaged. Initiate transport to an appropriate facility based upon the patient's clinical condition.

Always ensure that you have enough resources to safely carry a patient, especially over rough terrain. Ideally, you will have at least four rescuers to carry a patient, one on each corner of the basket or backboard.

Specific Types of Rescue Operations

You will be called to many types of environments to care for injured and ill patients. Patients will be found entangled in motor vehicles, at the bottom of a cliff, in a deep hole, or in water. In this section, you will become familiar with some of the various types of rescue operations you might be asked to participate in during your career.

Water Rescue

Water rescue is not only utilized in areas such as beaches or large bodies of water. In mountainous areas, heavy rains can lead to a significant amount of water flowing into canyons and flooding them. Normally shallow and calm water can become dangerous by increases in water flow. Do not underestimate the strength of water current. Moving water can be strong enough to move buildings, cars, and you. Conduct a scene size-up and determine the need for specific resources. Then request them through dispatch. Do not enter the water to access a patient unless you have been trained in water rescue and have the appropriate personal safety equipment.

An individual requiring water rescue may be any of the following:

- Stranded in water but not at risk
- In immediate danger of being washed away or caught in dangerous swift water
- Deceased, at which time the operation transitions from a rescue operation to a recovery operation

Upon arrival at the scene of an emergency where water rescue is required, immediately notify dispatch. Conduct a scene size-up, scanning the area and considering the following:

- *Water temperature.* Recall that the patient and rescuers are susceptible to hypothermia even in mild temperatures. In icy water, professional water rescue teams wear insulated suits to protect them from the freezing temperatures.
- *Moving water.* Water rescue involving moving water is the most dangerous. Swift water rescue teams are professionals who are extensively trained to understand how water depth, velocity, obstructions to flow, and changing tide affect the flow of water.
- *Debris.* The presence of debris in the water creates a risk for entrapment of an individual who is drifting downstream with a current. Current can be strong enough to pin someone against objects that are in the water. In some cases, an individual's foot will become pinned beneath debris in the water causing a loss of footing. If the water current is strong enough, it can hold the person beneath the water and drown him.

When floating in swift water, you should float on your back with your feet held at the surface and pointing downstream. This will reduce your risk of becoming pinned.

If you arrive on the scene to find a patient in calm (also called *flat*), water you should throw a flotation device with a line attached to it. Use the line to pull the patient to safety without entering the water yourself. Entering the water to rescue the patient without training and a PFD places your safety at significant risk. Patients in the water may be in a state of panic and can grab onto you or even pull you under the water as you attempt to rescue them.

Hazardous Atmosphere

Confined space rescues can present a number of life threats with the most serious being an oxygen-deficient space. A space is defined as oxygen deficient when the oxygen content is less than 19.5 percent at sea level (National Institute for Occupational Safety and Health, 2004). Confined spaces can appear to be safe but, once entered, pose a serious risk to the rescuer. The Bureau of Labor Statistics reported 20 confined space-related deaths in 2002 with nearly 50 percent of those who die being rescuers (Hoven, 2003).

When called to the scene where one or more individuals are unresponsive in a closed space, perform a scene size-up. *Do not enter* the space and do not allow others to enter it. Call for assistance. Trained rescuers will access the patient while wearing the appropriate PPE such as SCBA. Examples of spaces that may be oxygen deficient include storage tanks, transport containers, silos, manholes, cisterns, and mines.

In addition to a space becoming oxygen deficient, other hazards may be present including toxic or explosive materials, a risk of engulfment (or being buried), and electricity.

Vehicle Extrication

Of the various types of rescue operations, you will most frequently be involved in vehicle extrications. As discussed previously, you will likely be directed to stand by until the patient can be disentangled from the vehicle. At other times, you will enter the wreckage but only after donning the appropriate PPE. You will make sure the patient is protected and then initiate treatment.

Vehicle extrication is a skill that must be performed by trained professionals. In this section, you will learn how to manage an emergency where vehicle extrication is required.

Scene Size-Up

A good scene size-up of the incident is essential. It will inform your decisions related to the type of rescue techniques that are needed for quick and safe access to the patient. A **windshield survey**, or visual scanning of the collision scene, plus an on-scene briefing from the rescue unit leader will assist you in making critical decisions on what medical equipment will be needed, how the extrication will proceed, and what additional resources will be needed to perform a successful rescue with a viable patient. Additional resources to be considered include the following:

- Power company for control of power lines and poles
- Fire suppression units
- Hazardous materials team for fuel leaks or spills
- Law enforcement for traffic safety
- Air evacuation for critical patients or prolonged extrication
- Additional ambulances

Start your scene size-up as you arrive at the scene of a motor vehicle collision. The exterior condition of the automobile can provide many clues to the probable severity of the injuries sustained by the patient and to the equipment and additional resources you may need. (Recall what you have learned about mechanism of injury in Chapter 34.) When determining the amount of force involved in the collision, make note of the damage to the vehicle. Components that are considered to be part of the exterior of the vehicle include the following:

- Door posts are structural members that surround the door areas, and are also known as *pillars*. They are usually referred to alphabetically from front to rear as the *A, B,* and *C posts.*
- Quarter panels are from the tail edge of the back doors to the rear bumper.
- Kick panels and fender are from the leading edge of the front door or A post to the front bumper.
- Rocker panels are rounded areas below the doors between the fenders and quarter panels.

Extrication teams may focus on "rolling the dash" or cutting a post to "flap the roof" and forget that a person with injuries is inside the automobile. Providing optimum care for the injured person requires constant communication between you and the extrication officer. Be direct about how you wish the extrication to proceed or pause as the patient's condition dictates. Along with being the patient's advocate during the rescue, you must begin treatment of the patient according to your protocol. This is often a challenge because of the patient's entanglement, limited space to work in, and distractions such as noise.

Airway, breathing, and circulation treatment modalities may have to be performed from a compromising or contorted position. Techniques you learned in the classroom setting may have to be modified but must nevertheless be carried out in an aggressive manner to ensure the best outcome for the patient. For example, you may have to initiate an IV while in a significantly deformed vehicle with minimal access to the patient.

It must be noted that you may need to interrupt treatment during the attempt to free the patient and restart it when the rescue team resets the equipment and technique during the extrication attempt. Once the patient is extricated from the vehicle, all focus from those at the scene should be on continued patient care and patient packaging.

In rescue and extrication, the mechanism of injury plays an important part in your decision about how rapid assessments, treatment, and transport will be used. Speed and the choice of the most appropriate care facility are of the essence. You may need to make the decision to airlift the patient to the closest level 1 trauma center by helicopter inside the vehicle while you are directing the extrication and performing care.

Gaining Access

Removal of motor vehicle collision victims is a critical function of fire and rescue and ambulance services. Vehicle extrication can be a quite simple or an extremely complicated procedure. As a critical function that affects patient outcome, it requires individual proficiency in conjunction with teamwork. In most cases, your primary role will be patient care. Gaining access to the patient after controlling hazards and proper stabilization of the vehicle is critical. You must work with key personnel, such as the operations and safety officer, to ensure that everyone understands the plan for extrication and treatment.

During vehicle extrication, it is very common for access to be gained by the provider using whatever means necessary. It may be as simple as opening the opposite door and positioning yourself next to the patient to perform primary and secondary assessment, treatment, and reassessment or as difficult as crawling through a back windshield or window of an upside-down vehicle to perform the same care on an inverted patient.

Whatever the circumstances are, the patient's condition and the extent of entanglement must be relayed to the officers and clear objectives must be set. All involved must be aware of the "big picture," and often you will make the final decisions regarding how extrication will proceed. It is your responsibility to refocus the team on the true objectives of the mission: safe operation resulting in successful removal of a viable patient.

Many times during the rescue, the patient's condition will change quickly. Anticipation of changing conditions in both your patient and the environment will allow you to plan for the needed equipment and indicated treatment modalities. In some situations, the best approach may be rapid extrication and transport of the patient. The situation may call for this technique because of the need to get away from an immediate danger. In those cases, rapid movement of the patient to an area of safety before providing definitive care is justified.

Patient care during extrication will follow the same protocols that you operate within normal situations. However, deviations from, or alterations of, standing orders and protocols may occur due to special circumstances related to lengthy times, entrapment issues, or hazardous conditions. On-line medical direction may be required as time ticks away. Extended-care issues are not uncommon in heavy vehicle extrication situations.

Given your patient's exposure to the stress of the collision, pain from the injuries sustained, and treatments

PERSONAL PERSPECTIVE

Advanced EMT Mark Mendez: At 0130 on a very foggy morning, my partner and I were dispatched to a head-on collision on a busy two-lane highway. Knowing the posted speed limit on the highway is 55 mph, we requested an extrication team be dispatched to respond as well. Upon arrival at the scene, we saw a small pick-up truck and a full-sized pick-up truck with their front ends entangled together. After ensuring that the scene was safe to approach, we quickly found that the driver of one truck was DOA as was the passenger in the other. The surviving driver, a young woman in her 20s, was wedged on the floorboard of the truck by the steering column and dashboard. She was not responding and was exhibiting agonal respirations. With only enough space to pass an arm to where the woman's face was, my partner inserted an OPA and applied oxygen by way of a nonrebreather mask. All that could be done now was to wait for the extrication team to arrive so that they could access the patient and continue treatment.

In just a few minutes, the extrication team arrived on the scene. My partner began explaining the situation to the extrication team members and together they devised a plan to extricate the patient. Using spreaders and rams, the patient was freed in just a few minutes. With the assistance of the other responders, my partner and I were able to perform a rapid extrication of the patient from the vehicle, manage her airway, breathing, and circulation, and expedite transport to the nearest trauma facility. Even though the patient had sustained multiple long-bone fractures, a closed head injury, and multiple significant soft-tissue injuries, she survived.

The lesson is we recognized the potential for needing extrication and requested it early. Once on scene, an extrication plan was initiated, which resulted in the patient being freed quickly, allowing for treatment and transport to be initiated. This teamwork and appropriate use of resources provided the patient with her best chance of survival.

performed, establishing a rapport early will help in alleviating fears. Consider the following tips:

- Use the patient's name and be sure the patient knows yours.
- Make sure the patient knows that you will not abandon him.
- Explain treatments, extrication procedures, and any PPE that must be applied to the patient. Also, explain any delays in the extrication process.

Hazards

Modern automobile technology has created features that are meant to improve driver and passenger chances to survive a high-velocity impact. Some of those safety features present potential hazards to rescuers. The following segments describe relevant technologies and associated hazards.

Airbag Deployment

Along with the advent of the seat belt, supplemental restraint systems (SRS), or front-impact airbags, have provided increased collision protection. Many new automobiles on the market are equipped with additional airbags throughout the vehicle, including the following:

- Side-impact protection systems (SIPS)
- Head protection systems (HPS)
- Knee bolsters

Airbags have saved many lives and have reduced the injuries once realized during high-velocity collisions. It should be noted that accidental activation of those systems can occur during vehicle extrication, injuring you and your patient. Deactivation of the devices is essential for a safe extrication. Be aware of your surroundings.

In electrical restraint systems, an electrical impulse of as little as 0.5 volt may cause a system to be accidentally activated. For automobiles with mechanical systems, it is important to know where sensors are located and to avoid excessive pressure or force in those areas. There have been many reports of airbags that were not deployed in frontal or near-frontal crashes. Treat all nondeployed airbags as if they are live, even following proper disconnection. Proper distancing is the best way to reduce personal injury from a nondeployed airbag while you are providing care. Many rescue companies employ a rule-of-thumb airbag distance directive called the 5-10-20-inch rule:

- Keep 5 inches from a side-impact airbag.
- Double the figure for the driver's frontal airbag, or 10 inches.
- Double the figure again for a passenger-side front airbag, or 20 inches.

Nondeployed airbags pose a serious risk to you and your patient during extrication. Front-impact airbags can expand at speeds in excess of 200 mph. Side-impact airbags deploy at even higher rates.

Some common injuries that you may encounter during patient care after deployment of an airbag system are soft-tissue injuries to the upper extremities. Blunt force injuries to the face and head also are common. It is not unusual for a patient to experience fracture of the nose, especially if the patient was wearing glasses.

Fuel Leaks

Adding a flammable product to an MVC increases the potential for danger. Passenger vehicles run on a variety of fuels. Today, the most common are gasoline and diesel. Fuel cylinders are most likely to be found in the trunk area of a passenger car or the bed of a pickup truck. The extrication team must evaluate those areas for the presence of fuel and manage them. As a measure of safety related to fuel leaks during vehicle extrication, fire personnel will need to be used for potential fire suppression activity. A charged (filled with water) hand-line (fire hose) should be on standby if needed.

Animals and Extrication

A passenger traveling in any vehicle may very well be a dog or cat. Animals of all types may be traveling with their owners and may require special consideration during vehicle extrication. In some cases, wounded or scared animals pose a risk to your safety and the safety of others on the scene. This provides just one more reason to ensure that you wear *all* of your PPE during the rescue.

Other Hazards

Hazards at collisions can be caused by anything from road conditions to inclement weather. The following is a list of the most common hazards you may encounter at scenes:

- Ice
- Darkness
- Downed power lines. Consider all lines as charged with electricity ("live" or "hot") and avoid them.
- Damaged poles or trees
- Traffic
- Loaded bumpers are those with shock absorbers compressed after impact. Avoid them because they can spring with violent force at any time.
- Hazardous materials released from their containers, fluid leaks
- Debris, including jagged, sharp objects
- Glass
- Water

Vehicle Stabilization

One of the most important tasks before your patient can be extricated will be the stabilization of the vehicle. In the hurry to remove the patient, stabilization is sometimes overlooked. However, sudden movement caused by the use of tools and techniques or the shifting of weight can be dangerous and even fatal to the patient or rescuer. Stabilization by the rescue team will provide a stable environment that will assist you in treating your patient and prevent unnecessary movement that can exacerbate the patient's injuries. It must be emphasized that the most important concern of vehicle stabilization is safety—yours and that of your crew and your patient.

Stabilizing Techniques

Cribbing is filling void spaces to prevent the movement of the vehicle (Figure 47-2). Prefabricated wood, plastic, or metal pieces are stacked in void spaces between the base (ground) and the underside of the vehicle and arranged in a fashion to create a tight fit between the auto and base. Achieving a tight fit can be assisted with shims, which are thinner cribbing pieces used to fill the gaps between the bigger pieces.

Shoring is often used when cribbing cannot be accomplished in a practical way due to the opening or span being too large. Large timbers or pneumatic devices are used to stabilize the vehicle during rescue and extrication operations. The use of shoring is often used with vehicles found in precarious positions, such as a vehicle found on its side.

Rigging is used to further stabilize the vehicle. Some of the more common materials used for rigging are rope, chains, and webbing.

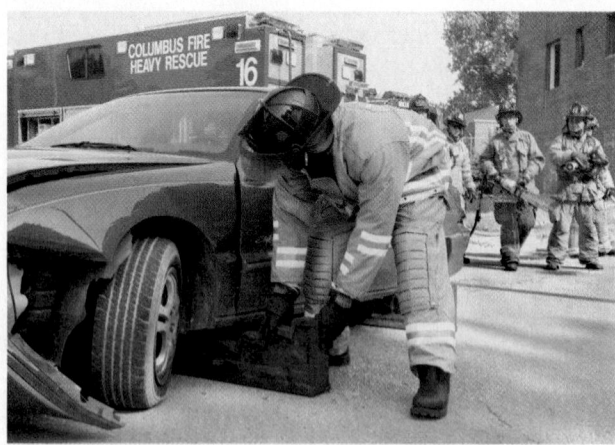

FIGURE 47-2

Cribbing is used to fill void spaces around a vehicle preventing movement.

Hybrid Vehicles

The number of **hybrid vehicles** on the road increases each day. Attention to proper identification of hybrid vehicles and some basic safety procedures should be all that you and your extrication team need in order to efficiently address the few differences between a hybrid and nonhybrid vehicle.

Knowing the location and construction of the battery compartments and components that isolate the electrical system will help you remain safe during extrication. Two of the most important aspects of disconnecting the electrical system of a hybrid vehicle, which contains high-voltage (HV) battery packs, are no different from those for a nonhybrid. First, turn the ignition off and remove the key. Second, disconnect the 12-volt battery system. The HV system has relays that automatically open and disconnect if the MVC is severe enough to deploy airbags. The HV system also is shut down as soon as the ignition is switched off or the 12-volt battery is disconnected.

Hybrid car manufacturers attempt to protect the HV systems from accidents by enclosing the HV batteries in metal cases and locating them near, under, or behind the rear seats. HV systems may remain powered for up to 10 minutes after the vehicle is shut off or the 12-volt system is disabled. To prevent serious injury or death, avoid touching, cutting, or breaching any HV power cable. The cables are bright orange in color.

The following are guidelines for working on or near a hybrid vehicle:

1. Identify the vehicle as a hybrid.
2. Stabilize the vehicle.
3. Access the passenger compartment.
4. Shift the gear selector to park.
5. Turn the ignition off.
6. Check the dash indicator for power.
7. Disconnect the 12-volt battery.

As with all vehicle collisions, a precautionary hand line (water-charged fire hose) from the first arriving pumper should be deployed. If fire is present, copious amounts of water should be used to cool the metal case that houses the HV battery pack.

Impact Damage and Extrication

Just as the type of collision and mechanism of injury provide you with clues to what types of injuries the patient may have sustained, you also can predict the types of hazards and level of difficulty expected during extrication. The following describes concerns that you should anticipate with various types of vehicle impacts:

- *Top impact.* Depending on how the vehicle came to rest, the top presenting part may or may not be the roof of the auto. You must be alert for potential difficulties involved in gaining access into the patient compartment related to how the auto came to rest. If the vehicle is on its roof, you and the extrication team must be aware of fluids that may be leaking into the patient compartment and contaminating the interior. You also must be aware of the ever-present danger of power lines that may be on or around the vehicle.

- *Bottom impact.* In most situations, the bottom of the wreckage will be the floor or the underside of the vehicle, and all or most wheels will be on a firm surface, which will ease access into the patient compartment. However, you must also be wary of what may be beneath the vehicle. Leaking fuel, battery acid, or other substances could pose safety issues that will need to be addressed.

- *Side impact.* Impacts to the sides of the vehicle are of great concern related to mechanism of injury. The sides are some of the least protected areas and should create a high index of suspicion for significant injuries. Advances have been made with the advent of side-impact airbags. However, any moderate-to-high-velocity impact to the side of the vehicle should alert you to the possibility of severe injuries.

- *Frontal impact.* If the vehicle is moving forward, the front is the aspect that should arrive first and, therefore, is the most commonly damaged part. A number of engine-related hazards should be of concern to you and the extrication team. The most common concern is fire. Broken fuel lines and a compromised electrical system can lead to a fire in the engine compartment. Attention to disconnection of the battery and control of the fuel leak should be part of any extrication team's standard operating procedures. A precautionary hand line from the first arriving pumper should be employed as a safety precaution.

- *Rear impact.* In most front-engine vehicles, the fuel tank is located in the rear of the vehicle. Most collisions that suffer rear-end damage do not result in ruptured fuel tanks. However, design flaws do occur, and the extrication team must be alert to potential fuel leaks. A precautionary hand line from the first arriving pumper should be employed as a safety precaution.

Interior of Vehicle

The interior is one of the most critical areas for removal of a patient from a vehicle. Interior components such as the dashboard, steering wheel, seats, and pedals may need to be removed from around the patient to accomplish extrication. The time it takes to remove the structures also means that you may have to spend extensive time with the patient inside the vehicle. You will be expected to perform life-sustaining and life-saving care even while the extrication is taking place. Ongoing assessment and monitoring of the patient during the extrication is of utmost importance. Continuing attention to airway management, fluid replacement, and spinal immobilization will be critical.

Extrication Tools

There are a variety of extrication tools. As an Advanced EMT, you may never use the tools to perform extrication. However, you will be working at incidents where those tools will be used, and you need to understand their purpose and use. One thing to note about tools needed for extrication: Extricating patients from vehicles may often be successful with basic hand tools and never require the use of more complex expensive power tools. Tools include the following:

- *Hand tools.* Common hand tools used during extrication are the same as those used in structural firefighting and other emergency or rescue work (Figure 47-3).

- *Striking tools.* The category of striking tools includes axes, hammers, mallets, battering rams, punches, and picks. They can be dangerous, and you must take precautions when using them near a patient. Wear PPE at all times to prevent serious injury when you are using striking tools.

- *Prying tools.* Prying tools are used to provide leverage and mechanical advantage by multiplying the force applied. They are used to open hoods, trunks, and doors. Common prying tools are the Halligan tool, crow bar, and pry bar. Used correctly, prying tools are safer than striking tools.

- *Cutting tools.* Used to cut through the different types of materials found at an extrication scene, common

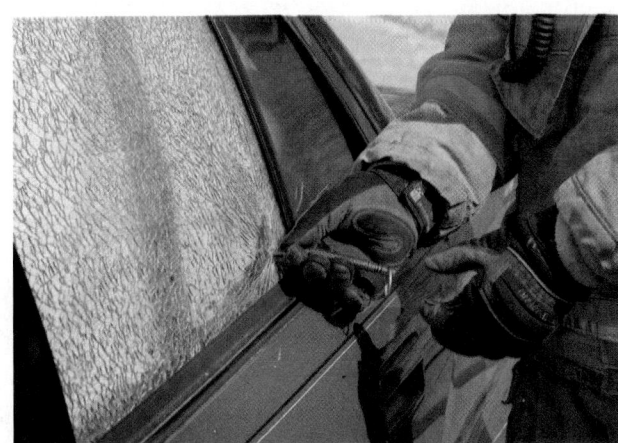

FIGURE 47-3

A window punch is an example of a hand tool used to access patients.

types of cutting tools are saws, knives, cutters, axes, and snipping tools. Because these tools are constructed with a sharp cutting edge, you must wear appropriate PPE to avoid injury.

- *Hydraulic tools.* Hydraulic tools are those in which force is exerted by a high-pressure liquid. They are many times called the *Jaws of Life*, which is a specific brand of hydraulic tool. However, hydraulic tools come in various forms and have various uses. It is critical for you as an Advanced EMT to understand the benefits and hazards associated with using hydraulic tools.

- *Manual hydraulic tools.* The manual hydraulic tool is powered by someone operating a pump lever to activate it. They work well in areas where space is limited. However, it must be noted that manual hydraulic tools operate more slowly and within a more limited range than their power-driven counterparts. Some common manual extrication devices used today are the Porta-power and other hydraulic jacks. The Porta-power comes with many accessories for various applications that will assist with extrication in limited spaces. It operates with pressure from a hand pump compressor, which allows for operation in narrow space.

- *Power-driven hydraulic tools.* These tools have a wide range of uses and power and speed superior to manual hydraulic tools. Most are operated by electric motors or gas-powered engines that keep the tool's hydraulic fluid under pressure for operation. Following are some of the more common power-driven hydraulic tools:
  - Spreaders, used for pushing or pulling (Figure 47-4)
  - Shears, used for cutting roof supports or posts (Figure 47-5)

- Pedal cutters, used for cutting pedal arms
- Extension rams, for pushing operations (Figure 47-6)

- *Pneumatic lifting tools.* These tools are used to lift or displace objects that cannot be lifted by conventional means. Pneumatic lifting bags are categorized as high, medium, or low pressure. As an Advanced EMT, you may find yourself working with a heavy rescue team with the pneumatic lifting bags. Common uses of the bags are to lift vehicles off patients. You will have to balance patient care with assisting in the rescue as the bags are inflated and deflated in order to free the patient from the entrapment. The bags also can assist with stabilization so other tools can be used to free the patient.

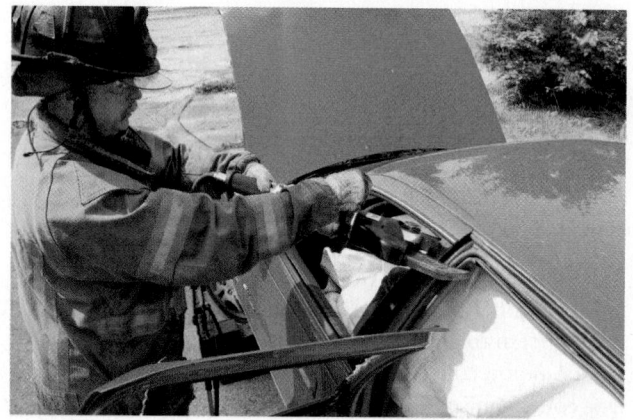

FIGURE 47-5

Hydraulic shears are used to cut vehicle posts and other structures.

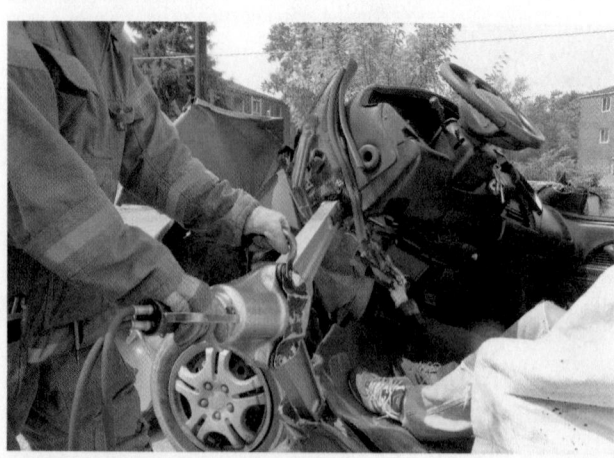

FIGURE 47-4

Hydraulic spreaders are used to separate vehicle parts to gain access to a patient.

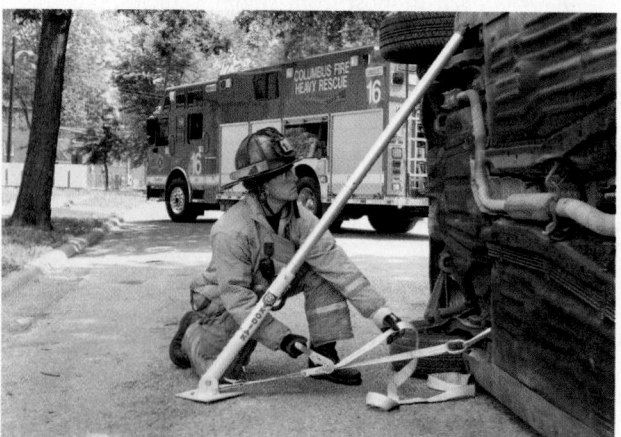

FIGURE 47-6

Hydraulic rams are used to stabilize vehicles and to separate vehicle parts, as when pushing a dashboard off of a patient.

Clinical-Reasoning Process

Advanced EMTs Al and Jay recognize that they will require additional assistance to access the patient and certainly to carry him up the embankment to the shoulder of the road. "Unit 3 to Dispatch. Please dispatch fire rescue for assistance," calls Al.

"Already on their way, Unit 3. ETA of 5 minutes," answers the dispatcher.

Al and Jay decide it is safe to walk down the embankment to the vehicle, so they grab their gear and a pry bar before heading toward the vehicle. Once safely at the vehicle, Al attempts to open the driver's door to assess the patient. He pulls but the door does not open. He can see the patient unconscious but breathing. As he grabs the pry bar and considers trying to pry the door open, Jay arrives at the passenger side door and opens it with ease. Jay enters the vehicle and begins to assess and treat the patient. Firefighters arrive on the scene and assist with packaging the patient and carrying him up the embankment.

CHAPTER REVIEW

Chapter Summary

You should begin performing patient care upon initial contact with the patient unless the scene is unsafe to do so. During extrication, patient care should continue uninterrupted to the best of your ability. There will be instances that extrication will supersede patient care. Treat the patient to the level that is safe for you, the patient, and the extrication crew. Any time you are providing patient care for the patient while he is still in the vehicle, you must wear the proper PPE. Also provide the patient with protection from sharp objects and flying debris.

Removal of the patient may be one of the most difficult tasks involved in extrication. Determinations about what means of egress you should use and the best method of patient packaging are critical. You will determine them by the patient's condition. Employ commercial devices for full spinal immobilization. As disentanglement occurs, you must provide additional care for soft-tissue and musculoskeletal injuries that are uncovered. Also, be prepared for issues related to hypovolemia, because blood and fluid loss may cause your patient to become hemodynamically challenged, resulting in shock.

This section examined motor vehicle extrication. Vehicles are more complicated and have more hazards than in past years. As technology evolves, you must keep informed about the safe and effective means to extricate and care for patients at the scene of a motor vehicle collision. The extrication process is typically performed by a designated rescue team. However, as an Advanced EMT, you must understand and, in certain instances, direct the extrication of patients from motor vehicles.

Review Questions

Multiple-Choice Questions

1. Many new automobiles on the market are equipped with additional airbags throughout the vehicle. They include all of the following EXCEPT:

   a. side-impact protection systems (SIPS).
   b. head protection systems (HPS).
   c. child impact protection systems (CIPS).
   d. knee bolsters.

2. You should consider the use of ___ to protect your patient during extrication.

   a. a tarp
   b. a blanket
   c. eye protection
   d. all of the above

3. Tools used to lift or displace objects that cannot be lifted by conventional means include which one of the following?

   a. Hand tools
   b. Cribbing
   c. Pneumatic lifting tools
   d. Shears

4. In a hybrid vehicle, the high-voltage systems will automatically disconnect EXCEPT:

   a. if the MVC is severe enough to deploy airbags.
   b. when the ignition is switched off.
   c. when the 12-volt battery is disconnected.
   d. when the vehicle comes to a stop.

5. Cribbing is:

   a. filling void spaces to prevent the movement of the vehicle.

   b. the use of cutting tools to free patients.

   c. prefabricated wood, plastic, or metal pieces used to extricate the patient.

   d. none of the above.

6. During the extrication of an animal involved in an MVC, it is important for the Advanced EMT to:

   a. get the animal out first.

   b. use all PPE when extricating the animal.

   c. leave the animal alone.

   d. call the police.

Critical-Thinking Questions

7. Describe what you would scan the area for during a windshield survey.

8. You arrive on the scene of an MVC where an unrestrained driver of a vehicle is pinned beneath the dashboard after striking a utility pole at approximately 60 mph. You notice electrical lines on the ground near the vehicle. Describe what additional resources may be needed at this scene.

9. You are called to the scene of an MVC where a hybrid vehicle was involved in a head-on collision with a pickup truck. The posted speed limit on the highway is 45 mph. Describe the guidelines for working in and around a hybrid vehicle on this scene.

References

Hoven, C. V. (2003). *Before entering that confined space…: ISHN.* Retrieved May 14, 2011, from http://www.ishn.com/Articles/Feature_Article/f2a5647b110c7010VgnVCM100000f932a8c0____

National Institute for Occupational Safety and Health. (2004). *NIOSH respirator selection logic 2004: NIOSH.* Retrieved May 14, 2011, from http://www.cdc.gov/niosh/docs/2005-100/chapter5.html

48

Hazardous Materials

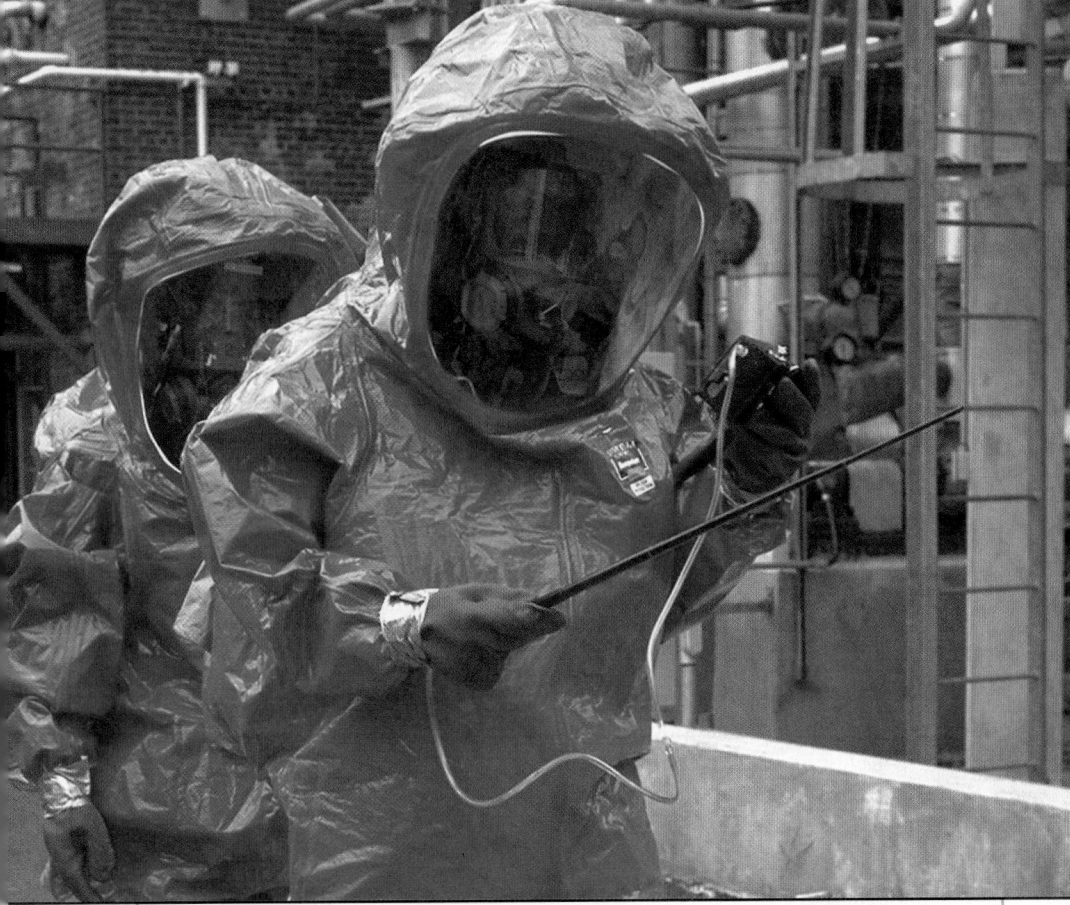

Content Area: EMS Operations

Advanced EMT Education Standard: The Advanced EMT applies knowledge and operational roles and responsibilities to ensure patient, public, and personnel safety.

Objectives

After reading this chapter, you should be able to:

48.1   Define key terms introduced in this chapter.

48.2   Explain the Advanced EMT's role in hazardous materials situations.

48.3   List indications that a hazardous materials situation may exist.

48.4   Describe the principle dangers and types of damage that can be caused by hazardous materials.

48.5   Given a scenario involving a hazardous materials incident, list specific actions you should take to minimize your chance of exposure to the materials.

48.6   Explain the U.S. Department of Transportation placard system and the National Fire Protection Association symbols for identifying hazardous materials.

(continued)

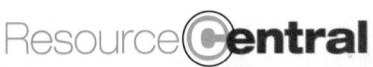

To access Resource Central, follow the directions on the Student Access Card provided with this text. If there is no card, go to www.bradybooks.com and follow the Resource Central link to Buy Access. Under Media Resources, you will find:

• *The NIMS Resource Center.* How to complete online training.

• *Hazardous Materials.* How prehospital professionals should prepare themselves for a possible exposure.

• *Common Toxidromes.* Common toxidromes, their presentations, and how to manage them.

CASE STUDY

Advanced EMTs John Parker and Julie Morin are about to end their shift when they are dispatched to the 1200 block of Industrial Park Avenue to respond to an "overturned truck." As they turn the corner to the street, they notice a large tanker truck lying on its side. It is a warm, sunny day, and a gash on the side of the truck is spilling a substance into an increasingly large pool of colorless liquid on the street. Two individuals are visible on the ground near the truck. One of them is wearing a green jumpsuit with what looks like industrial boots. The other is wearing jeans and a sport coat. Julie and John suddenly realize workers from nearby offices in the Industrial Park are beginning to congregate on the sidewalk, just as they notice what looks like evaporation spreading off the surface of the pool.

Problem-Solving Questions

1. What information should John and Julie provide to the dispatcher regarding the scene?
2. What kind of resources should they request to assist in the response to the scene?
3. What actions should they take to protect themselves, the workers, and the victims?

(continued from previous page)

48.7	Explain the purpose and limitations of shipping papers and material safety data sheets.
48.8	Identify resources that can be used in the identification and management of hazardous materials situations.
48.9	Differentiate among the levels of hazardous materials training levels identified by the Occupational Safety and Health Administration.
48.10	Discuss the components of hazardous materials incident management, including the following:

- Preincident planning
- Considerations in implementing the plan
- Establishing safety zones
- Decontamination

48.11	Differentiate between acute and chronic effects of hazardous materials exposure.
48.12	Describe the integration of patient care with the need for safety and patient decontamination when responding to hazardous materials incidents.
48.13	Describe special considerations in response to incidents involving radiation exposure and contamination.

Introduction

A **hazardous material**, sometimes called a *hazmat*, is any substance (solid, liquid, or gas) capable of harming people, property, or the environment. When hazardous materials are released through an industrial incident, highway collision, or other type of incident, people can be injured and require EMS response. Hazardous materials can cause injury through explosion, fire, release of harmful vapor, direct contact, and contamination of the environment. A hazardous materials incident is often a multiple casualty incident (MCI), necessitating implementation of the incident command system (ICS).

EMS personnel do not enter the immediate area of the release. Only highly trained hazardous material personnel can enter the area of the release, wearing specialized protective gear. There they can decontaminate patients so that they can receive medical care. Most EMS personnel are trained to the most basic of the hazardous materials training level identified by the Occupational Safety and Health Administration (OSHA), which is called the *Awareness* level. The Awareness level is designed to make sure that those who witness or identify an incident involving hazardous materials (a spill, leak, or collision, for example) are able to recognize the situation, take basic measures to protect themselves and others, and request needed resources.

Aside from recognizing potential hazardous materials incidents, protecting yourself and others from exposure, and reporting the incident, your role is to care for patients once they have been decontaminated by personnel who have special training and equipment. You should anticipate trauma, as well as problems caused by exposure to the hazardous materials. To manage decontaminated patients who have been exposed to hazardous materials, you must have a basic understanding of the types of hazardous materials and the problems they can cause.

The goals of this chapter are to help you recognize potential hazardous materials incidents, protect yourself and others from exposure, report key information while requesting additional resources, and provide emergency care for decontaminated patients.

Initial Recognition and Response

Hazardous materials can be found everywhere, including industrial sites, military bases, highway vehicles, trains, ships, aircraft, homes, and businesses that might not seem to be obvious places for hazardous materials. Of those locations, industrial centers, military bases, and transportation incidents have the highest likelihood of having large quantities of hazardous materials. However, with many substances, it takes very little to cause injury.

No matter the location of the incident, the actions of EMS personnel at a hazardous materials incident can be summarized by the mnemonic **RAIN**, described as follows:

R – Recognize the hazardous material.

A – Avoid the hazardous material.

I – Isolate the hazardous material.

N – Notify responders of the hazardous material.

Recognize the Hazardous Material

Sometimes, an incident is dispatched with the knowledge that hazardous materials are involved. For example, you may be dispatched to stand by at the scene of an industrial fire or explosion. In such cases, you will be dispatched to a designated safe staging area to await further instructions from incident command.

In other cases, dispatch information increases your suspicion of the potential for a hazardous materials incident. Fortunately, most hazardous materials incidents take place in a fixed location, such as industrial sites, where there are personnel who are trained to manage the specific materials involved. However, any time you respond to a factory or industrial site, keep in mind that the nature of the call, whether reported as a medical problem or trauma, could be related to a hazardous material exposure. Perform a thorough scene size-up to identify any signs of a hazardous materials incident.

Another potential site for exposure to hazardous materials at a fixed location involves clandestine drug labs in which a variety of toxic chemicals are used to manufacture illicit drugs. Know your community and be aware of areas where a clandestine drug lab may be operating.

Hazardous materials incidents also can occur during the transportation of chemicals. Hazardous materials are transported by ground, train, boat, and air. Often, in urban areas routes are designated for ground transport of hazardous materials to keep the vehicles carrying them as far away from the most densely populated areas as possible. Be suspicious of the potential for hazardous materials involvement whenever you are dispatched to a collision involving a tractor-trailer truck. Fortunately, in most cases, vehicles carrying hazardous materials display the required placard to identify the substance or substances being transported.

When you are the first to recognize a potential hazardous material incident, the timely and safe response of the appropriate resources depends on the actions you take.

The Preincident Phase

Part of recognizing the hazard depends on your knowledge of your community and your ability to anticipate the potential for hazardous materials incidents in the preincident phase.

It may not be possible to know ahead of time all of the hazardous materials risks in your community, but you can get a general idea of types of substances and their locations. Agricultural areas have a larger presence of anhydrous ammonia and organophosphate-containing pesticides, for example. In industrial areas, you might encounter chemical compounds such as those involving phosphorous (fireworks) or sodium chlorate (dye production). Many industries have unusual or trade-specific mixtures that may not be commonly known or might have unique chemical properties. Research parks and laboratories and military bases also are sites where you should anticipate the presence of hazardous materials.

Another source of information is the history of prior hazardous materials incidents in your area. What previous incidents has your agency responded to? What chemicals were involved? How was the situation handled? What lessons were learned? Those events, if kept in the organizational memory, can provide valuable information when responding to future incidents.

The On-Scene Phase

Once you are on the scene, you may see additional indications of a hazard materials incident as part of your scene size-up (Figure 48-1). Be extremely cautious. Remember the RAIN mnemonic: The second action is to *avoid* the hazard. Do not risk your personal safety to obtain information. Examine the overall scene, but never drive through the hazard

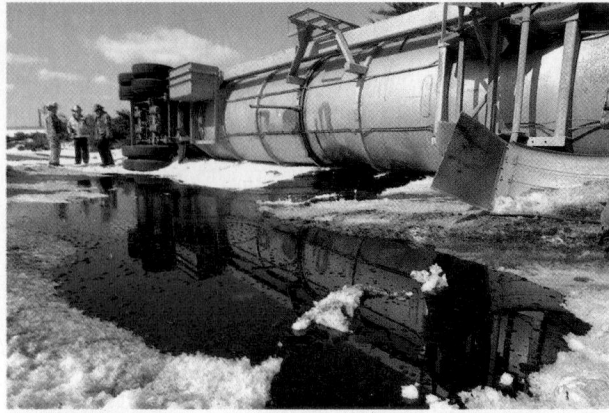

FIGURE 48-1

An overturned chemical tanker truck. (© Mark C. Ide)

or attempt to get closer to a suspected hazardous material incident. In fact, you may need to get further away from the scene immediately. You may be affected by a hazardous material very quickly, depending on its nature, and be unable to get away from it, resulting in severe injury or death. As part of its standard equipment, your vehicle may have a pair of binoculars to help you assess the scene from a distance.

Indications of a potential hazardous materials incident include the following:

- Smoke, vapors, or fumes
- Particulates or dust
- Fire
- Leaking liquids
- Unusual sounds, such as hissing, rumbling, or tearing metal
- A National Fire Protection Association (NFPA) 704 placard on a fixed storage container or a U.S. Department of Transportation placard on vehicles
- Unusual odors
- Multiple patients

Note the color of any smoke, particulates, vapors, or flames so you can report them when you notify dispatch. Also keep in mind that you might not notice signs of a hazardous materials incident until you are inside the building; be prepared to leave the structure immediately if you notice signs that a hazardous material is present.

Placards

Placards contain coded information that helps you identify what kind of material is involved and what your immediate actions should be. The NFPA 704 placard system is used on fixed chemical storage facilities. A different system, the U.S. DOT placard system, is used in the transportation industry. You have very likely seen both types of placards, but may not have paid much attention to them. However, both types

of placards can give you information that helps dispatch and incident command implement the correct response.

An NFPA 704 placard is diamond shaped with a different color in each of the quadrants. Each quadrant represents a different type of hazard associated with the chemical, as follows:

- Red—flammability
- Yellow—**reactivity**
- Blue—health effects
- White—other information, such as a precaution against using water on the substance, a radiation hazard, or **oxidation** hazard

The red, yellow, and blue quadrants each contain a number from 1 to 4 that represents the level of risk of each type of hazard. The numeral 1 is the lowest risk and 4 is the highest risk. For example, if the red quadrant is a 1, the yellow quadrant is a 3, and the blue quadrant is a 4, it means that the substance is not very flammable, but it is moderately reactive and very hazardous to health.

The white quadrant contains symbols that communicate more specific hazard information. A "W" denotes that the substance reacts with water, while the three-bladed radiation symbol indicates the presence of radiation.

The NFPA 704 system provides general information on hazards, but it does not give information that identifies the name of the substance, its specific effects or properties, initial isolation distances, or other information (Figure 48-2).

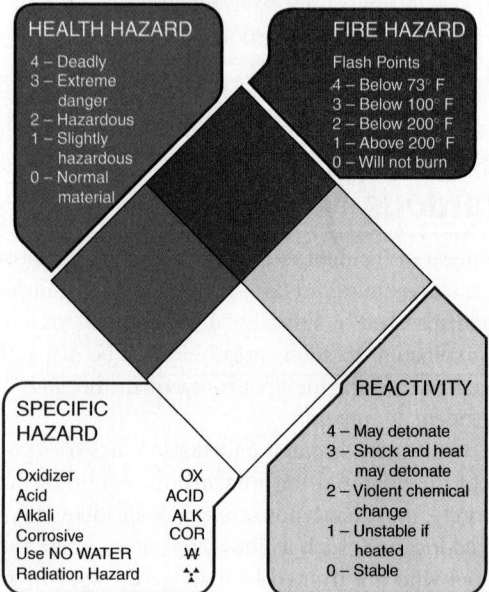

FIGURE 48-2

The key to a NFPA 704 placard.

TABLE OF PLACARDS AND INITIAL RESPONSE GUIDES TO USE ON-SCENE
USE THIS TABLE ONLY IF MATERIALS CANNOT BE SPECIFICALLY IDENTIFIED BY USING THE SHIPPING DOCUMENT, NUMBERED PLACARD, OR ORANGE PANEL NUMBER

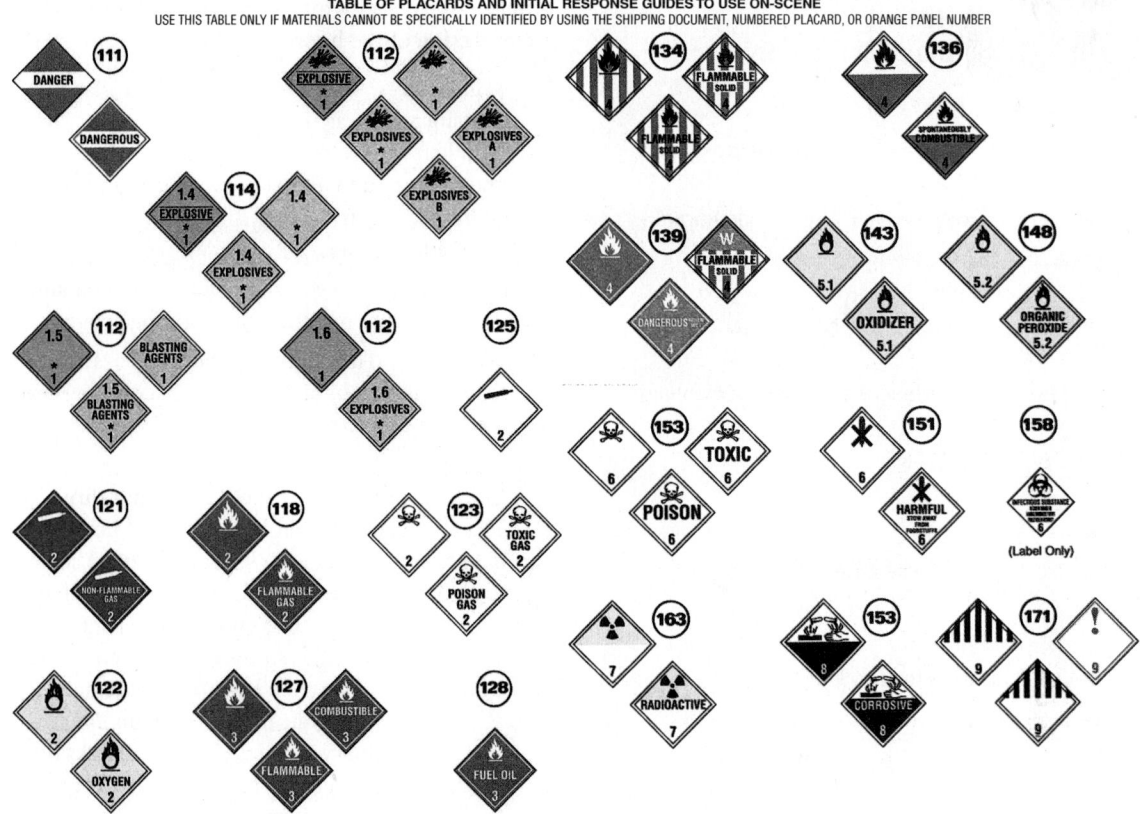

FIGURE 48-3

A DOT placard system.

DOT placards also are diamond shaped (Figure 48-3), but they give information different from the NFPA placards. DOT placards identify the International Hazard Classification System (IHCS) general classification of the substance, and list a United Nations (UN) number that serves as a reference for information about the substance in the *North American Emergency Response Guidebook*, usually called the **Emergency Response Guidebook (ERG)**.

The IHCS consists of nine classes of chemicals. Chemicals are classified based upon their most dangerous characteristic (Table 48-1). The nine classes are as follows:

Class 1 – Explosives

Class 2 – Gases

Class 3 – Flammable Liquids

Class 4 – Flammable Solids

Class 5 – Oxidizers

Class 6 – Poisonous and Infectious Substances

Class 7 – Radioactive Materials

Class 8 – Corrosives

Class 9 – Miscellaneous

The classifications provide a general idea of the type of precautions you must take on a scene involving chemicals in

each class. The classes use subclasses to differentiate among chemicals within the class. For example, there are four subclasses of gases: flammable, nonflammable compressed, poisonous, and corrosive.

The United Nations identification (UN ID) number is a unique identifier for each hazardous chemical. The **UN ID numbers** are used to reference additional information about the chemical in the *Emergency Response Guidebook*.

The *Emergency Response Guidebook* is published every four years (Figure 48-4). It provides information about

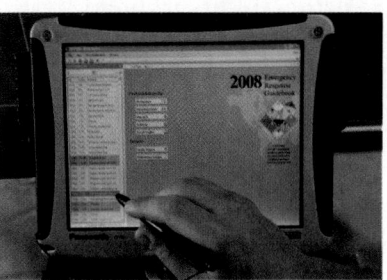

FIGURE 48-4

The *Emergency Response Guidebook* is a valuable resource for a hazardous materials response.

TABLE 48-1   Hazard Classification System

CLASS 1—EXPLOSIVES

Division 1.1	Explosives with a mass explosion hazard
Division 1.2	Explosives with a protection hazard
Division 1.3	Explosives with predominantly a fire hazard
Division 1.4	Explosives with no significant blast hazard
Division 1.5	Very insensitive explosives; blasting agents
Division 1.6	Extremely insensitive detonating articles

CLASS 2—GASES

Division 2.1	Flammable gases
Division 2.2	Nonflammable, nontoxic, compressed gases
Division 2.3	Gases toxic by inhalation
Division 2.4	Corrosive gases

CLASS 3—FLAMMABLE LIQUIDS AND COMBUSTIBLE LIQUIDS

CLASS 4—FLAMMABLE SOLIDS; SPONTANEOUSLY COMBUSTIBLE MATERIALS; AND DANGEROUS-WHEN-WET MATERIALS

Division 4.1	Flammable solids
Division 4.2	Spontaneously combustible materials
Division 4.3	Dangerous-when-wet materials

CLASS 5—OXIDIZERS AND ORGANIC PEROXIDES

Division 5.1	Oxidizers
Division 5.2	Organic peroxides

CLASS 6—TOXIC MATERIALS AND INFECTIOUS SUBSTANCES

Division 6.1	Toxic materials
Division 6.2	Infectious substances

CLASS 7—RADIOACTIVE MATERIALS

CLASS 8—CORROSIVE MATERIALS

CLASS 9—MISCELLANEOUS DANGEROUS GOODS

Division 9.1	Miscellaneous dangerous goods
Division 9.2	Environmentally hazardous substances
Division 9.3	Dangerous wastes

various common chemicals and dangerous goods that might be encountered in the highway transportation industry. The UN number or name of the chemical provides you with the information you need to guide your initial actions. The ERG has pages marked with different colors: yellow, blue, orange, green, and white. Each color corresponds to a different section of the book, as follows:

- *White pages.* These contain the DOT Hazard Classifications, as well as Emergency Response Phone Numbers, an overview of placards, a guide to railcars and tankers, and an overview of the guide itself.

- *Yellow pages.* These pages have a list of hazardous materials in sequential order by UN number. Each listing gives the name of the material and a corresponding reference in the orange pages.

- *Blue pages.* These have a list of the hazardous materials in alphabetical order. Each listing provides the UN number and a corresponding reference in the orange pages.

- *Orange pages.* The orange section has three parts: Potential Hazards, Public Safety, and Emergency Response. The orange pages are grouped according to chemical properties and characteristics that can impact responders. The same orange pages can apply to several chemicals that have similar characteristics.
  - *Potential Hazards.* Hazards associated with the type of chemical, such as flammability, combustibility, and specific health risks are listed in order from those most likely to occur to those least likely to occur.
  - *Public Safety.* This section includes measures that should be taken, such as suggested isolation distances, personal protective equipment (PPE), and other precautions.
  - *Emergency Response.* These pages provide first aid suggestions, emergency precautions against fire and other combustion, and procedures for handling a small or large spill of the chemical.

- *Green pages.* The green pages consist of tables of additional information, including more in-depth information about suggested isolation distances based on the time of day, the weather, and the size of the spill. The second table is a list of chemicals (sequential by UN number) that react to water to produce specific toxic gases.

Other Sources of Hazardous Material Information

Other sources of information about hazardous materials are the **material safety data sheets (MSDS)** and **shipping papers**. MSDS are written by chemical manufacturers in compliance with federal regulations, and are required to be stored in proximity to the location of the chemicals (Figure 48-5). The MSDS for a chemical provides detailed information about specific chemicals, including their properties, physical states, and health risks. The limitations of MSDS are that they rely on the manufacturers for information and that, since they must be stored close to the chemicals they describe, they might not be accessible when needed.

Health	2+
Flammability	0
Reactivity	1
Personal Protection	B

Material Safety Data Sheets

I – CHEMICAL IDENTIFICATION

| Name | regular Clorox Bleach | CAS No. | N/A |
| Description | clear, light yellow liquid with chlorine odor | RTECs No. | N/A |

Other Designations
EPA Reg. No. 5813-1
Sodium hypochlorite solution
Liquid chlorine bleach
Clorox Liquid Bleach

Manufacturer
The Clorox Company
1221 Broadway
Oakland, CA 94612

Emergency Procedure
• Notify your supervisor
• Call your local poison control center   OR
• Rocky Mountain Poison Center
  (303)573-1014

II – HEALTH HAZARD DATA

• Causes severe but temporary eye injury. May irritate skin. May cause nausea and vomiting if ingested. Exposure to vapor or mist may irritate nose, throat and lungs. The following medical conditions may be aggravated by exposure to high concentrations of vapor or mist: heart conditions or chronic respiratory problems such as asthma, chronic bronchitis or obstructive lung disease. Under normal consumer use conditions the likelihood of any adverse health effects are low. FIRST AID: EYE CONTACT: Immediately flush eyes with plenty of water. If irritation persists, see a doctor. SKIN CONTACT: Remove contaminated clothing. Wash area with water. INGESTION: Drink a glassful of water and call a physician. INHALATION: If breathing problems develop remove to fresh air.

III – HAZARDOUS INGREDIENTS

| Ingredients | Concentration | Worker Exposure Limit |
| Sodium hypochlorite CAS# 7681-52-9 | 5.25% | not established |

None of the ingredients in this product are on the IARC, NTP or OSHA carcinogen list. Occasional clinical reports suggest a low potential for sensitization upon exaggerated exposure to sodium hypochlorite if skin damage (e.g., irritation) occurs during exposure. Routine clinical tests conducted on intact skin with Clorox Liquid Bleach found no sensitization in the test subjects.

IV – SPECIAL PROTECTION INFORMATION

Hygienic Practices: Wear safety glasses. With repeated or prolonged use, wear gloves.

Engineering Controls: Use general ventilation to minimize exposure to vapor or mist.

Work Practices: Avoid eye and skin contact and inhalation of vapor or mist.

V – SPECIAL PRECAUTIONS

Keep out of reach of children. Do not get in eyes or on skin. Wash thoroughly with soap and water after handling. Do not mix with other household chemicals such as toilet bowl cleaners, rust removers, vinegar, acid or ammonia containing products. Store in a cool, dry place. Do not reuse empty container; rinse container and put in trash container.

VI – SPILL OR LEAK PROCEDURES

Small quantities of less than 5 gallons may be flushed down drain. For larger quantities wipe up with an absorbent material or mop and dispose of in accordance with local, state and federal regulations. Dilute with water to minimize oxidizing effect on spilled surface.

VII – REACTIVITY DATA

Stable under normal use and storage conditions. Strong oxidizing agent. Reacts with other household chemicals such as toilet bowl cleaners, rust removers, vinegar, acids or ammonia containing products to produce hazardous gases, such as chlorine and other chlorinated species. Prolonged contact with metal may cause pitting or discoloration.

VIII – FIRE AND EXPLOSION DATA

Not flammable or explosive. In a fire, cool containers to prevent rupture and release of sodium chlorate.

IX – PHYSICAL DATA

Boiling point...................................212°F/100°C (decomposes)
Specific Gravity (H_2O = 1).............1.085
Solubility in Water........................complete
pH..11.4

FIGURE 48-5

MSDS have specific chemical information.

As you gather information from the ERG, the MSDS, CHEM-TREC, ChemTel, and other sources, you may find that advice, such as protective action distances, is slightly different from source to source. Of the information you receive, use the one that provides the greatest safety for you and the public. You also must take into consideration the conditions at the location. If, even after keeping the suggested protective distance away, you still believe you are in the path of the hazardous materials, do not hesitate to move back even further.

Shipping papers, sometimes called a *manifest* or *bill of lading*, declare the contents on board a transport container (ship, trailer, train car). The description of the materials on board must contain, at a minimum, the proper shipping name, hazard class or division, the UN number, and the total quantity of the material. Because of their proximity to the hazard, the shipping papers may be inaccessible.

Emergency Assistance Numbers

There are at least three reliable sources of additional information about hazardous materials that you can access by phone. The Chemical Transportation Emergency Center, CHEMTREC, and ChemTel are staffed with specialists 24 hours a day. Both have toll-free numbers that are listed in the ERG. You also can contact a Poison Control Center. When calling for assistance, provide as much of the following information as possible:

- Your name and contact number
- Location and nature of the problem (fire, spill, explosion)

- Name and identification of the substances involved
- Shipper and point of origin (from the shipping papers)
- Carrier name, rail car, or truck number
- Container type and size
- Quantity of material
- Weather conditions
- Injuries and exposures
- Emergency services notified

Avoid the Hazardous Material

A hazardous materials scene may not be safe enough for you to enter for hours. In fact, in most cases, you will not enter the immediate vicinity. The hazardous materials team will decontaminate patients and bring them to you in the designated area called the **cold zone**. To prevent **exposure** to and **contamination** from hazardous materials, do the following:

- *Avoid the hazard.* Park uphill, upwind, and upstream to minimize chances of exposure and contamination. Inclement weather such as swirling winds, rain, or thunderstorms contribute to the unpredictability of hazardous materials scenes and you should consider these factors in your decision-making process. Wind direction and speed can change drastically, depending on the season and the area. Therefore, what may be safely upwind at one time may later become downwind. Remain carefully observant of weather conditions, and consider where you would re-stage your ambulance if those conditions were to change.
- *Avoid contaminated victims.* Do not touch anyone who was at the scene, no matter how much distress

Advanced EMT Mike Parish: I remember learning about hazardous materials events in class, but I never really thought too much about them because I work in a suburb where there are homes and office buildings and no industrial capacity whatsoever. However, one day we had an incident where a pipe below a gas station broke, and fuel had spilled in the station and onto the street. When we arrived on the scene, people were running around yelling and some were covered in gasoline. It was pure chaos! We decided to keep the ambulance about a block away so we would be far from it in case of an explosion. However, even being that distance away, a few ran up to the ambulance asking us to help them. A few looked a little wet, but other people seemed fine, but were a bit panicked. My partner grabbed my arm just as I was about to open the door for one, and he told me that we were going to have to wait for the hazardous materials team to arrive. I asked him why. After all, it was only gasoline!

That's when he reminded me of the potential for secondary contamination and also the flammability of even a small amount of gasoline fumes. So I had to tell them through the window that they would need to go talk to the Fire Department when they arrived. I could tell some were in possible respiratory distress, so having to drive away was one of the most difficult things I have had to do in my career. Thankfully, the Fire Department hazardous materials team arrived quickly, but we still had to wait another 45 minutes for them to set up their decontamination area so that we could see our first patients. My partner and I spoke to them, getting the latest information on additional hazards and numbers of patients.

It was a good thing that we asked, because we ended up having to call for additional ambulances, because we evaluated about two dozen patients, with five requiring transport. Thankfully, the gasoline was cleaned up without any additional injuries or illnesses, and without any additional contamination of the ambulance or on us."

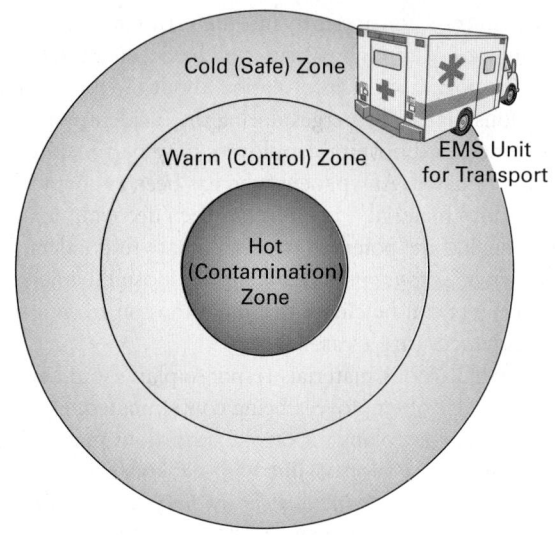

Hot (Contamination) Zone

Contamination is actually present.
Personnel must wear appropriate protective gear.
Number of rescuers limited to those absolutely necessary.
Bystanders never allowed.

Warm (Control) Zone

Area surrounding the contamination zone.
Vital to preventing spread of contamination.
Personnel must wear appropriate protective gear.
Lifesaving emergency care is performed.

Cold (Safe) Zone

Normal triage, stabilization, and treatment performed.
Rescuers must shed contaminated gear before entering the cold zone.

FIGURE 48-6

Hot, warm, and cold zones.

they are in, until they have been decontaminated. Although your first reaction may be to assist those who are injured, allowing yourself to become contaminated may result in you not being able to help at all, and divert additional responders from caring for patients so that they can care for you.

- *Avoid the outside.* Remain in your vehicle until the hazardous materials team declares that it is safe for you to exit. Roll up windows and recirculate the cabin air instead of opening the vents to outside air, which can contain particulates or vapors.

Isolate the Hazardous Material

Isolating the scene is a public safety action to prevent additional casualties and prevent spread of contamination. The public should be isolated uphill, upwind, and upstream of the hazard. The ERG provides specific recommendations on initial evacuation distances and other precautions.

The hazardous materials team will establish three zones at the scene. They are called the **hot zone**, **warm zone**, and cold zone (Figure 48-6):

- *Hot zone.* Also called the *exclusion zone*, this is the immediate area of the hazardous material. Only properly equipped and trained hazardous materials personnel enter this zone to retrieve patients and contain the hazard.
- *Warm zone.* The warm zone, or *contamination reduction zone*, is the area just beyond the hot zone. The hazardous materials team, equipment, and patients are decontaminated here as they are removed from the hot zone. There is an access corridor that serves at the point of entry and exit to the hot zone. A decontamination line provides for the orderly movement of individuals in and out of the hot zone.
- *Cold zone.* The cold zone is where support operations, such as triage and treatment areas, are staged to await decontaminated patients. Incident command is located in the cold zone. The cold zone also is where you will operate. It should be noted that the triage, treatment, and transport areas should not be located in the hot or warm zones. (See Chapter 49 for details on multiple-casualty incidents.) By the time you receive patients in the

cold zone, they will already have gone through a primary (and possibly secondary) decontamination, and traveled through the access corridor before being received in the cold zone.

Notify Responders of the Hazardous Material

You must communicate the information from your scene size-up to dispatch, initially, to determine the appropriate resources to be dispatched. From that point, you may communicate directly with the incoming hazardous materials team to relay additional information. The response time of the hazardous materials team varies. In urban and most suburban areas, the response time is usually short. In rural areas, you may have to wait an extended period of time for a fully equipped hazardous materials team to arrive.

The person who makes contact with the hospitals in the area is determined by protocol or your disaster plan, but the hospitals must be notified, as well, so they can prepare for the number of patients and the estimated severity of their injuries. Although patients will be decontaminated before transport, if more information about the nature of the hazardous material emerges during the incident, you, your ambulance, and hospital employees may be considered to be contaminated. Any patient who has been in contact with a hazardous material, even if he has been decontaminated at the scene, has the potential to contaminate responders. This is known as *secondary contamination*. Hospital emergency departments can be closed if contamination from a scene reaches patient care areas.

The hazardous materials response plan should address the possibility of employees being contaminated. Hospitals have contingency plans for on-site hazardous materials decontamination and for dealing with patients coming out of a hazardous materials incident. Providing as much information as possible as early as possible allows them to mobilize needed resources.

There are no specific antidotes to most hazardous materials. However, if there is a specific antidote, area poison control centers may maintain stocks of antidotes throughout the state, which can be made available for transport to hospitals. If provided with early enough notice, a hospital might receive the stock in time for the arrival of the first patients.

Hazardous Materials Operations

An overview of hazardous materials operations will help you work more effectively with hazardous materials teams.

Training Levels

OSHA recognizes five levels of hazardous materials training. They are as follows:

- *First Responder Awareness*. Those who are at this level are likely to witness a release. Their responsibilities are to notify the appropriate authorities and remain safely away. There is no minimum number of training hours, but FEMA and other organizations provide coursework for the awareness level.

- *First Responder Operations*. Responders with this level of training have completed an 8- or 16-hour course, and are trained to isolate an area and assist in maintaining protective action distances for the public in order to prevent the spread of contamination.

- *Hazardous Materials Operations*. Individuals trained to the operations level have taken a 40-hour training course, and can initiate defensive actions to prevent the spread of hazardous materials.

- *Hazardous Materials Technician*. Those who are at the level of technician have the knowledge and ability

to plug, patch, or stop the release of material. They use highly specialized PPE and are trained to make an area safe for entry by containing the incident. Typically, members of a hazardous materials team have been trained to this level.

- *Hazardous Materials Specialist*. Responders at this level have training in leadership and specialization in the support of hazardous materials operations. Most hazardous materials supervisors overseeing operations at an incident are trained to this level.

Incident Command

OSHA requires the use of the incident command system (ICS) during a hazardous materials incident. Review the material on incident command in Chapter 33.

Personal Protective Equipment

Hazardous materials response often requires the use of specialized personal protective equipment (PPE), which also requires training for proper use. The type of PPE is determined by the nature of the incident and can include respiratory protection, special garments, and barrier materials to protect personnel from exposure to biologic, chemical, and radioactive hazards. If the hazardous materials team requires you to use specialized PPE, you must be trained in its use. Do not use specialized gear that you are not trained to use. Using equipment without training can result in injuries and illnesses that may last weeks, months, or even years. Masks, for example, may require fit testing by a qualified fit tester, which will prevent you from simply putting it on and entering the scene. Many chemicals that have carcinogenic (cancer-causing) properties need only a single exposure to cause the illness later in life.

There are four levels of PPE for hazardous materials operations. Those levels are designed "A" through "D," with "A" offering the highest protection and "D" offering the least. They are as follows:

- *Level A*. This is a fully encapsulated suit with supplied air by a self-contained breathing apparatus (SCBA). Level A is worn when the type of chemical involved is unknown, or when it is known to be highly hazardous, requiring full body and respiratory protection.

- *Level B*. The suit is not fully encapsulated, but the responder still uses SCBA. The suit provides splash protection for the wearer.

- *Level C*. This level does not include SCBA, but does include a respirator mask with filter and a suit. Level C is used when the chemical is known, and its hazards do not require the use of SCBA or a fully encapsulated suit.

- *Level D*. The Level D is a regular work uniform, which is worn when the environment is considered safe for workers.

Decontamination

Decontamination must occur whenever a hazardous material contaminates patients or equipment. The decontamination process includes removing contaminated clothing and using copious amounts of water to remove contaminants from the skin. The water used for decontamination becomes contaminated in the process, and must be contained to prevent runoff from further contaminating the environment and posing a risk to others who come in contact with it. There are two points at which contamination can occur, known as *primary contamination* and *secondary contamination*. Regardless of how the contamination occurs, though, the patient—or EMS responder—must be decontaminated.

Contamination directly from the source itself is known as *primary contamination*. Primary contamination occurs in the hot zone, and is most likely to happen before, at the time of the release and before the isolation zones are established. Most primary contamination comes in the form of a liquid or a solid. Contamination is not as likely to occur with a hazardous gas. The risk with gases and vapors is respiratory exposure.

Secondary contamination comes from outside the hot zone, and is an indirect method of contamination. Secondary contamination is likely to occur from one of two sources coming out of the hot zone: patients or equipment. Secondary contamination occurs when ineffective or incomplete decontamination is performed in the warm zone.

Hazardous materials responses have unpredictable elements even when all necessary precautions are taken. It is possible that contaminated people can circumvent an organized evacuation and present themselves to you in the cold zone for assessment and treatment. If the patient looks contaminated, such as having a liquid or dust on him or his clothing, or the smell of chemicals, do not touch him. Direct him to report to the decontamination line. As a general rule, you will be positioned at the entrance to the access corridor at the junction of the warm and cold zones so that you will be able to triage, assess, and manage patients as they are decontaminated.

Be alert to indications that patients still have some of the hazardous material on them, even though they have gone through decontamination. Areas of the body that are prone to hidden contamination include the underarms, the groin, skin folds, the cleft of the buttocks, and between the fingers and toes. The risk of retained contaminants is higher in patients who are unconscious or incapacitated, because they are unable to follow instructions and assist in the decontamination process.

Rehabilitation

Areas called *rehabilitation areas* are set up to assess and treat hazardous materials responders. This is an important aspect of hazardous materials operations. The nature of working around hazardous materials requires wearing PPE, which poses particular health risks, including heat-related injuries. Hot temperatures, direct sunlight, and humidity make those injuries more likely. Your role may not only be to treat the initial patients, but also those who have responded to the emergency. You may be assigned a role as a medical monitor. OSHA regulations require that hazardous material entry team members have their vital signs taken before entering the hot zone and upon leaving it, to identify those who are at increased risk for injury in the hazardous environment.

Medical Aspects of Hazardous Materials

You learned about many poisons in Chapter 32. Much of that information applies to hazardous materials, but there are some additional considerations in toxicology related to hazardous materials. In particular, the term **toxicant** is used to refer to a poisonous substance not derived from the metabolism of an organism. Poisons, including those classified as hazardous materials, enter the body through inhalation, ingestion, injection, or absorption. Unlike other poisoning situations, inhalation is the most common way that hazardous materials gain access to the body.

The effects of a poison on the body depend on the time of exposure and the dosage of the substance. *Acute exposures* are abrupt, high-dose single exposures. Most of the patients you will encounter have experienced an acute exposure. *Chronic exposures* are longer term, typically a month or more, of lower levels of a substance. Assessment and treatment depend on the number of patients affected, the number of responders and resources available, and the severity of patients' injuries.

If the hazardous materials incident is a multiple-casualty incident in which the number of patients exceeds the resources available, patients will be prioritized for treatment and transport using a triage system. In cases where there are enough responders to treat the patients, you will take a more traditional approach. As the patient leaves the decontamination area, you will perform primary and secondary assessments, intervening to treat immediately life-threatening problems with the airway, breathing, and circulation. The treatment for toxicant poisoning depends on the patient's signs and symptoms. There rarely is a specific antidote.

Patient injuries can include blast trauma, thermal burns, chemical burns, and other injuries. Open wounds and burned skin can mean that there is chemical contamination in the wound and that absorption of the chemical through damaged skin is increased. As with other poisons, children, chronically ill patients, and the elderly are more susceptible to the effects of hazardous materials. They may show symptoms sooner and with greater severity, or their pre-existing conditions can be exacerbated.

Hazardous materials incidents can be frightening and the decontamination process can be emotionally traumatizing. If the emotional aspects of the situation are not handled properly, a hazardous materials scene can deteriorate quickly into chaos and instability.

Special Considerations in Radiation Incidents

Significant sources of radiation are usually identified with the universal symbol for radiation, a three-bladed icon called a *trefoil*. The concerns with radiation incidents depend on the type and amount of radiation involved, and whether a patient is exposed or contaminated.

Exposure occurs when radiation energy comes in contact with the body. An example of exposure is receiving an X-ray or being exposed to sunlight. The energy from the source penetrates your body, but the source does not actually come into contact with you. Contamination occurs when the particles that emit the radiation are on the person or in his body. A person who is exposed is not a danger to others because he is not the source of radiation. A person who is contaminated with radioactive material can contaminate anything he comes in contact with. A contaminated patient continues to receive exposure until he is decontaminated. Assume that all patients at a scene involving radiation are contaminated and must be decontaminated before medical treatment unless the **radiation safety officer** at the scene advises you otherwise.

Radiation is energy in the form of electromagnetic waves or subatomic particles. It is invisible and undetectable without special equipment. Low-level radiation is ubiquitous in the environment, but when higher levels are present radiation can disrupt cellular function. Nonionizing radiation is in the form of electromagnetic waves and includes infrared and ultraviolet light, radiofrequencies, microwave energy, and radar transmitters. There are two classifications of ionizing radiation: particulate and electromagnetic. Particulate radiation includes alpha and beta particles and neutron radiation. Electromagnetic ionizing radiation forms are gamma rays and X-rays. Ionizing radiation is found in hospitals and other health care facilities, nuclear reactors, and nuclear weapons. Sources of ionizing radiation may be transported and stored in many locations.

Alpha particles have a range of 1 to 2 inches from their source. These low-energy particles do not penetrate the skin, but they could cause damage if ingested or inhaled. Beta particles can range 10 feet from their source, but are also relatively low energy and thick clothing offers protection from beta particles. Gamma radiation is higher energy and its energy can range several hundred feet from its source and can easily penetrate the skin. Protection from gamma radiation requires a combination of time, distance, and shielding from the source. X-ray radiation is similar to gamma radiation, but is lower in energy. Neutron energy has the longest range, several hundred feet or farther. The same precautions must be used with neutron radiation as with gamma radiation.

Three factors affect the amount of biologic damage from radiation: total dose, the dose rate, and the type of radiation that caused the exposure. The Department of Energy unit of measurement for radiation dosage is the **radiation absorbed dose (rad)**. A rad is the application of 0.01 joule of energy in 1 kg of tissue. A **roentgen equivalent man (rem)** takes into consideration the amount of radiation and the likely biologic damage to occur. For emergency response, consider rad and rem as equivalent measurements.

People take in about 360 millirems (mrem) per year of radiation. Other activities can expose you to extra radiation. Cigarette smokers, for instance, are exposed to another 1,300 mrems/year, and those working in medical facilities take in about 54 mrems/year. The numbers may seem large, but radiation sickness requires a dose of about 100,000 mrems. Severe symptoms require an even higher dose of 250,000 mrems.

A person who receives a large dose of radiation, or even a smaller dose over a very short period of time, may develop acute radiation sickness (ARS). Signs and symptoms of ARS occur in four phases: prodromal, latent, illness, and recovery or death. In the prodromal stage, the patient experiences nausea and vomiting, loss of appetite, and diarrhea. Higher doses can cause fever, respiratory symptoms, and increased excitability. The symptoms last from hours to days. In the latent stage, the illness seems as if it is in remission and the patient appears to be healthy. The latent period is shorter than the prodromal phase. At higher dosages, the latent phase may not occur at all. In the illness stage, signs and symptoms recur. Depending on the dose, recovery or death occurs over the following weeks.

Radiation Injury

Radiation injury, also called *localized radiation injury (LRI)*, is a partial-body exposure. This situation can occur in individuals who work with or around radioactive substances. Usually, they are protected by special clothing and equipment, but failure to use the clothing or equipment properly can result in partial body exposure.

The integumentary system is a good indicator of LRI. At about 300 rad, hair loss occurs in one to three weeks. Erythema, or redness of the skin, occurs at a dosage of about 600 rad a few hours after exposure. The skin peels without blistering a few weeks after exposure to about 1,000 rad. Exposure to about 1,500 rad causes blistering and peeling two to five weeks after exposure, with large blisters occurring with 2,500 rad. A 5,000 rad exposure causes skin necrosis days or weeks after exposure.

Treatment for Radiation

Any patient who has been contaminated with a radioactive substance must be decontaminated before receiving emergency medical care. Remember, except in extremely high

Clinical-Reasoning Process

Advanced EMTs John Parker and Julie Morin are on a scene of an overturned truck containing a hazardous material. The contents of the truck are forming an increasingly large pool of colorless liquid that is beginning to evaporate. There are two known victims, but bystanders are congregating on the sidewalk.

The spilling liquid makes this an uncontrolled hazardous materials scene that requires specialized resources for containment and cleanup. The presence of bystanders indicates the possibility of additional victims if they do not act quickly to isolate them from the hazardous materials.

John looks for a placard on the truck and scans the scene to be sure the presence of the hazardous materials has not distracted them from other potential dangers at the scene.

Julie looks at a flag on top of a nearby building to check wind direction. The wind is blowing toward them, but away from the crowd of bystanders. Because they are downwind from the hazard, John and Julie drive around the block to the location of the bystanders. Even though the crowd is upwind of the hazard, Julie uses the PA system to instruct the bystanders to go back into the building and wait until the fire department notifies them that it is safe to leave.

Julie notifies dispatch that they are on the scene of a hazardous material spill with a DOT placard number of 1017 and requests a fire department and hazardous materials team response. She reports two patients and a crowd of about 25 bystanders and requests two transporting ambulances and law enforcement for traffic and crowd control. She advises dispatch that the wind is from the south and that all resources should stage on the access road on the south side of the industrial park.

Meanwhile, John uses the *Emergency Response Guidebook* to identify number 1017 as chlorine and that a good precautionary evacuation distance is at least 330 feet. Reading that the evaporating gas is heavier than air, John selects a spot higher than the pool of liquid and ensures they all are an adequate distance away.

Julie and John quickly sketch out hot, warm, and cold zones on a sheet of paper, and make recommendations for ingress and egress points for the responders. Within 10 minutes, another EMS crew and a hazardous materials truck arrive. John briefs the captain of the hazardous materials team. The captain takes the information and begins the setup for the emergency response, while John and Julie await their first patients.

doses, the signs and symptoms of radiation injury and sickness are delayed. A physician must evaluate all patients, even if they do not have immediate signs and symptoms. A patient with internal radiation contamination requires immediate hospitalization. Because there is no method of field decontamination for internal contamination, the patient continues to be exposed to the effects of radiation. Antidotes for certain types of radiation are available.

Transport patients to designated facilities according to your MCI plan. Specialized treatment may not be available at all facilities. Facilities also need to be notified that irradiated patients are being transported to their location so they can take necessary precautions against secondary contamination and be prepared to care for the patients' special needs.

CHAPTER REVIEW

Chapter Summary

While hazardous materials events can be unpredictable, the RAIN process provides a consistent, step-by-step framework for use on any scene. As you become more familiar with your jurisdiction, take the time to learn about the hazardous materials that you may encounter, and the resources available to you to identify and protect yourself on scene.

The ERG, MSDS, and telephone resources, such as CHEMTREC, ChemTel, and poison control centers can assist you in anticipating signs and symptoms and developing treatment plans for decontaminated patients. Remember, your personal safety is the most important consideration, so assume every chemical poses a health and safety risk to you, including risk of death.

Review Questions

Multiple-Choice Questions

1. You are on the scene of a hazardous materials incident, have recognized the chemical involved, and have avoided it. Your next step is to:
   a. notify the hazardous materials team.
   b. isolate the chemical from the public.
   c. begin patient decontamination.
   d. park uphill, upwind, upstream.

2. The minimum level of OSHA-required hazardous materials training for EMS providers is the ___ level.
   a. responder
   b. awareness
   c. technician
   d. specialist

3. You arrive at a hazardous materials incident involving a fixed storage container. Which one of the following types of information should you be able to find on the placard?
   a. IHCS classification
   b. UN ID number
   c. Name of the chemical
   d. General information on health risks

4. The yellow portion of an NFPA 704 placard gives information about the potential for:
   a. health risks.
   b. fire.
   c. reactivity.
   d. other effects not specified.

5. Which one of the following statements about a Material Safety Data Sheet is true?
   a. It is developed by the chemical manufacturer.
   b. It is the same as shipping papers.
   c. It must list the UN ID number.
   d. It is in the white pages of the *Emergency Response Guidebook*.

6. A patient approaches you with a dusty appearance and looks slightly disoriented. You suspect the patient is contaminated and do your best to avoid being touched. Where would you send this victim?
   a. Hot zone
   b. Decontamination line
   c. Cold zone
   d. Treatment sector

7. You have arrived on the scene of a motor vehicle collision to find that there is a tanker truck on its side. A liquid that is quickly evaporating is leaking from the tanker. You determine that the wind is from the northeast at about 15 mph. Without driving through the scene, you should locate your vehicle to the ___ of the tanker.
   a. southwest
   b. southeast
   c. northwest
   d. northeast

8. You have arrived on the scene of a tractor-trailer that has overturned and split open. Several 55-gallon drums have fallen out of the trailer and are leaking. The liquid is running down an incline on the easternmost side of the traffic lanes. The wind is from the northeast at about 25 miles per hour. Without driving through the scene, the safest place, of the following, to locate your vehicle would be to the ___ of the overturned trailer.
   a. north
   b. west
   c. south
   d. east

9. When providing emergency medical care at the scene of a hazardous materials incident, you should be located in the ___ zone.
   a. hazard reduction
   b. warm
   c. cold
   d. decontamination

10. You see from a distance that an overturned truck has a red and black three-bladed symbol on it. You should suspect that the material involved is:
    a. corrosive.
    b. highly reactive with water.
    c. radioactive.
    d. combustible.

Critical-Thinking Questions

11. Explain the steps associated with RAIN.

12. Why should you assume that any chemical can cause you serious harm or even kill you?

13. For each piece of information below, identify the corresponding color (or colors) of the *Emergency Response Guidebook* pages where you would find it.
    a. Protective action distances
    b. Emergency first aid suggestions
    c. Name of the chemical with the UN number "1114"
    d. Phone number for CHEMTREC
    e. Orange page numbers for "benzene"

Additional Reading

Arizona Board of Regents for the University of Arizona. (2003).
   Advanced hazmat life support (3rd ed.). Phoenix, AZ: Author.

49 Response to Terrorism and Disasters

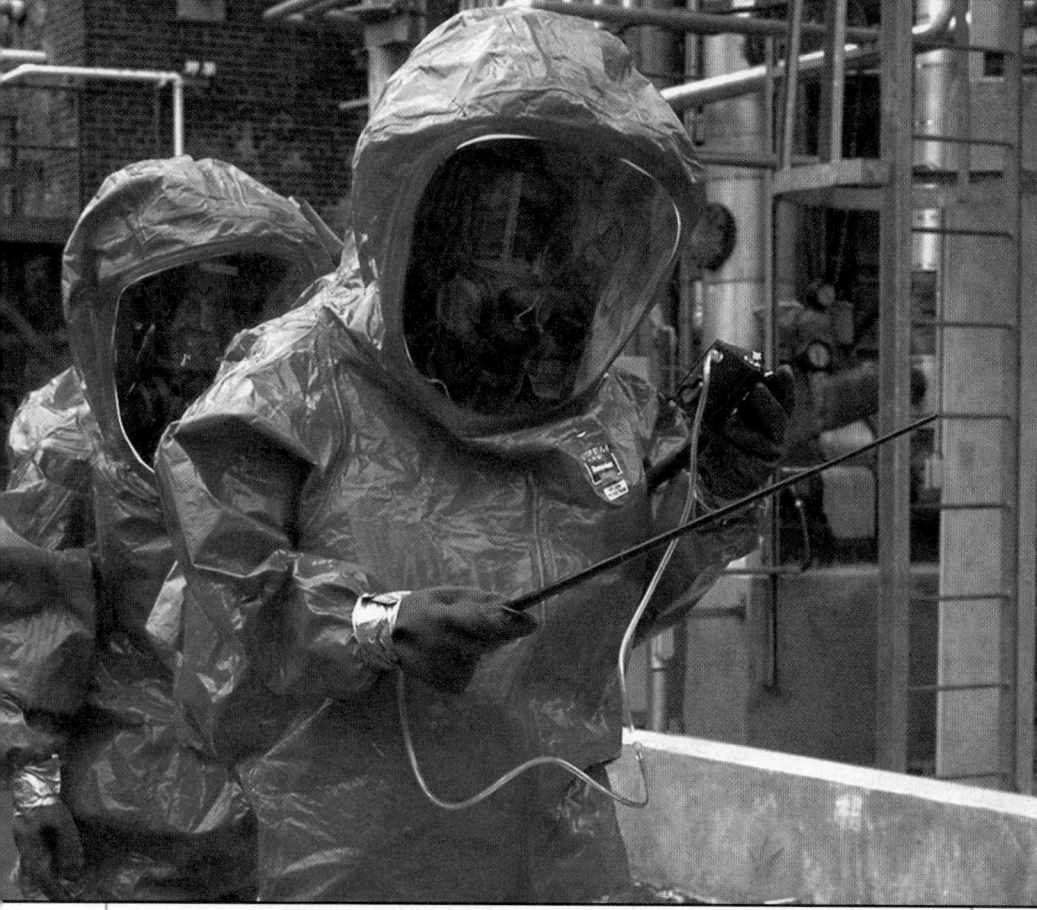

Content Area: EMS Operations

Advanced EMT Education Standard: Knowledge of operational roles and responsibilities to ensure patient, public, and personnel safety.

Objectives

After reading this chapter, you should be able to:

49.1 Define key terms introduced in this chapter.

49.2 Anticipate types of disasters to which you may respond as an Advanced EMT.

49.3 Identify the roles EMS providers play in response to disasters and terrorism incidents.

49.4 Identify the roles of other types of special teams that may be required in response to disasters and terrorism events.

49.5 Explain considerations in the planning phase of a disaster response.

49.6 Describe the purpose and process of windshield assessment in the response to a disaster.

49.7 Explain the purpose of the National Disaster Medical System.

(continued)

Resource Central

Advanced EMTs Bill Francis and Lucy Garcia are beginning their shift on a cold Tuesday morning when they are dispatched to the scene of an explosion that ripped through a small office down the street. When they arrive, a law enforcement officer tells them they are the first medical personnel on scene. Bill and Lucy notice bodies of at least a dozen individuals strewn on the street. As they look inside the broken glass front door of the office, they notice at least another four or five individuals either lying on the ground not moving or sitting down but covered in blood and glass.

Problem-Solving Questions

1. What assumptions should Bill and Lucy make about the safety of the scene?
2. What steps should Bill and Lucy take to establish an organized response?
3. How should they begin treatment of the patients?

(continued from previous page)

49.8	Discuss the relationship between multiple casualty incident response and post-traumatic and cumulative stress.
49.9	Anticipate psychological reactions of disaster survivors.
49.10	Describe the characteristics of each of the categories of weapons of mass destruction.
49.11	Recognize indications that a response may involve terrorism and weapons of mass destruction.
49.12	Given a series of scenarios of terrorism involving weapons of mass destruction, anticipate threats to responders, patients, and bystanders.
49.13	Predict patient injuries associated with various types of disasters and weapons of mass destruction.
49.14	Discuss the effects of exposure to various classifications of chemical agents that are likely to be used in a chemical terrorism event.
49.15	Give examples of biologic agents that are likely to be used in a bioterrorism event.
49.16	Discuss particular concerns with terrorism events involving radiation.

Introduction

Natural disasters and acts of **terrorism** are events that can result in multiple casualty incidents (MCI). As with all MCIs, EMS response can be impaired if the event overwhelms the available resources or because it requires specialized resources that are not immediately available. Natural disasters and acts of terrorism present unique challenges in how you carry out your responsibilities, but your basic responsibilities do not change (Figure 49-1).

Natural disasters such as earthquakes, volcanic eruptions, and storms have been as much a part of the human experience as civilization itself. As societies have organized and grown, the consequences of natural disasters have increased exponentially.

Acts of terrorism, like many natural disasters, can occur without warning. While natural disasters may randomly

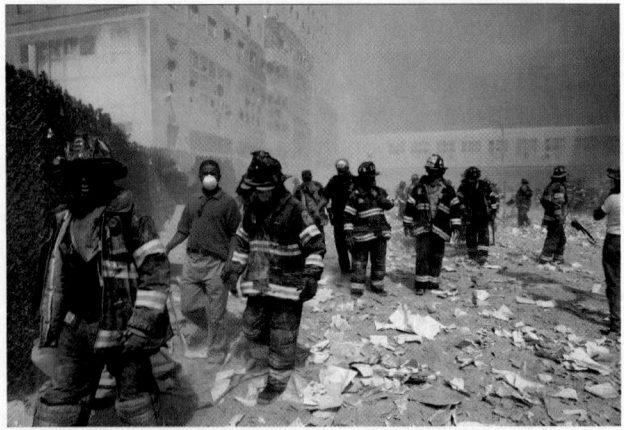

FIGURE 49-1

Catastrophic disasters can be isolated to a small region or impact an entire region. (© Allan Tannenbaum/The Image Works)

strike heavily populated areas, acts of terrorism are designed specifically to affect heavily populated areas. The tragic events of September 11, 2001, have forever changed the approach of emergency preparedness and response.

You may never be called upon to respond to an MCI created by a natural disaster or terrorist event, but you must always be prepared because the potential for those events always exists. On the other hand, many health care and public safety personnel choose to be ready to respond to such events, wherever they occur. You may become involved in an MCI outside your jurisdiction as part of mutual aid or because you opt to be active in the **National Disaster Medical System (NDMS)**. NDMS is a section of the U.S. Department of Health and Human Services that is responsible for managing the federal medical response to an emergency or disaster. It consists of locally based teams that respond jointly where disaster medical assistance is required.

General Considerations in Disasters and Terrorism

Always consider safety precautions the moment you are dispatched on a call. When an event, such as a hurricane, is anticipated, you can begin preparations ahead of time. In some cases, you might be involved in a large-scale response within or outside of your jurisdiction. Your response to the scene may unfold differently than during a typical call, so do not let the unusual circumstances distract you from performing a thorough scene size-up and remaining alert to the possibility of danger throughout your participation in the event.

When incident command has been established, you must work within the incident command system (ICS) structure and carry out the duties you are assigned. If you are first on the scene and see signs that the event is an MCI as a result of natural disaster or terrorism, stay in your vehicle and perform a *windshield assessment*. That is, ask yourself: What can I see from the windows of my vehicle? Relay the information to dispatch and establish command until the MCI or disaster plan can be implemented and you are relieved of command by designated personnel. Report the nature of the incident and, to the best of your ability, the number of patients involved and the need for additional resources. In cases where you are the first to respond, do not immediately rush to care for patients. Carefully assess the potential for danger at the scene. Depending on the nature of the situation, you must anticipate different hazards.

Hazards are inherent in the response to natural disasters and acts of terrorism. Carefully observe your surroundings to protect yourself, your coworkers, patients, and bystanders. Take an *all-hazards approach* to the situation, anticipating that multiple dangers are present. Geography and climate take on particular significance during the scene size-up of natural disasters and acts of terrorism. Flood waters, earthquake aftershocks, continuing storms, downed electrical lines, gas line leaks, unstable structures and vehicles, high winds, secondary explosions, and the potential presence of hazardous chemicals, radiation, or biologic agents can all pose hazards.

Other threats to your safety include the actions of desperate and disoriented patients and bystanders, or even the well-intentioned but unsafe actions of bystanders attempting to help. Anticipate behavioral emergencies and maintain awareness of the behaviors of those around you at all times.

PERSONAL PERSPECTIVE

Advanced EMT Melanie Williams: It was without question the largest scene I had ever been on. Early estimates put the numbers of those injured and missing in the earthquake at over 600 people. I thought I had prepared myself completely for this assignment: I was prepared mentally and physically for a long-term assignment, and I had received all my instructions from my supervisor at the ambulance service. But nothing could prepare me for what I was about to face when I arrived at the command area for check-in. There were hundreds of responders from all around the country who had been deployed to the area. I saw local, state, and even federal emergency personnel who were all preparing to assist in the disaster.

When I arrived at the check-in area, I gave my name and the name of my agency, and provided all the other information they requested. I couldn't believe all the paperwork I had to fill out! The check-in personnel also informed me of the cafeteria where I could eat after I returned from the field.

Once I had my assignment, which was patient treatment, I was told to go to a room at the command post for a safety briefing. When I entered the room, I found a seat in the back. The leader of the safety meeting was an emergency manager who called himself the "safety liaison" for the operational period. He went through all the various types of hazards in the area, and the types of injuries that other responders had experienced, and how to avoid those injuries. He also informed us that anyone going into the field would have to check in at the logistics table for assignment of response equipment and PPE. After he was done speaking, a person from the planning section informed us of our overall goals for the operational period, and the responsibilities of each branch for the next 12 hours.

Then we broke up. I reported to the staging area, as requested. There I met my unit leader as well as the others who were in our medical group. After the introductions, the leader went through a second safety briefing with us, and checked to be sure that everyone had their PPE and equipment. He told us that anyone who felt ill or injured in the group should report to him immediately. He then discussed on a grid map our area of responsibility. It was only after that that we finally entered the treatment area, which was in a large field with several tents. Though it took a long time, I appreciated all the safety precautions and the instructions on how to keep ourselves safe. I couldn't believe how many people were there, but was glad that I was able to be of assistance to those who needed us the most.

Use personal protective equipment (PPE) suited to the situation. In some situations, you must wear structural firefighting gear (turnout gear, including helmet, coat, bunker pants, and boots) for safety. If a chemical or biologic weapon is suspected, you might be issued special gear that requires training and fitting.

An additional element of response to natural disasters and terrorism events is the prolonged response that is often necessary. Be aware of the passage of time and feelings of fatigue, and take the opportunity to rest, drink fluids, and eat.

Response to the aftermath of an act of terrorism or natural disaster can be one of the most psychologically taxing events you experience in your career. Consider the images you have seen on television from recent disasters, such as the earthquake and tsunami on the coast of Japan and the tornadoes that devastated Joplin, Missouri, and other cities. Such scenes may expose you to disturbing visual images including large numbers of dead and decomposing bodies, disorientation and intense expressions of grief by survivors, and even violence resulting from the chaos.

Not everyone is well suited to operate during a major MCI outside their own jurisdiction where dozens or hundreds of patients are involved. If that includes you, it is okay. That does not make you any less qualified to be an EMS professional. But it does require you to communicate this to your supervisors *before* being deployed to an MCI outside your jurisdiction. Make sure you receive a complete briefing about the type of environment into which you will be placed. Do not be afraid to ask questions or express concerns. If possible, request an administrative assignment in the support sections, where you can assist on safety recommendations or in a liaison capacity.

Disaster mental-health services are a critical part of the response to natural disasters and terrorism events. Do not hesitate to make use of those services. The symptoms of acute and cumulative stress and post-traumatic stress disorder (PTSD) are covered in Chapter 3.

Even with all the necessary precautions, you might still become ill or injured while performing your duties. Do not attempt to continue "working through the pain," or ignore physiologic symptoms. If you are ill or injured you must report it to your immediate supervisor and seek medical treatment in a designated rehabilitation area.

Medical and psychological monitoring does not end when you leave the scene. Depending upon the type of event, you might be required to perform a follow-up physical at a doctor's office hours or even days after an event, particularly if you begin to experience unusual physiologic

signs and symptoms. For example, there are biologic agents such as smallpox or tularemia that have incubation periods from days to weeks after exposure.

Be aware of the nature of the weapon or destructive forces of a natural disaster when assessing patients in a natural disaster or terrorism event, and assume a high potential for multisystem trauma.

Natural Disasters

Natural disasters occur in all parts of the world. Many are caused by weather such as blizzards, floods, wildfires, hurricanes, and tornadoes. Some areas are more earthquake prone than others, but earthquakes also can occur in areas where people do not expect them. The destructive forces of nature can bring down power lines and rupture gas lines, creating the risks of electrocution, fire, and explosion. Buildings may be unstable and debris can cause risks for injury. Also keep in mind that pandemic illnesses, such as influenza or SARS, also can result in the need to activate an MCI or disaster plan.

Patients may have a variety of injuries, ranging from blast injuries and crush injuries to penetrating and blunt trauma, burns, and hypothermia. Caring for patients in the aftermath of disasters can be complicated by obstacles to getting to the scene and transporting patients, such as blocked or washed-out roads or damaged bridges or tunnels.

Hospitals may be damaged and unable to care for the patients who were already there at the time of the disaster, let alone receive new patients. Electricity may be interrupted, and therefore interfere with any kind of medical care that requires lights or electric-powered equipment. Water contamination, interruptions in water supply and waste disposal, lack of electricity, and infectious disease all can contribute to further injury and disease in the aftermath of a disaster. Those helping in the rescue and recovery efforts or attempting to access their homes or businesses can be injured or become ill and continue to contribute to the number of casualties after the initial event.

Man-made disasters, such as apartment building, hospital, or nursing home fires, gas pipeline explosions, airline or train crashes, building or bridge collapses, and other events also occur and require a response similar to responses to natural disasters.

Terrorism and Weapons of Mass Destruction

Terrorism is the use of violence to intimidate and incite fear in the population with the goal of social, political, or religious change, or in retaliation for acts of perceived threat or injustice. Targets of terrorism also may be symbolic structures such as national monuments or religious institutions. A common tool of terrorism is a **weapon of mass destruction**

IN THE FIELD

Acts of terrorism and the destructive forces of natural disasters have the potential for creating multiple casualties and multisystem trauma.

(WMD). WMDs are designed to kill and injure large numbers of people and cause damage to man-made and natural structures, including targets of symbolic value. WMDs may be **conventional explosives, nuclear weapons** or dispersion of radioactivity, chemical agents, and biologic agents.

Although prior terrorism events on a smaller scale had occasionally occurred in the United States and against U.S. interests in other parts of the world, the September 11, 2001, attacks changed the world forever. As a result, the United States has implemented measures for greater domestic preparedness in preventing and responding to terrorist attacks through cooperative efforts between local and state agencies and the Department of Homeland Security. Nonetheless, the threat of terrorism will likely always be present to greater and lesser degrees.

Terrorist Groups

Terrorist groups can be categorized by the nature of their organizational sponsorship as domestic or international. Lone wolf terrorists, acting alone or, when advantageous, cooperating with other groups, also exist.

Domestic terrorism is terrorism committed by citizens of the same country that is the target of the attacks. Some of the targets by U.S. groups have been facilities attached to the federal government. For instance, the Oklahoma City bombing that occurred in 1995 targeted the federal building that housed offices of the Internal Revenue Service (IRS), Federal Bureau of Investigation (FBI), and the Bureau of Alcohol, Tobacco, and Firearms (BATF), as well as other agencies. Controversial businesses also are targets. Animal testing facilities, family planning and abortion clinics, and companies that are viewed as posing a risk to the environment, such as logging companies, have been targets of domestic terrorism. For example, the Reserve Officers' Training Corps (ROTC) offices at the University of Wisconsin were struck by an explosion on August 24, 1970, by a group of protestors against controversial research being conducted at the university. The explosion killed a professor and nearly leveled an entire wing of the building.

International terrorism is terrorism committed by citizens of a different country from the target of the attacks. International terrorist groups generally fit into two major categories: state sponsored and unsponsored. State-sponsored groups are provided resources by a recognized government, while unsponsored groups do not have recognized government support. However, this does not mean that unsponsored groups are of little consequence. For example, the group Aum Shinrikyo did not receive any known government support, yet they were able to successfully organize and deploy attacks throughout Japan, including sarin gas attacks in the Tokyo subway in 1995. Al Qaeda is not officially a state-sponsored group, but it has received support from various governments that have provided weapons and safe haven for operatives.

A *lone-wolf terrorist* is a single individual who works alone and without the support of any particular group or government. Such individuals can be extremely effective, even if the scope of their attacks is limited by their personal resources. Typically, lone-wolf terrorists remain either unaffiliated, or are contracted by governments or other groups to commit certain attacks. Because lone-wolf terrorists work alone and without significant ties to other terrorists, they can be difficult to track. For example, Ted Kaczynski, the "Unabomber" (which stands for UNiversity and Airline BOMBER) sent devices to individuals for 18 years before he was captured. Centennial Park and serial abortion clinic bomber Eric Robert Rudolph was on the run for over six years before his capture in 2003.

In another example of lone-wolf terrorism, the awareness of biologic terrorism increased in the wake of the "Amerithrax" attacks in late 2001. Initially believed to be a follow-up by Al-Qaeda after the September 11, 2001, terrorist attacks, it was later determined by the FBI to most likely have been committed by a lone-wolf terrorist working for the U.S. Army as a bioscientist. The attack resulted in 5 deaths and 22 cases of anthrax infections.

Keep in mind that some types of crime scenes, such as police standoffs, hostage situations, mass shootings, and shoot-outs can bear some similarities to terrorist attacks.

Weapons of Mass Destruction

A number of different types of weapons could be used in a WMD event. They include conventional explosives, small arms (including high-power and automatic weapons), **incendiary devices**, chemicals, biologic agents, radiation, and nuclear weapons.

Incendiary Devices

Incendiary devices are designed to start fires and include gasoline or other fuels, Molotov cocktails, and other improvised devices. A smell of gasoline, kerosene, or other fuels may alert you to the possibility that such a device was used. A terrorist group may start several fires simultaneously. Such devices are easily made and deployed, so remain aware of the possibility of a second device aimed at rescuers, even after the initial fire has been extinguished.

Conventional Explosives

The materials used to create conventional explosives, such as a car bomb or pipe bomb, are relatively easy to obtain, instructions to create them are widely available, and they can detonate violently. They also can be used to disperse a load of shrapnel (shards of glass or nails, for example), chemicals, or radioactive material (a "dirty bomb"). When a conventional explosive is used to disperse radioactive material, it is called a **radiologic dispersion device (RDD)**. Although the heat of an explosion, theoretically, would destroy most biologic agents, a conventional explosive device could also potentially disperse them.

The safest assumption to make on the scene of a detonated device is that the detonation of the first device is evidence that the bomber has the material, expertise, and ability to deliver a secondary device. Look for backpacks, packages, boxes, and bags. Mailboxes, dumpsters, and the undercarriage of cars also are typical places to hide a conventional explosive device.

Biologic Weapons

A biologic WMD is a mechanism that deliberately disseminates a biologic agent, either a biologic toxin or a pathogen. A particular threat is the biologic agent that is readily available, that can survive the dispersal mechanism, is easily dispersed and spread through the population, and has the capability of creating widespread illness and death. Some pathogens that could be used occur naturally. Others are known only to be produced in laboratories. For example, *Yersinia pestis*, the biologic agent that causes the bubonic form of the plague, occurs naturally in parts of the United States and affects several people each year, particularly in the Southwestern United States. In contrast, the natural occurrence of smallpox was eradicated years ago, yet a supply of the virus could potentially be stockpiled for use as a biologic weapon.

In 1982, a cult in Oregon committed the largest, most organized act of bioterrorism known in U.S. history. They systematically contaminated salad bars in restaurants throughout the city. No one died, but 750 were sickened. However, government officials were unclear about an attack occurring until multiple victims presented at local hospitals with similar symptoms, meaning that it is not always possible to tell that a bioterrorism event has occurred until a pattern emerges.

Incubation periods for biologic agents vary, so the pattern may be difficult to determine at first, and the source of exposure may be difficult to track. In some cases, a potential exposure is more obvious, such as a powdered substance being sent through the mail in envelopes. In other cases, individuals may not be aware that they have been exposed until signs and symptoms occur. Also be aware that if the potential for an exposure is announced, public concern, even amongst those at low risk, can increase substantially and further overwhelm the health care system.

The Centers for Disease Control and Prevention (CDC, n.d.) categorize biologic agents by their virulence, with Category "A" agents being the most virulent, and Category "C" the least virulent (Table 49-1). The CDC has specific methods of handling different agents. Follow their recommendations for prevention and follow-up if you have been exposed or potentially exposed.

Chemical Weapons

Chemical terrorism uses the toxic properties of a chemical to cause illness or injury. Chemical weapons range from less lethal tear gas or riot gas to highly lethal chemical weapons such as organophosphates, ricin (derived from the castor bean), and mustard gas. Classifications of chemical WMDs include vesicants, asphyxiants (such as cyanide), **choking agents**, and **riot control agents** (such as tear gas or pepper

TABLE 49-1   CDC Categories of Bioagents

Category A	Category B	Category C
Anthrax (*Bacillus anthracis*)	Brucellosis (*Brucella* species)	Nipah virus
Botulism (*Clostridium botulinum* toxin)	Epsilon toxin of *Clostridium perfringens*	Hantavirus
Plague (*Yersinia pestis*)	Food safety threats (e.g., *Salmonella* species,	
Smallpox (variola major)	*Escherichia coli* O157:H7, *Shigella*)	
Tularemia (*Francisella tularensis*)	Glanders (*Burkholderia mallei*)	
Viral hemorrhagic fevers (filoviruses	Melioidosis (*Burkholderia pseudomallei*)	
[e.g., Ebola, Marburg] and arenaviruses	Psittacosis (*Chlamydia psittaci*)	
[e.g., Lassa, Machupo])	Q fever (*Coxiella burnetii*)	
	Ricin toxin from *Ricinus communis* (castor beans)	
	Staphylococcal enterotoxin B	
	Typhus fever (*Rickettsia prowazekii*)	
	Viral encephalitis (alphaviruses [e.g., Venezuelan equine encephalitis, eastern equine encephalitis, western equine encephalitis])	
	Water safety threats (e.g., *Vibrio cholerae*, *Cryptosporidium parvum*)	

Data from: Centers for Disease Control and Prevention. (n.d.). *Emergency preparedness and response: Bioterrorism agents/diseases A-Z.* Retrieved May 14, 2011, from http://www.bt.cdc.gov/agent/agentlist-category.asp

spray). Though the majority of countries have agreed to eliminate stockpiles of chemical weapons, some countries have not, so deployment by terrorist groups remains a possibility.

Response to a chemical terrorism event bears many similarities to a hazardous materials event. (See Chapter 48.) You should employ the acronym RAIN (recognize, avoid, isolate, and notify). However, recognizing a chemical terrorism event can be difficult, and determining the nature of the chemical can be even more difficult. There will not be any placards, MSDS, or other references accompanying the material. There may not be a recognizable source of the material, such as an overturned tanker or leaking fixed storage container.

A possible indication of chemical terrorism in your windshield survey is the presence of dead or incapacitated animals, such as livestock, flocks of birds, or fish kills. Although an unusual odor can tip you off to a possible chemical weapon, not all chemicals that could be used for a terrorism event have an odor or other physical properties that make recognizing the nature of the event easy. If you do notice an odor or other indications of a chemical release (such as a residue, vapor, or unusual liquid or powder), you are too close to the source and must evacuate further from the area.

Because you will not have the information needed, use the greatest isolation distances possible. The chemicals can persist in the environment, causing additional exposure. Follow the same rules of locating yourself, your vehicle, and others upwind, uphill, and upstream from any known source of a chemical weapon. If you are first on the scene, provide dispatch with as much information about the scene as possible, including sights, odors, the presence of possible dispersal mechanisms, signs and symptoms of patients, and the number of victims.

The signs, symptoms, and treatment depend on the chemical involved. Unfortunately, that information may not be immediately known. Once patients are decontaminated and triaged, treat them according to the type and level of distress present. Anticipate respiratory involvement and treat according to triage and treatment protocols.

Vesicants

Vesicants, or blister agents, were some of the most effective agents deployed during World War I. They produce burns and blisters on the skin. The fatality rate varies, but the agents can persistent in the environment for days to weeks. The blisters can be accompanied by pain and small vesicles

IN THE FIELD

Although chemical weapon attacks bear some similarities to hazardous materials incidents, you will not have the information about the chemical involved as you would in a typical hazardous materials incident. Use maximum isolation distances until hazardous materials personnel identify the nature of the chemical.

can become large blisters. They also can cause respiratory distress. The onset of symptoms can be delayed for 24 to 48 hours for some types of agents.

Asphyxiants and Choking Agents

The term "blood agent" was previously used to describe cyanide and similar cellular asphyxiants. Choking agents have an acute, severe effect on the respiratory system, particularly the lungs, and include phosgene. Signs and symptoms include dyspnea, tachypnea, coughing, pulmonary edema, chest pain, shock, and more generalized signs and symptoms such as headache, nausea and vomiting, altered mental status, and seizures.

Riot Control and Vomiting Agents

Although riot control agents have very low lethality, they can cause respiratory distress, burning of the eyes and other mucous membranes, coughing, nausea, and vomiting. It is more likely that you will encounter the use of a riot control agent in response to a police action than as a chemical WMD. The chemical does not respond well to attempts at decontamination with water, and, often, all that is needed for signs and symptoms to subside is time.

Vomiting agents are aerosolized and cause signs and symptoms when inhaled. They are potent and only a small dose is needed to cause distress. Contrary to the name, vomiting agents mostly cause irritation of the upper respiratory tract and the eyes, but the accompanying coughing and gagging can lead to vomiting.

Nerve Agents

Nerve agents can be among the most toxic chemical agents known to humankind. Exposure to some agents can result in death in minutes. Nerve agents inhibit the action of acetylcholinesterase, the enzyme that is necessary to break down acetylcholine in synapses in the nervous system. The result is unopposed, continuous stimulation of the functions of the affected target tissues. Nerve agents bind with acetyl choline and, after varying amounts of time, depending on the agent, the bond becomes irreversible. However, with prompt treatment, the effects can be reversed.

The two main categories of nerve agents are "G" agents, which persist for 24 hours, such as sarin; and "V" agents, such as VX, which is 100 to 150 times more toxic than sarin. While many government stockpiles of nerve agents, including those in the United States, have been destroyed, the raw materials and instructions for making them are readily available.

You can remember many of the signs and symptoms of nerve agents through the mnemonic SLUDGE, introduced in Chapter 32. SLUDGE stands for salivation, lacrimation, urination, defecation, gastric distress, and emesis. The mnemonic DUMBELS also is used, and stands for diarrhea, urination, miosis (constricted pupils), bradycardia (also, bronchorrhea [bronchial secretions] and bronchospasms), emesis, lacrimation, and salivation (also sweating and secretions). Muscle fasciculations (twitching) may occur.

As with all chemical exposures, protect yourself from contact with the substance. Allow specially trained personnel with the proper PPE to remove the patient from the source to minimize his continued exposure and decontaminate him before you begin treatment. Anticipate the need for supporting the airway, breathing, oxygenation, and circulation because manifestations of nerve agent poisoning include copious secretions, bronchospasm, and bradycardia.

The definitive treatment of nerve agent poisoning includes administering two medications. Atropine opposes the effects of the parasympathetic nervous system, which is overstimulated from the accumulation of acetylcholine. Pralidoxime (2-PAM) chloride prevents the bond between the agent and acetylcholinesterase from becoming irreversible, if it is administered in time. The two medications are packaged in kits called *Mark I kits* (available through the Chemical Stockpile Emergency Preparedness Program [CSEPP]) that can be used for self-administration or administration to a fellow responder who is exposed to a nerve agent. Both agents are recommended only for moderate to severe exposures. The amount of atropine needed can exceed the amount provided in the kit and you must transport the patient for additional treatment.

Radiologic and Nuclear Weapons

The use of nuclear and radiologic technology as a weapon is less than a century old, first used by the United States against Japan in World War II, but its destructive potential is well known. There are two types of hazards associated with radiologic and nuclear weapons. A radiologic hazard involves radiation emission and resulting radiation exposure or contamination. (See Chapter 48.) Nuclear hazards involve splitting or fusing atoms with release of massive amounts of energy along with radiation.

The use of nuclear technology in a terrorist event could be in the form of a nuclear detonation, an RDD, or an act of sabotage at a nuclear weapons or nuclear power facility. Depending upon the size and power of the weapon, the detonation of a nuclear warhead could instantly annihilate dozens of city blocks, killing most of its residents within a certain blast area and leaving unrivaled devastation. The release of radiation would continue to sicken and kill those exposed over a period of time. Depending on the selection of targets and the yield of the bomb, there could be tens of thousands to millions of casualties. While a nuclear launch would be an incredibly destructive event, the likelihood of its occurrence by a terrorist group is remote because of international cooperation in enacting high-security procedures to protect against the launch of nuclear weaponry.

Scene Size-Up

In most cases, you will be dispatched to a natural disaster or terrorism event as part of a large-scale response and will follow the instructions of incident command. Still, your safety is the highest priority and you must be observant for hazards at all times. Natural disasters and terrorism events are among the most hazardous of all scenes. If you are injured or ill at the scene, not only are your skills no longer available to those who need them, but other responders will have an additional patient to care for, potentially delaying care for other patients.

In a terrorism event, consider the possibility that a patient may not be an intended victim, but may be one of the perpetrators, who is either intentionally (intended suicide bombing) or unintentionally injured. Inexperienced bombers who create faulty devices could be injured in explosions they create. Considering the consequences of arrest and conviction, you may be dealing with a very dangerous, desperate person on the scene or in the ambulance. The perpetrator could have a second weapon or device on him. Follow law enforcement directions and take all precautions necessary to protect yourself, your partner, and the public.

Terrorism is a crime, and terrorism events are crime scenes. Follow evidence preservation protocols established by incident command. Make note of anything that could be of interest in the investigation by law enforcement. For example, gasoline cans, electrical components, or pieces of a cell phone may be evidence. During the investigation of the Pan Am Flight 103 explosion over Lockerby, Scotland, in 1988, a Scottish police officer discovered a piece of clothing close to where it was believed the explosion occurred (but not where the main wreckage was located) that was part of an 845-square-mile debris field. A piece of a circuit board the size of a thumbnail was discovered from the clothing and was traced to a batch sold to Libyan government.

As with all crime scenes, disturb the scene as little as possible and document anything you move or touch. Retain clothing removed from patients in a bag so it can be examined later by investigators. Unlike the paper bags preferred for most crime scene evidence, plastic bags are preferred in possible terrorism events. Once you have delivered a patient to the hospital, examine the ambulance for any items or debris that may have been dropped during transport.

Even items seemingly innocuous to the untrained eye can be of importance later, so good documentation as soon as possible after observation can be invaluable. If you have a few moments between tasks, jot down notes for later documentation. As with any criminal event to which you respond, it is possible that your documentation could be subpoenaed as evidence. Despite the challenges of documentation of MCIs, do your best to be complete and thorough.

Patient Care

The tasks you are most likely to perform are those you are most familiar with: triage, treatment, and transport. You also may be assigned to care for other responders in the rehabilitation area at a large-scale event. In chemical events, you must make sure that patients are decontaminated before beginning care, and in all cases, you must select the appropriate PPE for the situation.

The specific treatment depends on the nature of the injuries and the resources available. The scene size-up gives you an idea of the types of injuries your patients may have sustained. Suspect multisystem trauma and remember your priorities in patient care: establishing and maintaining an airway, ensuring adequate breathing and oxygenation, and controlling bleeding and ensuring adequate circulation. In some situations, the way you accomplish your priorities may require specific treatments, such as using a Mark I kit to treat a coworker for the effects of a nerve agent.

CASE STUDY WRAP-UP

Clinical-Reasoning Process

Advanced EMTs Bill Francis and Lucy Garcia find out that they are the first medical personnel to arrive on the scene of an explosion that ripped through a small office. The police officer who meets them informs them that there are a dozen patients outside the office and another half dozen or so inside, each with varying degrees of severity of injury.

Lucy, who drove the ambulance, immediately looks out her window to scan the area, as does her partner, Bill. They realize that a secondary device could be nearby, and so request a police officer to do a sweep of the area for other bombs. The officer has already called for backup units, who arrive quickly and in great numbers, and begin their sweep of the area while Bill and Lucy maintain a half-block distance from the scene of the explosion.

Lucy notices the road behind them has heavy traffic, so she parks the ambulance next to a side road that is clear of vehicles. Meanwhile, Bill contacts dispatch, provides the information about the scene, and requests additional EMS units, including a supervisor. Lucy goes into the back of the ambulance to get their disaster kit, which includes triage tags, bags to carry them, a clipboard, and other supplies. Within a few minutes, the commanding officer provides the "all clear," and approaches Bill and Lucy. He tells them that he will be assuming incident command of the scene, but that he will need them to run the medical operations until additional support arrives. Just as they collect the items from the ambulance, the EMS supervisor arrives. Bill and Lucy brief the supervisor, who tells them he wishes them to begin triage of the scene. He points out the area he has chosen for treatment, and Lucy tells the supervisor about the side road for ingress and egress from the scene. He agrees with her recommendation, and goes to talk to the incident commander.

Bill and Lucy take out the gloves and put on multiple pairs each, putting an "X" on the bottom pair. They agree Bill will perform the first triage shift while Lucy completes the documentation. They examine the scene once again for any hidden hazards such as downed power lines, large pieces of glass, or any suspicious objects. Finding none, they approach the area where the outside patients are located. Lucy says loudly, "Anyone who can hear me and understand, please stand up." Seeing no one do so, she walks up to her first patient. It is a woman in her mid-30s who is unconscious and bleeding from various laceration wounds. Lucy notices a large piece of glass embedded in her hand. She realizes the patient is breathing at a rate of less than 30 per minute. However, Lucy notes that the woman's perfusion is greater than 2 seconds, so Lucy puts an "Immediate" tag around the patient's wrist near the hand that has not been impaled, tears off the barcode located on the bottom of the tag, and hands it to Bill. Without touching her glove, he takes the barcode and places it in the bag. He makes notes as Lucy verbalizes them as she moves from patient to patient. She continues this process for five to six other patients until she notices that she is now on her last glove. She and Bill switch positions, Bill taking over triage responsibilities. As they complete their initial triage, they look out and notice additional responders who have begun the process of treating the patients who had been triaged.

CHAPTER REVIEW

Chapter Summary

At some point in your career as an Advanced EMT, you may respond to a disaster or terrorism event. Natural disasters are common events and include tornadoes, hurricanes, and earthquakes. Terrorism events are not as common, but are specifically targeted at densely populated areas with the intent of injuring or killing as many people as possible through the use of WMDs. WMDs include conventional explosives, small arms, incendiary devices, chemical agents, biologic agents, radiation, and nuclear weapons.

Disasters and terrorism involve many special considerations of the scene hazards and mechanisms of injury. In particular, the hazard may be ongoing due to continued inclement weather or secondary WMDs specifically targeting responders. Because most such events are MCIs, you must work within the ICS to carry out triage and transport. Though you will most likely respond as part of a large-scale response, you still must perform a scene size-up and remain vigilant to multiple and emerging hazards.

As an Advanced EMT, you have the tools to respond effectively and professionally to disasters and terrorism events. However, you must not ignore the physical and psychological toll such events can take on you. Take good care of yourself, as well as your patients.

Review Questions

Multiple-Choice Questions

1. Dispatch informs you that about a dozen victims have congregated near a dock outside of town. As you drive past the lake to the scene, you notice dead fish in the water and dew on some nearby tree leaves, even though it is a hot summer day. You immediately:

   a. get out to inspect the substance.
   b. continue to the scene.
   c. leave the area.
   d. select appropriate PPE.

2. Radiologic dispersion devices (RDDs) differ from nuclear weapons in that:

   a. their power is derived from atomic fission.
   b. nuclear weapons cause fewer casualties overall.
   c. their power is derived from atomic fusion.
   d. an RDD attack looks like a conventional bombing.

3. Your primary responsibility in response to disasters and terrorism incidents is:

   a. evidence preservation.
   b. your own safety.
   c. triage.
   d. assessing survivors for psychological symptoms.

4. The use of ammonium nitrate and diesel fuel to create a powerful blast capable of destroying large buildings is an example of a(n):

   a. nuclear device.
   b. biologic weapon.
   c. incendiary device.
   d. conventional explosive.

5. Sarin gas is a(n) ___ agent.

   a. nerve
   b. incendiary
   c. biologic
   d. radiologic

6. Anthrax is an example of a(n) ___ agent.

   a. nerve
   b. incendiary
   c. radiologic
   d. biologic

7. A group of people who immediately became ill when an individual released a gaseous substance inside a coffee shop have skin blisters and irritation and respiratory irritation. Of the following, their presentation is most consistent with a:

   a. riot control agent.
   b. vomiting agent.
   c. vesicant.
   d. cellular asphyxiant.

8. A group of office workers in a government building suddenly became ill with vomiting, stomach cramps, diarrhea, coughing, wheezing, and difficulty breathing. The description of their signs and symptoms to the dispatcher also includes muscle twitching, tearing of the eyes, and drooling. If the cause is related to terrorism, the most likely agent, based on this description, would be a:

   a. nerve agent.
   b. vesicant.
   c. riot control agent.
   d. choking agent.

Critical-Thinking Questions

9. Describe the characteristics of a scene that would indicate a WMD has been deployed against a civilian population. Then explain your general approach to the scene.

References

Centers for Disease Control and Prevention. (n.d.). *Emergency preparedness and response: Bioterrorism agents/diseases A-Z.* Retrieved May 14, 2011, from http://www.bt.cdc.gov/agent/agentlist-category.asp

Additional Reading

Federal Emergency Management Agency. (n.d.). *NIMS training.* http://www.fema.gov/emergency/nims/NIMSTrainingCourses.shtm

Endotracheal Intubation

Content Area: Airway Management; Respirations; and Artificial Ventilation

Advanced EMT Education Standard: The Advanced EMT integrates complex knowledge of anatomy, physiology, and pathophysiology into assessment to develop and implement a treatment plan with the goal of ensuring a patent airway, adequate mechanical ventilation, and respiration for patients of all ages.

Note: Endotracheal intubation is beyond the scope of practice expected of Advanced EMTs at the national level. However, some states may include endotracheal intubation in the Advanced EMT scope of practice. As with all skills, you may only perform endotracheal intubation if it is allowed in your scope of practice, you have been properly trained, and approved by your medical director to do so.

Objectives

After reading this appendix, you should be able to:

A1.1   Explain the indications, contraindications, and complications associated with oral endotracheal intubation.

A1.2   Identify the anatomic landmarks used for proper endotracheal tube placement.

A1.3   Identify the required and adjunctive equipment for endotracheal intubation.

A1.4   Perform oral endotracheal intubation under instructor supervision.

A1.5   Discuss current trends and controversies in prehospital endotracheal intubation.

Introduction

Endotracheal intubation is a procedure that secures the patient's airway by placing a cuffed, hollow ventilation tube into the trachea so that its tip rests just above the carina. A properly placed endotracheal tube isolates the airway for ventilation by bag-valve device or mechanical ventilator, avoiding the complication of gastric distention. The cuff prevents aspiration of blood, secretions, and emesis around the tube. An endotracheal tube is properly placed by achieving direct visualization of the glottis through a process called *laryngoscopy.*

Endotracheal intubation has long been considered the preferred procedure for definitive airway management in unresponsive patients. However, the availability of several safe, effective nonvisualized airway devices and studies that have identified patient safety issues with prehospital intubation have brought that assumption into question. The best way to secure a definitive airway in the prehospital setting is a current controversy in EMS.

As with all prehospital practices, you must consider the best evidence available when determining the usefulness and safety of any procedure. Although endotracheal intubation offers the advantage of isolating the trachea for ventilation and protecting the airway against aspiration, it also requires extensive training and regular opportunities for practice. Other disadvantages include worsening of patient hypoxia from prolonged attempts at placement and the potential for trauma to the teeth and soft tissues of the airway. Patients who are intubated are either ventilated by way of a bag-valve device or mechanical ventilator. The technique of endotracheal intubation is relatively simple, but the clinical decision-making process (the process by which you determine when to perform a skill) requires excellent assessment and critical-thinking skills. Once the skill is acquired, you must maintain proficiency through practice

Equipment

Before attempting endotracheal intubation, you must first gather the necessary equipment. Doing so helps avoid delays in the process that can result in patient hypoxia. Required equipment includes a laryngoscope (handle and blade), an appropriately sized endotracheal tube, a malleable stylet, a 10-mL syringe, Magill forceps, a suction device (preferrably a portable battery powered unit or fixed suction unit, because manual devices have limited vacuum and capacity), a mechanism for securing the tube (commercially manufactured or tape), a stethoscope, and a tube placement confirmation device, preferably capnometry.

Laryngoscope

A laryngoscope is an instrument used to lift the tongue and epiglottis in order to visualize the glottis during endotracheal intubation, or to remove foreign objects from the airway using Magill forceps.

The laryngoscope consists of two parts—a handle and a blade (Figure A1-1). The handle houses the batteries required to power a light source, which is mounted on the blade. The light illuminates the airway, making it easier to visualize the landmarks for passing the endotracheal tube.

The blade is attached to the handle by sliding the indention at the base of the blade onto the fitting bar located at the top of the handle until it locks into place (Figure A1-2). Once positioned on the fitting bar, the blade is lifted until it clicks into place at a right angle to the handle, which activates the light on the blade (Figure A1-3). The light should be bright and steady. If the light does not come on, is dim, or is flickering, the batteries in the handle may be low or dead, or the light bulb may be loose and require tightening. A loose bulb also can fall into the airway, creating the potential for foreign body aspiration. Always check to be sure the bulb is securely tightened prior to placing the blade in the patient's mouth.

Laryngoscope blades come in a variety of types and sizes. The two main types of blades are the curved blades, such as the MacIntosh blade, and straight blades, such as the Miller blade. Blade sizes range from size 0 for neonates to size 4 for larger adults. A size 3 blade is usually sufficient for most adult patients.

The curved blade is designed to lift the epiglottis indirectly. The tip of the blade is inserted into the vallecula. When the handle is lifted anteriorly, the tongue and epiglottis are elevated to expose the glottis (Figure A1-4). Because

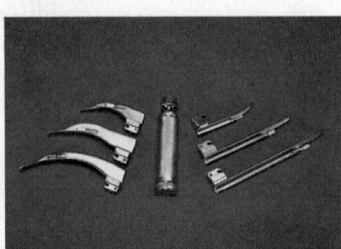

FIGURE A1-1

Laryngoscope handle with assorted blades.

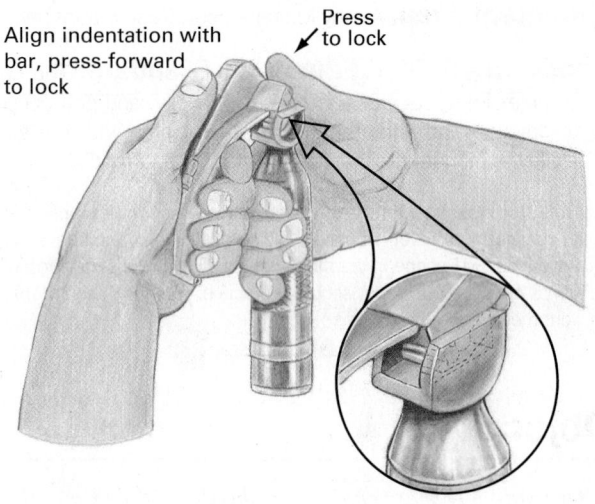

Align indentation with bar, press-forward to lock

Press to lock

FIGURE A1-2

The base of the laryngoscope blade attaches to the top of the handle.

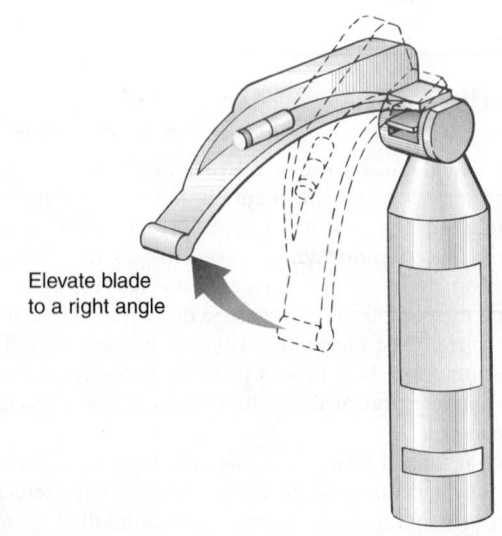

Elevate blade to a right angle

FIGURE A1-3

The laryngoscope blade light source is activated by lifting the blade.

Pediatric Care

Because the epiglottis in children is longer and more flexible than an adult's, straight blades, rather than curved ones, often work better because they lift the epiglottis directly.

of the curved design of the blade, you will find it easier to see around it to visualize endotracheal insertion through the vocal cords. The straight blade is designed to lift the epiglottis directly by placing the tip of the blade beneath it and lifting (Figure A1-5). Straight blades are sometimes used in a

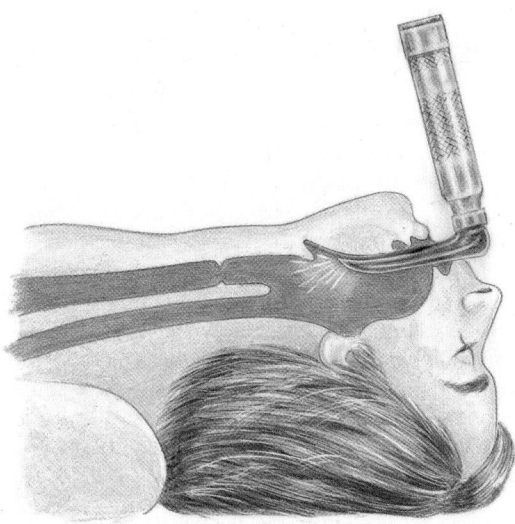

FIGURE A1-4

The tip of the curved blade is inserted into the vallecula and lifted.

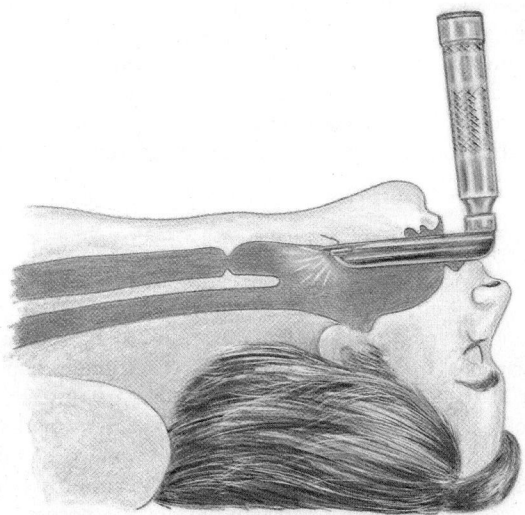

FIGURE A1-5

The straight blade is used to directly lift the epiglottis by placing the tip beneath it and lifting.

patient with a larger tongue because they can provide better displacement of the tongue.

Endotracheal Tube

An endotracheal tube is a flexible, translucent tube with a single lumen. It is available in a variety of lengths ranging from 12 to 32 cm. Each tube has centimeter markings running along its length. The proximal end of the tube is fitted with a standard 15-mm adapter to accommodate a bag-valve device for ventilating the patient. It also is available in varying diameters, ranging from an internal diameter of 2.5 to 4.5 mm (which may be uncuffed for pediatric patients) and 5.0 to 9.0 mm (cuffed for larger children and adults). The typical tube size for an average-size adult patient is from 7.0 to 9.0 mm (7.0 to 8.0 mm for female patients and 7.5 to 8.5 mm for male patients).

The end of the tube that is inserted into the trachea has a beveled tip, similar to that of a nasopharyngeal airway, which assists with smooth placement through the airway structures. Cuffed tubes have an inflatable 5- to 10-mL cuff a few centimeters above the beveled end, which forms a seal in the tracheal lumen. After the tube is placed, the cuff is inflated through a thin inflation line using a 10-mL syringe. The inflation line connects to the tip of the syringe at an adapter that contains a valve. The tip of the syringe opens the valve, allowing air to be injected or withdrawn from the cuff. For this reason, after the tube is placed and the cuff is inflated, you must remove the syringe to prevent air from leaking out into the syringe. A small pilot balloon on the inflation line reflects the inflation status of the cuff. When the pilot balloon is inflated, the cuff is inflated and vice versa (Figure A1-6).

Endotracheal tubes are supplied in a curved, sealed package. The curved shape of the tube facilitates insertion to the anteriorly located glottis.

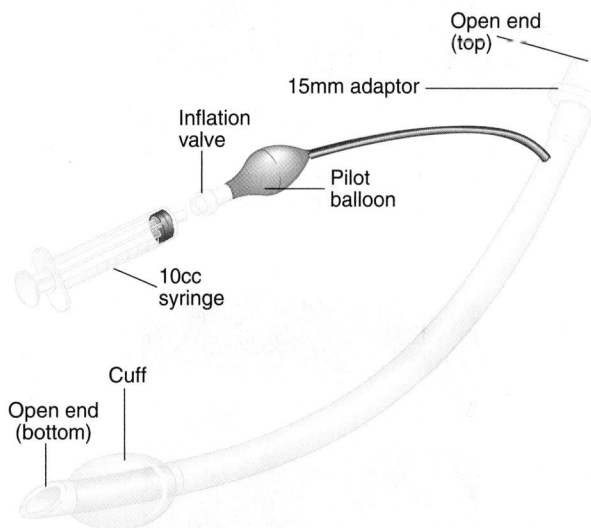

FIGURE A1-6

Endotracheal tube (ETT) and syringe.

Stylet

A stylet is a malleable, plastic coated wire used to mold the tip of the endotracheal tube at a slight angle (similar to that of a hockey stick) so that the tip of the tube is oriented toward the glottic opening. The tip of the stylet must not extend though the beveled end of the tube because this may result in injury to the airway tissues. The stylet should be recessed about 1 to 2 cm inside the tube. Some stylets have a stopper that prevents the stylet from slipping further into the tube once the stylet is properly placed. When using a stylet for a pediatric intubation, use a stylet made for pediatric tubes (Figure A1-7).

10-mL Syringe

A standard 10-mL syringe is used to inflate the cuff of the endotracheal tube, providing a seal within the trachea. The volume of air needed depends on the size of the tube and the size of the patient.

Magill Forceps

Magill forceps are angled forceps with circular tips that are used to remove foreign objects from a patient's airway or to guide the tip of the tube toward the glottic opening (Figure A1-8).

Suction Unit

Ensure that a suction unit is readily available when preparing to perform endotracheal intubation, because you may need to remove oral secretions, vomitus, or blood in order to

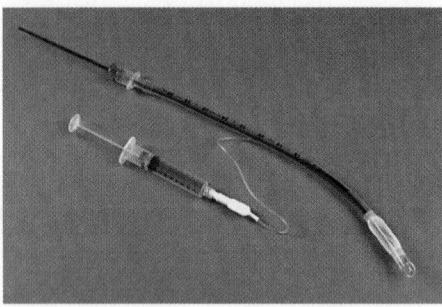

FIGURE A1-7

Endotracheal tube, stylet, and syringe.

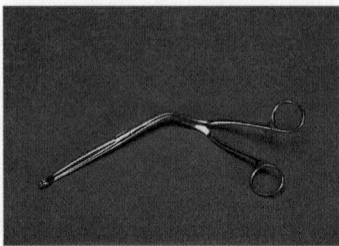

FIGURE A1-8

Magill forceps.

visualize the glottis. You may also need to perform endotracheal suctioning once the tube is in place.

Securing Device

Once you have successfully placed the tube within the patient's trachea, you must secure it to prevent it from becoming dislodged or slipping out of proper position. There are several types of commercially manufactured securing devices available, and some include an integrated bite block. You also can use tape to secure the device, but you should then place an oropharyngeal airway between the teeth to serve as a bite block. You should use a bite block in case the patient bites down on the tube, which would obstruct airflow through the tube. Once the tube is inserted and the cuff is inflated, this is the only route for air to enter the patient's lungs. If the tube is obstructed, there is no way for air to flow either through or around the tube and into the lungs.

Tube Placement Confirmation Devices

At a minimum, you must confirm tube placement by three methods. The first two methods are visualizing the tip of the tube as it passes through the glottic opening and auscultating breath sounds bilaterally as the patient is ventilated. The third method is either capnometry or the use of an esophageal detector device (EDD).

While there are several ways to confirm that the endotracheal tube is inserted into the trachea, capnometry is considered to be the most reliable. Follow your protocol for required methods of tube placement confirmation.

Anatomy

Endotracheal intubation requires the ability to recognize the anatomic landmarks used to identify the opening of the trachea (Figure A1-9). The epiglottis is the cartilaginous flap attached at the anterior side of the hypopharynx, just above the glottis. It closes during swallowing to prevent food and liquids from entering the trachea. The junction of the superior aspect of the epiglottis and the hypopharynx is called the *vallecula*. The posterior edge of the glottis is bordered by the arytenoid cartilage, sometimes called the *posterior cartilage*. The vocal cords are just inferior to the epiglottis and arytenoid cartilage, located on lateral borders of the glottis opening.

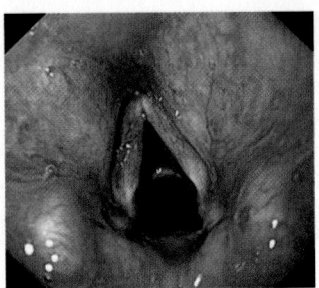

FIGURE A1-9

The glottis visualized through laryngoscopy. Note the landmarks: the epiglottis, arytenoid cartilage, and vocal cords.
(© Gastrolab/Photo Researchers, Inc.)

Indications

One of the most important aspects of performing endotracheal intubation is recognizing when a patient requires it, and also recognizing when a patient should *not* be intubated. In some cases, the patient will benefit best from more basic procedures, such as manual positioning, suctioning, basic airway adjuncts, or nonvisualized advanced airways.

When you are deliberating whether or not to perform endotracheal intubation, consider the following:

- *Is the patient's level of responsiveness adequate to allow him to maintain his airway?* Patients with a Glasgow Coma Scale (GCS) score of 8 or less are *not* able to maintain or protect their own airway. Therefore, endotracheal intubation is indicated. Remember this phrase, "GCS of 8, intubate." However, keep in mind that there are other methods of airway management that are safe and effective in unresponsive patients and a GCS of 8 does not mean you must intubate. It means you should consider it as one means of airway control.

- *Is the patient adequately ventilated and oxygenated? Is the patient exhibiting signs of respiratory failure?* If so, consider the need for intervention. If CPAP, oxygen administration, or bag-valve-mask device ventilations are not adequate to improve ventilation and oxygenation, consider the need for endotracheal intubation. Generally, patients who fit into this category are those who have become fatigued as a result of severe respiratory distress that has progressed to respiratory failure. Examples include patients with severe asthma attacks or those with exacerbation of CHF or COPD. Keep in mind that CPAP can be a good option to avert or delay the need for intubation in some patients with respiratory distress.

IN THE FIELD

When considering endotracheal intubation of a patient with an intact gag reflex, if your protocols allow, do so with extreme caution and have suction readily available because vomiting can result.

- *Do you expect a poor clinical course for the patient?* In some cases, you can reasonably anticipate that a patient's condition will deteriorate. Examples of such situations include those with airway burns, anaphylactic reactions that do not respond to epinephrine, and trauma to the neck resulting in edema. Stridor is a sign of upper airway obstruction, and, if present with edema, is an ominous sign. It may be necessary to secure an airway through endotracheal intubation before the opportunity to do so is lost as a result of severe laryngeal edema. But also be aware that an inexpert intubation attempt can convert a partial airway obstruction to a complete airway obstruction.

Complications

As with any medical procedure, there are potential complications with endotracheal intubation. You must be aware of those complications and pay close attention to details while performing the procedure to reduce their potential.

Hypoxia

Delays between positive pressure ventilations of the patient as a result of prolonged endotracheal intubation attempts may result in life-threatening hypoxia. You must limit the interruption in ventilations for each intubation attempt to no more than 30 seconds. Communicate with your team members and have someone start timing the instant the last positive pressure breath is delivered. When 30 seconds have elapsed, attach the bag-valve-mask device and deliver the next breath.

Equipment Malfunction

Test your equipment at the beginning of each shift to ensure it is in proper working condition. The moment you are preparing to perform endotracheal intubation is not the time to discover that the equipment does not work properly. Ensure each blade size is available, and that the light source of each works properly.

Damage to Teeth and Soft Tissues

Improperly performing endotracheal intubation can result in injury to the patient's lips, gums, deeper airway structures, and teeth. Rough handling of the laryngoscope can result in soft-tissue injuries, while improper lifting of the laryngoscope

IN THE FIELD

It is absolutely imperative that you avoid the temptation to prolong your intubation attempt "just a second longer" because you feel you are on the verge of passing the tube. Once your partner tells you that 30 seconds have elapsed since the patient's last ventilation, you must end the intubation attempt and ventilate the patient.

handle can result in broken teeth. When lifting the laryngo-scope handle to visualize the glottis, lift the handle and blade as one unit in a steady direction toward the patient's feet. *Do not pull* the handle toward the patient's head, using the teeth as a fulcrum. Doing so will not let you visualize the glottis, but it will provide great risk for breaking the patient's teeth.

Esophageal Intubation

Misplacement of the endotracheal tube into the esophagus of the patient will lead to life-threatening hypoxia and gastric distention if not immediately recognized. When the tube is in the esophagus, the patient's lungs are not being ventilated and he is becoming increasingly hypoxic. Forcing air into the stomach complicates that dire situation even further. Gastric insufflation often causes vomiting, which places the patient at risk for aspiration. Gastric distention also interferes with delivering full ventilations once the esophageal intubation is corrected. Indications of esophageal intubation include the following:

- Absence of chest rise and breath sounds upon ventilation
- Gurgling sounds auscultated over the epigastrium upon ventilation
- Cyanosis and persistent hypoxia
- Falling pulse oximetry readings
- Absence of monitored $EtCO_2$

If at any time you suspect the tube is not in the trachea, immediately deflate the endotracheal tube cuff, remove the tube, and ventilate the patient by bag-valve-mask device with high-flow oxygen.

Endobronchial Intubation

Insertion of the tube into the trachea does not guarantee proper placement. The airway branches into the right and left mainstem bronchi at the carina. If the tube is placed too deeply into the trachea, it will enter one of the mainstem bronchi and result in the ventilation of only one lung. The result is a ventilation–perfusion mismatch because both lungs are being perfused but only one is being ventilated. None of the blood circulating to the unventilated lung is being oxygenated or giving up carbon dioxide for exhalation. Because the right mainstem bronchi branches off at the carina in a much straighter direction than the left, excessively deep insertion of the endotracheal tube will nearly always result in intubation of the right mainstem bronchi. Follow these steps to avoid insertion of the endotracheal tube too deeply:

1. Advance the edge of the cuff of the tube no more than 2 cm past the vocal cords.
2. Hold the tube securely by hand after placement until it is secured with either tape or a commercial tube restraint device.
3. Note the depth to which the tube has been inserted by looking at the markings printed on the tube and frequently checking to see if it has moved.

Indications of endobronchial intubation include breath sounds heard only on one side of the chest and evidence of hypoxia despite adequate positive pressure ventilations.

Endotracheal Intubation Procedures

Endotracheal Intubation of a Patient with No Suspected Spine Injury

To properly perform endotracheal intubation of a patient without suspected spine injury, follow these steps (Scan A1-1):

1. Place the patient in a supine position with the head slightly elevated, sometimes called the *sniffing position*. You may elevate the head by placing a folded towel or blanket beneath the patient's head. In obese patients or patients with kyphosis, padding may be required beneath the shoulders to achieve proper airway alignment.

2. Insert an oropharyngeal airway and preoxygenate the patient with high-flow oxygen, providing positive pressure ventilation as needed.

3. While your partner preoxygenates the patient, gather and inspect the necessary equipment. Include the following in the inspection of your equipment:
   - Verify that the light source of the laryngoscope blade is functional.
   - Open the endotracheal tube package, but do not allow it to become contaminated. Remember: The end of the tube will be placed in the trachea, bypassing the protective mechanisms of the upper airway. Pneumonia is a common complication following endotracheal intubation and mechanical ventilation.
   - Insert a stylet into the endotracheal tube. Ensure that the tip of the stylet does not extend past the tip of the endotracheal tube.
   - Attach a 10-mL syringe and inflate the cuff with 5 to 10 mL of air. Remove the syringe. Ensure that the cuff does not leak by gently squeezing it.
   - Withdraw the air from the cuff and leave the syringe attached to the inflation tube.

4. Gently hyperextend the patient's neck, placing the head in the sniffing position, and open the mouth by pulling the mandible downward. Remove any dentures and suction the patient as needed.

5. Grasp the laryngoscope handle in your left hand (whether you are right or left handed, the laryngoscope is designed to be held in the left hand).

6. Insert the laryngoscope blade into the right side of the patient's mouth and use it to push the tongue to the left as you advance the tip of the blade.

7. Continue inserting the tip of the blade into the airway as you look for and identify the landmarks.

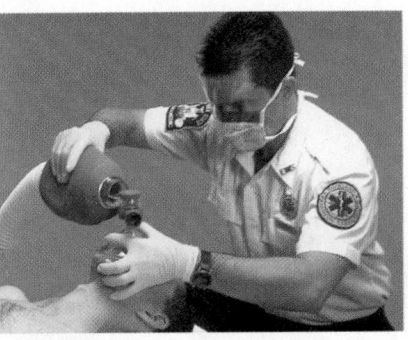

1. Ventilate the patient.

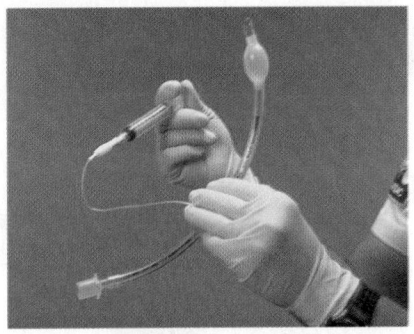

2. Prepare the equipment.

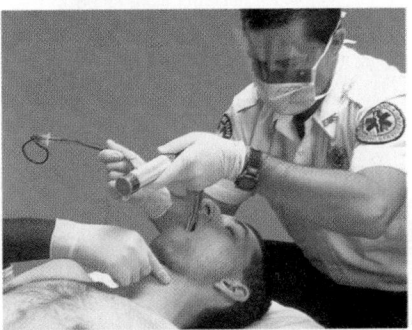

3. Apply Sellick's maneuver and insert the laryngoscope with the head slightly hyperextended into the sniffing position.

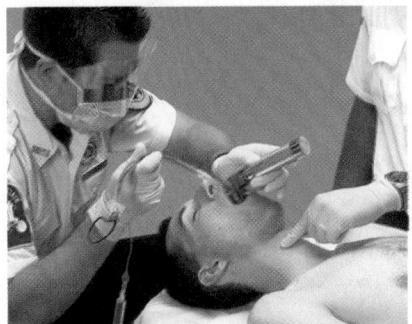

4. Visualize the larynx and insert the endotracheal tube.

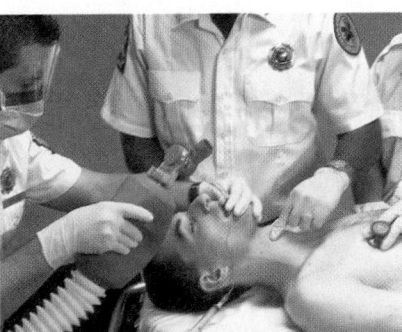

5. Inflate the cuff, ventilate, and auscultate.

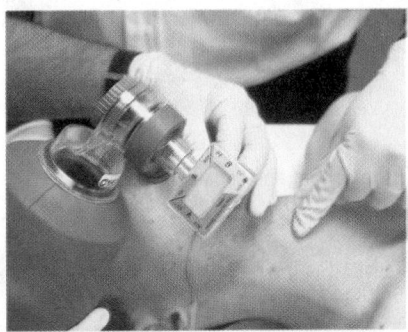

6. Confirm placement with an ETCO$_2$ detector.

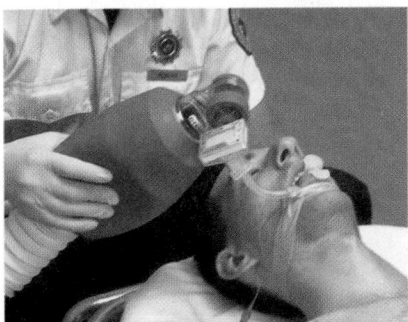

7. Secure the tube.

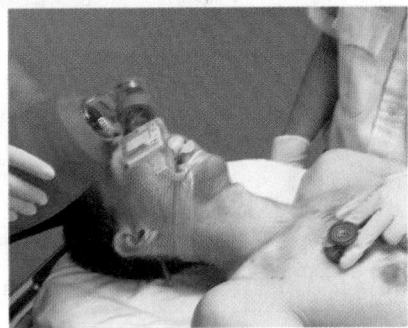

8. Reconfirm endotracheal tube placement.

Endotracheal Intubation in a Patient with Suspected Spine Injury

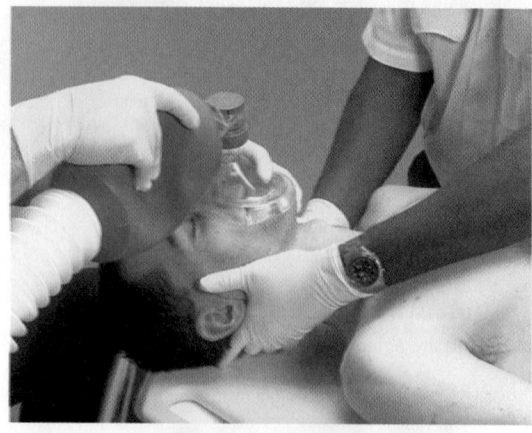

1. Ventilate the patient and manually stabilize the cervical spine, maintaining the head and neck in neutral alignment.

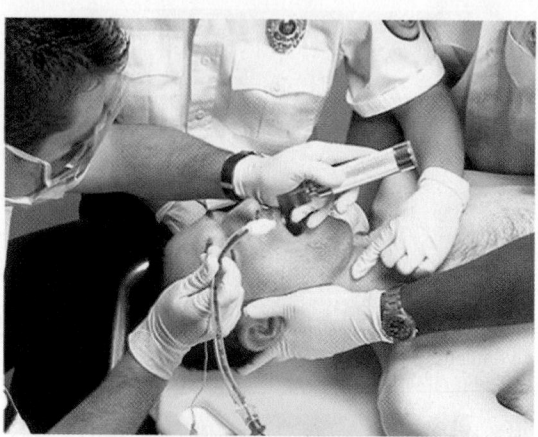

2. Apply Sellick's maneuver and intubate.

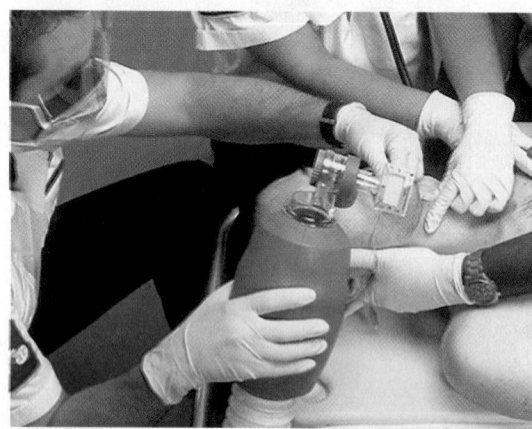

3. Ventilate the patient and confirm placement.

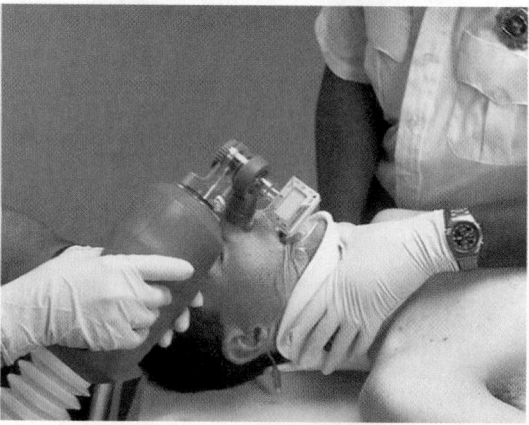

4. Secure the endotracheal tube and place a cervical collar.

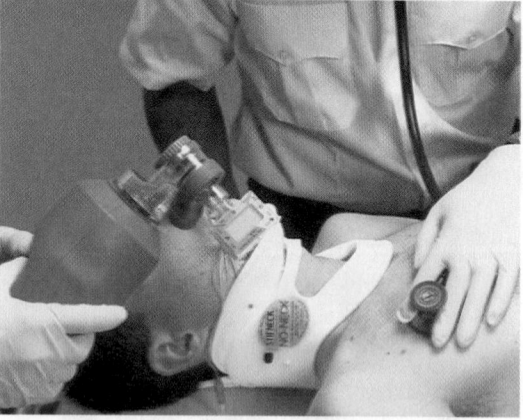

5. Reconfirm placement.

8. If using a curved blade, insert the tip of the blade into the vallecula and, using your arm and shoulder muscles, lift the handle toward the patient's feet. If using a straight blade, place the tip of the blade beneath the epiglottis and, using your arm and shoulder muscles, lift toward the patient's feet. Lift with a firm, steady motion until the vocal cords are visible. You may use Sellick's maneuver to assist with visualization of the vocal cords.

9. Grasp the endotracheal tube with your right hand and insert the tip of the tube from the right side of the patient's mouth, through the vocal cords.

10. Continue inserting the endotracheal tube until the cuff is 2 cm past the vocal cords.

11. Remove the laryngoscope blade from the patient's mouth while holding onto the endotracheal tube with your right hand to prevent it from being accidentally dislodged. Do not let go of it until it has been secured with tape or a commercial device.

12. Inflate the endotracheal tube cuff with 5 to 10 mL of air, and *remove* the syringe to prevent air leaking from the cuff back into the syringe.

13. Maintaining a hold on the endotracheal with your right hand, remove the stylet from the endotracheal and attach the bag-valve device.

14. Ventilate the patient and verify proper tube placement, using three methods, as previously discussed.

IN THE FIELD

If your patient has a cervical collar applied and the need for endotracheal intubation arises, remove the cervical collar. Leaving it secured in place will limit your ability to open the mouth to insert the laryngoscope blade and visualize the airway landmarks.

---

15. If the tube is properly placed, reinsert the oropharyngeal airway to act as a bite block. Secure the endotracheal tube with tape or a commercially manufactured tube restraint device.

Endotracheal Intubation of a Patient with Suspected Spine Injury

To properly perform endotracheal intubation of a patient with suspected spine injury, you must ensure the patient's head and neck remain in a neutral, in-line position throughout the procedure. This is accomplished by your partner grasping each side of the patient's head and holding manual stabilization of the head and neck as you perform the procedure. However, if the only way to establish and maintain a patient's airway is endotracheal intubation and you cannot accomplish it using a neutral position, use just the minimum amount of gentle hyperextension to gain visualization of the airway landmarks. Following the procedure, apply a cervical collar (Scan A1-2).

Summary

Prehospital endotracheal intubation is an invasive procedure that allows you to isolate the patient's airway for ventilation and protect against aspiration. Exercising excellent clinical judgment in making the decision to intubate is equally as important as having excellent skills in performing the procedure. When you must perform the skill, be sure the necessary equipment is readily available and in good working order. Follow the procedure for endotracheal intubation with attention to every detail, because improper placement of the endotracheal tube results in life-threatening hypoxia.

In recent years, there have been several journal articles published stating that endotracheal intubation should not be performed in the prehospital environment. This statement has been made as a result of several concerns such as the following:

- There is deterioration of skill proficiency as a result of infrequent skill performance.

- There is inadequate training.

- The performance of endotracheal intubation in the prehospital environment does not positively affect patient outcomes.

It is important that you understand each concern. As research evidence emerges, you may find that endotracheal intubation is either validated as a safe, effective prehospital intervention or that other methods of airway management are found to produce better outcomes and less harm. Remember: Your identity as a health care provider is not defined by what skills you are or are not allowed to perform. It is defined by doing what is in your patient's best interests, and doing it well no matter how simple or complex the skill.

Additional Reading

Davis, D. P., Peay, J., Sise, M. J., Vilke, G. M. Kennedy, F., Eastman, A. B., Velky, T., Hoyt, D. B. (2005). The Impact of Prehospital Endotracheal Intubation on Outcome in Moderate to Severe Traumatic Brain Injury. *Journal of Trauma-Injury Infection & Critical Care: 58:5*, 933–939.

Deacon, C. D, Peters, R., Tomlinson, P. & Cassidy, M. (2005). Securing the prehospital airway: a comparison of laryngeal mask insertion and endotracheal intubation by UK paramedics. *Emerg Med J 2005;22*, 64–67 doi:*10.1136/emj.2004.017178*

Stockinger, Z. T. & McSwain, N. E. Jr. (2004). Prehospital Endotracheal Intubation for Trauma Does Not Improve Survival over Bag-Valve-Mask Ventilation. *Journal of Trauma, 56:3*, 531–536.

Advanced ECG Recognition

Content Area: Assessment

Advanced EMT Education Standards: ECG recognition is supplemental to the Advanced EMT Education Standards. The information in this appendix is provided for programs that choose to teach advanced ECG recognition.

Objectives

After reading this appendix, you should be able to:

A2.1 Identify the indications, purpose, and limitations of continuous ECG monitoring.

A2.2 Relate the waves, segments, and intervals of the ECG to events in the cardiac cycle.

A2.3 Explain the clinical significance of common dysrhythmias.

A2.4 Demonstrate lead placement to obtain a Lead-II ECG.

A2.5 Use the rules for identifying normal sinus rhythm as the basis for comparison of ECGs.

A2.6 Identify the characteristics of, and recognize on an ECG strip, the following:
 - Accelerated junctional rhythm
 - Agonal rhythm
 - Asystole
 - Atrial fibrillation
 - Atrial flutter
 - Idioventricular and accelerated idioventricular rhythm
 - Junctional escape rhythm
 - Normal sinus rhythm
 - Premature atrial complex
 - Premature junctional complex
 - Premature ventricular complex
 - Sinus bradycardia
 - Sinus dysrhythmia
 - Sinus tachycardia
 - Supraventricular tachycardia (narrow complex tachycardia)
 - Ventricular fibrillation
 - Ventricular tachycardia

A2.7 Describe the purpose of prehospital 12-lead ECGs.

A2.8 Demonstrate lead placement to obtain a 12-lead ECG.

Introduction

There are several reasons ECG recognition can be important to Advanced EMTs. You may work with a paramedic partner and be called upon to assist in applying a cardiac monitor, you may be involved in the interfacility transport in which the patient's cardiac rhythm must be monitored (usually by a nurse or paramedic), or you may work as an emergency department technician, in which case cardiac monitoring is likely to be a routine part of your job. In some areas, Advanced EMTs may carry and use cardiac monitors as part of their patient assessment equipment. Prehospital 12-lead ECGs have been shown to be useful in reducing the time to treatment for acute myocardial infarction (AMI) in systems where there are hospital programs in place that use the results of prehospital 12-lead ECGs to make patient treatment decisions.

This appendix is provided as a reference to the Advanced EMT on the basic principles of electrocardiography. Do not consider it a substitute for a standard or advanced ECG course. Treatments are listed for informational purposes only. You must treat all patients according to the protocols approved by your medical director.

Standard ECG Monitoring

Electrocardiography offers a visual representation of electrical activity within the heart, called an *electrocardiogram (ECG)*. As an electrical impulse travels through the conduction system and myocardium, its direction and intensity is sensed by electrodes placed on the patient's skin. By utilizing a standard arrangement for ECG electrode placement, the tracings generated can be analyzed and compared to the characteristics that represent a normal ECG. The arrangement of the electrodes is referred to as *leads*. In electrocardiography, standard leads have been developed; the most frequently used in the field is Lead II, although other leads may be used, depending on protocol or preference (Figure A2-1). For consistency, the ECG examples given in this appendix are all Lead II unless otherwise noted.

Cardiac monitoring is a valuable assessment tool for the Advanced EMT in the field. ECG monitors can immediately reveal the nature of cardiac dysrhythmias. As a result, life-threatening dysrhythmias can be detected, documented, and treated.

ECG Monitors

There are many commercially available cardiac monitors. The most common ones provide four-electrode limb lead monitoring, so called because the electrodes are attached to or near the patient's limbs. With a four-electrode configuration, the monitor can display up to six different leads. One or more of them will be displayed on the monitor screen at any time, depending on the monitor features and options. Cardiac monitors also can record an ECG tracing, most commonly on paper, but also electronically. By incorporating an additional six electrodes that attach to the patient's chest, a monitor is capable of capturing a diagnostic quality 12-lead ECG. Many monitors with this capability provide some basic algorithms to assist in interpretation, and most include a feature to allow transmission to medical direction facilities through wireless phone systems or the Internet.

ECG Waveforms and Tracings

An ECG tracing (paper recording) permits close analysis of waveforms and measurements. Standard ECG paper is shown in Figure A2-2. Each small square is 1 square millimeter (mm). The paper moves through the monitor at 25 mm per second. Thus, each horizontal box represents 0.04 sec. This is useful in determining the duration of any component of the cardiac cycle (Figure A2-3). Relative voltage is determined by the

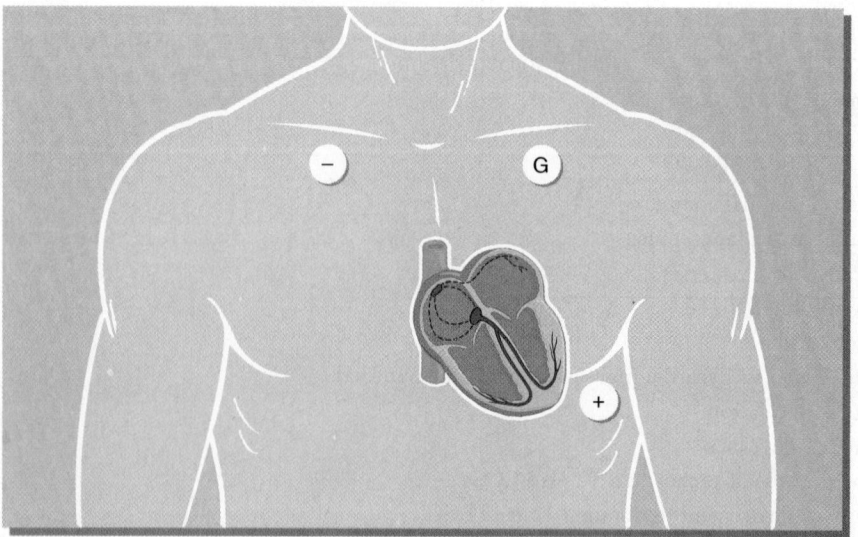

FIGURE A2-1

Placement of electrodes to monitor Lead II.

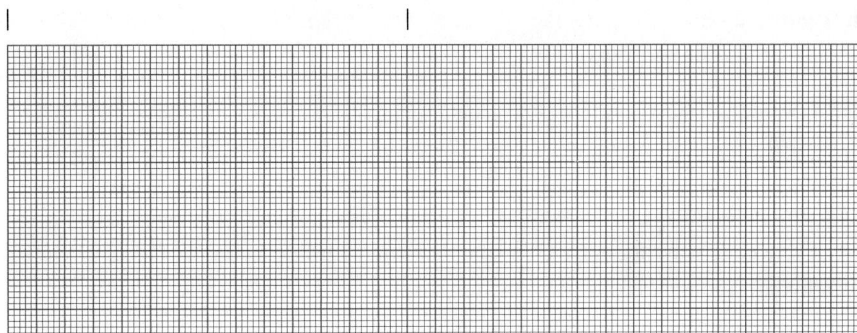

FIGURE A2-2

Sample ECG graph paper.

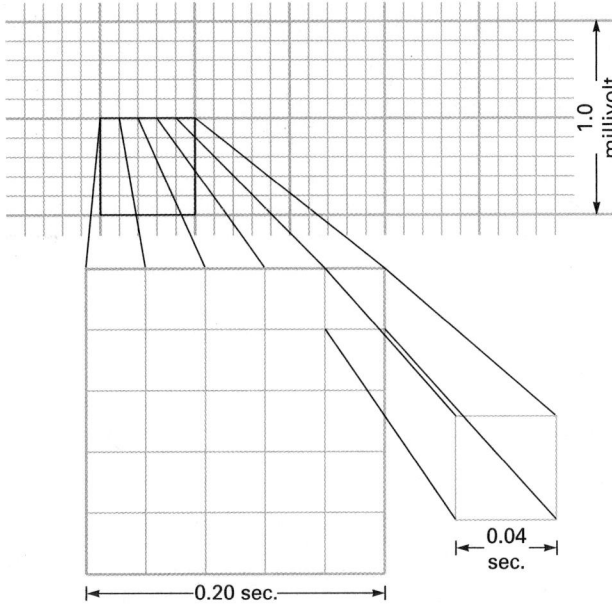

FIGURE A2-3

Using graph paper markings to measure voltage and time.

TABLE A2-1	**Normal Cardiac Cycle**	
ECG Feature	Normal Duration	Action Within the Heart
P wave	0.04–0.08 sec	Atrial depolarization
P-R interval	0.12–0.20 sec	"Pause" created by the atrioventricular node to allow full atrial contraction
QRS complex	Less than 0.12 sec	Ventricular depolarization
T wave	Not defined	Ventricular repolarization

direction and height (amplitude) of the vertical deflection of the wave. A positive (upright) deflection indicates electrical current flowing toward an electrode, and a negative (downward) deflection indicates current flowing away from an electrode.

Each feature of the ECG waveform can be related to an event in the cardiac cycle. While whole texts are devoted to the subject of electrocardiography, the basic events in the normal cycle are summarized in Table A2-1.

The normal cardiac cycle results in a rhythm called *normal sinus rhythm (NSR)*, reflecting its origin in the sinus (sinoatrial) node and its regular rhythm. Dysrhythmias are compared to the characteristics of normal sinus rhythm to define their features. A dysrhythmia occurs when the normal cardiac conduction cycle is disrupted. There are many causes for disruption, including ischemia (most common), electrolyte imbalances, toxic exposures, and others. The rhythm strips provided in Figures A2-4 through A2-22 should serve as examples of common dysrhythmias you will encounter. Each strip is noted with the following information: the name of the rhythm or dysrhythmia, along with an example; characteristics with respect to regularity, rate, and waveform; and additional notes on pathophysiology and treatment.

Normal Sinus Rhythm (Figure A2-4):

Regularity: Regular

Rate: 60 to 100 bpm

P waves: Uniform, upright

P-R interval: 0.12 to 0.20 sec

QRS complex width: Normally less than 0.12 sec

P-QRS relationship: There is a P wave for every QRS complex, and a QRS complex for every P wave.

Clinical notes: Sinus rhythm is considered a normal rhythm strip.

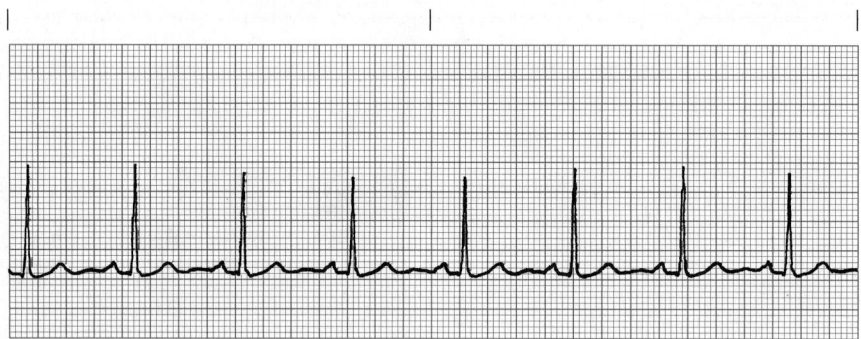

FIGURE A2-4

Rhythm strip: Normal sinus rhythm.

Sinus Tachycardia (Figure A2-5):

Regularity: Regular

Rate: 100 to 150 bpm

P waves: Uniform, upright

P-R interval: 0.12 to 0.20 sec

QRS complex width: Normally less than 0.12 sec

P-QRS relationship: There is a P wave for every QRS complex, and a QRS complex for every P wave.

Clinical notes: Sinus tachycardia has the same characteristics as a sinus rhythm, but with a rate greater than 100 bpm. Causes are many, but include exertion, fever, anxiety, and shock. Treatment is aimed at finding and correcting the underlying condition.

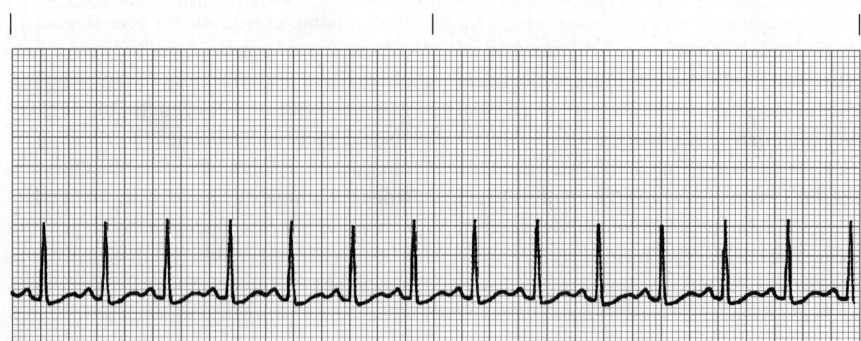

FIGURE A2-5

Rhythm strip: Sinus tachycardia.

Sinus Bradycardia (Figure A2-6):

Regularity: Regular

Rate: Less than 60 bpm

P waves: Uniform, upright

P-R interval: 0.12 to 0.20 sec; may be slightly longer at slower heart rates

QRS complex width: Normally less than 0.12 sec

P-QRS relationship: There is a P wave for every QRS complex, and a QRS complex for every P wave.

Clinical notes: Sinus tachycardia has the same characteristics as a sinus rhythm, but with a rate less than 60 bpm. Bradycardia may be normal in well-conditioned people; other causes include excessive vagal tone or medication toxicity. The preferred treatment is the administration of medications to increase the heart rate, but a cardiac pacemaker may be required. Transcutaneous cardiac pacemakers (TCP) use electrodes like those used to deliver defibrillation shocks to deliver a mild, regular, electrical current to the heart to stimulate myocardial contraction. TCP is a temporary solution. In cases where the heart rate cannot be increased, a permanent pacemaker is implanted.

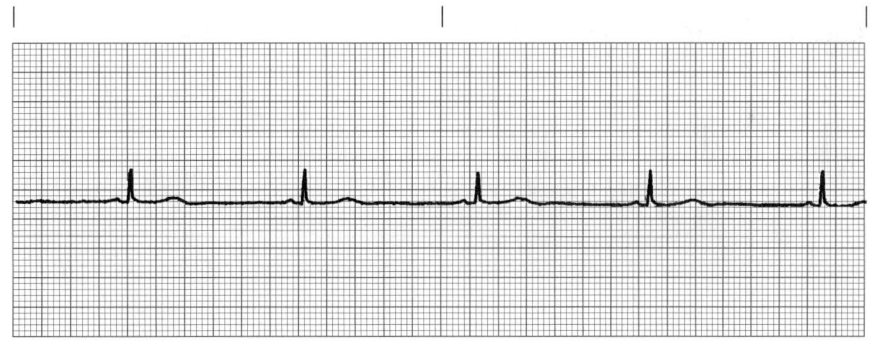

FIGURE A2-6

Rhythm strip: Sinus bradycardia.

Sinus Dysrhythmia (Figure A2-7):

Regularity: Irregular (regularly irregular)

Rate: Varies but averages between 60 and 100 bpm

P waves: Uniform, upright

P-R interval: 0.12 to 0.20 sec

QRS complex width: Usually less than 0.12 sec

P-QRS relationship: There is a P wave for every QRS complex, and a QRS complex for every P wave.

Clinical notes: Sinus dysrhythmia is caused by the action of the vagus nerve on the sinus node as it is stimulated by the respiratory cycle. You may observe a decrease in heart rate on expiration persisting through the end-expiratory phase, and a corresponding increase in heart rate during the inspiratory phase. This is common in young people and usually of no clinical significance. It is important to differentiate this dysrhythmia from atrial fibrillation by the presence of a P wave.

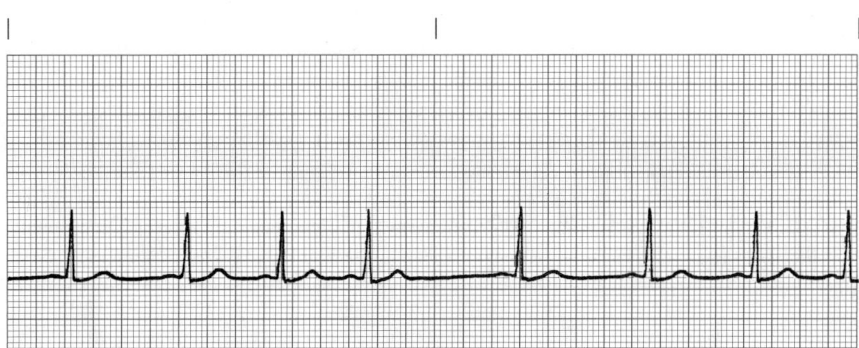

FIGURE A2-7

Rhythm strip: Sinus dysrhythmia.

Supraventricular Tachycardia (Figure A2-8):

Regularity: Regular

Rate: Greater than 150 bpm

P waves: May be present, but not discernable in very rapid rates, being obscured by the preceding T-wave

P-R interval: Not discernable

QRS complex width: Less than 0.12 sec

P-QRS relationship: Not reliable

Clinical notes: By definition, SVT is a narrow complex tachycardia with a rate greater than 150 bpm. This includes both sinus and junctional pacemakers. Because P waves are not visible, it is not possible to identify the pacemaker with certainty. Atrial fibrillation with rapid ventricular response is usually differentiated by its irregularity. Supraventricular tachycardia is treated with stimulation of the vagus nerve, medications, or delivery of an electrical shock synchronized with the cardiac cycle, called *synchronized cardioversion.*

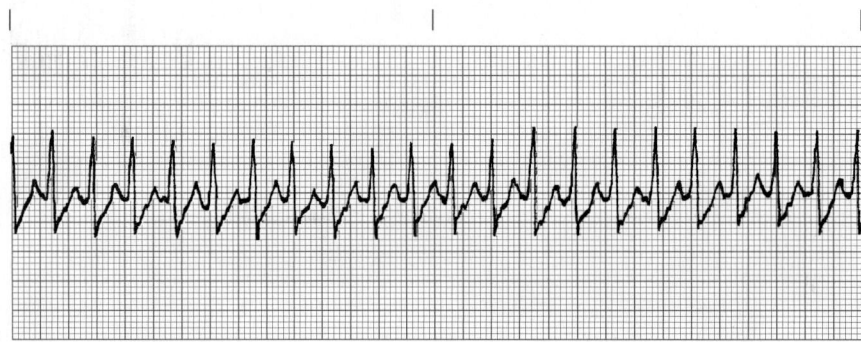

FIGURE A2-8

Rhythm strip: Supraventricular tachycardia.

Atrial Fibrillation (Figure A2-9):

Regularity: Irregular (irregularly irregular)

Rate: varies

P waves: Absent. *Fibrillatory waves* may be observed throughout the cardiac cycle (a "wavering baseline").

P-R interval: None

QRS complex width: Normally less than 0.12 sec

P-QRS relationship: None

Clinical notes: Atrial fibrillation is a common dysrhythmia, particularly in the elderly and in patients with heart failure and COPD. At normal rates (60 to 100 bpm) it is not life threatening, but may lead to complications such as thrombolytic strokes and pulmonary emboli. For that reason, patients with atrial fibrillation may take anticoagulant medications. Atrial fibrillation with ventricular rates over 150 bpm requires treatment with medications or the delivery of an electrical shock synchronized with the cardiac cycle, called *synchronized cardioversion.*

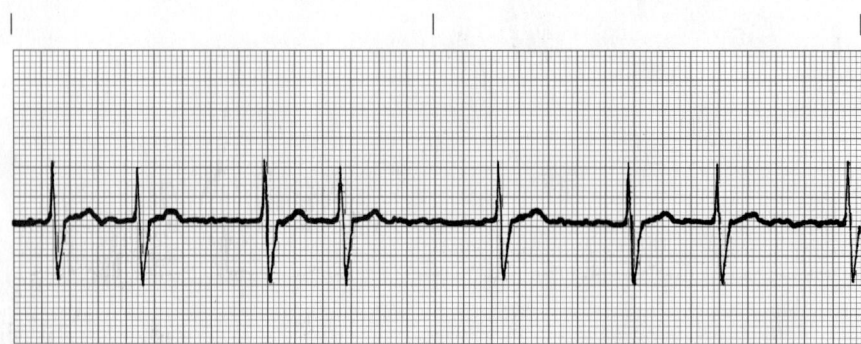

FIGURE A2-9

Rhythm strip: Atrial fibrillation.

Atrial Flutter (Figure A2-10):

> *Regularity:* Usually regular, but may be regularly irregular
>
> *Rate:* Varies upon conduction
>
> *P waves:* Absent. In their place are *flutter waves* representing repeated and continuous atrial depolarization.
>
> *P-R interval:* None
>
> *QRS complex width:* Normally less than 0.12 sec
>
> *P-QRS relationship:* None
>
> *Clinical notes:* Atrial flutter is characterized by a very rapid atrial rate of up to 300 bpm, and a ventricular rate that varies depending on the *conduction ratio* in the A-V node. For example, an atrial rate of 300 and a ventricular rate of 150 would represent a 2:1 conduction ratio, ventricular rate of 100 would be 3:1, and so on. The ratio may vary within the rhythm. Atrial flutter can be identified by its characteristic sawtooth baseline generated by the flutter waves.

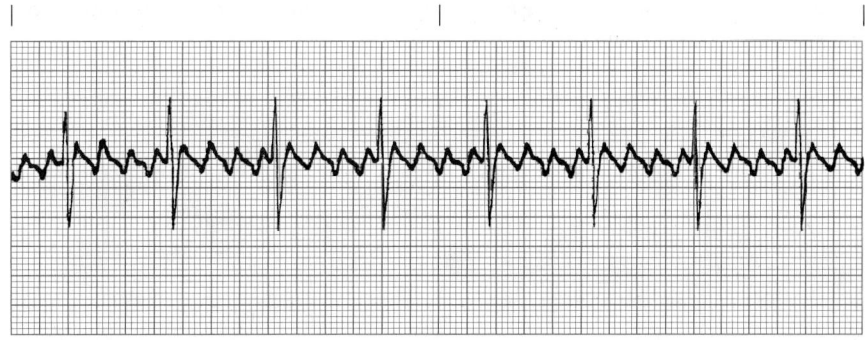

FIGURE A2-10

Rhythm strip: Atrial flutter.

Premature Atrial Complex (PAC) (Figure A2-11):

> *Regularity:* Irregular. Isolated PACs will interrupt the regularity of the underlying rhythm.
>
> *Rate:* Varies
>
> *P waves:* Present, usually upright and uniform and consistent with underlying rhythm
>
> *P-R interval:* Consistent with underlying rhythm, 0.12 to 0.20 sec
>
> *QRS complex width:* Normally less than 0.12 sec
>
> *P-QRS relationship:* There is a P wave for every QRS complex, and a QRS complex for every P wave.
>
> *Clinical notes:* PACs are atrial beats that look the same on the ECG as regular sinus beats, but occur early and cause irregularity in the overall rhythm. They have many causes, including exposure to caffeine and nicotine, but are often idiopathic and benign.

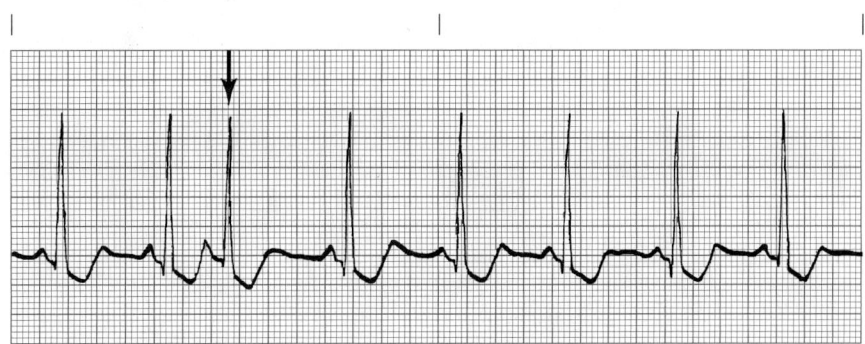

FIGURE A2-11

Rhythm strip: Premature atrial complex (PAC).

Junctional Escape Rhythm (Figure A2-12):

   Regularity: Regular

   Rate: Bradycardic, usually 40 to 60 bpm

   P waves: May be concealed by the QRS complex, or may appear inverted either before or after the QRS complex.

   P-R interval: If the P wave is discernable, the PRI will be short (greater than 0.12 sec).

   QRS complex: Normally less than 0.12 sec

   P-QRS relationship: If the P wave is discernable, there will be one P wave for every QRS complex and one QRS complex for every P wave.

   Clinical notes: The P wave (when visible) may be inverted due to retrograde conduction in the atria (impulse traveling from A-V node up through the atria). A pacemaker low in the atria may also cause an inverted P wave. However, in such a case, the P-R interval would be normal (0.12 to 0.20 sec). An *accelerated junctional rhythm* has the same characteristics as a junctional escape rhythm, but a rate of between 60 and 100 bpm. A *junctional tachycardia* has a rate of greater than 100 bpm, and rates of 150 bpm and greater are commonly called *supraventricular tachycardia*, because it is difficult to discern the presence of P waves at high rates.

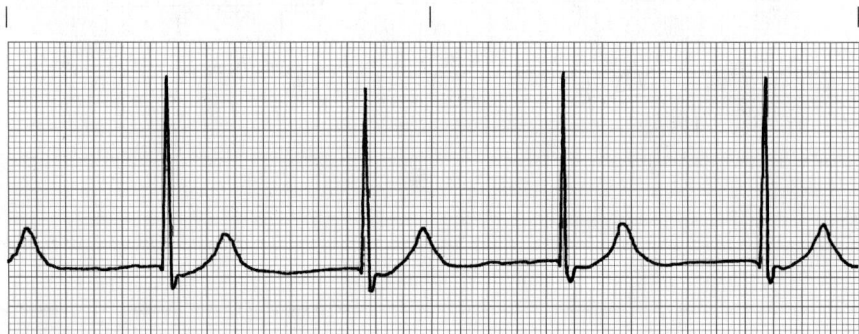

FIGURE A2-12

Rhythm strip: Junctional escape rhythm.

Premature Junctional Complex (PJC) (Figure A2-13):

   Regularity: Irregular

   Rate: Varies (ectopic beat)

   P waves: May be concealed by the QRS complex, or may appear inverted either before or after the QRS complex

   P-R interval: If the P wave is discernable, the PRI will be short (greater than 0.12 sec).

   QRS complex: Normally less than 0.12 sec

   P-QRS relationship: If the P wave is discernable, there will be one P wave for every QRS complex and one QRS complex for every P wave.

   Clinical notes: PJCs are similar to PACs. In this case, they are junctional beats that occur early and cause irregularity in the overall rhythm. Figure A2-13 shows a sinus bradycardia with two PJCs.

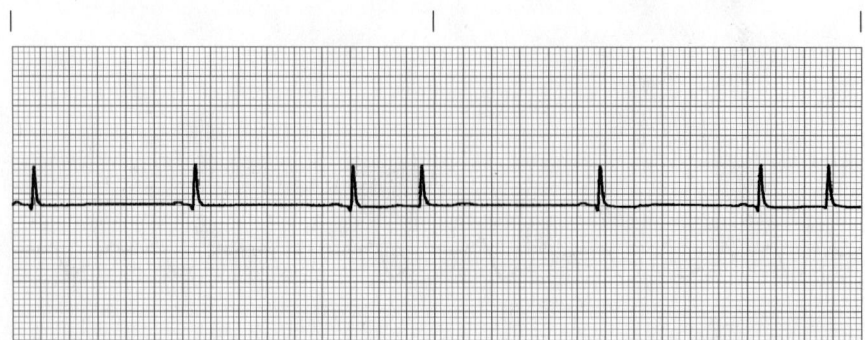

FIGURE A2-13

Rhythm strip: Premature junctional complex (PJC).

Idioventricular Rhythm (IVR) (Figure A2-14):

Regularity: Usually regular

Rate: Less than 40 bpm

P waves: Absent

P-R interval: None

QRS complex: 0.12 sec or greater, bizarre

P-QRS relationship: None

Clinical notes: Agonal refers to a "dying heart" rhythm. The ventricular pacemaker may take over when atrial and junctional pacemakers fail.

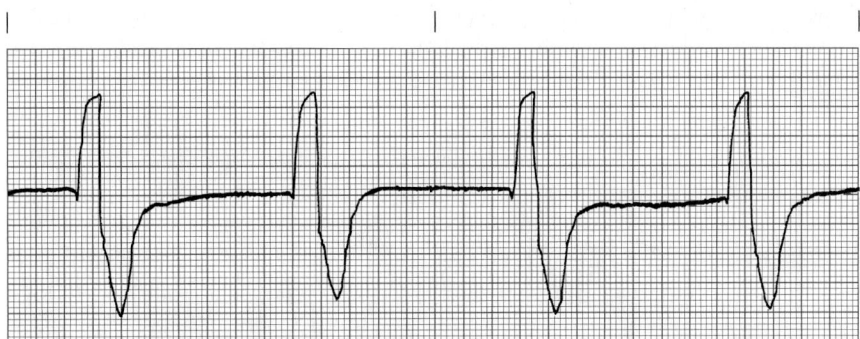

FIGURE A2-14

Rhythm strip: Idioventricular rhythm (IVR).

Premature Ventricular Complex (PVC) (Figure A2-15):

Regularity: Irregular

Rate: Varies (ectopic beat)

P waves: Absent

P-R interval: None

QRS complex: Wide (0.12 sec or greater) and bizarre

P-QRS relationship: None

Clinical notes: PVCs occur from an irritable focus in the ventricles, interrupting the normal rhythm of the heart. *Unifocal* PVCs originate from a single focus, and *multifocal* PVCs from two or more foci. The shape of the complexes is different in multifocal PVCs, whereas unifocal PVCs appear identical in shape. Figure A2-15 shows unifocal PVCs, and also demonstrates *bigeminal PVCs* or *ventricular bigeminy,* so named because of the occurrence of a PVC alternating with a normally conducted beat. PVCs may be a sign of ischemia or toxic exposure, or they may be benign. Oxygen is the treatment of choice for all PVCs.

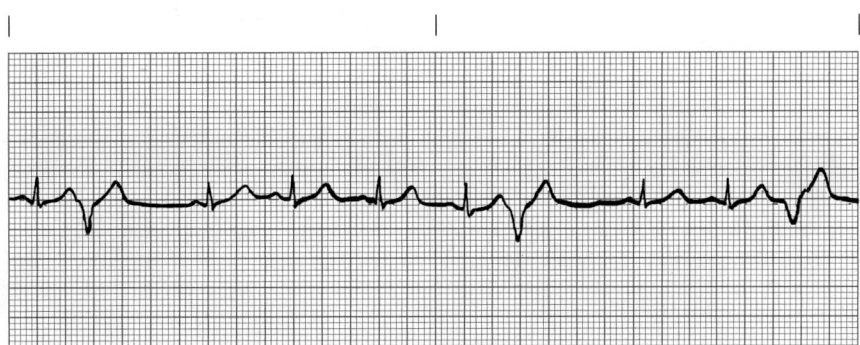

FIGURE A2-15

Rhythm strip: Premature ventricular complex (PVC).

Ventricular Tachycardia (VT) (Figure A2-16):

Regularity: Regular

Rate: 150 to 250 bpm

P waves: Absent

P-R interval: None

QRS complex: Wide (0.12 sec or greater) and bizarre

P-QRS relationship: None

Clinical notes: Ventricular tacycardia is one of the dysrhythmias associated with sudden cardiac arrest (SCA). VT results from a single irritable focus in the ventricles that takes over as the pacemaker for the heart. T waves, when seen, will usually be deflected in the opposite direction from the QRS complex in VT. This dysrhythmia may or may not be accompanied by a pulse. Pulseless ventricular tachycardia is treated the same as ventricular fibrillation, with CPR and immediate defibrillation. Even when a pulse is present, the dysrhythmia is considered serious because it can be a precursor to ventricular fibrillation. Ventricular tachycardia with a pulse is treated with medications or synchronized cardioversion.

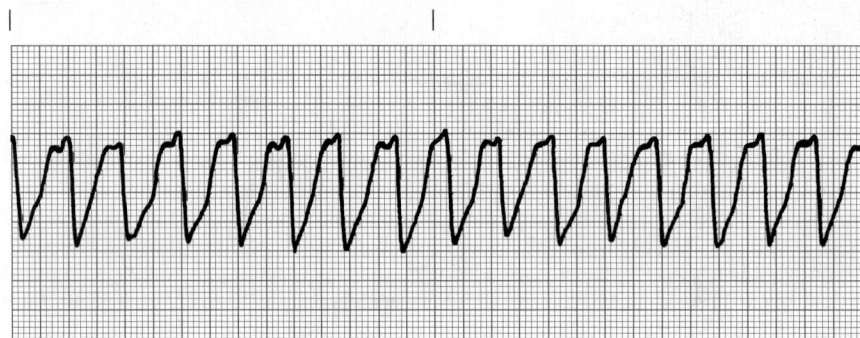

FIGURE A2-16

Rhythm strip: Ventricular tachycardia (VT).

Ventricular Fibrillation (VF) (Figure A2-17):

Regularity: Cannot be determined

Rate: Cannot be determined

P waves: None

P-R interval: None

QRS complex: None

P-QRS relationship: None

Clinical notes: VF is a preterminal rhythm arising from multiple irritable foci in the ventricles that fire randomly. It is one of the dysrhythmias associated with SCA. This causes the heart to "quiver" and cardiac output to fall to zero. It is characterized by fibrillatory waves, observed on the ECG as a wavering or chaotic baseline. The greater the size or amplitude of the waves, the "coarser" the VF is said to be. Untreated, VF will ultimately deteriorate into asystole. Ventricular fibrillation requires immediate treatment with CPR and defibrillation.

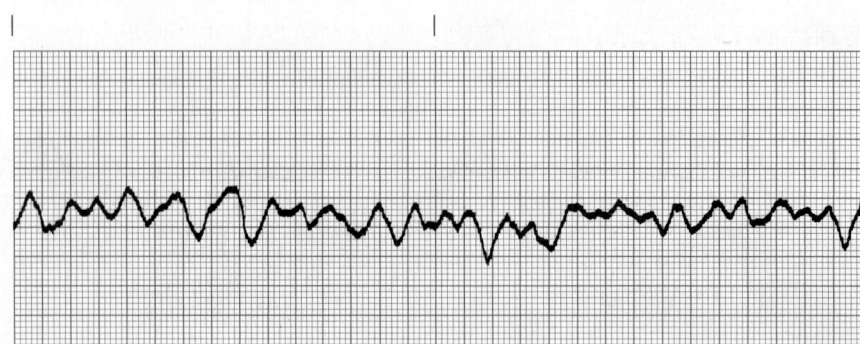

FIGURE A2-17

Rhythm strip: Ventricular fibrillation (VF).

Asystole (Figure A2-18):

In asystole, a straight line on the ECG tracing indicates an absence of electrical activity. There are no waveforms present. It is a lethal dysrhythmia and can be associated with SCA.

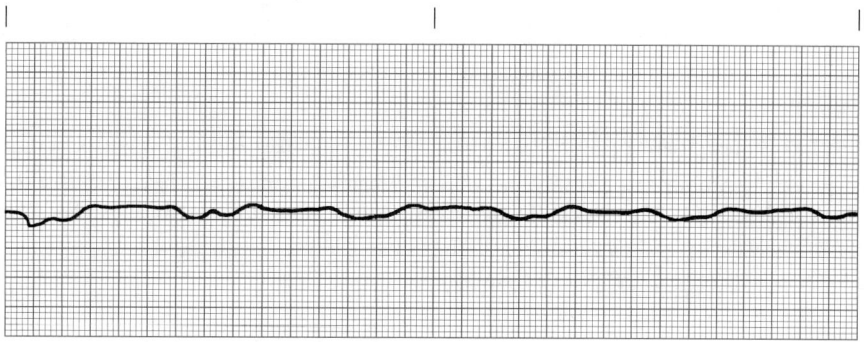

FIGURE A2-18

Rhythm strip: Asystole.

First-degree A-V Block (Figure A2-19):

Regularity: Regular

Rate: Depends on underlying sinus rate

P waves: Present, uniform, upright

P-R interval: Prolonged, greater than 0.20 sec

QRS complex: Normally less than 0.12 sec

P-QRS relationship: There is a P wave for every QRS complex, and a QRS complex for every P wave.

Clinical notes: First-degree A-V block is sinus rhythm with a prolonged P-R interval. There are a number of reasons for the dysrhythmias, the most frequent being medication toxicity, electrolyte disturbances, MI, and enhanced vagal tone. Treatment depends on the patient's perfusion status and the underlying cause of the dysrhythmia.

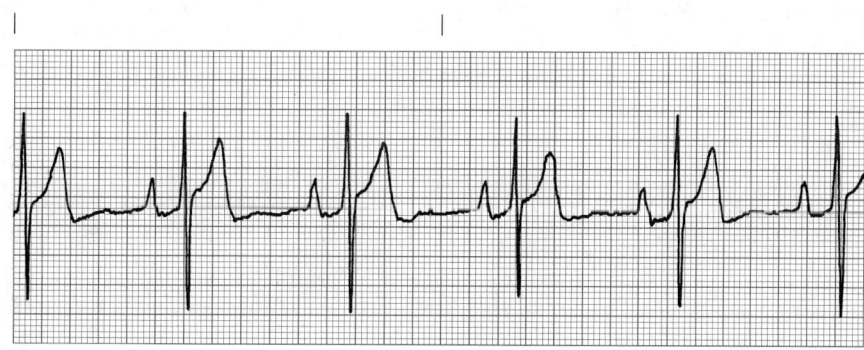

FIGURE A2-19

Rhythm strip: First-degree A-V block.

Second-degree A-V Block Mobitz Type I (Figure A2-20):

Regularity: Regularly irregular

Rate: Depends on underlying sinus rate

P waves: Present, uniform, upright

P-R interval: Varies, increasing in length over successive complexes until the R-wave is blocked, and then repeating the pattern

QRS complex: Normally less than 0.12 sec

P-QRS relationship: Inconsistent; there are more P waves than QRS complexes due to R waves periodically being blocked.

Clinical notes: Second-degree Mobitz I is relatively uncommon. When it occurs, it may be a precursor to a more serious dysrhythmia or a higher-degree heart block. If signs of cardiogenic shock are present, treatment may include atropine or transcutaneous pacing.

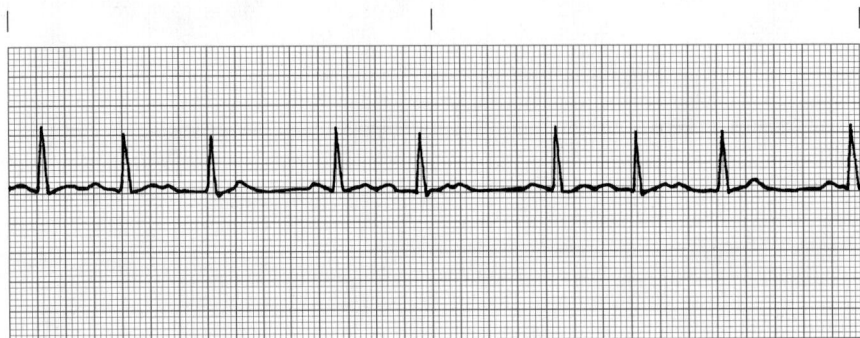

FIGURE A2-20

Rhythm strip: Second-degree A-V block Mobitz Type I.

Second-degree A-V Block Mobitz Type II (Figure A2-21):

Regularity: Irregular

Rate: Atrial rate is usually 60 to 100 bpm but may be slower. Ventricular rate is usually bradycardic and always less than the atrial rate.

P waves: Present, uniform, upright and usually regular in rhythm

P-R interval: May be normal or prolonged where it exists

QRS complex: Normally less than 0.12 sec

P-QRS relationship: While P waves occur consistently and regularly, QRS complexes are periodically missing due to periodically blocked conduction in the A-V node. The block may be regular (such as a 2:1 or 3:1 conduction) or irregular (no pattern of blocked versus unblocked complexes).

Clinical notes: Second-degree Type II block is considered a high-degree heart block and may progress to third-degree block if the underlying causes are not corrected. Bradycardia may lead to cardiogenic shock, requiring treatment with medications or transcutaneous pacing.

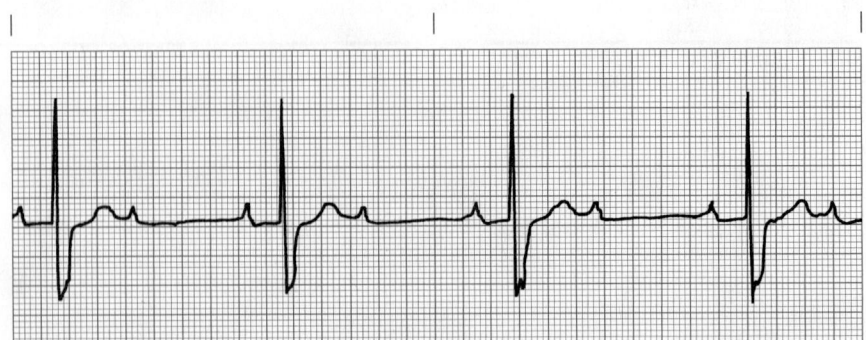

FIGURE A2-21

Rhythm strip: Second-degree A-V block Mobitz Type II.

Third-degree A-V Block (complete heart block) (Figure A2-22):

Regularity: Atrial and ventricular rates are regular.

Rate: Bradycardic. Atrial rate may range from near normal to as low as 30 bpm. Ventricular rates are consistent with the ventricular pacemaker rate of 30 to 40 bpm and may be even lower.

P waves: Present, uniform, upright

P-R interval: None discernable

QRS complex: Usually wide (0.12 sec or greater) and often bizarre appearing

P-QRS relationship: There is no correlation between P waves and QRS complexes.

Clinical notes: In a complete heart block, there is no conduction from the atria to the ventricles. Consequently, a ventricular pacemaker initiates. Third-degree heart block is always serious and usually requires treatment. Treatment may include medications, such as atropine, or transcutaneous pacing.

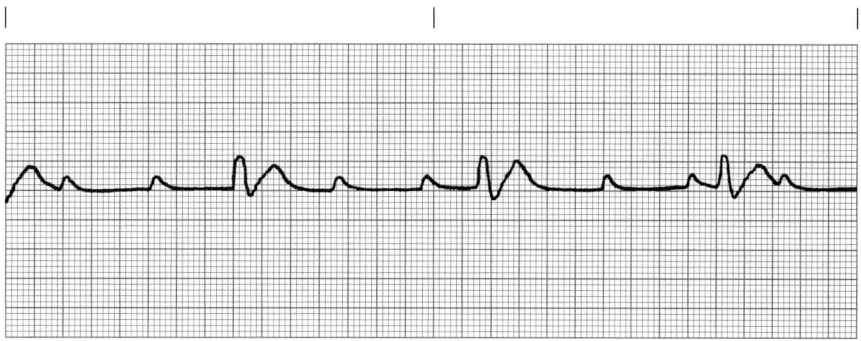

FIGURE A2-22

Rhythm strip: Third-degree A-V block.

Pulseless Electrical Activity

Pulseless electrical activity (PEA) is not a specific dysrhythmia, but is a condition in which there is an organized electrical rhythm that shows up on the monitor, but in which no pulse is generated. Despite the presence of electrical activity, the patient is in cardiac arrest and requires CPR. PEA sometimes has correctable underlying causes, such as hypovolemia, hypothermia, overdose, and other conditions. The treatment for PEA is to maintain perfusion while finding and correcting the underlying cause.

Reference

Walraven, G. (2010). *Basic Arrhythmias,* 7th ed. Upper Saddle River, NJ: Prentice Hall.

Appendix

3

Adult Intraosseous Infusion

Content Area: Pharmacology

Advanced EMT Education Standard: The AEMT applies fundamental knowledge of medications in the AEMT scope of practice to patient assessment and management.

Objectives

After reading this appendix, you should be able to:

A3.1 Explain the purpose, indications, contraindications, and complications associated with intraosseous access in adult patients.

A3.2 Demonstrate tibial or sternal intraosseous access using the device(s) chosen by your institution.

Introduction

The concept of intraosseous (IO) access has been around since the early 20th century (Drinker, Drinker, & Lund, 1922). But, following World War II, it became a forgotten resource for vascular access until it was reintroduced by pediatrician James Orlowski, M.D., in 1984 (Wayne, 2006). Since then, its use has become common in hospitals and in the prehospital setting for vascular access in pediatric and adult patients. In adults, IO access sites include the proximal and distal humerus, proximal and distal tibia, and manubrium of the sternum. The use of manual IO needles has been replaced by spring-loaded and battery-powered devices, which make accessing the medullary cavity of the bone much easier. Three devices have been approved by the U.S. Food and Drug Administration. The FAST1 (Pyng Medical Group, British Columbia, Canada) is a spring-loaded device that is inserted into the manubrium. The Bone Injection Gun (BIG) (WaisMed, Houston, Texas) is a spring-loaded device used for access at the proximal humerus or proximal tibia. The EZ-IO (Vidacare Corp, San Antonio, Texas) is a battery-powered device that is approved for use at the proximal and distal humerus and tibia. This appendix covers a common site of IO access used in the prehospital setting: the proximal tibia.

Follow the protocols set forth by your medical director regarding the indications, sites, approved devices, and procedures for obtaining intraosseous access.

Purpose of Intraosseous Access

Vascular access is a vital part of the resuscitation of any patient. Sometimes, obtaining peripheral IV access is difficult for a variety of reasons, including low intravascular volume and a patient's peripheral venous anatomy. In situations where you cannot quickly obtain reliable vascular access, the bone marrow within the medullary cavity of the bone offers an effective route for administering fluids and medications.

Bone marrow lies within the epiphysis and the medullary cavity of the diaphysis (Figure A3-1). When fluids and medications are infused into the spongy tissue of the medullary cavity, they are absorbed by way of the circulatory system within the bone, which leads to the systemic venous circulation (Alexander, Corrigan, Gorski, Hankins, & Perucca, 2009).

Indications

When you cannot readily obtain intravenous access, the intraosseous route can provide a fast, effective alternative means of delivering fluids and medications. Always follow protocol with regard to indications, and the device manufacturer's instructions. The primary indication for IO access is the inability to quickly obtain adequate peripheral venous access in a patient who requires an immediate route for administering intravenous fluids or medications, such as critical trauma patients and patients in cardiac arrest (Miller, Bolleter, & Philbeck, 2008).

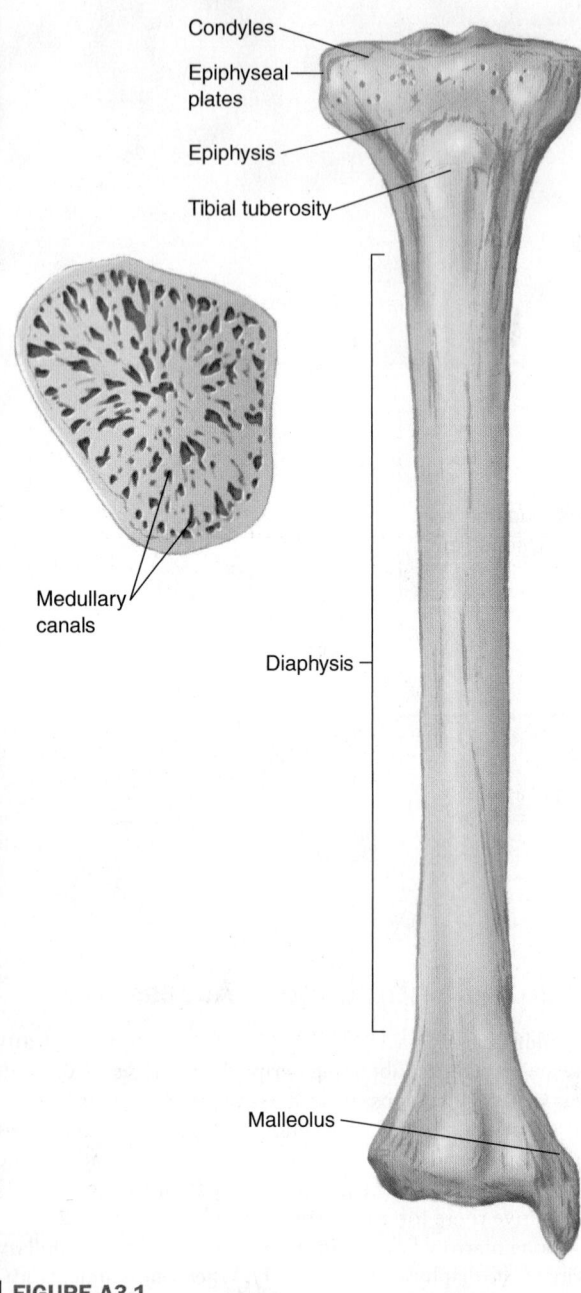

Condyles

Epiphyseal plates

Epiphysis

Tibial tuberosity

Medullary canals

Diaphysis

Malleolus

FIGURE A3-1

Tibia.

Contraindications

There are a few instances where intraosseous access is contraindicated. Before inserting the intraosseous needle, you must assess the patient and determine if any of the following contraindications exist (Miller et al., 2008):

- Fracture of the bone (including suspected fracture from a gunshot wound)
- Bone disease, such as severe osteoporosis
- Any previous orthopedic procedures near insertion site
- Prosthetic limb or joint near the insertion site
- IO placed within the past 24 hours in the same bone

- Infection, such as cellulitis, at the insertion site
- Inability to locate landmarks or excessive tissue over the intended site of insertion

Intraosseous access in patients with any of the listed conditions is only contraindicated in the affected insertion site. The presence of any of the listed contraindications does not exclude intraosseous access as a treatment option at another site.

Complications

Complications of intraosseous access can be reduced with proper training, including understanding the anatomy of the bone and how intraosseous infusion works. Complications of intraosseous access are as follows (Miller et al., 2008):

- *Infiltration.* Infiltration occurs when administered fluid collects within the tissues surrounding the insertion site rather than entering the medullary canal.
- *Osteomyelitis.* This is an infection of the bone. While a potential complication, infection rates are very low.
- *Pulmonary embolism.* Inserting an intraosseous needle could lead to bone, marrow, or fat entering the circulatory system.

Causes of complications of IO infusion include the following (Miller et al., 2008):

- Improper placement
- Not inserting the needle at a 90-degree angle
- Not maintaining and controlling pain after insertion in a conscious patient
- Not ensuring proper placement with a flush
- Not administering a 10-mL flush to open the medullary space prior to initial infusion
- Failure to maintain the right amount of pressure (greater than 35 mmHg) during the infusion
- Failure to use proper length or type of device in patients with excessive tissue at the target site
- Prolonged needle placement, longer than 24 hours

Procedure for Tibial Intraosseous Access

The proximal tibia is a common site of IO access in adults. A drill-like device (EZ-IO), consisting of a battery-operated driver and a sharp stylet that acts as a guide for the IO needle, or a manually triggered spring-loaded device (BIG) is used to obtain IO access in the proximal tibia.

1. Set up an IV of isotonic crystalloid solution.
2. Improper placement of the needle is the most common error when initiating intraosseous access. Palpate the tibial tuberosity (the raised ridge along the superior, anterior surface of the tibia, just below the knee). The proper insertion site is 2-cm medial and 1-cm proximal to the tibial tuberosity.
3. If using an EZ-IO, test the device to ensure that it is functioning. Attach the needle if it is not already attached.

4. Cleanse the site, preferably with a povidone iodine solution, using aseptic technique.

5. Prime the connecting tubing by using a 10-mL syringe to fill it with sterile normal saline solution for injection. Leave the 10-mL syringe attached. A short piece of extension tubing, sometimes called a "pigtail" is usually provided with the IO device. If it is not, you can use a short extension tubing, with or without a three-way stopcock as the connecting tubing to which you will attach the IV line once you have confirmed the IO needle placement.

6. Stabilize the leg and insert the needle at a 90-degree angle to the tibia, according to the device recommendations.

7. Always stabilize the needle hub while removing the insertion device and guide (trocar or stylet) from the needle.

8. Remove the stylet and discard it in a sharps container.

9. Attach the primed connecting tubing and 10-mL normal saline flush.

10. Administer a 10-mL normal saline flush to verify correct placement. Flushing may cause pain in conscious patients. If allowed by your protocols, injection of a topical anesthetic (1 or 2 percent lidocaine) prior to infusing IV fluids can diminish the discomfort.

11. Attach the IV tubing to the connecting tubing and set the fluid administration rate. You may require a pressure infusion device to achieve an adequate infusion rate when rapid infusion of fluids is required.

12. Dress the insertion site with 4" × 4" gauze squares or a commercial device supplied with the product to stabilize it and to prevent contamination.

Scan A3-1 illustrates the proper procedure for achieving intraosseous access using the EZ-IO device. Your instructor will demonstrate the proper insertion procedure for other intraosseous devices as necessary.

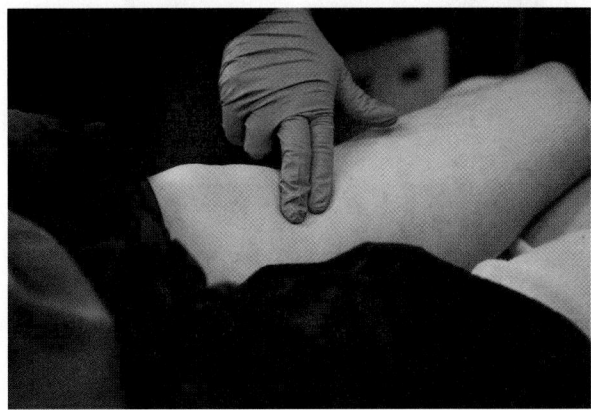

1. Palpate the tibial tuberosity (a raised bump on the anterior surface of the tibia). The proper insertion site is one finger width medial to the tibial tuberosity. Improper placement of the needle is the most common error when initiating intraosseous access.

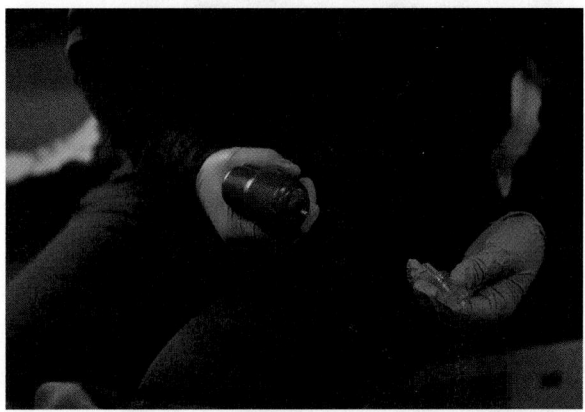

2. Test the device to ensure that it is functioning and attach the needle if it is not already attached.

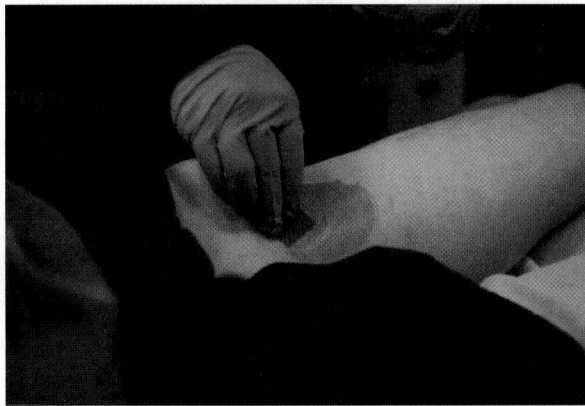

3. Cleanse the site using an aseptic technique.

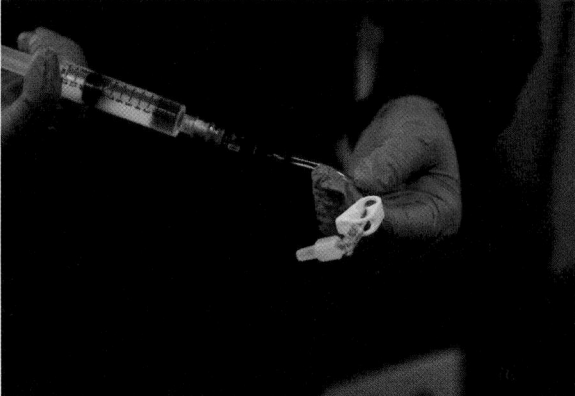

4. Prime the tubing with normal saline and leave the 10 mL syringe attached.

SCAN A3-1 Intraosseous Access Using the EZ-IO Device

(continued)

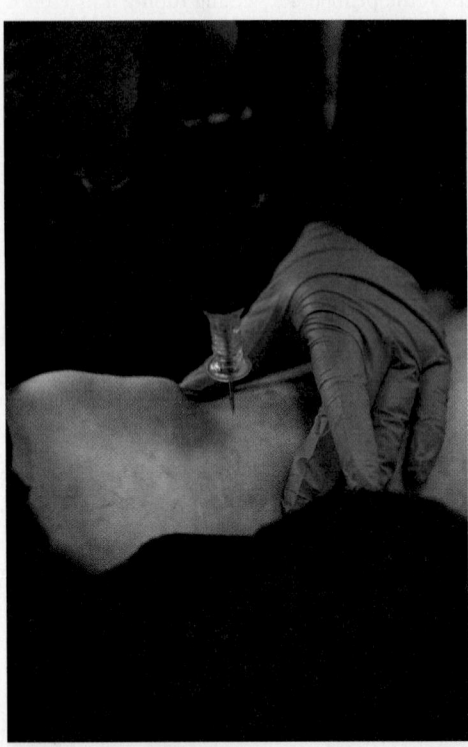

5. Stabilize the leg and insert the needle at a 90-degree angle to the tibia. Insert the needle according to the device's recommendations.

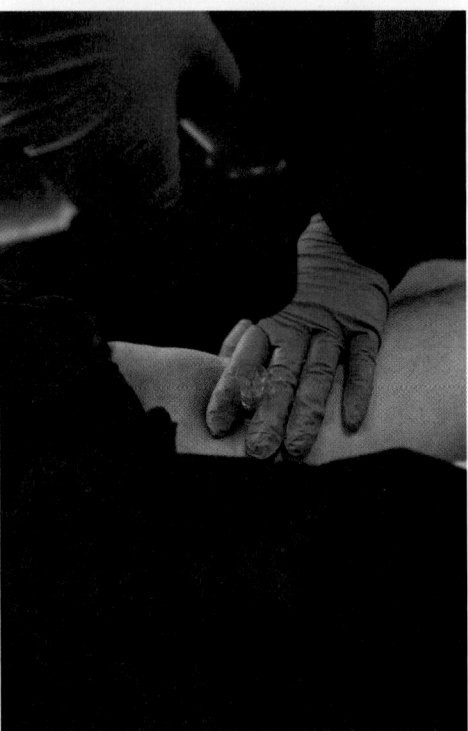

6. Always stabilize the needle hub while removing the device.

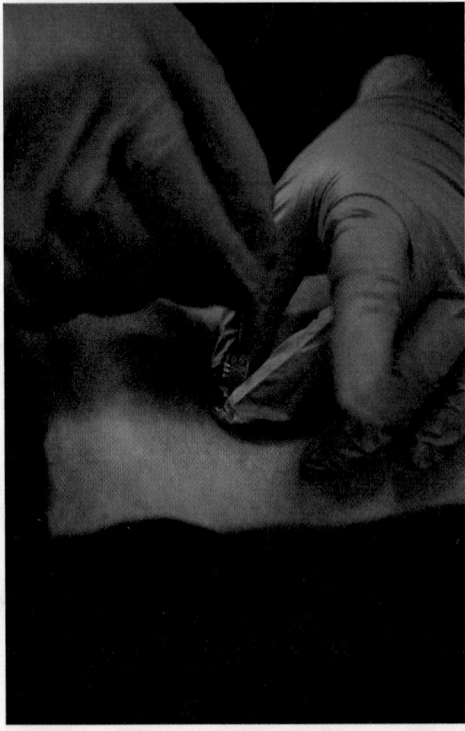

7. Remove the stylet and discard it in an appropriate sharps container.

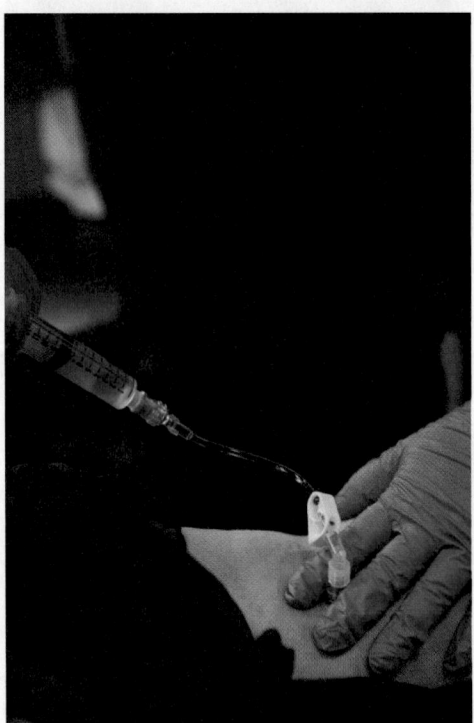

8. Attach the primed connector tubing and 10-mL normal saline flush. Administer a rapid 10-mL normal saline flush to verify correct placement. A rapid flush will ensure the opening of the medullary space allowing the intraosseous infusion to flow more freely. Note that flushing may cause pain to conscious patients. If using the EZ-IO device, it is recommended that you administer 2.5 mL of a 2-percent lidocaine solution through the needle prior to flushing. Follow your protocol for dosing.

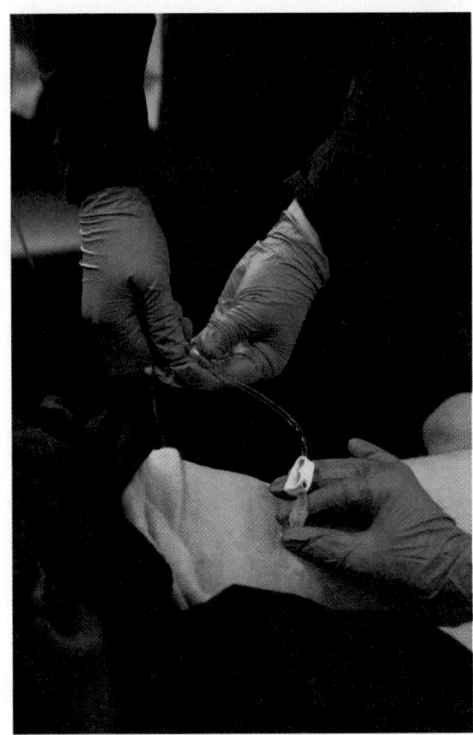

9. Attach IV tubing to the three-way stopcock connector tubing and set the fluid administration rate.

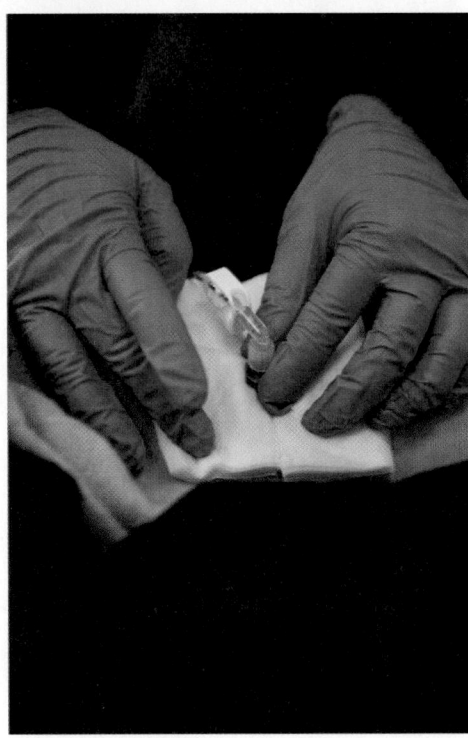

10. Dress the insertion site with a 4 × 4 gauze to prevent contamination.

Summary

In recent years, adult intraosseous access has proven effective and efficient as a route for administering fluids and medications. Currently, the EZ-IO, Bone Injection Gun (BIG), and the FAST 1 are the three FDA-approved adult intraosseous devices. The devices differ in their insertion sites and techniques. You must be familiar with the device or devices selected by your EMS service and become practiced in their use.

References

Alexander, M., Corrigan, A., Gorski, L., Hankins, J., & Perucca, R. (2009). *Infusion Nurses Society Infusion nursing: An evidence-based approach.* Retrieved January 9, 2011, from http://books .google.com/books?isbn[equals]1416064109

Drinker C., Drinker K., & Lund, C. (1922). The circulation in the mammalian bone marrow. *American Journal of Physiology, 62,* 1–92.

Miller, L., Bolleter, S., & Philbeck, T. (2008). *FAQ: Intraosseous vascular access and the EZ-IO®.*

Wayne, M. A. (2006). Adult intraosseous access: An idea whose time has come. *Israeli Journal of Emergency Medicine, 6*(2), 41–45. Retrieved January 9, 2011, from http://www.isrjem .org/April06_Intraosseous.pdf

Additional Reading

Blumberg, S. M., Gorn, M., & Crain, E. F. (2008). Intraosseous infusion: A review of methods and novel devices. *Pediatric Emergency Care, 24*(1), 50–56. Retrieved January 9, 2011, from http://pt.wkhealth.com/pt/re/merck/ fulltext.00006565-200801000-00013.htm

Buck, M. (2006). Intraosseous administration of drugs in infants and children. *Pediatric Pharmacotherapy, 12*(12), 1–4. Retrieved January 9, 2011, from http://medscape.com/ viewarticle/552022

Additional Emergency Medications

Content Area: Pharmacology

Advanced EMT Education Standard: Integrates comprehensive knowledge of pharmacology to formulate a treatment plan intended to mitigate emergencies and improve the overall health of the patient.

Note: These additional drug profiles are provided for informational purposes only. You must always work within your approved scope of practice and follow your EMS system's protocols for medication administration.

Objectives

After reading this appendix, you should be able to:

A4.1 Describe the drug profiles with respect to prehospital emergency use for the following drugs:

- Activated charcoal
- Adenosine
- Amiodarone
- Atropine
- Calcium chloride
- Diazepam
- Diltiazem
- Diphenhydramine
- Dopamine
- Epinephrine 1:10,000
- Fentanyl citrate
- Furosemide
- Ipratropium bromide
- Ketorolac
- Levalbuterol
- Lidocaine
- Lorazepam
- Magnesium sulfate
- Midazolam
- Morphine
- Ondansetron
- Sodium bicarbonate
- Thiamine

Introduction

There are several reasons you may need to be familiar with emergency medications other than those covered in the pharmacology chapters of this textbook. Your medical director may have approved additional medications based on needs in your community; you may work with and assist a paramedic partner; or you may work in an emergency department setting where the knowledge of additional medications is invaluable. This appendix provides drug profiles for medications commonly used in prehospital emergency care. The information in the appendix does not supply all of the information you must know to administer those medications. You must receive additional instruction through your training program or employer. As always, you must adhere to your protocols for approved medications and their indications and dosages.

Activated Charcoal, U.S.P.

Common trade name: Actidose-Aqua, Actidose with sorbitol

Class: Gastric **adsorbent**

Mechanism of action: Activated charcoal for emergency use consists of charcoal, ground into a fine powder and mixed with a liquid to form a slurry (suspension of solid particles in a liquid). The small particle size of activated charcoal provides a large surface area to adsorb (bind) certain toxins to the charcoal. Once bound, the toxins are carried through the GI tract for elimination. Sorbitol, a sugar alcohol with large molecules that cannot be absorbed from the GI tract, is often used as the liquid carrier in premixed activated charcoal preparations because it acts as a **cathartic** (has a laxative effect) to speed elimination of toxins through the GI tract.

Indications: Used for poisoning or overdose by ingestion.

Contraindications: Do not use in patients with inability to swallow or lack of a gag reflex. Do not use in infants. Do not give more than two doses of a preparation containing sorbitol because excessive fluid and electrolyte loss can occur (do not give more than one dose to pediatric patients). Do not use in patients who have ingested caustic substances.

Adverse reactions: Nausea and vomiting, constipation or diarrhea

Dosage: 1 to 2 grams/kg, PO or by gastric tube

Notes: Activated charcoal may not be effective for several toxins with low molecular weights, such as petroleum products, toxic alcohols, lithium, or heavy metals including mercury, lead, and iron. Give activated charcoal only as directed by medical direction or poison control.

Adenosine

Common trade name: Adenocard

Class: Cardiac antidysrhythmic, nucleoside (a biologic molecule that serves as a building block of RNA and DNA)

Mechanism of action: Decreases electrical conduction through the AV node. Also acts directly on the sinus node to decrease automaticity to slow the heart rate. *Adenosine has an immediate onset, but a duration of less than 10 seconds.*

Indications: Used for narrow complex tachycardia. Not indicated for atrial fibrillation with rapid ventricular response, atrial flutter, or ventricular tachycardia, because it is ineffective in converting these rhythms.

Contraindications: Do not use in patients with second- or third-degree AV node block, **sick sinus syndrome**, or hypersensitivity to adenosine.

Adverse reactions: Light-headedness, headache, chest pain, flushing, hypotension, shortness of breath, nausea, metallic taste, transient rhythm disturbances (bradydysrhythmia, sinus pause, ventricular ectopy, or asystole)

Dosage:

Adults: 6 mg rapid IV bolus through a proximal IV, followed by a 20 mL saline bolus to ensure that adenosine reaches the central circulation. If there is no change in rhythm after 1 to 2 minutes, give a 12-mg rapid IV bolus. If rhythm persists 1 to 2 minutes following the second dose, one additional 12-mg rapid IV bolus may be given. Do not exceed 30 mg total.

Pediatrics: 0.1 mg/kg (up to 6 mg) initial dose; may repeat in 1 to 2 minutes at double the initial dose; follow each dose with a 20-mL saline flush.

Notes: Due to its short half life (less than 10 seconds), administer adenosine through an IV that has been established as near as possible to the central circulation, such as in the antecubital fossa. Use as large a catheter as practical (minimum 18 gauge) to facilitate a rapid bolus. Place the patient supine prior to administration, and warn the patient of possible sensations such as flushing or transient chest tightness when the drug is administered. Push the medication as rapidly as possible, immediately following each bolus with a 20-mL bolus of normal saline. Activate the recorder on the cardiac monitor prior to administration to document any rhythm changes.

Amiodarone

Common trade name: Cordarone

Class: Cardiac antidysrhythmic

Mechanism of action: Slows depolarization of myocardial cells by blocking potassium and calcium channels. Amiodarone also has some properties similar to beta blockers.

Indications: Used for supraventricular tachycardia refractory to adenosine, ventricular tachycardia, or ventricular fibrillation that has not responded to defibrillation.

Contraindications: Do not use in patients with second- and third-degree heart blocks, severe bradycardia, pulmonary congestion, hypotension, or hypersensitivity to amiodarone.

Adverse reactions: Flushing, bradycardia, dizziness, hypotension, headache, AV node conduction abnormalities

Dosage:

Adults with perfusing rhythms: 150 mg infused over 10 minutes, followed by an infusion of 1 mg/min for 6 hours, and a 0.5 mg/min infusion over the next 18 hours.

Adults, with nonperfusing rhythms (cardiac arrest): 300-mg IV bolus, may follow with one bolus of 150 mg if rhythm persists, up to a maximum of 450 mg.

Pediatrics, with perfusing rhythms: Loading dose 5 mg/kg IV/IO over 20 to 60 minutes, up to 15 mg/kg/day.

Pediatrics, with nonperfusing rhythms (cardiac arrest): 5 mg/kg IV bolus.

Notes: Do not mix with sodium bicarbonate.

Atropine Sulfate

Common trade names: None, widely available generically

Class: Anticholinergic, parasympatholytic

Mechanism of action: Blocks the effects of acetylcholine, the principal neurotransmitter for the parasympathetic nervous system.

Indications: Used for symptomatic bradycardic rhythms, organophosphate poisoning, and certain specific nerve agent exposure.

Contraindications: No contraindications when indicated for emergency treatment of symptomatic bradycardia or organophosphate/nerve agent exposure. Use with caution in acute coronary syndromes; will not be effective in treating bradycardia in transplanted hearts.

Dosage for bradycardia:

Adults: 0.5 mg IV bolus; may repeat as needed up to a maximum of 3 mg.

Pediatrics: 0.02 mg/kg IV/IO/ET (diluted to 3 to 5 mL), minimum dose 0.1 mg, maximum single dose of 0.5 mg for a child and 1 mg for an adolescent. May repeat in 5 minutes for a maximum total dose of 1 mg for a child and 2 mg for an adolescent.

Dosage for organophosphate poisoning/nerve agents: 1 to 2 mg IV or IO; repeat every 1 to 5 minutes. Endpoint of administration is marked by drying of secretions. Determine dosing regimen based on the type of agent or poison, and the duration and amount of exposure. Consult medical direction or poison control.

Calcium Chloride

Common trade names: None, widely available generically

Class: Electrolyte

Mechanism of action: Calcium has a role in the function of the nervous system and voluntary muscle, cardiac contractility, and blood coagulation. Calcium chloride is dissociated and the calcium made available to the body.

Indications: Used for hyperkalemia, hypocalcemia, hypermagnesemia, and calcium channel blocker toxicity.

Contraindications: Do not use in patients with ventricular fibrillation, ventricular tachycardia, digitalis toxicity, renal failure, or hypercalcemia.

Side effects: Bradycardia, asystole, hypotension

Dosage:

Adults: 8 to 16 mg/kg IV of 10 percent solution, may repeat once in 10 minutes.

Pediatrics: 20 mg/kg IV of 10 percent solution, may repeat as needed for desired clinical effects.

Notes: Calcium chloride is extremely hypertonic and may cause severe necrosis in the event of extravasation; observe IV site closely while administering.

Diazepam

Common trade name: Valium

Class: Benzodiazepine, anticonvulsant, sedative

Mechanism of action: Depresses the neurons in the CNS. Raises the seizure threshold in the motor cortex of the brain.

Indications: Used for seizures, behavioral emergencies, and sedation prior to cardioversion or pacing.

Contraindications: Do not use in patients with pre-existing respiratory depression, CNS depression from head injury, hypotension, or hypersensitivity to diazepam.

Side effects: Respiratory depression, hypotension, confusion, nausea

Dosage:

Adults (for seizures): 5 mg IV/IO over 2 minutes, up to 10 mg per dose. May repeat every 10 to 15 minutes as needed up to a maximum of 30 mg.

Pediatrics (for seizures): 0.1 mg/kg every 5 to 10 minutes.

Sedation prior to cardioversion or pacing (adults): 5 to 15 mg IV 5 to 10 minutes prior to procedure.

Notes: Administer diazepam IV in the port closest to the vein to avoid precipitation (formation of particulate matter in the intravenous line). Be prepared for respiratory depression to occur, and have resuscitation equipment available.

Diltiazem

Common trade name: Cardizem

Class: Calcium channel blocker

Mechanism of action: Blocks calcium channels in smooth, voluntary and cardiac muscle, causing slowing of conduction in the AV node, and dilation of the coronary and peripheral vasculature.

Indications: Used for atrial fibrillation and atrial flutter with rapid ventricular response where slowing of heart rate is desired, supraventricular tachycardia refractory to adenosine, and multifocal atrial tachycardia.

Contraindications: Do not use in patients with sick sinus syndrome, hypotension, high-degree AV block (unless the patient has a pacemaker), Wolff-Parkinson-White syndrome, acute myocardial infarction, ventricular tachycardia, or wide complex tachycardia of unknown origin.

Side effects: Bradycardia, hypotension, chest pain, heart blocks (first and second degree), heart failure, syncope, nausea, dry mouth, shortness of breath, headache, atrial flutter, sweating, ventricular dysrhythmias

Dosage (adults only):

Bolus: 15 to 20 mg over 2 minutes, after 15 minutes if needed may repeat at 20 to 25 mg over 2 minutes.

Infusion: 5 to 15 mg/hr, titrate to effect for heart rate control.

Notes: The safety of diltiazem has not been established in pediatrics. Be alert for hypotension when administering. Do not mix with furosemide.

Diphenhydramine

Common trade name: Benadryl

Class: Antihistamine

Mechanism of action: Nonselectively blocks histamine (H_1 and H_2) receptors.

Indications: Used for allergic reactions, anaphylaxis, and acute dystonic reactions.

Contraindications: Do not use in patients taking MAO inhibitors, newborns, nursing mothers, or those with hypersensitivity to diphenhydramine.

Side effects: Drowsiness, coordination disturbances, hypotension, palpitations, tachycardia, bradycardia, thickening of bronchial secretions, and paradoxical excitement in pediatric patients. Rapid administration may cause seizures in pediatrics.

Dosage:

Adults: 10 to 50 mg IM or slow IV every 6 to 8 hours, up to 400 mg/day.

Pediatrics: 1 to 2 mg/kg slow IV or IO, up to 50 mg.

Notes: Be alert for sedation and respiratory depression. Because diphenhydramine increases viscosity of bronchial secretions. Use with caution in asthmatic patients.

Dopamine

Common trade name: Intropin

Class: Sympathomimetic

Mechanism of action: Acts on dopaminergic, $alpha_1$ and $beta_1$ receptors in a dose-dependent fashion. At doses below 5 mcg/kg/min, acts primarily on dopaminergic receptors, causing renal, mesenteric, and cerebral vasculature dilation. At dose ranges from 5 to 10 mcg/kg/min, $beta_1$ effects predominate, resulting in enhanced myocardial contractility, increased cardiac output, and increased systemic vascular resistance. At dosage ranges from 10 to 20 mcg/kg/min, $alpha_1$ effects predominate, producing peripheral vascular constriction.

Indications: Used for hypotension from vascular or cardiogenic origins.

Contraindications: Do not use in patients with hypovolemia, tachydysrhythmias, ventricular fibrillation, or pheochromocytoma.

Side effects: Tachycardia, hypertension, increased myocardial oxygen demand

Dosage: 2 to 20 mcg/kg/min, titrated to effect. See mechanism of action for dosage range and effects.

Notes: Use with caution in the presence of acute myocardial infarction, because increased myocardial oxygen demand may worsen ischemia. Use an infusion pump to ensure precise flow rates. Correct pre-existing hypovolemia prior to the use of dopamine.

Epinephrine, 1:10,000

Common trade name: Adrenalin

Class: Sympathomimetic

Mechanism of action: Acts directly and nonselectively on alpha and beta receptors. Effects are dose dependent. Causes bronchodilation and vasoconstriction. Epinephrine 1:10,000 is a concentration of 1 gram per 10,000 mL (1 mg/10 mL) for intravenous injection in cardiac arrest. An intravenous infusion of epinephrine in a concentration of 1 mcg/mL (made by adding 1 mg of epinephrine to 1,000 mL of normal saline) is used in some cases to treat severe, refractory bradycardia and refractory hypotension in anaphylactic shock.

Indications: Used for cardiac arrest (ventricular fibrillation, ventricular tachycardia, asystole, PEA); symptomatic bradycardia; hypotension refractory to other medications; anaphyaxis; and severe reactive airway disease.

Contraindications: No contraindications in cardiac arrest. Hypovolemic shock (correct hypovolemia first), hypersensitivity (relative – may use a lower dose in emergencies).

Side effects: Headache, nausea, restlessness, weakness, dysrhythmias, hypertension, chest pain, tachycardia

Dosage:

Adult cardiac arrest: 1 mg 1:10,000 solution IV/IO bolus every 3 to 5 minutes.

Adult bradycardia or hypotension: IV infusion at 2 to 10 mcg/min).

Pediatric cardiac arrest: 0.01 mg/kg (0.1 mL/kg of 1:10,000 solution) IV/IO every 3 to 5 minutes to a maximum of 1 mg per dose.

Notes: Patients taking beta blockers may have a reduced response to epinephrine. Do not mix with alkaline solutions such as sodium bicarbonate. Epinephrine may increase myocardial oxygen demand and may thus worsen ischemia in acute myocardial infarction. Elderly patients and patients with pre-existing cardiac disease should receive one half the indicated dose for anaphylaxis.

Fentanyl Citrate

Common trade name: Sublimaze

Class: Opioid analgesic

Mechanism of action: A synthetic opioid that rapidly crosses the blood–brain barrier and acts directly on the opiate receptors in the brain. Often given in concert with benzodiazepines for conscious sedation.

Indications: Used for analgesia.

Contraindications: Do not use in patients with respiratory depression, hypotension, head injury, cardiac dysrhythmia, myasthenia gravis, or hypersensitivity to opiates.

Side effects: Respiratory depression, hypotension, bradycardia, nausea, vomiting, itching

Dosage:

> *Adults:* 1 to 2 mcg/kg IV or IO slow bolus every 30 to 60 minutes prn.
>
> *Pediatrics:* Same as adults.

Notes: Be prepared for respiratory depression and have naloxone and resuscitation equipment available.

Furosemide

Common trade name: Lasix

Class: Loop diuretic

Mechanism of action: Inhibits the reabsorption of sodium and chloride in the kidney at the proximal tubule and the loop of Henle. IV administration also produces a modest vasodilatory effect, thus increasing venous capacitance.

Indications: Used for pulmonary edema associated with left-sided heart failure.

Contraindications: Do not use in patients with renal failure, dehydration, hypokalemia, hypersensitivity to furosemide, or hypersensitivity to sulfonamides.

Side effects: Hypotension, dysrhythmia, hypochloremia, hypokalemia, hyponatremia, hypercalcemia, and hyperglycemia. Transient deafness can occur in renal-impaired patients if IV bolus is given too quickly.

Dosage:

> *Adults:* 0.5 to 1 mg/kg slow IV bolus over 1 to 2 minutes (not to exceed 20 mg/min while delivering the bolus). May repeat in 1 to 2 hours.

Notes: Furosemide may worsen digitalis toxicity.

Ipratropium Bromide

Common trade name: Atrovent

Class: Anticholinergic

Mechanism of action: Inhibits interaction of acetylcholine at receptor sites on bronchial smooth muscle, resulting in bronchodilation.

Indications: Used for persistent bronchospasm and exacerbation of COPD.

Contraindications: Do not use in patients with hypersensitivity to ipratropium, atropine, alkaloid, soy protein, or peanuts.

Side effects: Nausea, vomiting, headache, tachycardia, dry mouth, blurred vision

Dosage:

> *Adults:* 500 mcg via nebulizer every 6 to 8 hours.
>
> *Pediatrics:* 125 to 250 mcg via nebulizer every 6 to 8 hours.

Notes: Not used as the sole agent in treating acute exacerbation of asthma or COPD. May mix with albuterol, levalbuterol, or other nebulized beta$_2$ agonist. In the prehospital environment, a single dose is considered effective and is usually not repeated with successive beta-agonist nebulizer treatments.

Ketorolac Tromethamine

Common trade name: Toradol

Class: Nonsteroidal anti-inflammatory (NSAID)

Mechanism of action: An anti-inflammatory drug, also inhibits prostaglandin synthesis and thus provides a peripherally acting non-narcotic analgesic effect.

Indications: Used for analgesia.

Contraindications: Do not use in patients with hypersensitivity to aspirin or other NSAID-type medications, bleeding disorders, renal failure, or peptic ulcer disease.

Side effects: Edema, sedation, bleeding, urticaria, headache, nausea

Dosage:

> *Adults:* 30 to 60 mg IM, 15 to 30 mg IV. Patients over 65, patients with renal impairment, and patients under 50 kg should receive one half this dose.
>
> *Pediatrics:* Not recommended.

Notes: Use with caution in patients taking anticoagulants and platelet inhibitors.

Levalbuterol

Common trade name: Xopenex

Class: Sympathomimetic

Mechanism of action: Selective beta$_2$ stimulation causes dilation of the smooth muscle of the bronchioles. Also relaxes all smooth airway muscle from the trachea to the terminal bronchioles.

Indications: Used for bronchospasm in adults, adolescents, and children over 6 years of age secondary to reversible obstructive airway disease.

Contraindications: Do not use in patients under 6 years of age, or those with hypersensitivity to levalbuterol or racemic albuterol.

Adverse reactions: Dysrhythmias, palpitations, anxiety, chest pain; may produce T wave and QT changes in the ECG

Dosage:

> *Adult acute asthma/status asthmaticus:* 1.25 mg/3 mL via nebulizer. May repeat up to two times.

Pediatric acute asthma/status asthmaticus:
(6 to 11 years): 0.31 mg via nebulizer every
6 to 8 hours.

Notes: Use with caution in patients taking MAO
inhibitors, diuretics, digoxin, or tricyclic
antidepressants. Beta blockers reduce the
bronchodilatory effect of beta$_2$ agonists.

Lidocaine Hydrochloride

Common trade name: Xylocaine

Class: Cardiac antidysrhythmic

Mechanism of action: Decreases ventricular irritability
to suppress ventricular ectopy and assist in the
management of ventricular tachycardia and ventricular
fibrillation. Slows conduction through the ventricles.

Indications: Frequent premature ventricular complexes
(PVCs) (>6/min), multifocal PVCs, PVCs that occur
in pairs or runs, PVCs that occur on the downslope
of the preceding T wave, refractory ventricular
fibrillation, pulseless ventricular tachycardia,
postelectrical defibrillation.

Contraindications: Second degree heart block, Type II,
third degree heart block, ventricular escape rhythms,
known hypersensitivity to local anesthetics, including
lidocaine.

Adverse reactions: Dizziness, drowsiness, seizures,
confusion, hypotension, nausea, vomiting, cardiac
arrest.

Dosage: 1.0 to 1.5 mg/kg of body weight as an
intravenous bolus, with half the original dosage
administered 20 minutes after the first dosage to
a maximum bolus dosage of 3.0 mg. A bolus that
successfully treats the dysrhythmia is followed by an
intravenous infusion of 2 to 4 mg/min. Reduce the
dosage by half for patients over age 70 years and
those with liver disease or heart failure.

Notes: Use caution in patients on beta blockers or other
antidysrhythmics. Amiodarone is the preferred
first line antidysrhythmic for refractory ventricular
tachycardia and ventricular fibrillation.

Lorazepam

Common trade name: Ativan

Class: Benzodiazepine, anticonvulsant, sedative

Mechanism of action: Depresses neuronal activity in the
CNS. Suppresses the propagation of seizure activity the
motor cortex, thalamus, and limbic areas of the brain.

Indications: Used for seizures, behavioral emergencies,
and sedation prior to cardioversion or pacing.

Contraindications: Do not use in patients with pre-
existing respiratory depression, CNS depression
from head injury, hypotension, or hypersensitivity
to benzodiazepines.

Side effects: Respiratory depression, hypotension,
confusion, nausea

Dosage:
Adults: 1 to 4 mg IV over 2 minutes. May repeat in
15 to 20 minutes as needed up to a maximum
of 8 mg.
Pediatrics: 0.05 to 0.1 mg/kg slow IV over 2 to
5 minutes, maximum 4 mg/dose. May repeat
0.05 mg/kg second dose in 10 to 15 minutes
if needed.

Notes: Be prepared for respiratory depression to occur
and have resuscitation equipment available.

Magnesium Sulfate

Class: Electrolyte

Mechanism of action: Relaxes smooth and voluntary
muscle by reducing acetylcholine release at the
myoneuronal junction.

Indications: Used for seizures secondary to eclampsia,
status asthmaticus refractory to beta agonist
therapy, **torsades de pointes**, ventricular
fibrillation that persists despite defibrillation and
first line antidysrhythmic therapy, and suspected
hypomagnesemia.

Contraindications: Do not use in patients with heart
block or myocardial damage. No contraindications
in cardiac arrest.

Side effects: Diaphoresis, hypotension, flushing, depressed
reflexes, hypothermia, reduced heart rate, respiratory
depression, diarrhea

Dosage:
Adult eclamptic seizures: 1 to 4 grams IV, maximum
30 to 40 grams/day.
Adult pulseless arrest: 1 to 2 grams/10 mL D$_5$W IV.
Adult torsades (nonarrest): Loading dose of 1 to
2 grams in 50 to 100 mL D$_5$W over 5 to 60
minutes IV. Follow with 0.5 to 1 gram/hr IV.
Titrate dose to control the dysrhythmias.
Pediatric pulseless arrest and torsades: 25 to 50 mg/kg
(maximum 2 grams) over 10 to 20 minutes.

Notes: When magnesium sulfate is used for treatment of
eclampsia, ensure that calcium gluconate or calcium
chloride is readily available as an antidote in case
respiratory depression occurs due to overdose of
magnesium sulfate.

Midazolam Hydrochloride

Common trade name: Versed

Class: Benzodiazepine, anticonvulsant, sedative

Mechanism of action: Depresses the neuronal activity
in the CNS. Suppresses the propagation of seizure
activity the motor cortex, thalamus, and limbic areas
of the brain.

Indications: Used for seizures, behavioral emergencies,
sedation prior to endotracheal intubation, and
cardioversion or pacing.

Contraindications: Do not use in patients with pre-existing respiratory depression, CNS depression from head injury, hypotension, or hypersensitivity to benzodiazepines. Glaucoma is a relative contraindication.

Side effects: Respiratory depression, hypotension, oversedation, nausea, vomiting

Dosage:

Adults: 1 to 2.5 mg IV over 2 minutes. May repeat as needed up to a maximum of 0.1 mg/kg.

Pediatrics: 0.1 to 0.15 mg/kg IV over 1 to 2 minutes, maximum 5 mg/dose.

Notes: Be prepared for respiratory depression or arrest to occur and have resuscitation equipment available. Hypotension is a common side effect.

Morphine Sulfate

Common trade name: Widely available generically for intravenous injection

Class: Opiate analgesic

Mechanism of action: Natural opiate alkaloid that acts directly on the opiate receptors in the brain. The primary effect is analgesia, but morphine also causes vasodilation, sedation, and euphoria.

Indications: Used for analgesia.

Contraindications: Do not use in patients with hypersensitivity to opiates, hypovolemia, hypotension, head injury, increased intracranial pressure, or severe respiratory depression.

Side effects: Respiratory depression, hypotension, sedations, tachycardia, bradycardia, palpitation, flushing, burning sensations, itching, euphoria, bronchospasm, dry mouth

Dosage:

Adults: 2 to 4 mg slow IV over 1 to 5 minutes every 5 to 30 minutes as needed to manage pain.

Pediatrics: 0.1 to 0.2 mg/kg IV (maximum total dose 15 mg).

Notes: Ensure that naloxone is available during administration. Use with caution in the elderly, asthmatics, and those susceptible to CNS or respiratory depression.

Ondansetron

Common trade name: Zofran

Class: Antiemetic

Mechanism of action: A selective serotonin receptor (5-HT$_3$ receptor) agonist. Its exact action is not well understood, but this type of serotonin receptor is present on the vagus nerve terminals and in the chemoreceptor trigger zone for vomiting located in the CNS.

Indications: Used for nausea and vomiting.

Contraindications: Do not use in patients with hypersensitivity to ondansetron.

Side effects: Hypotension, tachycardia, constipation, elevated liver enzymes, CNS depression

Dosage:

Adults: 4-mg slow IV bolus over 2 to 5 minutes every 4 to 6 hours.

Pediatrics: 0.1 mg/kg slow IV bolus every 4 to 6 hours.

Notes: Not recommended for children under 2 years of age.

Sodium Bicarbonate

Class: Electrolyte, alkalinizing agent

Mechanism of action: Reacts with free hydrogen ions to form water and carbon dioxide, thus raising pH levels. Provides sodium ion.

Indications: Used for tricyclic antidepressant overdose, known metabolic acidosis, alkalinization for treatment of specific intoxications, rhabdomyolysis, and crush syndromes.

Contraindications: Do not use in patients with metabolic or respiratory alkalosis, pulmonary edema, hypernatremia, or hypokalemia.

Side effects: Metabolic alkalosis, hypoxia, hypernatremia, seizures, increased intracellular CO_2

Dosage:

Adults: 1 mEq/kg IV, repeat 0.5 mEq/kg IV every 10 minutes.

Pediatrics: Same as adults.

Notes: Determine use based on arterial blood gas analysis. A patent airway and good alveolar gas exchange is required to eliminate the CO_2 produced by sodium bicarbonate administration.

Thiamine

Common trade name: Betaxin

Class: Vitamin (B$_1$)

Mechanism of action: Plays a vital role in carbohydrate metabolism.

Indications: Used for altered mental status, delirium tremens, and hypoglycemia.

Contraindications: Do not use in patients with hypersensitivity to intravenous thiamine.

Side effects: Hypotension, anxiety, nausea, vomiting, angioedema

Dosage (adults only): 100 mg slow IV injection over 1 to 2 minutes.

Notes: Consider thiamine administration prior to administration of dextrose in malnourished patients at risk for vitamin B$_1$ deficiency, but its use is not required for all patients.

Summary

Familiarity with commonly administered emergency medications will help you be more comfortable in situations in which those drugs are administered. In some cases, your scope of practice may be expanded by your state EMS office or medical director to include drugs that are not in the National Scope of Practice Model at the Advanced EMT level, based on the particular characteristics of your community and its emergency medical services needs. If you are allowed to administer any of the drugs in this appendix, you must receive additional training to ensure that you are knowledgeable about all components of the drug profiles.

Additional Reading

DailyMed. (n.d.). http://dailymed.nlm.nih.gov/dailymed/about.cfm

Medscape. (n.d.) *Drugs, OTCs, and herbals.* http://reference.medscape.com/drugs

Answers to Review Questions

Chapter 1

1. a
2. c
3. b
4. There is a defined body of specialized knowledge. There is a professional code of conduct, "The EMT Code of Ethics."
5. Example behaviors include taking the initiative to complete tasks without being prompted.
6. Example tasks include giving medications, and lifting and moving patients.
7. EMS providers are an important part of the health care team, providing a link between the prehospital setting and the hospital.

Chapter 2

1. c
2. d
3. a
4. b
5. d
6. a
7. b
8. c
9. d
10. a
11. The role of medical direction is to decide what care should be provided by each level of EMS provider in a system, what should be done prior to or without directly contacting medical direction, and what requires contact with the physician. Physicians play an active leadership role in EMS and EMS education and review care provided in the CQI process.
12. The use of ambulances and helicopters, and a variety of trauma care theories and techniques used in EMS today arose from military experience.
13. EMS was established in response to the recognition that there was an unacceptably high number of highway traffic deaths. The federal legislation that arose from this recognition called for a national agency (NHTSA) to address highway safety, including the provision of emergency medical services. EMS has since diversified to include response to many different types of emergencies. Arguments could be made for placing EMS under the direction of a more directly health-focused government agency to reflect this diversification. However, in the absence of a federal office of EMS, EMS is unlikely to be a perfect fit under any existing agency.
14. The IOM report made recommendations for EMS in the following areas:
    a. The evolving role of EMS as an integral component of the overall health-care system
    b. EMS system planning, preparedness, and coordination at the federal, state, and local levels
    c. EMS funding and infrastructure investments
    d. EMS workforce trends and professional education
    e. EMS research priorities and funding
15. EMS providers can make and report a number of observations about health and safety in their communities, and can take an active role in education and prevention programs.
16. To find out about issues and become involved in addressing them, you can subscribe to professional publications and journals and join local, state, and national EMS organizations and visit their websites.

Chapter 3

1. c
2. a
3. c
4. d
5. b
6. d
7. d
8. a
9. b
10. a
11. c
12. b
13. Consequences of chronically increased levels of cortisol include increased body fat, increased blood glucose levels, high blood pressure, impaired tissue maintenance and healing, and suppression of the immune system.
14. By reframing a stressor, you are looking at it from a different perspective to decrease its effect on you.
15. Gloves are the most appropriate PPE in this case, because it does not appear that there will be any spraying or splashing of blood. The most likely risk is hand contact with blood.
16. Although cleaning will remove gross contamination, you must use a hospital-grade disinfectant or 1:10 bleach solution to disinfect this piece of equipment.
17. Resources include http://www.mypyramid.com, various divisions of the Centers for Disease Control and Prevention (http://www.cdc.gov), and various divisions of the National Institutes for Health (http://www.nih.gov).
18. As an individual, you will have different strategies for enhancing your physical, emotional, environmental, social, occupational, spiritual, and intellectual wellness. You may decide to walk or cycle instead of drive at times, if feasible, to improve and maintain physical wellness. You may take a more active role with your employer or in a professional organization to enhance occupational wellness, and may look for various face-to-face or on-line courses, or commit to reading a book once a month to enhance intellectual wellness.

Chapter 4

1. c
2. a
3. b
4. d
5. a
6. c
7. d
8. a
9. c
10. b
11. c
12. b
13. Begin by trying to understand the basis of the patient's refusal. Perhaps he is in denial and does not understand the seriousness of the situation, or could be concerned about expenses, not being able to pick up his children from school, or a variety of other issues. Respond to those issues to the best of your ability. Your conversation with the patient, in addition to other components of assessment, will help you assess the patient's mental status. You should determine if he is alert and oriented to person, place, and time. Determine if he is showing appropriate concern for his circumstances. If possible, enlist the aid of family or coworkers (if the patient is at work) to convince the patient to accept treatment and transport. Consult with medical direction. If all efforts to inform the patient about his condition and the risks of refusing treatment fail, and he is competent to refuse, complete the documentation required by your service and have the patient sign the refusal in the presence of a witness. Document all of the circumstances of the refusal to support your assessment of the patient's competence and the adequacy of your attempts to persuade him to seek treatment.
14. Legally, your partner's actions constitute battery, at the least, but also may include assault and defamation. Ethically, your partner is violating a number of principles, such as nonmalfeasance, respect for dignity, concern for others, beneficence, and upholding the responsibilities of the profession. You must intervene to stop the battery on the patient, and assume control of the situation. Afterward, your partner's conduct must be reported to both your supervisor and medical director.
15. You do not have enough information to allow the coach to dismiss the need for care. You have a duty to respond and must make contact with the patient. While the coach may have the parents' permission to act in their absence (*in loco parentis*), you do not know at this point if the parents are present; if the patient is, in fact, a minor; or if the person you are speaking to is even the wrestler's coach. The patient is obviously injured and you must make contact and assess him, as well as obtain additional information. Explain to the coach that you are obligated to make contact with the patient.
16. Pay attention to the placement of items at the scene, and do not disturb anything unless it is necessary in order to care for the patient. If you must move or touch anything, inform law enforcement at the scene. Have as few providers as necessary enter the scene, and have everyone take the same path into and out of the scene. If you must

cut the patient's clothing, avoid cutting through any part of the clothing that may constitute evidence, such as punctures through the clothing.

Chapter 5

1. c
2. d
3. c
4. b
5. a
6. b
7. a
8. d
9. b
10. c
11. c
12. a
13. b
14. b
15. d
16. a
17. d
18. b
19. Some considerations include sounds of violence, unusual odors, lighting, temperature, barking dogs, a gathering crowd, and steps or stairs.
20. There is no set number. What constitutes an MCI is system dependent, and is based on available resources.
21. Using personal protective equipment, such as reflective vests; wearing seatbelts; exercising due regard in driving; defensive driving; having enough help to perform a lift; communicating during a lift; using proper body mechanics.
22. Do not make assumptions. Use a systematic approach to scene size-up, including assessment of the mechanism of injury/nature of illness; personal protective equipment/Standard Precautions; safety; number of patients; additional resources.
23. The cushion of safety is an area of clear space on each of the four sides of the ambulance that can provide room for error or evasive action. Drivers should ensure that there are no other vehicles within this space, and attempt to clear this space whenever possible.
24. Downgrading should be anticipated when your route of travel will include any of the following: traffic has nowhere to go; when approaching a blocked intersection at a red light; when entering or exiting a freeway; and when approaching a school zone or school bus.
25. Some conditions to be aware of include civilian driver confusion, ambulance operator adrenaline, speed, inexperienced drivers, vehicle size and weight, and driver inattention.

Chapter 6

1. a
2. c
3. d
4. a
5. a
6. b

7. d

8. d

9. c

10. a

11a. C

11b. R

11c. T

11d. H

11e. A

12. An abbreviated form of documentation, such as that provided by triage tags, would be used instead of full PCRs.

13. Empathy.

14. Focus on the patient. Do not assume he cannot communicate. If needed, follow up with family or bystanders.

15. Let the daughter know you understand she is concerned, but that it is important for you to hear what the patient has to say.

16. Your first concern is your safety. Stay back a safe distance, and check to make sure law enforcement is en route. If it is safe to do so, you can attempt to establish rapport with the patient by saying something like, "You sound upset, Mrs. Amos. I'd like to do what I can to help."

Chapter 7

1. d

2. b

3. b

4. c

5. a

6. c

7. a

8. b

9. d

10. c

11. a. Cervices, b. Renal calculi, c. Corpora, d. Indices

12. a. Gastrostomy, b. Hepatomegaly, c. Chondritis, d. Hypoxemia

13. a. Low carbon dioxide, b. Clotting cell (platelet), c. Inflammation of the sac surrounding the heart, d. Upper (outer) layer of skin

Chapter 8

1. a

2. b

3. a

4. d

5. b

6. d

7. a

8. d

9. b

10. a

11. c

12. b

13. c

14. a

15. d

16. c

17. d

18. b

19. a

20. a

21. b

22. d

23. b

24. d

25. c

26. b

27. c

28. a

29. b

30. a

31. d

32. b

33. The sodium/potassium pump keeps excess sodium out of the cell. If excess sodium enters the cell, water will follow, causing the cell to swell and eventually burst.

34. Oxygen is required for the Krebs cycle, which converts pyruvic acid (formed by anaerobic metabolism) into ATP and easily eliminated wastes (carbon dioxide and water). Without oxygen, only a small amount of ATP is produced and pyruvic acid cannot be broken down for elimination.

35. Skeletal muscles have an attachment along one bone and a tendon that crosses a joint to insert on another bone. When the muscle contracts, it shortens and moves the bone where the tendon is inserted to decrease the angle of the joint.

36. According to Boyle's law, the volume of a gas varies inversely with its pressure when the temperature is constant. When the muscles of the chest and the diaphragm contract and increase the volume of the thorax, the intrathoracic pressure decreases. Air flows from areas of higher pressure to areas of lower pressure. Therefore, air flows from the atmosphere into the lungs. When the chest muscles and diaphragm relax the volume of the thorax decreases, increasing the pressure within it. Air flows from the higher pressure in the lungs to the lower pressure of the atmosphere.

37. The respiratory membrane is the area in which an alveolar wall is in close proximity to the walls of the capillaries surrounding it. The walls of the alveoli and capillaries are a single cell-layer thick. This allows gases to diffuse across them.

38. The onloading of oxygen to hemoglobin is enhanced when the PaO_2 is high. Conversely, oxygen is offloaded more easily when the PaO_2 is low, such as at the cellular level.

39. An antigen is a substance recognized by the body as foreign. On first exposure to an antigen, the immune system can produce antibodies that are specific to the antigen. On subsequent exposure to the antigen, the body can react quickly to destroy it.

40. Blood pressure, as represented by mean arterial pressure, is determined by cardiac output and peripheral vascular resistance. In turn, cardiac output is determined by the stroke volume and heart rate. Peripheral vascular resistance is the degree of constriction of the arterioles.

41. After absorbing nutrients from the GI tract, blood in the veins leaving the GI tract is diverted to the liver by way of the hepatic portal vein. This allows the liver to remove

toxins and process nutrients before the blood returns to the systemic circulation.

42. The sympathetic and parasympathetic divisions of the autonomic nervous system balance each other to maintain homeostasis. The sympathetic nervous system responds to stressors, readying the body to fight or flee. Sympathetic response includes pupil dilation, increased cardiac output, dilation of blood vessels in the skeletal muscle but constriction of blood vessels in the GI tract, and dilation of the bronchioles. The parasympathetic nervous system controls everyday vegetative functions, such as digestion and reproduction.

43. The exocrine function of the pancreas is to secrete digestive enzymes and bicarbonate into the duodenum.

44. The special cells of the juxtaglomerular apparatus in the kidney monitor fluid levels and blood pressure. When blood pressure is low, the reninangiotensin-aldosterone system is activated. The results are vasoconstriction and decreased fluid loss through the kidneys.

Chapter 9

1. d
2. c
3. b
4. b
5. c
6. d
7. b
8. a
9. b
10. d
11. c
12. c
13. b
14. a
15. c
16. How an EMS provider decides to handle an ethical dilemma can be explained by Kohlberg's theory in terms of what the motivation is for the decision. For example, the person who makes a decision that is not in the patient's best interests in order to avoid punishment could be using preconventional moral reasoning, while the provider who reports a dog bite according to law may be using conventional moral reasoning.

17. As the function of the body declines, it becomes less able to respond to injury and illness. The maximum heart and respiratory rates are lower, so tachycardia and tachypnea may not be seen. Pre-existing hypertension may mask a drop in blood pressure. Impaired sympathetic nervous system response or the effects of medications may prevent the diaphoresis normally expected.

18. Children may have a range of feelings and exhibit a range of behaviors following the death of a loved one, including sadness, being withdrawn, crying, feeling vulnerable and insecure, constant thinking about the deceased, anxiety when separated from family members, anger, and nightmares.

19. Age-related changes in hearing and vision do not occur at the same rate or to the same degree in all patients, so do not assume impairment. However, be alert to signs that the patient is having difficulty seeing or hearing.

Offer to retrieve reading glasses or hearing aids. Speak clearly and be patient.

20. The patient may want to be cared for by a female Advanced EMT. Arrange this if at all possible. If it is not possible, ensure that the patient has a family member as a chaperone. Do your utmost to respect the patient's modesty.

21. Members of ethnic minority groups may have individually, or as a group, had negative experiences with the health care system. They may have been discriminated against, received inferior care (such as inadequate pain management), or their beliefs and customs may not have been respected.

Chapter 10

1. d
2. b
3. d
4. a
5. a
6. a
7. b
8. c
9. a
10. d
11. b
12. c
13. c
14. c
15. b
16. Glucose is required to produce ATP, which every cell needs for energy in order to carry out its functions, including maintaining its own integrity. Although some cells in the body can convert to using proteins and fats when glucose is not available, brain cells have no way of quickly doing that. If glucose is deficient, brain cells cannot function and will quickly lose their ability to maintain the cell membrane and begin to die.

17. When arterial oxygen levels are low, insufficient oxygen is delivered to the cells. The brain has a high need for oxygen to maintain normal function. In the presence of hypoxia, normal function is impaired because cellular energy production is impaired. Dysfunction of cells of the cerebrum causes confusion.

18. The amount of air delivered to the alveolar level in this patient is about 200 mL. To maintain the normal amount of alveolar ventilation, the patient's respiratory rate will have to increase to about 21 breaths per minute. Although this is possible, it is not likely with a narcotic overdose. It is likely that both the respiratory rate and tidal volume are decreased, resulting in hypoxia.

19. A pneumothorax causes part of the lung to collapse, resulting in areas of the lung that are not being ventilated. Circulation may continue through the affected area, but cannot pick up oxygen or lose carbon dioxide. A pulmonary embolism obstructs part of the pulmonary circulation, but the alveoli in the affected area continue to be ventilated. Again, a portion of the lung is not participating in gas exchange.

20. All patients in shock require general supportive treatment of the airway, breathing, and circulation, but

also require specific treatment aimed at reversing the cause of shock. The treatment that is beneficial for one patient in shock may be fatal for another. The weakened heart of a patient in cardiogenic shock cannot meet the increased demands that would be put on it by the administration of epinephrine, and IV fluids may result in pulmonary edema. On the other hand, epinephrine and fluids can be lifesaving in the patient with anaphylactic shock.

Chapter 11

1. a
2. c
3. a
4. b
5. a
6. b
7. a
8. a
9. c
10. These conditions all affect the integrity of the skin, reducing its ability to protect the body from the absorption of substances. The amount of drug absorbed may be much greater than intended.
11. The amount of water in the body and differences in the cardiovascular system, gastrointestinal system, amounts of body fat and plasma proteins, and skin affect how drugs are absorbed and distributed. Differences in the function of the liver and kidney affect how drugs are eliminated. The effects of drugs can be increased or decreased because of differences in the speed of metabolism and elimination.
12. The free drug levels of both drugs may increase, increasing the effects of both drugs.

Chapter 12

1. c
2. a
3. d
4. c
5. a
6. b
7. b
8. b
9. a
10. c
11. b
12. d
13. d
14. c
15. a
16. Although you usually deal with only one patient at a time in the prehospital setting, you still must make sure that the patient has the right indications for the drug and does not have any contraindications to the drug.
17. You must observe the patient for any adverse effects from the error, report the error to the receiving physician, notify your supervisor, document the error in the patient care report, and, most likely, complete a supplemental report documenting the error. The patient must

be informed of the error. Organizational policy determines who informs the patient. Once the patient has been informed, if policy allows, consider apologizing to the patient.
18. Several things can cause this problem. Check to see that you removed the constricting band, look for signs of infiltration, check to see that all clamps on the tubing are open, that the tubing is not crimped, that the patient's position is not interfering with IV flow, and that the IV bag is at an appropriate level above the patient's heart.

Chapter 13

1. c
2. b
3. c
4. d
5. b
6. a
7. d
8. b
9. d
10. d
11. A fluid that has the same tonicity as plasma is called *isotonic*. Solutions that have a higher tonicity than blood plasma are known as *hypertonic* and solutions that have a lower tonicity than blood plasma are known as *hypotonic*.
12. Glucagon works by stimulating the breakdown of glycogen stored in the liver into glucose. An alcoholic with advanced liver disease may have inadequate glycogen stores to be converted into glucose.

Chapter 14

1. b
2. c
3. b
4. a
5. d
6. Baseline vital signs are taken to get initial information about the patient's condition, which serves as a point of reference against which later sets of vital signs are evaluated. This allows you to determine the effects of treatment and identify trends in the patient's condition.
7. ABCD is used to remember to check the patient's airway, breathing, circulation, and disability (level of responsiveness). However, the mnemonic does not always represent the order in which they are assessed and managed. For example, you must have some idea of the patient's level of responsiveness (disability) in order to proceed appropriately in checking the airway, breathing, and circulation. While there is a check confirmation of level of responsiveness and absence of breathing in the cardiac arrest patient, the management priority is circulation–starting chest compressions.
8. a—P and R; b—S; c—S; d—R; e—S and R. Assessment is an iterative (repetitive) process in which initial findings are explored in more depth, additional findings are sought through the process, and findings are reassessed.

Chapter 15

1. c
2. a
3. d
4. c
5. b
6. c
7. b
8. a
9. c
10. b
11. A respiratory rate of 8 is inadequate, and must be corrected immediately. If an airway adjunct was not inserted when the airway was opened manually, consider inserting one now. Keep in mind that the patient may still have a gag reflex if he is responsive to pain. The patient requires assisted ventilations by bag-valve-mask with supplemental oxygen before completing the primary assessment or moving on to secondary assessment and treatment.
12. Decreased responsiveness can lead to relaxation of the jaw, allowing the tongue to obstruct the airway, and the patient's gag reflex may be diminished or absent.
13. The primary assessment is performed to identify and correct immediately life-threatening problems. Missing a problem with the airway, breathing, or circulation can result in harm or death.
14. Tidal volume is the amount of air moved in and out of the lungs in each breath. Without adequate tidal volume, not enough air reaches the lower airway for gas exchange. The tidal volume is not measured directly in the field, but is determined by the depth of respirations.
15. Airway obstruction by the tongue is managed by manual maneuvers and airway adjuncts, such as nasopharyngeal and oropharyngeal airways. Fluid or blood in the airway is managed by suctioning and positioning. Foreign bodies are managed by obstructed airway maneuvers.

Chapter 16

1. c
2. a
3. c
4. c
5. a
6. b
7. b
8. b
9. a
10. a
11. d
12. a
13. c
14. b
15. c
16. Hypoxia may have obvious signs or should be anticipated based on the patient's presentation and complaint. Indications of hypoxia include complaint of dyspnea, signs of respiratory distress (accessory muscle use, abnormal breathing noises, tachypnea or bradypnea, indications of airway obstruction, decreased tidal volume),

cyanosis, tachycardia or bradycardia, altered mental status, decreased or abnormal breath sounds, significant trauma or blood loss, chest pain, low SpO_2 (below 95 percent at lower elevations).

17. Look for signs that the patient's breathing efforts are not able to meet his metabolic needs. Exhaustion and altered mental status in addition to signs of respiratory distress indicate that the patient requires assisted ventilations.
18. CPAP is intended for patients with significant respiratory distress who are conscious and able to follow commands.
19. Inadequate ventilations occur when the rate and volume are either excessive or insufficient for the patient's age and size, there is inadequate chest rise, or significant resistance to ventilation (increased resistance to bag-valve-mask ventilations or generating excessive airway pressures with an ATV), or the patient's condition (skin color, SpO_2, and other signs of hypoxia) does not improve or deteriorates, gastric distention occurs, or cardiac output drops (tachycardia, hypotension).
20. Ensure that the patient's airway is open and clear. Determine if the airway adjunct being used is effective. Check the rate and volume of ventilation. Check that oxygen is connected to the bag-valve-mask and flowing.
21. Nasal cannulas are preferred for patients with mild distress and mild hypoxia. Any patient with moderate to severe respiratory distress, with chest pain, significant trauma or blood loss, or other critical conditions requires more oxygen than a nasal cannula can deliver. However, if a patient absolutely cannot tolerate a nonrebreather mask, a nasal cannula provides more oxygen than the patient would receive from ambient air.
22. Because a nonrebreather mask does not allow the entry of ambient air, the only source of air available to the patient comes from the reservoir bag. If the oxygen flow ceases or is insufficient, the patient can asphyxiate.
23. Normal cardiac output relies on the negative pressure ventilation that occurs naturally. The decrease in intrathoracic pressure reduces the resistance to blood returning to the heart, allowing adequate preload. In the absence of negative pressure and, worse, when intrathoracic pressure is excessive due to overventilation, blood return to the heart is reduced, reducing cardiac output and perfusion. This effect is even more profound in patients with already-low blood pressure, such as those in shock or receiving CPR.

Chapter 17

1. a
2. c
3. a
4. d
5. c
6. b
7. c
8. c
9. a
10. d
11. b
12. b
13. The patient's pale, cool, diaphoretic skin and rapid pulse are explained by the body's attempts to compensate for

shock. Sympathetic nervous system activation results in peripheral vasoconstriction, shunting blood away from the skin. The heart rate increases in an attempt to maintain cardiac output despite decreased blood volume. The weak pulse and unresponsiveness indicate that the body's compensatory mechanisms are failing and perfusion is decreased.

14. When cardiac arrest occurs, circulation ceases, yet some oxygen remains in the blood and in the lungs. Therefore, the most critical need is to restore circulation of the existing oxygen reserves. Health care providers begin ventilation after the first 30 chest compressions (in an adult) to provide additional oxygen. In contrast, airway management and ventilation procedures can significantly delay circulation of the oxygen present, further depriving cells of oxygen.

15. Yes, the patient is in shock, despite the warm, dry skin. He has a heart rate below 50 and signs of inadequate cerebral perfusion (altered mental status). Bradycardia can be the result of increased parasympathetic nervous system stimulation, which would also prevent sympathetic nervous system response that causes vasoconstriction (causing cool skin) and diaphoresis.

16. Survival from cardiac arrest depends on an intact Chain of Survival. A breakdown or weakness in any of the links decreases the patient's chances of survival. The public must be trained to recognize cardiac arrest, notify the EMS system, and begin CPR. EMS must be able to arrive promptly to provide defibrillation and other interventions. Quality advanced life support must be available to treat cardiac arrest and manage patients with ROSC. A continuous quality improvement program must be in place to collect data about where weaknesses are in the system. Possible solutions include public CPR training, public access defibrillation programs, changing ambulance deployment configurations, and additional EMS and hospital personnel training.

Chapter 18

1. a
2. d
3. d
4. b
5. c
6. d
7. b
8. c
9. d
10. b
11. c
12. d
13. b
14. a
15. b
16. d
17. d
18. b
19. a
20. d
21. There is no one right approach to the point at which you should take vital signs. You should consider the

patient's condition and priority for transport, what other tasks must be performed, and how much help you have available.

22. Forehead temperature strips are generally unreliable. You should select another method of obtaining the patient's temperature. In this patient, a four-year-old child, an oral or tympanic temperature would be most feasible and accurate. Oral temperatures are generally accurate, but can be affected if the patient has recently had something to eat or drink, or is unable to close his mouth. You can take axillary temperatures in patients who cannot hold a thermometer in the mouth, but they take longer and are less accurate. Tympanic temperatures are generally accurate, but you must align the light and sensor properly. The presence of excessive earwax can affect the reading. Most patients do not prefer to have a rectal temperature taken.

23. Palpating a blood pressure, or using obliteration of a pulse oximetry waveform, can be useful when background noise or a low blood pressure reading prevent auscultation, but you can only obtain a systolic pressure.

24. Anxiety, exertion, shock, hypoxia, cardiac dysrhythmia, and stimulant drugs are all potential causes of tachycardia.

25. A BGL should be obtained in diabetic patients and patients with altered mental status or neurologic deficits.

26. You should assess vital signs every 5 minutes or less for critical patients, and every 15 minutes for noncritical patients.

27. Patients with poor circulation or who are in cardiac arrest will have low exhaled carbon dioxide. When an endotracheal tube is placed in the esophagus, exhaled carbon dioxide will be low. Low exhaled carbon dioxide can also occur in some patients with hyperventilation syndrome.

28. SpO_2 is an adjunct to assessment skills and clinical judgment. It can tell you what percentage of hemoglobin is saturated, but you cannot determine if it is saturated with oxygen or carbon monoxide. It also cannot tell you how hard a a patient is working to maintain his oxygen saturation level. In general, a level of 95 to 99 percent is normal, 90 to 95 percent is mildly hypoxic, 85 to 90 percent is moderately hypoxic, and below 85 percent is severely hypoxic. If you work in a high-altitude area, lower SpO_2 levels are considered acceptable.

29. The pupils are assessed for size, equality, and reaction to light. Abnormalities in pupil size and reaction can be caused by drugs, hypoxia, eye trauma, and increased intracranial pressure. You must consider findings and decisions made on them in context.

Chapter 19

1. c
2. b
3. b
4. a
5. c
6. a
7. d
8. c
9. c
10. a

11. Mental status is a broad concept of which level of responsiveness is a part. In addition to level of responsiveness, mental status also includes the patient's thinking processes and content and emotions.

12. The signs and symptoms are the "five Ps" associated with compartment syndrome: pain, paralysis, paresthesia, pallor, and pulselessness.

13. Paradoxical motion of the chest wall suggests the presence of flail chest, which impairs ventilation and is a critical injury.

14. The odor of acetone, the ingredient in nail polish, is similar to the odor on the breath of some patients with diabetic ketoacidosis (diabetic coma).

Chapter 20

1. c
2. d
3. a
4. c
5. a
6. c
7. a
8. c
9. b
10. b

11. In addition to the dyspnea and diminished breath sounds on the affected side that would be expected with a simple pneumothorax, you should anticipate increasing respiratory distress, increased resistance to bag-valve-mask ventilations, hypoxia, altered mental status, hypotension, distended neck veins, and possible (late) deviation of the trachea away from the affected side.

12. Risk factors for pulmonary embolism include recent surgery, immobilization, long-bone fractures, estrogen replacement therapy, hormones taken for birth control, pregnancy, cancer, and deep venous thrombosis (DVT).

13. Noncardiogenic pulmonary edema can occur following severe infection, trauma, or shock (ARDS), or may occur in response to toxin exposure through inhalation or circulation.

14. Pneumonia and cardiogenic pulmonary edema both present with respiratory distress, which may progress to respiratory failure and respiratory arrest. Both conditions may result in altered mental status and other signs of hypoxia. Fever and chills are often present with pneumonia, but are not likely to be significant findings in acute pulmonary edema. The lung sounds in pneumonia would reflect the absence of air movement in the affected area, and rhonchi and possible wheezes in surrounding areas. In pulmonary edema, rales are most likely to be heard, but rhonchi and wheezes also may be present. The sputum in pneumonia is likely to be green, yellow, or rust-colored. The sputum in pulmonary edema is likely to be frothy and pink.

Chapter 21

1. d
2. c
3. c
4. d
5. a

6. c
7. b
8. a
9. b
10. d

11. To maintain cardiac output when the volume of blood decreases, the heart rate and systemic vascular resistance must increase.

12. During ACS, the ventricle may not empty effectively, decreasing cardiac output. The body attempts to compensate by increasing the heart rate. The underlying reason for tachycardia may also be anxiety, which can increase the heart's demand for oxygen.

13. Treatments that can open the obstructed artery must be implemented within a short period of time from the onset of signs and symptoms to prevent as much damage to the heart as possible. Ischemic areas of the heart can be reperfused, but once the tissue dies, it cannot be regenerated.

14. CPAP provides continuous positive pressure to the lower airways, making it more difficult for fluid to diffuse from the interstitial spaces of the lungs into the alveoli.

15. Both left-sided and right-sided heart failure occur when the affected ventricle is ineffective in pumping blood, resulting in a reduced ejection fraction. Left-sided heart failure may occur from AMI, or long-term increased work against increased systemic vascular resistance (hypertension), as well as other reasons. Right-sided heart failure most commonly occurs as a result of left-sided heart failure, but can also occur as a result of pulmonary disease (cor pulmonale). Left-sided heart failure results in backup of blood behind the left side of the heart, resulting in pulmonary edema. Right-sided heart failure results in backup of blood behind the right side of the heart, resulting in systemic edema.

Chapter 22

1. b
2. c
3. a
4. a
5. a
6. d
7. a
8. c
9. d
10. b
11. b
12. a
13. a
14. b
15. b

16. You should use initial manual maneuvers immediately. If there is no indication of a mechanism of injury that could cause cervical-spine injury, you should use a head-tilt/chin-lift maneuver. If you suspect cervical-spine injury, use a modified jaw-thrust maneuver. Use suction if needed. If it appears that there is an immediately reversible cause of unresponsiveness, such as a narcotic overdose or hypoglycemia, avoid using an oropharyngeal airway or advanced airway device until you have ruled those out as causes. Once you have ruled out immediately reversible causes,

consider the need for longer-term airway management and ventilation, in which case an advanced airway device may be the best choice.

17. Look beyond the obvious and consider serious and potentially life-threatening causes of back pain, including an abdominal aortic aneurysm, a kidney stone or pyelonephritis, pancreatitis, ulcers, or diverticulitis. The cause may also be traumatic, nontraumatic musculoskeletal, or neurologic.

18. First, clarify whether the patient is experiencing vertigo or faintness by asking her to describe the exact sensation she experienced. Then determine any associated symptoms and ask about her medical history, including medications.

19. Advanced EMTs may transport patients with a history of a variety of neurologic problems. Being familiar with the most common of them is important in establishing credibility and trust with the patient.

Chapter 23

1. d
2. c
3. a
4. c
5. b
6. a
7. c
8. d
9. When the blood glucose level rises above 180 mg/dL in untreated diabetes, the kidneys cannot reabsorb all the glucose in the filtrate. This makes the filtrate hyperosmolar, which draws more water in to the kidneys, causing large amounts of water to be lost in the urine (polyuria). The dehydration from increased water loss leads to thirst (polydipsia). Even though the blood glucose level is high, glucose cannot enter cells in sufficient amounts when insulin is inadequate. Inadequate fuel for cellular metabolism results in tissue starvation and hunger.

10.

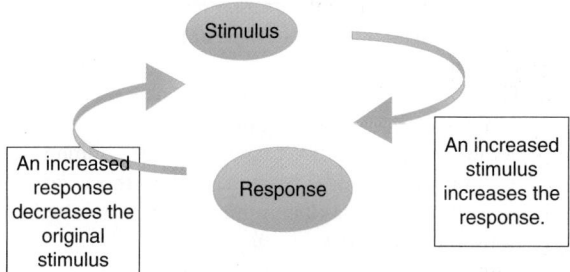

11. Complications of diabetes include cardiovascular disease, stroke, blindness, kidney disease, peripheral vascular disease, peripheral nerve disorders, delayed healing, infection, and lower extremity amputation.

12. In diabetic ketoacidosis (DKA), the diabetic has such insufficient insulin that the cells cannot use glucose for energy. Instead, fats are used for energy, but this results in production of ketones as a byproduct. Ketones lower the pH (cause acidosis). The respiratory system attempts to compensate for metabolic acidosis by excreting the carbon dioxide created by buffer systems by increasing the rate and depth of respiration. In nonketotic hyperosmolar coma (NKHC) insulin is decreased, but enough glucose is allowed to enter cells to prevent fats from being used for energy.

Chapter 24

1. d
2. b
3. b
4. d
5. a
6. b
7. d
8. a
9. c
10. a
11. b
12.

Feature	Appendicitis	Diverticulitis
Typical age of patients affected	10–30 years	>50 years
Character of pain at onset	Diffuse, periumbilical	Diffuse, periumbilical
Localization of pain	Right lower quadrant	Left lower quadrant
Associated signs and symptoms	Nausea, anorexia, constipation, fever	Diarrhea, lower gastrointestinal bleeding, fever

13. The patient is young, which decreases the suspicion of peptic ulcer disease and pancreatitis. His history of an illness with a fever, sore throat, and swollen glands prior to the onset of left upper quadrant pain is suspicion for mononucleosis, which can result in enlargement and inflammation of the spleen. It is very possible that this patient has splenomegaly, an enlargement of the spleen.

14. The patient's age and history of diabetes puts him at high risk for cardiovascular disease, which may include atherosclerosis of arteries supplying abdominal organs, resulting in ischemia. He is less able to fight infection, which could include diverticulitis or appendicitis. An additional cause of abdominal pain is diabetic ketoacidosis, although this patient would be more likely to have hyperglycemic hyperosmolar nonketotic coma. Regardless of the underlying cause, the diabetes and patient's age mean that he may not perceive pain as being severe, despite a serious underlying problem.

Chapter 25

1. c
2. d
3. b
4. a
5. c
6. b
7. b
8. b
9. a
10. d
11. b
12. b
13. Patients with a UTI may complain of urinary frequency, urgency, and dysuria; blood in the urine; cloudy or foul-smelling urine; and pain in the flank with tenderness at

the costovertebral angle. Patients also may be nauseated and have a fever. Female patients and patients with a Foley catheter are especially susceptible to UTIs.

14. Female patients with abdominal pain may have gynecologic, urinary, or digestive system disorders. Gynecologic causes of pain include dysmenorrhea, ovarian cyst, ectopic pregnancy, mittelschmerz, endometriosis, endometritis, or PID.

15. In addition to providing the care you normally would provide, based on the patient's complaints and presentation, you also must be especially aware of the patient's psychological needs and the importance of preserving evidence.

Chapter 26

1. d
2. d
3. b
4. c
5. a
6. b
7. c
8. c
9. Because the liver is responsible for manufacturing proteins such as albumin and clotting factors, you should suspect problems with edema from decreased blood osmotic pressure and with clotting because of decreased clotting factor synthesis. The liver also breaks down aged and damaged RBCs. The inability of the liver to get rid of the hemoglobin pigment bilirubin results in jaundice.
10. Vaso-occlusive crisis is exacerbated by low oxygen levels, which increases the number of sickled cells. Administering oxygen may help with tissues that are already ischemic and may prevent further microvascular occlusion.
11. The mechanism of injury could produce a shoulder injury, but pain from an injured spleen can be referred to the left shoulder. This patient may have excessive bleeding from even minor injuries. You should carefully assess him and monitor vital signs for changes. Administer oxygen if you suspect hemorrhage and obtain vascular access.
12. A number of conditions can impair blood clotting. You should obtain a list of the patient's medications, looking specifically for medications that can inhibit platelet activity or blood clotting. Medical problems such as leukemia or multiple myeloma could result in decreased platelet production, while liver disease can impair blood clotting. No matter what the contributing factors, use direct pressure to control the bleeding and administer oxygen. If the vital signs or other aspects of the assessment indicate significant blood loss, obtain vascular access.

Chapter 27

1. b
2. b
3. a
4. c
5. a
6. c
7. d
8. c

9. In shock, peripheral perfusion is decreased. Drugs administered subcutaneously have a slower onset than drugs administered intramuscularly, even when perfusion is normal. Subcutaneous administration will not be absorbed quickly or predictably. Intramuscular administration offers a better opportunity for absorption.

10. To prevent organ rejection, transplant patients take drugs that suppress the immune system. Keeping the ambulance clean, good hand washing and hygiene, and not coming to work when you are sick are ways to minimize transmitting infection to the patient. Do not perform unnecessary procedures, such as IVs, in the prehospital setting. Avoid putting the patient near others who may have infectious diseases. Communicate the history of organ transplant to hospital staff, even if it is not related to the immediate problem.

11. In autoimmune diseases, the immune system fails to recognize certain "self" molecules as part of the body. Instead, the molecules are recognized as foreign and are attacked by the immune system, resulting in tissue damage.

Chapter 28

1. d
2. a
3. c
4. a
5. c
6. a
7. b
8. d
9. a
10. c
11. c
12. b
13. MRSA is not generally a concern for healthy individuals. Your biggest concern is in preventing the spread of MRSA between patients. You should wear gloves, wash your hands thoroughly after patient contact, change linens, and clean and disinfect the ambulance, stretcher, and equipment.

14. The elderly are at increased risk because immune function diminishes with age. Children are more susceptible because they may not yet have developed immunity. Immunocompromised patients, such as those with HIV/AIDS or who are taking immunosuppressant medications, are also at risk.

15. Foreign body airway obstruction, croup, and epiglottitis are possible causes. The patient has a partial airway obstruction that could progress. A foreign body could be pushed further into the airway if there is an attempt to remove it or place anything in the mouth. In epiglottitis, anything placed in the mouth can result in complete airway obstruction. With both croup and epiglottitis, agitation and crying can increase oxygen demand and worsen airway edema. Consider the need for ALS or transport without delay to a facility with a pediatric emergency medicine service, if available.

16. Signs and symptoms of active pulmonary tuberculosis include fever, weight loss, night sweats, and coughing. Hemoptysis should increase suspicion. Tuberculosis is spread through the airborne route and you should wear

an N-95 mask when in close proximity to a patient with known or suspected active tuberculosis.

17. The history and presentation are most consistent with croup, but consider epiglottitis and other respiratory infections, as well. Keep the patient as calm as possible to avoid increasing airway edema, with humidified oxygen administered for hypoxia. For severe croup, consider requesting ALS or transporting without delay in anticipation of airway obstruction and asphyxia.

Chapter 29

1. c
2. b
3. a
4. d
5. c
6. a
7. The myoglobin released from damaged muscle cells is excreted by the kidneys, but is toxic to the kidney tubules. Promoting urination to eliminate myoglobin decreases the risk of renal failure. In addition, the damaged muscle swells and there is a significant shift of fluid from the intravascular space to the tissues, which can result in hypovolemia. The hypotension that occurs with hypovolemia will exacerbate the effects of myoglobin in the kidneys.
8. Patients with poor peripheral circulation are prone to slow healing and increased infection. The bacterium that causes gas gangrene is anaerobic, and thrives in the low oxygen environment provided by poor circulation. As infection increases, the tissue swells, causing more ischemia, which promotes further growth of the bacteria.

Chapter 30

1. c
2. c
3. b
4. a
5. a
6. Epiglottitis is unusual in a patient of this age, but it could occur. The absence of stridor makes it less likely, but the signs and symptoms still make airway obstruction a concern. The signs and symptoms are highly suggestive of peritonsillar abscess. However, do not attempt examination of the airway in the prehospital setting, especially without immediate access to intubation or a surgical airway. Transport the patient in a position of comfort. If there is no hypoxia, keep in mind that dry oxygen could further irritate the inflamed tissues. If the patient has signs of dehydration, IV fluids may be beneficial. The "hot potato" voice is actually an important piece of information to be relayed to the emergency physician, because this patient should be evaluated without delay. A simple report of a sore throat may not alert the physician to the potential seriousness of the situation.
7. Dental abscesses have the potential to lead to infection of other tissues, potentially resulting in sepsis or airway obstruction. Without transport, the patient will not otherwise have access to antibiotics in a timely manner. Although the emergency department physician can begin antibiotics and treat for pain, the patient needs a dental

referral so she can get the appropriate treatment and follow up.
8. Some causes of this problem, such as cerumen impaction, are benign and easily treated in the emergency department or physician's office. However, sudden hearing loss may also indicate stroke, or can be due to trauma. Obtain a good history and perform a physical exam that includes a neurologic assessment, and transport the patient for evaluation and treatment.

Chapter 31

1. c
2. a
3. d
4. b
5. b
6. a
7. c
8. Not all behavior that is undesirable in the eyes of another constitutes a behavioral emergency. In talking to both parties, with the assistance of law enforcement if necessary, determine if the patient's behavior or thinking is bizarre, delusional, paranoid, or in some other way disordered, and if he is a danger to himself or others.
9. Treat the patient with respect and empathy; maintain her personal space; do not argue with, invalidate, or minimize her perspective; and do not threaten or deceive her. Look around to be sure there are no items that can be used as weapons, and identify escape routes.

Chapter 32

1. d
2. c
3. c
4. a
5. a
6. b
7. b
8. a
9. d
10. d
11. c
12. b
13. a
14. a
15. b
16. d
17. a
18. Determine the names of the medications from the label and use a reference to identify their class, if you are not familiar with the medications. Note the concentration or strength of the medications, the date (for prescription medications), and the number of tablets or capsules originally in the containers. Determine whether other substances (such as alcohol or street drugs) were involved, and whether anything was done to try to treat the overdose. Consider the patient's current presentation and past medical history, and check for injuries. Determine whether the situation may be a suicide attempt.

19. Depending on the route of exposure and the nature of the toxin, the patient's level of toxin in the body may still be increasing, even though he is asymptomatic. Patients who are attempting suicide may not be honest about the nature of the exposure. Some toxins have fewer effects immediately, but potentially fatal effects develop over hours to days.
20. One of the determining factors in the method of suicide is availability. OTC drugs are relatively cheap and readily available, and antidepressants and cardiac drugs are prescribed to patients in high-risk groups: patients with depression and the elderly.

Chapter 33

1. d
2. c
3. b
4. c
5. d
6. c
7. b
8. d
9. b
10. The first of the three Es of injury prevention is education. An example is defensive driving courses. Enforcement is a strategy that uses the law to persuade individuals to behave in ways that reduce injuries, such as driving-while-intoxicated laws, mandatory helmet laws, child safety seat laws, and seatbelt laws. Engineering design features in manufacturing or construction to reduce the likelihood of injuries. Examples include passive vehicle restraint systems (airbags), guard rails along highways, and concrete barriers between traffic lanes.
11. An incident commander at an MCI may name the following officers to assist him:
    a. Safety officer (SO): The safety officer is responsible for the safety of responders and patients alike. This includes ensuring that all response activities are being carried out using the proper safety equipment.
    b. Liaison officer (LO): The liaison officer coordinates all activities with outside agencies, such as government agencies and private industry.
    c. Information officer (IO): The information officer is responsible for communicating information regarding the response to the public and press.
12. The public health approach consists of defining the problem, identifying risk and protective factors, developing prevention strategies, and implementing, evaluating, and sharing results. These steps are defined as follows:
    a. *Define the problem:* Before you can effectively address a problem, you must identify the scope of the problem. This is done by collecting data related to the problem from within the community.
    b. *Identify risk and protective factors:* This step involves identifying why a certain type of injury is occurring, what factors place people at risk for the injury, and what factors (if any) protect people from the injury.
    c. *Develop prevention strategies:* The knowledge gained from the two previous steps is used to identify prevention strategies.
    d. *Implement, evaluate, and share:* The prevention plan is put into action, the effects of the plan are evaluated for effectiveness, and results of the plan are shared either through public presentations or publication.

Chapter 34

1. a
2. d
3. a
4. b
5. a
6. b
7. Injuries the patient could have sustained include soft-tissue and musculoskeletal trauma to the head and neck, and left lateral side of the body including injury to the left arm, ribs, hip, and leg. In addition to the soft-tissue and musculoskeletal injuries, you should suspect internal injury, which could lead to internal bleeding.
8. Patients who have been ejected have the potential for soft-tissue, musculoskeletal, and internal injury to their entire body. Because ejection usually occurs with rollover collisions, the patient is thrown violently within the passenger compartment of the vehicle before being ejected. Once the patient is ejected, he is subjected to additional trauma until his body comes to rest.
9. Primary blast injury is injury caused by the pressure wave resulting from an explosion. This rapid increase in pressure produces injury to hollow organs such as the lungs, stomach, intestines, and inner ears. Secondary blast injury is injury caused by flying debris resulting from the explosion. Injuries include impaled objects, lacerations, musculoskeletal injury, and burns. Tertiary blast injury is injury caused as a result of being thrown by the pressure wave of an explosion. Injuries are similar to those resulting from ejection from a vehicle during an MVC. Quaternary injuries are injuries caused by environmental factors following an explosion.
10. The patient's GCS is E-2, V-2, M-5 for a total GCS score of 9.

Chapter 35

1. a
2. b
3. a
4. d
5. c
6. b
7. b
8. a
9. d
10. a
11. a
12. b
13. a
14. c
15. a
16. d
17. c
18. a
19. a

20. Burn center referral criteria: inhalation injury; partial-thickness burn greater than 10 percent BSA; full-thickness burn; burns of the hands, feet, face, genitalia, perineum, or major joints; electrical burns (including lightning strikes); chemical burns; or burns in patients with pre-existing medical conditions.

21. The patient is exhibiting signs and symptoms of hypoxia as a result of carbon monoxide poisoning. Pulse oximetry only reads a saturation percentage of hemoglobin. It cannot detect whether the hemoglobin is saturated with oxygen or carbon monoxide. You should treat the patient with high-flow oxygen by way of nonrebreather mask until his signs and symptoms are alleviated.

22. To control life-threatening external bleeding: Immediately apply direct pressure to the source of bleeding with a gloved hand. Apply a dressing to the wound and continue applying direct pressure. If bleeding is controlled, apply a pressure dressing. If you cannot control bleeding with direct pressure, you should apply a tourniquet.

23. The only definitive treatment for internal bleeding is surgery. It is vital to minimize on-scene times, because this will only delay definitive treatment for the patient. You should treat only life threats on scene and expedite transport to an appropriate facility.

Chapter 36

1. d
2. b
3. a
4. d
5. c
6. a
7. d
8. Joe and Lisa are delaying the transport of a critically injured patient to apply a traction splint. Even though femur fractures have the potential to produce significant hemorrhage, you should not delay transport, because internal bleeding has already led to shock in this patient. You should splint the femur fracture against the patient's other leg when he is immobilized to a long backboard.
9. The patient more than likely has sustained a fracture to the lower leg. Additionally, the patient has developed compartment syndrome as a result of pressure accumulation within the area of injury.
10. The application of a traction splint pulls the broken bone ends apart, immobilizing them and reducing the potential for broken bone ends to injure blood vessels within the leg. Additionally, when the thigh is pulled by traction, its diameter is reduced, which reduces the amount of space within the leg in which blood can accumulate.

Chapter 37

1. c
2. b
3. a
4. d
5. b
6. b
7. b
8. b

9. c
10. d
11. a
12. Hypertension occurs as ICP increases in an attempt to maintain cerebral perfusion. Increases in blood pressure must occur in order to compensate for increases in ICP. This increase in blood pressure is called Cushing's reflex. Treating this hypertension would result in a decrease in cerebral perfusion and cause further deterioration of the patient's condition.
13. When a patient presents with signs and symptoms of brain herniation—namely unequal pupils, posturing, and Cushing's triad—you should focus treatment on adequate ventilation of the patient. Proper ventilation of the brain-herniation patient is determined by hyperventilating the patient at a rate of 20 breaths per minute, or if capnography is available, ventilate the patient to maintain an $EtCO_2$ of 38 mmHg. This is done to ensure adequate oxygenation and that neither hypercapnea nor hypocapnea affect peripheral perfusion through either vasoconstriction or vasodilation.
14. Direct pressure to control a hemorrhage could cause additional injury to the brain if a depressed skull fracture or unstable skull fracture exists. Applying pressure to the site could force broken skull into the brain.

Chapter 38

1. c
2. d
3. c
4. b
5. a
6. a
7. c
8. Simple pneumothorax occurs when air enters the pleural space but pressure within the pleural space does not continue to rise. When injury allows air to accumulate in the pleural space, leading to collapse of the lung on the affected side and mediastinal shift, tension pneumothorax results.
9. When assessing a thoracic trauma patient's neck during the assessment process, be alert for subcutaneous emphysema, tracheal deviation, and jugular venous distention (JVD).
10. As blood accumulates within the pericardial sac, pressure also increases. This pressure is applied to the exterior walls of the heart, which will ultimately prevent normal expansion of the heart during diastole. Reduction of filling volumes of the heart leads to a decrease in cardiac output.

Chapter 39

1. d
2. c
3. A single stab wound to the RUQ of the abdomen with a 3-inch pocket knife blade can produce life-threatening injury to the underlying organs of the RUQ. Recall that the RUQ contains the majority of the highly vascular liver. Because the liver is a solid abdominal organ that is highly vascular, laceration may lead to massive hemorrhage.
4. Solid organs are highly vascular and may produce massive hemorrhage when injured. Hollow organs are much

less vascular; therefore, they do not pose much of a threat for massive hemorrhage. Instead, hollow organs pose a risk for serious infection if bacteria are released into the abdominal cavity as a result of injury.

5. Emergency care for abdominal evisceration is as follows: Expose the entire abdomen. Position the patient supine with knees flexed toward the chest if lower extremity or spinal trauma is not suspected. Transport with legs flat in the presence of these injuries. Apply a sterile dressing soaked with sterile water or normal saline directly over the eviscerated organs. Do not attempt to push eviscerated organs back into the abdominal cavity, because this may result in additional complications to the patient. Cover the dressing with an occlusive dressing to preserve moisture and heat. Administer high-flow oxygen. Monitor and treat for shock as indicated. Do not delay transport to initiate IV access on scene. Obtain IV access en route to an appropriate facility.

Chapter 40

1. b
2. c
3. a
4. d
5. c
6. c
7. Neurogenic hypotension resulting from spinal shock is called neurogenic shock. The dilation of vasculature is a result of loss of sympathetic nervous system function when there is injury to the spinal cord at the level of the cervical spine. The increased diameter of the peripheral vasculature results in a larger vascular container, for which the existing volume of blood is inadequate to fill. When this occurs, the patient becomes hypotensive. Ordinarily, the body is able to respond to hypotension with increased sympathetic nervous system influence on the heart and vasculature to cause increased heart and vasoconstriction. In contrast to the patient in hypovolemic shock who has pale, sweaty skin and an increased heart rate, the patient in neurogenic shock has warm, dry skin with a normal heart rate.
8. A patient with decreased level of responsiveness, diabetes, or neurologic impairment, suspected intoxication with alcohol or drugs, or a distracting injury may be less aware of symptoms of spine injury and the information he reports may be unreliable. It is also difficult to obtain reliable information from patients when there is a communication barrier or the patient is a pediatric patient.
9. The development of signs and symptoms of spine injury over time can occur from secondary spine injury as the spinal cord swells.
10. Rapid extrication is used when the patient is critical (has a problem with airway, breathing, or circulation), when the patient blocks access to a critical patient, or is in danger.
11. Partial spinal-cord injuries reflect the particular tract within the spinal cord that is affected. Some nerve tracts cross over, and some do not, and different sensations are carried by different tracts of nerve tissue in the spinal cord.

Chapter 41

1. d
2. c

3. c
4. a
5. d
6. b
7. a
8. b
9. Your initial actions should include ensuring that the patient's ABCs are intact while moving him to a warmer environment. Remove the wet clothes and dry the patient. Once the clothes are removed and the patient is dry, provide him with high-flow oxygen and rewarming.
10. Heat exhaustion is a heat-related illness that is characterized by inadequate perfusion resulting in a mild state of shock. This mild state of shock is the result of increased vasodilation in peripheral circulation, which leads to pooling of blood in the vessels of the skin. Prolonged and profuse sweating leads to loss of circulating blood volume and results in inadequate circulation. Heatstroke is a life-threatening emergency that occurs when the body's thermoregulatory mechanisms cease to work. Because the thermoregulatory mechanisms no longer work, the core body temperature rises uncontrollably resulting in the destruction of brain cells, which leads to permanent disability or death.
11. Pressure increases with the depth of a dive. This pressure results in compression of gases within the body. Specifically, gases such as nitrogen are compressed and dissolved into the blood. When ascending from a depth, the diver must do so at a controlled rate, making sure to breathe adequately while doing so. This is important because time must be provided for the pressure to slowly be decreased. Rapid decreases in pressure during an ascent results in nitrogen bubbles to form in the blood. The bubbles may form a gas embolism and cause pulmonary embolism or stroke.

Chapter 42

1. c
2. c
3. c
4. b
5. As an Advanced EMT, early identification of the life-threatening injuries; proper management of airway, ventilation, oxygenation, and perfusion; and rapid transport to an appropriate facility where definitive care is available can reduce morbidity and mortality associated with multisystem trauma. When the body's compensatory mechanisms are impaired in more than one way, for example having blood loss and impaired ventilations, the body is less able to compensate. For example, one of the early compensatory mechanisms for blood loss is an increase in ventilations. If the respiratory system is also impaired, the ability to increase ventilation is decreased, as well.
6. In order for adequate perfusion to take place, the patient must have an adequate number of red blood cells in circulation to carry oxygen to the tissues of the body. Additionally, the patient must have an adequate blood pressure to deliver oxygenated blood to the tissues of the body.
7. An adequate MAP is a better indicator of perfusion than the systolic blood pressure. In addition, MAP must be increased in the presence of increased intracranial pressure in order to perfuse the brain.

8. Trauma patients may already be at increased risk of
    heat loss because of blood loss (blood loss = heat
    loss), hypoxia (reduced metabolism = reduced heat
    production), and prolonged environmental exposure.
    Hypothermia can impair blood clotting, allowing further
    blood loss and anaerobic metabolism. Careless actions on
    the part of EMS providers, such as unnecessarily expos-
    ing the patient, failing to cover him up, delaying moving
    to the ambulance, not heating the back of the ambulance,
    and administering excess intravenous fluids can cause or
    worsen hypothermia and worsen the patient's outcome.

Chapter 43

1. c
2. b
3. b
4. c
5. b
6. a
7. a
8. c
9. c
10. d
11. b
12. d
13. b
14. b
15. c
16. d
17. a
18. d
19. b
20. d
21. Signs of imminent delivery include regular, strong contrac-
    tions 2 to 3 minutes apart, rupture of the amniotic mem-
    branes (with contractions), the mother feeling pressure as
    if she needs to have a bowel movement or saying that she
    feels she is about to deliver, and bulging of the perineum
    or crowning. Other things to take into consideration are
    the transport time, how quickly labor has progressed since
    its onset, and the number of previous deliveries.
22. In a breech delivery, the fetal shoulders or head may
    present an obstacle to delivery. If the fetus begins breath-
    ing before the head is delivered, you will need to create a
    space for him to breathe by inserting two gloved fingers
    into the vagina and making a "V" around the fetus'
    mouth and nose for him to breathe.
23. The first step is to dry the patient and use tactile stimula-
    tion, such as rubbing the back or flicking the soles of the
    feet. If that is not effective, apply supplemental oxygen.
    If that does not result in improvement, begin bag-valve-
    mask ventilations. If a few bag-valve-mask ventilations
    with supplemental oxygen are not effective and the heart
    rate is less than 60, begin chest compressions. Transport
    without delay, requesting ALS or air medical transport if
    transport time is long and those resources are available.

Chapter 44

1. d
2. c

3. b
4. a
5. b
6. c
7. a
8. d
9. b
10. d
11. a
12. c
13. c
14. b
15. b
16. d
17. The pediatric abdomen is less protected by the ribs and
    the weaker, thinner abdominal wall. The organs are pro-
    portionately large for the size of the abdominal cavity,
    increasing their exposure.
18. The higher respiratory rate increases the amount of water
    lost from the body with expiration. Fever, which may
    accompany respiratory distress, further increases fluid loss.

Chapter 45

1. d
2. b
3. a
4. c
5. a
6. c
7. b
8. b
9. c
10. a
11. You must suspect that a sudden change in mental status
    was caused by an underlying medical problem, instead
    of age-related cognitive decline (dementia). During the
    SAMPLE history, pay particular attention to medica-
    tions. The medications will give clues about current
    medical problems, as well as the possibility of medication
    side effects or interactions. Note recently prescribed med-
    ications. The physical exam should consider conditions
    likely to result in altered mental status, such as hypoxia,
    hypoperfusion, hypoglycemia, hyperglycemia, trauma,
    hypothermia, and hyperthermia.
12. The elderly are less able to compensate through
    homeostatic mechanisms, healing processes are slower,
    infection is more likely, and complications such as pul-
    monary embolism can occur due to pre-existing coagu-
    lopathies combined with major trauma, surgery, and
    immobility.

Chapter 46

1. b
2. c
3. d
4. b
5. c
6. b
7. In order to prevent breathing difficulty when transport-
    ing an obese patient, you should allow the patient to

assume a position of comfort or place rolled towels or sheets beneath the patient's shoulders and neck.

8. It is not your role to confront the potential abuser. It is your role to report your suspicions to the proper authorities according to your state's guidelines. Your goal is to remove the patient from the environment, care for him, and report your suspicions so that the authorities can intervene. Confronting the suspected abuser may lead to their refusal to allow you to transport the patient to the hospital.

9. There are two basic types of tracheostomy tubes used. A single-lumen tracheostomy tube is used for infants because of its small diameter. For larger children and adults, a tube is used that has an inner cannula and an outer cannula.

10. CPAP devices provide a continuous positive pressure during the inspiratory and expiratory phases of ventilation. BiPAP devices provide a higher positive pressure during inspiration and a lower positive pressure during expiration.

11. Both of these devices are designed to keep the lower airways open during expiration, which assists in ventilation and oxygenation.

12. If the tube is inserted through the nose, it is called a nasogastric (NG) tube. If the tube is inserted through the patient's mouth, it is called an orogastric (OG) tube.

Chapter 47

1. c
2. d
3. c
4. d
5. a
6. b
7. While performing a windshield survey, you will scan the scene and ask yourself: What has happened? What is happening? What hazards are present? What resources are needed? You will obtain this information in a matter of seconds and it will dictate how you will proceed.
8. Multiple agencies are required on this scene. First of all, you must notify the utility company to ensure that the downed electrical lines are not charged prior to approaching the area. Ensure that law enforcement is present and controlling traffic in the area where you will be working. The patient is pinned; therefore, you must request an extrication team to free the patient. The mechanism of injury suggests a high potential for life-threatening injuries. The patient must be transported to a facility where specialized services are available. You should consider aeromedical transport to reduce transport time to definitive care.
9. You will manage this scene as with any other MVC except for the manner in which you disconnect the power from the vehicle. Do not cut orange power cables because they can provide life-threatening electrical shock. When you identify the vehicle as a hybrid, ensure that the vehicle is stabilized before attempting to access the patient. Access the passenger compartment and shift the gear selector to park. Turn the ignition off and verify that dash lights are not illuminated. Lastly, disconnect the 12-volt battery.

Chapter 48

1. b
2. b
3. d
4. c
5. a
6. b
7. d
8. a
9. c
10. c
11. RAIN is a chronologic, four-step process of how to respond safely to a hazardous materials event. First, recognize that a hazardous materials event has occurred, and gather as much information as you can safely gather about the substance involved. Then, avoid the hazardous materials to prevent additional contamination from spreading to responders and equipment. It generally consists of avoiding the hazard, avoiding contaminated victims, and avoiding the outside. Then isolate. This is a safety measure that isolates the hazardous materials from bystanders and the public. Isolate the public uphill, upwind, and upstream. Finally, when you have completed the other steps, notify responders with specialized resources, as well as area hospitals. Also notify additional EMS resources if the event is an MCI.
12. Making the assumption that any chemical can harm or kill you provides a general guidance for responding to the scene, because it assumes that the chemical involved has the potential to inflict mortal damage on a responder. That psychological trigger will remind the responder to take the maximum safety steps possible.
13. Answers are as follows:
    a. orange, green
    b. orange
    c. blue
    d. white
    e. yellow

Chapter 49

1. c
2. d
3. b
4. d
5. a
6. d
7. c
8. a
9. The overall approach to a WMD scene is extreme caution. Safety is a paramount factor, and so, depending on the type of event being faced, you will have to take certain precautions, including avoiding the scene, donning PPE, and being observant of changing conditions. Characteristics to be aware of are indications of an explosion, dead animals, an oily residue, patterns of illness in patients, large groups of victims in a small area, uncontrolled fires, or armed suspects.

Glossary

A

abandonment termination of patient care without transferring care to a qualified health care provider, when the patient is still in need of and desires medical care.

abdominal evisceration a condition in which abdominal organs (usually the small intestines) protrude through an open or penetrating injury to the abdominal wall.

abortion loss of pregnancy from any cause prior to 20 weeks gestation.

abrasion an open injury that results from the skin being removed from the body by friction.

abruptio placentae premature separation of the placenta from the uterine wall.

abscess a pocket of pus (white blood cells and cellular debris) in the tissues.

absorption the process by which a medication moves from the site of administration into the vascular system.

accessory muscles of breathing muscles in the neck, torso, and abdomen that are not used in normal breathing, but are used to assist breathing in respiratory distress.

accreditation a formal process by which a professional body assesses whether or not a program or institution has met the established standards of the profession and formally recognizes that the standards have been met.

acetylcholine (ACh) a neurotransmitter in the somatic (voluntary) nervous system, in the preganglionic sympathetic division of the autonomic nervous system, and in the preganglionic and postganglionic parasympathetic division of the autonomic nervous system.

acids any substances that give up (donate) hydrogen ions in a solution and which have a pH below 7.

action potentials temporary changes in the electrical charge of the interior of a cell membrane (neuron or cardiac cell) from negative to positive, which allows an impulse to spread to adjacent cells. Electrical messages transmitted from one cell to another.

active listening listening beyond the sender's words for the meanings behind them.

acute coronary syndrome (ACS) a spectrum of coronary artery obstruction resulting from atherosclerosis; narrowing of coronary arteries leading to episodes of acute ischemia (stable and unstable angina) and acute myocardial infarction.

acute illness an illness with sudden onset, typically of short duration.

acute mountain sickness signs and symptoms that may occur when a person ascends to an altitude of 2,000 meters (6,600 feet) too rapidly.

acute myocardial infarction (AMI) sudden onset of coronary artery occlusion from a ruptured atherosclerotic plaque or clot, which results in obstruction of blood flow beyond the affected area, leading to death of heart muscle cells.

acute renal failure (ARF) the sudden inability of the kidney to produce urine, measured by levels of creatinine (Cr) and blood urea nitrogen (BUN).

acute respiratory distress syndrome (ARDS) a complication of shock and other critical illnesses that results in damage to the lungs, which allows leakage of fluid into the lung parenchyma , interfering with ventilation and oxygenation. ARDS has a high mortality rate. Also called *noncardiogenic pulmonary edema*.

acute stress reaction signs and symptoms that occur on exposure to a stressor. The effects may last up to four weeks.

Addison disease a condition that results from a failure of the adrenal cortices to produce adequate amounts of adrenal cortical hormones, which affects carbohydrate and protein metabolism and electrolyte and water balance.

adolescent a child from 12 to 18 years of age.

adrenal crisis a complication of Addison disease in which the body cannot maintain homeostasis because of a lack of adrenal cortical hormones.

adrenergic pertaining to the nerves that release the neurotransmitter norepinephrine and the receptors sites that it acts upon.

adrenocorticotropic hormone (ACTH) a hormone released from the anterior pituitary gland that acts on the adrenal glands, causing secretion of epinephrine and cortisol.

adsorbent a material to which substances can adhere or bind.

Advanced Emergency Medical Technician (Advanced EMT) a prehospital emergency care provider who uses basic and limited advanced life support skills to care for acutely ill and injured patients. Also called *AEMT*.

advanced life support (ALS) complex patient care assessments and interventions that require in-depth training.

AED short for automatic external defibrillator.

aerobic metabolism cellular production of energy that depends on the use of oxygen, and results in wastes (water and carbon dioxide) that are easily eliminated by the body.

affect a person's visible emotional state.

affinity a measure of attraction and degree of binding between a drug and a cellular receptor.

afterload the amount of resistance provided by the systemic vasculature, which the heart must overcome to effectively pump blood from the left ventricle.

agonal respirations ineffective, irregular, gasping breaths that occur as a patient enters cardiac or respiratory arrest.

agonists drugs that bind to a receptor and cause a response.

airway adjuncts devices inserted through the nose or mouth into the pharynx, esophagus, or trachea to maintain a passageway for air flow.

alkali a substance that can accept hydrogen ions in a solution and which has a pH greater than 7.

allied health care professionals health care providers other than nurses and physicians who provide specialized services, such as physical therapy, respiratory therapy, and emergency medical services.

alpha$_1$ receptor a molecule in certain cells that binds with specific substances to produce certain effects. Alpha$_1$ receptors in the blood vessels bind with epinephrine and norepinephrine to cause vasoconstriction.

ALS short for advanced life support.

alveolar ventilation the volume of air that actually reaches the air sacs in the lungs each minute.

Alzheimer's disease a common form of dementia; a progressive loss of cognitive function including memory loss, confusion, and alterations in emotions and behavior.

American Heart Association (AHA) a nonprofit organization that supports efforts to reduce death and disability from heart disease and stroke, and establishes standards for emergency cardiac care.

AMI short for acute myocardial infarction.

amputation the removal of a body part, usually a limb or digit, from the body either traumatically or surgically.

anaerobic metabolism cellular production of energy that takes place without oxygen, resulting in a small amount of energy with pyruvic acid as a waste product. Pyruvic acid requires oxygen to be converted to carbon dioxide and water.

analgesic a pain reliever; a medication that eliminates or reduces pain.

anaphylactoid reaction a life-threatening reaction to a substance that presents with signs and symptoms similar to anaphylaxis, but that is not mediated by the immune globulin IgE.

anaphylaxis a life-threatening allergic reaction that produces shock through vasodilation and fluid shifts, with the potential for asphyxia.

anatomic dead space the portion of the airway in which gases are present but in which there is no mechanism for exchange of gases with the blood.

anatomical position standing, facing forward, with the palms turned forward.

anemias conditions in which there is a decreased number of red blood cells or total blood cell volume.

angina pectoris chest pain that results from ischemia of the heart muscle, usually from coronary artery disease.

anginal equivalents signs and symptoms other than typical chest pain, such as shortness of breath, produced by myocardial ischemia.

angioedema dilation and increased permeability of blood vessels within the tissues that produces swelling.

angiotensin-converting enzyme (ACE) inhibitor a drug that prevents the production of angiotensin II, a hormone that causes vasoconstriction.

anisocoria a condition in which the pupils are unequal.

ankylosing spondylosis a form of arthritis of the spine, more common in men, in which the affected vertebrae can fuse.

anorexia a loss of appetite.

antagonists drugs that bind to receptor sites and prevent a normal response by the cell.

antecubital fossa the anterior, slightly depressed area of the arm over the elbow joint.

anterior-cord syndrome the set of signs and symptoms due to pressure or injury of the anterior spinal cord, such as from a bone fragment, or compression of the blood vessels of the anterior spinal cord.

antibodies immunoglobulins; substances synthesized by the immune system that can recognize specific foreign materials in the body and initiate a specific immune response against it.

anticholinergics drugs that block acetylcholine receptors, preventing the transmission of parasympathetic nerve impulses.

anticoagulant a medication that prevents blood clotting, reducing the risk of abnormal thrombi formation.

antigens any substances recognized by the body as foreign, or "not self."

antihyperglycemic agents medications taken by type 2 diabetics to lower blood glucose levels by a variety of mechanisms.

antioxidant a substance that limits cellular damage caused by the breakdown of molecules.

antiplatelet a medication that interferes with platelet aggregation.

aortic aneurysm a weakened area of the aortic wall that has dilated to more than 50 percent of the normal width of the aorta.

aortic dissection a condition in which blood enters through a tear in the tunica intima of the aorta and is forced between the layers of the aorta.

apnea absence of breathing.

apoptosis cell death caused by the genetic programming of the cell to eliminate damaged cells; essentially, suicide of damaged cells.

apparent life-threatening event (ALTE) an episode in an infant that involves some combination of gagging or choking, apnea, change in muscle tone and color change, and which is frightening to the observer.

arterial bleeding bright red, spurting blood from an injury to an artery.

arterial gas embolism (AGE) a condition caused by ascent barotraumas in which blood vessels are occluded by air bubbles.

arteriovenous malformation (AVM) an abnormal connection between an artery and a vein with a high risk for bleeding.

articulation disorder the inability to speak clearly resulting from impairment of muscles of the mouth and tongue. Also called *dysarthria*.

ascending spinal tracts bundles of nerve fibers in the spinal cord that carry impulses from the body to the brain.

aseptic without infection.

aseptic technique medical practices, such as preparing equipment or anatomic sites of procedures, in a manner to avoid contamination of the equipment and site in an effort to reduce the chances of infection caused by the procedure.

asphyxiation cellular deprivation of oxygen; suffocation.

assault placing a person in fear of imminent bodily harm.

assessment-based management providing treatments on the basis of the patient's signs and symptoms, without a specific diagnosis of the problem. For example, oxygen is given to patients who are hypoxic, without having to have a specific diagnosis of the underlying cause of hypoxia.

asystole the absence of electrical activity in the heart, resulting in cardiac standstill, evidenced by a flat line on an ECG.

ataxia a lack of motor coordination.

ataxic without motor coordination.

atelectasis an airless state in which the alveoli are collapsed.

atherosclerosis a condition in which fatty plaque builds up in arteries, eventually narrowing the lumen and restricting blood flow.

atlas the first cervical vertebra.

atrial fibrillation a cardiac dysrhythmia in which there are many ectopic (abnormal) pacemakers in the atria. A limited number of the ectopic impulses are conducted through the AV node on an irregular basis, resulting in an irregular pulse.

atrioventricular (AV) node a collection of conductive cells at the junction of the atria and ventricles; part of the cardiac conduction system.

aura an abnormal sensation that precedes some seizures and migraine headaches, and may involve any of the senses.

auscultation the process of listening to sounds inside the body, usually with the aid of a stethoscope.

autoimmune diseases conditions in which the immune system fails to recognize some of the body's molecules as its own, resulting in an immune response against the body's own tissues.

automatic external defibrillator (AED) a device that detects and analyzes specific lethal cardiac rhythms through electrode pads placed on the torso and delivers an electrical shock to correct abnormal rhythms.

automatic transport ventilator (ATV) a simple device that enables hands-free positive pressure ventilation through an advanced airway. The device is primarily limited to adjustment of rate and tidal volume.

automaticity a unique property of cardiac cells that allows them to initiate their own electrical impulse.

avulsion an injury in which a flap of skin and possibly underlying tissue, such as muscle, has been partly (partial avulsion) or totally (complete avulsion) torn away.

axis anatomically, the second cervical vertebra.

B

bag-valve-mask (BVM) device a manual piece of equipment used to deliver artificial ventilations through a sealed mask over the mouth and nose by squeezing the bag. The mask can be removed to deliver positive pressure ventilation through an advanced airway device.

bandage a material, such as roller gauze or self-adherent elasticized material, applied to hold a dressing in place.

barbiturates sedatives whose mechanism of action includes an increase in affinity between the receptor sites and the neurotransmitter GABA.

bariatric pertaining to the medical issues related to obesity.

barotrauma diving injuries that occur when air pressure in the hollow spaces of the body (such as the middle ear and sinuses) increases.

base stations high-power two-way radios in a fixed location, such as a dispatch center or hospital.

baseline vital signs the initial values of the patient's pulse, blood pressure, and respirations, which serve as a reference point to evaluate subsequent sets of vital signs.

basilar skull the floor of the cranial cavity, including portions of the temporal and occipital bones, as well as the sphenoid and ethmoid bones.

battery illegal physical contact with an individual.

Beck's triad the combination of jugular venous distention, hypotension, and muffled heart sounds that comprise the classic signs and symptoms of pericardial tamponade.

behavior a person's observable actions.

benign prostatic hypertrophy (BPH) a noncancerous enlargement of the prostate gland.

bereavement the experience of a loss.

beta blockers medications that block the cellular beta receptors for sympathetic nervous system actions, resulting in reduced rate and force of cardiac contraction and smooth muscle relaxation.

bicarbonate an anion (HCO_3^-) that can combine with other substances. The level of bicarbonate in blood is an indication of pH.

bile digestive fluid excreted from liver into the duodenum to emulsify fats. Excess bile is stored in the gallbladder.

bilevel positive airway pressure (BiPAP) a device that provides two levels of pressure: inspiratory positive airway pressure and a lower positive pressure during expiration, which prevents collapse of the alveoli during expiration, yet provides a lower pressure against which to exhale.

bioavailability the degree to which a drug becomes available at the site of physiological activity after it is administered.

biohazard any type of biologic substance that could produce harm or disease, such as medical equipment contaminated with infectious body fluids.

biotransformation the chemical alterations that a substance, such as a drug, undergoes within the body.

blood glucose level (BGL) the amount of the sugar glucose that is present in the circulating blood measured in units of milligrams of glucose per deciliter of blood. A normal BGL is 70 to 110 mg/dL.

blunt force injury trauma caused by mechanisms of injury that do not penetrate the body cavity. Also called *blunt trauma*.

body fluids with respect to infectious disease, includes fluids such as blood, plasma, respiratory secretions, breast milk, vaginal secretions, semen, synovial fluid (from joints), urine, and feces; tears and sweat are not included.

body mass index (BMI) a ratio of a person's weight to height, used as a measure of obesity.

body mechanics using the body properly (such as correct posture, correct muscle groups for lifting) in the performance of tasks to prevent injury.

body planes imaginary lines used to divide the body for anatomical reference.

body substance isolation (BSI) a form of Standard Precautions in which devices, such as gloves or goggles, are used to create a barrier between the skin and mucous membranes to prevent contact with the body fluids of another individual.

bolus a mass; in pharmacology, a single large dose of medication, usually intravenous.

Boyle's law states that at a constant temperature, the volume of a gas varies inversely with its pressure.

BPH short for *benign prostatic hypertrophy*.

bradycardia a slower-than-normal heart rate, which is a heart rate less than 60 beats per minute in adults.

brain herniation a condition that occurs when intracranial pressure increases to a point at which the brain tissue is forced toward the point of least resistance, which may be the incisura (opening) of the tentorium cerebelli (a tissue that divides the cerebrum and cerebellum) or the foramen magnum of the cranium.

Braxton-Hicks contractions mild, irregular uterine contractions prior to the onset of labor.

breach of duty failure to fulfill one's professional obligations.

breech position a fetal presentation in which the feet or buttocks are the presenting part.

bronchiolitis a viral illness that results in inflammation and sloughing of the bronchiolar lining, which can lead to respiratory distress in the pediatric population.

bronchoconstriction the narrowing or constriction of a bronchiolar passageway.

Brown-Séquard syndrome the set of signs and symptoms produced by hemitransection of the spinal cord.

BSI short for *body substance isolation*.

buffer system mechanisms in the body that prevent significant changes in pH.

burnout physical and psychological exhaustion occurring from prolonged stress.

BVM short for *bag-valve-mask device*.

C

calyx a term that means "cup." The renal calyces serve to collect urine.

cannulate to place a hollow tube (cannula) within a structure.

capillary bleeding slow oozing bright or dark red blood.

capillary refill time the time it takes for the capillaries of a superficial capillary bed, such as in the nailbeds, to refill with blood after the blood is emptied from them by applying pressure.

capnography the measurement and graphic representation over time of the level of carbon dioxide in an exhaled air sample.

capnometry the measurement of the level of carbon dioxide in exhaled air.

cardiac glycosides a class of plant molecule that has therapeutic value in the treatment of heart failure and atrial fibrillation, but which also is highly toxic.

cardiac tamponade a condition in which fluid or blood collects within the pericardium, compressing the heart and reducing cardiac output. Also called pericardial tamponade.

cardiomyopathy a disorder of the heart in which the muscle is enlarged and unable to function effectively.

carpopedal spasm involuntary contraction of the muscles of the hands and feet that occurs in hyperventilation syndrome.

carrier an asymptomatic individual who is infected with and can transmit a communicable disease.

cataracts clouding of the lens of the eye.

catatonic a motor disorder with extreme muscle rigidity or flaccidity due to a psychological cause.

cathartic a laxative.

cellulitis an inflammation of the skin, including the dermis and subcutaneous layers, usually caused by bacterial infection.

central intravenous catheters devices placed into a large vein, usually the subclavian vein that lies beneath the clavicle, allowing access to the central circulation to administer medications or total parenteral nutrition (TPN).

central pulses arterial pulses in the large arteries of the body, closer to the heart; specifically, the carotid and femoral pulses.

central-cord syndrome the set of signs and symptoms due to an injury to the center portion of the spinal cord; usually occurs with hyperextension of the cervical spine.

cerebrospinal fluid (CSF) fluid secreted from special cells in the ventricles of the brain that serves to cushion the brain and spinal cord, as well as provide a carefully regulated chemical environment around them. CSF also plays a role in the lymphatic system.

certification recognition of achievement of requirements, which can be granted by any agency.

cervical-spine precautions actions taken to restrict movement of the head and neck when injury to the cervical spine is suspected.

chalazion a chronic cyst in the eyelid.

Charles' law a law of physics that states that all gases will expand equally when heated and contract when cooled.

chemical burns tissue injury that occurs as a result of exposure of the tissue (eyes, skin, mucous membranes) to strong alkali or acid substances.

chemoreceptor sensory cells that respond to chemical changes in the body fluids, such as the level of carbon dioxide or oxygen, and send that information to the central nervous system to initiate changes that maintain or restore homeostasis. The taste buds and cells in the nasal mucosa also contain chemoreceptors that enable the senses of taste and smell.

Cheyne-Stokes respirations an irregular breathing pattern that alternates between periods of tachypnea and apnea, and which can be an indication of brain herniation.

chief complaint a patient's statement of the reason he is seeking medical attention.

child abuse any act or failure to act on the part of a parent or caretaker, which results in death, serious physical or emotional harm, sexual abuse, or exploitation of a child; or an act or failure to act that presents an imminent risk of serious harm to a child.

choking agents chemical weapons that cause severe respiratory distress.

cholecystitis inflammation of the gallbladder, most commonly due to gallstones (cholelithiasis).

cholinergics medications that stimulate the cellular acetylcholine (ACh) receptors.

chronic bronchitis a chronic obstructive pulmonary disease characterized by increased mucus production and repeated episodes of bronchial infection.

chronic homelessness the condition in which a person has been continuously without a home for a year or more or has experienced four or more episodes of homelessness over the past three years.

chronic illness a long-standing disease that changes or progresses slowly.

chronic obstructive pulmonary disease (COPD) long-term, progressive lung disease in which the airways are damaged, resulting in resistance to airflow. Includes both emphysema and chronic bronchitis.

chronic renal failure (CRF) the progressive loss of kidney function over time.

chronotropy pertaining to heart rate.

chyme the mixture of partially digested food and digestive fluids that leaves the stomach and enters the duodenum.

circadian rhythm a pattern of physiologic and behavioral changes that occur over a 24-hour period.

cirrhosis fibrotic scarring of the liver from chronic liver disease such as hepatitis or alcohol abuse.

civil law branch of law that deals with disputes between individuals and organizations, rather than with the commission of crimes.

clarification seeking feedback on your understanding of what a patient tells you.

classic heatstroke a life-threatening condition in which the body's heat dissipation mechanisms are overwhelmed by a hot environment, resulting in altered mental status and extremely high body temperature.

cleaning using soap or detergent and water to clean gross contamination from surfaces.

clinical impression a preliminary determination of the patient's problem based on the patient's history, signs, and symptoms and the application of the EMS provider's knowledge and process of clinical reasoning to the problem.

clinical problem solving engaging in a systematic reasoning process to identify and solve a patient's medical problem.

clinical training the portion of health care provider training that takes place in the medical setting, in particular, in the hospital.

clinical pertaining to observation of signs and symptoms or to a medical setting.

closed chest injury a traumatic condition in which the thoracic cavity has received blunt force injury but in which the integrity of the chest wall has not been breached and there is no opening from the environment into the thoracic cavity.

closed fracture a break in the continuity of a bone in which the overlying skin remains intact.

closed skull fracture a break in the continuity of one or more bones of the skull in which the overlying scalp remains intact.

closed soft-tissue injury injury to the soft tissues (skin, muscle, ligaments, tendons) in which the skin remains intact.

closed thoracic injury disruption of tissues of the chest wall or organs within the chest cavity in which the overlying skin remains intact.

closed-end questions questions with a narrow range of possible answers, such as "yes," or "no."

clotting cascade a complex series of events by which proteins in the blood are activated, leading to formation of a fibrin blood clot.

coagulation necrosis destruction of tissue that results in a thickened state of the skin as a result of exposure to strong acids.

coagulopathies defects in blood clotting with either inadequate or excessive blood clotting.

cognitive functions higher mental abilities, such as memory, reasoning, and problem solving.

cold zone the area at a hazardous materials incident that is at a safe distance from the chemical release where triage, treatment, and other operational support functions take place. Also called the *support zone.*

colloids IV fluids that contain proteins.

colostomy an opening on the surface of the abdomen to which the cut end of the colon is surgically connected to bypass the distal portion of the colon, which may have been removed surgically, or which may be healing from a surgical procedure. Fecal matter is collected in a pouch called a *colostomy bag.*

combining form a root word with a vowel added to connect it with another root word or a suffix.

comminuted fracture a condition in which a bone is broken into multiple pieces.

Commission on Accreditation of Ambulance Services (CAAS) an independent panel that encourages and promotes quality in medical transportation.

commotio cordis sudden cardiac arrest resulting from a blow to the center of the chest during a vulnerable portion of the cardiac cycle.

communicable illnesses infectious diseases that can be spread from person to person through direct or indirect contact; also called *communicable diseases.*

communication channels any mediums or means through which messages can be sent, such as body language, written documents, and verbal exchanges.

communication exchange of information between individuals using any means understood.

compartment syndrome a condition in which swelling within the enclosed space formed by the fascia surrounding a muscle causes an increase in pressure that compromises circulation, leading to tissue ischemia.

compensated shock a state of inadequate cellular perfusion in which the body can make adjustments to maintain perfusion to the vital organs, but at the cost of decreased circulation and oxygenation of the peripheral tissues.

competent having the mental capacity to make decisions.

complete spinal-cord injury the total disruption of the spinal cord; results in a total loss of neurologic function distal to the injury site.

compression with respect to spinal injury, a mechanism in which pressure is applied vertically to the spine, from either the cranial or caudal direction, which may lead to fracture of the vertebrae and injury of associated structures.

concurrent medical direction real-time physician supervision of emergency medical care. Also called *direct medical direction* or *online medical direction.*

concussion a brain injury in which neuronal function is temporarily disrupted, but in which no structural damage to the brain can be identified through imaging technology.

conduction with respect to environmental emergencies, heat loss from the body through direct contact with a cooler object.

conductivity a property of a structure that allows an electrical impulse to travel along it.

confabulate to unconsciously fill in gaps in memory with events that could have happened, but did not happen in that instance; a finding in some forms of dementia.

confrontation a therapeutic communication technique of pointing out inconsistencies in information to seek explanation.

conjunctivitis the inflammation of the conjunctiva, the outermost layer of the eye.

connective tissue one of the four basic tissue types in the body (in addition to muscle, epithelium, and nervous tissue). Connective tissue binds together and provides support for body structures.

contact burns burns that occur when the skin physically touches a hot surface.

contamination reduction zone See *warm zone.*

contamination with respect to hazardous materials, a condition in which a hazardous material is in contact with the patient's body.

continuing education instruction that takes place after initial competence has been established.

continuous positive airway pressure (CPAP) a device that delivers a constant level of increased air pressure to the airway through a mask sealed tightly on the face.

continuous quality improvement (CQI) a management process that uses benchmarks to ensure and better the value of a product or service.

contraindications the conditions under which administering an otherwise indicated medication would result in patient harm.

contusion a closed soft-tissue injury in which blood vessels beneath the surface of the skin or within deeper tissues are injured, causing bleeding within the tissues. With time, the blood takes on bluish-purple discoloration, which fades to green and then brown as the blood is broken down and reabsorbed by the body. In lay terms, a bruise.

convection heat transfer to air molecules that are passed across the skin due to a moving air current.

conventional explosives chemical materials that are specifically formulated to detonate violently.

COPD short for *chronic obstructive pulmonary disease.*

coping mechanisms psychological responses used consciously or unconsciously to reduce the effects of a stressor.

cor pulmonale right-sided heart failure resulting from increased resistance in the pulmonary circulation.

coronary artery disease (CAD) atherosclerotic disease of the coronary arteries.

cortisol a stress hormone released from the outer portion of the adrenal glands to help the body cope with stressors.

coup–contrecoup injury a condition in which the brain is traumatized at two points opposite of each other, usually anteriorly and posteriorly. The condition results from an initial blow to the head or sudden deceleration. An injury occurs at the initial point of impact and then, as the brain rebounds against the opposite side of the cranium, a second point of injury occurs.

CQI short for *continuous quality improvement.*

crackles noise heard in the lower airways when fluid is present, similar to the fizzing sound of a carbonated beverage. Also called *rales.*

credibility believability.

crepitus a crackling or grating sound within the body, such as from bone fragments rubbing together, arthritis, or subcutaneous air.

cribbing with respect to rescue operations, material designed to fill voids to stabilize objects from movement.

criminal law branch of law in which the government prosecutes individuals for the commission of crimes.

critical access hospitals small rural hospitals that provide 24-hour emergency care to stabilize critical patients for transfer to a facility that provides a higher level of care.

critical patients patients who require or are on the verge of requiring, immediate, lifesaving medical attention.

cross-tolerance a decrease in responsiveness to the effects of several related drugs.

croup laryngotracheobronchitis; a viral respiratory disease with a characteristic "seal bark" cough that is common in childhood.

crowning the visibility of the presenting part of the fetus at the vaginal opening during childbirth.

crush injuries tissue damage caused by application of tremendous pressure to the affected, such as being trapped between a fallen tree and the ground. The forces can rupture cells and blood vessels, resulting in open or closed wounds. Crushing injuries may or may not involve fractures.

crystalloid an intravenous fluid that consists of water and electrolytes or small carbohydrate molecules, such as glucose, but which does not contain proteins or large starch molecules.

Cullen's sign ecchymosis around the umbilicus, indicative of retroperitoneal hemorrhage.

cumulative effect the result of repeated doses of drug; occurs as more drug is administered than is eliminated from the body.

cumulative stress the sum of the effects of exposure to stressors over time.

Cushing reflex a decrease in heart rate in response to increased blood pressure, particularly systolic blood pressure, which results in a widened pulse pressure. The phenomenon occurs in response to severely increased intracranial pressure.

Cushing's syndrome a disorder caused by oversecretion of adrenal cortical hormones or by long-term corticosteroid therapy.

Cushing's triad Cushing's reflex (increased systolic blood pressure with a widened pulse pressure and bradycardia) in combination with an irregular breathing pattern.

cutaneous pertaining to the skin.

cyanosis dusky blue-purple discoloration of the tissues that occurs as a result of hypoxia; deoxygenated hemoglobin has a dark color that makes the tissues appear blue, rather than the normal pink color associated with oxygenated hemoglobin.

cystic fibrosis (CF) a genetic disease of the secretory glands that particularly affects the lungs, pancreas, and digestive tract.

D

Dalton's law a law of physics that states that the total pressure of a gaseous mixture is equal to the sum of the partial pressures of each individual gas that comprises the gaseous mixture.

DCAP-BTLS a mnemonic for the conditions to look for during the assessment of a trauma patient; letters stand for deformity, contusions, abrasions, penetrating trauma, burns, tenderness, lacerations, and swelling.

decompensated shock a state of inadequate cellular perfusion in which the body can no longer provide circulation of an adequate amount of oxygenated blood to the vital organs.

decompression sickness a condition that occurs as nitrogen gas bubbles are produced and accumulate in the blood and tissues as a result of rapid ascent during a dive. Also called *the bends.*

decontamination with respect to hazardous materials, the process of reducing or removing hazardous material from people and equipment.

decubitus ulcer a bedsore; pressure sore.

defamation injuring another person in reputation or occupation through the malicious communication of false information.

defendant the person against whom a legal action is brought.

defensive driving techniques of safe driving and crash avoidance that involve anticipating dangerous situations caused by adverse conditions or the mistakes of other drivers.

defibrillation an electrical current passed through the heart between two pads or paddles placed on the chest to terminate ventricular fibrillation and pulseless ventricular tachycardia.

delirium an acute state of confusion and agitation, usually due to an underlying medical cause. Delirium is usually reversible when the underlying problem is treated.

delirium tremens a syndrome that occurs due to the withdrawal of alcohol in a physically dependent individual.

delusions false beliefs maintained despite evidence to the contrary, such as the belief that one is being pursued by government agents or has special powers.

dementia the progressive, irreversible loss of cognitive function.

dependent lividity discoloration of the tissues after death caused by pooling of blood from the effects of gravity (livor mortis).

depolarization equalizing a difference in electrical charge across a cell membrane through the movement of ions.

depressed skull fracture broken cranial bones, usually from a severe blow to the head, in which bone fragments are pushed beneath the normal contour of the skull, resulting in a sunken area. Edema of the scalp over the injured area may obscure the sunken area, making it difficult to detect by palpation or inspection, or the area may be more obvious. Bone fragments may penetrate the brain tissue.

descending spinal tracts bundles of nerve fibers in the spinal cord that carry motor impulses from the brain to the body; their functions include controlling motor activity and muscle tone.

destination decision the determination of the most appropriate mode of transport to the nearest, most appropriate medical care facility based on the needs of the patient.

detailed physical exam careful, systematic examination of the body from head to toe. Also called a *head-to-toe exam*.

diabetes mellitus a disorder of glucose metabolism resulting from insufficient insulin.

diabetic ketoacidosis (DKA) a hyperglycemic diabetic emergency in which the patient suffers from dehydration, acidosis, and electrolyte imbalance.

Diagnostic and Statistical Manual (DSM IV TR) guidelines published by the American Psychological Association to provide criteria for the diagnosis of mental illnesses; currently in the fourth version with text revision.

dialysis the process of placing blood in contact with a semipermeable membrane (synthetic or peritoneum) that separates it from a dialysate to remove wastes from the blood.

diaphragmatic rupture an injury that occurs when a hole or tear in the diaphragm results in an opening between the thoracic and abdominal cavities, through which abdominal contents can herniate into the thoracic cavity.

diastolic blood pressure the force of blood against the arterial walls during relaxation of the left ventricle.

diffuse axonal injury non-focal trauma to the brain in which the axons of neurons are injured by shearing or tearing from acceleration/deceleration forces.

diffuse the movement of solutes from an area of higher concentration to an area of lower concentration.

digital radio equipment radio equipment that encodes voice signals into electronic data before sending, and decodes electronic data into voice signals at the receiving end.

dilation with respect to obstetrics, the opening of the os cervix in preparation for childbirth.

direct injury a wound that occurs at the point of contact with an object.

direct medical direction real-time physician supervision of emergency medical care. Also called *concurrent medical direction* or *online medical direction*.

direct pressure use of manual force to control bleeding, such as firmly pressing a dressing over a wound with the fingertips or hand.

direct transmission spread of a communicable disease from one person to another without an intermediary vector or fomite.

disability with respect to primary patient assessment, the patient's level of responsiveness.

disease period the phase of an infection in which the individual has signs and symptoms.

disinfecting using a hospital-grade chemical disinfectant product or 1:10 bleach-and-water solution to kill most micro-organisms on a surface.

dislocation a complete displacement of bone ends from a joint.

disseminated intravascular coagulation (DIC) a condition in which abnormal activation of the blood clotting mechanism results in blood clot formation within the vascular system. Consumption of the clotting factors by the process results in inability to control further bleeding.

distracting injury a painful or concerning condition that may make a patient less sensitive to the presence of other symptoms, such as tingling or numbness.

distraction a mechanism that places axial traction (pulling along the long axis) on the spine and can result in forceful separation of vertebrae or stretching of the spinal cord.

diuretics substances that promote the excretion of water through the kidneys.

diverticulitis infection and inflammation of a diverticulum, a blind pocket that protrudes from the wall of the colon.

DKA short for *diabetic ketoacidosis.*

DNR order short for *do not resuscitate order.*

do not resuscitate (DNR) order a physician's order that specifies what resuscitative care may and may not be provided to a patient.

documentation a record of an event.

domestic abuse violence used to intimidate a partner to gain power or control.

dorsiflex bending the ankle to bring the top of the foot closer to the anterior leg (shin).

dressing a material that is applied directly to an open injury to control bleeding, prevent contamination of the wound, or promote healing.

drip factor the number of drops of a particular size required to equal 1 mL of fluid in a specifically calibrated IV administration set.

dromotropy pertaining to the speed with which impulses travel through the electrical conduction system of the heart.

drowning suffocation from submersion in a liquid medium.

due regard appropriate caution and concern.

durable power of attorney legal permission granted to an individual to make health care decisions on behalf of a person who is not competent to make decisions for himself.

duty to act the legal obligation to provide emergency medical services.

dynamic ECG a real-time electronic display of the waveforms of the cardiac electrical cycle obtained by placing the electrodes of an electrocardiogram monitor on the patient's chest.

dysbarism a medical condition resulting from changes in atmospheric pressure, such as from high altitude or diving.

dysmenorrhea painful menstruation.

dyspnea difficulty breathing.

dysrhythmia a heart rhythm that may be irregular, too slow, too fast, or arise from a site other than the sinoatrial node. Dysrhythmia may or may not be life threatening.

dysuria painful urination.

E

ecchymosis a blue, purple, or black discoloration under the skin from bleeding; a bruise. The color may be red when fresh, and fade to green, yellow, and brown as it disappears.

ECG short for *electrocardiogram.*

eclampsia a hypertensive disorder of pregnancy characterized by the onset of seizure or coma.

ectopic pacemakers cells in the heart that have become irritable and create their own impulses, rather than being depolarized by the action potential initiated by the sinoatrial node.

ectopic pregnancy implantation of a fertilized ovum outside the uterus, usually in the fallopian tube.

effacement the thinning or flattening of the cervix.

ejection with respect to mechanisms of injury, being thrown from a vehicle during a collision.

ejection fraction the proportion of blood in the left ventricle at the end of diastole that is ejected during systole, expressed as a percentage.

elder abuse any act or failure to act on the part of a caretaker, which results in death, serious physical or emotional harm, sexual abuse, or exploitation of an elderly person; or an act or failure to act that presents an imminent risk of serious harm to an elderly person.

electrical burns tissue damage caused by the effects of electrical current passing through the body.

electrocardiogram (ECG) a graphic display of the waveforms of the cardiac electrical cycle obtained by placing electrodes on the chest to transmit the minute amount of electricity from the heart that reaches the skin to a device that gives a visual representation of electrical flow.

electrolyte a compound that dissociates into ions in a solution.

embryo a human organism from day four after fertilization of an ovum through the eighth week of development.

Emergency Medical Responder (EMR) an EMS provider who uses minimal equipment to provide immediate lifesaving care to critically ill and injured patients while awaiting the arrival of more highly trained EMS personnel.

emergency medical services (EMS) an organized network of resources and specially trained personnel that exists to provide lifesaving care to acutely ill and injured patients in the prehospital setting.

Emergency Medical Technician (EMT) an EMS provider who provides emergency medical care and transportation to the ill and injured, using the basic equipment supplied on an ambulance.

Emergency Medical Treatment and Active Labor Act (EMTALA) federal legislation that makes it illegal to refuse an appropriate screening examination and, if necessary, treatment or emergency transfer to patients with a medical emergency or in active labor, regardless of their ability to pay.

emergency moves techniques to quickly move a patient from a dangerous situation.

Emergency Response Guidebook (ERG) a directory published by the U.S. Department of Transportation every four years to assist in making initial decisions at the scene of a hazardous materials incident.

emergency response using visible (lights) and audible (siren) warning devices during ambulance operation to notify other drivers that you are requesting the right of way in order to minimize the time needed to arrive at the scene. Also called *emergent response.*

emesis the product of vomiting; vomit.

empathy insight into another person's feelings and situation.

emphysema a chronic obstructive pulmonary disease characterized by loss of elasticity of the airways and destruction of alveoli.

EMS provider an individual with one of four nationally recognized levels of training who provides lifesaving care to acutely ill and injured patients in the prehospital setting.

EMT short for *emergency medical technician.*

end-stage renal disease (ESRD) irreversible kidney damage requiring dialysis or transplant.

end-tidal carbon dioxide (ETCO$_2$) the amount of carbon dioxide in exhaled air at the end of expiration. Normal ETCO$_2$ is 35 to 45 mmHg.

endometriosis the presence of endometrium outside the uterine cavity.

endothelium epithelial tissue that lines the inner surface of a structure.

enhanced 911 a communication system through which the public can request emergency assistance using the universal telephone number 911; an enhanced 911 system displays the caller's location on the emergency operator or dispatcher's computer terminal. Also called *E-911.*

enteral pertaining to the gastrointestinal system.

epidermis the outermost layer of skin that serves as a barrier between the body and the environment.

epididymitis inflammation of the epididymis, the structure of the male reproductive system in which spermatozoa are stored.

epiglottitis swelling of the epiglottis, the leaf-shaped flap that protects the glottic opening during swallowing, most often caused by a bacterial infection. Airway obstruction can occur. The condition is now rare due to immunization, but can occur in unimmunized adults and children.

epilepsy a neurological disorder in which there are recurrent seizures.

epinephrine a stress hormone released from the inner portion of the adrenal gland to prepare the body to respond to a stressor in the fight-or-flight response. Also called *adrenaline.*

epistaxis bleeding from the nose.

epithelial tissue layers of cells that cover or line a structure, allowing for protection, absorption, secretion, and other specialized functions.

erythropoietin a hormone released, primarily from the kidneys, in response to hypoxia to stimulate bone marrow to increase red blood cell production.

eschar burned tissue that has no elasticity and takes on the appearance of dry leather.

esophageal varices distended, varicose veins in the esophagus due to portal vein hypertension.

ethics the principles of proper conduct within a profession; a branch of philosophy that addresses issues of what is right or good and what is wrong.

evaporation liquid turning to vapor; refers to perspiration vaporizing and dissipating from the skin, carrying body heat with it.

evidence-based practice using the best available research evidence to guide patient assessment and care. Also called *evidence-based medicine.*

excitability the property of being able to respond to a stimulus.

excited delirium syndrome (ExDS) an acute state of confusion accompanied by combative or aggressive behavior, insensitivity to pain, and unusual strength; may be provoked by use of cocaine or methamphetamine, as well as other causes, and can result in sudden death.

exclusion zone See *hot zone.*

exertional heatstroke an environmental emergency that occurs in individuals who are exercising or working in a hot environment and in which the core temperature rises rapidly.

expectoration removal of secretions from the lungs by coughing.

exposure a condition in which a person is affected by the properties of a hazardous material but has not directly come into contact with it, particularly in situations involving radiation; with respect to bloodborne pathogens, contact between a person's mucous membranes or nonintact skin with infectious blood or body fluids of another person.

expressed consent a patient's overt acknowledgement that he accepts the medical procedures that are going to be performed.

external bleeding hemorrhage in which blood is lost into the environment, as opposed to internal hemorrhage, which occurs within body cavities or tissues.

extracellular fluid (ECF) all fluid in the body that is not within cells.

extrication to free or remove a patient from entanglement, such as may be necessary in a motor vehicle collision or industrial setting.

exudate material that has seeped out of injured or inflamed tissues or blood vessels.

F

facilitation with respect to therapeutic communications, encouraging a patient to keep speaking.

false imprisonment unlawful detainment of an individual without just cause.

fascia the inelastic fibrous tissue that surrounds each muscle compartment.

febrile seizure abnormal discharge of neurons in the brain that occurs in the pediatric population and is caused by a sudden increase in body temperature associated with infection.

Federal Communications Commission (FCC) the U.S. government agency that regulates the standards and use of communication equipment.

feedback a message sent back to the original source of communication about how the message was received.

feeding tubes devices that are used to provide nutrition directly into the stomach or small intestine of patients who cannot chew or swallow.

fetus the developing human organism from 60 days gestation to birth.

fever a body temperature that is higher than normal due to internal body processes, such as infection or hyperthyroidism.

fibrin insoluble protein fibers that form the structure of blood clots.

fibrinolytic a substance that breaks down blood clots by initiating the body's normal mechanism for dissolving blood clots.

fibrous cap a thin layer of tissue over the top of an atherosclerotic plaque.

field impression an EMS provider's provisional diagnosis of a patient's medical problem upon which the medical treatment plan is based.

field training the portion of health care provider training that takes place in the practice setting; in EMS, refers to practical experience responding to EMS calls.

fight-or-flight response a sympathetic nervous system response to a stressor that causes physiologic changes, such as increased heart rate, increased blood flow to skeletal muscle, and other responses that prepare the body to react to the stressor.

filtrate a fluid that has passed through a filter, such as the filter created by the membranes of the nephron in the kidney. Kidney filtrate is similar to plasma, but with less protein.

finance/administration an incident command system section used in large-scale responses; responsible for accounting and administrative activities.

financial abuse the illegal or improper use of an individual's money, property, or resources; most often involves the elderly.

first-degree burns See *superficial burns.*

fixed-wing aircraft an airplane (prop or jet).

flail chest a condition that occurs when two or more adjacent ribs are each broken in two or more places, resulting in a bony segment being detached from the rib cage.

flame burns tissue damage that occurs when the body is exposed directly to fire.

flash burns tissue damage that occurs as a result of exposure to the heat and flame from a gas or liquid that ignites and burns very rapidly.

flat bones bones that have a width that is greater than their thickness; the sternum, scapula, and ribs.

flow-restricted oxygen-powered ventilation device (FROPVD) a high-pressure oxygen delivery system that is manually triggered to provide positive pressure ventilation.

fluency disorder stuttering speech.

focused physical exam a search for signs of illness or injury that is limited to the anatomical area or body system that is the source of the patient's chief complaint.

Foley catheter a clear plastic tube passed through the urethra and anchored in the bladder with an inflatable balloon to allow urine to drain into an external collection bag.

fomite an inanimate object that can transfer infectious material, resulting in disease.

fontanels areas where the immature skull bones of a fetus or infant are connected by membranous tissue to allow for compression of the bones during childbirth and rapid growth of the skull and brain after birth.

foramen magnum the large opening at the base of the skull that allows the brainstem to be continuous with the spinal cord.

Fournier's gangrene a serious infection of the subcutaneous tissues of the peritoneum.

Fowler's position a semi-sitting position with the head of the bed elevated; high Fowler's places the torso upright, regular (semi) Fowler's elevates the torso at a 45 degree angle or higher, and low Fowler's elevates the torso at 30 degrees.

fracture any disruption in the continuity of a bone.

French units (Fr.) units of measuring the diameter of medical devices such as suction and urinary catheters. 1 Fr. is equal to 0.33 mm.

frontal impact a vehicle collision that occurs when the object hit causes damage to the front of the vehicle. Also called a *head-on collision.*

full-thickness burns tissue destruction from thermal, chemical, electrical, or radiation energy that involves all layers of the skin. Also called *third-degree burns.*

fulminant severe, with a rapid onset.

G

gangrene the death of tissue; tissue necrosis.

gas burns tissue damage, including airway tissue, from exposure to hot gases.

gas gangrene tissue necrosis associated with gas-producing bacteria.

gastrostomy a surgical procedure performed to insert a feeding tube directly into the stomach.

GCS short for *Glasgow Coma Scale.*

general adaptation syndrome (GAS) a three-phase model (alarm, resistance, exhaustion) of the physiological response to stress.

generalized seizures seizure activity involving the entire cerebrum and which can result in loss of consciousness.

gestation the length of time from conception to birth; pregnancy.

Glasgow Coma Scale (GCS) a numeric rating scale to evaluate level of responsiveness.

glaucoma increased intraocular pressure leading to damage of the optic nerve and blindness.

glucagon a hormone secreted by alpha cells of the pancreas in response to low blood glucose levels. One of its primary actions is to stimulate breakdown of glycogen into glucose.

gluconeogenesis the synthesis (creation) of glucose from amino and fatty acids.

glycogenolysis the breakdown of glycogen stores into glucose.

glycolysis the breakdown of the sugar molecule glucose ($C_6H_{12}O_6$).

goiter an enlargement of the thyroid gland, which may be associated with both hypothyroid and hyperthyroid conditions.

Good Samaritan laws laws intended to protect those who volunteer assistance in an emergency against claims of negligence.

gout arthritis caused by uric acid crystals deposited in a joint.

governmental immunity statutory prohibition of legal action against government agencies.

gradient a graduated change in the degree of a property present.

Graves' disease a form of hyperthyroidism.

gravida a pregnant woman; number of pregnancies.

gravidity the total number of times a woman has been pregnant, regardless of the outcome. Also called *grava.*

greenstick fracture a partial break of a bone, typically seen in pediatric patients.

Grey-Turner's sign ecchymosis of the flanks, indicating retroperitoneal hemorrhage.

grief the emotional response to a loss.

gross negligence injury caused by a provider's disregard for the well-being of others.

gross refers to something that is obvious on physical examination without the use of magnification, stethoscope, or other devices.

H

habituation decreased response to a drug following repeated doses.

half-life the time that it takes for the level of a drug in the blood to decrease by 50 percent.

hallucinations perceptions of a sensation in the absence of actual stimuli.

hantavirus pulmonary syndrome (HPS) pulmonary edema, shock, and organ failure resulting from infection with a hantavirus.

hazardous material any substance (solid, liquid, or gas) capable of harming people, property, or the environment.

head-tilt/chin-lift maneuver a technique used to manually position the head and jaw to open the airway.

head-to-toe exam careful, systematic investigation of the body from head to toe to search for signs of illness or injury. Also called a *detailed physical exam.*

health a state of complete physical, mental, and social well-being and not merely the absence of disease or infirmity.

health care proxy a document in which the patient designates another individual to make health care decisions in the event he becomes incapacitated.

Health Insurance Portability and Accountability Act (HIPAA) federal legislation that regulates the security, distribution, and access to protected health information.

Healthy People 2010/2020 a report on the health status of people in the United States and recommendations for actions to improve health that is published every 10 years by the U.S. Department of Health and Human Services Office of Disease Prevention and Health Promotion.

hearing impairment partial or total loss of the ability to perceive sound. Also called *deafness*.

heat cramps the least severe of all heat-related emergencies; classified as muscle cramping caused by overexertion and dehydration in a hot environment.

heat exhaustion a condition considered to be a moderate heat-related illness that is characterized by inadequate perfusion that results in a mild state of shock.

heat stroke a life-threatening emergency that occurs when the body's thermoregulatory mechanisms cease to work as a result of exposure to a hot environment.

hematemesis vomiting blood, either fresh or partially digested.

hematochezia bloody stool.

hematoma a collection of blood in the tissues causing swelling.

hematuria blood in the urine.

hemoglobin an iron-containing protein molecule in red blood cells to which oxygen can bind reversibly.

hemolytic uremic syndrome (HUS) a serious condition resulting from toxins of *E. coli* strain 0157:H7. Manifestations include renal failure, pulmonary edema, and anemia.

hemophilias conditions characterized by a predisposition toward excessive or uncontrolled bleeding.

hemoptysis blood in the sputum.

hemorrhagic shock inadequate tissue perfusion caused by blood loss.

hemostasis the process by which the body stops bleeding. Hemostasis has three steps: vasoconstriction, platelet aggregation, and fibrin clot formation.

hemostatic agents substances that promote the clotting process when applied to a bleeding injury.

hemothorax the accumulation of blood in the pleural space.

Henry's law a law of physics that states the solubility of a gas in a liquid at a particular temperature is proportional to the pressure of that gas above the liquid.

hepatitis inflammation of the liver, either infectious or noninfectious.

hiatal hernia condition in which the stomach slides through the diaphragmatic hiatus (opening that allows the esophagus to pass through) into the thoracic cavity.

high-altitude cerebral edema (HACE) an swelling of the brain tissue in response to a high-altitude environment, leading to an increase in intracranial pressure.

high-altitude pulmonary edema (HAPE) an increase in lung interstitial fluid (noncardiogenic pulmonary edema) that occurs at altitudes of 2,500 meters (8,200 feet) or greater.

HIPAA short for *Health Insurance Portability and Accountability Act.*

histamine a substance released from certain white blood cells that causes vasodilation, smooth muscle constriction, increased gastric acid secretion, increased mucus production, and tissue swelling.

history of the present illness the sequence of events leading up to a patient's current problem.

homeostasis the state of dynamic equilibrium maintained by the body through processes of feedback and adjustment.

hordeolum an acute infection of a gland in the eyelid; a sty.

hormones any of a variety of molecules that act as chemical messengers when secreted into the blood by endocrine tissue.

hospice a philosophy of end-of-life care with a focus on palliative (relief of symptoms) care and social, spiritual, and emotional support for the terminally ill patient and his family.

hot zone the area of a hazardous materials incident where the chemical is released and contamination can occur. Also called the *exclusion zone.*

hybrid vehicles vehicles that use an on-board rechargeable energy storage system (RESS) and a fuel-based power source for propulsion.

hydrocephalus an increase in cerebrospinal fluid within the ventricles of the brain due to an imbalance between CSF production and drainage or absorption.

hydrostatic pressure the pressure exerted by nonmoving water.

hypercapnia an increased level of carbon dioxide in the blood.

hyperemesis gravidarum abnormally persistent, severe nausea and vomiting of pregnancy.

hyperextension movement of a joint beyond its normal range of motion to a greater angle of the opposing structures than possible under normal circumstances.

hyperflexion movement of a joint beyond its normal range of motion to a lesser angle of the opposing structures than possible under normal circumstances.

hyperglycemia a high level of glucose in the blood, greater than 140 mg/dL.

hyperpyrexia an extremely high fever, above 41.1°C or 106°F.

hypersensitivity an allergy.

hypertension high blood pressure.

hypertensive encephalopathy neurologic signs and symptoms resulting from acutely high blood pressure.

hyperthermia body temperature that is higher than normal, generally due to factors other than increased metabolism, such as prolonged exposure to an extremely hot environment.

hyperthyroidism the oversecretion of thyroid hormones, leading to signs and symptoms associated with increased metabolic rate.

hypertonic a solution that has a higher concentration of solutes than the solution to which it is being compared.

hyperventilation syndrome (HVS) condition in which ventilation exceeds metabolic needs, often resulting in hypocapnia.

hypocapnia a decreased level of carbon dioxide in the blood.

hypoglycemia a condition of low blood glucose, less than 70 mg/dL. (Treatment is usually not indicated unless blood glucose level is 60 mg/dL or less and the patient is symptomatic.)

hypotension low blood pressure.

hypothalamus a part of the brain involved in regulation of endocrine (hormonal) and autonomic nervous system functions.

hypothermia body temperature that is lower than normal.

hypothyroidism a condition in which an insufficient amount of thyroid hormones are secreted, resulting in signs and symptoms that reflect slowed metabolism.

hypotonic a solution that has a lower concentration of solutes than the solution to which it is compared.

hypoxia a decreased level of oxygen at the cellular level.

I

iatrogenic any adverse condition resulting from medical treatment provided.

icterus yellow discoloration of the sclera of the eye resulting from liver disease.

idiosyncratic reaction an unusual, unexpected reaction to a medication.

illusions misinterpretations of stimuli.

immunocompromise the suppression of immune system function resulting in increased susceptibility to infection and cancers.

impacted fracture a broken bone in which the overall length of the bone is decreased by compression of the bone ends toward each other.

impaled object an object, such as a knife, tree limb, or piece of metal, that has penetrated the tissues and remains embedded with a portion of the object protruding from the wound.

incendiary devices weapons intended to start a fire.

incident command system (ICS) a standardized management approach to organizing the response to an emergency by allowing for coordinated integration and management of all resources, equipment, personnel from multiple agencies, communications, and procedures. The five sections of an ICS are command, finance/administration, logistics, operations, and planning.

incident commander (IC) the individual responsible for the coordination of the entire incident response.

incomplete spinal-cord injury damage to the spinal cord that does not extend through the entire diameter of the affected area.

incontinence the loss of ability to control urination or defecation.

incubation period the time from exposure to an infectious disease to the onset of signs and symptoms.

indications the conditions that must be present for a medication to be administered.

indirect injury trauma that occurs away from the point of contact with an object due to forces transmitted through the tissues.

indirect medical direction physician guidance of emergency medical care through protocols or standing orders, rather than through direct, real-time contact with EMS providers; also called *offline medical direction*.

indirect transmission transfer of pathogens between two individuals by way of an intermediary fomite or vector.

infant a child from one month to one year of age.

infectious illnesses diseases caused by micro-organisms, such as bacteria, viruses, fungi, or parasites. Also called *infectious diseases*.

infiltration introduction of a substance not normally found in tissues.

inflammation the response of the body to injury as part of the repair and healing process.

information officer (IO) the person responsible for communicating information about a response to the public and press.

inotropy pertaining to the force of myocardial contraction.

insulin a hormone secreted by the beta cells of the pancreas in response to increased blood glucose levels. Insulin is necessary for adequate amounts of glucose to enter cells.

interfacility transfers ambulance transportation of patients between one health care facility and another, or between home and scheduled medical appointments.

interfacility transportation ambulance transportation of chronically or acutely ill patients from one health care institution to another.

interference anything that disrupts the transmission or receipt of a message.

interoperability the ability to exchange information between communication systems.

intervertebral disk a cartilagenous disk that separates the vertebrae from each other, acting as a shock absorber that prevents the vertebrae from damage.

intrinsic renal failure kidney failure caused by problems within the kidney, such as damage to the nephrons.

intussusception a telescoping of part of the bowel over itself.

involuntary guarding uncontrollable spasm of the abdominal muscle as a result of peritonitis.

ion a chemical particle that carries an electrical charge.

irreversible shock the state of shock in which, even with proper resuscitation, the patient ultimately cannot survive the amount of tissue damage done.

ischemia severely diminished or absent blood flow to tissues.

ischemic phase the phase of shock in which both the precapillary and postcapillary sphincters constrict to divert blood flow away from the peripheral tissues and gastrointestinal system.

ischemic stroke an obstruction of blood flow to a portion of the brain.

isotonic a solution that has the same solute concentration as the solution to which it is compared.

J

jaundice yellow pigmentation of the skin from the deposition of excess bilirubin that occurs in liver disease.

JumpSTART triage system the triage system that was created to be used on any patient who appears to be a child.

JVD short for *jugular venous distention* or *jugular vein distention*.

K

Kehr's sign referred pain to the shoulder caused by blood irritating the diaphragm; indicative of splenic injury.

ketones acidic substances that accumulate in the blood when fats are used for energy in large quantities.

kinetic energy the energy of objects in motion.

kinetics the physics of how objects in motion are affected by outside forces and how energy is distributed when objects collide.

Korotkoff sounds the series of tapping sounds that can be heard during auscultation of the blood pressure as blood under pressure returns to the artery that was occluded by the blood pressure cuff as the cuff is deflated.

Krebs cycle a complex series of reactions in the mitochondria of cells in which pyruvic acid (from anaerobic metabolism) is converted to energy. Also called the *citric acid cycle* or *tricarboxycilic acid (TCA) cycle*.

Kussmaul's respirations regular, deep, rapid respirations that reflect the body's attempt to compensate for metabolic acidosis in diabetic ketoacidosis (DKA).

kyphosis an abnormal convex curvature of the thoracic spine that can cause a hunchback appearance.

L

labyrinthitis the inflammation of the lining of the maze of canals in the inner ear.

lacerations open injuries to skin and, in some cases, underlying tissues that result from cutting or tearing. Lacerations can be caused by penetrating or blunt mechanisms of injury.

lactic acid a chemical formed from pyruvate in anaerobic metabolism; the cause of acidosis in shock.

language disorder the inability to understand spoken or written communication.

laryngitis inflammation of the larynx, often with hoarseness or loss of the voice.

laryngospasm the involuntary closure of the vocal cords over the glottis.

laryngotracheobronchitis croup.

latent inactive or dormant.

lateral impact a motor vehicle collision in which the vehicle is struck in the side. Also called a *T-bone collision*.

law of conservation of energy an law of physics that states that energy can neither be created nor destroyed, it can be changed from from one form to another.

law of inertia Newton's first law of motion, which states a body in motion will remain in motion and a body at rest will remain at rest unless acted upon by an outside force.

Le Fort criteria criteria for classifying fractures of the midface.

Le Fort I fractures breaks involving the maxilla only; may result in slight instability and deformity.

Le Fort II fractures break of the maxilla and nasal bones.

Le Fort III fractures a complicated set of breaks of the facial bones that results in separation of the facial bones from the underlying cranium.

Lead II the flow of cardiac electrical impulses along an axis between an electrode on the right upper chest (right arm) and the left lower chest (left leg).

leading questions questions phrased (usually inadvertently) to exert influence on the patient's answer.

left lateral recumbent (LLR) position a position in which the patient is lying on the left side with the arms and legs positioned to prevent rolling forward or backward. Also called *recovery position*.

lesions defined areas of injury or diseased tissue.

leukotriene inhibitors medications that prevent the release of certain chemicals that increase the body's inflammatory process; used to decrease lung inflammation in asthma.

level of responsiveness (LOR) a patient's ability to detect and respond to environmental stimuli, such as sound and pain. LOR is assessed as part of the mental status. Also called *level of consciousness*.

liability legal responsibility; being legally responsible.

libel defamation through a written document.

licensure the process through which a governmental agency grants permission for qualified individuals to engage in an occupation.

life expectancy the statistical calculation of the length of time a person can expect to live based on his year of birth, where he lives, ethnicity, and other factors.

life span the maximum biologically determined amount of time human beings could live under ideal conditions.

lightening the descent of the presenting part of the fetus into the maternal pelvis, which may occur up to three weeks prior to the onset of labor or not until after labor begins.

linear laceration an injury in which the tissues are separated in a straight line, such as a cut from a knife.

linear skull fracture the a break in a cranial bone that travels in a straight or nearly straight line.

liquefaction necrosis breakdown of tissues into fluid form as a result of exposure to a strong alkali substance.

living will an advance health care directive written by an individual who is competent to make decisions, which outlines his wishes regarding end-of-life care.

livor mortis discoloration of the skin after death caused by pooling of blood from the effects of gravity (dependent lividity).

logistics section the incident command system section responsible for acquiring and distributing essential supplies and equipment needed during the response.

long bones bones that have a greater length than diameter, such as the femur, humerus, radius, ulna, tibia, and fibula.

LOR short for *level of responsiveness*.

lumen the open channel within a structure, such as an artery or vein.

lymphadenopathy a swelling of the lymph nodes.

M

malfeasance performing an improper act that causes injury.

Mallory-Weiss tear laceration of the esophageal mucosa at the junction of the stomach and esophagus, usually due to forceful vomiting.

manual stabilization (of the cervical spine) placing the hands on either side of a patient's head to restrict movement of the head and neck when injury to the cervical spine is suspected.

mastoiditis an infection of the mastoid process of the temporal bone.

material safety data sheets (MSDS) an informational form created by the chemical manufacturer that describes the physical properties, hazards, and safe handling of a hazardous chemical.

mean arterial pressure (MAP) the average amount of pressure exerted against the walls of the arteries. Calculated as the diastolic blood pressure plus one third of the pulse pressure. MAP is determined by cardiac output and peripheral vascular resistance.

mechanism of action the way in a which drug has its therapeutic effect on the body.

mechanism of injury (MOI) the forces and energy that cause trauma.

meconium the contents of the first fetal or neonatal bowel movement.

Medicaid a program that funds medical care for eligible low-income families and individuals. Medicaid is jointly funded by the federal and state governments and administered by individual state governments.

medical priority dispatch systems (MPDS) methodical systems of call taking, allowing dispatchers to triage patients and send the appropriate EMS response.

Medicare a federally funded and administered program to fund medical care for patients over 65 years of age.

medium-duty ambulance an ambulance box mounted on a large truck chassis.

melena black, tarry stool due to the presence of blood exposed to digestive juices.

Ménière disease a condition of the inner ear leading to tinnitus, vertigo, and hearing loss.

meningismus signs reflective of inflammation of the meninges; includes headache, photophobia, and stiff neck.

mental status the degree to which a patient is aware of and able to respond to the environment, including higher cognitive functions and emotions.

metabolic acidosis a decreased blood pH and decrease in bicarbonate level in the blood.

metabolism the sum of all chemical and physical changes in the body.

micro-organisms microscopic living things, such as bacteria.

millimeters of mercury (mmHg) a measure of pressure as determined by the amount of pressure needed to raise a column of mercury 1 millimeter.

minute volume the amount of air moved in and out of the lungs over 1 minute; determined as the tidal volume multiplied by the respiratory rate.

misfeasance performing a legitimate act in a manner that causes injuries.

mobile data terminals electronic communication devices that send and receive a limited amount of data using a small screen that displays text information.

mobile radios radios mounted in a vehicle.

mode of transport the method utilized to move a patient from the scene to the closest, most appropriate medical facility.

modified jaw-thrust maneuver a technique used to manually position the jaw to open the airway in patients with suspected cervical-spine injury.

mourning the rituals and outward displays associated with grief.

mucous membranes mucus-secreting epithelial linings of body cavities exposed to the external environment, such as the oral cavity, around the eyes, genitals, and intestinal tract.

multiparous describes a woman who has given birth more than once.

multiple organ dysfunction syndrome (MODS) a complication of shock in which more than one organ system has been severely damaged by hypoxia and cannot carry out their functions.

multiple-casualty incident (MCI) any event in which the number of patients exceeds the capabilities of the resources on scene.

multisystem trauma a condition in which more than one body system has been injured.

myocardial contusion a bruise of the heart muscle due to blunt trauma.

myoclonus involuntary muscle jerking or twitching.

myoglobin the pigment in the muscle that can bind with oxygen.

myxedema coma a severe, life-threatening form of decreased metabolism resulting from hypothyroidism.

myxedema a doughy edema of the tissues in hypothyroid conditions; often associated with coarseness of the skin.

N

narrative report a written outline of the events of an EMS call, usually following one of several standard formats.

nasopharyngeal airway a short, flexible beveled tube inserted through the nose so that the beveled end rests in the pharynx to prevent the tongue from occluding the airway. Also called a *nasal airway*.

National Disaster Medical System (NDMS) a section of the U.S. Department of Health and Human Services responsible for managing the federal medical response to an emergency or disaster.

National Highway Traffic Safety Administration (NHTSA) a division of the U.S. Department of Transportation, which oversees many aspects of safety related travel on U.S. roads and highways, including the availability of emergency medical services.

national incident management system (NIMS) the uniform method of organizing the response and supervision of resources during a multiple casualty incident or disaster so different agencies (including fire, EMS, and law enforcement) can work together effectively under the same organizational structure using the same terminology.

National Registry of Emergency Medical Technicians (NREMT) a national organization that was established to ensure uniform credentialing standards for EMS personnel.

National Standard Curriculum (NSC) a document that prescribes the content, process, and structure for a particular level of EMS training; NSC at all levels is being phased out as the National EMS Education Standards are implemented.

nature of the illness the general type of medical problem a patient is suffering from on a given call.

NDMS short for *National Disaster Medical System*.

necrotizing fasciitis a rapidly spreading infection of fascia with tissue death and separation of tissues from the fascia.

neglect the failure of a caregiver to provide proper care to an individual for whom they are responsible.

neonate an infant from birth to one month of age. Also called *newborn*.

nephritis inflammation of the kidneys. Includes types affecting specific structures within the kidney, such as pyelonephritis, glomerulonephritis, and interstitial nephritis.

nerve agents chemical weapons with properties similar to organophosphate pesticides that produce severe cholinergic nervous system effects.

neural foramina openings between vertebrae through which nerves leave the spine and extend to other parts of the body. Also called an *intervertebral foramen*.

neurogenic hypotension hypotension as a result of vasodilation due to loss of sympathetic nervous control of blood vessel diameter.

neurogenic shock hypoperfusion due to neurogenic hypotension.

neurologic dysfunction abnormal neurologic function.

neurotransmitters any of several molecules that act as chemical messengers when secreted by the synaptic terminals of the axon of a neuron into the synapse between the neuron and an adjacent neuron, gland, or other tissue (such as muscle).

Newton's second law of motion a law of physics that illustrates how forces are distributed during a collision.

NHTSA short for *National Highway Traffic Safety Administration*.

NIMS short national incident management system.

nitrogen narcosis a diving emergency in which a state of stupor results from nitrogen's effect on cerebral function. Also called *rapture of the deep*.

nocturia frequent urination after going to bed.

noncritical patients patients who require medical attention, but who do not have an immediate threat to life or limb.

nonemergency (or nonemergent) response driving the ambulance under routine conditions that do not require that use of warning devices to clear traffic.

nonemergency moves use of a planned technique to move a patient from one location to another; generally from the position in which he was found to the wheeled ambulance stretcher, or from the stretcher to a hospital bed.

nonfeasance failure to perform an act that one is obligated to perform; wrongdoing by omission.

nonketotic hyperosmolar coma (NKHC) a complication of type 2 diabetes in which the blood glucose level may reach 1,000 mg/dL, resulting in diuresis, dehydration, thirst, and electrolyte disorders without ketoacidosis.

nonsteroidal anti-inflammatory drugs (NSAIDs) medications with pain-relieving and fever-reducing properties and which decrease the inflammatory response.

nonverbal cues messages conveyed by means other than spoken or written words.

normal flora micro-organisms that normally inhabit the body without producing disease.

normal sinus rhythm (NSR) the expected electrical pattern produced by a healthy heart; originates in the sinoatrial (sinus) node at a rate 60 to 100 beats per minute, producing a characteristic pattern of ECG waveforms.

nosocomial infection an infection acquired in a health care setting.

nuclear weapons explosive devices that derive their power from an atomic reaction such as fission or fusion.

nystagmus rapid, involuntary eye movements that can be lateral, vertical, or oscillating. Slight nystagmus can be normal, but it is often a sign of a neurologic or toxicologic problem.

O

oblique fracture a break that runs across the bone at an angle other than 90° to the axis of the bone.

obtunded having a decreased level of awareness and ability to respond to stimuli.

occult hidden; not obvious.

off-line medical direction physician guidance of emergency medical care through protocols or standing orders, rather than through direct, real-time contact with EMS providers. Also called *indirect medical direction* or *prospective medical direction*.

omega fatty acids a family of unsaturated fats that have a number of beneficial health effects, including decreasing heart disease and negative effects of inflammation; omega fatty acids are found in fish, nuts, flaxseed, fruits, and vegetables.

online medical direction real-time physician supervision of emergency medical care. Also called *direct medical direction* or *concurrent medical direction*.

open chest injury a traumatic condition in which either blunt or penetrating forces have caused a breach in the integrity of the chest wall, which may or may not be deep enough extend through the pleural cavity.

open fracture a break in the continuity of a bone in which there is an associated laceration or other open injury of the overlying tissues.

open injury a wound in which the integrity of the skin has been breached, such as a laceration, avulsion, or abrasion.

open pneumothorax a condition in which an opening in the chest wall is large enough to allow air to move through it into the pleural space with each inspiration. As the air accumulates within the pleural cavity, the lung is compressed, resulting in atelectasis of the affected area. Also called a *sucking chest wound* because air is sucked into the wound under negative pressure during inspiratory effort.

open skull fracture a break in the continuity of cranial bones in which the overlying scalp is lacerated or avulsed.

open thoracic injury trauma to the chest wall in which an opening is created between the environment and the pleural cavity.

open-ended questions questions that can lead to a broad range of possible responses.

opportunistic infections diseases that occur from pathogens that are normally destroyed by the immune system or kept in check by normal flora.

oropharyngeal airway a curved plastic device with two lateral or a single central channel that is inserted into the mouth with the tip resting in the pharynx to prevent the tongue from occluding the airway. Also called an *oral airway*.

orthostatic hypotension a decrease in systolic blood pressure by 20 mmHg or more, or an increase in heart rate by 20 beats per minute or more, after a patient rises from a supine to a standing position. Also called *postural hypotension*.

osmolarity the concentration of ions in a solution.

osmosis the movement of water across a semipermeable membrane from an area of lower solute concentration to an area of higher solute concentration to achieve equilibrium of solute concentration across the membrane.

osmotic pressure the force with which water passes through a semipermeable membrane.

osteoarthritis an age-related degenerative joint disease with loss of articular cartilage.

osteoporosis the loss of bone density resulting in fragile bones.

ostomy bags devices that are connected to an opening in the abdominal wall to collect feces directly from the patient's colon.

otitis externa an infection of the external ear canal.

otitis media an infection of the middle ear.

otoscope a lighted instrument used to inspect the ear canal and tympanic membrane.

ototoxic the property by which a substance, such as a drug, can cause temporary or permanent hearing loss.

over-the-counter (OTC) medication any drug that can be legally purchased without a prescription.

oxidation a particular type of chemical reaction in which the atoms of a substance lose electrons.

oxidative phosphorylation the cellular process by which adenosine triphosphate (ATP) is produced from adenosine diphosphate (ADP).

oxytocin the posterior pituitary hormone that plays a role in labor and lactation.

P

packaging (the patient) preparing the patient for transport using any of a number of devices for lifting and moving him, while ensuring that medical treatment is continued.

palliative care care aimed at making patients as comfortable as possible.

pallor pale skin.

palpate a physical examination technique in which the examiner uses his hands to feel for signs of illness or injury, or to obtain the pulse.

palpitations the sensation of feeling the heart beat within the chest.

para describes a woman who has delivered an infant of greater than 20 weeks gestation or weighing over 500 grams.

paradoxical movement (of the chest) the movement of a segment of the chest wall in a direction opposite that of the rest of the chest wall during inspiration and expiration.

Paramedic an allied health care professional who provides complex assessments and interventions for critical and emergent patients.

paranoid falsely believing that there is a threat to oneself, such as being spied on or having enemies that do not exist.

paraphimosis the constriction of the foreskin behind the glans penis, causing restriction in lymphatic drainage and circulation, resulting in pain, swelling, and potential necrosis of the glans.

parasympatholytics medications that reduce the actions of the parasympathetic nervous system.

parasympathomimetics classification of medications that are agonists to the parasympathetic nervous system.

parenteral outside the gastrointestinal system.

paresthesia tingling sensation.

parietal peritoneum the outermost lining of the abdominal structures that adheres to the inner walls of the abdominal cavity.

parity refers to the number of times a woman has given birth. Also called *para*.

Parkland formula a calculation used to determine the amount of fluid a patient with extensive burns should receive within the first 24 hours following the injury.

paroxysmal nocturnal dyspnea (PND) sudden waking at night with difficulty breathing, which is typically relieved by assuming an upright position; a classic sign of left-sided heart failure.

partial amputation condition in which a body part, usually a digit or limb, has been partly, but not completely, separated from the body.

partial pressure (Pa) the proportion of the total pressure of a mixture of gases that can be accounted for by an individual gas.

partial seizures abnormal neuronal discharge localized to a single area of the brain.

partial-thickness burns thermal, chemical, radiation, or electrical injury that involve the epidermis and dermis. Also called *second-degree burns.*

parturition the process of expelling a fetus through the birth canal; giving birth.

past medical history an account of a patient's previous and pre-existing health problems.

pathogens disease-causing micro-organisms.

pathologic fracture a bone that is broken with little force because of a diseased state of the bone.

pathology the study of disease states.

pathophysiology the study of the impact of disease on the body and the body's responses to the disease state.

patient assessment a systematic process of collecting relevant patient information in order to determine a patient's medical condition and establish priorities for treatment and transport.

patient care report (PCR) a written or electronic record of specific types of information that documents an EMS call.

peak expiratory flow rate (PEFR) the maximal rate at which air can be forcefully exhaled from the lungs, measured in liters per minute.

peak flow meter (PFM) a device to measure maximum expiratory flow rate.

peak load time at which the volume of EMS calls is the highest.

pediatric assessment triangle (PAT) a scheme for forming a general impression of the level of distress in a child by evaluating the general appearance, work of breathing, and circulation to the skin.

penetrating trauma an injury caused when an object, such as a knife or bullet is driven into the body creating an opening in the skin and, often, underlying tissues.

pepsin a powerful digestive enzyme in the stomach that breaks down proteins.

peptic ulcer erosion of the gastric or duodenal mucosa.

percutaneous through the skin.

perfusion provision of nutrients, oxygen, and other substances to the cellular level through adequate tissue capillary circulation.

pericardial tamponade see cardiac tamponade.

peripheral pulses the pressure waves felt in smaller arteries that are farther away from the heart, including the radial, brachial, popliteal, posterior tibial, and dorsalis pedis arteries.

peristalsis rhythmic smooth muscle contractions that propel the contents of hollow, tubular organs forward.

peritoneal cavity the space between the parietal and visceral peritoneum.

peritoneum the double-layer membrane that lines the abdominal cavity.

peritonitis irritation and inflammation of the peritoneal lining.

permissive hypotension maintaining a hemorrhagic shock patient's systolic blood pressure between 80 and 90 mmHg to avoid an increase in bleeding that is likely if the blood pressure is above this level.

personal protective equipment (PPE) articles worn for protection against safety risks; depending on the task, can include boots, safety goggles, hearing protection, and equipment used for body substance isolation (BSI).

pertinent negative signs or symptoms that are expected to accompany a particular problem, but are not present.

pertussis a respiratory infection that results in coughing fits that can interfere with breathing; characterized by a "whooping" sound as the patient tries to catch his breath after a fit of coughing. Also called *whooping cough.*

petechiae pinpoint hemorrhages in the skin.

pH the potential of hydrogen as measured by hydrogen ion concentration; a measure of the acidity or alkalinity of a substance on a scale from 0 to 14, with 0 being the most acidic, 7 being neutral, and 14 being the most alkaline.

pharmacodynamics the actions that drugs have on the body.

pharmacokinetics the branch of pharmacology concerned with the way drugs are absorbed, distributed, metabolized, and eliminated from the body.

pharmacology the study of the origin, nature, properties, and actions of drugs and their effects on living organisms.

pharyngitis a sore throat (inflammation of the throat).

phimosis a condition in which the foreskin is constricted and cannot be retracted from the glans penis.

phobias intense, unrealistic fears of a specific object or situation, such as flying, germs, or enclosed spaces.

photophobia hypersensitivity of the eyes to light.

physical abuse deliberate, unwarranted force that results in bodily injury.

physician medical director a licensed medical doctor or doctor of osteopathic medicine who assumes an oversight role in an EMS system to provide guidelines for medical treatment and continuous quality improvement activities.

phytonutrients naturally occurring plant substances that may play important roles in health through antioxidant and anti-inflammatory properties.

placenta the temporary organ of pregnancy that allows the exchange of nutrients, gases, and wastes between the fetus and the mother.

placenta previa a condition in which the placenta partially or completely covers the cervix.

plaintiff the party who brings a civil action against someone else.

planning section the incident command system division that analyzes data collected from responses and makes recommendations to change the response plans in order to improve future responses.

plantar flex bending the ankle in such a way as to move the bottom (plantar surface) of the foot downward.

plaque an abnormal collection of fatty tissue within the wall of a blood vessel.

pleuritic used to describe the pain characteristic of inflammation of the pleura; often described as sharp, well-localized, and worsened by inspiration.

pneumothorax an accumulation of air between the pleural layers that occupies space normally filled by the lungs.

polycystic renal disease a hereditary disease in which cysts form within the kidney, eventually destroying the nephrons.

polypharmacy the use of multiple medications.

portable radio a handheld two-way radio used by emergency personnel to communicate outside the vehicle.

portal hypertension increased pressure throughout the portal venous system of the digestive tract as a result of liver disease.

positive end-expiratory pressure (PEEP) maintaining positive pressure in the airway during expiration to prevent collapse of the smaller airways and alveoli.

positive pressure ventilation (PPV) artificial ventilation by forcing air into the airway.

post-traumatic stress disorder (PTSD) a severe, delayed response to a stressor that significantly interferes with functioning.

postictal the period of altered mental status following a seizure.

postrenal renal failure kidney failure caused by urinary obstruction, such as that from BPH or renal calculi.

postural hypotension a decrease in systolic blood pressure by 20 mmHg or more, or an increase in heart rate by 20 beats per minute or more, after a patient rises from a supine to a standing position. Also called *orthostatic hypotension.*

potentiation the enhancement of one medication as a result of being combined with another.

pre-eclampsia a hypertensive disorder of pregnancy characterized by high blood pressure, edema, protein in the urine, headache, visual disturbances, and hyperactive deep tendon reflexes. Untreated pre-eclampsia can progress to eclampsia.

precipitous delivery a delivery that occurs within 3 hours of the onset of labor.

prefix syllables or letters added to the beginning of a word to modify its meaning.

prehospital the environment and circumstances in which ill or injured patients are cared for by EMS providers between the onset of the emergency and arrival at the hospital.

preload the amount of blood in the left ventricle at the end of diastole.

premature newborn an infant delivered at 20 weeks gestation or greater and weighing at least 500 grams.

premature ventricular contraction (PVC) a depolarization of the myocardium earlier than expected because of an impulse generated by a cell in the ventricles.

prenatal prior to birth.

prerenal renal failure kidney failure caused by a problem outside the urinary system, such as hypotension resulting from shock or heart failure.

preschooler a child from three to six years of age.

presenting problems conditions that result in the patient's contact with the health care system.

pressure dressing a dressing that is secured snugly directly above the dressings used to control the bleeding to prevent a reoccurrence of bleeding.

preterm labor the onset of labor prior to 37 weeks gestation.

priapism a painful erection of the penis lasting more than 4 hours.

primary assessment a systematic process of determining the severity of a patient's medical condition, particularly with regard to airway, breathing, circulation, and level of consciousness.

primary blast injury trauma caused by the pressure wave from an explosion.

primary injury with reference to spine trauma, trauma to the spinal cord resulting from compression or shearing of the cord.

primary triage the immediate prioritization of patients by severity of injury performed by the firs EMS personnel on scene.

profession an occupation or vocation defined by a specialized set of knowledge and code of ethics or conduct.

prolapsed umbilical cord a condition in which the umbilical cord precedes the presenting part of the fetus into the birth canal.

pronator drift the involuntary pronation of the hand (turning the hand palm downward) when the patient's arms are held out in front of him due to weakness of muscles that oppose pronation.

proprioception the ability to sense the location, orientation, and movement of the body and its parts.

prospective medical direction physician guidance of emergency medical care through protocols or standing orders, rather than through direct, real-time contact with EMS providers. Also called *indirect medical direction* or *off-line medical direction.*

protocols written procedures that guide the management of specific emergency situations.

proximate cause an act or omission of an act that is the cause of injury; an event without which the injury would not have occurred.

psychological abuse the willful infliction of mental or emotional anguish through threat, humiliation, or other verbal or nonverbal means.

psychotic a mental state in which reality is distorted; often referred to as having lost touch with reality.

public access defibrillation a coordinated system in which AEDs are placed in public places where cardiac arrest may occur, such as airports, malls, and schools.

public safety answering point (PSAP) the dispatch center that receives calls requesting emergency services.

pulmonary contusion injury to the lung tissue in which blood leaks from damaged capillaries into the interstitial spaces of the respiratory membrane, decreasing gas exchange, potentially leading to hypoxia.

pulmonary edema an increase in interstitial fluid in the lungs resulting in a greater diffusion distance for oxygen and carbon dioxide across the respiratory membrane.

pulmonary embolism an obstruction of the pulmonary circulation by a blood clot or other material, resulting in ventilation of a nonperfused area of the lung and decreased oxygenation.

pulse oximetry the measurement of oxygen saturation of the hemoglobin using infrared light technology.

pulse pressure the difference between systolic blood pressure and diastolic blood pressure.

pulsus alternans a pulse that is alternately weaker and stronger.

pulsus paradoxus a drop of 10 mmHg or more in the systolic blood pressure during inspiration.

puncture/penetration injury an injury that results from an object being forced into the tissues of the body.

purpura small, blotchy areas of hemorrhage (greater than 3 mm in diameter) in the skin.

pyrexia fever.

pyrogenic reaction sudden onset of fever, chills, backache, headache, nausea, and vomiting as a result of being exposed to foreign proteins, such as those found in bacteria or fungi.

pyruvate the initial substance formed in the anaerobic phase of cellular metabolism, which, in the presence of oxygen, is then converted to acetyl coenzyme A for use in the Krebs cycle for further ATP production. In the absence of oxygen, pyruvate is converted to lactic acid.

Q

quaternary blast injury the fourth phase of injuries that occur from a blast, such as contamination with biological or nuclear materials.

R

radiation with respect to environmental emergencies, heat transfer from the body into still air.

radiation (of pain) the extension of pain from its origin to include other areas of the body.

radiation absorbed dose (rad) a measure of the disposition of 0.01 joules of energy in 1 kg of tissue; roughly equal to roentgen equivalent man (rem).

radiation safety officer a specially trained individual who directs the actions at a hazardous materials incident involving radiation.

radio frequency a specific portion of the electromagnetic field over which radio transmissions can be sent.

radiologic dispersion device (RDD) a conventional explosive such as TNT or dynamite wrapped with radiologic material.

RAIN an acronym that characterizes the response actions on a hazardous materials scene for a nonhazardous materials team member. The letters stand for recognize, avoid, isolate, and notify.

rales noise heard in the lower airways when fluid is present, similar to the fizzing sound of a carbonated beverage. Also called *crackles*.

rapid extrication a systematic procedure used to quickly remove a critical patient from a vehicle while minimizing movement of the spine.

rapid medical exam a quick physical exam of vital areas of the body performed on critical medical patients after the primary assessment.

rapid physical exam a quick physical exam performed on critical medical or trauma patients to identify potentially life-threatening conditions not found in the primary assessment. Includes both rapid medical exam and rapid trauma exam.

rapid trauma exam a quick physical exam of vital areas of the body that is completed on critical trauma patients after the primary assessment. Sometimes called *rapid trauma assessment*.

reactivity the ability of a substance to interact chemically with another substance; the ability to produce a chemical reaction.

rear impact a collision in which a vehicle is struck from behind.

reassessment re-evaluating previous components of the patient assessment process to identify trends in the patient's condition and response to treatments provided.

rebound tenderness pain felt when pressure from palpation is released from the area.

receiver the target of a communicated message.

reciprocity an agreement through which one state accepts the licensure of professionals from another state as evidence of competency for licensure.

recovery position position in which the patient, usually with a decreased level of responsiveness, is placed on his left side to help manage the airway. Also called *left lateral recumbent position*.

referred pain pain that occurs in another part of the body instead of the part in which the problem originates.

reflection mirroring a patient's words back to him to obtain further information.

reflexes an involuntary response to a stimulus.

refresher education instruction that takes place after initial competence has been established to ensure ongoing minimum competence.

registration having one's name listed in a database.

relatively contraindicated the situation in which a procedure or treatment is not usually advised but in which other factors may outweigh the risks or disadvantages associated with it.

renal calculus a stone formed in the kidney. May have various compositions. Causes pain on passing through the ureter, but can usually pass if less than 6 mm in diameter. Plural, *calculi*.

renal colic pain along the length of the ureter associated with renal calculi.

repeaters radio devices that receive low-power signals and rebroadcast them at higher power to increase the range of portable and mobile radios.

repolarization the return of a cell membrane to a polarized state following depolarization.

res ipsa loquitur a Latin term used legally to mean **the thing speaks for itself**; being self-evident.

research a systematic investigation that seeks to discover or revise facts, theories, or practical applications.

respiration the exchange of gases between the body and the environment.

respiratory arrest an absence of breathing; apnea.

respiratory distress difficulty breathing resulting in increased effort to maintain adequate ventilation and oxygenation.

respiratory failure the inability to maintain adequate ventilation and oxygen.

respiratory membrane the tissue layer created by the close proximity of the alveolar sacs and the walls of the capillaries surrounding them, which allows gases to diffuse between the lungs and blood.

respiratory syncytial virus (RSV) an infectious agent that causes bronchiolitis in the pediatric population.

responsibilities the obligations associated with a particular position or status.

resuscitation coordinated medical interventions to stabilize the condition of a critically ill patient, such as those in respiratory failure or arrest, shock, and cardiac arrest.

retro-reflective material specially manufactured textile that reflects nearly all light back to the source, or viewer, without diffusing it.

retrograde amnesia loss of memory for events preceding an injury to the brain, such as a concussion.

retroperitoneal cavity the portion of the abdominal cavity that lies behind the peritoneal tissue and which contains portions of the duodenum and pancreas as well as the kidneys, abdominal aorta, inferior vena cava, and ureters.

retroperitoneal space the posterior division of the abdominal cavity, which is separated from the rest of the abdominal organs by the parietal peritoneum.

retrospective medical direction physician review of the EMS care provided to a patient.

rhabdomyolysis the breakdown of skeletal muscle.

rhonchi coarse, rumbling sounds heard on auscultation, indicating the presence of secretions in the bronchi.

rigging the general term for the equipment used to stabilize crashed vehicles, such as rope, chains, and webbing.

right-sided heart failure inadequate function of the right side of the heart, resulting in redistribution of fluid to the interstitial spaces surrounding the systemic circulation, causing peripheral edema.

rigor mortis temporary muscular rigidity occurring after death, the onset of which may be affected by pre-existing metabolic, as well as environmental, conditions.

riot control agents low-toxicity chemicals, such as oleoresin capsaicin spray (pepper spray), designed for a short duration of action to cause temporary incapacitation in those exposed to it.

roentgen equivalent man (rem) the amount of radiation to which one is exposed and the likely biologic damage; roughly equivalent to radiation absorbed dose (rad).

roles the functions expected of individuals in particular situations.

rollover a type of motor vehicle collision in which the wheels of the vehicle leave the ground and the vehicle tumbles over before coming to a rest.

root word the part of a term that provides its basic meaning.

rotational impact a type of motor vehicle collision that occurs when an off-center collision (usually from the side) causes the vehicle to spin around.

rotor-wing aircraft a helicopter.

rule of nines a method that assigns multiples of 9 percent to regions of the body to determine the amount of body surface area affected by burns.

rule of palm a method of calculating the body surface area of burns that uses the size of the patient's palm as an approximate representation of 1 percent of the body surface area.

S

safety officer (SO) the person at an emergency response who is responsible for the safety of responders and patients alike. This includes ensuring that all response activities are being carried out using the proper safety equipment.

satisficing a blend of the terms *satisfying* and *sufficing*. A decision-making strategy in which the first acceptable, but not necessarily optimal, solution is accepted.

scalds burns caused by hot liquids.

scene size-up evaluating the setting in which a patient is found for the purposes of obtaining information about the operational (including safety) and clinical aspects of the call.

school age a child from 6 to 12 years of age.

sciatica neuralgia (nerve pain) of the sciatic nerve of the lower extremity.

scombroid fish poisoning toxicity due to ingestion of contaminated fish in which bacterial substances convert compounds in fish tissue to histamine. It is more correctly called *histamine fish poisoning* because affected fish can come from families other than *Scombroidei*.

scope of practice the defined tasks and skills that may be performed by licensed individuals with specific levels of training.

second-degree burns See *partial-thickness burns*.

secondary assessment systematically obtaining relevant patient information beyond the initial information obtained in the scene size-up and primary assessment.

secondary blast injury trauma caused by the debris that is thrown from an explosion as a result of the pressure wave.

secondary brain injury an injury caused by hypotension or swelling of the brain due to hypoxia or hypercapnia.

secondary injury with respect to spine trauma, damage to the spinal cord that occurs after the initial injury and is usually the result of swelling, ischemia, or movement of bone into or against the spinal cord.

secondary triage subsequent to primary triage, a re-evaluation of patients' priorities for treatment and transport at the scene of a multiple casualty incident; the patient's priority may remain the same, be increased, or be decreased.

semi-Fowler's position positioned with the head of the bed (ambulance stretcher) elevated at 45 degrees.

sender the individual who initiates a message in communication.

sensory impairment the dysfunction of one or more of the patient's senses such as hearing or speech.

serous fluid a watery serum-like fluid, such as that secreted by the serous membranes of the peritoneum lining the abdominal cavity.

sesamoid bones bones located within a tendon, referred to as sesamoid because of their resemblance to the shape of a sesame seed; include the patella and the pisiform of the wrist.

sexual abuse sexual contact of any kind with a non-consenting adult or any sexual contact with a person who is not legally capable of giving consent for sexual contact.

shipping papers documentation containing information on a particular hazardous material transported by land, sea, or air.

shock a state in which the level of perfusion to the tissues is not adequate to meet metabolic demands.

short bones bones that are not very long in relation to their diameter, such as metacarpals, metatarsals, and phalanges.

shoulder dystocia a condition in which labor and delivery are complicated by large fetal shoulders, which become wedged between the pubis and sacrum.

shunt graft an artificial tube connecting an artery and vein in the arm to allow for hemodialysis.

sick sinus syndrome dysfunction of the sinoatrial node of the heart.

significant blood loss blood loss that is 15 percent or greater of total blood volume.

significant MOIs forms of energy transfer to the body that are associated with life-threatening injuries.

signs indications of illness or injury that can be objectively observed.

silent MI a myocardial infarction that occurs without symptoms.

simple pneumothorax an accumulation of air within the pleural space.

Simple Triage and Rapid Treatment (START) a specific method of prioritizing patients, based on the severity of injury, at a mass casualty incident.

singular command a form of the incident command system used for smaller incidents, in which one agency assumes command of the response.

sinoatrial (SA) node the collection of pacemaker cells in the upper right atrium that serve as the primary pacemaker of the heart.

sinusitis infection of the sinuses.

slander spoken communication that defames another person.

sodium/potassium pump a mechanism of the cell membrane that uses energy to exchange sodium and potassium ions across the cell membrane.

sphygmomanometer a device used to noninvasively measure peripheral arterial blood pressure; a blood pressure cuff.

spinal shock a concussion-like injury to the spinal cord that causes temporary neurologic deficits below the level of injury.

spinal-column injury an injury to one or more vertebrae.

spinal-cord concussion a temporary disruption of normal spinal-cord function below the site of injury.

spinal-cord injury a traumatic condition that results in impairment of spinal cord function, with or without radiological evidence of injury.

spiral fracture a break that has a corkscrew pattern around the bone; commonly caused by rotational forces.

spirometry the measurement of various lung volumes and flow rates.

splint any device used to immobilize a body part.

spondylosis a form of arthritis that affects the vertebrae and intervertebral discs, particularly in the elderly.

spontaneous abortion the loss of a pregnancy from natural causes prior to 20 weeks gestation; miscarriage.

spontaneous pneumothorax accumulation of air in the thoracic cavity that occurs in the absence of trauma, usually due to lung disease (such as cancer or emphysema), but which can also occur in otherwise healthy individuals.

spotter a person who provides instructions and assistance to another individual who cannot see all possible hazards while carrying a patient or backing the ambulance.

sprain the stretching or tearing of the ligaments of a joint.

stable angina a pattern of ischemic chest pain that predictably comes on during exertion, goes away with rest or nitroglycerin, and has about the same duration and intensity from episode to episode.

stagnant phase (of shock) the phase of shock in which the precapillary sphincter fails, allowing blood to enter the microvasculature. The postcapillary sphincter remains closed, causing blood to pool in the capillary beds, where it collects lactic acid and microscopic blood clots are formed.

standard of care the degree of attention and caution that would be exercised by a reasonable person with the same training and in the same circumstances.

Standard Precautions safeguards taken to prevent exposure to communicable diseases based on the assumption that the body fluids of all patients are potentially infectious.

standing orders pre-existing written physician's orders that may be carried out by authorized health care providers without or prior to direct contact with the physician.

Star of Life a six-point (which stand for detection, reporting, response, on-scene care, care in transit, and transfer to definitive care) blue star in the center of which is the Rod of Asclepius, which represents medicine and healing; a symbol of emergency medical services.

static ECG a still image of ECG waveforms printed on graph paper as it moves through an ECG machine.

status asthmaticus a severe, prolonged asthma attack that cannot be broken with repeated doses of beta$_2$ agonists.

status epilepticus a sustained tonic–clonic seizure (greater than 5 minutes) or successive tonic–clonic seizures without an intervening period of consciousness.

statutes of limitations elapsed periods of time after which legal action cannot be pursued.

steam burns thermal injury from contact with superheated water vapor.

stellate laceration a jagged cut in the tissues, so-called because of the star-shaped appearance of such wounds.

sterilizing using a steam or chemical process to kill all micro-organisms on medical supplies, devices, and equipment.

stillbirth an infant of 20 weeks gestation or greater born without signs of life.

strain injury that occurs when muscle fibers are stretched beyond their limitations, resulting in tearing of the fibers.

stress the body's response to a stressor.

stressor something that places a demand on a person psychologically or physiologically.

stridor high-pitched inspiratory sound that indicates swelling in the airway.

subarachnoid hemorrhage bleeding between the brain and the arachnoid layer of the meninges.

subarachnoid space the space beneath the arachnoid mater in which the majority of cerebrospinal fluid is located.

subcutaneous emphysema air that has been trapped in the skin, resulting in tiny bubbles that can be seen and have a crackling feeling when palpated.

subcutaneous layer the innermost layer of skin, predominantly fatty tissue that assists with body temperature regulation.

subdural hematoma an accumulation of blood caused by bleeding between the dura mater and arachnoid mater.

subluxation a partial displacement of bone ends from a joint.

sucking chest wound see open pneumothorax.

sudden cardiac arrest (SCA) an abrupt, unexpected cessation of heart function that often occurs outside the hospital setting.

sudden infant death syndrome (SIDS) the unexpected, unexplained death of an infant younger than 12 months old.

suffix syllables or letters added at the end of a word to modify its meaning.

sulfonylurea a class of oral antihyperglycemic agents that act by stimulating the pancreas to increase insulin production.

summarization with respect to therapeutic communication, presenting the key points made by a patient back to him to check for understanding.

superficial burns tissue injury from thermal, radiation, electrical, or chemical energy that involve only the epidermis. Also called *first-degree burns*.

supine a position in which the patient is placed lying on his back.

supine hypotensive syndrome a decreased cardiac output and low blood pressure that occurs when the weight of the pregnant uterus compresses the inferior vena cava when the mother lays on her back in the third trimester of pregnancy.

support zone See *cold zone*.

surfactant a wetting agent that allows fluid to spread across a surface. Pulmonary surfactant changes the characteristics of the water of the alveolar surface to prevent the surface tension of the fluid from collapsing the alveoli.

sutures with respect to the musculoskeletal system, immovable joints that join the bones of the skull.

sympathetic beta$_2$ receptors proteins on the surface of some types of cells, including bronchiolar smooth muscle cells, that bind with specific substances, such as epinephrine and albuterol, to allow effects such as smooth-muscle relaxation.

sympatholytics medications that reduce the actions of the sympathetic nervous system.

sympathomimetics a classification of medications that mimic the effects of the sympathetic nervous system.

symptoms subjective sensations of an abnormality in body function.

syncope sudden loss of consciousness resulting from a temporary decrease in cerebral perfusion.

synergism the combined action of two drugs such that the effect is greater than the sum of the individual effects of the two medications.

system status management (SSM) a computerized ambulance and personnel deployment system.

systemic lupus erythematosus (SLE) an autoimmune disease that affects many tissues, including the kidneys.

systolic blood pressure the amount of force exerted against arterial walls during contraction of the left ventricle.

T

tachycardia a heart rate that is faster than normal, greater than 100 beats per minute in adults.

T-bone collision See *lateral* impact.

team a group of individuals working together to achieve a common goal.

tension pneumothorax a condition that occurs when air accumulates within the pleural space and cannot escape, leading increasing intrathoracic pressure that can collapse the lungs and shift the structures of the mediastinum, interfering with cardiac output.

teratogenic medication that when taken by a pregnant woman, may potentially deform, injure, or kill a fetus.

terrorism the use of violence to intimidate and incite fear in the population with the goal of social, political, or religious change, or in retaliation for acts of perceived threat or injustice.

tertiary blast injury trauma caused when a patient carried by the pressure wave of an explosion impacts the ground or surrounding structures.

therapeutic communication specific verbal and nonverbal techniques used by health care providers to establish rapport and elicit information from patients.

therapeutic hypothermia a condition in which the body temperature is actively lowered following return of spontaneous circulation after cardiac arrest. Research indicates that this may reduce organ damage following cardiac arrest.

therapeutic index a ratio comparing a medication's lethal dose, which would cause death in 50 percent of the population (LD_{50}), with an effective dose of the same medication for 50 percent of the population (ED_{50}). The closer the ratio is to 1, the less the difference is between the effective and lethal doses of a medication.

therapeutic threshold the level of medication in the blood that must be achieved in order for the medication to begin to have an effect.

thermal gradient the difference between body and environmental temperatures.

thermogenesis the process of generating heat.

thermolysis the process of transferring heat from the body to the environment.

thermoreceptors sensory nerve endings that monitor temperature within the body.

thermoregulation the process by which the body adjusts its internal or core body temperature to maintain it within normal range.

third service in EMS, a service that is a third branch of the city's or county's public safety services, in addition to the fire service and law enforcement.

third-degree burns See *full-thickness burns.*

thyrotoxicosis an extreme, life-threatening form of hyperthyroidism that includes tachycardia, hyperthermia, and altered mental status. Also called *thyroid storm.*

tidal volume (TV) amount of air (in milliliters) in a normal (unforced) exhalation following a normal inspiration.

tiered response an EMS system in which a greater number of BLS units distributed throughout the area can respond to emergencies quickly to provide initial care while awaiting response from a few strategically dispatched ALS units.

toddler a child from one to three years of age.

tolerance a decrease in susceptibility to the effects of a drug due to its prolonged use.

tonic–clonic seizures motor activity produced by a generalized neuronal discharge in the brain involving a state of rigid contraction of the muscles (tonic phase) followed by rhythmic muscle contractions (clonic phase).

torsades de pointes a type of ventricular tachycardia in which the abnormal pacemaker site in the ventricles moves between multiple sites. Also called *polymorphic ventricular tachycardia.*

tort law law pertaining to wrongdoing and harm done to one party by another.

tourniquet a wide band wrapped around an extremity used to constrict arterial and venous blood flow to stop bleeding.

toxicant any poisonous substance not derived from the metabolism of an organism.

toxidromes collections of signs and symptoms associated with a class of toxins.

toxins any substances that have a negative effect on the body.

tracheal deviation a shift of the trachea away from the midline, toward one side or the other; an indication of tension pneumothorax with substantial shift of the mediastinum.

tracheostomy a surgical opening into the trachea to establish an airway.

transient ischemic attack (TIA) an interruption of blood flow to a portion of the brain that lasts for less than 1 hour.

transverse fracture a break in a bone that is at a 90° angle to its long axis.

trauma an injury caused by the application of energy (such as kinetic, thermal, radiation, electric, chemical energy) to the tissues.

trauma chin lift a technique used to displace the mandible anteriorly to open the airway without hyperextending the cervical spine.

trauma system a network of resources specifically designed to provide definitive care for trauma patients.

traumatic asphyxia a condition that occurs as a result of sudden massive compression forces being applied to the chest resulting in retrograde blood flow from the heart to the upper body.

traumatic rhabdomyolysis breakdown of skeletal muscle, with release of potassium and myoglobin, due to crushing injury. Crush syndrome, a set of systemic complications that includes renal failure and cardiac dysrhythmias, may result from traumatic rhabodomyolysis.

triage the process by which the treatment of patients at a multiple casualty incident is prioritized.

triage desk the location in an emergency department in which arriving patients are first evaluated by medical care and assigned priority for care.

triage tags colored tags that correspond to the various categories into which injured patients may be sorted, based on the severity of their injuries: red (immediate), yellow (delayed), green (minor), and black (expectant).

tripod position a position in which a patient leans forward, supporting himself with his arms when experiencing respiratory distress.

tropic hormones chemical messengers (hormones) secreted by one endocrine gland that stimulate another endocrine gland.

turgor a measure of the hydration of the skin observed by the amount of time that it takes a fold of skin to return to its normal position after being pinched up from the underlying tissues.

TV short for *tidal volume.*

tympanic temperature a measurement of body temperature at the tympanic membrane (eardrum) with an infrared light and sensor placed in the ear canal.

type 1 diabetes a form of diabetes with onset at a younger age that requires insulin replacement therapy because of autoimmune destruction of pancreatic beta cells.

type 2 diabetes a form of diabetes with typical onset in middle-aged, obese individuals; usually controlled by diet, exercise, weight loss, and oral medications. Insulin may be required in severe cases.

type I ambulance an ambulance box mounted on a pick-up truck chassis.

type I decompression sickness a mild form of illness resulting from rapid ascent from a dive.

type II ambulance a van with a raised roof and modifications to allow emergency medical care.

type II decompression sickness a serious condition resulting from rapid ascent from a dive that produces signs and symptoms of the nervous, respiratory, and circulatory systems.

type III ambulance a modified van chassis with an ambulance box mounted on it.

U

UN ID numbers four-digit numbers that identify hazardous substances and products of commercial importance.

unified command the organization of the incident command system strucure used for large-scale incidents or disasters that are complex and require the concerted response of multiple agencies.

unstable angina a pattern of ischemic chest pain that progresses in duration, frequency, and/or severity.

upper respiratory infection (URI) any infectious illness that affects the structures of the upper airway, such as a cold.

uremia a condition including signs and symptoms of renal failure with an increase in blood urea nitrogen (BUN) and creatinine (Cr), which would normally be excreted by the kidneys.

uremic encephalopathy altered mental status caused by the accumulation of creatinine and blood urea nitrogen due to renal failure.

uremic frost flaky deposits of urea on the skin of severely uremic patients.

urticaria red, raised areas on the skin caused by swelling of, and release of fluid from, blood vessels in the skin in response to an allergic reaction. Commonly known as *hives.*

uterine fibroid benign tumor of the uterus.

V

vascular access device (VAD) an indwelling appliance that provides a means for delivering medications or fluids into a patient's circulation when repeated or on-going intravenous access is needed.

vasopressin a hormone released from the posterior pituitary gland that causes vasoconstriction and decreases urine output to increase blood pressure. Also called *antidiuretic hormone (ADH).*

vector an animal or insect that can spread diseases from one organism to another.

venipuncture a procedure in which a needle is inserted into the lumen of a vein.

venous bleeding loss of blood from an injured vein; the appearance of the blood is usually dark red with a steady (nonpulsating) flow.

ventilation the movement of air into and out of the lungs.

ventilation–perfusion (VQ) mismatch a condition in which either pulmonary circulation or alveolar ventilation is impaired.

ventricular fibrillation a lethal cardiac dysrhythmia in which multiple ectopic pacemakers in the ventricles create chaotic electrical activity that does not produce mechanical contraction of the heart.

ventricular tachycardia a cardiac dysrhythmia that produces a rapidly firing ectopic pacemaker in the ventricles. Typically regular with a wide QRS complex.

ventriculostomy shunt a drainage device placed in a ventricle in the brain to drains excess cerebrospinal fluid into the abdomen, heart, pleural space, or a blood vessel in the neck.

verbal cues meanings conveyed through written or spoken words.

vertigo a subjective sensation of spinning or moving while stationary; dizziness.

vigorous exercise physical activity at 74 to 88 percent of the peak heart rate.

villi fingerlike projections of certain cells, such as those lining the intestine, to increase their surface area for absorption.

virulent strong, able to overcome body defenses.

visceral peritoneum the innermost portion of a double membrane in the abdominal cavity, which is in contact with the abdominal organs.

vision impairment partial or total loss of the ability to see. Also called *blindness*.

vital signs the measurements of the pulse, respirations, blood pressure, and temperature.

voluntary guarding the tensing of the abdominal muscles by the patient in anticipation of palpation.

volvulus twisting of a loop of bowel around itself, cutting off circulation to the affected area.

vomiting agents chemical weapons that cause coughing, gagging, and, as a result, vomiting.

W

warm zone the area surrounding the hot zone of a hazardous materials scene, with the sole purpose of preventing the spread of contamination. Also called the *contamination reduction zone*.

washout phase (of shock) the phase of shock in which both the precapillary and postcapillary sphincters have failed and the blood that had stagnated in the capillary beds, along with lactic acid and microscopic blood clots, re-enters the circulation.

watts units of power used to measure the electronic strength of a radio transmitter.

weapon of mass destruction (WMD) a device designed to kill or injure a large number of people or other life forms as well as cause damage to structures.

wellness health and balance in mind, body, and spirit.

wheezing a high-pitched, usually expiratory sound caused by constriction of the bronchioles, such as that which occurs in an asthma attack.

white paper an authoritative government report that describes specific issues and makes recommendations for solving them.

window phase the period of time between infectious disease exposure and development of detectable amounts of antibody. The disease may be transmissible during this time.

windshield survey a scene size-up performed from inside emergency response vehicle as crews approach the scene to determine what has happened, what is happening, what hazards are present, and what resources are needed.

Y

Yankauer a hollow, rigid device that attaches to suction tubing to allow suctioning of the oropharynx.

Z

zone of coagulation the area of a burn that is necrotic.

zone of hyperemia the outermost zone of a burn, where an increase in blood flow causes edema to the tissues.

zone of stasis the area surrounding the zone of coagulation of a burn where blood flow is compromised but which may not become necrotic if blood flow is restored.

zygote a cell formed by the union of a sperm and egg.

Index

Page numbers followed by *f* indicate figures; those followed by *t* indicate tables.